DIAGNOSTIC NUCLEAR MEDICINE

THIRD EDITION

Volume One

DIAGNOSTIC NUCLEAR MEDICINE

THIRD EDITION

Volume One

MARTIN P. SANDLER, M.D., F.A.C.N.P.
PROFESSOR AND VICE CHAIRMAN
RADIOLOGY AND RADIOLOGICAL SCIENCES
DIRECTOR OF NUCLEAR MEDICINE/PET
VANDERBILT UNIVERSITY MEDICAL CENTER
NASHVILLE, TENNESSEE

JAMES A. PATTON, PH.D.
PROFESSOR
RADIOLOGY AND RADIOLOGICAL SCIENCES
PROGRAM DIRECTOR, NUCLEAR MEDICINE TECHNOLOGY
ADMINISTRATOR FOR RADIOLOGY ACADEMIC AFFAIRS
VANDERBILT UNIVERSITY MEDICAL CENTER
NASHVILLE, TENNESSEE

R. EDWARD COLEMAN, M.D.
PROFESSOR AND VICE CHAIRMAN
DEPARTMENT OF RADIOLOGY
DIRECTOR OF NUCLEAR MEDICINE
DUKE UNIVERSITY MEDICAL CENTER
DURHAM, NORTH CAROLINA

ALEXANDER GOTTSCHALK, M.D., F.A.C.R.
PROFESSOR OF RADIOLOGY
MICHIGAN STATE UNIVERSITY
EAST LANSING, MICHIGAN

FRANS J. TH. WACKERS, M.D.
PROFESSOR OF DIAGNOSTIC RADIOLOGY AND MEDICINE
DIRECTOR, CARDIOVASCULAR NUCLEAR IMAGING
AND STRESS LABORATORIES
YALE UNIVERSITY SCHOOL OF MEDICINE
NEW HAVEN, CONNECTICUT

PAUL B. HOFFER, M.D.
PROFESSOR
DIAGNOSTIC RADIOLOGY
DIRECTOR, NUCLEAR MEDICINE
YALE UNIVERSITY SCHOOL OF MEDICINE
NEW HAVEN, CONNECTICUT

SANS TACHE

Williams & Wilkins
A WAVERLY COMPANY

BALTIMORE • PHILADELPHIA • LONDON • PARIS • BANGKOK
BUENOS AIRES • HONG KONG • MUNICH • SYDNEY • TOKYO • WROCLAW

Editor: Charles W. Mitchell
Managing Editor: Marjorie Kidd Keating
Production Coordinator: Anne Stewart Seitz and Carol Eckhart
Copy Editor: Richard H. Adin
Designer: Dan Pfisterer
Illustration Planner: Ray Lowman
Typesetter: University Graphics, Inc.
Printer: Prestige Color, Inc.
Binder: Maple Press

351 West Camden Street
Baltimore, Maryland 21201-2436 USA

Rose Tree Corporate Center
1400 North Providence Road
Building II, Suite 5025
Media, Pennsylvania 19063-2043 USA

Accurate indications, adverse reactions, and dosage schedules for drugs are provided in this book, but it is possible that they may change. The reader is urged to review the package information data of the manufacturers of the medications mentioned.

Printed in the United States of America

First Edition 1976
Second Edition 1988

Library of Congress Cataloging in Publication Data

Diagnostic nuclear medicine / editors, Martin P. Sandler . . . [et al.].
—3rd ed.
p. cm.
Includes bibliographical references and index.
ISBN 0-683-07503-9
1. Radioisotope scanning. 2. Nuclear medicine. I. Sandler, Martin P.
[DNLM: 1. Radionuclide Imaging. 2. Nuclear Medicine. WN 445 D53455 1995]
RC78.7.R4D465—dc20
DNLM/DLC
for Library of Congress 94-32470
CIP

95 96 97 98 99
1 2 3 4 5 6 7 8 9 10

This book is dedicated to the scientists, physicians, and technologists who have been instrumental in the development of the speciality of nuclear medicine.

FOREWORD

The Third Edition of *Diagnostic Nuclear Medicine,* edited by Drs. Sandler, Coleman, Wackers, Patton, Gottschalk, and Hoffer clearly shows that the field of nuclear medicine is making remarkable progress in many directions! In light of such progress one of the most challenging aspects of editing a new edition of this classic work most certainly was the need to retain information of enduring importance while recasting the chapter outline and authorship to encompass new information and new concepts. As users of their book, we must congratulate the editors for their excellent judgment in defining its contents and their yeoman work in bringing such a multifaceted volume through the writing and editorial process.

Major books like *Diagnostic Nuclear Medicine* are important to every field of medicine and especially to ones like nuclear medicine that are both dynamic and diverse. Quite simply, experts can synthesize and document the knowledge base of the field in their respective areas in a way that none of us can do individually and more comprehensively than new knowledge is shared through journals and other periodicals.

There is always a sense of anticipation as one opens a major new book to the table of contents. To the neophyte, the contents page charts a course to new knowledge; those with experience in the specialty find old "friends" in the chapter titles but also see patterns of change that inevitably reshape the boundaries of the field. The important patterns of change for nuclear medicine are strongly and appropriately reflected in the Third Edition of *Diagnostic Nuclear Medicine.* For example, a familiar theme in nuclear medicine for the past decade and a half is the continued ascendancy of cardiovascular studies. No fewer than nine chapters are devoted to cardiovascular topics and it is fair to say that we find nuclear cardiology in robust middle age; myocardial perfusion imaging is well established as an important and standard test in health systems around the world. The value of cardiovascular procedures can be inferred from the number of continued new developments in instrumentation and new pharmaceuticals aimed at making the procedures even better.

Another striking trend in nuclear medicine practice illustrated by the selection of material for *Diagnostic Nuclear Medicine* is the continued renaissance of neurologic imaging. For years it appeared that brain imaging was lost to computed tomography and magnetic resonance imaging. We see in *Diagnostic Nuclear Medicine* that there is not only an unprecedented diversity of nuclear medicine techniques available for studying the brain, but in many cases, these are unique especially for assessment of receptor systems.

An area of nuclear medicine that is growing in both clinical practice and book content is nuclear oncology. In fact, if all of the chapters devoted to cancer were grouped together including those in the skeletal and endocrine sections, nuclear oncology would constitute the largest section of *Diagnostic Nuclear Medicine.* The specialty is converging in part on studies aimed at conditions representing the three most important causes of death in the United States; cardiovascular disease, neurologic (including neurovascular) disease, and cancer.

The continued importance of endocrine studies in both the culture and the practice of nuclear medicine is reflected in the Third Edition of *Diagnostic Nuclear Medicine.* In the case of the thyroid gland, the specialty is still involved in in vitro testing, imaging diagnostics, and radionuclide therapy. Even though the imaging studies are not as numerically important as they were 10 or 20 years ago and there has also been a fragmentation of responsibility for laboratory testing in many institutions, the use of radioiodine in diagnostic and therapeutic applications remains an exemplar for the entire specialty of nuclear medicine.

An enduring aspect of nuclear medicine practice is the importance of ventilation/perfusion imaging for the diagnosis of pulmonary embolism. The value of ventilation/perfusion imaging has been sustained over the years in spite of numerous challenges. What has changed in this edition of *Diagnostic Nuclear Medicine* is further refinement in our understanding of the significance of image findings and a continued refinement of clinical strategies for applying ventilation/perfusion imaging. Studies of the gastrointestinal tract and genitourinary tract have also remained important for selected indications.

Advances in imaging instrumentation are highlighted throughout *Diagnostic Nuclear Medicine.* It is noteworthy that many of the breakthroughs in computers and electronics necessary to achieve these advances have become available to nuclear medicine as a serendipity of general development in the commercial and industrial world. The rapidity and magnitude of these basic developments have greatly accelerated the ability to make progress in nuclear medicine and this trend is likely to continue.

Likewise, the expansion of knowledge about receptor systems, antibodies and molecular and cell biology have been convolved with new knowledge in chemistry to create what now appears to be an unlimited pharmacopeia of new radiotracers. The long-predicted paradigm of radiopharmaceuticals being first developed for positron emission tomography and then redeveloped by analogy for single photon imaging has also borne fruit.

During the time frame encompassed by the first two editions of *Diagnostic Nuclear Medicine,* the field was repeatedly rocked by competition from other new imaging methods including computed tomography, ultrasound, and magnetic resonance imaging. In retrospect, nuclear medicine lost out whenever the focus was anatomic imaging. Rather, the enduring strength of nuclear medicine at the beginning of its second half century, so well portrayed in the Third Edition of *Diagnostic Nuclear Medicine,* is the ability to use an increasingly rich variety of methods to study important functional parameters in virtually every organ system. Congratulations again to Drs. Sandler, Coleman, Wackers, Patton, Gottschalk, and Hoffer for presenting us with a book that encompasses both the scientific basis of nuclear medicine and thoroughly explores the utility and diversity of its contemporary clinical applications.

JAMES H. THRALL, M.D.
RADIOLOGIST-IN-CHIEF
MASSACHUSETTS GENERAL HOSPITAL
PROFESSOR OF RADIOLOGY
HARVARD MEDICAL SCHOOL

PREFACE

The impetus for producing the First Edition of *Diagnostic Nuclear Medicine* in 1976 was to provide a text "to be useful to the practicing radiologist with a significant commitment to nuclear medicine." The Second Edition was published 12 years later and had expanded to 11 sections with over 100 contributors and 75 chapters. The Foreword to the Second Edition described the text that had become a reference not only for "the practicing radiologist with a significant commitment to nuclear medicine," but also for those physicians who restrict their professional interest to this field as well. The Third Edition has now expanded to include six editors, 15 sections, 85 chapters, and over 150 contributors.

As the previous editors noted, nuclear medicine remains a vibrant and continually changing imaging modality. This is reflected by the fact that over 44 of the 84 chapters in the Third Edition are completely new. Since the last edition there have been significant advances in both imaging technology and radiopharmaceutical development. Included in the technological advances are improvements in scintillation camera design and specifications including the development of multidetector systems and the applications of digital technology. The widespread availability of this advanced technology has resulted in single photon emission computed tomography (SPECT) becoming the imaging procedure of choice in many diagnostic studies. Positron emission tomography has now expanded to over 65 centers in the United States, and its widespread clinical applications have been investigated extensively over the past 5–10 years. A significant advancement has been the development of 511 keV SPECT with simultaneous dual isotope acquisition, a technique that has the potential to enhance the growth of nuclear medicine. This technique will provide increased opportunities for investigation since imaging positrons will no longer require a uniquely defined positron camera, and long-lived positron emitters like ^{18}F-fluorodeoxyglucose can be obtained from sources some hours away.

Developments in radiopharmaceuticals since the last edition include the FDA approval of two technetium-labeled cardiac perfusion agents, ^{131}I-MIBG for diagnosing and treating patients with pheochromocytoma and neuroblastoma, detection of recurrent colon and ovarian cancer with an indium-labeled monoclonal antibody and the availability of octreoscan, a peptide hormone to diagnose carcinoid tumors and other apudomas.

In redesigning the Third Edition of *Diagnostic Nuclear Medicine*, the editors have attempted to provide a reference for those who are primarily involved in nuclear medicine, including both the generalist and specialist in nuclear cardiology. At the same time, we hope that this book will provide an encyclopedic reference for all who participate in nuclear medicine in any way.

Once again, it is tempting to predict the future with regard to the context of the next edition; however, it is clear from the previous editions that this is both foolhardy and unwise.

Finally, we hope that the readers of the Third Edition will use the portions of this text that are helpful to them while seeking current sources of information to keep abreast of new innovations. We remain confident that the excitement that has always been a part of nuclear medicine will continue to grow and increase in the future years.

MARTIN P. SANDLER, M.D.
R. EDWARD COLEMAN, M.D.
FRANS J. TH. WACKERS, M.D.
JAMES A. PATTON, PH.D.
ALEXANDER GOTTSCHALK, M.D.
PAUL B. HOFFER, M.D.

PREFACE TO THE FIRST EDITION

This book is designed to be useful to the practicing radiologist with a significant commitment to nuclear medicine. Many of the chapters about the current practice of nuclear radiology, such as those related to the use of cameras and scanners as well as those describing imaging of various organ systems, have a combination of useful "tricks of the trade," and a miniatlas with key illustrations available for study of reference.

It is inevitable, however, that nuclear medicine will become progressively more inclusive and therefore more complicated. As a result, several chapters have a more sophisticated bent. It is difficult, if not impossible, to take topics like collimator design; compartments, pools and spaces; and flow measurements; and couch them in terms of "2 × 2" arithmetic. In spite of this, it seems to us that these chapters are necessary both as reference material and for those instances in which the radiologist may be actually involved in utilizing the techniques or principles described. In short, this volume was written to help the radiologists practice better nuclear radiology now, and in the future.

ALEXANDER GOTTENSHALK, M.D.
E. JAMES POTCHEN, M.D.

CONTRIBUTORS

Hakan Ahlstrom, M.D., Ph.D.
Department of Diagnostic Radiology
PET Center
University Hospital
Uppsala, Sweden

Abass Alavi, M.D.
Professor of Radiology, Neurology and Psychiatry
Chief, Division of Nuclear Medicine
Department of Radiology
Hospital of University of Pennsylvania
Philadelphia, Pennsylvania

Bruce J. Barron, M.D.
Assistant Professor of Radiology
University of Texas Medical School
Houston, Texas

Robert N. Beck, B.S.
Professor
Department of Radiology
Franklin McLean Memorial Research Institute
Director, University of Chicago Argonne National Laboratory Center for Imaging Science
Chicago, Illinois

David V. Becker, M.D.
Professor
Departments of Radiology and Medicine
Cornell University Medical College
Director, Division of Nuclear Medicine
The New York Hospital-Cornell Medical Center
New York City, New York

Lewis C. Becker, M.D.
Professor, Department of Medicine
The Johns Hopkins Medical Institutions
Baltimore, Maryland

Mats Bergstrom
PET-Center
University Hospital
Uppsala, Sweden

Daniel S. Berman, M.D.
Co-chairman, Department of Imaging
Cedars-Sinai Medical Center
Professor of Medicine
UCLA School of Medicine
Los Angeles, California

Manu M. Bhattathiry, M.B., B.S., S.A.C.N.P.
Fellow in Pediatric Nuclear Medicine
Children's Hospital, Los Angeles
Los Angeles, California

Robert O. Bonow, M.D.
Chief, Division of Cardiology
Northwestern University Medical School
Chicago, Illinois

Frederick J. Bonte, M.D.
Cain Distinguished Chair in Diagnostic Imaging
Director, Nuclear Medicine Center
University of Texas Southwestern Medical Center
Dallas, Texas

Robert J. Boudreau, M.D., Ph.D.
Professor of Radiology
Director, Division of Nuclear Medicine
University of Minnesota
Minneapolis, Minnesota

Manuel L. Brown, M.D.
Chief, Director of Nuclear Medicine
Department of Radiology
University of Pittsburgh Medical Center
Pittsburgh, Pennsylvania

Thomas F. Budinger, M.D., Ph.D.
Professor
Lawrence Berkeley Laboratory
University of California at Berkeley
Berkeley, California

Jerrold T. Bushberg, Ph.D.
Clinical Associate Professor of Radiology
Director of Health Physics Program
University of California, Davis Medical Center
Sacramento, California

Henry S. Cabin, M.D.
Professor of Medicine and Pathology
University Director of Coronary Care Unit
Associate Director of Cardiac Catheterization Laboratory
Associate Chief of Cardiology
Yale University School
Chief of Clinical Cardiology Services
Yale-New Haven Hospital
New Haven, Connecticut

Michelle G. Campbell, M.D.
Department of Radiology and Radiological Sciences
Vanderbilt University Medical Center
Nashville, Tennessee

Martin Charron, M.D.
Head, Division of Nuclear Medicine
Department of Radiology
Children's Hospital of Pittsburgh
Assistant Professor of Radiology
University of Pittsburgh
Pittsburgh, Pennsylvania

Simon R. Cherry, Ph.D.
Assistant Professor
Department of Molecular & Medical Pharmacology & Crump Institute for Biological Imaging
UCLA School of Medicine
Los Angeles, California

K. Soni Clubb, M.D.
Clinical Instructor in Surgery
Yale University School of Medicine
New Haven, Connecticut

Marvin B. Cohen, M.D.
Chief, Nuclear Medicine Service
Veterans Affairs Medical Center
Sepulveda, California
Professor, Department of Medicine and Radiological Science
University of California Los Angeles
Los Angeles, California

R. Edward Coleman, M.D.
Professor and Vice Chairman
Department of Radiology
Director of Nuclear Medicine
Duke University Medical Center
Durham, North Carolina

Frederick L. Datz, M.D.
Professor of Radiology
Department of Nuclear Medicine
University of Utah Health Sciences
Salt Lake City, Utah

Dominique Delbeke, M.D., Ph.D.
Associate Professor
Clinical Director PET
Department of Radiology & Radiological Science
Vanderbilt University Medical Center
Nashville, Tennessee

Michael D. Devous, Sr., Ph.D.
Associate Professor
Department of Radiology
Associate Director
Nuclear Medicine Center
University of Texas Southwestern Medical Center
Dallas, Texas

Eva Dubovsky, M.D., Ph.D.
Professor of Radiology (Nuclear Medicine)
University of Alabama School of Medicine
Director and Attending Physician Division of Nuclear Medicine
University of Alabama Hospital
University of Alabama at Birmingham Medical Center
Birmingham, Alabama

Bonnie B. Dunn, Ph.D.
Radiochemist
Division of Medical Imaging
Food and Drug Administration
Rockville, Maryland

Howard J. Dworkin, M.D.
Director
Department of Nuclear Medicine
William Beaumont Hospital
Royal Oak, Michigan

William C. Eckelman, Ph.D.
Chief, PET Department
National Institutes of Health
Bethesda, Maryland

Peter J. Ell, M.D., M.Sc., Ph.D.
Head of Department
Institute of Nuclear Medicine
University College London Medical School
London, United Kingdom

Barbro Eriksson, M.D., Ph.D.
Associate Professor
Department of Internal Medicine
University Hospital
Uppsala, Sweden

Theo H.M. Falke, M.D.
Professor of Radiology
Department of Diagnostic Radiology
Free University
Amsterdam, The Netherlands

J. Douglas Ferry, Ph.D.
Director
Nuclear Medicine Radioimmunoassay Lab
William Beaumont Hospital
Royal Oak, Michigan

Darlene M. Fink-Bennett, M.D.
Vice Chief
Department of Nuclear Medicine
William Beaumont Hospital
Royal Oak, Michigan

Alan J. Fischman, M.D., Ph.D.
Director, Nuclear Medicine Division
Department of Radiology
Massachusetts General Hospital
Boston, Massachusetts

Mathews B. Fish, M.D.
Nuclear Medicine Physician
Department of Nuclear Medicine
Sacred Heart General Hospital
Director and CEO
Oregon Medical Laboratory
Eugene, Oregon

John E. Freitas, M.D.
Director, Nuclear Medicine Services
Department of Radiology
St. Joseph Mercy Hospital
Clinical Associate Professor of Internal Medicine
University of Michigan Medical School
Ann Arbor, Michigan

Anne E. Freitas, M.D.
Acting Assistant Professor of Radiology
University of Washington Medical Center
Seattle, Washington

Michael J. Gelfand, M.D.
Chief, Section of Nuclear Medicine
Department of Radiology
Children's Hospital Medical Center
Professor of Radiology
University of Cincinnati
Cincinnati, Ohio

Guido Germano, Ph.D.
Assistant Professor
Department of Radiological Sciences
UCLA School Of Medicine
Director, Nuclear Medicine Physics
Medical Physics & Imaging
Cedars-Sinai Medical Center
Los Angeles, California

S. Julian Gibbs, D.D.S., Ph.D.
Professor
Department of Radiology & Radiological Sciences
Vanderbilt University Medical Center
Nashville Tennessee

David L. Gilday, M.D., F.R.C.P.C., B.Eng.
Professor of Radiology
University of Toronto
Head Division of Nuclear Medicine
The Hospital for Sick Children
Toronto, Ontario
Canada

Alexander Gottschalk, M.D., F.A.C.R.
Professor of Radiology
Department of Radiology
Michigan State University
East Lansing, Michigan

L. Stephen Graham, Ph.D.
Medical Physicist
Nuclear Medicine Service
Veterans Affairs Medical Center
Sepulveda, California
Adjunct Professor
Biomedical Physics
UCLA School of Medicine
Los Angeles, California

Milton D. Gross, M.D.
Professor
Department of Internal Medicine
Division of Nuclear Medicine
University of Michigan Medical Center
Director/Chief, Nuclear Medicine Service
Department of Veterans Affairs
Ann Arbor, Michigan

Donald L. Gunter, Ph.D.
Research Associate (Assistant Professor)
Department of Radiology
Franklin McLean Memorial Resarch Institute
The University of Chicago
Chicago, Illinois

C. Craig Harris, M.S.
Associate Professor Emeritus of Radiology
Duke University Medical Center
Durham, North Carolina

D.J. Hawkes, Ph.D., F.I.P.S.M.
Reader in Radiological Sciences
United Medical and Dental Schools
Guy's Hospital
University of London
London, United Kingdom

Randall A. Hawkins, M.D., Ph.D.
Professor of Radiology
Chief, Nuclear Medicine Program
Vice Chairman, Department of Radiology
University of California, San Francisco
San Francisco, California

Sydney Heyman, M.D.
Director of Nuclear Medicine
Children's Hospital of Philadelphia
Professor of Radiology
University of Pennsylvania School of Medicine
Philadelphia, Pennsylvania

Carl K. Hoh, M.D.
Assistant Professor
Department of Molecular and Medical Pharmacology and Radiological Sciences
UCLA Medical Center
Los Angeles, California

Lawrence E. Holder, M.D.
Professor of Radiology
Director, Division of Nuclear Medicine
Department of Diagnostic Radiology
University of Maryland Medical System
Baltimore, Maryland

B. Leonard Holman, M.D.
Chairman, Department of Radiology
Brigham and Women's Hospital
Philip H. Cook Professor of Radiology
Harvard Medical School
Boston, Massachusetts

James R. Hurley, M.D.
Associate Professor
Department of Medicine and Radiology
Cornell University Medical College
Associate Director
Division of Nuclear Medicine
The New York Hospital-Cornell Medical Center
New York, New York

Roger A. Hurwitz, M.D.
Professor
Department of Pediatrics (Cardiology), Radiology (Nuclear Medicine)
Indiana University School of Medicine
Indianapolis, Indiana

A. Everette James III, M.B.A., J.D.
CEO, President United Medical International
Palm Beach, Florida

A. Everette James, Jr., Sc.M., J.D., M.D.
Senior Project Officer
Institute of Medicine
National Academy of Sciences
Washington, D.C.
Visiting Scientist, National Institutes of Health
National Cancer Institute
Bethesda, Maryland

Lynne L. Johnson, M.D.
Division of Cardiology
Rhode Island Hospital
Providence, Rhode Island

William D. Kaplan, M.D. *(deceased)*

John D. Kemp, M.D.
Professor
Department of Pathology, Microbiology, and Immunology
University of Iowa College of Medicine
Associate Director
Department of Immunopathology Laboratory
University of Iowa Hospitals
Iowa City, Iowa

Robert M. Kessler, M.D.
Professor
Vanderbilt University Medical Center
Director of Neuroradiology
Department of Radiology and Radiological Sciences
Nashville, Tennessee

Hosen Kiat, M.D., F.R.A.C.P., F.A.C.C., F.C.C.P.
Director of Nuclear Medicine Research
Assistant Professor of Medicine
UCLA School of Medicine
Los Angeles, California

E. Edmund Kim, M.D., M.S.
Professor of Radiology & Medicine
Nuclear Medicine & Diagnostic Radiology
University of Texas M.D. Anderson Cancer Center
Professor of Radiology
University of Texas Medical School
Houston, Texas

Eric P. Krenning, M.D., Ph.D.
Professor of Nuclear Medicine
Head, Department of Nuclear Medicine
University Hospital
Rotterdam, The Netherlands

Marvin W. Kronenberg, M.D.
Professor of Medicine and Radiology
Departments of Internal Medicine and Radiology
Wayne State University
Detroit, Michigan

Christopher C. Kuni, M.D.
Department of Radiology
University of Minnesota
Minneapolis, Minnesota

Alvin Kuruc, M.D., Ph.D.
Postdoctoral Fellow
Center for Functional Imaging
Lawrence Berkeley Laboratory
Berkeley, California

Dik J. Kwekkeboom, M.D.
Department of Nuclear Medicine
University Hospital of Rotterdam
Rotterdam, The Netherlands

Steven W.J. Lamberts, M.D., Ph.D.
Professor of Medicine
Erasmus University
Rotterdam, The Netherlands

Lamk M. Lamki, M.D.
Professor of Radiology
Chief, Division of Nuclear Medicine
Department of Radiology
University of Texas Medical School
Houston, Texas

Bengt Langstrom, Ph.D.
Professor
PET Center
Uppsala University
Uppsala, Sweden

Sandra Lawrence, M.D.
Department of Radiology and Radiological Sciences
Vanderbilt University Medical Center
Nashville, Tennessee

Edwin M. Leidholdt, Jr., Ph.D.
Clinical Associate Professor of Radiology
University of California, Davis
Regional Radiation Safety Program Manager
VHA Western Region
U.S. Department of Veterans Affairs
San Francisco, California

Anders Lilja
University Hospital
Uppsala, Sweden

Karen E. Linder, Ph.D.
Senior Research Investigator
Chemical and Biological Evaluation
Bracco Research USA Inc.
Princeton, New Jersey

Bruce R. Line, M.D.
Professor of Radiology
Albany Medical Center
Albany, New York

Val J. Lowe, M.D.
Medical Director, PET Imaging
Assistant Professor of Medicine
Nuclear Medicine Department
St. Louis University Health Sciences Center
St. Louis, Missouri

Massoud Majd, M.D.
Director, Section of Nuclear Medicine
Diagnostic Imaging and Radiology
Children's National Medical Center
Professor of Radiology and Pediatrics
George Washington University School of Medicine
Washington, D.C.

Leon S. Malmud, M.D.
Herbert M. Stauffer Professor of Diagnostic Imaging
Senior Vice President for Health Sciences
Temple University Hospital
Philadelphia, Pennsylvania

Ronald G. Manning, Ph.D.
Associate Professor
Department of Radiology and Radiological Sciences
Vanderbilt University Medical Center
Nashville, Tennessee

William H. Martin, M.D.
Assistant Professor
Department of Radiology and Radiological Sciences
Vanderbilt University Medical Center
Nashville, Tennessee

John G. McAfee, M.D., F.R.C.P.(C)
Chief, Section of Radiopharmaceutical Research
Department of Nuclear Medicine
The National Institutes of Health
Bethesda, Maryland
Professor, Department of Radiology
George Washington University Medical Center
Washington, D.C.

Barbara J. McNeil, M.D., Ph.D.
Division of Nuclear Medicine
Brigham & Women's Hospital
Ridley Watts Professor of Health Care Policy and Professor of Radiology
Harvard Medical School
Boston, Massachusetts

John H. Miller, M.D.
Head, Division of Nuclear Radiology
Children's Hospital of Los Angeles
Professor of Radiology
University of Southern California School of Medicine
Los Angeles, California

Gerd Muehllehner, Ph.D.
President
UGM Medical Systems
Philadelphia, Pennsylvania

Dieter Munz, M.D.
Professor and Chairman
Department of Nuclear Medicine
Charite Hospital
Berlin, Germany

Patrick B. Murphy, M.D.
Attending Cardiologist
Mid Central Cardiology
Bloomington, Illinois

Conrad E. Nagle, M.D., F.A.C.N.P., F.A.C.S.M.
Chief
Department of Nuclear Medicine
William Beaumont Hospital
Troy, Michigan

Ronald D. Neumann, M.D.
Chief
Department of Nuclear Medicine
The National Institutes of Health
Bethesda, Maryland

Andrew Newberg, M.D.
Department of Internal Medicine
Graduate Hospital
Philadelphia, Pennsylvania

Adrian D. Nunn, C.Chem., F.R.S.C.
Senior Director
Chemical & Biological Evaluation
Bracco Research USA, Inc.
Princeton, New Jersey

Robert E. O'Mara, M.D.
Professor, Department of Radiology
Head, Division of Nuclear Medicine
University of Rochester Medical Center
Rochester, New York

Kjell E. Oberg, M.D., Ph.D.
Head Endocrine Oncology Unit
Department of Internal Medicine
University Hospital
Uppsala, Sweden

Bernard E. Oppenheim, M.D.
Professor
Department of Radiology
Indiana University School of Medicine
Indianapolis, Indiana

Alan B. Packard, Ph.D.
Senior Research Associate
Division of Nuclear Medicine
Children's Hospital
Assistant Professor
Department of Radiology
Harvard Medical School
Boston, Massachusetts

Chang H. Paik, Ph.D.
Head, Radiochemistry
Department of Nuclear Medicine
The National Institutes of Health
Bethesda, Maryland

J. Anthony Parker, M.D., Ph.D.
Radiologist
Division of Nuclear Medicine
Beth Israel Hospital
Associate Professor of Radiology
Department of Radiology
Harvard Medical School
Boston, Massachusetts

C. Leon Partain, M.D., Ph.D.
Professor and Chairman
Department of Radiology and Radiological Sciences
Vanderbilt University Medical Center
Nashville, Tennessee

James A. Patton, Ph.D.
Professor
Radiology and Radiological Sciences
Program Director
Nuclear Medicine Technology
Administrator for Radiology Academic Affairs
Vanderbilt University Medical Center
Nashville, Tennessee

Michael E. Phelps, Ph.D.
Jennifer Jones Simon Professor & Chairman
Department of Molecular & Medical Pharmacology
Director, Crump Institute for Biological Imaging
Chief, Division of Nuclear Medicine
UCLA School of Medicine
Los Angeles, California

David R. Pickens, Ph.D.
Associate Professor of Radiology and Radiological Sciences
Vanderbilt University Medical Center
Nashville, Tennessee

Donald A. Podoloff, M.D.
Professor and Chairman
Department of Nuclear Medicine
University of Texas
M.D. Anderson Cancer Center
Houston, Texas

Myron Pollycove, M.D.
Professor Emeritus
Departments of Laboratory Medicine and Radiology
University of California, San Francisco, School of Medicine
San Francisco, California

Steven Port, M.D.
Professor of Medicine
University of Wisconsin Medical School
Director of Nuclear Cardiology
Milwaukee Heart Institute
Milwaukee, Wisconsin

Thomas A. Powers, M.D.
Associate Professor of Radiology and Radiological Sciences
Director of Abdominal Imaging
Vanderbilt University Medical Center
Nashville, Tennessee

Ronald R. Price, Ph.D.
Professor of Radiology and Radiological Sciences
Director of Radiological Sciences Division
Vanderbilt University Medical Center
Nashville, Tennessee

Jean-Claude Reubi, M.D.
Professor of Pathology
Head, Division of Cell Biology and Experimental Cancer Research
Institute of Pathology
University of Berne
Berne, Switzerland

Henry D. Royal, M.D.
Associate Director
Division of Nuclear Medicine
Department of Radiology
Mallinckrodt Institute of Radiology
Professor of Radiology
Washington School of Medicine
St. Louis, Missouri

Robert H. Rubin, M.D.
Chief of Transplantation Infectious Disease
Massachusetts General Hospital
Director, Center for Experimental Pharmacology and Therapeutics
Harvard-M.I.T.
Boston, Massachusetts

Charles D. Russell, M.D., Ph.D.
Professor of Radiology (Nuclear Medicine)
University of Alabama School of Medicine
Attending Physician, Nuclear Medicine Service
V.A. Medical Center—Birmingham
Birmingham, Alabama

Martin P. Sandler, M.D., F.A.C.N.P.
Professor and Vice Chairman
Radiology and Radiological Sciences
Director of Nuclear Medicine/PET
Vanderbilt University Medical Center
Nashville, Tennessee

Salil D. Sarkar, M.D.
Associate Professor
Department of Radiology
SUNY Health Science Center at Brooklyn
Brooklyn, New York

Jaap Schipper, M.D.
Department of Radiology
Leyehburg Hospital
Den Haag, The Netherlands

Marcus Schwaiger, M.D.
Professor of Medicine
Department of Nuclear Medicine
Technical University of Munich
Munich, Germany

Aldo N. Serafini, M.D.
Professor of Radiology and Medicine
University of Miami-Jackson Memorial Medical Center
Sylvester Comprehensive Cancer Center
Miami, Florida

Braham Shapiro, M.B., Ch.B., Ph.D.
Professor of Internal Medicine
Division of Nuclear Medicine
University of Michigan
Physician
Department of Nuclear Medicine
Veterans Affairs Medical Centers
Ann Arbor, Michigan

Barry L. Shulkin, M.D.
Associate Professor
Director, Pediatric Nuclear Medicine
Department of Internal Medicine
University of Michigan Medical Center
Ann Arbor, Michigan

Barry A. Siegel, M.D.
Professor of Radiology and Medicine
Director, Division of Nuclear Medicine
Mallinckrodt Institute of Radiology
Washington University School of Medicine
St. Louis, Missouri

Edward B. Silberstein, M.D., F.A.C.N.P.
Professor
Department of Radiology & Medicine
University of Cincinnati Medical Center
Director, Nuclear Medicine Service
The Jewish Hospital
Cincinnati, Ohio

James C. Sisson, M.D.
Professor of Internal Medicine
Division of Nuclear Medicine
University of Michigan Medical Center
Ann Arbor, Michigan

Andrea Soricelli, M.D.
Department of Nuclear Medicine
University of Naples—Federico II
Naples, Italy

H. Dirk Sostman, M.D.
Professor and Director of Academic Affairs
Department of Radiology
Duke University
Durham, North Carolina

Richard P. Spencer, M.D., Ph.D.
Professor and Chairman
Department of Nuclear Medicine
University of Connecticut Health Center
Farmington, Connecticut

Michael G. Stabin, C.H.P.
Radiation Internal Dose Information Center
Oak Ridge Institute for Science and Education
Oak Ridge, Tennessee

Joseph Steigman, Ph.D.
Emeritus Professor of Radiology
Division of Nuclear Medicine
State University of New York
Health Science Center at Brooklyn
Brooklyn, New York

H. William Strauss, M.D.
Division of Nuclear Medicine
Department of Radiology
Stanford University School of Medicine
Stanford, California

Mary Tono, B.A.
Department of Nuclear Medicine
University of California
San Francisco General Hospital
San Francisco, California

S.T. Treves, M.D.
Chief, Division of Nuclear Medicine
The Children's Hospital
Boston, Massachusetts

Kevin Tse, M.D.
Department of Nuclear Medicine
University of Hong Kong
Hong Kong

Benjamin M.W. Tsui, Ph.D.
Professor
Department of Biomedical Engineering
University of North Carolina
Chapel Hill, North Carolina

Jean-Luc Urbain, M.D.
Associate Professor
Department of Diagnostic Medicine
Temple University Hospital
Associate Professor
Fels Institute for Cancer Research and Molecular Biology
Philadelphia, Pennsylvania

Kenneth F. Van Train
Director, Computer Research and Development
Medical Imaging and Physics
Cedars-Sinai Medical Center
Los Angeles, California

Marie-Christiane M. Vekemans, M.D.
Co-Chairman, Internal Medicine Department
Centre Hospitalier du Grand Hornu
Belgium

Frans J.Th. Wackers, M.D.
Professor of Diagnostic Radiology and Medicine
Director, Cardiovascular Nuclear Imaging and Stress Laboratories
Departments of Diagnostic Radiology and Nuclear Cardiology
Yale University School of Medicine
New Haven, Connecticut

Henry N. Wagner, Jr., M.D.
Professor of Medicine and Radiology
Departments of Nuclear Medicine and Radiation Health Sciences
The Johns Hopkins Medical Institutions
Baltimore, Maryland

Heinz W. Wahner, M.D., F.A.C.P.
Professor of Radiology
Consultant, Nuclear Medicine
Department of Diagnostic Radiology
Mayo Clinic
Rochester, Minnesota

Alan D. Waxman, M.D.
Director, Department of Nuclear Medicine
Cedars-Sinai Medical Center
Los Angeles, California

Ronald E. Weiner, Ph.D.
Associate Professor of Nuclear Medicine
Department of Nuclear Medicine
University of Connecticut Health Center
Farmington, Connecticut

Gil Wernovsky, M.D.
Director, Cardiac Intensive Care Unit
Associate in Cardiology
Children's Hospital of Philadelphia
Associate Professor of Pediatrics
University of Pennsylvania School of Medicine
Philadelphia, Pennsylvania

Jeannette James Whitson, J.D.
Berry and Sims
Nashville, Tennessee

George A. Wilson, M.D. *(deceased)*

Robert M. Witt, Ph.D.
Assistant Professor
Department of Radiology
Indiana University School of Medicine
Indianapolis, Indiana

Daniel Worsley, M.D.
Assistant Professor of Nuclear Medicine
Department of Radiology
Vancouver General Hospital
University of British Columbia Faculty of Medicine
Vancouver, British Columbia
Canada

Robert K. Zeman, M.D.
Professor and Clinical Director of Diagnostic Radiology
Georgetown University Medical Center
Washington, D.C.

Sibylle I. Ziegler, Ph.D.
Department of Nuclear Medicine
Technical University of Munich
Munich, Germany

Harvey A. Ziessman, M.D.
Professor, Department of Radiology
Director, Division of Nuclear Medicine
Georgetown University Hospital
Washington, D.C.

CONTENTS

SECTION XII. ONCOLOGY

SECTION XIII. TRANSPLANTATION

SECTION XIV. PEDIATRICS

SECTION XV. INFLAMMATION

SECTION XVI. LEGAL ISSUES

SECTION I. HISTORICAL CONSIDERATION

1 Beginnings of Nuclear Medicine

MARVIN B. COHEN and L. STEPHEN GRAHAM

In the 5th century B.C., Leucippus and his pupil Democritus postulated that all material things were composed of small, indivisible units, which Democritus called atoma (atoms). Another 5th century B.C. Greek philosopher, Empedocles, argued that all matter was composed of four "elements," fire, earth, air, and water (1). At that time theories were accepted or rejected, not on the basis of evidence, but on the prestige of the proponent. The prestige of the four element theory's main advocate, Aristotle (384–322 B.C.), was so great that it was accepted for over 2000 years. Ancient alchemists labored to manipulate the four elements in their efforts to transmute base metals into gold.

The four element theory was not seriously questioned until 1774, when the French chemist Antoine L. Lavoisier demonstrated that air was a mixture of at least two gases, which today are known as nitrogen and oxygen. In 1781, English chemists Joseph Priestley and Henry Cavendish helped to finally overturn the four element theory by demonstrating that water was composed of oxygen and hydrogen. By 1789, Lavoisier had laid the groundwork for a modern concept of elements, which he defined as "The last point which analysis is capable of reaching." He also listed 33 known elements, 20 of which are still accepted as correctly classified (1). The discoveries of the chemists, and those of astronomers Copernicus, Kepler, and Galileo, helped to overthrow the influence of Aristotle. While Isaac Newton and the Irish chemist Boyd W. Higgins had written of atoms, John Dalton is considered the father of the modern theory of atoms and molecules because his 1803 theory was quantitative. This English schoolteacher stated that all atoms of a given element are identical, are unchanged by chemical reaction, and combine in a ratio of simple numbers. Dalton measured atomic weights by reference to hydrogen to which he assigned a value of unity. Dalton did not have a clear idea of the difference between atomic weights and molecular weights. Because he considered the formula for water to be HO and ammonia to be NH, he had determined "equivalent weights" rather than the atomic weight (1).

In 1811, the Italian physicist Amedeo Avogadro stated that under equal conditions of temperature and pressure, equal volumes of different gases contain equal numbers of molecules. Confusion over the differences between atoms and molecules continued until 1858 when another Italian, Stanislao Cannizzaro, explained the significance of Avogadro's statements. It was then rapidly accepted that a gram-molecular weight of any ideal gas occupied 22.4136 liters at 0°C and 1 atmosphere of pressure and contains 6.0225×10^{23} molecules. The latter, called Avogadro's number, is one of the fundamental constants in the universe and has been independently confirmed by several other means (1). Cannizzaro demonstrated that atomic and molecular weights were readily explainable and measurable by using Avogadro's number.

Meanwhile, the list of elements grew and could not be related to their physical and chemical properties. Several proposed schemes of the elements had obvious faults. Dmitri Mendelyeev recognized the periodic regularity of chemical elements and their relationship to atomic weights. This Russian scientist proposed the first modern periodic table of the elements in 1869. He boldly left gaps in his table for undiscovered elements. He also was able to predict the properties of these missing elements. His idea began to excite real interest in 1875 when the newly discovered element gallium had the predicted properties. The discovery of scandium in 1879 and germanium in 1886 provided further confirmation of his proposal. The periodic table of the elements has been modified and amended several times, but the basic ideas of Mendelyeev have been confirmed (1).

The phenomenon of static electricity was known by the ancient Greeks, who also speculated on the nature of light. The Pythagorean theory of particles or corpuscles of light was revived in the 17th century by Isaac Newton. In 1704, he published "Opticks" and speculated that the corpuscles of light may also be associated with waves. The particle versus wave debate continued for the next 200 years. The demonstration of optical interference or diffraction patterns favored the wave theory. The first reasonably accurate measurements of the velocity of light in the mid-19th century demonstrated that light travels faster in air than in water. This finding also favored the wave theory, because the corpuscular theory of light predicted the opposite results. It was also known early in the 19th century that electricity and magnetism were interrelated and could be explained by a wave theory. It was known that sound waves were propagated through air. Nineteenth century physicists, therefore, believed that light waves required a media for their transmission and postulated the existence of an all pervading stationary "ether" that carried light waves. The brilliant Scottish scientist J. Clerk Maxwell demonstrated that light is associated with a varying electromagnetic field and that electromagnetic waves traveled with the same velocity as light. These ideas, published in his 1873 "Treatise on Electricity and Magnetism," strengthened belief in light waves and the hypothetical ether (1). The American physicist Albert A. Michelson devised an experiment to measure the velocity at which the earth traveled through the stationary ether. In 1881, he utilized a system of mirrors to measure the time it took for two rays from a split beam of light to travel at right angles to each other and return to the point of origin. He was startled when the difference predicted by the ether theory was not found. He, therefore, repeated the experiment in collaboration with

Edward W. Morley. Again the velocity of light appeared to be independent of the direction of travel, which meant that the earth could not be traveling through a stationary ether. The Michelson-Morley experiment not only led to the demise of the ether theory, but also laid the foundation for later work by Albert Einstein (1).

Other physicists in the second half of the 19th century were interested in the properties of electrical discharges in gas at low pressures. These studies were greatly facilitated by the English physicist William Crookes, who designed a greatly improved vacuum discharge tube. These Crookes' tubes, which we now call cathode-ray tubes, led to a virtual explosion of research in many areas. Crookes concluded that a stream of electrically charged particles were discharged from the negative electrode or cathode at extremely high velocities. This also caused the opposite end of the tube to glow, which could be amplified by coating the end of the tube with various chemical substances. Such improvement in the studies of fluorescence and phosphorescence led to many important basic discoveries (1).

This year is the centennial of one of the most famous discoveries, Wilhelm Conrad Roentgen's discovery of the x-ray. He had noticed that there were stray radiations coming out of the sides of a Crookes' tube. These radiations were capable of fogging or exposing photographic plates, even if he covered them with lightproof paper or placed them in a lightproof box. On November 8, 1895, Roentgen, at the laboratory adjacent to his home in Wurzberg, Germany, had his wife place her hand between the side of a Crookes' tube and a photographic plate in a light proof container. When he developed the plate, he was amazed to see not just an outline of her hand, but all of the bones in fine detail. Roentgen performed additional experiments and sent some of the photographic plates to a few colleagues in Vienna, Austria. One of them, Professor Lecher of Prague, was the son of the publisher of the "Wiener Presse." The next day the image of Frau Roentgen's hand was front page news in Vienna and immediately caused a worldwide sensation. Such nonscientific publication can be excused in this case, as Roentgen refused to patent his discovery of x-rays or their medical use. He believed it was too important and belonged to mankind (2).

Two months after Roentgen's discovery of x-rays, the Frenchman Antoine Henri Becquerel began a series of experiments to determine if phosphorescent materials such as uranium salts could be excited by sunlight to give off x-rays. He considered this as a possible alternative to the use of Crookes' cathode-ray tube. He prepared his photographic plates and lightproof covering. Becquerel then exposed the uranium salts to sunlight for several hours before placing them overnight in a dark drawer containing the lightproof photographic plates. He developed the plates and found what today we would call an autoradiograph of the uranium salts. This convinced him that sunlight had caused the production of x-rays by the phosphorescent uranium salts, but he was a good scientist and realized the importance of verifying his discovery before publishing. He prepared new photographic plates, but was unable to expose the uranium salts to sunlight because of the overcast cloudy weather in Paris, so the salts were placed back in the drawer on the photographic plates. It was not sunny in Paris for several days, but Becquerel decided to prepare fresh photographic plates and develop the old ones. To his astonishment the unactivated uranium salts produced an autoradiograph of equal intensity to that produced by sunlight activation (Fig. 1.1). Becquerel realized that the uranium salts themselves were giving off penetrating radiation similar to Roentgen's x-ray. He presented his results to the French Academy and also suggested to his good friend Pierre Curie that the study of the nature of these radiations from uranium salts would be a good subject for the doctoral dissertation of his young Polish wife, Marie Sklodowska (3).

As Madame Curie initiated her research, important discoveries were being made in England. In 1897, Joseph J. Thomson, at the Cavendish Laboratory at Cambridge University, applied a scale to the end of a cathode-ray tube, which permitted measurements of the deflection of charged particles in magnetic and electric fields. This apparatus permitted the calculation of the velocity of these particles and led to the discovery of the electron. Thomson called them corpuscles, a name he used for the next 20 years. This identification of the first subatomic particle permitted Thomson to develop the first theory of the structure of the atom. He theorized that these negative corpuscles or electrons were imbedded in a positive charged mass (4).

Marie Curie's research progressed rapidly and produced such exciting results that Pierre, who was already a well-known professor of physics, dropped his own work on piezoelectricity and magnetism to collaborate with his wife. They discovered, in 1898, two new elements in the uranium ore pitchblende. These were a trace element, which Marie named polonium after her homeland, and a more radioactive one, radium. Marie also coined the terms radioactive and radioactivity. The radiation from the two new elements was measured using a piezoelectric device developed by Pierre, who was an expert at measuring small currents. The many conservative members of the French

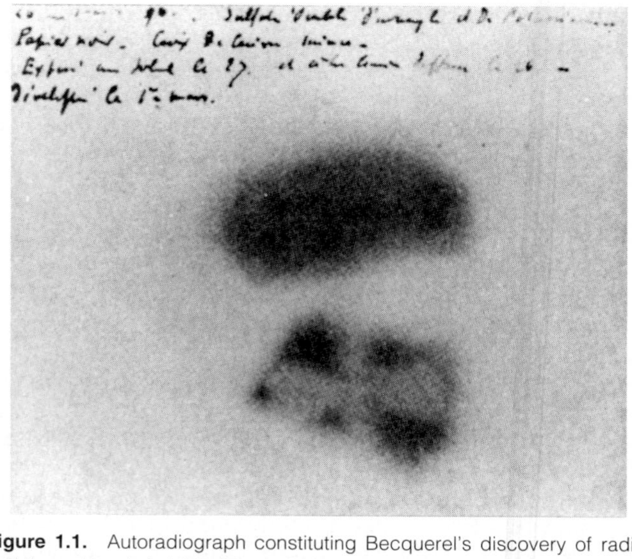

Figure 1.1. Autoradiograph constituting Becquerel's discovery of radioactivity on March 1, 1896. (Reproduced by permission from Nobel lectures: Physics 1901–1921. Amsterdam. Elsevier Publishing Company.)

Academy would not accept the two new elements based merely on a few physical properties such as their radiations. More traditional identification was demanded, and Madame Curie was forced to begin the Herculean task of reducing tons of pitchblende to a few milligrams of polonium and radium, which was to win her and Pierre the Nobel Prize (1, 5). Pierre died in 1906 and the unit of radioactivity in a gram of radium (a Curie) was so named as a tribute to him. Marie won a second Nobel Proze in 1911, but the French Academy of Science refused to admit a woman.

Becquerel received the first radiation burn in 1901 after he carried a vial of the Curie's radium in his vest pocket during a trip to England. Pierre Curie heard of this incident and confirmed the cause by exposing his arm to a similar sample of radium. He also recognized the potential medical use of radium and gave a sample to Henri Danlos, who performed the first radiation therapy using radium in Paris in 1901. Robert Abbe in New York obtained a radium needle in 1905, and cured an exophthalmic goiter by placing the needle into the thyroid for 24 hours. William Duane, an American, worked as a fellow in the Curie's laboratory and recognized that the most effective agent for radiation therapy was radon. Radon was called "radium-milk" and it had to be separated from the "radium-cow" (6). Brucer states that an editor later considered the term "cow" to be undignified and changed it to generator.

Becqueral switched from using photographic plates to the new gold leaf electroscope (Fig 1.2), which was more sensitive than the piezoelectroscope of the Curies. The Spinthariscope ("spark viewer") was described by Crookes in 1903 and may be considered a forerunner to the detectors used in modern scintillation cameras. It used a microscope eyepiece to view flashes of light produced in zinc sulfide when struck by α particles from a radium solution (7). Wilson developed the cloud chamber, a device containing supersaturated water vapor that permitted visualization of the tracks produced by events caused by ionizing radiation (1). J.J. Thomson continued basic research at Cambridge, as did his first postdoctoral student, Ernest Rutherford. Ten of J.J. Thompson's students went on to win Nobel Prizes. One of these was his son, George P. Thomson. J.J. Thomson won his Nobel Prize for discovering the electron

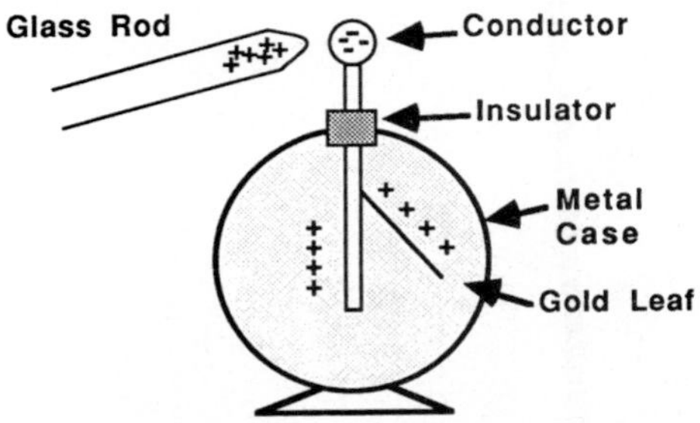

Figure 1.2. Diagram of a gold leaf electroscope. Addition of static electrical charge causes the gold leaf to deflect because of the repulsion of like charges. The gold leaf collapses when radiation passing through the chamber produces ionization which neutralizes the charge. (Reproduced by permission from Graham LS, et al. Nuclear medicine from Becquerel to the present. Radiographics 1989:9;1189.)

and demonstrating that it was a particle (4). G.P. Thomson was rewarded later for proving that it was a wave (1).

Rutherford's illustrious career included many important fundamental discoveries during his collaboration with J.J. Thomson and as Professor of Physics at McGill University in Montreal, Canada, and later at Manchester University in England. Thomson had already demonstrated that the cathode ray beam in a Crookes' tube could be deflected by a magnet. Thomson and Rutherford demonstrated that Roentgen's rays caused gas to be a conductor of electricity at ordinary pressures. Thomson called this phenomenon "ionization" and was able to separate and measure the charge of these "ions." Rutherford then utilized a magnet to demonstrate that two different types of "rays," which he called α and β, were emitted by uranium (5). The discovery of the γ ray awaited the Frenchman Paul Villard in 1900 (8). Rutherford used the Greek letter λ in 1899 to designate the disintegration rate (decay constant) and he developed the fundamental formula for radioactive (Marie Curie's term) decay, $A_t = A_0 e^{-\lambda t}$. In 1900, he took a boat to his native New Zealand to get married. This long journey allowed him to evaluate previously obtained data. From this study, Rutherford formed the concepts of half-life and radioactive decay. Marshall Brucer, the first medical director at the Oak Ridge National Laboratory, points out that Rutherford used various circumlocutions such as half-value period and that the term half-life only came into common use during the World War II Manhattan Project (9). Rutherford used the old alchemist term "transmutation" for radioactive decay. Brucer emphasizes that around the turn of the century radiation and radioactivity were subjects understood by only a small group of scientists who were considered heretics by many. J.J. Thomson claimed there was something smaller than an atom, Becquerel made a discovery that appeared to violate the law of conservation of energy, and now Rutherford was using alchemy concepts and claiming that one element was turned into another element (5, 10). The confusion increased when Albert Einstein published his "Special Theory of Relativity" in 1905. Incidently, Einstein won his Nobel Prize for his explanation of Brownian motion and the photoelectric effect, not for his theories of relativity.

Experiments performed by Rutherford at Manchester involved the use of thorium, which was the most powerful source of α rays then available. These "scatter" experiments, plus those of his students Hans Geiger and Ernest Marsden, proved to Rutherford that the atom was mostly empty space. In 1911, he abandoned the J.J. Thomson model of the atom and postulated an atom composed of a central positive charge, which he soon called a "nucleus," that was surrounded by electrons. Niels Bohr came from Copenhagen to study with J.J. Thomson and then with Rutherford. In a series of papers in 1913, he revised the Rutherford model of the atom to the Rutherford-Bohr model and later to the Bohr model of the atom (1). Bohr envisioned electrons orbiting in shells around the nucleus, and he related the energy of the electrons to the German Max Planck's "energy elements," which Einstein had renamed "Quantum" in 1905.

A number of researchers investigated the emissions and decay of the five known radioactive elements: uranium, thorium, actinium, radium and polonium. This led to five confusing families of elements. For example, there was radium-A, B, C, D, E, and F. Physical and chemical investigations established α and β as particles, but did not clarify the multiple bewildering decay series. This was accomplished by another of the many future Nobel Laureates to come out of Rutherford's laboratory, the Polish-born German chemist, Kasimir Fajans. Fajans went to the opera on November 23, 1912, to see "Tristan und Isolde." His mind wandered to the periodic table of elements and his upcoming dissertation on radioactive transformation by α decay and to Neils Bohr's recent theory that the β particle was emitted from the nucleus of the atom. During the second act he had a sudden insight, and the concept of isotopes was born. Fajans wrote that "alpha particle emission is accompanied by a transition from right to left in a horizontal row of the periodic table. . . . In a similar fashion beta disintegrations caused a transition to the next higher group: i.e., from left to right in a horizontal row." Fajans wrote about these "displacement laws" and used the term "pleid" (11, 12). The term "isotope" was actually coined a year later by Dr. Margaret Todd of Glascow, Scotland, at a dinner party given by another of Rutherford's students, Frederick Soddy (12). Atomic number was finally established as the basis for the Periodic Table.

Rutherford continued his own research at Manchester where Dalton had developed the atomic theory over 100 years earlier. In 1919, Rutherford demonstrated nuclear transformation using a powerful radium source for α particles, which irradiated a nitrogen target to produce oxygen and a particle he identified as a proton (Fig. 1.3). In 1920, he postulated the existence of the neutron, which would be discovered in 1932 by one of his British students, James Chadwick (13). As one of the many rewards for their monumental research and leadership both J.J. Thomson and

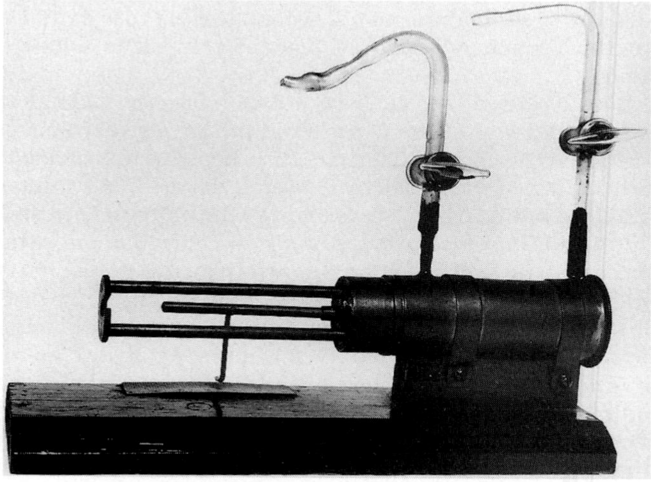

Figure 1.3. Rutherford was the first to "split" the atom and identify the proton. This relatively simple device held the radium source and nitrogen target in a $N_2(a,p)O_2$ reaction. (Reproduced by permission from Sterland EG. Energy into power. New York: Natural History Press, 1967:85.)

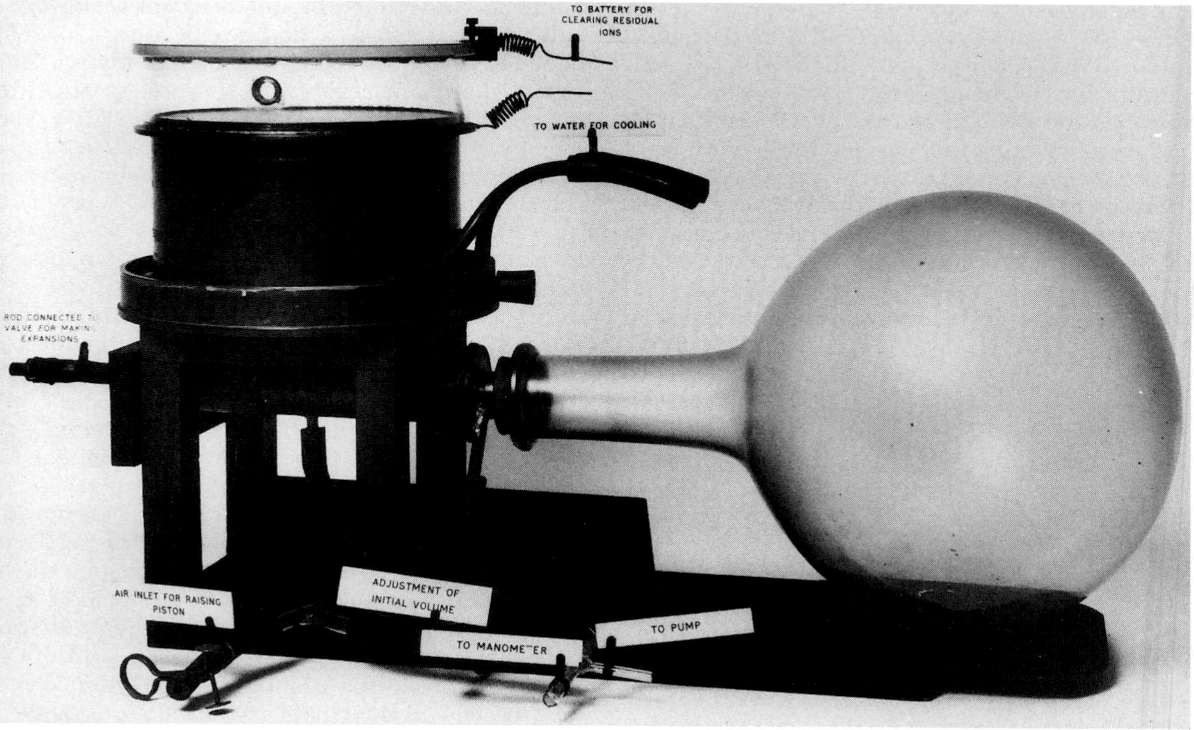

Figure 1.4. Wilson cloud chamber contains supersaturated water which visually can be seen to condense on the ionization path produced by charged particles passing through its globe. Used by Blumgart and Weiss and many basic researchers including Rutherford's demonstration of the proton and Anderson's discovery of the positron in cosmic rays. (Reproduced by permission from Sterland EG. Energy into power. New York: Natural History Press, 1967:84.)

Ernest Rutherford were later to be buried in Westminster Abbey, a few feet away from Isaac Newton.

Georg Charles de Hevesy was a multilingual Hungarian student of Rutherford. He participated in many research studies and acted as interpreter for many of Rutherford's foreign students. Hevesy is often called the "Father of Nuclear Medicine." He performed studies of plant metabolism in 1923 using 10.6 hour lead-212 and a gold leaf electroscope. This experiment demonstrated the thousand-fold or more increase in sensitivity over chemical methods, as well as the fact that because such minute quantities were required the toxic effects of lead could be avoided (14). These important advantages of the isotope methodology were used by Hevesy in 1924 in the first radioindicator studies in animals. In 1911, while a student of Rutherford, Hevesy lived in a boarding house where he suspected the landlady of making fresh food only once a week on Saturday and then recycling the leftovers in various forms. When the landlady denied this accusation, Hevesy added some lead-212 to the food the following Saturday and then took samples of subsequent meals for analysis with his gold leaf electroscope. He confronted the landlady with the evidence to prove his accusation. She acknowledged the power of the radioindicator methodology by saying "This is magic," but she evicted Hevesy. He did not publish this incident or consider it to be the first tracer experiment. He considered it as "just a radioactive measurement like many hundreds done before" (1). Hevesy did develop the dilution principle and used deuterium, shortly after its discovery by the American Harold Urey in 1932, to study body water in man.

Hevesy was the first to use the manmade isotope ^{32}P in animals and later in humans. He produced his first ^{32}P in 1935 by utilizing the neutrons produced from the 600 mg of radium that Neils Bohr had received as a 50th birthday present. Measurements of ^{32}P were made using the device perfected by Geiger in 1928. These studies suggested to Hevesy that body composition, including the skeleton, were not static, but were in a dynamic equilibrium which he later emphasized in his Nobel acceptance speech (15).

Two Americans, Herrman Blumgart and Soma Weiss, were the first to intravenously inject a radioactive substance into humans (16). In 1924, they injected radium-C (^{214}Bi) in one arm and measured the "velocity of the circulation" by detecting its arrival in the other arm using a Wilson cloud chamber (Fig. 1.4). They went on, with multiple coauthors, to measure various circulation times in health and several diseases using different methodologies. Blumgart also laid the foundation for the modern therapy of acute myocardial infarction by demonstrating in dogs that the extent of myocardial infarction was strongly related to the duration of occlusion (17).

Ernest O. Lawrence built the first cyclotron in Berkeley, California, in 1931, for the performance of high energy physics experiments (18). The same year, Carl Anderson, another American, discovered the positron at the California Institute of Technology in Pasadena, California (19). They, and the rest of the world, were startled when Marie Curie's daughter Irene and her husband Frederick Joliot published a method for the artificial production of radioactive elements. The Curies utilized 100 mCi of polonium as a powerful source of α particles, which were used to bombard various targets. The targets remained radioactive and emitted positrons after the polonium was removed. They had produced nitrogen-13, phosphorus-30, and silicon-27. In their February 1934 article in "Nature," the Curies suggested that "radio-elements" could be obtained by bombarding appropriate targets with neutrons, deuterons, or protons (20). The Italian physicist Enrico Fermi obtained 800 mCi of radon from the Rome "radium-cow" and mixed it with beryllium powder to obtain what, for 1934, was an extremely powerful source of neutrons. He bombarded targets of every pure element he could find and published the results in "Nature" 3 months after the original article of Curie and Joliot. He confirmed their findings and extended the number of artificial isotopes to 14, including ^{32}P and ^{128}I (21).

Lise Meitner described a new method of decay in 1936 called "isomeric transition," which became clinically important after the discovery of technetium-99 (1). Another,

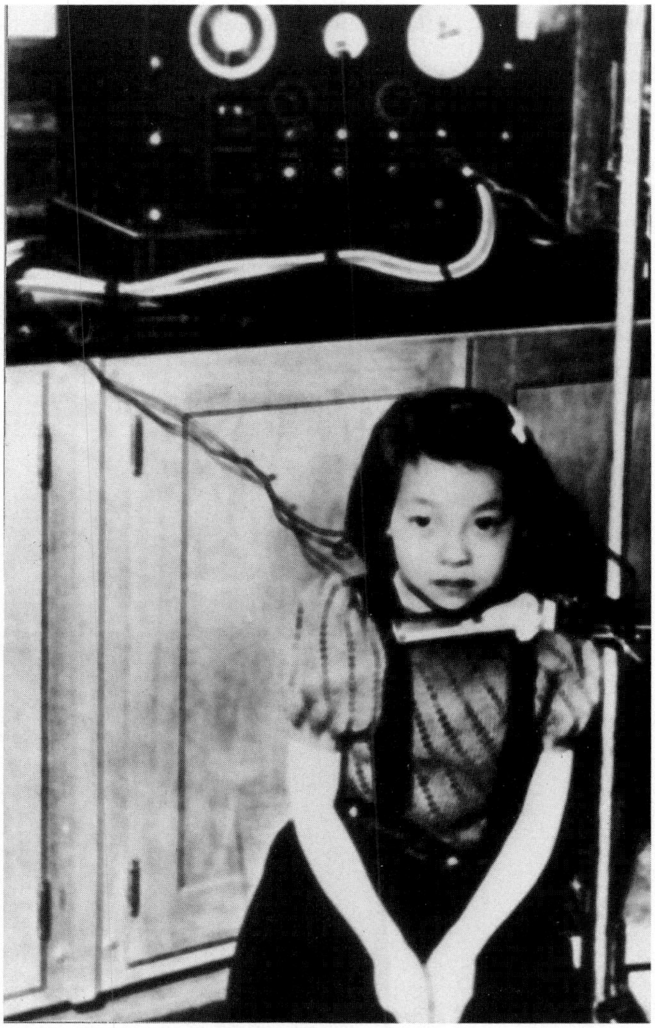

Figure 1.5. Measurements of thyroid uptake were originally performed using a Geiger counter. (Reproduced by permission from Myers WG. Introduction: Historical perspectives, nuclear medicine in clinical pediatrics. New York: Society of Magnetic Resonance, 1925.)

somewhat obscure, discovery in 1936 was the identification of the muon by Carl Anderson and others. According to the current Standard Model of Fundamental Particles and Interactions, which developed from Murray Gell-Mann's discovery of quarks, the first elementary particle to be discovered was the electron and the second was the muon. The neutron and proton are not currently considered as elementary particles because they are composed of quarks (1).

In Boston, in 1936, a group of physicists from the Massachusetts Institute of Technology (MIT) and clinicians from the Massachusetts General Hospital (MGH) became aware of Fermi's paper describing the production of a radioisotope of iodine and began a collaboration for applying radioiodine to the study of thyroid physiology and disease (22). That same year, in Berkeley, Joseph Hamilton and Robert Stone used ^{24}Na from the cyclotron to treat three patients with leukemia. A third physician, John Lawrence, Ernest's brother, performed preclinical studies and began therapeutic trials in chronic leukemia with ^{32}P (23).

Saul Hertz, Arthur Roberts, and Robley Evans of the MIT/MGH group used radon as a source of neutrons for the bombardment of natural ^{127}I to produce the 25-minute half-life ^{128}I in 1937 (Fig. 1.5). This was injected into the ear veins of rabbits in the first study of thyroid physiology using radioiodine (22). Joseph Hamilton and Mayo Soley of the Berkeley group recognized the significance of this work and proceeded directly to human studies (24). They complained about the shortcomings of 25-minute ^{128}I to Glenn Seaborg, which in 1 week led to Seaborg's and Jack Livingood's development of a method for the production of the 8-day half-life ^{131}I by bombardment of a tellurium target with 8 Mev deuterons in the Berkeley cyclotron (25). Hamilton and Soley used this ^{131}I in a few patients, but it was not pure and the method of production was not very practical, so they had to settle for the use of the 12-hour half-life ^{130}I. Forty-six different isotopes were synthesized and characterized in Berkeley between 1934 and 1940 (Fig. 1.6), including the discovery by Martin Kamen and S. Ruben of ^{14}C, which revolutionized biologic research (26). The MIT/MGH group built the first cyclotron dedicated to biomedical use and began the production of ^{131}I in 1940, which was used by Hertz and Roberts to treat 29 patients with hyperthyroidism (22).

The idea of using radioiodine for the treatment of thyroid cancer originated with Samuel Seidlin, a New York endocrinologist, who had a patient with classical hyperthyroidism despite a total thyroidectomy several years earlier for a "malignant adenoma." Seidlin obtained biopsy proof of metastatic thyroid tumor and he enlisted the assistance of the MIT/MGH group in the successful treatment of the patient with ^{130}I (27).

All of this was prologue. Nuclear medicine entered the modern era after The Manhattan Project Headquarters, Washington, DC, announced, in the June 14, 1946, issue of "Science," that many radioactive isotopes were available

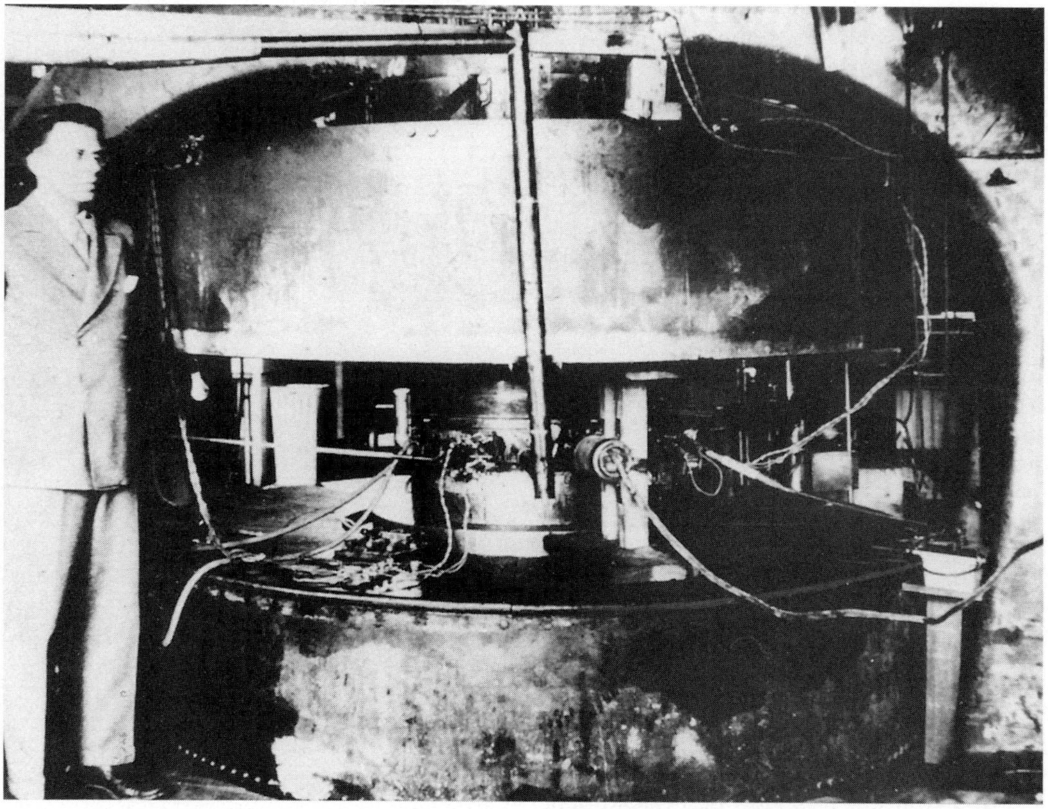

Figure 1.6. Invention of the cyclotron by Ernest O. Lawrence (pictured here) in Berkeley, California, led to a rapid expansion in the number of radionuclides available as tracers. (Reproduced by permission from Myers WG, Wagner HN Jr. Nuclear medicine: How it began. Hospital Practice 1974:9;1192.)

for public sale from the "uranium chain-reacting pile" (28). The widespread availability of radioactive isotopes led to the invention of new equipment and the development of many new clinical applications.

REFERENCES

1. Glasstone S. Sourcebook on atomic energy. 3rd ed. Princeton: Van Nostrand, 1967.
2. Glasser O. William Conrad Roentgen. Springfield, IL: Charles C. Thomas, 1933.
3. Becquerel AH. Nobel lectures: Physics 1901–1921. Amsterdam: Elsevier Publishing Co., 1967:47–73.
4. Thomson JJ. Recollections and reflections. Cambridge: Cambridge University Press, 1937.
5. Brucer M. Becquerel breaks the law. Vignettes in nuclear medicine No. 94. St. Louis: Mallinckrodt, 1979.
6. Brucer M. William Duane and the radium cow: An American contribution to an emerging atomic age. Med Phys 1993;20:1601–1605.
7. Graham LS, Kereiakes JG, Harris C, Cohen MB. Nuclear medicine from Becquerel to the present. Radiographics 1989;9:1189–1202.
8. Villard P. Sur le rayonnement du radium. Comptes Rendus 1900; 130:1010–1012.
9. Brucer M. Half-life. Vignettes in nuclear medicine No. 34. St. Louis: Mallinckrodt, 1968.
10. Brucer M. Rutherford resurrects transmutation. Vignettes in nuclear medicine. No. 96. St. Louis: Mallinckrodt, 1980.
11. Fajans K. Inaugural dissertation to Karlsrule faculty. Verk Naturist-Med Verein Heidelberg 1912;12:173.
12. Brucer M. Fajans triggers Soddy's isotopes. Vignettes in nuclear medicine. No 98. St. Louis: Mallinckrodt, 1981.
13. Boorse HA, Motz L, eds. The world of the atom. New York: Basic Books Inc., 1966.
14. Hevesy G. The absorption and translocation of lead by plants. Biochem J 1923;17:439–445.
15. de Hevesy G. Noble lecture. Stockholm, December 12, 1944.
16. Blumgart HL, Weiss S. Studies in velocity of blood flow. J Clin Invest 1927;4:15.
17. Blumgart HL, Gilligan R, Schlesinger MJ. Experimental studies on the effect of temporary occlusion of coronary arteries. II. The production of myocardial infarction. Am Heart J 1941;22:374–389.
18. Lawrence EO, Livingston MS. Production of high speed light ions without the use of high voltages. Phys Rev 1932;40:19–35.
19. Anderson CD. The positive electron. Phys Rev 1933;43:491–494.
20. Joliot F, Curie I. Artificial production of a new kind of radio-element. Nature 1934;133:201.
21. Fermi E. Radioactivity induced by neutron bombardment. [Letter]. Nature 1934;133:757.
22. Chapman EM. History of the discovery and early use of radioactive iodine. JAMA 1983;250:2042–2044.
23. Aebersold PC. The development of nuclear medicine. In: Blahd WH, Bauer FK, Cassen B, eds. The practice of nuclear medicine. Springfield, IL: Charles C Thomas, 1958.
24. Hamilton JG, Soley MH. Studies in iodine metabolism by use of a new radioactive isotope of iodine. Am J Physiol 1939;127:557–572.
25. Livingood JJ, Seaborg GT. Letter to the editor. Phys Rev 1939; 53:1015.
26. Kamen MD. Isotopic tracers in biology. 3rd ed. New York: Academic Press, 1957.
27. Brucer M. From surgery without a knife to the atomic cocktail. Vignettes in nuclear medicine No 2. St. Louis: Mallinckrodt, 1966.
28. Announcement. Science. June 14, 1946;103:697.

2 Basic Physics of Nuclear Medicine

JAMES A. PATTON

Nuclear medicine imaging techniques are performed by administering pharmaceuticals that are labeled or tagged with radionuclides so that they are preferentially accumulated in the organs of interest. Images are then obtained using detection systems that are sensitive to the γ-radiation emitted from the administered radiotracers. These images do not possess the spatial resolution of other imaging modalities such as computed tomography and magnetic resonance imaging; however, the information provided to the clinicians is generally of a different type, namely functional information. To successfully utilize these techniques, a knowledge of the basic physical principles of nuclear medicine is required. The specific topics include the basic concepts of the atom, the fundamentals of radioactive decay, and the mechanisms by which radiations interact with matter.

ATOMIC PHYSICS

Early Greek philosophers postulated that all matter was composed of fundamental units arranged in specific patterns to form different types of matter. It is now known that molecules are the smallest subdivisions of matter that retain the original physical and chemical properties of the matter. Molecules can be further broken down into basic fundamental building blocks, termed atoms, of which all matter is composed. A basic group of substances exist that cannot be broken down into different substances except by the processes of radioactive decay or nuclear reactions. These substances are termed elements and each element is composed of a single type of atom. Two or more chemical elements can combine chemically to form compounds by bonding of the atoms composing the individual elements. Thus the atom is the fundamental constituent of matter and the understanding of its anatomy is the first step in obtaining knowledge of nuclear medicine physics.

The current simplified concept of the atom was proposed by Bohr in 1913 and is shown in Figure 2.1. It is composed of a positively charged nucleus containing positively charged protons and electrically neutral neutrons, collectively termed nucleons. Surrounding the nucleus in discrete orbits or shells are enough negatively charged electrons to make the atom electrically neutral. Thus the proton number equals the electron number in the electrically neutral atom. The electron orbits were described as circular by Bohr, but in fact are elliptical. The atomic particles and their fundamental characteristics are shown in Table 2.1. Since the masses of these particles are very small, another scale, based on the atomic mass unit (amu), is often used. One amu is defined as 1/12 of the mass of the ^{12}C atom. Recall that 1 g atomic weight (mole) of ^{12}C has a mass of 12 g and contains 6.023×10^{23} atoms (Avogadro's Number). One amu thus has a mass of 1.66×10^{-24} g. Using this definition, the masses in amu's of the subatomic particles are also shown in Table 2.1. The shells of the atom are denoted by letters of the alphabet, with the innermost shell being the K shell. The next shell is identified by the letter L, the next M, and so forth. The shells are also identified by an integer number referred to as the principle quantum number, n. For the K shell $n = 1$, for the L shell $n = 2$, for the M shell $n = 3$, and so forth. In 1925, a modification to the Bohr model of the atom was presented by Pauli which stated that no two electrons can exist in the same energy state. This principle placed a limit on the number of electrons that can reside in each shell. Simply stated, Pauli's principle yields the statement that each shell can only contain a maximum of $2n^2$ electrons, and is actually composed of $2n-1$ subshells, each with slightly different characteristics. These factors are determined by selection rules, a topic which is beyond the scope of this text.

The electrons are held in their orbits by the Coulomb attractive force between them and the positively charged nucleus, and balanced by centrifugal forces as the electrons move around the nucleus. The atom is in its most stable configuration or lowest energy state when the electrons are positioned as closely as possible to the nucleus in the allowed inner orbits. This configuration is termed the ground state. It is in these positions that the force of attraction on the electrons is greatest, and it is here that the

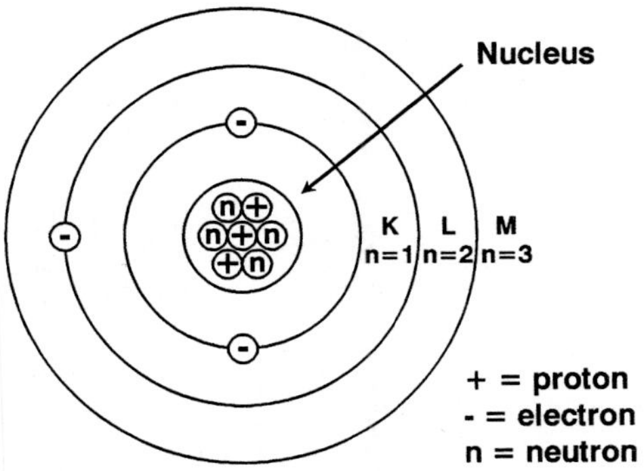

Figure 2.1. Current simplified concept of the atom.

Table 2.1.
Subatomic Particles

Name	Symbol	Charge	Mass (gm)	Mass (amu)	Relative Mass
Electron	e^-	−1	0.9108×10^{-27}	0.000549	1
Proton	p	+1	1.6724×10^{-24}	1.007277	1836
Neutron	n	0	1.6747×10^{-24}	1.008665	1840

electrons are most tightly bound. The energy required to completely remove an electron from a particular shell within an atom is defined as the binding energy of that shell. Binding energies for a particular shell increase with increasing positive charge of the nucleus. For a given atom, binding energies decrease in moving from inner to outer shells. Thus, in order to move an electron from an inner shell to an outer shell, energy must be supplied to the electron. This process is called excitation, and the energy supplied must be at least equal to the difference in binding energies of the two shells involved in the transition. Conversely, when an electron moves from an outer shell to an inner shell, this same amount of energy must be released in the process. This de-excitation process results in the emission of either a characteristic x-ray or an Augér (pronounced oh-zhay) electron (Fig. 2.2**A**). The characteristic x-rays are photons whose energies are equal to the difference in binding energies of the two shells involved in the transition. They are identified on the basis of the shell in which the original vacancy existed. For example, an electron dropping down from the L shell to fill a vacancy in the K shell will result in the emission of a K x-ray.

Augér electron emission is an alternative to characteristic x-ray emission. In this process, the energy released by an outer-shell electron when filling an inner-shell vacancy is transferred to another orbital electron, usually an outer-shell electron, which is then ejected from the atom. The kinetic energy of this electron is equal to the binding energy of the shell being filled minus the sum of the binding energies of the two shells ending up with vacancies after the process is complete. Characteristic x-ray emission or Augér electron emission occurs after each transition. The fluorescent yield is defined for each shell of each element as the probability of characteristic x-ray emission per shell vacancy, and increases with increasing positive charge of the nucleus.

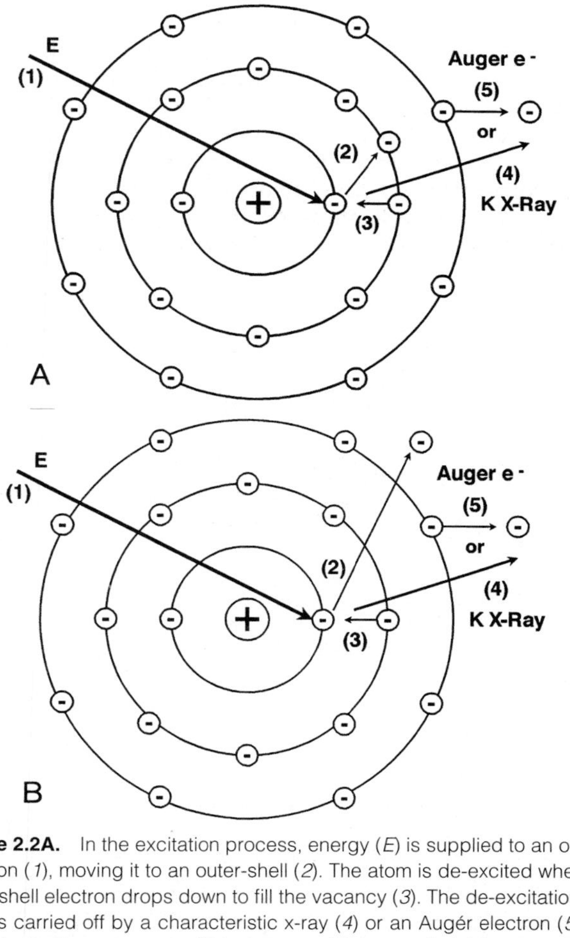

Figure 2.2A. In the excitation process, energy (*E*) is supplied to an orbital electron (*1*), moving it to an outer-shell (*2*). The atom is de-excited when an outer-shell electron drops down to fill the vacancy (*3*). The de-excitation energy is carried off by a characteristic x-ray (*4*) or an Augér electron (*5*). **B**. In the ionization process, sufficient energy (*E*) is supplied (*1*) to completely remove an electron from the atom (*2*). The vacancy is then filled by the de-excitation process described above.

The binding energies of electrons in their shells and the energies of characteristic radiation are relatively small. These values are usually stated in terms of the electron volt (eV). This unit is defined as the kinetic energy acquired by a single electron when accelerated through a 1 volt potential difference. Outer shells of light atoms have binding energies of a few electron volts, whereas inner shells of heavy atoms have binding energies that approach 100 keV (1 keV = 1000 eV). Nuclear processes discussed later involve higher energy values which are measured in terms of millions of electron volts (1 MeV = 1000 keV = 1,000,000 eV).

If sufficient energy is absorbed by an orbital electron to completely remove it from the atom, the process is termed ionization (Fig. 2.2**B**). The electron then has a kinetic energy equal to the energy absorbed minus the binding energy of the shell from which it was removed. The atom is left in an excited state and it is de-excited by outer-shell electrons dropping down to fill the vacancies, again resulting in characteristic x-ray or Augér electron emission as previously described. This process continues until the vacancy moves to the outermost shell, where a free electron is captured to return the atom to its ground state and make it electrically neutral again.

NUCLEAR PHYSICS

As previously stated, the nucleus of an atom is composed of positively charged protons and neutrons with no charge. Coulomb's law predicts that there would be very strong electrostatic forces of repulsion between the positive charges when brought together. However, within the nucleus, the presence of neutrons in combination with the protons provide an environment in which short-range attractive nuclear forces exist that are many times stronger than the repulsive electrostatic forces, and thus a very dense, compact nucleus is created. In fact, the neutrons may be thought of as glue that helps hold the nucleus together. If the mass of the nucleus is subtracted from the sums of the masses of the individual nucleons, a positive mass difference remains. This difference, termed the mass deficit or mass defect, is explained by the fact that each nucleon gives up a small amount of mass when they are bound within the nucleus. In actuality, this mass is converted to energy and determines the magnitude of the nuclear binding energy which holds the nucleons together. The nuclear binding energy can be calculated by the equation developed by Einstein when he proposed that mass is simply another form of energy. This equation is given by

$$E = \Delta mc^2$$

where E is the binding energy, Δm is the mass defect, and c is the velocity of light. In practice, the mass defect can be calculated using atomic mass units and converted to energy units by using the energy definition of 1 amu (931.5 MeV). Nuclear binding energies are significantly higher than electron binding energies (on the order of millions of electron volts (MeV)). A relationship that is commonly quoted is the binding energy per nucleon and is directly related to the stability of the nucleus.

The most fundamental characteristic of an atom is its atomic number (Z), which is the number of protons within the nucleus (also the number of electrons in the electrically neutral atom). Each element has a unique atomic number and the chemical symbol for the element is synonymous with the atomic number. The number of neutrons within the nucleus is denoted by N. The atomic mass number (A) is the total number of nucleons (neutrons + protons) within the nucleus, thus $A = Z + N$. The atomic mass number is approximately equal to, but not to be mistaken for, the atomic weight, which is the average of the atomic mass numbers of all the naturally occurring atoms of an element weighted according to their natural percentages of abundance.

Any nucleus plus its orbital electrons (i.e., any atom) is termed a nuclide. Nuclides are classified on the basis of their nuclear composition and arrangement of nucleons within the nucleus. A nuclear shorthand exists for the characterization of nuclides and is of the form ${}^{A}_{Z}X_{N}$ where X is the chemical symbol of the element to which the nuclide belongs. Since Z is synonymous with the chemical symbol and $N = A - Z$, the shortened form ^{A}X is generally used, as in ^{131}I ($Z = 53$, $N = 78$) and ^{57}Co ($Z = 27$, $N = 30$). Another form that is acceptable, but now less widely used, is *X-A*, as in I-131 and Co-57.

Nuclides that have similar characteristics are often grouped into nuclear families. Isotopes are nuclides that have the same atomic number (Z) and thus are nuclides of a particular element. Isobars are nuclides with the same atomic mass number (A). Isotones are nuclides with the same number of neutrons (N). Isomers are nuclides that are identical in all characteristics except the energy state of the nucleus. An easy way to remember these definitions is: isoto*p*es have the same *p*roton number, isob*a*rs have the same *a*tomic mass number, isoto*n*es have the same *n*eutron number, and isom*e*rs differ only in *e*nergy state. These nuclear families, along with examples, are summarized in Table 2.2.

Table 2.2.
Nuclear Families

Name	*A*	*Z*	*N*	Energy State	Examples
Isoto*p*e	Dif.	Same	Dif.	Dif.	^{127}Xe, ^{129}Xe, ^{131}Xe
Isob*a*r	Same	Dif.	Dif.	Dif.	^{131}I, ^{131}Xe, ^{131}Te
Isoto*n*e	Dif.	Dif.	Same	Dif.	^{131}I, ^{132}Xe, ^{133}Ce
Isom*e*r	Same	Same	Same	Dif.	^{99m}Tc, ^{99}Tc

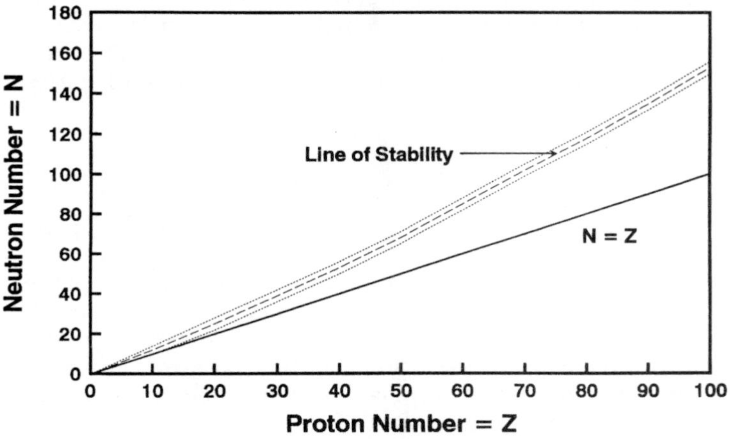

Figure 2.3. Neutron number (N) versus proton number (Z) for stable nuclei. The line of stability deviates from the $N = Z$ line (*dashed line*) due to a necessary excess of neutrons. Nuclei to the left and right of the line of stability are radioactive.

RADIOACTIVE DECAY

It has been observed that most nuclei existing in nature are stable and have high binding energies per nucleon. On the other hand, certain nuclei have lower binding energies per nucleon and are not stable. These nuclei transform themselves randomly and spontaneously to form more stable configurations. These transformations can result in the emission of particles or photons and energy from the nuclei. One important factor in the stability of the nucleus is the neutron:proton ratio. Figure 2.3 shows a plot of neutron number, N, versus proton number (atomic number), Z, for the relatively stable nuclei. The stable nuclei fall along a narrow band called the line of stability. Light nuclei tend to contain the same number of neutrons and protons, and thus the slope is initially approximately unity. As Z increases, the N:Z ratio increases to about 1.5. The extra neutrons serve to increase the average distance between protons within the nucleus, thereby reducing the repulsive Coulomb force acting between these particles. If the N:Z ratio deviates to either side of the line of stability due to an excess of protons or neutrons, the nuclides become unstable. Stability is achieved by emission of particles from the nucleus, resulting in a change in the identity of the nuclide and a more favorable N:Z ratio.

Radioactive decay is a random and spontaneous nuclear process in which an unstable parent nucleus transforms into a more stable daughter nucleus through the emission of particles or γ-rays. Energy is also released and carried off by the radioactive emissions. The process is totally unaffected by changes in temperature, pressure, or chemical combinations. The term radioactive "decay" was coined in the early 1900s by investigators who noted that some elements lost their radioactive properties in a consistent fashion that varied from one element to another. It was reasoned that some radioactive atoms were "disintegrating" and producing other atoms. The rate at which the atoms were "decaying" was measured in "disintegrations per second." Any unstable or radioactive atom is referred to as a radionuclide. The most important factors determining stability are a favorable N:Z ratio, pairing of nucleons, and a high binding energy per nucleon. The greater the variance from these three factors, the greater the tendency of a nuclide to be unstable.

Radionuclides either occur naturally or are artificially produced. The naturally occurring radionuclides are those that exist in an unstable state in nature. They emit radiation spontaneously with no external influence necessary to produce radioactive decay. Most of the naturally occurring radionuclides have atomic numbers greater than 82. Two notable exceptions are ^{14}C and ^{40}K. The artificial radionuclides are manmade, unstable nuclides produced by bombarding stable nuclides with high-energy particles in a cyclotron, linear accelerator, or nuclear reactor. All of the radionuclides used in nuclear medicine fall into the latter category.

DECAY SCHEMES

All radioactive decay processes can be described using decay schemes that present a detailed analysis of how a radioactive parent is transformed into the ground state of the daughter. Figure 2.4 illustrates the standard format used. An arrow is drawn from the parent to the daughter with the *D-U-I* mnemonic used to indicate that an arrow drawn to the left indicates a decrease in atomic number (positive particle emission), straight down indicates unchanged atomic number (γ emission), and to the right indicates an increase in atomic number (negative particle emission). Several horizontal lines may be drawn to indicate the various energy states of the daughter. Additional information, usually supplied on the diagram, includes energies and percent abundances of the transitions and half-lives of the energy states. The decay scheme is actually an energy level diagram with energy represented by the vertical axis and the lowest energy state or ground state at the bottom of the diagram.

Radioactive decay processes can also be described using nuclear equations. These are of the general form:

$$^{A}_{Z}X \rightarrow {}^{A'}_{Z'}Y + W + Q$$

where X represents the parent radionuclide with atomic mass number A and atomic number Z, Y represents the daughter nuclide with atomic mass number A' and atomic number Z', W is the radiation type emitted (may be more than one), and Q is the total energy released in the nuclear transition. These nuclear equations must be balanced as chemical equations so that total charge, total number of nucleons (A), and total energy (remember that mass is one form of energy) are the same on both sides of the equation. Since this equation describes a nuclear decay process, Q is determined by the differences in the mass of the parent nucleus and the sums of the masses of the daughter nucleus and the particles produced in the decay process. This mass difference is converted to energy and released as the daughter products are produced. The magnitude of the energy released in the process can be calculated by Einstein's mass-energy equation.

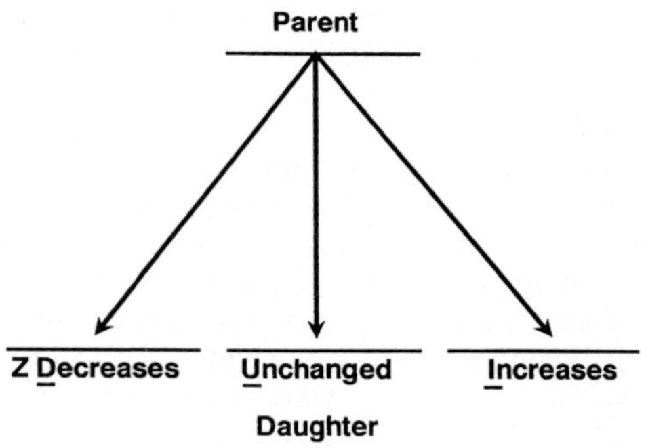

Figure 2.4. Standard format used to illustrate decay schemes.

DECAY PROCESSES

There are seven basic nuclear decay processes, which may be grouped into three major categories. These are α transitions, isobaric transitions (including β emission, positron emission, and electron capture), and isomeric transitions (including excited and metastable state transitions and internal conversion). The kinds of radiation emitted in these processes are summarized in Table 2.3. The transformation of a radioactive parent to the ground state of the daughter may involve one or more of these transitions. Of these seven, only six are of importance in nuclear medicine imaging. These are β emission, positron emission, electron capture, and the isomeric transitions.

α Decay

The α decay process may be described by the equation:

$$^{A}_{Z}X \rightarrow {}^{A-4}_{Z-2}Y + {}^{4}_{2}\alpha + Q$$

The α particle is the nucleus of the ^{4}He atom, which consists of two protons and two neutrons, and therefore has a charge of +2 and a mass of approximately 4 amu's. α-Particles usually possess high energy and short range (a few centimeters in air, a fraction of a millimeter in tissue) and are emitted primarily from extremely heavy nuclei (atomic numbers greater than 82). An example of α decay is shown in Figure 2.5 and is described by the equation:

$$^{226}_{88}Ra \rightarrow {}^{222}_{86}Rn + {}^{4}_{2}\alpha$$

Because of the large size, high energy, and short range of α particles, they cannot escape body tissues, and, therefore, they deposit very high radiation doses internally. α-Emitters also have very long lifetimes and thus have no use in nuclear medicine imaging procedures.

β Decay

Isobaric transitions are decay processes in which the parent and daughter are isobars—members of a nuclear fam-

Table 2.3.
Emissions from Radioactive Decay Processes

Name	Symbol	Charge	Mass (gm)
Alpha	α	+2	6.6394×10^{-24}
Beta	β^-	−1	0.9108×10^{-27}
Positron	β^+	+1	0.9108×10^{-27}
Neutrino	υ	0	0
Gamma	γ	0	0

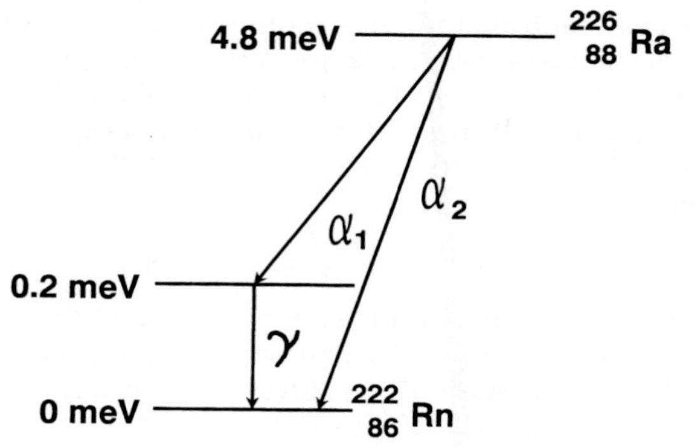

Figure 2.5. ^{226}Ra decay scheme illustrating α decay.

ily that have the same atomic mass number A but different Z and N. Three isobaric processes are possible: β decay, positron decay, and electron capture. In β-emission the nuclear reaction is of the form:

$$^{A}_{Z}X \rightarrow \, ^{A}_{Z+1}Y + \beta^- + v + Q$$

The β particles (β^-) are negatively charged electrons that originate in the nucleus and have the same mass and charge as orbital electrons. They have a broad distribution of energies, their velocities approach the speed of light, and they are classified as medium range particles (several hundred centimeters in air, a few millimeters in tissue). β^- Emission occurs in unstable nuclides that have an unfavorably high N/Z ratio due to an excess of neutrons. Greater stability is obtained in these nuclides by the conversion of a neutron into a proton and the emission of a β particle. This conversion may be written as:

$$^{1}_{0}n \rightarrow \, ^{1}_{1}p + \beta^- + v + Q$$

It was originally thought that Q, the energy of the transition, was exactly equal to the energy of the β particle plus that of any associated γ-rays. However, when measurements of β energies were made from a large number of atoms of a particular radionuclide, it was observed that the β particles had a continuous range of energies from zero to a maximum value that was equal to Q when there were no γ-rays involved in the decay process. A typical β spectrum is shown in Figure 2.6. The average β energy is approximately equal to 1/3 the maximum energy. To explain the variance in both energies, a new particle was postulated by Pauli in 1931, and its existence was later verified experimentally. This particle, the antineutrino ($\bar{v}$), has no mass and no charge. It carries off the excess energy in each β decay process ($E_{max} = E_{\beta} + E_{v}$). In some nuclides, after β decay the nucleus may be left in an excited state, with the excess energy carried away by one or more γ-rays as the nucleus moves to the most stable configuration or the ground state.

An example of β decay is the transformation of ^{131}I to ^{131}Xe by the nuclear equation

$$^{131}_{53}\mathrm{I} \rightarrow \, ^{131}_{54}\mathrm{Xe} + \beta^- + \bar{v}$$

The corresponding decay scheme is shown in Figure 2.7.

Positron Decay

Positron emission is a second type of isobaric transition. In this decay process, unstable nuclides that have an unfavorably low N/Z ratio, because of an excess of protons, are transferred to a more stable configuration by the nuclear equation

$$^{A}_{Z}X \rightarrow \, ^{A}_{Z-1}Y + \beta^+ + v + Q$$

The positron (β^+) has the same mass as an orbital electron but is positively charged. The decay process may be described by the conversion of a proton to a neutron with the emission of a positron as indicated by

$$^{1}_{1}p \rightarrow \, ^{1}_{0}n + \beta^+ + v + Q$$

Although this reaction appears impossible because the mass of the neutron is greater than the mass of the proton, the equation describes the restructuring of the nucleus and, therefore, it is understood that part of the energy necessary to form the neutron is supplied by the other nucleons. Positrons decay with a continuous spectrum of energies, as with β decay, and the difference between the expected energy, E_{max}, and the observed energy in each decay process is carried off by the neutrino.

A unique characteristic of the positron is that it cannot exist at rest in nature. Once it loses its kinetic energy, it immediately combines with a negatively charged electron and undergoes an annihilation reaction in which the masses of the two particles are completely converted into

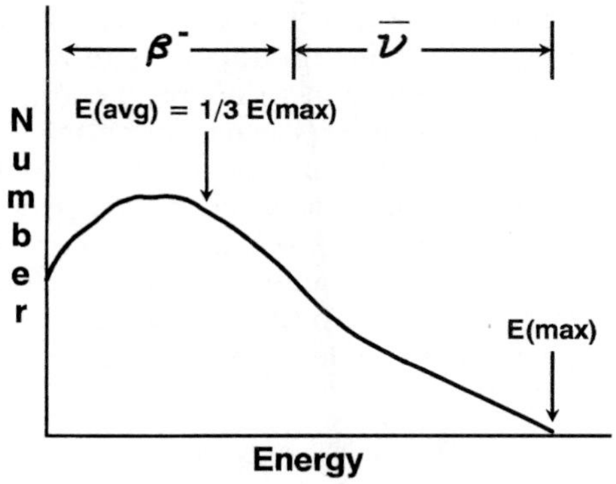

Figure 2.6. Typical spectrum of β energies for a particular β decay process. The sum of the energies of the β particle and the neutrino is equal to the total energy given off in the decay process if no γ-rays are involved in the process.

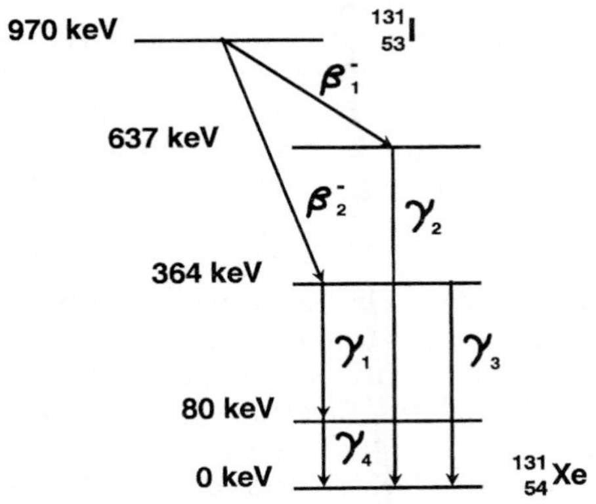

Figure 2.7. ^{131}I decay scheme illustrating β decay.

energy in the form of two 0.511 MeV γ-rays or annihilation photons, which leave their production site at 180° from each other (Fig. 2.8). There is a minimum energy of 1.022 MeV that must exist between the parent and the daughter before positron emission can occur. The excess energy above that value is divided between the positron and the neutrino. As with other processes, the daughter may be left in an excited state, with γ-emission being the process by which the daughter moves to the ground state.

An example of positron decay is the decay of ^{15}O to ^{15}N given by the equation:

$$^{15}O \rightarrow {}^{15}N + \beta^{+} + \upsilon$$

The corresponding decay scheme is shown in Figure 2.9.

Electron Capture

The third isobaric transition possibility is electron capture. Like positron emission, electron capture occurs in unstable nuclides that have an unfavorably low N/Z ratio. Electron capture is a nuclear decay process in which the nucleus captures one of the inner-shell orbital electrons (most probably from the K shell) of the atom, as illustrated in Figure 2.10. The general nuclear equation is of the form

$$^{A}_{Z}X + e^{-} \rightarrow {}^{A}_{Z-1}Y + \upsilon + Q$$

The daughter produced by electron capture is the same as that resulting from positron decay. In fact, positron emission and electron capture are competing decay processes in certain radionuclides. Electron capture may be thought of as reverse β decay in that the electron unites with a proton to form a neutron with excess energy carried off by the neutrino. The equation may be written as

$$^{1}_{1}p + e^{-} \rightarrow {}^{1}_{0}n + \upsilon + Q$$

The process may leave the nucleus in an excited state, which subsequently leads to γ-emission. After electron capture the atom is also left in an excited state due to the vacancy created in the inner-shell of the atom. The atom is de-excited by outer-shell electrons dropping down to fill the vacancies, resulting in characteristic x-ray or Augér electron emission as shown in Figure 2.10. The detection of the characteristic x-rays is the primary mechanism for the identification of electron capture decay processes. An example of electron capture is the decay of ^{201}Tl to ^{201}Hg by the equation

$$^{201}_{81}Tl + e^{-} \rightarrow {}^{201}_{80}Hg + \upsilon + \gamma$$

The γ-ray is included in this equation because the daughter nucleus is left in an excited state and is immediately de-excited by γ-emission. The corresponding decay scheme is shown in Figure 2.11.

γ-EMISSION

Excited State Transitions

As stated in each of the earlier descriptions of the various decay processes, in many instances the daughter nuclide is left in an excited state. It subsequently is de-excited through the release of energy in the form of γ-rays. Many times the transition through the excited state is virtually instantaneous, i.e., the lifetime of the excited state is too short to measure (less than 10^{-12} seconds). In general the nuclear equation for excited state transitions can be written as:

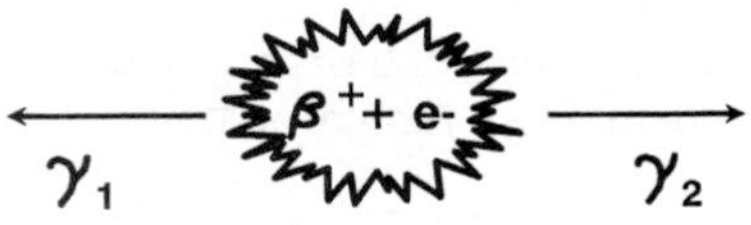

Figure 2.8. In the annihilation process, an electron and a positron combine to form two 511 keV γ-rays that leave their production site at 180° from each other.

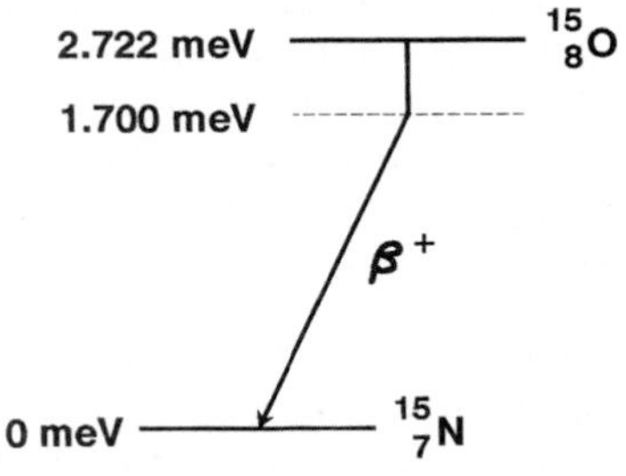

Figure 2.9. ^{15}O decay scheme illustrating positron decay.

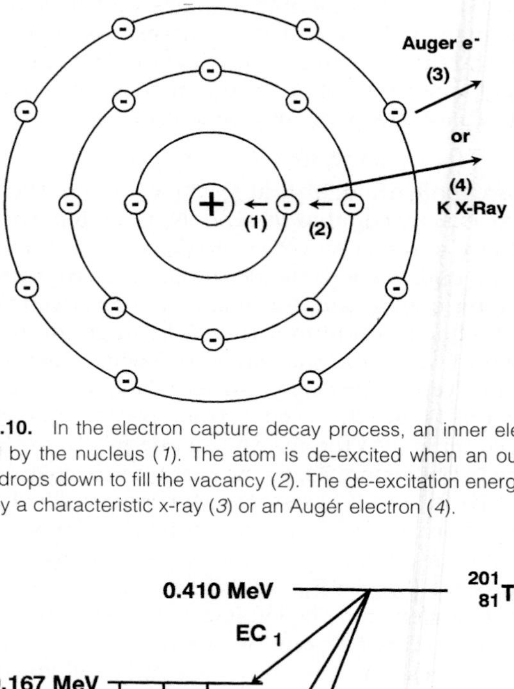

Figure 2.10. In the electron capture decay process, an inner electron is captured by the nucleus (*1*). The atom is de-excited when an outer-shell electron drops down to fill the vacancy (*2*). The de-excitation energy is carried off by a characteristic x-ray (*3*) or an Augér electron (*4*).

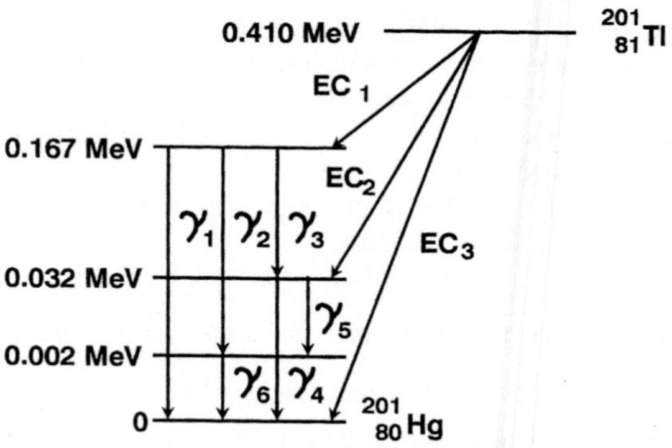

Figure 2.11. ^{201}T1 decay scheme illustrating decay by electron capture.

$${}^{A}_{Z}X \rightarrow [{}^{A'}_{Z'}Y]^{*} + W + Q \rightarrow {}^{A'}_{Z'}Y + W + Q + \gamma$$

Since the excited state has no measurable lifetime, the middle section of this equation is usually deleted. An example is the decay of ^{123}I to ^{123}Te as illustrated by the equation

$${}^{123}_{53}\text{I} + e^{-} \rightarrow {}^{123}_{53}\text{Te} + \upsilon + \gamma$$

Thus ^{123}I decays to an excited state of ^{123}Te by electron capture. The nucleus immediately goes from the excited state to the ground state by the emission of a γ-ray. In γ-emission, the de-excitation process may be very simple (only one γ-ray emitted) or very complicated. For example, ^{206}Bi has 74 γ-ray transitions in its decay scheme. γ-Rays may appear on a decay scheme in parallel (side-by-side) to represent alternate modes of decay or in cascade (one after the other) to indicate passage through multiple excited states. The decay scheme for ^{123}I is shown in Figure 2.12.

Metastable State Transitions

If the excited state of the nucleus exists for a measurable lifetime (more than 10^{-12} seconds), the state is referred to as an isomeric or metastable state. The metastable state and ground state of the daughter are called isomers since they have the same Z and N and differ only in energy state. The general nuclear equations for this decay process may be written as

$${}^{A}_{Z}X \rightarrow {}^{A'm}_{Z'}Y + W + Q$$

$${}^{A'm}_{Z'}Y \rightarrow {}^{A'}_{Z'}Y + \gamma$$

An "m" is added to the atomic mass number of the first state of the daughter to indicate a metastable state with a measurable lifetime. The metastable state moves to the ground state through de-excitation by γ-emission. The only difference between metastable and excited state transitions is the measurable lifetime of the metastable state. An example is the decay of ^{99}Mo to ^{99}Tc through the metastable state, ^{99m}Tc. The decay equations are

$${}^{99}_{42}\text{Mo} \rightarrow {}^{99m}_{43}\text{Tc} + \beta^{-} + \upsilon$$

$${}^{99m}_{43}\text{Tc} \rightarrow {}^{99}_{43}\text{Tc} + \gamma$$

The corresponding decay scheme is shown in Figure 2.13.

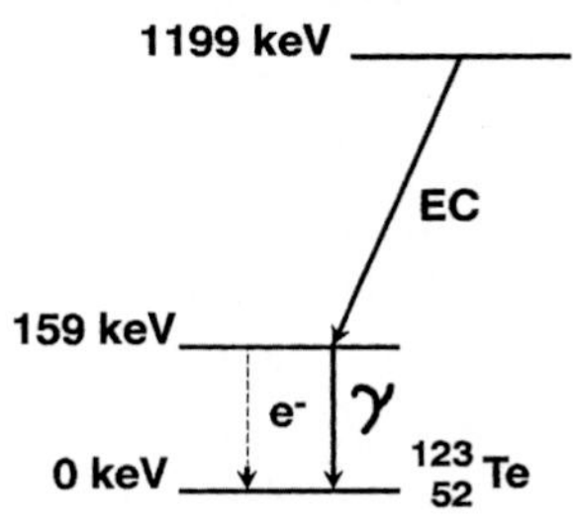

Figure 2.12. ^{123}I decay scheme illustrating γ-emission through an excited-state transition.

Internal Conversion

In many nuclides that undergo de-excitation by emitting γ-rays, there is a process that competes with γ-emission. This is the process of internal conversion and it occurs primarily in metastable state transitions. In this process, the nucleus, while changing energy states, may occasionally transfer energy from the nucleus to inner-shell orbital electrons, which are subsequently ejected from the atom. We may think of this process as if the γ-ray from the nucleus is internally absorbed by the electron, as illustrated in Figure 2.14. This conversion electron exits the atom with a kinetic energy equal to the original γ-ray energy minus the binding energy of the electron in its shell. This process leaves the atom in an excited state due to the vacancy created, and the atom is de-excited by an outer-shell electron dropping down to fill the vacancy and is, therefore, followed by characteristic x-ray or Augér electron emission.

The percentage of internal conversion electrons and γ-rays emitted is given by the internal conversion coefficient, which is defined experimentally for each radionuclide decaying by the two processes. This coefficient is the ratio of conversion electrons emitted from the atom to

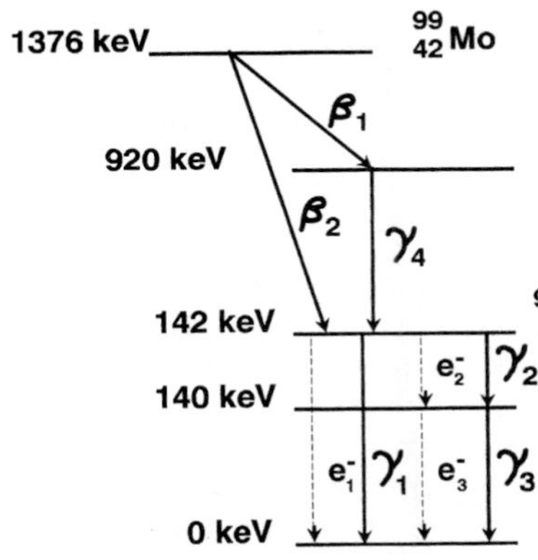

Figure 2.13. ^{99}Mo decay scheme illustrating γ-emission through a metastable state transition.

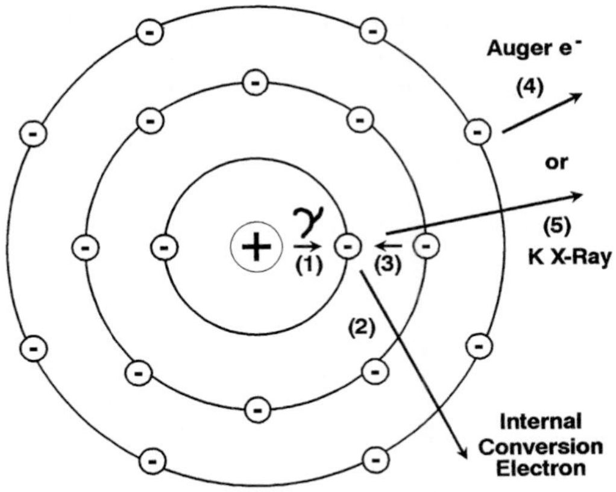

Figure 2.14. In the internal conversion process, a γ emitted from the nucleus is captured by an inner-shell electron (*1*) which is then ejected from the atom (*2*). The atom is de-excited when an outer-shell electron drops down to fill the vacancy (*3*). The de-excitation energy is carried off by a characteristic x-ray (*4*) or an Augér electron (*5*).

γ-rays emitted from the nucleus. It is usually defined for each shell, with the highest probability being the K shell coefficient. The decay schemes in Figures 2.11, 2.12, and 2.13 illustrate how internal concession competes with γ-emission.

In selecting a radionuclide for imaging, one must consider, in addition to the half-life, the modes of decay, the energies of the transitions, and the percentage of occurrence of each transition. Table 2.4 details all of the radiation types that result from each of the seven basic processes. Table 2.5 lists the primary radiations from the most common radionuclides used in nuclear medicine imaging.

DECAY EQUATIONS

Radioactive decay has been considered on a microscopic scale in the past several sections in order to examine the various types of radioactive decay processes that are possible. Radioactive decay can also be considered on a macroscopic scale by writing decay equations to describe the processes independent of the types of decay.

In a given group of identical atoms of a radionuclide, we cannot predict when a particular atom will decay. However, if there are N radioactive atoms present and ΔN atoms decay in a small increment of time Δt, we can say that the average rate of decay, R, is $\Delta N/\Delta t$. This value is also referred to as the activity, A. The decay rate or activity is directly proportional to the number of atoms present and is given by

$$R = A = -\lambda N$$

The proportionality constant, λ, is the decay constant and is the fractional number of atoms decaying per unit of time. The decay constant thus has units of (1/time). The decay constant is a unique value characteristic for each radionuclide. The minus sign in the decay equation indicates that N is decreasing with time. It must be noted that R is the average decay rate. Measurements of decay rate will fluctuate about the average decay rate since radioactive decay is statistical in nature and based on Poisson statistics.

Units of decay rate are disintegrations per second (dps) or disintegrations per minute (dpm). Since these values are usually relatively large, activity is generally measured using an alternative scale. The basic conventional unit of activity that has been used in the past is the curie (Ci), which is based on an early observation that 1 g of ^{226}Ra had a decay rate of 3.7×10^{10} dps (only approximately correct). Other units of activity are defined in Table 2.6. Fractional units of activity are specific activity (activity per unit mass) and concentration (activity per unit volume).

Table 2.4.
Radioactive Decay Processes

Process	Possible Radiation Types Emitted
Alpha decay	α
Beta decay	β^-, υ
Positron decay	β^+, υ, 2γ
Electron capture	ν, x-ray, Augér electron
Gamma emission	γ
Internal conversion	IC electron, γ, x-ray, Augér electron

IC = internal conversion

A new system of units, the Systeme Internationale (SI) has been introduced and is now the preferred system. The basic unit of activity in this system is the Becquerel (Bq) which corresponds to a decay rate of one disintegration per second. The units of this system are also shown in Table 2.6.

Since the number of atoms, N, remaining to decay at any time, t, is always less than the original number, N_o, present at time t=0, an equation is needed to specify the number of atoms remaining to decay. This equation is

$$N = N_o e^{-\lambda t}$$

This equation says that the number of atoms, N, remaining to decay at any time, t, is equal to the original number, N_o, reduced by the exponential $e^{-\lambda t}$. This exponential is known as the decay factor and "e" ($\bar{v}$ 2.7) is the base of the natural system of logarithms (recall that $e^x = y$ implies that $\ln y = x$).

Two other forms of this equation are

$$R = R_o e^{-\lambda t}$$

$$A = A_o e^{-\lambda t}$$

There are several ways to solve problems with these equations. In the past, graphic solutions were performed using semilogarithmic graph paper since plots of exponentials on this type of paper are straight lines. Values of e^x and e^{-x} are tabulated so that mathematic solutions can be easily obtained. Most pocket calculators have natural logarithm calculation capability, making mathematic solutions relatively simple. Often decay factors are tabulated for commonly used radionuclides to simplify activity calculations for technologists.

Physical Half-life

It was previously stated that the decay constant, λ, is uniquely defined for each radionuclide. However, a term related to the lifetimes of radionuclides has a more physical meaning in their routine use. The most commonly used factor is the physical half-life ($T_{1/2}$). This is the time required for one-half of a group of radioactive atoms to decay or the time for an activity or a decay rate to be reduced to one-half its original value. It can be shown that the half-life and the decay constant are related by

$$\lambda T_{1/2} = 0.693$$

Thus, the decay equation may be written as

$$N = N_o e^{-\frac{0.693t}{T_{1/2}}}$$

The decay rate and activity equations can be modified accordingly to yield their most widely used forms.

$$R = R_o e^{-\frac{0.693t}{T_{1/2}}}$$

$$A = A_o e^{-\frac{0.693t}{T_{1/2}}}$$

Table 2.5.
Nuclear Decay Data for Radionuclides used in Clinical Nuclear Medicine Imaging

Nuclide	Half-Life	Transition	Energy (keV)	Abundance (%)
^{67}Ga	78 hrs	EC[a] (9 KeV x-rays)		100
		Gamma 1[b]	93	38
		Gamma 2[b]	185	24
		Gamma 3[b]	300	16
		Gamma 4	394	4
		IC[c] electron 1	93	33
		IC[c] electron 2	185	<1
		IC[c] electron 3	300	<1
^{111}In	68 hrs	EC[a] (23 KeV x-rays)		100
		Gamma 1[b]	172	90
		Gamma 2[b]	247	94
		IC[c] electron 1	172	10
		IC[c] electron 2	247	6
^{123}I (Fig 2.12)	13 hrs	EC[a] (27 KeV x-rays)		98
		Gamma[b]	159	84
		IC[c] electron	159	16
^{131}I (Fig 2.7)	8 days	Beta 1	333	7
		Beta 2	606	90
		Gamma 1	284	6
		Gamma 2	637	7
		Gamma 3[b]	364	84
		Gamma 4	80	7
^{99}Mo (Fig 2.13)	66 hrs	Beta 1	456	18
		Beta 2	1234	80
		Gamma 4	778	5
^{99m}Tc (Fig 2.13)	6 hrs	Gamma 1	142	<1
		Gamma 2	2	1
		Gamma 3[b]	140	88
		IC[c] electron 1	142	1
		IC[c] electron 2	2	99
		IC[c] electron 3	140	11
^{201}Tl 100 (Fig 2.11)	73 hrs	EC[a] (70 KeV x-rays)[b]		
		Gamma 1	167	10
		Gamma 3	135	<3
		IC[c] electron 1	167	15
		IC[c] electron 3	135	8
^{133}Xe	5 days	Beta	346	99
		Gamma[b]	81	37
		IC[c] electron	81	52
^{11}C	20 min	Positron[d]	960	100
^{13}N	10 min	Positron[d]	1198	100
^{15}O	122 sec	Positron[d]	1732	100
^{68}Ga	68 min	Positron 1[d]	822	1
		Positron 2[d]	1899	88
		EC[a] (9 KeV x-rays)		11
^{18}Fl	110 min	Positron[d]	633	97
		EC[a] (0.5 KeV x-rays)		3
^{82}Rb	1.3 min	Positron 1[d]	2375	12
		Positron 2[d]	3150	83
		EC[a] (13 KeV x-rays)		5

[a]EC = Electron Capture (characteristic radiation secondary)
[b]Transition used for imaging
[c]IC = Internal Conversion (Note! The energies stated for the internal conversion electrons include those of the resulting characteristic x-rays and/or Augêr electrons.)
[d]511 keV γ-rays result from position annihilation and are used for imaging

Mean Life

Another useful lifetime measurement is the mean life or average life. This is the period of time that it would take for all of the atoms of a radionuclide to decay if the false assumption is made that they decay with the initial decay rate until all of the atoms have decayed. The mean life, $\overline{T}$, is then given by

$$\overline{T} =, 1.44\ T_{1/2}$$

The mean life is a useful relationship to use in radiation dose calculations, since the total number of disintegrations occurring in an administered dose is the product of the administered activity and the mean life.

Effective Half-life

In radiation dose calculations based on internally administered radionuclides and in imaging situations, the most important factor to be considered is the rate of disappear-

Table 2.6.
Units of Decay Rate (Activity) Standard Units and System Internationale (SI) Units

Standard Units	dis/sec	SI Units	dis/sec
Curie (Ci)	3.7×10^{10}	Becquerel (Bq)	1
Millicurie (mCi)	3.7×10^{7}	Kilobecquerel (KBq)	10^3
Microcurie (μCi)	3.7×10^{4}	Megabecquerel (MBq)	10^6
Nanocurie (nCi)	3.7×10	Gigabecquerel (GBq)	10^9
Picocurie (pCi)	3.7×10^{-2}		

1 Ci = 37 GBq
1 Bq = 27.03 pCi

ance of the radioactivity from the target organ and the body due to both radioactive decay and biologic excretion. An effective disappearance probability (λ_{eff}) can be defined which is equal to the probability of excretion (λ_b) plus the probability of decay (λ). Thus

$$\lambda_{eff} = \lambda_b + \lambda$$

If the biologic excretion is also exponential in form, then

$$\lambda_b T_{1/2b} = 0.693$$

The effective disappearance is then measured by the effective half-life ($T_{1/2eff}$) which is given by

$$T_{1/2eff} = (T_{1/2b} \times T_{1/2})/(T_{1/2b} + T_{1/2})$$

where $T_{1/2b}$ and $T_{1/2}$ are the biologic and physical half-lives, respectively. The mean effective life that can be used in dosimetry calculations (T_{eff}) is then defined as

$$\overline{T}_{eff} = 1.44\ T_{1/2eff}$$

RADIOACTIVE EQUILIBRIUM

The decay equations may become more complicated when the radioactive parent decays to a daughter that is also radioactive. This problem arises because the daughter is decaying at the same time it is being formed by the decay of the parent. A differential equation can be written to characterize this process, and its solution yields the Bateman equation, which provides an expression for the activity of the daughter at any time. This equation in its general form is:

$$A_d = F\left(\frac{\lambda_d}{\lambda_d - \lambda_p}\right)A_{po}(e^{\lambda_p t} - e^{-\lambda_d t}) + A_{do}(e^{-\lambda_d t})$$

where:

A_d = Activity of the daughter at time t
A_{po} = Initial activity of the parent
A_{do} = Initial activity of the daughter
F = Fraction of the parent decaying to the daughter
λ_p = Decay constant of the parent
λ_d = Decay constant of the daughter

There are three special cases that simplify this equation. The first case occurs when the half-life of the daughter is greater than the half-life of the parent ($\lambda_d < \lambda_p$). In this case, the parent decays very rapidly to the daughter which then decays slowly away. There is never any fixed relationship between the parent and the daughter. In the remaining two cases, where the half-life of the parent is greater than the half-life of the daughter, a constant relationship can exist between them which is defined as the condition of radioactive equilibrium.

The second case occurs when the half-life of the parent is many times greater (i.e., approaches infinity) than the half-life of the daughter ($\lambda_p\ \lambda_d$). In this case, the Bateman equation simplifies to:

$$A_d = FA_{po}(1 - e^{-\lambda_d t})$$

If we begin with a pure parent, after several half-lives the daughter activity builds up to the point where it reaches an equilibrium condition, termed secular equilibrium, with the parent activity as shown in Figure 2.15. When equilibrium is reached, the decay rate (activity) of the daughter is equal to the decay rate (activity) of the parent, and the daughter will continue to have the same decay rate as the parent as long as no daughter nuclei are removed. An example of secular equilibrium is the decay of ^{226}Ra with a 1622 year half-life to ^{222}Rn with a 3.8 day half-life.

The third case is of special interest in nuclear medicine and occurs when the half-life of the parent is greater than the half-life of the daughter ($\lambda_p < \lambda_d$) but does not approach infinity. In this case, the Bateman equation simplifies to:

$$A_d = F\left(\frac{\lambda_d}{\lambda_d - \lambda_p}\right)A_{po}(e^{-\lambda_p t} - e^{-\lambda_d t})$$

If we begin with a pure parent, after a few half-lives, the daughter's activity builds up to a point where a constant relationship exists between the parent and daughter. The activity of the daughter can then be calculated from

$$A_d = F(A_p \times T_{1/2p})/(T_{1/2p} - T_{1/2d})$$

The daughter then decays with the half-life of the parent as shown in Figure 2.16. This condition is defined as transient equilibrium. An example is the decay of ^{99}Mo with a 66-hour half-life to ^{99m}Tc. Transient equilibrium forms the basis for the radioisotope generator as shown in Figure 2.17. In the ^{99}Mo to ^{99m}Tc generator, the activity of ^{99m}Tc builds up to approximately that of ^{99}Mo in about four half-

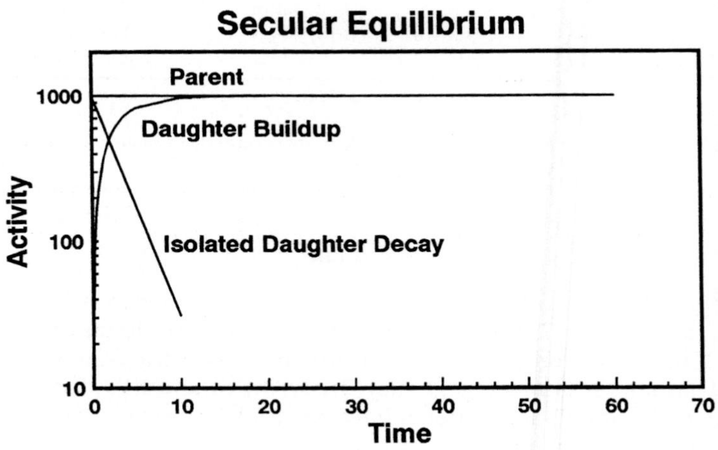

Figure 2.15. Plot of activity versus time on semilog scale for a parent and daughter satisfying the conditions for secular equilibrium.

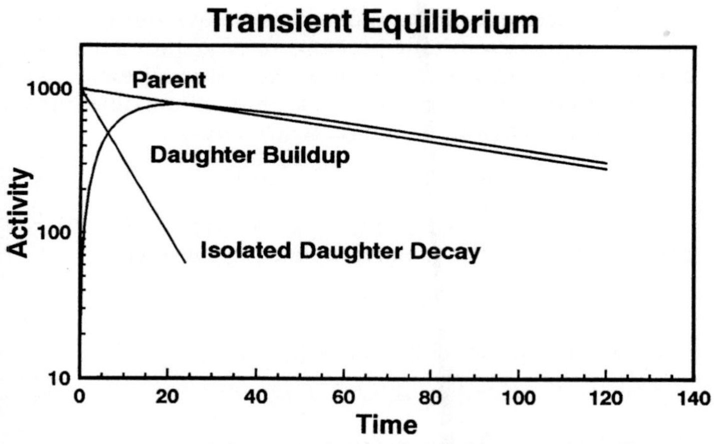

Figure 2.16. Plot of activity versus time on semilog scale for a parent and daughter satisfying conditions for transient equilibrium.

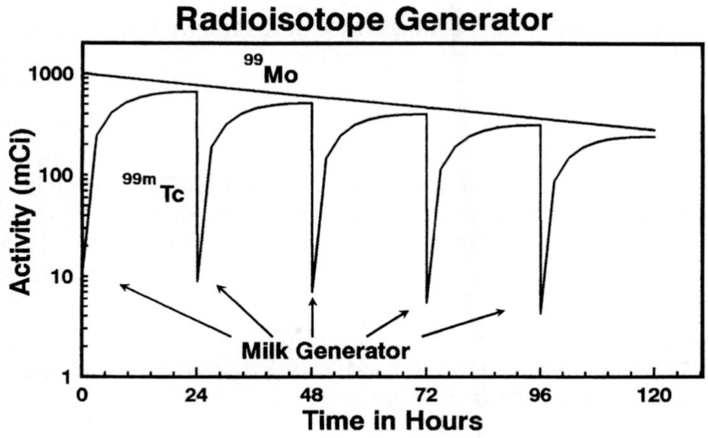

Figure 2.17. Plot of activity versus time on semilog scale of ^{99}Mo and ^{99m}Tc in secular equilibrium illustrating the principle of the radioisotope generator.

lives. If the ^{99m}Tc is removed (by "milking" the generator), the process of buildup begins immediately, with equilibrium being approached in another four half-lives, at which time the generator may be "milked" again. Thus, it is possible to receive a 1 Ci generator calibrated at 8:00 a.m. on Monday morning, "milk" it once each day, and obtain about 3.2 Ci for nuclear medicine procedures during the week.

STATISTICS

Generally, any type of measurement that is performed has some deviation in the accuracy of the value obtained. If mistakes are excluded from the discussion, then there are two basic types of deviations or errors that may contribute to the inaccuracy of a measurement. *Systematic errors* are deviations that appear in every measurement and cause the experimental values obtained to be biased either above or below the actual value by some consistent amount. Repeated measurements yield the same value with the same error. A simple example would be the measurement of a specific length using a ruler that is improperly labeled such that 1-inch is actually only 15/16-inch. Consistent measurements would yield reproducible values but all values would be shorter than the actual length. The term *accuracy* is used to characterize systematic errors and measurements that contain systematic errors are said to be *biased*.

Random errors are variations that occur in measurements generally due to factors over which the observer has no control. These errors may be due to physical constraints imposed by the methods used to perform the measurements or to actual differences in the variable being measured at the time of each measurement. For example, the measurement of a long length with a very short ruler will result in random errors due to the limitations of the measurement device. Another example is the measurement of the diameter of beans with a micrometer resulting in random errors due to the variability in the diameter of the beans. The terms *precision* and *reproducibility* are used to characterize random errors, and the term *uncertainty* is used as a measure of the random error associated with a measurement.

If a large number of measurements containing random errors are made on a variable and the number of like values versus the measured values are plotted in a frequency distribution, the result is a bell-shaped or Gaussian curve as shown in Figure 2.18. The peak of this curve is the average value or *mean*, and the width of the curve is determined by the magnitude of the random errors associated with the measurements. If a large number of measurements are made and only random errors are associated with the measurements, the actual value should be the mean of the distribution. If N measurements are made and the values obtained are $n_1, n_2, n_3, \ldots, n_N$, then the mean is given by

$$mean = (n_1 + n_2 + n_3 + \ldots + n_N)/N$$

$$mean = \bar{n} = \sum \frac{n_i}{N}$$

The Gaussian distribution is characterized by the following equation

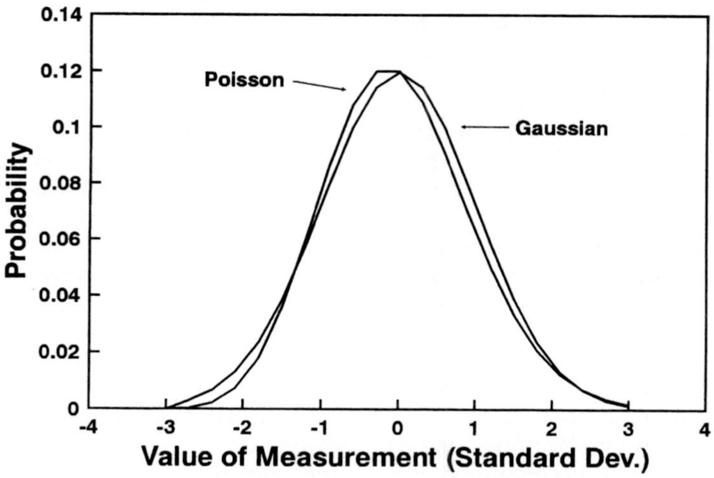

Figure 2.18. Plot of Poisson and Gaussian distributions. Measured values are plotted as a function of standard deviations about the mean. Note that the Poisson distribution is defined only for positive values.

$$P(n) = \frac{1}{\sigma\sqrt{2\pi}} e^{\frac{1}{2}\left(\frac{n-\bar{n}}{\sigma}\right)^2}$$

where $P(n)$ is the probability of measuring n, and σ is defined as the standard deviation and is a measure of the width of the Gaussian distribution. Since the width of the distribution is determined by the random errors associated with the measurements, the standard deviation is used to characterize the random errors. For the set of measurements above, the standard deviation can be calculated by

$$\sigma = \sqrt{\sum \frac{(n_i - \bar{n})^2}{n - 1}}$$

For the Gaussian distribution, there is a 68% probability that a measurement will fall within a range about the mean of one standard deviation (mean $\pm 1\sigma$). If the ranges are extended to two and three standard deviations (mean $\pm 2\sigma$ and mean $\pm 3\sigma$) the probabilities are increased to 95% and 99% respectively. These probabilities are referred to as *confidence intervals*.

Radioactive decay is a classic example of random errors being associated with a measurement. This is because radioactive decay is completely random. The decay equations defined earlier actually refer to average values of N (number of atoms decaying) and R (decay rate). Multiple measurements of N and R will yield different values which vary about some average or mean values. Radioactive decay is described by Poisson statistics and is represented by the Poisson distribution. Figure 2.27 shows that the Poisson and Gaussian distributions are very similar and essentially overlap when the mean value is large. When a single measurement of N counts is made from a radioactive sample, it is important to know the random error, also known as the *uncertainty*, associated with the measurement. Since it has been stated previously that the standard deviation (σ) is the best measure of random error, this value can be extracted from the Poisson distribution if the mean value is approximated by N and is given by

$$\sigma = \sqrt{N}$$

The result of the measurement with its associated error may then be reported as

$$N \pm \sigma = N \pm \sqrt{N}$$

The significance of the confidence intervals defined above can now be described. If there are only random errors associated with the decay process to be considered, then there is a 68% probability that the average value will fall within the measured value $\pm 1\sigma$. Similarly there is a 95% probability and a 99% probability that the average value will fall within the mean $\pm 2\sigma$ and the value $\pm 3\sigma$ respectively. Thus, these ranges define the confidence that appropriate measurements are obtained.

It is often more useful to know the percent error associated with a measurement. In general the percent error (percent uncertainty or percent standard deviation) is given by 100 times the error divided by the value in which the error is calculated. For N, this value is

$$\%\ \sigma = \frac{\sigma}{N} \times 100 = \frac{\sqrt{N}}{N} \times 100 = \frac{100}{\sqrt{N}}$$

A measurement of the differences in two decay measurements in a given time period is often required, for example when a measurement is to be adjusted for background. In general, the error in the sum or the difference of two measurements, A and B, is given by

$$\sigma_{A+/-B} = \sqrt{(\sigma_A)^2 + (\sigma_B)^2}$$

If two measurements, N_1 and N_2, are obtained, the difference between the two measurements N_n is given by

$$N_n = N_1 - N_2$$

and the error in the difference is given by

$$\sigma_{N_n} = \sqrt{N_1 + N_2}$$

The percent error in the difference is given by

$$\%\ \sigma_{N_n} = \frac{\sigma_{N_n}}{N_n} = \frac{\sqrt{N_1 + N_2}}{N_1 - N_2} \times 100$$

If N counts are measured in a time interval t, the count rate R from the sample is given by

$$R = \frac{N}{t}$$

The error in the time measurement is usually extremely small and generally can be ignored. The error in the count rate is then the error in the counts and is given by

$$\sigma_R = \frac{\sqrt{N}}{t} = \sqrt{\frac{R}{t}}$$

The percent error (100 times the error divided by the value) in the count rate is then given by

$$\%\ \sigma_R = \frac{\frac{\sqrt{N}}{t}}{\frac{N}{t}} \times 100 = \frac{100}{\sqrt{N}} = \frac{100}{\sqrt{Rt}}$$

Occasionally, a measurement is made from a sample in one time interval and a measurement of background is made in a longer time interval. In this situation, it is necessary to determine the difference in two count rates and the error associated with this difference. In general, if N_1 counts are measured in t_1 minutes and N_2 counts are measured in t_2 minutes, the net count rate R_n in counts per minute is given by

$$R_n = \frac{N_1}{t_1} - \frac{N_2}{t_2} = R_1 - R_2$$

The error in the net count rate is given by

$$\sigma_{R_n} = \sqrt{(\sigma_{R_1})^2 + (\sigma_{R_2})^2} = \sqrt{\frac{R_1}{t_1} + \frac{R_2}{t_2}}$$

The percent error in the net count rate is given by

$$\%\ \sigma_{R_n} = \frac{\sigma_{R_n}}{R_n} = \frac{\sqrt{\frac{R_1}{t_1} + \frac{R_2}{t_2}}}{R_1 - R_2} \times 100$$

INTERACTIONS OF RADIATION WITH MATTER

In general, radiation is an outward flow of energy from some energy source. The radiation may be in the form of either particles or electromagnetic radiation propagating through space. The particles may be either charged or uncharged and possess kinetic energies ranging from a few electron volts (eV) to billions of electron volts (BeV). Similarly, electromagnetic radiation may possess small amounts of energy per photon (low-energy x-rays and light photons) or relatively large amounts of energy (γ-rays). Radiation interacts with matter through the transfer of energy to its surroundings. Knowledge of these interactions is important because these mechanisms are the means by which radiation dose is delivered to tissues and also the means by which radiations are detected. Radiation may interact with nuclei, electrons, or total atoms, with energy being transferred totally or in part to nuclei, electrons, atoms, or even molecules.

Radiation interactions with matter are often classified in terms of *specific ionization, linear energy transfer,* and *range*. Specific ionization is defined as the number of ion pairs produced along each unit of path length of the trajectory of the particle (i.e., ion pairs per millimeter or ip/mm). The linear energy transfer (LET) is a related quantity and is defined as the amount of energy that a particle loses to its surrounding medium for each unit of path length it travels (i.e., keV/mm). The range of a particle is defined as the distance the particle travels before giving up enough of its kinetic energy so that it no longer interacts with the medium through which it travels. All three of these factors depend on the type of particle (mass and charge), the energy of the particle, and the interacting medium. In general, an average of 34 eV is required to produce one ion pair.

CHARGED-PARTICLE INTERACTIONS

Charged-particle interactions are generally due to the Coulomb force between charged particles rather than direct physical contact. Charged-particle interactions may result in ionization in which orbital electrons are dislodged from atoms to form positive and negative ions; atomic excitation in which orbital electrons are excited to higher energy levels in the atoms; molecular excitation in which vibrations are produced in molecules; molecular collisions in which atoms or parts of atoms are dislodged from the molecule, resulting in a break in the molecular chain; and bremsstrahlung, which is the production of photons due to deceleration and deflection of particles. Ionized electrons often receive enough energy to produce secondary ionizations.

Charged particles may be classified as heavy (protons, deuterons, α particles, and ionized atoms) or light (electrons and positrons). Heavy charged particles generally travel in relatively straight lines and are characterized by high specific ionization, high LET, and short range. In general, a small amount of energy is lost in each interaction, but many interactions occur in a short distance. Heavy-charged-particle interactions have very little application in nuclear medicine other than in the production of radioisotopes.

Light-charged-particle interactions are important because the interactions of x-rays and γ-rays with matter generally result in the production of free electrons with enough kinetic energy to produce secondary interactions. Electron interactions are similar to those of heavy charged particles. However, since electrons are much smaller, they must travel at high speed to possess the same kinetic energy and their velocities may approach the speed of light. Also, because their masses are small, a large amount of energy may be transferred to another particle in a single interaction. Thus, the path of an electron may be very tortuous as it travels through a medium due to the large angles of deflection that may result from some interactions. Electrons generally have a much smaller specific ionization and LET and longer range than heavy charged particles.

PHOTON CHARACTERISTICS

γ-Rays and x-rays are forms of electromagnetic radiation that transport energy through space as a combination of electric and magnetic fields. Some interactions of these electromagnetic radiations with matter are explained using the theories of wave propagation. Others are explained only by assuming that the radiation consists of discrete bundles of energy or photons with particle-like characteristics because of their short wavelength and high frequencies. If a photon has at least 15 eV of energy, it is capable of ionizing atoms and it is referred to as ionizing radiation. Thus, x-rays, γ-rays, and some ultraviolet rays are types of ionizing radiation.

When a beam of photons is reduced in intensity during its passage through a material, the process is referred to as attenuation. Photon attenuation can occur in two ways. Photons may be absorbed or completely removed from the beam and cease to exist, or they may be scattered or deflected from their original line of travel. Photons may interact with matter primarily by one of five basic processes. These are coherent scattering, photoelectric absorption, Compton scattering, pair production, and photodisintegration. Of these possibilities, only photoelectric absorption and Compton scattering are of significant consequence in nuclear medicine.

ATTENUATION EQUATION

When a photon traverses a medium, there is a probability of interaction associated with each of the listed five processes. In general, this probability is a function of the energy of the photon and the thickness and composition of the material with which the photon interacts.

An equation can be written which describes the attenuation of photons by matter. If I_o is the number of photons incident upon an absorber of thickness, Δx, as shown in Figure 2.19, and I is the number of transmitted photons, then the number of photons absorbed is given by:

$$\Delta I_o = I_o - I$$

The fraction of photons absorbed is $\Delta I_o/I_o$ and is directly proportional to the thickness of absorber, Δx. An equation can then be written by inserting a proportionality constant μ as follows:

$$\Delta I_o / I_o = -\mu \Delta x$$

The minus sign indicates that the number of transmitted photons decreases with increasing thickness of absorber. Applying the techniques of integral calculus, this relation yields the general attenuation equation

$$I = I_o e^{-\mu x}$$

which states that the number of photons transmitted through an absorber I is equal to the number of photons incident upon the absorber I_o reduced by $e^{-\mu x}$, the attenuation factor for the absorber. The quantity μ is the total linear attenuation coefficient and has the units of (1/distance). This factor is defined as the fraction removed from the beam per unit of thickness of the absorber or the probability of interaction in the absorber. The total linear attenuation coefficient, μ, is actually the sum of the linear attenuation coefficients for each of the five possible interactions. Thus

$$\mu = \Omega + \tau + \sigma + \kappa + \pi$$

where Ω, τ, σ, κ, and π are the linear attenuation coefficients for coherent scattering, photoelectric absorption, Compton scattering, pair production, and photodisintegration, respectively. The value of μ is dependent on the energy of the photon (monochromatic radiation only) and the type of absorbing material and its physical state (solid, liquid, or gas).

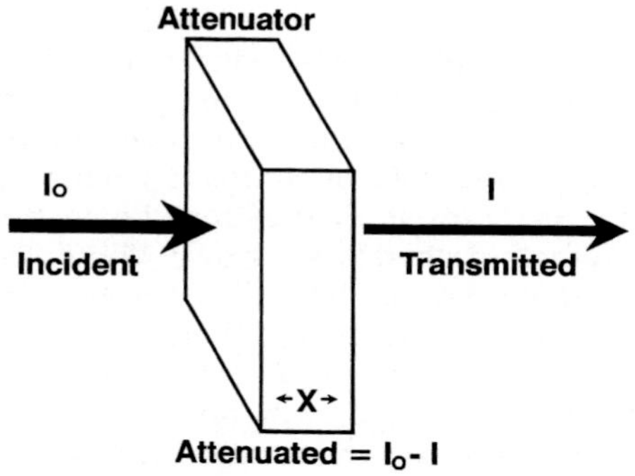

Figure 2.19. Attenuation of a beam of photons by an absorber.

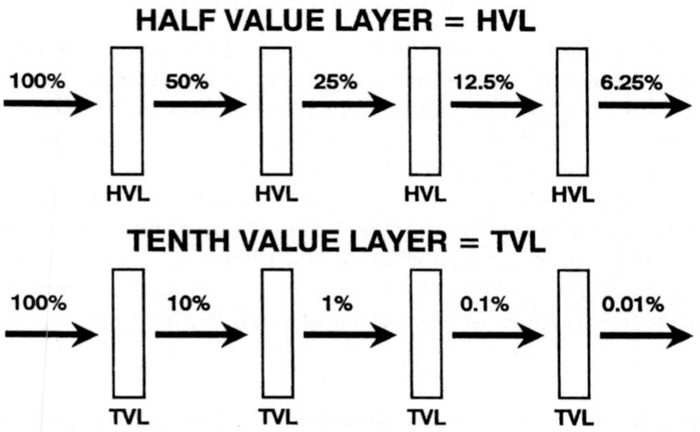

Figure 2.20. A thickness of absorber equal to one-half-value layer (HVL) or one-tenth-value layer (TVL) reduces the intensity of a photon beam to 50% and 10% respectively.

To simplify attenuation descriptions, the concept of the half-value layer (HVL) has been defined as the thickness of absorber that will reduce the number of transmitted photons in a beam to one-half of the incident number. The HVL is related to μ by

$$\mu \text{HVL} = 0.693$$

and is similar in concept to the half-life in the decay equation. In shielding calculations, the concept of the tenth-value layer (TVL) is often used. The TVL is related to μ by

$$\mu \text{TVL} = 2.30$$

The use of the HVL and TVL are shown diagrammatically in Figure 2.20.

Occasionally, it is useful to eliminate the physical state of the absorber in attenuation problems. To accomplish this, the concept of the mass attenuation coefficient, μ_m, has been defined by the relation

$$\mu_m = \mu / \rho$$

where ρ is the density of the absorber, and μ_m has the units of cm^2/g. Thus, the mass attenuation coefficient of a material is the same whether it is a solid, liquid, or gas.

Coherent Scattering

Coherent or classical scattering (also known as Rayleigh scattering) results from the interaction of a photon with the total atom as shown in Figure 2.21. In this process, virtually no energy is transferred to the atom, and the effect is a change in direction of the photon with no loss in energy. Coherent scattering is a low energy interaction occurring only at energies below 50 keV. Thus, in the diagnostic energy range for imaging (70–400 keV) the probability of coherent scattering (Ω) is zero, and therefore is of no importance in nuclear medicine applications.

Photoelectric Absorption

Photoelectric absorption is an extremely important ionization process and is shown diagrammatically in Figure 2.22. When a photon undergoes photoelectric absorption, the to-

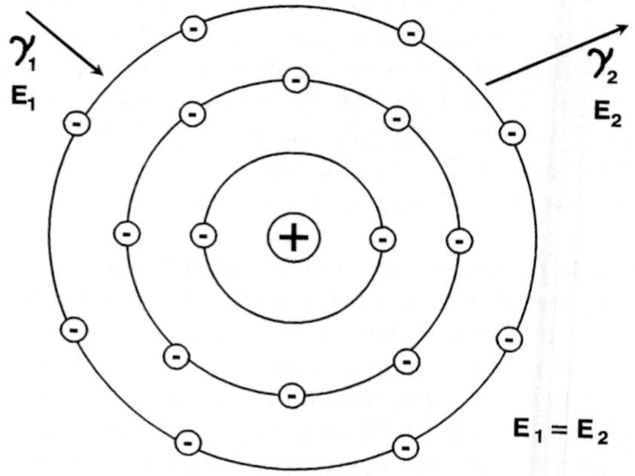

Figure 2.21. In coherent scattering (Rayleigh scattering), the incident photon is effectively absorbed by an atom and then reemitted in a new direction with no loss in energy.

tal energy of the incident photon is transferred to an inner-shell electron. The electron (called the photoelectron) is then ejected from the atom with a kinetic energy, E_e, equal to the difference between the energy of the incident photon, E_γ, and the binding energy of the electron in its shell, BE,

$$E_e = E_\gamma - BE$$

In general, the most tightly bound inner-shell electrons are involved in the process. However, this is a threshold interaction in that photoelectric absorption cannot occur with an electron unless the energy of the photon is greater than the binding energy of the electron. Thus, a photon with an energy greater than the binding energy of the K shell most probably will interact with a K shell electron. It can also interact with electrons in the L, M, etc., shells, but with decreasing probabilities. However, if the photon has an energy less than the K shell binding energy, but greater than the L shell binding energy, it can only interact with L, M, etc., shell electrons.

After photoelectric absorption, the remainder of the atom is left as a positive ion due to the vacancy created in the inner-shell. This vacancy is filled by an outer-shell electron dropping down to take the place of the photoelectron, and the resulting de-excitation energy is emitted as a characteristic x-ray or Augér electron as previously described. Thus, photoelectric absorption produces an ion pair as shown in Figure 2.23 (negative ion = the photoelectron and positive ion = the atom minus 1 electron), and characteristic radiation (x-rays or Augér electrons due to de-excitation of the positive ion). The photoelectron possesses sufficient energy to ionize other atoms as previously described.

Photoelectric absorption is a low energy interaction and the probability (τ) decreases very rapidly with increasing photon energy (proportional to $1/E^3$) as shown in Figure 2.24. Since photoelectric absorption with a particular shell requires the photon energy to be equal to or greater than the binding energy of the shell, there are discrete changes in the probability at the binding energy of each shell. The probability of photoelectric absorption is strongly dependent on the atomic number (Z) of the absorber (proportional to Z^4) and increases very rapidly with increasing Z.

Figure 2.25 combines the two dependencies described and demonstrates the significance of photoelectric absorption in nuclear medicine. For sodium iodide detectors (Z =

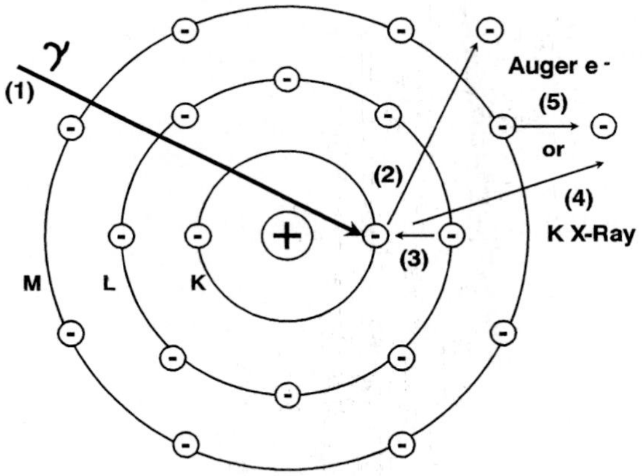

Figure 2.22. In the process of photoelectric absorption, a photon is absorbed by an inner-shell electron (*1*), which is then ejected from the atom (*2*) with an energy equal to the incident proton energy minus the binding energy of the electron. The atom is then de-excited by an outer-shell electron filling the vacancy (*3*), followed by characteristic x-ray (*4*) or Augér electron emission (*5*).

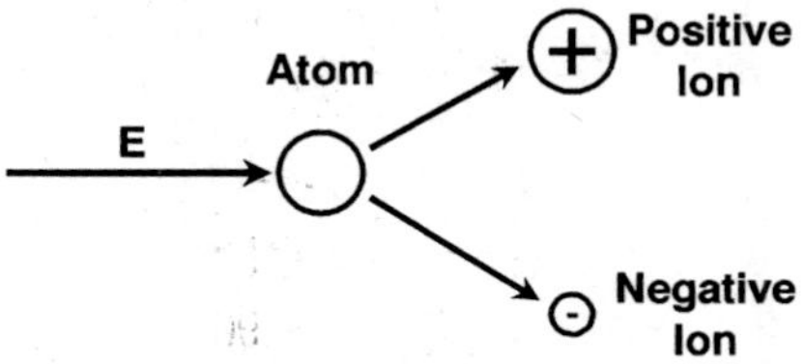

Figure 2.23. The end result of photoelectric absorption and Compton scattering is the production of an ion pair (an atom minus 1 electron and the freed electron).

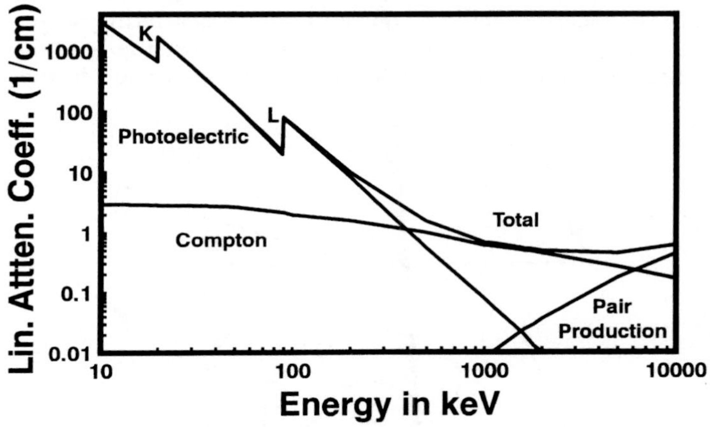

Figure 2.24. Plot of linear attenuation coefficients for photoelectric absorption (τ), Compton scattering (σ), and pair production (κ), and the total linear attenuation coefficient ($\mu = \tau + \sigma + \kappa$) versus photon energy.

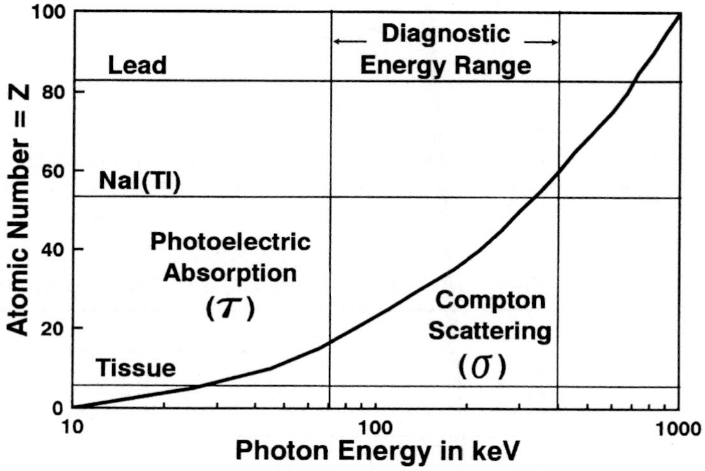

Figure 2.25. Plot of atomic number (Z) versus photon energy (E) illustrating the combinations of Z and E in which photoelectric absorption (*left of curved line*) and Compton scatter (*right of curved line*) predominate. Three examples are shown (tissue, sodium iodide, and lead). The diagnostic energy range for imaging shown is 70–400 keV.

53), the primary interaction in the diagnostic energy range for imaging (70–400 keV) is photoelectric, implying total absorption which is important for photon detection. For lead collimators (Z = 82), the primary interaction is also photoelectric, again implying total absorption which is important in shielding applications, but also yielding a source of the characteristic x-rays of lead which must be taken into consideration in patient and sample counting procedures.

Compton Scattering

The other interaction important in nuclear medicine is Compton scattering, shown diagrammatically in Figure 2.26. Compton scattering is the process whereby a photon interacts with a loosely bound electron, with the electron receiving energy from the photon. The electron recoils at an angle, θ, with respect to the direction of travel of the incident photon. The photon also has its direction of travel altered by an angle, ϕ. The amount of energy transferred to the electron depends on the angle of scattering of the photon. In Compton scattering interactions, the binding energies of the electrons are small in comparison to the photon energies and, therefore, the electrons are considered to be free. Conservation of energy thus yields the equation

$$E_\gamma = E_{\gamma'} + E_e$$

which states that the energy of the incident photon, E_γ, is equal to the sum of the energies of the scattered photon, $E_{\gamma'}$, and the recoil electron, E_e. Conservation of momentum yields an equation relating the energy of the scattered photon, $E_{\gamma'}$, in keV, to the angle of scatter of the photon, ϕ:

$$E_{\gamma'} = E_\gamma/[1 + (E_\gamma/511)(1 - \cos\phi)]$$

In this equation, 511 is the rest mass of the electron in kilo electron volts. The scattering angle, ϕ, of the photon ranges from 0° (no interaction) to 180° (backscatter). Since the electron is assumed to be at rest before interaction, its scattering angle ranges from 0–90°. Both θ and ϕ tend to decrease as the energy of the incident photon increases. The products of Compton scattering are an ion pair as shown in Figure 2.23 (positive ion = atom minus 1 electron and the electron), and a photon of reduced energy and having a new direction of travel. Table 2.7 illustrates the energies of the scattered photon and electron versus scattering angle of the photon for selected radionuclides used in nuclear medicine.

The probability of Compton scattering (τ) decreases slowly with increasing energy (approximately proportional to $1/E$) and is directly proportional to the atomic number (Z) of the absorber. The latter statement is due to the fact that the probability of a photon interacting with an atom is determined by the number of electrons in the atom which is equal to its atomic number.

Figure 2.24 shows that Compton scattering is the dominant interaction for photons within the body (Z = 8 for tissue, crossover point is 25 keV; Z = 20 for bone, crossover point is 45 keV) throughout most of the diagnostic energy range. Thus, if a photon interacts within the body, it will most likely be by Compton scattering with the original photon being replaced by another photon with decreased energy traveling in a new direction.

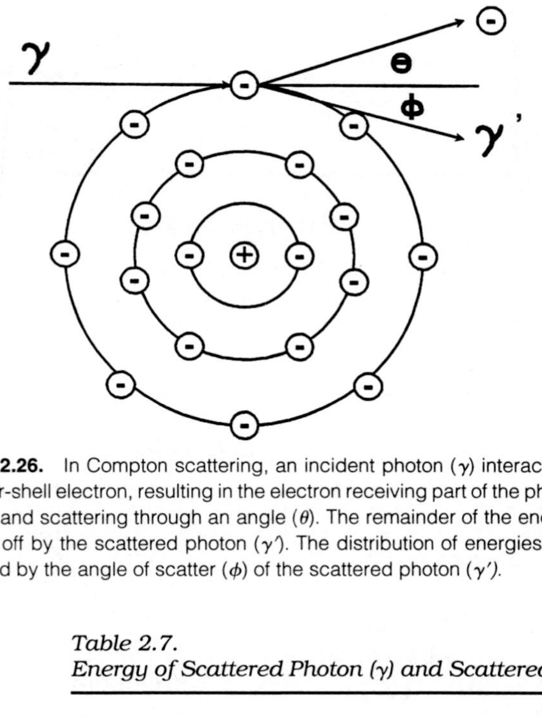

Figure 2.26. In Compton scattering, an incident photon (γ) interacts with an outer-shell electron, resulting in the electron receiving part of the photon's energy and scattering through an angle (θ). The remainder of the energy is carried off by the scattered photon (γ'). The distribution of energies is determined by the angle of scatter (ϕ) of the scattered photon (γ').

Pair Production

Pair production is a threshold interaction resulting from the photon interacting primarily with the strong electric field of the nucleus of an atom as shown in Figure 2.27. In

Table 2.7.
Energy of Scattered Photon (γ) and Scattered Electron (e^-) vs. Scattering Angle in Compton Scattering

Photon Energy[a] (keV)	Scattering Angle 0°		30°		45°		90°		180°	
	γ	e^-	γ	e^-	γ	e^-	γ	e^-	γ	e^-
70	70	0	69	1	67	3	62	8	55	15
140	140	0	135	5	130	10	110	30	90	50
364	364	0	332	32	301	63	213	151	150	214
511	511	0	451	60	395	116	255	256	170	341

[a]Primary photon energies of ^{201}Tl, ^{99m}Tc, ^{131}I, and annihilation radiation respectively.

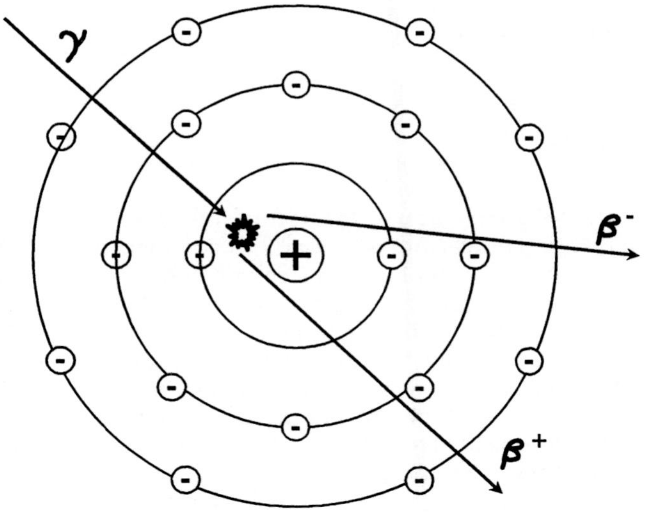

Figure 2.27. In a pair-production interaction of a photon with energy greater than 1.022 MeV occurring with the electric field of the nucleus, 1.022 MeV of energy is converted to mass in the form of a positive and a negative electron. The remaining energy is carried off as kinetic energy by the two electrons.

this interaction of the photon, energy is converted to mass in the form of a positive and a negative electron ($e^+ + e^-$). Since the rest mass energy of the electron is 0.511 MeV, the photon must have at least 1.022 MeV of energy for the interaction to occur. The energy in excess of this value is transferred to the two electrons as kinetic energy. The electrons interact with the medium as previously described until this energy is lost. The positive electron then annihilates with a negative electron as previously described and illustrated in Figure 2.8. Since pair production is only possible for photons with energies greater than 1.022 MeV, this interaction is of no consequence in nuclear medicine applications.

Photodisintegration

When the photon has a very high energy (7 MeV) it has sufficient energy to produce a photonuclear reaction resulting in the ejection of a nucleon from the nucleus. The probability of this interaction is very small and, because of the high energy required, it is also of no consequence in nuclear medicine.

SUGGESTED READINGS

Bushberg JT, Seibert JA, Leidholdt EM Jr, Boone JM. The essential physics of medical imaging. Chs. 1, 2, 14. Baltimore: Williams and Wilkins, 1994.

Chandra R. Introductory physics of nuclear medicine. 4th ed. Chs. 1–3, 6. Philadelphia, PA: Lea & Febiger, 1992.

Johns HL, Cunningham JR. The physics of radiology. 4th ed. Chs. 1, 3–5. Springfield, IL: Charles C. Thomas, 1974.

Sorenson JA, Phelps ME. Physics in nuclear medicine. 2d ed. Chs. 1–3, 6, 8, 9. Orlando, FL: Grune and Stratton, Inc., 1987.

3 Physics of MRI, CT, and Ultrasound

DAVID R. PICKENS, JAMES A. PATTON, and RONALD R. PRICE

MAGNETIC RESONANCE IMAGING

Magnetic resonance imaging (MRI) is a diagnostic technique for imaging the human body that has evolved from nuclear magnetic resonance (NMR) chemical assay methods, which have been in routine use for many years. MRI makes use of magnetic fields and radiofrequency (RF) waves to generate intensity-modulated images from specific sections of the body. The intensity of a point within a conventional MR image is determined by the number of hydrogen nuclei (protons) at the corresponding point in the patient, and also by the chemical makeup of the tissue at that point. Signal intensity is measured by placing the patient in a strong magnetic field, irradiating the region of interest with RF waves, and recording the radiation reemitted from the patient. Variations in the time interval between excitation and measurement can produce drastic differences in image appearance. Thus, not only does MRI produce high-quality images of body anatomy, but it also provides the capability for measuring in vivo body chemistry.

BASIC PHYSICAL PRINCIPLES

The principle of nuclear magnetic resonance is based on the fact that certain nuclei have an odd number of neutrons or protons, creating a charge distribution that results in each nucleus possessing a characteristic called spin angular momentum, and, thus, a magnetic moment. This concept can be understood by thinking of the nucleus as a small spinning top as shown in Figure 3.1. Since the nucleus has a positive charge and is in motion, it becomes a magnetic dipole, generating a magnetic field similar to that of a small bar magnet. The magnetic field is characterized by the magnetic moment μ, which is a vector quantity because the magnetic field has both a specific strength and direction (toward the north pole). There are many atoms existing naturally in nature whose nuclei exhibit a net magnetic moment (i.e., ^{1}H, ^{13}C, ^{19}F, ^{23}Na, ^{31}P, and ^{39}K). Since hydrogen atoms constitute the vast majority of the atoms in the human body, this abundance makes in vivo proton (^{1}H) MRI possible.

When no magnetic field is present, the nuclei in the region of interest are oriented at random, as shown in Figure 3.2**A**. However, when placed in a static magnetic field (B_0), the nuclei experience a torque that causes a majority of them to tend toward an alignment with the magnetic field (Fig. 3.2**B**). This tendency is disturbed to some extent by thermal motion effects, but these effects are ignored here. As the nuclei align themselves, they begin to oscillate or precess about the direction of the applied magnetic field. This motion is very similar to the wobbling of a child's spinning top that is trying to maintain its alignment with the gravitational field of the earth.

The frequency at which the nuclei precess is different for different nuclei, but is the same for identical nuclei, and is directly proportional to the strength of the applied magnetic field. This precessional frequency is called the Larmor frequency, and is the fundamental basis for NMR. The magnetic field strengths used in imaging range from about 0.05–4.0 tesla, where 1 tesla (T) equals 10,000 gauss (G), compared to the earth's magnetic field of approximately 0.5 G. At these field strengths, the Larmor frequency falls in the RF band. The Larmor equation:

$$\omega_0 = \gamma B_0$$

provides the relationship between the precessional frequency, ω_0, and the applied static magnetic field strength, B_0. The proportionality constant, γ, is called the gyromagnetic ratio and is unique for each type of nucleus (1). For hydrogen nuclei, γ is approximately 42.58 MHz/T or 4258 Hz/G.

In general, the application of a magnetic field to a quantity of identical nuclei results in their orientation in the direction of the magnetic field. Some nuclei align themselves antiparallel, but a majority align parallel to the field with their precession about that direction. These nuclei all precess at the Larmor frequency but with random phase (Fig. 3.2**B**) where the directions of the magnetic moments are random. However, since their individual magnetic moments (μ) are tending toward the direction of the applied magnetic field (B_0), the individual moments sum together

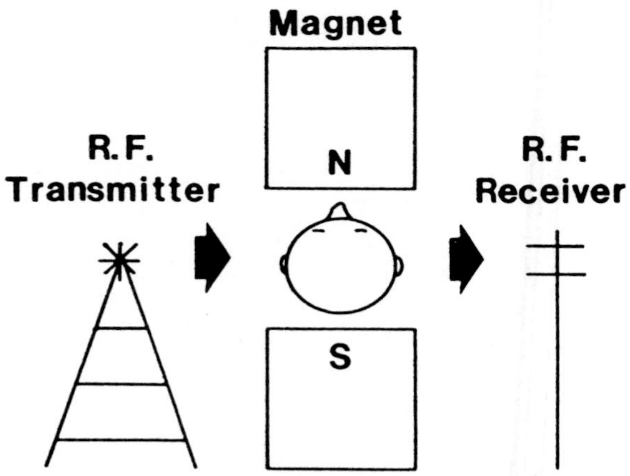

Figure 3.1. A nucleus with an odd number of neutrons or protons possesses spin angular momentum and thus generates a magnetic field, like a small bar magnet, with a magnetic moment μ pointing in the direction of the magnetic field and functionally with a north pole (*N*) and a south pole (*S*). (Reproduced by permission from Sandler MP, Patton JA, Shaff MI, Powers TA, Partain CL. Correlative imaging: nuclear medicine, magnetic resonance, computed tomography, ultrasound. Baltimore: Williams and Wilkins, 1989.)

by vector addition to produce a net magnetization or net magnetic moment M along that direction (Fig. 3.3). The magnitude of M is determined by the number of hydrogen nuclei present, and also by the strength of the static magnetic field. There is no net precession of M in this orientation because the phases of the μ's are random; therefore, their components in the X and Y directions cancel each other. Thus, no signal can be detected from the precession of the nuclei in this equilibrium orientation.

To cause the nuclei to generate a detectable NMR signal, it is necessary to change the orientation of the net magnetic moment. This is accomplished by the application of external energy so that M is no longer parallel to the static magnetic field (2). This external energy is applied by an RF pulse emitted from a coil that serves as a transmitting antenna. This pulse varies with time and is perpendicular to the direction of the static magnetic field. For energy to be absorbed so that the net magnetic moment can be tilted away from the direction of the static magnetic field, the frequency must exactly match the resonant frequency, ω_0, or Larmor frequency of the nuclei. The effect of this coherence is that the individual magnetic moments, μ, begin to align themselves to each other, and precess in phase as they absorb energy from the RF excitation. When the RF pulse is turned on, the net magnetic moment begins to spiral away from the direction of the static magnetic field, as shown in Figure 3.4. It will then have both a longitudinal or parallel component (M_L), and a transverse or perpendicular component (M_T) (3). If the pulse is left on long enough, the net magnetic moment will be rotated 90° and lie in the transverse plane (plane X-Y perpendicular to the static magnetic field) (Fig. 3.5). This would place it in the transverse plane $M_L = 0$ and $M_T = M$.

Since the net magnetic moment has been rotated (flipped) 90°, the applied pulse is called a 90° pulse. At the

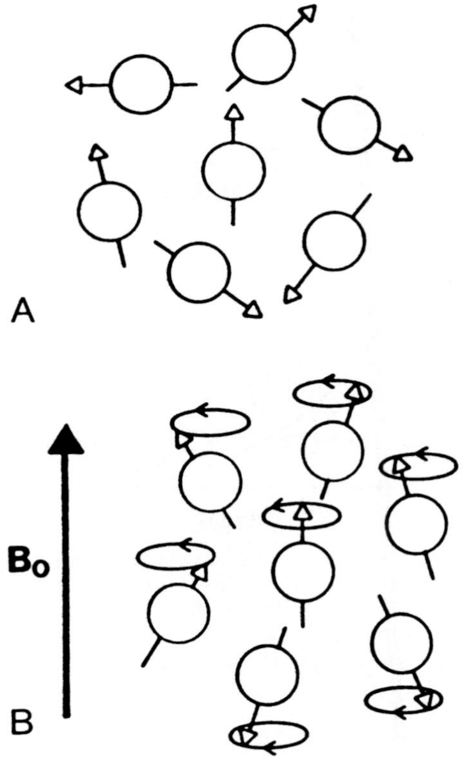

Figure 3.2. **A.** With no magnetic field present, nuclei are oriented at random. **B.** When a static field is applied (B_0), the magnetic moments begin to oscillate or precess about the direction of the field, with a majority of the nuclei aligning themselves with the field. (Reproduced by permission from Sandler MP, Patton JA, Shaff MI, Powers TA, Partain CL. Correlative imaging: nuclear medicine, magnetic resonance, computed tomography, ultrasound. Baltimore: Williams and Wilkins, 1989.)

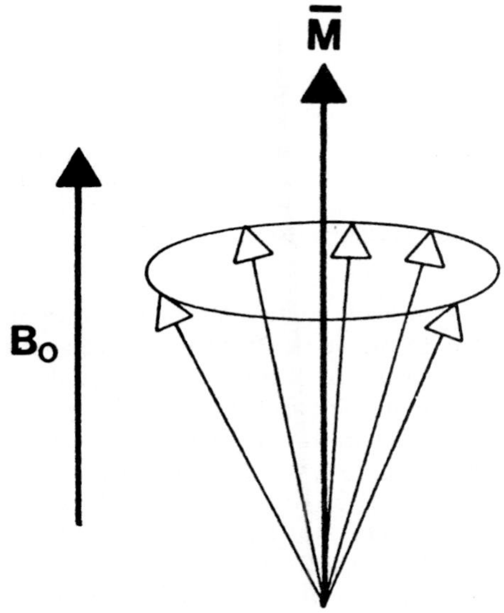

Figure 3.3. Since a majority of the nuclei are aligned with the field, the magnetic moments sum together to produce a net magnetic moment or net magnetization (M) along the direction of the field. (Reproduced by permission from Sandler MP, Patton JA, Shaff MI, Powers TA, Partain CL. Correlative imaging: nuclear medicine, magnetic resonance, computed tomography, ultrasound. Baltimore: Williams and Wilkins, 1989.)

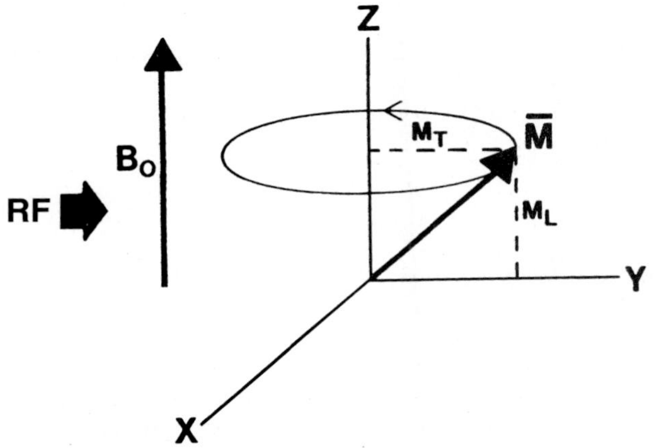

Figure 3.4. The application of RF energy perpendicular to the net magnetic moment M causes M to spiral away from the direction of the applied field, B_0. M will then have a longitudinal (M_L) or parallel component and a transverse (M_T) or perpendicular component. (Reproduced by permission from Sandler MP, Patton JA, Shaff MI, Powers TA, Partain CL. Correlative imaging: nuclear medicine, magnetic resonance, computed tomography, ultrasound. Baltimore: Williams and Wilkins, 1989.)

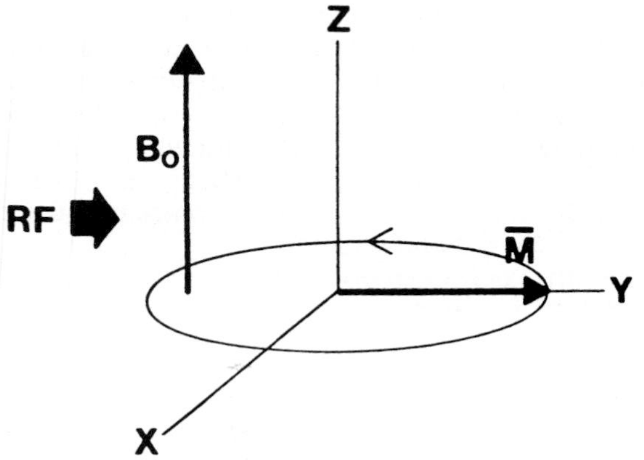

Figure 3.5. The application of a 90° *RF* pulse (a burst of RF energy applied long enough to rotate *M* by 90°) results in *M* oscillating in the *X-Y* plane perpendicular to the static magnetic field. (Reproduced by permission from Sandler MP, Patton JA, Shaff MI, Powers TA, Partain CL. Correlative imaging: nuclear medicine, magnetic resonance, computed tomography, ultrasound. Baltimore: Williams and Wilkins, 1989.)

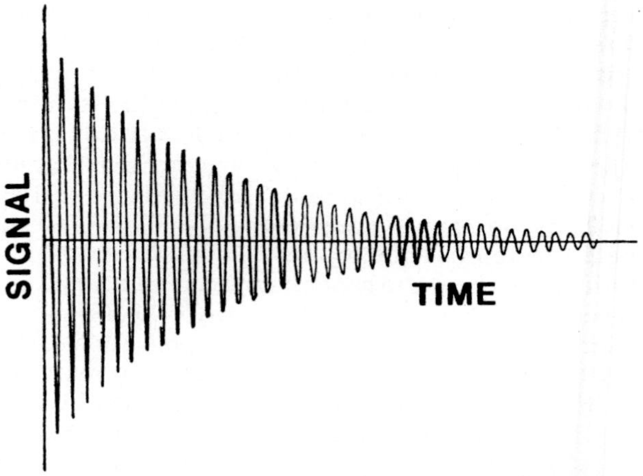

Figure 3.6. Signal from free-induction decay generated by the precessing net magnetic moment (M) as it returns from the transverse plane to a position parallel to the applied field. (Reproduced by permission from Sandler MP, Patton JA, Shaff MI, Powers TA, Partain CL. Correlative imaging: nuclear medicine, magnetic resonance, computed tomography, ultrasound. Baltimore: Williams and Wilkins, 1989.)

instant the RF pulse is turned off, all the individual nuclei are precessing in phase so that the net magnetic moment is precessing about the static magnetic field in the *X-Y* plane. The nuclei immediately begin to dephase because of localized differences in the magnetic field due to molecular environments, giving up the absorbed RF energy. The net magnetic moment begins to return to its previous state parallel to the applied static field because of the tendency of nuclei to align themselves with the RF field. This moving magnetic moment can induce a voltage in a receiver coil, also perpendicular to the static magnetic field, that varies with the same frequency as the applied field and decays with time as the net magnetic moment returns to its original state. This phenomenon of relaxation is called free-induction decay; the magnitude of the generated signal is shown in Figure 3.6. The initial amplitude is proportional to the number of hydrogen nuclei present in the sample and, therefore, is a measure of proton density (ρ). M_L and M_T can be plotted as a function of time, t, as M returns to its original state, yielding exponential growth and decay curves, respectively (Fig. 3.7).

The equations for these two curves as a function of t are given by:

$$M_L = M[1 - e^{-t/T_1}]$$
$$M_T = Me^{-t/T_2}$$

The quantities T_1 and T_2 mathematically are time constants that are generally called relaxation times. T_1 is the time required for M_L to recover to 63% of the magnitude of *M*. It is called the spin lattice or longitudinal relaxation time, and is affected by the molecular composition in which the hydrogen nuclei reside. T_2 is the time required for M_T to fall to 37% of the magnitude of *M*. It is called the spin-spin or transverse relaxation time, and is affected by slight changes in the magnetic field due to the presence of neighboring nuclei. Since water is a major component of biologic systems, it is the measurement of T_1, T_2, and density of hydrogen nuclei that yield MR images of tissues.

Some generalized comments can be made concerning T_1 and T_2 of hydrogen nuclei. T_1 values are determined primarily by interactions between macromolecules and a single hydration layer. T_2 values are determined primarily by exchange diffusion of water between the bound layer and a free water phase (4). The magnitude of T_1 depends on the strength of the magnetic field, while T_2 is apparently independent of field strength (Fig. 3.8). T_1 values are typically

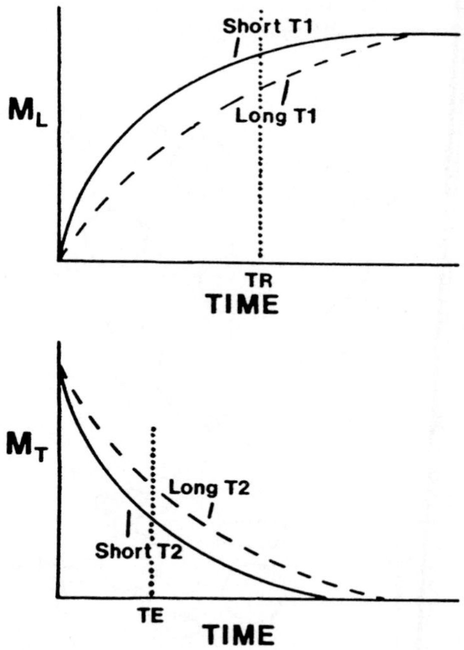

Figure 3.7. Plots of the longitudinal (M_L) and transverse (M_T) components of M as it returns from the transverse plane to a position parallel to the applied field. (Reproduced by permission from Sandler MP, Patton JA, Shaff MI, Powers TA, Partain CL. Correlative imaging: nuclear medicine, magnetic resonance, computed tomography, ultrasound. Baltimore: Williams and Wilkins, 1989.)

on the order of 1 second, while T_2 values are generally less, as illustrated in Table 3.1 (5). Small molecules tend to have greater T_1 and T_2 values, whereas large molecules tend to have lesser T_1 and T_2 values. Different tissue types (both normal and abnormal) differ in T_1 and T_2 contrast. It is the utility of imaging techniques that emphasize these tissue differences that determines the diagnostic capability of MRI.

IMAGING PRINCIPLES

The signals arising from different tissues at different locations within the body are of great interest. The position of these signals can be determined by using gradient coils to linearly change the magnetic field in one or more directions. Since the Larmor frequency is determined by the strength of the magnetic field, establishment of field gradients causes the resonant frequency to be different for each location within the field. To image a plane, gradients are established to select the plane and to separate individual points within the plane. RF pulses are applied, and a complex series of frequencies are received. Then the individual frequencies, phases, and amplitudes are determined using the mathematical techniques of Fourier analysis. By using three gradient coils corresponding to the X, Y, and Z orthogonal directions that can alter the magnetic field linearly in those directions, images of individual transverse, sagittal, and coronal planes within the body can be obtained.

In general, MR images have contributions from three NMR parameters: ρ, T_1, and T_2. Each of these three parameters may be selectively emphasized in a specific region through the appropriate selection of the combinations of 90° and 180° RF pulses and gradient values, all in a predetermined time sequence. Proper pulse sequence selection in MRI is the key to obtaining high-quality diagnostic information.

The most frequently used pulse sequence for imaging uses the spin-echo technique. It begins with the application of a 90° pulse to move the net magnetic moment into the transverse or X-Y plane (Fig. 3.9**A**). When the net magnetic moment begins to return to its original position, individual nuclei immediately begin to dephase due to localized differences in magnetic field strength (Fig. 3.9**B**). The

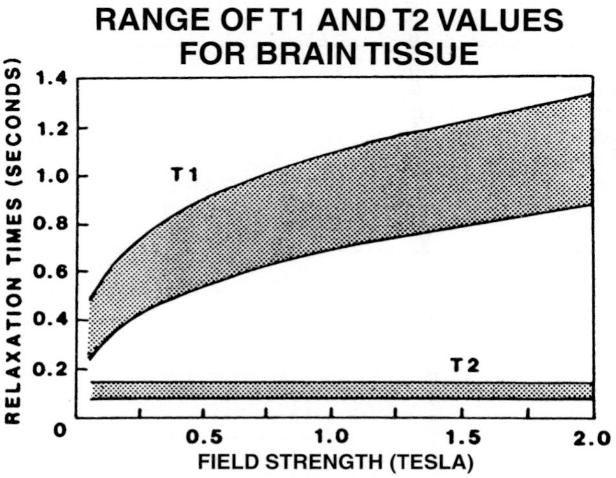

Figure 3.8. Plot of ranges of T_1 and T_2 values for brain tissue (normal and abnormal) versus magnetic field strength. (Plots were developed from data published in Bottomley PA, Hardy CJ, Argersinger RE, et al. A review of 1H nuclear magnetic resonance relaxation in pathology: are T_1 and T_2 diagnostic? Med Phys 1987;14:25.)

Table 3.1.
*T_1 and T_2 Values for Normal Brain Tissues and Selected Brain Abnormalities at 1.5 Tesla (T)**

Tissue Type	T_1[a]	T_2[a]
	msec	msec
Normal brain		
Gray matter	917 ± 156	101 ± 13
White matter	782 ± 133	92 ± 22
Unspecified	880 ± 167	76 ± 21
Misc tumors	1068 ± 385	121 ± 63
Meningioma	974 ± 175	103 ± 31
Glioma	956 ± 335	111 ± 33
Edema	1210 ± 278	141 ± 73
Astrocytoma		
Grades I, II	913 ± 46	141 ± 4
Grades III, IV	1107 ± 89	[b]

[a]Values are calculated from data published in Bottomley PA, Hardy CJ, Argersinger RE, et al. A review of ^{1}H nuclear magnetic resonance relaxation in pathology: are T_1 and T_2 diagnostic? Med Phys 1987;14:25.

[b]Data not available.

*Reproduced by permission from Sandler MP, Patton JA, Shaff MI, Powers TA, Partain CL. Correlative imaging: nuclear medicine, magnetic resonance, computed tomography, ultrasound. Baltimore: Williams and Wilkins, 1989.

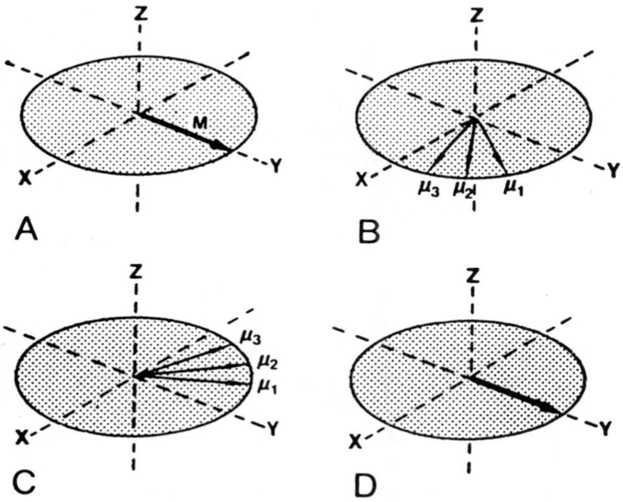

Figure 3.9. A. After the application of a 90° pulse in the spin-echo technique, the net magnetization lies in the transverse plane. **B.** The net magnetization begins to return to its original position and individual nuclei begin to dephase due to localized differences in magnetic field strength, with those in areas of higher field strengths precessing at higher frequencies, i.e., frequency μ_3 is higher than frequency μ_2 which is higher than frequency μ_1. **C.** The application of a 180° pulse flips the individual magnetic moments, providing a mirror image about the *Y-X* plane. **D.** The individual moments then rephase and generate an NMR signal or echo. (Reproduced by permission from Sandler MP, Patton JA, Shaff MI, Powers TA, Partain CL. Correlative imaging: nuclear medicine, magnetic resonance, computed tomography, ultrasound. Baltimore: Williams and Wilkins, 1989.)

signal from free induction decay appears and fades away. However, the RF receiver is not turned on during this process. Instead, after time τ, a 180° pulse is applied to flip the individual magnetic moments, providing a mirror image using the Y-Z plane as the mirror (Fig. 3.9**C**). As the individual moments come back into phase (Fig. 3.9**D**) at time τ after the 180° pulse, an NMR signal (echo) is generated that disappears as the individual nuclei once again dephase. This echo is "read out" by the receiver coil and used for imaging purposes.

The equation that describes the image brightness or MRI signal intensity at a point in an image using the spin echo technique is given by:

$$S = D[1 - e^{-TD/T_1}]e^{-TE/T_2}$$

where D is a function of proton density, and T_1 and T_2 are the NMR relaxation times. The delay time, *TD*, is the time after the signal (echo) is received before the sequence is repeated, and the repetition time, *TR*, is the total time for a single pulse sequence (sequence interval). The echo time, *TE*, the time between the 90° pulse and the echo, is equal to 2τ where τ is the time between the 90° and 180° pulses. τ also represents the time between the 180° pulse and the signal (echo) received in the receiver coil. The parameters *TE* and *TD*, which define *TR*, can be set in the data collection process to control the amount of T_1 and T_2 contribution to the images and to enhance the difference in T_1 or T_2. For example, by making TE short with respect to T_2, the effects of T_2 can be reduced because the value of e^{-TE/T_2} approaches 1. On the other hand, by making T_D long with respect to T_1, the effects of T_1 are reduced because the value of e^{-TD/T_1} approaches 0. If *TE* is lengthened while *TD* remains long, then the contribution of T_2 is increased. If *TE* remains short while *TD* is shortened, then the contribution of T_1 is increased (Table 3.2).

Some additional observations to be made concerning the equation for the spin echo signal intensity are that for a given TD and TE, the signal intensity, S, is proportional to *M*, which is a function of proton density; S increases as T_1 decreases, and S increases as T_2 increases. Thus, it is important in imaging to use pulse sequences that isolate T_1 and T_2 as much as possible. Table 3.3 provides a summary of these relationships.

Signal intensities at specific points in an imaging volume are most commonly measured with the spin echo technique using the two-dimensional Fourier transform (2DFT) method. Choosing the coordinate system shown in Figure 3.10 for transverse slice imaging as an example, slice selection is chosen in the *Z* direction, frequency is encoded in the *X* direction, and phase is encoded in the Y direction, by the techniques illustrated by the pulse sequence in Figure 3.11. For imaging of sagittal and coronal planes, the *X* and *Y* gradients, respectively, would be used for plane selection, with the other two gradients being used to encode frequency and phase. First, the *Z* gradient is turned on to select the slice to be imaged, while the 90° *RF* pulse, which contains a range of frequencies appropriate for the selected plane, is triggered to move the magnetic moments in the *X-Y* plane. At the termination of the 90° pulse, all the magnetic moments in that slice are precessing in phase at the same frequency, so no spatial information can be obtained.

Spatial locations can be obtained from within the slice, however, by frequency and phase-encoding of the precessing nuclei. Phase can be encoded in the *Y* direction by turning off the slice-selection gradient and turning on the

Table 3.2.
*Effect on NMR Parameters of Varying Echo Time (TE) and Delay Time (TD) in a Spin-Echo Sequence**

Signal Intensity[a]	TE	TD
f (proton density)	TE $<T_2$	TD $\gg T_1$
f (proton density, T_2)	TE $>T_2$	TD $\gg T_1$
f (proton density, T_1)	TE $<T_2$	TD $<T_1$
f (proton density, T_1, T_2)	TE $>T_2$	TD $<T_1$

[a]The signal is a function of proton density, T_1, or T_2 if TE and TD have the values shown.
*Reproduced by permission from Sandler MP, Patton JA, Shaff MI, Powers TA, Partain CL. Correlative imaging: nuclear medicine, magnetic resonance, computed tomography, ultrasound. Baltimore: Williams and Wilkins, 1989.

Table 3.3.
*Effect on Signal Intensity of Spin-Echo Technique by Varying NMR Parameters**

Signal Intensity	Proton Density	T_1	T_2
Increases	Increases	Constant	Constant
Increases	Constant	Decreases	Constant
Increases	Constant	Constant	Increases
?	Increases	Decreases	Constant
?	Constant	Decreases	Increases

*Reproduced by permission from Sandler MP, Patton JA, Shaff MI, Powers TA, Partain CL. Correlative imaging: nuclear medicine, magnetic resonance, computed tomography, ultrasound. Baltimore: Williams and Wilkins, 1989.

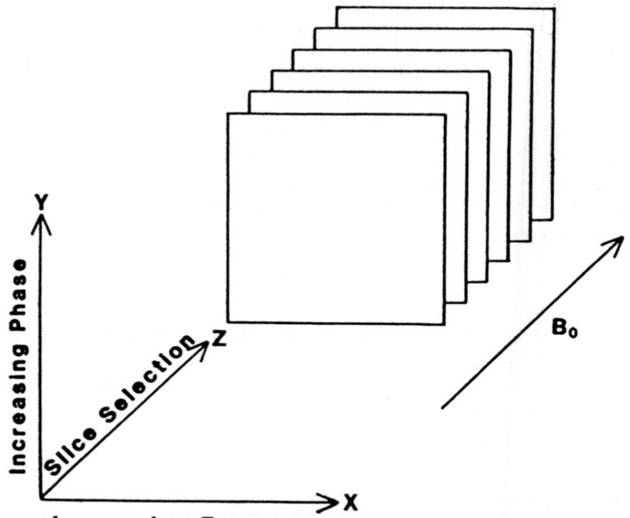

Figure 3.10. In transverse slice imaging, slice selection is made in the *Z* direction, phase is encoded in the *Y* direction, and frequency is encoded in the *X* direction. (Reproduced by permission from Sandler MP, Patton JA, Shaff MI, Powers TA, Partain CL. Correlative imaging: nuclear medicine, magnetic resonance, computed tomography, ultrasound. Baltimore: Williams and Wilkins, 1989.)

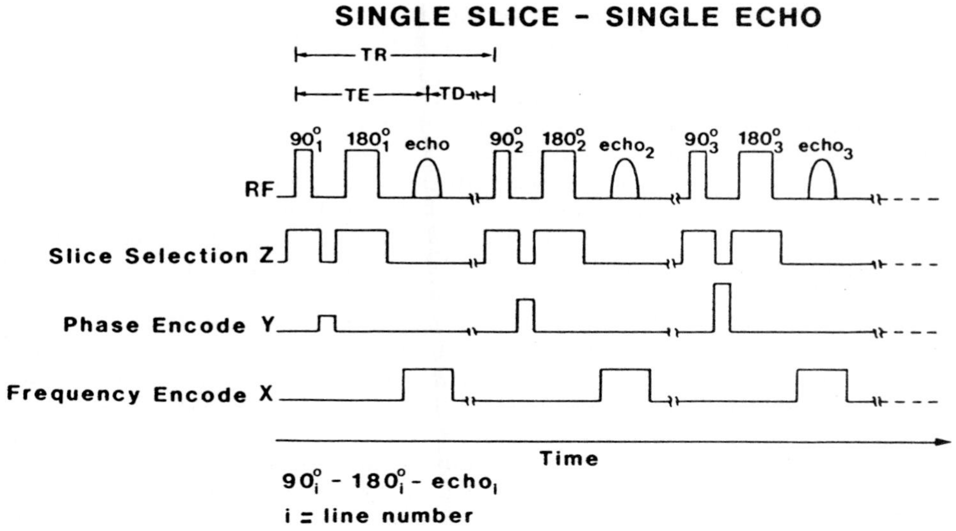

Figure 3.11. Pulse sequence for performing spin-echo, single transverse slice, single-echo imaging. (Reproduced by permission from Sandler MP, Patton JA, Shaff MI, Powers TA, Partain CL. Correlative imaging: nuclear medicine, magnetic resonance, computed tomography, ultrasound. Baltimore: Williams and Wilkins, 1989.)

phase-encoding (*Y*) gradient. While the phase-encoding gradient is on, the precessional frequencies will increase linearly in the *Y* direction in proportion to the applied gradient field strength. When this gradient is turned off, the precessional frequencies will again be the same; however, the phase angles will be different along the Y direction. For readout, the slice-selection gradient is again turned on, the 180° *RF* pulse is triggered, the slice-selection gradient is turned off, and the frequency-encoding (*X*) gradient is turned on while the echo is received. The gradient in the *X* direction increases the frequencies of the received echoes linearly in that direction so that spatial information can be obtained in the *X* direction.

The received echo consists of a series of frequencies of specific amplitude and phase where frequency determines the *X* coordinate, phase determines the *Y* coordinate, and amplitude determines the signal intensity. This information is retrieved from the echo by applying the Fourier transform. In practice, because of the high resonant frequencies associated with the technique, a single phase-encoding step is not adequate. Typically, 128, 192, 256, or 512 phase-encoding steps are used to obtain a single slice. Thus, the sequence in Figure 3.11 would be repeated 128, 192, 256, or 512 times, although only three are shown. Frequency is typically encoded in 256 or 512 increments, yielding array sizes of 256×128, 256×192, 256×256, or more pixels. In actual imaging applications, it is often necessary to alter the *X*, *Y*, and *Z* gradient signals shown in Figure 3.11 to perform corrections for phase changes induced by gradient switching; however, these alterations have been ignored for simplicity.

Magnetic resonance imaging systems are able to take advantage of pulse sequence delay times to accomplish multislice and multiecho imaging. Multislice imaging may be accomplished by using the recovery time *TD* after the first slice acquisition to collect data from other slices. The data are collected one line at a time from each slice. The number of slices that can be obtained is determined by the length of the recovery time. In practice, it is necessary to leave a small space between the selected slices to prevent overlap or crosstalk between adjacent slices. The multiecho sequence can also be implemented with multislice sequences to simultaneously obtain multiple echo images from multiple slices. Again, the technique is to use the recovery time from the first slice after the last echo to collect echoes from additional slices. The same restrictions discussed for the multislice technique also apply here.

In routine imaging, one pulse sequence and data collection process for each line often does not provide sufficient signal for generating high quality images. Therefore, manufacturers provide the capability for repetitive pulse sequences so that multiple data sets from a single line may be collected and averaged before image reconstruction. These repetitive acquisitions affect the length of the imaging study, however, by increasing the required imaging time.

Imaging time can be calculated by using the following equation:

$$T = TR \times n \times NY$$

where *TR* is the sequence repetition time, *n* is the number of signals averaged into one line, and *NY* is the number of gradient steps in the *Y*, or phase-encoding, direction. For a technique using a *TE* of 30 milliseconds and a TR of 500 milliseconds with two signal averages and 128 *Y*-gradient steps:

$$T = 0.500 \times 2 \times 128$$

$$T = 2.1 \text{ minutes}$$

During that time, it would be possible to collect images of $TD/(1.5 \times TE)$ or $(0.500)/(1.5 \times 0.030) = 11$ slices using a multislice technique.

It is also possible to perform true volume imaging instead of multislice imaging by using the three-dimensional Fourier transform (3DFT). With this technique, the *Z* gradient is used to encode phase in the *Z* direction instead of being used as a slice-selection gradient. Both the *X* and *Y* gradients are used to encode frequency and phase, respectively, as is done in single slice imaging. Then, the 3DFT is used to decode the complex frequency distribution that is collected into images of slices in any projection. If the *Z* gradient step size is the same as that used for the *X* and *Y* gradients, then the volume collection is isotropic. If the *Z* gradient step size differs from that of the *X* and *Y* gradients, then the volume collection is anisotropic.

One of the primary imaging problems associated with MRI is the time required to acquire images. Imaging times of 2–20 minutes are common. Three-dimensional acquisitions can be longer still. An examination of the imaging time equation shows that the most significant method of reducing imaging time is to reduce the *TR*. This is true because the smallest number of averages (*n*) that can be used is one. Reducing the number of phase-encoding gradient steps (*NY*) would degrade resolution in the phase-encoding direction. However, as stated earlier, *TR* must be longer than T1 in the conventional spin echo technique to allow for complete relaxation before initiating the next pulse sequence.

This problem can be circumvented by using tip angles that are less than 90°. For example, referring to Figure 3.4, if the net magnetization were moved only 20° from the vertical, then only a very small change in the longitudinal magnetization, M_L, would be accompanied by a substantial change in the transverse magnetization, M_T, since in the equilibrium state M_L = M and M_T = 0. Thus, using small tip angles results in significantly less time for nuclei to return to equilibrium and permits the use of significantly smaller *TR*'s.

A problem with this technique is that the 180° rephasing pulse will invert the longitudinal magnetization, resulting in an equilibrium state in which the magnetization goes to zero. This problem can be eliminated by using a gradient reversal or gradient echo technique instead of the 180° rephasing pulse. The gradient echo technique uses a bipolar frequency-encoding gradient to alternately dephase all the nuclei across the selected slice with the negative lobe of the bipolar gradient and rephase with the positive lobe. A rephased echo is created at the center of the positive lobe of the bipolar gradient. Thus, it is possible to acquire 128 gradient steps with a TR of 40 milliseconds and two averages in 10.2 seconds.

Some systems are equipped with specialized gradient systems and drivers that support very high speed gradient switched imaging modes, called echo-planar imaging (EPI). Systems so equipped can produce images as quickly as 40–50 msec each, enabling ungated studies of the heart and other dynamic processes. Additionally, the very rapid acquisition capabilities are useful for more conventional studies where motion is often a problem, such as lung imaging. Acquisition of data is by means of gradient echo sequences where a single *RF* pulse is followed by rapid switching of the phase encoding gradient to produce a string of echoes that are used to reconstruct an image.

The clinical utility of echo planar imaging is under investigation, so this capability is not widely available. Additionally, the cost can be substantially more than a conventionally equipped instrument.

MRI EQUIPMENT

A block diagram of a typical MRI system is shown in Figure 3.12. The static magnetic field is established by a large magnet that may be one of four types (8, 9). One, which is currently available in commercial systems, is the permanent magnet (Fig.3.13**A**). Permanent magnet designs offer a relatively simple way to generate magnetic fields and have the advantage of limited fields external to the imaging system. The latter characteristic is due to the pole pieces of the magnet being physically connected to each other, providing a return path for the magnetic lines of flux. In the past, the application of permanent magnet technology to image applications has been hampered by the extremely

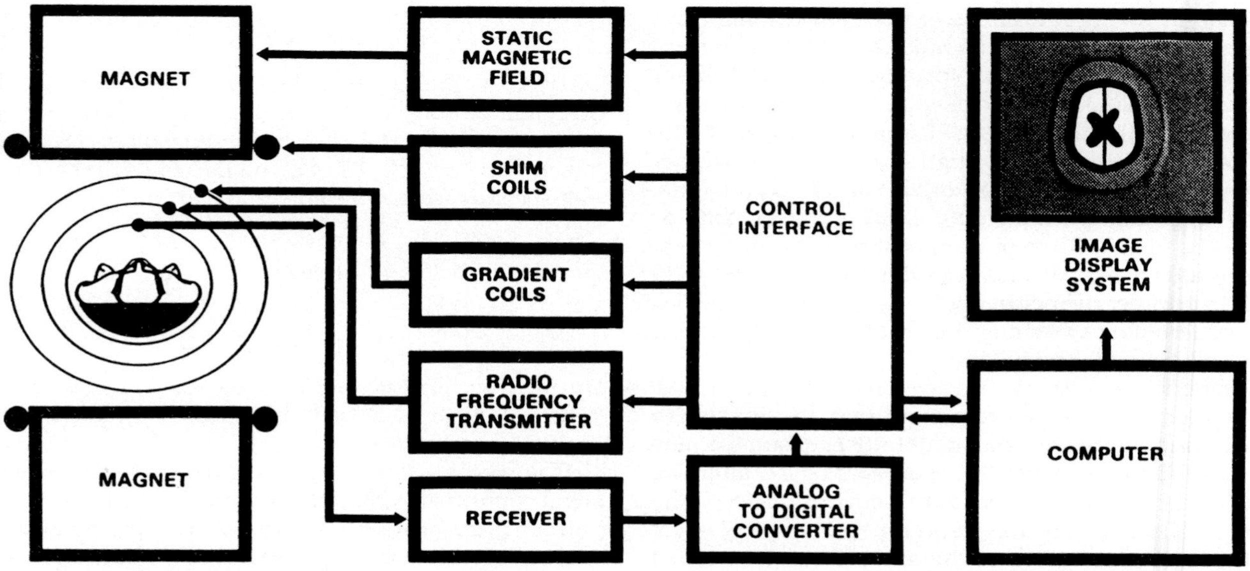

Figure 3.12. Block diagram of a typical MRI system. (Reproduced by permission from Sandler MP, Patton JA, Shaff MI, Powers TA, Partain CL. Correlative imaging: nuclear medicine, magnetic resonance, computed tomography, ultrasound. Baltimore: Williams and Wilkins, 1989.)

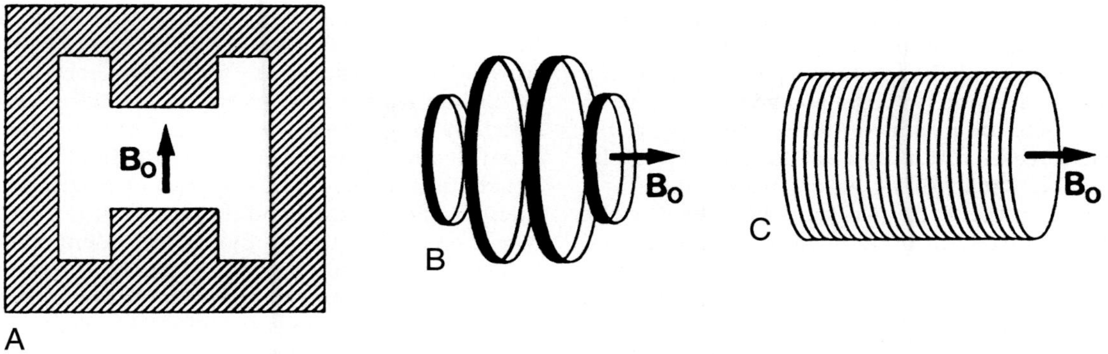

Figure 3.13. Schematics of a permanent magnet **(A)**, a resistive magnet **(B)**, and a superconducting magnet **(C)** that can be used to establish the static magnetic field (B_0) necessary for MRI. (Reproduced by permission from Sandler MP, Patton JA, Shaff MI, Powers TA, Partain CL. Correlative imaging: nuclear medicine, magnetic resonance, computed tomography, ultrasound. Baltimore: Williams and Wilkins, 1989.)

large size required (weighing 250,000 lbs.), thermal instability, and the relatively poor uniformity of the fields that are generated. However, the use of new lightweight magnetic alloys has reduced the weight problem, while the addition of coils for shimming purposes has significantly improved uniformity and reduced the thermal effects.

Resistive magnets were the first types of electromagnets used for MRI. Resistive magnets generally consist of four coils of hollow copper tubing wound to roughly approximate the shape of a sphere (Fig. 3.13**B**). When current flows through the coils, a magnetic field is established in the center of the coils, which is directly proportional to the magnitude of the current flow. Copper is an excellent conductor; however, it does have some resistance that results in heat production because of the large amount of current flowing through the coils. In practice, this heat is dissipated by deionized cooling water flowing through the center of the copper tubing. Disadvantages of these systems include the need for cooling and the associated deionizer and heat exchanger, the large power requirements necessary to maintain the magnetic field, and a practical limitation in field strength to about 1500 G (0.15 T) because of a heat dissipation problem. The advantages of these magnets are that they are relatively inexpensive to manufacture and maintain. Additionally, they can be shut down quickly, when necessary, simply by turning off the electrical power.

Hybrid magnets are now being constructed that use the permanent magnet configuration, as shown in Figure 3.13**A**, with the addition of current-carrying coils around the pole pieces. Current flowing through these coils augments the field of the permanent magnet, yielding a larger field than would be available with the permanent magnet alone. Electric shim coils stabilize the field and make it more uniform.

The magnet design with the most appeal for imaging is the superconducting magnet, which is based on the principle that certain materials lose their resistance completely and become perfect conductors when they are cooled to temperatures approaching absolute zero. Once a current is introduced into such a material at or below its superconducting temperature, it will continue to flow indefinitely with no applied voltage and no heat dissipation, as long as the low temperature is maintained. A superconducting magnet for imaging purposes is constructed by wrapping several miles of small-diameter niobium-titanium wire in a cylinder (solenoid) (Fig. 3.13**C**). To maintain the extremely low temperatures necessary for superconductivity, the coils are surrounded by a Cryostat containing liquid helium. Because of the relatively high cost of liquid helium, a Cryostat containing liquid nitrogen surrounds the liquid helium Cryostat to keep the loss of helium to a minimum. The need for cooling is a disadvantage because of the high fabrication costs associated with the complex cryogen system, the costs of liquid nitrogen and helium, and the need for external venting of the gases. Helium refrigeration systems are available on some recently designed systems that eliminate the need for the nitrogen cryostat and reduce helium consumption to a very low level.

Advantages of superconducting magnets are significant. The field is maintained at all times with no applied voltage. High field strengths of excellent stability and uniformity can be produced. Small-bore superconducting magnet systems for small animal studies are currently available with field strengths of 4.7 T or higher; however, clinical imaging is generally limited to systems below 2.0 T, with the majority of systems operating at 1.0 T or 1.5 T.

Other important components of the imaging system are the various coils used for different purposes. Currently available magnets alone cannot provide the uniformity necessary for imaging. However, by placing coils of wire, called shim coils, at various locations around the imaging volume, and carefully adjusting the amount of current flowing through each coil, the field uniformity can be corrected or "shimmed" so that variations of no more than a fraction of a part per million over the imaging volume are achieved. Gradient coils are used to selectively alter the magnetic field in one or more directions, resulting in different Larmor frequencies at different positions in the imaging field. To accomplish this task, three separate coils, termed the X, Y, and Z gradient coils, are present, and are constructed so that passage of current through each of the coils will linearly alter the magnetic field in the direction controlled by that coil.

The actual signal transmission and reception are accomplished through the use of an RF transmitter coupled to a transmitting coil or antenna within the imaging unit and an RF receiver coupled to a receiving coil or antenna, also located in the imaging unit and positioned as close as possible to the patient for maximum sensitivity. Some manufacturers have used the same coil for both transmission and reception, while others use separate coils.

In most systems, there are two transmit-receive coils. One is optimized for use in body imaging and is permanently installed within the bore of the magnet. A second coil, optimized for head imaging, can be placed on the bed so that the patient's head can be positioned within the coil. Then, the entire bed and head coil are positioned in the bore of the magnet. When imaging the head, the body coil is usually made inactive.

Another category of coils often used to image selected regions of the body is surface coils, which are usually receive-only. These coils can be placed close to the region of interest, providing increased sensitivity for imaging in that region, while decreasing coil noise that results from patient-coil loading (10). The increased signal-to-noise ratio that results from this technique can be used to decrease 5slice thickness and also to decrease pixel size, providing magnified images with improved spatial resolution. It is usually necessary to increase the number of signal averages in order to take full advantage of these capabilities. Circular, square, or rectangular-shaped single-loop coils, and various coil arrays have been used for imaging of the spine, orbits, and temporomandibular joints. All of these coils have their maximum sensitivity and signal-to-noise ratio in the center of the plane of the coil, and these variables decrease rapidly with distance.

Finally, a powerful computer system with a large memory, substantial storage capabilities, an array processor, and a high quality multiformat imager are necessary to acquire, process, and display the large volume of data associated with the imaging process. The system usually can be connected to an image network so that images can be distributed electronically.

ULTRASOUND

Diagnostic ultrasound systems use sound waves having frequencies greater than 20,000 Hz. Ultrasound waves are mechanical rather than electromagnetic, requiring a medium for propagation. The physical characteristics of the medium, especially its density and compressibility, are the most important determinants of the speed at which the ultrasound wave travels. These differences in physical properties constitute the interfaces within a medium that produce sound wave reflections or echoes.

Medical ultrasound techniques are derived from the military development called SONAR (sound navigation and ranging), which was used extensively during World War II to detect underwater objects. By measuring the time interval between the transmitted pulse and the reflected echo, it is possible to calculate the distance between the transmitter and the object by the following equation:

$$S = (V \times t)/2$$

where S is the distance between transmitter and object, V is the velocity of sound in the medium, and t is the time interval. In medical imaging applications, it is the echoes from interfaces at organ surfaces and from internal structures that are responsible for the observed image features.

Sound waves used in medical applications are generated by a piezoelectric crystal or "transducer" that is mounted in a specially constructed holder. When an electric field is applied across a piezoelectric crystal and suddenly removed, the crystal vibrates at a frequency, called the resonant frequency, that is dependent on its thickness. When the vibrating crystal is placed in contact with the body, a longitudinal compression sound wave at the same frequency will be projected into the body.

The same crystal can be used to produce an ultrasonic wave and to detect the returning echoes. During detection, the transducer produces an electrical signal by the inverse piezoelectric effect, in direct proportion to the echo intensity. The electrical signal that produces the ultrasonic wave is applied for only 1–10 microseconds out of every millisecond. The rest of the time, the transducer is available to receive sound waves that reflect off of internal organs in the body. In diagnostic units, sound typically is being produced only 1% of the time or less.

The three basic modes of interaction with the medium are reflection, refraction, and absorption. When the ultrasonic beam encounters a boundary between two tissues, part of the wave is reflected back toward the transducer, and part is transmitted into the second medium. The fraction of incident beam intensity that is reflected depends on the fundamental property of the material called its acoustic impedance. Additionally, part of the transmitted wave can be refracted, i.e., move through the interface and enter another material at an angle that is different from the original direction. The transmitted component of the beam becomes the new incident beam for all interfaces located at other depths.

Ultrasound imagers have evolved from instruments that produced only A-mode (amplitude-mode) displays of the reflected echo amplitude versus position. From these instruments evolved B-mode (brightness-mode) systems, which display the echoes in a brightness-modulated, two-dimensional image format. The first of these B-mode systems were called static B-mode scanners, since the image was created by manually moving the transducer over the body for a period of 10–20 seconds. During this time, an image was "painted" into an analog scan converter and displayed on a video monitor. Since the image creation took so long, these systems were relegated to imaging static or nonmoving structures. More recently, the practice of ultrasonography has rapidly moved away from the slower static scanners to a variety of different designs of "real-time" scanners (9–12). Real-time scanners can be divided into two design categories: those that use mechanical beam steering and those that employ electronic steering.

MECHANICALLY STEERED SCANNERS

Most mechanically steered scanners produce a sector or pie-shaped format image. The sector opening angles may range from 30–90°, and in some cases may be somewhat larger. The ultrasonic beam may be steered by moving the transducer itself (Fig. 3.14) or by reflecting the beam from an oscillating "acoustic mirror" (Fig. 3.15). Because of the difficulty of maintaining good direct skin contact with either the moving transducer or the moving mirror, most mechanically steered scanners use a fluid-filled case with an acoustically transparent window to contain the moving parts. In this manner, skin contact is made with the acoustic window case rather than directly with the moving components. This configuration ensures adequate acoustic coupling, even at relatively large steering angles.

Mechanically steered scanners have two main advantages over electronically steered scanners: (a) the use of a single-element transducer requires less sophisticated electronics and generally allows for a more simple transducer head design, and (b) image artifacts due to side lobes and grating lobes, unique to electronically steered beams, are less frequent.

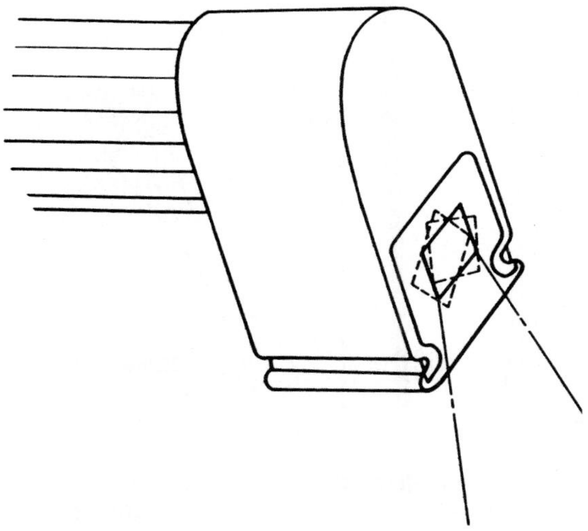

Figure 3.14. Diagram of a mechanical real-time scanner that uses a single-element oscillating transducer. (Reproduced by permission from Fleischer AC, James AE Jr, eds. Real-time sonography. East Norwalk, CT: Appleton-Century-Crofts, 1984:19.)

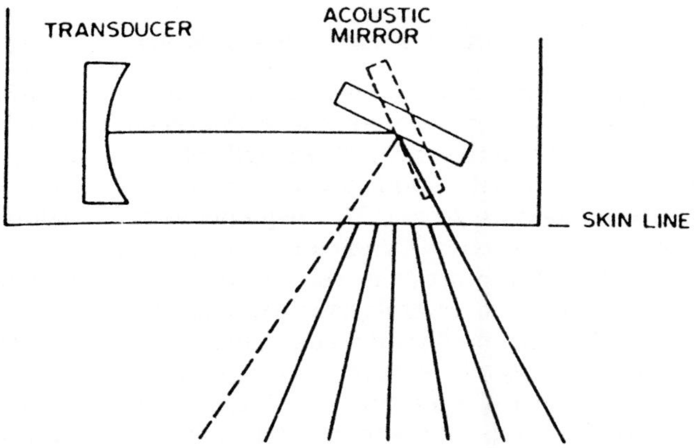

Figure 3.15. Diagram of a mechanical real-time scanner that uses an oscillating mirror for beam steering. (Reproduced by permission from Fleischer AC, James AE Jr, eds. Real-time sonography. East Norwalk, CT: Appleton-Century-Crofts, 1984:17.)

There are several disadvantages to the use of mechanical scanning methods: (a) The beam focus and beam pattern are fixed for a given transducer. To change the focus, one must change the entire transducer head. (b) The image framing rate depends on how rapidly the transducer is oscillated. The framing rate is governed by the line density needed to produce an image of diagnostic quality and the depth of the field of view. The velocity of ultrasound in tissue is the ultimate factor governing the oscillation rate of the transducer. Thus, the framing rate may become quite low when using large fields of view, which require large excursions of the transducer element. (c) Field of view and image frame rates are in competition when the total number of scan lines per image is kept constant. Therefore, large opening angles are needed for large field sizes and small opening angles are required for high resolution. In other words, the sector angle must decrease if higher line density is desired. This problem is not unique to mechanical scanners, however, and is discussed again in regard to electronically steered scanners.

Oscillating-Transducer Scanner

Although many variations on the oscillating-transducer design have been built, the most common design is a transducer that oscillates about a single fixed point and yields a sector-shaped image format (Fig. 3.14).

When a single-element "wobbler" transducer is placed in contact with the skin surface, it is rocked from side to side in a small arc by means of an electric motor. Each individual line of the B-mode image is produced and displayed as a radius of a circle with the transducer at the center.

Early commercial systems of this design employed an exposed transducer coupled directly to the skin surface with large quantities of coupling gel. Because of the difficulty of keeping adequate skin contact, such designs were forced to use small sector angles (30–45°). Most currently available scanners enclose the transducer in a fluid-filled case with a flexible membrane that touches the skin, eliminating much of the contact problem.

Beam formation in mechanical scanners is achieved in the same manner as with static or manual B-mode scanners. The transducers are mechanically focused, using either a shaped transducer (internal focus) or an acoustic lens attached to the transducer surface (external focus). One disadvantage of this design is that to change the focal zone, one must physically replace the transducer. Consequently, the focal zone cannot conveniently be changed during scanning. Electronically focused scanners focus by delayed pulse sequences, allowing the focal zone to be changed without physically altering the scanner.

Stationary Transducer with Oscillating Acoustic Mirror

An alternative approach to beam steering in a mechanical scanner is to keep the transducer stationary and use an oscillating acoustic mirror to move the beam in a sector format (Fig. 3.15). This design requires that the mirror and transducer be contained within a fluid-filled housing so that the moving mirror does not make direct contact with the patient.

The oscillating-mirror design offers an advantage over the oscillating-transducer design by eliminating the need to move an electrically active component (the transducer). Additionally, the mirror is usually lighter and can be moved more easily and rapidly. Therefore, a smaller motor can be used, resulting in a lighter, more compact scanner.

A plane mirror only changes the direction of the beam and does not affect the beam focus. Thus, the focal characteristics are entirely determined by the transducer and its mechanical construction. The angle at which the beam is reflected from the mirror surface is equal to the angle of beam incidence analogous to light reflection with essentially no energy loss in the reflection process. The fluid path length, by necessity, is slightly longer (approximately 1 cm) than in scanners using an oscillating transducer without a mirror, thus making the image field of view more trapezoidal in format. This is not necessarily a disadvantage, however, since the additional offset of the skin line usually results in better lateral resolution by moving the poor skin line away from the transducer face and closer to the focal zone of the transducer. Scanners of this design typically operate at 15–30 frames per second.

Rotating-Wheel Transducer

The most common design of rotating-wheel transducers consists of three transducers mounted 120° apart on a wheel that is rotated by an external motor (Fig. 3.16). The wheel is always rotated in the same direction, making the mechanical assembly simpler. The wheel and transducer are housed in a fluid-filled case with an acoustic window at the lower surface that makes contact with the patient. As the transducers rotate, the output is switched from one transducer to the next in sequence, depending on which transducer has rotated in front of the acoustic window. This design allows for rapid framing without significant flicker—typically 30 frames per second. The design produces a sector-shaped field of view and allows a wide opening angle of 90° or more.

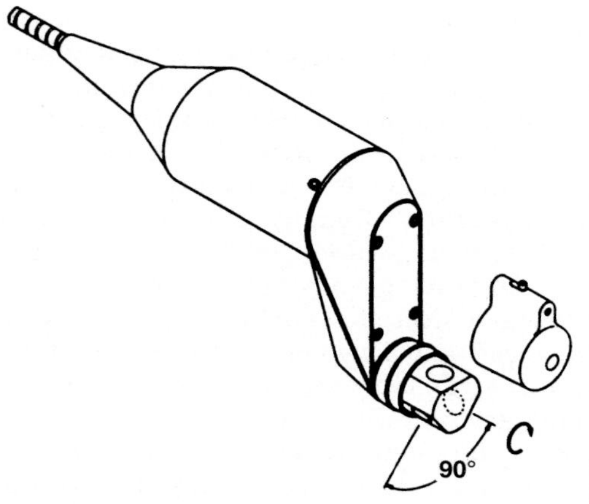

Figure 3.16. Diagram of a real-time scanner that uses a rotating-wheel design. (Reproduced by permission from Price RR, Rollo FD, Monahan WG, James AE Jr, eds. Digital radiography: a focus on clinical utility. New York: Grune & Stratton, 1982:378.)

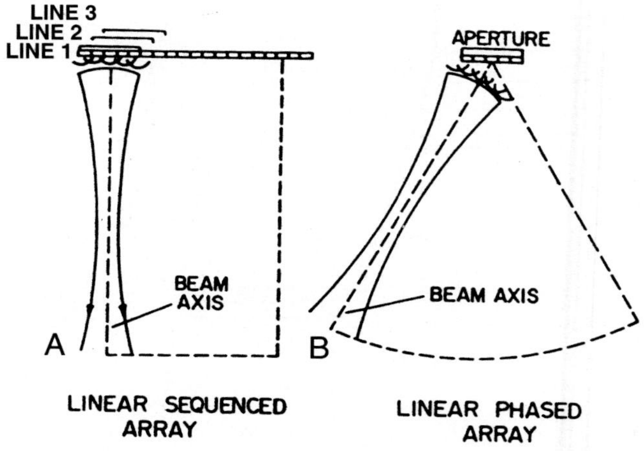

Figure 3.17. **A.** Linear sequenced array. Each scan line is produced by pulsing a small group of elements simultaneously and sequentially moving through the entire group to produce an image. **B.** Linear phased array. Each scale line uses all elements in the array. Steering is achieved electronically. (Reproduced by permission from Fleischer AC, James AE Jr, eds. Real-time sonography. East Norwalk, CT: Appleton-Century-Crofts, 1984:24.)

ELECTRONICALLY STEERED SCANNERS

Electronically steered scanners include linear phased arrays, multielement linear sequenced arrays, and multielement annular arrays. Through the proper phasing of the transmit-receive timing of the transducer elements used to fabricate the arrays, a composite ultrasonic beam can be created. In this manner, the beam can be focused and steered electronically. Fundamental to electronic focusing is that each element of the array generates an ultrasonic wave that has a definite phase relationship with the waves from the other elements. The ultrasonic waves generated by each element can be superimposed precisely to create the effect of a single wave front (Figs. 3.17**A** and **B**). In addition to "transmit focusing," array scanners also are capable of focusing on receiving an echo. By assessing the relative arrival times of an echo to the various array elements, only echoes arriving from a prescribed depth can be processed, providing a dynamic focusing capability. The combination of transmit and receive focusing has resulted in significant improvements in lateral resolution in current scanners.

Multielement Linear Sequenced Array

Multielement linear scanning arrays are pulsed to produce a wave front that moves normal to the transducer face, yielding a rectangular field. The length of the transducer array may vary with frequency; at 3.5 MHz, transducers may be as long as 20 cm. The sequencing of transducer activation can be chosen and can occur in groups.

The transducer array is usually composed of many small piezoelectric crystals (M) arranged in a row (Fig. 3.17**A**). Since the field from a single small crystal element diverges very rapidly, several elements (N) are driven simultaneously, and electronic focusing is used. In the subgroup of N crystals, the outer crystals may be pulsed first, with the inner crystals delayed. In this circumstance, the field from the N elements will be focused at a depth that depends on the magnitude or time interval of the delays. By changing the magnitudes of the delays, the transmit focal zone can be scanned through a specified range of depths. The elements may also be designed to be sensitive to the returning waves so that delay differences, upon receipt, are used to constitute a focusing effect on the returning signals. A single scan line in the real-time image is formed in this manner. The next adjacent scan line is generated by using another group of N crystals formed by shifting from the previous N crystals, one crystal position along the transducer array. The same transmit-receive pattern is then repeated for this set of N crystals, and subsequently for all other sets of N crystals along the array, in a cyclical manner. Focusing in the plane of the transducer elements improves lateral resolution, as well as sensitivity, by increasing the amount of energy in the focal zone by constructive interference. Focusing in the plane perpendicular to the scan lines determines the slice thickness, and is accomplished by mechanically focusing the elements in the slice thickness direction, a technique known as double focusing.

Linear Phased Array

The linear phased array is frequently termed an electronic-sector scanner, since the resulting field is pie-shaped, with the field diverging as the distance from the transducers is increased (Fig. 3.17). How this field shape is created is illustrated in Figure 3.18. The outside transducers are activated first and the inner transducers are delayed in time, with the central transducer having the greater delay, to yield a wave axis perpendicular to the plane of the transducer (Fig. 3.18**A**). By varying the order of the delay, the wave can be focused at a specified depth (Fig. 3.18**B**) and the wave axis can be scanned through a sector of 60–90° (Fig. 3.18**C**). Properly selected delays can produce steering and focusing simultaneously (Fig. 3.18**D**).

Phased Annular Array

The phased annular array scanner represents a hybrid system that possesses characteristics of both mechanical and electronic designs. The transducer comprises a series of independent transducers, each element in the shape of an annular ring, and multiple elements are arranged in concentric rings about a central transducer element (Fig. 3.19).

Beam formation and focusing are achieved electronically by proper phasing of the transducer elements. An advantage of this design is that focusing is achieved in two dimensions similar to a single focused element; but, unlike mechanically focusing transducers, the focal zone can be changed without physically changing the transducer. Beam steering, on the other hand, must be done mechanically. The beam is swept through a trapezoidal field of view with an oscillating mirror or by physically moving the transducer. As with other mechanically steered scanners, the transducer and mirror, if present, are contained within a fluid-filled housing. In this design, the transducer may be quite large, if desired. Commercially available annular-array scanners offer a variable focal zone option.

DISPLAY AND STORAGE OF REAL-TIME IMAGES

The number of gray shades displayed in the ultrasound image depends upon the type of "scan converter" used to

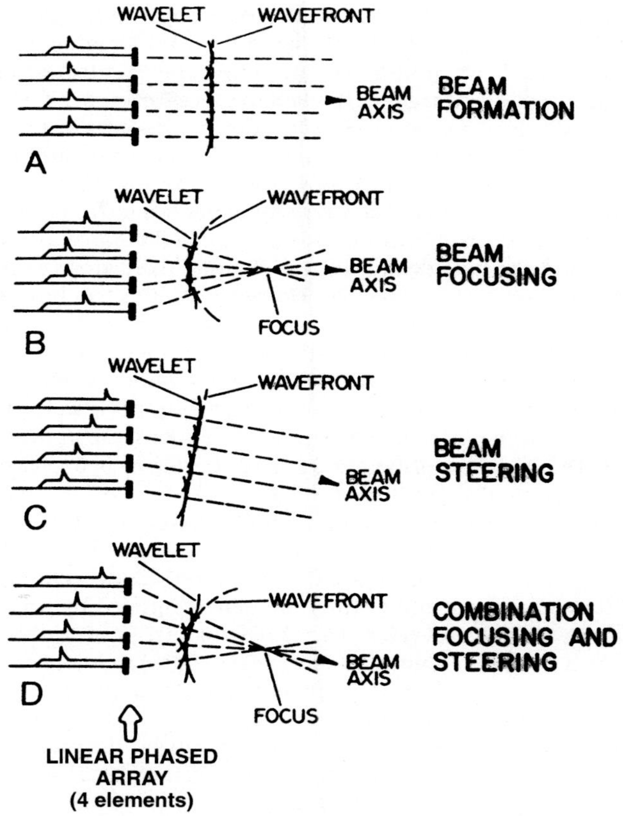

Figure 3.18. Beam formation and steering with a linear phased array. **A.** Wavefront formed to move perpendicular to transducer axis. **B.** Focusing by center symmetric transmit delays. **C.** Steering by sequential delay patterns. **D.** Steering and focusing by asymmetric delay sequences. (Reproduced by permission from Fleischer AC, James AE Jr, eds. Real-time sonography. East Norwalk, CT: Appleton-Century-Crofts, 1984:25.)

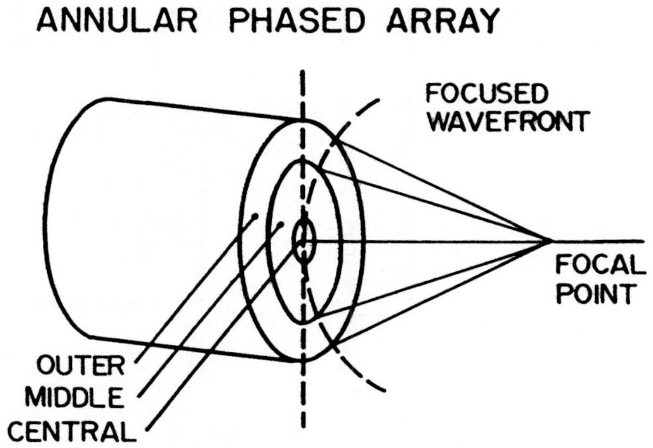

Figure 3.19. Diagram of an annular array. The outer rings are pulsed before the inner rings to produce a beam focused in two dimensions. (Reproduced by permission from Fleischer AC, James AE Jr, eds. Real-time sonography. East Norwalk, CT: Appleton-Century-Crofts, 1984:26.)

translate the pressure change received by the transducer to electrical impulses. Early systems used "analog" scan converters. In an analog system, scan converter tubes consisting of silicon targets are used to store information electronically by "charging" the targets in proportion to the echo amplitude. Once an image has been stored, the scan converter tube is "read," and the results displayed on a video monitor. Since the intensity of each picture element of the stored image varies with the applied voltage, a relatively infinite gray scale, without definite fixed steps or levels, is theoretically possible. However, due to tracking errors and noise, the scan converter tube has resolution limitations. Scan converter tubes need periodic alignment and are temperature sensitive. Systems using analog scan converters generally require long warm-up periods for the equipment to perform properly, and frequently drift during use. This drift is subtle and difficult to detect before it becomes clinically significant.

Current instruments for B-mode imaging use "digital scan converters" (Fig. 3.20). In these systems, the analog voltage levels that correspond to the returning echo amplitudes for each line of the image are digitized by an analog-to-digital converter. The generated array of numbers is then stored in digital memory. The digital memory is divided into a number of picture elements or pixels. Typically, a pixel element depicts a region in the body of 1–2 mm or less. The size of the memory can be described by the number of pixel elements, such as 512×512. The memory can then be interrogated and the image displayed on a video monitor. The brightness of the video signal representing each picture element is controlled by the value stored in the corresponding digital word at each pixel location. The number of shades of gray available is determined by the size of the digital word used to store the information. The size of the word is measured in terms of the number of bits and is frequently referred to as the "depth" of the memory. Three-bit words provide the capacity for displaying eight shades of gray, four bits provide 16 shades of gray, and five bits provide 32 shades of gray. Most digital memories used for real-time scanners are at least 512×512 by 6–8 bits deep (64–256 shades of gray).

The discreteness of digital systems for both the spatial information and the gray-scale shades provides an image that may not be as "smooth" as the analog image. The appearance of the image will be different and the margin between picture elements (pixels) more definite than with analog displays; however, as the number of pixels increases and the pixels become smaller, it becomes more difficult to distinguish between the two types of images. Images are frequently processed by linear interpolation to produce more aesthetically pleasing images. Interpolation fills in between picture elements without altering the original image data.

The all-digital system has many advantages over the older analog technology. The digital system is more stable, does not drift, is less sensitive to heat, and allows preprocessing and postprocessing of the digital images. Additionally, many functions that were impossible to implement in analog systems are standard features of current instruments. Furthermore, by imbedding a computer in the imager, many functions can be reprogrammed to reflect the requirements of users and new developments.

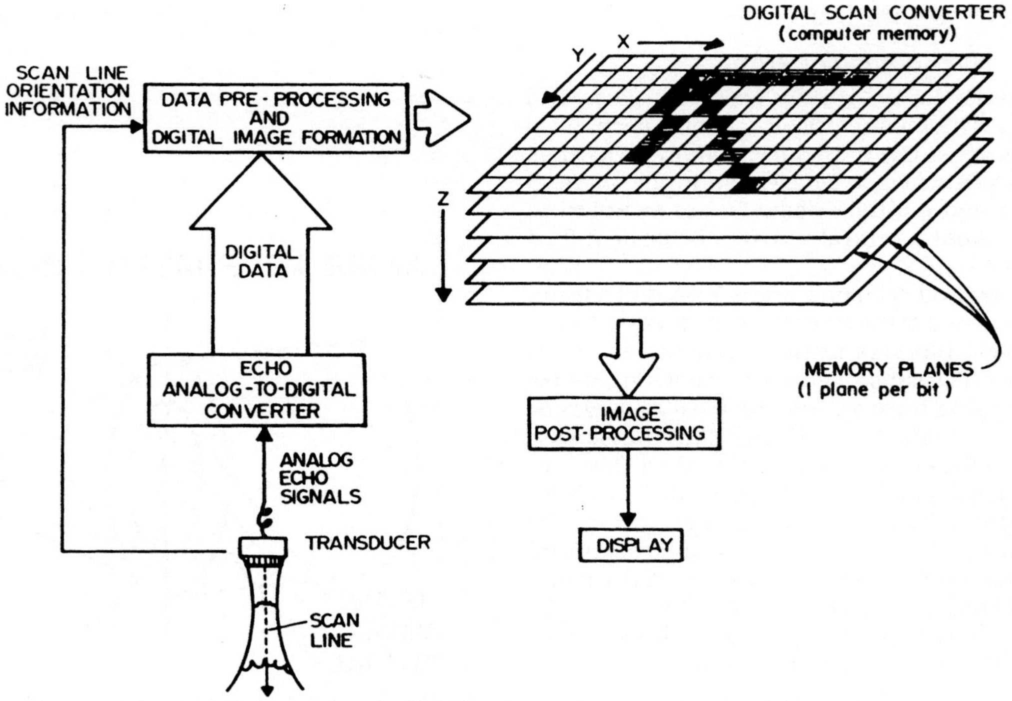

Figure 3.20. Echoes received by the transducer are digitized by an analog-to-digital converter and then stored in digital memory (often called a digital scan converter) at a location determined by the orientation of the transducer. (Reproduced by permission from Fleischer AC, James AE Jr, eds. Real-time sonography. East Norwalk, CT: Appleton-Century-Crofts, 1984:31.)

DOPPLER PHYSICS AND INSTRUMENTATION

The basic Doppler phenomenon is relatively familiar to most people (13–19) involved with medical imaging. However, the manner in which it is manifest in real-time color-flow imaging (CFI) systems remains a mystery to many. One source of the mystery derives from the number of different implementations of CFI. Furthermore, CFI has increased the number of machine controls and scan parameters, leading to additional confusion.

The Doppler Effect

Ultrasound, when scattered from moving objects such as red blood cells, experiences a shift in frequency relative to the transmitted pulse. This frequency change is called the Doppler shift. When the red blood cells are moving toward the receiver, the echo frequency will be shifted to a higher frequency. When the red blood cells move away from the transducer, the echo frequency will be shifted lower. The magnitude of the Doppler shift (δf) is proportional to the velocity of the reflecting blood and to the angle from which the receiver views the blood vessel:

$$\delta f = \frac{2Vf_o}{C} \cos \theta$$

frC

where V = the velocity of the reflecting object, f_o = the frequency of the transmitted pulse, C = the velocity of sound in soft-tissue, and θ = the angle between the direction of blood flow and the line-of-sight of the receiver transducer.

Since f_0, C, and θ are all constants for a given image, the velocity can be related directly to the measured Doppler shift. Table 3.4 lists Doppler shifts for a range of velocities and transducer frequencies that may be encountered in the human body.

Pulsed Doppler

The first step in the evolution from traditional pulse-echo gray scale ultrasound imaging to CFI was the development of the multigate pulsed Doppler technique. In pulsed Doppler (PD) systems, a burst of ultrasound is transmitted; then, following a selected time delay, the receiver is turned on for a short time interval. Thus, the PD system will be listening for Doppler shifts arriving only from a predetermined depth. A new burst can be transmitted as soon as the signal from the desired depth is received. The pulse repetition frequency (PRF), therefore, must be reduced as the depth increases, to allow additional time for the echo to return.

The length of the transmitted burst and the time interval during which the receiver is active determine the length of the sampled volume. Since the transmitted burst is usually at least three wavelengths long to assure reasonable accuracy in the frequency measurement, the length of the volume will be on the order of 1 mm. The width of the sampled volume will depend upon the beam width at the selected depth. The beam width, in turn, is determined by the transducer focus.

Since the echo is sampled at the rate determined by the PRF in PD systems, one is only able to accurately measure frequency shifts that are less than 1/2 of the PRF. Shifts that are actually greater than this maximum value will be displayed erroneously as very small shifts. This phenomenon is referred to as "aliasing." Thus, PD systems, unlike continuous-wave (CW) Doppler systems, are limited in their ability to accurately measure large velocities. For example, for a PRF of 5 kHz, which corresponds to a depth of 15 cm, the maximum shift frequency would be 2.5 kHz. From Table 3.4 one can see that this corresponds to a velocity below about 50 cm/sec for a 5 MHz transducer.

Table 3.4.
*Doppler Shift (Doppler Angle 45°)**

	Frequency (MHz)		
Velocity (cm/sec)	3	5	7
1	27 Hz	46 Hz	65 Hz
10	275 Hz	459 Hz	643 Hz
50	1.37 kHz	2.29 kHz	3.15 kHz
100	2.75 kHz	4.59 kHz	6.43 kHz

*Reproduced by permission from Sandler MP, Patton JA, Gross MD, Shapiro B, Falke THM. Endocrine imaging. Norwalk, CT: Appleton & Lange, 1992.

Color-Flow Imaging

Conventional pulse-echo gray-scale imaging and Doppler flow mapping, for the most part, are complementary. That is, when imaging a vessel, it is the vessel wall that contributes to the gray-scale image and not the lumen contents. Similarly, the Doppler shift information comes from the lumen contents primarily and not the vessel wall. Thus, the combination of the two methods is a logical extension of the methodologies. Table 3.5 from Evans (18) shows a typical resolution for CFI.

CFI systems are essentially multigate pulsed Doppler systems with simultaneous real-time gray-scale imaging. Digital Fast-Fourier Transforms (FFT), used in duplex pulsed Doppler systems to compute a complete spectrum of shift frequencies from a selected region in a gray-scale image, take about 5 msec. Therefore, the FFT is too slow to be useful for real-time color imaging where the number of Doppler samples along a line is equal to the number of gray-scale picture elements. If, for example, an image is composed of 50 scan lines and is refreshed at a rate of 20 times per second, the time available for one line is only 1msec, which implies that the spectral resolution is about 1 kHz at best.

The problem of computing spectra at high speed, however, has been overcome by two elegant techniques. The first was developed in 1981 by Nowicki and Reid called "in-

Table 3.5.
*Typical CFI Resolution**

Resolution (mm)	3	5	7
Axial	1.5	1	0.7
Lateral	3.5	2	1.5

*Reproduced by permission from Sandler MP, Patton JA, Gross MD, Shapiro B, Falke THM. Endocrine imaging. Norwalk, CT: Appleton & Lange, 1992.

finite gate" pulsed Doppler, which is a moving target indicator method, and the second, developed in 1983 by Namekawa, is based on a real-time autocorrelation method (20, 21). In each of these methods, quadrature-encoded echoes received from pairs of transmitted pulses are compared for phase differences. In quadrature detection, the returning signal is divided into two parts that are shifted by 90° with respect to one another. Quadrature detection is used to tell the direction of the phase shift. From the two pulse pairs, the second set is delayed in time by an amount equal to the time between transmission of the first and second pulses. The resulting echoes should be in phase unless something has moved. This phase shift can be related to the mean Doppler shift frequency. As an added bit of information, the variance in the mean is also available. To provide reliable estimates of the mean frequency and its variance, measurements of several pulse pairs are generally made. The larger the number of pulse pairs used to estimate the mean and variance, the better the estimates will be. Unfortunately, using more pulse pairs slows the imaging rate. Typically, eight or more pulses per line are required for reliable CFI. Thus, the result is to reduce the frame rate by that factor (1/8) relative to conventional grayscale ultrasound for the same field-of-view. Some instruments reduce the CFI field-of-view to a selected portion of the gray scale field-of-view in order to improve frame rate.

CFI Controls

CFI introduces a number of scan parameters and system controls in addition to those found on conventional grayscale and duplex systems. Since the same echo information is used for both imaging and flow, a threshold based upon the backscattered echo amplitude can be used as a method to discriminate flowing reflectors from stationary reflectors. Color gain is related to sensitivity and separate from overall system gain. The color display is generally chosen to display flow toward the probe as red and flow away from the probe as blue, with slow flow toward the probe being red, tending to yellow at faster flows. Slow flow away from the probe is displayed as blue, tending to lightblue for faster flow. If the color gain is too high, red and blue noise will be generated.

Other display modes used with CFI include variance display and power display. Variance, a measure of turbulence, is often displayed in shades of green added to the more traditional color display. Unlike the other modes of display, the turbulence display is independent of flow direction. Specifically, the display is dependent on the degree of turbulence. In the power display mode, the brightness of the display indicates the intensity of the received echoes.

COMPUTED TOMOGRAPHY

The foundations for computed tomography (CT) were set in the early 1900s with the mathematical concepts formulated by Radon. He proved that a density distribution could be found from processing the projections of the distribution collected at a sufficient number of angles (22). The problem, however, was deemed unsolvable until Cormack of the United States and Hounsfield of Great Britain independently proved that the practical application of Radon's mathematics could produce images of distributions of sufficient detail for use in medicine. These developments, and the availability of inexpensive digital computers, led to the development of the first commercial CT scanner, the EMI 800 series manufactured by Electronic Music Industries, Ltd., of England (23).

Computed tomography uses x-rays to produce transverse thin-sectional images of the body. These x-rays are carefully collimated so that they impinge only on a section of the body. The collimation is designed so that the usable beam from the x-ray tube is either pencil-shaped or fanshaped and very thin. The x-ray tube is mounted on a gantry so that it can be moved in a circular path around the body. In this manner, the x-ray beam can pass through the body section from a large number of angles.

Opposite the x-ray tube is an array of detectors. These detectors, and their associated electronics, convert the x-ray energy incident on them into a varying signal that is processed by the reconstruction computer system. The number of detectors depends on the design of the particular scanner. In some cases, only a few detectors are mounted, so that they move with the x-ray tube. In other designs, over 1000 detectors circle the patient and are fixed in position. A typical configuration is illustrated in Figure 3.21.

Several types of detectors are suitable for use in CT systems. Among them are scintillation crystals coupled to photomultiplier tubes or solid-state photodiodes and gas-filled ionization chambers (24, 25). Sodium iodide (NaI) crystal detectors suffer from the phenomenon of afterglow, but are very efficient in detecting the x-ray photons. Afterglow is the persistence of the scintillation light after the

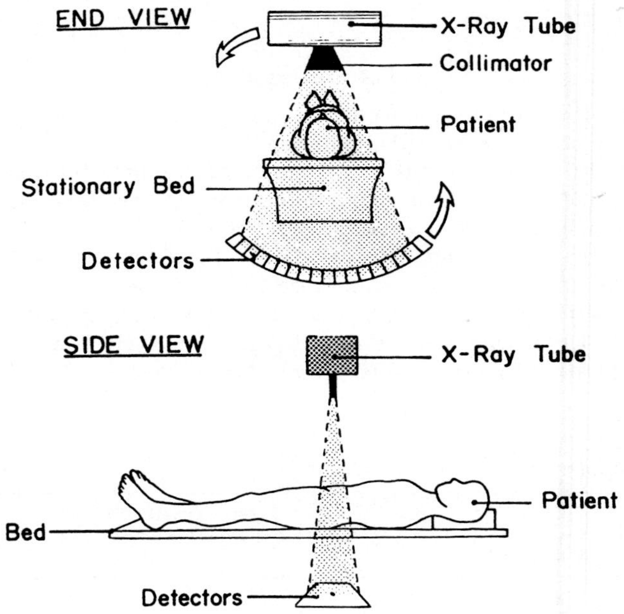

Figure 3.21. Diagram of a typical CT scanner showing the relationship between the x-ray tube, the detectors, and the patient. (Reproduced by permission from Sandler MP, Patton JA, Shaff MI, Powers TA, Partain CL. Correlative imaging: nuclear medicine, magnetic resonance, computed tomography, ultrasound. Baltimore: Williams and Wilkins, 1989.)

x-ray has been detected. It is a property of all scintillators, but is especially noticeable with NaI crystals. To reduce the problems with afterglow, bismuth germinate, cadmium tungstate, or cesium iodide can be used. The amount of afterglow affects the rate at which information can be collected from a detector, which, in turn, affects the speed of acquisition of the scanner.

The scintillation crystal-photodetector system is very similar to that found in a nuclear camera. However, each crystal-photodetector pair is separated from the other detectors, and usually is collimated separately, so there is no specific position sensitivity within the scintillation assembly. Position information is provided by the mechanical alignment of each detector with respect to its neighbors.

Ionization chambers as detectors avoid the afterglow problems of scintillators, responding very rapidly to each event. These detectors usually are filled with xenon gas under high pressure and exhibit linear current output response to x-ray exposure. Ionization detectors are not as sensitive as the scintillation crystal-photomultiplier tubes, but their high-speed response and low cost make them attractive for use in scanners.

The transmitted x rays that strike the detectors are the result of the interaction of the x-ray beam with the material through which it is passing (25–27). The equation that relates the intensity of the incoming x-ray beam to the intensity of the x-ray beam that strikes the detector is an exponential relationship of the form:

$$I = I_o e^{-\mu x}$$

where I_o is the intensity of the x-ray beam before it strikes the patient and I is the intensity of the beam after it has passed through the patient. The intensities of the x-ray beam can be measured, as can x, the thickness of the body. Therefore, only the linear attenuation coefficient, μ, is left to be calculated. μ represents the summation of the linear attenuation coefficients of all materials through which the x-ray beam passes. Thus, CT measures the linear attenuation coefficients of the body. Each detector produces a signal that reflects the absorption of the x-ray photons in a linear path through the body at a particular position of the x-ray tube and the detector (Fig. 3.22).

SYSTEM DESIGN

The mechanism that positions the x-ray system and the detectors is very elaborate. In the original EMI scanners, a motion called scan-rotate was used (25, 28). In this design, the x-ray beam was heavily collimated into a pencil shape and was detected by a pair of NaI detectors mounted on the opposite side of the scanning area. The scanner was designed to collect information for two contiguous slices during each complete scan. Furthermore, the system performed head studies only. This was, in part, due to limitations in the capability of the instrument to scan quickly and limitations in the densities of material the system could process. Since the original scanner took about 5 minutes to perform a scan, any motion was likely to create severe artifacts. The scanner was equipped with a water bag that fit around the patient's head to avoid reconstruction problems caused by the sudden change in density from air to bone and to provide a continuous water calibration during the scan.

The EMI scanner (Fig. 3.23) collected 160 measurements along a line by moving the coupled x-ray tube and detectors. The x-ray beam passed through the head and was detected at each of 160 points, representing a single

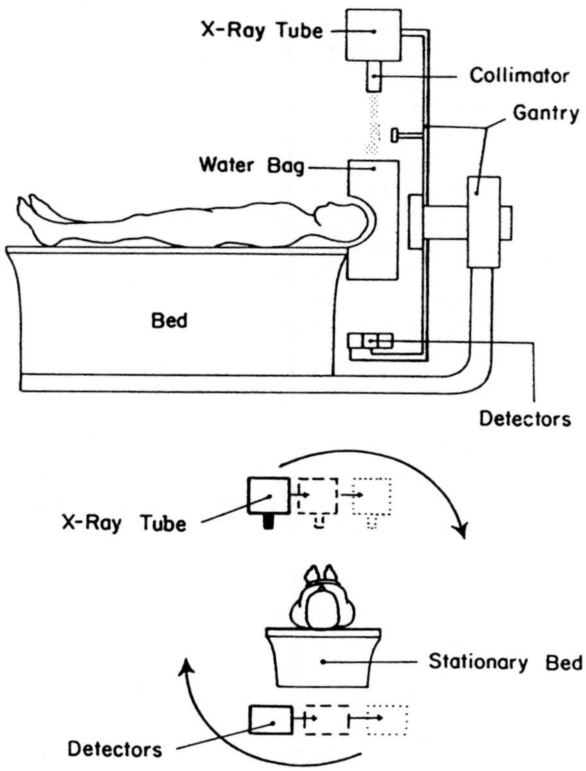

Figure 3.22. The interaction of x-rays as they pass through the body can be described by the linear attenuation equation relating the intensity of the incoming x-rays to the resulting x-ray intensity.

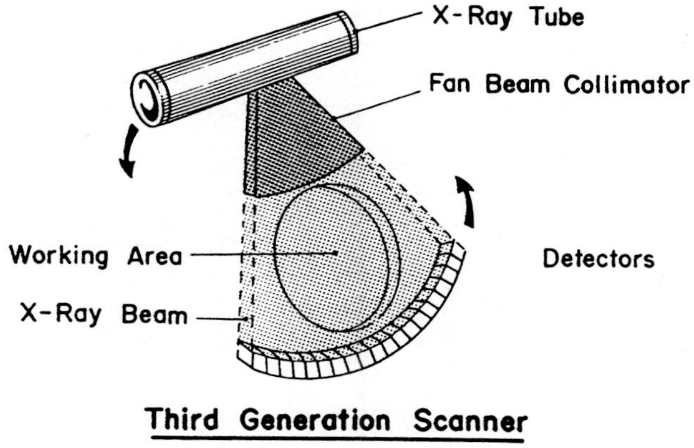

Figure 3.23. The early CT scanners were designed to be head-only units in which the patient's head was surrounded by a water bag in the gantry. The scans typically took about 5 minutes per slice pair, producing 180 attenuation profiles through the head. (Reproduced by permission from Sandler MP, Patton JA, Shaff MI, Powers TA, Partain CL. Correlative imaging: nuclear medicine, magnetic resonance, computed tomography, ultrasound. Baltimore: Williams and Wilkins, 1989.)

projection. Measurements were stored for use during reconstruction, and the detectors were calibrated at the end of each line. The gantry rotated 1°, and the linear collection was repeated. This motion continued until 180 projections were collected. The scan time required for this was about 5 minutes, with reconstruction requiring another 4 or 5 minutes. The resulting images were displayed in an 80×80 matrix. In a typical imaging session, 10 or more slices were collected, so the imaging time could be 25 minutes or more.

Improvements quickly led to the second-generation scanner. The primary objective was to speed the collection process so that fewer patient-motion artifacts would arise and the system could be used more efficiently. The approach to improving speed was to increase the number of detectors used to collect the information for each slice. With a larger number of detectors, less linear motion was required to collect the same amount of information as the original scanner. The x-ray beam collimation was changed so that the beam became fan-shaped in the transverse dimension and very thin axially (3–13 mm, determined by collimation). This configuration used much more of the available photons from the x-ray tube and permitted higher scan speeds due to increased data acquisition rates from a larger number of detectors. Since the rotational steps were bigger, the system was able to complete a scan in 10–90 seconds. The water bag was eliminated by using a varying-thickness absorber to compensate for the changes in thickness of the head.

Third-generation scanners (Fig. 3.24), currently available commercially, offer further refinements to the system design, once again providing reduced scan times. These instruments are capable of collecting data in less than 1–10 seconds. In this design, the x-ray beam is collimated to a fan subtending an arc of as much as 50° that covers the entire active transverse scanning region. A sufficient number of detectors are mounted on the opposite side from the x-ray tube so that all the measurements are collected at once. Designs vary, but as many as 750 detectors may be used. The entire apparatus can rotate more than 360° during the scan operation with no linear motion at all. Many medium- and high-performance systems employ this design. A disadvantage is that calibration of the detectors cannot be performed during the scan as in other designs, so the reconstruction algorithm must assume that the detectors remain balanced. Additionally, third-generation scanners have had to incorporate elaborate cable-handling mechanisms into the designs because both the x-ray tube and the detectors are on the moving gantry.

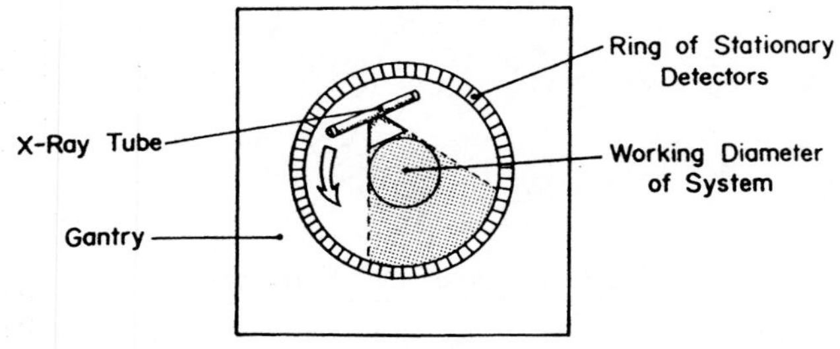

Figure 3.24. Third-generation scanners use fan-beam geometry that enables them to collect a whole profile in one position of the tube-detector assembly. (Reproduced by permission from Sandler MP, Patton JA, Shaff MI, Powers TA, Partain CL. Correlative imaging: nuclear medicine, magnetic resonance, computed tomography, ultrasound. Baltimore: Williams and Wilkins, 1989.)

A variation of the third-generation scanner approaches the limitations to gantry motion by using slip-ring technology instead of cable mechanisms to manage the electrical signals. Similar to x-ray tubes needing application of very high voltages to function, each detector must receive power and control signals and must supply the detector signals. Slip-ring technology permits these signals to be transmitted to the moving gantry through specialized contactors riding on continuous-ring conductors. Some variations use optical coupling of signals in place of direct contact for the detector and control signals. This design permits the gantry to rotate continuously in one direction without the need to scan in the opposite direction for the purpose of unwrapping the cables. The advantages of this approach are that the scanner, with high speed detectors and associated electronics, as well as high heat-capacity x-ray tubes, can perform single slice acquisitions in less than 1 second because the gantry is already rotating and is simply boosted to scan speed as needed. Multiple images can be acquired rapidly, so breath-hold imaging is very practical for most patients.

Fourth-generation scanners do not provide any increase in speed over the third-generation designs but can be calibrated during the scan. In these systems, the detectors surround the entire imaging region (Fig. 3.25). Only the x-ray tube moves in an arc around the patient, so there are fewer mechanical constraints with this system. Disadvantages include the cost of thousands of detectors, and the increased complexity of the data acquisition system. Additionally, the x-ray tube must move within the arc of detectors, causing increased focal spot magnification and increased patient exposures. Some machines have detector rings that nutate or wobble out of the way as the x-ray tube passes, reducing the exposure and magnification effects. Cable handling problems exist with fourth generation scanners, since the x-ray tube and its controls move with respect to the stationary detectors. However, manufacturers of fourth-generation machines have incorporated slip-ring systems into their most expensive machines, permitting continuous rotation high-speed scans.

Third- and fourth-generation scanners using slip-ring technology can employ a helical scanning mode. Because the slip-rings permit continuous rotations, data can be collected as the patient bed moves continuously into the gantry of the scanner. This motion produces profiles that are not collected from 360° around a single slice. The resulting helical data set must be reformatted and interpolated prior to reconstruction to produce approximations of contiguous transverse planes. The advantage to helical scanning is that pauses in data collection for bed indexing are not required, enabling the system to scan entire sections of the body in seconds, a capability that is significant in trauma applications. Also, because of the interpolation and reformatting, there is great flexibility in how the images are reconstructed. Most of the limitations to helical scanning are related to heat capacity of the x-ray tube and practical limits to data storage and reconstruction times.

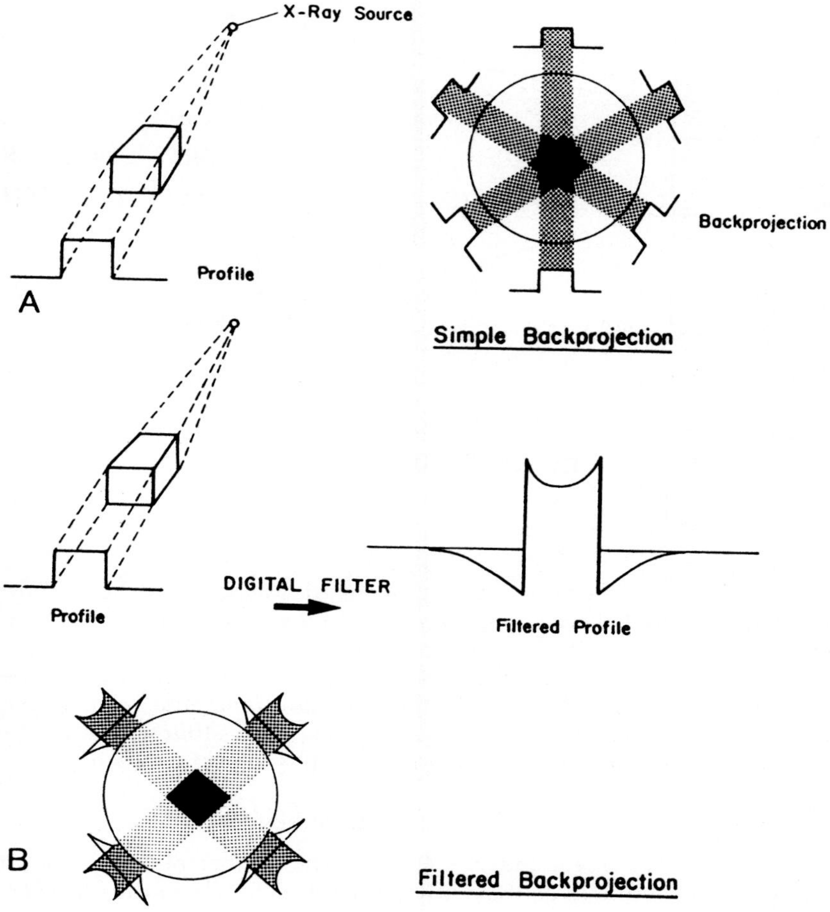

Figure 3.25. Fourth-generation scanners use a fixed set of detectors surrounding the patient and a moving x-ray tube. (Reproduced by permission from Sandler MP, Patton JA, Shaff MI, Powers TA, Partain CL. Correlative imaging: nuclear medicine, magnetic resonance, computed tomography, ultrasound. Baltimore: Williams and Wilkins, 1989.)

Another commercially available scanner uses a magnetically controlled beam of electrons that sweeps 210° around a shaped tungsten ring, producing x-rays transversely across the opening of the ring. The resulting fan-beam of x-rays strikes the detectors the same way as with the third-generation mechanical systems. The device is capable of 50-msec acquisitions and is used for collecting images of the heart in motion, as well as for conventional imaging. This type of machine has also been successful in emergency room installations because of its ability to scan almost any patient with no motion artifacts. However, the installation costs of this instrument are significantly higher than for more conventional mechanical designs.

IMAGE RECONSTRUCTION

Scanning the x-ray beam across the acquisition area produces a series of one-dimensional profiles that represent the attenuation of the beam as it passes through the body. Each profile is composed of the contributions from one detector moved in a line (first-generation system) or from the contributions of a number of detectors (second-, third-, and fourth-generation systems). These profiles together provide the raw data set that will be processed into an image.

There are several ways that the profiles can be processed to yield clinically useful images (29, 30). Techniques using the Fourier transformation have been applied commercially, as have methods employing iterative reconstruction, in which successively better approximations to the actual image are produced by the reconstruction algorithms. However, virtually all current commercial machines use filtered backprojection because it is simple and effective, can be easily implemented in hardware, and permits fast reconstruction times.

In backprojection, the profiles that have been collected at many positions around the body are assumed to have individually come from somewhere in the active area of the image field and represent the integrated attenuation of the x-ray beam measured by each detector. However, exactly where these attenuations occurred cannot be described from the single projection. During the reconstruction process in the computer's memory, the profile is "spread" or "projected back" across this area from where it is assumed to have originated. Each profile is processed in this way, and the overlapping of each of the spread profiles is algebraically summed. The resulting image is a blurred representation of the actual attenuation coefficients in the body. This blur renders the simple backprojection method relatively useless because of the lack of detail in the images (Fig. 3.26**A**).

However, backprojection (Fig. 3.26**B**) can be made to function very well by the addition of a processing step that

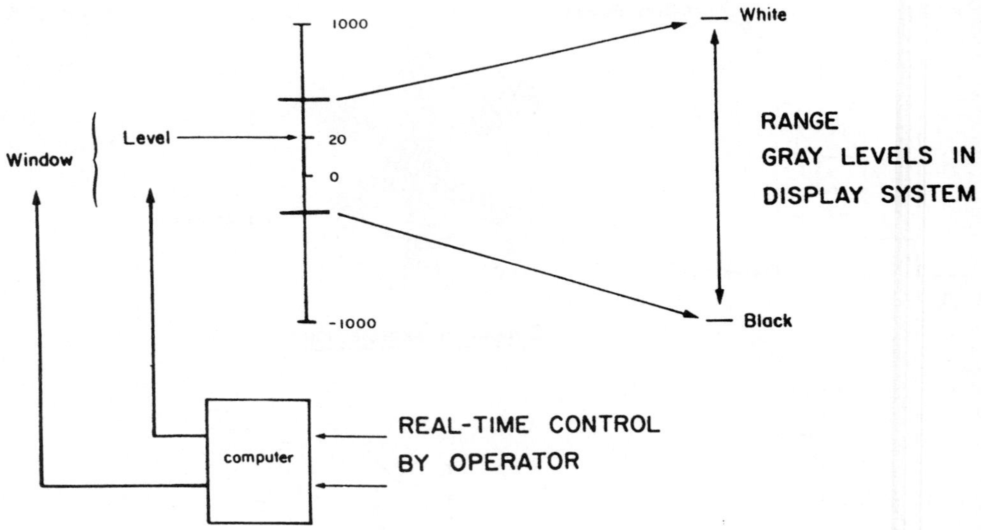

Figure 3.26. A. Simple backprojection projects profiles back across the region from where they are assumed to have originated, summing all profiles to make an image. A large star artifact exists around the edge and the image is so blurred as to be unusable. **B.** In filtered backprojection, the profiles are filtered before the backprojection process, resulting in positive and negative components that cancel each other, yielding excellent reconstructions of the image. (Reproduced by permission from Sandler MP, Patton JA, Shaff MI, Powers TA, Partain CL. Correlative imaging: nuclear medicine, magnetic resonance, computed tomography, ultrasound. Baltimore: Williams and Wilkins, 1989.)

results in a modification to each profile. Each profile is "filtered" in the computer's memory before backprojecting it, resulting in an alteration of the profile information so that it contains both positive and negative components. The filter function is one-dimensional, like the profiles, and is applied to the entire profile in a mathematical process called convolution. During backprojection, the common points are summed into the image algebraically. Since the modified profiles contain both positive and negative components, some contributions cancel out others, resulting in an image with much better resolution and far fewer blurring artifacts than an image produced by simple backprojection. Furthermore, the physician can select from several different filter functions or kernels, which enhance resolution at the expense of noise, or display smoother, more noise-free images at the expense of resolution.

The filtered backprojection method lends itself to implementation in special-purpose hardware in the reconstruction computer. Each profile can be filtered when it is available and backprojected, even while the system is collecting other profiles. Thus, it is possible to have a CT system that exhibits nearly instantaneous reconstruction of images. This is in contrast to Fourier reconstruction, which can only be partially completed until all profiles are collected, or iterative methods, which must work with a set of profiles.

IMAGE QUALITY

The ability of the physician to visualize diagnostically important structures in an image is, in part, a function of the quality of the images produced by a CT scanner. Those factors that directly influence image quality are spatial resolution, inherent noise, energy of the beam, quantum mottle present, contrast differential between materials, and the slice sensitivity profile (31–33).

Design parameters of the system that can generally be controlled by the manufacturer are density resolution, spatial resolution, and the slice sensitivity profile. These parameters describe how well a scanner is able to image tissues with nearly identical attenuation coefficients, how well the scanner can image small structures or sudden density transitions in the body, and how well the system can maintain the uniformity of a tissue that lies within the section. Noise in the form of quantum mottle and contrast differential between materials is more a function of the operation of the instrument and the object being scanned.

IMAGE DISPLAY

The image that results from the reconstruction is not an actual map of the attenuation coefficients of the body (23, 34). The attenuation coefficients are converted to "CT numbers" or "Hounsfield units." CT numbers are the result of comparing the attenuation of the x-ray beam by living tissue to the attenuation of the beam by water. The calibration of the system usually specifies a CT number of 0 for water. The most dense material, such as dense bone, is assigned a value of +3000, while air is assigned a value of −1000. Such a range, however, does not mean that the CT system can distinguish between 4000 different densities. The capability to distinguish between different densities, called the accuracy of the system, is a function of the system design. Increasing the range of the CT numbers by using a different constant does not improve the accuracy, which is usually in the range of 0.2%. The original EMI scanner, by comparison, had a CT number range of −500 to +500, with an accuracy of about 0.5%.

With a wide range of possible CT numbers for each pixel in the CT image, those levels to be presented on the video screen by the display must be selected from the range of available gray levels in the image. This is due to limitations in the design of video displays, which can present no more than about 60 levels of gray, as well as the inability of the human eye to distinguish more than 40–60 shades at once. If the information in the image has a range from −1000 to +3000 CT numbers, and the CT numbers each could be presented as a gray level in the image, 4000 individual gray levels would need to be displayed. Much of the subtle detail would be lost trying to present such a range of values on a monitor. The problem's solution is to use window and level controls to adjust the mapping of the CT numbers to the display, providing optimum contrast for the tissues of interest.

The window and level controls permit the operator of the scanner to select a narrower range of CT numbers to display on the screen. A level in the entire range of values in an image is selected around a window or range of larger and smaller values. Only those values that fall within the window are presented on the screen. Values that fall outside the window are mapped to either white or black. White usually represents all values above the maximum value in the window, while black represents all values below the minimum in the window. If the window is set narrow enough, individual CT numbers are presented as single gray levels in the image. However, one must keep in mind the accuracy of the machine and realize that differentiations seen between adjacent gray levels on the screen may not provide additional information.

Images are displayed in different formats that are usually related to the cost of the machine. High-performance CT scanners produce images in a matrix that is 512×512 or 1024×1024. Head scanners and lower-performance (less expensive) units may provide a 320×320 or 256×256 image matrix. Likewise, the thin slice capabilities of the system are related to the cost. High-performance systems can produce images with slices as thin as 1mm, while a less expensive machine might be limited to 3 or 4 mm. Thicker slices can be specified by the operator during a study.

PATIENT RADIATION DOSE

The dose a patient receives from a CT scanner is dependent on the design parameters of the instrument and can vary from machine to machine. Dose may also vary from image set to image set if the radiologist specifies different types of image acquisitions. Patient dose may vary from a few mGy to 70 mGy or more at the skin, as determined in measurement studies. Differences are due to the machine type, single or multiple contiguous slices, the presence of contrast media, and whether high accuracy acquisitions are performed (28, 32, 35, 36). When comparing the dose from CT to that of conventional screen-film radiography, one must appreciate the fact that the dose distribution is quite different due to the tomographic nature of the scan. In general, a patient receives considerably more integrated dose from CT studies than from a conventional x-ray study of the same part of the body.

SUMMARY

We described the basic operation and physics of three of the computerized electronic imaging modalities that are available in most hospitals. In each case, the clinical usefulness of the instrument was brought about by the availability of inexpensive, powerful computers and their associated software. In the future, significant benefits will be realized in resolution, ease of use, speed, and costs for these systems, as computer and electronic technologies continue to evolve. More and more functions will be made possible by computer software working with high-speed hardware to form highly versatile integrated imaging systems.

REFERENCES

1. NMR, a perspective on imaging. Milwaukee: General Electric Company, 1982.
2. Bottomley PA. The basis of imaging and chemical analysis by NMR. In: Partain CL, ed. Nuclear magnetic resonance and correlative imaging modalities. New York: Society of Nuclear Medicine, 1984:37–44.
3. Crooks LE, Kaufman L. Basic physical principles. In: Margulis AR, Higgins CB, Kaufman L, Crooks LE, eds. Clinical magnetic resonance imaging. San Francisco: Radiology Research and Education Foundation, 1983:13–24.
4. Bottomley PA, Foster TH, Argersinger RE, Pfeifer LM. A review of normal tissue hydrogen NMR relaxation times and relaxation mechanisms from 1–100 MHz: dependence on tissue type, NMR frequency, temperature, species, excision, and age. Med Phys 1984;11:425.
5. Bottomley PA, Hardy CJ, Argersinger RE, Allen-Moore G. A review of 1H nuclear magnetic resonance relaxation in pathology: are T_1 and T_2 diagnostic? Med Phys 1987;14:25.
6. Oldendorf W. Magnetic systems: resistive, superconducting and permanent. In: Partain CL, ed. Nuclear magnetic resonance and correlative imaging modalities. New York: Society of Nuclear Medicine, 1984:45–54.
7. Kaufman L, Crooks LE. Instrumentation. In: Margulis AR, Higgins CB, Kaufman L, Crooks LE, eds. Clinical magnetic resonance imaging. San Francisco: Radiology Research and Education Foundation, 1983:31–39.
8. Schenck JF, Hart HR, Foster TH, et al. Improved MR imaging of the orbit at 1.5 *T* with surface coils. AJR 1985;144:1033–1036.
9. Fleischer AC, James AE Jr. Real-time sonography. East Norwalk, CT: Appleton-Century-Crofts, 1984.
10. Sanders RC, James AE Jr. The principles and practices of ultrasonography in obstetrics and gynecology. 3rd ed. Norwalk, CT: Appleton-Century-Crofts, 1985.
11. Hykes D, Henrick WR, Starchman DE. Ultrasound physics and instrumentation. New York: Churchill Livingstone, 1985.
12. Fullerton GD, Zagzebski JA, eds. Medical physics of CT and ultrasound: tissue imaging and characterization. New York: American Association of Physicists in Medicine, 1980.
13. Merritt CRB. Imaging blood flow with Doppler. Diagnostic Imaging 1986;(Nov):146–159.
14. Thieme GA, Price RR, James AE Jr. Ultrasound instrumentation and its practical applications. In: Sanders RC, James AE, eds. The principles and practice of ultrasonography in obstetrics and gynecology. Chapter 3. Norwalk, CT: Appleton-Century-Crofts, 1985.
15. Taylor KJW. Gating to the depths with duplex Doppler ultrasound. Diagnostic Imaging 1987;(Oct):106–116.
16. Baker J, Marich K, Bluth R, et al. Standardized imaging and Doppler criteria for cerebrovascular diagnosis using duplex sonography. J Ultrasound Med 1986;5:159.
17. Powis L. Angiodynography: a new real-time look at the vascular system. Applied Radiology 1986;15:55–59.
18. Evans DH, McDiken WN, Skidmore R, Woodcork JP. Doppler ultrasound: physics instrumentation and clinical applications. New York: John Wiley & Sons, 1989.
19. Taylor KJ, Holland S. Doppler ultrasound. Part 1: Basic principles, instrumentation and pitfalls. Radiology 1990;174:297–307.
20. Namekawa K, Kasai C, Tsukamoto M, Koyano A. Real-time blood flow imaging system utilizing auto-correlation techniques. In: Ler-

ski RA, Mosley P, eds. Ultrasound 1982. New York: Pergamon, 1982.
21. Nowicki A, Reid JM. An infinite gate pulse Doppler. Ultrasound Med Biol 1981;1:41–50.
22. Mackay RS. Medical images and displays. New York: John Wiley & Sons, 1984:46.
23. Hounsfield GN. Computerized transverse axial scanning (tomography). Part 1. Description of system. Br J Radiol 1973;46:1016–1022.
24. Walmsley B. Computed tomography—equipment. In: Kreel L, Steiner RE, eds. Medical imaging. Chicago: Year Book, 1979:15–22.
25. Curry TS III, Dowdey JE, Murry RC Jr, eds. Computed tomography. In: Christensen's introduction to the physics of diagnostic radiology. Philadelphia: Lea & Febiger, 1984.
26. Coulam CM, Erickson JJ. Equipment considerations in computed tomography. In: Coulam CM, Erickson JJ, Rollo FD, James AE Jr, eds. The physical basis of medical imaging. East Norwalk, CT: Appleton-Century-Crofts, 1981.
27. Winter J, King W III. Basic principles of computed tomography. In: Greenberg M. Essentials of body computed tomography. Philadelphia: W.B. Saunders, 1983.
28. McCullough EC, Payne JT. Patient dosage in computed tomography. Radiology 1978;129:457–463.
29. Brooks RA, Di Chiro G. Theory of image reconstruction in computed tomography. Radiology 1975;117:561–572.
30. Coulam CM, Erickson JJ. Image considerations in computed tomography. In: Coulam CM, Erickson JJ, Rollo FD, James, AE Jr, eds. The physical basis of medical imaging. East Norwalk, CT: Appleton-Century-Crofts, 1981.
31. Pullan BR. Computed tomography limits and resolution. In: Kreel L, Steiner RE, eds. Medical imaging. Chicago: Year Book, 1979:10–14.
32. Allemand R. Basic technological aspects and optimization problems in x-ray computed tomography (CT). In: Guzzard R, ed. Physics and engineering of medical imaging. Hingham, MA: Martinus Nijhoff, 1987:207–217.
33. Barrett HH, Swindell W. Computed tomography. In: Radiological imaging: the theory of imaging formation, detection, and processing. Vol. 2. New York: Academic Press, 1981.
34. Miraldi F. Imaging principles in computed tomography. In: Haaga JR, Alfidi RJ, eds. Computed tomography of the whole body. Vol. 1. St. Louis: C.V. Mosby, 1983.
35. Hobday P, Parker RP. Radiation exposure to the patient in computerized tomography. Br J Radiol 1978;51:925–926.
36. Bushberg JT, Seibert JA, Leidholdt EM Jr, Boone JM. The essential physics of medical imaging. Baltimore: Williams and Wilkins, 1994.

4 Scintillation Detector

BERNARD E. OPPENHEIM, ROBERT N. BECK, and ROBERT M. WITT

Detector systems used in nuclear medicine serve to intercept, measure the energy of, and count the γ-ray and x-ray photons that are emitted from a volume, the boundaries of which are defined by a collimator or well. They provide information about the concentration of a radionuclide within the volume, since the rate of photon emission is proportional to this concentration.

Some photons pass directly to the detector from their point of origin and are referred to as *primary photons*. Others reaching the detector have undergone Compton scattering, and are referred to as *predetector scattered photons*. Still others are *background photons*, and bear no relationship to the radioactivity being measured. As a rule, primary photons are the only reliable indicators of radionuclide concentration; it is, therefore, desirable to distinguish them from the other photons. This is done based on the photon energy.

Photons emitted during radioactive decay have discrete energies characteristic of the radionuclide from which they originate. The primary photons have carried all of this energy to the detector. The predetector scattered photons have lost a part of this energy in accordance with the angle of scatter: the greater this angle, the greater the energy loss. The background photons, which are usually due to cosmic rays or radioactive contaminants in the detector materials or surroundings, may have any energy, depending on their origin.

The detector converts the photon energy into an electric signal, which is then amplified. Every step in the detection process is essentially *linear* (that is, the output is a fixed fraction or multiple of the input), but is also subject to some random variation. Therefore, the amplitude of the electric signal produced by the detector is approximately proportional to the energy of the photon. From the amplitude one can thus infer, with reasonable accuracy, whether or not the photon was a primary photon. Incorrect inferences will be made, however, whenever a small-angle scattered photon (which has lost little energy) or a background photon with energy very near that of the primary photon is detected, because the amplitude of the resulting electric signal will correspond to that of a primary photon. Also, the energy of the primary photon is not always completely converted by the detector. Incomplete conversion results in a low-amplitude electric pulse, causing the primary photon to be misclassified as a scatter photon. These situations are discussed later under Pulse Height Spectrum.

The efficiency of a detector is an important characteristic. This is a measure of the fraction of the emitted photons that it detects. A large number of primary photons must be detected to measure radionuclide concentration accurately, but this is practical only if it can be accomplished within a reasonably short time interval. The efficiency increases as the size, thickness, and density of a detector increase.

With rare exceptions, the scintillation detector equipped with a thallium-activated sodium iodide crystal (NaI(Tl)), is the instrument used for photon detection in nuclear medicine. It is moderately priced, easy to operate and maintain, reliable, and reasonably efficient. Semiconductor detectors (1) are capable of measuring photon energy more precisely, but because of high cost, inefficiency, and technical problems in operation and maintenance (e.g., the crystal must be cooled by liquid nitrogen), these detectors have found only limited application in nuclear medicine.

The scintillation detector has three basic components: the *scintillation crystal* that converts the energy of the γ-photon into visible light, the *photomultiplier tube* that converts the light into an electronic pulse, and the *processing unit* that amplifies the pulse and, by means of *pulse height analysis*, selects it for recording or rejects it. The operation of each component will be described.

The purpose of the scintillation crystal is to stop the γ-photon and convert its energy into a brief burst (scintillation) of visible light. A high-energy photon entering the crystal may pass through without interacting (and remain undetected), or may interact with and transfer energy to one of the electrons within the crystal, either by a photoelectric or a Compton interaction (a third type of interaction, pair-production, may occur at very high photon energies, but is rarely encountered in nuclear medicine). A complete description of what happens next is far beyond the limits of this discussion (see Curran (2) and Birks (3)), and only a simplified summary can be given (Fig. 4.1). The energized electron is ejected from the region that it had occupied and travels a short distance through the crystal, exciting (transferring energy to) other electrons along the way. These "excited" electrons can lose their excess energy in two ways: either by transferring it to other electrons or through the release of photons of visible light. In a pure sodium iodide crystal at room temperature, the first process is far more likely than the second, so that nearly all energy transferred to the crystal appears as increased molecular activity or heat. If a small amount of thallium is present, however, some of the excited electrons migrate to the regions of the thallium atoms, where they are trapped, and lose their excess energy through the release of a light photon having an energy of about 3 eV. These light photons appear within a fraction of a microsecond after the initial interaction of the high-energy photon, and form the scintillation. About 20–30 of the 3-eV light photons are produced per thousand electron volts of energy transferred to the crystal (4). They pass freely through the sodium iodide

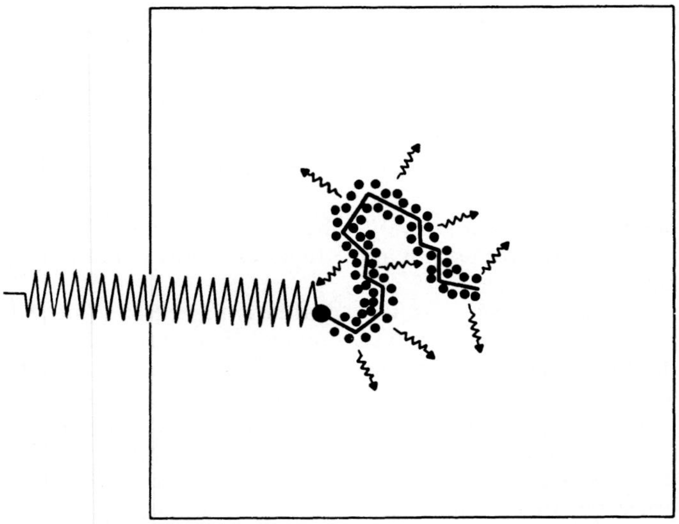

Figure 4.1. Energy transfers within scintillation crystal. The entering photon (*heavy jagged line*) transfers energy to an electron (*large dot*) within the crystal, which leaves its orbit and moves through the crystal (*irregular line*), exciting other electrons (*small dots*) along its path. These electrons usually lose their excess energy in the form of crystal lattice vibrations or heat (not illustrated), but sometimes through the release of 3 eV light photons (*small jagged arrows*). These light photons comprise the scintillation. The number of light photons, on the average, is proportional to the energy absorbed in the crystal.

This illustration represents a photoelectric interaction, in which the entering photon gives up all of its energy to a bound electron, part of the energy being used to eject the electron from its orbit (filling of the resulting vacancy may give rise to an x-ray or Auger electron, which are not shown), and the remainder transferred to the electron as kinetic energy. Alternatively, a Compton interaction may occur, in which the entering photon gives up only part of its energy to an electron, carrying away the remainder as a Compton-scattered photon, which may or may not undergo further interactions in the crystal.

crystal, which is quite transparent to light photons of this energy.

The mean number of light photons contained in the scintillation is proportional to the energy that the original photon transfers to the crystal. It is desirable that as many of these light photons as possible enter the photomultiplier tube. Therefore, the surface of the crystal facing the tube is highly polished and optically coupled to the tube by means of a transparent cement with an appropriate index of refraction, so that light photons reaching this surface usually pass into the tube. In contrast, the other surfaces of the crystal are rough-ground and are covered with a reflecting powder of aluminum oxide, so that light photons reaching these surfaces are reflected back into the crystal (Fig. 4.2). In an efficient detector, about 30% of the light photons will reach the photocathode of the photomultiplier tube (5).

The sodium iodide crystal is housed in a light-tight, watertight aluminum container (Fig. 4.2) that has three functions: (a) it excludes room light, which would obscure the light produced in the scintillation process; (b) it excludes moisture (since sodium iodide is highly hygroscopic, and is discolored by water, the transparency of the crystal is reduced when it is exposed to moisture); and (c) it serves to protect the crystal from physical damage. The surface of the crystal facing the photomultiplier tube is usually sealed by an optical window of glass or quartz (Fig. 4.2).

One point must be emphasized: The number of light photons formed in the scintillation represents only that portion of the original photon energy transferred to the crystal. Three situations are possible. First, the original photon may undergo a photoelectric interaction in the crystal, in which case the energy transfer is complete (unless iodine x-ray escape occurs—see "Pulse Height Spectrum," later) and the photon is totally absorbed in the crystal. Second, the original photon may undergo one or more Compton interactions, followed by a photoelectric interaction. In a Compton interaction, only part of the incident photon energy transfers to the crystal—the remainder appears as a Compton-scattered photon (not to be confused with the predetector scattered photons that have undergone Compton scattering *before* reaching the detector). As long as the series of Compton interactions culminates in a photoelectric interaction, however, the energy transfer is complete within the crystal, and the original photon is totally absorbed. Third, the original photon may undergo one or more Compton interactions, and the final Compton-scattered photon may escape from the crystal. In this instance, the energy transfer is incomplete, and the original photon is only partially absorbed within the crystal, so that the detector assigns to it a lower energy than it actually possessed. The percentage of partially absorbed photons are kept low by using crystals of sufficient size to minimize the escape of the Compton-scattered photons.

PHOTOMULTIPLIER TUBE

Within the photomultiplier tube the light photons transfer their energy to electrons, which then undergo a series of multiplications, resulting in a large stream of electrons at the output of the tube (Fig. 4.3). The number of electrons in this stream is, on the average, proportional to the number of light photons and, in turn, to the energy of the original photon.

The photomultiplier tube is a vacuum tube containing a *photocathode* and a series of *dynodes*. As light photons enter the photomultiplier tube they immediately encounter the photocathode, a thin film on the inside face of the tube, usually consisting of an alloy of cesium and antimony, in which the outer orbital electrons are loosely bound. Some fraction of the light photons interacts with electrons in the photocathode, causing them to be ejected from their orbits as *photoelectrons*. The fraction of light photons producing photoelectrons varies randomly from scintillation to scintillation, but has an average value that is determined by the composition of the photocathode, ranging from 15% for some photocathodes to nearly 30% for others (6, 7). This value is the *quantum efficiency* of the photocathode.

Near the photocathode is the first dynode, a metal electrode at a potential of about +300 volts. Since the photocathode is at ground, or zero volts, the negatively charged photoelectrons accelerate toward the first dynode. The fraction of the photoelectrons that reach the first dynode depends mainly on tube construction. A typical value is 75% (8). As each photoelectron strikes the dynode it dis-

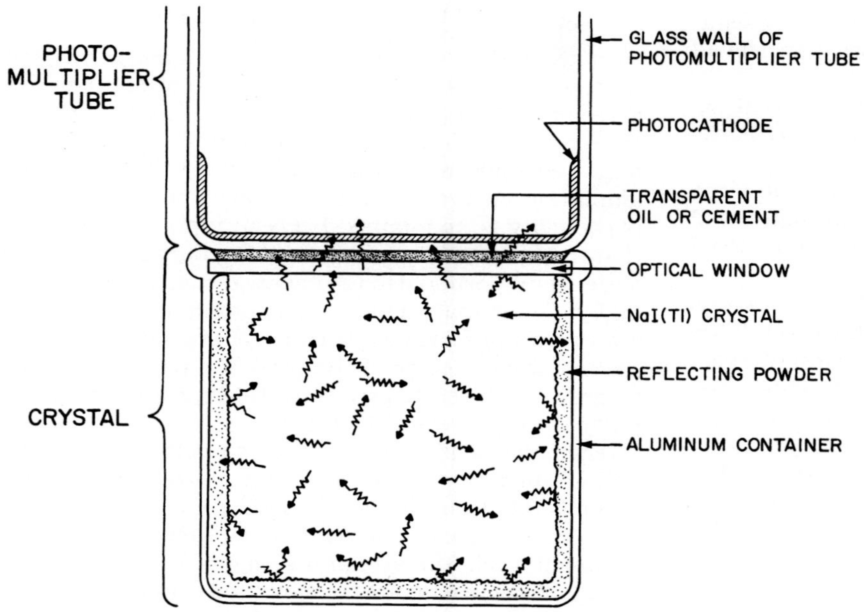

Figure 4.2. Fate of 3 eV light photons. These photons (represented by *short jagged arrows*) pass freely through the crystal. When they reach the highly polished surface of the crystal facing the photomultiplier tube, they tend to exit from the crystal, but when they reach any of the other surfaces (which are rough-ground and covered with reflecting powder) they tend to be reflected back into the crystal. About 30% of the light photons reach the photocathode of the photomultiplier tube.

The crystal is sealed in an aluminum container, and the surface facing the photomultiplier tube is sealed by an optical window. A transparent oil or cement is used to join the crystal and the tube.

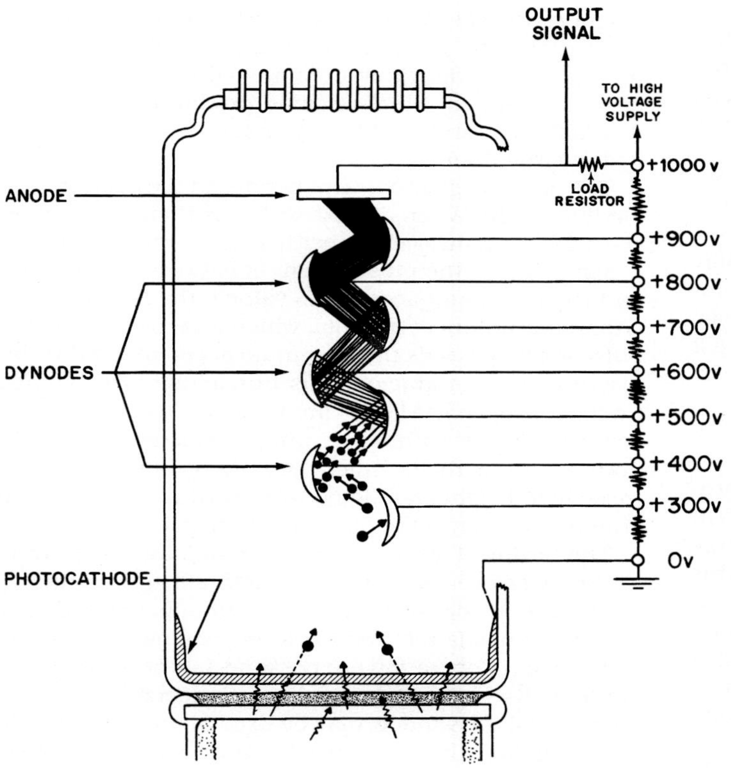

Figure 4.3. Operation of photomultiplier tube. This is a vacuum tube containing the photocathode, a series of dynodes, and the anode, each maintained at a progressively higher voltage. Some of the 3 eV light photons eject photoelectrons (*dots with arrows*) from the photocathode. These are attracted to the first dynode by the positive voltage difference and eject secondary electrons from it, which are attracted to the second dynode and eject more secondary electrons from it, and so on. About 10^6 or 10^7 electrons reach the anode for each photoelectron released from the photocathode. These electrons flow through a load resistor to produce a voltage pulse, which is the output signal.

The photocathode, dynodes, and anode are connected to the pins at the top of the tube, which are in turn connected to a string of voltage-dividing resistors. Direct connections to the resistor string have been drawn in for simplicity.

lodges several secondary electrons from the dynode surface, which is coated with a material similar to that of the photocathode. These secondary electrons are, in turn, accelerated toward the second dynode, which is about 100 volts more positive than the first dynode, producing additional secondary electrons. This process continues over a total of 6–14 dynode stages. At each stage, many secondary electrons, averaging about four (4), are released for each incident electron. This results in an overall *gain* ranging from 10^5–10^8 electrons produced per photoelectron, depending on the number of stages and the operating voltage. A value of 2×10^6 is typical.

If the high voltage increases by 1%, then at each stage the mean number of secondary electrons per incident electron also increases by about 1%, and the overall increase over 10 stages is about 10%. For this reason, the *high volt-*

age supply that operates the tube must be closely regulated so that the voltage does not vary by more than a small fraction of a percent.

It is instructive to examine each step in a typical example of the conversion of a 140 keV photon into an electric pulse, as shown in Table 4.1.

The electrons reaching the *anode*, the last dynode of the photomultiplier tube, are collected and flow through a load resistor to form a voltage pulse, which is the output signal for the photomultiplier tube (Fig. 4.3).

Although each of the totally absorbed 140 keV photons transfers an identical amount of energy to the crystal, the voltage pulse at the anode of the photomultiplier tube varies from one photon to another (see Fig. 4.6**B**). This is because each of the above processes is a random process whose output, for a given input, will vary purely by chance. In the example in Table 4.1, the energy of the 140 keV photon is represented by a different number of photons or electrons at each stage of the conversion process. This number is lowest at step 4 where, on average, 185 photoelectrons reach the first dynode. Since the conversion process is governed by Poisson statistics, the number of photoelectrons reaching the first dynode is actually 185 $\pm$13.6 (mean $\pm$1 standard deviation). Although this number is increased a millionfold in step 5, the relative variation about the mean remains about the same. As a result of this variation the *energy resolution* of the detector described by Table 4.1, as measured by its *full width at half-maximum* (see "Pulse Height Spectrum," later), is 17%.

ELECTRONIC PROCESSING UNIT

The functions of the electron processing unit are to amplify and shape the voltage pulse at the output of the photomultiplier tube, to determine (by pulse height analysis) whether the pulse represents an acceptable photon, and if it is acceptable, to make some record of it.

AMPLIFICATION AND PULSE-SHAPING

The voltage pulse has an amplitude or "height" that is proportional to the number of electrons leaving the photomultiplier tube, and hence is proportional to the energy that the original photon transfers to the crystal. Since this pulse amplitude is too small to be measured accurately, an *amplifier* is used to increase it. If a cable separates the photomultiplier tube from the electronic processing unit, a preamplifier connected to the photomultiplier output may be used to make the signal large enough to pass through the cable. Each stage of amplification should be linear, that is, the output should be proportional to the input as nearly as possible.

A *pulse-shaping circuit* is inserted before the main amplifier. The primary function of this circuit is to cut off pulse tails abruptly (soon after each pulse reaches its maximum) in order to avoid "pulse pileup" (9). This condition is due to long pulse tails, and may occur in the absence of such a circuit whenever photons are detected in rapid succession, because the pulse generated for each one may be superimposed on the tails of previous pulses. When this happens pulse height no longer reflects energy.

PULSE HEIGHT ANALYZER

As noted earlier, we need to distinguish the *primary* photons, which pass directly from their point of origin to the detector, from the photons that have undergone *predetector scatter* and from the *background* photons. The *pulse height analyzer* makes this distinction on the basis of pulse amplitude. At every step in the detection process, a proportionality is maintained between input and output, so that the height of the pulse reaching the pulse height analyzer is proportional to the energy transferred to the crystal by the original (high energy) photon. Even though it is not *exactly* proportional because of statistical factors operating at each stage of the detection process, the pulse height is sufficiently precise so that most of the primary photons are correctly identified.

The pulse height analyzer consists of two *discriminators* and an *autocoincidence circuit* (Fig. 4.4**A**). Each discriminator is an electronic device that produces a signal only when the voltage of the input signal exceeds some predetermined level. The size and shape of the output signal, when one is present, are constant and unrelated to the size of the input signal. The two discriminators operate in tandem. The *lower level discriminator* is set to the minimum height of an acceptable pulse, whereas the *upper level discriminator* is set to the maximum acceptable height. Signals from both discriminators are fed into the anticoincidence circuit, in which signals produced by the latter discriminator serve to block passage of signals produced by the former one.

The pulse height analyzer operates in the following fashion (Fig. 4.4**B**). When a pulse with less than the minimum acceptable height occurs, neither discriminator produces a signal. When the pulse height is between the minimum and the maximum acceptable values, the lower level discriminator produces a signal, which is recorded. When the pulse height exceeds the maximum acceptable value, both discriminators produce signals, but, in this case, the signal from the upper level discriminator blocks that from the lower level one within the anticoincidence circuit, and nothing is recorded. Thus, the only pulses recorded are those with heights falling between settings of the two discriminators (hence the term *pulse height analysis*).

The setting of the lower level discriminator is referred to as the lower level, baseline, threshold, sill, or E setting, and the *separation* between the lower and upper level discriminator settings is referred to as the window or δE setting. Two modes of operation are possible: (a) the lower and upper level discriminators may be set independently of each other, or (b) the window may be fixed at any desired value, and changing the lower level setting will automatically change the upper level setting so that the window is maintained at its fixed value. The latter mode is generally more convenient, because it facilitates accurate location of energy peaks.

RECORDING DEVICES

A variety of recording devices is available, each device serving a specialized function. For quantitative studies, pulses are counted by a *scaler* that does the actual counting and a *timer* that turns the scaler off after some preset time. A

Table 4.1.
Example of Conversion of 140-keV Photon into Electrical Pulse

Step	VProcess	Efficiency	No. of Photons or Electrons Resulting from Process
1	Conversion of 140-keV photon into 3-eV light photons [assume total absorption within the NaI(Tl) crystal]	About 30 photons/keV of energy transferred to the crystal	About 4200 light photons
2	Light photons leave NaI(Tl) crystal and reach photocathode	About 30%	About 1250 light photons
3	Light photons eject photoelectrons from photocathode	About 20%	About 250 photoelectrons
4	Photoelectrons reach first dynode	About 75%	About 185 photoelectrons
5	Electrons are multiplied in photomultiplier tube	About 2×10^6 electrons per electron reaching the first dynode	About 4×10^8 electrons reach anode

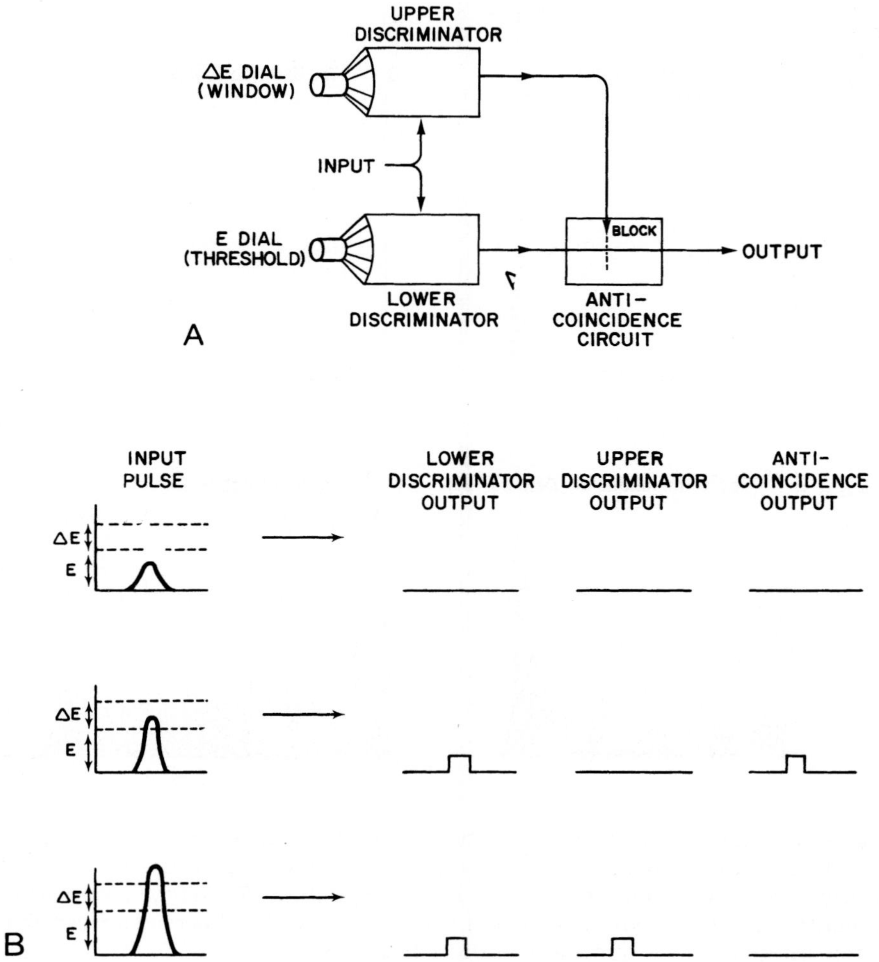

Figure 4.4. Pulse height analyzer. The values E and δE are set by the respective potentiometer dials. If the height of the input pulse is greater than E+δE, the upper discriminator also produces an output, which blocks that from the lower discriminator within the anticoincidence circuit. Therefore, an output pulse occurs only when the height of the input pulse is between E and E+δE. **A**: Block diagram. **B**: Anticoincidence output for various input pulses.

rate meter is used to indicate the count rate during a short time interval. The length of the interval can be varied by changing the *time constant* of the rate meter. When a long time constant is used, the meter reading is determined by a relatively large number of counts and tends to be steady, but responds sluggishly to a changing count rate. A *strip recorder* that plots count rate as a function of time can be used to obtain a permanent record of a changing count rate (e.g., a renogram). Finally, if the detector is designed to provide information on the spatial distribution of radioactivity (e.g., the scintillation camera), the detected events are recorded by appropriately placed marks on film or by incrementing appropriate locations in computer memory.

PULSE HEIGHT SPECTRUM

A scintillation detector may be used to generate a *pulse height spectrum*, which is a graph of the relative abundance

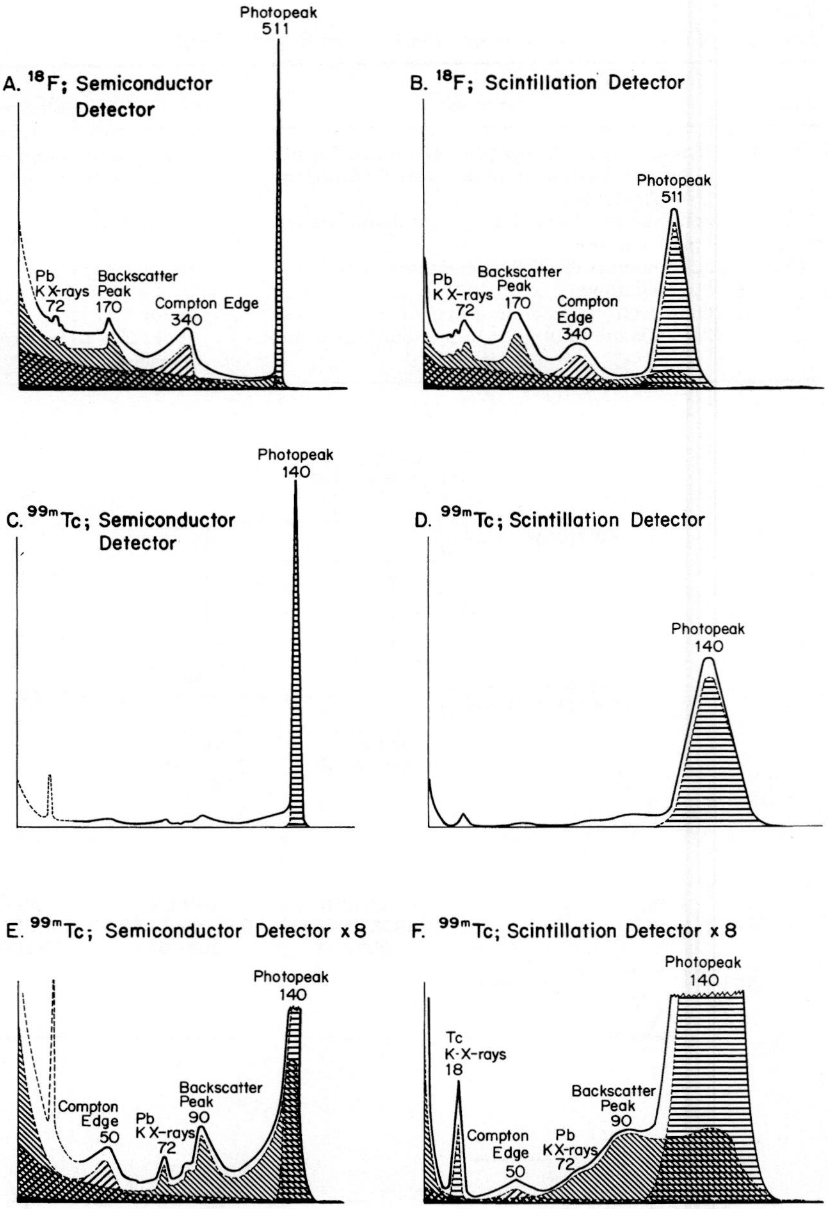

Figure 4.5. Pulse height spectra for ^{18}F and ^{99m}Tc, made with semiconductor detector and scintillation detector. In each instance, a point source and a 19-hole focused collimator were used, with the point source at the focal point of the collimator and surrounded by water density scattering material. The *upper solid line* is the observed spectrum; the *dashed lines* are hypothetical spectra for the different components of the observed spectrum: totally absorbed primary photons (*horizontal crosshatch*); partially absorbed primary photons (*heavy diagonal crosshatch*); predetector scattered photons (*light diagonal crosshatch*); and background photons (*solid line at bottom*). The lowest energy range for the semiconductor detector is also hypothetical and represented by a *dashed line*, because the detector was very inefficient in this range. The Compton edge occurs at the maximum energy that a partially absorbed primary photon transfers to the crystal in a single Compton interaction. The back-scatter peak occurs at the energy of a photon scattered 180°, the minimum energy of a predetector scattered photon after one scattering interaction. The lead K shell x-rays arise from photoelectric interactions in the lead collimator. **A** and **B**: ^{18}F. **C** and **D**: ^{99m}Tc. **E** and **F**: Magnification ×8 of C and D.

of pulses of all possible heights (energies) (Fig. 4.5). A narrow, fixed window is used. The lower level setting is advanced by small and equal increments from the lowest to the highest setting (after proper gain adjustment), and at each setting counts are collected for a fixed time interval.

Because this procedure is quite tedious and time-consuming, a *multichannel analyzer* is often used to generate pulse height spectra. In this device, the total range of pulse heights is divided into many small windows (channels) of equal width, each of them associated with its own counter. The incoming pulses are sorted according to height and routed to the appropriate channels, where they are counted; in this way, pulses of all possible heights can be counted simultaneously.

The photons interacting with the detector may be classified into four types: totally absorbed primary photons, partially absorbed primary photons, predetector scattered photons, and background photons. Each type produces its own pulse height spectrum, and the observed spectrum is a composite of these (Fig. 4.5).

The pulse height spectrum has one or more prominent peaks corresponding to the characteristic photon energies of the radionuclide under observation. These peaks are produced by the totally absorbed primary photons, and are called *photopeaks*, since total absorption involves a photoelectric interaction in the NaI(Tl) crystal (Fig. 4.5, *horizontal crosshatch*). The photopeaks are bell-shaped (approximately Gaussian) curves centered on pulse heights that correspond to the primary photon energies. If the detector had perfect energy resolution, generating a pulse *ex-*

actly proportional to the energy transferred to the crystal, totally absorbed photons of the same energy would give rise to pulses of the same height, so that each photopeak would be a narrow spike (Fig. 4.6**A**). It was noted earlier, however, that photons transferring identical amounts of energy to the crystal usually give rise to pulses of slightly different heights, because of random variation at each step of the detection process. This variation accounts for the broadening of the photopeaks (Fig. 4.6**B**).

The *energy resolution* of a detector is its ability to distinguish between photons of similar energies, and it depends on the shape of the photopeak: the broader the photopeak the poorer the energy resolution. The most commonly used measure of energy resolution is the *full width at half-maximum (FWHM)*, which is simply the number of thousands of electron volts corresponding to the width of a photopeak measured at half its height (under conditions of minimal predetector scattering and background), and is usually expressed as a percentage of the energy of the photopeak. (For a Gaussian curve the FWHM is 2.36 × standard deviation ÷ mean.) The smaller the FWHM, the better the energy resolution of the detector. The FWHM is energy dependent, its absolute value increasing and the percentage value decreasing with increasing energy of the photopeak; therefore, it is always necessary to know at what energy it was measured. If the energy is not noted, it is assumed to be the 662 keV peak of ^{137}Cs, which has been adopted as the standard reference energy. Eight percent is a typical value for the resolution of a sodium iodide crystal at this energy (10). Semiconductor detectors, however, often have an energy resolution below 1%, resulting in much narrower photopeaks (Figs. 4.5**A** and **C**).

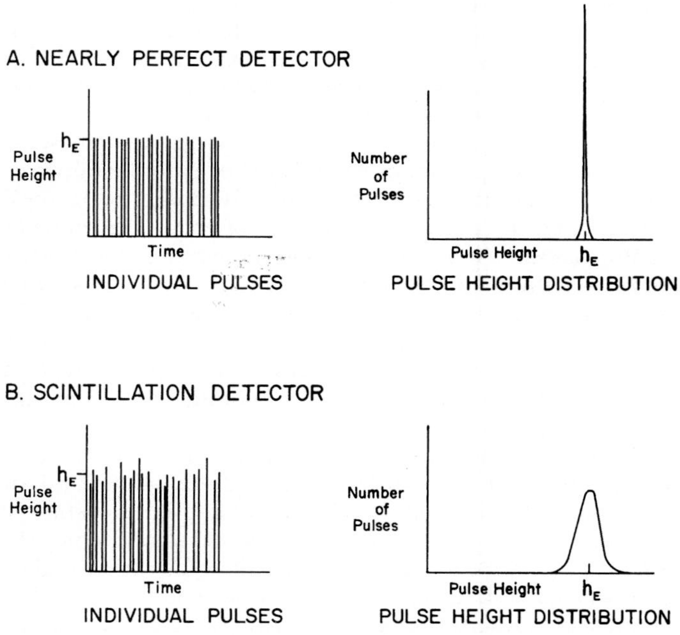

Figure 4.6. Pulse height distribution for totally absorbed monoenergetic photons of energy E. If the detector were nearly perfect, as in **A**, all of the totally absorbed photons would produce pulses of about the same height, and the distribution of these pulse heights would be represented by a narrow spike centered on the mean height h_E (the pulse height corresponding to energy E). In the scintillation detector, however, these photons produce pulses of varying heights, as shown in **B**, because of the random nature of the various steps in the detection process. The distribution of these pulse heights is a bell-shaped curve centered on the mean height h_E.

The partially absorbed primary photons are those that transfer only a portion of their energy to the crystal, the remainder usually escaping as Compton-scattered photons (Fig. 4.5, *heavy diagonal crosshatch*). The maximum energy that a primary photon of energy E can transfer to an electron in the crystal during a single Compton interaction is given by the expression E •= (E/(E + 256 keV)) (see ref. 11, Section 5.08). This maximum energy appears in the pulse height spectrum as the *Compton edge*. When a primary photon undergoes a Compton interaction in the crystal, and the resulting scattered photon escapes from the crystal, a pulse is produced falling at or below the Compton edge. When the scattered photon undergoes additional Compton interactions and then escapes from the crystal, a much less frequent occurrence, the resulting pulse usually falls between the Compton edge and the photopeak. Finally, the scattered photon may undergo a photoelectric interaction and be completely absorbed, in which case the entire energy of the primary photon will have been transferred to the crystal, and the corresponding pulse will be a part of the photopeak. The larger the crystal, the greater the fraction of totally absorbed primary photons.

Partial absorption may occur following a photoelectric interaction. Such interactions involve "bound" electrons, and part of the energy of the photon is used to overcome the binding energy of the electron. For photons with an energy greater than 33 keV, the most likely photoelectric interaction is with a K shell electron of iodine. When this electron is ejected, another one, usually from the L shell, fills the vacancy, and either a 28.5 keV x-ray (representing the difference in the binding energies of K and L shell electrons of iodine) or an Auger electron is produced. In the former case, if the 28.5 keV x-ray escapes from the crystal, the energy absorbed in the crystal is reduced by this amount. Partial absorption of this type gives rise to an "iodine escape peak" which is 28.5 keV below the total absorption peak.

Predetector scattering is always present (Fig. 4.5, *light diagonal crosshatch*) the amount depending on the size, shape, and density of the source; the structures surrounding the source; and the other structures separating it from the detector. The amount is minimal for a small source in air. The spectrum of the predetector scattered photons usually includes a *backscatter peak*, representing those photons that have been scattered through angles that approach 180°. It also may include K shell x-rays of lead produced by photoelectric interactions in the collimator.

Finally, some portion of the detected activity represents background radiation (Fig. 4.5, *solid line at bottom*). This includes all high-energy radiation that does not arise from the radioactivity introduced to carry out the study. Cosmic rays and radionuclides within building materials are a constant source of low-level radioactivity. Inadequately shielded radiation sources, contamination from spillage, and other patients and samples in the area result in a moderate and somewhat variable level of background activity. High background activity may be present if the patient under study has had a recent injection of a radionuclide.

The composite pulse height spectrum (Fig. 4.5, *solid lines*), which is the spectrum actually observed, is the sum of the separate spectra.

PRACTICAL CONSIDERATIONS

The pulse height analyzer is used to separate the primary photons from the predetector scattered photons and the background photons. This is accomplished by adjusting the settings on the analyzer so that the window brackets the photopeak. The window will include most of the primary photons, as well as some fraction of the predetector scattered and background photons. This fraction is very small with a semiconductor detector, since the photopeak can be bracketed by a very narrow window. It is much larger with a scintillation detector, however, since the window must be considerably wider because of the poorer energy resolution of the detector.

Predetector scattering is quite undesirable in radionuclide imaging procedures because it obscures the margins of structures and reduces image contrast so that small lesions are hard to identify. In well counting procedures, however, one accounts for predetector scattering by counting the standard (containing a known quantity of radionuclide) and the sample under identical geometric conditions (see Chapter 5). Predetector scattering can largely be accounted for in *in vivo* procedures, such as thyroid uptake studies, if the standard is placed in a phantom that simulates the anatomy of the body region being counted.

Background activity is much less of a problem. In radionuclide imaging the effect of background is to decrease image contrast, but seldom to an annoying extent, and it can usually be ignored. In counting procedures, one corrects for background activity by counting the patient (or some sample obtained from the patient) *before* the radionuclide is administered, and subtracting the value thus determined from subsequent patient or sample counts, and similarly counting an empty vial and subtracting the resultant value from the standard counts.

NEWER DEVELOPMENTS

In recent years there has been considerable improvement in sodium iodide crystal-photomultiplier tube combinations as a result of increased efficiency of the various steps described in Table 4.1 (12, 13). A more typical value for scintillation photon yield (*step 1*) is 50 photons/keV, and light collection efficiency (*step 2*) is now about 50%, but the quantum efficiency (*step 3*) remains at about 20% (13). There are a variety of new photomultiplier designs, no one of which is clearly superior to the others (12). Most of the improvement in these designs is in the cathode-to-first dynode region (*step 4*) and in the electron multiplier structure, principally the first dynode (*step 5*) (12). With these improvements we would expect new sodium iodide scintillation detectors to yield about 550–600 photoelectrons reaching the first dynode (*step 4*) for 140 keV photons, which corresponds to an energy resolution of about 10% FWHM in contrast to the 17% value for the example in Table 4.1. This is consistent with reported values (12). This improvement translates into improved intrinsic spatial resolution and predetector scatter rejection for scintillation cameras; the former because of less random variation in the signals entering the positioning circuitry, and the latter because narrower energy windows may be used. In the last 10 years, additional improvements in photomultiplier tubes (PMT) led to the development of a variety of shapes and sizes especially for application in positron emission tomography (PET) scanners (14). The introduction of position-sensitive PMT led to new methods to increase the spatial resolution of the detector arrays in PET systems (14) and to the development of a novel SPECT system for dynamic studies (15).

Although sodium iodide remains the scintillator of choice for most probe counters and the Anger camera, the designers of ring detectors for PET are turning to two other scintillators, bismuth germanate (BGO) and cesium fluoride (CsF). These scintillators have a much lower photon yield (*step 1* in Table 4.1) than sodium iodide, which leads to very poor energy resolution. Energy resolution is not as critical for PET ring detectors as it is for scintillation cameras, however, since it has little effect on spatial resolution, which is determined primarily by the size of the crystals in the ring (16). Moreover, PET ring detectors with sodium iodide crystals are forced to use wide energy windows since a large fraction of 511 keV photons interacting in a crystal are only partially absorbed as a result of the small size of the crystal, and most of these partially absorbed photons must still be accepted to permit reasonably efficient coincidence detection (see Chapter 10). Crystals made of BGO, because of its higher density and effective atomic number, will absorb a much higher fraction of the energy of 511 keV photons, on the average, than those of equal size made of sodium iodide. This allows the use of narrower energy windows, resulting in better rejection of predetector scatter while still maintaining efficient coincidence detection (15, 17). Spatial resolution improves with BGO, since smaller crystals can be used with acceptable coincidence detection efficiency (15, 17). An additional advantage of BGO is that it is not hygroscopic (15).

Cesium fluoride has a low detection efficiency for 511 keV photons very similar to that of sodium iodide, and an even lower photon yield than BGO, but has a much shorter scintillation decay time than the other two scintillators (15, 18). This allows the PET detector to handle much higher count rates without incurring an unacceptably high percentage of random coincidences (which are due to simultaneous detection of photons from two different annihilations and which degrade the images) (19, 20). The most promising aspect of CsF crystals, however, is the potential for time-of-flight detection. In normal coincidence detection, one determines the path of a pair of 511 keV photons but the site of origin of these photons along this path is unknown. In time-of-flight detection, the site of origin is inferred from the time interval between detection of each photon of the annihilation pair. Positron emission tomography systems utilizing CsF crystals are capable of measuring intervals between detection as short as 500 psec, which allows them to localize the site of origin of an annihilation to within about 7.5 cm (18). This positional information can produce as much as a fourfold improvement in the signal-to-noise ratio of reconstructed PET images of large objects (18), although the actual improvement is a complicated function of the object size, the detector spatial resolution, the timing resolution of the time-of-flight circuitry, and the spatial resolution of the reconstructed image (21).

NEWER SCINTILLATION MATERIALS

During the last decade, considerable effort has been made to discover and develop new scintillation materials. Several new types of inorganic scintillation materials have been discovered and intensively investigated. Many of these materials have applications in the field of medical imaging especially in nuclear medicine. Some of these newer materials potentially may replace the detectors currently used in positron emission tomography (PET) but have less application as detectors for traditional nuclear medicine imaging devices such as the Anger camera.

The two major scintillators used for PET are BGO and barium fluoride (BaF_2). BGO has become the work horse for non-time-of-flight PET and BaF_2 has become the scintillator of choice for time-of-flight PET (22). While CsF initially showed promise as the scintillator for time-of-flight PET, the discovery of BaF_2 with its very fast decay time (0.8 ns) made it the fastest inorganic scintillator known (23).

The interest in discovering new scintillation materials remains high. A novel method to rapidly screen potential materials for their scintillation properties uses synchrotron radiation from the facility at Los Alamos Laboratories (24). The high intensity of the radiation allows the screening of materials still in powdered form eliminating the need to develop the sometimes difficult methods to grow single crystals of sufficient size to allow measurements. To be suitable as scintillation radiation detectors, the materials must be single crystals or compressed to form ceramics.

The new materials discovered and investigated can be separated into two types, single crystals and ceramics, with single crystals representing the majority. The single crystal materials include simple and complex fluorides; orthophosphates; oxyorthosilicates; and others not as easily grouped. The ceramics are not readily classified, but include inorganic compounds that have rare-earth elements such as gadolinium, europium, and yttrium. Some of the compounds are similar to the "rare-earth" materials in modern screens used in radiology screen-cassette systems.

To challenge the existing scintillation materials, any new material must have at least two of the following three properties: (a) high stopping power; (b) high light output; and (c) a fast decay time. Ideally, one wants a material that has the light output of NaI(Tl), the stopping power of BGO, and the fast decay time of BaF_2. The physical properties of many of these new scintillation materials include high effective atomic number, high physical density resulting in a high stopping power, stability at room temperature, and no hygroscopicity. The characteristics of the scintillation process include emission wavelengths between 300 nm and 400 nm, a fast decay time, efficient energy transfer to scintillation centers, and sufficiently high intensity.

Many of the promising new scintillation materials include the element cerium (Ce). There are the concentrated or stoichiometric compounds with cerium in ionic form as a chemical constituent such as in cerium trifluoride (CeF_3) (25), and there are those compounds with cerium as a dilutant or a dopant as in gadolinium oxyorthosilicate (GSO) and lutetium oxyorthosilicate (LSO). Doped compounds are currently superior. The concentrated compounds show a reduced light output apparently due to a lack of transfer of the primary electron-hole excitations to the active ion, in this case Ce^{3+}.

One group of single crystal, scintillation materials investigated includes simple fluorides and complex fluorides. Cerium trifluoride (CeF_3) shows promise as a replacement for BGO. It has similar attenuation characteristics as BGO, but a much faster decay time at 27 ns. Its disadvantage is it only has about 20% of the light output of BGO (26, 27). Attempts to improve its light output by doping with dysprosium (Dy), erbium (Er), and praseodymium (Pr) proved unsuccessful as they all tended to decrease the light output. Studies continue to increase knowledge of the mechanism of the scintillation processes in order to improve the total light output (25). The principal disadvantage of BaF_2 is that the wavelength of its scintillation light is 220 nm and requires the use of expensive photomultiplier tubes with quartz glass windows. Attempts to shift the wavelength of the light output of barium fluoride crystals by doping with Ce cause the fast and slow components of pure BaF_2 to disappear and be replaced by a single component with a decay time of about 100 ns. The wavelength of the output light is shifted to a value greater than 300 nm to allow the use of PMT's with ordinary glass windows (28). Complex fluorides, such as $CsGd_2F_7$ and K_2YF_5, when doped with cerium or praseodymium also show promise as useful scintillators (29). Of the two complex fluorides studied, $CsGd_2F_7$ had the better scintillator characteristics, but its light output is too low to be a useful scintillation detector for PET.

Another group of single crystal, scintillation materials include rare-earth oxyorthosilicates (30). The 1982 discovery of cerium-doped gadolinium oxyorthosilicate (GSO) appears to have begun the investigations into many of these new scintillation materials (31, 32). Oxyorthosilicate crystals display two structures: one that is stable for large rare-earth elements and another that is stable for smaller rare-earth elements such as Dy and lutetium (Lu) (29). Cerium-doped gadolinium oxyorthosilicate ($Gd_2(SiO_4)O:Ce$ (GSO)) and cerium-doped lutetium oxyorthosilicate ($Lu_2(SiO_4)O:Ce$ (LSO)) belong to the latter structure type. LSO possesses the desirable physical properties of an ideal scintillation material including high density and a high effective atomic number. It possesses a combination of high emission intensity and a fast decay time that together are superior to any other known single crystal scintillator (33).

Other oxyorthosilicates investigated include yttrium oxyorthosilicate (YSO).

A newer group of inorganic scintillators includes orthophosphates doped with cerium. Some orthophosphates investigated include lutetium and other rare-earth elements such as lanthanum (La) and gadolinium (Gd), all doped with cerium (34). These crystals possess many of the desirable properties of scintillators including a high density and a fast decay time with a light output greater than BGO. These scintillation materials are physically hard, durable at room temperature, and not attacked by water, water vapor, organic solvents, or most of the common concentrated acids. They have a high melting point (2000°C), and are resistant to radiation damage (i.e., "radiation hard"). The rare-earth orthophosphates represent another example of compounds containing cerium as a dopant with remarkable scintillator performance. They serve as good host crystals for scintillators because they do not compete for scintillation sites when doped with cerium. With its high atomic number of 71 and a fast decay time of 24 ns, lutetium orthophosphate doped with cerium (($LuPO_4$:Ce) (LOP)) shows the most promise.

The second type of scintillation material is luminescent ceramics or ceramic scintillators. They fill the gap between powders and crystals. Luminescent ceramics include rare-earth-doped oxides, oxysulfides, garnets, and silicates. For tests, the powdered materials were cold-pressed to form polycrystalline structures. Methods of processing the powders strongly affect the conversion efficiency, afterglow, and energy resolution. The processing methods can affect the microstructure, final optical quality, and the defect structure. These materials exhibit long scintillation decay times. Rare-earth dopants could provide faster optical transitions as with the oxyorthosilicates. Presently, ceramic scintillation materials work best as an x-ray detector operating in current mode similar to those used in x-ray computed tomography (35).

Of all the newer scintillators investigated, LSO appears the most promising for applications in nuclear medicine. With a greater light output and a faster decay time than BGO, LSO becomes a potential replacement for BGO in PET scanners (36). For small crystals (2×2×10 cm), LSO has better energy resolution than BGO because of a 4–5 times greater light output. With its higher light output, it still has sufficient light output even when coupled to PMT's with light guides. The use of light guides allows packed crystal arrays in PET detector designs employing continuous rings. With a fast decay time, LSO detectors allow the use of narrower timing windows, reducing the ratio of random to true coincident count rates. LOP also has many of the desirable properties of scintillation materials. Discovered recently, LOP is less well-developed as a scintillation material. However, with its fast decay time and with a light output twice that of BGO, LOP will undoubtedly soon appear as a detector material in an experimental PET system.

REFERENCES

1. Hoffer PB, Beck, RN, Gottschalk A. Semiconductor detectors in the future of nuclear medicine. New York: Society of Nuclear Medicine, 1971.
2. Curran SC. Luminescence and the scintillation counter. New York: Academic Press, 1953.
3. Birks JB. Scintillation counters. London: Pergamon Press, 1953.
4. Hine GJ. Sodium iodide scintillators. In: Hine GJ, ed. Instrumentation in nuclear medicine. Vol. 2, Chap. 6. New York: Academic Press, 1967.
5. Ramm WJ. Scintillation detectors. In: Attix FH, Roesch WC, eds. Radiation dosimetry. 2nd ed. Vol. 2, Chap. 11. New York: Academic Press, 1966.
6. Lavoie L. Comparison of radiation detector materials for imaging applications in nuclear medicine. Phys Med Biol 1973; 18:120.
7. "EMI Photomultiplier Tubes." Brochure ref: 3M/6-67 (PMT), Issue 1. Hayes Middlesex, England: EMI Electronics Ltd., 1967.
8. Young AT, Schild RE. Photoelectron collection efficiency in photomultipliers. Appl Optics 1971;10:1668.
9. Fairstein E, Hahn J: Nuclear pulse amplifiers—fundamental design practice. Nucleonics 1965;23:81.
10. Ross DA, Harris CC. Measurement of radioactivity. In: Wagner HN, ed. Principles of nuclear medicine. Chap. 5. Philadelphia: WB Saunders, 1968.
11. Johns HE, Cunningham JR. The physics of radiology. 3rd ed. Springfield, IL: Charles C. Thomas, 1969.
12. Persyk DE, Moi TE. State-of-the-art photomultipliers for Anger cameras. IEEE Trans Nucl Sci NS-1978;25:615.
13. Derenzo SE. Monte Carlo calculations of the detection efficiency of arrays of NaI(Tl), BGO, CsF, and plastic detectors for 511 keV photons. IEEE Trans Nucl Sci NS-1981;28:131.
14. Hayashi T. New photomultipliers tubes for medical imaging. IEEE Trans Nucl Sci NS-1989;36:1078.
15. Singh M, Leahy R, Brechner R, Yan X. Design and imaging studies of a position sensitive photomultiplier base dynamic SPECT system. IEEE Trans Nucl Sci NS-1989;36:1132.
16. Muehllehner G, Colsher JG. Instrumentation. In: Ell PJ, Holman BL, eds. Computed emission tomography. Chap. 1. New York: Oxford University Press, 1982.
17. Cho ZH, Farukhi M. Bismuth germanate as a potential scintillation detector in positron cameras. J Nucl Med 1977;19:840.
18. Ter-Pogossian MM, Mullani NA, Ficke DC, Markham J, Snyder DL. Photon time-of-flight-assisted positron emission tomography. J Comput Assist Tomogr 1981;5:227.
19. Allemand R, Gresset C, Vacher T. Potential advantages of cesium fluoride scintillator for a time-of-flight positron camera. J Nucl Med 1980;21:153.
20. Mullani NA, Ficke DC, Ter-Pogossian MM. Cesium fluoride: a new detector for positron emission tomography. IEEE Trans Nucl Sci NS-1980;27:572.
21. Wong WH, Mullani NA, Phillippe EA, Hartz R, Gould KL. Image improvement and design optimization of the time-of-flight PET. J Nucl Med 1983;24:52.
22. Wong WH. PET camera performance design evaluation for BGO and BaF_2 scintillators (non-time-of-flight). J Nucl Med 1988; 29:338.
23. Laval M, Moszynski M, Allemand R, et al. Barium fluoride—inorganic scintillator for subnanosecond timing. Nucl Instr and Meth 1983;206:169.
24. Derenzo SE, Moses WW, Cahoon JL, Perera RCC. Prospects for new inorganic scintillators. IEEE Trans Nucl Sci NS-1990;37:203.
25. Wojyowicz AJ, Berman E, Koepke C, Lempicki A. Stoichiometric cerium compounds as scintillators. Part I: CeF_3. IEEE Trans Nucl Sci Ns-1992;39:494.
26. Derenzo SE, Moses WW. Cerium fluoride—a new, fast, heavy scintillator. IEEE Trans Nucl Sci NS-1989;36:173.
27. Anderson DF. Properties of the high-density scintillator cerium fluoride. IEEE Trans Nucl Sci NS-1989;36:137.
28. Visser R, Dorenbos P, van Eijk CWE, Hollander RW. Scintillation

properties of Ce^{3+} doped BaF_2 crystals. IEEE Trans Nucl Sci NS-1991;38:178.
29. Dorenbos P, Visser R, van Eijk CWE, Khaidukov NM, Korzhik MV. Scintillation properties of some Ce^{3+} and Pr^{3+} doped inorganic crystals. IEEE Trans Nucl Sci NS-1993;40:388.
30. Takagi K, Fukazawa T. Cerium-activated Gd_2SiO_5 single crystal scintillator [Letter]. App Phys 1983;42:43.
31. Ishibashi H, Shimizu K, Susa K, Kubota S. Cerium doped GSO scintillators and its application to position sensitive detectors. IEEE Trans Nucl Sci NS-1989;36:170.
32. Melcher CL, Schweitzer JS. Scintillation properties of GSO. IEEE Trans Nucl Sci NS-1990;37:161.
33. Suzuki H, Tombrello TA. Light emission mechanism of $Lu_2(Si)_4)O$:ce. IEEE Trans Nucl Sci NS-1993;40:380.
34. Lempicki A, Berman E, Wojtowicz AJ, Balcerzyk M. Cerium-doped orthophosphates: new promising scintillators. IEEE Trans Nucl Sci NS-1993;40:384.
35. Rossner W. Bödinger H, Lepert J, Grabmaier BC. The conversion of high energy radiation to visible light by luminescent ceramics. IEEE Trans Nucl Sci NS-1993;40:376.
36. Daghighian F, Shenderov P, Pentlow KS, Grahm MC, Eshaghian B. Evaluation of cerium doped lutetium oxyorthosilicate (LSO) scintillation crystal for PET. IEEE Trans Nucl Sci NS-1993; 40:1045.

5 Gamma Well Counter

JAMES A. PATTON and C. CRAIG HARRIS

Nuclear medicine applications involving the detection and counting of radionuclides may be divided into imaging and nonimaging techniques. Nonimaging techniques may be further divided into *in vivo* and *in vitro* procedures. *In vitro* procedures involve the measurement of radioactivity in a sample either directly or, more commonly, as a relative measurement in comparison to a standard of known activity. Because most procedures utilize γ-emitters, the scintillation detector is typically the detector of choice for performing these measurements. The samples generally contain very small amounts of radioactivity. It is, therefore, necessary to utilize a scintillation detector with a very high detection efficiency, which is accomplished by using a special purpose scintillation detector, a well counter that is constructed with a hole in the center of the crystal (Fig. 5.1). This geometry permits the sample to be inserted within the crystal so that the sample is almost completely surrounded by detector material. Utilizing low energy γ-emitters and scintillation well counters, it is possible to detect as many as 95% of the emitted photons.

Quantitative assays of radioactivity at the nanocurie (10^{-9} Ci) level in sample volumes of 1–3 ml may be performed using a well counter by counting the samples in the same fixed source location in comparison with the counting of standards of radioactive sources of the same radionuclide in the same physical size and configuration.

PHYSICAL CONSIDERATIONS

CONSTRUCTION

Well-type scintillation crystals are fabricated exactly as are conventional "solid" crystals. The only difference is that a hole (well) is made in the crystal, usually on the face opposite to that to be coupled to the photomultiplier tube (see Chapter 4). The well is constructed by drilling directly into the sodium iodide crystal and lining the hole with the same thin aluminum covering that houses the outside of the crystal. Reflective material is placed between the well section of the can and the cavity in the crystal, just as it is on the outer surfaces. The crystal may be housed in a separate can with a glass exit pane for scintillations, or it may be mounted integrally on a photomultiplier tube (integral line assembly) as shown in Figure 5.1 (1).

Because of the presence of the well, light collection from the crystal is less efficient than that from an undrilled crystal, and pulse height resolution is, therefore, reduced. A light guide is often employed to improve pulse height resolution. Alternatively, the well may be formed in the side of the crystal for convenience with a horizontally mounted detector assembly. However, this geometry also yields poor pulse height resolution unless two photomultipliers are used (one at each end of the crystal). Under many circumstances of well counter use, pulse height resolution is not an overwhelmingly important consideration; however, it is important in multiple-radionuclide counting.

Most well counters in use today are available in two sizes (Table 5.1). Two sizes of well allow use of small (13 mm) and large (24 mm) sample tubes, even with a protective liner in place in the well.

HANDLING PRECAUTIONS

A sodium iodide well counter is fragile and subject to the same precautions against rough handling and thermal shock as any other scintillation counter. The counter must be shielded from sources of background radiation (usually samples waiting to be counted). Most importantly, it should be protected from radioactive contamination that may come from the outside of sample tubes. A thin-wall plastic liner (or even plastic film) placed in the well may be used to minimize the possibility of introducing contamination into the well by a sample tube. A plastic liner also helps to protect the can and crystal at the bottom of the well from the impact of samples dropped or forced suddenly into the well.

SYSTEM CHARACTERISTICS

ELECTRONIC COMPONENTS

Even the simplest systems require certain minimum electronic circuits to convert the output of the scintillation counter into useful information. Hence, available systems range from those with minimum electronics and manual controls to "semi-intelligent" systems using microprocessor control of instrument settings, automated data reduction, and hardcopy printing services. A generic block diagram of a well counter system illustrating the multiple components that may be utilized is shown in Figure 5.2.

Scintillation detectors require a well-regulated source of steady voltage (usually 700–1200 volts DC), a preamplifier (to convert the charge output of the photomultiplier tube to voltage pulses), a linear amplifier (to adjust the level of the voltage pulses in a linear fashion for optimum pulse height analysis), a pulse height analyzer (to eliminate voltage pulses due to the detection of unwanted photons), a scaler in which to store acceptable counts, and a timer to control the data acquisition process. The use of a pulse height analyzer allows reduction of the effects of background radiation and facilitates the assay of two or more radionuclides in the same sample. The use of multiple energy windows, either by using multiple pulse height analyzers and scalers or by using a multichannel analyzer, greatly reduces the time required for multiple-radionuclide activity determinations, but a single window can be used

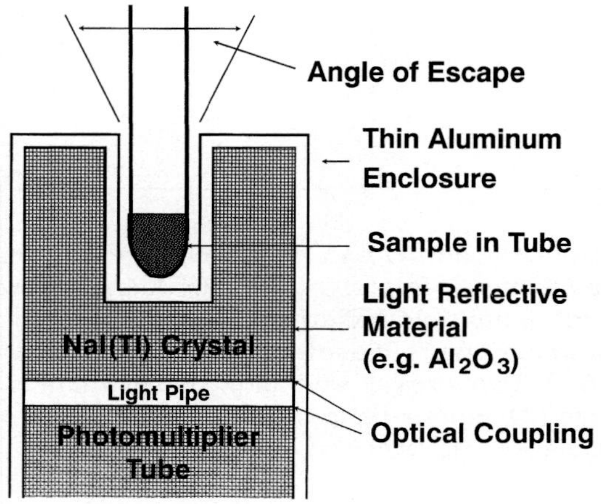

Figure 5.1. Well detector construction. A longitudinal section drawing of a typical well detector shows essential elements and their relationships. In this type of construction, the crystal, light guide, and photomultiplier tube (PMT) are integrally assembled. The aluminum can provides a hermetic seal, light-tight integrity, mechanical rigidity, and good transmission for γ- and x-ray photons. Alternatively the crystal may be canned with a glass faceplate, which is then coupled to a PMT. External means of excluding ambient light must then be provided, such as wrapping with vinyl electrical tape.

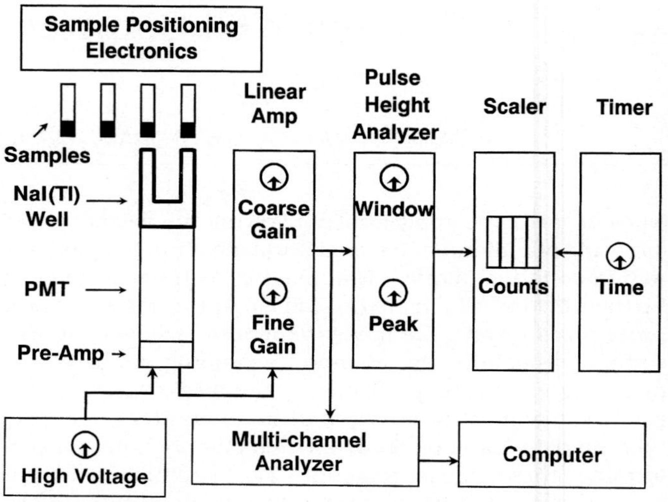

Figure 5.2. Block diagram of a well counting system. Specific systems may use single or multiple pulse height analyzers/scalers for single or multiple window counting. Modern day systems utilize a multichannel analyzer and computer system for simultaneous multiple window counting and automated calculations of assayed values.

Table 5.1.
Common Sizes of Well Counters and Usual Well Configurations.

Crystal Size (Outer Dimensions)	Well Dimensions (Inside Diameter × Depth)
1¾-in diameter × 2-in high	0.656 × 1.546 in (16.7 × 39.2 mm)
2-in diameter × 2-in high	1.00 × 1.546 in (25.4 × 39.2 mm)
3-in diameter × 3-in high	0.656 × 2.046 in (16.7 × 52 mm)
3-in diameter × 3-in high	1.00 × 2.046 in (25.4 × 52 mm)

with multiple passes with the window set for different energies. Current systems typically use a multichannel analyzer and computer system so that the entire energy spectrum from a sample may be captured and pulse analysis performed after data collection using computer programs to determine counts from selected photopeaks.

PHYSICAL AND MECHANICAL CONFIGURATIONS

System configurations range from very simple units made for manual insertion of a single sample and with manually operated electronic controls, to devices with an apparatus for automatic serial counting of hundreds of samples. Older designs accommodated a variety of sample vial sizes, in an endless conveyor chain-type sample changer. More current systems are designed for a mass market in radioimmunoassay (RIA) and have changers that use only small tubes in special racks similar to test tube racks. More recent designs are only for low-energy (<500 keV) photon counting, with reduced shielding of detector crystals, whereas older systems had massive shielding for use with all radionuclides. Some have refrigeration systems for samples and detector(s). Systems for high energy photon counting may be fabricated to user specifications by some manufacturers. Multiple detectors facilitate large throughput in laboratories performing large numbers of procedures daily. A computer is generally used at present to coordinate positioning of samples and the acquisition of data from each sample.

SYSTEM LIMITATIONS

Well counter systems are limited by the properties of the internal components and by certain deliberately chosen design factors. The most usual limitation encountered is in counting of high-activity samples because totally incorrect results will be obtained if sample activities are excessive. Another common limitation, particularly in newer RIA-oriented counting systems, is a lack of flexibility in selecting different energy windows. Often, only preselected windows are available, and it is difficult to find systems designed for counting high-energy radionuclides. For example, a modified Schilling test (Dicopac; Amearsham Corp., Arlington Heights, IL 60005) uses ^{58}Co (811 keV) and cannot be performed properly on many current designs. Obviously, radioactive microspheres labeled with high energy emitters cannot be used with such instruments.

Limitations in counting high-activity samples are not caused by pulse height analyzers with their typical time resolution for paired pulses (events) of 1–5 microseconds. It is the slow decay of the scintillations in NaI(Tl) (mean life 0.23 microseconds) that causes overlap and pileup of events that limit counting rates. Poor amplifier design and pulse-shaping with long time constants aggravate this problem. The difference between true and observed count rates using a scintillation counter with a 5 microsecond deadtime is shown in Figure 5.3.

Most well counter systems should not be used at apparent counting rates higher than 5000 counts per second (cps) or 300,000 counts per minute (cpm) unless sample and standard have comparable activity. Above this rate, effects of pileup and deadtime losses can become excessive, and electronic malperformance can appear. Well-designed high-quality systems can operate usefully up to 100,000 cps or 6,000,000 cpm with reasonable accuracy except for coincidence and deadtime losses. Hence samples containing about 0.2 μCi (7.4 kBq) of ^{125}I, 0.3–0.4 μCi (11.1–14.8 kBq) of ^{131}I, 6–10 μCi (222–370 kBq) of ^{51}Cr, or 1–3 μCi (37–111 kBq) of ^{59}Fe represent reasonable upper limits on many well counter systems. This is not a common problem, however, because most RIA samples typically contain less activity than these upper limits and standards are usually made to approximate typical sample activities by dilution techniques.

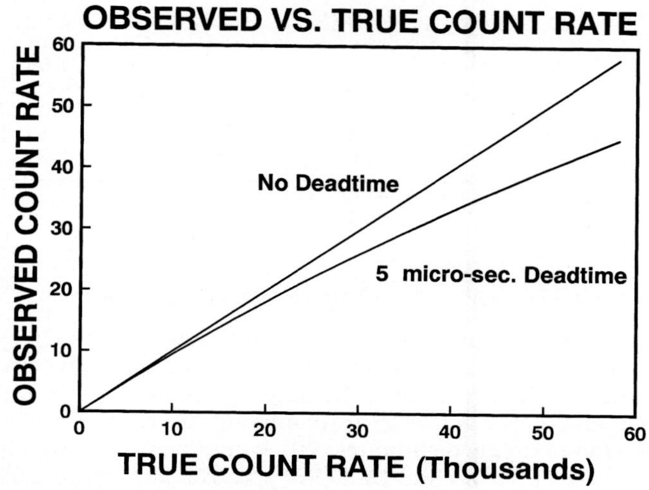

Count Rates in CPS x Thousand

Figure 5.3. Observed versus true count rate for a scintillation counter with a 5 microsecond deadtime. Measured count rates above 6000 cps deviate from actual count rates for this system.

APPLICATIONS

SYSTEM RESPONSE TO COMMONLY USED RADIONUCLIDES

The most typical applications of the well counter in nuclear medicine studies or radiobioassay procedures involve only a few radionuclides (Table 5.2). Iodine-125, perhaps the most often encountered, is used in thyroid function tests and glomerular filtration rate (GFR) determinations and several competitive binding assay (RIA) procedures.

Investigations of blood flow are greatly facilitated by the use of radiolabeled microspheres. Many of these have photon energies in excess of 500 keV, requiring the use of older or specially fabricated, more flexible counting systems. A variety of labeled microspheres are commercially available.

The attractiveness of large well counters (3×3-inch) lies in their increased efficiencies at high energies. Figure 5.4 (2) shows that for 1–2 ml samples, counting rates from ^{59}Fe samples are over three times higher with a 3×3-inch well counter than with the typical smaller one. This factor is important when sample activities are very low or when reduced counting times are required for large numbers of samples.

Although the counting rates given in Table 5.2 are typical and not absolute, serious departures from these approximate values are indicative of errors associated with the counting process. Occasionally, the radiopharmaceutical manufacturer's labeled activity may be in error, and the stated activity should be verified. Counting rates from samples containing ^{125}I are subject to the thickness of the aluminum enclosure, since absorption of photons in the

Table 5.2.
Radionuclides Used in γ Well Counters[a]

Radionuclide	Useful γ (or x) Radiation: $T_{1/2}$[b]	Application[c]	Weighted Mean Energy (keV)	No. per 100 Dis.	Typical Window (keV)	Counting Efficiency: 1¾ × 2 In (%)	3 × 3 In (%)	Typical Background: 1¾ × 2 In (cpm)	3 × 3 In (cpm)	Typical Counting Rate per 0.1 μCi (0.37 kBq), 1¾ × 2 In: cps	cpm
^{125}I	60.2 d	R,M	28.3	143	15–80	72	72	20	40	2600	156,000
^{57}Co	270 d	M	123	97	100–160	86	88	35	150	3000	180,000
^{99m}Tc	6.02 h	C	140	88	110–170	85	87	30	140	2700	162,000
^{141}Ce	32.5 d	M	145	48	120–175	84	86	30	140	1500	90,000
^{51}Cr	27.8 d	M,C	322	9	270–330	36	64	65	125	120	7,200
^{131}I	8.04 d	C	364	84	314–414	28	55	60	120	780	46,800
^{113}Sn	115 d	M	393	64	350–440	27	51	50	110	620	37,200
^{103}Ru	39.8 d	M	497	88	450–550	19	42	40	100	600	36,000
^{85}Sr	64.7 d	M	514	100	465–565	18	40	40	100	650	39,000
^{137}Cs	30 y	C	662	84	600–720	12	30	30	75	370	22,200
^{95}Nb	35 d	M	770	100	650–900	9.5	27	20	60	350	21,000
^{58}Co	71.3 d	C	811	100	700–930	8.8	26	20	60	320	19,200
^{46}Sc	84 d	M	955	200	800–1200	6.4	21	18	45	470	28,200
^{59}Fe	45 d	C	1200	99	1000–1400	5.5	19	12	30	200	12,000
^{60}Co	5.26 y	C	1250	199	1000–1500	5.2	17	12	30	380	22,800

[a]A listing of some radionuclides available or in common use, with applications, radiation properties, typical efficiencies (window counting of 1–2 ml samples in 12 mm tubes in 16.7 mm well), and typical counting rates per unit of activity. "Counting efficiency" is overall, and equal to geometric efficiency × can transmission × crystal intrinsic peak efficiency

[b]h = hours, d = days, y = years

[c]R = radioimmunoassay, M = microspheres, C = clinical or standards

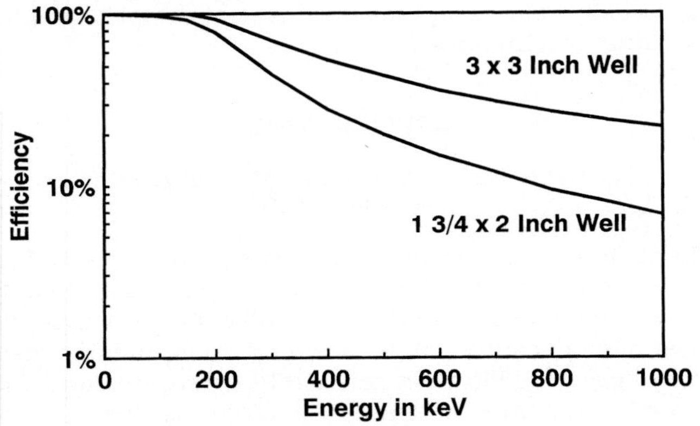

Figure 5.4. Intrinsic peak efficiency versus energy for certain NaI(Tl) crystals. Intrinsic peak efficiency is the ratio of total energy absorption ("photopeak") detection events to γ-ray photons incident on the entrance surface of the crystal. This quantity is shown plotted versus photon energy for two well crystals. Intrinsic peak efficiency approaches 100% at about 120 keV for both crystals shown.

Table 5.3.
Relative Counting Rates and Volume Correction Factors for Sources of Different Volumes[a]

Radionuclide (Window)	Source Volume (ml)	Relative Counting Rate: 1¾ × 2 in	Relative Counting Rate: 3 × 3 in	Correction Factor: 1¾ × 2 in	Correction Factor: 3 × 3 in
^{125}I (15–40 keV)	1	1.00	1.00	1.00	1.00
	2	1.00	0.985	1.00	1.015
	3	0.99	0.975	1.01	1.025
	4	0.90	0.935	1.11	1.07
	5	0.75	0.865	1.33	1.16
^{125}I (15–80 keV)	1	1.00	1.00	1.00	1.00
	2	0.98	0.98	1.02	1.02
	3	0.95	0.96	1.05	1.04
	4	0.85	0.92	1.18	1.09
	5	0.75	0.85	1.33	1.18
^{51}Cr (280–360 keV)	1	1.00	1.00	1.00	1.00
	2	0.97	0.975	1.03	1.025
	3	0.89	0.94	1.12	1.06
	4	0.79	0.88	1.27	1.13
	5	0.675	0.815	1.48	1.23

[a]Source volumes contain some activity for the two radionuclides given, in 12 mm test tubes

enclosure reduces the measured counting rates, but typically not lower than 200 cps/0.1 μCi (3.7 kBq). With ^{125}I, counting only the photopeak from detection of single events (15–40 keV) can reduce counting rates to 70% of those obtained in 15–80 keV windows. Additional discussion of ^{125}I counting considerations is presented in a later section. The values listed in Table 5.2 should be useful in assessing system performance.

EFFECT OF SAMPLE VOLUME

Sample volumes in radiobioassay procedures are typically about 1–2 ml and sample and standard volumes should be approximately equal. When sample volumes are larger, however, counting efficiencies are reduced because portions of the source are farther from the well crystal and attenuation in the sample may be increased. Table 5.3 gives the relative counting rates for the same activity in volumes of 1, 2, 3, 4, and 5 ml in 12 mm test tubes in both 1 3/4×2-inch and 3×3-inch crystals (16.7 mm well). For both crystals, response to the same activity diminishes as the sample volume increases. The smaller correction in counting of ^{125}I for the larger crystal is due more to a slightly larger, flat-bottomed source vial than to the well configuration. In this case, the 5 ml sample is not as tall in the vial as it is in the ordinary test tube, and thus has a more optimum configuration for counting. The smaller correction at 320 keV (^{51}Cr) in the larger crystal, although chiefly due to tube configuration, also shows the higher efficiency of the larger crystal for photons of this energy.

Table 5.3 shows that minor variations in sample volume below 2 ml do not cause serious counting errors. Samples larger than this value should have their counting rates corrected by the factors shown. The correction factors are not necessary if samples and standards have precisely the same (even if large) volume. This is the primary advantage of comparative counting, requiring only that the sample and standard be counted under similar conditions of placement (geometry and window setting).

ASSAY OF TWO OR MORE RADIONUCLIDES

A mixture containing two or more different radionuclides can be assayed (by comparative techniques) for each component in the presence of the others. Mixtures of ^{125}I and ^{51}Cr, and of ^{59}Fe and ^{51}Cr, are commonly assayed by simple two-radionuclide techniques. When energies are so widely separated (^{125}I, 28 and 56 keV; ^{51}Cr, 322 keV; ^{59}Fe, 1.09 and 1.295 MeV) the spectroscopic properties of NaI(Tl) are sufficiently good to facilitate simple procedures.

If all detected events represented total absorption of γ-rays leading to photopeak counts, dual radionuclide counting would consist simple of "tuning" to each photopeak with a suitable window (e.g., 15–80 keV for ^{125}I and 270–370 keV for ^{51}Cr). However, the response of NaI(Tl) is not perfect and, in fact, the partial absorption of higher energy photons interferes with counting of the lower energy photons. Therefore, quantitative determination of the constituents of a sample containing two or more radionuclides requires measurement (or calculation) of the higher energy emitters. To illustrate this process, an example will be presented in which a quantitative separation of the components of a sample containing ^{51}Cr, ^{57}Co, and ^{125}I is explained in detail.

Refer to Figure 5.5, which shows the pulse height spectrum that may be obtained from a source containing the three named radionuclides. (It is not necessary to generate this plot to make the calculations. The illustration is offered to facilitate understanding of the basis for the calculations, and to indicate how the process would work for any number of radionuclides.) In this composite spectrum, it is seen that the ^{57}Co spectrum is "sitting on" the ^{51}Cr spectrum, and that, in turn, the ^{125}I spectrum is "sitting on" the other two. The "crosstalk" or "downscatter" contributions from the higher energy photons to the lower are thus defined as regions (*M1*, *L1*, and *L2*). Other information, such as total counts in the windows (*L*, *M*, and *H1*), is also shown.

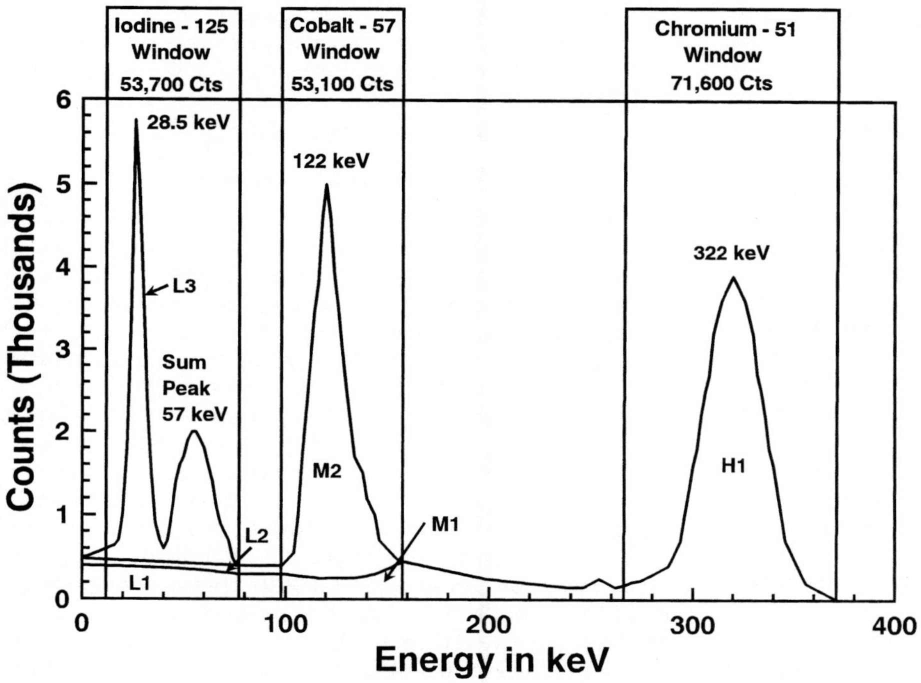

Figure 5.5. Simultaneous assay of multiple radionuclides. The pulse height spectrum resulting from detection of a mixture of ^{125}I, ^{57}Co, and ^{51}Cr in a well counter is shown. In this example the following photopeaks exist: ^{51}Cr at 322 keV; ^{57}Co at 122 keV; and ^{125}I (28.4 keV single peak and 57 keV sum coincidence peak). The counts in the ^{51}Cr window are due entirely to ^{51}Cr. The counts in the other windows, however, contain contributions from ^{51}Cr and ^{57}Co. The counts associated with a given spectral feature is related to the area of that feature.

From Figure 5.5, the following variables are defined: *H1, M,* and *L* are the total counts in the high (^{51}Cr), middle (^{57}Co), and low (^{125}I) windows, respectively.

H1 = ^{51}Cr counts in high window
M1 = ^{51}Cr counts in middle window
L1 = ^{51}Cr counts in low window
M2 = ^{57}Co counts in middle window
L2 = ^{57}Co counts in low window
L3 = ^{125}I counts in low window
X1 = M1/H1 (or ^{51}Cr in M window/^{51}Cr in H window)
Y1 = L1/H1 (or ^{51}Cr in L window/^{51}Cr in H window)
X2 = L2/M2 (or ^{57}Co in L window/^{57}Co in M window).

The last three variables (*X1, Y1,* and *X2*) are the interference factors. The values of *X1* and *Y1* are determined by counting a pure ^{51}Cr source in all three windows, and *X2* is found by counting a pure ^{57}Co source in the middle and low windows. These factors are reasonably constant for constant window settings and similar source volumes.

The desired net counts from each radionuclide are *H1, M2,* and *L3* and are calculated for each sample as follows:

1. H1 (net ^{51}Cr counts): *H1* = *H1*, direct measurement
2. M2 (net ^{57}Co counts): $M2 = M-[X1 \times H1]$
3. L3 (net ^{125}I counts): $L3 = L-[(Y1 \times H1) + (X2 \times M2)]$.

Note that the order is from highest energy radionuclide to lower, and that *M2* must be calculated before *L3*.

From Figure 5.5, *H1* = 71,600, *M* = 53,100, and *L* = 53,700. From prior measurements, *X1* = 0.109, *Y1* = 0.177, and *X2* = 0.022. The calculation then becomes:

1. *H1* = 71,600
2. *M2* = 53,100−(0.109×71,600) = 45,296
3. *L3*= 53,700 = [(0.177×71,600) + (0.022×45,296)] = 40,030.

If actual activities are desired, the net counts obtained must be related to counting rates, which are then compared to counts per microcurie per unit time as obtained from the system (with identical energy windows) from standard sources of comparable volumes. See Table 5.2 for approximate typical values.

If, in this example, the counts of Figure 5.5 had been obtained in a 1 minute count, Table 5.2 indicates that the activities would be approximately:

^{51}Cr: 71,600 cpm/(72,000 cpm/μCi) = 0.99 μCi (36.6 kBq)
^{57}Co: 45,296 cpm/(1,800,000 cpm/μCi) = 0.025 μCi (0.93 kBq)
^{125}I: 40,030 cpm/(1,560,000 cpm/μCi) = 0.026 μCi (0.95 kBq)

In a computer-based counting system, the spectrum for the individual standards and the unknown sample would be collected, the regions of interest identified, and the mathematics performed above would be duplicated in a simple algorithm to produce the same results.

Other mixtures of radionuclides can be treated in a similar fashion. The calculations for a mixture of six radionuclides are extended, but are no less straightforward. Where there is clear separation between the photopeaks of the radionuclides, as in this example, the technique outlined above is adequate. However, if the photopeaks overlap, as in the case of an ^{131}I-^{51}Cr mixture, the assay is more difficult but can be managed using spectrum stripping techniques(3).

SPECIAL EFFECTS—COINCIDENCE SUMMING

A special consequence of well counting, called *coincidence summing*, can be both damaging and beneficial, depending on the circumstances. Certain radionuclides, in the decay process, can emit two γ- or x-ray photons essentially simultaneously. When only one of these interacts in the crystal, an ordinary detection event occurs. When both interact, however, an event carrying the combined energy of both photons is the result. When a source is outside a crystal, coincidence summing occurs with low probability since the probability of detecting both photons is the product of their individual detection probabilities. However this combined detection probability can be large when a source is in a well counter. Hence ^{125}I in a well counter shows in its spectrum, in addition to a photopeak at 28.5 keV, a "sum peak" at 2×28.5, or 57 keV. This sum can contain up to 30% of the available counts and, therefore, a window of 15–80 keV is usually set to include both peaks (see Fig. 5.5).

The 15–80 keV setting should be used in counting ^{125}I for maximum efficiency since this is the best technique for recovering the counts that would be lost if only the "singles" peak (15–42 keV) were counted. (Summing causes two events to be removed from the 15–42 keV region, but only provides one count in their place, in the 42–80 keV region.) Use of the 15–80 keV window also increases source volume corrections (Table 5.3).

Whereas several radionuclides have decay properties that result in coincidence summing, ^{125}I is almost uniquely well-suited to a method of absolute assay (4). The only essential requirements are the ability to count in 15–42 keV and 42–80 keV windows, and geometry large enough to get a good coincidence count in the 42–80 keV window. Spectrometric well counters meet both requirements adequately. If the counting rate (in counts/second) in the 15–42 keV window is designated R_s ("singles") and the counting rate in the 42–80 keV window is designated R_c ("coincidence"), then the absolute disintegration rate (R_o) is given by:

$$R_o = \frac{(R_s + 2R_c)}{4R_c} \qquad (5.1)$$

The units of R_o are disintegrations/second (Becquerels). R_o may be divided by 37 or 37,000 to yield activity in nanocuries or microcuries, respectively.

Certain other radionuclides, notably ^{24}Na, ^{46}Sc, ^{60}Co, and ^{111}In, have simple cascade photon emissions that make it possible to perform absolute activity assays. However, the expressions by which the activities are calculated are much more complicated.

Well counting of samples of isotopes like ^{75}Se, which have multiple γ emissions, causes problems of accuracy because of coincidence summing, but the problems can be circumvented by requiring equality of sample and standard volumes and a suitable energy window (100–450 keV) encompassing all emitted photons (5).

Well counting of blood samples containing positron-emitting isotopes is important in evaluating blood flow by positron emission tomography. These samples can cause count rate-dependent nonlinearities (nonconstant deadtime) due to random coincidence summing of single 511 keV annihilation photons, as well as true coincidences enabled by well counter geometry. Narrow window (511 keV ±10%) counting leads to large and variable deadtimes. However, a threshold-only window (on high-quality systems) with a lower level of 400 keV, yields small, near-constant deadtimes that can be used to provide count-loss correction at observed counting rates up to 100,000 cps (6).

OPERATING CONSIDERATIONS

PERFORMANCE AND CALIBRATION

Fortunately, a properly installed and adjusted well counter system should operate consistently for very long periods, barring catastrophic failure of some component. Additionally, the inherent properties of comparative counting can provide immunity from even serious malfunctions of certain kinds. The most important single criterion of instrument performance is that counts be observed when a source is present and that the counting rate drop to reasonable background levels when the source is removed.

For high-confidence use, however, a counting system should meet the additional requirements of (a) consistent response to a long-lived check source, and (b) consistent response to known levels of activity as indicated in Table 5.2. A γ well counter used over a large photon energy range should be "calibrated" daily by "peaking" it on both the 662-keV and 32-keV peaks from the decay of ^{137}Cs-^{137}Ba. Sources for this purpose are readily available. Amplifier gain and photomultiplier voltage required should be noted and recorded since sudden changes generally indicate trouble. After calibration, a wider window should be set and a count for a standard time taken and recorded. A result outside of normal statistical expectations indicates trouble.

A well counter used primarily to count ^{125}I samples may be calibrated on the 32-keV x-ray photons from ^{137m}Ba (^{137}Cs), but requires careful peaking. An alternative is a source of ^{129}I, a very long half-life substitute for ^{125}I. Its principal radiations are the x-rays from the daughter ^{129}Xe (30.44 keV-weighted mean) instead of the ^{125}Te x-rays from the decay of ^{125}I (28.4 keV mean). In any event, a well counter used extensively with ^{125}I should be calibrated every day with ^{125}I (or ^{129}I) and the results recorded and examined for consistency. Background measurements from a well counter should be reasonably constant. Increasing background counts, in the absence of contamination of the well, particularly when associated with increasing photomultiplier tube high voltage, usually indicates instrument malfunction.

PITFALLS

There are common pitfalls to be avoided in routine γ well counting, but reasonable sample counting procedures should eliminate them. Daily calibration will avoid gross maladjustments. Examination of test results for plausibility, in the light of expected counting rates, can detect errors of operator and instrument performance.

Detector contamination can be avoided by simply exercising caution in the handling of samples and the use of a liner for the well, as noted earlier. Lack of proper concern will be evidenced in increased "background" counts.

One common error, usually resulting from hasty manual sample placement, is failure to properly seat a test tube completely into the well. Occasionally, when maladjusted, automatic sample changers will also fail to seat samples properly.

Failure to observe maximum limits on activity (and counting rates) is perhaps the most common operator error. Avoidance of the problem requires operator knowledge and understanding, because there is nothing about the (almost certainly) erroneous result to warn the operator. If counting losses from deadtime are less than 20% they may be corrected by use of the approximate expression

$$R = \frac{R_o}{(1 - R_o t)} \qquad (5.2)$$

where R is the corrected counting rate (or counts/unit time), R_o is the observed counting rate, and t is the deadtime of the system, expressed in the unit time. Unfortunately, this latter term varies with window setting, and must be determined experimentally for each radionuclide.

An appropriate method uses two sources, the activities of which do not need to be known (7).

SUMMARY

The NaI(T1) scintillation well counter is the basic tool for assay of radioactivity in test tube samples. Most well counter systems, once properly operating, are inherently reliable. By comparative counting of samples against a known standard in the same geometry and energy-selective counting conditions (windows), consistent quantitative results may be obtained from samples with very low levels (10^{-5} μCi (3.7×10^{-1} Bq)) of radioactivity. Techniques are straightforward even for assay of mixtures of radionuclides. Commonsense, care, and regular calibration can provide reproducible results over long periods of time.

REFERENCES

1. Lindow JT, Shrader E, Farukhi MR, et al. Harshaw scintillation phosphors. 3rd ed. Solon, OH: The Harshaw Chemical Company, 1975.
2. Harris CC, Hamblen DP, Francis JE. Basic principles of scintillation counting for medical investigators (technical manual). ORNL 2808 (with ORINS 30). Washington, DC: Office of Technical Services, Department of Commerce, 1958.
3. Francis JE, Bell PR, Harris CC. Medical scintillation spectrometry. Nucleonics 1955;13:8882.
4. Eldridge JE, Crowther P. Absolute determination of Iodine-125 activity. Nucleonics 1965;22:56.
5. Ross DA, Rohrer RH, Harris CC. Quantitative counting in the presence of coincidence summing scintillations. J Nucl Med 1967; 8:502.
6. Harris CC, Warren LP, Estrada MC, Coleman RE. Problems in scintillation well-counting of blood samples containing positron emitting radionuclides. J Nucl Med 1987;28(Suppl):697–698.
7. Adams R, Hine GJ, Zimmerman CD. Deadtime measurements in scintillation cameras under scatter conditions simulating quantitative nuclear cardiography. J Nucl Med 1978;19:538.

6 Physics of Collimator Design

BENJAMIN M.W. TSUI, DONALD L. GUNTER, ROBERT N. BECK, and JAMES PATTON

The collimator of a radiation detector used for radionuclide imaging is analogous to the lens of a camera in that each of these components strongly affects the sensitivity, spatial resolution, and depth of field of an image-forming device. However, unlike the glass lens, which changes the direction of light rays by refraction to achieve a focusing effect, the collimator is entirely passive, consisting of one or more holes in a dense high-Z (atomic number) material, such as lead or tungsten, that is relatively opaque to γ-rays encountered in nuclear medicine. If a γ photon is emitted so that it happens to travel in a direction that enables it to pass through a collimator hole, then it is regarded as a properly collimated photon, which may contribute to the *geometric* component of the detector response. If the photon travels in a direction that impinges on a collimator septum, it may either be absorbed by, or penetrate through, the septal material. The photons that have penetrated one or more septa before reaching the detector contribute to the *penetration* component of the detector response. A small fraction of the photons may experience Compton interactions with the septal material, resulting in scattered photons with reduced energy. A larger fraction undergo Compton scattering within the patient. The detected photons that experience single or multiple scattering constitute the *scatter* component of the detector response. Both the penetration and the scatter components reduce image contrast. In the design of collimators, the goal is to maximize the geometric component of response while reducing the penetration component to a negligible level, so that adequate spatial resolution and image contrast can be obtained.

There are two main categories of collimator design. The first consists of collimators that are used with scanning and multiple detector systems. Although these systems have become largely obsolete in conventional nuclear medicine imaging, they are still found in a few single photon emission computed tomography (SPECT) systems. Collimators for scanning and multiple detector systems usually consist of multiple holes to maximize detection efficiency. Each hole is tapered and the axes of all the holes are focused to the same point in order to maintain adequate spatial resolution. All photons that pass through collimator holes are detected by a single scintillation crystal and produce pulses that are associated with the location of the collimator axis. An image is formed by recording these events while mechanically scanning the detector-collimator assembly over the area of interest.

The second category of collimators consists of those designed for scintillation cameras, which are used almost exclusively in planar imaging and in most SPECT systems. The detector of a scintillation camera consists of a large-area scintillator viewed by an array of photomultiplier tubes (PMTs). The location on the crystal of each detected photon that passes through the collimator is determined from the PMT output pulses. Thus, the detected image can be obtained without any motion of the scintillation camera. The most common camera-type collimators consist of straight holes with parallel axes. This type of collimator provides a one-to-one projection of the object onto the detected image plane. In imaging small objects, converging hole collimators are often used to produce a magnified projection of the object onto the image plane. Here, the collimator holes are arranged such that all the hole axes converge to the same point beyond the object. The converging hole design provides increased detection efficiency for the same spatial resolution, when compared with the parallel-hole design, by maximizing the use of crystal area. Conversely, to image objects that are larger than the crystal area, diverging hole collimators may be used with resulting minification and loss of detection efficiency.

In this chapter, the physical principles of collimator design are described. The most important concepts are detection efficiency and spatial resolution. First, the properties of single-hole collimators are described. The single-hole collimator is important to our understanding of collimator design because it constitutes the basic unit of collimators with multiple holes. Second, we discuss multiple-hole collimators for scanner and multiple detector systems and scintillation camera systems. The geometric components of both detection efficiency and spatial resolution are derived in terms of the design parameters and the imaging conditions. Finally, the effects of the penetration and scatter components on the total collimator response are described. The penetration component is especially important in imaging high energy photons. In short, this chapter provides the basic concepts necessary for the design of optimum collimators for specific diagnostic applications using conventional nuclear medicine and SPECT imaging systems.

SINGLE HOLE COLLIMATORS

Since the geometric response of a multiple-hole collimator used in a scanner, a multiple detector system or a scintillation camera is simply the sum of responses of single holes, we first examine the single-hole collimator (Fig. 6.1), and summarize the essential factors regarding collimator response, described in terms of efficiency and spatial resolution.

GEOMETRIC RESPONSE TO A POINT SOURCE

Referring to Figure 6.1, consider first the case of a point source placed on the collimator axis and at a distance z

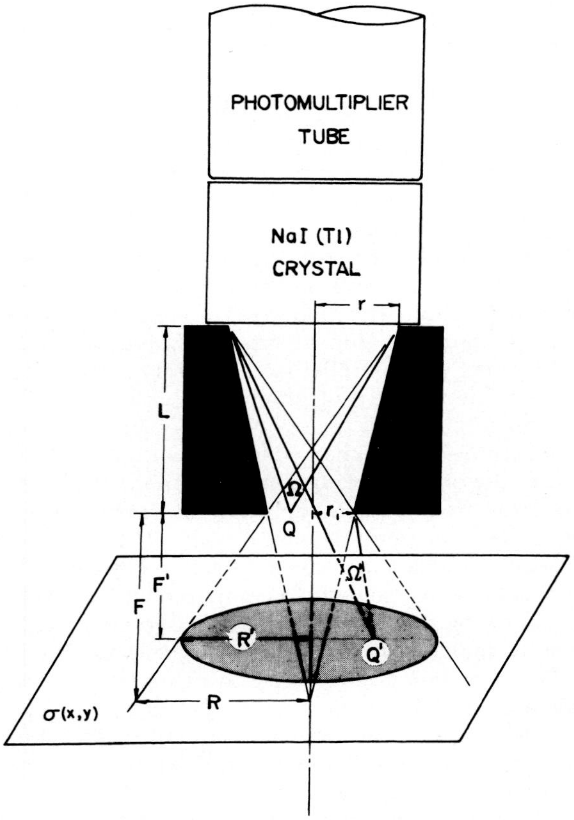

Figure 6.1. Single-Hole Collimator. Scintillation detector with a single-hole collimator that defines a circular field of view with radius R' at a distance F'. The response to a uniform sheet distribution of radioactivity σ (photons emitted/cm^2-sec) is independent of F'.

from the collimator face. If n_E is the number of γ-rays with energy E emitted per second by the point source, the expected count rate (C) is given by

$$C = g(0,\ 0,\ z)\eta\psi n_E = p_G(0,\ 0,\ z)n_E \left[\frac{\text{count}}{\text{sec}}\right] \tag{1}$$

where η is the probability that a γ-ray will be totally absorbed in the detector to produce a "photopeak pulse," and ψ is the probability that the window setting of the pulse height analyzer will pass such a pulse. The *geometric factor* $g(x, y, z)$ is defined as the fraction of radiation that will pass through the collimator. For a point source located at position (0, 0, z), where $z = F' < F$ (F = the focal distance), it is given by the fraction of the spherical surface that is covered by the crystal seen by the point source, i.e.,

$$g(0,\ 0,\ z) = \frac{\pi r^2}{4\pi(L + z)^2} = \frac{a_D}{4\pi(L + z)^2} \tag{2}$$

where L is the collimator hole length, and r is the radius and $\sigma = \pi r^2$ is the aperture of the collimator hole at the back plane. The factor $p_G(0, 0, z)$ is the value of the geometric component of the point source response function for a point source at $(x, y, z) = (0, 0, z)$ and has the unit of

$$\left[\frac{\text{counts}}{\text{sec}} \Big/ \frac{\gamma\text{-rays emitted at }(0,\ 0,\ z)}{\text{sec}}\right].$$

Beyond the focal point, that is, $z \geq F$, the crystal that can be seen by the point source is limited by the entrance aperture of the collimator; thus, the geometric factor is given by

$$g(0,\ 0,\ z) = \frac{a_1}{4\pi z^2} = \frac{\pi r_1^2}{4\pi z^2} \tag{3}$$

where r_1 is the radius and $a_1 = \pi r_1^2$ is the aperture of the collimator hole at the front plane.

GEOMETRIC RESPONSE TO A UNIFORM PLANAR SOURCE

To obtain adequate spatial resolution for imaging, the field of view of the single-hole collimator must be comparable to or smaller than the size of the object to be imaged. The geometric response to a uniform planar source provides a useful measure of the efficiency and is an important property of the collimator.

Consider the response of a single hole collimator to a planar source,σ(γ-rays emitted/cm^2-sec), placed against the collimator face, that is, at $z = 0$. The number of γ-rays emitted per second within the entrance aperture is $a_1\sigma = \pi r_1^2\sigma$, and for each γ photon the solid angle of view through the collimator is given by $a_D/L^2 = \pi r^2/L^2$ [steradians] (1–3). Thus the number of γ-rays passing through the collimator per second is given approximately by

$$C\left[\frac{\text{counts}}{\text{sec}}\right] = G_0\eta\psi\sigma \tag{4}$$

where

$$G_0\left[\frac{g\text{-rays collimated}}{\text{sec}} \Big/ \frac{g\text{-rays rays emitted}}{\text{sec-cm}^2}\right] = g_0 a_1 = \frac{a_1 a_D}{4\pi L^2} \tag{5}$$

is the *geometric efficiency* of the single-hole collimator for a uniform planar distribution of radioactivity at the collimator face (4) and $g_0 = g(0, 0, 0)$ is the geometry factor at the collimator face given by equation 2.

As the planar source is moved away from the collimator face, the geometry factor decreases according to the inverse square law. If the source is large enough to cover the collimator field of view, the amount of radioactivity within the area of this field increases as the square of the distance. This compensates precisely for the inverse square decrease in the geometry factor. As a result, the *geometric efficiency* is given by integrating the geometric factor over the collimator field of view at any distance z, i.e.,

$$G = \int\int_{-\infty}^{+\infty} g(x,\ y,\ z)dxdy = \frac{a_1 a_D}{4\pi L^2} \tag{6}$$

which is independent of z (5).

The validity of equation 6 is not limited to round tapered holes such as that in Figure 6.1; it is equally valid for square, triangular, hexagonal, or irregularly shaped collimator holes, provided only that the entire aperture area at the back plane can be seen from every point within the aperture at the front plane.

For a focused hole collimator as shown in Figure 6.1, the geometric efficiency can be written as

$$G = \frac{\pi r^2}{4L^2}\left(\frac{LR' - F'r}{F' + L}\right)^2 = \frac{\pi r^2 R^2}{16F^2[(2r/R) + 1]^2} \qquad (7)$$

where R' is the radius of view at a distance $z = F'$. For a multihole focused collimator, it is most convenient to employ holes that taper to a common focal point at distance F, at which a particular value of radius of view, R, is required. From equation 7, we find that for fixed values of r and R, G is proportional to the inverse square of the focal length (F) or collimator length (L). It is also clear that G is proportional to the detector area (πr^2) or to the area of view (πR^2) only if $2r/R \ll 1$. From simple geometric relationships, this condition is equivalent to the condition $L/F \ll 1$. Since this is not the case for most collimators in use, one must be cautious in discussing the dependence of G on the detector area or the collimator area of view.

Additionally, for fixed values of R and F, it is clear from equation 7 that G increases with r and approaches a limit

$$G = \frac{\pi R^4}{64F^2} \qquad (8)$$

as r approaches ∞. In this case, L also increases without limit. This unattainable value of G, which requires an infinitely large detector and a collimator with infinitely length, is exactly four times the geometric efficiency of the optimum cylindrical collimator that has the same radius of view at the same distance from the collimator face (6). The impracticality of this approach to increased detector sensitivity led to the introduction of multihole focused collimators (7) of reasonable length, so that large-diameter detectors could be used.

SPATIAL RESOLUTION

All measures of spatial resolution can be derived from the image of a point source or the point source response function for the collimator. In the process of image formation with a scanning system, γ-rays detected at all points on the crystal are recorded at the position of the axis of the focused collimator at the time of detection. Stated more explicitly, if a point source is located at the point $\mathbf{r}_o = (x_o, y_o, z_o)$ in object space, and the detector axis is at the point $\mathbf{r}_D = (x_D, y_D)$ on the detector-image plane, the geometry factor can be written as $g(\mathbf{r}_D; \mathbf{r}_o)$. (Note that we have assumed the detector axis to be at $(x_D, y_D) = (0, 0)$ in the earlier, less explicit, notation.)

The geometric component of the point source response function for the scanner can be written as

$$p_{SG}(\mathbf{r}_D; \mathbf{r}_o) = \left[\frac{\text{counts at } \mathbf{r}_D}{\text{sec}} \Big/ \frac{\text{photons emitted at } \mathbf{r}_o}{\text{sec}}\right] = g(\mathbf{r}_D; \mathbf{r}_o)\eta\psi \qquad (9)$$

If an area A(cm^2) is scanned in a total time of T (sec), the scanning time per unit area is t (sec/cm^2), and the geometric component of the numeric image of the point source is given by

$$n_G(\mathbf{r}_D)\left[\frac{\text{counts}}{\text{cm}^2}\right] = C\left[\frac{\text{counts at } \mathbf{r}_D}{\text{sec}}\right]t\left[\frac{\text{sec}}{\text{cm}^2}\right] = n_E(\mathbf{r}_o)p_{SG}(\mathbf{r}_D; \mathbf{r}_o)t = n_E(\mathbf{r}_o)g(\mathbf{r}_D; \mathbf{r}_o)\eta\psi t \qquad (10)$$

Therefore, the geometric component of the image of a point source at (x_o, y_o, z_o) formed by a scanner has the same shape as the geometry factor for the z_o plane.

An exact expression for the point source response function is rather complex. However, the geometric component of the collimator transfer function, $\text{CTF}_G(\vec{\nu})$ of a single-hole collimator can be derived in relatively simple form (8). This function describes the spatial frequency response of the collimator and is given by the Fourier transform of the geometric point spread function (or normalized point source response function).

The geometry factor or the geometric component of the point source response function is proportional to the area of overlap of the back aperture, $a_b(\mathbf{r})$ and the projection of the front aperture onto the collimator back plane, $a_f^p(\mathbf{r})$. Figure 6.2 shows the geometric relationship for a single-hole focused collimator in the image forming process. The aperture of the collimator hole is concave. Letting ρ be the distance of the point source from the axis of the collimator hole, the area of overlap can be described by the convolution

$$a(\rho) = \int\int_{-\infty}^{+\infty} a_f^p(\mathbf{r} - \vec{\rho})a_b(\mathbf{r})d\mathbf{r}. \qquad (11)$$

In general, when the point source is placed at distance Z from the collimator face and out of the focal plane, the two disk functions $a_b(\mathbf{r})$ and $a_f^p(\mathbf{r})$ are different. From Figure 6.2, we find $a_f^p(\mathbf{r}) = a_b\{[(F + Z)/Z(L + F)]\mathbf{r}\}$, where L is the collimator hole length and F is the focal length of the collimator hole. The displacement (d) between the centers of $a_b(\mathbf{r})$ and $a_f^p(\mathbf{r})$ is given by $\rho L/Z$. The point spread function expressed in terms of the point source location $\vec{\rho}$ is pro-

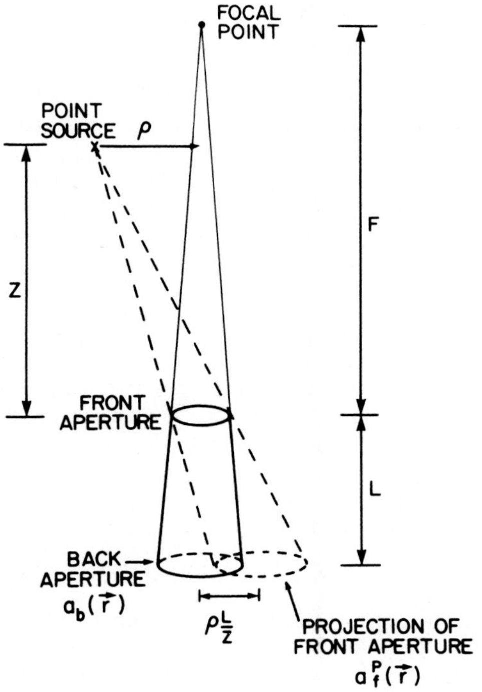

Figure 6.2. Scanner-Type Collimator. Geometric relationship in the image-forming process of a scanner-type single-hold focused collimator.

Table 6.1
Geometric Factors and Aperture Functions of Typical Collimators with Different Hole Shapes

	ROUND	SQUARE	EQUILATERAL TRIANGLE	HEXAGONAL
HOLE SHAPE	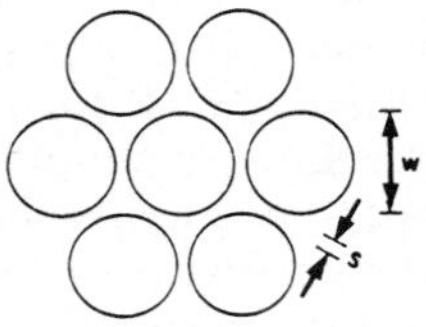	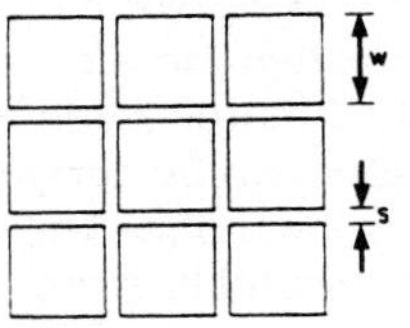	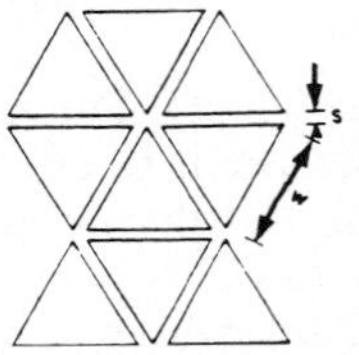	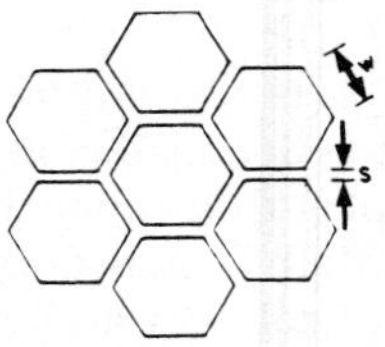
HOLE OPEN AREA a_{open}	$\frac{\pi w^2}{4}$	w^2	$\frac{\sqrt{3}}{4} w^2$	$\frac{3\sqrt{3}}{2} w^2$
UNIT HOLE AREA a_{total}	$\frac{\sqrt{3}}{2}(w + s)^2$	$(w + s)^2$	$\frac{\sqrt{3}}{4}(w + \sqrt{3}s)^2$	$\frac{3\sqrt{3}}{2}\left(w + \frac{s}{\sqrt{3}}\right)^2$
GEOMETRIC FACTOR g_o	$\frac{\pi}{32\sqrt{3}}\left[\frac{w^2}{L_e(w + s)}\right]^2$	$\frac{1}{4\pi}\left[\frac{w^2}{L_e(w + s)}\right]^2$	$\frac{\sqrt{3}}{16\pi}\left[\frac{w^2}{L_e(w + \sqrt{3}s)}\right]^2$	$\frac{3\sqrt{3}}{8\pi}\left[\frac{w^2}{L_e(w + s/\sqrt{3})}\right]^2$
APERTURE FUNCTION $A(\nu)$	$\frac{J_1(\beta)}{\beta}$	$\frac{2\sin(\beta_c)\sin(\beta_s)}{\beta^2\sin(2\theta)}$ when $\theta \neq \pi/2$ $\left(\frac{\sin\beta}{\beta}\right)$ when $\theta = n\pi/2$	$\frac{2}{\beta^2}\left(\frac{\cos\theta}{\cos3\theta}\right)\{[\cos(\beta_c) - \cos(\sqrt{3}\beta_s)]^2 + [\sqrt{3}\tan\theta\sin(\beta_c) - \sin(\sqrt{3}\beta_s)]^2\}^{1/2}$ when $\theta \neq (2n + 1)\pi/6$ $\frac{2}{\beta_3}\left\{1 + \left[\mathrm{sinc}\left(\frac{\beta_3}{2}\right)\right]^2 - 2\mathrm{sinc}(\beta_3)\right\}^{1/2}$ when $\theta = (2n + 1)\pi/6$	$\frac{2}{\beta_3^2}\left(\frac{\cos\theta}{\cos3\theta}\right)\{\cos(\beta_c)\cos(\sqrt{3}\beta_s) - \cos(2\beta c) - \sqrt{3}\tan\theta\sin(\beta_c)\sin(\sqrt{3}B_s)]\}$ when $\theta \neq (2n + 1)\pi/6$ $\frac{1}{3}\left\{2\mathrm{sinc}(\beta_3) + \mathrm{sinc}\left(\frac{\beta_3}{2}\right)\right\}$ when $\theta = (2n + 1)\pi/6$

where $\beta = \pi w\nu$, $\beta_c = \beta\cos\theta$, $\beta_s = \beta\sin\theta$, $\beta_3 = \sqrt{3}\beta$, $\mathrm{sinc}(x) = \sin(x)/x$
L_e is the effective length of the collimator hole
$J_1(x)$ is the first order Bessel function of the first kind

portional to the convolution of the two disk functions $a_b(\mathbf{r})$ and $a_f^p(\mathbf{r})$. The corresponding geometric transfer function of the collimator is given by

$$CTF_G(\vec{\nu}) = A_b[(Z/L)\vec{\nu}] \cdot A_b\{[F(L + Z)/L(L + F)]\vec{\nu}\} \quad (12)$$

for the plane located at a distance Z from the collimator face. The function $A_b(\vec{\nu})$ is the Fourier transform of the aperture function $a_b(\mathbf{r})$. Equation 12 is normalized to 1 at 0 frequency. The convolution expression for the point spread function and the corresponding transfer function are rigorously correct only if the inverse square and cosine law effects are negligible; that is, only if

$$\left(\frac{D_a}{L}\right)^2\left[\frac{2F + L}{F + L}\right]^2 \ll 1 \quad (13)$$

where D_a is the diameter of the aperture function $a_b(\mathbf{r})$. In practical collimator design, the condition expressed by equation 13 is satisfied to a good approximation.

When the point source is located in the focal plane (i.e., $Z = F$), the functions $a_b(\mathbf{r})$ and $a_f^p(\mathbf{r})$ are identical for a tapered hole. Equation 12 then is reduced to

$$CTF_G(\vec{\nu}) = A_b[(F/L)\vec{\nu}]^2 \quad (14)$$

Similarly, the condition expressed by equation 13 must be satisfied for equation 14 to be rigorously correct. The aperture functions for typical collimator hole shapes are given in Table 6.1.

Since camera collimators are almost exclusively of multiple-hole design, we defer the discussion of the spatial resolution of camera collimator to a later section.

MULTIPLE-HOLE FOCUSED COLLIMATORS

For the traditional scanning system, multiple-hole focused collimators, such as that shown in Figure 6.3, were suggested by Newell, et al. (7), as a means for making efficient use of large-diameter NaI(Tl) crystals to achieve good spatial resolution while preserving a reasonable collimator length (L). If the exposed crystal diameter (D) is approximately equal to or less than $(L + F)/2$, then the N holes comprising the collimator are essentially identical. These types of collimators have also been found in multiple-detector based SPECT systems. The response characteristics of these collimators can be described in terms of the geometry factor and the derived measures of geometric efficiency, spatial resolution, and depth of field.

GEOMETRY FACTOR

The geometry factor, $g(x, y, z)$ of multiple-hole collimators, such as those shown in Figure 6.3, can be described as a superposition or spatial summation of the geometry factors for all holes which are identical.

At $z = 0$, the geometry factor $g(x, y, 0)$ is essentially constant over each collimator hole and zero over the septa. At a short distance from the face of the multiple-hole collimator, where the fields of view of neighboring holes overlap

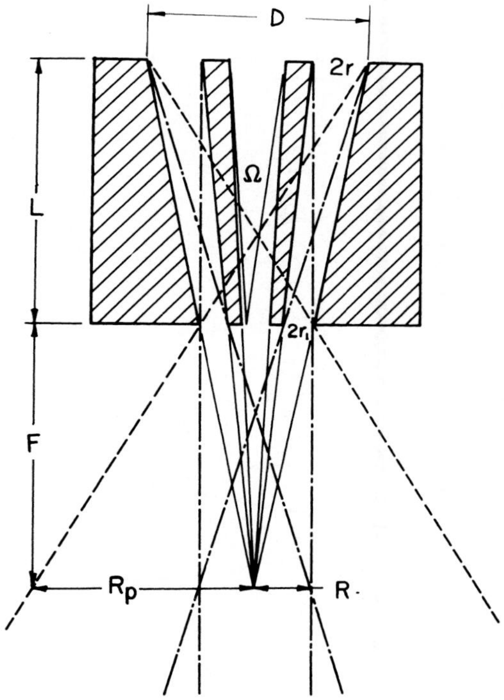

Figure 6.3. Multiple-Hole Focused Collimator. A focused collimator with practical length, high efficiency, and good spatial resolution can be designed for a relatively large-diameter crystal by use of an array of small holes with overlapping fields of view.

appreciably, the magnitude of $g(x, y, z)$ is essentially independent of (x, y) over the entire aggregate field of view, and falls to 0 fairly abruptly at the periphery of this field.

GEOMETRIC EFFICIENCY FOR PLANAR SOURCE

The discussion of geometric efficiency for single-hole collimators can be extended to multiple-hole collimators. For a uniform planar source that covers the geometric field of view of a collimator with N holes that are essentially identical, it follows from equation 6 that the geometric efficiency is given by

$$G = \frac{Na_1a_D}{4\pi L^2} \tag{16}$$

SPATIAL RESOLUTION

For multiple-hole focused collimators, the geometry factor is a superposition of the geometry factors for all holes. At the focal plane, the fields of view of the individual holes coincide with each other; that is, the field of view of the multiple-hole collimator is the same as that of the single hole. When the point source is not in the focal plane, the fields of view of the individual holes do not coincide. Here the field of view of the multiple array is larger than that of any individual hole.

If the largest distance between the hole centers in the collimator plane is small enough so that the condition expressed in equation 13 is satisfied, the point source response functions of various holes are essentially the same. Then the superposition of the point source response functions from the individual holes can be expressed mathematically by convolution of the functions with an appropriately scaled array of impulse functions. The latter represent the centers of the collimator holes and are usually arranged in a hexagonal array. From the convolution theorem, the geometric component of the transfer function of a multiple-hole collimator with holes in a completer hexagonal array is given by (8)

$$CTF_G^{\text{m.h.}}(\vec{\nu}) = CTF_G^{\text{s.h.}}(\vec{\nu}) \cdot H_M(\vec{\nu}, \theta; s) \tag{16}$$

where $CTF_G^{\text{s.h.}}(\vec{\nu})$ is the transfer function of a single hole as given by equation 12, $H_M(\vec{\nu}, \theta; s)$ is the normalized two-dimensional Fourier transform with $(M + 1)$ points on a side, s is the spacing between the impulses, and θ is the orientation of the hexagonal array with respect to the direction of the measured line spread function.

MULTIPLE-HOLE CAMERA COLLIMATORS

For scintillation cameras (9, 10), parallel-hole collimators, such as the type shown in Figure 6.4, have been the most widely used. However, collimators with converging-hole axes (6, 11, 12) and a single pinhole (13, 14) have been introduced to provide increased detector sensitivity and improved spatial resolution for imaging small organs such as the thyroid. Additionally, collimators with diverging-hole axes have been introduced (15) which provide a larger field of view for imaging the lungs, with some sacrifice in sensitivity and spatial resolution. Figure 6.5 shows the configurations and fields of view of four typical camera collimators. The diameters of the useful field of view of these collimators as a function of distance from the collimator face are shown in Figure 6.6. A review of the design and characteristics of the different camera collimator types is available (16).

GEOMETRIC FACTOR

For parallel-hole camera collimators, the magnitude of $g(x, y, z)$ is essentially independent of z because the area of the crystal that is seen through the collimator increases with distance z. This compensates for the decrease due to the inverse square law for each hole. For a practical collimator, the hole length is much larger than the diameter of the hole, and the geometry factor can be written as (17)

$$g(x, y, z) = g_0\left(\frac{a_{\text{open}}}{a_{\text{total}}}\right) = \left(\frac{a_{\text{open}}}{4\pi L^2}\right)\left(\frac{a_{\text{open}}}{a_{\text{total}}}\right) \tag{17}$$

where a_{open} is the area of the hole aperture at the back plane and a_{total} is the total area of a unit hole aperture including the septa. The first term on the right hand side of equation 17 represents the solid angle subtended by a collimator hole, and the second term represents the fraction of the camera crystal that is not covered by the septa. Explicit expressions of the hole open area a_{open}, unit hole area a_{total}, and geometric factor g_0 for collimator holes with different shapes areas, are shown in Table 6.1.

If the holes of the camera collimator have diverging axes, the magnitude of $g(x, y, z)$ decreases with z, as shown in Figure 6.7 for the response to a 3-inch disk source, for which these general statements are nevertheless valid.

Figure 6.4. Multiple-Hole Collimator for Scintillation Camera. Radius of view of a single hold is R' at focal distance F'; however, the image of a point source placed at this distance has a somewhat larger radius, R, on the crystal.

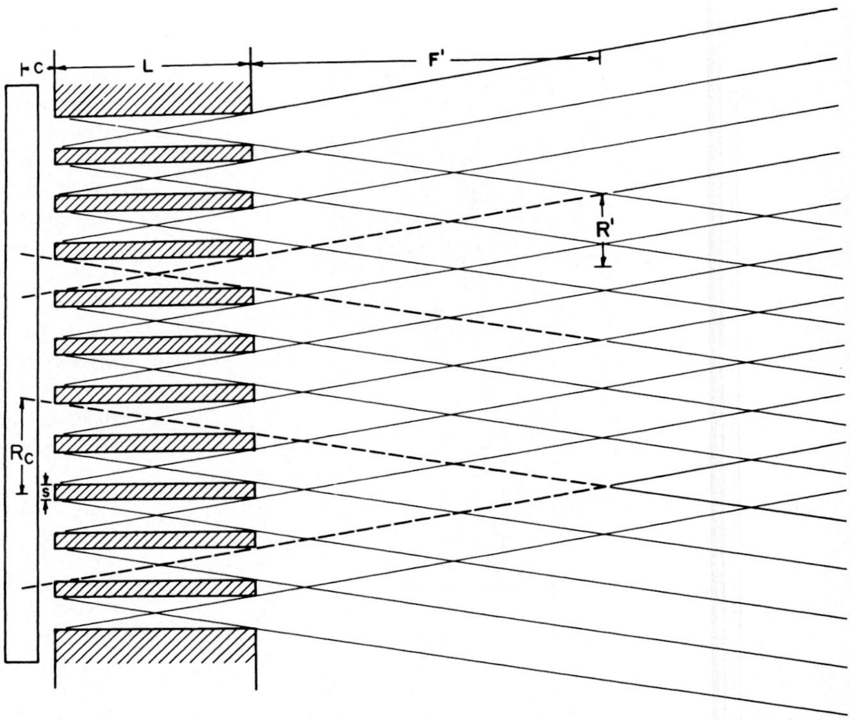

For converging camera collimators or focused collimators for scanners, $g(x, y, z)$ actually increases with increasing z, despite the inverse square law, because of the increasing overlap of the fields of view. For a focused collimator, $g(0, 0, z)$ is maximum at an axial point just inside the focal distance, that is, at a value of $z \lesssim F$. Beyond the focal distance, the geometry factor decreases in magnitude and spreads laterally.

GEOMETRIC EFFICIENCY

Unlike the situation for a multiple-hole focused collimator with a single detector system, the fields of view of collimators for scintillation camera systems are generally larger than the object to be imaged. Here the useful geometric efficiency is proportional to the fraction of the total collimator field of view that is covered by the object to be imaged. Thus, if the object has an area A_0 and the collimator of the scintillation camera has a field of view with area $A_C \leq A_0$, then the effective geometric efficiency of the collimator is

$$G_0 = \frac{A_0}{A_C} G = \left(\frac{A_0 N}{A_C}\right)\left(\frac{a_1 a_D}{4\pi L^2}\right) = \frac{N_0 a_1 a_D}{4\pi L^2} = N_0 a_1 g_0 \quad (18)$$

where N_0 is simply the number of holes covered by object and g_0 is defined by equation 2 with $z = 0$. This statement applies not only to parallel-hole collimators, but also to those with holes that diverge or converge.

SPATIAL RESOLUTION

In the process of image formation with a stationary scintillation camera, γ-rays detected at each position on the detector crystal are recorded essentially at the position of detection. The geometry factor $g(\mathbf{r}_0)$ is essentially constant for all points within the field of view on the z_0 plane, whereas the spatial density distribution of these events over the detector area (A_D), or the fraction per unit area at each point r_D, is described by

$$g'(\mathbf{r}_D; \mathbf{r}_0) \times \left(\frac{\text{photons directed toward } \mathbf{r}_D}{\text{cm}^2 - \text{sec}} \Big/ \frac{\text{photons emitted at } \mathbf{r}_0}{\text{sec}}\right]$$

which might be called the *differential geometry factor*. The geometry factor $g(\mathbf{r}_0)$ is simply the sum of the integral of the differential geometry factor over the entire detector area (A_D); that is,

$$g(\mathbf{r}_0) = \int\int_{-\infty}^{+\infty} A_D g'(\mathbf{r}_D; \mathbf{r}_0) d\mathbf{r}_D \quad (19)$$

The geometric component of the point source response function of a scintillation camera, due to collimator effects, is described by

$$p_{CG}(\mathbf{r}_D; \mathbf{r}_0) = \left[\frac{\text{counts at } \mathbf{r}_D}{\text{cm}^2 - \text{sec}} \Big/ \frac{\text{photons emitted at } \mathbf{r}_0}{\text{sec}}\right] = g(\mathbf{r}_D; \mathbf{r}_0)\eta\psi \quad (20)$$

If the total observation total is T(sec), the image of a point source at $\mathbf{r}_0$ that emits n_E (photons/sec) is described by

$$n_G(\mathbf{r}_D)\left(\frac{\text{counts}}{\text{cm}^2}\right) = c\left[\frac{\text{counts at } \mathbf{r}_D}{\text{cm}^2 - \text{sec}}\right] T[\text{sec}] = n_E(\mathbf{r}_0) p_{CG}(\mathbf{r}_D; \mathbf{r}_0) T = n_E(\mathbf{r}_0) g'(\mathbf{r}_D; \mathbf{r}_0)\eta\psi T \quad (21)$$

Therefore, the geometric component of the image of a point source at (x_0, y_0, z_0) formed by a scintillation camera,

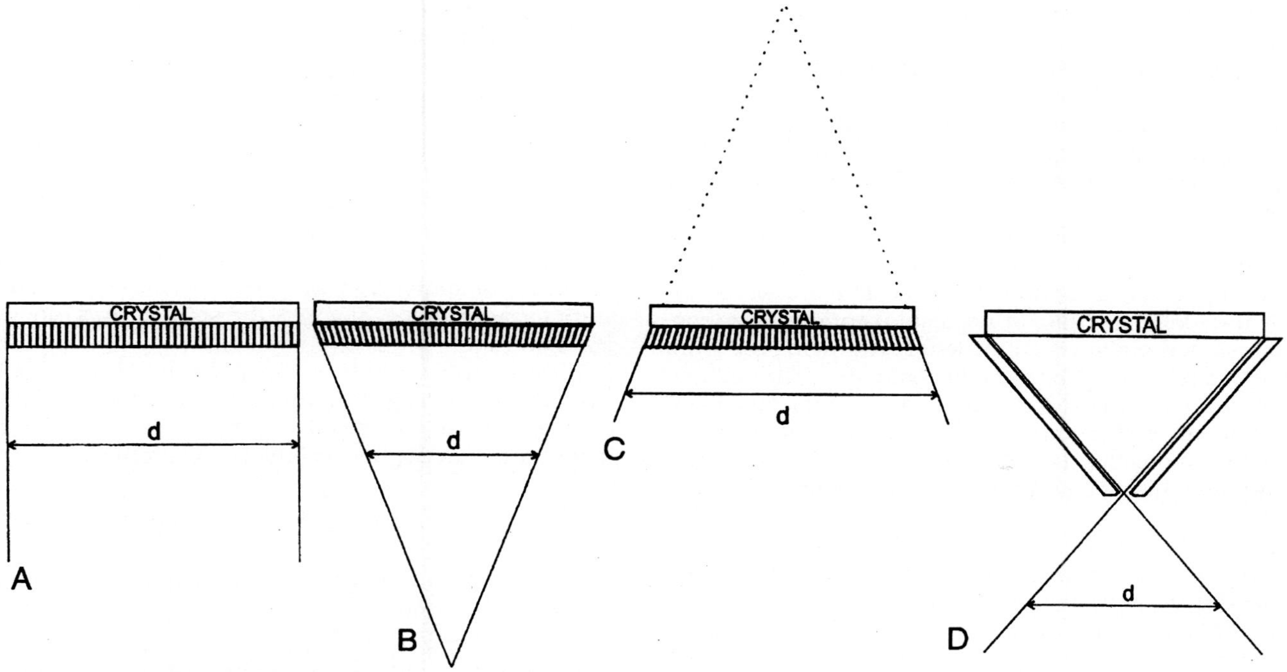

Figure 6.5. Schematic diagrams of the fields of view, *d*, of **(a)** parallel-hole, **(b)** converging-hole, **(c)** diverging-hole, and **(d)** pinhole camera collimators.

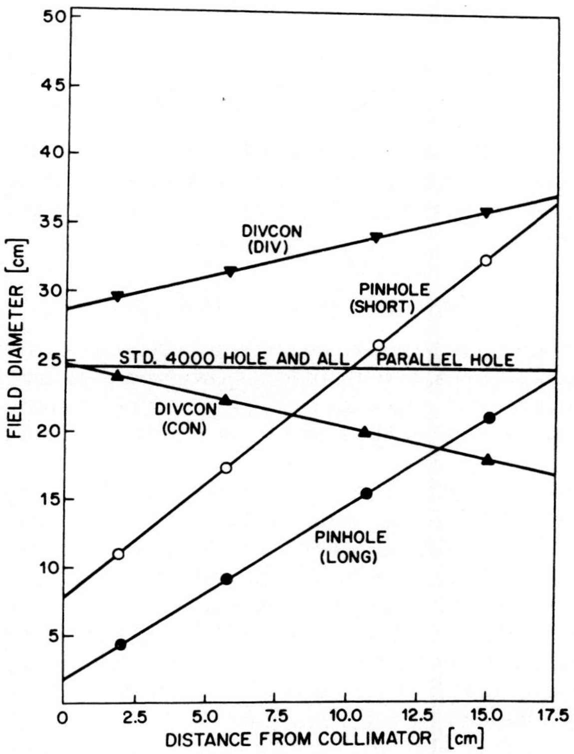

Figure 6.6. Collimator Fields of View. The useful field of view of collimators for scintillation cameras is essentially constant if the holes are parallel, and increases with distance for diverging and pinhole collimators. (DIV) = diverging, (CON) = converging.

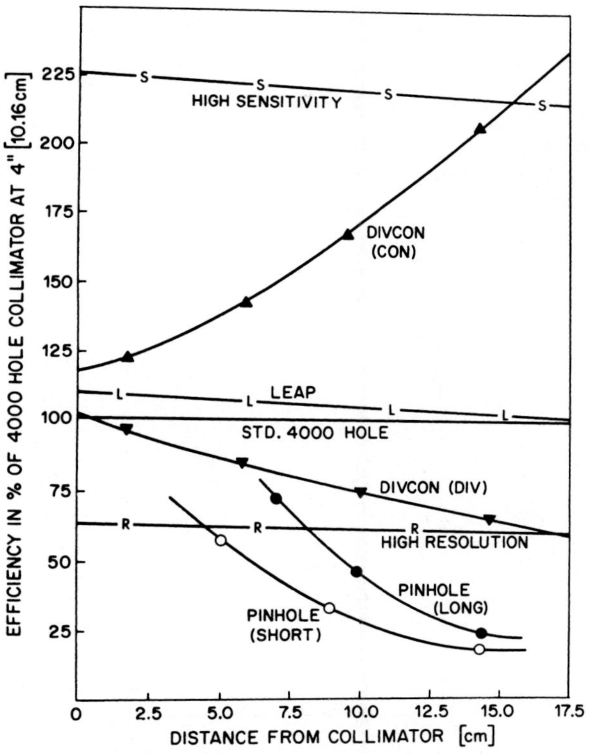

Figure 6.7. Collimator Efficiency. For most camera collimators, the response to a point source of Tc-99m is essentially constant or decreases with increasing distance from the collimator; however, if the axes of a multiple-hole collimator are made convergent, the geometry factor, and thus the response to a point source, increases with distance. Results shown here were obtained with a 3-inch disk source, for which these general statements are also valid. (CON) = converging, (DIV) = diverging.

has the same shape as $g'(\mathbf{r}_D; \mathbf{r}_0)$, the differential geometry factor.

The point source response function of a multiple-hole camera collimator depends on the position of the point source relative to the pattern of the hole array. For example, the point source response functions are different when the point source is directly in front of a collimator hole or a septum. To eliminate this positional dependence we can define an effective collimator point source response function of a parallel hole collimator to be the image of a point source that would be obtained if the collimator were uniformly translated (9, 18). For negligible septal penetration, the translation motion is equivalent to averaging the point source images formed for various positions of the collimator hole array relative to the point source. Thus, for a camera collimator with congruent straight parallel holes, we need only to consider the geometric effects of a single hole to determine the effective geometric point source response function.

Figure 6.8 shows the image formation of a point source by a single hole of arbitrary congruent shape. Without loss of generality we assume that the point source is located at $\mathbf{r}_0 = (0, 0, Z)$ or on the z axis and at a distance Z from the collimator face. Let $a(\vec{\xi})$ be the aperture function of the collimator hole at the front and back planes. When the axis of the collimator hole is centered over position $\mathbf{r}'$, the projections of the front and back apertures onto the image plane are given by

$$a_f^p(\mathbf{r}_D, \mathbf{r}) = a\{[Z/(Z + L + B)]\mathbf{r}_D - \mathbf{r}'\} \quad (22)$$

and

$$a_b^p(\mathbf{r}_D, \mathbf{r}') = a\{[(Z + L)/(Z + L + B)]\mathbf{r}_D - \mathbf{r}'\} \quad (23)$$

respectively, where L is the length of the collimator hole and B is the distance from the collimator back plane to the image plane.

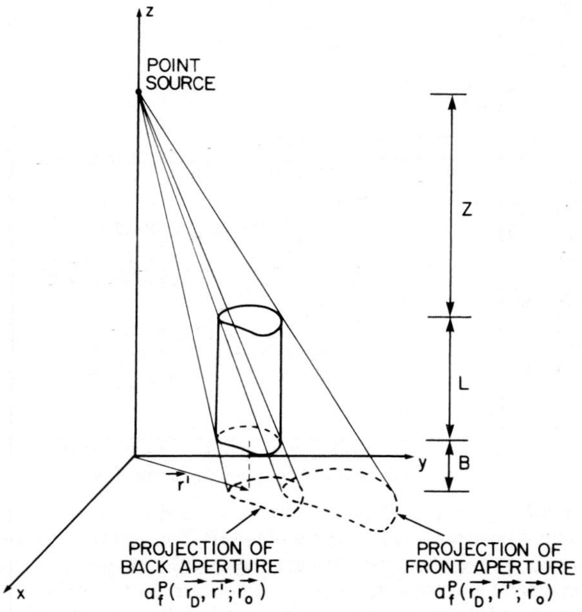

Figure 6.8. Camera-Type Collimator. Geometric relationship in the image-forming process of a single hole in a camera-type collimator.

The photon fluence reaching position r in the image plane due to a point source at r is given by (18)

$$\phi(\mathbf{r}_D, \mathbf{r}') = ka\left[\left(\frac{Z}{Z + L + B}\right)\mathbf{r}_D - \mathbf{r}'\right] \cdot a\left[\left(\frac{Z + L}{Z + L + B}\right)\mathbf{r}_D - \mathbf{r}'\right] \quad (24)$$

where k is proportional to $[(Z + L + B)^2 + |\mathbf{r}_D - \mathbf{r}_0|^2]^{-3/2}$ because of inverse square and cosine law effects. For most practical collimator designs, the value k is essentially constant for positions $\mathbf{r}_D$ at which the point spread function is non-zero.

If the collimator hole is translated to all possible locations $\mathbf{r}'$ during image formation, the resulting total photon fluence at $\mathbf{r}_D$, or the effective point source response function of the multiple hole collimator, is given by

$$\bar{\phi}(\mathbf{r}_D) = \int\int_{-\infty}^{+\infty} \phi(\mathbf{r}_D; \mathbf{r}')d\mathbf{r}' \quad (25)$$

By substitution of equation 24 in equation 25 and a change of variable, we find

$$\bar{\phi}(\mathbf{r}_D) = k\int\int_{-\alpha}^{+\alpha} a\left[\left(\frac{L}{Z + L + B}\right)\mathbf{r}_D - \mathbf{r}'\right] \cdot a(-\vec{\rho})d\vec{\rho} \quad (26)$$

The right hand side of equation 26 can be recognized as a convolution integral. Thus, the effective geometric transfer function is given by

$$CTF_G(\vec{\nu}) = \Phi(\vec{\nu})/\Phi(0) \quad (27)$$

where

$$\Phi(\vec{\nu}) = \text{F.T.}[\bar{\Phi}(\mathbf{r}_D)] \cong k \,\|\, A\left[\left(\frac{Z + L + B}{L}\right)\vec{\nu}\right]\Big|^2 \quad (28)$$

and $A(\vec{\nu})$ is the two-dimensional Fourier transform (F.T.) of the aperture function. Explicit expressions of $A(\vec{\nu})$ for four typical hole shapes can be derived (18) and are given in Table 6.1.

Measures of Spatial Resolution

It is convenient to regard an object as a spatial distribution of point sources, and its image as the superposition of images of these sources. In this sense, the point source response function enables one to account for the resultant image.

The degree of smoothing introduced by the imaging system depends on the shape of the point source response function, and increases with the width of this function. The degree of image smoothing that can be attributed to the collimator is determined by the shape (and especially the width) of $g(\mathbf{r})_D; \mathbf{r}_0)$ for scanners and by $g'(\mathbf{r}_D; \mathbf{r}_0)$ for cameras, at each distance from the collimator face. Commonly used measures of spatial resolution due to collimator geometry alone include

1. The maximum radius (R') of g or g' (4).
2. The full width at the half maximum height (FWHM) of g or g' (19).
3. The FWHM of the collimator image of a line source of radio-

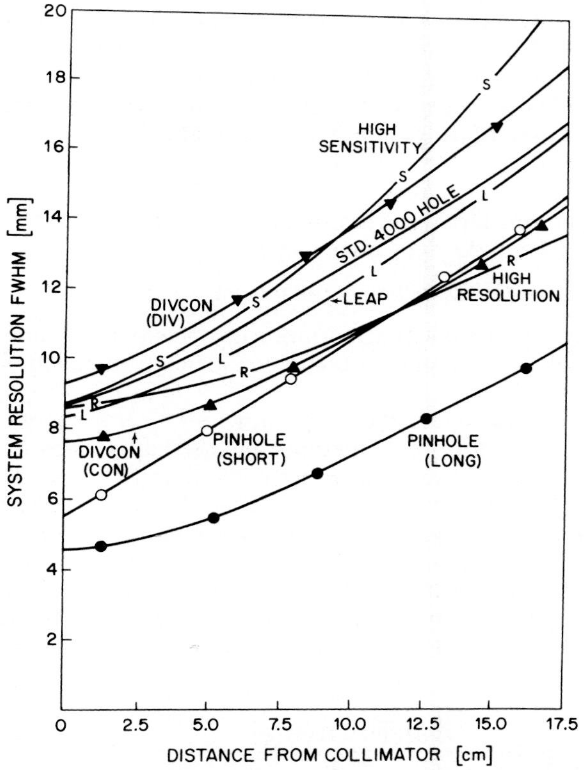

Figure 6.9. Measures of Spatial Resolution. The collimator resolution distance—that is, the full width at half-maximum height (FWHM) of a line source imaged with multiple-hole collimators, or the distance between two points sources imaged as tangent disks with pinhole collimators—is smallest near the collimator face. A scintillation camera with an intrinsic resolution of 8 mm FWHM for Tc-99m (140 KcV) was used. (DIV) = diverging, (CON) = converging.

activity, the shape of which, for a camera collimator, is described by

$$L(x_D;\ z_0) \propto \int_{-\alpha}^{+\alpha} g'(x_D,\ y_D;\ x_0,\ z_0)dy_D \tag{29}$$

for a line source parallel to the y axis (see Fig. 6.9).

4. The geometric component of the collimator transfer function $CTF_G(\vec{\nu})$, or spatial frequency response of the collimator (20), is defined by the normalized two-dimensional Fourier transform (F.T.) of g or g'; that is

$$CTF_G(\vec{\nu}) = \frac{\text{F.T.}[g'(\mathbf{r}_D;\ \mathbf{r}_0)]}{\int g'(\mathbf{r}_D;\ \mathbf{r}_0)d\mathbf{r}_D} \tag{30}$$

For scanner-type collimators with given hole size and shape, explicit expressions for $CTF_G(\nu)$ can be derived from equations 11 and 15 for single-hole and multiple-hole designs, respectively. For camera-type collimators with straight and parallel holes, the geometric component of the collimator transfer function is given by equations 27 and 28.

If g' is symmetric, then the normalized one-dimensional F.T. of $L(x_D;\ z_0)$ is adequate to describe the spatial frequency response in all directions (21, 22).

Clearly, to describe the spatial resolution of the entire imaging system, one can generalize all of these measures of collimator spatial resolution to include the effects of septal penetration, scattering, the intrinsic spatial resolution of the detector, and the recording device.

PRACTICAL CALCULATIONS OF RESOLUTION AND EFFICIENCY OF COLLIMATORS FOR THE SCINTILLATION CAMERA

In practice the spatial resolution of a collimated scintillation camera is generally measured with a line source that is small with respect to the resolution that is being measured, as shown in Figure 6.10. The FWHM of the profile or line spread function (LSF) across the line source is the measured system spatial resolution. For a parallel hole collimator with circular holes, the geometric resolution of the collimator alone can be calculated by

$$R_g = \frac{d(l_s + h)}{l_s} \tag{31}$$

where h is the distance from the center of the line source, d is the hole diameter, and $l_s = L - 2/\mu$ is the actual hole length L reduced by the effects of septal penetration of the collimator constructed of material with linear attenuation μ. To calculate the geometric resolution of converging, diverging, and pinhole collimators, additional factors must be added to equation 6.31 (23).

The geometric resolution of the collimator is only one of the two major factors that determine the spatial resolution of the scintillation camera system. The other factor is the intrinsic resolution of the scintillation detector R_i. The system resolution R_s is given by

$$R_s = \sqrt{R_i^2 + R_g^2} \tag{32}$$

This calculated value can be compared to the measured FWHM of the LSF to verify construction parameters.

For a parallel hole collimator, the efficiency G may be calculated by

$$G = K^2(d/l_s)^2[d^2/(d + s)^2] \tag{33}$$

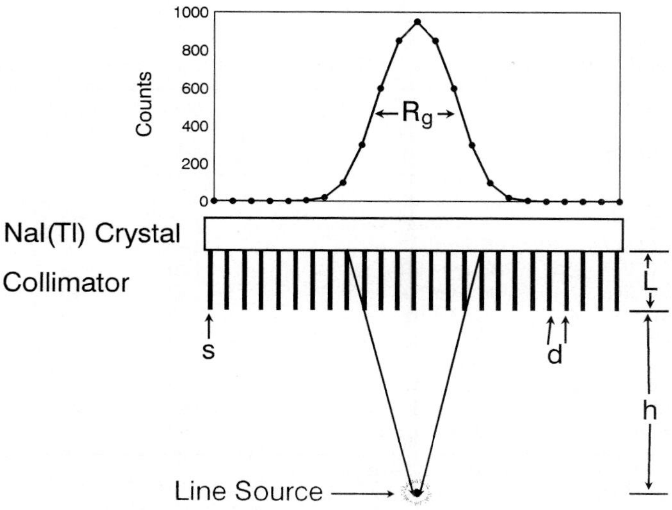

Figure 6.10. Measurement of spatial resolution. In practice, the FWHM of a count profile measured across a small line source is used to determine the spatial resolution of a collimated detector system.

where s is the septal thickness and K is a constant that takes into account the shape of the holes ($K = 0.24$ and 0.26 for round and hexagonal holes respectively in a hexagonal array, $K = 0.28$ for square holes in a square array). As with geometrical resolution calculations, additional geometric factors must be added for other collimator types (23).

DEPTH OF FIELD

The concept of depth of field is associated with the range of depths in object space ($z_{min} \leq z_0 \leq z_{max}$) over which the spatial resolution is regarded as being adequate; therefore, any quantitative measure of depth of field must depend not only on the measure of spatial resolution that is adopted, but also on the notion of adequacy. Universal agreement on these issues has not been achieved. It is, nevertheless, possible to discuss the qualitative implications of the depth of field concept.

For example, for focused collimators, all of the earlier mentioned measures of spatial resolution imply that the best resolution occurs at the focal distance. If the spatial resolution rapidly becomes worse for planes a short distance away from the focal plane, the collimator is said to have a short depth of field and will produce images in which only those structures near the focal plane are adequately resolved. This is typical of high resolution focused collimators designed for large-diameter crystals, and can be used to produce a tomographic effect that reduces the interference due to structures in other planes.

For multiple-hole camera collimators, the best resolution is near the collimator face. The resolution is degraded slowly with distance from the collimator face if the ratio of collimator length to hole diameter ($L/2r$)b is large (24).

EFFECTS OF SEPTAL PENETRATION

Septal penetration is commonly specified for a single septal thickness, as shown in Figure 6.11. If an incident γ-ray passes through a single septum only, the shortest path length through the septum for the γ-ray to pass from one hole to the next is w. From geometric considerations, the relationship between the septal thickness s, the length L, diameter d of the collimator holes, and w is given by

$$s = 2dw/(L - w) \quad (34)$$

For a given septal thickness w, the fraction of γ-rays passing through the septum is given by

$$\textit{Fraction Transmitted} = e^{-\mu w} \quad (35)$$

where μ is the linear attenuation coefficient of the material from which the collimator is constructed (typically lead) (23).

Table 6.2 shows typical parameters for low energy collimators (<200 keV), medium energy collimators (<400 keV), and an ultra-high energy collimator (511 keV). These data show how the factors previously discussed determine spatial resolution and efficiency of collimators. Although septal penetration is quoted for a single septum, the Figure may be misleading. For example, it is estimated that the plane source sensitivity shown in the Table for the ultra-high energy collimator includes approximately 50% pene-

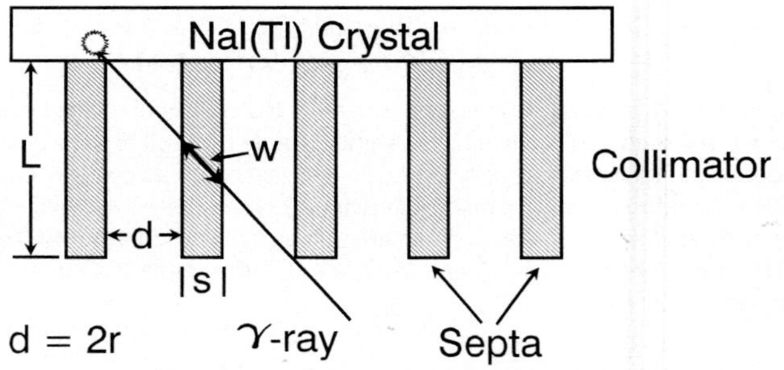

Figure 6.11. Calculation of single-hole septal penetration. Septal penetration for a single septum between two adjacent holes is determined by calculating w from geometric considerations and using the attenuation equation.

Table 6.2.
Collimator Specifications of Selected Collimators for Routine Clinical Use

Collimator	Application	Maximum Energy (keV)	Core Length (mm)	Hole Diameter (mm)	Septal Thickness (mm)	Septal Penetration (%)	System Res. FWHM (mm) @ 100 mm	Sensitivity Cts/min/μCi
LEUHS	Cardiac 1st Pass	140	25.4	3.31	0.356	2.6	19.4	1520
LEMS	Thallium & Multi-gated	140	25.4	1.75	0.205	2.1	10.8	430
LEGP	General	140	35	1.9	0.2	0.9	9.0	270
LEHR	Bone Scans	140	35	1.5	0.2	0.2	7.2	160
LEUHR	Brain SPECT	140	40	1.5	0.2	0.1	6.8	120
MEGP	$^{67}Ga/^{111}In$	300	58	3	1.05	2.0	10.0	160
HEGP	^{131}I	360	66	4	1.8	2.0	11.7	190
UHEGP	Positrons	511	80	4	2.5	3.9	14.9	110
LEUHR—FB	Brain SPECT	140	40	1.5	0.2	0.1	6.3	220
LEGP—FB	Cardiac SPECT	140	29	1.9	0.2	0.8	10.3	490
Pinhole	Small Organs	360	—	6	—	—	7.0	136

LEUHS = Low Energy Ultra High Sensitivity
LEMS = Low Energy Medium Sensitivity
LEGP = Low Energy General Purpose
LEHR = Low Energy High Resolution
LEUHR = Low Energy Ultra High Resolution
MEGP = Medium Energy General Purpose
HEGP = High Energy General Purpose
UHEGP = Ultra High Energy General Purpose
LEUHR—FB = Low Energy Ultra High Resolution Fan Beam
LEGP—FB = Low Energy General Purpose Fan Beam
Collimator Data provided by Elscint, Inc., Hackensack, NJ.

tration events. This results in a significant reduction in image contrast. However, even with this significant penetration, acceptable image quality is attainable with this collimator in imaging 511 keV γ-rays from positron emitters and clinically acceptable diagnostic images of the heart can be obtained with ^{18}FDG (25).

In a well-designed multiple-hole collimator, the septa between holes block most of the γ-rays that fail to travel through a collimator hole. However, some γ-rays will always penetrate septa and appear in the image. For low energy radiation, the penetration is not a significant design problem, but for γ-rays greater than about 200 keV, septal penetration can be an important consideration in collimator design. As the photon energy increases, the attenuation coefficient of the septal materials decreases, and more γ-rays penetrate through the septa to degrade the image. In extreme cases of septal penetration, a distinctive pattern appears in the image. For a point source image, spokes appear to project symmetrically from the point image. These spokes give the overall image a star-like appearance. Where more complicated sources are imaged, the star patterns overlap to create streaks through the image. The star like pattern appears because the penetrations occur preferentially through the thinnest portion of the collimator septa. For collimator holes set in a regular array, the septa will always appear thinnest in the direction aligned with the rows of holes. In less extreme cases of septal penetration, the star-like pattern may not be visible; nonetheless, the penetration effect appears as a diffused background to the image. The response function for penetrating photons is very broad and unpeaked compared to the geometric response. Thus, the penetration response has little effect on the spatial resolution as measured by either the FWHM or the high frequency cutoff f, at which the collimator transfer function $CTF_G(\vec{\nu})$ is equal to 0. Rather, the effect is primarily to reduce the detector *MTF* in the midfrequency range, which reduces image contrast (21).

Septal penetration makes the design of a collimator for high energy γ-rays a difficult task. The simple geometric argument described earlier does not account for the exponential attenuation of radiation passing through the collimator material. Attempts to analyze penetration generally begin with the definition of the penetration fraction (f_p) as the ratio

$$f_p = \frac{\text{No. of primary photons that penetrate the septa}}{\text{No. of primary photons that pass through the holes}} \quad (31)$$

for a uniform planar source that covers the field of view. Clearly, the penetration fraction is a function of septal thickness, γ-ray energy E, attenuation coefficient λ_E (cm^{-1}) of the collimator material, and the hole dimensions. Although the exact dependence of f_p on these parameters is not known precisely, formulas for estimating f_p have been proposed by various workers (4–6, 26–28). In most of these approaches to collimator design, the goal is to maximize sensitivity for fixed geometric collimator resolution and some acceptable penetration fraction. Typically, values of $f_p \leq 0.1$ are regarded as acceptable.

In principle, septal penetration can be reduced by use of a collimator material with a large attenuation coefficient. For example, a collimator can be made from gold or tungsten, rather than lead, to reduce penetration. Unfortunately, there are only a limited number of such dense, high-Z, materials available, and few of these are economical. A second method is to increase the septal thickness, while scaling other collimator dimensions to preserve the required spatial resolution. Unfortunately, this simple scaling is of limited value when the hole size and separation exceed the intrinsic resolution of the camera, resulting in a visible hole pattern in the image. This hole pattern may degrade the image worse than the penetration it is intended to cure.

Over the last decade, the demand for collimators suitable for high energy γ-rays (particularly 511 keV annihilation radiation) has spurred considerable effort in collimator design. Sophisticated computer programs have replaced crude analytic estimates of septal penetration (29–31). The idea of these programs is to trace individual γ-rays through the collimator. The probability of attenuation of each ray is determined by the distance traversed within the septal material. The point source response function is then reconstructed by combining the attenuated intensity from many (10^5) rays to form an image. The resultant point source response function is the most accurate predictor of collimator performance presently available. Figure 6.12 shows the point source response function for a 511 keV source located at 10 cm above a collimator designed for imaging ^{82}Rb (31). The central peak represents the geometric response of the collimator, while the long exponential tail represents the septal penetration. The collimator sensitivity, determined by integrating the point source response function is 1.34×10^{-4}. The penetration tail for radii greater than 1.2 cm contributes less than 10% of the counts in the point source response function. Fifty percent of the counts lie within 0.6 cm of the center of the point source response functions. Such detailed predictions of collimator performance will assist significantly in developing new designs of collimator design for high energy radiation. Even with such programs, optimizing collimator design for high energy γ-rays will continue to be limited by the materials available and by the visibility of the hole pattern in the image.

EFFECTS OF SCATTERED RADIATION

Mather (32) has shown that the response due to scattered radiation from the walls of a lead collimator is negligible compared to the geometric response, even for collimators with a large ratio of hole length to diameter. Conversely, the response to photons that have been scattered within the patient may be appreciable with scintillation detectors (30), which have relatively poor energy resolution. The scatter fraction (f) is defined by the ratio

$$f_S = \frac{\text{No. of recorded events due to scattered photons}}{\text{No. of recorded events due to primary photons}} \quad (32)$$

As with septal penetration, the response to scattered photons, which may be due to γ-rays emitted in all parts of the source, is very broad and unpeaked relative to $g(x,$

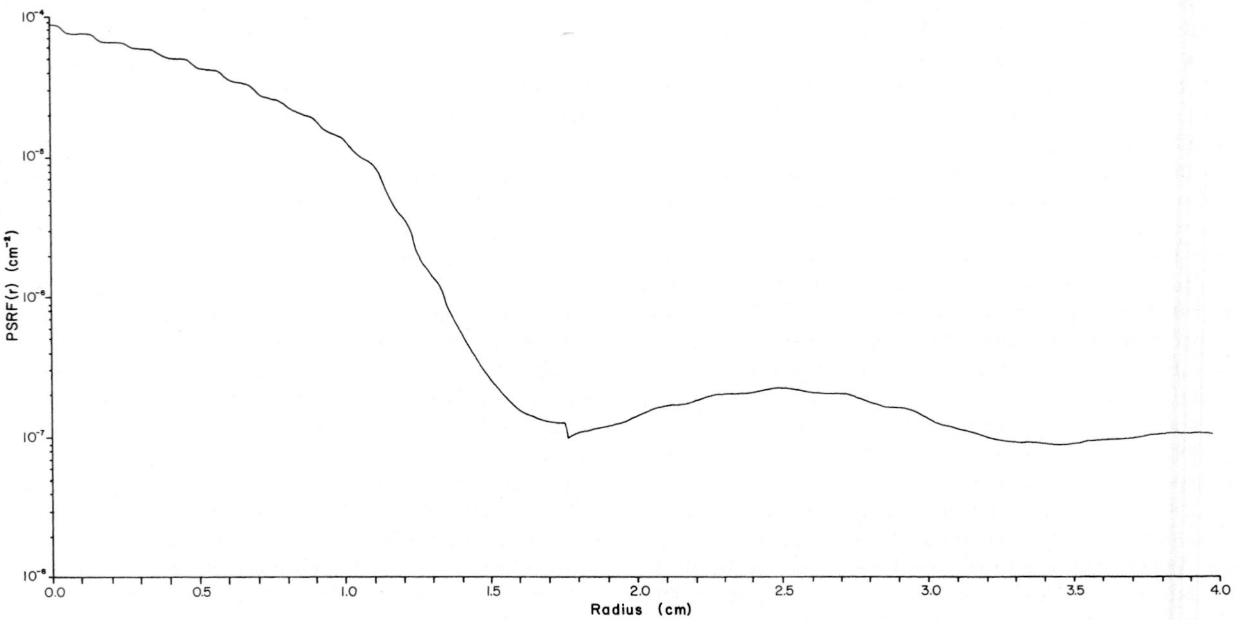

Figure 6.12. Point Source Response Function at 511 keV. The point source response function of an experimental collimator at 511 KeV. A long penetration "trail" is due to the high-energy radiation passing thorugh many septa.

y, z). Consequently, the principal effect of the recording of scattered photons is reduced image contrast, not increased FWHM (34–35).

For a detector system with a given energy resolution, the scatter fraction can be reduced by raising the baseline discriminator level. However, above a certain level the detection of primary radiation will be decreased concurrently. Based on the figure-of-merit criterion, an optimum baseline setting can be determined, which results in a compromise between increased image contrast and decreased detection efficiency (36). A more effective method of minimizing scattered radiation is the use of detectors with good energy resolution (34). For example, solid state semiconductor detectors have much better energy resolution that NaI(Tl) detectors; however, their detection efficiency is too low to be practical.

The effects of scattered radiation can be reduced by subtracting the scatter component from the detected image (37). This technique is only approximate because scatter fraction is a function of the depth of the source. Scatter subtraction techniques can increase image contrast, but only at the expense of the loss of detected counts. Since the scatter component of the detector response is broadly peaked instead of flat, the scattered radiation carries a certain amount of spatial information. Appropriate utilization of such information should enhance the detected image while maintaining the detection efficiency (21).

A more complete understanding of the effects of scattered radiation can be obtained using the Monte Carlo method of computer simulation (38, 39). Through such simulation studies, detailed descriptions of the spatial and energy distributions of the scattered radiation can be produced. This detailed information is useful in an understanding of the effects of scattered radiation and is important in the design of scatter correction and utilization methods that improve the detected image quality.

SUMMARY

In general, we may conclude that

1. Focused collimators do not bend or refract γ-rays as lenses refract light.
2. Focused collimators do not respond solely or even preferentially to radioactivity in the focal plane, in terms of the magnitude of response; however, the spatial resolution tends to be best for this plane.
3. The geometric efficiency tends to increase with increased detector area and area of view, and to decrease with increased focal length, collimator length, and γ-ray energy. In general, the functional dependence depends upon which parameters are assumed to be fixed.
4. The collimator does not selectively accept or reject photons from a large-volume distribution of radioactivity that are scattered at any particular angle or range of angles.
5. The effect of septal penetration, as well as scattering in the patient, is primarily to reduce image contrast.
6. The collimator is perhaps the weakest link in the image-forming chain of components for both scanners and cameras in that it limits detector sensitivity, spatial resolution, and depth of field. For these reasons, an understanding of the effects of the collimator on the image is of special importance.

ACKNOWLEDGMENTS

The authors are especially grateful to Dr. Robert A. Moyer of Searle Radiographics, Incorporated, for permission to publish the data contained in Figures 6.5, 6.6, and 6.8.

REFERENCES

1. Garrett MW. Solid angle subtended by a circular aperture. Rev Sci Instr 1954;25:1208.

2. Jaffey AH. Solid angle subtended by a circular aperture at point and spread sources: formulas and some tables. Rev Sci Instr 1954;254:349.
3. Masket AVH, Rogers WC. Tables of solid angles. Chapel Hill, NC: University of North Carolina, 1962.
4. Beck RN. A theoretical evaluation of brain scanning systems. J Nucl Med 1961;2:314.
5. Beck RN Collimators for radioisotope scanning system. In: Medical radioisotope scanning. Vol. 1. Vienna: IAEA, 1964:211.
6. Beck RN. Collimation of gamma rays. In: Gottschalk A, Beck RN, eds. Fundamental problems in scanning. Ch. 6. Springfield, IL: Charles C. Thomas, 1968.
7. Newell RR, Saunders W, Miller E. Multichannel collimators for γ-rays scanning with scintillation counters. Nucleonics 1962;10:36.
8. Metz CE, Tsui BMW, Beck RN. Theoretical prediction of the geometric transfer function for focused collimator. J Nucl Med 1974; 15:1078.
9. Anger HP. Scintillation camera with multichannel collimators. J Nucl Med 1964;5:515.
10. Anger HP. Radioisotope cameras. In: Hine GJ, ed. Instrumentation in nuclear medicine. Vol. 1. New York: Academic Press, 1967:485–552.
11. Dowdey JE, Graham KD, Bonte FJ. Collimator magnification of scintillation camera images. J Nucl Med 1971;12:352.
12. Moyer RA: A low-energy multihole converging collimator compared with a pinhole collimator. J Nucl Med 1974;15:59.
13. Anger HO, Rosenthal DJ. Scintillation camera and positron camera. In Medical Radioisotope Scanning. Vol. 1 Vienna: IAEA, 1959:59.
14. Mallard JR, Myers MJ. The performance of a gamma camera for the visualization of radioactive isotope in vivo. Phys Med Biol 1963;8:165.
15. Muehllehar G. A diverging collimator of γ-ray imaging cameras. J Nucl Med 1969;10:197.
16. Tsui BMW. Collimator design, properties, and characteristics. In: Simmons GH, ed. The scintillation camera. Ch. 2. New York: The Society of Nuclear Medicine, 1988.
17. Muehllehar G, Dudeh J, Moyer R. Influence of hole shape on collimator performance. Phys Med Biol 1976;21:242.
18. Metz CE, Atkins FB, and Beck RN. The geometric transfer function component for scintillation camera collimators with straight parallel holes. Phys Med Biol 1980;25:1059.
19. Borwnell GL. Spatial resolution. In: Gottschalk A, Beck RN, eds. Fundamental problems in scanning. Ch. 4. Springfield, IL: Charles C. Thomas, 1968.
20. Beck RN. Nomenclature for Fourier transforms of spread functions of imaging systems used in nuclear medicine. J Nucl Med 1972;13:704.
21. Beck RN, Zimmer LT, Charleston DB, Harper PV, Hoffer PB. Advances in fundamental aspects of imaging systems and techniques. In: Medical Radioisotope Scintigraphy. Vol. 1. Vienna: IAEA, 1973:3.
22. MacIntyre WJ, Fedoruk SO, Harris CC, Kuhl DE, Mallard JR. Sensitivity and resolution in radioisotope scanning, In: Proceedings of the IAEA Symposium on Medical Radioisotope Scintigraphy. Vienna: IAEA, 1969.
23. Sorenson JA, Phelps ME. The Anger camera: performance characteristics. In: Physics in nuclear medicine. 2d ed. Orlando, FL: Grune & Stratton, Inc., 1987:331–345.
24. Gottschalk A. Modulation transfer function studies with the gamma scintillation camera. In: Gottschalk A, Beck RN, eds. Fundamental problems in scanning. Ch. 27. Springfield, IL: Charles C. Thomas, 1968.
25. Martin WH, Delbeke D, Patton JA, et al. ^{18}FDG-SPECT: correlation with ^{18}FDG-PET. J Nucl Med, 1995, in press.
26. Husak V, Perinova V, Kleinbauer K. Design of multichannel focused collimators for scintillation scanning. In: Proceedings of the IAEA Symposium on Medical Radioisotope Scintigraphy. Vienna: IAEA, 1969.
27. Keller EL. Optimum dimensions of parallel-hole multi-aperture collimators for gamma-ray cameras. J Nucl Med 1968;99:233.
28. Walker WG. Design and analysis of scintillation camera lead collimators using a digital computer. In: Proceedings of the IAEA Symposium on Medical Radioisotope Scintigraphy. Vienna: IAEA, 1969.
29. Muehllehar G, Luig H. Septal penetration in scintillation camera collimators. Phys Med Biol 1973;18:855.
30. Jahns MF. The influence of penetrating radiation in collimator performance. Phys Med Biol 1981;26:113.
31. Beck RN, Retung LD. Collimator designs using ray-tracing techniques. IEEE Trans Nucl Sci, 1985;NS31:865.
32. Mather RL. Gamma-ray collimator penetration and scattering effects. J Appl Physics 1957;28:1200.
33. Beck RN, Schuh MW, Cohen TD, Lembares N. Effects of scattered radiation on scintillation detector response. In: Proceedings of the IAEA Symposium on Medical Radioisotope Scintigraphy. Vienna: IAEA, 1969.
34. Beck RN, Zimmer LT, Charleston DB, Hoffer PB, Lembares N. The theoretical advantages of eliminating scatter in imaging system. In: Hoffer PB, Beck RN, Gottschalk A, eds. Semiconductor detectors in the future of nuclear medicine. Ch. 7. New York: The Society of Nuclear Medicine, 1971.
35. Ehrhardt JC, Oberley LW, Lensink SC. Effect of a scattering medium on gamma-ray imaging. J Nucl Med 1974;15:943.
36. Atkins FB, Beck RN, Hoffer PB, Palmer D: Dependence of optimum baseline setting on scatter fraction and detector response function. In: Medical radionuclide imaging. Vol. 1. Vienna: IAEA, 1977:101.
37. Bloch P, Sanders T. Reduction of the effects of scattered radiation on a sodium iodine imaging system. J Nucl Med 1973;14:67.
38. Dresser M. Scattering effects in radioisotope imaging [Dissertation]. Ann Arbor, MI: University of Michigan, University Microfilms, 1972: MI #73-6821.
39. Atkins FB. Monte Carlo analysis of photon scattering in radionuclide imaging [Dissertation]. Chicago: The University of Chicago, 1978.

7 Anger Scintillation Camera

L. STEPHEN GRAHAM and GERD MUEHLLEHNER

The Anger scintillation camera is the standard instrument of choice for imaging both static and dynamic radionuclide distributions in vivo. Since its commercial introduction in 1964 (1), it has improved dramatically in all of the basic performance parameters: field-of-view, uniformity, spatial resolution, energy resolution, and the ability to handle high incident count rates. Its evolution was shaped by the need to faithfully image the 140 keV γ-rays emitted by ^{99m}Tc. The combination of this generator-produced radionuclide and the Anger camera has provided the nuclear medicine physician with a powerful tool that has contributed to the continued growth of the field of nuclear medicine.

While other approaches to imaging low-energy γ-rays were explored (e.g., image intensifiers, solid-state detectors, or position-sensitive proportional chambers), changes in the Anger camera have kept it as the instrument of choice for a wide variety of clinical studies. One of the major milestones occurred in 1977, when the original prototype of today's SPECT cameras was introduced by Jaszczak (2), based on principles described in 1963 by Kuhl and Edwards (3). Apart from continued improvement in detector performance and stability, recent developments have focused on increases in sensitivity (multiple detectors and the use of magnifying collimators), the addition of features which enhance image quality, such as the ability to perform noncircular orbits, and the use of extremely powerful computers for analysis and display of images. In many state-of-the-art systems operation of the camera is fully integrated into the computer.

This chapter outlines the principles of operation of the modern Anger scintillation camera, describes its fundamental performance parameters, and summarizes recent improvements.

PRINCIPLES OF OPERATION

Figure 7.1 shows a block diagram of an Anger camera. An image of the radionuclide distribution is formed in a thin thallium-activated sodium iodide [NaI(Tl)] scintillation crystal by the action of the collimator. γ-Rays can reach the detector primarily by passing through holes in the collimator. Visible and ultraviolet light produced in the crystal at the site of interaction travels outward in all directions and is detected by an array of photomultipliers that converts the light distribution into a set of electronic signals. The position logic circuit converts these voltage pulses into x and y position signals by calculating the centroid of the light distribution. The position signals are then divided by the energy signal so that image size will be independent of the incident γ-ray energy. This subset of the electronics is called the ratio circuit. Only those events that fall within a specific energy range corresponding to the photon energy(ies) of the administered radionuclide are used for further processing. The position and energy signals are then corrected by digital processors that compensate for imperfections in the crystal/photomultiplier assembly and in the position logic circuit. Finally, the processed x and y position information is used to form an image of the radionuclide distribution one event at a time either on an analog display system such as a high resolution cathode ray tube (CRT) or in digital memory. A number of vendors also include special circuits that automatically balance the photomultiplier tubes. This operation minimizes the effect of drift and aging of electronic components.

COLLIMATION

The collimator projects an image of the radionuclide distribution onto the scintillation crystal by absorbing γ-rays that do not travel in the desired direction. Although collimation is covered in considerable detail in a later chapter, it is appropriate to present a brief overview here. The first cameras were fitted with pinhole collimators (4). An inverted, mirror image was formed on the detector with the image size determined by the position of the object relative to the aperture. Because of its low sensitivity due to the small aperture size (3–10 mm), it is now commonly used only for imaging small objects such as the thyroid or lachrymal glands. In these cases high resolution images can be obtained because of magnification.

Markedly higher sensitivity for larger objects is provided by parallel hole collimators, the most commonly used type (1). The image of a radionuclide distribution is projected onto the detector without magnification. These collimators can be modified to provide the appropriate spatial resolution/sensitivity for a wide variety of clinical needs and properly handle photons from many different radionuclides. A variant of this design is the slant hole collimator used for gated blood-pool imaging. By setting the holes at an angle of 30° compared to the normal configuration, the collimator face can be positioned closer to the patient in the left anterior oblique (LAO) view.

Diverging collimators are used when the object is larger than the field-of-view of parallel hole collimators. Because the holes are aligned so they focus to a point behind the detector, the image is minified. These collimators were developed primarily to accommodate large organs, such as the liver, spleen, or both lungs, with a small-field-of-view camera (5). The increased field of view must, however, be traded for decreased resolution and/or lower sensitivity. With the advent of large-field-of-view circular and rectangular detectors, the need for these collimators has largely been eliminated. However, single-axis diverging collimators are still used on a few systems for whole body imaging.

Figure 7.1. Anger scintillation camera.

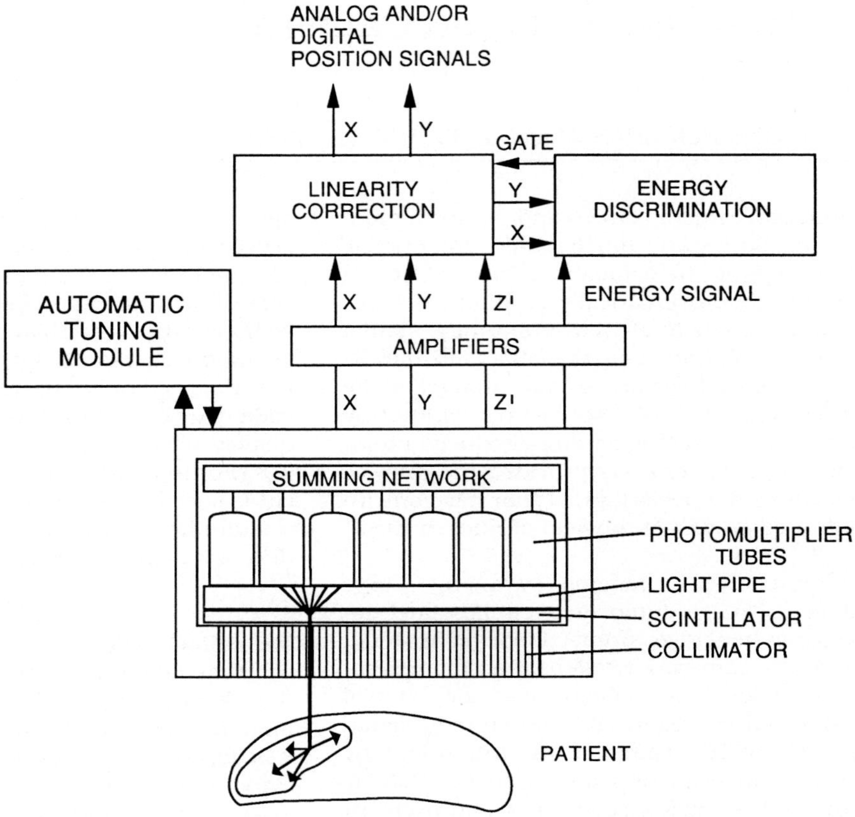

Converging collimators are similar to diverging collimators except that the holes are focused to a point in front of the detector. As such, they magnify the object—usually to a lesser degree than pinhole collimators—and provide better resolution and sensitivity than a comparable parallel-hole collimator (6). Because the magnification changes as a function of distance from the surface of the collimator, the projected image will have a different appearance than the image obtained with a parallel-hole collimator (7). Objects that are farther from the collimator face are more highly magnified.

γ-RAY DETECTION

After passing through the collimator holes the γ-rays may interact with the NaI(Tl) scintillation crystal. At low energies (<100 keV) the primary mode of interaction is photoelectric and the stopping power is essentially 100% (Table 7.1). As photon energy increases the probability of Compton scatter in the crystal increases and the stopping power decreases rapidly. When a γ-ray is scattered in the crystal, it may either escape from the crystal, interact by a photoelectric event, or undergo multiple scattering and finally be totally absorbed within the crystal. If all the energy is deposited in the crystal by one or more events, the energy signal will fall within the photopeak and the photon will be used in the image formation process. Table 7.1 shows the probabilities of a photoelectric interaction and total photopeak interaction as a function of crystal thickness and γ-ray-energy (8). If the first interaction in the crystal is a single photoelectric event, all the light is emitted from a region less than 1 mm in diameter. However, if the γ-ray first interacts by one or more Compton scatter interactions and finally deposits all of its energy in the crystal, the position logic circuit will calculate a set of x,y coordinates that does not correspond to the point of entry into the crystal. This scenario produces a loss of spatial resolution which is even more serious at high energies (8, 9). At lower energies (<140 keV), loss of spatial resolution is primarily due to the limited amount of light emitted by the crystal, as discussed later. Thus, there are two competing effects. As the energy of the γ-ray increases, more energy is deposited in the crystal and more light is emitted. Because the amount of light is approximately proportional to the energy of the γ-ray (10), this should produce improved spatial resolution. However, as the energy of the γ-ray increases, a larger fraction of the total photopeak interactions are of the Compton-photoelectric type, which produces inaccurate positional information. As spatial resolution has improved over the years, the change has been more significant at lower energies, as can be seen from the data presented in Figure 7.2.

LIGHT DISTRIBUTION AND EVENT LOCALIZATION

The light released from thallium in a NaI crystal spreads out in all directions. Because NaI is hygroscopic, it is enclosed in a container that has an aluminum entrance "window" and a glass exit window. To minimize the loss of light at interfaces, a silicon compound or special bonding ma-

Table 7.1.
Probabilities of Photopeak and Photoelectric Interactions in Sodium Iodide for Various Crystal Thicknesses[a]

γ-Ray Energy (keV)	Photopeak			Photoelectric		
	6.25 mm	9.52 mm[b]	12.5 mm	6.25 mm	9.52 mm[b]	12.5 mm
100	0.965	0.97	0.900	0.863	0.87	0.882
150	0.707	0.85	0.909	0.568	0.66	0.707
200	0.452	0.60	0.715	0.332	0.43	0.487
280	0.236	0.34	0.444	0.148	0.20	0.245
360	0.143	0.22	0.298	0.078	0.11	0.136
511	0.071	0.12	0.169	0.034	0.045	0.056

[a]Data from Anger HO, Davis DH. Gamma-ray detection efficiency and image resolution in sodium iodide. Rev Sci Instr 1964;35:693.
[b]Values determined by nonlinear interpolation of data from Anger HO, Davis DH. Gamma-ray detection efficiency and image resolution in sodium iodide. Rev Sci Instr 1964;35:693.

terial is used to optically couple the glass exit window of the detector "can" to the "light pipe" and/or photomultiplier tube (many newer cameras no longer have "light pipes"). When light reaches the photomultiplier tube many photons interact with the photocathode which releases electrons. This signal is then amplified by a series of electrodes called dynodes set at increasingly higher voltages. In the photocathode plane, the light intensity has a bell-shaped distribution with its center directly above the point of scintillation. The photomultipliers sample this distribution at discrete intervals. When the photomultipliers are moved closer to the crystal, the bell-shaped distribution becomes narrower, but at the same time, fewer tubes provide useful signals. Because the limiting factor in spatial resolution—at least for a γ-ray energy of 140 keV—is the statistical accuracy of each photomultiplier tube signal, bringing the photomultipliers closer to the crystal produces larger, more accurate signals. Because the light distribution is narrower in this design, the number of photomultiplier tubes is usually increased to provide finer sampling of the "light."

Two different approaches are currently used to determine the position of *x*- and γ-ray interactions. The basic analog Anger positioning circuit finds the centroid of the samples taken by the photomultipliers. It has two inherent shortcomings: (a) the centroid of the samples taken by the photomultipliers does not necessarily correspond to the centroid of the light distribution, resulting in mispositioning of the event and in general compressing the counts toward the centers of the photomultipliers (11), and (b) each signal is treated as if it carried equal position information, thus summing the contributions from the photomultipliers in a less than optimum manner. The end result of positioning the photomultipliers closer to the crystal is an improvement in spatial resolution but at the cost of positional distortion and poor flood-field uniformity because of incorrect centroid determination.

Light that reaches the photomultipliers after an *x*- or γ-ray interacts with the NaI is converted into weak electronic signals in the photocathode which are subsequently amplified, first by internal multiplication in the photomultiplier tube itself, and then by external electronic preamplifiers. These signals are combined in a position logic circuit which gives each photomultiplier signal different weights

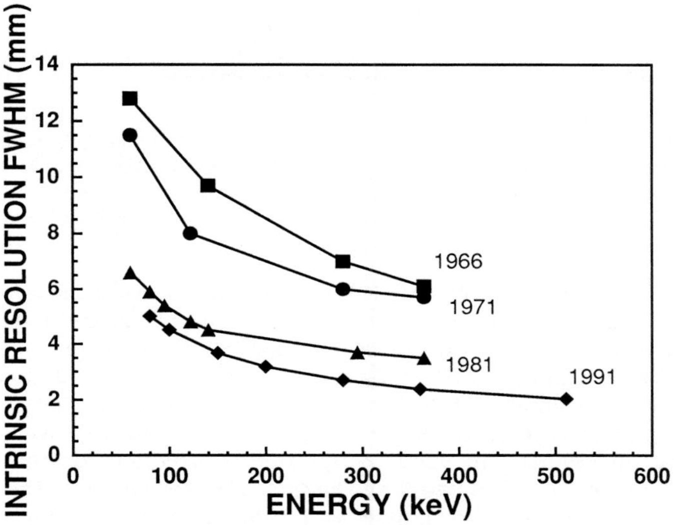

Figure 7.2. Anger camera intrinsic spatial resolution. Resolution of the Anger camera as a function of energy from: 1966 (■) (25 cm field-of-view camera with 12.5 mm crystal); 1971 (●) (25 cm field-of-view camera with 12.5 mm crystal); 1981 (▲) (38 cm field-of-view camera with 9.5 mm crystal); 1991 (♦) (calculated for a 38 cm field-of-view camera with 9.5 mm crystal).

to derive the position information, or, as is the case in some newer systems, calculated from the digitized output of the preamplifiers (described later).

Changes in the crystal configuration and light pipe design affect the light distribution and, thereby, the relative signals received by the photomultipliers. By placing opaque masks between the crystal and light pipe, light can be redirected, and the shape of the light response function can be altered to achieve more uniform spatial resolution across the image and better flood-field uniformity (12). These masks are not commonly used on today's cameras because they limit the intrinsic spatial resolution.

In an analogous fashion, the signals from the photomultipliers can be amplified in a nonlinear preamplifier (13, 14) to change the contributions that the photomultiplier signals make to the position signals (Fig. 7.3**B**). These nonlinearities take two forms: (a) small signals that are statistically poor in information are eliminated by using

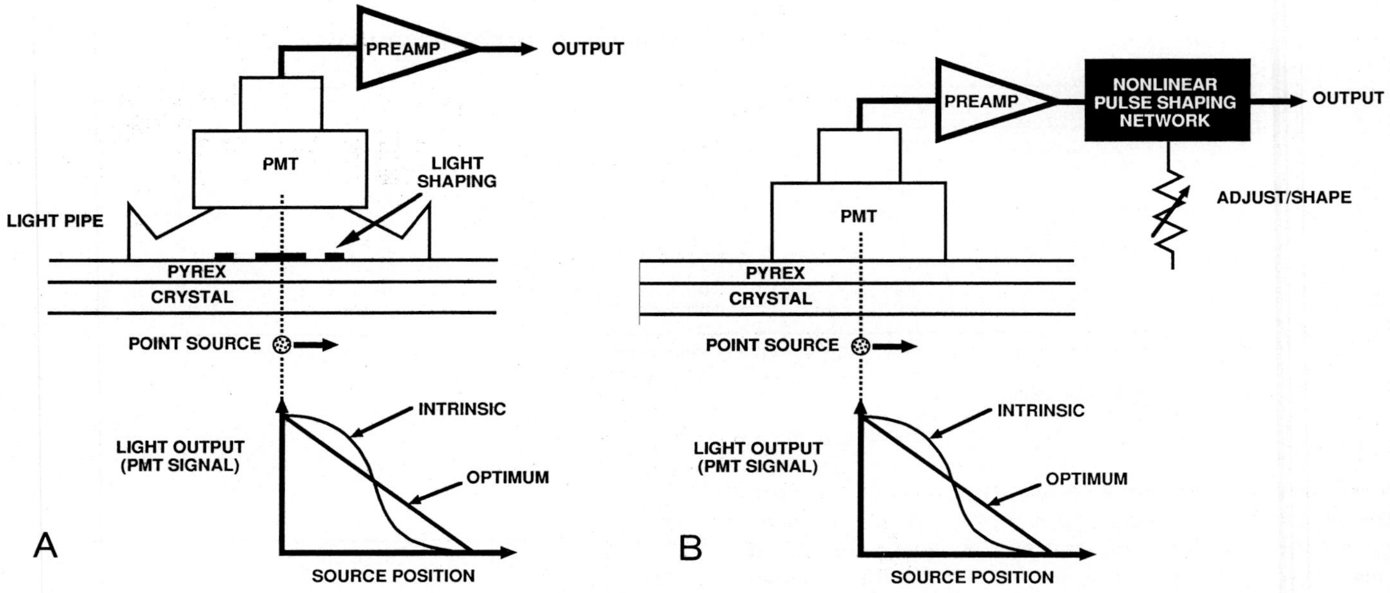

Figure 7.3. Light collection from an Anger camera with and without a light pipe. **A.** The optimum response is a linear decrease in signal intensity as a source is moved away from the central axis of the photomultiplier tube. Without a light pipe a sigmoidal response is obtained. Use of a light pipe and masks to produce light shaping gives a nearly linear response. **B.** When a light pipe is not present, a nonlinear pulse shaping network is used to "linearize" the intrinsic response. (Reproduced with permission from Eric Woronowicz, Ph.D., 1989.)

threshold preamplifiers (13), and (b) large signals are reduced in amplitude (14). Figure 7.3**A** illustrates the photomultiplier tube output in a camera with a light pipe. If the scintillation occurs directly under the center of the photomultiplier, that tube receives the largest signal. Small displacements about the center cause only relatively small changes in signal amplitude. Correction for this problem is complicated by the fact that the shape of the nonlinear response changes with interaction depth, which varies with incident photon energy. On average, low energy photons interact nearer the crystal entrance surface than do high energy photons. However, this does not significantly change the light distribution because of reflections from the MgO that coats the aluminum entrance window.

A number of years ago, Genna, et al. (15), proposed a digital technique that essentially corresponded to nonlinear amplification with optimum weights in which the photomultiplier signals are digitized and, depending on their amplitude, are transformed into weighted signals that sharply reduce the contribution of the photomultiplier directly above the scintillation. This general approach is now used by several vendors. The signal from each photomultiplier tube is digitized by a high speed analog-to-digital converter (ADC). Event position is then calculated by algorithms that can incorporate threshholding and nonlinear response as a function of energy. This approach also provides the opportunity to use sophisticated algorithms for optimizing the final determination of the interaction site.

Energy Discrimination and Correction

After a scintillation event is detected, the energy pulse is examined to assure that only events falling in the photopeak are accepted. As suggested by Svedberg (16), two different approaches can be used to generate the energy pulse (these are shown in Figure 7.1 as the Z' and ENERGY signals). One is to use the same signal that is used for position pulse normalization (Z'). This pulse is optimized to provide the best overall linearity. A second approach is to generate an energy signal that is optimized for uniform signal amplitude over the entire detector area, especially near the edge of the crystal. Even when the latter is used, local variations in light output or light collection efficiency require the use of a digital correction method, as described below.

Good energy discrimination is essential to reduce the amount of radiation that undergoes Compton scattering in the patient and reaches the detector with reduced energy. Because the energy resolution at 140 keV has improved from approximately 16% in 1975 to 8–10% today, the energy window must be reduced by an equivalent amount (from 20–12%) to take full advantage of the improvement. It is also important to note that on an angle-for-angle basis, low energy photons lose less energy when they are scattered than do high energy photons. Therefore, scattered radiation is more of a problem for low energy photons than for high.

When a collimated point source is moved across the detector face there is a variation in point source sensitivity (counts/unit time) largely caused by shifts in the photopeak relative to the energy acceptance window. These variations can be produced by improper gain setting of the photomultiplier tubes due to incorrect tuning or changes in the electronic components with time. They can also be due to an optical design in which light collection efficiency varies as a function of position.

Using a simple spatially invariant energy window has a number of disadvantages: (a) the energy resolution is worse than it should be because all regions of the camera are treated in common, (b) the point source sensitivity will vary from region to region as the photopeak shifts relative to the window, and (c) the design must be compromised to minimize energy variation at a sacrifice in spatial resolution.

Because shifts in the position of the photopeak are weak functions of distance, it is possible to measure and record the location of the photopeak in regions corresponding to the pixels in a 128 × 128 or finer matrix, and use this information to correct for variations. An event-by-event processor uses the x,y coordinates to look up the photopeak information for that position, and then either moves the energy window (17) or adjusts the energy signal amplitude to compensate for spatial variations in photopeak amplitude. It was shown (17) that this correction is valid over a wide range of energy window widths, γ-ray energies, incident count rates, and scatter conditions. A further refinement of this technique involves changing the width of the energy window to compensate for positional variations in energy resolution (18), but this method is not used on current cameras.

Correction for Spatial Nonlinearity

Spatial nonlinearities are systematic errors in the positioning of scintillation events. Such distortions are caused by nonlinear changes in the light distributions in the scintillator as a function of location. Because the linear Anger camera arithmetic scheme is not adequate to compensate for these effects, events are not recorded in their true location. The errors are small compared to the event-by-event error resulting from statistical uncertainties in the number of photons received by each photomultiplier. However, these small distortions cause visible changes in intensity because the displacements are applied to *all* events in a particular region.

Nonuniformities resulting from spatial distortion are caused by local count compression or expansion (19). To be visually noticeable in an image of a line pattern phantom or orthogonal-hole pattern, such distortions must exceed several millimeters in spatial displacement; to be seen in clinical images, the distortions must be even more severe. However, nonlinearity may cause unacceptable flood-field variations even when the displacement is less than 1 mm. As an example, if a circular area of 20 mm is compressed toward its center from all directions (as would be the case under the center of a photomultiplier) by 0.4 mm, the effective area is reduced from 100π mm^2 to 92π mm^2. This causes an 8% increase in count density in the surrounding area. Thus, spatial distortions cause noticeable flood-field nonuniformities well before displacements are visually apparent in line pattern images. Nonlinearity is the primary cause of flood-field nonuniformity, although local shifts of the photopeak do contribute to this problem (20).

Distortion can be corrected through event-by-event processing during data collection. First the displacements must be measured accurately using a line or orthogonal hole test pattern and a fine matrix (at least 128 × 128, or as high as 512 × 512). Because the true location is known and the actual (distorted) location in the image is measured, a displacement correction can be calculated. This calculation is performed for all source locations in the field. As data are collected, the original x and y digital coordinates of each event are corrected in live-time by the displacement factors and repositioned. With both energy and nonlinearity correction applied, the result is excellent uniformity. However, it must be noted that in some cameras this operation is not totally energy independent. When nuclides other than ^{99m}Tc are used, renormalization maps must also be applied. These are usually based on high count intrinsic flood images acquired using the radionuclide of interest.

If a scintillation camera is designed for good spatial resolution, large distortions are present. Figure 7.4 shows an example of a large-field-of-view camera both before and after distortion removal. This clearly shows that distortions can be the major factor in producing flood-field nonuniformities. Because these distortions are inherent in the design, they *generally* are independent of energy window width, incident count rates, and scatter conditions (11).

AUTOMATIC TUNING

For the energy and linearity correction circuits to work properly, it is imperative that the photomultiplier tubes be properly balanced, as they were when the correction factors were generated, and that all electronic circuits be stable with respect to time. Temporal changes in the gain of the photomultiplier tubes and drifts of electronic components can partially or completely invalidate the corrections and produce significant nonuniformity (21). Environmental influences on the detector, such as changing magnetic fields and temperature, can also produce a loss of uniformity. To minimize this problem, a number of camera manufacturers have added circuits to monitor photomultiplier tube gain and automatically "tune" the detector. Different techniques are used, but they can be divided into two general categories: on-demand and "continuous."

On-Demand Tuning

The ARC series of cameras marketed by ADAC Laboratories utilizes a radionuclide source for tuning (22). After removing the collimator, a special lead mask with holes centered on the photomultiplier tubes is mounted on the detector. A ^{99m}Tc point source is then placed directly in front of the detector and the tuning sequence initiated. The tubes are checked one at a time, starting with tube 61. After acquiring a spectrum the centroid is calculated. If the photopeak has shifted by more than 1%, the preamplifier gain is adjusted; if not, the microprocessor steps acquisition to the next tube, etc. The tuning sequence requires approximately 30 minutes and is usually initiated when the intrinsic uniformity exceeds specification. For typical cameras, tuning is required no more frequently than once every 3 months.

In the XP Series of cameras, Picker International analyzes the balance of the photomultiplier tubes during the daily quality control intrinsic uniformity tests. With the aid of split windows, tubes that have drifted are identified and the amount of gain shift is quantitated (23). These tubes are subsequently recalibrated to restore their output to reference values. A chronologic record of the adjustments is

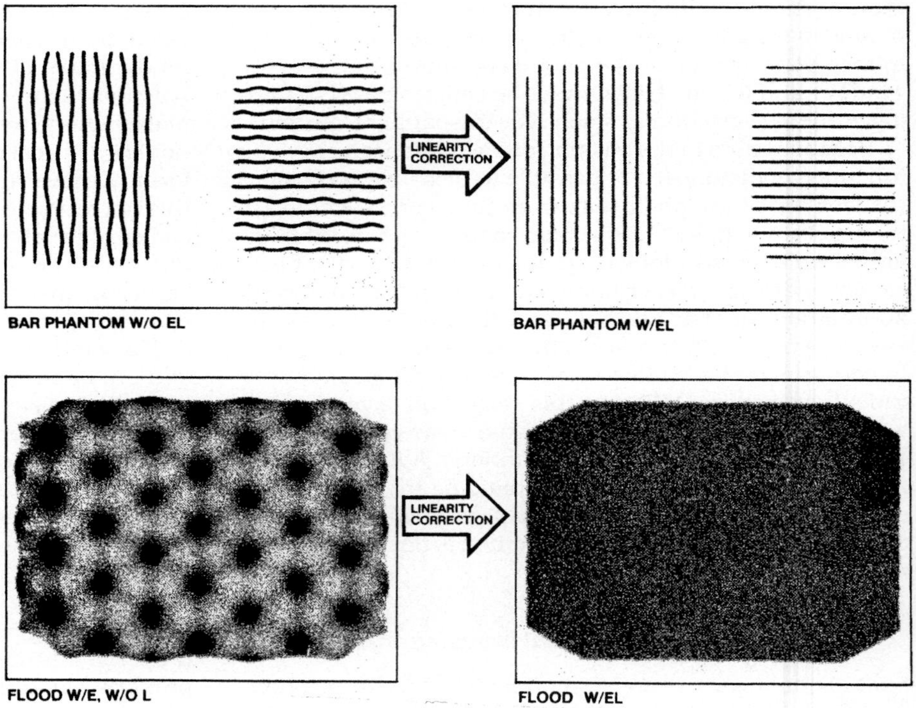

Figure 7.4. Nonlinearity without and with energy and linearity correction. **A.** Intrinsic slit pattern image with energy and linearity correction turned off (*top left*); intrinsic slit pattern image with energy and linearity correction turned on (*top right*). **B.** Intrinsic flood with energy correction on and linearity correction off (*bottom left*); intrinsic flood with energy and linearity correction turned on (*bottom right*). (Reproduced by permission from Technicare Introduces Sentinel Electronics. Solon Ohio: Technicare Corporation, 1984.)

maintained in an on-board database. Any tube that requires frequent adjustments triggers the microprocessor to signal service. These systems can also be accessed via a modem to monitor (or even adjust) PMT gain and to remotely evaluate other service problems. This enables service personnel to identify components that may need replacement prior to leaving for the job site.

A totally different approach is used to tune Elscint cameras. A multistage calibration procedure is implemented, involving weekly and daily procedures. Once a week, the camera is tuned with a radioactive source. Small software windows are opened in front of each photomultiplier which is then tuned. Following this step, the crystal is illuminated by a light-emitting-diode (LED) optical system, and the response of the photomultiplier tubes is recorded for reference. Thus, by activating the optical system which compares the measured photomultiplier response with the reference ones, the camera can be quickly returned to the tuned state without the need for a radiation source (24).

The optical system consists of a single LED placed in the detector housing and optical fibers are used to transfer light to the crystal which is sensed by the photomultiplier tubes. The signals of each tube are compared to the reference values previously measured with the radioactive source. If a significant shift has occurred, the gain on the tube is adjusted. One cycle requires approximately 20 seconds to complete. The vendor recommends that this be done at least once per day (25).

"Continuous" Tuning

LEDs are also used to tune General Electric cameras. Technically speaking, the tuning is not "continuous," but from a practical standpoint it is. Each photomultiplier contains an LED mounted in the neck of the tube. At a high frequency (hundreds of times per second), the LED is pulsed and light travels down the glass and illuminates the photocathode. Some light also enters the crystal and is seen by surrounding tubes. The signals from the photomultiplier tubes are fed to individual capacitors (one for each tube) with a time constant of approximately 1 second. The voltages on the capacitors are compared to a reference voltage and the gain of the tube is adjusted if necessary (26).

A similar approach is used by Toshiba Medical Systems (27). An LED is incorporated in each tube and is pulsed for 0.2 microseconds, one tube at a time in sequence. One cycle is completed every 200 microseconds. This process is repeated 255 more times and the output of each tube averaged. After 256 cycles the average output for each tube is compared to reference values and the preamplifier gain adjusted if necessary. If radiation from the patient strikes the crystal at the same time the LED is pulsed, the γ-ray event takes precedence because of a difference in pulse height. Once the tuning sequence is complete, the data are erased and the process is repeated.

The "Digitrac" series, manufactured by Siemens Medical Systems, utilizes radiation emitted by the patient to tune the camera although it can also be calibrated automatically using a point source of ^{99m}Tc (28). During clinical studies, counts are acquired in two narrow tuning windows set on the high side of the photopeak to minimize the acceptance of scatter events. Each tube has two registers (buffers), one for each window, which record the total number of counts. Tuning is initiated when a statistically adequate number of counts is collected in the tuning windows of several tubes. Photomultiplier tube gain adjustment is based on the ratio of the counts in the tuning windows of each tube. A ratio of 1 means the gain is the same as it was when the energy and linearity correction maps were prepared. Each radionuclide requires specific tuning window sizes and positions. These data are stored in lookup tables that are automatically loaded when automatic peaking is initiated.

A simpler approach, used by Summit Nuclear (Hitachi), utilizes a microprocessor to continuously monitor the high voltage input to the photomultiplier tube (29). The circuit includes a temperature sensor in the detector housing. As needed, the voltage is adjusted back to a set of reference values stored at the time the correction maps were prepared.

Additional details concerning some of the methods used for automatic tuning can be found in a review by Graham (21).

IMAGE FORMATION

Images of radionuclide distributions are formed by recording the location of each scintillation event-by-event. A persistence CRT displays each event in its appropriate x and y location, but the brightness fades slowly. Thus, an image can be observed in real-time as the patient is positioned under the camera. However, the image has relatively poor contrast and detail, and persistence CRTs are only used for patient positioning.

Permanent images are formed on film by recording the events displayed on a high-resolution CRT either for a predetermined number of counts or for a fixed exposure time. Alternately, each event can be recorded in a digital memory by adding each count at the appropriate x and y location in a two-dimensional matrix that is subsequently displayed as a gray-scale or color image.

SYSTEM PERFORMANCE

The Anger scintillation camera has progressively improved over the 30 years since it became available commercially and has now reached a state of development in which uniformity is very good and system spatial resolution is largely determined by the characteristics of the collimator. This section describes the most important performance parameters, stressing recent improvements.

RESOLUTION AND SENSITIVITY

Intrinsic Spatial Resolution

Intrinsic detector resolution has improved to the point where it now makes a relatively minor contribution to the system resolution except when ultra-high resolution collimators are used. A number of factors have contributed to the improvement: (a) increase in the number of photomultipliers, (b) the use of thinner scintillation crystals, (c) improved design freedom through spatially varying energy windows and spatial distortion removal for uniformity correction, and (d) direct digitization of photomultiplier tube signals. Manufacturers of scintillation cameras use various combinations of these improvements, with the result that the best intrinsic resolution of present-day large field-of-view cameras is 2.9–4.5 mm as measured by the full-width-at-half-maximum (FWHM).

Since 1974, the Anger scintillation camera has evolved from a device with 19 photomultipliers and a 10-inch field-of-view, to either a high resolution (3–4 mm FWHM), 10-inch field-of-view camera with 37 photomultipliers (2-inch diameter), or a medium resolution (5–6 mm FWHM), 15-inch field-of-view camera with 37 photomultiplier tubes (3-inch diameter). Although there were a number of variants, this pattern predominated with intrinsic resolution slowly changing from the high end of the range to the low end over the years. As alternative methods for resolution improvements were exhausted, a new family of large circular and rectangular field-of-view cameras with 61, 75, 91, or 107 photomultipliers were developed. This brute force technique and other refinements improve resolution by approximately 1–2 mm so that these large field-of-view cameras now have approximately the same intrinsic resolution as 10-inch diameter cameras.

With the widespread use of ^{99m}Tc radiopharmaceuticals and ^{201}Tl, the performance of scintillation cameras at low energies has become increasingly important. Reducing the scintillation crystal thickness from 12.5 mm (1/2-inch) to either 9.6 mm (3/8-inch) or 6.3 mm (1/4-inch) improves spatial resolution by approximately 1 mm FWHM for energies of 140 keV and below. Although various publications on this subject are not in complete agreement (30–32), Table 7.2 presents the expected resolution gain and sensitivity loss at low energies (31).

The reason for improved intrinsic spatial resolution with a thinner crystal is not as obvious as appears at first glance. It is a popular misconception (32) that the improvement results from moving the photomultipliers closer to the origin of the light in a 6.3 mm crystal. If this were true, the same result could be achieved by reducing the thickness of the glass covering by 6.3 mm. This reduction in glass thickness, however, does not achieve the desired result. A better explanation is that the reduced thickness changes the light distribution in the photomultiplier tube array.

One of the prime requirements of the analog Anger positioning electronics is the "proper" shape of the light response function. The light response function is the light intensity measured by a photomultiplier as a function of distance from the center of the photomultiplier (Fig. 7.3). Much effort has been spent on analytic approaches to this problem (34, 35), on methods to achieve the proper re-

Table 7.2.
Resolution and Sensitivity Change as a Result of Crystal Thickness Reduction from 12.5 mm to 6.25 mm

Radionuclide	Intrinsic Resolution Improvement[a]	Loss of Sensitivity
^{201}Tl	1.3 mm FWHM	negligible
^{99m}Tc	1.0 mm FWHM	15%

[a]The resolution improvement is stated in terms of millimeters of full-width-at-half-maximum (FWHM) changes for a line spread function; bar pattern resolution must be multiplied by 1.8 to give comparable numbers.

sponse by manipulation of the light distribution (12) and the use of nonlinear preamplifiers (13), and on delay-line methods (36). In each case, the designer tries to optimize spatial resolution with the constraint of uniform (or nearly uniform) light collection for good energy resolution and of good linearity for acceptable flood-field uniformity. Through the introduction of digital techniques for spatially varying energy discrimination and spatial distortion removal, as discussed previously, a major constraint has been removed from scintillation camera design. Figure 7.4 shows, as an intermediate step, the highly distorted but high resolution image of the analog processor before the digital processor corrects for nonlinearities. This increased design freedom can lead to improved spatial resolution compared with an analog processor. By replacement of the analog positioning circuitry with ADCs and software techniques, even more complex position determination can be done, as well as compensation for changes in photon energy.

Collimator and System Resolution

As described earlier, better collimator spatial resolution can only be achieved at a sacrifice in sensitivity. High sensitivity collimators are typically only used for fast dynamic studies in which short imaging times preclude collection of an adequate number of counts with higher resolution and therefore lower sensitivity collimators.

Overall system resolution (*Rs*) is determined by both collimator (*Rc*) and intrinsic spatial resolution (*Ri*). It can be represented by the formula

$$R_s = \sqrt{R_c^2 + (MR_i)^2} \tag{7.1}$$

where *M* is the magnification factor when converging or diverging collimators are used ($M = 1$ for parallel hole collimators). This relationship implies that close to the surface of the collimator where Rc is low, system resolution is dominated by the intrinsic resolution, whereas at large distances from the collimator—say 15 cm—system resolution is largely determined by the collimator performance, particularly for low (large FWHM) values of intrinsic resolution. System resolution cannot be improved significantly by reducing the intrinsic resolution below 3 mm.

UNIFORMITY

If the scintillation camera is exposed to a uniform flux of γ-radiation, the resulting image should have uniform intensity. Because any deviation from this condition can potentially interfere with accurate interpretation of patient images, it is extremely important to verify camera uniformity by acquiring daily flood field images. This can be done either with a point source of activity if the collimator is removed or with a "sheet" source (i.e., a large uniform source) if the collimator is in place. Many of the digital correction methods (energy and linearity corrections) were developed to improve uniformity, with the result that most modern scintillation cameras exhibit only negligible uniformity variations for most planar imaging situations. State-of-the-art cameras have integral uniformity values ranging from 2–4.5% when measured using the NEMA protocol (37). However, it should be noted that those cameras with the best uniformity (2%) include a separate renormalization step that is not used by other vendors.

Unfortunately, photomultipliers (and sometimes associated analog electronic components) tend to be unstable with time. If one or several photomultipliers "drift," hot or cold spots may appear in the flood image. Furthermore, photomultiplier gain can be affected by magnetic fields such as the earth's magnetic field (or a nearby nuclear magnetic resonance unit), which can cause the uniformity to change as a function of detector orientation. This is particularly detrimental in emission computed tomography where data from a complete detector rotation (360°) are used to generate an image. For this reason, almost all companies now incorporate "self-tuning" circuitry that adjusts the photomultiplier gain periodically when a change in amplification is detected. Great care must be used in the design of the gain adjustment processor to avoid shifts of the energy spectrum under varying scatter conditions such as are encountered in emission computed tomography.

ENERGY RESOLUTION

With improved photomultiplier tubes and the use of energy correction circuits, energy resolution of state-of-the-art Anger scintillation cameras now falls in the range of 8–11%. This means that better elimination of scatter radiation can be achieved by the use of narrower (12–15%) pulse height analyzer windows without the loss of a significant percentage of photopeak events. A decrease in the scatter fraction with improved energy resolution has been documented (38). The work of Kojima, et al. (38), did reveal, however, that proper selection of the optimum window was strongly dependent on the relationship between the scatter fraction and the number of primary counts in the image.

In integrated camera-computer systems, several vendors now offer elaborate techniques for "elimination" of scatter radiation. Elscint uses a method based on the Klein-Nishina formula for Compton scattering (39, 40). Up to 32 images are collected using narrow pulse height analyzer windows (41). For ^{99m}Tc SPECT, 16 images are often acquired for each projection. From this set of images, spectra are generated for each pixel. Figure 7.5**A** shows the photopeak plus single, double, and triple scatter components for ^{99m}Tc. Figure 7.5**B** presents the multiple, narrow analyzer windows that are used to "measure" the spectrum at each pixel in the image. Each spectrum is decomposed into the contribution of the photopeak and the summed contribution of several orders of Compton scattering. By separating scatter events from photopeak events, this methodology makes it possible to remove scatter in different patients and even from different locations within the same patient. The resulting images show markedly improved contrast but there is usually an increase in noise. However, increased amounts of computer storage are required and high speed processing is needed to remove the scatter in each projection of a multiple view SPECT study.

A computationally simpler method is available for the removal of scatter (42). A conventional pulse height analyzer window is surrounded by two narrow 3% subwindows—one positioned just above and one just below the

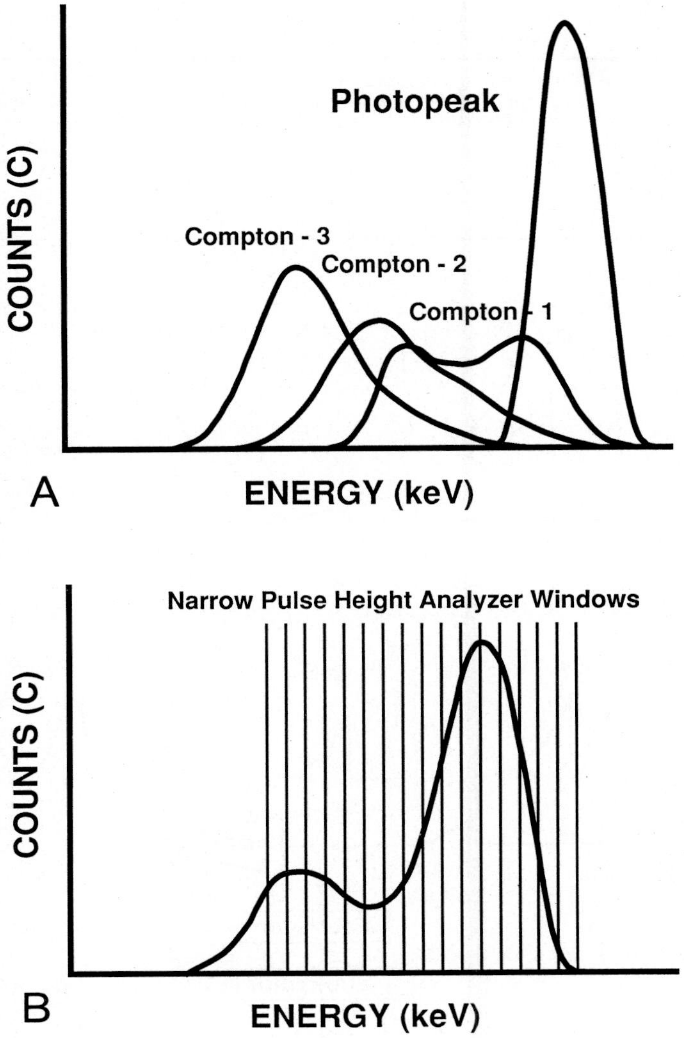

Figure 7.5. Elimination of scatter using multiple windows. **A.** The first three Kline-Nishina probability coefficients for Compton scattering (single, double, and triple scatter) and the photoelectric peak in a NaI(Tl) crystal. **B.** ^{99m}Tc spectrum in scatter media showing the positioning of 16 narrow pulse height analyzer windows used to measure the spectrum on a pixel-by-pixel basis. For ^{99m}Tc, the windows cover the energy range from 95–161 keV.

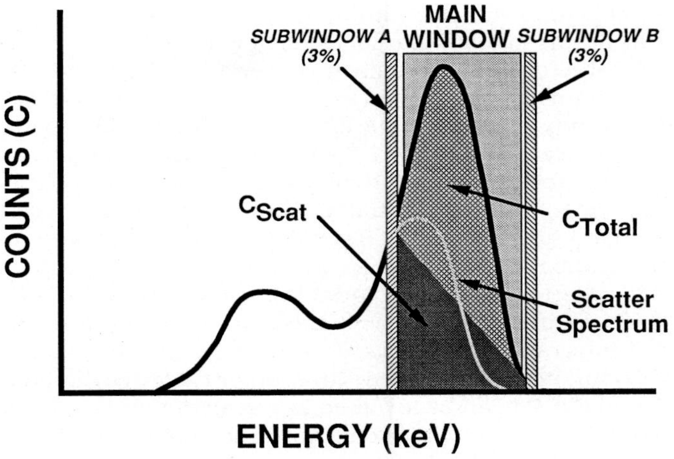

Figure 7.6. Triple-energy window method for scatter removal. Narrow subwindows are positioned just above and below the main window to "measure" the amount of scatter that is present in the photopeak on a pixel-by-pixel basis. These counts are subtracted from the total counts to "eliminate" scatter and improve contrast. (Modified by permission from Ichihara T, Ogawa K, Motomura N, Kubo A, Hashimoto S. Compton scatter compensation using the triple-energy window method for single- and dual-isotope SPECT. J Nucl Med 1993;34:2216–2221.)

main window. A trapezoid, defined by the baseline and the number of counts in each of the subwindows, is used as an estimate of the scatter superimposed on the photopeak. A schematic diagram is shown in Figure 7.6. The number of counts within the trapezoid is subtracted from the counts in the main window on a pixel-by-pixel basis. Contrast in clinical studies is improved and image noise is increased.

COUNT RATE CAPABILITY

The ability to handle high count rates is often a limiting performance parameter in first-pass cardiac studies. For example, if 4 mCi (148 mBq) of ^{99m}Tc are injected as a bolus with a general purpose collimator on the camera, then a maximum of 10,000 counts/second (cps) are recorded (assuming a 50% attenuation). If it is assumed that no counts are lost at such a relatively low count rate, it is easy to calculate that a 20 mCi (740 mBq) injection with a high-sensitivity collimator on the camera (i.e., a typical first-pass situation) should yield 100,000 cps. Yet, many Anger cameras will show a significant loss of counts at this rate.

The count rate capability of the Anger scintillation camera is limited by the decay time of NaI(Tl) and by the processing and display electronics. If new ultra-short-lived radionuclides are developed, e.g., ^{178}Ta (43), count rate capability will become more important and the processing and display electronics will need to be redesigned to reduce count losses.

After a γ-ray interacts in NaI(Tl), the resulting light is emitted with a decay time of 240 nsec; 1000 nsec are required to collect 98% of the light. If the γ-rays arrive at regular time intervals, and if every detected event falls in the energy acceptance window, then 1 million events/second could be handled. However, in clinical studies, one-half to two-thirds of the incident counts are due to scattered radiation and are discarded. Nevertheless, every event must be analyzed and this increases the total dead-time. Because the incident radiation arrives at random time intervals, the maximum data rate is further reduced. Typical maximum count rates in older cameras were approximately 100,000 cps with a source in air and less than 30,000 cps in clinical situations.

All modern cameras utilize four to five stages of derandomizer buffers to improve count rate performance. If two or more events arrive before the camera completes processing the first event, sample-and-hold circuits preserve them until they can be processed.

Other techniques are also used to significantly increase the count rate capability of Anger cameras. One method involves shortening the time during which the electrical signals from the photomultiplier tubes is integrated, but this means that only part of the light emitted by the crystal is captured. This technique was previously described (44–46) and has been applied to Anger cameras (46, 47). Because only a fraction of the light is used, there will be some loss of resolution. Table 7.3 summarizes calculated count rate capability and resolution loss as a function of integration time. It is assumed that the pulse is shortened to correspond to the listed integration time. Note that with an integration time as short as 240 nsec, 63% of the light is still collected. By using a variable integration time (47, 48), the resolution loss can be limited. At low count rates the full integration time is used; at high count rates shorter integration times are used. Thus, an intrinsic resolution of 5 mm FWHM can be achieved in a system that has 4 mm FWHM resolution with a long integration time. Pulse shortening with variable integration time offers one useful option by which the count rate capability of Anger cameras can be improved significantly with only a small loss of intrinsic resolution.

A serious problem still remains. It must be determined whether the event of interest is either preceded or followed by an event that occurs close enough in time to prevent accurate position and energy determination. This loss of accuracy occurs because one pulse stands on the tail of another pulse. A number of techniques have been developed to deal with this problem and fall under the general category of *pulse pile-up rejection.* An example of pulse pile-up is shown in Figure 7.7**A**. If one of the piled-up events is a photopeak event, then the composite pulse is likely to be eliminated because it will not fall in the energy selection window. This is called "coincidence loss." More seriously, if two scattered events are summed, they may combine to fall into the energy window and will be recorded as a single event that will be localized somewhere *between* the two actual events. As mentioned previously, this is called a misplaced event; image quality is degraded without pile-up rejection (49, 50).

Pile-up rejection circuits generally operate in one of two ways. One approach is to process only the first part of the pulse, as described earlier. This strategy diminishes the effects on the pulses that follow, but degrades energy and spatial resolution because the signals are smaller (46). Pulse pile-up is not eliminated, but higher counting rates are required before it is prominent (51). A second approach is to measure the length of the output pulse. If it does not return to a value close to the baseline level by a preset time, the pulse is discarded (52). Under this condition, increasing numbers of events are discarded as the count rate increases. While cameras with this type of pile-up rejection will have better image quality at high count rates, they will also have apparently longer deadtimes because they do not count these mispositioned events. It has been shown (50, 53) that some cameras with apparently high count rate capability achieve this "good" performance by including misplaced events due to pile-up.

Recently, high speed electronics have led to the development of a better solution to the problem of pulse pile-up (51, 54). The incoming pulse to the amplifier is monitored and the decay of the pulse tail is followed with a circuit called an estimator (Fig. 7.7**B**). If a second pulse arrives before the first pulse has returned to the baseline, the input to the amplifier is immediately switched to a second channel. The estimator extrapolates the first pulse to complete the tail. The extrapolated tail is also routed to the second channel and subtracted from the second pulse. This operation removes the pedestal on which the second pulse is sitting. The cameras that currently use this technique may have multiple levels of extrapolation. Tail ex-

Table 7.3.
Effect of Pulse Shortening on Camera Performance

Output Count Rate, 20% Data Loss (cps)	Integration Time (nsec)	% Light Emitted	Resolution FWHM (mm)
89000	1000	98	4.0
223000	400	81	4.4
372000	240	63	5.0
890000	100	34	6.9

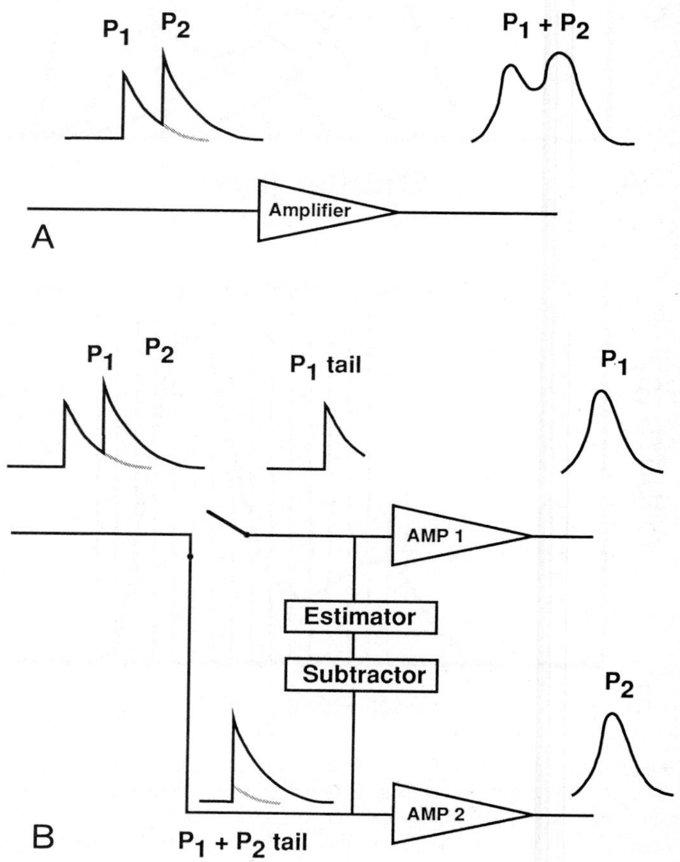

Figure 7.7. Pulse pile-up. **A.** Effect of pulse pile-up when a second pulse (P_2) arrives before the first pulse (P_1) has been completely processed. The height of the composite pulse ($P_1 + P_2$) is larger than that of P_1 alone. **B.** Tail extrapolation circuit which removes the effect of pulse pile-up. (Modified by permission from Lewellen TK, Pollard KR, Bice AN, Zhu JB. A new clinical scintillation camera with pulse tail extrapolation electronics. IEEE Trans Nucl Sci 1990 37:702–706.)

trapolation is particularly attractive because it significantly reduces the number of misplaced events (51).

SUMMARY

For planar imaging of radionuclide distributions in humans, the Anger scintillation camera remains the instrument of choice. Although its principal components have not changed significantly, it has been perfected and enhanced to the point where its system resolution is now largely limited by the collimator and uniformity is excellent. Count rate capability has improved in many cameras, but this performance parameter is extremely variable from vendor to vendor.

The limitations imposed by the collimator are severe. Compared to other imaging modalities, nuclear medicine images have poor resolution and are limited in image quality because of poor statistics in the number of γ-rays detected. However, the availability of multiple detector systems and magnifying collimators has produced significant improvements in image quality. In part this is due to better statistics; in part it is due to the ability to use collimators with higher resolution (55). In some clinical studies, the improved sensitivity can be used to increase throughput; in others, it may be used to improve image quality. One method for overcoming these limitations is positron emission tomography, which is becoming practical for clinical use. Major improvements in radionuclide imaging are possible with single photon emission computed tomography using both dedicated imaging instruments and multiple detector rotating scintillation cameras.

REFERENCES

1. Anger HO. Scintillation camera with multichannel collimators. J Nucl Med 1964;5:515–531.
2. Jaszczak RJ, Murphy PH, Huard D, and Burdine JA. Radionuclide emission computed tomography of the head with Tc-99m and a scintillation camera. J Nucl Med 1977;18:373–380.
3. Kuhl DE and Edwards RQ. Image separation radioisotope scanning. Radiol 1963;80:653–662.
4. Anger HO, Rosenthall DJ. Scintillation camera and positron camera. In: Medical Radioisotope Scanning. Vienna: International Atomic Energy Agency, 1959:59.
5. Muehllehner G. A diverging collimator for γ ray imaging cameras. J Nucl Med 1969;10:197–201.
6. Moyer, RA. A low-energy multihole converging collimator compared with a pinhole collimator. J Nucl Med 1974;15:59–64.
7. Bonte FJ, Graham KD, Dowdey JE. Image aberrations produced by multichannel collimators for a scintillation camera. Radiol 1971;98:329–334.
8. Anger HO, Davis DH. Gamma-ray detection efficiency and image resolution in sodium iodide. Rev Sci Instr 1964;35:693–697.
9. Svedberg JB. Computed intrinsic efficiencies and modulation transfer functions for gamma-camera. Phys Med Biol 1973; 18:658–664.
10. Birks JB. The theory and practice of scintillation counting. New York: MacMillan, 1964:432.
11. Muehllehner G, Colsher JG, Stoub EW. Correction for nonuniformity in scintillation cameras through removal of spatial distortion. J Nucl Med 1980;21:771–776.
12. Martone RJ, Goldman SC, Heaton CC. Scintillation camera with light diffusion system. U.S. Patent No. 3784819, 1974.
13. Kulberg GH, Van Dijk N, Muehllehner G. Improved resolution of the Anger scintillation camera through use of threshold preamplifiers. J Nucl Med 1972;13:169–171.
14. Stout KJ. Radiation sensing device. U.S. Patent No. 3911278, 1975.
15. Genna S, Pang S, Smith A. Digital scintigraphy: principles, design and performance. J Nucl Med 1981;22:365–371.
16. Svedberg JB. On the intrinsic resolution of a gamma-camera system. Phys Med Biol 1972;17:514–524.
17. Steidley JW, Kearns DS, Hoffer PB. Uniformity correction with the Micro-Z processor. J Nucl Med 1978;19:712.
18. Knoll GF, Bennet MC, Koral KF, Strange DR. Removal of gamma-camera nonlinearity and nonuniformities through realtime signal processing. In: Di Paola R, Kahn E, eds. Information processing in medical imaging. Paris: INSERM, 1980:187–200.
19. Cradduck TD, Fedoruk SO, Reid WB. A new method of assessing the performance of scintillation cameras and scanners. Phys Med Biol 1966;11:423–435.
20. Wicks R, Blau M. Effect of spatial distortion on Anger camera field-uniformity correction: concise communication. J Nucl Med 1979; 20:252–254.
21. Graham LS. Automatic tuning of scintillation cameras: a review. J Nucl Med Tech 1986;14:105–110.
22. ADAC digital gamma-camera detectors. Milpitas, CA: ADAC Laboratories, 1982.
23. Valentino F, Picker International. Personal communication, 1994.
24. Wainer N, Elscint Inc. Personal communication, 1994.
25. Bernstein T. Image quality by automatic corrections and calibrations. Boston, MA: Elscint Inc. (no date).
26. H3000BD Product Data, Starcam 500A Imaging Detector. General Electric Company, Medical Systems Division, 1984.
27. Ichihara T, Toshiba Medical Systems. Internal Report (no date).
28. ZLC with Digitrac. Siemens Medical Systems, #917–00000014A-b, 1/84.
29. Enos G. Personal communication, 1994.
30. Sano RM, Tinkel JB, La Vallee CA, Freedman GS. Consequences of crystal thickness reduction on gamma-camera resolution and sensitivity. J Nucl Med 1978;19:712–713.
31. Chapman D, Newcomer K, Berman D, Waxman A. Half-inch vs quarter-inch Anger camera technology: resolution and sensitivity differences at low photopeak energies. J Nucl Med 1979;20:610–611.
32. Royal HD, Brown PH, Claunch BC. Effects of a reduction in crystal thickness on Anger camera performance. J Nucl Med 1979; 20:977–980.
33. Muehllehner G. Effect of crystal thickness on scintillation camera performance. J Nucl Med 1979;20:992–993.
34. Baker RG, Scringer JW. An investigation of the parameters in scintillation camera design. Phys Med Biol 1967;12:51–63.
35. Svedberg JB. Image quality of a gamma-camera system. Phys Med Biol 1968;13:597–610.
36. Hiramoto T, Tanaka E, Nohara N. A scintillation camera based on delay-line time conversion. J Nucl Med 1971;12:160–165.
37. Performance measurements of scintillation cameras. Standards Publication/No. NU 1–1994. Washington, DC: National Electrical Manufacturers Association, 1994.
38. Kojima A, Matsumoto M, Takahashi M, Uehara S. Effect of energy resolution on scatter fraction in scintigraphic imaging: Monte Carlo study. Med Phys 1993;20:1107–1113.
39. Maor D, Berlad G, Chrem S, Soil A, Todd-Pokropek A. Klein-Nishina based energy factors for Compton Free Imaging (CFI). J Nucl Med Suppl 1991;32:1000.
40. Berlad G, Maor D, Natanzon A, Shrem Y, Todd-Pokropek A. Compton Free Imaging (CFI): validation of a new scatter correction method. J Nucl Med Suppl 1994;35:143P.
41. Elscint Helix Procedure Manual. Elscint, Inc. (no date).

42. Ichihara T, Ogawa K, Motomura N, Kubo A, Hashimoto S. Compton scatter compensation using the triple-energy window method for single- and dual-isotope SPECT. J Nucl Med 1993;34:2216–2221.
43. Adams R, Lacy JL, Ball ME, Martin LJ. The count rate performance of a multiwire gamma-camera measured by a decaying source method with 9.3-minute tantalum-178. J Nucl Med 1990; 31:1723–1726.
44. Asmsel G, Bosshard R, Zajde C. Shortening of detector signals with passive filters for pile-up reduction. Nucl Instr Meth 1969; 71:1–12.
45. Brasshard C. Fast counting with NaI spectrometers. Nucl Instr Meth 1971;94:301–306.
46. Muehllehner G, Buchin MP, Dudek JH. Performance parameters of a positron imaging camera. IEEE Trans Nucl Sci 1976;23:528–537.
47. Tanaka E, Nohara N, Murayama H. Variable sampling-time technique for improving countrate performance of scintillation detectors. Nucl Instr Meth 1979;158:459–466.
48. Kastner M. A high speed stabilized gated integrator. IEEE Trans Nucl Sci 1984;NS31:447–450.
49. Strand S, Larsson I. Image artifacts at high photon fluence rates in single-crystal NaI(Tl) scintillation cameras. J Nucl Med 1978; 19:407–413.
50. Lewellen TK, Murano R. A comparison of countrate parameters in gamma-cameras. J Nucl Med 1981;22:161–168.
51. Lewellen TK, Pollard KR, Bice AN, Zhu JB. A new clinical scintillation camera with pulse tail extrapolation electronics. IEEE Trans Nucl Sci 1990;37:702–706.
52. Nicholson PW. Nuclear electronics. London: John Wiley & Sons, 1974.
53. Johnston AS, Gergans GA, Kim I, Barnes E, Kaplan E, Pinsky SM. Deadtime of computers coupled with Anger cameras: counting losses and false counts. In: Sorenson IAJA, ed. Single photon emission computer tomography and other selected topics. New York: Society of Nuclear Medicine, 1980:219–237.
54. Lewellen TK, Bice AN, Pollard KR, Zhu JB, Plunkett ME. Evaluation of a clinical scintillation camera with pulse tail extrapolation electronics. J Nucl Med 1989;29:1554–1558.
55. Muehllehner G. Effect of resolution improvement on required count density in ECT imaging: a computer simulation. Phy Med Biol 1985;30:163–173.

8 Basic Principles of Computers

HENRY D. ROYAL, J. ANTHONY PARKER, and B. LEONARD HOLMAN

Many nuclear medicine physicians received their formal training before computers had such a great impact on all activities of everyday life. The incredibly rapid growth in the use of computers has made adults who grew up before the advent of video games anxious. One reason for the anxiety that computers create is that they perform numeric calculations at previously inconceivable rates, using number systems and techniques that are decidedly inhuman. Some tasks that are impossible for humans to perform can be done with remarkable ease by the computer. With the mystery surrounding how computers "think" and with the insidious invasion of this fascinating technology, it is no surprise that many wonder, partly in awe and partly in fear, what computers will "do" next (1).

This chapter is divided into five major sections. The first presents important preliminary concepts of computer operations. The second discusses general purpose computer functions such as word processing and spreadsheets. The third describes the hardware used in a nuclear medicine computer system. The fourth discusses the software necessary for acquisition and analysis of nuclear medicine studies. The final section outlines the integrated package of hardware and software that is necessary to perform specific functions in nuclear medicine.

PRELIMINARY CONCEPTS

Since computers are physical devices, abstract concepts such as numbers must be represented by electronic states. The simplest, most reliable, and fastest method of electronically representing numbers is to use a sequence of "switches" that are either "on" or "off." Limiting the position of the switch to either on or off greatly facilitates the speed and reliability with which the position of the switch can be checked. The binary number system is used to mimic the electronic design. A 0 can be used to represent the "off" state and a 1 can represent the "on" state. Large numbers can be symbolized by a series of 1's and 0's. Each binary digit in the number is called a bit. Since computers use the binary number system, numbers that represent powers of 2 take on new significance and repeatedly occur in discussions of computers (Table 8.1). The largest number (32 bits in modern computers) that a computer can conveniently use affects fundamental characteristics of the computer such as the amount of memory and disk space that can be used and the speed with which data can be transferred.

Computers are called digital devices since quantities are represented by integers (whole numbers) that are exactly denoted using a specified number of binary digits. In contrast, electronic analog devices often use the magnitude of a voltage to represent a value. In this latter case, the voltage may have any value between the maximum and minimum possible voltage. Digital devices are often more accurate than analog devices since their accuracy is not affected by fluctuations in voltages.

Table 8.1.
Significant Computer Numbers

Number (Base 10)	Comment
255 ($2^8 - 1$)	Largest integer that can be stored in 8 binary digits (BYTE)
1024 (2^{10})	Power of 2 most nearly equal to 1000; referred to as 1 kilobyte or 1 K
65,635 ($2^{16} - 1$)	Largest integer that can be stored in 16 binary digits (WORD)
1,048,576 (2^{20})	Power of 2 most nearly equal to 1,000,000; referred to as 1 megabyte or 1 M
1,073,741,824 (2^{30})	Power of 2 most nearly equal to 1,000,000,000; referred to as 1 gigabyte or 1 G
4,294,967,295 ($2^{32} - 1$)	Largest integer that can be stored in 32 binary digits (DOUBLE WORD)

Computers are designed to rapidly perform a sequence of operations (a program). Repetitive tasks that can be unambiguously, simply, and completely defined can be better performed by computers than by humans. Unfortunately, most tasks are difficult to unambiguously, simply, and completely define. Although computers can perform repetitive numeric calculations very rapidly, the current generation of computers cannot perform many tasks that humans perform with ease. For example, a human can identify objects in a photograph quickly and accurately, whereas this task is extremely difficult for computers to perform. An even simpler task, such as recognizing the letters on an image of a printed page, is just becoming possible with computers.

Most computer systems use an 8-bit number, or byte, as the smallest convenient way to represent data. The 8-bit byte became the standard because much of the information that computers need to process are alphanumeric characters. Since 128 (27) different letters, numbers, special characters, and control characters can be symbolized by a 7-bit number, this size binary number can be conveniently used to represent character data. One of the standard systems for representing these alphanumeric codes, the American Standard Code for Information Interchange (ASCII, pronounced "ask key") (Table 8.2), uses a 7-bit number. In the early years of computer development, an eighth bit was added so that error checking could be performed internally. This eighth bit was called a parity bit. Data were made internally consistent by setting the parity bit to 1 or 0 depending on whether there was an even or

Table 8.2.
ASCII and Equivalents

Decimal	Octal	Hex	ASCII	Decimal	Octal	Hex	ASCII	Decimal	Octal	Hex	ASCII	Decimal	Octal	Hex	ASCII
0	000	00	NUL	32	040	20	SP	64	100	40	@	96	140	60	
1	001	01	SOH	33	041	21	!	65	101	41	A	97	141	61	a
2	002	02	STX	34	042	22	"	66	102	42	B	98	142	62	b
3	003	03	ETX	35	043	23	#	67	103	43	C	99	143	63	c
4	004	04	EOT	36	044	24	$	68	104	44	D	100	144	64	d
5	005	05	ENQ	37	045	25	%	69	105	45	E	101	145	65	e
6	006	06	ACK	38	046	26	&	70	106	46	F	102	146	66	f
7	007	07	BEL	39	047	27	'	71	107	47	G	103	147	67	g
8	010	08	BS	40	050	28	(	72	110	48	H	104	150	68	h
9	011	09	HT	41	051	29	)	73	111	49	I	105	151	69	i
10	012	0A	LF	42	052	2A	*	74	112	4A	J	106	152	6A	j
11	013	0B	VT	43	053	2B	+	75	113	4B	K	107	153	6B	k
12	014	0C	FF	44	054	2C	,	76	114	4C	L	108	154	6C	l
13	015	0D	CR	45	055	2D	-	77	115	4D	M	109	155	6D	m
14	016	0E	SO	46	056	2E	.	78	116	4E	N	110	156	6E	n
15	017	0F	SI	47	057	2F	/	79	117	4F	O	111	157	6F	o
16	020	10	DLE	48	060	30	0	80	120	50	P	112	160	70	p
17	021	11	DC1	49	061	31	1	81	121	51	Q	113	161	71	q
18	022	12	DC2	50	062	32	2	82	122	52	R	114	162	72	r
19	023	13	DC3	51	063	33	3	83	123	53	S	115	163	73	s
20	024	14	DC4	52	064	34	4	84	124	54	T	116	164	74	t
21	025	15	NAK	53	065	35	5	85	125	55	U	117	165	75	u
22	026	16	SYN	54	066	36	6	86	126	56	V	118	166	76	v
23	027	17	ETB	55	067	37	7	87	127	57	W	119	167	77	w
24	030	18	CAN	56	070	38	8	88	130	58	X	120	170	78	x
25	031	19	EM	57	071	39	9	89	131	59	Y	121	171	79	y
26	032	1A	SUB	58	072	3A	:	90	132	5A	Z	122	172	7A	z
27	033	1B	ESC	59	073	3B	;	91	133	5B	[	123	173	7B	{
28	034	1C	FS	60	074	3C	<	92	134	5C	/	124	174	7C	|
29	035	1D	GS	61	075	3D	=	93	135	5D	]	125	175	7D	}
30	036	1E	RS	62	076	3E	>	94	136	5E	^	126	176	7E	~
31	037	1F	US	63	077	3F	?	95	137	5F	–	127	177	7F	DEL

odd number of 1's or 0's in the 7-bit number. Using this convention, malfunctions that involved only 1 of the 8 bits could be easily detected. Today the eighth bit is often used to identify additional symbols.

If computers could only perform arithmetic operations, their utility would be severely limited; however, computers can also perform logical operations that enable them to make simple decisions (conditional branching). The rules for some of the logical operations (AND, OR, XOR, and NOT) that computers perform were developed in the mid-1800s by George Boole. In Boolean logic, a variable can have only one of two possible values, true or false. Boolean logic is thus perfectly compatible with the fundamental binary design of computers. Relational operators (EQUAL, GREATER THAN, and LESS THAN) are used to compare the value of numbers. These operators have two ordered numbers as their input value and their output value is simply a logical value, true or false.

The source of the enormous power of the computer flows from its ability to perform simple logical and relational operations that provide the capability to perform repetitive tasks and conditional branching. A simple pseudoprogram to subtract a constant background from each picture element (pixel) in a digital image (Table 8.3) provides insight into why computers perform repetitive tasks so well. First, the values for the number of pixels in the image ("num pixels") and the array or matrix of values for each pixel ("pixel val") are read into main memory (line 1). The user is asked how much background to subtract ("bkg counts") (line 2). The repetitive part of the program is listed in lines 3–5. The "FOR" statement in line 3 controls the number of repetitions, and the statement consists of four parts. First, the initialization segment ("I = 1") sets a variable named "I" to its starting value; the second segment states the condition ("I < = num pixels") that must be true for line 4 to execute; the third segment denotes how much to increment the counter ("I = I + 1") each time lines 3–5 execute; and the fourth segment (enclosed in brackets) contains the statement (line 4) or statements to execute. A program to subtract a million numbers is no longer or more complicated than a program to subtract two numbers; only the value of the variable "num pixels" needs to be changed. Once the task is defined, repetitions are trivial.

Table 8.3.
Program to Subtract a Constant from an Image

```
1. READ (num__pixels, pixel__value)
2. INPUT ("How much background to subtract? ",bkg__counts)
3. FOR (I = 1; I < num__pixels; I = I + 1) [
4. pixel__value(I) = pixel__value(I) − bkg__counts
5.  ]
```

GENERAL COMPUTER CAPABILITIES

Computers have become a very useful general tool. The computer shy reader might ask "Why are computers use-

A.

	A	B
1	Half life of the	radionuclide:
2	6	Hours
3		
4	Time (hours)	% Remaining
5	0	=EXP((-LN(2)*A5)/$A$2)
6	1	=EXP((-LN(2)*A6)/$A$2)
7	2	=EXP((-LN(2)*A7)/$A$2)
8	3	=EXP((-LN(2)*A8)/$A$2)
9	4	=EXP((-LN(2)*A9)/$A$2)
10	5	=EXP((-LN(2)*A10)/$A$2)
11	6	=EXP((-LN(2)*A11)/$A$2)
12	7	=EXP((-LN(2)*A12)/$A$2)
13	8	=EXP((-LN(2)*A13)/$A$2)
14	9	=EXP((-LN(2)*A14)/$A$2)
15	10	=EXP((-LN(2)*A15)/$A$2)
16	11	=EXP((-LN(2)*A16)/$A$2)
17	12	=EXP((-LN(2)*A17)/$A$2)

B.

	A	B
1	Half life of the radionuclide:	
2	6	Hours
3		
4	Time (hours)	% Remaining
5	0	100.00%
6	1	89.09%
7	2	79.37%
8	3	70.71%
9	4	63.00%
10	5	56.12%
11	6	50.00%
12	7	44.54%
13	8	39.69%
14	9	35.36%
15	10	31.50%
16	11	28.06%
17	12	25.00%

Figure 8.1. A simple spreadsheet to determine the percentage of a radionuclide remaining as a function of time. **A.** The actual contents of each cell in the spreadsheet is shown. Formulas are identified by the initial = sign. Repetitive formulas such as the one occurring in cells B5–B17 do not have to be entered individually. Clever copy commands can be used to increment the desired variables in the formulas. The *$* signs in *$A$2* (cell b5) indicate that this part of the formula should not be incremented when the formula is copied. A sequence of numbers such as those in cells A5–A17 can also be entered automatically. Once the spreadsheet has been designed, complex calculations can be performed quickly and easily. For example, the results shown in cells B5–B17 will automatically be recalculated when the value for the half-life (cell A2) is changed. **B.** The results of the spreadsheet are shown.

ful?" Most of the utility of computers falls into a few categories—word processing, spreadsheets, databases, image manipulation, and communications. The relatively seamless ability to combine these capabilities adds to the utility of each.

Word Processors

Word processing software is one of the most mature computer applications. When word processing software first appeared, it was considerably more difficult to use than current generation software. Special symbols and commands had to be embedded in the text by the user to make the typed characters appear on the page in a specific fashion. The user had to learn an abstract word processing language for describing the appearance of the final text. Modern word processors show the user exactly how the printed page will look. The computer jargon for this is "What You See Is What You Get" (WYSIWYG, pronounced "wiziwig"). Modern word processing programs are very complicated, having a large number of options—fonts, sizes, styles, page layout, inclusion of other objects, mail lists, etc. However, these complexities are due to the application, not due to inadequacies in the design of the software.

Compared to word processing software, nuclear medicine specific software is much less mature. The user often has to deal with inadequacies in the design of the software. Hopefully, the progression with nuclear medicine software will be similar to the progression with word processing software.

Spreadsheets

Spreadsheets provide a simple method for doing repetitive calculations. Each cell in a spreadsheet can hold a number or a formula. The number or the result of the formula can be referenced by another cell. Quite complicated calculations can be built in a simple stepwise fashion. The simple layout of the spreadsheet came from the business world where row and column totals were often the only calculation. With a computer it is possible to put many much more complicated mathematic functions in the cells of the spreadsheet. Spreadsheets are a desirable replacement for a calculator and a pencil and paper any time the calculations are tedious or repetitive. For example, only a few key strokes are set up a chart of decay factors (Fig. 8.1). A well-written spreadsheet can be easily modified to perform other similar calculations. In Figure 8.1, the percent of the radionuclide remaining is automatically recalculated when a new physical half-life is entered into cell A2.

Database Programs

Database programs provide rapid access to large and often complicated data structures. The data in a database are stored in one or more tables. Tables have a simple two-dimensional structure (Fig. 8.2.) consisting of rows called records and columns called fields. For example, each row (record) could represent one patient; the columns (fields) might be medical record number, name, sex, date of birth, etc. The complexity of the database structure comes from the relationships between the tables. For example, there might be a second table which was the studies done in nuclear medicine. Each study would be represented by one row (record); columns (fields) in that table might be medical record number, study number, date of study, type of study, etc. Tables are related to each other by having a common field. The studies table is related to the patients table by the medical record number. A patient could have none, one, or many studies done in nuclear medicine.

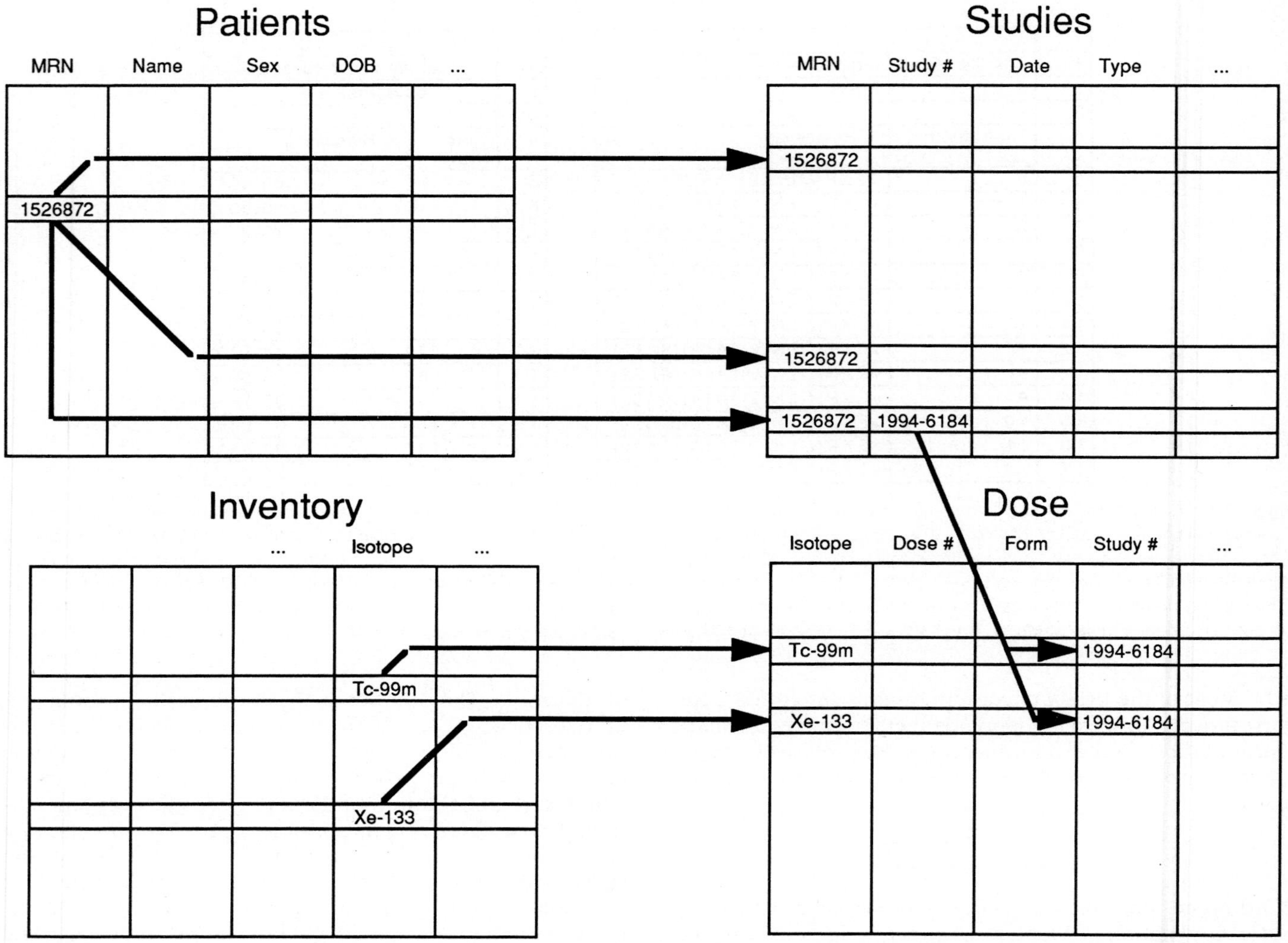

Figure 8.2. Structure of a database. Unique patient data is included once and only once in the patient database table. Each patient is assigned a unique medical record number (*MRN*). The *MRN* is then used as the unique link to the studies database. In turn, the studies database table is linked (related) to dose database table by the unique *Study #* field. The dose is not kept in the studies database table because one study may have more than one dose. The dose table can also be related to the radiopharmacy inventory table.

In addition to the study table, there might be a dose table. Each row (record) in the dose table would represent one dose; the columns (fields) in the table might be isotope, dose number, form, study number, etc. The dose table is related to the studies table by the study number which is stored in both tables. The doses are also related to the patients tables via the link (medical record number) between the studies table and the patients table. Additionally, the dose table might be related to a radiopharmacy inventory control system.

The database system can become quite complicated. Database programs allow the database to be easily accessed. For example, a report might show the nuclear medicine studies for 1 day with patient name and isotopes. The report would appear to be a simple list, but in fact the data comes from three tables. The advantage of a well-constructed database is that many different types of reports can be constructed from the database. The referring clinician, the technologist, and the radiopharmacist can all have a different view of the data using their respective reports.

Because the structure of each table is very simple, it is possible to develop fast algorithms to access the records using one or more fields or combinations of fields. At the same time the relationships between the tables allow a complicated structure to be represented by the database.

Learning to design a database properly requires some experience. There are a few rules of thumb. A single piece of data, like the patient's name, should only be entered in a single place in the database. Rather than having separate fields for isotope #1, isotope #2, isotope #3, and isotope #4, there should be a separate table which has one record for each isotope. Accession numbers, e.g., the study number, are important for uniquely identifying a record in the database, but in general, the user should never see these numbers. An exception is the medical record number; the medical record number (or possibly a Unique Patient Identification Code) is an important tool for uniquely identifying patients.

Image Manipulation

Drawing and painting programs are useful for making diagrams and other pictures. Several image processing programs allow for relatively complex image manipulations. Images can be combined with text and be made into slides or computer presentations. Integration of video with text and still images is becoming widely available and will allow for interesting multimedia presentations. Multimedia materials on CD discs are becoming an important source of continuing medical education. Multimedia capability combined with emerging communications capabilities will open new methods of working, learning, and playing (2).

Communications

The most rapidly expanding computer capability is communications. Communications covers a broad range of capabilities—point-to-point, Local Area Networks (LAN) (3), Wide Area Networks (WAN) (4), or Internet—based on various types of connections—voice grade telephone (using a modem), Integrated Services Digital Networks (ISDN), Ethernet, or Asynchronous Transfer Mode (ATM). The type of network and the quality of the connection often determine what functions are possible and reasonable.

A discussion of these capabilities is beyond the scope of this chapter. However, the Internet is currently the most widespread and most capable network. The Internet network is a collection of interconnected networks which use the TCP/IP (Transmission Control Protocol/Internet Protocol) protocols. (The TCP/IP protocols are also useful for networks which are not connected to Internet.) A direct Ethernet quality connection to Internet is desirable for picture communications; however, many Internet capabilities can be used with a good dial up connection.

Some of the functions supported by communications—electronic mail (e-mail), remote log-in, file sharing, file transfer, gopher and the World Wide Web (WWW)—are briefly described.

Electronic Mail. Electronic mail, particularly international electronic mail over the Internet, has opened a new method of communication. Electronic mail is different from telephone, FAX, and written communications, but shares some characteristics of all three. It is sent immediately, but recipients read it on their schedule. It is more structured than telephone conversations, but less formal than written communications. Group interaction is facilitated by easy copying and forwarding of electronic mail. In short, it does not supplant other methods of communications, but provides a new communications window.

Remote Log-in. Remote log-in is the oldest form of communications. It allows a terminal to communicate with a remote computer and function as if it were directly connected to the computer (5). Initially, the connection was almost always via voice-grade phone lines emulating a serial terminal. Currently, the terminal is typically a personal computer which is emulating a full screen character terminal. A variety of links are used. An Internet protocol, Telnet, allows a user at one computer on the network to log-in to another computer anywhere in the world.

File Sharing. File sharing allows a file system on one computer to appear to be located on another computer or computers. This technique is particularly useful in local area networks where a group of computers need rapid access to the same data. For example, this method can be used in a nuclear medicine picture archive and communications system (PACS). Image data is available to all of the computers without any special image sending or receiving software.

File Transfer. There is a special Internet protocol, file transfer protocol (FTP), which allows transfer of files from one computer to another computer. There are several other protocols for file transfer between computers, but the Internet's FTP protocol is by far the most widely available method. File transfer is more complicated than file sharing, but can be used to accomplish many of the same goals for more loosely coupled computers. FTP is a very important tool for sharing programs and data over the Internet. The FTP protocol is a hacker's delight—lots of unfriendly commands. (More sophisticated programs such as Mosaic, discussed later, make FTP more friendly.) Many of the uses of FTP are being supplanted by a more sophisticated mail protocol, multipurpose internet mail extensions (MIME), which allows mailing of both messages and attached files.

Gopher. A very popular protocol, Gopher, was developed at the University of Michigan and allows the user to search through a tree structure on the Internet. Gopher is a client/server protocol. A client program running on the user's computer requests services (typically information) from a server somewhere on the network. The user can hop from gopher server to gopher server around the world, following the trail of information. The user can also get lost—a problem with surfing the Internet.

World Wide Web. An even more powerful client/server protocol is the World Wide Web (WWW). Gopher is one of several World Wide Web protocols. The World Wide Web was developed at CERN, the European high energy physics laboratory. Use of the World Wide Web received a large boost with the development of Mosaic, a set of World Wide Web clients, by the National Center for Supercomputer Applications at the University of Illinois–Urbana/Champagne. Mosaic clients exist for Macintosh, PC Windows, and a host of X-terminal machines, especially Unix machines. Mosaic provides a uniform, cross-platform look and feel to a vast array of Internet services.

The World Wide Web uses hypertext for navigation. A highlighted portion of text is linked by a uniform resource locator (URL) to another resource—a text file, an image, a movie, a sound recording, a Gopher search, a Telnet log-in, a file transfer protocol, etc. The user points at the highlighted text and clicks, and the client program goes out on the network to get the new resource. That resource can be located on the server that was last accessed or on any other server in the world. By pointing and clicking on highlighted text the user can surf the resources on the Internet.

World Wide Web nuclear medicine services are just beginning to appear; however, in a short period of time the World Wide Web will be essential for practice (4, 6–16). Many societies, such as the RSNA, have home pages which list services (17). The Computer and Instrumentation Council of the Society of Nuclear Medicine has a home page which points to several educational resources of special interest to the nuclear medicine community.

The client/server paradigm is being used more and more for hospital-based systems. Security and encryption will provide the means for transfer of confidential medical information along with nonconfidential information on the information superhighway. The doctor's desktop of the future will be largely an electronic desktop. Client programs will access various general purpose information services—weather, references—as well as hospital information sources. Multimedia (text, images, cine, and voice) reports will improve communication to the referring clinician. The World Wide Web provides a convenient protocol for sending this information.

HARDWARE

All nuclear medicine computer systems consist of a CPU (central processing unit), internal storage locations (memory), external storage locations (floppy disks, etc.), a camera-computer interface, and a display system. Simple, inexpensive computer systems can be used for most computer tasks in nuclear medicine. Specialized software and hardware (analog to digital converters) often add significant costs to the system. More powerful computers are available to perform additional tasks such as sophisticated image processing and picture archiving and communications systems (PACS).

Central Processing Unit

The CPU is appropriately named since it is the control center for the computer system. The CPU consists of a control unit, an arithmetic-logic unit, and, in most computers, several general-purpose registers (Fig. 8.3).

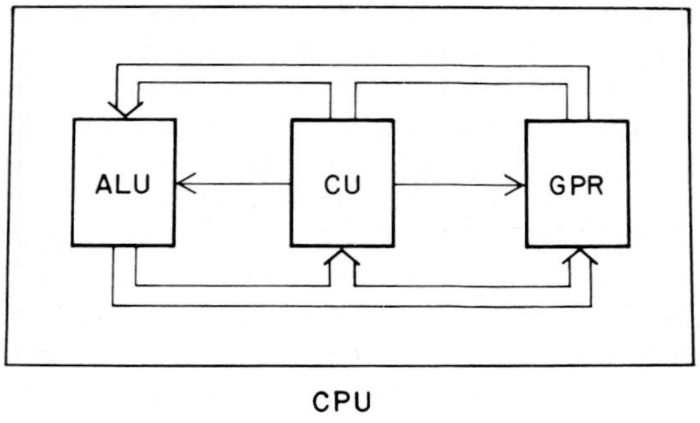

Figure 8.3. The central processing unit (CPU) of a computer consists of an arithmetic-logic unit (*ALU*), a control unit (*CU*), and general-purpose registers (*GPR*). The *CU* interprets instructions and transfers data to the *ALU* and the *GPR* when necessary. (Reproduced by permission from Holman BL, Parker JA. Computer-assisted cardiac nuclear medicine. Boston: Little, Brown & Co., 1981.)

The control unit of the CPU reads instructions from memory and rapidly executes them in sequence. Recently, reduced instruction set computers (RISC) have become popular. In contrast to complex instruction set computers (CISC), RISC computers perform only a limited set of basic instructions. This limited set of instructions has several implications in terms of CPU design. The result is that speed of operation is significantly increased. The penalty for this speed increase is that more complicated multistep instructions are needed to program certain advanced functions. Since these advanced functions are used infrequently, the penalty imposed by requiring multistep instructions is minimal. Central processing units typically used in nuclear medicine can add about 50 million numbers in 1 second. Some computer systems can service multiple users. Since the speed at which the CPU can operate is usually much greater than the needs of any individual user, multiple tasks appear to be occurring simultaneously even though the CPU services each user in sequence.

The results of arithmetic operations are stored in a general-purpose register. The number of general-purpose registers varies from one CPU to the next. These general-purpose registers are used by both the control unit and the arithmetic unit because they are storage locations that can be accessed more quickly than storage locations in memory.

Computer systems are often described by the size of the largest binary number that they can conveniently access. Modern nuclear medicine computer systems use 32-bit CPUs.

Main Memory

The program instructions and data that a computer requires are temporarily stored in main memory. Although information stored in memory is not as readily available to the CPU as is information stored in the general-purpose registers, it is much more accessible than information saved on peripheral storage devices such as disks or tapes.

Main memory size has increased enormously as the cost of memory has fallen greatly. The electronic circuits used in main memory must permit the storage and retrieval of data. This read/write (R/W) memory differs from read only memory (ROM) and programmable read-only memory (PROM). ROMs can only be written to once and therefore are used for programs and data that are unlikely to change. For example, ROMs are used to store parts of the computer's operating system. Proms allow for increasing amounts of adaptation by the manufacturer.

Since the CPU executes instructions very quickly, the speed with which main memory can be read from and written to is important. The access time for devices used in main memory is short (typically 100 nsec) and is independent of location (random access memory (RAM)). One method of improving memory performance is to have a small amount of very fast memory which is often located on the CPU chip. This cache memory (Fig. 8.4) becomes loaded with parts of the program that are used frequently by the CPU. Cache memory allows the CPU to minimize access times and can speed the execution of programs by factors of 2 or greater.

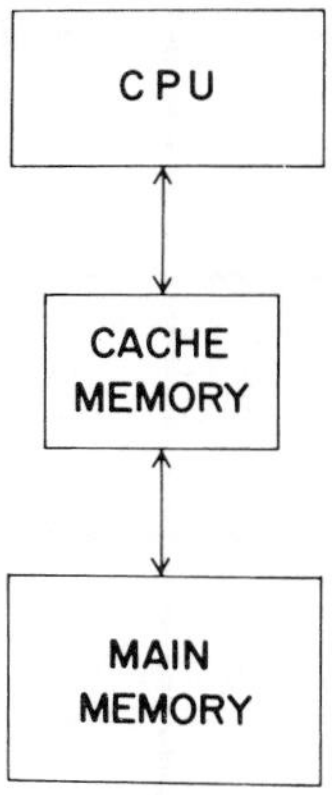

Figure 8.4. Cache memory is fast but expensive memory. The cache memory becomes loaded with the instructions and data that the CPU repeatedly uses. A small amount of cache memory results in faster execution times with a minimum of expense. (Reproduced by permission from Holman BL, Parker JA. Computer-assisted cardiac nuclear medicine. Boston: Little, Brown & Co., 1981.)

Bus

The different components of the computer are connected by one or more buses. The term bus is used because the computer's bus transports data (instead of people). In physical terms, a bus is rather uninteresting; it typically consists of just a set of wires. However, conceptually a bus is very important. The rules used to communicate over the bus provide a hardware interface between the components. This interface allows each of the hardware devices to be independent. The manufacturer of one component only needs to follow the bus rules; it does not need to know the specifics of the other components. Additionally, the speed of a computer is often affected by the speed with which the bus can transport data.

External Storage Devices

Data and programs are usually saved on external storage devices since these devices are less expensive than main memory. Magnetic tapes, floppy disks, hard disks, and optical disks are the most commonly used external storage devices. Each of these devices has found its own niche as an external storage device.

Magnetic tape is the oldest external storage technology still in use. Magnetic tape is used primarily for archival storage and backup because the access time (the time to find the data of interest) is long. Tapes are read sequentially and all the data stored on the tape prior to the desired data must be read first. Once the desired data are reached, the transfer rate (the time to transfer the data to main memory) can approach that of other media (e.g., hard disk). Its popularity as an archival media is due to the fact that large amounts of information can be stored in a small space at low cost.

To minimize the long access times imposed by magnetic tapes, hard magnetic disks were introduced as external storage devices. Disk packs have been replaced by nonremovable sealed hard disk drives (Winchester disks). Before using a disk, the disk must be formatted and initialized.

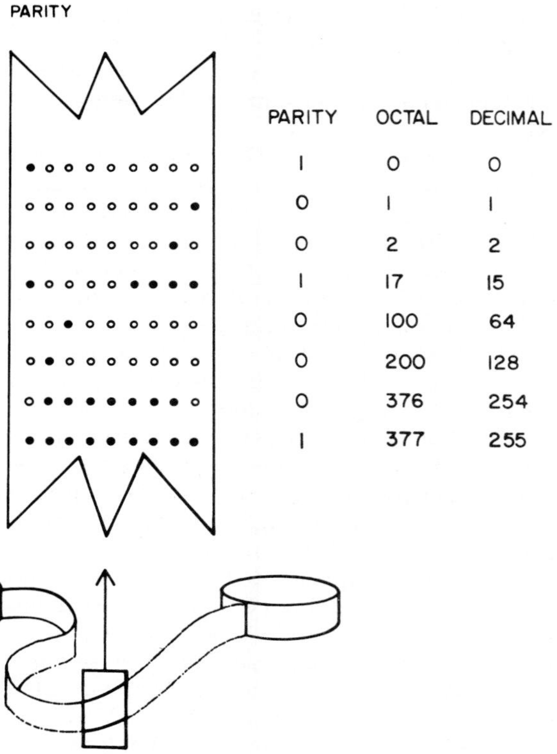

Figure 8.5. Data are written on magnetic disk in numerous closed circles called tracks. The tracks are further subdivided into sectors. One block of data is stored on each sector. Entire blocks of data are read or written at one time. The size of a block varies greatly depending on the computer system and the capacity of the hard disk. The location of the tracks on the disk is indicated by magnetic marks that are written to the disk when it is formatted. (Reproduced by permission from Holman BL, Parker JA. Computer-assisted cardiac nuclear medicine. Boston: Little, Brown & Co., 1981.)

Formatting involves writing special marks to the disk that identify the tracks and sectors on a disk. Data is written on tracks that encircle the disk (Fig. 8.5). Direct (random) access of any data on the disk is possible and greatly reduces access times. The tracks are divided into a number of pie-shaped sectors each of which holds a block of data. This division may be done optically (hard sectored) or can be done by writing magnetic landmarks on the disk (soft sectored). The number of tracks and sectors on a physically identical disk can vary depending on the formatting software that is used. The start of the sectors on each track may be offset to allow time for the read/write head of the disk drive to switch tracks (interleaving). The number of bytes in one block of data is not standard. The physical arrangement of data on the disk is determined by circuitry called a controller. Initializing the disk consists of writing special files such as the disk directory. The protocols for the way this information is organized on the disk vary and are dependent on the operating system that is used.

Hard disk drives can have single or multiple disks of magnetic media. The read/write heads of these types of disks are aerodynamically designed to fly in the swirling air a fraction of an inch above the recording surface. Since no contact is ordinarily made, the recording surface does not become worn, making these devices very reliable. Very reliable does not, however, mean failure-proof. The reliability of hard drives lulls the user into a false sense of security. Eventually, even the most reliable disk fails. A strategy to back up all valuable data on hard disk is essential.

The storage capacity of hard disk drives have increased dramatically as the price of drives have plummeted. High capacity (1 gigabyte) hard disk drives can be purchased for around $500. A group of high capacity disk drives can be used together to provide high transfer rates and redundancy (called a redundant array of inexpensive disks (RAID)). These arrays are often combined with a tape system for backup. RAIDs are now inexpensive enough to be used for archival storage in nuclear medicine. Tape is still useful for backup and/or long-term off-site storage.

Optical disks use lasers to encode data by burning small holes on the surface of disks. Although some schemes for making this medium erasable have been proposed, its relative irreversibility and high capacity may make it an ideal archival medium. A juke box of optical disks can be used to increase the capacity. CD ROM disks are a form of optical disk that store about 650 megabytes of data. They use the same format as audio discs. CD ROM drives are relatively inexpensive ($200–$300) and are included as standard devices on most computer systems. CD-ROM disks can be produced very cheaply in large quantities so software is often distributed on CD-ROM. Inexpensive ($4000) CD-ROM disk writers can produce single copy CD-ROM disks, although they use relatively expensive blanks ($20). A patient study archive could be stored and retrieved using one CD-ROM writer and an array of inexpensive CD-ROM readers.

Flexible (floppy) disks were introduced in the late 1970s. Because they revolve at much slower rates than hard disk, they have access times that are several times longer than hard disks. Their slower revolution also limits the rate at which data can be transferred to 1/10 to 1/20 of the speed that is achievable with a hard disk. Floppies are less reliable than hard disks for two reasons. First, the physical protection provided for these disks is much less than the protection provided for a hard disk. Second, the read/write head of a floppy disk drive actually makes physical contact with the magnetic recording media. This contact will gradually wear the recording surface. The life expectancy of a frequently used floppy disk is less than a year. Despite these limitations, floppy disks have become exceedingly popular because they are an inexpensive, convenient, easily transportable device to store small amounts of data.

Camera-Computer Interface

The x and y signals produced by most gamma-cameras are analog signals that indicate the two-dimensional coordinates of a scintillation within the crystal of the detector. When these analog signals are digitized, the field of view of the camera is divided into discrete rows and columns of boxes (picture elements or pixels) (Fig. 8.6). The exact location of the event is no longer recorded; only the digital coordinates of the scintillation are tabulated. This digital representation of the image can then be processed by a computer. The storage requirements of the matrix increase geometrically with the size of the matrix (Table 8.4).

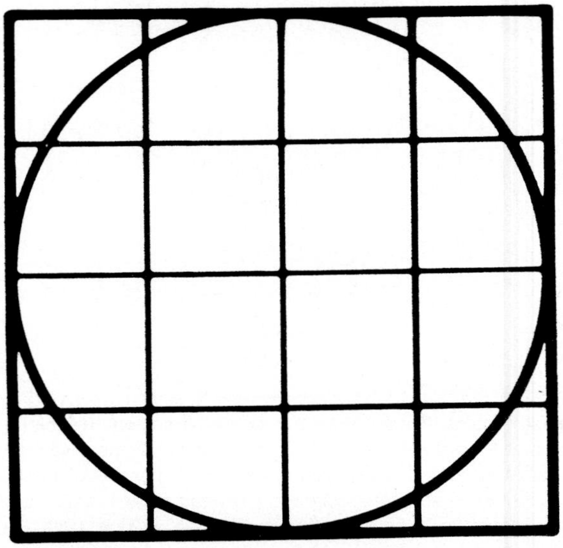

Figure 8.6. Image matrix. The field of view of a gamma-camera can be divided into discrete rows and columns of picture elements (pixels). If the number of scintillations that occur in each pixel is stored as the value of that pixel, a digital image can be produced. For illustrative purposes, only a 4×4 matrix is shown. Clinically used matrix sizes range from 322–5122. (Reproduced by permission from Holman BL, Parker JA. Computer-assisted cardiac nuclear medicine. Boston: Little, Brown & Co., 1981.)

Table 8.4.
Matrix Storage Requirements

Matrix Size	Number of Pixels	Frames per Megabyte	
		8-Bit Pixel	16-Bit Pixel
64 × 64	4K	250	125
128 × 128	16K	64	32
256 × 256	64K	16	8
512 × 512	256K	4	2
1024 × 1024	1M	1	0.5

To connect an analog gamma-camera to a digital computer, analog-to-digital converters (ADCs) with support circuitry are required. The support circuitry provides the proper scaling and buffering of the analog signals, as well as providing signals which notify the ADCs when conversions can take place. Older gamma-cameras only needed to digitize the analog x and y position signals, but now it is common to digitize the analog z or energy signal as well. Choosing an ADC is usually a compromise between resolution (number of bits in the output), speed (input sample rate), and cost. ADCs used to digitize x and y analog position signals in gamma-cameras need a resolution which matches the largest digital image matrix expected at the maximum zoom factor to be used and a minimum speed to match the largest count rate expected. For example, the minimum ADC resolution needed for a 1024×1024 nuclear medicine digital image for a zoom factor of unity is N = 10 bits ($2^N = 1024$) and the minimum speed for a maximum expected count rate of 100,000 counts per second is 100,000 samples per second (assuming one ADC dedicated

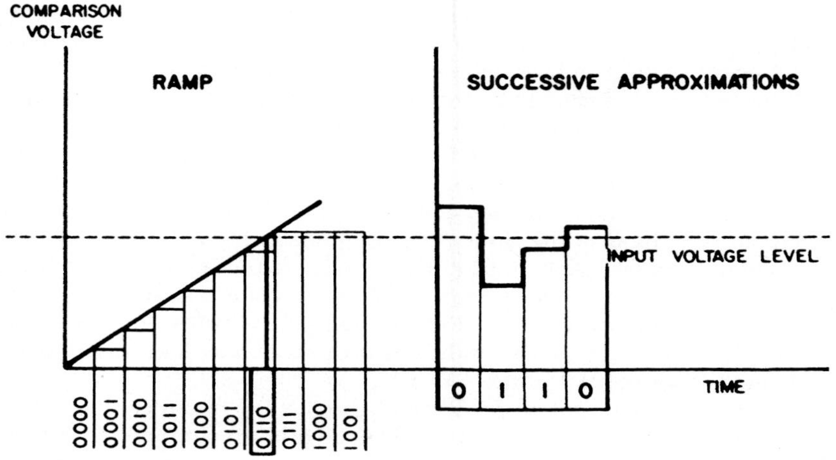

Figure 8.7. Two types of analog-to-digital converters are shown. Ramp-type converters compare the input voltage level with a series of monotonously increasing test voltages. When the test voltage exceeds the input voltage, the value of the input voltage is known. Note that the time required for the test voltage to exceed the input voltage varies with the magnitude of the input voltage. Successive approximation converters compare the input voltage to a series of test voltages that are determined by the bits in the test voltage number that has been set. Starting with the bit that has the highest value, a test voltage corresponding to that bit being equal to 1 is compared with the input voltage. If the input voltage is less than the test voltage then the bit is set to 0. This comparison continues for all bits therefore the time required for digitization is independent of the magnitude of the input voltage. (Reproduced by permission from Holman BL, Parker JA. Computer-assisted cardiac nuclear medicine. Boston: Little, Brown & Co., 1981.)

to each analog x and y position signal and that there is analog derandomizing circuitry).

The two main architectures that are used to implement ADCs are serial and parallel. High-resolution ADCs are generally built using serial architectures that most often determine one output bit at a time in a sequence of measurements. Examples of popular serial architecture ADCs include ramp (or integrating), delta-sigma, and successive approximation (Fig. 8.7). Ramp ADCs are designed for very high resolution at the expense of speed (due to the time required to compare the integrated input voltage with a reference voltage). Ramp ADC's are not used in today's high-performance gamma-cameras as they once were in the early days of gamma-cameras. Delta-sigma ADCs also offer high resolution and at a low cost but are used in audio-band signal processing applications (usually up to 44 kHz) which is below the possible high count rates encountered in procedures such as first pass studies. Successive approximation ADCs offer good resolution and speed at a reasonable cost and are the ADC of choice in gamma-camera applications. High-speed or flash ADCs are generally built using parallel architectures from which all the bits are determined simultaneously in a single measurement. Flash ADCs are usually not used in gamma-cameras due to the high cost and limited resolution as compared with successive approximation ADCs.

With the ramp ADC, the test voltage begins at 0 and is increased linearly with time. The input voltage is assigned a value based on the time required to be surpassed by the test voltage. The conversion time increases exponentially as the precision increases. The deadtime of the ramp ADC varies with the magnitude of the input value; this complicates deadtime corrections. Usually a relatively long fixed deadtime is imposed to simplify this problem.

The successive approximation ADC determines the value of each bit of the input value by comparing the input voltage with the appropriate test voltage. Since each cycle determines the value of a bit, the conversion time increases linearly as the precision required increases. The deadtime for this type of ADC is constant since it is proportional to the number of bits of precision desired, not the magnitude of the input value.

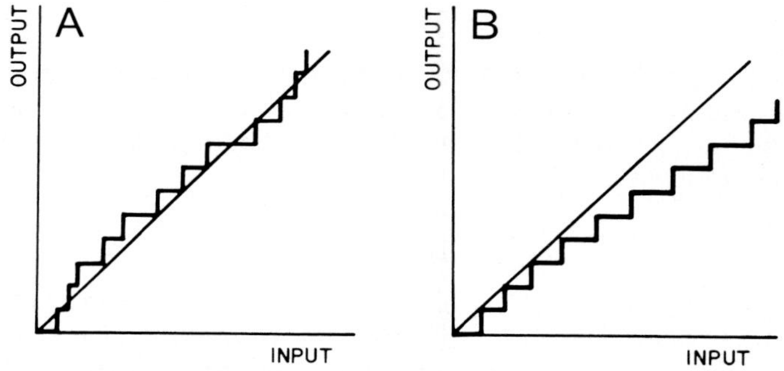

Figure 8.8. Linearity of ADCs. **A.** Poor differential linearity occurs when the bin sizes vary considerably. The differential linearity of successive approximation ADCs is poorer than ramp ADCs. **B.** Poor integral linearity occurs when there is a systematic error in bin size. This is a greater problem with ramp ADCs than with successive approximation ADCs. (Reproduced by permission from Holman BL, Parker JA. Computer-assisted cardiac nuclear medicine. Boston: Little, Brown & Co., 1981.)

Linearity is an important specification for describing the performance of ADCs. Two types of linearity, differential and integral, are measured (Fig. 8.8). Differential linearity quantifies the uniformity of the size of the analog voltage steps (bin size), which correspond to successive digital values. Integral linearity relates the analog voltage to the digital value over the entire range of analog values. It is possible to have good integral linearity and poor differential linearity and vice versa. Ramp ADCs are more likely to have good differential linearity and successive approximation ADCs tend to have better integral uniformity. Satisfactory differential linearity for successive approximation ADCs is achieved by selecting an ADC that has several bits greater precision than is needed. Fourteen bits of accuracy are sufficient to provide a matrix resolution of 512^2.

Since the shape and duration of the x and y signals varies from camera to camera, the analog input to the ADCs must be adjusted to obtain a uniform response from the ADCs. Camera-computer interfaces that have multiple individually adjustable input ports are optimal. Special provisions must be made to interface cameras that are more than a few hundred feet from the computer (13).

User-adjustable ADCs give the user the ability to employ any amount of magnification. Very high magnification may be necessary to perform certain quality control procedures such as measurement of a line spread function. Multiple preset ADC settings will allow the user to acquire studies in multiple magnification modes.

Once the analog x and y signals are converted to their digital counterparts, an address maker in the interface rapidly calculates the address in memory that is to be incremented when a study is collected in matrix mode. When studies are collected in list mode, the address maker is bypassed and the x and y values of the event are explicitly stored.

Gamma-cameras with digital outputs are becoming more common. These cameras present new interfacing problems since the digital output from the camera cannot input directly to an ADC. If digital data are passed through a digital-to-analog converter (DAC) and then through an ADC patterning, artifacts will result because of aliasing. One solution is to provide a digital pathway that bypasses the ADCs.

In addition to the ADCs for the x and y signals, camera-computer interfaces often have additional ADCs for interfacing a joystick and/or an electrocardiogram (ECG) to the computer.

Display Systems

Once digital images are obtained, a display screen (14, 15, 18) is required to view them. To avoid degrading the image, display systems are designed to avoid adding distracting artifacts (19). For example, interpolation of images obtained in a 64×64 matrix to a 256×256 matrix makes the individual pixels of the image less noticeable; therefore, the viewer is able to concentrate on the information content of the images. At least 80 levels of gray are necessary so that the viewer will not perceive the transition of one level of gray to another. If transitions between levels of gray are perceivable, artificial edges are created (Fig. 8.9). Many displays provide 256 (2^8) levels of gray since most computers are optimized to use 8-bit bytes.

If photographs are to be obtained from the display, it is important to realize that the eye responds differently to the display than does film. Two video devices are usually necessary to accurately photograph and view the displayed images.

When displaying a sequence of images, the same gray scale should be used on all images. Occasionally, the viewer may want to display each image in a sequence with a gray scale that optimizes the contrast within each image. That is, the levels of gray are assigned according to the range of pixel values in each image. This results in a sequence of images in which the meaning of any given gray level changes throughout the sequence of images. If this type of gray scale assignment is incorrectly used on studies such as gated radionuclide angiocardiograms, structures that have a constant activity level (e.g., the pulmonary blood pool) may change intensity because the gray scale assignment keeps changing from frame to frame.

Color should be used with care. An observer will equate similar colors in different portions of an image. By contrast, an observer will compare gray levels to surrounding values. Color may be useful for functional images or cross-sectional images where values in different portions of the image need to be compared. For example, in brain scintigraphy the cortex on one side of the image is often compared to the opposite side. However, the observer needs to be aware that he or she may attribute more significance to the change from one color to another than to a change in one shade of the same color to another shade. Color is particularly likely to produce the appearance of artificial edges. Use of color is appropriate when color transitions have a special meaning. For example, if the transition from one color to another indicates pixels that have a normal and an abnormal value.

Human engineering of the display is critical since the display is the most widely used human-computer interface in the nuclear medicine computer system. The display needs to be carefully adjusted so that the display intensities appear equally spaced to the observer. Nonlinear contrast enhancement can be applied to the image, but the display itself should appear linear. One of the most important functions of the computer is the ability to change the background and window. These display parameters should be easily changed on the whole image or part of the image for both static and cine mode display.

SOFTWARE

One of the characteristics of computer systems is that they are potentially very versatile. Computer technology is now used to determine if your car door is open, your bank account is overdrawn, or the reentry path of the space shuttle is correct. Often the same physical components are used for markedly dissimilar tasks. The malleability of computers is largely due to the fact that they are programmable. The list of instructions that is used to direct the computer can be changed without physical modification of the computer, hence the name software.

The software required for a nuclear medicine system can be broadly divided into three general categories. First, there is general-purpose software called the operating system, which provides the programs needed to perform common nonspecialized computer tasks. These tasks include keyboard command interpretation, file maintenance, input and output operations, and programming.

Second, there is special-purpose software supplied with the computer system that provides programs to perform image acquisition and analysis. In nuclear medicine, the software and computer needed to provide image acquisition and minimal image analysis has become an integral part of most cameras. These integrated systems are likely to serve the computational needs of many nuclear medicine users. Larger independent computer systems will be needed to perform sophisticated image processing and PACS functions.

The third type of software used in nuclear medicine is user-written applications software. This type of software is usually least well thought out, least field tested, and least supported of all the software available to nuclear medicine, yet it is on the basis of this software that clinical decisions are usually made.

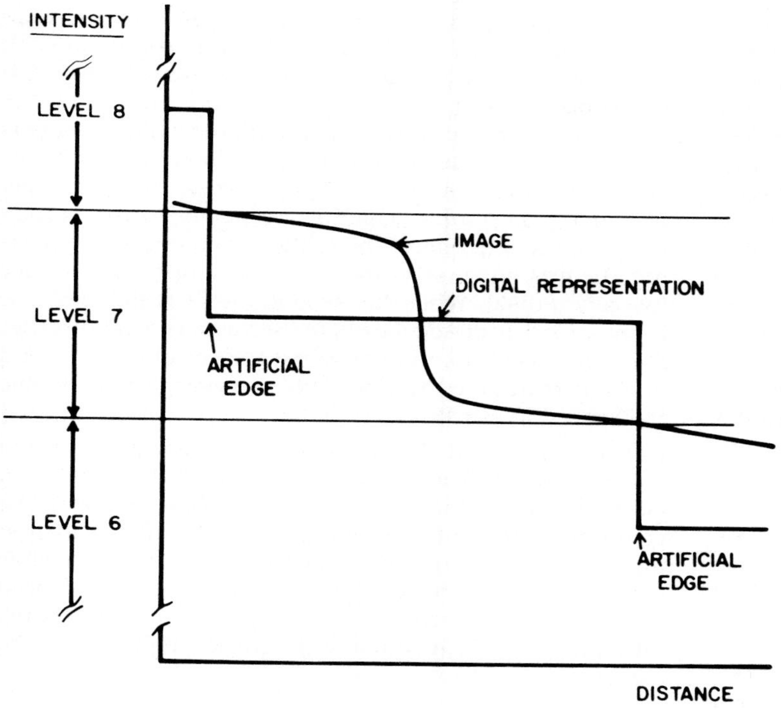

Figure 8.9. Artificial edges are created when there is an inadequate gray scale. (Reproduced by permission from Holman BL, Parker JA. Computer-assisted cardiac nuclear medicine. Boston: Little, Brown & Co., 1981.)

Operating System

The casual user of the nuclear medicine computer system may be unaware of the operating system that is used on his or her computer system. Some older nuclear medicine systems have no operating system at all, but rather have functions normally provided by a general-purpose operating system provided by the image acquisition and analysis software. For any user who wants to use the computer for anything other than the routine nuclear medicine applications, an unmodified general-purpose operating system is best. A general-purpose operating system that has been modified by the nuclear medicine system vendor is less desirable since there is often a considerable lag in modifying subsequent versions of the operating system. As a result, features incorporated into new versions of the general-purpose operating system may be unavailable to the nuclear medicine user.

The performance of the computer system is greatly affected by the operating system as well as the hardware that is used. Macintosh and PC-based computers each use their own hardware-dependent operating systems. There are number of efforts, which will succeed by necessity, to make operating systems hardware-independent (UNIX and Windows NT are examples). Machine-independent software makes it possible to have a uniform computer environment. If different computer hardware used the same machine-independent software, only one basic set of commands need be mastered. Since versatility is an important design factor, these systems can usually be easily customized to meet the needs of individual markets.

One reason that operating systems have such a great impact on computer performance is that they determine basic human-computer interactions. In the past, a keyboard and simple text was used as the primary human-computer interface. Modern interfaces include the extensive uses of graphics and pointing devices (mouse or a track ball).

General aspects of the filing system, such as how the directory of files is structured, are controlled by the operating system. The file maintenance facilities provided by the operating system have become increasingly important as the storage capacity of peripheral storage devices has increased. After a period of time, a confusing mass of files may accumulate. A tree-structured file directory is desirable since it allows groups of files to be associated.

The final major elements of the operating system are programming aids, including compilers for programming languages, text editors, and debugging tools. The importance of these programs depends on whether the computer system user plans to develop his or her own programs. The desirable features of the programming environment that are provided by the operating system are discussed in detail under "User-written Software."

Nuclear Medicine Software

Acquisition Software. Acquisition software allows the user to define preset protocols for routinely performed studies. Different types of image collection include static, dynamic, gated, list mode, and tomographic studies.

Static Study. A pulmonary perfusion study is an example of a static study. One view is obtained, data acquisition stops, and the patient is repositioned for the next view. A start button is used to begin each acquisition. Collection parameters that are specified when collecting a static image include matrix size, number of frames, method of ending the study, and method for handling overflow conditions. The matrix size used in a static study should be large enough not to degrade image resolution. Image resolution is preserved if the pixel size of the matrix that is used is less than at least one-half the size of the smallest object that can be seen in the analog image. The smallest lead bar that can be resolved under ideal conditions with a state-of-the-art camera at the face of a high-resolution collimator is 2–3 mm; therefore, under ideal conditions, a 512×512 matrix should be used. The pixel size of a 512×512 matrix obtained on a large-field-of-view (400-mm diameter) camera is less than 1 mm. In clinical practice, a number of factors (scatterer, depth, general-purpose collimator, physiologic motion, low count images, decreased target-to-background ratio) degrade the practical resolution of the camera by at least a factor of 2–4, making a 128×128 matrix acceptable for many routine images. For high-count, high-resolution images, a 256×256 matrix may be useful. The 512×512 matrix is necessary to collect the high-resolution images of bar phantoms, which are used for quality control.

Most acquisition software does not allow the user to change the number of frames in the study after acquisition is begun. This is unfortunate since additional views may be requested. Two inadequate solutions have been to routinely include one or two extra frames in the predefined protocols or to save the extra frames as a second study on the same patient. Facilities to delete and reuse a frame during the acquisition of a study are useful since it is sometimes necessary to repeat a view because the patient has moved.

Four possible methods of ending image acquisition include preset total counts, preset acquisition time, preset count density, and manual. The manual end of acquisition is useful when a patient moves. When a byte matrix is used, the user must decide what to do when a pixel in the matrix overflows (exceeds its maximum value of 255). If the collection proceeds, the relative values of the pixels in the image are no longer maintained since pixels with the maximum counts cannot be incremented. Structural detail in the region of these pixels is lost (20). Loss of detail may be acceptable if these pixels are not located in an area of clinical interest, such as the bladder on a bone scan. In quantitative studies, overflow may invalidate the results. The user should have the option to end the acquisition when one pixel in the frame reaches its maximum value (close frame on overflow). An alternative solution is to collect the frame in a word matrix rather than a byte matrix. A pixel of a 16-bit word matrix can store a number as large as 65,535. The disadvantage of always using a word matrix is that it requires twice the storage space of a byte matrix.

Dynamic Study. A dynamic study is one in which a continuous series of images is acquired. Continuous acquisition prohibits the repositioning of the patient once acquisition has begun. A ^{99m}Tc-MAG3 renal study is an example of a dynamic study. Even though the patient's position cannot be changed during a dynamic study, the frame rate and matrix size of the study can be changed. This capability is quite helpful since high temporal resolution (1 frame every 1–2 seconds) is often required for only the first minute or so following the injection. Subsequent images can be obtained at lower frame rates (1 frame every 20–60 seconds). When high temporal resolution images are obtained, spatial resolution will be poor since the total counts in each image will be relatively small, allowing a smaller (64×64) image matrix to be used.

When a dynamic study is acquired, the main memory is used to store two sequential images. When the first image is finished, the input stream is directed to the second set of memory locations, which corresponds to the second image in the sequence. While this second image is collecting, the first image is written to an external storage device (usually a disk). When the second image is finished, the input stream is directed back to the memory locations that had been used for the preceding image and the second image is written to the disk. This process is called double buffering (Fig. 8.10).

Gated Studies. Gated studies use a physiologic signal to synchronize data acquisition. The term gate refers to an electronic "gate" that "opens" to allow data to flow to the computer. When gated cardiac blood pool studies were first introduced they consisted of 2 images, one at end-diastole and one at end-systole. The electronic gate only allowed data to flow to the computer during these time intervals. These 2-frame acquisitions were quickly replaced by the

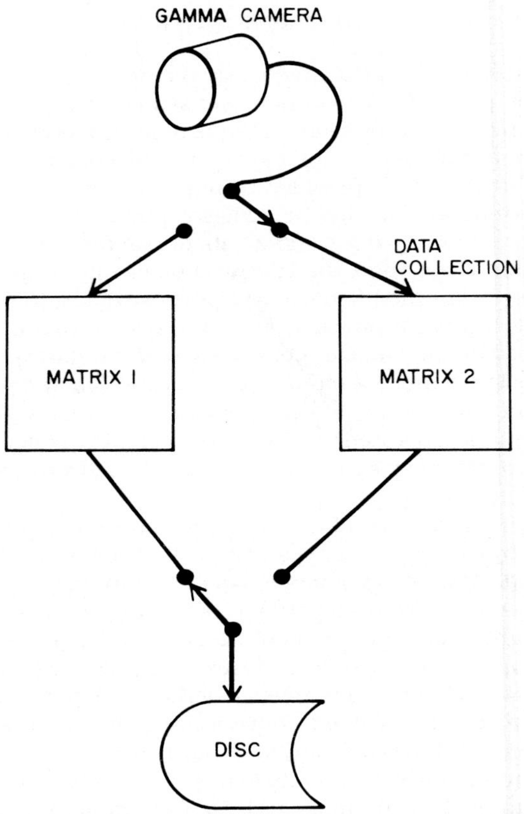

Figure 8.10. When dynamic studies are acquired, memory is divided into two sections that store two frames (matrices of the study). When one of the matrices is being acquired (*matrix 2*) the other (*matrix 1*) is written to the disk. This technique is called double buffering. (Reproduced by permission from Holman BL, Parker JA. Computer-assisted cardiac nuclear medicine. Boston: Little, Brown & Co., 1981.)

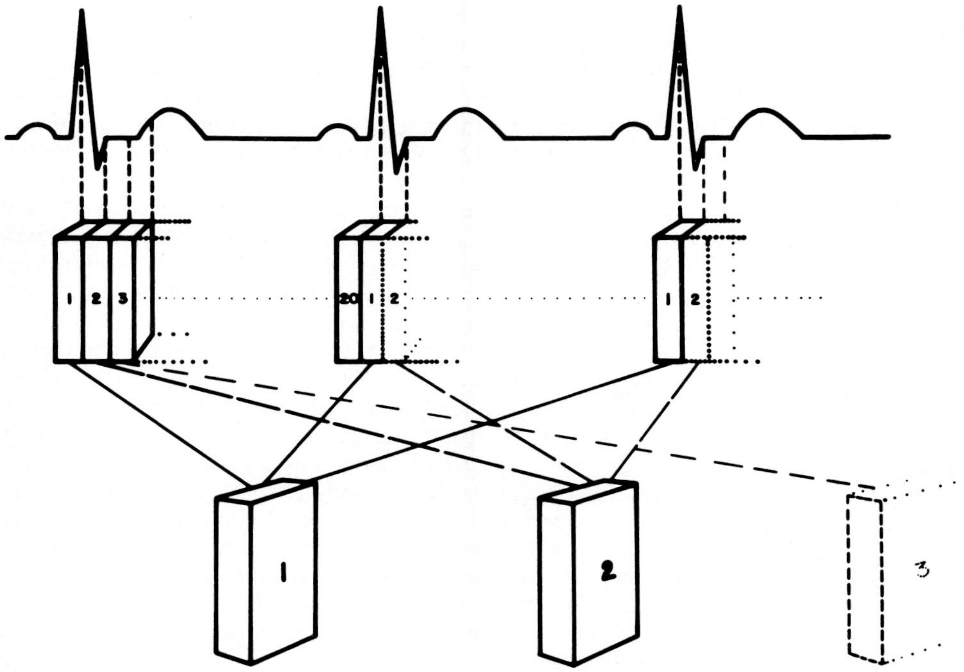

Figure 8.11. Electrocardiographic gating. In a gated cardiac study, image acquisition is synchronized using the R wave of the patient's ECG. In this example, the average R-R interval was divided into 20 frames. Counts from the same time frame of hundreds of cardiac cycles are added together to form a composite or average heartbeat. (Reproduced by permission from Holman BL, Parker JA. Computer-assisted cardiac nuclear medicine. Boston: Little, Brown & Co., 1981.)

continuous acquisition of data in multiple sequential images (multiple gated acquisition or MUGA).

With gated cardiac blood pool scans, the R wave of the ECG is used to synchronize image acquisition (Fig. 8.11). Before the acquisition of the study begins, the computer monitors successive R waves and determines the average R-R interval. Once the average R-R interval is calculated, the frame duration is determined by dividing this interval by the number of frames in the study. For example, if a patient has a heart rate of 60 beats/sec (1000 msec/R-R interval) and 20 frames are collected per R-R interval, then each frame will have a duration of 50 msec. Alternatively, some systems allow the user to enter the desired frame duration and the desired number of frames. Some computers have the capability to continuously average the RR interval and can dynamically change the frame duration to match any change in heart rate.

Since the count rate during a gated cardiac study is about 10,000–20,000 counts/sec, only 500–1000 counts would be collected during the 50-msec frame duration. Since many more counts are needed to form an image, the computer sums hundreds of low-count 50-msec images from each of the 50-msec intervals or frames of the cardiac cycle using the R wave as a reference point. Since hundreds of heartbeats are summed, the gated study represents an average heartbeat.

The minimum number of frames needed in a gated study varies depending on which physiologic parameters are being measured. Ejection fraction can be measured with as few as 20 frames/R-R interval since there is an isovolumic period during end-diastole and end-systole. Higher temporal resolution studies are needed to accurately measure instantaneous rates of change such as peak emptying or filling rates (21–31).

The main memory of the computer is used to store all the frames of a gated cardiac study during acquisition. Traditionally, matrix sizes of 64×64 have been used, but larger matrix sizes can be used with modern computers.

Patients who have variable R-R intervals present special problems during the acquisition of a gated cardiac blood pool study. Shorter than average R-R intervals will cause the computer to redirect the input stream to the first frame of the study; therefore, frames toward the end of the cardiac cycle will have fewer total counts (Fig. 8.12). Fortunately, the duration of the systolic portion of the cardiac cycle is less variable than the diastolic portion. When the R wave is used to synchronize the beginning of systole of the many heartbeats, the end of systole will also be reasonably synchronous even with moderate variations in R-R interval. On the other hand, the fidelity of the diastolic portion of the volume curve is more severely affected by arrhythmias because the duration of the diastolic portion varies more than the systolic portion of the cardiac cycle. The fidelity of the diastolic portion of the curve can be better preserved using backwards gating (see hybrid list mode study later).

Acquisition programs for gated cardiac studies usually provide some arrhythmia rejection capability. Typically the user will enter the maximum variability in the R-R interval that is acceptable (gate tolerance). When a premature (or prolonged) R wave that is outside the gate tolerance occurs, the input stream is ignored for the next two R waves. The beat interrupted by the PVC has a short R-R interval. This beat with the short R-R interval is included in the representative average heartbeat. No retrospective correction is possible since the incoming data has already been added to the matrix data in memory by the time the abnormal R-R interval is detected. At first, this method of handling ectopic beats seems suboptimal. However, upon further reflection, the method is satisfactory. Beat 1 in Table 8.5 has

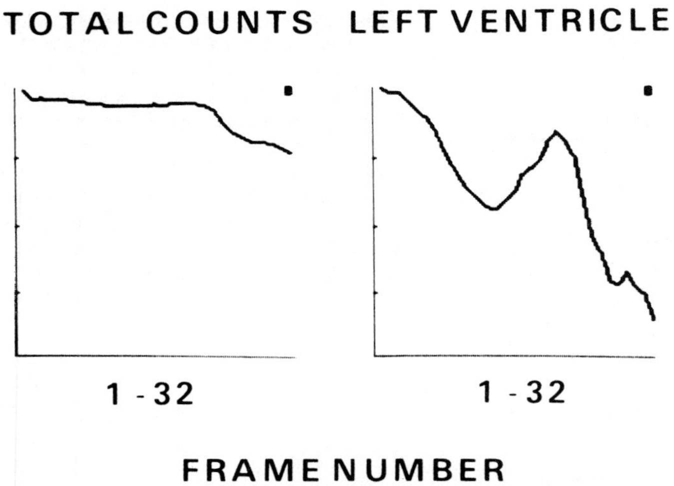

Figure 8.12. Effect of arrhythmia on the volume curve. *Left:* The total counts for each frame in a cardiac cycle are shown for a patient with atrial fibrillation. The lost of total counts at the end of the cardiac cycle is due to the fact that when each R wave is detected the subsequent counts are redirected to the first frame in the study. Frames late in the cycle will have fewer counts because only some beats have long enough R-R intervals to deposit counts in these frames. *Right:* The background-corrected left ventricular volume versus time curve from the same patient. The volume curve provides an important quality control tool to indicate that the gating was adequate.

Table 8.5.
Effect of a PVC on RR Interval and Ejection Fraction.

	Beat 1 NSR	Beat 2 PVC	Beat 3 NSR	Beat 4 NSR
RR Interval	Short	Long	Normal	Normal
Ejection Fraction	Normal	Decreased	Increased	Normal

a short R-R interval because diastole was interrupted by a premature ventricular contraction; however, the ejection fraction was normal because its filling time and mode of depolarization was normal. Beats 2 and 3 (the PVC and the postextrasystolic potentiated beat) are rejected. Their ejection fractions are decreased and increased, respectively, primarily because of decreased (beat 2) and increased (beat 3) ventricular filling. It is important to note that a homogeneous population of beats can not be selected on the basis of its RR interval alone; the RR interval of the preceding beat must also be considered.

List Mode Study. Another approach to data acquisition that enables the user to retrospectively format the data is to use a list mode study (29, 31–36). With list mode, the x and y location of each scintillation is recorded along with millisecond timing marks. Many x,y pairs are available for coding nonscintillation data (e.g., timing marks). For example, if the round field of view of the camera is mapped into a matrix that is an exscribed square, corner pixels can be used to save nonimage data. The data on this list can be reformatted after collection to provide frame rates with a temporal resolution of up to 1 msec. A gated list mode study can be acquired by using a second unique x,y pair to record the R wave in the data stream.

Using this technique, the list mode study could be reformatted using only the counts from beats that had specified characteristics. Ideally, the user would want to be able to specific the RR interval of the current beat and the preceding beat. Identifying the R-R interval of the preceding beat is important because the R-R interval of the preceding beat determines the loading conditions of the heart. As discussed earlier, beats with a normal R-R interval that have been preceded by a beat with a prolonged R-R interval will have a higher than normal ejection fraction (postextrasystolic potentiation). Additional physiologic information such as inspiration and expiration could be encoded, using a respiratory gate, to determine their effects on cardiac or lung function (37).

List mode has not been routinely used because of two disadvantages. First, the storage requirements of a list mode study are much greater than the storage requirements of a matrix mode study. Two bytes are required to store each x and y pair. A typical gated list mode study consists of 10 million counts and requires 20 megabytes of storage. If the same 10 million count study is collected as a gated cardiac study consisting of 32 64×64 word frames, it requires only 256 kilobytes of storage. In this example, the storage requirement of the gated matrix mode study is approximately one-eightieth of the list mode study and is dependent only on the size of the matrix and the number of frames in the study. Disks with the large capacity needed to conveniently perform a list mode study are now widely available.

The second disadvantage of list mode studies is the clinical relevance of reporting ejection fraction for different population of beats. A routine gated cardiac blood pool study already gives a frequency-weighted average of all populations of beats. It is unclear what unique clinical information is gained by performing a separate analysis of each population of beats.

A hybrid list mode and matrix mode study can be used for better arrhythmia rejection and to achieve better fidelity in the diastolic portion of the volume curve. To select beats with a constant R-R interval, the x,y data are kept in list mode for a few R-R intervals. They are then added to the matrix mode data only if they meet the established R-R criterion. To achieve better fidelity in the later diastolic portion of the curve, the x,y values are kept in the list mode until the R-R interval is known. The systolic portion of the cardiac cycle is lined up as usual (forward gating) but the late diastolic portion of the cardiac cycle is generated by calculating the time backward from the R wave (backward gating) (34). This provides maximum synchrony in the first and last frame of the study. This type of hybrid study is not routinely available on most computer systems.

Tomographic Studies. Software for acquisition of standard single photon emission computed tomographic (SPECT) studies performed with rotating gamma-cameras was introduced in the mid-1980s (38). It is often necessary to use the camera manufacturer's software to acquire these studies since more sophisticated systems have hardware communications to control and record the position of the rotating gantry. Two acquisition modes are in common use, continuous acquisition and step and shoot. Continuous acquisition has the advantage that no counts are lost while the camera head moves from one position to the next. However, some investigators have expressed concern that blurring of the projection data occurs. Blurring is not a significant problem if there is sufficient angular sampling. Typically, SPECT studies are acquired in a format that is similar to the dynamic study.

Recently, software to acquire gated myocardial perfusion or cardiac blood pool SPECT studies was introduced. Gating considerably increases the storage and processing requirements of a SPECT study. A minimum of 8–12 frames per cardiac cycle are necessary, making the storage and processing requirements of each SPECT study 8–12 times greater than a standard SPECT study (39, 40).

Analysis Software. Analysis of digital images is a much more complex task than the acquisition of these images. Analysis software has been designed to provide a wide range of elementary image processing commands. Typically, these commands allow the user to alter the image display, perform numeric operations on the image, draw regions of interest, and generate activity-time curves.

The display commands provided by most nuclear medicine systems allow the user to display images in a variety of formats. Usually images are displayed by using a look-up table that linearly maps the counts per pixel with the intensity of the pixel over the entire range of counts per pixel. Displays with at least 256 gray levels have become standard.

A great advantage of digital displays over film is that images can be displayed using different look-up tables that assign gray levels to pixel values in different ways. For example, instead of distributing the gray levels over the entire range of counts per pixel, they can be distributed over a smaller range of counts per pixel by using threshold commands that identify the range of counts that pixels must have in order to be displayed. The range is selected either as a percentage of the maximum counts per pixel or as the actual counts per pixel. This technique is valuable since it distributes the gray scale over the range of pixels of interest (contrast enhancement). Most systems provide commands to use a variety of nonlinear mapping (e.g., logarithmic) of gray level to counts per pixel. Other display formats include isocount (isoband) displays that depict only pixels with equal, user-selected count levels.

Display commands allow the user to choose a color or black-and-white intensity scale, display multiple static images or a rapid sequence of images, and change the size and/or orientation of the displayed image. Commands for displaying multiple whole-body images as large as 256×1024 are necessary when interpreting bone scintigraphy.

When multiple images are displayed, the user should have the option to use the same gray scale on all images or a different gray scale on each image. Viewing rapid sequences of individual images is often very useful in analyzing dynamic studies. The user should have dynamic control over the rate at which the images are displayed and the contrast enhancement used. Simultaneous display of multiple cines with the display parameters being individually adjustable is necessary when interpreting multiple views of a gated cardiac study. Zooming all or parts of an image should be possible by changing the physical size of the image, the matrix size, or both. Increasing the matrix size of the image is usually done with linear interpolation where the value of the pixels of the new rows and columns of the expanded matrix are calculated by averaging the values of the pixels in the adjacent rows and columns. Interpolation after data collection may improve the quality of the image but not as much as collection in a higher resolution matrix (Fig. 8.13). The display command for interpolation does not change the raw data. Having commands that will expand and compress the matrix size of the raw data is helpful since many analysis programs require a particular matrix size and will not work with other matrix sizes. Simple image orientation commands should be provided to rotate images in multiples of 90°, translate images in pixel increments horizontally and vertically, and display mirror images. More sophisticated image rotation and translation capabilities allow the user to rotate images any number of degrees and translate images by fractions of pixels. These functions, which are available on more sophisticated image processing systems, are useful in nuclear medicine to superimpose images obtained at different times, such as initial and delayed thallium images.

Commands to manipulate images include image-arithmetic commands and smoothing and other filtering commands. Image-arithmetic commands provide facilities for adding, subtracting, multiplying, or dividing images by a constant or by another image. These commands are very useful for generating simple functional images such as those used in nuclear cardiology (41–44). Smoothing can be used to eliminate some of the noise in an image. A simple 9-point smoothing algorithm is common (Fig. 8.14). Although smoothing decreases noise, it also decreases image resolution (Fig. 8.15). Many other more sophisticated filters are used in image processing to enhance various components of the image. These filters have not been routinely used with planar imaging. The exact choice of filters for tomography remains controversial (45, 46).

Two types of regions of interest, regular and irregular, are supported by most nuclear medicine computer systems. Regular regions of interest are square, rectangular, circular, or elliptical. Their standard shape makes them more reproducible; however, they usually do not conform to anatomy. On the other hand, irregular regions of interest can have any shape but are more difficult to reproduce. Reproducibility can be greatly aided by the use of edge-detection algorithms. Edge detection (47, 48) is a complex task for which nuclear medicine systems provide only the most rudimentary tools (isocount lines). Slightly more complex algorithms to detect edges use count profiles to identify edges as the point at which the instantaneous change in the number of counts is greatest (second derivative method). Edges defined using this technique are often jagged because of the noise in the image. Some of the non-anatomic irregularities in the edges can be removed using smoothing algorithms.

Even the best edge-detecting algorithms used in nuclear medicine are only able to automatically define the left ventricular region of interest on a gated blood pool study 80–

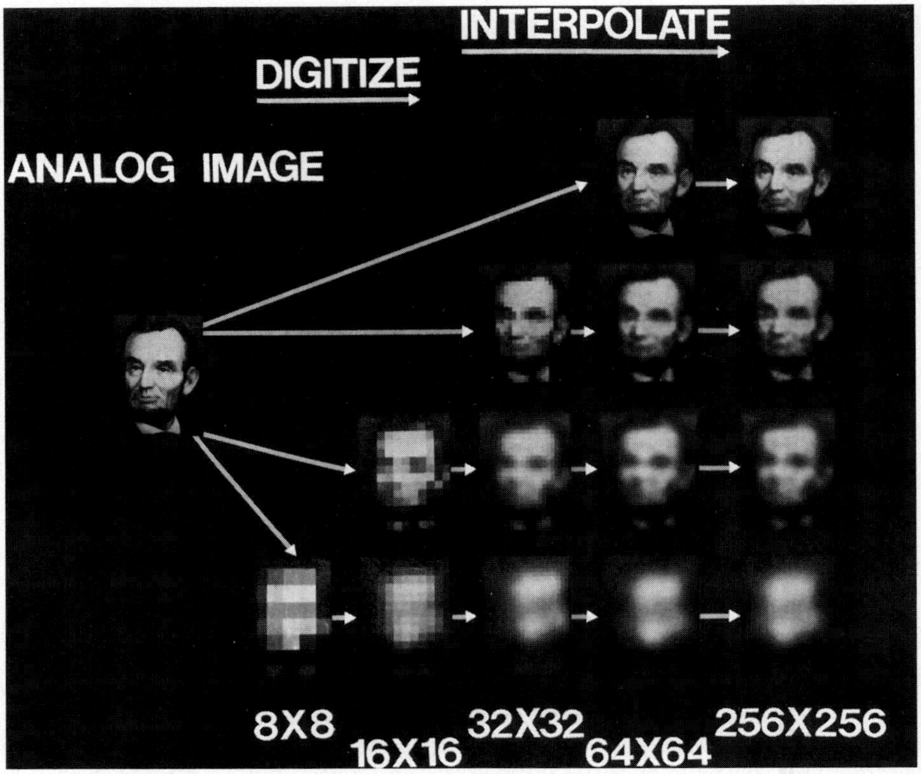

Figure 8.13. The effects of the acquisition matrix size and linear interpolation are shown. Interpolation improves image resolution but not as much as acquiring the image with a higher resolution matrix. (Reproduced by permission from Holman BL, Parker JA. Computer-assisted cardiac nuclear medicine. Boston: Little, Brown & Co., 1981.)

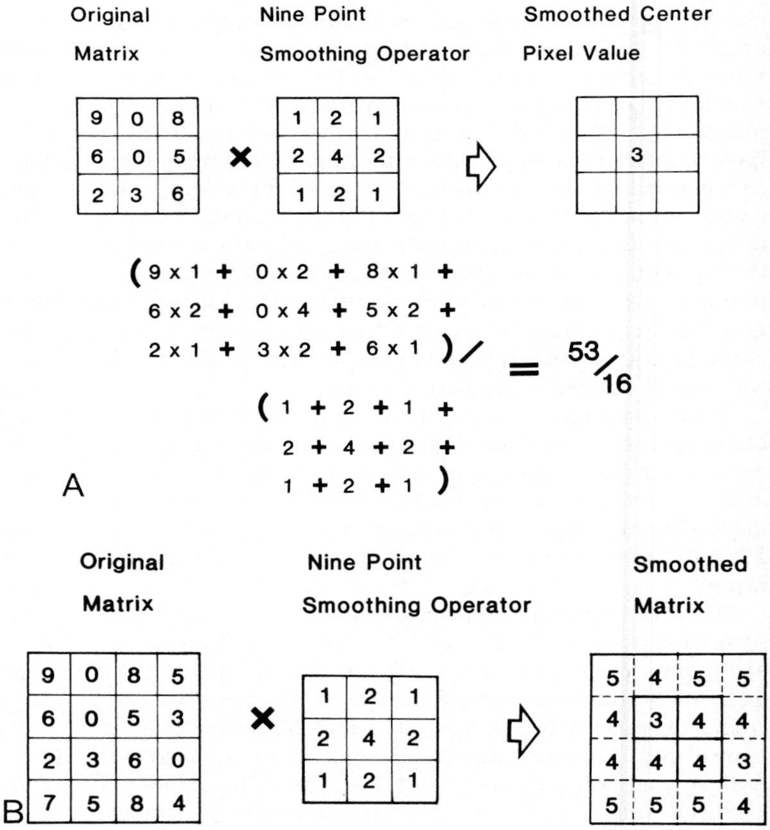

Figure 8.14. Smoothing. **A.** The smoothed value of the center pixel of the left-hand (*original matrix*) is calculated by multiplying each value in the matrix by the corresponding value in the *9-point smoothing operator matrix*, summing the products, and dividing by the sum of the weights used. **B.** When the same smoothing operator is used on a larger matrix (4×4), the smoothed values for each of the four central pixels is calculated using the procedure shown in A. A modified smoothing operator must be used for the edge and corner pixels. Note how smoothing eliminates much of the random variability in the original matrix.

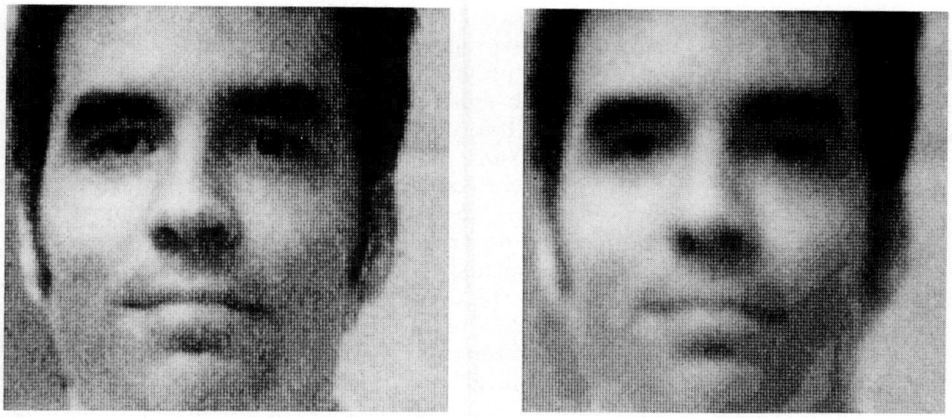

Unsmoothed Smoothed

Figure 8.15. Effects of smoothing. Smoothing decreases the resolution of the image as well as decreasing the noise. Smoothing prior to finding edges is helpful since it partially eliminates nonanatomic variations in edges that are due to noise.

90% of the time (49, 50). Failures are due to three factors. First, when a person defines a region of interest they have a preconceived notion of anatomy. Based on past experience, they can "fill in the edges" when the edges do not exist on the image. Second, a person can use the sequence of images to help decide where the edge is on any one image. Most edge-detection schemes use only the information on one image to determine the edge. Third, the parts of organs that we would like to separate (the chambers of the heart) are not separated by two-dimensional planes that are perpendicular to the face of the crystal. Because of this, perfect edge-detection algorithms will not perfectly separate organs or parts of organs. Despite these limitations, sophisticated edge-detection algorithms in nuclear medicine are an asset since they promote reproducibility and remove the tedium from quantitative analysis.

A complementary approach to edge detection is background (organ crosstalk) correction (51–54). Perfect background correction eliminates the need for edge detection since only counts from the organ of interest remain. The first step in background correcting a region of interest is to identify the region. A first approximation to background can be obtained by examining the counts in pixels adjacent to the region and performing a bilinear interpolation where the background counts in each pixel of the region of interest are assumed to be equal to the average of a linear interpolation between the two background pixels in the horizontal and vertical direction. Further modification of the bilinear interpolated background may be necessary because the organ of interest displaces some of the structures that contributed to background.

Once regions of interest have been selected, activity-time curves can be generated from the regions. Typically, these curves can be displayed in a variety of formats including absolute total counts or average counts per pixel versus frame number or time. Display of multiple curves with individual axes or on the same axis is desirable. Commands for adding, subtracting, dividing, and multiplying curves and constants are helpful. Routines for fitting lines, exponentials, γ-variates, polynomials, and splines to curves should be provided (12). Tools for linking ROI, curve, and other derived data to the patient's study are necessary.

A powerful feature of any analysis system is to provide the user with a method for easily combining the general-purpose image processing commands discussed above into relatively complex analysis programs for specific applications. An editor can be used to create or modify a file of commands that are used to analyze a particular type of study. This file of commands is often called a macro. Unfortunately, even sophisticated image processing systems cannot anticipate and provide all of the functionality that a user may want in an analysis program. Some modern sophisticated computer systems do not provide the simple building blocks (e.g., simple commands to add frames of a study) that are necessary for image manipulation and analysis. Ironically, these building blocks were provided by older less sophisticated systems. Certain specific mathematic functions and report generation usually must be provided by the user. These specific needs led to the development of user-written software.

User-Written Software

Most software, especially user-written software, comes with a disclaimer indicating that the supplier does not take responsibility that the software works. Physicians must take this to heart! Much of the software available for use in nuclear medicine is unreliable. It is the responsibility of the physician who uses the software to determine whether it gives reliable results. Failure to take this responsibility seriously will quickly and justifiably discredit the potential value of quantitative analysis.

Two minimum steps must be taken to assure the reliability of the software. First, the algorithms used to perform the analysis must be known. Programs must not be black boxes that input numbers in one end and output numbers at the other end. Most programs are only reliable when the simple assumptions upon which they are based are true. The user must recognize when the assumptions are not met. Second, the results produced by the program must be validated. The new user of the program should be supplied with a number of test cases so that he or she can compare his or her results with the results obtained by an experienced user. These cases should be analyzed multiple times by one observer and once by several observers to determine the intra- and interobserver variability. Ideally, the results of the analysis program should also be compared with some independent reference measurement (e.g., ejection fraction from contrast ventriculography); however, this comparison is not always feasible. In the near future, data banks of actual patient studies should be available so that medical centers can compare the results of their analysis program with the results from other medical centers.

At institutions where user-written software is developed, the physician must unambiguously communicate to the programmer what the program is to do. The most important part of any programming project is carefully defining the goals and methods. Wasted effort can be avoided if a program is carefully planned from the beginning. Good algorithm design will decrease the overall difficulty of the project. To minimize development time, it is often best to start by designing a simple implementation of the program. Modularity of design should allow for enhancement of the program with time.

Since the cost of software development is great, tools that increase programming efficiency should be available. The most important tool is a good programming language. Other useful tools include a good editor and debugging aids.

Languages are divided into high-level languages and low-level languages. High-level languages are easier for humans to understand, whereas low-level languages are closer to the numerically coded instructions that the computer will execute. For image processing tasks, the image processing commands form the highest level language. C, C++, Pascal, FORTRAN (an acronym for FORmula TRANslation), and BASIC (Beginner's All-purpose Symbolic Instruction Code) are the most widely used general-purpose high-level languages. The popularity and availability of these language continue to promote their use.

Low-level languages are assembly language and machine code. Machine code is the actual binary numbers that are used to code the computer instructions. Obviously, programming in machine language is extremely difficult and inefficient for humans. Assembly language uses mnemonics instead of numbers to code programs. Programs written in assembly language execute more quickly and take up less space than programs written in higher level languages. The increased difficulty in programming in assembly language, however, is rarely outweighed by its advantages. If a program is time critical, only a small portion (usually much less than 5%) of the program needs to be rewritten in assembly language since typically only a small portion of a program accounts for its execution speed. Both machine language and assembly language are CPU specific (nonretargetable).

When programs are written in languages other than machine language, the program must be first translated (interpreted or compiled) into machine language. Traditionally, BASIC language translators are interpreters. Each BASIC instruction is translated into machine language and executed immediately. Every time the program is run it has to be retranslated. Since this translation process takes time, traditional BASIC programs run several times slower than programs written in other languages where the translation process, called compilation, occurs only once prior to running the program. BASIC interpreters can be easier for beginning programmers to use and to debug since the effects of each instruction can be observed immediately. Newer BASIC interpreters also give the option to compile a program.

An often overlooked aspect of program development is documentation, which is crucial for both the nonprogrammer user and for programmers who will be responsible for future enhancements and software maintenance. Documentation for the nonprogrammer user should include (a) the names of all the files necessary to compile and run the program, (b) what the program does and what algorithms are used, (c) the format and location of the necessary input values, (d) a detailed description of any user interactions, (e) the format of the output values, and (f) the programmer's name and location. It is also useful to have a text file on the disk in which the user can write the dates and description of program malfunctions. This "bugs" file can be edited by the programmer to reflect revisions of the program that correct these documented dysfunctions.

Documentation for programmers is intended to make software maintenance and enhancement less difficult. In addition to the documentation described for the user, programmer documentation should include (a) an overview of the program's structure to provide a quick guide to what parts of the program perform which functions (e.g., input, calculations, output), (b) program design features that were selected to facilitate future enhancements, and (c) a brief summary of the function of each module/subroutine with a description of the necessary input and output. Frequent comments within the body of the program are very helpful in making the program more readable. Parts of the program that are clear to the programmer at the time that the program is written may become foggy in the future. Modern programming languages provide simple facilities for making programs self-documenting. For example, languages that allow the use of long variable names can be very helpful since the statement "average counts per pixel = sum counts per pixel/number of pixels" is much clearer than "x = y/z."

As programs become longer, the difficulty in making them work often grows exponentially. Newer programming methods have attempted to limit complexity as programs grow larger. Although most user written programs are short, these methods can still be helpful. A key concept is modularity. Different portions of the program are written as separate modules with well-designed software interfaces between modules. A concept called object oriented software divides a program into well-defined objects. In addition to clearly defined interfaces, new software objects can be defined in terms of other objects inheriting many of their properties. For example, a child window in a graphical user interface may inherit the properties of the parent window. Object oriented programming provides a natural structure for expressing these relations.

Nuclear medicine computer systems may have higher level programming languages. Data collection, analysis, or even display can be defined in these higher level languages. The concepts used in these languages are very similar to the concepts used in any programming language. Documentation, modularity, and object orientation are important in these languages.

NUCLEAR MEDICINE COMPUTER SYSTEMS

Types of Systems

One way to simplify the choice of a computer (55) is to divide nuclear medicine computer systems into three basic types: integrated camera-computer systems, vendor-designed standalone nuclear medicine computer systems, and user-adapted general-purpose computer systems. These systems provide for increasing amounts of adaptability by the user at the expense of increased complexity.

Acquisition computers are an integral part of many modern gamma-cameras. The computer not only acquires image data but also often controls other camera functions such as gantry movement.

Integrated camera computer systems offer a number of advantages to nuclear medicine computer users. First, since the camera and computer may share electronic components, the cost of the integrated unit is often significantly less than if the camera and the computer were purchased separately. Second, the integrated design allows for optimization of the camera/computer interface (a single console controls both the camera and the computer). Third, negotiation of a sales agreement and maintenance of the system is simpler if there is only one vendor involved. Fourth, each integrated camera-computer functions independently, permitting simultaneous acquisition of multiple studies. Fifth, multiple camera-computer systems in a department provide the redundancy that is needed for the department to continue to function when one system fails. Finally, administratively it is often easier to obtain approval for the purchase of a integrated camera-computer system than for a gamma-camera and a separate computer system.

Despite their advantages, the computers provided by integrated camera-computer systems certainly will not meet the needs of all users. Since the computer in the integrated camera-computer system, is responsible for controlling the camera, it cannot be customized by the user. If an integrated camera-computer system is expected to provide all of the department's computing needs, the buyer must be reasonably certain that the necessary functions are currently implemented.

The second type of nuclear medicine computer system is the vendor-designed standalone nuclear medicine computer system. Such a system is typically not used to acquire studies. Its primary function is image analysis, archival storage, and communications. This type of system should use a standard computer that is readily expanded and modified by the user. A great variety of general-purpose software is available for this type of system. User-written programs, word processing, spreadsheet, statistics, and graphics programs are simple to implement when a general-purpose operating system is available. Unfortunately, some of the advantages of using a general-purpose operating system are lost when vendors modify a general-purpose operating system so that the nuclear medicine software runs more efficiently.

Since the user base of a general-purpose computer system is great, a wide selection of hardware (e.g., external storage devices) is available for the system from the nuclear medicine vendor, from the original computer manufacturer, and from third-party manufacturers. Generally, enhancements purchased from the nuclear medicine vendor will be the most expensive since the vendor will take responsibility for integrating the hardware into the system. Often hardware and software enhancements can be installed by users who have some computer expertise. Additionally, these computers can often serve as clients for other systems within the hospital.

The third type of system available is the user-adapted general-purpose computer system, which gives the user the most freedom in the design and functionality of the system. This type of system requires the most in-house expertise and is best suited for academic institutions where the pursuit of research interests leads to unique applications. Since the user integrates the system, the latest technologic advances can be used in the system. With vendor-adapted systems, there is often considerable delay in the integration of new technology. The price paid for this increased flexibility is that unique hardware often requires unique software. The cost of this software frequently is underestimated. If standard hardware-software interfaces are defined and hardware-independent software becomes more available, software development costs will stabilize.

Some user-adapted general-purpose computer systems are relatively easy for users to implement. For example, the National Institutes of Health has written a relatively powerful image processing program called NIH Image. Because this program was developed using taxpayer money, it is free. Using this software and an inexpensive Macintosh computer (<$2500), images can be viewed and analyzed. Similar packages are available for IBM-compatible computers. Because of their low cost these user-adapted general-purpose computer systems are often used as inexpensive display stations in physicians' offices and homes.

If more than one computer is available, studies that are acquired from one computer system should be transferable to another for analysis and for archival storage. Unfortunately transfer of studies is still not a trivial task (3, 56–59). Several standards are used to facilitate the transfer of data between computers. The ethernet standard describes the physical requirements for a communications network. TCP/IP, the standard used for the Internet, deals with how packets of data are sent on the network. More and more, these basic levels of communication are provided by the hospital information services much as the telephone is provided.

Functional Requirements

The functions to be served by a nuclear medicine computer system vary greatly from one department to the next. The complicated task of choosing a computer system can be simplified by first composing a list of the essential needs to be filled by the system (55). After this list of essential needs is prepared, an expanded prioritized list that includes desirable but optional uses should be made.

Increased functionality usually entails an increase in

the initial cost and complexity of a system. The hidden costs of more complex systems (i.e., the need for a systems manager) must be realistically planned for if the system is to be used to its potential.

Cardiac Applications. Certainly the most common use of a nuclear medicine computer system is the acquisition and analysis of cardiac studies (Table 8.6). A computer is essential for quantitative cardiac blood pool studies, first-pass angiocardiograms, and myocardial perfusion studies.

In addition to the usual camera-computer interface, acquisition of gated studies requires an interface that is able to accept the ECG signal. The ECG interface should provide feedback so that the user knows which part of the ECG signal the computer is detecting as the R wave (Fig. 8.16). Additional feedback that is helpful is a constantly updated display of a histogram of the R-R intervals. Some interfaces are more sophisticated than others and allow for the detection of multiple physiologic signals (cardiac and respiratory gating).

A 12-frame 64×64-matrix 64-projection gated SPECT cardiac study requires greater than 3 megabytes of memory for the images alone. The operating system and the acquisition program require additional memory. Gated cardiac list mode studies also require considerable storage space (10–20 megabytes) for the initial data. Once the list mode study has been reformatted into the desired matrix mode study or studies, the storage requirements are markedly reduced. Fortunately, most modern computers greatly surpass these memory and storage requirements.

Table 8.6.
Cardiac Applications

- Types of acquisition
  - Gated (blood pool)
  - List mode (blood pool)
  - Slow dynamic (shunts)
  - Fast dynamic (quantitative first-pass)
  - Static planar (myocardial perfusion imaging)
  - Static SPECT (myocardial perfusion imaging)
  - Gated SPECT (myocardial perfusion/blood pool imaging)
- Types of analysis
  - Blood pool
    - Cine generation for regional wall motion
    - Ejection fraction (global, regional, right, left)
    - Functional image generation (stroke volume, regional ejection fraction, and paradox volume and/or phase and amplitude images)
    - Stroke volume ratio
    - Ventricular volumes
    - Cardiac output
    - Ventricular ejection and filling rates
    - Trend analysis
    - R-R interval histogram
    - R wave feedback
  - Shunts
    - Pulmonary blood flow to systemic blood flow ratio (QP/QS)
  - First-pass
    - Cine generation for regional wall motion
    - Ejection fraction (global, regional, right, left)
    - Functional image generation (stroke volume, regional ejection fraction, and paradox volume and/or phase and amplitude images)
    - Ventricular volumes
    - Cardiac output
    - Ventricular ejection and filling rates
    - Trend analysis
  - SPECT
    - Bull's-eye analysis
      - Standard display of tomographic slices
    - Quality control
      - Sinogram
      - Linogram
      - Cine of projection images
  - Gated SPECT

Archival storage of studies, especially gated cardiac data, in digital form is very useful because the sequential studies on patients can be more easily compared. In the past, many departments used one floppy disk to store each patient's study. A typical 3.5-inch floppy disk can store about 1 megabyte of data; therefore, a three-view 40-frame 64×64-word matrix gated study can be stored on one floppy disk (3×40×64×64×2 bytes/word = 0.960 megabytes). The cost of storage (about $1/megabyte) is considerably greater for floppy disks than for digital audio tapes (DAT) (about $0.01/megabyte). Archival storage on tape can be automated so that backup of patient studies (and other important computer files) to tape occurs with minimal operator intervention. Tape has the minor disadvantage of requiring more retrieval time (5–15 minutes) than individual floppy disks.

Quantitative analysis of gated cardiac blood pool studies has included the measurement of many functional parameters. By far the most common measurement is the ejection fraction (24, 33, 36, 41, 60–62). Numerous algorithms to measure ejection fraction have been described. Variations include operator-defined versus computer-defined ventricular regions of interest, operator-selected versus computer-selected background regions of interest, and variable versus fixed ventricular regions of interest. Remarkably, despite their variations, most analysis programs have worked well when employed by experienced users.

Other software useful in the analysis of gated studies are programs to generate functional images (either the simple stroke volume and paradox volume images or the computationally more complex phase and amplitude images (41–44)) and to measure other parameters of cardiac

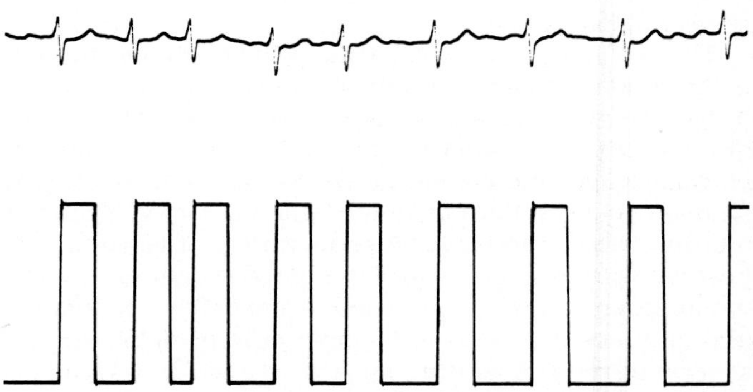

Figure 8.16. R wave feedback. A computer-ECG interface that outputs a square wave when an R wave is detected provides an inexpensive feedback mechanism. Quality control of gated studies is simplified since the user can see what part of the ECG the computer is detecting as the R wave.

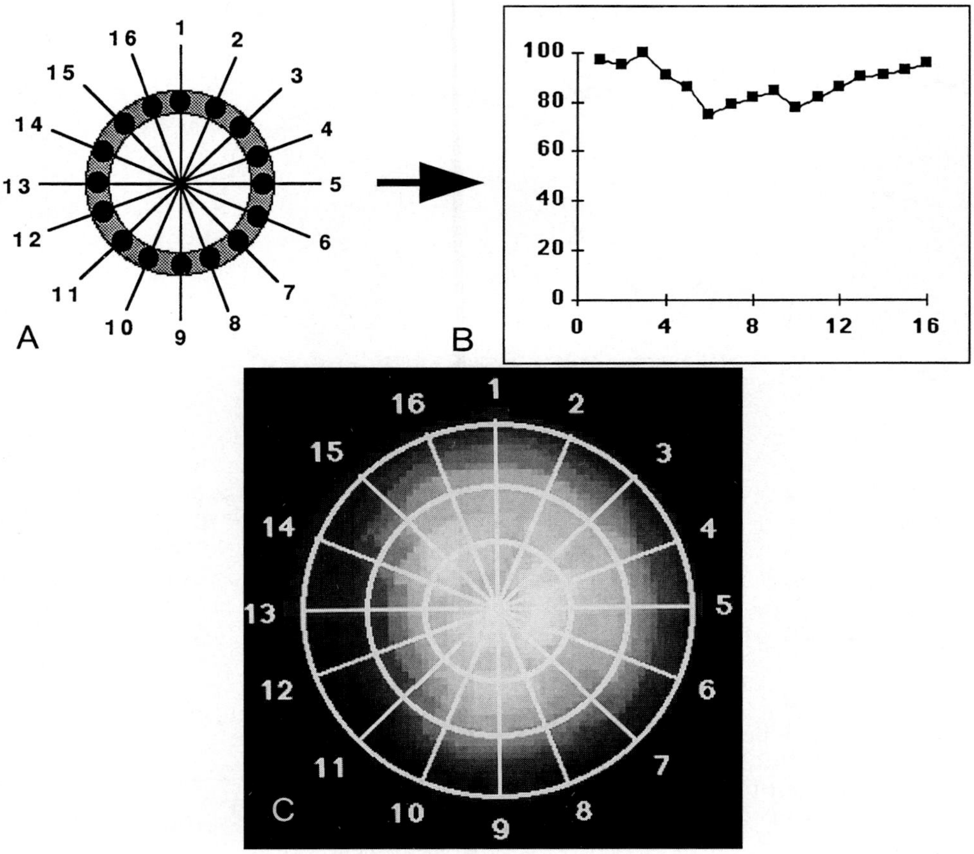

Figure 8.17. Bull's-eye analysis. The short axis slices are used to construct a bull's-eye plot of the activity from a myocardial perfusion study. The bull's-eye is created by determining the peak activity along radii for selected short axis slices (**A**). Rather than attempting to interpret multiple circumferential profiles (**B**), the bull's-eye combines all the circumferential profiles into a single image (**C**). The distance from the center of the bull's-eye corresponds to the distance from the apex to the base of the heart, the direction from the center corresponds to the myocardial wall (1 = anterior; 5 = lateral; 9 = inferior; 13 = septal), and the intensity corresponds to the amount of activity.

function, such as the left ventricular-to-right ventricular stroke volume ratio (63) and the peak ventricular filling rate (21, 24, 27–31, 35, 36). Additionally, a number of techniques have been described to measure absolute left ventricular volume (64) from gated studies. Once absolute volumes are known, absolute cardiac output can be measured.

Software that produces quantitative results should not replace subjective analysis. Despite their aura of accuracy, quantitative results may be erroneous for a variety of reasons. Proper interpretation of studies should include both quantitative and subjective analysis. No analysis of a gated cardiac study is complete without subjective analysis of the study in a movie or cine format. Simultaneous display of the multiple views facilitates the subjective analysis. When discrepancies between the subjective analysis and the quantitative measures arise, the experienced user can usually identify the cause. Errors in the quantitative measures are just as likely as errors in the subjective impression.

A variety of programs are available for the quantitative analysis of myocardial perfusion scintigraphy (42, 46, 65–75). The most popular approach (bull's-eye analysis) determines the peak activity along a number of radii (typically every 6°) projected on the short axis slices. For each slice a circumferential profile is generated. The circumferential profiles are then plotted on a bull's-eye where the intensity of the point represents the magnitude of activity and the location of the point represents the location of the slice (based on the distance from the center of the bull's-eye) and the location of the radius (based on the angle from the center of the bull's-eye) (Fig. 8.17). When the bull's-eye was introduced, it was created using the short axis slices. Because of partial volume effects, the magnitude of activity at the apex was originally calculated from the midvertical long axis slice. Today, a variety of approaches are used. When bull's-eyes are generated for the immediate and delayed images of a myocardial perfusion scan, fixed areas of decreased activity and areas of redistribution can be identified. Additional images can be derived from the bull's-eye images to show the size of the defect and the amount of redistribution.

Table 8.7.
Other SPECT Applications

Types of acquisition
Continuous
Stop and shoot
Types of analysis
Iterative vs. analytic reconstruction
Attenuation correction
Quality control (linearity, uniformity, center of rotation)
Dynamic display of slices
Volume rendering

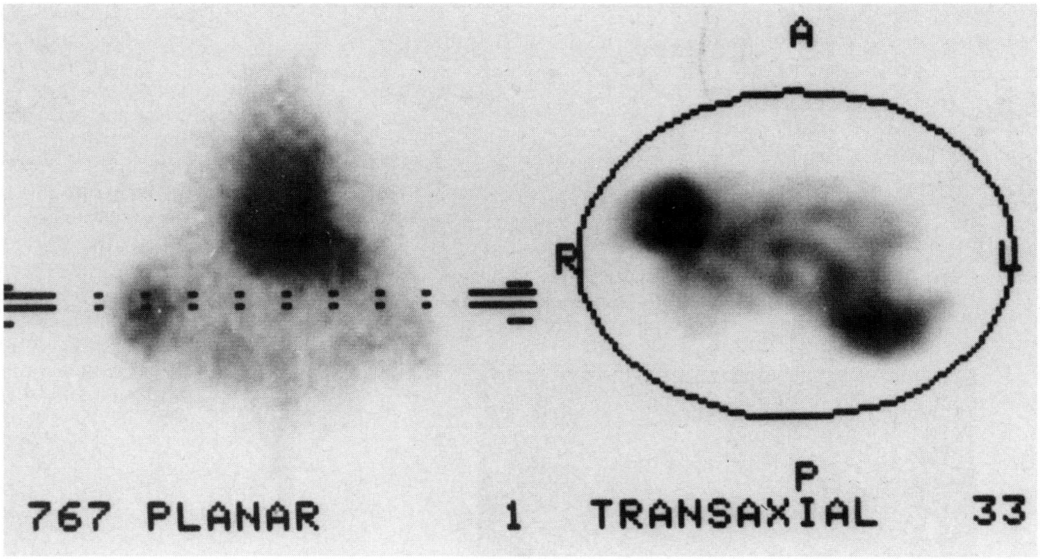

Figure 8.18. Planar and SPECT images of a blood pool study of the liver indicating an abnormal blood pool in the lateral aspect of the right lobe of the liver. Simultaneous display of the planar image with a line indicating the level of the tomographic slice greatly aids the interpretation of the myriad of tomographic images.

The bull's-eyes that are generated by quantitative programs are very useful in confirming the subjective interpretation of myocardial perfusion scans and are useful in research to more objectively measure the results of the myocardial perfusion scans. Bull's-eyes must be interpreted cautiously since asymmetries in myocardial perfusion distribution caused by overlying soft tissue (breast and diaphragm) and changes in positioning cannot be distinguished from true asymmetries unless the images themselves are carefully analyzed.

Single Photon Emission Computed Tomography. Hardware requirements for gated SPECT (39, 40) are the most demanding of the applications in nuclear medicine. As many as 12 64×64 matrices in 60 projections may be acquired (one view every 6°), requiring over 3 megabytes of storage for the raw data. Attenuation correction data requires an additional 3 megabytes. Reconstruction is computationally intense, since complex calculations, using many data points, are performed. Fortunately, modern computers can perform reconstruction of even complex gated SPECT studies in 10 minutes or less. Some systems will simultaneously acquire the raw data and reconstruct the tomographic images so that there is little delay in viewing the final images.

The interface between the rotating gamma-camera and the computer is particularly complex. Data acquisition and camera rotation need to be synchronized. Therefore, a method for conveying the position of the rotating gantry to the computer is helpful. If an elliptical orbit is used to more closely follow the body contour, the computer must control the gantry. Camera-computer integration simplifies the user's task by providing one console for the camera and computer. The complexity of the camera-gantry-computer interface usually limits the user to the specific SPECT package provided by a gamma-camera manufacturer.

Table 8.8.
Additional Applications

Miscellaneous nuclear medicine
Absolute and relative renal function
Renal obstruction
Ureteral reflux
Renal vascular hypertension
Relative pulmonary function
Gastric and gallbladder emptying
Cines for GI bleeding, HIDA, etc.[a]
Organ flow
Quality control
Archival storage of studies
Other functions
Word processing
Scheduling, billing
Patient demographics
Spreadsheet
Statistics
Graphics
Literature searches

[a]GI = gastrointestinal; HIDA = hepatobiliary iminodiacetic acid scan

Unique software is required for SPECT acquisition and reconstruction (Table 8.7). Since gamma-camera performance is critical with SPECT, programs that facilitate measurement and evaluation of the performance of the gamma-camera are necessary (76, 77). Uniformity, linearity, and center of rotation need to be measured and visual feedback needs to be provided. Changes in camera performance with time can be displayed using histograms and by displaying quality control images as a cine.

Software necessary for reconstruction includes a selection of filters to process the raw data prior to reconstruction and several reconstruction algorithms (45, 46). Different filters are necessary, depending on which components

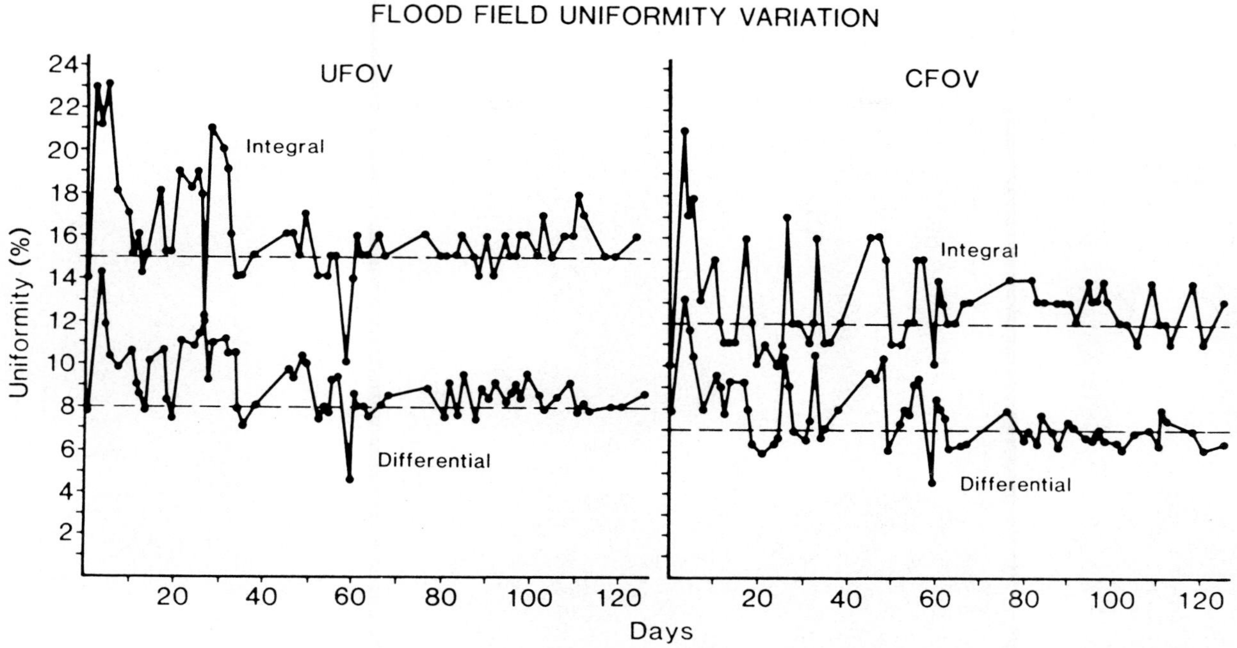

Figure 8.19. Quality control of gamma-cameras is aided by programs that display changes in various performance specifications over time. *UFOV* = useful field of view, *CFOV* = central field of view (75% of UFOV radius). (Reproduced by permission from Raff U, Spitzer VM, Hendee WR. Practicality of NEMA performance specification measurements for user-based acceptance testing and routine quality assurance. J Nucl Med 1984;25:679–687.)

Table 8.9.
Interfile Header

In the original file, the keys are listed sequentially. In this table, to save space, the keys are listed in three columns. The keys should be read from left to right, then row by row. Note that the keys are self-descriptive. (Courtesy of Andrew Todd-Pokropek.)

!INTERFILE :=	!imaging modality :=nucmed	!originating system :=uclim
!version of keys :=3.2	!date of keys :=1989:11:18	!conversion program :=uclim
!program author :=a. todd-pokropek	!program version :=3.01	!program date :=1991:07:30
!GENERAL DATA :=	original institution :=ucl	contact person :=a. todd-pokropek
!data starting block :=0	!name of data file :=stat.img	patient name := joe doe
!patient ID := 12345	patient dob := 1968:08:21	patient sex := M
!study ID := test	data compression :=none	data encode :=none
!GENERAL IMAGE DATA :=	!type of data :=Static	study date := 1991:08:21
study time := 10:00:00	!imagedata byte order :=LITTLEENDIAN	!number of windows := 1
window A :=	flood corrected :=N	decay corrected :=N
!STATIC STUDY (General) :=	number of images/window :=2	!Static Study (each frame) :=
!image number :=1	!matrix size (x) :=64	!matrix size (y) :=64
!number format :=signed integer	!number of bytes per pixel :=2	!image duration (sec) :=100
image start time :=10:20: 0	!maximim pixel count :=22	total counts := 7781
!Static Study (each frame) :=	!image number :=2	!matrix size (x) :=64
!matrix size (y) :=64	!number format :=signed integer	!number of bytes per pixel :=2
!image duration (sec) :=200	image start time :=11:10: 0	!maximum pixel count :=21
total counts :=8512	!END OF INTERFILE :=	

of the image are to be emphasized and on the counting statistics of the image. A number of reconstruction algorithms have been described, including iterative and analytic techniques. A continuing problem with quantitative tomographic imaging is correction for attenuation (67, 78–80). Different approaches to the problem of attenuation may be needed depending on which part of the body is being imaged.

Until now, iterative reconstruction algorithms have not had a major impact on clinical nuclear medicine. The speed of modern computer systems and the appearance of attenuation correction data and scatter correction algorithms

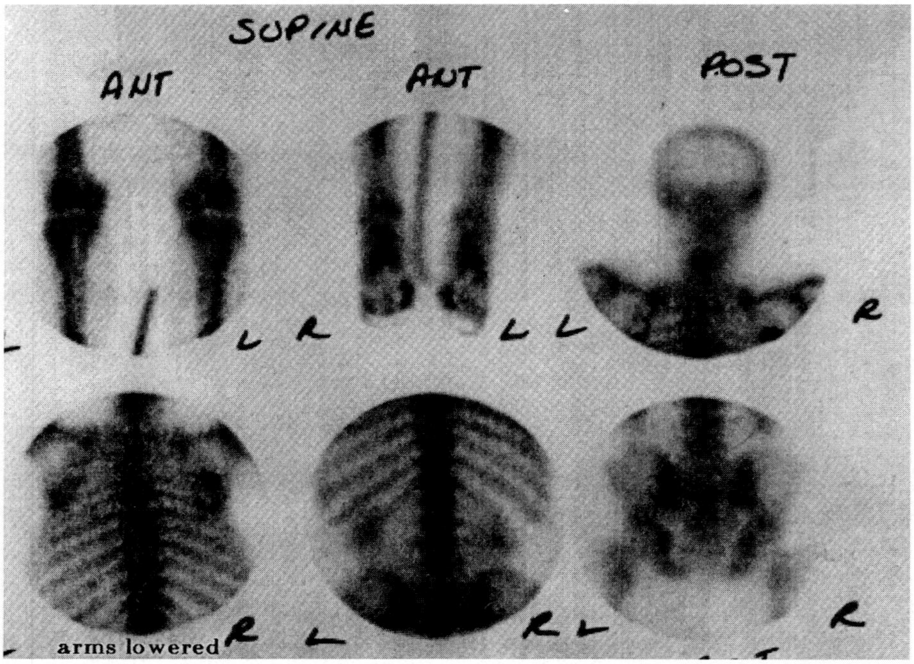

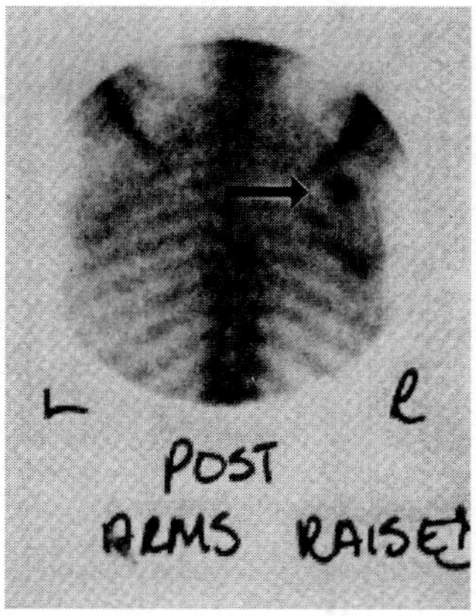

Patient Information:

Name: Henry Royal

Number: 12 34 56

Date of Birth: January 15, 1945

Send Report To:

Dr. Anthony J. Parker
25 Walnut Cove
Boston, MA 02215

Scan Date	Scan	Form	Dose
1/12/85	BONE	MDP	750 MBq

report:

Abnormal bone scan with increased uptake in T-8 and in the 4th rib in the lower left figure (image with arms down). Images with arms up show that the lesion is in the rib and not the scapula as indicated by the arrow in the figure on the right.

Figure 8.20. Laser printers produce high-quality, inexpensive images on hardcopy along with the written report, making communication of the results of tests more efficient and effective. (Courtesy of Demonics, Cambridge, MA.)

may change this. Faster computer systems may be required to make these algorithms practical for clinical application.

Since data are acquired from a large volume of the body, reconstructed slices can be oriented in any of the three standard anatomic planes (transverse, coronal, sagittal). Additionally, software to orient a slice in a nonstandard plane is essential to analyze tomographic thallium scans since the desired planes should be parallel or perpendicular to the long axis of the heart. Interpretation of the myriad slices that can be generated can be facilitated by simultaneously displaying the conventional two-dimensional image with a line indicating the slice that is being displayed (Fig. 8.18). Multiple slices in parallel planes can be viewed conveniently as a movie in which the user can view all the slices in rapid sequence or can select the slice to be viewed using a joystick.

Routine Nuclear Medicine Applications. Computer acquisition of dynamic studies is very valuable (Table 8.8), since the study can be replayed continuously at varying speeds and using multiple contrast levels. Additionally, software has been developed for measurement of various objective physiologic indexes for dynamic studies such as renal blood flow, renal function (51, 53, 81), and gastric and gallbladder emptying studies. Acquisition and analysis of static images are used routinely to measure relative renal and pulmonary function.

One underutilized application of computers in nuclear medicine is in the area of quality control of gamma-cameras (82). Programs to quantitatively measure uniformity, linearity, and spatial resolution are invaluable in acceptance testing, day-to-day quality control, and documenting improvements in camera performance following service. Software to conveniently display longitudinal changes in each camera's daily performance specifications helps to indicate when service should be requested for a camera (Fig. 8.19).

The dramatically increased storage capacity of new devices has made digital archival storage of patient studies very feasible (57). Database management programs are necessary to keep track of patients' studies. For example, a 1 gigabyte disk will store hundreds of patient studies. Paging through the disk's directory using a terminal that displays 10–20 patient studies per page to find a patient's study is tedious at best. A program to automatically find a patient's study using the patient's name, number, study date, and/or type of study is very useful (56). Such a program can be expanded to find studies that are located in the digital archive.

To archivally store studies that are acquired on multiple computer systems on one central system, a method for transferring the data from one system to another is needed. High-speed networks are now common (3, 58, 59). Unfortunately the data format used to store studies varies from vendor to vendor. In the past, translation programs were needed to convert the data format of one vendor to a data format that another vendor could read. Recently, vendors are providing software that translates their own file format to interfile format (a standard image format developed by a working group of scientists to facilitate the exchange of image data in nuclear medicine) (83). The interfile format has a header which includes information about the patient and about the data. All of the header information is stored in ASCII format so that it can be viewed (or even edited) with a simple text editor (Table 8.9).

When choosing a system that will be used for archival storage, it is important to have duplicates of the archival drives. Two drives are necessary so that the essential backup copies of patient studies can be conveniently obtained. A number of data compression techniques are available to reduce the storage requirements of backup copies of the patient studies by factors of 2.

The additional cost of storing all studies digitally can be offset by eliminating the use of film as hardcopy (57). Very inexpensive hardcopy can be obtained by using a laser printer and plain paper (Fig. 8.20). Although this image will not be of high enough quality to be used exclusively for diagnostic purposes, it is very useful for widespread dissemination of the image, such as with the dictated report.

REFERENCES

1. Honeyman JC, Dwyer SJD. Historical perspective on computer development and glossary of terms. Radiographics 1993;13:145–152.
2. Chen CC, Hoffer PB, Swett HA. Hypermedia in radiology: computer-assisted education. J Digit Imaging 1989;2:48–55.
3. Lummis RC, Wexler JP. Networks in nuclear medicine. [Review]. Semin Nucl Med 1994;24:66–74.
4. Andreessen M. Getting Started with NCSA Mosaic. file://ftp.ncsa.uiuc.edu/Web/Mosaic/Papers/getting-started.ps.Z.
5. Orlin JA, Tal I, Parker JA, Front D, Israel O, Kolodny GM. Evaluation of routine telephone transmission of nuclear medicine studies. Clin Nucl Med 1989;14:22–27.
6. Andreessen M. A beginner's guide to URLs. file://ftp.ncsa.uiuc.edu/Web/Mosaic/Papers/url-primer.ps.Z.
7. Andreessen M. NCSA Mosaic technical summary. file://ftp.ncsa.uiuc.edu/Web/Mosaic/Papers/mosaic.ps.Z.
8. Andreessen M. A beginner's guide to HTML. file://ftp.ncsa.uiuc.edu/Web/Mosaic/Papers/html-primer.ps.Z.
9. Schatz BR, Hardin JB. NCSA Mosaic and the World Wide Web: global hypermedia protocols for the Internet. Science 1994;895–901.
10. Hayes B. The World Wide Web. Am Scientist 1994;416–420.
11. Schiller JI. Secure distributed computing. Sci Am 1994;271:72–76.
12. Wallis JW, Miller MM, Miller TR, Vreeland TH. An Internet-based nuclear mdicine teaching file. J Nucl Med 1995;(in press).
13. World Wide Web home. http://info.cern.ch/.
14. Berners-Lee T. World Wide Web initiative. http://info.cern.ch/hypertext/WWW/TheProject.html.
15. Berners-Lee T. WWW bibliography: papers. http://info.cern.ch/hypertext/WWW/Bibliography/Papers.html.
16. Cradduck TD. The wide world of Internet. J Nucl Med 1994;30N–35N.
17. RSNA. http://www.rsna.org.
18. D'Alessandro MP, Lacey DL, Galvin JR, Erkonen WE, Santer DM. The networked multimedia textbook: distributing radiology multimedia information across the internet. AJR 1994;1233–1237.
19. Arnstein NB, Chen DC, Siegel ME. Interpretation of bone scans using a video display. A necessary step toward a filmless nuclear medicine department. Clin Nucl Med 1990;15:418–423.
20. Bunker SR, Handmaker H, Torre DM, Schmidt WP. Pixel overflow artifacts in SPECT evaluation of the skeleton. Radiology 1990; 174:229–232.

21. Archer SL, Mike DK, Hetland MB, Kostamo KL, Shafer RB, Chesler E. Usefulness of mean aortic valve gradient and left ventricular diastolic filling pattern for distinguishing symptomatic from asymptomatic patients. Am J Cardiol 1994;73:275–281.
22. Marzullo P, Parodi O, Sambuceti G, et al. Does the myocardium become "stunned" after episodes of angina at rest, angina on effort, and coronary angioplasty? Am J Cardiol 1993;71:1045–1051.
23. McCallister SH, Juni JE, Hibbelin JF, Starling MR. Effects of alterations in systolic pressure on radionuclide measurements of left ventricular filling dynamics. J Nucl Med 1993;34:747–753.
24. Pace L, Cuocolo A, Stefano ML, et al. Left ventricular systolic and diastolic function measurements using an ambulatory radionuclide monitor: effects of different time averaging on accuracy. J Nucl Med 1993;34:1602–1606.
25. Levy WC, Cerqueira MD, Abrass IB, Schwartz RS, Stratton JR. Endurance exercise training augments diastolic filling at rest and during exercise in healthy young and older men. Circulation 1993; 88:116–126.
26. Perrone-Filardi P, Bacharach SL, Dilsizian V, Bonow RO. Effects of regional systolic asynchrony on left ventricular global diastolic function in patients with coronary artery disease. J Am Coll Cardiol 1992;19:739–744.
27. Villari B, Betocchi S, Pace L, et al. Assessment of left ventricular diastolic function: comparison of contrast ventriculography and equilibrium radionuclide angiography. J Nucl Med 1991; 32:1849–1853.
28. Sheikh KH, Davidson CJ, Honan MB, Skelton TN, Kisslo KB. Bashore TM. Changes in left ventricular diastolic performance after aortic balloon valvuloplasty: acute and late effects. J Am Coll Cardiol 1990;16:795–803.
29. Chikamori T, Dickie S, Poloniecki JD, Myers MJ, Lavender JP, McKenna WJ. Prognostic significance of radionuclide-assessed diastolic function in hypertrophic cardiomyopathy. Am J Cardiol 1990;65:478–482.
30. Bareiss P, Facello A, Constantinesco A, et al. Alterations in left ventricular diastolic function in chronic ischemic heart failure. Assessment by radionuclide angiography. Circulation 1990; 81:III71–77.
31. Stewart RA, McKenna WJ. Assessment of diastolic filling indexes obtained by radionuclide ventriculography. Am J Cardiol 1990; 65:226–230.
32. Miller TR, Wallis JW, Landy BR, Gropler RJ, Sabharwal CL. Measurement of global and regional left ventricular function by cardiac PET. J Nucl Med 1994;35:999–1005.
33. Vainio P, Jurvelin J, Kuikka J, Vanninen E, Lansimies E. Analysis of left ventricular function from gated first-pass and multiple gated equilibrium acquisitions. Int J Card Imaging 1992;8:243–247.
34. Lear JL, Pratt JP. Real-time list-mode processing of gated cardiac blood pool examinations with forward-backward framing. Eur J Nucl Med 1992;19:177–180.
35. Clements IP, Sinak LJ, Gibbons RJ, Brown ML. O'Connor MK. Determination of diastolic function by radionuclide ventriculography. Mayo Clin Proc 1990;65:1007–1019.
36. Bacharach SL, Bonow RO, Green MV. Comparison of fixed and variable temporal resolution methods for creating gated cardiac blood-pool image sequences. J Nucl Med 1990;31:38–42.
37. Karam M, Wise RA, Natarajan TK, et al. Mechanism of decreased left ventricular stroke volume during inspiration in man. Circulation 1984;69:866–873.
38. Greer KL, Jaszczak RJ, Coleman RE. An overview of a camera-based SPECT system. Med Phys 1982;9:455–463.
39. Fischman AJ, Moore RH, Gill JB, Strauss HW. Gated blood pool tomography: a technology whose time has come [Review]. Semin Nucl Med 1989;19:13–21.
40. Gibson CJ. Real time 3D display of gated blood pool tomograms. Phys Med Biol 1988;33:569–581.
41. Boudreau RJ, Loken MK. Functional imaging of the heart [Review]. Semin Nucl Med 1987;17:28–38.
42. Datz FL, Gabor FV, Christian PE, Gullberg GT, Menzel CE, Morton KA. The use of computer-assisted diagnosis in cardiac-perfusion nuclear medicine studies: a review [Review]. J Digit Imaging 1992; 5:209–222.
43. Santinelli V, Fazio S, Turco P, De Paola M, Santomauro M, Chiariello M. Phase image analysis in Wolff-Parkinson-White syndrome. Role of transesophageal pacing. Acta Cardiol 1991;46:43–50.
44. Sychra JJ, Pavel DG, Olea E. Radionuclide synthetic Fourier images of cardiac wall motion abnormalities. Med Phys 1989; 16:537–543.
45. Links JM, Jeremy RW, Dyer SM, Frank TL, Becker LC. Wiener filtering improves quantification of regional myocardial perfusion with thallium-201 SPECT. J Nucl Med 1990;31:1230–1236.
46. Garcia EV, Cooke CD, Van Train KF, et al. Technical aspects of myocardial SPECT imaging with technetium-99m sestamibi. Am J Cardiol 1990;66:23E–31E.
47. Pretorius PH, van Aswegen A, Lotter MG, Herbst CP, Nel MG, Otto AC. Verification of a varying threshold edge detection SPECT technique for spleen volume: a comparison with computed tomography volumes. J Nucl Med 1993;34:963–967.
48. Cios KJ, Sarieh A. An edge extraction technique for noisy images. IEEE Trans Biomed Eng 1990;37:520–524.
49. Reiber JHC, Lie SP, Simoons M, et al. Clinical validation of fully automated computation of ejection fraction from gated blood-pool scintigrams. J Nucl Med 1983;24:1099–1107.
50. Goris ML, McKillop JH, Briandet PA. A fully automated determination of the left ventricular region of interest in nuclear angiocardiography. Cardiovasc Intervent Radiol 1981;4:117.
51. Hurwitz GA, Champagne CL, Gravelle DR, Smith FJ, Powe JE. The variability of processing of technetium-99m DTPA renography. Role of interpolative background subtraction. Clin Nucl Med 1993;18:273–277.
52. Erwin WD, Groch MW, Ali A, Fordham EW. Image normalization and background subtraction in Tl-201/Tc-99m parathyroid subtraction scintigraphy. Effect on lesion detection. Clin Nucl Med 1992;17:81–89.
53. Moonen M, Granerus G. Subtraction of extra-renal background in 99mTc-DTPA renography: comparison of various regions of interest. Clin Physiol 1992;12:453–461.
54. Koster K, Wackers FJ, Mattera JA, Fetterman RC. Quantitative analysis of planar technetium-99m-sestamibi myocardial perfusion images using modified background subtraction. J Nucl Med 1990;31:1400–1408.
55. Graham MM, Links JM, Lewellen TK, et al. Considerations in the purchase of a nuclear medicine computer system. J Nucl Med 1988;29:717–724.
56. Brown PH, Krishnamurthy GT. Design and operation of a nuclear medicine picture archiving and communication system. Semin Nucl Med 1990;20:205–224.
57. Cohen AM, Parker JA, Donohoe K, Jansons D, Kolodny GM. Three years' experience with an all-digital nuclear medicine department. Semin Nucl Med 1990;20:225–233.
58. Sampathkumaran KS, Miller TR. An efficient and cost effective nuclear medicine image network. Eur J Nucl Med 1987;13:161–166.
59. Miller TR, Jost RG, Sampathkumaran KS, Blaine GJ. Hospital-wide distribution of nuclear medicine studies through a broadband digital network. Semin Nucl Med 1990;20:270–275.
60. Makler PT Jr, McCarthy DM, Bergey P, et al. Multiple-hospital survey of ejection-fraction variability using a cardiac phantom. J Nucl Med 1985;26:81–84.
61. Massardo T, Gal RA, Grenier RP, Schmidt DH, Port SC. Left ven-

tricular volume calculation using a count-based ratio method applied to multigated radionuclide angiography [published erratum appears in J Nucl Med 1990;31(9):1449]. J Nucl Med 1990; 31:450–456.
62. Nichols K, DePuey EG, Gooneratne N, Salensky H, Friedman M, Cochoff S. First-pass ventricular ejection fraction using a single-crystal nuclear camera. J Nucl Med 1994;35:1292–1300.
63. Stewart RE, Gross MD, Starling MR. Mechanisms for an abnormal radionuclide left ventricular ejection fraction response to exercise in patients with chronic, severe aortic regurgitation. Am Heart J 1992;123:453–461.
64. Levy WC, Cerqueira MD, Matsuoka DT, Harp GD, Sheehan FH, Stratton JR. Four radionuclide methods for left ventricular volume determination: comparison of a manual and an automated technique. J Nucl Med 1992;33:763–770.
65. Datz FL, Rosenberg C, Gabor FV, et al. The use of computer-assisted diagnosis in cardiac perfusion nuclear medicine studies: a review (Part 3) [Review] [published erratum appears in J Digit Imaging 1993;6(4):240]. J Digit Imaging 1993;6:67–80.
66. Datz FL, Gabor FV, Christian PE, Gullberg GT, Menzel CE, Morton KA. The use of computer-assisted diagnosis in cardiac perfusion nuclear medicine studies: a review (Part 2). J Digit Imaging 1993; 6:1–15.
67. Garvin AA, Cullom SJ, Garcia EV. Myocardial perfusion imaging using single-photon emission computed tomography. Am J Card Imaging 1994;8:189–198.
68. Maddahi J, Kiat H, Van Train KF, et al. Myocardial perfusion imaging with technetium-99m sestamibi SPECT in the evaluation of coronary artery disease. Am J Cardiol 1990;66:55E–62E.
69. Klein JL, Garcia EV, DePuey EG, et al. Reversibility bull's-eye: a new polar bull's-eye map to quantify reversibility of stress-induced SPECT thallium-201 myocardial perfusion defects. J Nucl Med 1990;31:1240–1246.
70. Mannting F, Morgan-Mannting MG. Gated SPECT with technetium-99m-sestamibi for assessment of myocardial perfusion abnormalities. J Nucl Med 1993;34:601–608.
71. Van Train KF, Areeda J, Garcia EV, et al. Quantitative same-day rest-stress technetium-99m-sestamibi SPECT: definition and validation of stress normal limits and criteria for abnormality. J Nucl Med 1993;34:1494–1502.
72. Van Train KF, Garcia EV, Maddahi J, et al. Multicenter trial validation for quantitative analysis of same-day rest-stress technetium-99m-sestamibi myocardial tomograms. J Nucl Med 1994; 35:609–618.
73. Minoves M, Garcia A, Magrina J, Pavia J, Herranz R, Setoain J. Evaluation of myocardial perfusion defects by means of "bull's eye" images. Clin Cardiol 1993;16:16–22.
74. Cooper JA, Neumann PH, McCandless BK. Effect of patient motion on tomographic myocardial perfusion imaging. J Nucl Med 1992; 33:1566–1571.
75. Garcia EV, DePuey EG, Sonnemaker RE, et al. Quantification of the reversibility of stress-induced thallium-201 myocardial perfusion defects: a multicenter trial using bull's-eye polar maps and standard normal limits. J Nucl Med 1990;31:1761–1765.
76. O'Connor MK, Vermeersch C. Critical examination of the uniformity requirements for single-photon emission computed tomography. Med Phys 1991;18:190–197.
77. Maniawski PJ, Morgan HT, Wackers FJ. Orbit-related variation in spatial resolution as a source of artifactual defects in thallium-201 SPECT. J Nucl Med 1991;32:871–875.
78. Bateman TM, Kolobrodov VV, Vasin AP, O'Keefe JH, Jr. Extended acquisition for minimizing attenuation artifact in SPECT cardiac perfusion imaging. J Nucl Med 1994;35:625–627.
79. DePuey EGR. How to detect and avoid myocardial perfusion SPECT artifacts. J Nucl Med 1994;35:699–702.
80. Kemp BJ, Prato FS, Dean GW, Nicholson RL, Reese L. Correction for attenuation in technetium-99m-HMPAO SPECT brain imaging [published erratum appears in J Nucl Med 1992;33(12):2250]. J Nucl Med 1992;33:1875–1880.
81. Dey HM, Hoffer PB, Lerner E, Zubal IG, Setaro JF, Black HR. Quantitative analysis of the technetium-99m-DTPA captopril renogram: contribution of washout parameters to the diagnosis of renal artery stenosis. J Nucl Med 1993;34:1416–1419.
82. Raff U, Spitzer VM, Hendee WR. Practicality of NEMA performance specification measurements for user-based acceptance testing and routine quality assurance. J Nucl Med 1984;25:679–687.
83. Todd-Pokropek A, Cradduck TD, Deconinck F. A file format for the exchange of nuclear medicine image data: a specification of Interfile version 3.3. Nucl Med Commun 1992;13:673–699.

9 Single Photon Emission Computed Tomography

THOMAS F. BUDINGER

HISTORICAL PERSPECTIVES

The three major categories of emission imaging are projection or planar imaging, longitudinal or laminar tomography, and transverse section tomography (Fig. 9.1). Conventional planar imaging is almost universally conducted by a gamma-camera attached to a computer image enhancement and data reduction system. Longitudinal tomography involves sampling over a limited range of angles and usually involves motion of a detector system or collimator arrangement in a plane parallel to the long axis of the body. Transverse section tomography involves rotation of the detector system around the body, with presentation of transaxial sections or arbitrary sections (e.g., coronal, sagittal, oblique) by reformatting transverse section data. The two classes of emission tomographic studies are known as positron emission tomography (PET) and single photon emission computed tomography (SPECT).

The major work in longitudinal or limited angle tomography commenced with Anger's tomoscanner (1), which was an analog device designed to yield a series of in-focus planes and was a modification of conventional x-ray longitudinal tomography (laminography), which used moving guns and moving film. About 10 years after introduction of this method it, too, was combined with computer methods for data manipulation.

SPECT dates from the early 1960s, when the idea of emission transverse section tomography was presented by Kuhl and Edwards (38). They used a rectilinear scanner to detect emissions from a series of sequential positions transverse to the cephalad-caudad axis of the body. The data collection from multiple angles was facilitated by employing up to four banks of detectors. The method of simple backprojection was used with optical superposition methods using a cathode ray tube and photographic film. In the early 1970s, digital computers were employed to compensate for both the blurring caused by the process of simple superposition and the attenuation problem of SPECT. These early approaches are still the known contemporary methods of computed tomography (CT) (11, 12, 23, 24, 39, 47, 55, 56).

This chapter presents an explanation of emission tomography by describing longitudinal and transverse section tomography. In principle, all modes of tomography can be considered under the general topic of coded apertures, wherein the code ranges from translation of a pinhole collimator to rotation of a parallel hole or focused collimator array. The problems and physical solutions for SPECT differ significantly from those of x-ray, computed tomography (CT), magnetic resonance imaging (MRI), and positron emission tomography (PET), mainly in the areas of spatial variation in resolution, photon attenuation, and photon scattering.

LONGITUDINAL TOMOGRAPHY

PINHOLE ARRAYS

The basic idea of longitudinal tomography can be shown by moving a pinhole aperture (Fig. 9.2). The image of two sources at different depths will appear shifted by amounts that are proportional to their depths and the amount the pinhole camera is displaced (P_x) from the original position. Because the "box" is closer to the aperture, its image is displaced more than that of the ball. The amount of displacement is proportional to the ratio of the movement distance to the depth of the object and to the distance between the camera and the aperture. The relevant equations are derived by similarity of the triangles as shown in Figure 9.2.

Initially the position of the image of the "box" is given by

$$\frac{x_1}{h} = \frac{-a}{Z_1} \qquad (1)$$

where x_1 is the distance from the center of the image to the "box" image, h is the distance from the camera to the pinhole, a is the true distance of the box source from the axis of the imaging system, and Z_1 is the depth of the source from the pinhole. After a move of the pinhole by a displacement P_x,P^y the image moves from x_1, to a new position $x_1 + \delta_x$ in accord with

$$\frac{x_1 + \Delta_x}{h} = \frac{-(a + P_x)}{Z_1} \qquad (2)$$

In general, for a given depth Z_1 we find that for each displacement there will be a corresponding image displacement δ_x, δ_y.

Suppose there are a multitude of sources at various depths and positions; the pinhole image will represent the superpositions of these sources, but their positions and magnification in the image will depend on the actual depth and planar position of these sources. Thus, if all the sources were at depth Z_1, then the displacement of the image of each source on a second image corresponding to a pinhole displacement of P_{x1},P^{y1} would be described by

$$\Delta_{x1} = \frac{H}{Z_1} P_{x1}$$
$$\Delta_{y1} = \frac{H}{Z_1} P_{y1} \qquad (3)$$

Suppose a third image is formed for another displacement from the original image. The source image will move by δ_{x2}, δ_{y2} from the position in the original image in accord with equation 3.

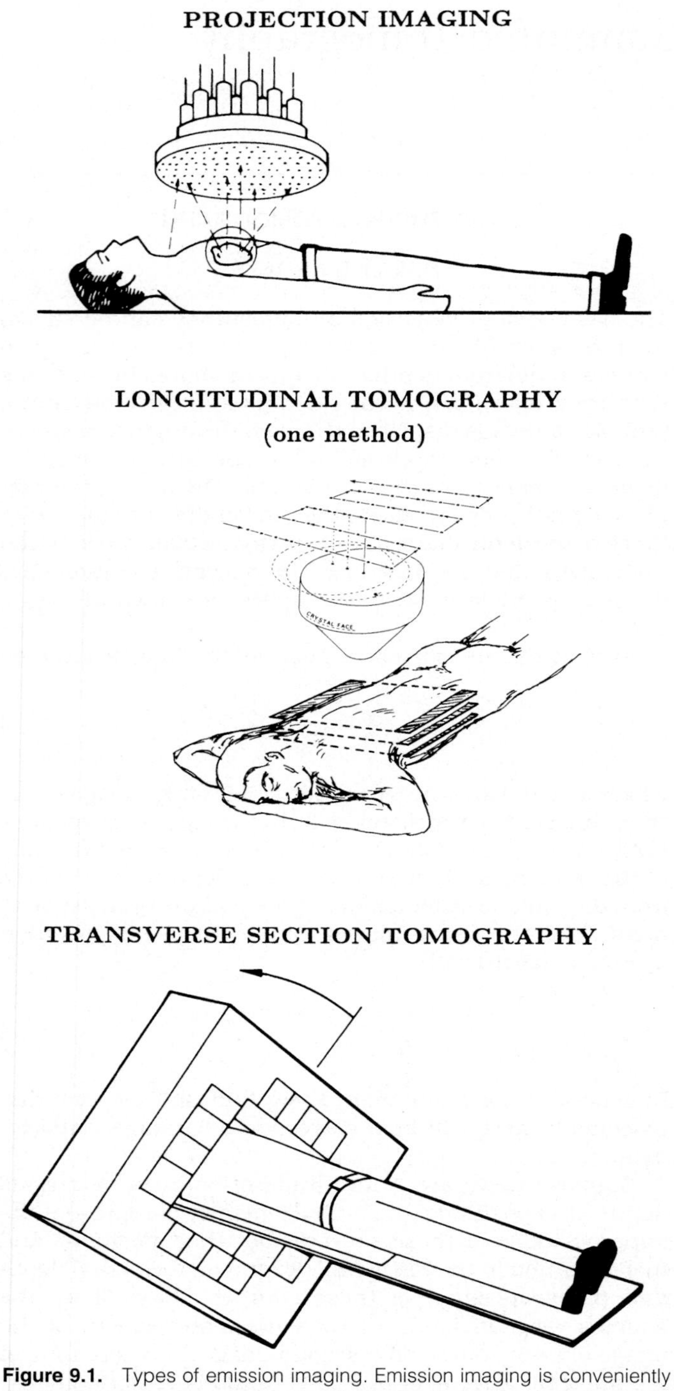

Figure 9.1. Types of emission imaging. Emission imaging is conveniently divided into projection imaging, longitudinal or limited-angle tomography, and transverse section tomography (SPECT).

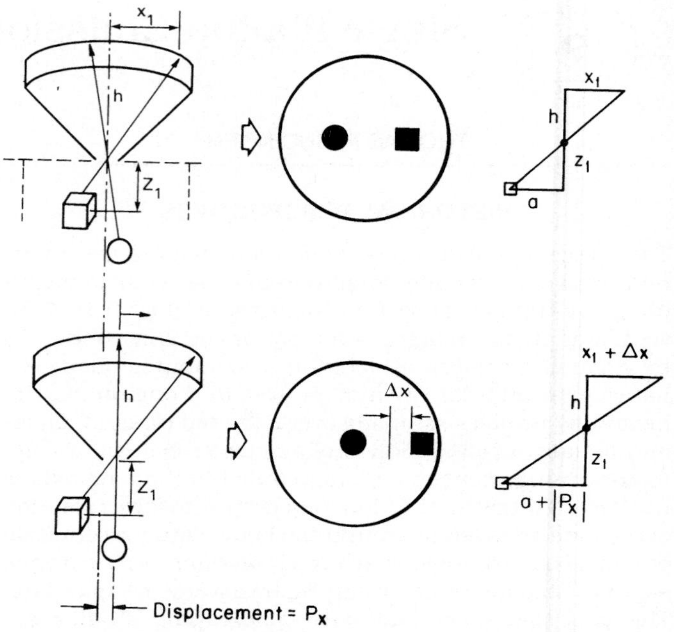

Figure 9.2. Longitudinal tomography. Depth information is reflected by relative displacement of sources for different positions of pinhole aperture. Relationship between amount of displacement and depth of source is derived by noting the similarity of triangles formed by ray optics.

Now let us create a tomograph by reversing the process of equation 3, that is, by shifting each picture element value to a new picture element using $-\delta_{xi}$, $-\delta_{yi}$, for each displacement image I. We sum the resultant images to get a perfect image of the sources exactly as if the pinhole camera had not been moved, as long as the actual depth of the sources was actually Z^1. However, suppose we erred in our estimate or did not know the true depth of Z^1 in equation 3; the result of shifting and summing will be a blurred image of the sources. Next, suppose we do not know at what depth the sources lie but guess at three successive depths and perform the operation of equation 3 to calculate the $-\delta_{xi}$, $-\delta_{yi}$ for each set of images, by using different Z^1 for the three assumed depths. The sources that happen to lie at the properly guessed depth will be in focus, whereas those at other depths will be out of focus. The blurred tomograms are similar to the simple backprojection images of transverse section computed tomography, discussed later, and are the same as the images from Anger's ingenious longitudinal tomographic device (the Pho/con).

Methods for deblurring these tomograms have not shown dramatic improvements. One method is that of successive approximations, whereby the data in each image are corrected by factors derived from a comparison of the *reprojected* images with the observed images. The *reprojections* are obtained by computing what the image data should be if the tomographic result is the true result (Fig. 9.3); that is, the tomographic process is reversed in a computational simulation. The data in the source space are adjusted until the differences between the reprojected images and true images are small. The most recent embodiment of this approach is known as the 7-pinhole system (58). This operation is similar to the early methods of computer-assisted tomography, such as the arithmetic reconstruction technique (ART).

STOCHASTIC CODED APERTURE

A second class of multiple pinhole imaging is the stochastic coded aperture (35, 61). Instead of moving an individual

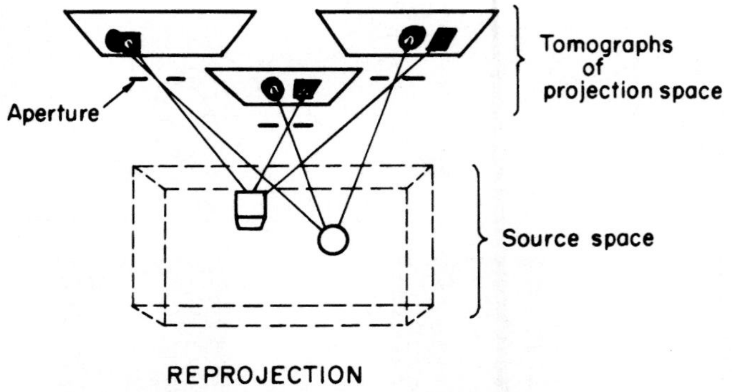

Figure 9.3. Deblurring longitudinal tomograms. One method of removing blur from multiple pinhole imaging system is to reproject simple superposition or backprojection images and make corrections to these images based on difference between reprojected images and actual data.

pinhole or providing many separate imaging chains, which look at the object from different directions as is done in the independent pinhole systems such as the 7-pinhole collimator, the multiple aperture method collects the superposition of many pinhole views on each image. A sequence of images is recorded, each with a somewhat different arrangement of pinholes (Fig. 9.4). Suppose five images are taken, each with a uniquely different pinhole pattern. Recall that each pinhole represents a different angular view. After recording five or more images, we must "decode" the image data to obtain projection data corresponding to each angular view. To do so we solve the set of simultaneous equations shown in Figure 9.4. In this particular case, the angular view A_1, corresponding to pinhole 1 projection only, is determined by adding and subtracting various images (I); thus

$$\begin{aligned} A_1 &= \frac{I_1 + I_3 + I_4 - I_2 - I_5}{2} \\ &= \frac{(A_1 + A_2) + (A_3 + A_4) + (A_1 + A_5) - (A_2 + A_3) - (A_4 + A_5)}{2} \qquad (4) \\ &= A_1 \end{aligned}$$

A_1 is the two-dimensional pinhole projection image obtained from the object distribution viewed from the No. 1 aperture. After this decoding, we have data corresponding to various angular views and the reconstruction problem becomes similar to that for multiple pinhole systems or general computed tomography. This approach combines depth coding with good sensitivity because many apertures are "looking" at the subject at one time. Coded aperture techniques can be extended to complete angular sampling (61). The Fresnel pattern has been used as a coding system for tomography wherein a series of concentric lead rings is used as the collimator (7, 43). But here also the result is limited angle tomography without any signal to noise advantages over pinhole coding.

Six problems associated with the longitudinal tomography techniques are: (a) noise propagation occurs during

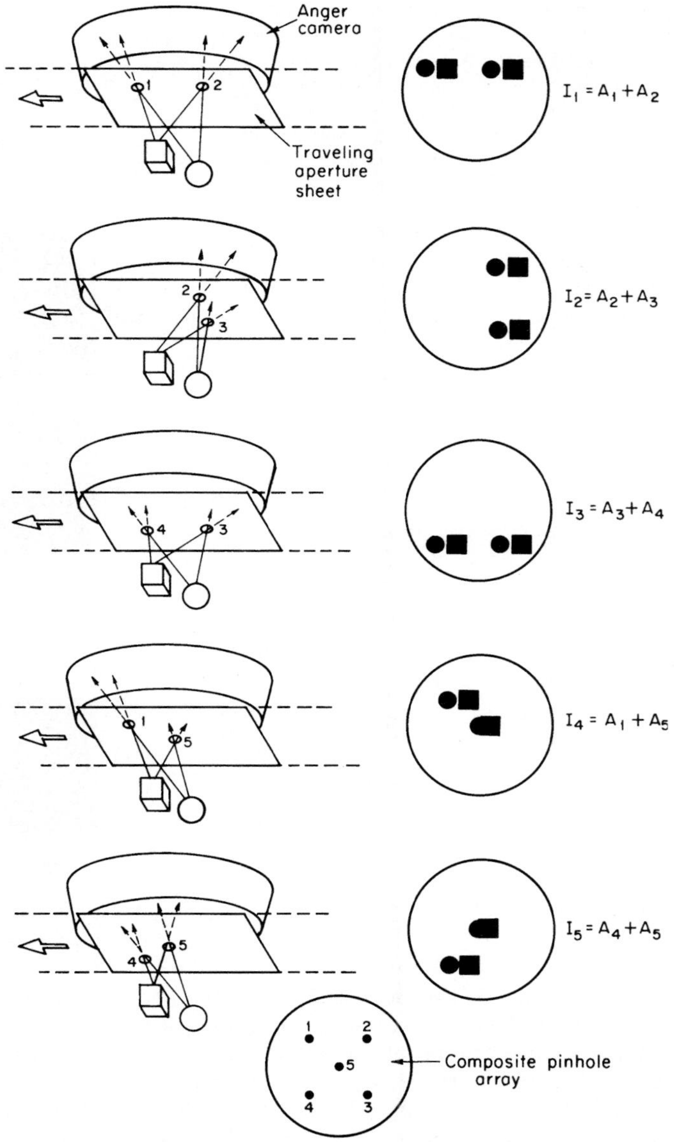

Figure 9.4. Stochastic coded aperture imaging. Schematic of concept of stochastic aperture imaging wherein successive images are obtained, each representing a different combination of views. By solving the set of simultaneous equations shown at the *right*, information corresponding to particular aperture or angle can be "decoded."

the decoding stage (e.g., the variance in A_1 data is the sum of the variances of each image); (b) attenuation compensation is complex and further amplifies errors; (c) the decoding calculation is tractable but computationally costly; (d) variable geometric magnification will cause distortion for pinhole systems; (e) a significant sensitivity nonuniformity exists for pinhole systems; and (f) the data set lacks complete angular sampling.

The limitations imposed by collection of data over a limited angular range are illustrated in Figure 9.5, which shows that the results of a reconstruction are dependent on the shape and orientation of the object being reconstructed. The reason the 7-pinhole technique gives such

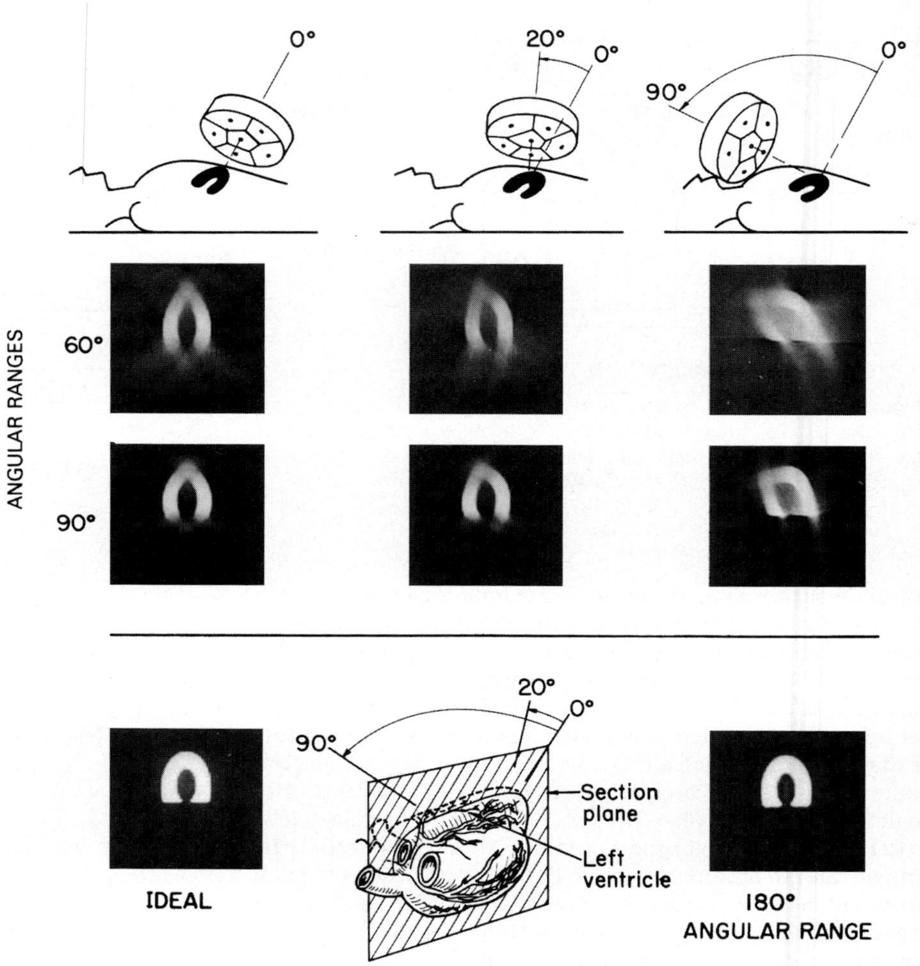

Figure 9.5. Effect of limited angular tomography. Simulation of dependence of reconstructed results on orientation of a tomographic imaging system relative to multiple pinhole or parallel-hole system that has axis of symmetry of object. Angular sampling was limited to 60° and 90° for comparison with 180° of sampling without attenuation. Optical axis of imaging system is varied by 20° and 90° to demonstrate dependence of results on orientation of object relative to imaging axis.

remarkably good images of the heart with only seven views over a limited angular range is, in good part, due to the symmetric orientation of the detector array relative to the axis of the left ventricle's cylinder-like shape. Note in Figure 9.5 that a change of only 20° in the tilt of the detector array relative to the long axis of the left ventricle results in distortions, and a change of 90° results in useless data. Sagittal sections are shown to illustrate the distortion problem and the magnitude of interplane errors due to the shape compared with the aperture orientation problem. When attenuation is added to the problem, even worse results are found. This example was calculated using an iterative reconstruction technique (63) (conjugate gradient iterative least squares) with noiseless nonattenuated data and exact weighting for pixel geometry.

METHODS OF DEBLURRING FOR LIMITED ANGULAR SAMPLING

Attempts to overcome the problem of limited angle in computed tomography by mathematic approaches have been made. One approach, now successfully employed in optical microscopy, is the use of a predetermined or known deblurring operator that relates data at one position to their blurred representation or false data on other planes. This idea has been formulated and implemented in theoretic papers (7, 43, 57), but no practical procedures have emerged from the preliminary experiments, even though the ideas have been discussed for over 15 years. The reason is that it is not possible to reconstruct data that have not been adequately sampled.

A major potential of coded aperture methods is the promise for dynamic emission tomography with single photons when employed in concert with full angular sampling and new detector designs. For example, if the bulk of the detector system can be reduced in a pinhole design by very high resolution crystal arrays and position readout electronics, then the distance between the pinholes surrounding an object can be significantly reduced, thus allowing a system of detectors to surround the body with adequate angular sampling (Fig. 9.6), as recently suggested by Barrett and coworkers (48).

TRANSAXIAL COMPUTED TOMOGRAPHY

The general concept of transaxial CT involving complete angular sampling around the patient is shown relative to longitudinal tomography in Figure 9.6. Projections of emission data made at regular angular intervals around 360° are detected and these projections are then backprojected to form the superposition image (Fig. 9.7). Figure 9.8 illustrates some specialized instruments used to acquire these

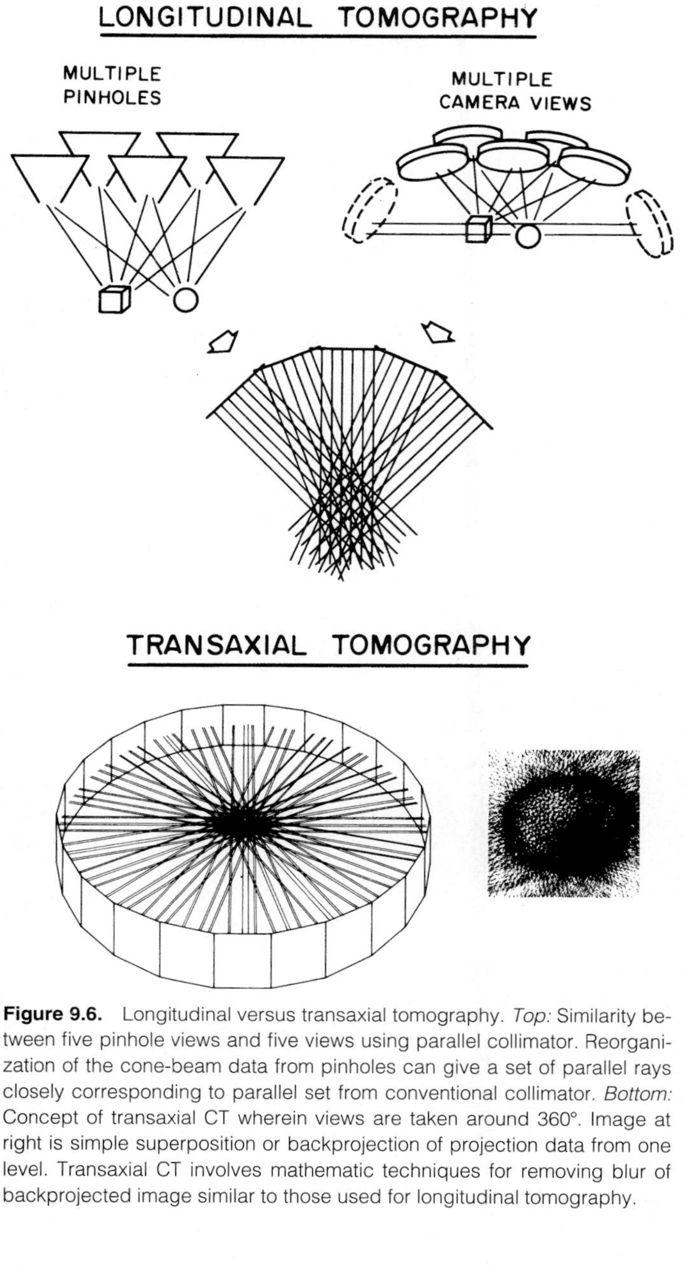

Figure 9.6. Longitudinal versus transaxial tomography. *Top:* Similarity between five pinhole views and five views using parallel collimator. Reorganization of the cone-beam data from pinholes can give a set of parallel rays closely corresponding to parallel set from conventional collimator. *Bottom:* Concept of transaxial CT wherein views are taken around 360°. Image at right is simple superposition or backprojection of projection data from one level. Transaxial CT involves mathematic techniques for removing blur of backprojected image similar to those used for longitudinal tomography.

data. For both longitudinal and transaxial tomography the backprojected image is blurred as a result of superposition of activity. This blurring is removed by the reconstruction procedures discussed later. Though the methods are similar to those used in other forms of reconstruction tomography, problems unique to emission tomography (PET and SPECT) are the need to compensate for photon attenuation and scattered events. Transaxial emission tomography using single photon emitters can be as quantitative as PET if corrections for these factors are employed.

Seven physical science aspects of SPECT (reconstruction strategies with attenuation compensation, angular sampling requirements, variable spatial resolution, scattered radiation, quantitative capability, sensitivity, and dynamic emission tomograpy) are discussed in the next sections. Comparisons to PET are made where instructive.

RECONSTRUCTION STRATEGIES WITH ATTENUATION COMPENSATION

The importance of methods for compensating for attenuation is illustrated in Figure 9.9. The ideal constant distribution is shown in the upper left, with examples of the distortion caused by attenuation of the photons of different energies. The lower two panels correspond to the effects for 140 keV ($\mu = 0.15$) and 511 keV ($\mu = 0.09$) photons in a disc of 20 cm diameter. The reconstruction activity in the center of the disc is erroneously low by a factor of 3.5.

In emission tomography, we seek the position and strength of a radionuclide distribution; therefore, the mathematic algorithm must include some method to account for the attenuation between the unknown sources and the detectors. This task is far more difficult than that of x-ray tomography, wherein the source position and strength are known at all times and only the attenuation coefficients need to be determined. The reconstruction algorithms are similar to those for x-ray CT with the exception of the need to compensate for attenuation. Attenuation effects have until recently been ignored in commercial SPECT. To some extent clinical results were acceptable because the resulting reconstruction, although not quantitative, shows relative concentrations if the activity distribution is concentrated in the central portion of the section. The usual strategy for gamma-camera techniques is to organize the data into a series of slice projections, each corresponding to a section of 10–20 mm thickness. Each section is computed separately. Before reconstruction, compensation for field uniformity must be made (30, 32); then one of several methods for attenuation compensation is employed. A comprehensive discussion of the mathematics is found in Budinger, et al. (9), and a listing of the computer programs with examples in Huesman, et al (63).

Although the methods of correcting for this attenuation error are conveniently implemented in PET, the techniques are more cumbersome for SPECT. Nevertheless, over the past few years convenient methods have evolved using iterative approaches (11, 13) and direct convolution techniques (16, 25, 26). Thus, for situations of constant attenuation, the mathematic intractability has been overcome. Three methods are described below.

Modification of the Geometric Mean (Method I)

The results of reconstructing projection data that have been modified by forming the geometric mean (square root of the product of opposite detected rays) are better than those when no such maneuver is used; however, serious data distortion still occurs. By applying a correction factor that takes into account the thickness and average activity distribution, it is possible to improve these results. First, the geometric mean of projection bin data is formed by multiplying opposing projection rays by one another, then taking the square root. To this modified projection value, a hyperbolic sine correction (sinh) is applied, and then the convolution reconstruction method is used. The sinh correction factor is

$$\frac{e^{\mu}fx}{\sinh(x)}$$

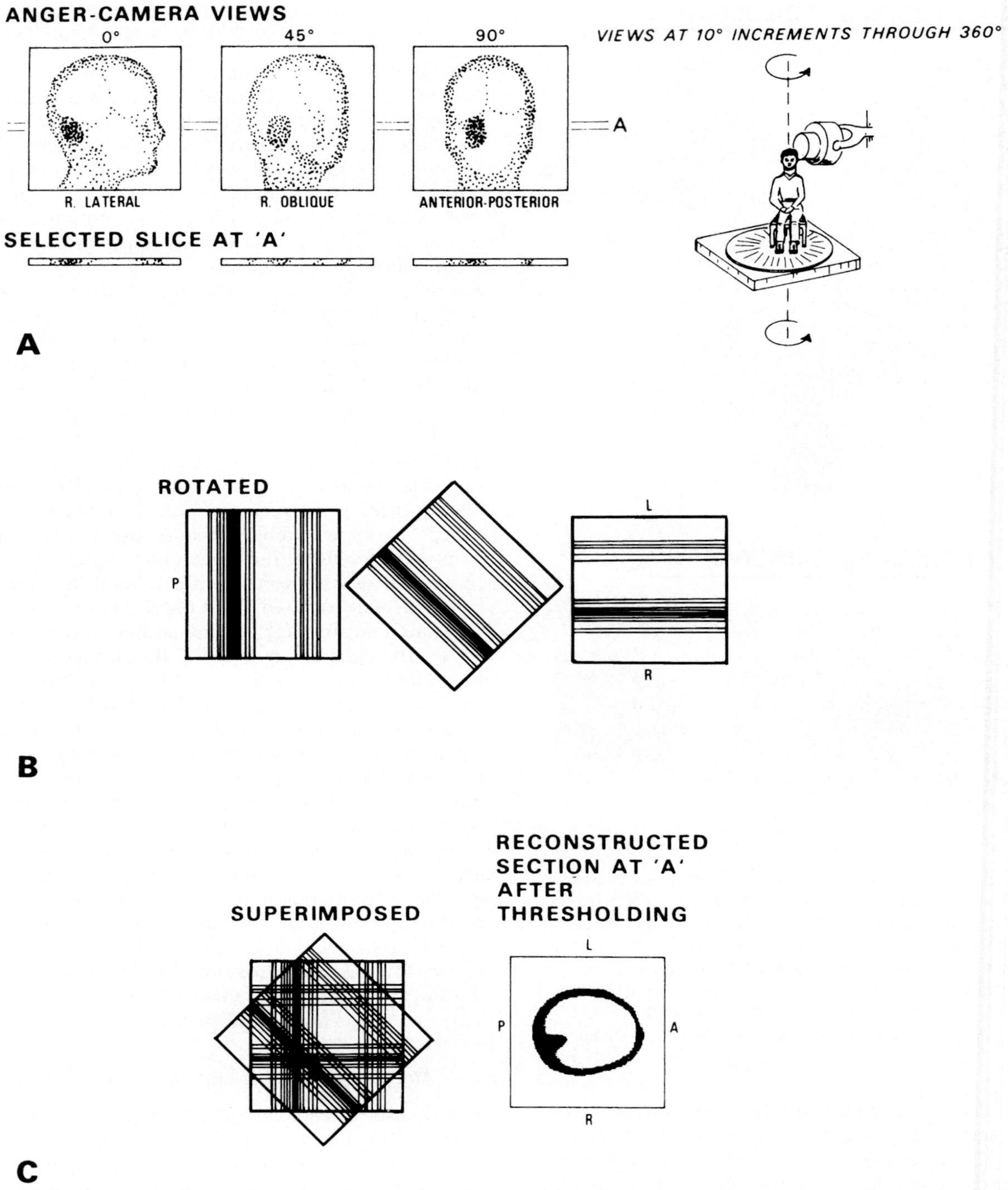

Figure 9.7. Emission tomography reconstruction. The basic idea of emission tomography reconstruction is the initial separation of projection data into slices corresponding to a particular level (**A**). These projections are back-projected and superimposed as illustrated in **B** and **C**. Compensation for attenuation and mathematic techniques for removing the image blur complete the basic concept of reconstruction in SPECT.

where μ is the attenuation coefficient, x is the thickness/2, and f is set from 0.5–0.75 depending on the relative amount of activity along the projection line being modified (8). The method of finding the thickness of the object for each projection line involves estimation of the edges of the object from an initial reconstruction before applying the sinh correction. This method works well for sources distributed near the center of the object; however, if the data are statistically poor as in ^{201}Tl imaging of the heart, the data projections through the posterior thorax contain only a few percent of the actual photons from the heart. Multiplication of these posterior projections with the less noisy anterior projections can lead to worse results than to use only 180° of anterior projections alone.

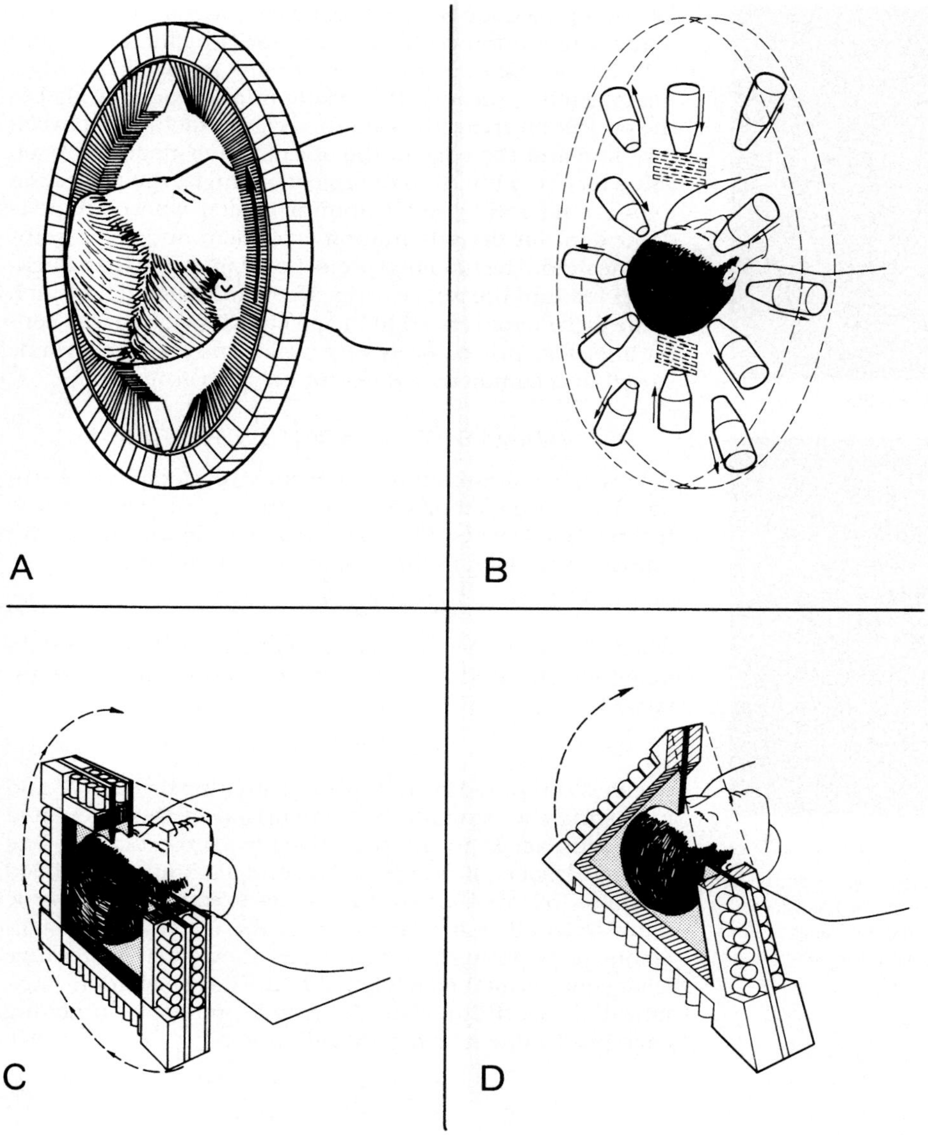

Figure 9.8. New instrument concepts for SPECT. **A** and **B** are types of instrumentation that have been applied to transaxial SPECT. **C** is a potential configuration for a head system. **D** is a schematic of the multiple pinhole system wherein the camera is a small, high resolution detector, which allows multiple pinholes to be positioned without bulky detectors controlling the number of pinholes (48).

Iterative Modification of Pixels (Method II)

If SPECT is performed without consideration of attenuation, the value of each pixel is low because the projected values were modified by an attenuation in accord with the distance between the pixel and the object edge along each ray that passes through that pixel. This modulation is given by $e^{-\mu d_i}$, where d_i is the distance along a particular ray denoted by i (Fig. 9.10).

The overall modification of the source in a particular pixel is merely the sum of these separate modifications divided by the number of projections M:

$$\frac{1}{M}\sum_i e^{-\mu d_i}$$

The method of correction suggested by Chang (13, 14) involves first performing a reconstruction to give the distribution $\rho_{i,j}$, modified by

$$\rho_{\text{new } i,j} = \rho_{\text{old } i,j} \frac{1}{\left(\frac{1}{M}\sum_i e^{-\mu d_i}\right)} \quad (5)$$

Then the modified data are reprojected and the differences between the reprojected bin values and the measured projection data are determined. These "difference projections" are used to reconstruct an error image that, when added to the modified image, gives a good result for constant μ. These techniques work well for objects, such as the head, that have more or less constant attenuation coefficients with the exception of 1.5 cm of bone.

Modification of Bin Values Before Convolution (Method III)

This procedure was originally developed by Bellini (4) and subsequently evaluated for SPECT (26). First, bin values

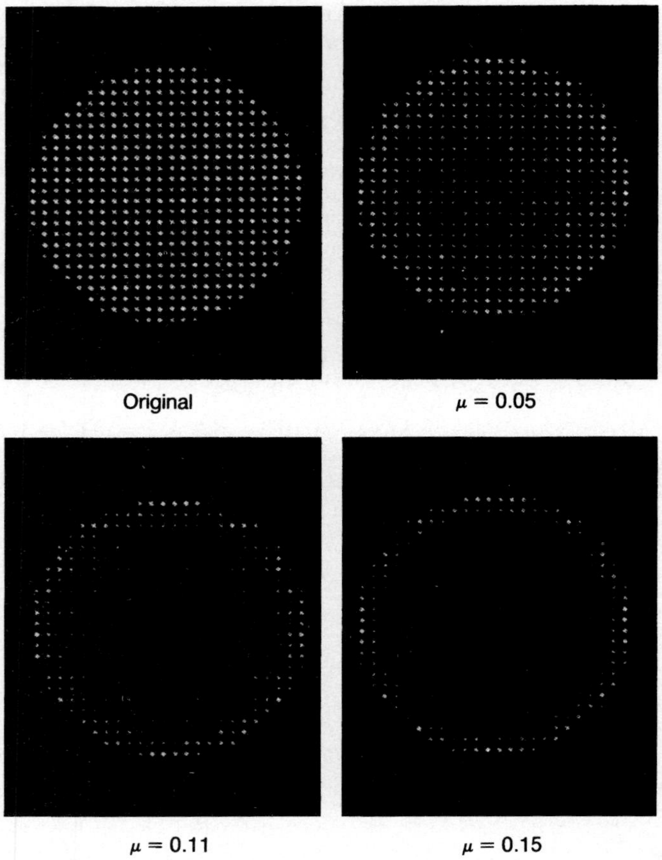

Figure 9.9. Effects of attenuation. The effects of attenuation are shown for a 20 cm diameter disc whose uniform activity is reconstructed as if there is less activity in the center because of the attenuation of photons emitted from sources in the center. $\mu = 0.11$ and $\mu = 0.15$ correspond to the attenuation of tissue for photons of 511 keV and 140 keV, respectively.

for each projection are multiplied by a factor $e^{\mu dk}$ where μ is the attenuation coefficient and dk is defined in Figure 9.11 as the distance from a center line to the object edge. Imagine a line through the axis of rotation and parallel to the projection array; the value of dk is the distance between that line and the edge of the object. After modifying each value for every bin of each projection angle, the projection data are filtered by application of a filter whose shape is dependent on the attenuation coefficient and the resolution desired. The modified projection values are then back-projected into the image array after multiplication of each value by a factor related to the pixel distance from the center line. This procedure is very rapid, and the filter can be varied to accommodate different noise environments.

VARIABLE ATTENUATION DISTRIBUTION

For variable attenuation coefficient situations, two methods have been employed using iterative reconstruction techniques. The iterative reconstruction algorithms involve iterative solutions to the classic inverse problem

$$P = FA \qquad (6)$$

where P is the projection matrix, A is the matrix of true data being sought, and F is the projection operation. The inverse is

$$A = F^{-1}P$$

which is computed by iteratively estimating the data A' and modifying the estimate by comparison of the calculated projection set P' to the true observed projections P. The iterative least squares method (8) and maximum likelihood methods (52) are the two approaches to estimating the true data. Both allow incorporation of the attenuation coefficients as weighting factors such as shown for the iterative least squares method in Figure 9.12. The expectation-maximization algorithm solves the inverse problem by updating each pixel value a_i in accord with

$$a_i^{k+1} = \sum_j p_j \frac{a_i^k f_{ij}}{\sum_i a_i^k f_{ij}} \qquad (7)$$

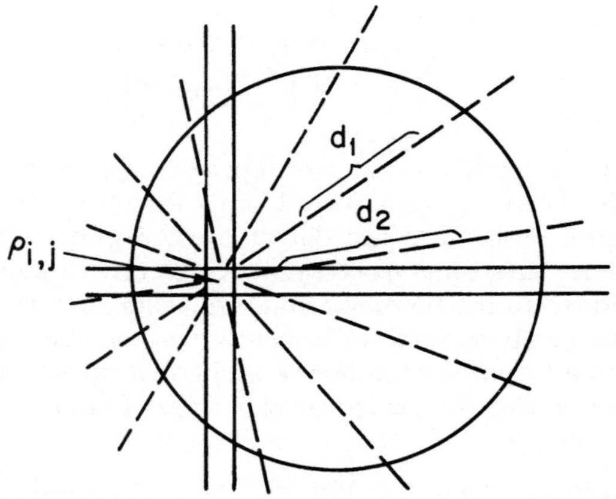

Figure 9.10. Iterative method of attenuation correction. Activity in a pixel i,j is detected as different event rates depending on the distance between activity and edge of attenuating object. From analysis of average attenuation for all views, compensation for distortion can be made by iterative technique.

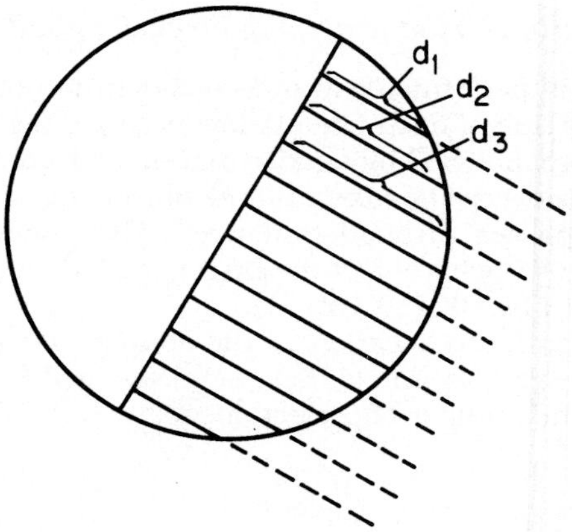

Figure 9.11. Attenuation correction using the convolution method. First stage of the method is to modify each projection before application of special filter in implementing convolution-type SPECT to compensate for attenuation involves modification of projection data by $e^{\mu d_k}$.

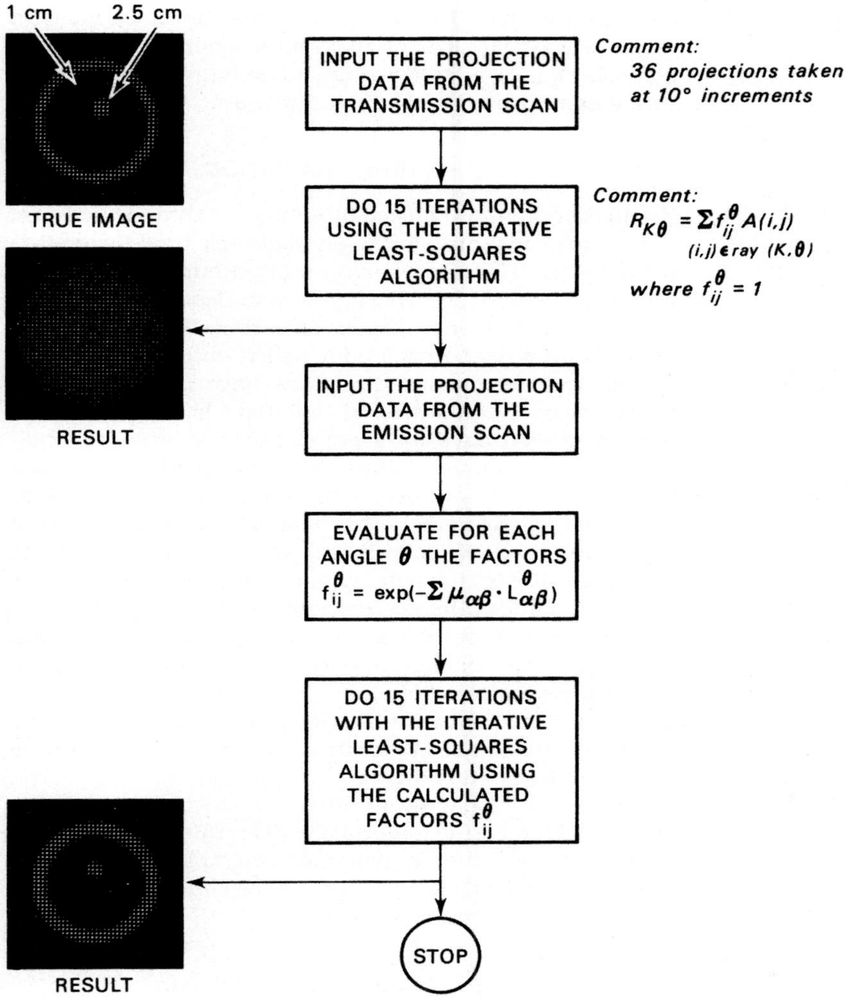

Figure 9.12. Attenuation-corrected iterative least-squares algorithm. A method for attenuation compensation using prior experimental information on the distribution of attenuation coefficients.

where P is the measured projection, f_{ij} is the probability a source at pixel i will be detected in projection detector j, and k is the iteration. Although first described in 1974 (11) and 1982 (52), these methods have only recently attracted interest, probably because the computational task has only recently been simplified by computer technology.

The attenuation coefficients are determined from a transmission scan. A second approach uses a map of attenuation coefficients estimated from the outline of the soft tissues and lungs obtained from the first emission reconstruction and assumed values of the attenuation coefficients. This method is presently under evaluation for practical clinical applications in cardiac nuclear medicine.

ANGULAR SAMPLING REQUIREMENTS

Data distortion from limited angular sampling was shown in Figure 9.5. Another type of distortion occurs when there is 360° coverage but an inadequate number of views (Fig. 9.13). Both of these sampling problems result in streaks and artifacts that are identified as the aliasing problem of undersampling (9, 15). Figure 9.13 gives some semiquantitative idea of the number of views needed for an image consisting of 64×64 resolution units. We note that angular sampling of about 3° is adequate. This corresponds to 120 projections. A more quantitative analysis (Fig. 9.14) uses the projection theorem, which states that the Fourier coefficients corresponding to the Fourier transform of a projection are found along a line that passes through the center of the two-dimensional Fourier transform and is parallel to the line of projection bins. We see that the number of angles is 2π times the number of resolution lengths across the image.

VARIABLE SPATIAL RESOLUTION

An important aspect of SPECT is the nonuniformity of resolution with depth for parallel-hole collimation (Fig. 9.15). Positron emission tomography has a similar, but less severe, problem. In SPECT, this problem can be solved partially by forming the geometric mean (square root of the product of opposing rays), and then treating the data as parallel projections for an angular range of 180°. This method, however, is inferior to other techniques that require projections over 360° (13, 26).

Other methods to solve the resolution uniformity problem include use of collimators that give a uniform resolution over the range of the object (32), moveable focused col-

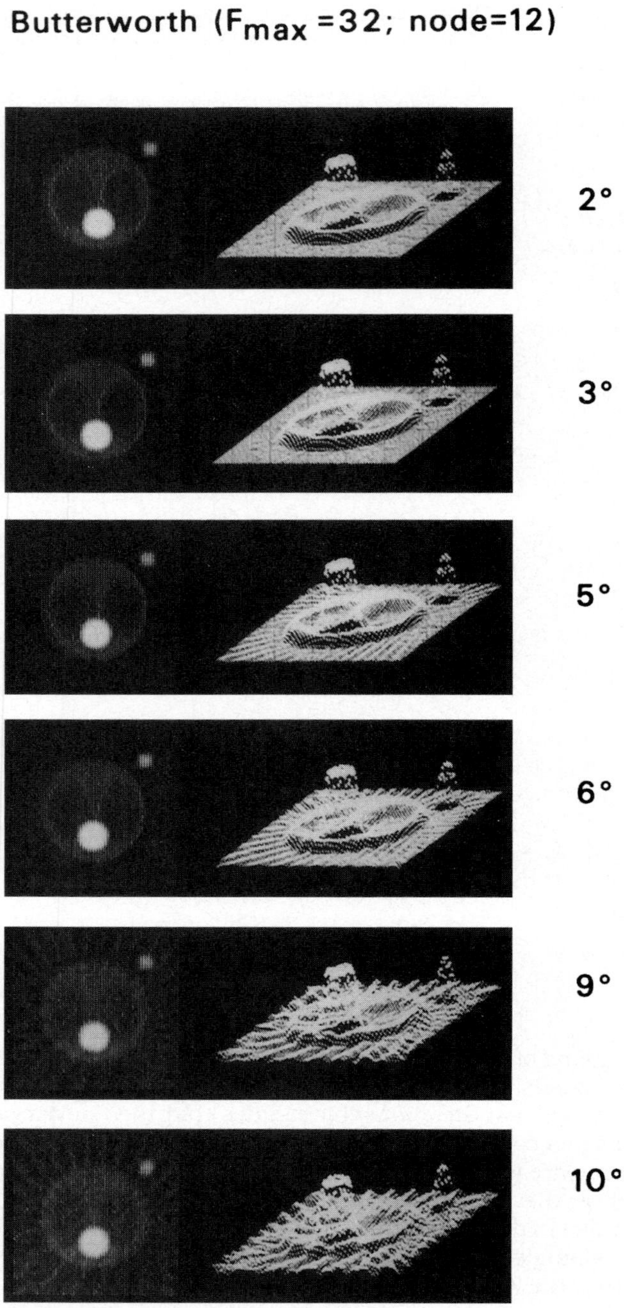

Figure 9.13. Angular sampling requirements determined by resolution elements. The number of angular views necessary for 360° coverage in transverse section CT is approximately equal to the number of resolution elements across the image. In this case, for 64 resolution elements across the image, aliasing artifact accompanying coarsely-sampled data disappears for sampling with less than 3° increments.

limators (used in the Cleon scanner (54)), and incorporation of the spread function data in the reconstruction algorithm (20). Use of measured or theoretic spread function data in an iterative algorithm by modifying the weighting factors as done initially for the effect of attenuation (11) is a promising method for dealing with the collimator problem. The computational approach using an iterative least-squares or maximum likelihood approach might become available on clinical systems in the near future with improved computing hardware.

SCATTERED RADIATION

Recall that photons emitted by sources within the body are either absorbed through the photoelectric process or scattered by the electrons surrounding atoms of the tissue (Compton scattering). These processes lead to the serious attenuation problems discussed earlier. Those scattered photons from deep in the body which enter the detection system from erroneous directions have less energy per photon than the unscattered radiation; however, detector systems do not have sufficient energy resolution to eliminate all these photons. Thus, scattered photons can contribute as much as 50% of the total collected events in SPECT as well as in PET. This means that a true void deep in a phantom or subject will have an observed false activity that is 20–40% of the activity in contiguous regions of the object (3). Unless the scatter contribution is removed before the attenuation correction is applied, an amplification of this unwanted background will occur as shown in Figure 9.16. These scattered photons contribute to inaccuracy in quantitating the amount of radioactivity and degrade the reconstructed images by blurring fine detail and lowering image contrast and to errors in quantitation (Fig. 9.16). The extent and magnitude of scatter increases with the amount of scattering material between the source and the detector. Hence, the fraction of detected photons in a projection is a function of the source depth and distance from the edges of the scattering medium.

Scatter Compensation Methods

Simple methods of merely subtracting an estimated background are not applicable generally because Compton scattering depends on the shape of the scattering material (the distribution of attenuation coefficients) and on the distribution of the radionuclide. Additionally, the scatter contribution is very much dependent on the collimator and the energy window. For example, the contribution of scatter from sources deep in the subject might be 5 times greater than the scatter from the sources at the surface near the collimator.

Scatter compensation techniques fall into four general categories: multiple energy window subtraction, energy weighted compensation, convolution-subtraction technique, and patient specific scatter modeling.

The method of Compton window subtraction is based on using a second "scatter" energy window placed below the photopeak window during data acquisition (33). It is assumed that the data obtained from this energy window are an estimate of the scatter component in the photopeak window. The scatter compensation consists of subtracting an empirically determined fraction of the "scatter" data from the photopeak image. A variant on this energy window method is the dual photopeak window method (34). Here two abutting energy windows are used to span the photo-

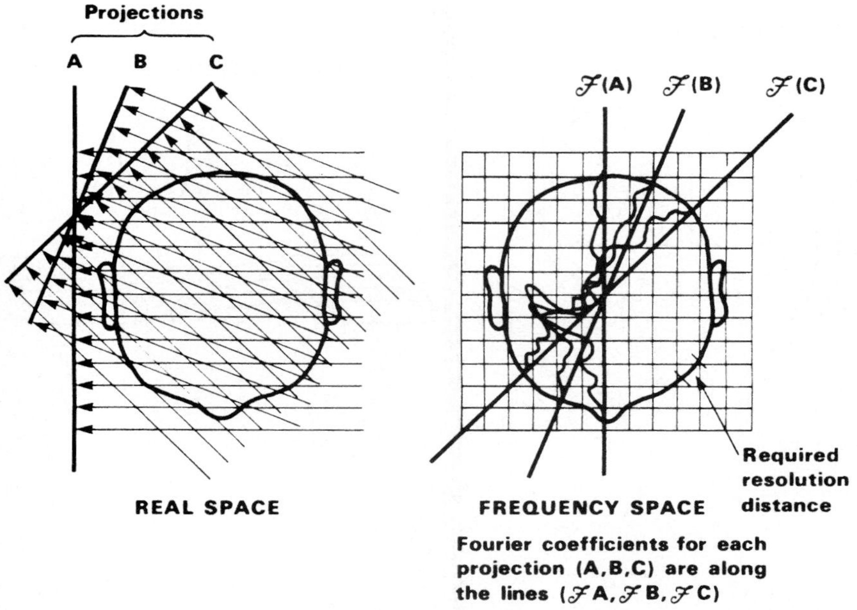

Number of resolution distances around circumference:

M = 3.14 x (number of resolution distances across the object)

For X-ray CT:

Number of angles = M/2 x 2

(Projections at 180° are identical but sampling theorem requires 2 samples per resolution distance)

For Emission CT

Number of angles = M x 2

(Attenuation causes projections at 180° to be different and 2 samples per resolution are required)

XBL 8510-8527

Figure 9.14. Projection theorem for angular sampling requirements. The number of angles required for reconstruction can be determined by an analysis of adequate sampling, which depends on the number of resolution elements across the image space. In this analysis, we rely on the projection theorem to arrive at a simple formula that is applicable to SPECT.

peak of the energy spectrum. These methods have provided some image improvement and improved quantitation (22). The use of multiple energy windows below or even straddling the photopeak window have resulted in image improvements. However, these methods suffer from the fact that the scattered photons arriving at a particular energy window depends on patient geometry, source distribution, and the type of collimator used (21).

The energy weighted compensation methods seek to estimate the scatter correction by analyzing the energy spectrum detected at each pixel (17). These spectra are weighted by an energy-weighted function designed to minimize the scatter contribution. This method has been implemented in one commercial system (Siemens, Hoffman Estates, IL).

A third class of methods estimates the scatter by blurring the projection data, usually by convolution of the measured projections with a smoothing kernel (42, 45). Subsequently, some fraction of this blurred projection "profile" is subtracted from original measured projections. This method requires an estimate of the scatter fraction multiplier to be applied to the smoothing data before subtraction.

The scatter modeling methods are patient specific and therefore able to take into account the fact that the scatter response function varies as a function of both depth inside the scatter medium and distance from the edge of the scatter medium. Exact scatter response derived from Monte Carlo simulation (2, 3) has been used in both subtraction and iterative reconstruction methods for accurate compensation for scatter. However, the extensive computations and large memory required for Monte Carlo simulation or other exact methods of scatter modeling (21) on every patient is not practical at the present time.

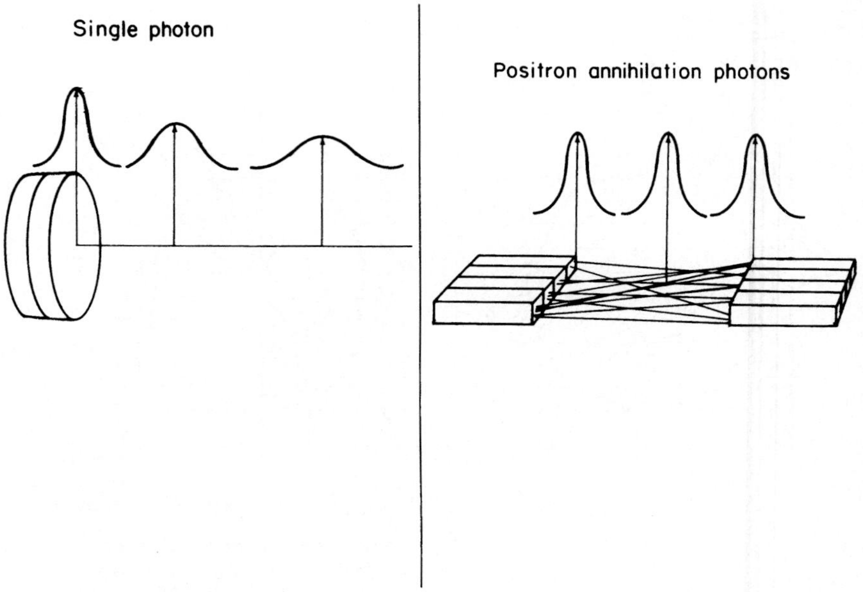

Figure 9.15. Uniformity of resolution. Uniformity of resolution is generally poor with SPECT systems unless special collimation is used.

QUANTITATIVE CAPABILITY

Statistical Precision

The statistical precision of SPECT is dependent on the number of detected events and the volume of interest. In conventional planar imaging, the signal-to-noise ratio is estimated as the square root of the number of detected events per pixel. However, the act of reconstruction results in a propagation of noise that decreases the expected signal-to-noise ratio by factors of eight or more, depending on the resolution sought and the size of the object. The reason for this increase in statistical uncertainty due to reconstruction is illustrated by Figure 9.17. The variance of a value detected in one projection bin is equal to the number of events detected and the signal-to-noise is therefore given by $S/\sqrt{S}$ because the square root of the variance is the expected noise, and of course, S (the detected number of events) is the signal. Now, during the reconstruction, each pixel will receive a contribution from all pixels lying along the particular projection ray (because the ray sum value for all the pixels is placed back in each pixel during back-projection). Under the condition that there are n pixels across the image, the noise in any particular pixel is proportional to the sum of the values of the n pixels (Fig. 9.14). Thus, instead of a signal-to-noise of $S/\sqrt{S}$, we have $S/\Sigma\sqrt{S}$ or a decrease in signal-to-noise by the square root of the average number of pixels or resolution elements in projection rays. The formula that deals with the general case is

$$\%\ \text{uncertainty} = \frac{1.2 \times 100\ (\text{no. resolution cells})^{3/4}}{(\text{total no. events})^{1/2}} \quad (8)$$

The factor 1.2 is based on the convolution kernel, (rms = root mean square). Figure 9.18 shows the relation between the total number of events and the number of resolution cells in an image for four levels of uncertainty. Figure 9.17 shows the relationship between detected events and volume of interest. If we collected 300,000 events for a section with 300 pixels (1000 events/pixel), the rms uncertainty is 13.2%. A naive prediction based on $1/\sqrt{S} \times 100$ would give only 3.2% uncertainty. The discussion above assumes a uniform distribution. If the activity is concentrated in a small region of the image the tomographic uncertainty decreases, thus in cases of a single object in a uniform field (10):

$$\%\ \text{uncertainty} = \frac{1.2 \times 100\ (\text{total no. events})^{1/4}}{(\text{average no. events per resolution cell in the target})^{3/4}} \quad (9)$$

The importance of this modification can be appreciated by evaluation of the uncertainty for cardiac imaging wherein the effective number of resolution elements is almost 10 times less than the total number of pixels in a transverse section. Thus, for an image of the thorax with 500,000 detected events, the expected uncertainty for heart distribution occupying about 135 resolution elements is 7%, but that calculated for the whole thorax of about 2500 resolution elements would be erroneously estimated at 50%. The new heart-seeking agents using ^{99m}Tc allow SPECT of the heart to give more reliable data than ^{201}Tl from a statistical standpoint because as much as five times more activity is injected.

The arguments presented favor the importance of the effective number of resolution elements when imaging the heart, but indicate the difficulty of imaging the distribution of radionuclides in organs like the lungs, which occupy most of the resolution elements. Thus, the effective number of elements is close to the actual number of image picture elements.

If the resolution cell size decreases by two, the required number of events for constant uncertainty increases by eight. Thus, an important goal for instrument design is to increase sensitivity and an important goal of reconstruc-

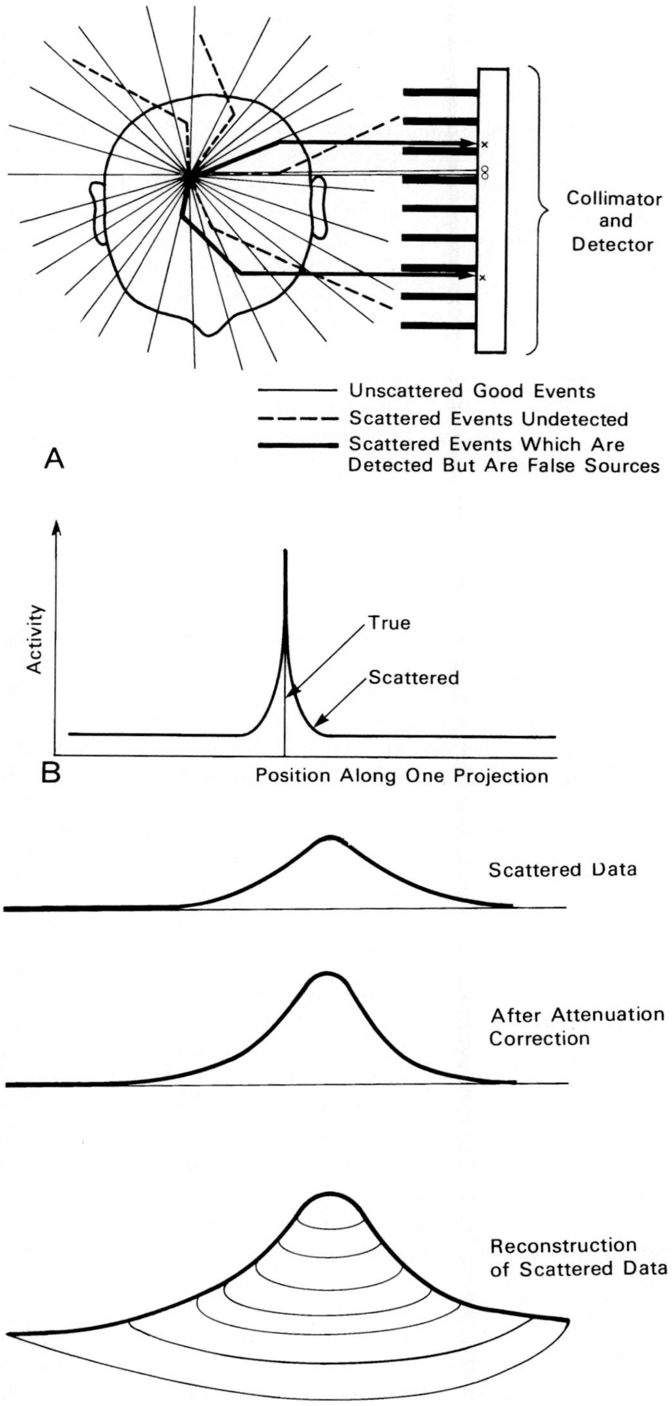

Figure 9.16. Effect of scattered radiation. The occurrence of scattered photons in emission imaging can lead to background that is spread throughout the image space, and is dependent on the source position and amount of scattering material between the source and the detector.

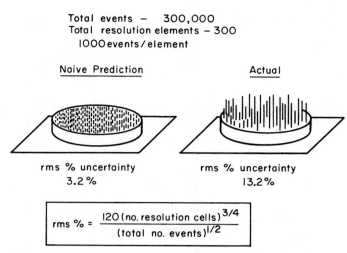

tion algorithms is to optimize resolution recovery and suppress noise artifacts.

Another aspect of noise propagation peculiar to SPECT (and PET) is the influence of errors in the attenuation coefficients used to correct the attenuation of projection data. If variable attenuation coefficients are present in the region

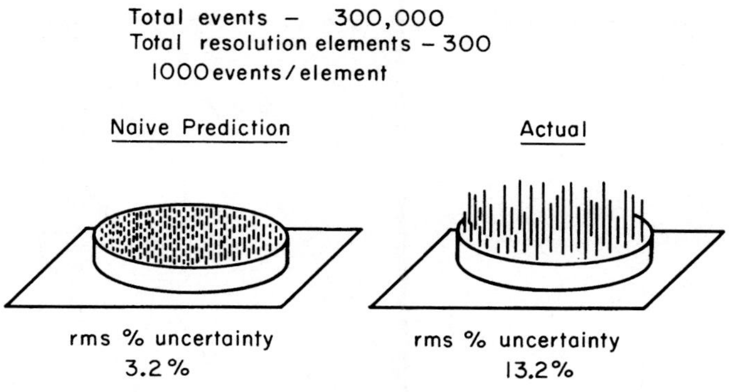

$$\text{rms } \% = \frac{120\,(\text{no. resolution cells})^{3/4}}{(\text{total no. events})^{1/2}}$$

Figure 9.17. Statistical precision. Demonstration of magnitude of decrease in statistical reliability expected from projection image and that after computation of transverse section. *rms* = root mean square.

to be imaged, a transmission study is required to provide the attenuation. But if the transmission data used to correct for variable attenuation have poor statistics, the statistical uncertainty in the resulting SPECT image will be adversely affected.

Quantitative Concentration Recovery (Accuracy)

The quantitative accuracy in a transverse section reconstruction with attenuation compensation depends on the size of the object relative to the resolution. In fact, the accuracy or bias related to correct sampling of data is quite different from the precision of a measurement that is dependent on statistics, as discussed earlier. This important concept can be seen from the simulations shown in Figure 9.19. As the sampling resolution decreases from 10 mm to 2 mm, the reconstruction data have more statistical fluctuation (less precision), but in a region of interest corresponding to the region of the source, the mean value becomes closer to the actual value (more accuracy). For SPECT, collimation is necessary to increase the in-plane resolution, and this results in a decrease in the solid angle and a loss in sensitivity by a larger factor than is the case for PET, as discussed later. Commercially available instruments have resolution of 7–10 mm. Thus, objects less than 15 mm in size will not be quantitatively imaged. This problem is particularly important for tracers which localize in the cerebral gray matter wherein activity in the 3.5 mm-wide cerebral cortical ribbon cannot be quantitatively compared to activity in the much larger central gray regions (e.g., caudate nucleus, putamen).

SENSITIVITY

Quantitative precision requires an adequate number of detected events. Thus, for clinically useful SPECT, instrument sensitivity is extremely important, and is the major design feature for most instrument development efforts. Sensitivity is the number of events detected for a given

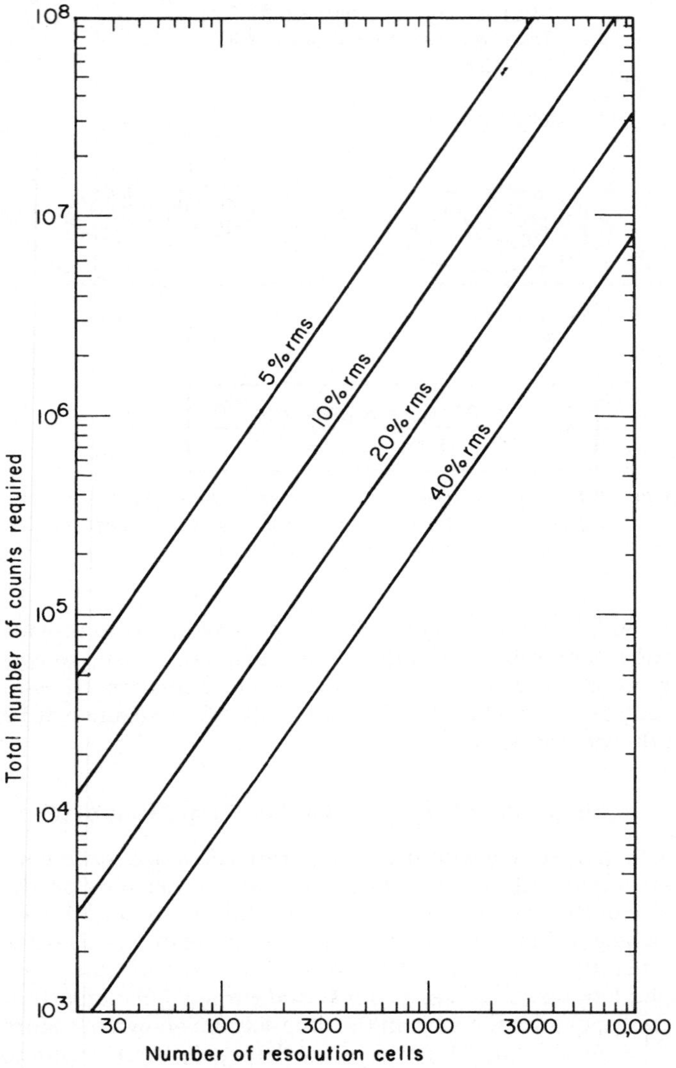

Figure 9.18. Statistical certainty in emission tomography. Relationship between the number of detected events and number of resolution elements in image for various degrees of statistical certainty.

source of radiation, and depends mainly on the solid angle of detection. The solid angle is defined as the ratio of area of detector available to a source anywhere in the imaging volume to the area of a sphere with radius R from the center of the volume to the imaging detectors. For example, if 1 cm × 1 cm is the area of detection for a single gamma-camera for an object with a radius of 15 cm from the detector, the single photon solid angle factor is

$$\frac{1\ \text{cm}^2}{4\pi R^2 \text{cm}^2} = \frac{1}{2835} \quad (10)$$

Because the positron device can have a ring of detector area, for example, 1 cm thick around the entire circumference, the solid angle factor is

$$\frac{1 \times 2\pi R}{4\pi R^2} = \frac{1}{30} \quad (11)$$

or almost 100 times better than that of the single photon system for 1 cm resolution. It was on the basis of this incomplete argument that many concluded that SPECT would never compete with PET. However, there are many other factors that must be taken into account, as shown in Figure 9.20. First, if four arrays of detectors are placed around the object this advantage is reduced to 25. Secondly, for PET, the probability of positron detection is the product of the probability of detection by each opposing crystal; thus a crystal efficiency of 80% leads to a PET efficiency of 0.8^2, which is only 64%. The attenuation losses are associated with the total path length through the object in PET and are greater in PET than in SPECT. In addition to the efficiency and attenuation differences, PET requires a larger diameter (e.g., 60 cm for PET and 30 cm for SPECT for the head). Instead of a sensitivity ratio of 100, the expected sensitivity ratio for 1 cm resolution in an instrument for head imaging, as derived from Figure 9.20, is:

$$\frac{S(\text{PET})}{S(\text{SPECT})} = \frac{15}{a} \quad (12)$$

where S is sensitivity and a (cm) is the resolution in three dimensions. Having 15 times less sensitivity is not a serious deterrent to SPECT of the brain, but the relative sensitivity for a resolution of 5 mm is 30 and this difference makes SPECT less practical at high resolution. Figure 9.21 shows the relative sensitivity for head and whole-body instruments. An instrument for imaging the thorax or abdomen has much less sensitivity than the head instrument because of the R^2 influence, as shown in Figure 9.21 (*right*).

Multiple Layer Instruments

Early work with multiple-section SPECT was done on patients rotated relative to a large-field-of-view Anger camera at Donner Laboratory (11), but the sensitivity was only a few events per second per microcurie. An important commercial design employs three gamma-cameras arranged in a triangular fashion (41). This design and the square or four-sided design appear to be optimal at present; however, available dual-headed gamma-camera systems can provide tomographic data for multiple levels, but with a sensitivity about one-half that of the three- or four-sided systems.

A high-sensitivity, single-section, single photon device, such as the old Cleon scanner (62), cannot be extended easily to a multisection instrument, because the crystal area used to gain the sensitivity obviates packing adjacent detector layers in the axial direction without large shielding gaps between layers. A three-sided fan-beam system or a four-sided parallel-beam arrangement has been considered optimal for SPECT because more detectors would require an increase in R to accommodate the projection geometry for more detectors (Fig. 9.22). To obtain multiple angles, the single photon device must rotate. However, the multiple pinhole design using high resolution detectors close to the pinhole aperture can provide volumetric data without the need to rotate (48).

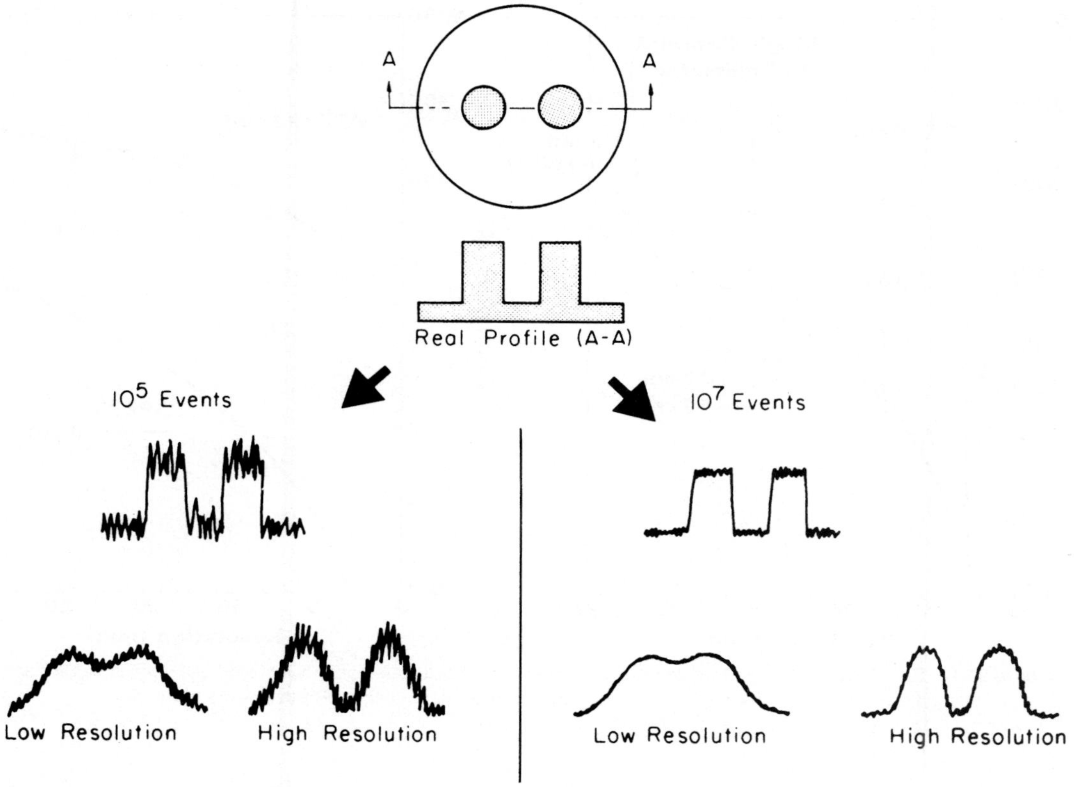

Figure 9.19. Quantitative accuracy dependence on resolution. The quantitative accuracy of the images is controlled by the sampling resolution. A system with good resolution will channel the events into the regions of interest from which they originate. However, a system with poor resolution will spread the data outside the anatomic region of interest, owing to blurring in the poor-resolution system. Statistical uncertainty is a separate consideration.

$$S_{T_{c-99m}} \propto \frac{no.\,detector\ arrays \times resolution^2 \times packing \times efficiency \times attenuation(\gamma)}{4\pi R_1^2}$$

$$S_{\beta^+} \propto \frac{2\pi R_2 \times resolution \times packing \times efficiency^2 \times attenuation(\beta^+)}{4\pi R_2^2}$$

Radius of detector array:

$$R_1 = 200mm$$

$$R_2 = 300mm$$

Attenuation:

$$T_{c-99m} \sim e^{-\mu d/2}$$

$$\beta^+ \sim e^{-\mu d}$$

Figure 9.20. PET versus SPECT sensitivity. The basic parameters that enter into a calculation of sensitivity for single photon detector systems (SPECT) ($S_{Tc\text{-}99m}$) versus those for PET ($S_{\beta+}$).

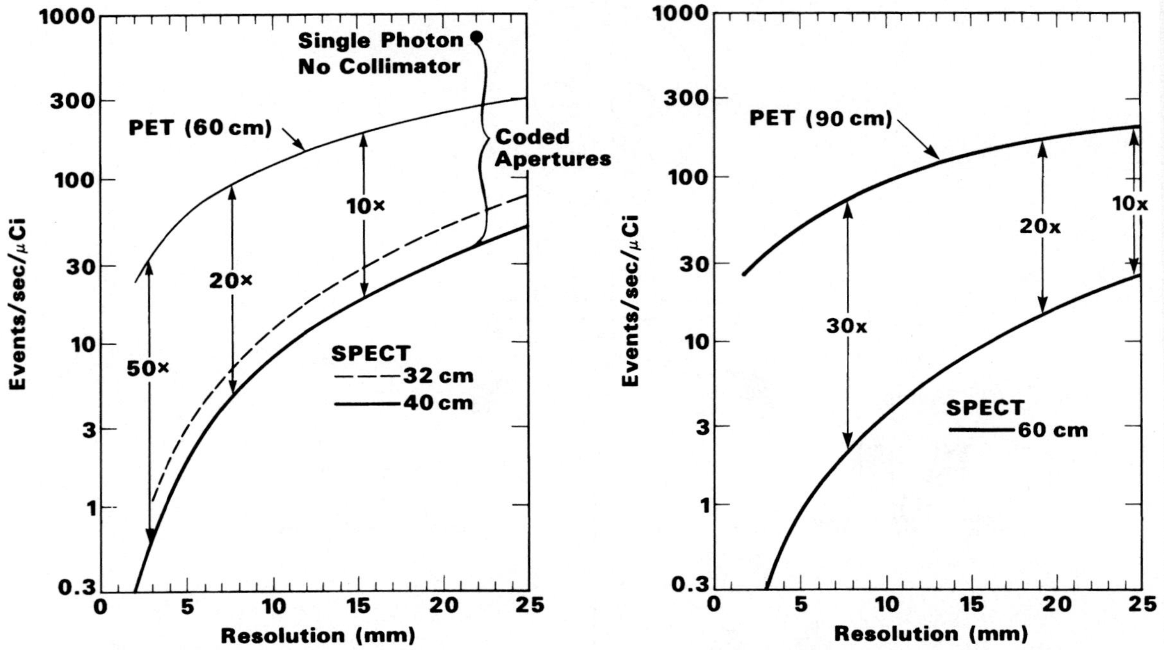

Figure 9.21. Sensitivity of head and whole-body instruments. The calculated sensitivity for SPECT versus PET for an instrument designed to image the head (*left*) and an instrument designed to image the body (*right*).

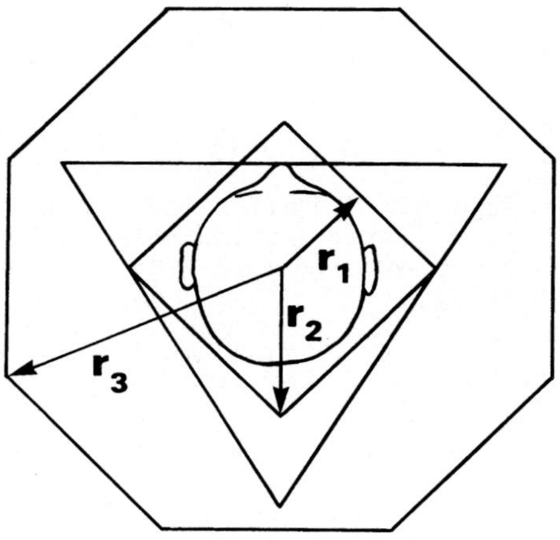

$$r_3^2 \gg r_2^2 > r_1^2$$

$$S \propto \frac{1}{r^2}$$

Figure 9.22. Effect of imaging instrument radius on sensitivity. Sensitivity (S), is inversely proportional to the radius squared of the imaging instrument. The sensitivity for SPECT increases with more detector material around the subject; however, the decrease due to the radius squared effect outweighs this increase in area unless special geometries are used (Fig. 9.8A, B, and D).

SPECT with Positron Emitters

The potential of SPECT systems for detection of the 511 keV photons from ^{18}F in fluorodeoxyglucose studies of organ metabolism and applications to lesion detection, can be evaluated by an examination of the equations relative to sensitivity and the physical principles of collimation. As shown in equation 12, the sensitivity relative to PET for a resolution of 10 mm is decreased by 15, but this equation is derived for collimator conditions of low-energy photons associated with ^{201}Tl, ^{99m}Tc, and ^{123}I. The lead septa of the collimator for 10 mm resolution for 511 keV photons occupies at least 50% of the area, and the efficiency of the usual gamma-camera crystals is more than two times less than that for the single photon emitters commonly used, further reducing the relative sensitivity. In summary, instead of a sensitivity difference between a three- or four-sided SPECT and PET of 15, we can expect a sensitivity penalty of 45 for 10 mm resolution and about 100 for 5 mm resolution. This is needed, for example, in axillary node detection in breast cancer clinical studies. Despite this large sensitivity difference, FDG SPECT has clinical potentials for detection of lesions about 2 cm in diameter and for evaluation of cardiac FDG intake versus perfusion mismatches. The absence of washout and the 1.8-hour half-life of ^{18}F allow time to collect adequate statistics for this positron emitter.

CLINICAL APPLICATIONS

Applications of SPECT to clinical studies preceded x-ray CT, and the first quantitative physiologic studies with SPECT were reported in 1975 (36, 40). At present, the main interest in SPECT is in heart perfusion imaging with ^{201}Tl and ^{99m}Tc-sestamibi and brain imaging using ^{99m}Tc and ^{123}I flow agents and some neuroreceptor ligands. SPECT agents in common use for cerebral blood flow are N-isopropyl-p-(^{123}I)iodoamphetamine (IMP) (28, 37, 49) and the ^{99m}Tc-labeled hexamethylpropyleneamine oxime (HMPAO). The diffusible gas ^{133}Xe is also being used (18, 27). The possibility for revival in brain imaging using SPECT appears to be great because the new compounds concentrate in the brain in proportion to flow (46, 60) and can be imaged over short periods of time (5 minutes) with a resolution of 7 mm full-width at half-maximum (FWHM) with appropriate instrumentation. SPECT can provide clinical information similar to perfusion, permeability, and blood volume information obtainable by PET, but with somewhat less resolution, as discussed earlier.

With the advent of new compounds that concentrate in the heart (44, 59) there is renewed interest in SPECT of the heart. A machine designed to do dynamic SPECT of the heart is not yet commercially available; however, rotating three-headed gamma-camera systems have demonstrated the clinical potential for perfusion imaging using ^{99m}TC-labeled agents (6, 51, 53).

Examination of liver and kidneys with SPECT was shown to be more specific and sensitive in the detection of lesions than conventional projection imaging (5, 31, 50). However, the studies require data acquisition time in the range of 30 minutes for available devices to obtain adequate statistics to allow reconstruction with distributed sources. An appreciation of the problem is gained if one considers the fact that because of attenuation only two of 100 photons directed toward the collimator from a source on one side of a 40 cm diameter abdomen will be detected. Yet, for a quantitative reconstruction, all sources must be detected from all positions with good statistics.

SUMMARY

Single photon emission computed tomography and positron emission tomography comprise emission tomography. Single photon tomography uses collimator systems for detection of γ photons from radionuclides, and is divided into longitudinal or limited-angle tomography and transverse section tomography. The majority of new developments and practical applications use transverse section tomography, which gives results similar to those of PET and shares with PET the physical problems of attenuation, angular sampling requirements, nonuniformity of resolution, scatter, and statistical limitations. The severity of these problems is greater for SPECT than for PET; however, they can be compensated for through instrument design and mathematic treatment of the data. Whereas the SPECT sensitivity, in terms of detected events for a given amount of radionuclide in the patient, is one-tenth that of PET, the availability of new SPECT radiopharmaceuticals, particularly for the brain and head, and the practical and economic aspects of SPECT instrumentation make this mode of emission tomography attractive for clinical studies of the heart and brain.

REFERENCES

1. Anger H. Tomography and other depth discrimination techniques. In: Hine GJ, Sorenson JA, eds. Instrumentation in nuclear medicine. New York: Academic Press, 1974:61–100.
2. Axelsson B, Msaki P, Israelsson A. Subtraction of Compton-scattered photons in single-photon emission computerized tomography. J Nucl Med 1984;25(4):490–494.
3. Beck JW, Jaszczak RJ, Coleman RE, Starmer CF, Nolte LW. Analysis of SPECT including scatter and attenuation using sophisticated Monte Carlo modeling methods. IEEE Trans Nucl Sci 1982; 29:506.
4. Bellini S, Piacentini M, Cafforio C, Rocca F. Compensation of tissue absorbtion in emission tomography. IEEE Trans Acoust Speech Signal Processing 1979;27(3):213–218.
5. Biersack HF, Koischwitz D, Lackner K, Reske SN, Knopp R, Winkler C. Single-photon emissions-computertomogiraphie (SPECTS) der leber mit einerm rotierenden γ-kamerasystem. Eur J 1981; 10:205.
6. Budinger T, Araujo L, Ranger N, et al. Dynamic SPECT feasibility studies [Abstract]. J Nucl Med 1991;32(5):955.
7. Budinger TF. Three-dimensional imaging of the myocardium with isotopes. In: Harrison DC, Sandler H, Miller HA, eds. Cardiovascular imaging and image processing, theory and practice. Palos Verdes Estates, CA: Society of Photo-Optical Instrumentation Engineers, 1975:263–271.
8. Budinger TF, Derenzo SE, Gullberg GT, et al. Emission computer assisted tomography with single-photon and positron annihilation photon emitters. J Comput Assist Tomogr 1977;1:131.
9. Budinger TF, Derenzo SE, Gullberg GT, et al. Trends and prospects for circular ring positron cameras. IEEE Trans Nucl Sci 1979;26:2742.
10. Budinger TF, Greenberg WL, Derenzo SE, et al. Quantitative potentials of dynamic emission computed tomography. J Nucl Med 1978;19:309.
11. Budinger TF, Gullberg GT. Three-dimensional reconstruction in nuclear medicine emission imaging. IEEE Trans Nucl Sci 1974; 21:2–20.
12. Budinger TF, Gullberg GT, Huesman RH. Emission computed tomography. In: Herman GT, ed. Topics in applied physics: image reconstruction from projections: implementation and applications. Berlin: Springer-Verlag, 1979:147–246.
13. Chang L. A method for attenuation correction in radionuclide computed tomography. IEEE Trans Nucl Sci 1978;25:638.
14. Chang L. Attenuation correction and incomplete projection in single photon emission computed tomography. IEEE Trans Nucl Sci 1979;26:2780.
15. Crawford CR, Kak AC. Aliasing artifacts in computerized tomography. Appl Opt 1979;18:3704.
16. Derenzo SE, Zaklad H, Budinger T. Analytical study of a high-resolution positron ring detector system for transaxial reconstruction tomography. J Nucl Med 1975;16(12):1166–1173.
17. DeVito RP, Hamill JJ. Determination of weighting functions for energy-weighted acquisition. J Nucl Med 1991;32(2):343–349.
18. Devous MDS, Payne JK, Lowe JL. Dual-isotope brain SPECT imaging with technetium-99m and iodine-123: clinical valida-fjtion using xenon-133 SPECT. J Nucl Med 1992;33(11):1919–1924.
19. Ell PJ, Holman BL, eds. Computed emission tomography. Oxford: Oxford University Press, 1982.
20. Formiconi AR, Pupi A, Passeri A. Compensation of spatial system response in SPECT with conjugate gradient reconstruction technique. Phys Med Biol 1989;34(1):69–84.
21. Frey EC, Tsui BMW. A comparison of scatter compensation methods in SPECT: subtraction-based techniques versus iterative reconstruction with an accurate scatter model. Orlando, FL: Proceedings of The Conference Record of the 1992 Nuclear Science

Symposium and the Medical Imaging Conference, 1992:1035–1037.
22. Gilardi MC, Bettinardi V, Todd-Pokropek A, Milanesi L, Fazio F. Assessment and comparison of three-scatter correction techniques in single photon emission computed tomography. J Nucl Med 1988;29(12):1971–1979.
23. Gilbert P. Iterative methods for the three-dimensional reconstruction of an object from projections. J Theor Biol 1972;36:105.
24. Gordon R, Herman GT. Three-dimensional reconstruction from projections: a review of algorithms. Int Rev Cytol 1974;38:111–151.
25. Gullberg G. The attenuated radon transform: theory and application in medicine and biology [PhD Thesis]. University of California, Berkeley: Lawrence Berkeley Laboratory, 1979.
26. Gullberg GT, Budinger TF. The use of filtering methods to compensate for constant attenuation in single-photon emission computed tomography. IEEE Trans Biomed Eng 1981;28:142.
27. Hellman RS, Collier BD, Tikofsky RS, et al. Comparison of single-photon emission computed tomography with (^{123}I)iodoamphetamine and xenon-enhanced computed tomography for assessing regional cerebral blood flow. J Cereb Blood Flow and Metab 1986; 6(6):747–755.
28. Hill TC, Holman BL, Lovett R, et al. Initial experience with SPECT (single photon computerized tomography) of the brain using n-isopropyl I-123-*p*-iodoamphetamine. J Nucl Med 1982;23 191.
29. Lawrence Berkeley Laboratory. Donner algorithms for reconstruction tomography. Pub. 214. Berkeley, CA: Lawrence Berkeley Laboratory, 1977.
30. Jaszczak RJ, Chang L-T, Stein NA. Whole-body single-photon emission computed tomography using dual, large-field-of-view scintillation cameras. Phys Med Biol 1979;24:1123.
31. Jaszczak RJ, Coleman RE, Lim CB, Whitehead FR. Lesion detection with single photon emission computed tomography (SPECT) and conventional imaging. J Nucl Med 1982;23:97.
32. Jaszczak RJ, Coleman RE, Lim CB, Whitehead FR. Physical factors affecting quantitative measurements using camera-based single photon emission computed tomography (SPECT). IEEE Trans Nucl Sci 1981;28:69.
33. Jaszczak RJ, Floyd CE, Coleman RE. Scatter compensation techniques for SPECT. IEEE Trans Nuclear Sci 1985;32:786.
34. King MA, Hademenos GJ, Glick SJ. A dual-photopeak window method for scatter correction. J Nucl Med 1992;33(4):605–612.
35. Koral KF, Rogers WL. Application of ART to time-coded emission tomography. Phys Med Biol 1979;24:879.
36. Kuhl DE, Alavi A, Hoffman EJ, et al. Local cerebral blood volume in head-injured patients. Determination by emission computed tomography of 99m-Tc-labeled cells. J Neurosurg 1980;52:309.
37. Kuhl DE, Barrio JR, Huang SC, et al. Quantifying local cerebral blood flow by N-isopropyl-*p*-(^{123}I)iodoamphetamine (IMP) tomography. J Nucl Med 1982;23(3):196–203.
38. Kuhl DE, Edwards RQ. Image separation radioisotope scanning. Radiology 1963;80:653.
39. Kuhl DE, Edwards RQ, Ricci AR, Reivich M. Quantitative section scanning using orthogonal tangent correction. J Nucl Med 1973; 14(4):196–200.
40. Kuhl DE, Reivich M, Alavi A, Nyary I, Staum M. Local cerebral blood volume determined by three-dimensional reconstruction of radionuclide scan data. Circ Res 1975;36:610.
41. Lim CB, Walker R, Pinkstaff C, et al. Triangular SPECT system for 3-D total organ volume imaging: performance results and dynamic imaging capability. IEEE Trans Nucl Sci NS-1986;33(1): 501–504.
42. Ljungberg M, Strand S-E. Scatter and attenuation correction in SPECT using density maps and Monte Carlo simulated scatter functions. J Nucl Med 1990;31:1560.
43. MacDonald B, Chang L-T, Perey-Mendez V, et al. γ-Ray imaging using a Fresnel zone-plate aperture, multiwire proportional chamber detector, and computer reconstruction. IEEE Trans Nucl Sci 1974;21:678.
44. Maddahi J, Merz R, Van Train KF, Roy L, Wong C, Berman DS. Tc-99m MIBI (RP-30) and Tl-201 myocardial perfusion scintigraphy in patients with coronary disease: quantitative comparison of planar and tomographic techniques for perfusion defect intensity and defect reversibility. J Nucl Med 1987;28:654.
45. Maski P, Axelsson B, Larson S. Some practical factors influence the accuracy of convolution scatter correction in SPECT. Phys Med Biol 1989;34:283.
46. Mayberg HS, Lewis PJ, Regenold W, Wagner HNJ. Paralimbic hypoperfusion in unipolar depression. J Nucl Med 1994;35(6):929–934.
47. Oppenheim BE. More accurate algorithms for iterative three-dimensional reconstruction. IEEE Trans Nucl Sci 1974;21:72.
48. Pang I, Barrett HH, Chen J-C, et al. Physical evaluation of a four-dimensional brain imager [Abstract]. J Nucl Med 1994;35(5):28P.
49. Podreka I, Baumgartner C, Suess E, et al. Quantification of regional cerebral blood flow with IMP-SPECT. Reproducibility and clinical relevance of flow values. Stroke 1989;20(2):183–191.
50. Raynaud C, Syrota A, Soussaline F, Todd-Pokropek A, Kellershohn C. Single photon emission computed tomography in diagnosis of liver metastasis [Abstract]. J Nucl Med 1981;22:P31.
51. Sasaki M, Ichiya Y, Kuwabara Y, et al. Rapid myocardial perfusion imaging with ^{99m}Tc-teboroxime and a three-headed SPECT system: a comparative study with ^{201}Tl. Nucl Med Communications 1992;13(11):790–794.
52. Shepp LA, Vardi Y. Maximum likelihood reconstruction for emission tomography. IEEE Trans Med Imaging 1982;1:113–122.
53. Smith AM, Gullberg GT, Christian PE, Datz FL. Kinetic modeling of teboroxime using dynamic SPECT imaging of a canine model. J Nucl Med 1994;35(3):484–495.
54. Stoddard HF, Stoddart HA. A new development in single gamma transaxial tomography: Union Carbide focused collimator scanner. IEEE Trans Nucl Sci 1979;26:2742.
55. Tanaka E, Shimizu T, Iinuma TA, et al. Digital simulation of section image reconstruction. Natl Inst Radio Sci (Jpn) 1973;12:3.
56. Todd-Pokropek AE. The formation and display of section scans. In: Proceedings of Symposium of American Congress of Radiology. Amsterdam: Excerpta Medica, 1972:545.
57. Townsend D, Piney C, Jeavons A. Object reconstruction from focused positron tomograms. Phys Med Biol 1978;23:235.
58. Vogel RA, Kirch D, LeFree M, et al. A new method of multiplanar emission tomography using a seven pinhole collimator and an Anger scintillation camera. J Nucl Med 1978;19:648.
59. Watson DD, Smith WH, Teates CD, Beller GA. Quantitative myocardial imaging with Tc-99m MIBI: comparison with Tl-201. J Nucl Med 1987;28:653.
60. Wilhelm KR, Schroder J, Henningsen H, Sauer H, Georgi P. Preliminary results of ^{99m}Tc-HMPAO-SPECT studies in endogenous psychoses. J Nucl Med 1989;28(3):88–91.
61. Williams JJ, Knoll GF. Initial performance of SPRINT: a single photon system for emission tomography using a seven pinhole collimator and an Anger scintillation camer. J Nucl Med 1978; 19:648.
62. Zimmerman RE, Kirsch CM, Lovett R, Hill TC. Single photon emission computed tomography with short focal length detectors. In: Sorenson JA, ed. Single photon emission computed tomography and other selected topics. New York: Society of Nuclear Medicine, 1980.
63. Huesman RH, Gullberg GT, Greenberg WL, Budinger TF. Users manual—Donner algorithms for reconstruction tomography. Lawrence Berkeley Laboratories PUB-214, 1977.

10 Positron Emission Tomography: Methods and Instrumentation

SIMON R. CHERRY and MICHAEL E. PHELPS

POSITRON EMISSION TOMOGRAPHY

Positron emission tomography (PET) is a unique biologic imaging tool which can be used to obtain functional information from the living human body (1). Modern commercial PET systems now have the ability to simultaneously image the whole brain or heart with 4–5 mm spatial resolution and a temporal resolution of seconds. Methods have also been developed to image the entire body in one imaging session. This chapter provides an overview of the methods and instrumentation used in PET, including the fundamentals of PET imaging, the production and characteristics of commonly employed positron emitters, a description of the modern PET scanner and the process of image reconstruction, a look at the correction factors necessary to achieve quantitative PET images, and the use of tracer kinetic models to turn PET images into biologic assays.

BIOLOGIC IMAGING WITH POSITRON EMISSION TOMOGRAPHY

In contrast to other radionuclide imaging techniques, the count density in reconstructed PET images is directly proportional to the local radioactivity concentration allowing absolute quantification of tracer uptake. In addition to having superior spatial resolution and quantitative potential, PET also has much greater sensitivity (i.e., number of γ-rays detected per unit injected dose) than single photon emission computed tomography (SPECT) due to the use of electronic collimation. Furthermore, the biologic ubiquity of the elements which are available as positron emitters gives PET an unprecedented power to image the distribution and kinetics of natural and analog biologic tracers. Because of the exquisite sensitivity of detection systems to γ-ray emission, these biologic probes can be introduced in trace amounts (nano- or even picomolar concentrations) such that they do not disturb the biologic process under investigation. By combining a tracer which is selective for a specific biochemical pathway, an accurate tracer kinetic model and a dynamic sequence of quantitative images from the PET scanner, it is possible to estimate the absolute rates of biologic processes in that pathway. Examples of such processes which have been successfully measured with PET include regional cerebral and myocardial blood flow, rates of glucose utilization, rates of protein synthesis, cerebral and myocardial oxygen consumption, synthesis of neurotransmitters, enzyme assays, and receptor assays (2–4).

There is also a growing realization of the power of combining PET with pharmacology and drug development (5–8). The synergism of this relationship results from the common requirements in the development of a drug and a biologic imaging probe. Each is designed to target a single step in a biologic process, the drug to modify the process and the biologic imaging probe to measure the function of that process. Each is designed to be administered systemically, with minimum breakdown by enzyme systems or sequestering by the immune system, and to cross membranes to reach their target. Because of this commonality, many of the new biologic imaging probes will be labeled drugs originating out of the merger of modern biology, biotechnology, and drug development. These new generations of drugs and biologic imaging probes will focus on the fundamental processes regulating biologic systems, such as signal transduction, second messengers, transcription, and translation. With PET, not only can the modifying effects of drugs on a particular biologic process be monitored, but the drugs themselves can be labeled and introduced in trace amounts, allowing the biodistribution to be safely determined in the living human body. As PET technology continues to mature, we are seeing the beginnings of a powerful merger between biology, pharmacology, and imaging, and with it the true birth of in vivo biologic imaging.

ROLE OF POSITRON EMISSION TECHNOLOGY IN MEDICAL IMAGING

PET, like SPECT, plays a complementary, but quite distinct role from other commonly employed medical imaging modalities such as magnetic resonance imaging (MRI) or x-ray computed tomography (CT). These methods mainly provide anatomic information and will be the method of choice where disruption to normal anatomy by disease is to be expected. There are many situations, however, where anatomic changes may be completely absent, or where functional changes precede anatomic changes. Examples in the brain include neurodegenerative diseases, such as Alzheimer's, Parkinson's, and Huntington's diseases, neurodevelopmental disorders, epilepsy, psychiatric disorders, and drug abuse (9, 10). In patients with coronary artery disease and cardiomyopathies, PET is able to distinguish between ischemic (but viable) and infarcted myocardium (11, 12). In cancers throughout the body, PET is capable of detecting early developing disease, grading degree of malignancy, staging and differentiating residual tumor or recurrence from necrosis, surgical scarring, and edema (13–16). PET is also effective at monitoring patient response to cancer therapy. Thus, PET can examine a wide range of biologic processes in vivo and is increasingly providing unique information not available from other modalities.

FUNDAMENTALS OF POSITRON EMISSION TOMOGRAPHY

The nucleus of an atom contains both neutrons and protons (collectively known as nucleons). The number of protons and neutrons in a stable nucleus is such that the repulsive electrostatic force between the positively charged protons is balanced by the attractive strong nuclear forces which act on all nucleons. Using nuclear reactors or cyclotrons, it is possible to create isotopes which have an excess of protons and are, therefore, unstable. These proton-rich isotopes can decay by two modes: electron capture and positron emission. The net result of either decay mode is to convert one of the protons into a neutron, thus decreasing the atomic number of the atom by one, resulting in a better balance between the forces acting on the nucleus.

ELECTRON CAPTURE

In electron capture, the nucleus captures one of the atomic electrons from the inner shells and combines this with a proton to form a neutron. In terms of the nucleus, this can be written as:

$$ {}^{A}_{Z}N \rightarrow {}_{Z-1}^{\ A}N + \nu \qquad (1)$$

where Z is the atomic number, A is the mass number and ν is a neutrino. Energy is released in the decay process because the final daughter-state has a lower total energy than the parent-state, and this energy is carried off by the neutrino. The likelihood of electron capture increases with atomic number, because the inner shell electrons tend to find themselves closer to the nucleus and are thus easier to capture. Since this mode of decay does not lead to any detectable particles or γ-radiation, it is of no use for imaging purposes and will not be discussed further.

POSITRON EMISSION

An alternative decay mode is positron emission whereby a proton in the nucleus is considered to be transformed into a neutron and a positron. The positron (e^+) has the same mass as the electron, but has a positive charge of exactly the same magnitude as the electron's negative charge. The nuclear equation for positron emission can be written as:

$$ {}^{A}_{Z}N \rightarrow {}_{Z-1}^{\ A}N + e^+ + \nu \qquad (2)$$

In order for positron emission to be energetically feasible, the difference in total energy between the parent and daughter states has to be at least 1.022 MeV. It turns out that positron emission is favored in low Z elements (in contrast to electron capture). In some higher Z elements, positron emission is actually energetically forbidden because of the 1.022 MeV requirement, and decay can only proceed by electron capture. In many intermediate Z, proton-rich nuclei, the two decay modes are competing processes. An example of this, the decay of ^{18}F into ^{18}O is shown in Figure 10.1. The energy difference between the parent and daughter states (1.65–1.022 MeV) is shared between the positron and the neutrino. Emitted positrons therefore have a spectrum of energies (Fig. 10.2), with the maximum energy, E_{max}, equal to:

$$E_{max} = E({}^{A}_{Z}N) - E({}^{\ A}_{Z-1}N) - 1.022 \text{ MeV} \qquad (3)$$

POSITRON ANNIHILATION

The positron has a very short lifetime in solids and liquids. It rapidly loses kinetic energy by scattering interactions with atomic electrons. Eventually, when it reaches thermal energies (essentially at rest), it will combine with an electron and the two particles will annihilate, converting their mass into energy in the form of γ-rays. The energy released by the annihilation process is 1.022 MeV. To simultaneously conserve both momentum and energy, the annihilation must produce two γ-rays with 511 keV energy which are emitted at 180° to each other (Fig. 10.3). The detection of the two 511 keV γ-rays forms the basis for imaging with PET.

COINCIDENCE DETECTION AND ELECTRONIC COLLIMATION

There is a relatively high probability that both 511 keV γ-rays will escape from the body without scattering. If both

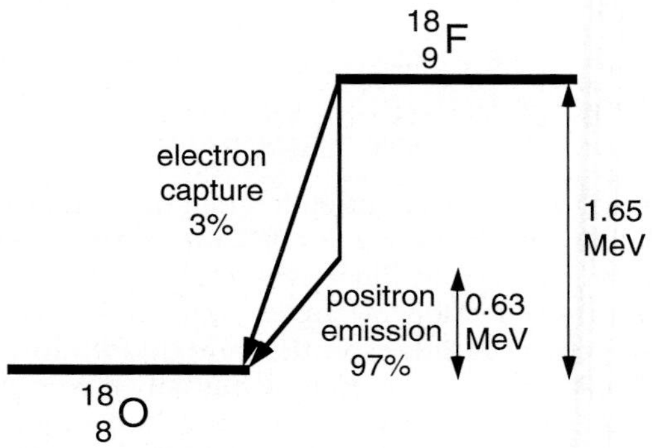

Figure 10.1. Decay scheme and energy levels for fluorine-18 showing competition between positron emission (97%) and electron capture (3%). The total energy of the transition is 1.65 MeV, of which 0.63 MeV is available for positron emission.

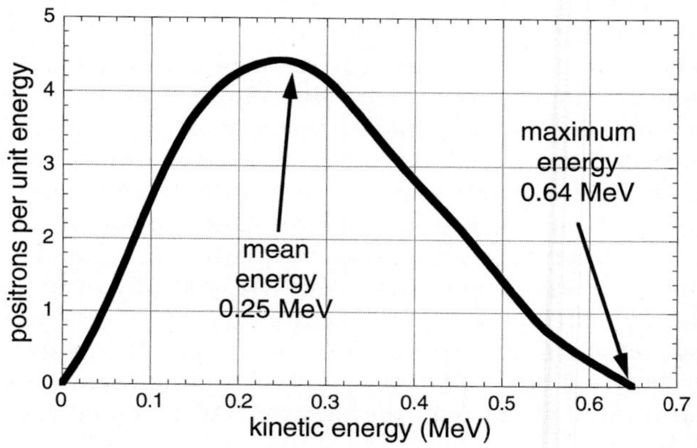

Figure 10.2. Typical energy distribution of positrons after emission. The mean energy is roughly one-third the maximum energy. The higher the positron energy, the further it is likely to travel before annihilation, setting limits on the spatial resolution attainable with PET.

γ-rays can subsequently be detected, we can define the line along which the annihilation must have occurred. Since the distance the positron travels before annihilation is generally small, this is a good approximation to the line along which the emitting atom must be located. By having a ring of detectors surrounding the patient, it is possible to build up a map of the distribution of the positron-emitting isotope in the body.

One major advantage of PET is that it employs electronic collimation. By using coincidence detection (i.e., simultaneous or coincident detection of two γ-rays on opposite sides of the body), we can define the direction that the γ-rays came from. In conventional nuclear medicine techniques, where only one γ-ray is available, this can only be achieved by use of a lead collimator, drilled with small holes, which mechanically collimates the arriving γ-rays. Obviously, the absorption of many photons in the lead leads to a large reduction in sensitivity compared to PET. Another advantage is that all positron-emitting isotopes lead to 511 keV γ-rays, so the PET scanner can be optimized for detection at this energy. In other nuclear medicine techniques, the γ-ray energy varies from isotope to isotope, so it is not easy to optimize imaging for all isotopes.

PHYSICAL LIMITS OF SPATIAL RESOLUTION IN POSITRON EMISSION TOMOGRAPHY

There are two factors which ultimately limit the spatial resolution attainable with PET. First, as mentioned earlier, the positron will travel a short distance between the site of emission and site of annihilation. This distance is referred to as the positron range and can vary from fractions of a millimeter up to several millimeters, depending on the energy spectrum of the emitted positrons and the tissue in which the emission occurs. For most positron emitting isotopes, this effect leads to a blurring of the data which is characterized by an exponential function with a full width at half-maximum (FWHM) of the order of 0.2–3 mm. The positron range for some commonly employed isotopes is shown in Table 10.1.

The other factor which can limit spatial resolution is caused by the residual kinetic energy and momentum of the positron and electron at the moment they annihilate. This leads to the angle between the two γ-rays deviating slightly from 180°. The blurring effect caused by this component depends on the diameter of the PET scanner under consideration. For a typical clinical system with a ring diameter on the order of 80 cm, the resolution degradation due to this effect is 1.8 mm. By convolving the noncolinearity and positron range effects, it becomes apparent that the absolute resolution limit in clinical PET scanners is approximately 2 mm. As shown later, current clinical systems are capable of 4–5 mm spatial resolution.

Table 10.1.
Characteristics of Common Positron-Emitting Isotopes

Isotope	Half-life	β^+ fraction	β^+ E_{max} (MeV)	Range (mm)
Carbon-11	20.4 min	0.99	0.96	0.28
Nitrogen-13	9.96 min	1.00	1.19	0.45
Oxygen-15	2.07 min	1.00	1.72	1.04
Fluorine-18	1.83 hr	0.97	0.64	0.22
Copper-62	9.74 min	0.98	2.94	2.29
Gallium-68	68.3 min	0.88	1.90	1.35
Rubidium-81	1.25 min	0.96	3.35	2.6

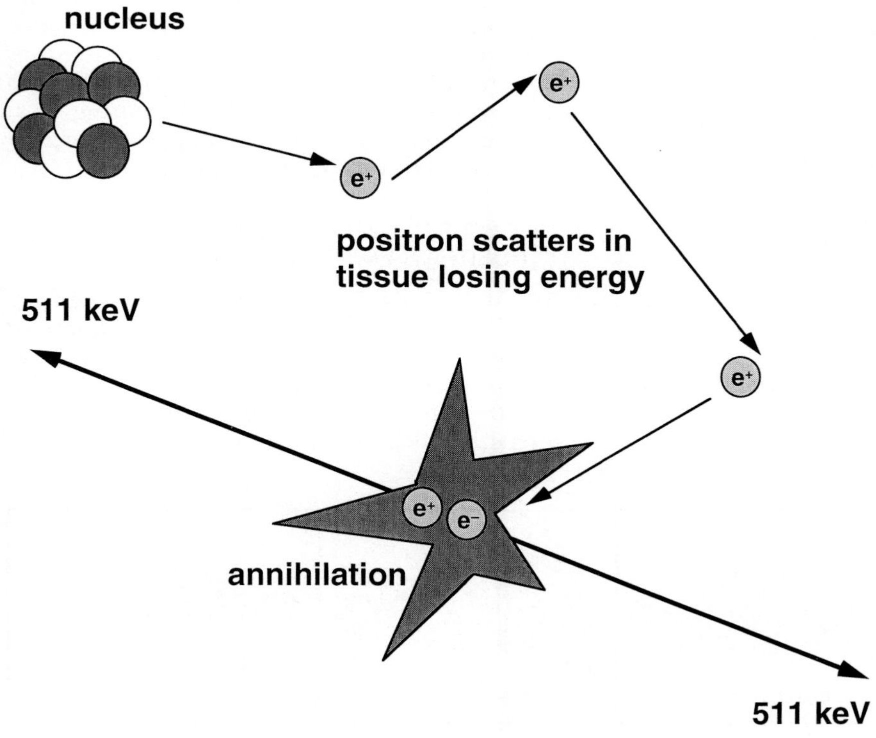

Figure 10.3. Proton-rich isotopes can decay by positron emission. The positron rapidly loses kinetic energy, scattering off atomic electrons. Eventually it slows down sufficiently to combine with an electron, and the two particles annihilate, converting their mass into energy in the form of two 511 keV γ-rays which are emitted back to back.

RANDOM AND SCATTERED COINCIDENCE EVENTS

In addition to detection of the true coincidence events, PET imaging with coincidence detection can result in two other undesirable types of events. Scattered coincidences occur when one or both of the γ-rays undergo a Compton scatter interaction inside the body. This changes their direction and reduces the energy of the photon. The change in direction results in a misidentification of the γ-ray origin as shown in Figure 10.4. The fraction of γ-rays which get scattered depends on the scattering media and the path length through the body. Therefore, the contribution from scattered events is more evident in abdominal imaging than in brain imaging. Although the γ-rays that are scattered have their energy reduced below 511 keV, the energy resolution of most PET systems is insufficient to use this as an effective means of scatter rejection. Thus, many of the scattered events are accepted and subsequently lead to mispositioned data. However, a number of scatter correction or reduction schemes are available to limit the impact of scattered events (17–21).

Although each annihilation produces two γ-rays, it is common for only one of the two to be detected (the opposing γ-ray may not intersect the detection system or may be scattered out of the system). Random (or accidental) coincidence events (22) occur when two unrelated single 511 keV γ-rays (i.e., not from the same annihilation) strike opposing detectors within the coincidence resolving time of the system (Fig. 10.4). This is accepted as a valid event since it is indistinguishable from a true coincidence event. The random coincidence rate is roughly proportional to the square of the activity in the field of view and is, therefore, a particular problem for high count rate studies. Fortunately, the correction for these events is relatively straightforward.

POSITRON-EMITTING TRACERS AND THEIR PRODUCTION

POSITRON-EMITTING ISOTOPES

One of the unique attributes of PET lies in the availability of isotopes of elements which are the building blocks of all organic molecules. The most important of these are carbon-11, nitrogen-13, and oxygen-15. Fluorine-18 is another very important isotope, as fluorine is considered the "master-element" in drug design. It also has very similar chemical properties to hydrogen, allowing it to substitute for hydrogen atoms to create positron-labeled tracers. The properties of these positron-emitting isotopes are shown in Table 10.1. Using these isotopes, it is, in theory, possible to label just about any compound of biologic interest. Indeed, to date, over 500 positron-emitting compounds have been synthesized (23). These include substances found naturally in the body such as substrates, proteins, amino-acids, hormones, and neurotransmitters, or close analogs of these which isolate specific pathways of biochemical interest. Drugs can also be labeled, and because of the exquisite sensitivity of PET, the biodistribution can be imaged using nano- or picomolar concentrations which are well below the concentrations at which pharmacologic effects become important. It becomes possible, therefore, to look at potentially toxic compounds in the living human body.

There are also many other positron-emitting isotopes available (e.g., ^{62}Cu, ^{68}Ga, ^{124}I), but like many of the single photon isotopes used in conventional nuclear medicine (e.g., ^{99m}Tc, ^{123}I, ^{67}Ga), they are not isotopes of elements that are commonly found in the human body. Therefore, it is only with great difficulty that they can be synthesized into tracers with real biologic meaning.

PRODUCTION OF POSITRON-EMITTING ISOTOPES

Positron emitters are produced in a cyclotron. Here stable nuclei are bombarded with protons or deuterons (hydrogen with an added neutron) to create the proton-rich state necessary for positron emission. Some positron emitters which have parent states which also decay, but with a longer half-life, can be produced in generator form. The parent is produced by a cyclotron and slowly decays into the daughter positron emitter in the generator. Doses of the positron emitter can then be eluted from the generator at regular intervals for use in the PET center. Examples of generator-produced positron emitting isotopes include ^{62}Cu, ^{68}Ga, and ^{82}Rb (24, 25). ^{62}Cu-PTSM and ^{82}RbCl can be used as blood flow tracers (26–28), and [^{68}Ga]EDTA is used to measure blood-brain barrier permeability (29, 30).

The ^{68}Ge-^{68}Ga parent/daughter combination is also used as a calibration source and in the sources used for attenuation correction. The slow decay of ^{68}Ge (half-life 273 days) provides a steady supply of positron-emitting ^{68}Ga, allowing these sources to be used continually over a period of many months before needing replacement.

CYCLOTRON PRODUCTION OF POSITRON-EMITTING ISOTOPES

The most useful positron emitters, however, come from stable parent isotopes and, therefore, cannot be produced in generator form. Because of their relatively short half-lives, it is necessary that they be produced close to the PET scanner; therefore, most PET facilities have their own cyclotrons or receive labeled compounds from regional dis-

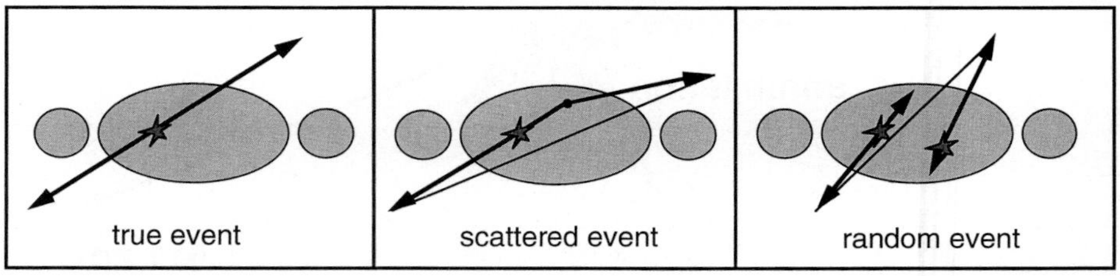

Figure 10.4. Three types of events are detected by the PET scanner: true, scattered, and random coincidence events. Only true events are part of the desired signal; random and scattered coincidences are misplaced and add low spatial frequency noise to the image. Corrections for random and scattered coincidences must be applied to maximize quantitative accuracy.

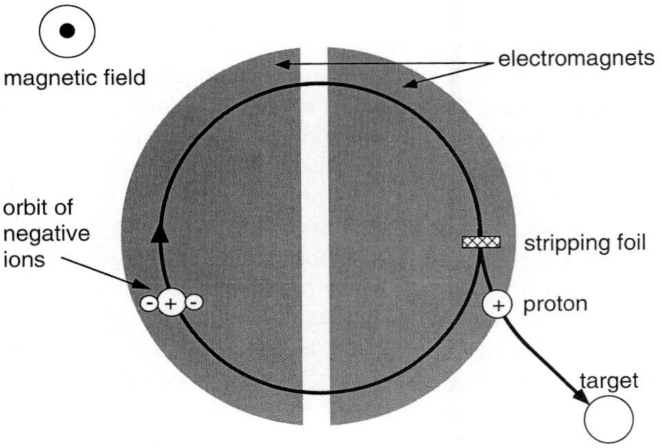

Figure 10.5. Schematic figure showing operation of a negative ion cyclotron. The H^- ions are stripped of their electrons after passing through a thin carbon foil. The resulting proton is extracted from the beam because it has positive charge and strikes the target to produce the positron-emitting isotope.

tribution centers. The technology for medical cyclotrons has advanced dramatically in the last decade (31). What started out as large, complicated research machines for nuclear physics groups requiring experienced staff and a large, well-shielded vault, have now become compact, automated, self-shielding, and reliable medical devices which can be operated by a single technician.

The radioisotope delivery system (RDS) made by Siemens is typical of a modern PET cyclotron. It accelerates negative hydrogen ions (1 proton, 2 electrons) to 11 MeV. Once the beam of hydrogen ions has reached the desired energy, it is extracted from the cyclotron by passing it through a thin carbon foil which strips off the two electrons. The resulting proton feels the cyclotron's magnetic field acting in the opposite direction, and the proton leaves the cyclotron and strikes the target (Fig. 10.5). The great advantages of this system are that it is possible to have multiple ports on the cyclotron each set up to produce a different isotope and that the beam can be extracted simultaneously into two ports, allowing two isotopes to be produced simultaneously. Other advantages of negative ion cyclotron designs include easy control, simplified beam-shaping, very little beam loss (giving rise to less prompt radiation and induced activity, thus reducing shielding requirements), and uniform beam intensity distribution. The RDS device can deliver a 50 μA proton beam through a 1 cm collimator at the target entrance, yielding 2–3 Ci of ^{18}F, ^{11}C, or ^{15}O, and 0.6 Ci of ^{13}N. The whole system can be operated by a single technician sitting at a workstation or personal computer.

POSITRON EMISSION TOMOGRAPHY TRACER SYNTHESIS

There are a number of important considerations in tracer design for PET (31, 32). Obviously, the availability of isotopes which do not alter the biochemical behavior of the compound of interest is an enormous advantage. However, the half-life of these isotopes is relatively short; therefore, the synthesis of the labeled product must be rapid. In practice, complex tracers can only be labeled with either ^{18}F, ^{11}C, or ^{13}N, since ^{15}O has just a 2-minute half-life and its use is limited to simple tracers such as H_2O, CO, O_2, and CO_2. Another issue is whether to produce a natural substrate (direct substitution of a positron-emitting atom for a stable atom) or an analog (modification of natural substrate at one or several key locations). The advantage of the analogs is that they can be targeted and limited to interactions in a small section of complex biochemical reaction sequences. This can facilitate subsequent analysis and interpretation of the PET data. The position at which the positron-emitting label is placed (there is often a choice) is also critical. The best labeling position is generally dictated by the biochemical result desired and minimizes the number and amount of labeled metabolites appearing. Often, this requires detailed knowledge of the biochemical reaction sequence for the tracer under consideration.

Taking the positron-emitting isotope from the cyclotron target and synthesizing the labeled tracer of interest can be a labor- and dose-intensive task. A great deal of innovative work centers around the design of automated devices for taking the positron-emitting precursor and turning it into labeled compound ready for injection into the patient. Such devices, which draw heavily on technology developed for automated gene sequencing and peptide synthesis, are now available for producing some of the more commonly used PET tracers such as ^{18}F-fluorodeoxyglucose (a glucose analog) and L-6-[^{18}F]Fluoro-DOPA (a precursor to dopamine). These devices are referred to as biosynthesizers and are integrated directly into the cyclotron, allowing sterile, pyrogen-free labeled compounds to be produced automatically without any user intervention.

POSITRON EMISSION TOMOGRAPHY INSTRUMENTATION: DESIGN PRINCIPLES

To image the distribution of positron-emitting isotope in the body, it is necessary to detect both of the 511 keV γ-rays emitted from the positron annihilation in coincidence. To achieve high quality images, it is important that the detectors used in a PET scanner have high intrinsic spatial resolution, high detection efficiency, and high count-rate capability (minimizing deadtime losses). The ultimate sensitivity of the device (the number of events detected for a given concentration of positron emitter) is strongly related to the product of the detector efficiency and the solid angle coverage of the scanner. Therefore, PET scanners typically consist of multiple rings of detectors surrounding the subject. The current detector of choice in all commercially available PET scanners is a scintillating material coupled to a photomultiplier tube. The 511 keV γ-ray interacts via the photoelectric effect or Compton scattering in the scintillator and deposits all or part of its energy. The scintillator converts this energy into a flash of visible light, which is detected by the photomultiplier tube and converted to a small current pulse. If the subsequent coincidence circuitry determines that two γ-rays were detected simultaneously from opposite sides of the body, then an event is registered and stored. These events are subsequently reconstructed by a computer into tomographic (cross-sectional) images of the body.

INTRINSIC SPATIAL RESOLUTION

The intrinsic spatial resolution of a PET system is largely determined by the spatial resolution of the detectors, although for very high resolution systems, there may be a contribution from either the positron range or noncolinearity effects described earlier. Consider passing a point source of radioactivity along a line centered between two detectors of width D. The resulting coincidence point spread function is triangular, with an FWHM of D/2 (Fig. 10.6). In practice, the resolution in the reconstructed images may not be as good as this, due to effects related to data sampling, statistical noise, and the reconstruction algorithm. The reconstructed image resolution is discussed later. However, it is readily apparent that building a high resolution PET scanner requires the use of very small detector elements or a larger detector with very good position resolution.

DETECTOR EFFICIENCY

The efficiency of the detector depends on the stopping power of the scintillator material (strongly related to the effective atomic number) and the depth of the scintillator used in the detector. Table 10.2 lists the properties of some commonly available scintillators. Bismuth germanate (BGO) is used in the majority of PET systems because of its unrivalled stopping power for 511 keV γ-rays. Even with BGO, a 3-cm depth of material is required to get 90% of the incoming 511 keV γ-rays to interact. Since both γ-rays must be detected, the overall efficiency for a pair of 3-cm thick detectors is $(0.9)^2$, or 0.81. Despite its good stopping power, BGO has disadvantages relative to other scintillators in that its decay time (the amount of time after the γ-ray interacts over which scintillation light is produced) is quite long, causing count-rate limitations, and its light output (the amount of scintillation light generated when a 511 keV γ-ray interacts) is low.

ENERGY RESOLUTION AND SCATTERED EVENTS

Events which undergo a Compton scatter in the body will be misplaced (Fig. 10.4). Fortunately, the γ-ray loses some energy upon scattering, potentially allowing scatter to be rejected by the use of energy discrimination. This is made possible by the fact that the amount of scintillation light produced is directly proportional to the energy deposited in the scintillator. There are, however, a number of factors which conspire to make the rejection of scatter by energy discrimination a difficult problem in PET. Firstly, the amount of scintillation light produced by BGO is not very high, thus the energy resolution, which is proportional to the square root of the number of scintillation photons produced, is typically only 20–30%. Secondly, γ-rays, when they scatter in the body, tend to only lose a small amount of energy. Thus, the energy of the scattered photons is not much less than 511 keV, and with only 20% energy resolution, these cannot be distinguished from unscattered photons. Thirdly, some unscattered γ-rays interact in the detector by the Compton interaction and only deposit part of their energy. Therefore, they have the signature of a scattered event but are, in fact, true unscattered events. Thus, setting an energy threshold too high results in the loss of true events. In a typical BGO PET system, the energy threshold is set around 350 keV, which is effective in removing some of the scattered events. Still, on the order of 12–16% of the events detected in a brain study will have been scattered. The effect is to add a low spatial frequency background to the PET images, resulting in a slight loss of contrast.

COINCIDENCE TIMING AND RANDOM EVENTS

To register a valid event, the PET scanner must detect two γ-rays on opposite sides of the body simultaneously. The condition of simultaneity must, in practice, be relaxed a little to account for differences in arrival times of the two γ-rays, the finite time taken to produce scintillation light in the detector, and differences in time delays caused by the processing electronics. The coincidence window for each event is usually set to 12 ns, thus requiring that both events occur within ± 12 ns of each other for an event to be registered. The finite width of the coincidence window,

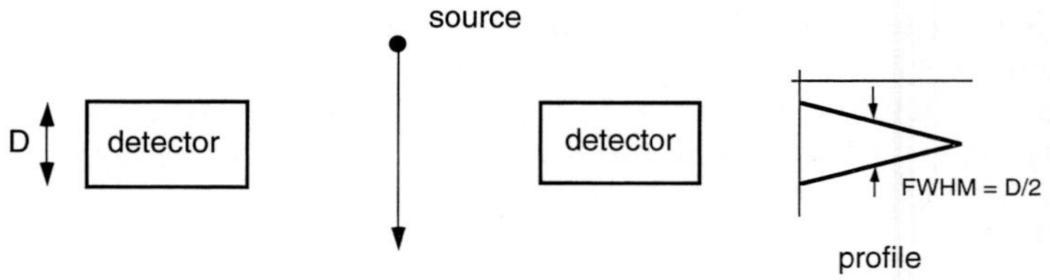

Figure 10.6. Line spread function resulting from two detectors in coincidence. The profile is triangular with a FWHM of half the detector size, thus the resolution in PET is strongly influenced by the size of the detectors utilized.

Table 10.2.
Characteristics of Scintillating Materials for PET

Scintillator	Effective *Z*	Decay (μs)	Index of refraction	Rel. light yield	Peak (nm) wavelength
Sodium iodide	50	0.23	1.85	100	410
Bismuth germanate	74	0.30	2.15	13	480
Lutetium oxyorthosilicate	66	0.04	1.82	65	420
Gadolinium oxyorthosilicate	59	0.06	1.85	25	430
Barium fluoride	52	0.62	1.49	13	310
		0.0006		3	220

however, allows for the detection of random (or accidental) events where the two detected γ-rays come from unrelated annihilations. The rate of random coincidences, R, is given by:

$$R = 2\tau S_1 S_2 \quad (4)$$

where τ is the coincidence time window and S is the singles rate on the detectors. The optimal width of the coincidence time window can be determined experimentally by plotting the true and random events as a function of τ. If τ is too small, then many true events will be discarded; if τ is too big, many random events will be accepted. Random events, if not corrected for, add a low frequency background very much like scattered events, leading to a loss of image contrast, and can also cause image artifacts (22). The fraction of random events increases as the activity in the field of view increases. Doubling the activity doubles the number of true counts, but since the randoms are proportional to the square of the singles rate (which in turn is roughly proportional to activity), it quadruples the randoms rate.

SENSITIVITY

To achieve high sensitivity, the detectors must subtend a large solid angle to the subject. This is why in conventional two-dimensional PET imaging, a ring of detectors is used to capture all the γ-ray pairs emitted from a given slice of the body. To make even better use of the injected dose, modern PET systems consist of multiple rings of detectors, thus allowing multiple slices of the body to be imaged simultaneously (Fig.10.7). Thin metal collimators, called septa, are placed between the rings of detectors to help reduce the number of scattered and random coincidences. A modern PET system typically produces 15–64 slices, from an axial field of view of 10–15 cm, which can be stacked to provide volumetric image data from the entire heart or brain.

The sensitivity of a single slice of such a system can be calculated as the product of the detector efficiency and the solid angle. For a ring of detectors of diameter d, each D cm in width (in the axial direction), the sensitivity (in the absence of any scattering or attenuation of γ-rays in the body) at the center of the field of view is:

$$S = 4\pi \sin(\tan^{-1}(D/d)) \quad (5)$$

For a typical whole-body PET system with d = 80 cm and D = 6 mm, this results in an absolute sensitivity of just 0.7%. Thus, even using complete rings of detectors, slice-based imaging makes very poor use of the injected dose. For this reason, the resolution attainable in a reconstructed PET image with sufficiently high signal-to-noise for diagnostic purposes is limited by the number of counts detected rather than by the intrinsic spatial resolution of the detector.

SYSTEM DEADTIME AND COUNT-RATE CAPABILITY

It takes a finite amount of time to process an event after a 511 keV γ-ray strikes a detector. The rate determining process is usually the collection of the scintillation light by the photomultiplier tubes. The integration time is usually 2–3 times the decay time of the scintillator. For BGO, an integration time of 1 μsec allows 90% of the scintillation light to be collected. Electronic multiplexing of signals and the coincidence circuitry can, however, also have nonnegligible deadtime components. While an event is being processed, the detector is essentially inactive and cannot perceive another incoming event as a separate event. This event is therefore lost, and the effective sensitivity of the scanner is reduced (33). A very simplistic model for deadtime in a PET scanner is given by:

$$S = S_o \exp(-\sigma S_o) \quad (6)$$

where S_o is the actual singles rate on the detector, σ is the deadtime and S is the detected singles rate. Using this model, σ is approximately 1–3 μsecs for most PET systems. Deadtime is no problem when the PET system consists of a very large number of individual detectors. However, in most PET systems, the detectors employ some form of multiplexing which effectively increases the area which becomes dead when an event is processed. Thus, in some studies employing high doses of short-lived isotopes, deadtime can become a limiting factor. Deadtime leads to a reduction in the number of counts recorded per unit injected dose and can thus be seen as effectively lowering the sensitivity of the system at high count rates. The count-rate performance of a particular PET system is easily determined by monitoring the count rate as a function of the activity within the object of interest.

NOISE EQUIVALENT COUNT RATE

A useful concept in determining the count rate performance of a PET scanner is the noise equivalent count (NEC) rate. This is the number of counts detected as a function of the activity concentration, after correcting for the effects

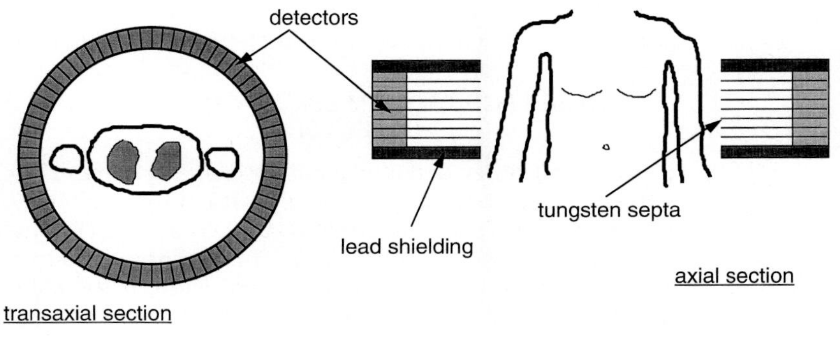

Figure 10.7. Transaxial and axial cross-sections through a multiring PET scanner showing the interplane septa and lead shielding which help to reduce the singles rate, thus improving count-rate performance and decreasing the fraction of random events detected.

of random and scattered events and taking into account deadtime losses. The noise equivalent count rate has been shown to be directly proportional to the signal-to-noise in the final reconstructed PET images, and is thus a good guide to scanner performance (34). It is defined as:

$$NEC = \frac{T^2}{T + 2kR + S} \quad (7)$$

where T is the true count rate, R is the random count rate and S is the rate of scattered coincidence events. S is defined to include only scattered events which fall within the field of view of the object being imaged. The factor k takes into account that random events are spread rather broadly across the field of view, and only those in the field of view of the object contribute to noise in the image. The factor 2 arises from the use of the delayed coincidence method of correcting for randoms events, which will be discussed later. A plot of the NEC against activity for a standard 20-cm uniform cylinder is often the easiest way of comparing performance among scanners and predicting the signal-to-noise that will be achieved in the final images. It is important that the object used to obtain the NEC rates be identical if any comparisons are to be made, because the NEC rate is very sensitive to the size and shape of the object in the field of view.

BLOCK DETECTOR

To achieve high spatial resolution, small detectors must be used. Many commercial PET systems today employ "block" detectors which consist of a segmented block of BGO, coupled to four photomultiplier tubes (35, 36). Typically, the BGO is 3 cm in depth and is segmented into a 6×8 or 8×8 array of elements, each approximately 4 mm in size (Fig. 10.8a). The element in which a γ-ray interacts is determined by looking at the relative light output from the four photomultiplier tubes. Anger-type logic is used to obtain

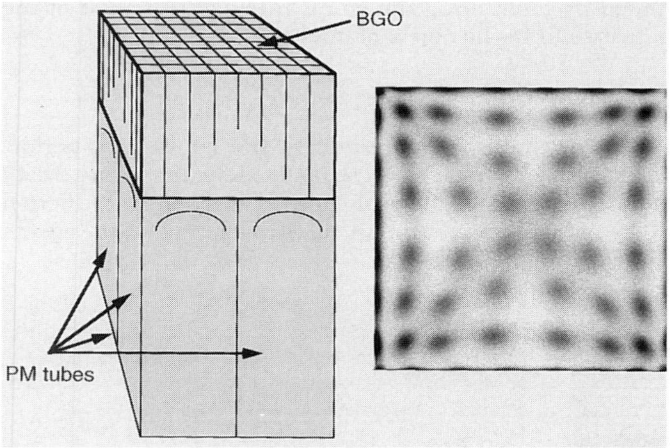

Figure 10.8. **A.** Schematic figure showing the BGO block detector commonly used in commercial PET systems. The element in which the γ-ray interacts is determined by looking at the relative outputs of the four photomultiplier tubes. **B.** An image of X_{pos} and Y_{pos} (determined from the four photomultiplier tube outputs as shown in equation 8) following flood illumination of a block detector. The individual block elements are clearly visualized.

an X position and a Y position from the four photomultiplier tube outputs (P_i) as:

$$X_{pos} = \frac{P_a + P_b - P_c - P_d}{P_a + P_b + P_c + P_d} \qquad Y_{pos} = \frac{P_a + P_c - P_b - P_d}{P_a + P_b + P_c + P_d} \quad (8)$$

The sharing of the scintillation light between the photomultiplier tubes is controlled by the depth of the cuts in the BGO, or by the use of a light guide. The aim is to make X_{pos} and Y_{pos} a linear function of the source position, thus enabling adjacent elements to be separated. Figure 10.8b shows the result of irradiating such a block detector with a flood source of 511 keV γ-rays. The individual elements of the 8×8 array are visualized, although there is some nonlinearity towards the edges of the block, which makes the outer elements more difficult to separate.

The great advantage of the block detector over using single crystal/PM tube combinations is that the crystal size is no longer limited by the size of the smallest PM tube available (currently 1 cm), and the cost per detector element is also reduced. Thus, the block detector allows a dramatic improvement in spatial resolution to be realized, while still maintaining a very high packing fraction of detectors. A further advantage is that by reducing the output from 64 crystals into just two signals, the electronic requirements are automatically multiplexed to a more manageable scale.

However, there are drawbacks to the block detector design. Perhaps the most important of these is the increase in effective area of the detector unit, leading to an increase in deadtime. Each block has just one set of processing electronics and cannot distinguish between two events which strike different elements in the block within the integration time set to collect the scintillation light. In this situation, only one event is detected (despite the interaction of two γ-rays), and the position of the event will be an average (weighted according to the amount of energy deposited by each γ-ray) of the locations of the two γ-rays. This effect, known as pileup, leads both to a loss of events and to a mispositioning of events (37).

BGO block detectors also fail to reach the spatial resolution predicted by the simple point spread function of Figure 10.6. This is because the position is determined by the relative distribution of light among the four PMTs. Since the scintillation light output of BGO is quite low (it is estimated that each 511 keV interaction leads to the production of approximately 150 electrons at the photocathode of the PMT), the PMT outputs are subject to statistical fluctuations. This shows up as fluctuations in the position estimations X_{pos} and Y_{pos} and leads to a degradation in spatial resolution. The effect is to add approximately 2 mm in quadrature to the predicted FWHM spatial resolution (38).

OTHER POSITRON EMISSION TOMOGRAPHY DETECTORS

A number of other detector configurations are under investigation for PET. The most successful of these alternatives is the use of a large area (50×16×2.5 cm) NaI(Tl) crystal coupled to 40 PM tubes (39). This position-sensitive detector is effectively a gamma-camera without the collimator. The complete PET system uses a hexagonal ring of six NaI detectors. Because of the large area, such a detector is susceptible to count rate limitations; however, quite high count rates have been obtained by the use of pulse clipping and a centroid method (which uses just a few PM tube outputs) for position determination. This system is now available commercially through a joint venture between General Electric and UGM Medical Systems.

The concept of time of flight PET is very attractive. The basis for this method is to use a very fast scintillator and time the difference in arrival of the two 511 keV photons at the detectors to find the position of the annihilation (40). Unfortunately, there are many inherent difficulties in this approach. The fast scintillators, such as barium fluoride (see Table 10.2), have much lower stopping power than BGO, thus the sensitivity of such a machine is lower. Furthermore, the best timing resolution achieved to date is only sufficient to locate the annihilation to within about 10 cm. There is a small signal-to-noise gain in using time of flight; however, this is negated by the lower efficiency of the fast scintillators and the complex electronics required for such accurate timing. At this time, there are no time of flight PET machines being produced commercially.

Other detector technologies, such as multiwire proportional chambers (41) and scintillating fibers (42), are being investigated for PET; although they can obtain high spatial resolution, their sensitivity is generally an order of magnitude lower than BGO-based PET systems.

DESIGN OF A CLINICAL POSITRON EMISSION TOMOGRAPHY TOMOGRAPH

The majority of modern clinical PET tomographs utilize multiple rings of BGO block detectors to simultaneously achieve high spatial resolution and sensitivity. We will take the ECAT EXACT HR (CTI/Siemens, Knoxville, TN) as an example of a modern PET tomograph (43), although a similar configuration is also offered by the GE ADVANCE (44) system (General Electric Medical Systems, Milwaukee, WI). A low-cost, rotating PET system consisting of partial rings of BGO block detectors is also produced by Siemens/CTI and is suitable for a wide range of clinical applications (45).

The ECAT EXACT HR scanner (Fig. 10.9) has 18,816 BGO elements and 1344 PM tubes configured as 24 rings of 784 detectors per ring. Translated into block units, this is 3 rings of 112 blocks. Each block has 7×8 BGO elements of size 2.9×5.9×30 mm. The ring diameter is 82 cm and the axial field of view is 15 cm, thus the whole brain or heart can be scanned simultaneously. The coincidence time window is $2\tau = 24$ ns and the energy window is typically set from 350–650 keV. The septa on this scanner can be retracted under computer control, allowing three-dimensional data acquisition as well as the standard two-dimensional acquisition. Two-dimensional data acquisition leads to datasets of 12.4 MBytes, whereas three-dimensional datasets can be as large as 152 MBytes. Data acquisition methods are discussed in the next section. Reconstructed image datasets typically consist of 47 transaxial planes of data, with a plane-to-plane spacing of 3.125 mm. The image volume can naturally be resliced into coronal or sagittal sections, or sections of any arbitrary orientation relative to the scanner axis. ^{68}Ge-filled rod sources

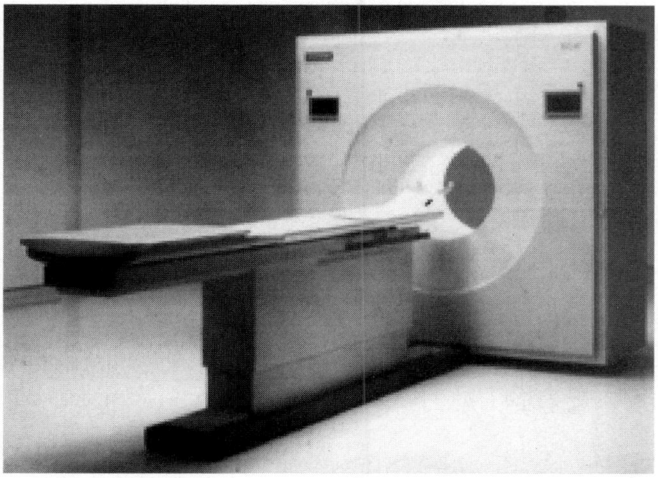

Figure 10.9. Photograph of the Siemens/CTI ECAT Exact HR PET system. (Reproduced with permission from Siemens Medical Systems, Nuclear Medicine Group.)

are used for attenuation and calibration purposes. The extraction of these sources from their shielding and subsequent rotation around the field of view is also computer controlled.

Measurements of the performance of the ECAT EXACT HR system have been carried out in accordance with the recommended performance standards for PET (43). The transaxial spatial resolution has been measured as 3.4 mm FWHM at the center of the field of view, degrading to just under 5 mm at 10 cm from the center. The axial resolution is 4 mm FWHM at the center of the field of view, degrading to 5 mm at a radius of 10 cm. The total sensitivity of the system to a uniform 20 cm diameter system is 177 kcps/μCi/cc in two-dimensional acquisitions, increasing to 1460 kcps/μCi/cc in three-dimensional mode. For this same cylinder, the fraction of events which have been scattered, and will therefore be mispositioned, is 12% in two-dimensional mode and 38% in three-dimensional mode. The peak noise equivalent count rate is approximately 110,000 cps at an activity concentration of 2.25 μCi/cc in the cylinder. Some representative data from an [^{18}F]fluorodeoxyglucose (FDG) brain study from a normal subject obtained with the ECAT EXACT HR are shown in Figure 10.10. Transverse, coronal, and sagittal cross-sections are shown, the latter obtained by stacking the set of two-dimensional images and reslicing. Notice the clear delineation of small subcortical structures, the high gray white matter contrast and the delineation of the cortical ribbon.

POSITRON EMISSION TOMOGRAPHY DATA ACQUISITION

Many modern PET scanners are capable of acquiring data in two different modes: two-dimensional acquisition with the septa in place and three-dimensional acquisition with the septa removed. Additionally, total body imaging acquisition protocols which extend the axial scan length by moving the patient sequentially through the scanner have be-

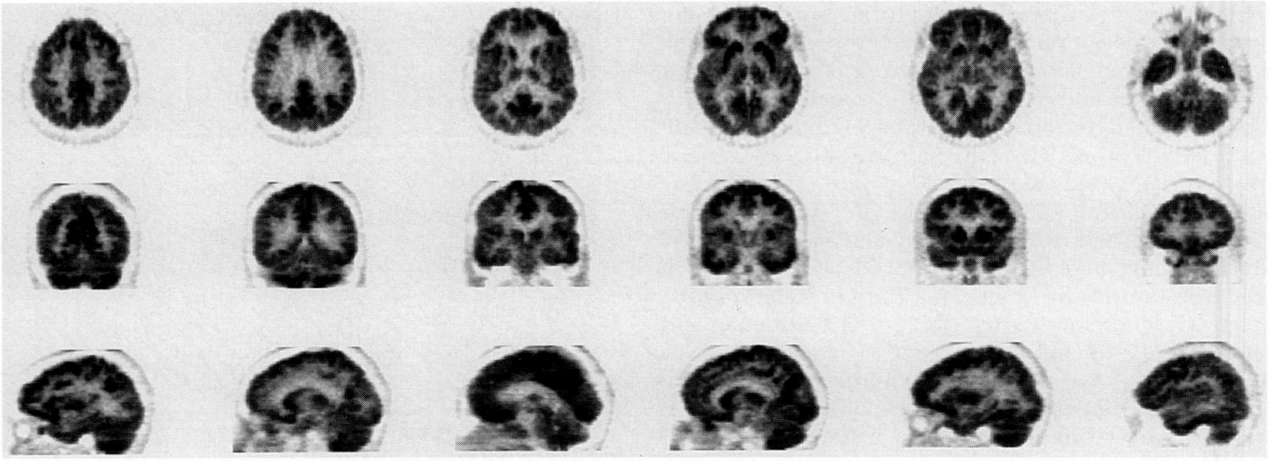

Figure 10.10. Representative [^{18}F]fluorodeoxyglucose images from the brain of a normal subject acquired on the ECAT Exact HR PET system. Scan length was 60 minutes. (Reproduced with permission from Klaus Wienhard, Ph.D, Max-Planck Institute, Cologne, Germany.)

come an important tool. In this section, we examine different data acquisition strategies and discuss how the raw data is stored in the form of projection matrices known as sinograms.

STORING RAW POSITRON EMISSION TOMOGRAPHY DATA AS SINOGRAMS

Each detector pair records the sum of activity along a given line through the body. The data for all possible combinations of detector pairs in a given ring are stored in what is called a sinogram. This is more efficient than storing each recorded event separately, since each detector pair will usually record multiple events in a PET study. A typical sinogram from a human FDG brain study is shown in Figure 10.11. Each point in the sinogram represents the sum of all events that occur between a particular pair of detectors. The sinogram matrix is organized such that each row represents the projected activity of parallel detector pairs at a given angle relative to the detector ring. The sinogram itself provides little information on the activity distribution. The data in the sinograms must be reconstructed using CT or iterative algorithms to convert the projection data into an interpretable image.

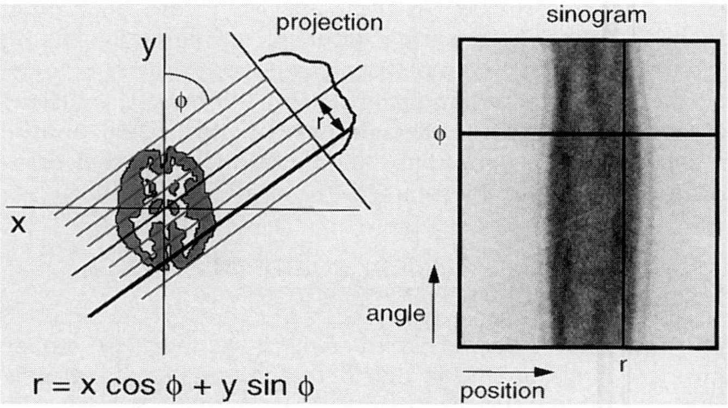

Figure 10.11. PET projection data is conventionally stored in the form of sinograms. Each element in the sinogram represents the activity seen by a pair of detectors (the projection or sum of all the activity along the line joining the two detectors). This figure shows the relationship between the projection line and its placement in the sinogram.

TWO-DIMENSIONAL (SLICE) DATA ACQUISITION IN POSITRON EMISSION TOMOGRAPHY

The basic principle of two-dimensional imaging is to take coincidences within a given ring of detectors and form a sinogram from these data, which is then reconstructed to form an image for that detector ring. In this way, we would expect a system with n detector rings to produce n image planes. In practice, to improve sensitivity and axial sampling, coincidences between nearby detector rings are also acquired and averaged together. These are assigned to the slice corresponding to their average axial position. For example, if coincidences between ring 8 and ring 6 are combined, they are assumed to originate from a slice centered on ring 7. Coincidences between immediately adjacent detector rings (e.g., rings 4 and 5) lead to image slices which fall halfway between detector rings. In this way, we actually obtain $2n$-1 image planes, spaced by 1/2 the detector width, from an n-ring PET scanner. Each image plane is formed from an average of several projection datasets, which are combined together into a single sinogram. This approach is limited to small ring differences, because, as the differences get larger, eventually the interplane septa get in the way and prevent detection of events. Additionally, the averaging process leads to a blurring of the data in the axial direction, especially toward the edge of the field of view, where the averaged coincidence lines diverge significantly (Fig. 10.12). This effect becomes intolerable for large ring differences. After considering the trade-offs between sensitivity and resolution loss, most modern systems use a maximum ring difference of ±5 in forming the two-dimensional dataset (Fig.10.12). Two-dimensional data acquisition leads to $2n$-1 sinograms, each of which is reconstructed independently to form $2n$-1 transaxial images, which can be stacked on top of each other to form a three-dimensional image volume.

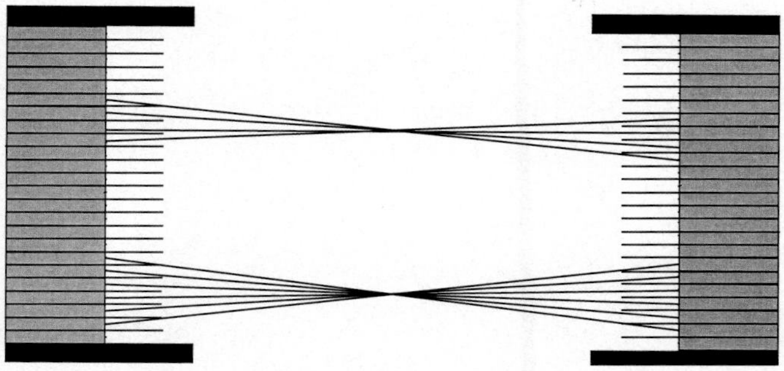

Figure 10.12. Axial cross-section through a 24-ring PET scanner showing the standard two-dimensional acquisition mode, where ring differences of up to ±5 are utilized. Using some of the oblique lines of response helps improve sensitivity but leads to a degradation in axial resolution, since all the data contributing to a given slice is assumed to come from within the plane.

TWO-DIMENSIONAL TOTAL BODY ACQUISITION IN POSITRON EMISSION TOMOGRAPHY

In cancer patients, it is vital to assess whether the disease has metastasized, as this is the critical factor in the choice of therapy and in determining prognosis. The PET scanner, however, only covers 10–15 cm of the body at any one time. The development of total-body PET (46, 47) overcomes this limitation by moving the bed under computer control and acquiring data at a number of adjacent bed positions, thus achieving coverage of the entire body. To improve axial sampling (leading to better quality coronal and sagittal sections), the datasets are often interleaved, that is to say that for each axial section of the body, two datasets are acquired spaced by 1/4 of a detector width. When the two datasets are combined, the separation between adjacent images is just 1/4 of the detector width (compared to 1/2 the detector width with the standard acquisition). Covering the entire body (length *L*) in interleaved mode with a PET scanner with axial field of view *A*, requires $2L/A$ separate acquisitions and results in several hundred transaxial images, which can be stacked and resliced into coronal or sagittal views. A typical total-body dataset obtained using $^{18}F^-$ as the tracer is shown in Figure10.13. This data was acquired at 16 different bed positions, imaging for 4 minutes per position. Total-body data acquisition has become a very important tool in the management of cancer patients.

THREE-DIMENSIONAL (VOLUME) DATA ACQUISITION IN POSITRON EMISSION TOMOGRAPHY

Even with the addition of neighboring ring coincidences, the sensitivity of PET systems is less than 3%. A new mode of PET imaging, called three-dimensional PET acquisition, can be used to dramatically improve sensitivity by removing the interplane septa and allowing coincidences between all detector rings (Fig. 10.14). This leads to a fivefold increase in true sensitivity but also results in a higher fraction of scattered coincidence events (48, 49). This is reflected in the performance data for the ECAT EXACT HR presented earlier (43). A further complication of three-dimensional imaging is that the sinogram data cannot be averaged together in the manner described for two-dimensional imaging. Because of the large ring differences acquired in three-dimensional datasets, this would result in a very severe blurring in the axial direction. Rather, it is now necessary to employ a fully three-dimensional image reconstruction technique which reconstructs the data volumetrically, taking into account the precise direction of each projection line (50, 51). Although this is computationally intensive, it does result in all the data being reconstructed in the correct location. The longer reconstruction times, together with the larger size of the three-dimensional raw projection datasets (there are now n^2 sinograms, rather than the $2n$-1 sinograms in two-dimensional imaging), has limited the use of three-dimensional PET. However, the evolution of faster workstations with rapid data transfer capability onto extremely large disks and multiprocessor boards for reconstruction (52) is turning three-dimensional PET into a viable proposition. A number of scatter correction schemes have been proposed which reduce the scatter to acceptable levels, and three-dimensional acquisition and reconstruction has recently become available on commercial scanners.

The gain in sensitivity afforded by three-dimensional acquisition is particularly beneficial in low count rate studies (e.g., neuroreceptor studies and total-body studies), where the full sensitivity gain can be realized irrespective of deadtime considerations. Figure 10.15 shows a comparison between 20-minute two-dimensional and three-dimensional acquisitions of data from a normal subject, 2 hours after the administration of 6 mCi of [^{18}F]fluoroDOPA. This tracer is concentrated in the caudate and putamen in healthy individuals, and these structures are easily identified in the images. The noise level in the three-dimensional dataset is clearly much lower than in the two-dimensional study. Three-dimensional data acquisition can lead to signal-to-noise gains of a factor of 2–3 for low count rate studies or, alternatively, can be used to reduce the imaging time (thus improving patient throughput in the clinical environment) or the injected dose (useful for pediatric studies), while maintaining equivalent image statistics to the two-dimensional case.

SIMETRY

The majority of the dose in a PET study comes from the deposition of energy by the positron, rather than from the 511 keV γ-rays. The doses are, therefore, isotope-dependent, and for dosimetry purposes, the dose from the transmission scan can be safely ignored. Table 10.3 shows the dose for a range of common PET studies per mCi of injected tracer. In general, around 10 mCi of ^{18}F-labeled tracers are used, up to 20 mCi of ^{11}C or ^{13}N-labeled tracers, and up to 180 mCi of ^{15}O-labeled tracers may be injected while still staying within recommended federal dose limits.

IMAGE RECONSTRUCTION

In this section, we qualitatively describe how to get from the raw PET data in the form of sinograms to a reconstructed image. We concentrate on the reconstruction of a single sinogram representing a single image plane. Reconstruction of a three-dimensional PET dataset is somewhat more complicated, but many of the principles are the same.

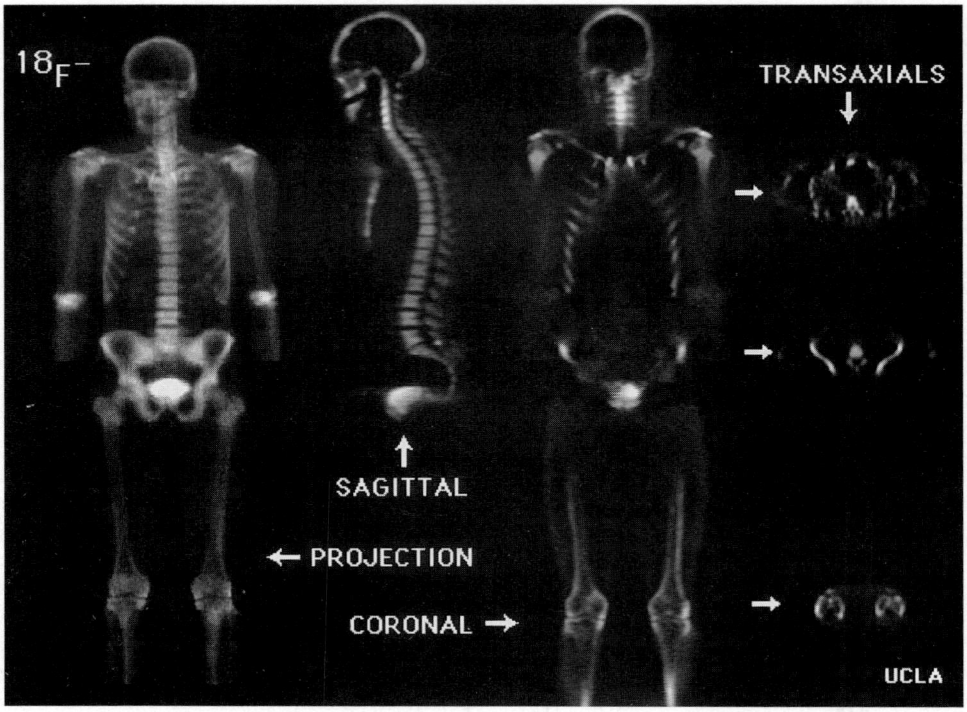

Figure 10.13. Total body images of the skeletal system obtained using $^{18}F^-$ ion. Total scan time was 64 minutes. The dataset can be viewed as a projection dataset or, after image reconstruction, the transaxial slices may be stacked and resliced into sagittal and coronal cross-sections as shown. (Reproduced with permission from Magnus Dahlbom, Ph.D, UCLA.)

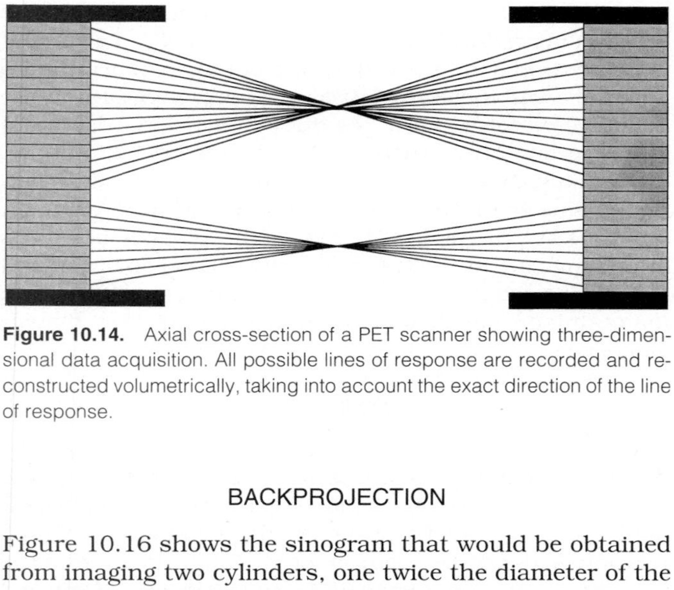

Figure 10.14. Axial cross-section of a PET scanner showing three-dimensional data acquisition. All possible lines of response are recorded and reconstructed volumetrically, taking into account the exact direction of the line of response.

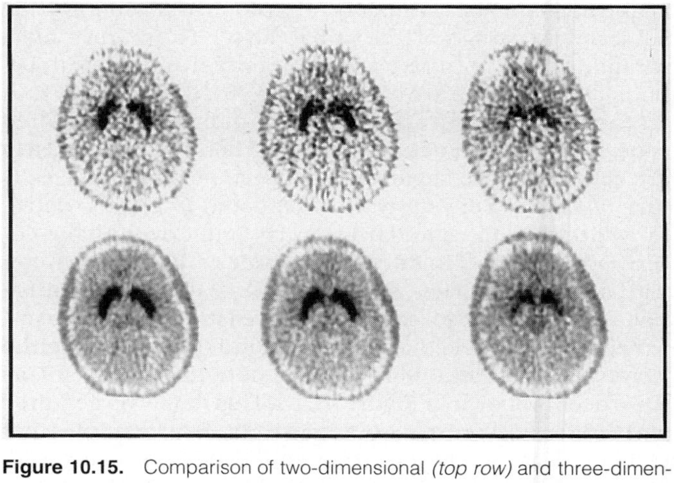

Figure 10.15. Comparison of two-dimensional *(top row)* and three-dimensional *(bottom row)* acquisitions in a normal subject after the injection of 6 mCi of [^{18}F]fluoroDOPA. The acquisition time was 20 minutes in each case. Notice the dramatically improved signal-to-noise in the three-dimensional dataset due to the higher sensitivity.

BACKPROJECTION

Figure 10.16 shows the sinogram that would be obtained from imaging two cylinders, one twice the diameter of the other, but both containing the same activity concentration. Each element in the sinogram represents the sum of activity along a line (the line of response) joining two detectors. Each row in the sinogram forms a one-dimensional projection representing a view of the object from a particular angle (Fig. 10.11). An intuitive approach to image reconstruction is to take each sinogram element and backproject it along the line from which the detected events came (Fig. 10.17). In other words, the events detected for a given detector pair are spread uniformly along a line joining the detector pair. Figure 10.16 shows the outcome of this process after all angles have been backprojected. The resulting image is a crude approximation of the actual object. However, the backprojection process is clearly incorrect, as it results in activity being placed outside the object.

FILTERED BACKPROJECTION

To get the correct image, it can be shown mathematically that each projection has to be filtered prior to backprojecting (56). The filter is a convolution filter, so it is most conveniently applied in frequency (Fourier) space, where the convolution becomes a simple multiplication. In broad terms, the filtered backprojection reconstruction process is described by the following steps:

Table 10.3
Dosimetry for Commonly Used PET Tracers[d]

Tracer	Typical Dose (mCi)	Critical Organ	Critical Organ Dose (rad/mCi)	Whole-Body Dose (rad/mCi)
[^{18}F]fluorodeoxyglucose	10	Bladder wall	0.241[a]	0.041
[^{18}F]fluoroDOPA	10	Bladder wall	0.380[b]	0.033
[^{15}O]water	120–300[c]	Lungs	0.002	0.002
[^{13}N]ammonia	20	Bladder wall	0.03	0.006

[a]Voiding schedule required
[b]With carbidopa
[c]Total dose injected over multiple runs
[d]Data from references (53–55)

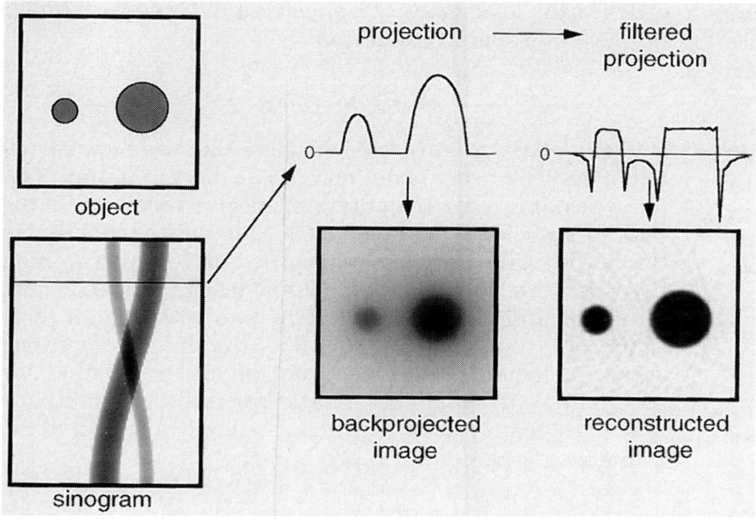

Figure 10.16. The principles of image reconstruction. The sinogram obtained from imaging two cylinders of equal activity is shown. The profile of a single projection line is also shown. Simple backprojection of all the projection data leads to a blurred representation of the object. To obtain a faithful representation, the projection must be filtered prior to backprojection.

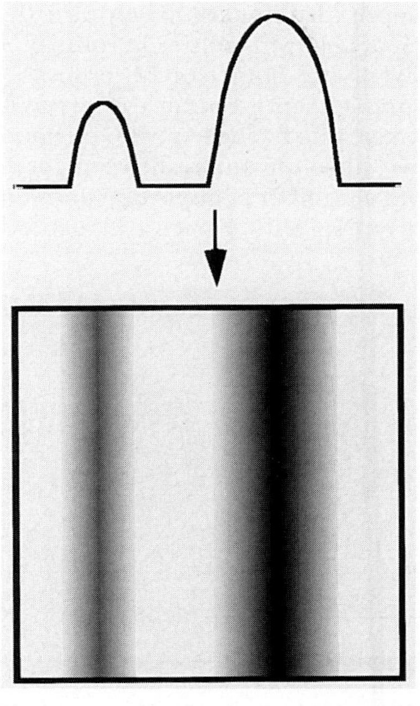

Figure 10.17. The process of backprojection involves taking each projection and spreading it across the image matrix at the appropriate angle.

1. Take projection for angle 1 (row 1 in the sinogram)
2. Take the Fourier transform of this projection
3. Multiply by the reconstruction filter
4. Take the inverse Fourier transform of the filtered projection
5. Backproject the data for angle 1
6. Repeat for all other angles in the sinogram.

Figure 10.16 shows a single projection before and after filtering. The negative numbers introduced by the filtering process remove activity placed outside the object by the backprojection process. The result of backprojecting all the filtered projections (Fig. 10.16) is a faithful representation of the original object.

RECONSTRUCTION FILTER

The functional form of the reconstruction filter can be derived intuitively from the following argument. Look at the projection data in Figure 10.16a. The larger cylinder contributes more counts to the projection data, because the path length (and thus the amount of activity along the line) is larger. Using simple backprojection of the data apparently leads to higher activity in the larger cylinder, even though it has the same activity concentration as the small cylinder. The process of simple backprojection amplifies the activity in large structures relative to smaller structures. Looked at in spatial frequency terms, high frequencies (corresponding to small structures) are underrepresented relative to low frequencies (corresponding to large structures). To correct for the effects of backprojection, we need to weight the lower frequencies less than the higher frequencies. The correct mathematically-derived filter (Fig. 10.18) turns out to be a ramp in frequency space (hence the term ramp filter). The form of the filter is in agreement with our intuitive argument that higher frequencies should be weighted more than lower frequencies.

RECONSTRUCTION FILTER AND IMAGE NOISE

One unfortunate side effect of the ramp filter is that it also amplifies noise, because statistical fluctuations from one sinogram element to the next are inherently a high frequency phenomenon. To counteract this effect, it is often desirable, unless the statistical quality of the data is very good, to attenuate the reconstruction filter at high frequencies. This can be achieved by using a number of different window functions, such as the Shepp-Logan or the Hann window, which modify the basic ramp filter shape at higher frequencies. Several different filter forms are shown in Figure 10.18. A filter factor (typically in the range of 0–0.5) further characterizes these functions by indicating the point at which the curve turns over or reaches zero. Although these window functions help to control image noise, they must also reduce spatial resolution, because reducing the high frequencies is equivalent to smoothing the data. Figure 10.19 shows an FDG brain image reconstructed using the filters shown in Figure 10.18. The trade-off between increasing signal-to-noise but decreasing resolution can clearly be seen as the filter function is changed. Ultimately, the reconstruction filter chosen depends on the number of counts in the study and the personal preferences of the investigator or physician in trading off image noise versus spatial resolution.

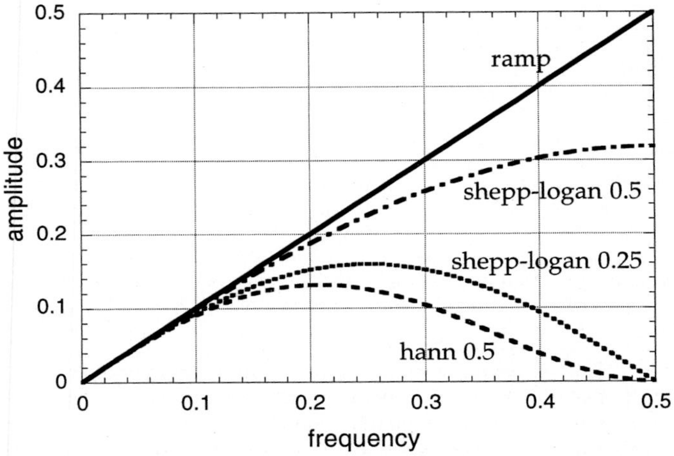

Figure 10.18. Some common reconstruction filters shown in frequency space. The ramp filter can be derived mathematically as the appropriate filter to apply. However, it amplifies high frequency noise components; therefore, in practice, the ramp is usually multiplied by a window function, which attenuates the magnitude of the filter at high frequencies.

IMAGE ARTIFACTS

It is quite easy to introduce artifacts into the reconstruction if sufficient care is not taken. The most important factor in avoiding reconstruction artifacts is to ensure that the data is sufficiently sampled (57). Sampling theory states that if the highest resolution recorded in the data is R mm, then the data must be sampled at least every $R/2$ mm. Thus, for a PET system with detectors with spatial resolution of 6 mm, the sampling (i.e., the distance between adjacent elements in the sinogram) should be <3 mm. Additionally, sufficient angular sampling is also required. Artifacts are readily demonstrated when only a subset of the available angular data is used.

QUANTITATIVE POSITRON EMISSION TOMOGRAPHY IMAGING

One of the unique features of PET is the potential to achieve accurate, quantitative images which directly express the concentration of positron emitter in units of μCi/cc. Once this is achieved, the data can be processed through a mathematic model representing the process studied, to convert the image into biologic units (i.e., nanomoles/min/g). To achieve absolute quantification, or even relative quantification, a number of important corrections must be made to the raw PET data. Errors still result however, par-

Figure 10.19. Effects of reconstruction filters on a [^{18}F]fluorodeoxyglucose study of the brain. Notice the trade-off between spatial resolution and signal-to-noise as smoother filters (increasing attenuation at higher frequencies) are used.

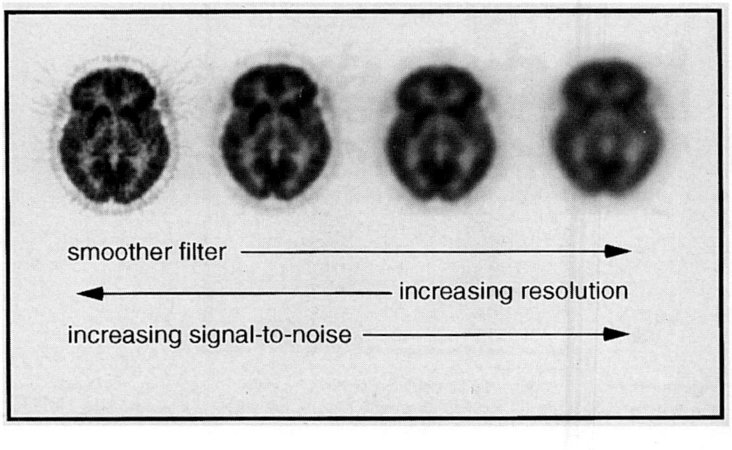

ticularly in structures which have dimensions which are similar or smaller than the image resolution. Cross-registration to high resolution anatomic images such as MRI can help to quantify these partial volume errors, as well as provide a convenient means for defining anatomically-based regions of interest for application to the PET data.

DETECTOR NORMALIZATION

A modern PET scanner consists of many thousands of individual detector elements. Because of differences in the exact dimensions of the detectors, the optical coupling to the photomultiplier tube and a whole host of other factors, there can be a considerable variation in efficiency among different detectors. In practice, this means that different detector pairs will register different count rates when viewing the same activity. To remove these efficiency variations, it is necessary to apply detector normalization factors. These normalization factors are measured by allowing each detector pair to see essentially the same activity. This can be achieved using a thin plane source which is rotated to different angles in the field of view, or by using a rotating rod source of activity, orbiting at the edge of the field of view. Adequate counts must be acquired so the normalization is not statistics-limited (i.e., the normalization should contain many more counts per detector pair than is actually registered during a clinical scan); otherwise, noise from the normalization scan will be propagated into the reconstructed image. Typically, normalization files are acquired weekly to account for possible changes in photomultiplier tube gains over time.

ATTENUATION CORRECTION

This is the largest correction factor applied in PET. As the two 511 keV γ-rays pass through the body, there is a high likelihood that one or both of the γ-rays will be absorbed or will be scattered away from the two detectors they would have hit. Attenuation is an exponential process and depends both on the attenuation coefficient of the material and the amount of tissue the γ-rays must pass through. Typical attenuation coefficients at 511 keV are 0.095 cm^{-1} for soft tissue, 0.031 cm^{-1} for lungs, and 0.151 cm^{-1} for bone. The magnitude of the error caused by attenuation can be appreciated by realizing that typically only 1 in every 5 γ-ray pairs escapes from the brain and only 1 in 30 or 40 escapes from the torso. The attenuation correction factors are, therefore, very large and must be estimated accurately to recover the original isotope concentration.

Fortunately, the unique nature of the annihilation radiation makes it possible to measure the attenuation correction factors directly. Consider the attenuation in a cylinder of cross-section D, with attenuation coefficient μ as shown in Figure 10.20. If the positron-emitter is concentrated at position x, and the number of γ-ray pairs emitted is N_O, the number of γ-ray pairs, N, which escape without being attenuated is given by:

$$N = N_O \exp(-\mu x) \exp(-\mu(D - x)) = \exp(-\mu D) \quad (9)$$

This is just the product of the probability of escape for each of the two γ-rays. The important thing to notice is that

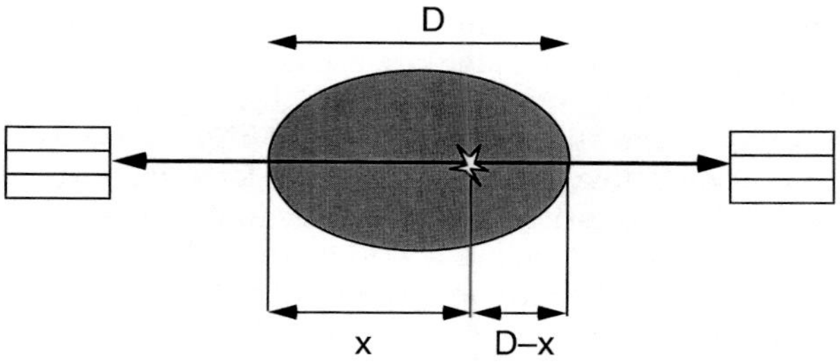

Figure 10.20. Attenuation for a given line of response is independent of the source position along the line, because both γ-rays must escape the body (see equation 9). The combined path length through the body is thus always equal to the width of the body for that projection line.

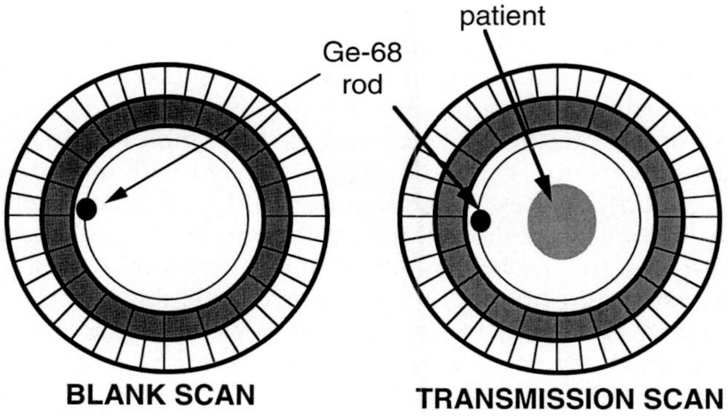

Figure 10.21. Illustration of blank scan *(left)* and transmission scan *(right)* used for measuring attenuation correction in PET. The source is either a ring or a rotating rod of ^{68}Ge. Blank and transmission scans are generally acquired before activity is injected into the patient.

the attenuation is independent of the source position x. This remains true when the attenuation coefficient is variable within the cross-section under study. Thus, wherever the source is along the line joining two detectors, the attenuation is the same. Even if the activity is outside the patient, the attenuation will still be the same. We can, therefore, use an external positron-emitting source (usually a ring source or a rod source orbiting just inside the field of view) to measure the attenuation correction factors in the following manner:

Blank Scan: Acquire data with the external source, but nothing else in the field of view. This measurement represents the unattenuated flux N_O (Fig. 10.21).

Transmission Scan: Now position the patient in the scanner (the patient has not been injected with positron-emitter at this stage) and acquire another scan with activity from the external source. This represents the attenuated flux N (Fig. 10.21).

Attenuation correction factors are calculated for each detector pair by taking the ratio of the blank and the transmission sinograms. High statistics are preferable (but not always practical) in transmission images because the noise associated with statistical fluctuations in the blank and transmission image can propagate through to the final image and may also introduce biases (58). The transmission scan increases the amount of time a study takes and the time during which the subject must lie still. In areas of the body where the attenuation coefficient is reasonably homogeneous (e.g., in the brain and in parts of the abdomen), it is possible to calculate the attenuation correction based on the body outline (59). This has the advantage of speeding up the study and not propagating noise into the reconstructed image. It is, however, less accurate than measured attenuation correction because of the assumptions which have to be made and is, therefore, of most use when scans are being used in a qualitative or semiquantitative way.

DEADTIME CORRECTION

It takes a finite time to collect and process the scintillation light from each γ-ray interaction in the detector. During this period, the block detector is effectively dead and cannot process another event. If another event does arrive, it will be combined with the first event resulting in a loss of data (two events turn into one) and mispositioning (the block will calculate the position of the event based on the centroid of all the light received). If the combined energy of the two events is high enough, the event will fall outside the energy window of the scanner, and both events will be lost. The loss of data is referred to as deadtime. In most systems, the fraction of time that the detector is "dead" is measured on-line and used to correct the data. This correction adjusts for the events that were lost while the system was busy, but it cannot reposition those events which were misplaced. In practice, other components of the PET system, such as the coincidence processor, also have deadtime, so the overall deadtime correction is a complex function of several different factors (33). Although the deadtime correction only becomes a large factor (>1.5) in high count rate studies such as O-15-water studies and some three-dimensional studies, it is still important to ensure that it is accurate over the range of count-rates encountered in practical imaging situations.

RANDOM CORRECTION

Random or accidental coincidences which occur when two unrelated γ-rays are detected within the coincidence time window can be corrected in one of two ways (22). The most common correction method makes use of two coincidence circuits. The first of these measures the true coincidences plus the randoms (collectively referred to as prompt coincidences) in the standard way. The second circuit has a delay (several hundred ns) inserted so all true coincidences are thrown out of coincidence and are not registered. The singles rate on each detector is, however, still the same, thus the randoms rate (given by eq. 4) remains, apart from statistical fluctuations, unaltered. To correct for randoms, the counts from the delayed circuit are simply subtracted, usually on-line, from those obtained from the prompt circuit. It should be noted that the randoms detected in the prompt coincidence circuit are not the same as those detected in the delayed circuit. Because of this, the subtraction of random events increases the statistical noise. Consider a sinogram element which registers T true counts and R random counts. The corrected number of counts, N, is given by:

$$\begin{aligned} N &= \textit{prompts} - \textit{delayeds} \\ &= (T + R) - R \end{aligned} \tag{10}$$

Assuming Poisson statistics, the noise, ΔN, is:

$$\Delta N = \sqrt{(T + 2R)} \tag{11}$$

The second correction method involves measuring the singles rate for each detector and calculating the random rate using equation 4. Because the singles rate is high, this correction adds little noise, but requires accurate knowledge of the coincidence timing window. This is not trivial, as small differences in transit time through the electronics will vary the width of this narrow 24 ns window. The random rates in any given study depend on the rate at which single events are detected. Typically, the fraction of random events is below 20%.

SCATTER CORRECTION

Scatter remains one of the most intractable problems in PET. Some degree of scatter rejection is accomplished by energy thresholding, as discussed earlier. Of the residual scatter, the contribution to the reconstructed image is quite small and, in many cases, is neglected. The most popular correction method is to use a deconvolution approach (20), although simple background fitting procedures can also yield surprisingly good results. Scatter becomes a bigger problem in three-dimensional PET acquisitions, where the scatter fraction (true events divided by scattered events) may be as high as 40% in a brain study. Fortunately, much of this scatter falls outside the reconstructed brain image, and the low spatial frequency scatter distribution is further suppressed by the reconstruction filter. However, there is still a measurable bias in the reconstructed image values due to scatter. A number of approaches are being explored for scatter correction in three-dimensional PET, all of which are likely to provide adequate correction in all but the most demanding situations (17–19, 21).

CALIBRATION

To reconstruct images in absolute units of μCi/cc, it is necessary to calibrate the PET scanner against a standard source. This is commonly done by imaging a uniform cylinder. An aliquot from the same cylinder is placed in a vial and well counted against a source of known activity to obtain the absolute activity concentration, which is then related to the counts in the reconstructed PET images (after all corrections have been applied) to obtain the appropriate calibration factor.

ACCURACY LIMITS IN POSITRON EMISSION TOMOGRAPHY

In addition to the corrections outlined earlier, corrections for decay of the isotope are usually applied during image reconstruction. The accuracy of the quantitative pixel values in the final reconstructed PET images depends critically on how well all the corrections are applied. In the best case, it is estimated that the absolute activity in a region in a PET scan can be measured to around 5% (60). Relative accuracy within an image may be as good as 1–2%. If any of the corrections are neglected or inappropriately applied, however, the errors can be much larger.

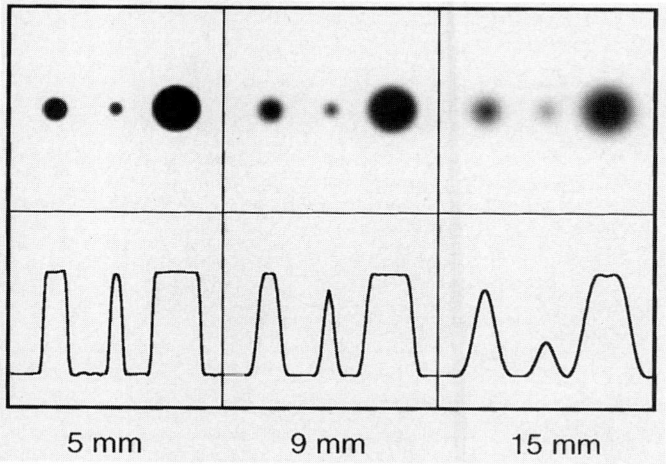

Figure 10.22. Illustration of the partial volume effect. Reconstructed images and profiles through cylinders of diameter 1 cm, 2 cm, and 4 cm—each containing equal activity. Notice how the resolution of the scanner degrades, the recovery of activity in the smaller structures becomes incomplete, and activity is underestimated.

PARTIAL VOLUME EFFECTS

It is possible to produce highly quantitative PET images provided all correction factors are appropriately applied. This approach works well for all structures that have dimensions greater than twice the spatial resolution of the PET scanner. As the dimension of a structure gets smaller than this, the activity concentration is progressively over- or underestimated, depending on the activity distribution. This is illustrated in Figure 10.22, which shows a profile through different sized structures—all containing the same activity concentration relative to a cold background. The resolution in these images is 6 mm. As the size of the structure decreases, the apparent activity concentration also decreases, and this effect, known as the partial volume effect, is solely due to the limited spatial resolution of the PET scanner. The correction factor required to obtain the correct value is known as the recovery coefficient. Since many structures of interest have dimensions less than twice the resolution of current clinical systems (e.g., 8–10 mm), this is a serious problem and, unfortunately, one which is not easy to remedy. For simple geometric shapes, it is possible to calculate the recovery coefficients if the activity distribution is known. This has been applied with some success in cardiac studies, where the myocardial wall is modeled as a uniform bar. In most other applications, it is not possible to calculate recovery coefficients, and interpretation of the images must account for the underestimation of activity in small structures which contain high activity levels relative to the background, and the overestimation of activity in small structures containing little activity relative to the background.

TRACER KINETIC MODELING

The distribution of a labeled tracer in the body following intravenous injection is a dynamic process. By obtaining a dynamic sequence of quantitative PET images starting from the time of injection, it is possible to observe the transport and metabolism of the tracer by organ systems in the body. Figure 10.23 illustrates this, showing a time series of PET scans in a single transaxial slice of the brain after the injection of [^{18}F]FDOPA. The distribution evolves from a nonspecific distribution reflecting blood volume and blood flow at early times, to one representing the specific location of dopamine synthesizing neurons. Figure 10.24 shows time activity curves for three different brain regions: cortex, striatum, and cerebellum. The aim of tracer kinetic modeling is to mathematically model the fate of the tracer after injection and to relate parameters in the model to biologically relevant information. Observables include the total tissue tracer concentration as a function of time (from the PET data) and blood or plasma concentration as a function of time (from blood sampling). Known information can also be used to constrain the model. Tracer kinetic models have been widely applied with great success in the biologic sciences and in pharmacology. PET, for the first time, allows quantitative biologic assays to be performed in vivo.

COMPARTMENTAL MODELS

Most kinetic models employed to date are linear compartmental models, where compartments are used to represent different spatial locations for the tracer (i.e., blood, interstitial space, intracellular) as well as different products involving the initial tracer (61). An example is shown in Figure 10.25, again for [^{18}F]FDOPA. The arrows between compartments represent the rate at which tracer in one compartment diffuses and is transported or metabolically transformed into a second compartment. These rate constants are usually represented by k_i, where i identifies the particular rate constant for exchange from one compartment to another. A number of assumptions are made about the compartments. Mixing within the compartment is assumed to be complete and the concentration homogeneous. The rate at which tracer leaves a compartment is assumed to be proportional to the amount of tracer in the compartment. This leads to first order differential equations which govern the exchange of the positron-emitting label from one compartment to another as a function of time. Even with fairly simple tracers, extensive knowledge of the transport and metabolism of tracers is required to help formulate the model. With this understanding, it is often possible to relate the rate constants to biologically meaningful parameters. In the example in Figure 10.25, k_3 is the rate constant for converting [^{18}F]FDOPA into its metabolic products, and K_1 is related to the product of blood flow and first pass extraction of FDOPA from blood to tissue. To estimate these rate constants, we must take a time series of data (Fig. 10.23), extract the time activity curve for structures of interest (Fig. 10.24), and then fit the compartment model for the individual rate constants.

INPUT FUNCTION

One compartment we have external access to is the vascular compartment. This can be seen as the input stage to the model, as the tracer is delivered through the blood; the blood time activity curve is, therefore, known as the input

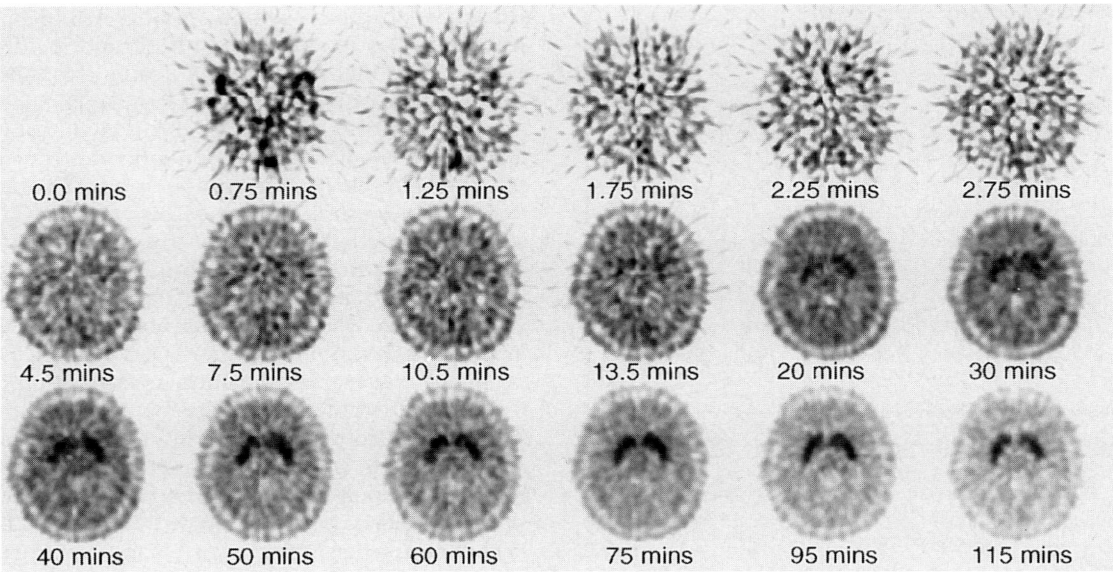

Figure 10.23. Time sequence of PET scans following the injection of [^{18}F]FDOPA. The initial distribution reflects blood volume, but changes over a period of an hour to finally reflect the distribution of dopamine storage sites in the brain.

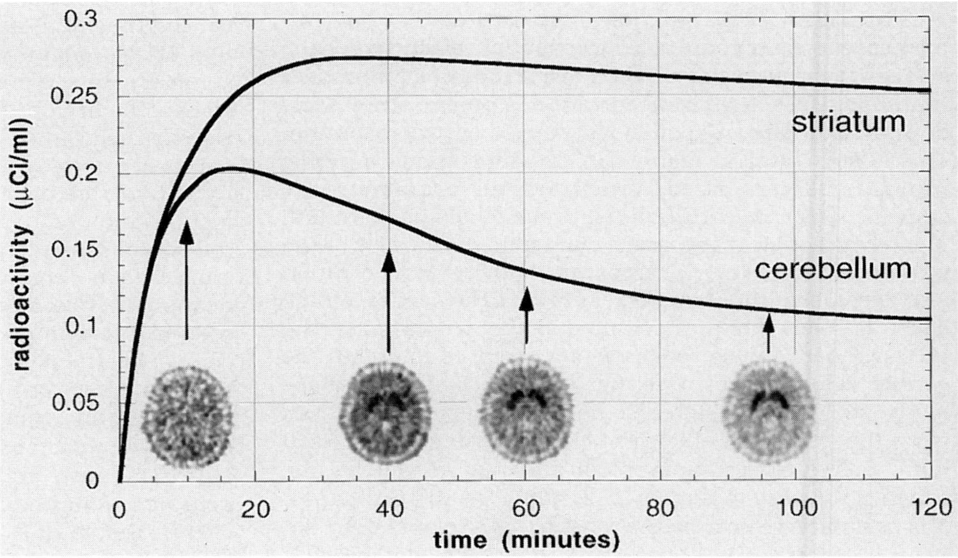

Figure 10.24. Time activity curves from the study in Figure 10.22 for the cerebellum, the striatum, and blood. This information is used, together with a mathematic model, to determine the regional rate of specific uptake of [^{18}F]FDOPA into the brain.

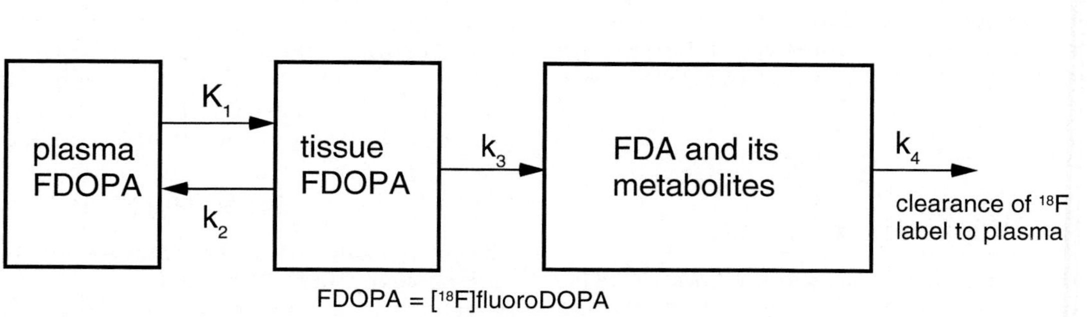

Figure 10.25. Compartmental model for transport and metabolism of [^{18}F]FDOPA.

function. By taking arterial blood samples over time, we have a good approximation of the time course of tracer delivery to the region of interest. This is not exact because of delay and dispersion effects between the point at which arterial blood is sampled (usually the radial artery) and the arterial blood actually supplying the region of interest. The input function is very important, as it can be considered to drive the model. Both the magnitude and the time course of the input function can have a dramatic effect on the time activity curves for a given region of interest.

To avoid the relatively invasive procedure of taking arterial blood, it is possible in some circumstances to substitute venous blood samples. These are often taken from the back of the hand, with the hand being heated to open up arteriovenous shunts, such that the blood is more "arterial" in nature. Venous blood samples are a good approximation when the extraction of the tracer on any one pass through a capillary bed is low. In certain circumstances, where a large volume of blood is inside the PET field of view (e.g., cardiac studies or studies including the aorta), it is possible to obtain the input function from rapid dynamic PET imaging, thus eliminating the need for blood sampling. However, the temporal sampling of the PET data can be a limitation, as are partial volume effects from adjacent tissues.

OPERATIONAL EQUATION

For any linear compartmental model, one can describe the activity seen by the PET scanner as the convolution of the input function with a set of exponential functions describing tracer exchange between compartments. Because the PET data has limited temporal resolution, and due to the half-life of available positron emitters, we are limited to measuring changes which happen on the time scale of seconds to several hours. Furthermore, because PET sees the sum of activity in multiple compartments and produces relatively noisy data, it is not possible to unambiguously calculate rate constants from a large number of compartments. The practical limit in PET is three compartments, measuring up to four separate rate constants. Often, models can be simplified by using analog tracers, rather than the natural substrate itself. These analog tracers are carefully designed such that they only follow a limited segment of a complicated biochemical pathway. FDG, which is an analog for glucose, is a good example of this. It has analogous transport and phosphorylation to glucose but is not further metabolized after entering the cell and becomes effectively trapped. The uptake is proportional to that tissue's metabolic rate for glucose. For tracers such as FDG, labelled amino acids, and ligands or drugs that react in near irreversible ways, even simplified integral equation models based upon accumulation of tracer in proportion to the process measured can be employed (62).

MODEL DEVELOPMENT AND VALIDATION

Any model applied to PET data must be carefully developed and validated using prior knowledge of the diffusion, transport, and metabolism of the tracer of interest (61). In some cases, it is possible to directly measure the biologic parameter of interest in animal studies and compare this with the values obtained through tracer kinetic modeling. Some measure of confidence in how well the model describes the data can be obtained by looking at the residuals. These are the difference between the predicted tissue time activity curves using the rate constants estimated from the PET data and the PET data itself. If any bias is detected in the residuals (i.e., they do not appear random over the time course examined), then the model is clearly insufficient to explain the data.

PARAMETRIC IMAGING

Over recent years, efforts have been made to integrate the image reconstruction process and the biologic model process into a single operation for well-established models. The result is an image of the rate of the process being measured (i.e., metabolic rate for glucose, blood flow, and receptor binding). These parametric images directly display biologic information in quantitative units for the entire imaging field of view, obviating the need to define regions of interest and apply the model to these one at a time. Increasingly, high resolution MRI images are being used in conjunction with PET data. By coregistering the two studies (63), regions of interest can be defined on the MRI scan and then copied onto the PET data. This should lead to more systematic region of interest definition based on anatomy.

SUMMARY

There are now over 150 PET centers worldwide, performing a wide range of studies. Modern PET tomographs are capable of producing high resolution, high quality images, which are used both as a diagnostic or prognostic tool and also in clinical and basic science research. In the patient care setting, PET is often used semiquantitatively with high signal-to-noise images of biologic processes, forming the basis for diagnosis. In clinical research, where the goal is often to obtain more fundamental information on the rate of biologic processes in the body, the full quantitative analysis with kinetic modeling and blood sampling is justified. Ultimately, however, the quantitative accuracy of the results are limited primarily by partial volume effects which relate to the resolution limits of PET and the signal-to-noise in the data which is related to the sensitivity of the PET scanner.

The challenge in PET instrumentation is to find techniques to improve both spatial resolution and system sensitivity, without pushing the cost of the instrument dramatically higher. Research continues into developing ever more compact and reliable accelerator devices for producing positron-emitting isotopes, and into automated synthesizer units which produce the labeled biologic probes ready for injection into the patient without requiring intervention from a skilled radiochemist. Another active area of research is in reconstruction algorithms. The filtered backprojection methods described earlier, while fast, are far from ideal. Iterative algorithms which accurately model the imaging system and the statistical nature of the data have been shown to improve signal-to-noise in the images, although their relative complexity and subjectivity, the potential to introduce bias, the long reconstruction times and their variable performance when compared with filtered backprojection remain as obstacles to their routine implementation. The challenges in tracer kinetic modeling, apart from developing models for new tracers, are to find ways to handle the image noise optimally and to further refine models. Image registration techniques which allow for correction of patient movement in long dynamic studies and for registration to MRI scans for ROI definition are also an important area of development. Technology and methods for PET continue to mature as we reach the stage where PET begins to realize its enormous potential.

REFERENCES

1. Phelps ME, Mazziotta JC, Schelbert HR. Positron emission tomography and autoradiography. New York: Raven Press, 1986.
2. Phelps ME, Mazziotta JC, Huang S-C. Study of cerebral function with positron emission tomography. J Cerebr Blood Flow Metab 1982;2:113–162.
3. Schelbert HR, Schwaiger M. Positron emission tomography studies of the heart. In: Phelps ME, Mazziotta JC, Schelbert HR, eds. Positron emission tomography and autoradiography. New York: Raven Press, 1986:581–661.
4. Mazziotta JC, Phelps ME. Positron emission tomography studies of the brain. In: Phelps ME, Mazziotta JC, Schelbert HR, eds. Positron emission tomography and autoradiography. New York: Raven Press, 1986:493–579.
5. Boles Ponto LL, Ponto JA. Uses and limitations of positron emission tomography in clinical pharmacokinetics/dynamics (part I). Clin Pharmacokinet 1992;22:211–222.
6. Boles Ponto LL, Ponto JA. Uses and limitations of positron emission tomography in clinical pharmacokinetics/dynamics (part II). Clin Pharmacokinet 1992;22:274–283.
7. Tilsey DWO, Harte RJA, Jones T, et al. New techniques in the pharmacokinetic analysis of cancer drugs. IV. Positron emission tomography. Cancer Surv 1993;17:425–442.
8. Sadzot B, Franck G. Noninvasive methods to study drug deposition: positron emission tomography. Eur J Drug Metab Pharmacokinet 1990;15:135–142.
9. Maziere B, Maziere M. Where have we got to with neuroreceptor mapping of the human brain? Eur J Nucl Med 1990;16:817–835.
10. Phelps ME. PET: a biological imaging technique. Neurochem Res 1991;16:929–940.
11. Schelbert HR. Positron emission tomography for the assessment of myocardial viability. Circulation 1991;84(Suppl I):I122–I131.
12. Bergman SR. Use and limitations of metabolic tracers labeled with positron-emitting radionuclides in the identification of viable myocardium. J Nucl Med 1994;35(Suppl):15S–22S.
13. Hawkins RA, Hoh C, Glasby J, et al. The role of positron emission tomography in oncology and other whole-body applications. Semin Nucl Med 1992;22:268–284.
14. Glasby JA, Hawkins R, Hoh CK, Phelps ME. Use of positron emission tomography in oncology. Oncology 1993;7:41–46.
15. Strauss LG, Conti PS. The applications of PET in clinical oncology. J Nucl Med 1991;32:623–648.
16. Wilson CB. PET scanning in oncology. Eur J Cancer 1992;28:508–510.
17. Grootoonk S, Spinks TJ, Jones T, Michel C, Bol A. Correction for scatter using a dual energy window technique with a tomograph operated without septa. IEEE Trans Nucl Sci 1991;38:1569–1573.
18. Cherry SR, Meikle SR, Hoffman EJ. Correction and characterization of scattered events in three-dimensional PET using scanners with retractable septa. J Nucl Med 1993;34:671–678.
19. Ollinger JM, Johns GC. Model-based scatter correction for fully 3D PET. IEEE Trans Nucl Sci 1993;40:1264–1268.
20. Bergström M, Eriksson L, Bohm C, Blomqvist G, Litton J. Correction for scattered radiation in a ring detector positron camera by integral transformation of the projections. J Comput Assist Tomogr 1983;7:42–50.
21. Bailey DL, Meikle SR. A convolution-subtraction scatter correction method for 3D PET. Phys Med Biol 1994;39:411–424.
22. Hoffman EJ, Huang SC, Phelps ME, Kuhl DE. Quantitation in positron emission tomography. 4. Effect of accidental coincidences. J Comput Assist Tomogr 1981;5:391–400.
23. Fowler JS, Wolf AP. Positron emitter-labeled compounds: priorities and problems. In: Phelps ME, Mazziotta JC, Schelbert HR, eds. Positron emission tomography and autoradiography. New York: Raven Press, 1986:391–450.
24. Grant PM, Erdal BR, O'Brien HA. A 82Sr-82Rb isotope generator for use in nuclear medicine. J Nucl Med 1975;16:300–304.
25. Robinson GD, Zielinski FW, Lee AW. Zn-62/Cu-62 generator: a convenient source of copper-62 radiopharmaceuticals. Int J Appl Radiat Isot 1980;31:111–116.
26. Mathias CJ, Welch MJ, Raichle ME, et al. Evaluation of a potential generator-produced PET tracer for cerebral perfusion imaging: single-pass cerebral extraction measurements and imaging with radiolabeled Cu-PTSM. J Nucl Med 1990;31:351–359.
27. Budinger TF, Yano Y, Derenzo SE, et al. Infarction sizing and myocardial perfusion measurements using rubidium-82 and positron emission tomography [Abstract]. Am J Cardiol 1979;45:39.
28. Herrero P, Markham J, Weinheimer CJ, et al. Quantification of regional myocardial perfusion with generator-produced 62Cu-PTSM and positron emission tomography. Circulation 1993; 87:173–183.
29. Hawkins RA, Phelps ME, Huang S-C, et al. A kinetic evaluation of blood-brain barrier permeability in human brain tumors with [^{68}Ga]EDTA and positron computed tomography. J Cerebr Blood Flow Metab 1984;4:507–515.
30. Webb S, Ott RJ, Cherry SR. Quantitation of blood-brain barrier permeability by positron emission tomography. Phys Med Biol 1989;34:1767–1771.
31. Saha GB, MacIntyre WJ, Go RT. Cyclotrons and positron emission tomography radiopharmaceuticals for clinical imaging. Semin Nucl Med 1992;22:150–161.
32. Barrio JR. Biochemical principles in radiopharmaceutical design and utilization. In: Phelps ME, Mazziotta JC, Schelbert HR, eds. Positron emission tomography and autoradiography. New York: Raven Press, 1986:451–492.
33. Eriksson L, Wienhard K, Dahlbom M. A simple data loss model for positron camera systems. IEEE Trans Nucl Sci 1993;40:1548–1552.
34. Strother SC, Casey ME, Hoffman EJ. Measuring PET scanner sensitivity: relating countrates to image signal-to-noise ratios using noise equivalent counts. IEEE Trans Nucl Sci 1990;37:783–788.
35. Tornai MP, Germano G, Hoffman EJ. Positioning and energy response of PET block detectors with different light sharing schemes. IEEE 1993;40:1126–1130.
36. Casey ME, Nutt R. A multicrystal two-dimensional BGO detector system for positron emission tomography. IEEE Trans Nucl Sci 1986;33:460–463.
37. Germano G, Hoffman EJ. A study of data loss and mispositioning due to pileup in 2-D detectors in PET. IEEE Trans Nucl Sci 1990; 37:671–675.
38. Moses WW, Derenzo SE. Empirical observation of resolution degradation in positron emission tomographs utilizing block detectors [Abstract]. J Nucl Med 1993;34:P101.
39. Karp JS, Muehllehner G, Mankoff DA, Ordonez CE, Ollinger JM, Beerbohm DJ. PENN-PET: a positron tomograph with volume imaging capability. J Nucl Med 1990;31:617–627.

40. Ter-Pogossian MM, Mullani NA, Ficke DC, Markham J, Snyder DL. Photon time-of-flight-assisted positron emission tomography. J Comput Assist Tomogr 1981;5:227–229.
41. Wells K, Ott RJ, Suckling J, Bateman JE, Stephenson R, Connolly JF. The status of the ICR/RAL BaF2-TMAE positron camera. IEEE Trans Nucl Sci 1992;39:1475–1479.
42. McIntyre JA. Design for an 80-ring optical-fiber PET. IEEE 1990; 37:1355–1363.
43. Wienhard K, Dahlbom M, Erikkson L, et al. The ECAT EXACT HR: performance of a new high resolution positron scanner. J Comput Assist Tomogr 1994;18:110–118.
44. DeGrado TR, Turkington TG, Williams JJ, Stearns CW, Hoffman JM, Coleman RE. Performance characteristics of a new generation PET scanner. J Nucl Med 1993;34:101P.
45. Townsend DW, Wensveen M, Byars LG, et al. A rotating PET scanner using BGO block detectors: design, performance and applications. J Nucl Med 1993;34:1367–1376.
46. Dahlbom M, Schiepers C, Hoffman EJ, et al. Evaluation of PET for whole body imaging. J Nucl Med 1990;31:749.
47. Guerrero T, Hoffman EJ, Dahlbom M, Cutler PD, Hawkins RA, Phelps ME. Characterization of a whole-body imaging technique for PET. IEEE Trans Nucl Sci 1990;37:676–680.
48. Cherry SR, Dahlbom M, Hoffman EJ. Three-dimensional positron emission tomography using a conventional multislice tomograph without septa. J Comput Assist Tomogr 1991;15:655–668.
49. Townsend DW, Geissbuhler A, DeFrise M, et al. Fully three-dimensional reconstruction for a PET camera with retractable septa. IEEE Trans Med Image 1991;10:505–512.
50. Defrise M, Townsend DW, Geissbuhler A. Implementation of three-dimensional image reconstruction for multi-ring tomographs. Phys Med Biol 1990;35:1361–1372.
51. Cherry SR, Dahlbom M, Hoffman EJ. Evaluation of a 3D reconstruction algorithm for multislice PET scanners. Phys Med Biol 1992;37:779–790.
52. Guerrero TM, Cherry SR, Dahlbom M, Ricci AR, Hoffman EJ. Fast implementations of 3D PET reconstruction using vector and parallel programming techniques. IEEE Trans Nucl Sci 1993; 40:1082–1086.
53. Kearfott KJ. Absorbed dose estimates for positron emission tomography (PET): C15O, 11CO, and CO15O. J Nucl Med 1982; 23:1031–1037.
54. ICRP. Publication 53: Radiation dose to patients from radiopharmaceuticals. Annals of the ICRP 1988;18(1–4):67–68.
55. Brown WD, Oakes TR, Nickles RJ. Revised dosimetry for fluorodopa with carbidopa pretreatment [Abstract]. J Nucl Med 1993; 34:157P.
56. Brooks RA, Di Chiro G. Principles of computer assisted tomography (CAT) in radiographic and radioisotopic imaging. Phys Med Biol 1976;21:689–732.
57. Huang S-C, Hoffman EJ, Phelps ME, Kuhl DE. Quantitation in positron computed tomography. 3. Effect of sampling. J Comput Assist Tomogr 1980;4:819–826.
58. Meikle S, Dahlbom M, Cherry SR. Attenuation correction using count-limited transmission data in positron emission tomography. J Nucl Med 1993;34:143–150.
59. Siegel S, Dahlbom M. Implementation and validation of a calculated attenuation correction for PET. IEEE Trans Nucl Sci 1992; 39:1117–1121.
60. Hoffman EJ, Cutler PD, Guerrero TM, Digby WM, Mazziotta JC. Assessment of accuracy of PET utilizing a 3-D phantom to simulate the activity distribution of 18-F FDG uptake in the human brain. J Cereb Blood Flow Metab 1991;11:A17–A25.
61. Huang S-C, Phelps ME. Principles of tracer kinetic modeling in positron emission tomography and autoradiography. In: Phelps ME, Mazziotta JC, Schelbert HR, eds. Positron emission tomography and autoradiography. New York: Raven Press, 1986:287–346.
62. Patlak CS, Blasberg RG. Graphical evaluation of blood-to-brain transfer constants from multiple-time uptake data. J Cereb Blood Flow Metab 1985;5:584–590.
63. Woods RP, Mazziotta JC, Cherry SR. MRI-PET registration with automated algorithm. J Comput Assist Tomogr 1993;17:536–546.

11 Quality Assurance

JAMES A. PATTON

Quality assurance is an extremely important aspect of any patient-related procedure and must be included in the routine performance of diagnostic imaging studies. Quality assurance in nuclear medicine involves many aspects in addition to the routine quality control procedures associated with the preparation of radiopharmaceuticals and the evaluation of instruments. Quality assurance is a state of mind that must involve all personnel associated with the procedure. Their goal must be to ensure that the correct patient, properly prepared, is administered the correct amount of the prescribed radiopharmaceutical. The patient should also be studied at the appropriate times in the required positions with the correct instrumentation which has been properly calibrated, and the referring physician should be given the correct results based on appropriate evaluation of the data obtained from the study. All of these quality assurance procedures should be documented, along with the results of periodic evaluations of the procedures. Everyone involved in the performance of a study has both a moral and a legal obligation to follow good quality assurance practices in conducting the study. In fact, the guidelines provided by the Joint Commission on Accreditation of Healthcare Organizations (JCAHO) state that there shall be documented quality assurance procedures that ensure the safety of the patient and the appropriateness of the study. Additionally, records shall be maintained to document the constant monitoring of these procedures. If these procedures are not documented and adhered to, a healthcare organization can be cited and its accreditation placed in jeopardy. Thus, in simple terms, the goal of a quality assurance program is to see that no mistakes are made in the performance of a patient procedure.

PATIENT PREPARATION

Most nuclear medicine imaging procedures require very little, if any, patient preparation. However, there are some factors that affect the normal uptake and distribution of radiopharmaceuticals and may therefore affect the quality of the images that are obtained. For example, several factors affect the uptake of the thyroid and result in poor-quality or nondiagnostic images (1). These factors are discussed in the chapters on the different organ systems. Patients should be carefully screened and studies appropriately postponed if any of the interfering factors are present.

A second point to be stressed, even though it may appear on the surface to be trivial, is to be absolutely certain that the correct patient is about to be studied before commencing the study. On a referral basis, no patient should be studied without a signed requisition from the referring physician. Additionally, the person performing the study should obtain written documentation as to the identity of the patient, including a hospital unit number or a Social Security number. Patient mixups caused by such rare situations as two patients with the same name occupying the same hospital room have been documented. Careful attention to details can prevent the administration of a radiopharmaceutical to the wrong patient.

Women should be carefully screened to make sure that they are not pregnant before a radiopharmaceutical is administered because of the potentially high radiation doses that the fetus may receive from the procedure. If there is any doubt, the study should be postponed until a pregnancy test is performed or until the patient is in the first 2 weeks of her menstrual cycle.

Finally, every dose to be administered to a patient should be assayed using a radionuclide dose calibrator to ensure that the correct level of activity has been prepared. In an ideal situation, the dose would be prepared and assayed by radiopharmacy staff and double-checked by a technologist before the dose is administered. The latter is especially important in the preparation of therapy doses. Some nuclear medicine laboratories require the presence of a physician when a therapy dose is assayed so that three people are involved in the dose verification process. In facilities utilizing unit doses from an external radiopharmacy with no mechanism for validation of the dose, a careful review of the documentation accompanying the dose must be performed before the dose is administered.

RADIOPHARMACEUTICAL PREPARATIONS

As with any drug that is administered to a patient, radiopharmaceutical preparations must be carefully tested for sterility and the presence of pyrogens. These preparations must also be evaluated for the presence of chemical impurities. Additionally, radiopharmaceuticals must be carefully screened to make sure they do not contain radionuclide impurities. Although the presence of these impurities may not alter the chemical performance of the drugs, they may result in the presence of interfering decay processes that affect imaging capabilities or significantly increase the radiation dose associated with the drug administration. Results of these evaluations are generally documented by radiopharmaceutical manufacturers in brochures or labels accompanying the drugs. However, if radiopharmaceuticals are prepared in-house, testing must be performed and the results documented.

An interesting aspect of imaging radiopharmaceuticals distribution is the fact that some organs may actually be used as quality assurance reference organs for procedures involving other regions of the body. For example, in performing imaging studies with ^{99m}Tc-labeled compounds, an increased concentration of activity may be observed in the region of the stomach. The question then arises as to whether this is free pertechnetate or actually an abnormality. Because pertechnetate (the chemical form of ^{99m}Tc before preparation of these pharmaceuticals) is trapped by the thyroid, an image of the neck with the scintillation camera will provide the answer to that question.

INSTRUMENTATION QUALITY CONTROL

DOSE CALIBRATOR

To ensure the administration of the correct amount (activity) of radiopharmaceutical, quality control procedures must be performed routinely using a dose calibrator to measure activity. Daily measurements should include background levels to check for contamination and sources close to the calibrator, and precision tests to check for reproducibility of measurements performed with the instrument. The latter is performed by daily measurements of a long-lived source of known activity with an energy close to that of the radionuclides used for routine imaging. An ideal calibration standard is ^{57}Co with an energy of 122 keV and a half-life of 270 days. For quality control applications, a standard of known activity is obtained from a radiopharmaceutical manufacturer, and its activity is measured in the dose calibrator daily. These standards are directly traceable to National Bureau of Standards calibration sources and are warranted by the manufacturer to specific accuracies (usually $\pm 5\%$). The results of the measurements are then compared with the known activity. Variations of no more than $\pm 5\%$ are acceptable on a daily basis with state-of-the-art dose calibrators. The data generally are recorded on a graph, as shown in Figure 11.1. The decay of the source is plotted along with the $\pm 5\%$ error ranges. Any measurement falling outside the error ranges should be considered unacceptable and explained (i.e., service of the calibrator may be necessary). Some departments are equipped with computer systems with automated quality assurance programs that maintain these records on a daily basis.

Verification of the accuracy of measurements over the useful range of the calibrator should be performed at least annually, and preferably every 6 months. Accuracy is evaluated by measuring the activity of several known long-lived standards of different energies (e.g., ^{133}Ba, ^{137}Cs, ^{57}Co, and ^{129}I) and comparing the results with the known values. Variations of no more than $\pm 5\%$ are acceptable.

Linearity should be evaluated quarterly and can be measured in two ways. One method is to begin with several hundred millicuries of ^{99m}Tc and make repeated measurements of activity until only a few microcuries remain. The values are then plotted as a function of time on semilog graph paper. This plot should yield a straight-line curve with a half-life of 6 hours (Fig. 11.2). Variations from this expectation indicate nonlinearities, and the dose calibrator must be recalibrated or repaired. To obtain enough data points to adequately evaluate the instrument throughout its functional range, it may be necessary to extend the measurements over 3 or 4 days. Another method is to use aliquots of the known volume to measure different activity levels. Alternatively, linearity can be measured using a single, high-activity source and calibrated shields that attenuate the source by known amounts (2). These shields are commercially available for quality control procedures. With this technique, the shields are calibrated by using them to make measurements simultaneously with a linearity check performed as described above. They can then be used with a source of high activity to quickly perform a linearity test.

Geometry correction factors should be obtained when the dose calibrator is first placed into operation to eliminate the effects of dose volume on dose activity. These calibrations are performed by preparing samples with the same activity in a wide range of volumes and assaying each sample in the dose calibrator. By plotting measured activity versus volume, correction factors can be obtained to adjust the measured activity to the true activity. These factors can then be used for future measurements. Geometry

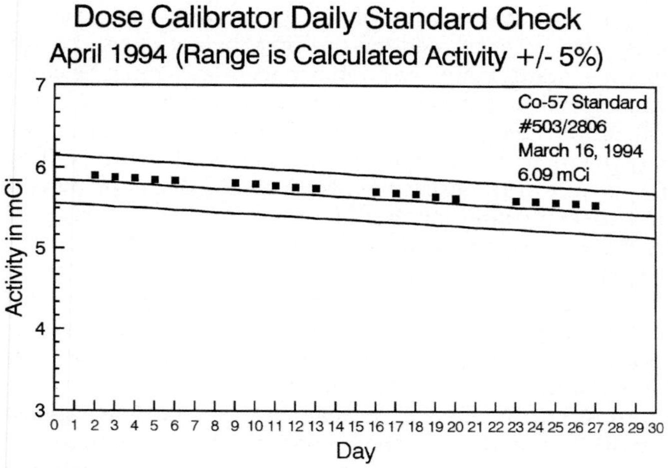

Figure 11.1. Precision or reproducibility measurements on a dose calibrator are performed daily using a long-lived standard such as ^{57}Co, and the data are recorded in graphical form. Measurements falling outside of the acceptable ranges ($\pm 5\%$) must be explained.

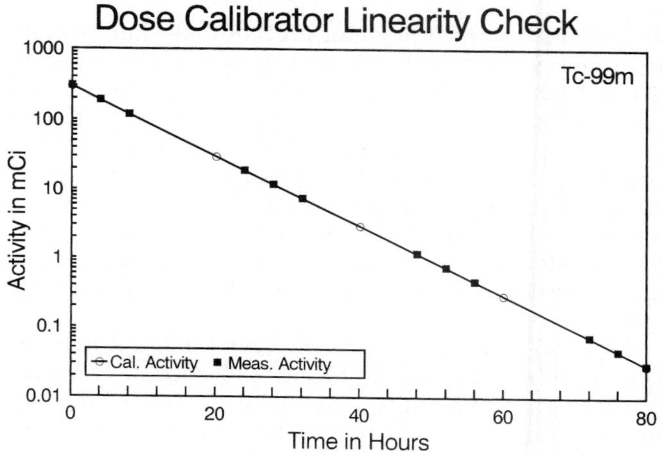

Figure 11.2. Linearity measurement performed on a dose calibrator beginning with a high-activity source of ^{99m}Tc and making multiple measurements of activity as the source decays.

correction factors should be obtained for those radioisotopes that are anticipated to be measured with widely varying volumes.

SCINTILLATION WELL COUNTERS

Scintillation well counters used for routine sample counting in glomerular filtration rate (GFR), blood volume, Shilling tests, radioimmunoassay (RIA), and other in vitro procedures, require routine quality control procedures to ensure the accuracy and precision of the tests. Daily measurements of background and precision should be performed and the results recorded. It is generally recommended that precision be evaluated using two long-lived, calibrated standards, one in the low energy range such as ^{129}I (mock ^{125}I source) at about 30 keV and one in the high energy range such as ^{137}Cs at 662 keV. Daily precision measurements should be within ±3 standard deviations of the mean counts for each standard. Measurements falling outside this range may be indicative of contamination, abnormal room background, or electronic problems such as window, peak, or high-voltage shifts.

At least annually, a measurement of linearity should be performed using prepared samples of a commonly used radionuclide with varying and known activities. The samples are counted and a linearity plot is obtained relating measured counts to sample activity. The straight-line portion of this curve denotes the useful linear range of the instrument.

A useful test for detecting equipment malfunctions is the chi-square test. This test should be performed every 3 months in the following manner. A series of counting measurements (20 is usually sufficient) is collected, and the mean (n) of these measurements is calculated. The chi-square is then calculated using the formula

$$Chi\text{-}Square = \sum_{i=1}^{N} \frac{(n_i - n)^2}{n}$$

where n_i is each individual measurement and N is the number of measurements. The chi-square value is then found in a table of P values. If the corresponding P value is less than .01 or greater than .99, there is cause to doubt the reliability of the instrument.

Most automated sample counters have electronic circuitry for performing selected tasks such as push buttons for window and peak selection and dials for background subtraction and ratio corrections. Current systems are now computer-based and programmable for specific functions, including peak selection. It is important that quality control procedures be routinely performed to ensure the proper function of this equipment.

IN VITRO LAB EQUIPMENT

In addition to the nuclear counting equipment routinely used for in vitro sample measurements, quality control procedures must be in place for all the other commonly used lab equipment. Temperatures of refrigerators, freezers, and water baths must be monitored, pipettes must be checked routinely for precision and accuracy, balances must be evaluated and calibrated for weight measurements, and centrifuges must be calibrated routinely for accuracy of speed selections. All these practices are in keeping with the goal of ensuring the proper and correct performance of patient-related procedures.

IMAGING SYSTEMS

There are many aspects of quality assurance associated with nuclear medicine imaging instrumentation that should be considered to obtain high-quality images. However, before an imaging system is placed into operation, it is important to verify that the system meets the specifications stated by the manufacturer in the purchase agreement. This acceptance testing procedure can also be used to establish standards of performance that can then be monitored on a regular basis by quality control procedures.

Acceptance Testing

After the manufacturer has completed the installation procedure and before the first clinical use of an imaging system, acceptance testing of the equipment should be performed. It is advisable to reach an agreement with the manufacturer on how acceptance testing will be accomplished and what criteria will be used for acceptance before the purchase agreement is completed. There are several established specifications that describe the performance of nuclear medicine imaging systems. The National Electrical Manufacturers Association (NEMA) established methods for measuring these performance parameters and published these methods in a document entitled *Performance Measurements of the Scintillation Camera*. Most manufacturers have adopted these standards of measurement and use them to report the specifications of their equipment so that meaningful comparisons of equipment may be made by prospective buyers. The techniques utilized in these measurements often require specialized equipment and typically cannot be used to verify performance in acceptance testing. However, the American Association of Physicists in Medicine (AAPM) has established acceptance testing methods for verifying performance which may be used to establish acceptance testing criteria.

There are three methods for performing acceptance testing. The first method is simply to require the manufacturer to provide the buyer with a set of measurement results performed on-site, verifying that the system meets specifications. The second method is to perform measurements using qualified personnel employed by the purchasing institution. Often it is preferred by all parties to employ an outside consultant to perform the acceptance testing to eliminate any possibility of bias in the measurements.

Once the buyer is satisfied with the results of acceptance testing, and identified problems have been resolved, selected acceptance testing results may be used to establish baseline criteria for daily quality control.

Scintillation Camera

Quality control procedures should be performed daily at a specific time—ideally at the beginning of the workday. This begins with a general checkout of the camera to look for dents or scratches in the collimators or crystal housing, unusual noises during movement of the camera head, excessive play in the motion of the detector head, or any other factor that may affect the performance and/or safety of the system. This inspection should also include a superficial cleaning of the system.

The next step is to peak the camera. The radionuclide energy peak should be checked at the beginning of the day and each time there is a change in the radionuclide to be imaged. This procedure is performed by using a source placed beneath the uncollimated detector. A source of ^{99m}Tc is generally chosen with an activity of about 300 μCi to provide a count rate of no more than 30,000 counts per second. By adjusting the window and radionuclide energy peak settings, a 20% window (15% for newer cameras) is placed symmetrically about the photopeak. On older cameras, this is accomplished by manually adjusting two dials controlling the peak and window positions while viewing a display of superimposed energy (Z) pulses with a dark rectangle representing the window being overlaid on top of the display. Newer cameras use a multichannel analyzer (MCA) to display the energy spectrum of the radionuclide with the window being represented by data points of increased intensity. On cameras with autopeaking, the position of the window should always be verified. A symmetric window is necessary to provide a uniform response, because scintillation cameras are tuned to provide a uniform response only with a symmetric window. Placing the window asymmetrically above or below the photopeak without retuning the camera will result in hot or cold spots in the images. The window position should always be checked before each patient study. If a different radionuclide is to be used, the camera must be peaked before the study is begun. The radionuclide distribution in the patient should not be used for the peaking process because the presence of scatter will result in positioning of the window below the actual photopeak position. Figure 11.3 illustrates this point using a thyroid phantom in a simulated neck geometry. The increase in background and the loss in contrast and edge detail can be observed in Figure 11.3 with the camera window placed below the photopeak in the scatter region.

After the peaking process, a daily flood image should be obtained by placing the source a distance of three camera diameters (standard field of view (SFOV): 30 inches; large field of view (LFOV): 45 inches) from the center of the uncollimated detector and collecting an image to assess the uniformity of response. Typically, 1 million counts are collected for a SFOV camera, 2 million counts for an LFOV camera, and 3 million counts for a rectangular field-of-view camera. Tripod source holders are commercially available to center the source above the detector at a reproducible standard distance, but these should be used only when the crystal is protected by a plexiglass shield. The flood image should be compared to one obtained immediately after the camera was last tuned and in acceptable working condition, to look for changes in detector response that may indicate the presence of, or potential for equipment malfunctions. The flood image evaluates the crystal, light pipe, photomultiplier tubes, preamplifiers, pulse height analyzer, position electronics, and display system. Figure 11.4 shows an acceptable flood image, along with three flood

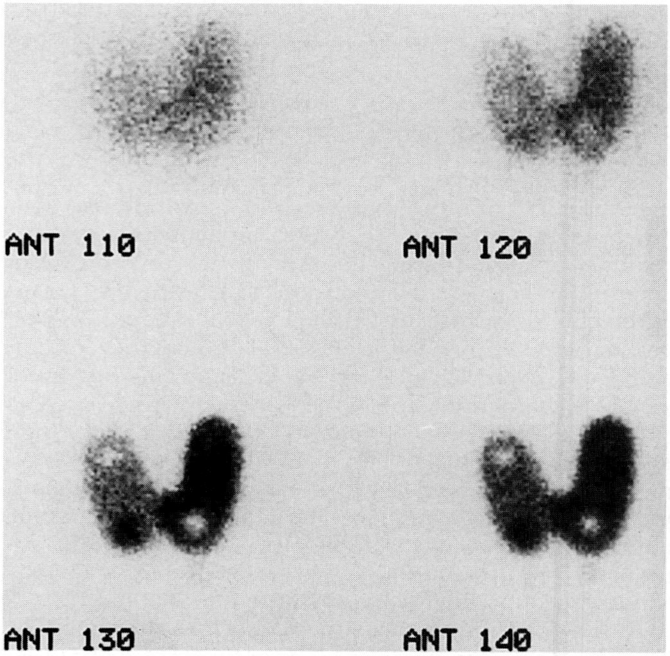

Figure 11.3. Images of a thyroid phantom containing ^{99m}Tc in a scattering medium using a 20% window with the peak placed at 110, 120, 130, and 140 keV, respectively.

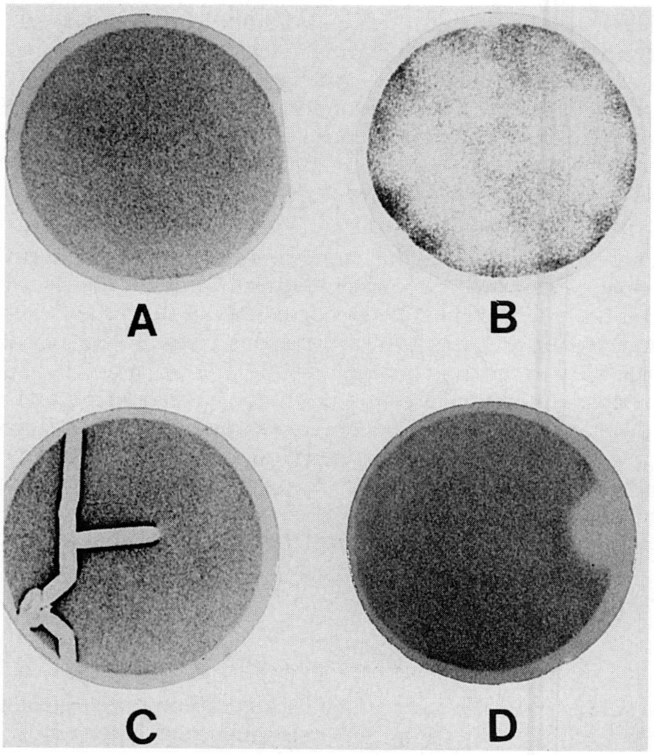

Figure 11.4. Flood images from a scintillation camera demonstrating (**A**) acceptable uniformity, (**B**) shift in high voltage, (**C**) broken crystal, and (**D**) nonfunctioning photomultiplier tube. (Reproduced by permission from Sandler MP, Patton JA, Partain CL, eds. Thyroid and parathyroid imaging. East Norwalk, CT: Appleton-Century-Crofts, 1986:83.)

images that are not acceptable. If obvious nonuniformities are present, the camera should not be used for patient studies until it is serviced. The flood image, along with the collection time, display intensity, isotope peak, and window settings, should be recorded daily in a log book.

Resolution and linearity checks should be performed weekly by placing a phantom of parallel lead bars in contact with the uncollimated camera face and irradiating it with the point source in the same position as for the flood image. The image should contain 1, 2, or 3 million counts, depending on whether the camera is an SFOV, LFOV, or rectangular field of view, and should be carefully assessed for nonlinearities or distortions in the regular phantom pattern. The size and spacing of the pattern should approach the spatial resolution of the camera (Fig. 11.5). For 4-quadrant bar patterns, an image should be obtained with the smallest bars placed in each of the 4 quadrants of the camera to test the limit of resolution of the camera. Slight regional variations in resolution can be detected using this technique, and repairs can be performed before major problems result.

Because of the fragile nature of the collimators used in nuclear medicine, a monthly evaluation of all collimators should be performed to look for possible damage by performing a flood with the collimator on the camera using a ^{57}Co plane source or a refillable plexiglass phantom containing a well-mixed solution of ^{99m}Tc.

Every 3 months, a detailed assessment of camera performance should be made, at which time selected parameters measured during acceptance testing should be verified. These include sensitivity, linearity, integral uniformity, count rate capability, and multiple energy window registration.

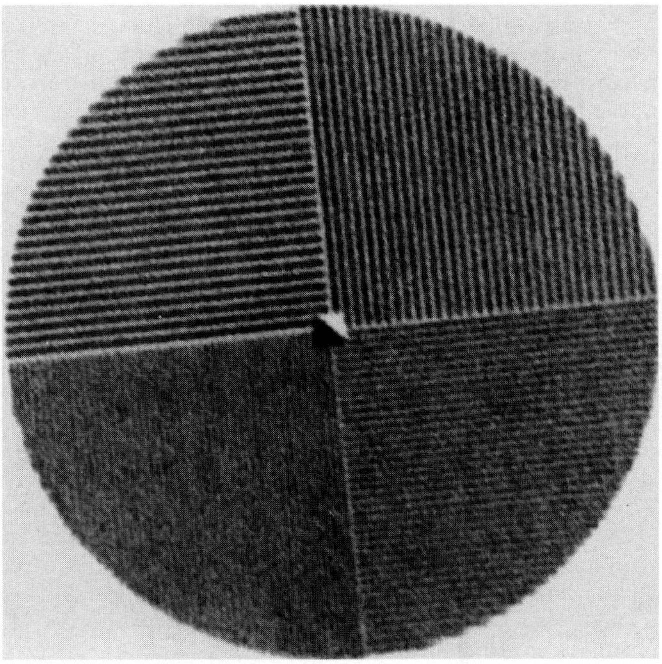

Figure 11.5. Linearity and spatial resolution measurements from a scintillation camera performed with a 4-quadrant bar pattern.

Digital Scintillation Cameras. The commercial availability of digital scintillation cameras, where analog signals are digitized either at the base of the photomultiplier tubes or at the analog position circuitry, has resulted in altered protocols for camera quality control and expanded capabilities. Radionuclide energy peak and window adjustments are made under computer control, and digital images are acquired in computer memory so that a programmed mathematic analysis of image quality can be easily performed. Current digital cameras have the capability for acquiring linearity and uniformity maps in each functional energy range so that automated correction processes are implemented, resulting in improved camera specifications. These capabilities permit the uniformity corrections process to be extended to include the collimator so that the effects of small localized differences in collimator sensitivity can be eliminated. The results of typical automated daily quality control procedures for a digital camera are shown in Figure 11.6. A plane source of ^{57}Co is placed over the collimated detector (the source must be larger than the collimated field of view) and an energy spectrum is collected. The position of the photopeak is measured using the energy calibration of the camera as a baseline for the measurements. A flood image is then collected before and after uniformity correction, and a calculation of integral uniformity is performed. The images and quantitative measurements can be plotted in a graph format and automatically updated (Fig. 11.7). Using this protocol, quality control history of imaging systems can be easily maintained and limits defined for acceptable performance.

Single Photon Emission Computed Tomography

The increased clinical use of single photon emission computed tomography (SPECT) procedures has placed additional burdens on the performance of quality assurance programs. The presence of nonuniformities, nonlinearities, and misalignments is of even more concern than in routine imaging, because artifacts that are generated by these problems are propagated and even amplified during the data collection and image reconstruction process. Thus, quality assurance plays an important role in the performance of SPECT procedures.

SPECT systems utilizing scintillation cameras should exhibit excellent linearity and uniformity, and these factors should be evaluated regularly with the combined scintillation camera-computer system. Computer systems for SPECT imaging have the capability for correcting nonuniformities before reconstruction is initiated. This is done by collecting a flood with excellent counting statistics (10–30 million counts), which is used to generate a uniformity correction matrix that is applied to each image collected in the study. Additionally, it is important to verify that the uniformity of response of the system does not change with orientation. Early scintillation cameras with SPECT capability had poor magnetic shielding of the photomultiplier tubes, resulting in variations in response as the detector head position was changed with respect to the earth's magnetic field. After a SPECT system is installed, the absence of these variations should be verified during acceptance testing by collecting floods with the detector positioned at

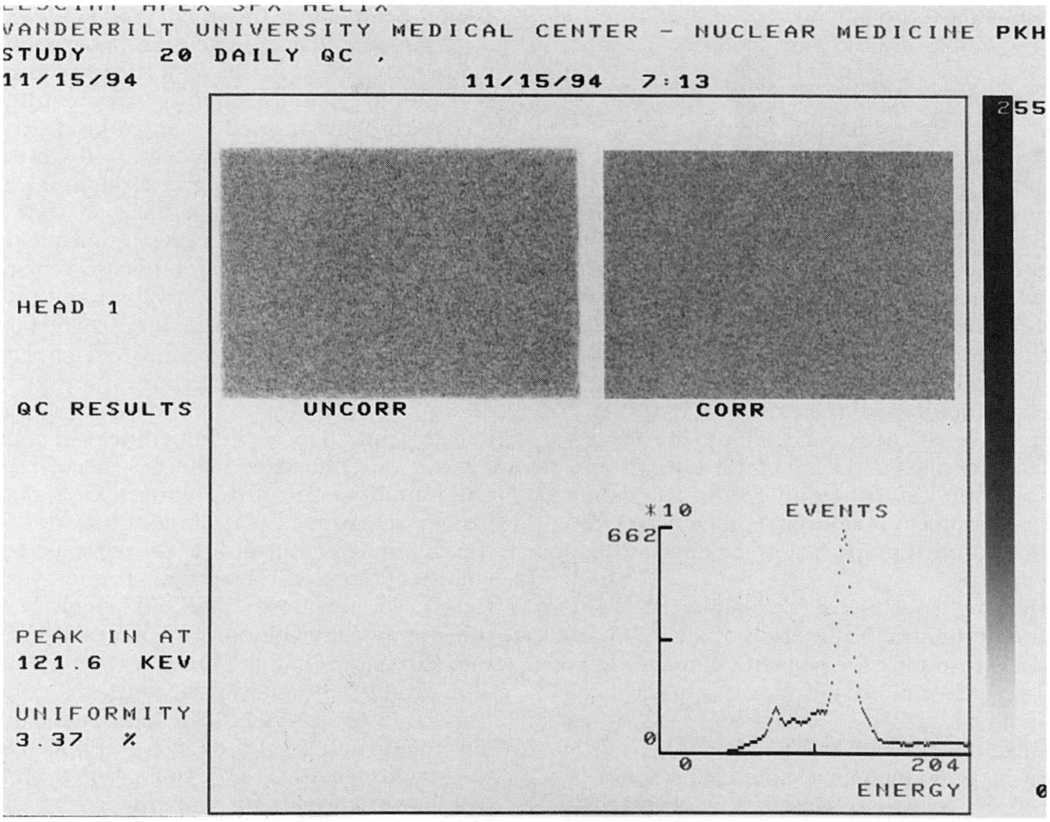

Figure 11.6. Quality control report from a digital scintillation camera showing an energy spectrum from ^{57}Co, the position of the photopeak, a flood from the collimated camera obtained with a plane source of ^{57}Co before and after uniformity correction, and the results of a calculation of integral uniformity.

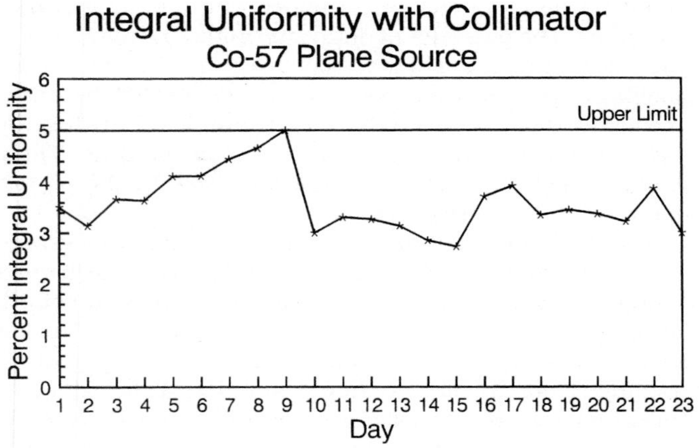

Figure 11.7. Results of a plot of calculated integral uniformity measurements obtained as described in Figure 11.6. The camera was serviced when the integral uniformity exceeded the upper limit of acceptability.

0°, 90°, 180°, and 270°. All floods should be identical. These measurements should be repeated whenever any change in the environment occurs that might alter the magnetic field where the system is located, such as the installation nearby of a magnetic resonance imaging system.

Another important factor that should be evaluated regularly is the measured center of the axis of rotation (3). For perfect geometry in the reconstruction process, the center of the field of view should correspond exactly to the center of the digitized image array accumulated in the computer. Positional variations due to errors in the calibration of the analog-to-digital converter used to digitize position will result in artifacts in the reconstruction process (i.e., point sources may be reconstructed as rings). This situation can be evaluated manually by positioning a point source precisely at the center of rotation and collecting images at 0°, 90°, 180°, and 270°. The center of the point source should be at the center of the digitized array in each image. Current systems have the capability for automated measurement and correction of errors in center-of-rotation positioning. This is done simply by scanning a point source near the center of rotation and then generating correction factors for each frame based on the measured movement of the source in relation to the center of rotation. Limits are established which determine when service is required. Evaluation of errors in the center of rotation should be performed on a weekly basis. Figure 11.8 shows images of a cardiac phantom obtained with a system with a gross error in the center of the rotation and images after the error was corrected. On a monthly basis, the imaging capability of

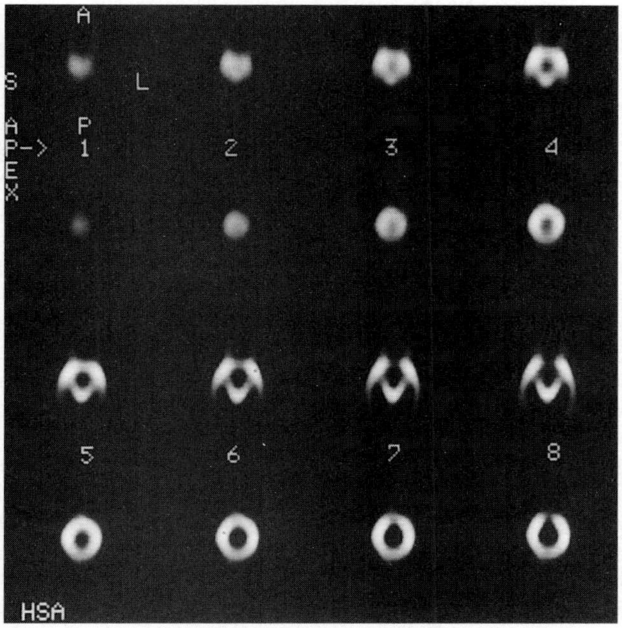

Figure 11.8. SPECT images obtained with a Data Spectrum cardiac phantom from a scintillation camera with a center-of-rotation error (*rows 1 and 3*) and with the error corrected (*rows 2 and 4*).

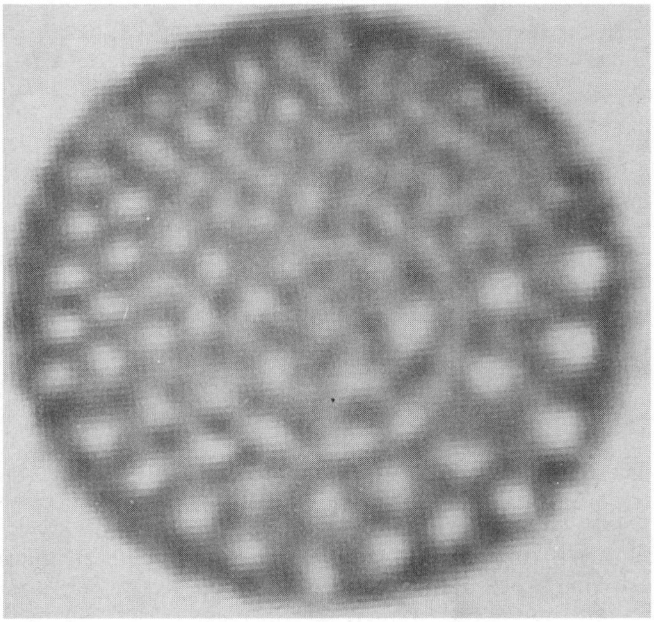

Figure 11.9. SPECT images with a Data Spectrum cold rods phantom from a scintillation camera utilizing inadequate uniformity correction.

the entire SPECT system should be measured by collecting a high count image from a volume phantom containing structures to evaluate the resolution of the imaging system. An example of a SPECT phantom evaluation is shown in Figure 11.9. The phantom consists of a set of cold rods (Data Spectrum phantom) and illustrates a ring artifact in the center due to inadequate uniformity correction.

Computers

In addition to routinely evaluating the performance of the scintillation camera, it is also important to perform quality assurance testing with the camera-computer systems in routine use to verify the validity of images and numeric data that are obtained from the computer and reported for diagnostic purposes (4). Data acquisition performance of an independent camera and computer system can be evaluated by collecting images in the computer at the same time the camera is being evaluated for nonuniformities and comparing the two sets of data that are obtained. Analysis software can be evaluated on a routine basis by processing a standard set of data to verify reproducibility of results. Cardiac phantoms also are available to evaluate both data acquisition and processing techniques. Although each of the commercially available phantoms has limitations, they have all proven to be of use in routine quality assurance evaluations. Software used to provide quantitative measurements should always be validated using phantoms with known characteristics. Whenever a change is made in the software, the validation process should be repeated.

Action Criteria

Of equal importance to the performance of routine quality control of instrumentation is the development of procedures to be followed in the evaluation of measurements performed. A responsible person (technical supervisor, physicist, physician, or quality assurance technologist) should evaluate the measurement results immediately after they are performed and determine whether the equipment is acceptable for use. It is important to establish action criteria based on defined limits. This is easily accomplished with quantitative measurements (e.g., integral uniformity above 6%—repeat measurement and if still above 6%, call service) but may be more difficult for subjective evaluations (viewing and evaluating floods from analog cameras). Thus, it is important that the person responsible for quality control be knowledgeable, trained, and experienced in the procedures performed and the measurements obtained. In larger, multicamera departments, especially in academic institutions, it is useful to display the daily quality control measurements on the viewing board with reference measurements displaying acceptable results. These images may then be reviewed by physicians during the reading session and also used for instructional purposes. Previous measurements should be filed away in log books and maintained for 3 years.

Maintenance

A final factor that should be mentioned in the quality assurance of instrumentation is maintenance. A service log of repairs and maintenance should be maintained for each instrument in routine use. The log should indicate the problems encountered, the service performed, service response time, and downtime. This log is useful in documenting equipment reliability, as well as providing valuable information to service personnel. It is also useful in developing a database to be used when it is necessary to justify the replacement of equipment.

IMAGING QUALITY ASSURANCE

COLLIMATION

Collimator selection is extremely important in nuclear medicine imaging procedures. A low-energy, all-purpose, parallel-hole collimator is used for most diagnostic imaging applications. The high-sensitivity collimator is used only for first-pass or bolus studies because of its high efficiency but poor spatial resolution. The high-resolution collimator is generally used for difficult imaging situations where improved spatial resolution is desired and photon detection efficiency is not a problem, especially in cold-lesion or deep-lesion detection problems such as those encountered in liver imaging. Converging collimators offer magnification capabilities for SFOV cameras but may yield distorted images, especially at the periphery of the field of view. Because of their minification properties, diverging collimators provide the capability for imaging large organ structures with a small field of view camera. However, they suffer from degraded spatial resolution with distance from the collimator face. Slant, parallel-hole collimators are used in some laboratories for cardiac-gated blood pool studies and SPECT studies of the brain to improve spatial resolution through better detector positioning. Medium-energy collimators are used for imaging radionuclides with energies from 200–400 keV. These collimators also can be used in some low-energy imaging situations, such as dual-isotope studies when the patient cannot be moved between images to change collimators. Spatial resolution generally is sacrificed in this situation because of the thicker septa and larger hole diameters used in medium-energy collimators. However, low-energy collimators cannot be used to image radionuclides with energies greater than 200keV because of septal penetration. Ultra-high energy collimators are now available for imaging 511 keV photons from positron emitters.

Collimator positioning is also extremely important in nuclear medicine imaging. Since the spatial resolution of any collimator falls off with distance from the collimator face, it is important to place the detector as close as possible to the region of interest while maintaining the region of interest within the field of view.

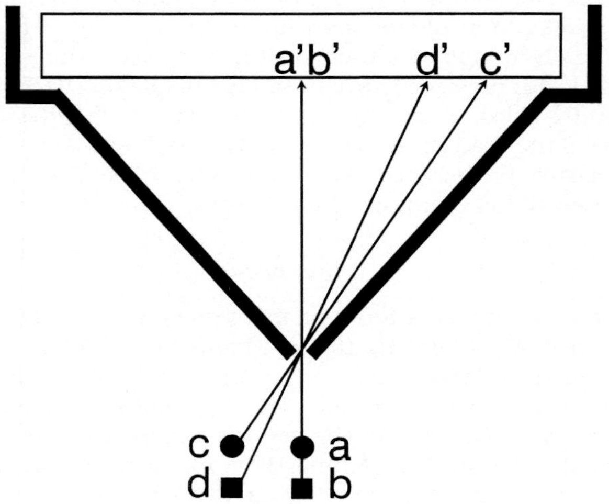

Figure 11.10. Diagram of a pinhole collimator illustrating sources of image distortion.

The pinhole collimator provides the capability for magnification while sacrificing counting efficiency. Some manufacturers offer different aperture sizes, with a diameter of 4–6 mm considered optimum. It should be noted that smaller aperture sizes provide improved resolution at the expense of reduced efficiency. Although the pinhole provides high spatial resolution because of its magnification property, the mechanism by which magnification is achieved also provides the potential for image distortion (Fig. 11.10). Photons from the center of the field of view pass through the collimator aperture and strike the crystal at a 90° angle. However, photons originating from areas other than the center pass through the aperture only if they are traveling at angles less than 90°. The angle decreases with increasing distance from the center of the field. This results in variations in superimposed information from the depth dimension that become very pronounced at the periphery of the field of view. Thus, apparent distortions in nodule location may result, and difficulties in precise nodule markings may be encountered (see section on Anatomic Markers).

PATIENT SCREENING

Before imaging a patient, it is important to screen the patient for necklaces, earrings, buttons, zippers, belt buckles, or other items of clothing that might interfere with the study. Since the photons used for diagnostic imaging studies are commonly low in energy (70–400 keV), these photons are attenuated easily by external objects, and this attenuation could result in the formation of artifacts in the final images. Additionally, any previous surgery related to the region of interest should be noted. Interpretation of images from a surgically altered organ is often difficult, and any information pertaining to the previous surgery that can be obtained from the patient may be helpful in the final image analysis.

PATIENT POSITIONING

Another factor affecting the quality of diagnostic imaging is patient positioning. Since typical nuclear medicine imaging procedures require 1–30 minutes of immobility at a time, it is important to make the patient as comfortable as possible to prevent movement during the study. Very often, patient immobilizers such as sandbags, Velcro strips, or adhesive tape are used to prevent movement. During imaging, the patient should be discouraged from any physical movement while the image acquisition is in progress to prevent degradation of the final images. Pediatric and uncooperative adult patients may require sedation. The use of VCRs for viewing by pediatric patients during imaging procedures has proven useful in occupying their attention to prevent excessive movement.

As stated in the previous section, it is desirable to image with the detector as close as possible to the patient because

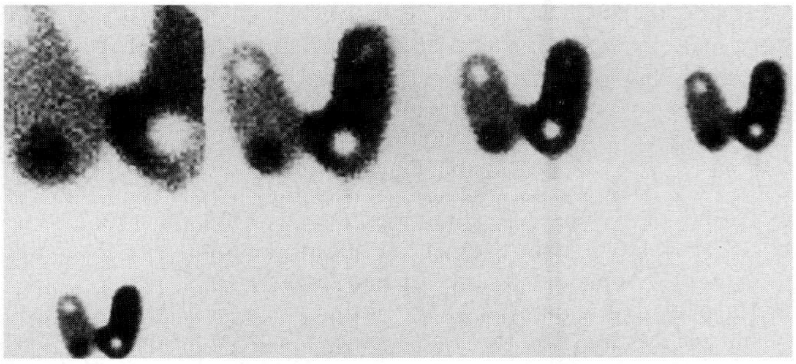

Figure 11.11. Images of a thyroid phantom with the pinhole collimator at distances of 0–4 inches from the collimator face.

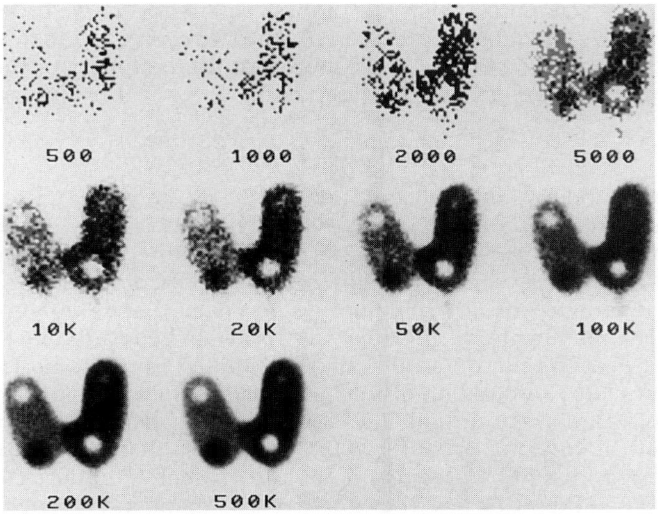

Figure 11.12. Images of a thyroid phantom with total counts of 500–500,000 illustrating the importance of adequate counts in thyroid imaging.

the resolution of any collimator decreases with distance. However, if the patient is positioned too close to a pinhole or converging collimator, the periphery of the region of interest may be distorted (Fig. 11.11). Many imaging laboratories use a standard distance marker for thyroid positioning. This distance is always used to obtain a reference image so that evaluations of gland size may be performed.

IMAGE ACQUISITION

High-quality diagnostic images can be obtained only when radiopharmaceutical distributions are imaged at the appropriate times. Important factors to consider in selecting the optimum time for imaging are the organ uptake characteristics of the radiopharmaceutical and its effective half-life in the organ. For example, thyroid uptake of ^{99m}Tc pertechnetate peaks at 20 minutes postinjection. This is the optimum time for imaging. In the case of orally administered ^{123}I, a delay of 4–8 hours is required before imaging for the radiopharmaceutical to be trapped by the thyroid. Trapping of ^{99m}Tc-labeled macroaggregated albumin by the lungs occurs on the first pass through the organ, so imaging may begin immediately after administration of the radiopharmaceutical.

In any imaging technique it is important to collect enough counts in an image to eliminate statistical variations and characterize as accurately as possible the radionuclide distribution. However, almost every imaging procedure in nuclear medicine involves a conflict between spatial resolution and counting efficiency. Thus, imaging generally becomes a matter of establishing a trade-off between the desired statistical image quality and the amount of imaging time that can be tolerated. Figure 11.12 demonstrates the effects of total counts on image quality using a thyroid phantom in a scattering medium. It can be observed from these images that image quality improves with increased counts—up to a point. In some situations, adequate counts can be obtained in a reasonable length of time (e.g., bone and liver). In other situations, statistics must be sacrificed for spatial resolution or acceptable imaging times (e.g., thyroid and exercise cardiac studies).

Diagnostic reports of imaging procedures in nuclear medicine are generated by physicians after viewing images of radiopharmaceutical distributions in the patient. Although this statement may appear trivial, the importance of good technique in imaging should be noted. Anterior, posterior, and lateral views should be true anterior, posterior, and lateral views and not modified obliques. Supplementary oblique views should be obtained and labeled when suspected abnormalities are not clearly identified and localized on routine views. For example, in imaging patients with suspected thyroid nodules, it is important to supplement the routine and labeled anterior view with left and right anterior obliques. These images provide additional information about the extent of the nodule and can be used to identify nodules that lie above or below normal thyroid tissue.

ANATOMIC MARKERS

Nuclear medicine imaging differs from computed tomography, magnetic resonance imaging, and ultrasound in that anatomic landmarks may not be obvious in the images because of preferential and specific uptake of the radiopharmaceutical. Thus, it becomes important to mark specific portions of the anatomy with "hot" or "cold" markers to provide anatomic references to aid physicians in interpreting the images. These markers also may be used for size determinations by having them calibrated for distance. It is a good practice to use a "hot" marker to label one side of the patient in views of symmetric organs, such as anterior or posterior brain and kidney images, to eliminate the possibility of mistaking left for right. All images should be clearly labeled by the technologist as to position and orientation. If there is any doubt as to orientation, checks should be made with "hot" markers to verify them. Marking of palpable thyroid nodules on radionuclide scans is a process that warrants careful attention. With the patient positioned for imaging, the physician should palpate the thyroid and outline with a marking pen any suspicious area. The technologist then may use a "hot" or "cold" marker placed over the nodule to determine its precise location. In both situations, when the pinhole collimator is used, the nodule should be centered in the field for one image so that the distortion effects associated with the periphery of the pinhole field of view are eliminated.

REPORTING RESULTS

On a referral basis, it is important for the consulting physician to discuss signs and symptoms of disease with the patient, explore the potential for conflicting medication, and possibly conduct a limited physical examination (e.g., of patients with thyroid nodules or localized sites of pain). The results of this endeavor may prove to be invaluable in the interpretation of the images obtained from the radionuclide examination. Clinical or surgical follow-up also is of value in continually assessing the diagnostic accuracy of the imaging procedures (5). In the new managed care environment, "outcomes data" are extremely important. Data evaluating how the course of treatment and response to therapy are altered by the information obtained from diagnostic procedures are essential in identifying proper procedures to be performed and in eliminating procedures which do not provide useful information (6).

It is only with careful attention to every detail in the diagnostic process that the physician can feel comfortable in his analysis, interpretation, and reporting of study results.

REFERENCES

1. Patton JA, Sandler MP. Quality assurance. In: Sandler MP, Patton JA, Partain CL, eds. Thyroid and parathyroid imaging. East Norwalk, CT: Appleton-Century-Crofts, 1985:77–93.
2. Davis DA, Giomuso CA, Miller WH, et al. Dose calibrator activity linearity evaluations with ALARA exposures. J Nucl Med Tech 1981;9:188–200.
3. Jaszczak RJ, Greer K, Coleman RE. SPECT system misalignment: comparison of phantom and patient images. In: Esser PD, ed. Emission computed tomography. New York: Society of Nuclear Medicine, 1983:57–70.
4. Erickson JJ, Rollo FD. Quality control of nuclear medicine computer systems. In: Erickson JJ, Rollo FD, eds. Digital nuclear medicine. Philadelphia: J.B. Lippincott, 1983:218–231.
5. Wagner HN. Standardization in medical diagnosis and reporting of results. In: Rhodes B, ed. Quality control in nuclear medicine. St. Louis: CV Mosby, 1977:45–52.
6. Lamki LM, Haynie TP, Podoloff DA, Kim EE. Quality assurance in a nuclear medicine department. Radiology 1990;177:609–614.

12 Quality Assurance of Correlative Systems

DAVID R. PICKENS, JAMES A. PATTON, and RONALD R. PRICE

QUALITY ASSURANCE

When a medical imaging procedure is performed, the technologists who operate the systems, the patients on whom the procedure is performed, and the physicians who review the images all assume that the instrumentation is performing at its design specifications and that the instrument has produced the best images it is capable of producing, given the selected imaging parameters, the positioning of the patient, and other factors. Furthermore, the same group of people who use and depend on the instrument assume that it will perform in the same fashion each time it is used, if the set circumstances of the imaging procedure are the same. The collected testing procedures and the documentation of those procedures and results to ensure consistency are known as the quality assurance program.

The purpose of a quality assurance (QA) program is to ensure that the diagnostic suitability of all images is maintained. A QA program includes monitoring all imaging procedures to ensure the proper and consistent operation of all equipment on a day-to-day basis, and includes standard tests designed to evaluate specific parameters of operation. These tests must be distinguished from equipment acceptance tests, which must be performed on delivery of new equipment and then repeated following major repairs. QA testing will detect deviations from baseline acceptance test results and long-term trends that could influence system performance. One should keep in mind that QA is the joint responsibility of the physician, the medical physicist, the technologist, and the service support personnel.

MAGNETIC RESONANCE IMAGING

IMAGING EVALUATION

As with any imaging modality, magnetic resonance imaging (MRI) requires a quality assurance program to ensure the maintenance of high-quality imaging performance. A variety of different types of phantoms (objects of known imaging characteristics) and techniques have been suggested for evaluating the daily performance of these systems (1). The American Association of Physicists in Medicine has produced guidelines for quality assurance programs in MRI with the goal of acquainting users with currently available phantoms and techniques for routine evaluations of image quality and equipment performance (2). Similar efforts are underway in conjunction with the American College of Radiology, which is seeking to standardize and accredit MRI facilities. Here we will acquaint the reader with the various parameters that should be evaluated on a routine basis in an ongoing QA program.

Performance parameters that must be evaluated routinely are:

1. Resonant frequency
2. Signal-to-noise ratio
3. Image uniformity
4. Spatial linearity
5. Spatial resolution
6. Slice thickness
7. Slice location.

Other parameters, such as quantitative determination of T_1, T_2, and proton density, may have clinical utility in the future, so routine evaluation of these parameters may be necessary as well. Also, as with any complex imaging system, the presence of artifacts should be noted and the cause determined before continuing to use the system clinically.

Frequency Check

Daily measurements of the resonant frequency should be performed to evaluate the stability of the primary magnetic field. This is done by tuning the system for maximum signal using a phantom that produces a strong nuclear magnetic resonance (NMR) signal. Several types of materials, primarily consisting of oils (1) and water solutions of various paramagnetic ions (3), have been used. The NMR parameters should approximate those of human tissue (i.e., $100 < T_1 < 1200$ msec, $50 < T_2 < 400$ msec, and proton density approximating that of water), noting that relaxation times are dependent on temperature and on field strength. Some typical examples of materials are shown in Table 12.1.

The Larmor equation can be used to calculate the magnetic field strength from the resonant frequency. Deviation of resonant frequency by more than 50 parts per million (ppm) between daily measurements requires that the cause of the change be investigated. Note that superconducting magnets normally exhibit a very slow downward trend in the resonant frequency due to the slow decay of the magnetic field; this is on the order of a few parts per million (<10) per day.

Signal-to-Noise Ratio

An important parameter that strongly affects image quality is signal-to-noise ratio, which can be influenced by a number of factors related to system calibration, gain, coil tuning and loading, and scan parameters. Generally, signal is defined as the difference in the average signal intensity over a signal-producing area (S_v) and the average background signal intensity measured in air (S_a). A measure of noise (N) often used is the standard deviation of signal intensity over the background area (air). Signal-to-noise ratio

Table 12.1.
NMR Parameters of Typical Phantom Materials at 0.5 Tesla

Material	Concentration	T1 msec	T2 msec
$CuSO_4$	1–25 mM	860–40	625–38
NiC_{12}	1–25 mM	806–59	763–66
1,2 Propanediol in distilled water	0–100%	2134–217	485–72

(S/N) is calculated by dividing the signal value by the noise value:

$$S/N = (S_v - S_a)/N$$

Since background may vary in the frequency and phase encoding directions, an alternative definition of noise that can be used is the standard deviation of signal intensity over the signal-producing area ($SD\ S_v$). Signal-to-noise ratio may then be calculated by:

$$S/N = S_v/(SD\ S_v)$$

Signal-to-noise ratio usually is calculated by imaging a disk phantom that is at least twice as long as the slice thickness and covers at least 80% of the image field, or 10 cm, whichever is larger (2). For multislice measurements, the recommended phantom length is the length of the volume to be imaged plus two slice thicknesses. If the phantom is filled with nonconducting material, as recommended by the AAPM Task Group No. 1 report, the measurements will be made in an "unloaded" coil and will, therefore, not simulate a clinical situation. Parameters specific to coil loading and coil tuning will require a special phantom designed to simulate the conductive/electric properties of the human body.

The measurement of signal-to-noise ratio is very sensitive to variations in overall system status and serves as an excellent technique for monitoring magnetic resonance image quality. The recommended method described by Task Group No. 1 is likely to be the method of choice for most sites.

Image Uniformity

Currently available MRI systems provide highly uniform magnetic fields with nonuniformities of a few parts per million throughout the imaging volume. The use of specialized equipment is required to directly measure the uniformity of the magnetic field. However, of more importance in imaging is the uniformity of the images that are routinely obtained. Image uniformity can be evaluated subjectively on a regular basis by imaging a uniform disk phantom (Fig. 12.1). An inspection of the image obtained gives a visual estimate of uniformity. Numerical data can be obtained by analyzing the phantom images using the region of interest (ROI) function available on all imagers. Routine measurements such as these should be performed using a reproducible geometry and a constant technique such as a spin-echo 500/30 pulse sequence. A measure of integral uniformity (2) can be calculated from the data in Figure 12.1**A** by:

$$\text{Image Uniformity} = \left(1 - \frac{S_{max} - S_{min}}{S_{max} + S_{min}}\right) \times 100\%$$

where S_{max} and S_{min} are the maximum and minimum signal intensities in the image. Using this relationship, 100% represents perfect integral uniformity. Estimates of S_{max} and S_{min} can be obtained manually using the window and level functions on the scanner console.

The measurement of operating frequency and image uniformity are the minimum recommendations for routine daily quality assurance. They do not begin to evaluate all of the imaging capabilities of any instrument; however, they provide a quick analysis of the operational status of the system.

Spatial Linearity

Spatial linearity is the ability of an imaging system to precisely reproduce a distribution without geometric distortions. Suggested phantoms for evaluating this parameter center on the concept that images of straight-line distributions should yield straight lines. Deviations from straight lines are documentation of spatial nonlinearities or distortions. Orthogonal holes, line grids, and bar patterns may be used to evaluate spatial linearity in both two-dimensional and three-dimensional imaging techniques.

The percent distortion can be found by subtracting the value found for the dimensions of the phantom measured on the image from the known dimensions divided by the known dimension times 100%. In general, for relatively large fields of view, the distortions would be expected to be less than 5%.

Spatial Resolution

Spatial resolution refers to the ability of an imaging system to separate (resolve) small objects placed close together. In MRI, spatial resolution is determined by pixel size. For example, using a 256 mm field of view and imaging by encoding frequency and phase in 256 increments, the size of a pixel is 256/256 or 1 mm in both the frequency- and phase-encoding directions. Spatial resolution can be measured using phantoms with multiple signal-producing cylinders or lines of varying sizes and separations (Fig. 12.2). The spatial resolution is defined as the smallest objects that can be visually separated.

AAPM Task Group No. 1 recommends that high-contrast spatial resolution be measured using a phantom having either collections of rods or holes of varying sizes spaced so the appearance is of alternating signal and non-signal-producing material. The recommended sizes range from 5 mm to 0.5 mm or smaller, depending on the capabilities of the instrument and the design of the phantom. The rods should be at least twice as long as the slice thickness to be measured. In use, the phantom should be aligned so that the rods are perpendicular to the specified slice. The resolution of the machine is determined by the smallest full line of rods that can be seen in the image.

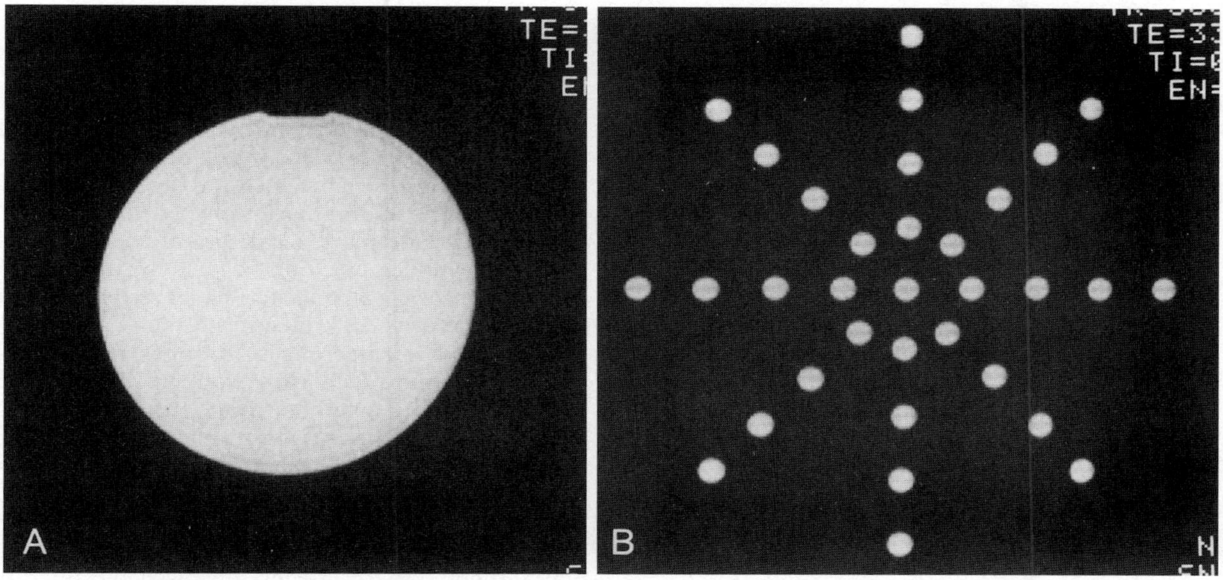

Figure 12.1. Images of a uniform disk phantom (**A**) and a phantom of discrete signal-producing cylinders (**B**) for uniformity measurements. (Reproduced by permission from Sandler MP, Patton JA, Shaff MI, Powers TA, Partain CL. Correlative imaging: nuclear medicine, magnetic resonance, computed tomography, ultrasound. Baltimore: Williams and Wilkins, 1989.)

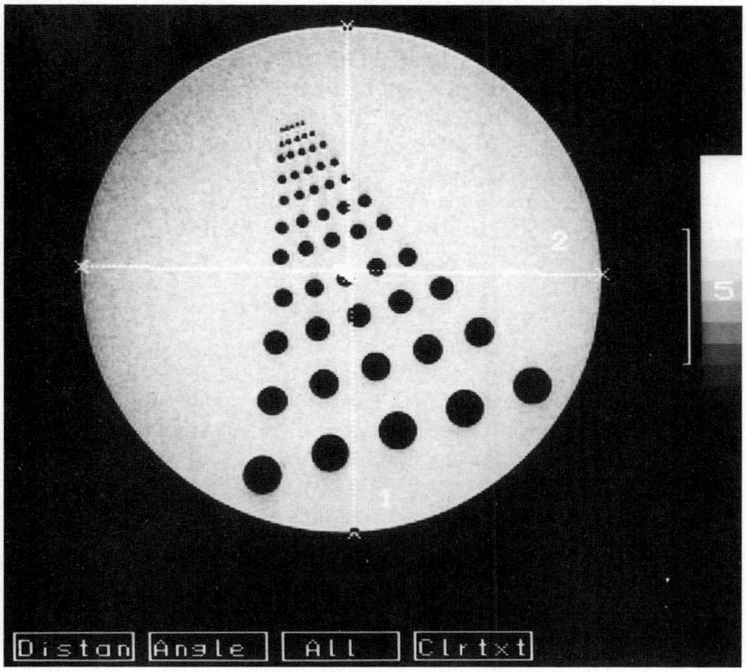

Figure 12.2. Measurement of spatial resolution using a phantom consisting of plastic rods of decreasing size and spacing.

Slice Thickness

The correct slice thickness, defined as the full width at half maximum (FWHM) of a slice profile, is important in routine imaging to interpret patient studies and evaluate potential abnormalities. Variations of the slant-line, slant-plane, continuous-wedge, and step-wedge concepts have been used for these measurements. The step-wedge measurement entails imaging a phantom that contains incremental steps of a signal-producing material (2 mm steps, for example) and plotting the difference in signal intensity between adjacent steps. The FWHM of this plot yields a measure of slice thickness (Fig. 12.3).

The AAPM Task Group No. 1 recommendation is for the use of opposing ramp pairs oriented at a fixed angle with respect to each other (Fig. 12.4). If the orientation angle is 90°, the calculation of the slice thickness at FWHM is the geometric mean of the slice profiles seen on the image. In general, the slice thickness should be within ±1 mm for slice thicknesses >5 mm.

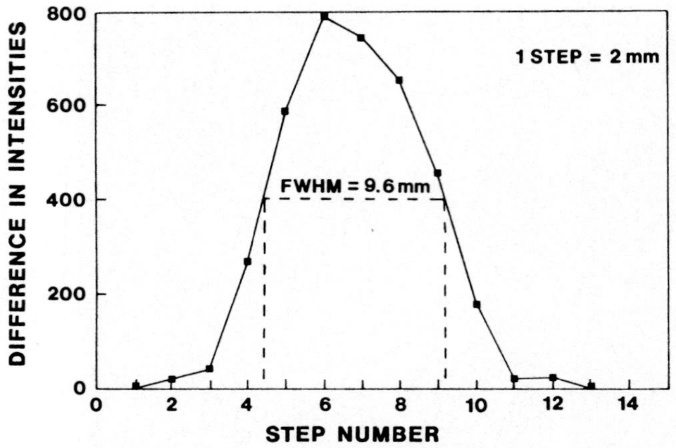

Figure 12.3. Measurement of slice thickness using a discrete step-wedge phantom. (Reproduced by permission from Sandler MP, Patton JA, Shaff MI, Powers TA, Partain CL. Correlative imaging: nuclear medicine, magnetic resonance, computed tomography, ultrasound. Baltimore: Williams and Wilkins, 1989.)

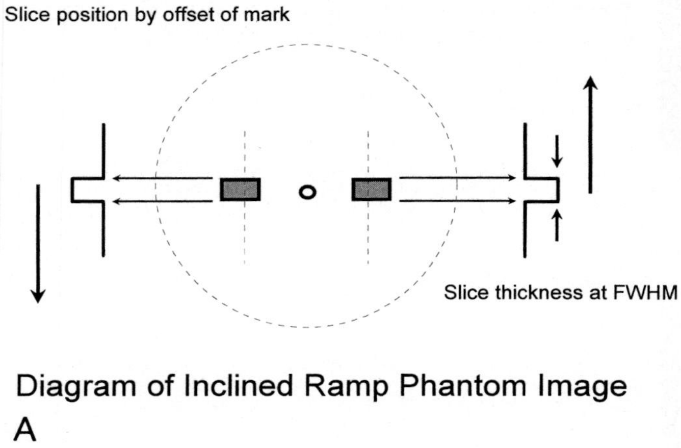

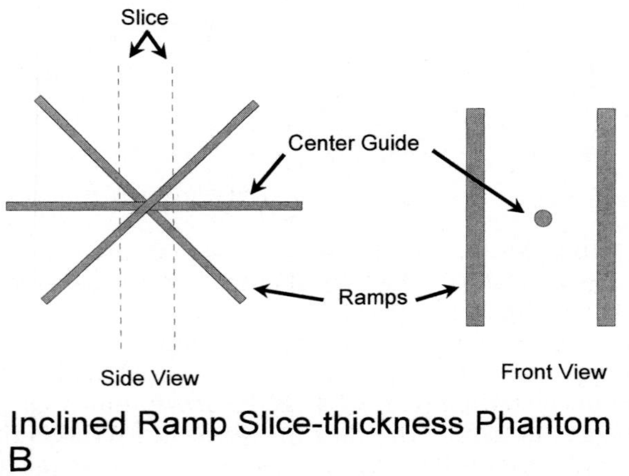

Figure 12.4. **A.** Inclined ramp phantom recommended by AAPM Task Group No. 1. **B.** Diagram of image from inclined ramp phantom.

Slice Location

The accuracy of slice localization and distance between slices for multislice techniques is also of great importance for image interpretation. One method used in nuclear medicine tomography, as well as in computed tomography, for performing these measurements is the spiral-line phantom (Fig. 12.5). This phantom consists of a double-helix formed with tubing containing signal-producing material wound around a cylinder 18 cm in height. The helix is wound so that 10° of arc corresponds to 1 cm of vertical distance. Two vertical lines are placed on opposite sides of the cylinder to serve as position references. A transverse section image through the phantom yields two high-intensity spots corresponding to the points at which the image plane passes through the two arms of the helix, as well as two additional spots corresponding to the intersections with the vertical lines (Fig. 12.6). In images of subsequent slices, the line connecting the first two spots will rotate about the center in direct proportion to the displacement of each slice. The actual displacement of each slice is determined by measuring the amount of rotation and calculating the slice position from the known pitch (1 cm/10°) of the phantom.

The AAPM recommends using an inclined ramp phantom, which can also be used for slice thickness measurement. To use the dual ramp, alignment marks must be available on the phantom so that it can be properly positioned in the magnet with respect to the external alignment systems. The displacement of the ramp image from the center alignment rod will indicate the slice position. In general, the external reference markers should agree with the slice position within ±2 mm. Slice separation, which can be measured as well, should be within 20% of the specified separation or ±1 mm, whichever is greater.

ARTIFACTS

There are many causes of artifacts in MRI procedures that may present problems in the interpretation of images from routine patient procedures. Some sources of artifacts can be tested for as part of a QA program, while others are related to individual scan conditions and individual patients. The causes of all of these artifacts must be understood and

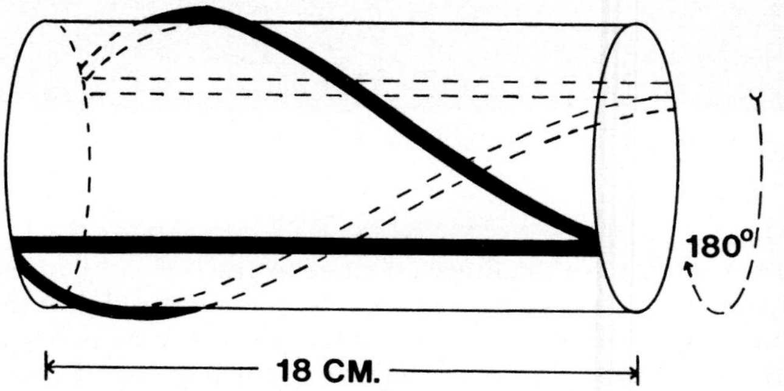

Figure 12.5. Spiral-line phantom for slice localization measurements. (Reproduced by permission from Sandler MP, Patton JA, Shaff MI, Powers TA, Partain CL. Correlative imaging: nuclear medicine, magnetic resonance, computed tomography, ultrasound. Baltimore: Williams and Wilkins, 1989.)

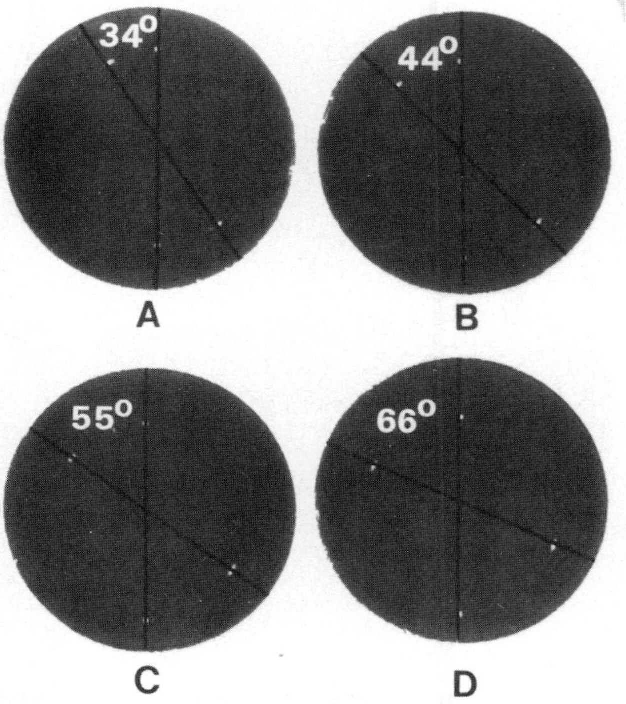

Figure 12.6. Four adjacent transverse slices (**A-D**) through the spiral-line phantom in Figure12.5. (Reproduced by permission from Sandler MP, Patton JA, Shaff MI, Powers TA, Partain CL. Correlative imaging: nuclear medicine, magnetic resonance, computed tomography, ultrasound. Baltimore: Williams and Wilkins, 1989.)

eliminated, if possible, so that correct interpretations may be obtained. Artifacts may be grouped into three categories: those internal to the patient, those external to the patient, and those that are due to system failures or are inherent in the data collection and image reconstruction techniques that are used with MRI systems.

Internal Sources

As with most imaging modalities, patient motion degrades magnetic resonance images. It is extremely important that the patient does not move while data collection is in progress, a timeframe of 1–15 minutes. The effect of patient motion is an overall reduction in image quality with a marked blurring or ghosting in the y or phase-encoding direction. Respiratory and cardiac motion can also severely degrade image quality during an MRI study. Physiologic motion in the frequency-encoding or x direction results in a blurring between the limits of excursion. Periodic physiologic motion results in multiple ghost structures in the phase-encoding or y direction, due to the development of a coherence between the number of gradient steps being used in the imaging procedure and the frequency of the motion. It has been shown that the higher the frequency of motion or the longer the time between changes in the phase encoding, the farther apart the ghosts. On the other hand, the separation is decreased by decreasing either the length of the phase-encoding gradient or the amount by which the phase-encoding gradient is incremented (4).

External Sources

Sources of artifacts that are external to the patient generally are due to items of clothing. All patients should be screened for jewelry, metal buttons, zippers, belt buckles, etc. that may alter the uniformity of the magnetic field and distort the images obtained. For body imaging, it usually is advisable to have the patient disrobe and put on a hospital gown or pajamas.

Placement of ECG leads also is of importance in MRI. Although nonferromagnetic leads are available, they still should be placed as far from the imaging volume as possible to eliminate the possibility of interference.

System Sources

There are many potential sources of artifacts that may be caused either by malfunctions of the imaging system or simply by peculiarities of the data acquisition and image reconstruction process.

Several phase artifacts that can be evaluated with phantoms should be looked for during routine QC programs. These errors are "ghosting" due to phase-encoding gradient errors and due to transmit and receive radiofrequency quadrature phase problems. These ghosts appear as increases in signal in areas where none was expected.

RF receiver quadrature errors can be identified using a disk phantom with a signal-producing object that is offset from the center of the disk. The errors appear to be objects similar to the real object with reduced intensity, but located on the diagonal on the opposite side of the image field. Evaluation of the artifact is made by finding the percent difference from the true object. The ghost should be less than 5% of the true (2).

ULTRASOUND

Ultrasound QA measurements can be separated into those that evaluate imaging performance and those that evaluate the ultrasound beam. This section will consider overall image production parameters that can be evaluated during daily QA.

PERFORMANCE PARAMETERS

Performance parameters that should be measured on a routine basis are:

1. Gray scale photography
2. Relative sensitivity
3. Axial resolution
4. Lateral resolution
5. Dead zone
6. Depth and distance accuracy
7. Time-gain-compensation accuracy.

Numerous test objects and instruments are now available for assessing the performance of ultrasonic equipment. Various documents contain detailed protocols for establishing a QA program (5). At present, the single most versatile and complete test object to be used in these studies is the American Institute of Ultrasound in Medicine

(AIUM) Standard 100 mm Test Object (Fig. 12.7). The AIUM phantom consists of five sets of wire groups (sets A-E), each designed to test a specific image parameter: set A, axial resolution; set B, lateral resolution; set C, vertical distance accuracy; set D, dead zone; and set E, horizontal distance accuracy. In addition to evaluation of the gray scale system, the AIUM Test Object may be used to assess each of the other system parameters. The minimal QA program provides relative parameter values. Relative values are useful for detecting early changes in image system characteristics. Absolute measurements of system parameters are more difficult and may require additional test objects and equipment. These standards should be developed and published, and equipment should be monitored to determine if specifications are met.

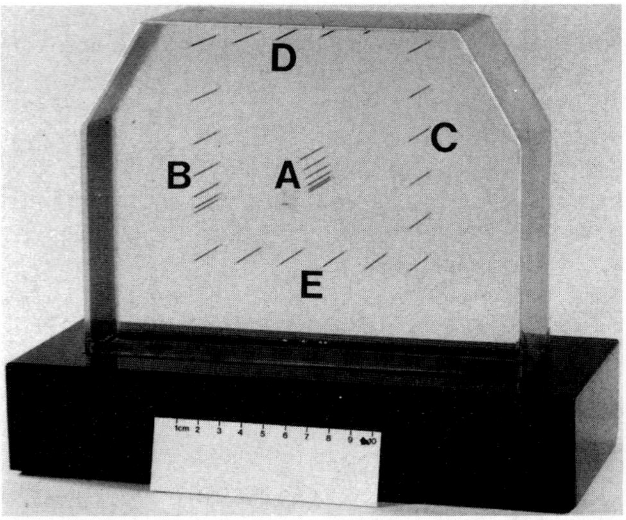

Figure 12.7. AIUM test phantom for use with ultrasound imagers. (Reproduced by permission from Sandler MP, Patton JA, Shaff MI, Powers TA, Partain CL. Correlative imaging: nuclear medicine, magnetic resonance, computed tomography, ultrasound. Baltimore: Williams and Wilkins, 1989.)

Gray Scale Photography

The initial camera settings or scan converter output controls depend largely on individual points of reference. Once a baseline has been established, a daily evaluation should be made to ensure that the same range of echo amplitudes can be seen as on previous test exposures. Most systems now generate gray scale bars that are displayed to one side or at the bottom of the image. This bar should be examined daily for consistency of step distribution and display. A comparison can be made either by visual inspection or, more accurately, with the aid of an optical densitometer.

Relative Sensitivity

A simple test for sensitivity stability can be performed with the aid of the AIUM phantom. After carefully positioning the transducer directly above the reference wires spaced 2 cm apart (wire set C) with the transducer face flat against the phantom surface, the system gain (attenuation or output) settings should be adjusted to display a one-division echo from the most distant wire. The gain settings required to yield a discernible echo in the B-mode image should not change with time. By this method, the stability of the instrumentation over time can be determined.

Dead Zone, Resolution, and Other Parameters

A single B-mode image of the AIUM phantom (Figs. 12.8**A-C**) will provide data regarding dead zone and axial resolution, as well as the accuracy and linearity of the distance in the set of diagonal wires at the center of the phantom. The dead zone is defined as the depth of the wire nearest to the surface that can be resolved in the image (set D). Axial resolution is defined as the minimum separation of wires in set A that can be detected.

Lateral resolution is defined in a similar manner; however, a second scan taken along the vertical face next to wire set B is required. Current state-of-the-art instruments should present axial and lateral resolutions in the focal zone that are 2 mm or better. The accuracy and linearity of the system-generated distance markers can be evaluated by a direct measurement of the distances of the vertical and horizontal wires from a B-mode image (wire sets C and E). The distance between the uppermost and bottom wires in the 2-cm-spaced group actually is 10 cm, and this distance, estimated by the markers, should not differ by more than 2 mm (20%).

In addition to the AIUM phantom (which uses a relatively nonattenuating medium), there are a number of tissue-equivalent phantoms on the market that can be used to check the performance of the instruments when presented with a more realistic attenuating material. These phantoms are particularly good for evaluating instrument output, depth of penetration, and calibration of the time-gain-compensation controls.

DOPPLER SYSTEMS

Doppler ultrasound systems require additional measurements beyond those discussed for conventional systems. The parameters that should be verified in the operation of Doppler systems include Doppler sensitivity, Doppler frequency resolution, and Doppler time resolution. Additionally, display of fluid acceleration and deceleration and time versus ECG misalignments should be evaluated. For color Doppler imaging systems, proper performance in the presence of rapidly changing particle (blood) velocity is important. These additional measurements require phantoms simulating flowing blood in some way.

Phantoms that simulate moving blood and the appropriate variations in the velocity waveform that would be found in a clinical situation are available commercially. Many of these phantoms use a moving string immersed in a water bath. This design permits evaluation of continuous wave and pulsed Doppler systems at continuous and varying velocities consistent with pulsatile flow, which can be specified from front panel controls. In general, these moving string phantoms have been found to be more accepta-

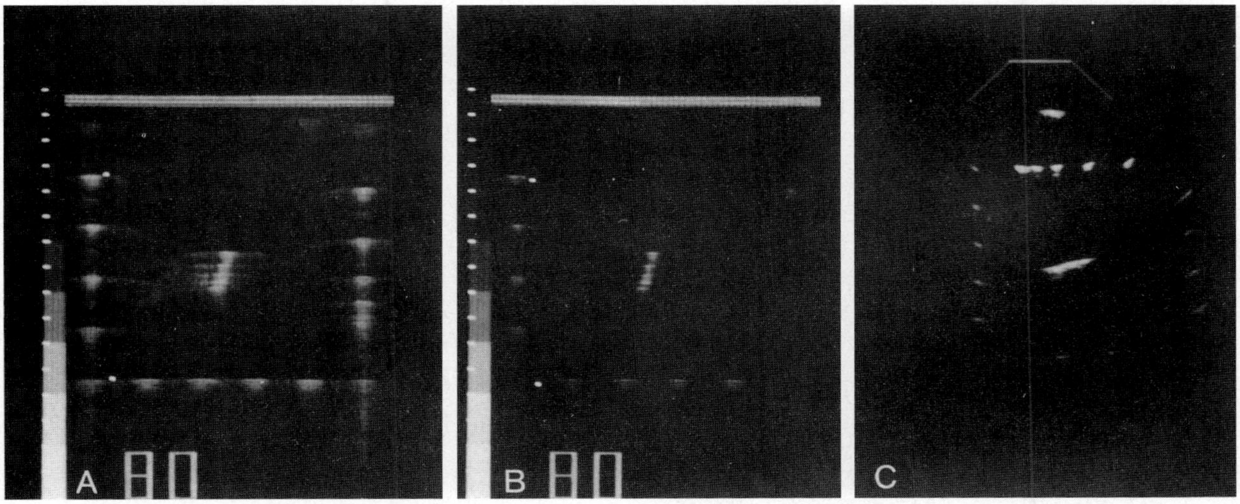

Figure 12.8. **A.** Image of AIUM phantom showing dead zone measurements using wire group D. **B.** Axial resolution using wire group A. **C.** Lateral resolution using wire group B with scan rotated 90°. (Reproduced by permission from Sandler MP, Patton JA, Shaff MI, Powers TA, Partain CL. Correlative imaging: nuclear medicine, magnetic resonance, computed tomography, ultrasound. Baltimore: Williams and Wilkins, 1989.)

ble for QA purposes and much less trouble than older systems using simulated blood pumped through tubing. Designs based on moving fluids suffer from difficulties in determining the magnitude and direction of echogenic particles in the simulated blood. Additionally, the distribution of particles cannot be determined during operation of the phantom, and particles can lose their echogenic properties over time.

COMPUTED TOMOGRAPHY

IMAGING EVALUATION

Several parameters are considered to be of importance in evaluating the performance of a CT system for routine quality assurance (7–16). Some of these evaluations are performed as part of the startup procedures each morning and are designed to detect changes in performance characteristics before they become clinically significant problems.

Performance characteristics that should be checked regularly are:

1. System noise and water value (daily)
2. Uniformity of CT values (daily)
3. Slice thickness and position (weekly)
4. Spatial resolution (weekly)
5. Low-contrast deductibility (weekly)
6. Presence of artifacts (daily).

The characteristics of the scanner are evaluated using phantoms designed for one or more tests of the system. Often the manufacturer of the scanner will provide a set of phantoms for QA testing. If this is not the case, phantoms are available from several companies specializing in radiographic imaging support equipment. The American Association of Physicists in Medicine (AAPM) phantom has been widely used in the evaluation of CT scanners, but it is bulky and must be filled with water. Other phantoms are available commercially that use plastic materials designed to have x-ray attenuation characteristics similar to water.

In most cases, the QA procedure can be performed very quickly once the appropriate phantom is positioned. For those phantoms designed to work with a particular scanner, there usually is an alignment jig that holds them properly. Otherwise, the person performing the tests must follow the recommendations of the phantom manufacturer to position the phantom.

System Noise and Water Value

System noise is important to understand and measure, because noise often is the limiting factor in CT images. Noise refers to random fluctuations in the image and is usually due to the statistical nature of the generation and absorption of x-rays. Such noise is called quantum noise. Other sources of noise include electronic noise in the analog sections of the imaging chain and round-off errors in the reconstruction algorithms. The low-frequency characteristics of the convolution filter selected by the operator also affect the noise content.

To evaluate noise in the image, a uniform water phantom is usually specified. The water phantom consists of a cylindrical container about 22 cm in diameter (30 cm for body imaging) and several centimeters thick. The phantom is scanned using the recommended radiographic technique specified by the manufacturer of the scanner. The standard deviation of the pixel values within an ROI in the water is computed using the ROI program available on all scanners (Fig. 12.9). This value ordinarily is multiplied by 100% and divided by the range of the CT scale to obtain the noise value, often called the precision of the machine. For a standard deviation of 20 on a scanner with a range of values of −1000 to 3000, the noise value is ±0.25%, a value typical of many CT scanners.

From the same image, the value can be obtained for the CT number assigned to water. This calibration is checked

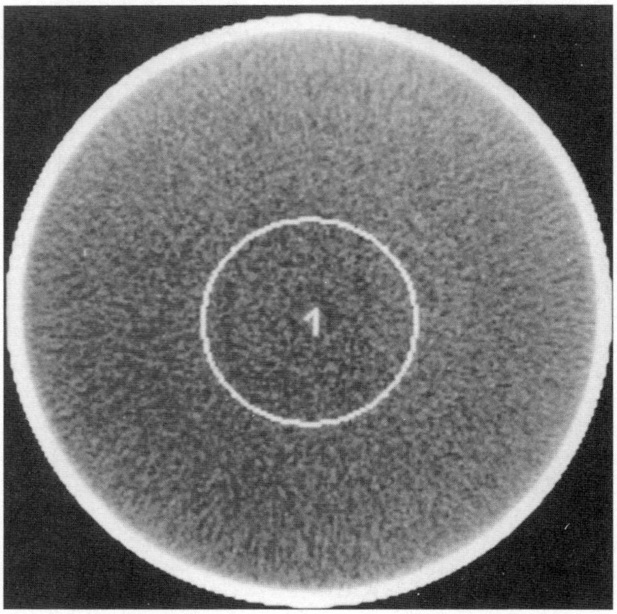

Figure 12.9. Image of CT water phantom with a circular region of interest selected in the center. (Reproduced by permission from Sandler MP, Patton JA, Shaff MI, Powers TA, Partain CL. Correlative imaging: nuclear medicine, magnetic resonance, computed tomography, ultrasound. Baltimore: Williams and Wilkins, 1989.)

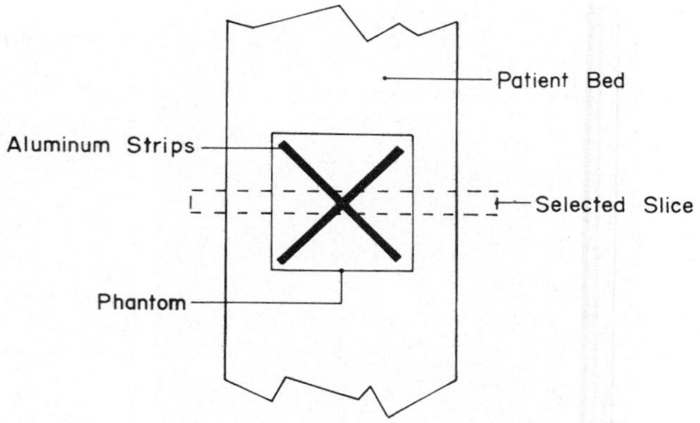

Figure 12.10. Orientation of the crossed aluminum strips in a phantom designed to measure the slice thickness of a CT scanner. (Reproduced by permission from Sandler MP, Patton JA, Shaff MI, Powers TA, Partain CL. Correlative imaging: nuclear medicine, magnetic resonance, computed tomography, ultrasound. Baltimore: Williams and Wilkins, 1989.)

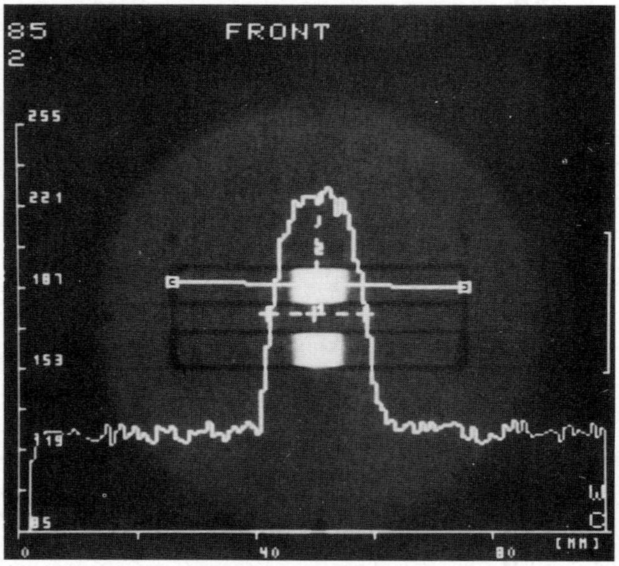

Figure 12.11. Image of slice thickness phantom during slice thickness determination. The full width at half maximum (FWHM) is taken from the profile of intensities across the top strip in this image. (Reproduced by permission from Sandler MP, Patton JA, Shaff MI, Powers TA, Partain CL. Correlative imaging: nuclear medicine, magnetic resonance, computed tomography, ultrasound. Baltimore: Williams and Wilkins, 1989.)

easily and is important to verify because all attenuation values are normalized to the attenuation value of water. The center of the CT number scale (also called the Hounsfield scale) is specified as 0.0 plus or minus a range that is a characteristic of the scanner design. With some systems, it is also appropriate to obtain a value for air by scanning an open gantry. This value can be used with the value for water to check the calibration of the CT numbers.

Also from the same image, information about the spatial linearity of the system can be obtained. This is found by taking several regions across the water bath image, usually vertically and horizontally, recording the mean pixel value for each region, and plotting the regions on a graph of position versus mean value. There should be little or no difference in the mean values at any comparable-size region in the image. Deviation of the values around the periphery of the phantom is an indication of problems requiring further evaluation by a service engineer.

Slice Thickness Evaluation

Slice thickness determination is an important part of the QA procedure, since slice thickness affects both the quantum noise present in the image and the voxel resolution due to partial volume effects. Slice thickness phantoms commonly are crossed aluminum or plastic strips mounted at a known angle with respect to one another (usually 90°), immersed in water. The *X* formed by the strips is positioned parallel to the patient bed so that the slice to be measured falls within the body of the *X* (Fig. 12.10). The full width at half maximum (FWHM) of the density of the strip in the image is measured on the screen using the ROI. An intensity profile is generated, and the FWHM intensity is found. An image of such a phantom is shown in Figure 12.11. The FWHM multiplied by a scale factor related to the inclination of the strips is a measure of the slice thickness. For a 90° opening angle of the *X*, the strips are mounted at 45° with respect to the slice. In this case, the scale factor is equal to 1, and the FWHM is the slice thickness. When using a system that does not provide the capability to produce a profile plot, it is possible to set the window controls for a very narrow window (1 gray level) and to move the level up and down while observing the change in the width of the image. An approximation of the FWHM value can be obtained this way. Changes in slice thickness values can indicate problems with collimation of the system or with component alignment.

Spatial Resolution

Spatial resolution can be estimated visually from scan images of line-pair phantoms. Line-pair phantoms are constructed of alternating radiopaque and radiotranslucent strips embedded in plastic or water. These phantoms have several line-pair groups of different widths to provide several spatial frequencies. Scans are performed, and the smallest line-pair section that can be resolved in an image is taken as an estimate of the spatial resolution of the system (Fig. 12.12). Instead of line-pairs, groups of holes of decreasing sizes can be used. The holes are filled with air and are drilled in acrylic plastic, so they represent moderately high contrast. Spatial resolution is estimated by the size of the smallest holes that can be seen by an observer. Neither type of phantom will provide the true limiting spatial resolution for the system.

As part of the QA procedure on some scanners, the modulation transfer function (MTF) can be calculated. The MTF is a graph of the ratio of the output (image) information to the input (object) information for all spatial frequencies. The MTF provides an indication of the response of the system to increasing spatial frequencies and is a more accurate indicator of the ultimate spatial resolution of the scanner than line-pair phantoms. The MTF is derived from the scan of a thin wire. A profile across the wire provides the line spread function necessary for calculation of the MTF. On scanners that compute the MTF, software is provided to assist the user. If such software is not available, finding the MTF will not be practical as a routine QA procedure.

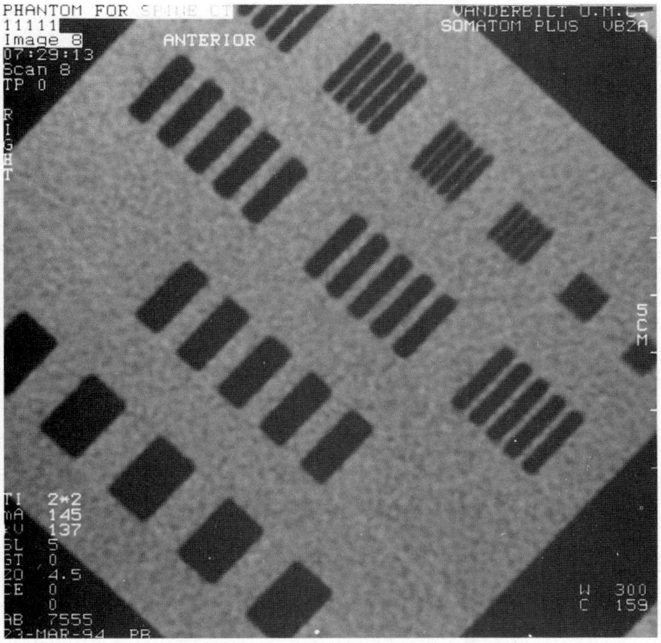

Figure 12.12. Line-pair section of CT phantom used for determining the spatial resolution of the system. The estimated spatial resolution is determined from observing the most closely spaced line-pairs that can be seen distinctly.

An example of a thin-wire image and the resulting MTF plot is shown in Figure 12.13.

Low-Contrast Detectability

Low-contrast detectability is an important parameter that should be measured regularly, because it reflects the ability of the scanner to provide visualization of subtle differences in tissue and is directly related to the noise levels in the scan. A phantom design for performing low-contrast detectability studies consists of water-equivalent plastic into which a series of plastic pins, which have attenuation characteristics similar to those of the surrounding material, are inserted. These pins are arranged in groups of varying sizes, the smallest of which is 2 or 3 mm in diameter. Pins in a group often are arranged so that the center-to-center distance between like-sized pins is twice the pin diameter. Contrast differences between the surrounding medium and the pins typically are about 0.5% ±0.1%. Often a range of contrasts is provided by using different densities of pins. Comparison is made between the pins that can be seen in the scan and the surrounding regions under specified acquisition conditions. An example of the type of image provided by this phantom is shown in Figure 12.14. An alternate design uses plastic with water-filled holes of varying sizes. Sometimes, provision is made to fill the holes with different solutions to simulate a variety of contrasts.

Artifacts

Throughout the QA procedures and during routine imaging, the operator should be aware of image artifacts. Artifacts are observed for a variety of reasons and should be identified as not being related to a machine malfunction before the scanning is resumed. Different designs of systems will exhibit characteristic artifacts under certain conditions of patient geometry and scan protocol. These should be recognized by the operators. Other artifacts are characteristic of a malfunction in the system (such as the ring artifacts seen in third-generation systems with a failed detector). An awareness of the expected appearance of images, whether they are from a phantom or a patient, will help in the detection of problems that require service of the system.

FILM IMAGERS

Film imagers are integral parts of CT systems, as well as of other digital imaging systems. These devices are usually based on a digitally controlled laser with the appropriate film-handling equipment that transfers selected images from collected data sets to film for later viewing on a light box. The typical laser imager is adjusted at the time of scanner installation to match the characteristics of the film that will be used and the type of data available from the CT scanner's computer. Since film imagers are an important part of the CT scanner and receive significant use, it is important to assess their performance routinely.

In the early 1980s, the Society of Motion Picture and Television Engineers (SMPTE) formed a committee to evaluate medical imagers and the films developed for them.

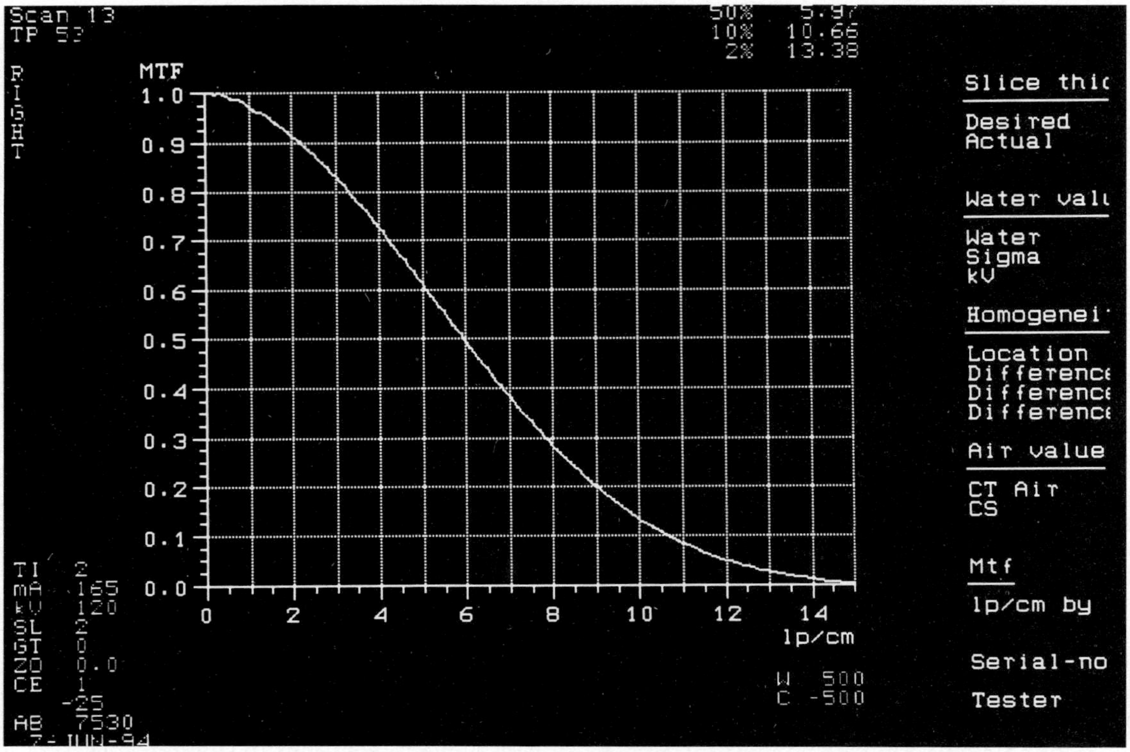

Figure 12.13. Scan of thin wire (**A**) and MTF plot (**B**) which is calculated from the wire image. The MTF plot is a good indicator of system resolution performance.

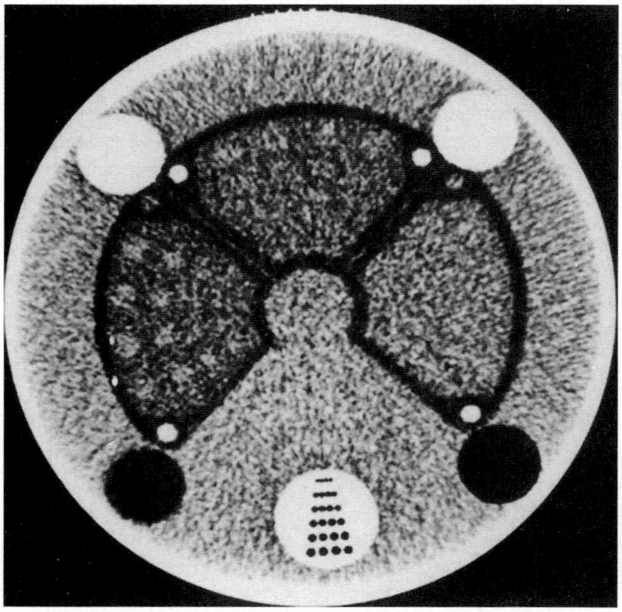

Figure 12.14. Low-contrast deductibility phantom showing decreasing sizes of plastic pins in a plastic block. A spatial resolution insert consisting of holes of decreasing sizes is seen at the bottom of the image. (Reproduced by permission from Sandler MP, Patton JA, Shaff MI, Powers TA, Partain CL. Correlative imaging: nuclear medicine, magnetic resonance, computed tomography, ultrasound. Baltimore: Williams and Wilkins, 1989.)

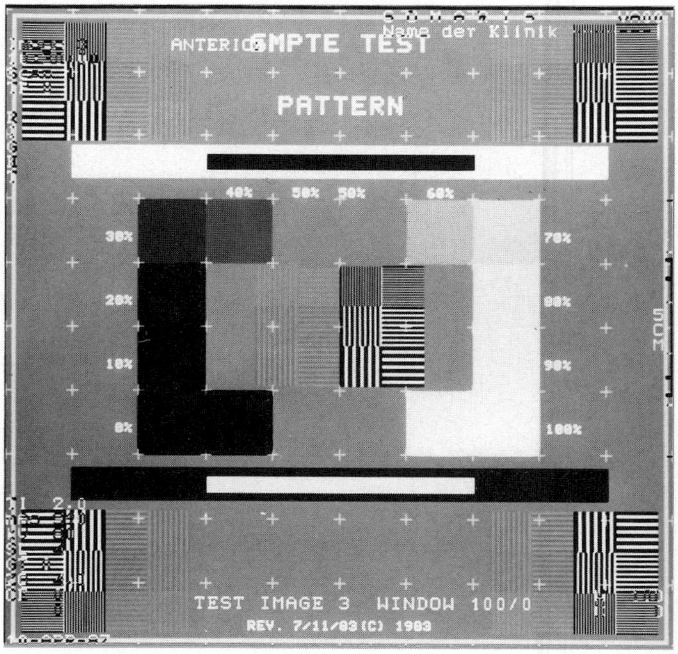

Figure 12.15. Image of STMP test pattern generated by CT scanner as part of routine QA test procedures. Normal identifying text from the CT scanner is superimposed on the test pattern.

This committee designed a test pattern, usually known as the SMPTE test pattern, that can be used for acceptance testing and routine QA of the imager and film. The pattern contains high and low contrast areas arranged in symmetric patterns to enable quick evaluation of the image quality being produced by the imager. This pattern has been accepted widely and is often incorporated as part of an automated test procedure on CT systems. Many laser cameras internally generate the test pattern. Figure12.15 shows the SMPTE test pattern produced by a scanner for testing the connected film imager.

The use of the SMPTE test pattern should be part of any QA program. It is recommended that the pattern be produced on film daily and the image be reviewed for artifacts and other problems (16, 17). Additionally, a densitometer should be used to evaluate parts of the image with known densities for some of the formats that are used routinely. On a monthly basis, a more comprehensive evaluation of the pattern at different formats can be performed. These values can be plotted daily on control charts for continuous monitoring of image quality.

A good QA program must be in place for the processors used for developing film. Such programs evaluate the consistency and operational characteristics of processor systems by evaluating temperature, processing speed, replenisher operation, and other parameters related to proper film processing. Improper development can degrade image quality significantly and render other efforts at QA useless.

MECHANICAL PROPERTIES AND RADIATION DOSE

Attention to the mechanical operation of the CT scanner is important as part of ongoing QA procedures. In particular, the functioning of the patient alignment system and the patient bed index should be observed each time the system is used. Routine evaluation of patient positioning is especially important when thin-slice modes of operation are part of the clinical protocols. Systems with automatic QA procedures often will include measurement of bed index and position accuracy. Most of the other electromechanical systems will be tested in the course of performing the QA phantom studies.

It is important to know the expected radiation exposure for a variety of examinations performed by the system, but the dosage is not measured during routine QA procedures. Likewise, scattered radiation ordinarily is not evaluated in the course of routine QA, although it is relatively easy to measure using an ionization chamber positioned near a phantom that is being scanned. Both dosage and scatter should be evaluated during acceptance testing and after major repairs to the system.

Quality assurance should be performed on a regular basis and records should be kept to enable the operators to detect long-term trends. Most of the procedures and tests mentioned earlier can be done daily, and should certainly be done at least weekly. In particular, system noise, water value, uniformity of CT values, and spatial resolution can be tested daily with the proper phantoms without taking a significant amount of time. Most modern instruments will perform routine QA scans automatically once the QA phantom that comes with the machine is properly placed. At the end of the procedure, the results can be transferred to film or printed so that QA records can be reviewed at a later date. Other evaluations, such as low-contrast detectability, can be performed on a daily or weekly basis as recommended by the manufacturer or as a matter of institutional policy.

SUMMARY

The actual schedule of performing the QA tests on individual instruments will depend on the machine usage and other factors, but under no circumstances should routine tests be ignored. Quality assurance requires that the users of the systems think about what they are doing and monitor the system's performance with phantoms. Observation and awareness of the way the machine functions are the hallmarks of a satisfactory operating environment and enable the system to provide the best possible clinical performance.

Of equal importance to the actual performance testing is documentation of results. These recorded data are essential for accurate monitoring of equipment performance and are useful to both the service personnel and equipment manufacturer. Additionally, documentation of the results of all QA procedures is required by government regulatory and certifying agencies.

Finally, the QA procedures and documentation must be viewed as only part of a total quality management approach within the imaging environment. QA procedures describe tests that determine how the imaging machines are functioning on a regular basis, but also of importance is the documentation of the actions to be taken as a result of a QA evaluation that is outside of documented action levels. The methods for evaluating the instrument are described, the point at which the evaluations are not within specifications are documented, the actions to be taken in the event of an unsatisfactory QA evaluation are described, and the documentation of the actions taken to bring the QA evaluation back into the normal operating range, all are critical parts for maintaining a properly functioning imaging system. The ultimate goal of total quality management is to maintain action levels as tight as possible in order to obtain the best imaging performance.

REFERENCES

1. Price RR, Patton JA, Erickson JJ, et al. Concepts of quality assurance and phantom design for NMR systems. In: Thomas SR, Dixon RL, eds. Medical physics monograph No. 14, NMR in medicine: the instrumentation and clinical applications. New York: American Institute of Physics, 1985:414–444.
2. Price RR, Axel L, Morgan T, Newman R, et al. Quality assurance methods and phantoms for magnetic resonance imaging: report of AAPM nuclear magnetic resonance Task Group No. 1. Med Phys 1990;17:287–295.
3. Bucciolini M, Ciraolo L, Renzi R. Relaxation rates of paramagnetic solutions: evaluation by nuclear magnetic resonance imaging. Med Phys 1986;13:298–303.
4. Wood ML, Henkelman RM. MR image artifacts from periodic motion. Med Phys 1985;12:143–151.
5. Phillips DJ, Hossack BS, Beach KW, Strandness DE Jr. Testing ultrasonic pulsed Doppler instruments with a physiologic string phantom. J Ultrasound Med 1990;9:429–436.

6. Pulse echo ultrasound imaging systems: performance tests and criteria. AAPM Report No. 8. New York: American Association of Physicists in Medicine, 1980.
7. McCullough EC, Payne JT, Baker HL, et al. Performance evaluation and quality assurance of computed tomography scanners, with illustrations from the EMI, ACTA, and delta scanners. Radiology 1976;120:173–188.
8. McCullough EC. Specifying and evaluating the performance of computed tomography (CT) scanners. Med Phys 1980;7:291–296.
9. Droege RT. A quality assurance protocol for CT scanners. Radiology 1983;146:244–246.
10. Cohen G, DiBianca FA. The use of contrast-detail-dose evaluation of image quality in a computed tomographic scanner. J Comput Assist Tomogr 1979;3:189–195.
11. McCullough EC, Payne JT. Patient dosage in computed tomography. Radiology 1978;129:457–463.
12. Functional tests to comply with FDA regulations. Supplement to operating instructions for the Siemens DRH Computed Tomography Scanner. Islen, NJ: Siemens Medical Systems, Inc., 1985.
13. Showalter CK, McCrohan JL, Burkhart RL, et al. Quality assurance for computer assisted imaging systems. In: Fullerton GD, Hendee WR, Lasher JC, Properzio WS, Riederer SJ, eds. Electronic imaging in medicine. New York: American Association of Physicists in Medicine-American Institute of Physics, 1984:439–458.
14. Description of the AAPM CT performance phantom. In: Catolog G-6, Radiology instruments and accessories. New York: Nuclear Associates, 1992:28–29.
15. Coulam CM, Erickson JJ. Image considerations in computed tomography. In: Coulam CM, Erickson JJ, Rollo FD, James AE Jr, eds. The physical basis of medical imaging. Chap. 14. East Norwalk, CT: Appleton-Century-Crofts, 1981.
16. NCRP Report No. 99: quality assurance for diagnostic imaging equipment. Bethesda, MD: National Council on Radiation Protection and Measurement, 1988.
17. Gray JE. Multiformat video and laser camera acceptance testing (and quality control). In: Proceedings, Volume II, AAPM 1991 Summer School: specification, acceptance testing, and quality control of diagnostic x-ray imaging equipment. Santa Cruz, CA: University of California, 1991.

13 Evaluation and Impact of Diagnostic Tests

HENRY D. ROYAL and BARBARA J. MCNEIL

Recognition that healthcare dollars are limited has provided much of the motivation for developing techniques to evaluate the usefulness of various diagnostic and therapeutic endeavors. A new federal agency, the Agency for Health Care Policy and Research, was created to encourage research on patient outcomes and evidence-based practice guidelines for diagnosis and treatment are becoming increasingly common (1–7). Healthcare planners are becoming more influential in determining the behavior of healthcare providers. Then practicing physicians must gain a better understanding of costs associated with diagnostic testing, and nuclear medicine physicians must be prepared to educate others of the benefits and risks of new and existing diagnostic procedures.

Throughout this chapter, we describe both the usefulness of the techniques that are applied to study the role of tests and their limitations. In many instances, complex tasks must be oversimplified to use currently available analytic tools. Certain tools, such as decision analysis (8–11), are useful because they can provide insight regarding the most favorable diagnostic/therapeutic strategies, and because they can identify areas where present knowledge is inadequate and help put priorities on areas of research.

A generalized scheme for evaluating the value of performing a diagnostic test on patient outcomes is presented in Figure 13.1. First, patients must be recruited for the study and a decision made to perform or not perform the test. If no test is performed, the clinician makes a decision to treat or not treat a patient on the basis of all the information he or she has at the time. If the test is performed, the test result is used in making a treatment decision. Presumably a positive test result will influence the clinician to act differently than a negative test result. Finally, the value of performing the test is determined by comparing the patient outcomes when the test was performed versus when the test was not performed.

This process can be conceptualized as having three distinct components. To perform a proper evaluation of a test, each component must be performed correctly. This chapter discusses each component of the process in the order it is performed. The first, and frequently overlooked, component of the process is *patient recruitment and assignment.* Which patients are included in a study can greatly affect both the information content of the test and its impact on health outcomes. The second component of the process is an *evaluation of the information content* of the test. The test may add unique additional information, it may add no additional information, or it may add erroneous information. Many evaluations of diagnostic tests are limited to this component of the evaluation process. The final, and most difficult, component involves an *evaluation of the impact of the test on patient outcomes.* In its broadest sense, this evaluation includes all the costs and benefits that directly or indirectly affect not only the individual patient but society as a whole.

PATIENT RECRUITMENT AND ASSIGNMENT

In the course of designing a study to determine the value of a diagnostic test, it is necessary to predict the number of patients needed to detect a change in information content or in health outcome if a change really exists (12, 13). This estimate requires an understanding of the term *statistical significance* and *power.* In general, an observed difference that has a less than 1 in 20 chance ($P \le 0.05$) of occurring as a result of chance alone is called a *significant*

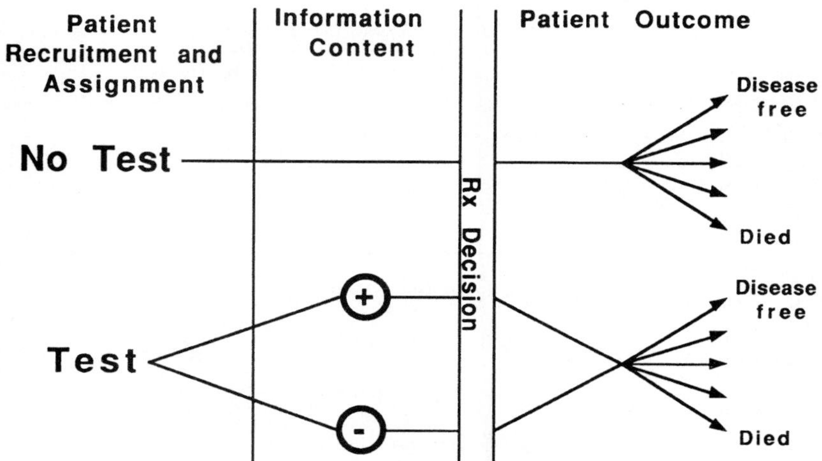

Figure 13.1. Value and impact of a diagnostic test on patient outcome. This schematic of the process of evaluating the value and impact of a diagnostic test consists of three distinct components. In the past, most studies of diagnostic tests have concentrated on the information content of the test. In the future, studies will be required to determine the impact of the test on patient outcome.

difference (14). With this criterion, there is 1 chance in 20 of calling a difference that occurred by chance alone a significant difference even though no real difference exists. This error is called a *type I* or *alpha error.*

A second error (called a *type II* or *beta error*) is possible (14). A real difference may in fact exist but it may not be detected as a statistically significant difference because the sample size was too small. The sample size that is needed to detect a real difference will vary depending on the expected difference in the means, the standard deviations of the means, the experimental design, and the type of data used. The likelihood of committing a type II error is equal to 1 minus the power of the statistical test.

Since sample size has such a great effect on the likelihood of committing a type II error, the chances of recognizing a real difference when one exists greatly decrease as the sample population is subdivided. This fact puts the statistician at odds with the clinician. The clinician, recognizing the complexity of patients (and imaging results), would like to subdivide the subjects studied and the imaging results obtained into more homogeneous subgroups. The statistician is often forced to reject a complex analysis of many subgroups because the statistical power of such an analysis will be unacceptable. The only solution to this conflict is to encourage large multicenter studies.

Once the necessary sample size, and hence the feasibility of the study, has been estimated, patient recruitment can begin (15). In their seminal article, Ransohoff and Feinstein (16) enumerated a number of characteristics that should be routinely included in the description of the patient population that is used to evaluate a test. These include pathologic, clinical, and comorbid components. The pathologic component includes information such as the histology, location, and extent of disease. The clinical component includes factors such as the chronicity of disease, the severity of symptoms, and prior or current treatment regimens. The comorbid component includes coexisting ailments that might affect the test outcome. For example, a test that requires the measurement of some exhaled metabolite might not work as well with patients with chronic obstructive lung disease. It is equally important that the nondiseased subject be well-characterized. Ideally, these nondiseased patients should be matched by symptoms, age, sex, and comorbid ailments. For example, when evaluating a test that is to be used clinically to diagnose malignant diseases of the liver, subjects with benign disease of the liver should be included in the "nondiseased" group.

It is important to note that the population initially used to evaluate a test may be different from the population on which the test ultimately will be performed (17). In the initial studies of a new test, the investigator usually tries to perform the test on subjects who can independently and easily be determined to be unequivocally disease free or unequivocally diseased. These subjects tend to be the very sick and the very healthy. If a new test appears promising with these groups, it is then appropriate to assess the test in a more rigorous fashion using as a patient sample all patients presenting with a particular set of signs and symptoms (e.g., low back pain) suspected of having a particular disease (e.g., herniated disc). This population should be described in sufficient detail so that readers are able to determine if the results obtained in a study are applicable to their patients.

EVALUATION OF THE INFORMATION CONTENT OF A TEST

DECISION MATRICES

Once a test has been performed, a simple framework is used to evaluate the results. A 2×2 matrix is used to tabulate the test results (Fig. 13.2). The binary outcome of the test result (abnormal versus normal) is indicated by the row, and the binary description of disease status (present or absent) is indicated by the column. In each of the four cells of the matrix, the number (not the percentage) of outcomes that correspond to that test result-disease state pair is indicated.

The test result is a **true-positive** (*TP*; cell *A* in Fig. 13.2) when the test outcome is abnormal and the disease is present. A **false-positive** (*FP*; cell *B*) occurs when the test is abnormal and the disease is absent. A **false-negative** (*FN*; cell *C*) result occurs when the test is normal despite the presence of disease. Finally, a **true-negative** result (*TN*; cell *D*) occurs when the test is normal and disease is absent. Often, the sums of the rows and columns are also indicated since this facilitates the calculation of the derived ratios described later.

From this simple matrix, seven ratios can be derived to indicate the information content of the test (Table 13.1). Many synonyms have been used to describe these ratios and other important concepts (Table 13.2).

Sensitivity is the number of true-positive results divided by the total number of test subjects with disease [*A*/(*A* + *C*)]. Note that only patients with the disease need to be studied to determine the sensitivity of the test. Sensitiv-

		DISEASE		
		Present (D+)	Absent (D−)	
TEST	Abormal (T+)	A (TP)	B (FP)	A+B
	Normal (T−)	C (FN)	D (TN)	C+D
		A+C	B+D	

Figure 13.2. The decision matrix. *TP* = true-positive, *FP* = false-positive, *FN* = false-negative, *TN* = true-negative.

Table 13.1.
Derived Ratios

$$\text{Sensitivity } (P[T+|D+]) = \frac{A}{A + C} = \frac{TP}{TP + FN}$$

$$\text{Specificity } (P[T-|D-]) = \frac{D}{D + B} = \frac{TN}{TN + FP}$$

$$\text{False negative ratio (FNR)} = \frac{C}{A + C} = \frac{FN}{TP + FN}$$

$$\text{False positive ratio (FPR)} = \frac{B}{D + B} = \frac{FP}{TN + FP}$$

$$\text{Accuracy} = \frac{A + D}{A + B + C + D} = \frac{TP + TN}{TP + FP + FN + TN}$$

Table 13.2.
Decision Making Synonyms

Sensitivity
True-positive ratio (TPR)
True-positive fraction (TPF)
Accuracy in disease
$P(T+\|D+)$
Specificity
True-negative rate (TNR)
True-negative fraction (TNF)
Accuracy in nondisease
$P(T-\|D-)$
False-negative ratio
False-negative fraction
1-Sensitivity
1-True-positive ratio
$P(T-\|D+)$
False-positive ratio
False-positive fraction
1-Sensitivity
1-True-negative ratio
$P(T+\|D-)$
Prior probability
A priori probability
Disease prevalence
Pretest probability
$P(D+)$
Predictive value
Posttest probability
$P(D+\|T+)$ or $P(D-\|T-)$

ity indicates nothing about the results in nondiseased patients; therefore, by itself it does not indicate the test's ability to separate normal and diseased patients. In probability notation, sensitivity is expressed as $P(T+|D+)$, which is read "The probability of obtaining a positive test result given the condition that the patient has the disease."

Specificity is the number of true-negatives divided by the total number of patients without the disease $[D/(B + D)]$. Specificity can be determined by tabulating test results in patients without disease. Like sensitivity, by itself specificity does not indicate how well the test will separate patients with and without disease.

The **false-negative ratio** is the number of false-negative results divided by the total number of test subjects with disease $[C/(A + C)]$. The true-positive ratio (sensitivity) plus the false-negative ratio must equal 1. The **false-positive ratio** is the number of false-positive ratio results divided by the total number of test subjects without disease $[B/(B + D)]$. Specificity plus the false-positive ratio equals 1.

The first four ratios listed in Table 13.1 are independent of disease prevalence $[(A + C)/(A + B + C + D)]$ and characterize the test itself.

At first glance, the most important ratio describing the information content of a test might appear to be the number of true-positive and true-negative outcomes divided by the total number of outcomes $[(A + D)/(A + B + C + D)]$. This ratio is called the *accuracy* of the test. Unfortunately, accuracy can be affected by the disease prevalence and, therefore, is not always a good measure of the information content of the test. The effect of disease prevalence on the accuracy of a test is shown in Figure 13.3, where accuracy has been calculated for a constant sensitivity and specificity (90% and 60%, respectively) and for two different disease prevalences (10% and 90%). For convenience, an arbitrary number (1000) of studies were used in the sample calculations. In Figure 13.3**A**, the number of diseased studies [sum of first column: $(A + C)$] can be calculated by multiplying the total number of studies by the disease prevalence ($1000 \times 0.10 = 100$). The number of nondiseased studies [sum of second column: $(B + D)$] equals the total number of studies minus the number of diseased studies ($1000 - 100 = 900$). Once the number of diseased studies and nondiseased studies is known, the values for each cell in the 2×2 matrix can be calculated. The number of true-positives (cell A) equals the number of studies in diseased patients times the sensitivity ($100 \times 0.90 = 90$). The number of false-negatives can be calculated by subtracting the number of true-positives from the total number of studies in diseased patients ($100 - 90 = 10$). Likewise, the number of true-negative outcomes (cell D) can be calculated by multiplying the number of nondiseased studies times the specificity ($900 \times 0.60 = 540$). The number of false-positives (cell B) equals the number of studies in nondiseased patients minus the number of true-negatives ($900 - 540 = 360$). Once the 2×2 matrix is completed, accuracy can be determined.

In Figure 13.3**B**, accuracy has been calculated for a disease prevalence of 90%. Note that the accuracy was 87% with a disease prevalence of 90% and was only 63% with a disease prevalence of 10%. In this example, the accuracy increased as the disease prevalence increased because the sensitivity was greater than the specificity. If the specificity of a test is greater than the sensitivity, then the overall accuracy would be greater for a low disease prevalence compared to a high disease prevalence.

A limitation in the use of sensitivity and specificity to summarize the information content of a diagnostic test is that the results will vary depending on the test interpretation criteria that the investigators use. The researcher is forced to reduce the complex results of an imaging test to a binary result (normal or abnormal). This data reduction makes subsequent data analysis much simpler. However, the obvious drawback is that significant information from the test is ignored. This problem is often exacerbated because the actual interpretation criteria used in a diagnostic accuracy study are poorly described.

Unfortunately, the 95% confidence intervals for sensitivity and specificity are rarely reported. This omission hides the fact that sensitivity and specificity measurements often are inexact simply because of the small number of subjects used to measure these two parameters (Table 13.3).

RECEIVER OPERATING CHARACTERISTIC CURVES

Many evaluations of diagnostic tests report only the sensitivity and specificity of the test. The "sensitivity" and "specificity" of a diagnostic test is affected by many important factors in addition to the information content of the test. One important factor is the criteria that are used to arbitrarily divide the continuous spectrum of results obtained from a complex imaging test (18, 19). When interpreting the results of a complex imaging test, an observer

Figure 13.3. Effect of prevalence on accuracy. Accuracy has been calculated for a constant sensitivity (90%) and specificity (60%). **A.** A 10% disease prevalence. **B.** A 90% disease prevalence.

A

Test Results	Disease Status: Disease Present D+	Disease Status: Disease Absent D-
Abnormal T+	90 (A)	360 (B)
Normal T-	10 (C)	540 (D)

$$\text{Accuracy} = \frac{TP + TN}{TP + FP + FN + TN} = \frac{A + D}{A + B + C + D} = \frac{90 + 540}{1000} = 63\%$$

$$\text{Predictive Value of a Positive Test} = \frac{TP}{TP + FP} = \frac{A}{A + B} = \frac{90}{90 + 360} = 20\%$$

$$\text{Predictive Value of a Negative Test} = \frac{TN}{FN + TN} = \frac{D}{C + D} = \frac{540}{540 + 10} = 98.2\%$$

B

Test Results	Disease Status: Disease Present D+	Disease Status: Disease Absent D-
Abnormal T+	810 (A)	40 (B)
Normal T-	90 (C)	60 (D)

$$\text{Accuracy} = \frac{TP + TN}{TP + FP + FN + TN} = \frac{A + D}{A + B + C + D} = \frac{810 + 60}{1000} = 87\%$$

$$\text{Predictive Value of a Positive Test} = \frac{TP}{TP + FP} = \frac{A}{A + B} = \frac{810}{810 + 40} = 95.3\%$$

$$\text{Predictive Value of a Negative Test} = \frac{TN}{FN + TN} = \frac{D}{C + D} = \frac{60}{90 + 60} = 40\%$$

Table 13.3.
Calculation of 95% Confidence Intervals for a 90% Proportion

Number of Subjects (N)	95% Confidence Intervals
10	71.4%–100%
20	76.9%–100%
50	81.7%–98.3%
100	84.1%–95.9%

$$\text{Standard error (SE) of a proportion (P)} = \sqrt{\frac{P \times (1 - P)}{N}}$$

$$\text{95\% confidence interval} = P \pm 1.96 \times SE$$

will express varying degrees of certainty regarding whether the test result is normal or abnormal. Five categories (definitely normal, possibly normal, possibly abnormal, probably abnormal, and definitely abnormal) are often used to describe these levels of certainty (Fig. 13.4). From these five categories, four sets of sensitivities and specificities can be calculated by using a different category as the dividing point for a normal and an abnormal study. For example, if all test results except those that were "definitely normal" are considered abnormal (lax threshold), the test will have a high sensitivity at the expense of a lower specificity. On the other hand, if only the test results that are "definitely abnormal" are considered abnormal (strict threshold), the test will have a high specificity at the expense of a lower sensitivity. Analysis of the information content of every complex test should result in a family of sensitivity and specificity pairs rather than a single sensitivity and specificity.

When these four sets of sensitivities and specificities are plotted as sensitivity versus 1 minus specificity, a receiver operating characteristic (ROC) curve is produced (Fig. 13.5) (20–26).

The further to the left and upward the ROC curve, the better the test. The advantage of the curve is that it defines the performance of the test independently of the threshold that is used. For example, if test *A* has a reported sensitivity of 70% and a specificity of 85%, and test B has a reported sensitivity of 40% and a specificity of 95%, little can be said about the relative information content of the tests (Fig. 13.6). Test A may be better than test B, or they may be equally efficacious if the same threshold had been used. Use of a ROC curve will eliminate this confusion.

The optimal threshold to separate the normal and abnormal results of a test varies with the disease prevalence. Intuitively, many physicians recognize this principle. They are reluctant to call a test positive when the clinical setting makes disease unlikely, and are more easily convinced that the test is abnormal if they know the pretest probability

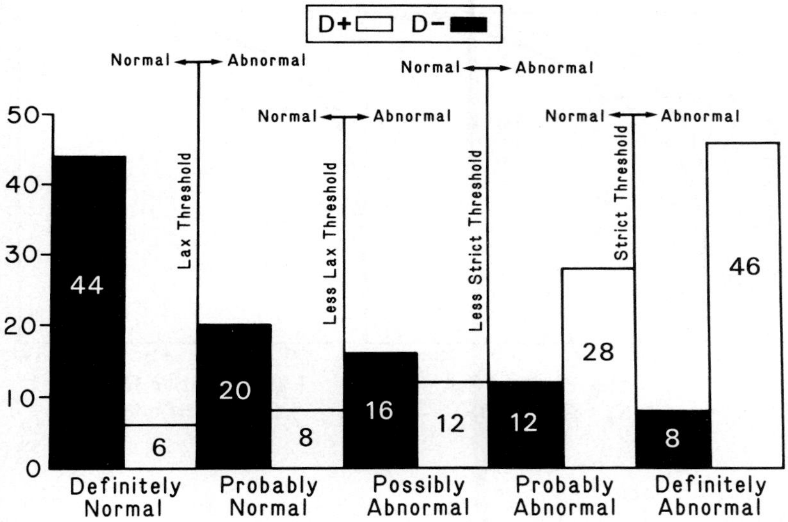

Figure 13.4. Levels of certainty regarding test results. This bar histogram graphically shows the distribution of categorical test results in 100 normal and 100 abnormal subjects. The better the test, the less overlap of test results in the intermediate categories. The four possible dividing lines (thresholds) that can be used to separate "abnormal" and "normal" test results are shown. Use of a strict threshold results in a test that has a high specificity at the expense of a lower sensitivity, whereas a lax threshold results in a higher sensitivity at the expense of a lower specificity. (Reproduced by permission from Royal HD, McNeil BJ. Quantitative analysis in clinical nuclear medicine. In: Maissey MN, Britton KE, Gilday DL, eds. Clinical nuclear medicine. London: Chapman and Hall, 1983:457–479.)

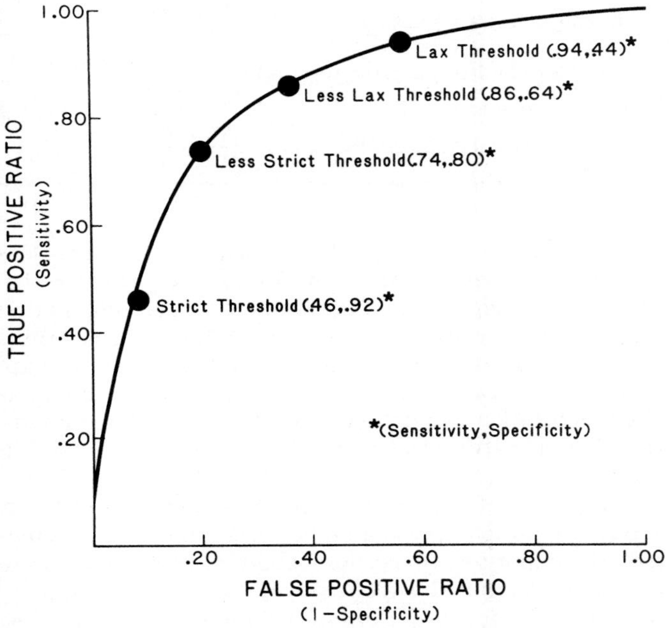

Figure 13.5. Receiver operating characteristic curve. The four pairs of sensitivities and specificities generated from the four possible thresholds depicted in Figure 13.4 are plotted as sensitivity (*y*-axis) versus 1 − specificity (*x*-axis). The resulting graph is called a receiver operating characteristic curve. (Reproduced by permission from Royal HD, McNeil BJ. Quantitative analysis in clinical nuclear medicine. In: Maissey MN, Britton KE, Gilday DL, eds. Clinical nuclear medicine. London: Chapman and Hall, 1983:457–479.)

that the patient has the disease is high. The idea that the threshold used to interpret tests should be influenced by the disease prevalence means that when tests are used clinically, their interpretation can be maximized only if the interpreter has all the clinical information available to him or her at the time of the interpretation. An example of this principle at work would be the interpretation of a bone scan abnormality in a man with newly diagnosed prostate carcinoma. Since the prevalence of metastatic bone disease in patients with a PSA of less than 20 mg/l is less than 1% (27), abnormalities in this group of patients must be cautiously interpreted. Of course, when clinical information is used to interpret a test, this fact should be clearly indicated in the report to prevent important clinical information being counted twice (i.e., once by the test interpreter and once by the clinician).

Another factor that determines the optimum threshold to use on the ROC curve is the relative value of the four possible (*TP*, *TN*, *FP*, and *FN*) outcomes. For example, if effective treatment exists for a potentially serious disease (e.g., neonatal hypothyroidism), a threshold that maximizes sensitivity at the expense of specificity should be used. This threshold corresponds to a point on the ROC curve where the slope is less steep. On the other hand, if treatment is hazardous and/or not very effective (e.g., asymptomatic bone metastasis), a less sensitive, more specific threshold is optimal.

Significant differences between ROC curves can be determined by comparing the differences in the areas under the curves (28). The number of normal and abnormal subjects (Table 13.4) that are needed to detect differences in ROC curves can be estimated for given alpha and beta errors and for a given standard error of the area (29). If the same patients have both tests, as is experimentally desirable (i.e., a paired design), the number of patients required for a given statistical power can, depending upon the correlation between the tests, be reduced considerably (Table 13.5).

LIKELIHOOD RATIOS

An especially useful way to express the diagnostic accuracy of complex imaging tests is to use likelihood ratios (30). This approach forces investigators to develop a detailed list of potentially important image features (15, 31). For example, in a study to determine the diagnostic accuracy of a test in distinguishing benign from malignant lung nodules, the size of a lung nodule, whether its borders are smooth or poorly defined, whether it is calcified, and so on, may be important image features (32). How often these fea-

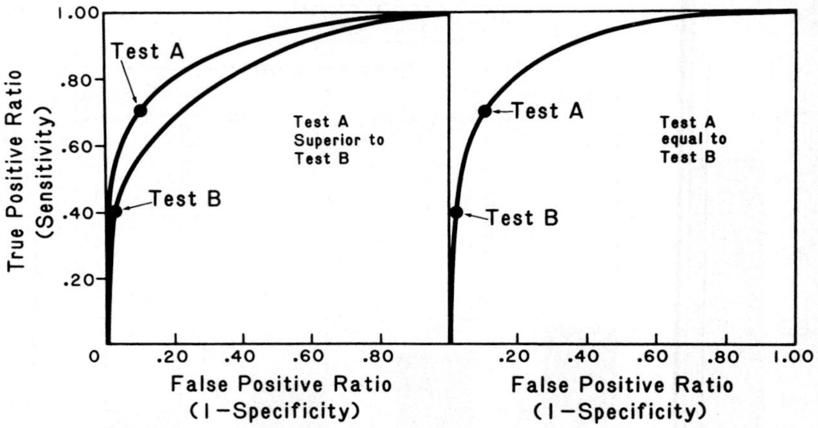

Figure 13.6. Comparison of tests using ROC curves. With ROC curves, it is much easier to determine if one test performs better than another (*left graph*) or if the difference in the cited sensitivities and specificities is due to the use of a different threshold (*right graph*). (Reproduced by permission from Royal HD, McNeil BJ. Quantitative analysis in clinical nuclear medicine. In: Maissey MN, Britton KE, Gilday DL, eds. Clinical nuclear medicine. London: Chapman and Hall, 1983:457–479.)

Table 13.4.
Number of Normal and Abnormal Subjects Required to Provide a Probability of 80%, 90%, or 95% of Detecting Various Differences Between the Areas Under Two ROC Curves (Using a One-Sided Test of Significance with P = .05)

		Percent Probability		
Δ Area	Average Area	80	90	95
.05	.825	463	634	797
.05	.875	350	477	597
.05	.925	228	308	383
.10	.850	110	149	185
.10	.900	81	108	134
.15	.875	46	61	75

Table 13.5.
Comparison of the Number of Normal and Abnormal Patients Needed for a Paired and an Unpaired Study to Have an 80% Probability of Detection of Difference Between Areas Under Two ROC Curves When the Correlation Between the Tests is .60

Δ Area	Average Area	Unpaired	Paired
.05	.825	463	213
.05	.875	350	168
.05	.925	228	116
.10	.850	110	52
.10	.900	81	40
.15	.875	46	22

tures are present in the disease of interest (malignant lung tumors) is compared with an appropriate "nondisease" group (benign lung nodules).

The likelihood ratio is calculated by dividing the probability of finding that particular image feature in patients with disease by the probability of finding that identical image feature in patients without the disease (Table 13.6). If the likelihood ratio for a particular image feature is much greater than 1.0 (the feature is much more common in patients with the disease than in those without the disease), the feature greatly increases the chances that the patient has the disease. If the likelihood ratio is equal to 1, that image feature does not help distinguish patients with and

Table 13.6.
Likelihood Ratios

For a test with a binary outcome

$$\text{Likelihood ratio of a positive test result} = \frac{\text{Sensitivity}}{1 - \text{Specificity}}$$

$$\text{Likelihood ratio of a negative test result} = \frac{1 - \text{Sensitivity}}{\text{Specificity}}$$

General definition

$$\text{Likelihood ratio of the nth test result} = \frac{P(T_n|D+)}{P(T_n|D-)}$$

without the disease. If the likelihood ratio is much less than 1, that image feature is useful for excluding the disease. Useful diagnostic tests should have test results that have likelihood ratios of >10 or <0.1. When image features are listed with their likelihood ratios, it becomes very apparent which features have the most diagnostic value. The likelihood ratios can be determined not only for the individual image features but also for combinations of features.

The results of complex imaging tests often cannot be adequately characterized using the constraints of a 2×2 matrix. The importance of certain image features is widely appreciated and must be taken into account when evaluating the information content of an imaging test. For example, the significance of perfusion abnormalities on a lung scan will vary depending on their number, size, character, and location. The presence or absence of an associated x-ray or ventilatory abnormality must also be considered. As shown in Table 13.7, a 2 × n decision matrix was be used to tabulate the results of the PIOPED study (33). The investigators reported the results in terms of sensitivity and specificity, but reporting the results of a 2 × n decision matrix this way can be confusing. Clinicians are not used to thinking about tests with multiple outcomes—with each outcome having a unique sensitivity and specificity. A better way to report the results is to use likelihood ratios (Table 13.8).

A likelihood ratio is calculated for each of the four categories of test readings (high, intermediate, low probability, and normal). For example, the reading (Table 13.8) of "high probability" occurs in the minority (41% [102/251]) of patients with pulmonary embolism. The usefulness of a

Table 13.7.
PIOPED Results

Test Result	PE Present	PE Absent
	A. Raw Data	
High	102	14
Intermediate	105	217
Low	39	199
Near normal/normal	5	50
Total	251	480
	B. Sensitivity and Specificity as originally reported	
Test Result	Sensitivity	Specificity
High	41% (102/251)	97% ([50 + 199 + 217]/480)
Intermediate	82% ([102 + 105]/251)	52% ([50 + 199]/480)
Low	98% ([102 + 105 + 39]/251)	10% ([50]/480)

Table 13.8.
Calculation of Likelihood Ratios from the PIOPED Results

Test Result	$P(T+\|D+)$	$P(T+\|D-)$	Likelihood Ratio
High	0.406 (102/251)	0.0292 (14/480)	13.9
Intermediate	0.418 (105/251)	0.452 (217/480)	0.925
Low	0.155 (39/251)	0.415 (199/480)	0.375
Near normal/ normal	0.0200 (5/251)	0.104 (50/480)	0.191

high probability test result is that it rarely (3% [14/480]) occurs in patients without pulmonary embolism. The likelihood ratio of a high probability result is 13.9 (0.406/0.0292).

The data from PIOPED would be more useful if the likelihood ratios were reported for particular image features (e.g., 3–5 moderate size mismatched segments and no matched scintigraphic abnormalities) rather than for categories of interpretations (high, intermediate, low, and normal). Additionally, the current PIOPED criteria confuse the information provided by the test result and the posttest probability. As used by PIOPED, "low probability" result should be reported as "low likelihood" ratio result to distinguish the test result from the posttest probability. Posttest probability can only be obtained by combining the pretest probability with the test results.

LIMITATIONS OF DIAGNOSTIC ACCURACY STUDIES

Despite their widespread use, diagnostic accuracy studies have a number of glaring deficiencies that are rarely emphasized (34). Ideally, the summary statistics used to convey the information content of a diagnostic test is a function solely of the accuracy of the diagnostic test. In reality, these summary statistics are often greatly affected by many other factors. First, summary statistics are affected by the case mix of the study population. Better results are expected if the study population consists of easy cases (e.g., obvious disease) than if it consists of difficult cases (e.g., early disease).

Table 13.9.
Calculation of the Kappa Statistic

Observed Agreement 95%			Expected Agreement 82%		
	Observer 2			Observer 2	
Observer 1	$T+$	$T-$	Observer 1	$T+$	$T-$
$T+$	75	25	$T+$	10	90
$T-$	25	875	$T-$	90	810

Note—$T+$ = Test Positive
$T-$ = Test Negative

$$\text{Kappa Statistic} = \frac{\text{Observed Agreement-Expected Agreement}}{\text{1-Expected Agreement}}$$

$$= \frac{.95-.82}{1-.82} = \frac{.13}{.18} = 72\%$$

Second, the results vary depending on the observational skills of the interpreter. A number of techniques are used to quantify the amount of variability due to two different readers interpreting the same test (interobserver variability) or to the same reader interpreting the same test twice (intraobserver variability). The variability of the readings is an important factor that must be measured in a complete evaluation of test performance. Interobserver variability is often reduced by first performing a pilot study to determine which findings on an image are reproducibly identifiable. Reducing observer variability is important since the power of statistical tests increases as the variability decreases. Unfortunately, interobserver and intraobserver variabilities of diagnostic tests are infrequently reported. When reported, they are often reported incorrectly as the percentage of cases for which observers agree. The fallacy of this approach is shown by the following example. If observer 1 and observer 2 both interpret a test as showing the absence of disease 90% of the time (partly because they know the disease is relatively uncommon), they will "agree" 82% of the time by chance alone (Table 13.9). The correct way to report observer agreement is the kappa statistic, which indicates the fraction of interpretations that agree beyond what one would have expected from chance alone (30, 35–37).

Third, the presence or absence of the disease is often determined by another imperfect test, and therefore does not necessarily represent truth. In most cases, it is unrealistic to expect that two independent tests (e.g., myocardial perfusion scintigraphy and coronary arteriography) will agree with each other more than 90% of the time, especially if the reference test agrees with itself (interstudy variability) only 90% of the time and if it measures a different pathologic marker of the disease (luminal narrowing vs. stress-induced relative regional hypoperfusion).

Fourth, the results depend on the quality of the instrumentation and the imaging protocol used. Less accurate results are expected with suboptimal instrumentation or an inferior protocol for image acquisition.

Fifth, biases (workup bias, diagnostic review bias, test review bias, and incorporation biases) may be introduced when associating the test result with the disease status (16, 31). *Workup bias* occurs when the results of a test influence the subsequent workup of the patient. If the disease is sought less vigorously in patients with a negative test result, then the disease is less likely to be found. Workup bias is difficult to avoid in a retrospective study since the results of tests normally will influence the subsequent workup of patients. Workup bias can be more readily avoided in prospective studies. Hopefully, prospective studies will become much more common in the future. *Diagnostic review* bias may occur if the test result is known by the individual making a subjective review of the data used to establish the diagnosis. Knowledge of the test result may influence the decision regarding the disease status. The simplest way of avoiding this bias is to prevent the diagnostician from knowing the test result. *Test review* bias occurs when the diagnosis is known at the time that the test is interpreted. If the results of pertinent other tests, as well as the history and physical findings, are available to the test interpreter, the interpreter may arrive at the correct test result because of this ancillary data. Although it is appropriate in a clinical setting to use all data possible when interpreting a test, this information is usually withheld when evaluating a test. This approach may cause the test to perform differently during the evaluation than it will perform clinically. *Incorporation bias* occurs when the test results are overtly used to categorize patients' disease statuses. Although this error is obvious when pointed out, patients' disease-free statuses are guaranteed in many studies since negative test results are not pursued by any additional tests.

Sixth, when tests are evaluated under an ideal setting (i.e., state-of-the-art equipment and expert observers), they may yield good results. This measures the efficacy of the test. What is clinically important is how the test performs in a more realistic setting (i.e., average equipment and observers). This measures the effectiveness of a test.

Seventh, some diagnostic studies are technically unsatisfactory for a number of reasons (e.g., patient motion on a SPECT study), necessitating an additional row for unsatisfactory exams in the $2 \times n$ matrix. These studies must be included for accurate calculation of summary statistics.

PREDICTIVE VALUE OF A TEST

Sensitivity, specificity, ROC curves, and likelihood ratios are useful when evaluating the information content of a test. Unfortunately, none of these summary statistics directly answer the clinician's question ("How often will patients with a positive (negative) test actually have disease (nondisease)?"). The answer requires calculation of the **predictive value** of a positive (negative) test. The predictive value of a test indicates the probability that a patient has or does not have disease after obtaining an abnormal or a normal test result. This probability is also called the *posterior probability* to distinguish it from the probability of disease before performing the test (*prior probability*). In probability notation, the predictive values of a positive and negative test are written $P(D+|T+)$ and $P(D-|T-)$, respectively. To calculate the predictive value of a test, the test result must be combined with the pretest probability of disease.

The predictive value of a positive test result can be calculated from the 2×2 decision matrix and is equal to the number of true-positives divided by the total number of positive test results $[A/(A + B)]$ (Fig. 13.3). Likewise, the predictive value of negative test equals the number of true-negatives divided by the number of true-negatives and false-negatives $[D/(C + D)]$. Note that since the calculation of predictive values requires numbers from each column of the 2×2 matrix, it will be affected by the disease prevalence.

The predictive value of a test can be calculated in one step using Bayes' theorem. When written in probability notation, Bayes' theorem often looks complex to the novice; however, it is easily mastered if the predictive values are first written as ratios of *TP*, *TN*, *FP*, and *FN* and then the probability notation is substituted. Bayes' theorem is most useful when written in terms of probability notation since the predictive values can then be calculated if the sensitivity, specificity, and disease prevalence are known. For a positive test result, Bayes' theorem is

$$P(D+|T+) = \frac{TP}{TP + FP} = \frac{P(T+|D+) \times P(D+)}{[P(T+|D+) \times P(D+)] + [P(T+|D-) \times P(D-)]} \quad (1)$$

Likewise, for a negative test result, Bayes, theorem, is

$$P(D-|T-) = \frac{TN}{TN + FN} = \frac{P(T-|D-) \times P(D-)}{[P(T-|D-) \times P(D-)] + [P(T-|D+) \times P(D+)]} \quad (2)$$

To calculate predictive value using likelihood ratios the following formula can be used.

$$\text{Posttest Odds}(D+) = \text{Pretest Odds}(D+) \times \text{Likelihood Ratio} \quad (3)$$

The predictive values for a positive test for the data presented in Figure 13.3 have been recalculated using Bayes theorem and likelihood ratios. These calculations are presented in Table 13.10. Calculations using likelihood ratios are less complex than calculations using Bayes' theorem, once the method for converting probabilities to odds and odds to probabilities is mastered. The odds of having disease can be related to the probability of having disease by the following formula.

$$\text{Odds}(D+) = \frac{P(D+)}{1 - P(D+)} = \frac{\text{Chances of Disease}}{\text{Chances of No Disease}} \quad (4)$$

If the pretest probability of disease is 10%, the pretest odds are 1 chance of having disease to 9 chances of not having disease (1:9 or 0.11 [0.10/0.90]). The formula for converting odds back to probability is

$$P(D+) = \frac{\text{Odds}(D+)}{\text{Odds}(D+) + \text{Odds}(D-)} = \frac{\text{Chances of Disease}}{\text{Chances of Disease} + \text{Chances of No Disease}} \quad (5)$$

Therefore, if the odds of disease are 0.11 (1:9), the probability of disease is

$$P(D+) = \frac{1}{1+9} = 10\% \quad (6)$$

If the pretest probability of disease is 90%, the pretest odds of disease are 9 chances of having disease to 1 chance of not having disease (9:1 or 9 [9/1]). Using the formula for converting odds back to probability is

$$P(D+) = \frac{9}{9+1} = 90\% \quad (7)$$

In Table 13.10, note again that the predictive value of a positive test is greatly influenced by the prevalence of the disease. In the example given, the predictive value of a positive test was 20% with a disease prevalence of 10% and was 95.3% with a disease prevalence of 90%.

In Table 13.11, the predictive value of a negative test is calculated. To keep the likelihood method simple, the same formula was used to calculate the posttest Odds($D+$) of a negative test result (equation 3). The following formula is needed to convert the resulting probability ($P[D+|T-]$) to the predictive value of a negative test ($P[D-|T-]$).

$$P(D-|T-) = 1 - P(D+|T-) \quad (8)$$

A common way to graphically illustrate the predictive value of a test for all prior probabilities and for a constant sensitivity and specificity is to plot the prior probability on the x-axis and posterior probabilities for a negative and positive test result on the y-axis (Fig. 13.7). If the test provides no useful information, the posterior probability of disease will not change; therefore, a graph of the predictive value versus the prior probability will be the line of identity. As the sensitivity and specificity of the test improve, the graph of predictive values moves further and further from the line of identity.

Some authors suggested that tests are most useful when they are used in a population of patients who have a disease prevalence that maximizes the difference between the pretest and posttest probability of disease (38). Although this approach may yield the correct answer in some clinical settings, it does not always do so. Tests are potentially useful when the posttest probability of disease causes the clinician to change course of action. For example, patients who have a 90% or greater chance of having a hypothetical disease might be treated for that disease; patients with less than a 10% chance of having the disease might be observed and not treated; and patients with between a 10% and a 90% chance of having the disease might have an invasive procedure to establish the diagnosis. In some patients with between a 10% and a 90% chance of having the disease, a noninvasive test performed prior to the invasive test may change the probabilities sufficiently so that the invasive test can be avoided. Note that in this example a single noninvasive test (with a sensitivity and specificity of 90% and 80%, respectively) is not warranted in patients who have the maximum difference in their pre- and posttest probability (Fig. 13.7, *shaded area, left graph*) since their posttest probability of disease will still be be-

Table 13.10.
Calculation of P(D+|T+) Using Bayes Theorem and Likelihood Ratios (Sensitivity = 90%; Specificity = 60%)

I. Disease Prevalence = 10%

Bayes Theorem

$$\frac{P(T+|D+) \times P(D+)}{P(T+|D+) \times P(D+) + P(T+|D-) \times P(D-)} = \frac{0.90 \times 0.10}{(0.90 \times 0.10) + (.40 \times .90)} = \frac{0.09}{0.09 + 0.36} = 20\%$$

Likelihood Ratio

Pretest Odds($D+$) × Likelihood Ratio = Posttest Odds($D+$)

$$1{:}9X\frac{0.9}{0.4} = 2.25{:}9$$

$$P(D+|T+) = \frac{2.25}{2.0 + 9.25} = 20\%$$

II. Disease Prevalence = 90%

Bayes Theorem

$$\frac{P(T+|D+) \times P(D+)}{P(T+|D+) \times P(D+) + P(T+|D-) \times P(D-)} = \frac{0.90 \times 0.90}{(0.90 \times 0.90) + (.40 \times .10)} = \frac{0.81}{0.81 + 0.04} = 95.3\%$$

Likelihood Ratio

Pretest Odds($D+$) × Likelihood Ratio = Posttest Odds($D+$)

$$9{:}1X\frac{0.9}{0.4} = 20.25{:}1$$

$$P(D+|T+) = \frac{20.25}{20.25 + 1.0} = 95.3\%$$

Table 13.11.
Calculation of P(D−|T−) Using Bayes Theorem and Likelihood Ratios (Sensitivity = 90%; Specificity = 60%)

I. Disease Prevalence = 10%

Bayes Theorem

$$\frac{P(T-|D-) \times P(D-)}{P(T-|D-) \times P(D-) + P(T-|D+) \times P(D+)} = \frac{0.60 \times 0.90}{(0.60 \times 0.90) + (0.10 \times 0.10)} = \frac{0.54}{0.54 + 0.01} = 98.2\%$$

Likelihood Ratio

Pretest Odds(D+) × Likelihood Ratio = Posttest Odds(D+)

$$1{:}9 \times \frac{0.1}{0.6} = 0.1667{:}9$$

$$P(D+|T-) = \frac{0.1667}{9.1667} = 1.81\% \text{ Therefore}$$

$$P(D-|T-) = 100 - 1.81 = 98.2\%$$

B. Disease Prevalence = 90%

Bayes Theorem

$$\frac{P(T-|D-) \times P(D-)}{P(T-|D-) \times P(D-) + P(T-|D+) \times P(D+)} = \frac{0.60 \times 0.10}{(0.60 \times 0.10) + (0.10 \times 0.90)} = \frac{0.06}{0.06 + 0.09} = 40.0\%$$

Likelihood Ratio

Pretest odds × Likelihood Ratio = Posttest Odds

$$9{:}1 \times \frac{0.1}{0.6} = 1.5{:}1$$

$$P(D+|T-) = \frac{1.5}{1.5 + 1.0} = 60\% \text{ Therefore}$$

$$P(D-|T-) = 100 - 60 = 40\%$$

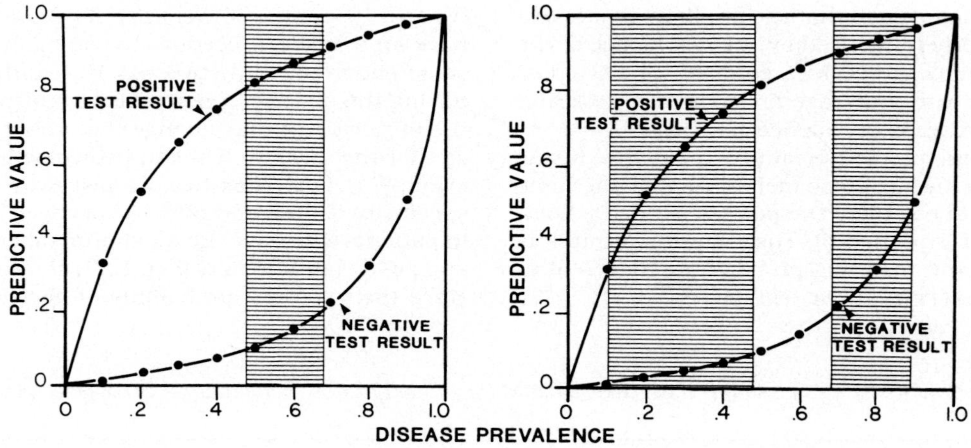

Figure 13.7. Predictive value of a test. The predictive value of a positive and a negative test result (*y*-axis) is plotted as a function of disease prevalence (*x*-axis). Note that the predictive value of a test is greatly affected by the disease prevalence. In this example, the predictive value of a positive or negative test never exceeds 90% nor falls below 10% in the region where the difference in the predictive value is maximized (*shaded area, left graph*). On the other hand, predictive values of greater than 90% and less than 10% can be obtained in regions where the difference in predictive values is not maximized (*shaded areas, right graph*). (Reproduced by permission of the Association for the Advancement of Medical Instrumentation from Royal HD. Clinical evaluation of diagnostic tests. Part II: The pitfalls. Med Instr 1984;18:75–77.)

tween 10% and 90%. The posttest probabilities of disease may change sufficiently in patients with a moderately low or moderately high pretest probability (*shaded area, right graph*) so that the invasive test can be avoided.

In Figure 13.8, the posttest probability of disease for a positive and negative test result is plotted as a function of the disease prevalence for representative likelihood ratios. Note that with a likelihood ratio of 1, the pretest probability of disease (disease prevalence) equals the posttest probability of disease (predictive value).

The level of certainty that is necessary to make a clinical diagnosis varies. If one assumes that a probability of disease of 90% is sufficient to make a clinical diagnosis, one can calculate the likelihood ratio that is necessary to obtain this predictive value of a test for any disease prevalence (Fig. 13.9). Note how rapidly the likelihood ratio necessary to yield a 90% predictive value increases when the disease prevalence decreases. For a disease prevalence of 0.1 and 0.2, likelihood ratios of 81 and 36, respectively, are needed to obtain a predictive value of 90%. Test results with likelihood ratios this large are very uncommon.

One major problem with the practical applications of Bayes' theorem is that there is both uncertainty in knowing the sensitivity and specificity of a test and uncertainty in knowing the probability of the patient having the disease prior to the performance of the test (prior probability). The

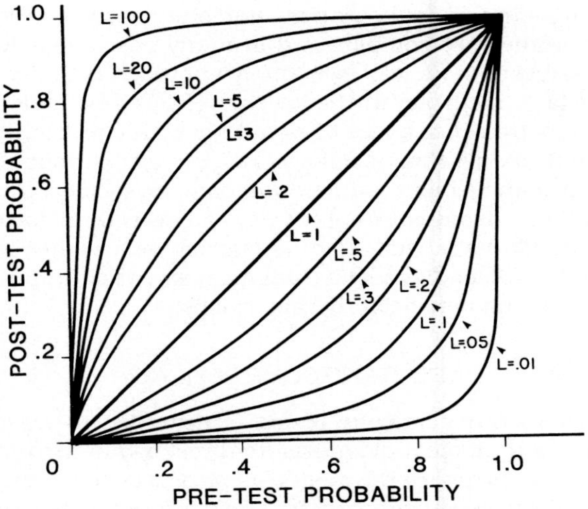

Figure 13.8. Posttest probability of disease. The predictive value of a test result is plotted for a series of likelihood ratios (*L*). Note that it is the predictive value of having disease that is plotted for a negative test result [*P*(*D*+|*T*−)].

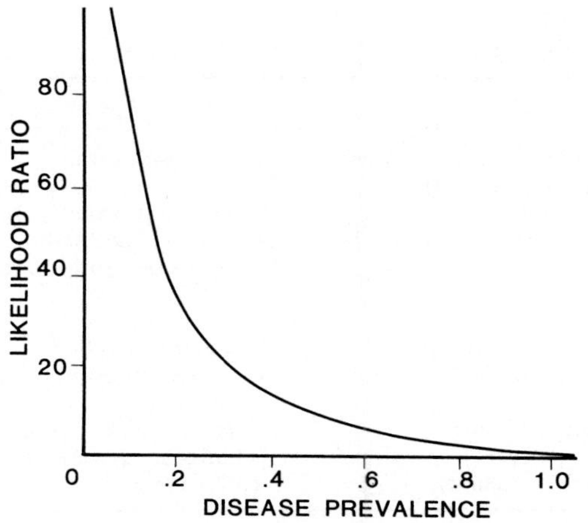

Figure 13.9. Likelihood ratio necessary for a *P*(*D*+|*T*+) of ≥90%. The likelihood ratios (*y*-axis) necessary to obtain a 90% positive predictive value are plotted as a function of disease prevalence (*x*-axis).

effects of these uncertainties increase as they are combined, so the predictive value of a test may be associated with a large range of possible results.

Bayesian analysis is applied most extensively in clinical medicine in the subspecialty of cardiology. Diamond and Forrester have developed tables that provide the prior probability of coronary artery disease based on a limited number of factors (39). Although Diamond and Forrester are unable to account for all factors, they have shown that, on average, their estimates of the prior probability of disease are usable with sensitivity and specificity values for several diagnostic tests to accurately predict posterior probabilities (40).

Since virtually all tests have likelihood ratios of less than 20 or 30 (and usually less than 10), when the prevalence of disease is low multiple tests must be used serially to obtain a predictive value of greater than 90%. For example, a test that has a sensitivity and specificity of 91% has a positive likelihood ratio of approximately 10 [.91/(1−.91] and would only yield a predictive value greater than 90% when the disease prevalence is greater than approximately 50%.

The posttest probability of multiple independent tests can be calculated using the following formula based on likelihood ratios.

$$\text{Posttest Odds}(D+) = \text{Pretest Odds}(D+) \times LR_1 \times LR_2 \times LR_3 \times LR_n \quad (9)$$

where

LR_1 is the likelihood ratio of the first test,
LR_2 is the likelihood ratio of the second test,
LR_3 is the likelihood ratio of the third test, and
LR_n is the likelihood ratio of the *n*th test.

The fact that the likelihood ratios are multiplicative means that two independent tests with likelihood ratios of 10 have an effective likelihood ratio of 100 when the test results agree. When test results are not independent of each other, then this formula does not apply. In radiology, because many imaging tests are based on similar principles, dependency is likely to be large.

MEASURING EFFICACY

Efficacy is when the "usefulness" of a diagnostic test is measured under ideal conditions (e.g., experts evaluating the test using the best equipment in a research setting). Effectiveness is the measure of the test's usefulness under nonideal clinical conditions. The effectiveness of the test is always less (sometimes much less) than its efficacy. Healthcare planners are generally more interested in effectiveness than efficacy, but efficacy is what is most commonly measured.

To state that a test is "useful" is ambiguous. Table 13.12 lists levels of "usefulness" (efficacy) according to Thornbury (41). These levels of efficacy have a natural hierarchy. Demonstration that a technology is "better" at a lower level of efficacy is a necessary, but insufficient, requirement to show that the technology is "better" at a higher level of efficacy.

The lowest level measures the technical quality of the image. These performance characteristics (e.g., intrinsic and extrinsic spatial resolution) are used by physicists to compare similar instruments. Measurable differences in instrument performance do not necessarily translate into diagnostic utility (42).

The next higher level of efficacy measures diagnostic accuracy. The most rudimentary study of diagnostic accuracy is to compare the findings in the patients with obvious disease with the findings in healthy subjects. This initial rough assessment determines whether further evaluation of the technology should be pursued. Unfortunately, promising but preliminary assessments are often misconstrued as indicating that the technology is clinically useful.

The third level attempts to determine how the information provided by the test changes the probability that the patient has a disease (diagnostic thinking efficacy). This level can be prescriptive or descriptive. Using the information content (sensitivity and specificity) of a diagnostic test, prescriptive analysis uses Bayes' theorem to estimate

Table 13.12.
Levels of Efficacy

Level[1]	Example
1. Technical characteristics	Spatial resolution
2. Diagnostic accuracy	
Descriptive	Findings in normals/abnormals
Quantitative	Sensitivity/specificity
	Receiver operating characteristic curve
	Likelihood ratio
3. Diagnostic certainty	Posttest probability
4. Patient management	Treatment changed because of test result
5. Patient outcome	Patient outcome changed due to change in treatment
6. Societal outcome	Cost/benefit

[1]Lower number indicates lower level of efficacy

the change in probability that occurs based on a given test result and disease prevalence. Descriptive analysis attempts to measure the change in diagnostic thinking directly by querying physicians regarding their estimates of the probability of disease before and after a test is performed.

The fourth level of efficacy determines the effect of a test on treatment (management efficacy) by quantifying the number of times that treatment is changed because of the test results. Less specific measures of management efficacy would be to tabulate how often a test was considered "helpful" in the subsequent management of a patient. Although documenting actual changes in treatment strategies is attractive from a number of perspectives, there are three difficulties. First, such documentation ignores intangible benefits that may result (e.g., greater sense of certainty about the disease state for the physician and greater peace of mind for the patient) regardless of the therapeutic plans. Second, it is extremely difficult to measure accurately and objectively changes in treatment plans. Techniques for this purpose are usually subjective and involve querying the referring physician with questions like: "In the absence of this test, what would you have done in terms of treatment or additional diagnostic tests?" These questions are very hard to answer. Third, these studies may simply identify the biases of practicing physicians. A physician is more likely to act on the basis of a test result that he is familiar with and believes in. This faith is not necessarily based on scientific evidence.

The fifth level of efficacy, measuring the value of a diagnostic test in terms of its impact on the patient's health (patient outcome efficacy), is, at first glance, the most attractive measure. Because of the potential importance of this measure it is discussed in detail later.

The sixth level of efficacy measures the costs and benefits of a test to society (societal efficacy). A lifesaving procedure is invaluable to the patient who benefits from it. However, in the context of limited resources, society must maximize the benefits it receives from the resources that it expends. Increasingly, the benefits and costs of medical technology are being compared with the benefits and costs of other nonmedical endeavors.

Even though we are ultimately interested in demonstrating efficacy at the patient outcome or societal level, such studies are complex and in many cases logistically impossible to do. A less formidable approach is to demonstrate lack of efficacy at the lower levels. For example, if it can be shown that a test does not have an effect on diagnostic thinking, then it follows that the test cannot affect patient management, patient outcome, or society. On the other hand, demonstrating efficacy at a lower level does not necessarily mean that there is efficacy at a higher level. Tests that affect diagnostic thinking may not affect patient outcome if no beneficial therapy exists.

PATIENT OUTCOME EFFICACY

Physicians order imaging tests for a number of reasons, including to make a diagnosis, to direct a therapeutic intervention, to determine prognosis, to accede to a patient's demands, to reassure a patient, and to prevent malpractice litigation. The ultimate justification, however, must be improved patient outcome.

Measuring improved patient outcome is difficult for many reasons. First, the complexity of medical care makes a cause-and-effect relationship between the performance of a single test and the improved patient outcome hard to establish. Second, there may be a long delay between the time when the test is performed and the time when the improved outcome is observed. Third, patient outcomes are varied and often involve tradeoffs such as decreased mortality at the expense of increased morbidity.

The simplest and most common approach to quantify patient outcomes involves the measurement of survival, expressed either as a survival rate at one or several points in time or as a cumulative value-life expectancy. The latter index obviously provides, in simple form, more information than does the former, but has two major limitations. First, it fails to consider that, for some patients, survival over the short-term may be more valuable than survival over the long-term. For example, use of radiation therapy for stage 1 lung cancer may be more appealing to some patients than use of surgery because of the higher probability of survival in the first 2 years after treatment with radiation therapy than with surgery (43). Second, life expectancy does not include any measure of morbidity (44, 45). Given these problems, the best measure of outcome currently in use today is the "quality adjusted life year" (QALY) (46). This measure explicitly adjusts for morbidity by decreasing life expectancy by some fraction that reflects the fact that a year of survival with morbidity is worth less to a patient than a year without morbidity. For example, a patient might say that he or she would find 1 year of survival with severe chest pain so disabling that 6 months of survival without chest pain is of equivalent value (47).

Determining QALYs is complicated by four factors. First, variability in an individual's preferences is likely to occur when the estimates are determined under different conditions, for example, when an individual is healthy or unhealthy. Second, conveying the true character of the disability may be difficult since it is likely that neither the physician nor the patient may have experienced a similar morbid event in the past. Third, the patient (or the physician) may be unfamiliar with or may react negatively to the experimental technique (basic reference gamble or proportional tradeoff method) used to determine the weight that the patient gives to the disability. Finally, the physician may unconsciously bias the patient whose preferences are being sought.

The experimental design of studies used to determine the effects of diagnostic tests on patient outcome is important since each of the three types of studies in common use have their own advantages and disadvantages. The first type is the *nonrandomized study*. Two versions of this type of study exist. In one version, patient outcomes before the introduction of a test are compared to patient outcomes after the test was introduced. This before-after comparison can be flawed since differences in therapy or patient selection may have occurred simultaneously with the introduction of the test. The second version of this type of study compares contemporaneous groups of patients who have and have not had the test. This comparison assumes a correct experimental design, otherwise the results may be misleading because the two groups of patients may not be truly comparable.

The second type of study usable to determine patient outcomes is an *analytic* one that uses decision trees and existing data from several studies to determine the expected values of various diagnostic/therapeutic strategies (8–11). When the necessary data needed to calculate the expected value of a strategy are not available from the literature, experts can be consulted to determine the best estimate of the probability of a particular event. If experts cannot agree on the probability of an outcome, a sensitivity analysis can be performed to determine if the optimal strategy would change depending on which reasonable estimate of an outcome was used. Sensitivity analysis is very useful in identifying areas where further research is needed to improve our ability to identify optimal strategies.

The final type of study used to determine the effect of tests on patient outcomes is a *randomized control study*. This experimental design can be more readily applied to screening tests than to diagnostic tests since ethical problems arise when a diagnostic test is randomly withheld from patients who have a significant chance of having disease. Randomized controlled studies have been used to demonstrate the value of mammography as a screening modality (48–52). Only a few randomized controlled studies have been done on diagnostic tests and none have been done in nuclear medicine.

COSTS

Consideration of healthcare costs adds further complexity to the measurement of the impact of diagnostic tests. When estimating total costs, both the cost of testing (diagnosis) and the cost of treatment must be considered.

The total cost of performing the test cannot be estimated simply from the price charged by the supplier. Both the production costs and the induced costs must be considered. The production costs include direct costs (equipment, labor, and expendable materials) and indirect costs (rent/building depreciation, space preparation and upkeep, utilities, support and administrative services). Many of these costs are fixed costs that do not decrease if fewer studies are performed. Maximum savings are only realized if less equipment is purchased, less space is allotted, fewer personnel are employed, and so forth.

Induced costs include diagnostic tests added or averted, treatments administered or avoided, and health benefits provided or lost. These induced costs will vary depending on the number of true-positive, true-negative, false-positive, and false-negative test results.

Determining the health benefit of diagnostic tests is more complicated when the benefit derived occurs at a future time. Such delayed benefits are less valuable than immediate benefits; they must be discounted to account for the fact that the money invested to obtain the benefit will be worth considerably more (if invested in some other enterprise) when the benefits are realized. Economists do not agree on any universal discount rate. When benefits occur at a time long after the costs have been incurred (e.g., prevention of coronary artery disease through diet modification), the total cost varies greatly depending on the discount rate used.

Once the total cost of a diagnostic/therapeutic strategy is known, a cost-effectiveness ratio, usually expressed in terms of dollars per QALYs saved, can be calculated. How much society is willing to pay to extend life is controversial, but some guidelines exist.

The cost incurred to save a life-year in nonmedical settings is generally much higher than the cost to save a life-year in most medical settings (Table 13.13) (53). For medical interventions, the median cost per life-year saved (1993 dollars) is $19,000. In contrast, the median cost per life-year saved is $48,000 and $2,782,000 for interventions to reduce fatalities due to accidents and toxins, respectively. Society appears to be willing to spend considerably more money to avoid involuntary risks (e.g., carcinogen exposure) than voluntary risks (e.g., smoking).

In medicine, it is sometimes necessary to compare the cost of a diagnostic/therapeutic strategy with and without a given diagnostic test. The marginal cost-effectiveness ratio of the test is equal to the difference of the costs (with and without the test) divided by the difference in the effectiveness measures (with and without the test). The concept

Table 13.13.
Representative Cost Effectiveness Programs

Life-Saving Program	Cost per Life-Year (1993 Dollars)
Medical programs	
Childhood immunization	≤ $0
β-Blockers following MI	$2,000
Cervical cancer screening	$12,000
Hypertension screening	$20,000
Renal dialysis	$46,000
Heart transplantation	$54,000
Nonmedical programs	
Seat belts	$32,000
Highway improvements	$64,000
Radon control	$141,000
Asbestos control	$1,865,000
Radiation control	$27,386,000
Radiation control at NRC-licensed & non-DOE facilities	$2,612,903,000

Figure 13.10. Costs and benefits of different screening strategies for colorectal cancers. Diagnostic options considered were testing stool for presence of occult blood (*TS*), barium enemas (*BE*), sigmoidoscopies (*SG*), and colonoscopies (*CL*). Numbers next to letters represent the time interval between screening tests in years.

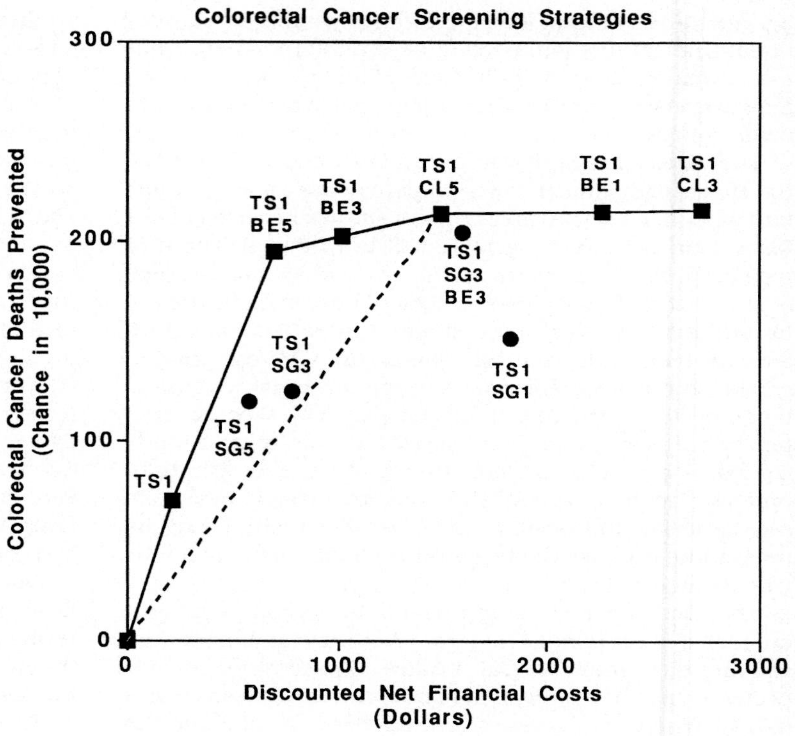

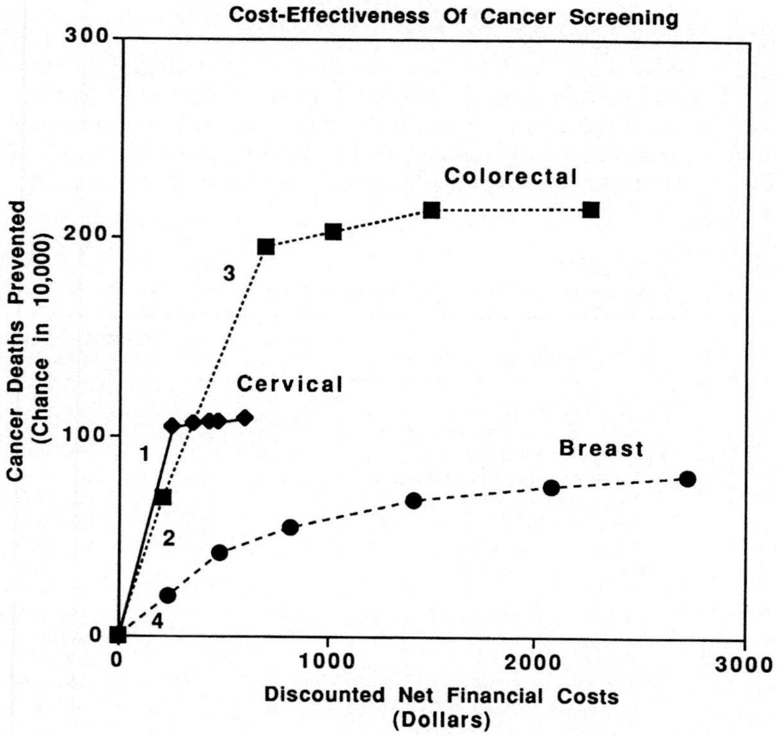

Figure 13.11. Costs and benefits (cancer deaths prevented in this example) for different cancer screening strategies. The marginal cost effectiveness of different cancer screening strategies is determined by the slope of the line connecting screening strategies that fall on the efficient frontier. Given limited resources, health benefits are maximized when healthcare dollars are spent on screening strategies in order of their marginal costs. In this example, healthcare dollars would first be spent on pap smears, then on testing stool for blood, then on a barium enema every 5 years, then on mammography.

of marginal cost effectiveness can be best understood through a concrete example (34). Assume that a finite number of dollars are available to prevent cancer deaths by screening the population to detect early curable cancers. How can we prevent the most cancer deaths with finite resources?

To determine the best course of action, the cost and benefits of different diagnostic strategies must be determined. Eddy has estimated the benefits and cost of different diagnostic strategies for screening for colorectal, cervical, and breast cancers (1). His estimates are used in following examples.

Figure 13.10 depicts the possible benefits and costs of different strategies for screening for colorectal cancer. The costs and benefits differ depending on (a) the diagnostic test or the combination of diagnostic tests that is used; (b) the frequency with which the test is used; and (c) the population of patients that is screened. The y-axis represents the benefits (in this case the number of cancer deaths prevented), and the x-axis represents the cost. From this graph, one can readily appreciate which screening strategy prevents the greatest number of deaths for the least amount of money. The screening strategies (*squares* in Fig. 13.10) that fall on the solid line are said to lie on the "efficient frontier." The strategies that do not fall on this line (*circles* in Fig. 13.10) are not considered because more deaths are preventable for the same amount of money by using a different strategy.

The marginal cost effectiveness is the slope of the line segment connecting a screening strategy on the efficient frontier with the preceding strategy. When trying to maximize health benefits, it is the marginal cost effectiveness that should be considered—not the cost per cancer death prevented for a particular screening strategy (*dotted line* in Fig. 13.10). The latter approach is misleading (the slope of the dotted line is much greater than the slope of the line representing the real marginal cost effectiveness) and may result in the use of very inefficient diagnostic strategies.

The efficient frontier for different screening strategies for colorectal, breast, and cervical cancer, is shown in Figure 13.11 (1). If there are finite resources and if the goal is solely to prevent the maximum number of cancer deaths, then expenditures should be prioritized on the basis of their marginal costs. Money should be spent on line segments where the slope is steepest, because that would indicate where the greatest number of deaths are preventable for the least amount of money. The line segments in Figure 13.11 have been numbered according to their slope to indicate the order in which monies to prevent cancer deaths should be spent to use limited resources most efficiently.

Cost-effectiveness analysis is much more difficult than this simple example indicates. Costs and benefits are difficult to measure accurately. Ideally, costs should include both the direct and indirect economic costs as well as physical and psychologic costs. Benefits must be measured in some universally applicable units. In the example given, the number of cancer deaths avoided may seem like a reasonable measure of benefit; however, not all avoided deaths are equal. Preventing the death of a young person and gaining many healthy years of life is of greater benefit than gaining only a few years of healthy life. For this reason, cost per year of quality-adjusted life gained are the preferred units for cost effectiveness analysis.

SUMMARY

In the past, generous financial resources have been available for most aspects of medical care. Society has always highly valued health and there is no reason to believe that this fundamental concern will diminish. What is apparent is that there is a limit to how much society is willing to spend on healthcare. The proportion of the Gross National Product spent on healthcare costs in the United States has tripled from 5% in 1960 to approximately 15% in 1993 (54). Healthcare professionals have an obligation to ensure that the public gets its money's worth.

Clearly, the greatest savings can be achieved in the areas of greatest expense. Nationally supported studies on the efficacy of various diagnostic/therapeutic strategies should be directed at the most common or expensive diseases. Efficacy studies that document underutilization of innovative, new, technologically advanced cost-effective therapies are as important as those that document overutilization (55).

Generally, the healthcare system of the past resulted in unparalleled advances for the patient; therefore, it is not surprising that physicians are anxious about the inevitable future changes. The danger that future changes will interfere with our goal of providing optimal healthcare will be lessened if all physicians help to guide these changes. This chapter has provided physicians with the basic tools to more actively participate in this process of optimizing healthcare.

REFERENCES

1. Eddy DM. A manual for assessing health practices & designing practice policies. The explicit approach. Philadelphia: American College of Physicians, 1992.
2. Evidence-based medicine group. Evidence-based medicine. A new approach to teaching the practice of medicine. Evidence-Based Medicine Working Group. JAMA 1992;268:2420–2425.
3. Sox H Jr, Woolf SH. Evidence-based practice guidelines from the US Preventive Services Task Force [Editorial]. JAMA 1993; 269:2678.
4. Woolf SH. Practice guidelines: a new reality in medicine. I. Recent developments. Arch Intern Med 1990;150:1811–1818.
5. Woolf SH. Interim manual for clinical practice guideline development. AHCPR Pub. No. 91–0018. Washington, DC: Public Health Service, Agency for Health Care Policy and Research, 1991.
6. Woolf SH. Practice guidelines, a new reality in medicine. II. Methods of developing guidelines. Arch Intern Med 1992;152:946–952.
7. Woolf SH. Practice guidelines, a new reality in medicine. III. Impact on patient care. Arch Intern Med 1993;153:2646–2655.
8. Wong JB, Kaplan MM, Meyer KB, Pauker SG. Ablative radioactive iodine therapy for apparently localized thyroid carcinoma. A decision analytic perspective. Endocrinol Metab Clin North Am 1990;19:741–760.
9. Thornton JG, Lilford RJ, Johnson N. Decision analysis in medicine. BMJ 1992;304:1099–1103.
10. Habbema JD, Bossuyt PM, Dippel DW, Marshall S, Hilden J. Analysing clinical decision analyses. Stat Med 1990;9:1229–1242.
11. Eckman MH, Levine HJ, Pauker SG. Decision analytic and cost-

effectiveness issues concerning anticoagulant prophylaxis in heart disease. Chest 1992;102:538S–549S.
12. Carpenter LM. Is the study worth doing? Lancet 1993;342:221–223.
13. Oxman AD, Sackett DL, Guyatt GH. Users' guides to the medical literature. I. How to get started. The Evidence-Based Medicine Working Group. JAMA 1993;270:2093–2095.
14. Glantz SA. What does "not significant" really mean? In: Glantz SA, ed. Primer of biostatistics. Ch. 6. New York: McGraw-Hill, Inc., 1992:155–187.
15. Jaeschke R, Guyatt GH, Sackett DL. Users' guides to the medical literature. III. How to use an article about a diagnostic test. B. What are the results and will they help me in caring for my patients? The Evidence-Based Medicine Working Group. JAMA 1994;271:703–707.
16. Ransohoff DF, Feinstein AR. Problems of spectrum and bias in evaluating the efficacy of diagnostic tests. N Engl J Med 1978; 299:926–930.
17. Hulley SB, Feigal D, Martin M, Cummings SR. Designing a new study. IV. Experiments. In: Hulley SB, Cummings SR, eds. Designing clinical research. Ch. 11. Baltimore: Williams and Wilkins, 1988:110–127.
18. Popma JJ, Dehmer GJ, Walker BS, Simon TR, Smitherman TC. Analysis of thallium-201 single-photon emission computed tomography after intravenous dipyridamole using different quantitative measures of coronary stenosis severity and receiver operator characteristic curves. Am Heart J 1992;124:65–74.
19. Brismar J. Understanding receiver-operating-characteristic curves: a graphic approach. Am J Roentgenol 1991;157:1119–1121.
20. Vining DJ, Gladish GW. Receiver operating characteristic curves: a basic understanding. Radiographics 1992;12:1147–1154.
21. Sainfort F. Evaluation of medical technologies: a generalized ROC analysis. Med Decis Making 1991;11:208–220.
22. Van der Schouw YT, Verbeek AL, Ruijs JH. ROC curves for the initial assessment of new diagnostic tests. Fam Pract 1992;9:506–511.
23. Obuchowski NA. Computing sample size for receiver operating characteristic studies. Invest Radiol 1994;29:238–243.
24. Hilden J. The area under the ROC curve and its competitors. Med Decis Making 1991;11:95–101.
25. Harrington MB. Some methodological questions concerning receiver operating characteristic (ROC) analysis as a method for assessing image quality in radiology. J Digit Imaging 1990;3:211–218.
26. Hanley JA. Receiver operating characteristic (ROC) methodology: the state of the art. Crit Rev Diagn Imaging 1989;29:307–335.
27. Chybowski F, Keller J, Bergstrahl E, Oesterling J. Predicting radionuclide bone scan findings in patients with newly diagnosed, untreated prostate cancer: prostate specific antigen is superior to all other clinical parameters. J Urol 1991;145:313–318.
28. Metz CE. Some practical issues of experimental design and data analysis in radiological ROC studies. Invest Radiol 1989;24:234–245.
29. Hanley JA, McNeil BJ. Comparing the area under two ROC curves derived from the same sample of patients. Radiology 1983; 148:839.
30. Altman DG. Some common problems in medical research. In: Altman DG, ed. Practical statistics for medical research. London: Chapman and Hall, 1991:403–409.
31. Jaeschke R, Guyatt G, Sackett D. Users guides to the medical literature. 3. How to use an article about a diagnostic test. a. Are the results of the study valid? JAMA 1994;271:389–391.
32. Gurney JW. Determining the likelihood of malignancy in solitary pulmonary nodules with Bayesian analysis. Radiology 1993; 186:405–413.
33. PIOPED I. Value of the ventilation/perfusion scan in acute pulmonary embolism. Results of the prospective investigation of pulmonary embolism diagnosis (PIOPED). JAMA 1990;263:2753–2759.
34. Royal HD. Technology assessment: scientific challenges. AJR 1994;163:503–507.
35. The clinical examination. In: Sackett DL, Haynes RB, Guyatt GH, et al., eds. Clinical epidemiology: a basic science for clinical medicine. Ch 2. Boston: Little, Brown and Company, 1991:25–34.
36. Kopans DB. The accuracy of mammographic interpretation. N Engl J Med 1994;331:1521–1522.
37. Elmore JG, Wells CK, Lee CH, Howard DH, Feinstein AR. Variability in radiologists' interpretations of mammograms. N Engl J Med 1994;331:1493–1499.
38. Hamilton G, Trobaugh GB, Ritchie JL, Gould L, DeRouen TA, Williams DL. Myocardial imaging with thallium-201: an analysis of the clinical usefulness of Bayes' theorem. Semin Nucl Med 1978; 8:358.
39. Diamond GA, Forrester JS, Hirsch M, et al. Analysis of probability as an aid in the clinical diagnosis of coronary artery disease. New Engl J Med 1979;300:1350–1358.
40. Hlatky M, Botvinick E, Brundage B. Diagnostic accuracy of cardiologists compared to probability calculations using Bayes' rule. Am J Cardiol 1982;49:1927–1931.
41. Thornbury JR. Clinical efficacy of diagnostic imaging: love it or leave it. AJR 1994;162:1–8.
42. Hoffer PB, Neumann R, Quartararo L, Lange R, Hernandez T. Improved intrinsic resolution: does it make a difference? J Nucl Med 1984;25:230–236.
43. McNeil BJ, Weichselbaum R, Pauker SG. Fallacy of five-year survival in lung cancer. New Engl J Med 1978;299:1397–1401.
44. McNeil BJ, Pauker SG, Sox HCJ, Tversky A. On the elicitation of preferences for alternative therapies. New Engl J Med 1982; 306:1259–1262.
45. McNeil BJ, Weichselbaum R, Pauker SG. Speech and survival tradeoffs between quality and quantity of life in laryngeal cancer. New Engl J Med 1981;305:982–987.
46. Keeney RL, Raiffa H. Decision making with multiple objectives: preferences and value tradeoffs. New York: John Wiley & Sons, 1976.
47. Cleary PD, Greenfield S, McNeil BJ. Assessing quality of life after surgery. Control Clin Trials 1991;12:189S–203S.
48. Shapiro S. Evidence for screening for breast cancer from a randomized trial. Cancer 1977;39:2772.
49. Miller AB. Mammography screening guidelines for women 40 to 49 and over 65 years old. Ann Epidemiol 1994;4:96–101.
50. Nystrom L, Rutqvist LE, Wall S, et al. Breast cancer screening with mammography: overview of Swedish randomised trials [Published erratum appears in Lancet 1993;342:1372]. Lancet 1993; 341:973–978.
51. Burhenne LJ, Burhenne HJ. The Canadian National Breast Screening Study: a Canadian critique. AJR 1993;161:761–763.
52. Eddy DM. Screening for cancer: theory, analysis and design. Englewood, NJ: Prentice -Hall, 1980.
53. Tengs TO, Adams ME, Pliskin JS, et al. Five-hundred life-saving interventions and their cost-effectiveness. Risk Analysis 1995;(in press).
54. McNeil BJ. Socioeconomic forces affecting medicine: times of increased retrenchment and accountability. Semin Nucl Med 1993; 23:3–8.
55. Doubilet P, Abrams HL. The cost of underutilization. Percutaneous transluminal angioplasty for peripheral vascular disease. New Engl J Med 1984;310:95–102.

14 Radiopharmaceuticals

WILLIAM C. ECKELMAN, J. STEIGMAN and C. PAIK

Since the first tracer study by George C. de Hevesy in 1923, in which he used the tracer principle to study the absorption and translocation of lead nitrate with ^{212}Pb (1), many radionuclides have been used both in vitro and in vivo to trace various biologic processes. Suitable radionuclides have γ-ray energies between 60 and 600 keV and have physical properties such that a usable photon flux is available for the diagnostic study without excessive absorbed radiation dose to the patient. Additionally, ready availability and low cost are important. The ability to incorporate radionuclides with optimal decay characteristics into tracer molecules has been the foremost consideration in the development of most radiopharmaceuticals. However, many of these radionuclides were chosen because they were inexpensive, which usually means reactor produced, and easily converted to the intended chemical form. The radioisotopes of iodine in particular have played an important role in the development of nuclear medicine since their early use in thyroid metabolism studies (^{131}I) and radioimmunoassay (^{125}I). Although ^{131}I does not have ideal nuclear properties for external imaging with the Anger camera, it was used extensively because of its ready availability and easy conversion to the appropriate chemical form. Most of the iodine-labeled radiopharmaceuticals for imaging were eventually replaced by biologically equivalent ^{99m}Tc radiopharmaceuticals.

TECHNETIUM CHEMISTRY

A turning point for nuclear medicine occurred in the late 1950s at Brookhaven National Laboratory. In the process of separating the fission product ^{132}Te, the daughter radionuclide, ^{132}I, was contaminated with ^{99m}Tc. This observation and subsequent experiments led to the development of the ^{99}Mo-^{99m}Tc generator. When the long-lived parent ^{99}Mo ($t_{1/2}$ = 66 hours) was adsorbed to alumina, the short-lived daughter ^{99m}Tc ($t_{1/2}$ = 6 hours) could be eluted with isotonic saline (2). The first generators used fission product ^{99}Mo and hence used high specific activity ^{99}Mo (specific activity $>10^4$ Ci/g), whereas ^{99}Mo was later produced in a reactor by irradiating ^{98}Mo with thermal neutrons. This produced lower specific activity material. Because of the demand for Curie-level generators and the shielding requirements associated with large generators, fission-produced ^{99}Mo is once again used. With high specific activity, fission-produced ^{99}Mo, smaller alumina columns can be used with satisfactory chromatographic properties (i.e., low ^{99}Mo breakthrough). Of the conveniently available radionuclides, ^{99m}Tc has by far the best nuclear properties for imaging with the Anger camera. The 6-hour physical half-life and absence of β particle result in a low equilibrium dose constant ($D = 0.303$ γ-rad/μCi-hr) (3). The 140-keV γ emission has satisfactory tissue penetration (50% is absorbed in 4.6 cm of tissue), and yet the energy is low enough to be collimated easily.

With Curie-level generators, attention must be given to the total mass of technetium present. The label of "carrier-free ^{99m}Tc" is a misnomer because 13% of the ^{99}Mo disintegrations produce ^{99}Tc directly, whereas 87% of the disintegrations go through the ^{99m}Tc metastable state. Because of the parallel paths and the use of Curie-level generators, micromolar concentrations of ^{99}Tc ($t_{1/2} = 2 \times 10^6$ years) can be detected (4). The ^{99}Mo-^{99m}Tc generator system is described mathematically by a simplification of the general decay equation for the particular situation known as transient equilibrium (5).

REDUCING AGENTS FOR Tc(VII)

The chemical form of ^{99m}Tc eluted from the generator is usually TcO_4^-, the most stable chemical state of technetium in aqueous solution (6). With the advent of the ^{99}Mo-^{99m}Tc generator in the 1960s (2), the development of "instant" kits (7), and innovations in the type of chelating agents, the use of ^{99m}Tc-labeled compounds has expanded. But pertechnetate does not bind to chelating agents necessary for bone and renal imaging procedures, nor does it coprecipitate with particles necessary for pulmonary imaging procedures. Consequently, a less stable lower oxidation state of ^{99m}Tc capable of reacting with various chelating agents must be formed. The only exception to this is ^{99m}Tc sulfur colloid, which is considered to have the Tc(VII) oxidation state, because the insolubility of the technetium sulfide stabilizes the ^{99m}Tc in this oxidation state (6). Reduced states of technetium can be achieved by treatment with such reducing agents as stannous ion, the combination of ferric chloride and ascorbic acid, ferrous ion, sodium borohydride, concentrated hydrochloric acid, sodium dithionite, hypophosphorous acid, and hydrazine. The sulfhydryl group and the aldehyde group have been used as reducing agents, but both require heat and time to produce reasonable yields, which makes them somewhat less convenient. Pertechnetate can also be reduced electrolytically; that is, electrons can be supplied by a voltage applied to inert electrodes. With zirconium and tin electrodes, metallic-reducing species probably are responsible for the reduction. In the reduced state, the technetium binds readily to chelating agents, forming compounds such as ^{99m}Tc diethylenetriaminepenta acetic acid (DTPA), ^{99m}Tc methylene diphosphonate (MDP), and ^{99m}Tc glucoheptonate, which are commonly used in diagnostic imaging. Reduced technetium also coprecipitates with colloids to produce compounds such as ^{99m}Tc stannous oxide or ^{99m}Tc microaggregates, and with particles to produce ^{99m}Tc stannous macroaggregated albumin (MAA).

Many of the first ^{99m}Tc chelates were formed using ferric chloride and ascorbic acid as the reducing agent (8). Although these agents produced a suitable radiopharmaceutical, the need to use special equipment, such as a pH meter, and to prepare sterile buffers prevented their routine use in most nuclear medicine laboratories. The introduction of stannous ion as a reducing agent permitted pertechnetate to be added to the reaction vial with no pH adjustment or addition of other substances. Pertechnetate is reduced at pH 4–7 and then bound by the chelating agent (7). On a practical level, this use of stannous ion was a key development; most current radiopharmaceutical kits employ the stannous reduction technique. For blood cells, which are sensitive to changes in pH, stannous ion is ideal.

OXIDATION STATE OF ^{99m}Tc RADIOPHARMACEUTICALS

Although there have been considerable efforts to characterize Tc compounds (9), many studies have been carried out in nonaqueous solutions and therefore are not directly applicable to clinical ^{99}Tc radiopharmaceuticals. On the other hand, recent work on ^{99}Tc compounds in aqueous solution has involved thiol compounds that are not used routinely (10). The following oxidation states have been established for the carrier preparation (^{99}Tc) of the clinically useful radiopharmaceuticals:

- Tc(III)
  - Tc-Sn-DTPA
  - Tc-Sn-phosphonate
  - Tc-Sn-phosphate
  - Tc-teboroxime
  - Tc-HIDA (hepatobiliary agents)
- Tc(IV)
  - Tc-Sn-phosphonate
  - Tc-Sn-phosphates
- Tc(V)
  - Tc-gluconate
  - Tc-DMSA
  - Tc-MAG3
  - Tc-exametazime (HMPAO)
- Tc(I)
  - Tc-sestamibi

Whether the ^{99m}Tc-labeled compounds exist in these oxidation states, however, has not been determined absolutely, although for teboroxime and sestamibi the evidence is very strong.

CHELATING AGENTS FOR TECHNETIUM

Technetium chelates are used to varying degrees in the study of three organ systems: the kidney, the liver, and bone (Table 14.1). The kidney agents can be divided into three groups: (a) those that measure glomerular filtration, (b) those that measure tubular secretion, and (c) those that measure multiple functions including filtration, secretion, and absorption. The exact mechanisms of localization and excretion of many of the agents in the third category are unknown (Table 14.1).

Technetium-99m DTPA is the best example of a kidney agent that is filtered by the glomeruli (11). ^{99m}Tc DADS (*N*, *N*'-bis(mercaptoacetamido)-ethylenediamine) and derivatives thereof have been shown to be cleared primarily by tubular secretion (12), and then have been replaced by ^{99m}TcMAG3 which has fewer stereoisomers (13).

Table 14.1.
Chelating agents for ^{99m}Tc

Kidney	Liver	Bone
Glomerular filtration		
DTPA	Penicillamine	Polyphosphate
EDTA	Pyridoxylidene glutamate	Tripolyphosphate
Cyclam	Dihydrothioctic acid	Pyrophosphate
Tubular secretion		
DADS	Tetracycline	Diphosphonates
Multiple function		
Mannitol	Mercaptoisobutyric acid	
Caseidin	6-Mercaptopurine	
Citrate	HIDA	
Tetracycline	BIDA	
Inulin	PIPIDA	
Ascorbate	DISIDA	
Gluconate		
Glucoheptonate		
Dimercaptosuccinic acid		

Renal extraction efficiencies were determined by McAfee, et al., for many of the kidney agents in Table 14.1 (14). Orthoiodohippurate had the highest extraction efficiency, whereas the ^{99m}Tc complexes of DTPA and glucoheptonate have extraction efficiencies of only 27–29%. ^{99m}Tc dimercaptosuccinic acid (DMSA) and ^{197}Hg chlormerodrin have lower extraction values of 8% and 14%, respectively. DTPA and DADS form stable chelates with ^{99m}Tc so that the radiochemical purity in vivo is high. Chromatography of either plasma or urine confirms this high radiochemical purity.

In 1971, Subramanian and McAfee published the first studies of the use of a ^{99m}Tc bone-imaging agent (15). Up to that time ^{85}Sr strontium chloride and ^{18}F sodium fluoride had been used for bone imaging. In general, the quality of images obtained with the ^{99m}Tc bone agents has been closely correlated with rapid blood clearance. In this respect, ^{99m}Tc MDP appears to be one of the most rapidly cleared bone-imaging agents and is the most widely used clinically. Later, emphasis was placed on relative bone uptake. A hydroxy group on the central carbon of the diphosphonate moiety appears to enhance that property. Both ^{99m}Tc MDP (no hydroxy group) and ^{99m}Tc HMDP (1-hydroxy group) appear to clear the blood rapidly. Although ^{99m}Tc HMDP has lower bone concentration, it has a higher differential uptake between areas of bone with different metabolic rates (16, 17).

Buja, et al. (18), have shown that the soft tissue uptake of ^{99m}Tc HEDP is positively related to tissue calcium levels. Other proposed uptake mechanisms, such as high-affinity binding to organic matrix, to tissue phosphatases, or to various proteins of damaged tissue, may play minor roles in ^{99m}Tc localization in the bone (19).

Autoradiographic studies confirm that the growing face of the apatite crystal is the point of uptake of ^{99m}Tc bone-imaging agents (20, 21); the chemical form could not be distinguished from ^{99m}Tc MDP (22). Earlier theories had proposed that ^{99m}Tc would be displaced on the bone surface by calcium to produce TcO_2 (19, 23, 24). Pinkerton, et al., have shown that ^{99m}Tc HEDP prepared with sodium borohydride contains many components before injection (25, 26), and Steigman, et al., have suggested the possibility of polymeric species (27). Therefore, in vivo radiochemical purity is difficult to assess.

The localization mechanism of ^{99m}Tc phosphate radiotracers in myocardial infarcts and in other soft-tissue abnormalities probably involves microcalcification. Of the bone tracers, ^{99m}Tc pyrophosphate (PYP) is the most widely used in clinical evaluation of myocardial infarcts (28). The reasons for the discrepancies between the relative uptakes of ^{99m}Tc PYP and ^{99m}Tc MDP in damaged myocardial tissue and the relative uptakes of these complexes in bone are not known.

^{99m}Tc chelates that are taken up by the hepatocytes in the liver are a recent class of ^{99m}Tc chelates used in the clinic. The hepatocytes in the liver remove the ^{99m}Tc hepatobiliary agents from plasma by an active transport process. Most current ^{99m}Tc hepatobiliary agents are cleared by the same general anionic mechanism operative for bilirubin. Therefore, in hyperbilirubinemia, there is competitive inhibition for transport of the ^{99m}Tc agents. All hepatobiliary agents appear to have certain chemical characteristics that distinguish them from substances excreted by the kidney (29). The molecular weight of hepatobiliary agents is usually between 300 and 1000; the molecules contain at least two lipophilic structures and a polar group. Neither ^{99m}Tc pyridoxylidene glutamate (PG) nor ^{99m}Tc *N*-(2,6-dimethylphenol-carbamoylmethyl)-iminodiacetic acid (HIDA) is extensively protein bound in plasma (30).

To optimize these chemical properties, many ^{99m}Tc agents have been prepared and evaluated. As early as 1974, hepatobiliary ^{99m}Tc chelates were proposed as possible replacements for ^{131}I Rose Bengal (31) for evaluation of hepatobiliary excretion disorders. The early ^{99m}Tc hepatobiliary agents were excreted by both kidney and liver. The first improvements focused on decreasing the kidney component of clearance; later efforts centered on accelerating blood clearance. The search continues for derivatives that are cleared from the blood and liver at a faster rate. Both ^{99m}Tc HIDA and ^{99m}Tc PG radiopharmaceuticals are bis chelates of ^{99m}Tc (32). Other stannous ion instant kits leading to disofenin (33), lidofenin, and mebrofenin (34) have been produced.

Recent Advances in ^{99m}Tc Chelate Chemistry

^{201}Tl, as the +1 thallous ion, has been the agent of choice for myocardial perfusion studies (35). Since 1980, technetium cations have been proposed as myocardial perfusion agents (36). These agents contain lipophilic groups complexed to the technetium in such a way that there is a formal charge of +1 for the complex. The complexing agents contain arsine- or phosphine-containing ligands and are identified by the acronyms of Tc-DIARS and Tc-DMPE. Although these agents distributed in the canine myocardium as a function of blood flow and superior images of perfusion defects were obtained, the same results could not be obtained in humans. The species differences observed earlier by Carr, et al. (37), for bretylium were again evident in these technetium cations. Carr, et al. (37), proposed an uptake-2 mechanism in animals that was absent in humans as an explanation for the lack of bretylium concentration in the human heart, whereas Ichimura, et al. (38), proposed a redox mechanism to explain the low concentration of the technetium cations in the human heart. In the latter hypothesis the Tc(III) (net charge +1) is reduced to Tc(II) (net charge 0), and this neutral species is not retained by the myocardium.

The next group of technetium complexes to be tested were those with technetium in a lower oxidation state, Tc(I) (also containing a net charge of +1). The technetium hexakis (isonitrile) (CNR) complexes (39) and the technetium tris-DMPE (40) complexes are examples of such potential myocardial perfusion agents. Whereas technetium $DMPE_3^+$ disappears from the blood of humans much slower than it does in animals, $Tc(CNR)_6^+$ showed high uptake in the human lung. Both of these problems led to delayed imaging times. Improvements in the pharmacokinetic properties by producing esters and other derivatives of the isonitriles have led to better myocardial imaging agents (41, 42).

Other ^{99m}Tc cations, such as hexakis (2-methoxy-2-methylpropyl) isonitrile (also known as sestamibi and RP-30) and neutral ^{99m}Tc complexes such as bis[(1,2-cyclohexane dionedioximato(1)-O], [(1,2-cyclohexanedione-dioximato(2●) - O)]methylborato(2●) - N,N′,N″,N‴,N⁗,N‴″) - chlorotechnetium (one of a class of boron adducts of technetium dioximes (BATOs) also known as teboroxime, SQ 30,217 or CDO-MeB) (43–45) have been evaluated to determine their suitability as myocardial perfusion agents. Although these two radiopharmaceuticals are both indicated for use as myocardial perfusion agents, their biologic properties differ substantially. Sestamibi is a positively charged, lipid soluble ^{99m}Tc complex that appears to be bound in the mitochondria of myocytes by virtue of the transmembrane potential (46). Sestamibi is taken up by the myocardium and retained with a half-life of greater than 12 hours, whereas ^{99m}Tc-labeled teboroxime is taken up rapidly and released rapidly (47, 48). With teboroxime, the imaging must be completed within the first 10 minutes after injection. This latter compound is more characteristic of xenon than of thallium, and can be used to obtain rapid repeat studies. Teboroxime is a neutral compound that is more highly extracted than thallium and/or sestamibi and should, therefore, be more sensitive to small changes in flow, especially during a stress test. Both ^{99m}Tc radiopharmaceuticals do not "redistribute" to the extent that ^{201}Tl does and, therefore, two injections are required to obtain a stress and a rest study. There have been recent efforts to view the net efflux of teboroxime from the heart as "redistribution" (49, 50) and obtain both stress and rest information from a single injection. A recent review of cardiac imaging with sestamibi and teboroxime by Leppo, DePuey, and Johnson, which crowns an excellent series of 10 articles on these two heart agents, appears in the October, 1991 edition of the Journal of Nuclear Medicine (51). Both heart agents were approved by the Federal Drug Administration (FDA) at the end of 1990 and are rapidly expanding the type of information obtained in diagnostic myocardial perfusion studies. Sestamibi is more widely utilized than teboroxime because of the rapid clearance of teboroxime from the myocardium and the difficulty this clearance poses for imaging.

^{133}Xe is approved by the FDA for the measurement of cerebral perfusion. ^{123}I-labeled N-isopropylamphetamine (52) (Spectamine), in 1989, became the second commercially available agent that crosses the intact blood-brain barrier. The distribution immediately after injection is flow related, but the immediate uptake and later distribution are dependent on amine uptake processes. Recently, several neutral ^{99m}Tc-labeled compounds were proposed for measuring cerebral blood flow in disease states in which the blood-brain barrier is intact. The series of propyleneamineoximes are interesting cerebral perfusion agents. Whereas ^{99m}Tc PNAO (propyleneamine oxime) is taken up efficiently and released from the cerebrum rapidly, a derivative, ^{99m}Tc exametazine (d,l hexamethylpropylene-amine oxime (HMPAO)) is taken up and retained. The mechanism of retention is thought to be binding to glutathione in the brain, although this is far from proven (53). Because the available single-head rotating SPECT instruments are relatively insensitive to emitted photons, the latter compound is being studied in the clinic after approval by the FDA in 1989. However, with the proliferation of multihead SPECT machines, those compounds with fast pharmacokinetics may be more useful because repeat studies can be carried out with minimal delay. The analogy with myocardial imaging agents is important. Finally, there is an ester derivative of the diamino, disulfide chelation system (N,N′-1,2 ethylenediyl-bis-L-cysteine diethylester, Neurolite and Tc-ECD) that is taken up in the human brain (54). This compound depends on the slow hydrolysis of the ester groups in the blood and the rapid hydrolysis of ester groups in the brain to give high cerebral uptake and retention of the more hydrophilic metabolite. It appears that a series of first generation ^{99m}Tc compounds have been developed to measure perfusion in the brain and hold great promise for establishing the usefulness of nuclear medicine studies of cerebral perfusion in diseases that do not disrupt the blood-brain barrier. Dementia and stroke are the two most frequently mentioned abnormalities that can be evaluated by cerebral perfusion imaging. In general, the preparation of teboroxime, sestamibi, Tc-HMPAO, and Tc-ECD is more complicated than that needed for the previously established kits, but still falls under the general concept of "instant kits."

COLLOIDS AND PARTICLES LABELED WITH ^{99m}Tc

Numerous radiolabeled colloids for use in hepatic scintigraphy have been reported. The one most commonly used is ^{99m}Tc sulfur colloid prepared from the acid decomposition of sodium thiosulfate in the presence of a variety of stabilizing agents. Among these are gelatin (the most popular), albumin, polyvinylpyrrolidone and polyhydric alcohol. Stabilizer-free preparations also have been proposed, as well as compounds with the carriers rhenium and antimony. Other types of colloids include stannous oxide, technetium oxide, and microaggregated albumin (55).

Determination of the particle size of colloids is important because the size may be related to the distribution. Methods of determining particle size differ, depending on whether the colloids are radioactive or nonradioactive. Warbick, et al. (56), assuming no differences between labeled and nonlabeled colloid particle size distribution, compared several sizing methods. ^{99m}Tc sulfur colloid prepared with perrhenate carrier showed at least three major size components: 22% of particles were $<$100 nm; 39% between 200 and 400 nm; and 24% $>$400 nm (56). Davis, et al. (57), also showed that such cellulose membrane filters as Millipore do not filter particles according to size because of the filter thickness and irregular path. For the technetium sulfur colloid analyzed by Warbick, et al. (56), electron microscopy revealed the presence of aggregates as the cause of the bimodal distribution observed with Nuclepore filters. They have demonstrated that technetium antimony sulfur colloid has a smaller particle size (average = 10 nm) than thiosulfate-prepared sulfur colloid. Billinghurst and Jette (58) proposed gel filtration for colloidal particles below 100-nm diameter because larger particles are above the maximum operating range. Additionally, based on the relationship between percentage radioactivity and number of particles, they proposed that the surface area, not the volume, is the relevant variable. Only certain particle size ranges can be analyzed on these columns, and the elution time is long (58).

Pedersen and Kristensen (59) used several techniques, including filtration, photon correlation spectroscopy, and light microscopy for evaluating colloid preparations. They confirmed by these methods that several ^{99m}Tc colloid preparations change with time. They reemphasized that the Nucleopore filtration technique measures the distribution of radioactivity in particles of different sizes, whereas photon correlation spectroscopy (Nanosizer) measures particle size.

Recently, Subhani, et al. (60), compared 14 commercially available colloids. They used Nucleopore filters with various pore sizes to determine the distribution of the ^{99m}Tc colloids. Colloids ranged from those having greater than 97% passing through a 0.2 mm filter to those which had $>$49% of the particles larger than 3 mm. The amount in the liver of mice for the preformed colloids ranged from 73–93%. The albumin-based colloids showed similar distribution in mice, but a broader range of liver uptake in rabbits.

In some preparations of ^{99m}Tc sulfur colloid, the colloid adheres to the walls of the glass vial in which it has been prepared. If the total vial is assayed, an aliquot removed may not represent the true fraction removed. It is, therefore, necessary to assay the dose in the syringe. Unless the syringe containing colloid is flushed with the patient's blood, a substantial fraction of the dose can remain in the syringe.

Several ^{99m}Tc-labeled particles can be used for lung scanning. Methods and types of preparations include macroaggregation of ^{99m}Tc-labeled albumin, the conversion of technetium sulfur colloid into human serum albumin (HSA) macroaggregates, coprecipitation of ^{99m}Tc with iron hydroxide, macroaggregation of albumin in the presence of colloid, and incorporation of ^{99m}Tc sulfur colloid or reduced technetium into microspheres. Macroaggregates are the most commonly used (61).

Microspheres are particles formed by extrusion of albumin into hot oil, as opposed to macroaggregates which are formed by heating albumin in water (62). Other microspheres of various compositions are valuable for diagnostic and therapeutic purposes (63).

It is important that labeled particles be of nearly uniform size and that only a small proportion of unbound radionuclide exists. Microspheres are supplied presieved and have a narrow size range. The fraction of unbound radionuclide may be determined by washing or incubating with the fluid to be used, filtering the mixture of spheres and fluid through a 0.45-μm filter to retain the spheres, and determining the activity of the filtrate. The U.S. Pharmacopeia (USP) specifies that no less than 90% of ^{99m}Tc MAA have diameters between 10 and 90 μm and none may have a diameter greater than 150 μm (64). On some occasions, the particles may break under rough handling. They may also form large aggregates if they are mixed with blood before injection.

LABELING OF CELLS AND BLOOD ELEMENTS WITH ^{99m}Tc

The erythrocytes and albumin (HSA) have received the most attention in radiolabeling with ^{99m}Tc (65). Although in vitro labeling of red blood cells (RBCs) appears to be superior to in vivo labeling (injecting tin intravenously, followed 20 minutes later by injecting ^{99m}Tc pertechnetate), many laboratories still use the latter technique because of technical ease. In vitro methods, especially those using the pretinning kit developed by Brookhaven National Laboratory, appear to produce quantitative retention of radioactivity in the RBCs (66, 67). The problem with the in vivo labeling technique described by Pavel and Zimmer (68), is the low labeling yield in some patients (69). Gottschalk, et al. (70), have suggested that the two techniques can be combined as follows. Stannous pyrophosphate is injected as in the in vivo technique, but instead of injecting ^{99m}Tc pertechnetate 15 minutes later, blood is withdrawn and labeled in vitro. This modification permits determination of the labeling yield before reinjection (70).

Attempts have also been made to label leukocytes, lymphocytes, and platelets using this technique, although little success has been achieved in the clinic. Tumor cells that have been labeled with ^{99m}Tc include murine fibrosarcoma, human carcinoma of the breast, lung and colon, and malignant melanoma. Thymocyte labeling with ^{99m}Tc also has been reported.

Because of the frequency of thromboembolic disorders, great interest has surrounded labeled fibrinogen and urokinase for thrombus localization. Streptokinase, although not found in humans, has been studied for the same reasons, as has plasmin. For these and all other blood products and cells mentioned, the labeling procedure is based on the stannous chloride method developed for RBCs and HSA.

METHODS TO RADIOLABEL PROTEINS WITH ^{99m}Tc

Most iodinated radiopharmaceuticals used in nuclear medicine have been replaced by ones labeled with ^{99m}Tc. The inferior nuclear properties of ^{131}I for imaging, and the chemical instability of the iodine-carbon bond, are usually given as the reasons for this. In the case of ^{131}I-labeling of antibodies, the logic is complicated by its therapeutic properties. Therefore, this comparison is valid only for radiolabeled antibodies used for diagnosis. Soon after the discovery of ^{131}I in a tellurium target bombarded in the Berkeley cyclotron, Hamilton and Soley (71), in 1939, used this radionuclide in its simplest chemical form, iodide, to study iodine metabolism. In the following years, various molecules were radioiodinated. The ability to radioiodinate proteins at high specific activity was a major factor in the development of the insulin radioimmunoassay by Berson and Yalow (72). Antibodies were also first radiolabeled with ^{131}I (73). As early as 1957, Pressman, et al. (73), were able to localize tumors by scanning using radiolabeled antibodies. With the development of the ^{99}Mo-^{99m}Tc generator system in the late 1950s, there has been a continuous effort to first label proteins and later to label antibodies with ^{99m}Tc.

Because ^{99m}Tc-labeled antibodies is used for diagnosis, the ideal radiolabeled antibody is the one for which the ^{99m}Tc "traces" the distribution of the antibody. However, the clinical importance of antibody radiolabeled with ^{99m}Tc is still not well-documented. Nuclear medicine is competing with other imaging modalities that are capable of much higher information density. Although the use of ^{99m}Tc-labeled antibodies will increase the specificity of the nuclear medicine study, no studies have been published showing that the sensitivity is comparable to computed tomography (CT) or magnetic resonance imaging (MRI) in establishing the size, shape, and position of a tumor. In general, nuclear medicine's strength lies in its ability to map either perfusion or biochemical changes. The contrast agents used to enhance CT or MRI are at relatively high concentrations and therefore not suited for measuring biochemical processes.

In general, CT and MRI have higher resolution than the planar scintillation camera or SPECT. If the general location of the primary tumors or the metastases can be specified, CT or MRI should be superior in detecting small tumors. High tumor to nontumor ratios and high count ratios are necessary to detect even 1 cm^2 tumors at depths of 1–5 cm using the planar Anger camera (74). In the very important case where the metastases are extensive and a whole body survey is indicated, the radiodiagnostic technique has an advantage.

Larson, et al. (75), have also suggested staging and monitoring therapeutic response as important goals of cancer diagnosis with radionuclides. Another important use is to characterize the tumor by using antibodies specific for a particular tumor marker such as a growth hormone receptor. SPECT offers some improvement in resolution, especially when overlying structures are involved but the need for information density is increased. Most SPECT studies to date are carried out with 5–10% of the injected dose in the target organ, whereas antibody concentrations rarely reach the level of 0.1% dose localized in the tumor (76).

Based on the energy or the γ-ray emission, ^{123}I is similar to ^{99m}Tc. Given that ^{123}I is easier to manipulate chemically than ^{99m}Tc, the former should be the radionuclide of choice for labeling antibodies. However, pure ^{123}I is only produced at a high energy cyclotron, whereas ^{99m}Tc is available from a generator system. Thus, ^{123}I is not competitive with ^{99m}Tc either from availability or cost standpoint. Even with the rather complicated chemistry needed to label antibodies with ^{99m}Tc, the overall advantage still lies with ^{99m}Tc.

Direct labeling, that is, using the amino acids of the antibody to complex the metal, may result in a labile chemical bond because of the stereochemistry of the functional groups in the tertiary structure of the antibody. Only when the protein is known to bind the metal with high affinity is direct labeling useful. Even in those cases, the protein is usually labeled by injecting a soluble salt that exchanges with the protein. The injection of ^{67}Ga-citrate and ^{111}In-chloride are examples of direct labeling of proteins (e.g., transferrin) in vivo. On the other hand, ^{99m}Tc has been directly labeled to proteins, and particularly to antibodies (77–79), but the stability and inertness of the bond are in question. Although the investigators utilized different buffer systems, pH, and incubation times, a common feature is the use of stannous ion as a reducing agent. The advantage of direct labeling is its experimental simplicity. However, in at least one case, the resulting antibody complex with ^{99m}Tc has been reported to be unstable, necessitating the use of an elaborate molecular permeation chromatographic system to purify the ^{99m}Tc-labeled antibodies. This observation is consistent with that of Eckelman, et al. (80), who published in 1971, that albumin binding of ^{99m}Tc is so weak, multiple chromatographic purifications resulted in further radiochemical impurities as a result of dissociation. The competitive binding of ^{99m}Tc by stannous oxide also was a source of radiochemical impurities. Since then, other reviews have documented the same instabilities. Steigman, et al. (81), suggested that the mechanism of binding was related to sulfhydryl groups, but Hnatowich's group (82) proposed the importance of a helix structure. Paik, et al. (83), suggested that ^{99m}Tc is bound by both a high affinity, low capacity site and a low affinity, high capacity site. Their study suggests that the high affinity site is, indeed, related to the presence of sulfhydryl groups. However, the extent of high affinity site-binding is not quantitative and depends on the antibody fragment used. For IgG and $F(ab')_2$ which contain disulfide bridges between the heavy chains, high titers of reduced disulfide groups are detected in the presence of stannous ion. For Fab, which does not have a disulfide bridge between heavy chains, very few sulfhydryl groups could be detected. This trend parallels the percentage binding of ^{99m}Tc when binding to the low affinity site is prevented by the presence of excess DTPA. For IgG, about 24% of the ^{99m}Tc binds to high affinity sites, whereas for $F(ab')_2$ only 16% of the ^{99m}Tc is bound to the high affinity sites. Very little ^{99m}Tc is bound to Fab with high affinity. These results are useful in interpreting other data. For instance, Rhodes, et al., probably increased the high affinity binding by long incubation of antibodies with stannous ion. Khaw, et al. (84), probably had a small percentage of directly bound antibody because they used Fab fragments, whereas Lanteigne, et al. (85), showed binding via DTPA and directly to IgG. The best solution to the problem of low affinity binding of ^{99m}Tc has been put forth by Paik, et al., who suggest that all radiolabeling with ^{99m}Tc or with ^{111}In should be done in the presence of excess DTPA. Even though that may decrease the radiochemical yield, it guarantees an inert chemical bond either directly to the protein through the high affinity sites for ^{99m}Tc, or through the bifunctional chelate for Tc and In.

It has been more than 14 years since Rhodes developed the direct labeling method of pretinning the antibody by overnight incubation with stannous chloride (86). This procedure is the basis for the many "direct labeling" methods being pursued today. In Rhodes' current method, 0.67 ml of a solution containing 5 mm $SnCl_2$, 40 mm potassium phthalate, and 13.4 mm sodium potassium tartrate at pH 5.6 is added to 1 ml of 1 mg/ml antibody and incubated for 21 hours at room temperature (87). The pretinned antibody can be stored frozen at $-70°C$. Pertechnetate is added and incubated for 1 hour at room temperature. The radiochemical purity was determined using a TSK G3000SW column eluted with phosphate buffer. A transchelation challenge test used either 3 mm EDTA, 100 μg of pretinned antibody in phosphate buffer, 100 μg of pretinned antibody in 1% human serum albumin, or phosphate buffer. Equal volumes were mixed and incubated at room temperature for 1 hour or more before HPLC analysis. HPLC analysis of technetium labeled IgG mixed with one of the four challenge solutions showed that the technetium remains bound to the IgG. If the antibody has not been pretinned, the exchange with the challenge agent is rapid. The antibody must be rigorously purified before radiolabeling or low molecular weight components will be radiolabeled. Others have shown that the presence of citrate, for example, can reduce the radiochemical purity of labeled proteins (88).

Reno and Bottino (89) refined and expanded on Rhodes' approach by suggesting a series of reducing agents, weak chelating agents for ^{99m}Tc, and stabilizers for the preformed sulfhydryl groups. They showed that untreated antibody binds only 24% of added ^{99m}Tc, whereas DTT treated antibody binds 85%. Zinc stabilized antibody has a longer shelf-life than a reduced but unprotected antibody. Pak, et al. (90), in a patent, used a reducing agent such as dithiothreitol along with stannous chloride and a water-soluble ligand. Saccharic acid, glucoheptonic acid, tartaric, or another polyhydroxy carboxylic acid capable of complexing technetium were proposed as stabilizing agents.

In most cases, the direct labeling technique is a combination of an approach to increase the number of sulfhydryl groups in an antibody with a reducing agent and the use of a ligand capable of solubilizing Tc(V), yet still able to undergo rapid metal exchange with the antibody. Steigman, et al. (91), had proposed Tc(V) gluconate as the ideal exchange ligand after studying a series of polyalcohols and polyhydroxy carboxylic acids. A recent variation on this theme was presented by Bremer, et al. (92), who used propylenetetraphosphonate as the solubilizing ligand. They also preincubated the protein with a reducing agent such as 2-mercaptoethanol or 2-aminoethanethiol to increase the sulfhydryl concentration. Hansen, et al. (93), proposed a similar procedure whereby the freshly prepared Fab fragment is mixed with their reducing agent for 24 hours before adding pertechnetate.

DeFulvio and Thakur titrated free sulfhydryl groups using ninhydrin. Using molar ratios of between 1000 and 5000 of dithiothreitol (DTT), dierythritol (DTE), or 2-mercaptoethanol (2-ME) to IgG, they observed less than 2% reduction of the available 35 disulfide groups in IgG. Stannous chloride at molar ratios of 500–2500 reduced up to 1.8% of the available disulfide groups. The highest percentage reduction was obtained with molar ratios of 3500–17,500 of ascorbic acid. All reducing agents were mixed with IgG for 30 minutes. Radiolabeling with ^{99m}Tc led to various yields with a maximum of 96% for an ascorbic acid ratio of 3500. Incubation of the radiolabeled protein with 500 molar excess of DTPA or with HSA did not result in transchelation. Blocking the sulfhydryl groups with iodoacetate or cysteine decreased ^{99m}Tc binding. This most comprehensive report relates reducing agents to the number of sulfhydryl groups produced and radiochemical yield. More recently, John, Wilder, and Thakur (94) compared the fragmentation products from human polyclonal IgG after treatment with the various reducing agents. All reducing agents produced fragmentation with the least being seen with the authors' ascorbic acid procedure and the greatest with 2-mercaptoethanol procedure. The subsequent labeling with ^{99m}Tc produced a spectra of radiolabeled IgG and fragments.

There have been few comparisons in vivo of different methods of radiolabeling (95). The direct method of radiolabeling used was that of Rhodes (96). The indirect method was that of Abrams (97) using the hydrazine nicotinamide chelator. Direct labeling reduced the immunoreactivity to a greater extent than indirect labeling. Electrophoresis showed that direct labeling led to lower molecular weight species. The in vivo distribution showed the direct method produced more radioactivity in the kidney and less in the liver compared to the indirect method. However, there was no difference in clearance in patients using radiolabeled fragments (98), presumably because of the greater renal clearance of the fragments and the increased difficulty in observing increased renal radioactivity.

Another approach to binding ^{99m}Tc directly to antibodies is to increase the sulfhydryl groups using 2-iminothiolane (99). A molar ratio of 50 of 2-iminothiolane to IgG mixed for 30 minutes led to a 94% radiochemical yield with ^{99m}Tc using 1.4 μg tin(II). Using DTPA in a molar excess of 764 did not decrease the yield after 2.5 hours. Challenge experiments with cysteine led to 50% transchelation after 4 hours. Serum did not remove ^{99m}Tc. Goedemans, et al. (99), quote earlier work on Pb protein labeling as the basis for their approach. IgG has sufficient exposed lysine groups so that 6–9 attached sulfhydryl groups are introduced. Joiris, et al. (100), studied the same reaction for directly labeling antibodies. They state that this procedure is superior to the –use of a disulfide reducing agent because the latter produces fragments. For example, Fab is produced from $F(ab')_2$ whereas 1-iminothiolane does not produce such fragmentation.

The direct labeling of proteins in general and antibodies in particular is progressing with a number of these approaches being used in clinical trials. There is no doubt that the ^{99m}Tc is bound to the antibody. Nevertheless, identification of the binding site, the oxidation state of Tc, and the stability of the site(s) needs to be pursued. With the low percentage of the injected dose in the tumor and the photon-poor nature of nuclear medicine imaging, the search for these answers is of utmost importance.

The early indirect labeling methods mostly involved the use of DTPA conjugated to the protein. DTPA is considered a bifunctional chelate in that it binds to the protein and to ^{99m}Tc. Other chelating agents, derivatives of dimercaptoacetamide (DADS) (101), bis-N-methylthiosemicarbazone (102), metallothionein, thiolactone diaminedithiol, hydrazinonicotinic acid, and diaminetetrathiol have been conjugated to antibodies for ^{99m}Tc labeling.

Because both the direct labeling methods, which apparently depend on free sulfhydryl groups for binding ^{99m}Tc, and the bifunctional chelate approach, which depends on a competition between weak and strong direct binding and binding by the covalently bound chelating agent, do not achieve high radiochemical purity, investigators have turned to prelabeling the ligand and then reacting this ^{99m}Tc chelate with the antibody. Fritzberg, et al. (103), has prelabeled the DADS ligand and then bound the ligand to the antibody via an activated ester. Likewise Franz, et al. (104), have prelabeled a N-propylamine derivative of cyclan with ^{99m}Tc and then reacted that chelate with an activated antibody. Recently, BATO derivatives were used for a preformed ^{99m}Tc chelate approach to label antibodies. This method assumes that the ^{99m}Tc is bound to the chelating agent and, therefore, a single radiochemical is produced. On the other hand, the development of an "instant kit" will be difficult with this approach.

QUALITY CONTROL OF ^{99m}Tc RADIOPHARMACEUTICALS

The aim of quality control in radiopharmaceutical chemistry is to assure radionuclide and radiochemical purity, as well as sterility and apyrogenicity. Specific data on radionuclide impurities in the ^{99m}Tc generator are presented by Colombetti (105); the USP XXV also contains the acceptable limits of radionuclide impurities. In practice, ^{99}Mo impurity is limited to 0.15 μCi (5.55 kBq)/mCi of ^{99m}Tc at the time of administration. Tests for sterility and apyrogenicity are not required if sterile components such as nonradioactive kits and generator eluates are used. Reference texts on all aspects of quality control in nuclear medicine have been published (106, 107), but in general, the test for ^{99}Mo and tests for radiochemical purity are the major concerns. A chemical test for alumina being eluted from the ^{99m}Tc generator should also be a routine clinical procedure.

Radiochromatographic quality control of ^{99m}Tc radiopharmaceuticals has been relatively unsophisticated. Only recently has high performance liquid chromatography (HPLC) been applied to detect subtle impurities. Most systems are capable of detecting only one radiochemical impurity-pertechnetate. Likewise, most of the earlier systems for radioiodinated tracers were designed to detect iodide. For the newer iodinated products, especially receptor binding radiotracers, HPLC has become a necessity (107).

Most radiopharmaceuticals cannot be studied by ultraviolet or infrared spectroscopy, nuclear magnetic resonance, or elemental analysis because they are either no-carrier-added or carrier-free. Accordingly, chromatography has become the major analytic tool for determining their radiochemical purity. However, the term radiochemical purity is much maligned. The strict definition is the percentage of the radionuclide in question in the desired chemical form. The common mistake is to use a chromatographic system that can only separate one radiochemical impurity, usually pertechnetate, and then to report the radiochemical purity on that basis. Certainly, pertechnetate is the most obvious impurity, but a second impurity, commonly called reduced unbound ^{99m}Tc or reduced hydrolyzed ^{99m}Tc, has been identified (108). The exact nature of this species is not known and it may be a combination of impurities, but nevertheless, it is an impurity that must be separated from the required radiopharmaceutical.

Chromatographic Techniques

The most common method of separating a ^{99m}Tc radiopharmaceutical from its radiochemical impurities is chromatography. Paper chromatography and thin-layer chromatography (TLC) are simple methods of separation with closely related techniques for sample application, development, and detection. Column chromatography, including HPLC, is a more complicated technique that offers the choice of a wider variety of solid supports (absorption, gel filtration and permeation for molecular size, ion exchange, etc.) and is more adaptable to large-scale separations and to quantitation of the species present (109, 110). Recently, HPLC has been used for the less polar ^{99m}Tc chelates. This sensitive technique promises to make the definition of radiochemical purity more restrictive. With TLC and paper chromatography, only unchelated ^{99m}Tc species have been identified as radiochemical impurities, but with HPLC various chelated species have already been identified.

Paper and thin layer chromatography, used primarily to determine the presence of pertechnetate in radiopharmaceuticals, may be completed within 1 hour, are simple to perform, and do not require expensive equipment. The procedure consists of the application of microliter amounts of the radiochemical to the plate covered with a thin layer of adsorbent, or to the paper chromatogram, at a point approximately 1 inch from the end that is to be immersed in the eluting solution. This point is called the origin and is marked at the lateral surface of the strip or plate with pencil or some other identifying marker. The chromatogram is then immersed in the preferred solvent and the chromatographic tank is tightly covered. The solution level must be clearly below the point at which the radioactive sample is spotted. The solution ascends the strip by capillary action, carrying each radiochemical component according to its partition between the solid support material (e.g., the paper or silica gel) and the solution. When the solution has traveled the desired distance, the solvent front (S_f) is marked and the plate or strip is removed from the container and allowed to dry.

The distance traveled by each radioactive component of the solution under analysis is the most important factor in these determinations. This distance, termed the R_f value, is defined as the ratio of the distance traveled by a given radiochemical component compared to the solvent front. It is dependent upon conditions such as temperature, quality of the support material, and preequilibration of the solution; because of these variables, R_f values are not always reproducible. For this reason, a separate control strip with a pure sample of the suspected radiochemical impurity (e.g., pertechnetate) should be chromatographed simultaneously in the same container.

The radioactivity associated with the various components can now be determined by counting cut up portions of the chromatogram in a well counter or by counting using a radiochromatogram scanner, which gives the distribution of the radioactivity as a function of distance. Since glass-backed thin-layer strips must be scraped before counting the sectioned pieces, thus lengthening the procedure, fiber-backed or aluminum-backed thin-layer plates are preferable when cutting is necessary. Some clinics use the γ-camera to measure radioactivity as a function of distance on the chromatographic strip. Whatever analytic technique is used, the clinician must be certain that the counting is done with no counting losses due to coincidence at high count rates (see Chapter 7).

Generator Chromatography

The most important factor in the preparation of ^{99m}Tc radiopharmaceuticals is the radiochemical purity of pertechnetate eluted from the generator.

Two primary paper chromatography systems, based on the original work of Shukla (111), have been suggested to identify the various technetium species present in the generator eluate. These systems contrast with the majority of chromatographic systems in which the sole purpose has been the identification of pertechnetate in ^{99m}Tc chelate and colloid preparations. Here, one may separate reduced states of ^{99m}Tc that act as impurities with paper chromatography (in 0.3 M HCl or 90% methanol solutions), identifying the technetium species IV, V, and VII.

Although these systems are capable of identifying the Tc(IV), Tc(V), and Tc(VII) states, only the Tc(V) state can be eluted with Tc(VII)-TcO_4 directly from the alumina column in the generator (112). This species does not bind to certain chelates (e.g., DTPA), and has been implicated in certain instances of nonbonding by the effluent of the ^{99}Mo generator (113).

Pertechnetate Impurity Chromatography

Another major problem is reoxidation of the reduced state of $^{99m}TcO_4^-$ which can be rapidly determined by several chromatographic systems. No information, however, is provided regarding the radiochemical purity of the reduced compound. In most cases, nonradioactive kits for the various compounds are properly prepared; as a result, labeling problems that develop are most likely a result of pertechnetate formed by oxidation of the reduced technetium in one's own laboratory. Simple systems such as silica gel in acetone or methyl ethyl ketone are designed to adsorb all nonpertechnetate compounds at the origin in TLC or on the support in column chromatography. Only the presence or absence of TcO_4 is evaluated (Table 14.2).

Radiochemical Purity Chromatography

To assure that a ^{99m}Tc radiopharmaceutical contains only the desired reduced species, at least two chromatographic

Table 14.2.
Chromatographic Systems for the Determination of Pertechnetate

Radiopharmaceutical	Tc-DPTA, Tc-SC, Tc-Sb_2S_3, Tc-HSA, Tc-PP_i, Tc-HEDP, Tc-glucoheptonate, Tc-DMSA, Tc-MDP
Supports	Silicia gel TLC
Solvent	Acetone or methyl ethyl ketone
R_f values	Tc chelate, R_f = 0
	Tc reduced, hydrolyzed, R_f = 0
	TcO_4,−, R_f = 1

Table 14.3.
Chromatographic Systems for the Determination of Pertechnetate and Reduced Hydrolyzed Tc

Radiopharmaceutical	Tc-DTPA, Tc-HEDP, Tc-MDP
Support	Paper
Solvent	Saline
R_f values	Tc chelate, R_f = 1.0
	TcO_4−, R_f = 0.7–0.8
	Tc reduced, hydrolyzed, R_f = 0

systems should be used. Both systems used to assay for radiochemical purity should demonstrate a single band of radioactivity and possess a partition coefficient such that the compound is not freely eluted nor strongly adsorbed. Because of the complexity of these techniques, they are primarily utilized as research tools. Since pertechnetate is the most frequent impurity in ^{99m}Tc chelate degradation, the previously described chromatographic systems for pertechnetate will usually suffice. The most common paper chromatographic system uses saline as the solvent. Polar ^{99m}Tc chelates travel near the solvent front, $Tc0_4$ travels to an R_f of 0.7, and reduced, hydrolyzed ^{99m}Tc stays at the origin (Table 14.3).

Other systems are also capable of separating radiochemical impurities and new systems will, by necessity, be developed with the ever-increasing number of chelating agents. These systems can often be adapted from methods used to purify the nonradioactive chelating agent. The need for more advanced techniques in this field is emphasized by the absence of any report demonstrating the separation of a chelating agent (DTPA) and its radioactive metal chelate counterpart (Tc-DTPA). This has been true despite the obvious difference between these compounds. Separations may be possible with compounds that show slow dissociation by the use of HPLC.

The more polar ^{99m}Tc chelates have been difficult to analyze on HPLC because of their poor retention. Russell and Majerik (114), using a weakly-basic, anion-exchange column eluted with buffer, separated pertechnetate from polar chelates such as DTPA, HEDP, and glucoheptonate, but since the chelates are not retained, they appeared to be radiochemically pure. Wong, et al. (115), also studied a number of ^{99m}Tc chelates on HPLC using a μ-Bondagel column eluted with buffer and a μ-Bondapak C-18 column eluted with buffer and acetonitrile. There was good separation between Tc-HIDA or Tc-HSA and pertechnetate, but minimal separation between polar chelates (DTPA, MDP, and pyrophosphate) and pertechnetate. The nonpolar chelates such as ^{99m}Tc-HIDA are more easily retained, especially on reversed-phase columns, as first shown by Loberg and Fields (116). They were able to separate Sn-HIDA, HIDA, and Tc-HIDA on an HPLC μ-Bondapak C-18 column eluted with acetonitrile and buffer. In a subsequent study they were able to separate a number of chelate-containing ^{99m}Tc HIDA radiochemical impurities when analogs were used with pK_a values for the imino nitrogen of greater than 7. Fritzberg and Lewis (117) have also discovered radiochemical impurities other than pertechnetate and reduced-hydrolyzed technetium in ^{99m}Tc HIDA derivatives that have large substituents in the *ortho* position. These impurities convert to the major component, either as a function of time or increased pH. Pinkerton, et al. (25), were the first to develop an HPLC system to separate bone imaging agents. Using an anion-exchange column eluted with buffer, they found up to seven components in Tc-HEDP, in addition to pertechnetate and reduced hydrolyzed technetium. This result was observed using ^{99}Tc, whereas with ^{99m}Tc only one major peak was found. However, Srivastava, et al. (118), using reversed-phase HPLC, found multiple peaks for ^{99m}Tc. High performance liquid chromatography (HPLC) is state of the art for analysis of radiopharmaceuticals. Wieland, Tobes, and Mangner (119), edited a series of papers dealing with the technique and applications of HPLC to radiopharmaceutical research. Various contributors covered not only the basic technique but applications to the development of organic and metal chelate radiopharmaceuticals. Recently, Boothe and Emran (120) reviewed the current methods for a series of SPECT and PET radiopharmaceuticals. Pike, et al. (121), in the same textbook give similar information on various PET radiopharmaceuticals.

Chromatographic Pitfalls

There are two main sources of error in the chromatographic analysis of ^{99m}Tc radiochemical purity. The first derives from the ease of oxidation of certain reduced states of technetium. For this reason, compounds should not be dried on the TLC plate or paper strip before elution in either chromatographic system. In the event this is done inadvertently, oxidation may ensue with subsequent formation of pertechnetate not originally present in the radiopharmaceutical. Additionally, nonspecific adsorption of the compound, as has been reported with ^{99m}Tc-Sn-HSA (122), may occur because of the small number of highly active sites on the chromatography strip or plate. This phenomenon has also been observed in the preparation of high-specific activity iodinated hormones used for radioimmunoassay (123).

The second source of error results from interaction of the solid phase of the chromatography system with the radiopharmaceutical. In this instance, there is competition for the ^{99m}Tc by the solid support itself, because of its own chelating ability. For example, the polysaccharide Sephadex can compete favorably for certain weak chelates, such as ^{99m}Tc gluconate and ^{99m}Tc mannitol (124, 125), thus a ^{99m}Tc radiopharmaceutical analyzed on such a chromatographic system would appear to contain a radiochemical impurity (a reduced form of technetium) that is not bound to the chelating agent. This shortcoming has been demonstrated for a number of weak chelates analyzed with Sephadex column chromatography. To avoid this artifact, the inert solid-phase polyacrylamide Bio Gel P10, with which there is no competitive adsorption of ^{99m}Tc to the base support, may be used (126). Alternatively, the Sephadex column can be eluted with the same concentration of chelating agent that is used in the preparation of the radiopharmaceutical (124, 127). Both options provide reasonable assurance that the determination of radiochemical purity is accurate.

This same phenomenon may also occur with paper chromatographic systems. When radiochemically pure ^{99m}Tc pyrophosphate is eluted with saline, most of the reduced ^{99m}Tc appears to be unbound; however, if the paper is eluted with a pyrophosphate solution, the chelate is found to be radiochemically pure (128). With the dilutional effect of the saline solvent and the rapid dissociation of technetium pyrophosphate, the chelate can release the ^{99m}Tc to another chelating compound. This property must be considered when evaluating radiochemical purity determinations with these systems.

Finally, chelate stability on Sephadex and paper does not imply in vivo stability of the compound. This merely serves as an index of the competition (at the specific concentrations used) between their respective groups and the chelating agent.

As more lipid-soluble ^{99m}Tc radiopharmaceuticals are prepared, new chromatographic systems must be developed. Certainly, the simple systems suggested for a polar compound such as ^{99m}Tc DTPA will not be useful in the analysis of ^{99m}Tc HIDA (129).

RADIOPHARMACEUTICAL CHEMISTRY OF IODINE

Radioisotopes of iodine have been vital to the development of nuclear medicine. The major advantage in many situations has been their availability, low cost, and relatively long half-lives.

The radionuclides of iodine with the best nuclear properties for γ-ray detecting systems are ^{123}I, ^{125}I, and ^{131}I. Both ^{125}I and ^{131}I are reactor-produced and therefore less expensive and more readily available than the cyclotron product ^{123}I. The radiation absorbed dose to the patient from both ^{131}I and ^{125}I is high; however, ^{123}I is a superior radionuclide for imaging systems, with a 159 keV γ-ray and low radiation absorbed dose. This γ-ray has a half-value layer in water of 4.7 cm and therefore affords satisfactory tissue penetration, yet its energy is low enough to be easily collimated. Unfortunately, this radionuclide can be produced only in a cyclotron and currently cannot be easily made free of ^{124}I and/or ^{125}I contamination. High-energy protons or helium particles produce the purest ^{123}I, but are not readily available (130). The most frequently used reaction to produce ^{123}I of high purity is the ^{127}I(p,5n)^{123}I reaction.

Iodine-124 is an undesirable radionuclide impurity because of its long half-life (4.2 days) and its positron and high-energy photons (511 keV and 723 keV). A 1% concentration of ^{124}I at time of production usually results in 4–5% contamination at 24 hours. The ^{124}I degrades resolution because a significant fraction of the collimated high-energy γ-rays are detected as Compton scatter radiation in the 159 keV energy window. With a low-energy collimator, the contribution is about 28%. With a high-resolution, medium-energy collimator, the contribution is 10%. With a high-energy collimator, only 3% is Compton-scattered radiation, but the sensitivity is greatly reduced. The need for high radionuclidic purity is obvious (131).

CHEMISTRY OF IODINE

Of the halogens, iodine is most likely to support a positive charge and thus is the least reactive toward electrophilic addition or substitution. Nevertheless, electrophilic substitution of activated aromatic rings such as a phenol in tyrosine and imidazole in histidine can be carried out rapidly and with high yield. Most often iodine is present as iodide in basic solution so that an oxidizing agent must be used to label activated aromatic rings. The most popular iodinating agents used to produce electrophilic addition or substitution are (a) iodine, (b) iodine monochloride, (c) chloramine-T, (d) lactoperoxidase, (e) electrolytically generated iodine, and (f) prelabeled ligands (132). Of these, chloramine-T and lactoperoxidase are unique in that they produce high-yield, no-carrier-added iodination. The chloramine-T method has been used extensively to radiolabel proteins.

One of the strengths of nuclear medicine is its ability to detect and quantify physiologic function rather than to record fixed anatomic properties, which are often better detected by other imaging techniques (133). Although ^{99m}Tc has superior physical properties and is readily available compared to iodine, it does not readily allow study of biochemical pathways because of poor chemical properties and the necessity of combining a relatively large ^{99m}Tc chelate with the parent structure. In some cases, the chemistry of ^{99m}Tc is well-defined so that an inert chelate can be prepared, but the perturbation caused by a ^{99m}Tc chelate may be difficult to overcome. In those cases of relatively low molecular weight biochemicals and drugs, iodine, especially ^{123}I, has been a reasonable substitute for ^{99m}Tc.

An early review enumerated the iodinated radiopharmaceuticals that have been tested (134). Labeled dyes, macromolecules, steroids, heterocyclics, and other compounds have been studied as tracers of the parent molecule. Few have been used routinely.

^{125}I is used most often as a label for in vitro radioimmunoassays and radioreceptor assays. Its long half-life, high specific activity, and low energy make it ideal for this application. The list of radioiodinated tracers for in vitro tests has grown because of the ease of counting ^{125}I compared to ^{3}H.

In addition to these radiopharmaceuticals that have been actually used in the clinic, there are a number of radiotracers that have been validated in animal models but have not been used extensively in humans.

The concentration of radiotracer in white matter is a complex function of blood-brain barrier permeability, metabolism, and lipophilicity. Iodinated benzene appears to fill the criteria of a myelin imaging agent based on the work of Frey, et al. (135). Benzene has been labeled with ^{123}I in 20% yield.

Several agents have been suggested for myocardial imaging, but few have successfully imaged the myocardium in humans (37). One compound based on guanethidine did, however, show myocardial uptake in humans. This compound, m-iodobenzylguanidine (mIBG), undergoes the same uptake, storage, and release mechanisms as norepinephrine, but is not metabolized (136). Radioactive mIBG is prepared by an iodide exchange procedure using ammonium sulfate (137).

One of the most heavily studied groups of radioiodinated tracers are those that bind to the estrogen receptor because of the obvious clinical demand for such a radiotracer (138). Many iodinated estrogens have been evaluated (for a review see Katzenellenbogen, et al. (139)), but few bind with high affinity to the estrogen receptor. Hochberg (140, 141) demonstrated that 16α-iodoestradiol binds to the rat uterus and that the uptake is blocked by preinjection of diethylstilbestrol. This compound can be labeled at high specific activity with either ^{125}I or ^{131}I. The uterus of the squirrel monkey has been imaged using a γ-camera (141). 17α-Iodovinyl,11β-methoxyestradiol has recently been reported to give one of the highest uterus-to-blood ratios recorded to date (142).

Kung and Blau (143) have proposed a method of localization based on pH differences between blood and brain. They have prepared various iodinated species containing amines, the best of which is N,N,N-trimethyl-N-(2-hydroxy-3-methyl-5-iodobenzoyl)-1,3-propanediamine (HIPDM) which is labeled by an exchange technique (144). Earlier, Winchell, et al. (145), proposed an iodinated amphetamine (IAMP) that has similar distribution to HIPDM. The mechanism of localization of iodoamphetamine is not known, but is presumed to be by the pH shift mechanism in part, and binding to low-affinity, high-capacity proteins. IAMP has a higher net extraction in the brain, but HIPDM reaches maximum concentration faster (146). Technetium-99m-labeled cerebral perfusion agents have been proposed, but none have the pharmacokinetic properties of HIPDM or IAMP (147).

Another radioiodinated receptor-binding radiotracer is 3-quinuclidinyl-4-iodobenzilate, a muscarinic-cholinergic receptor-binding radiotracer (148). This agent was designed to study the change in receptor as a function of disease (149). 3-Quinuclidinyl-4-iodobenzilate (4-IQNB) is prepared using the triazine reaction. Although the side reactions are numerous, radioiodinated 4-IQNB can be prepared at specific activities approaching 2200 Ci (81,400 GBq)/mmol. One study in humans defining the location of muscarinic receptors by external imaging has been reported (150).

Most of the early iodinated radiopharmaceuticals have been replaced by a biologically similar ^{99m}Tc compound. However, in the field of labeled biochemicals and drugs used to trace a portion of a biochemical pathway, it is likely that ^{123}I will be the radionuclide of choice among single photon-emitting nuclides. The major competition comes rather from ^{18}F-labeled biochemicals and drugs. Fluorine-18-labeled fluoro-2-deoxyglucose is the prime example of such a radiotracer (151). But until an inexpensive source of ^{18}F becomes available and positron imaging devices become less expensive, it is likely that ^{123}I will prevail. A recent chapter (152) describes the in vitro and in vivo chemistry of this class of compounds.

OTHER RADIONUCLIDES

SELENIUM-75

Selenium-75 is incorporated into methionine by replacing the sulfur atom with selenium (153). The product ^{75}Se selenomethionine has been used for pancreas imaging. The synthesis can be done either chemically or by biosynthesis. Selenium-75 has a 120-day half-life and decays by electron capture.

GALLIUM-67

Gallium-67 is produced by many nuclear reactions from targets of enriched stable zinc isotopes using protons or deuterons (154). It decays with a 78-hour half-life by electron capture with no particle emission and emits a number of γ-rays with energies ranging from 93–395 keV.

Gallium is a member of the group IIIA metals in the periodic table and exists primarily as a trivalent species. It is injected as either the chloride or citrate and rapidly complexes with plasma proteins, especially transferrin. Since the gallium-transferrin complex is more stable than gallium citrate, injected gallium citrate should have similar behavior independent of the citrate concentration. The major purpose of citrate appears to be to keep the gallium in a soluble chemical form until it binds to transferrin by exchange labeling. The mechanism of uptake of gallium in tumors is thought to be via a transferrin receptor (155).

Gallium-67 citrate is one of the few efficacious general tumor imaging agents (156). Most other radiopharmaceuticals used for tumor detection localize in a specific target organ. Although ^{67}Ga citrate is a general tumor imaging agent, it is not tumor specific; that is, it can be used for either tumor or abscess detection (157).

INDIUM-111

Indium-111 has been prepared by cyclotron bombardment of enriched silver or cadmium isotopes (158). Indium-111 decays by emission of two cascading photons of 173 and 247 keV with 89% and 94% abundances, respectively. It thus yields 183 photons for every 100 disintegrations compared to only 93 for ^{67}Ga. Indium-111 chloride has been injected directly as a bone marrow imaging agent. Indium appears to follow iron kinetics in some aspects, but apparently is not a true tracer for iron (159, 160). It has also been converted to various other compounds for use as radiopharmaceuticals. These include indium citrate, indium ferric hydroxide colloid, indium DTPA, indium bleomycin, and indium hydroxyquinoline. Indium bleomycin, indium DTPA, and indium 8-hydroxyquinoline oxine are formed easily, since these complexes are more stable than the chloride or citrate complexes. Indium 8-hydroxyquinoline has been used to label leukocytes, lymphocytes, and platelets.

Indium-111-labeled leukocytes have been used for abscess detection, and ^{111}In-labeled platelets have been used for the detection of arterial lesions, coronary artery thrombi, atherosclerosis, and vascular grafts (161, 162).

Indium-111 has been used most extensively to radiolabel antibodies using the bifunctional approach. The first attempts were with the cyclic anhydride approach, but more recent approaches have used substituted DTPA molecules that retain the amine and carboxylate binding groups of the DTPA (163).

THALLIUM-201

Thallium-201 is most conveniently produced by irradiating naturally occurring thallium metal foils with protons, producing the ^{203}T1(p,3n)^{201}Pb reaction (164). The lead can be separated from the target thallium and decays with a 9.4-hour half-life to daughter ^{201}Tl in a pure and carrier-free form. Thallium-201 decays by electron capture with a half-life of 73 hours. It emits a cluster of x-rays between 69 and 83 keV, somewhat below the optimum energy for current in vivo imaging techniques. Thallium has been used to measure myocardial perfusion.

COBALT-57

Carrier-free ^{57}Co is produced by cyclotron irradiation of iron or manganese (165). It decays by electron capture with convenient emissions at 122 keV (87%) and 136 keV (11%).

Cobalt-57 has been used as a radiolabel for vitamin B_{12} in Shilling's test (166) and as a label for bleomycin (167). Cobalt-57 bleomycin is more sensitive in the detection of certain tumors than is ^{67}Ga citrate. Although the absorbed dose for patients with good renal function is low, the contamination hazards posed by a 270-day half-life radionuclide have prevented its widespread use. Unlike ^{67}Ga citrate, ^{57}Co bleomycin is filtered by the kidneys with no localization in normal tissue (168).

BONE PALLIATION AGENTS

In addition to the advances in diagnostic radiopharmaceuticals, several new therapeutic radiopharmaceuticals are approaching clinical reality. Therapy has always been a major part of nuclear medicine and, with a new series of radiopharmaceuticals being developed, promises to expand the field considerably. Recently, Volkert et al. (169), reviewed these therapeutic radionuclides. While the community awaits a number of diagnostic monoclonal antibodies to be approved and then extended to therapy, the next class of compounds closest to routine clinical use are the agents designed to treat bone pain from skeletal metastases. They are ^{89}Sr chloride, which is now FDA-approved, ^{186}Re-HEDP, and ^{153}Sm-EDTMP. The important considerations for these therapeutic agents is the energy of the β particle and the physical and biologic half-life. The β energy should be such that adjacent cells are destroyed, but should not be high enough to cause radiation damage to the sensitive bone marrow. The biologic half-life should be such that the radiopharmaceutical localizes quickly in the bone, but clears the rest of the body rapidly. The shortest physical half-life that is consistent with the biologic half-life will deliver the maximal dose rate to the bone. In addition to these therapeutic agents, there is interest in the β-emitting colloids for radiation synovectomy and the radiolabeled particles for intra-arterial treatment of tumors.

GENERATOR SYSTEMS

Strontium-82—Rubidium-82

Strontium-82, the parent of ^{82}Rb, is produced in highest yield by a spallation reaction on rubidium and decays with a 25-day half-life. Rubidium-82 decays with a half-life of 1.3 minutes by positron emission (96%). The parent and daughter radionuclides are separated by a number of solid adsorbents that retain ^{82}Sr but permit the elution of ^{82}Rb with ammonium acetate or saline solutions (170). Generator-produced ^{82}Rb is a monovalent cation that has been used for myocardial imaging as a potassium congener (171).

Germanium-68—Gallium-68

Gallium-68 is the daughter of ^{68}Ge, which is produced by proton irradiation of stable gallium (172). The parent and daughter half-lives, 275 days and 1.14 hours, respectively, are convenient for generator preparation and storage and for patient imaging studies. Gallium-68 decays by positron emission (88%) and is thus particularly useful for positron tomographic imaging. The gallium generator consists of an alumina column that retains the parent ^{68}Ge and allows the ^{68}Ga to be eluted with ethylenediaminetetraacetic acid (EDTA) as the gallium-EDTA chelate. The eluate is useful for brain tumor imaging; however, the preparation of other ^{68}Ga radiopharmaceuticals is complicated by the need to dissociate gallium from gallium-EDTA as the first step of any labeling procedure. Recently, other elution systems have been developed (173). Many gallium radiopharmaceuticals can be prepared in a manner similar to that used to prepare the ^{113m}In radiopharmaceuticals described later.

Rubidium-81—Krypton-81m

A radionuclide with a very short half-life (13 seconds) can be used by a nuclear medicine laboratory only through a generator system. Multimillicurie quantities of ^{81}Rb can be produced by bombarding sodium bromide with particles or by proton bombardment of an enriched ^{82}Kr gas target. The ^{81}Rb is adsorbed on a small ion-exchange column and the ^{81}Kr is eluted with water or with air if gas-phase samples are needed (174). The major use has been to study lung ventilation and to measure blood flow in various tissues.

Tin-113—Indium-113m

The ^{113}Sn parent is produced by thermal neutron bombardment of enriched ^{112}Sn. An acid solution of ^{113}Sn tin chloride is adsorbed by a zirconium oxide column. The ^{113}In daughter is eluted with dilute acid solution. The predominant species is In(III), which is cationic in acid solution and can be easily chelated or coprecipitated with colloids and particles without a change in oxidation state as is required for pertechnetate (175).

The long half-life of the parent ^{113}Sn guarantees an available source of radionuclide. The radiation dose from

^{113m}In is equivalent to that from ^{99m}Tc compounds because the former has a shorter half-life but greater number of conversion electrons.

Because the commercially available scintillation camera was designed for the 140-keV emissions of ^{99m}Tc, detection efficiency for the 392-keV γ-rays of ^{113m}In is low, and special high-energy collimators are required. With rectilinear scanners, the sensitivity is similar for both radionuclides.

Indium compounds are readily made for imaging the brain (^{113m}In DTPA), the liver and spleen (colloidal ^{113m}In phosphate), the lung (^{113m}In iron hydroxide), and bone (^{113m}In diethylenetriaminepentamethylenephosphonic acid). Indium-113m chloride injected directly at the eluted pH of 1.6 binds to transferrin to give a blood pool agent.

RADIOLABELED PHYSIOLOGIC TRACERS OR BIOCHEMICAL PROBES

Single photon-emitting radionuclides have a range of half-lives and γ-ray emissions (Table 14.4). These radionuclides provide variation in both nuclear and chemical properties. This variation has been used to develop physiologic tracers. Physiologic tracers are defined as probes for a particular portion of a particular biochemical pathway (133). Most of the ^{99m}Tc radiotracers, such as ^{99m}Tc MAA and ^{99m}Tc DTPA, do not follow major biochemical pathways in vivo.

Because of the rather large steric perturbation caused by introducing a ^{99m}Tc chelate, the ideal nuclear properties of ^{99m}Tc have not been used in this particular application. Rather, investigators have used either ^{123}I or ^{77}Br to label physiologic tracers. Tomographic methods have been developed for single photon-emitting radiotracers, but the ability to use tomography (SPECT) is dependent on the kinetics of the radiotracer and the speed of the SPECT device. In many situations, the time constraints do not match. One situation in which they do match is brain flow determination using the agents iodoamphetamine or HIPDM with the SPECT device (146). Both radiotracers are taken up rapidly by the brain and remain in the brain for sufficient time to allow a tomographic image to be taken either by one of the multicrystal devices or by a rotating γ-camera. A similar kinetic behavior is observed for ^{201}Tl (176) and for the routine ^{99m}Tc radiopharmaceuticals ^{99m}Tc MAA and ^{99m}Tc-sestamibi (177, 178), although all three are considered to be agents to measure flow rather than biochemistry. A number of biochemical tracers have been developed to date. Consequently, there are now numerous ^{123}I-labeled receptor binding radiotracers. Most of the effort to map biochemical reactions with both SPECT and PET, outside of the seminal work on ^{18}F-FDG (179) and later on ^{18}F-6-FluoroDOPA (180), has been directed toward receptor binding radiotracers. There are three steps in the development of a biochemical probe. The first is to develop a diagnostic agent that binds preferentially to a chosen enzyme or receptor or takes part in a single biochemical step. Single-step reactions such as receptor-or enzyme-binding are preferred because interpretation of the data by external imaging is more straightforward. This approach has been designated metabolic trapping (181). We now have several receptor binding radiotracers labeled with either single photon emitting or position emitting radionuclides that bind to the receptor, fulfilling the first criterion of a biochemical probe (182, 183). The second step is to determine the sensitivity of the diagnostic agent to a change in the biochemistry. Although many excellent pharmacokinetic analyses have been published (184), use of collected data at one time point after injection, where the distribution reflects the biochemical change and not flow or transport, is simplest (185).

Table 14.4.
Single Photon-emitting Radionuclides

Radionuclide	Half-life	Major γ radiation (keV)
Technetium-99m	6 hr	140 (88%)
Iodine-123	13.3 hr	159 (86%)
Bromine-77	56 hr	240 (30%)
Gallium-67	78 hr	93 (40%), 184 (24%), 296 (22%)
Indium-111	67 hr	173 (89%), 247 (94%)
Cobalt-57	270 days	122 (87%), 136 (11%)
Thallium-201	73 hr	69–83 (98%)

One of the major goals of positron emission tomography is the in vivo measurement of biochemistry. Perhaps the most famous of the measurements is that for glucose metabolism using 2-fluoro-2-deoxyglucose labeled with ^{18}F. This radiotracer has been used to measure changes in glucose metabolism in a large number of brain dysfunctions and in tumors (186). The measurement of in vivo biochemistry is one of the major areas of emphasis in nuclear medicine. Very few other imaging modalities have the capability of mapping biochemical processes by external imaging.

REFERENCES

1. Professor George C. de Hevesy [Editorial]. J Nucl Med 1961; 2:167.
2. Richards P, Tucker WD, Srivastava SC. ^{99m}Tc: an historical perspective. Int J Appl Radiat Isot 1982;33:793.
3. Dillman LT. Radionuclide decay schemes and nuclear parameters for use in radiation dose estimation. J Nucl Med 1969; 10(Suppl 2):7.
4. Deutsch E, Heineman WR, Zodda JP, Gilbert TW, Williams CC. Preparation of "no-carrier-added" technetium-99m complexes: determination of the total technetium content of generator eluents. Int J Appl Radiat Isot 1982;33:843.
5. Lamson M, Hotte CF, Ice RD. Practical generator kinetics. J Nucl Med Technol 1975;4:21.
6. Richards P, Steigman J. Chemistry of technetium as applied to radiopharmaceuticals. In: Subramanian G, Rhodes BA, Cooper JF, Sodd VJ, eds. Radiopharmaceuticals. New York: Society for Nuclear Medicine, 1975:23–35.
7. Eckelman WC, Richards P. Instant ^{99m}Tc-DTPA. J Nucl Med 1970;11:761.
8. Harper PV, Lathrop K, Gottschalk A. Pharmacodynamics of some technetium-99m preparations. In: Radioactive pharmaceuticals. Washington, DC: U.S. Atomic Energy Commission, 1964:335.
9. Cotton FA, Wilkinson G. Advanced inorganic chemistry. 3rd ed. New York: Interscience, 1972.
10. Johannson B, Spies H. Chemie and radiopharmakologie von technetium komplexen. Dresden: Akademie der Wissenschaften der DDR, 1981.
11. Atkins HL, Cardinale KG, Eckelman WC, Hauser W, Klopper JF, Richards P. Evaluation of ^{99m}-Tc-DTPA prepared by three different methods. Radiology 1971;98:674–677.

12. Fritzberg AR, Klingensmith WC, Whitney WP, Kuni CC. Chemical and biological studies of Tc-99m N,N-Bis(mercaptoacetamido)-ethyl-enediamine: a potential replacement for I-131 iodohippurate. J Nucl Med 1981;22:258.
13. Fritzberg AR, Kasina S, Eshima D, Johnson DL. Synthesis and biological evaluation of technetium-99m-MAG_3 as a hippuran replacement. J Nucl Med 1986;27:111.
14. McAfee JG, Grossman ZD, Gagne G, et al. Comparison of renal extraction efficiencies for radioactive agents in normal dog. J Nucl Med 1981;22:333–338.
15. Subramanian G, McAfee JG. A new complex of ^{99m}Tc for skeletal imaging. Radiology 1971;99:192.
16. Bevan JA, Tofe AJ, Benedict JJ, Francis MD, Barnett BL. Tc-99m HMDP (hydroxymethylene diphosphonate): a radiopharmaceutical for skeletal and acute myocardial infarct imaging. II. Comparison of Tc-99m hydroxymethylene disphosphonate (HMDP) with other technetium labeled bone-imaging agents in a canine model. J Nucl Med 1980;21:967.
17. Bevan JA, Tofe AJ, Benedict JJ, Francis MD, Barnett BL. Tc-99m HMDP (hydroxymethylene disphosphonate): a radiopharmaceutical for skeletal and acute myocardial infarct imaging. I. Synthesis and distribution in animals. J Nucl Med 1980;21:961.
18. Buja LM, Tofe AJ, Kulkarni PV, et al. Sites and mechanisms of localization of technetium-99m phosphorus radiopharmaceuticals in acute myocardial infarcts and other tissues. J Clin Invest 1977;60:724.
19. Jones AG, Francis MD, Davis AM. Bone scanning: radionuclide reaction mechanisms. Semin J Nucl Med 1976;6:3.
20. Dewanjee MK, Kahn PC. Mechanism of localization of ^{99m}Tc-labeled pyrophosphate and tetracycline in infarcted myocardium. J Nucl Med 1976;17:639.
21. Francis MD, Ferguson DL, Tofe AJ, Bevan JA, Michaels SE. Comparative evaluation of three diphosphonates: in vitro absorption (C-14 labeled) and in vivo osteogenic uptake (Tc-99m complexed). J Nucl Med 1980;21:1185.
22. Christensen SB, Krogsgaard OW. Localization of Tc-99m MDP in epiphyseal growth plates of rats. J Nucl Med 1981;22:237.
23. Tofe AJ, Francis MD. Optimization of the ratio of stannous tin:ethane-7-hydroxy-1,1-diphosphonate for bone scanning with ^{99m}Tc pertechnetate. J Nucl Med 1974;15:69–74.
24. Van Langevelde A, Driessen OMJ, Pauwels EKJ, Thesingh CW. Aspects of ^{99m}technetium binding from an ethane-1-hydroxy-1,1-diphosphonate-^{99m}Tc complex to bone. Eur J Nucl Med 1977;2:47.
25. Pinkerton TC, Heineman WR, Deutsch E. Separation of technetium hydroxyethylidene diphosphonate complexes by anion exchange high performance liquid chromatography. Anal Chem 1980;52:1106–1110.
26. Wilson GM, Pinkerton TC. Determination of charge and size of technetium diphosphonate complexes by anion-exchange liquid chromatography. Anal Chem 1985;57:246–253.
27. Steigman J, Meinken G, Richards P. The reduction of pertechnetate-99 by stannous chloride-II. The stoichiometry of the reaction in aqueous solutions of several phosphorus (V) compounds. Int J Appl Radiat Isot 1978;29:653–660.
28. Lyons KP, Olson HG, Aronow WS. Pyrophosphate myocardial imaging. Semin Nucl Med 1980;10:168.
29. Firnau G. Why do ^{99m}Tc chelates work for cholescintigraphy? Eur J Nucl Med 1976;1:137.
30. Loberg MD, Porter DW. Review and current status of hepatobiliary imaging agents. In: Sorenson J, ed. Radiopharmaceuticals II. New York: Society of Nuclear Medicine, 1979:519.
31. Tubis M, Krishnamurthy GT, Endow JS, Blahd WH. ^{99m}Tc penicillamine, a new cholescintigraphic agent. J Nucl Med 1972; 13:652.
32. Fritzberg AR. Advances in the development of hepatobiliary radiopharmaceuticals. In: Fritzberg A, ed. Radiopharmaceuticals: progress and clinical perspectives. Vol. I. Boca Raton, FL: CRC Press Inc, 1986:89–116.
33. Winston BW, Subramanian G, Gagne GM, et al. Experimental and clinical trials of new ^{99m}Tc hepatobiliary agents. Radiology 1978;128:793.
34. Nunn AD, Loberg MD, Conley RA. A structure-distribution relationship approach leading to the development of Tc-99m mebrofenin: an improved cholescintigraphic agent. J Nucl Med 1983;24:423.
35. Strauss HW, Buchner CA. Myocardial perfusion studies: lessons from a decade of clinical use. Radiology 1986;160:577–584.
36. Deutsch E, Glavan KA, Ferguson DL, Lukes SJ, Nishiyama H, Sodd VJ. Development of a Tc-99m myocardial imaging agent to replace Tl-201 [Abstract]. J Nucl Med 1980;21:56.
37. Carr EA Jr, Carroll M, Counsell RE, Tyson JW. Studies of uptake of the bretylium analogue, iodobenzyltrimethylammonium iodide, by nonprimate, monkey, and human hearts. Br J Clin Pharmacol 1979;8:425.
38. Ichimura A, Heineman WR, Vander Heyden JL, Deutsch E. Technetium electrochemistry 2. Electrochemical and spectroelectrochemical studies of the bis (tertiary phosphine) (D) Complexes trans-(TcIIID2–$_2^+$) (X=C1, Br) and ($TcID_3^+$). Inorg Chem 1984; 23:1272–1278.
39. Jones A, Abrams MJ, Davison A, et al. Biological studies of a new class of technetium complexes: the hexakis (alkylisonitrile) technetium (I) cations. Int J Nucl Med Biol 1984;11:225–234.
40. Ketring AR, Deutsch E, Libson K, et al. The Noah's ark experiment. A search for a suitable animal model for the evaluation of cationic Tc-99m myocardial imaging agents. J Nucl Med 1983; 24:9.
41. Sporn V, Perez-Balina N, Holman BL, et al. Myocardial imaging with Tc-99m CPI: initial experience in the human. J Nucl Med 1976;27:878.
42. McKusick K, Holman BL, Jones AG, et al. Comparison of 3 Tc99m isonitriles for detection [of] ischemic heart disease in humans. J Nucl Med 1986;27:878.
43. Johnson LL, Seldin DW, Muschel MJ, et al. Comparison of planar SQ 30,217 and TI-201 myocardial imaging with coronary anatomy [Abstract]. Circulation 1987;76:IV-217.
44. Seldin DW, Johnson LL, Blood DK, et al. Myocardial perfusion imaging with technetium-99m SQ 30,217: comparison with thallium-201 and coronary anatomy. J Nucl Med 1989;30:312.
45. Meerdink DJ, Thuber M, Savage S, et al. Comparative myocardial extraction of two technetium-labeled boron oxime derivatives (SQ 30,217, SQ 32,014) and thallium. J Nucl Med 1988; 29:972.
46. Piwnica-Worms D, Kronauge JF, Chiu ML. Uptake and retention of hexakis (2–methoxy isobutyl isonitrile)technetium (I) in cultured chick myocardial cells. Mitochondrial and plasma membrane potential dependence. Circulation 1990;82:1826.
47. Coleman RE, Maturi M, Nunn AD, Eckelman WC, Juri PN, Cobb FR. Imaging of myocardial perfusion with Tc-99m SQ 30,217: dog and human studies. J Nucl Med 1986;27:893–894.
48. Narra RK, Nunn AD, Kuczynski BL, et al. A neutral ^{99m}Tc complex for myocardial imaging. J Nucl Med 1989;30:1830.
49. Kim AS, Akers MS, Faber TS, et al. Dynamic myocardial perfusion imaging with Tc-99m-teboroxime in patients; comparison with thallium-201 and arteriography [Abstract]. Circulation 1990;82:111.
50. Gewirtz H. Differential myocardial washout of Technetium-99m tebotroxime: mechanism and significance. J Nucl Med 1992; 32:2009.
51. Leppo JA, DePuey EG, Johnson LL. A review of cardiac imaging with sestamibi and teboroxime. J Nucl Med 1991;32:2012.
52. Winchell HS, Horst WD, Braun L, et al. N-isopropyl-

(^{123}I)piodoamphetamine: single pass brain uptake and washout, binding to brain synaptosomes, and localization in dog and monkey brain. J Nucl Med 1980;21:947.

53. Neirinckx RD, Burke JF, Harrison RC, et al. The retention mechanism of ^{99m}Tc-HMPAO; intracellular reaction with glutathione. J Cereb Blood Flow Metab 1988;S4:12.
54. Vallabhajosula S, Zimmerman RE, Picard M, et al. Technetium-99m ECD: a new brain imaging agent: in vivo kinetics and biodistribution studies in normal human subjects. J Nucl Med 1989;30:599.
55. McAfee JG, Subramanian G, Aburano T, et al. A new formulation of ^{99m}Tc minimicroaggregated albumin for marrow imaging: comparison with other colloids, In-111 and Fe-59. J Nucl Med 1982; 23:21–23.
56. Warbick A, Ege GN, Henkelman RM, Maier G, Lyster DM. An evaluation of radiocolloid sizing technique. J Nucl Med 1977; 18:827.
57. Davis MA, Jones AG, Trindale H. A rapid and accurate method for sizing radiocolloids. J Nucl Med 1974;15:923.
58. Billinghurst MW, Jette D. Colloidal particle size determination by gel filtration. J Nucl Med 1979;20:133.
59. Pedersen B, Kristensen K. Evaluation of methods for sizing of colloidal radiopharmaceuticals. Eur J Nucl Med 1981;6:521.
60. Subhani M, Van Nerom C, Bormans G, Hoogmartens M, DeRoo M, Verbruggen, A. Comparative evaluation of fourteen ^{99m}Tc-colloids. In: Nicolini M, Bandoli G, Mazzi U, eds. Technietium and Rhenium in chemistry and nuclear medicine. Verona, Italy: Cortina International, 1990:667.
61. Davis MA. Particulate radiopharmaceuticals for pulmonary studies. In: Subramanian G, Rhodes BA, Cooper JF, Sodd VJ, eds. Radiopharmaceuticals. New York: Society for Nuclear Medicine, 1975:267–281.
62. Rhodes BA, Zolle I, Buchanan JW, Wagner HN Jr. Radioactive albumin microspheres for studies of the pulmonary circulation. Radiology 1969;92:1453.
63. Tubis M. Hospital preparation and dispensing of radiopharmaceuticals. In: Tubis M, Wolf W, eds. Radiopharmacy. New York: Wiley Interscience, 1976:421.
64. The United States Pharmacopeia. 20th rev. Rockville, MD: U.S. Pharmacopeial Convention, 1975.
65. Eckelman WC. Technical considerations in labeling of blood elements. Semin Nucl Med 1975;5:3.
66. Smith T, Richards P. A simple kit for the rapid preparation of ^{99m}Tc red blood cells. J Nucl Med 1974;15:534.
67. Hegge FN, Hamilton GW, Larson SM, Ritchie JL, Richards P. Cardiac chamber imaging: a comparison of red blood cells labeled with Tc-99m in vitro and in vivo. J Nucl Med 1978;19:129.
68. Pavel DG, Zimmer AM. In vivo labeling of red cells with ^{99m}Tc pertechnetate. J Nucl Med 1978;19:972.
69. Leitl GP, Drew HM, Kelly ME, Alderson PO. The interference with Tc-99m labeling of red blood cells (RBCs). J Nucl Med 1980; 21:P44.
70. Gottschalk A, Armas R, Thakur ML. Reply to spleen scanning with Tc-99m-labeled red blood cells (RBC). J Nucl Med 1980; 21:1000.
71. Hamilton JG, Soley MH. Studies in iodine metabolism by the use of a new radioactive isotope of iodine. Am J Physiol 1939; 127:557.
72. Berson S, Yalow RS, Rauman A, Rothschild M, Newerly K. ^{131}I metabolism in human subject: demonstration of insulin binding globulin in the circulation of insulin treated subjects. J Clin Invesr 1956;35:170.
73. Pressman D, Eisen HN. The zone of localization of antibodies. V. An attempt to saturate antibody-binding sites in mouse kidney. J Immunol 1950;64:273.
74. Rockoff SD, Goodenough DJ, Mclntire KR. Theoretical limitations in the immunodiagnostic imaging of cancer with computed tomography and nuclear scanning. Cancer Res 1980;40:3054.
75. Larson SM, Carrasquillo JA, Reynolds JC. Radioimmunodetection and radioimmunotherapy. Cancer Invest 1984;2:363.
76. Keenan AM, Harbert JC, Larson SM. Monoclonal antibodies in nuclear medicine. J Nucl Med 1985;26:531.
77. Pettit WA, DeLand FH, Bennett SJ, Goldenberg DM. Improved protein labeling with stannous tanrate reduction of pertechnetate. J Nucl Med 1980;21:59.
78. Rhodes BA, Torvestad DA, Breslow K, Burchiel SW, Reed KA, Austin RK. ^{99m}Tc labeling and acceptance testing of radiolabeled antibodies. In: Burchiel SW, Rhodes BA, eds. Tumor imaging. New York: Masson, 1982:111.
79. Sundrehagen E. Formation of ^{99m}Tc immunoglobulin G complexes free from radionuclides, quality controlled by radioimmunoelectrophoresis. Eur J Nucl Med 1982;7:549.
80. Eckelman WC, Meinken G, Richards P. ^{99m}Tc-human serum albumin. J Nucl Med 1971;12:707.
81. Steigman J, Williams HP, Solomon NA. The importance of the protein sulfhydryl group in HSA labeling with ^{99m}Tc. J Nucl Med 1975;16:573.
82. Lanteigne D, Hnatowich DJ. The labeling of DTPA coupled proteins with ^{99m}Tc. Int J Appl Radian Isot 1984;35:617.
83. Paik CH, Pham LNB, Hong JJ, et al. The labeling of high affinity sites of antibodies with ^{99m}Tc. Int J Nucl Med Biol 1985;12:3.
84. Khaw BA, Strauss HW, Carvalho A, Locke E, Gold HK, Haber E. ^{99m}Tc labeling of antibodies to cardiac myosin Fab and to human fibrinogen. J Nucl Med 1982;23:1011.
85. Lanteigne D, Hnatowich DJ. The labeling of DTPA-coupled proteins with ^{99m}Tc. Int J Appl Radiat Isot 1984;35:617.
86. Rhodes BA, Torvestaad DA, Burchiel SW, Austin RK. A kit for direct labeling of antibody and antibody fragments with Tc-99m. J Nucl Med 1980;21:54.
87. Hawkins EB, Pant KD, Rhodes BA. Resistance of direct Tc-99m-protein bond to transchelation. Antibody Immuno Conj Radiopharm 1990;3:17.
88. Pszona A, Sakowicz A. The influence of citrate ions on the radiochemical purity of ^{99m}Tc-human serum albumin. Int J Radiat Isot 1981;32:349.
89. Reno JM, Bottino BJ. Radiolabeled proteins, especially antibodies, and their preparation and use as diagnostic and therapeutic agents. European Pat Appl EP 237150 A2, 1987.
90. Pak KY, Dean RT, Mattis JA, Buttram S, Lister-James J. Method for labeling antibodies with isotopic technetium or rhenium, their use in immunotherapy and scintigraphy, and kits for performing the method. International Patent WO 8807382, 1988.
91. Steigman J, Richards P. Chemistry of technetium as applied to radiopharmaceuticals. In: Subramanian G, Rhodes BA, Cooper J, Sodd V, eds. Radiopharmaceuticals. New York: Society for Nuclear Medicine, 1975:23–35.
92. Bremer KH, Kuhlmann FL, Schwarz A, Steinstraesser A. Preparation of a technetium-99m-labeled organ-specific substance. European Pat Appl EP 271806 A2, 1988.
93. Hansen HJ, Jones AL, Sharkey RM, et al. Preclinical evaluation of an "instant" ^{99m}Tc-labeling kit for antibody labeling. Cancer Res 1990;50(Suppl):794s.
94. John E, Wilder S, Thakur ML. Structural perturbations of monoclonal antibodies following radiolabeling: in vitro evaluation of different techniques. Nucl Med Commun (In press, 1994).
95. Hnatowich DJ, Mardirossian G, Rusckowski M, Fogarasi M, Virzi F, Winnard P Jr. Directly and indirectly technetium-99m-labeled antibodies—a comparison of in vitro and animal in vivo properties. J Nucl Med 1993;34:109–119.
96. Rhodes BA, Zamora PO, Newell KD, et al. Technetium-99m-labeling of murine monoclonal antibody fragments. J Nucl Med 1986;27:685–693.

97. Abrams MJ, Juweid M, tenKate CI, et al. Technetium-99m-human polyclonal IgG radiolabeled via the hydrazino nicotinamide derivative for imaging focal sites of infection in rats. J Nucl Med 1990;31:2022–2028.
98. Hnatowich KJ, Mardirossian G, Roy S, et al. Pharmacokinetics of the FO23C4 anti-CEA antibody fragment labeled with technetium-99m and indium-111: a comparison in patients. Nucl Med Commun 1993;52–63.
99. Goedemans W Th, Panek KJ, Ensing GJ, deLong M Th. A new, single method for labeling of proteins with ^{99m}Tc by derivatization with 1-imino-4–mercaptobutyl groups. In: Nicolini M, Bandoli G, Mazzi U, eds. Technetium and rhenium in chemistry and nuclear medicine. Vol 3. Verona, Italy: Cartino Int., 1990:595.
100. Joiris E, Bastin B, Thornback JR. A new method of labeling of monoclonal antibodies and their fragments with Technetium-99m. Nucl Med Biol 1991;18:353.
101. Kasina S, Vanderheyden JL, Fritzberg AR. Application of diamide dimercaptide N2S2 bifunctional chelating agents for ^{99m}Tc labeling of proteins. Boston: Proc 6th Int Symp Radiopharmaceutical Chemistry, 29 June-3 July 1986;269.
102. Arano Y, Yokoyama A, Magata Y, Saji H, Horiuchi K, Torizuka K. Synthesis and evaluation of a new bifunctional chelating agent for ^{99m}Tc labeling proteins: p-carboxyethylphenyl-glyoxal-di(N-methylthiosemicarbazone). Int J Nucl Med Biol 1985;12:425.
103. Fritzberg AR. Advances in ^{99m}Tc-labeling of antibodies. Nucl Med 1987;26:7.
104. Franz J, Volkert WA, Barefield EK, Holmes RA. The production of technetium-99m-labeled conjugated antibodies using a cyclam-based bifunctional chelating agent. Nucl Med Biol 1987; 14(6):569.
105. Colombetti L. Performance of ^{99m}Tc generating system. In: Rhodes BA, ed. Quality control in nuclear medicine—radiopharmaceuticals, instrumentation, and in vitro assays. St. Louis: CV Mosby, 1977:183–196.
106. Rhodes BA. Quality control in nuclear medicine—radiopharmaceuticals, instrumentation, and in vitro assays. St. Louis: CV Mosby, 1977.
107. Wieland DM, Tobes MC, Mangner T, eds. Analytical and chromatographic techniques in radiopharmaceutical chemistry. New York: Springer-Verlag, 1986.
108. Richards P, Atkins HL. ^{99m}Tc technetium-labeled compounds. In: Proceedings of the 7th Annual Meeting of the Japanese Society of Nuclear Medicine, Tokyo, Japan, Nov. 17–18, 1967. Tokyo: Tokyo Radioisotope Association, 1968:165–170.
109. Brown PR. High pressure liquid chromatography: biochemical and biomedical applications. New York: Academic Press, 1973.
110. Mikes O, ed. Laboratory handbook of chromatography and allied methods. New York: Halsted Press, 1979.
111. Shukla SK. Ion exchange paper chromatography of Tc(IV), Tc(V) and Tc(VII) in hydrochloric acid. J Chromatogr 1966;21:92–97.
112. Cifka J, Vesely P. Some factors influencing the elution of technetium-99m generators. Radiochim Acta 1971;16:30–35.
113. Eckelman WC, Meinken G, Richards P. The chemical state of ^{99m}Tc in biomedical products. II. The chelation of reduced technetium with DPTA. J Nucl Med 1972;13:577–581.
114. Russell CD, Majerik J. Tracer electrochemistry of pertechnetate chelation of ^{99m}Tc by EDTA after controlled potential reduction at mercury and platinum cathodes. Int J Appl Radiat Isot 1978; 29:109–114.
115. Wong SH, Hosain P, Zeichner SJ, Spitznagle LA, Hosain F. Quality control studies of ^{99m}Tc-labeled radiopharmaceuticals by high performance liquid chromatography. Int J Appl Radiat Isot 1981; 32:185–186.
116. Loberg MD, Fields AT. Chemical structure of technetium-99-labeled N-(2,6-dimethylphenylcarbamoylmethyl)-iminodiacetic acid (Tc-HIDA). Int J App Radiat Isot 1978;29:167–173.
117. Fritzberg AR, Lewis D. HPLC analysis of Tc-99m iminodiacetate hepatobiliary agents and a question of multiple peaks: concise communication. J Nucl Med 1980;21:1180–1184.
118. Srivastava SC, Bandyopadhyay D, Meinken G, Richards P. Characterization of Tc-99m bone agents (MDP, EHDP) by reverse phase and ion exchange high performance liquid chromatography. J Nucl Med 1980;22:P69–P70.
119. Wieland DM, Tobes MC, Mangner TJ. Analytical and chromatographic techniques in radiopharmaceutical chemistry. New York: Springer-Verlag, 1986.
120. Boothe TE, Emran AM. The role of high performance liquid chromatography in radiochemical/radiopharmaceutical synthesis and quality assurance. In: Emran AM, ed. New trends in radiopharmaceutical synthesis, quality assurance, and regulatory control. New York: Plenum Press, 1991:409.
121. Pike VW, Waters MJ, Kensett MJ, et al. Radiopharmaceutical production for PET: quality assurance, practice, experiences and issues. In: Emran AM, ed. New trends in radiopharmaceutical synthesis, quality assurance, and regulatory control. New York: Plenum Press, 1991:433.
122. Lin MS, Kruse SL. Goodwin DA, Kriss JP. Albumin-loading effect: a pitfall in saline paper analysis of ^{99m}Tc albumin. J Nucl Med 1974;15:1018–1020.
123. Yalow RS, Berson SA. Immunoassay of plasma insulin. In: Glick D, ed. Methods of biochemical analysis. Vol. 12. New York: Wiley Interscience Publications, 1964:69–96.
124. Steigman J, Williams HP. Gel chromatography in the analysis of ^{99m}Tc-radiopharmaceuticals [Letter]. J Nucl Med 1974;15:318–319.
125. Valk PE, Dilts CA, McRae J. A possible artifact in gel chromatography of some ^{99m}Tc-chelates. J Nucl Med 1973;14:235–237.
126. Billinghurst MW, Palser RF. Gel chromatography as an analytical tool for ^{99m}Tc radiopharmaceuticals. J Nucl Med 1974; 15:722–723.
127. Schneider PB. A simple "electrolytic" preparation of a ^{99m}Tc (Sn) citrate renal scanning agent. J Nucl Med 1973;14:843–845.
128. Eckelman WC, Reba RC, Kubota H, Stevenson JS. ^{99m}Tc-pyrophosphate for bone imaging. J Nucl Med 1974;15:279–283.
129. Zimmer AM, Majewski W, Spies SM. Rapid miniaturized chromatography for Tc-99m IDA agents: comparison with gel chromatography. Eur J Nucl Med 1982;7:88–91.
130. Lambrecht RM, Wolf AP. Cyclotron and short-lived halogen isotopes for radiopharmaceutical applications. In: Radiopharmaceuticals and labeled compounds. Vol. 1. Vienna: IAEA, 1973:275.
131. Wellman HN, Anger RT Jr, Sodd V, Paras P. Properties, production and clinical uses of radioisotopes of iodine. CRC Crit Rev Clin Radiol Nucl Med 1975;6:81.
132. Eckelman WC. The development of single-photon-emitting receptor-binding radiotracers. In: Nunn A, ed. Radiopharmaceuticals. New York: Marcel Dekker, 1989.
133. Wagner HN Jr. Nuclear medicine in motion. J Nucl Med 1977; 18:2–4.
134. Wolf AP, Christman DR, Fowler, JS, Lambrecht RM. Synthesis of radiopharmaceuticals and labeled compounds using short-lived isotopes. In: Radiopharmaceuticals and labeled compounds. Vol. 1. Vienna: IAEA, 1973:345.
135. Frey KA, Wieland DM, Brown LE, Rogers WL, Agranoff BW. Development of a tomographic myelin scan. Ann Neurol 1981; 10:214–221.
136. Wieland DM, Brown LE, Rogers WL, et al. Myocardial imaging with a radioiodinated norepinephrine storage analog. J Nucl Med 1981;22:22–31.
137. Mangner TH, Wu J, Wieland DM. Solid-phase exchange radio iodination of aryl iodides. Facilitation by ammonium sulfate. J Org Chem 1982;47:1484–1488.

138. Edwards DP, Chamness GC, McGuire WL. Estrogen and progesterone receptor proteins in breast cancer. Biochim Biophys Acta 1979;560:457–486.
139. Katzenellenbogen JA, Heiman DF, Carlson KE, Lloyd JE. In vivo and in vitro steroid receptor assays in the design of estrogen radiopharmaceuticals. In: Eckelman WC, ed. Receptor binding radiotracers. Vol. 1. Boca Raton, FL: CRC Press, 1982:93–126.
140. Hochberg RB. Iodine-125-labeled estradiol: a γ-emitting analog of estradiol that binds to the estrogen receptor. Science 1979; 205:1138–1139.
141. Hochberg RB, Rosner W. Interaction of 16-(125I)iodo-estradiol with estrogen receptor and other steroid-binding proteins. Proc Natl Acad Sci USA 1980;77:328–332.
142. Jagoda EM, Gibson RE, Goodgold H, et al. ^{125}I-17-α-iodovinyl-1, 1 β-methoxyestradiol; in vivo and in vitro properties of a high affinity estrogen-receptor radiopharmaceutical. J Nucl Med 1984;25:472–477.
143. Kung HF, Blau M. Regional intracellular pH shift: a proposed new mechanism for radiopharmaceutical uptake in brain and other tissues. J Nucl Med 1980;21:147–152.
144. Kung HF, Tramposch KM, Blau M. A new brain perfusion imaging agent: (^{123}I)HIPDM: N,N,N-trimethyl-N-(2-hydroxy-3-methyl-5-iodobenzyl)-1,3-propanediamine. J Nucl Med 1983; 24:66–72.
145. Winchell HS, Horst WD, Braum L, Oldendorf WH, Hattner R, Parker H. N-isopropyl-(^{123}I)-p-iodoamphetamine: single pass brain uptake and washout; binding to brain synaptosomes, and localization in dog and monkey brain. J Nucl Med 1980;21:947–952.
146. Holman BL, Lee RGL, Hill STC, Bovett RD, Lister J. A comparison of two cerebral perfusion tracers, N-isopropyl I-123 p-iodoamphetamine and I-123 HIPDM, in the human. J Nucl Med 1984; 25:25–30.
147. Kung HF. Brain radiopharmaceuticals. In: Fritzberg A, ed. Radiopharmaceuticals: progress and clinical perspectives. Vol. 1. Boca Raton, FL: CRC Press, 1986:21–39.
148. Rzeszotarski WJ, Eckelman WC, Francis BE, et al. Synthesis and evaluation of radioiodinated derivatives of 1–azabicyclo (2,2,2) oct-3-yl α-hydroxy-α-(4-iodophenyl) phenylacetate as potential radiopharmaceuticals. J Med Chem 1984;27:156–159.
149. Gibson RE. Quantitative changes in receptor-concentration as a function of disease. In: Eckelman WC, ed. Receptor binding radiotracers. Vol. II. Boca Raton, FL: CRC Press, 1982:185.
150. Eckelman WC, Reba RC, Gibson RE, et al. External imaging of cerebral muscarinic acetylcholine receptors. Science 1984; 223:291–293.
151. Gallagher BM, Fowler JS, Gutterson NI, MacGregor RR, Won CN, Wolf AP. Metabolic trapping as a principle of radiopharmaceutical design. Some factors responsible for the biodistribution of ^{18}F 2-deoxy-2-fluoro-D-glucose. J Nucl Med 1978;19:1154–1161.
152. Eckelman WC. The testing of putative receptor binding radiotracers in vivo. In: Diksic M, Reba RC, eds. Radiopharamceuticals and brain pathology studied with PET and SPECT. Boca Raton FL: CRC Press, Inc., 1991:41.
153. Blau M, Manske RF. The pancreas specificity of ^{75}Se selenomethionine. J Nucl Med 1961;2:102.
154. Helus F, Maier-Borst W. A comparative investigation of methods used to produce ^{67}Ga with a cyclotron. Vol. I. In: Radiopharmaceuticals and labeled compounds. Vienna: IAEA, 1973:317–324.
155. Larson SM. Mechanisms of localization of gallium-67 in tumors. Semin Nucl Med 1978;8:193–204.
156. Jones SE, Salmon SE. The role of radionuclides in clinical oncology. Semin Nucl Med 1976;6:331–346.
157. Staub EV, McCartney WH. Role of gallium-67 in inflammatory disease. Semin Nucl Med 1978;8:219.
158. Silvester DJ. Accelerator production of medically useful radionuclides. In: Radiopharmaceuticals and labeled compounds. Vol. I. Vienna: IAEA, 1973:197–222.
159. McNeil BJ, Holman BL, Button LN, Rosenthall DS. Use of indium chloride scintigraphy in patients with myelofibrosis. J Nucl Med 1974;15:647–651.
160. McIntyre PA, Larson SM, Eikman EA, et al. Comparison of metabolism of iron transferrin (Fe-Tf) and indium transferrin (In-Tf) by the erythropoietic marrow. J Nucl Med 1973;14:425–426.
161. Mathias CJ, Welch MJ. ^{111}In-labeled platelets for the detection of vascular disorders in animal models. In: Lambrecht RM, Eckelman WC, eds. Animal models in radiotracer design. New York: Springer-Verlag, 1983:149–177.
162. Thakur ML. Radiolabeled leukocytes and platelets. In: Fritzberg A, ed. Radiopharmaceuticals: progress and clinical perspectives. Vol. III. Boca Raton, FL: CRC Press Inc, 1986:1–23.
163. Gansow O. Newer aproaches to the radiolabeling of monoclonal antibodies by use of metal chelates. Nucl Med Biol 1991;18:369.
164. Lebowitz E, Greene MW, Bradley-Moore P, et al. Thallium-201 for medical use. J Nucl Med 1973;14:421.
165. Clark JW, Fulmer CB, Williams IR. Excitation functions for radioactive nuclides produced by deuteron-induced reactions in iron. Phys Rev 1969;197:1104.
166. Schilling RF. The absorption and utilization of vitamin B_{12}. Am J Clin Nutr 1955;3:45–49.
167. Renault H, Rapin J, Rudler M, et al. Labeling method using the chelation of various radioactive cations by some polypeptides. Application to bleomycin. Chem Ther 1972;7:232–235.
168. Reba RC, Eckelman WC, Poulose KP, et al. Tumor specific radiopharmaceuticals. In: Subramanian G, Rhodes BA, Cooper JF, Sodd VJ, eds. Radiopharmaceuticals. New York: Society for Nuclear Medicine, 1975:464–473.
169. Volkert WA, Goeckeler WF, Ehrhardt GJ, et al. Therapeutic radionuclides: production and decay property considerations. J Nucl Med 1991;32:174–185.
170. Gennaro GP, Neirinckz RD, Bergner B, et al. A radionuclide generator and infusion system for pharmaceutical quality Rb-82. In: Knapp FF Jr, Butler TA, eds. Radionuclide generators. American Chemical Society Symposium Series 241. Washington, DC: American Chemical Society, 1984:135–150.
171. Gould KL, Goldstein RA, Mullani NA, et al. Noninvasive assessment of coronary stenosis by myocardial perfusion imaging during pharmacologic coronary vasodilation. VIII. Clinical feasibility of positron cardiac imaging without a cyclotron using generator-produced rubidium-82. J Am Coll Cardiol 1986;7:775–789.
172. Finn RD, Molinski VJ, Hopt HB, Kramer H. Radionuclide generators for biomedical applications. Technical Information Center, USDOE [NAS-NS-3202]. Washington DC: U.S. Department of Energy, 1983.
173. Neirinckx RD, Davis MA. Development of a chromatographic Ge-68–Ga-68 generator yielding ionic gallium. In: Sorenson J, ed. Radiopharmaceuticals II. New York: Society for Nuclear Medicine, 1979:791–799.
174. Philip MS, Ramsey CE, Ma JM, Lamb JF. A Rb-81/Kr-81m perfusion generator. In: Knapp FF Jr, Butler TA, eds. Radionuclide generators. American Chemical Society Symposium Series 241. Washington DC: American Chemical Society, 1984:67–73.
175. Welch MH, Welch TJ. Solution chemistry of carrier-free indium. In: Subramanian G, Rhodes BA, Cooper JF, Sodd VJ, eds. Radiopharmaceuticals. New York: Society for Nuclear Medicine, 1975:73–79.
176. Holman BL, Kirsch CM, Zielonka JS. The heart. In: Ell PJ, Holman BL, eds. Emission computed tomography. Oxford: Oxford University Press, 1983:475–494.
177. Khan O, Ell PJ. Liver and spleen. In: Ell PJ, Holman BL, eds. Emission computed tomography. Oxford: Oxford University Press, 1983:438–474.

178. Macey DJ, Marshall R. The lungs. In: Ell PJ, Holman BL, eds. Emission computed tomography. Oxford: Oxford University Press, 1983:495–520.
179. Phelps ME, Huang SC, Hoffman EJ, et al. Tomographic measurement of local cerebral glucose metabolic rate in humans with (F-18) 2-fluoro-2-deoxy-glucose: validation of a method. Ann Neuro 1979;6:371.
180. Martin WRW. Dopa metabolism in quantitative imaging. In: Frost JJ, Wagner HN Jr, eds. Neuroreceptors, neurotransmitters. New York: Raven Press, 1990:167.
181. Fowler JS, Wolf AP. 2-deoxy-2-(18-F)fluro-D-glucose for metabolic studies. Int J Appl Radiat Isot 1986;37:663.
182. Eckelman WC. Radiopharmaceuticals and brain pathology studied with PET and SPECT. Chap. 4. In: Diksic M, Reba RC, eds. The testing of putative receptor binding radiotracers in vivo. Boca Raton, FL: CRC Press, Inc. 1990:41.
183. Kilbourn M. Radiotracers for PET studies of neurotransmitter binding sites: design considerations. In: Kuhl DE, ed. In vivo imaging of neurotransmitter functions in brain, heart and tumors. Washington, DC: American College of Nuclear Physicists, 1991:47.
184. Gjedde A, Wong DF. Modeling neuroreceptor binding of radioligands in vivo in quantitative imaging. In: Frost JJ, Wagner HN Jr, eds. Neuroreceptors, neurotransmitters. New York: Raven Press, 1990:51.
185. Eckelman WC. The status of radiopharmaceutical research. Nucl Med Biol 1991;18:iii–vi.
186. Phelps ME, Mazziotta JC, Huang SC. Study of cerebral function with positron computed tomography. J Cerebral Blood Flow Metab 1982;2:113–162.

15 Radiopharmaceuticals for Cardiac Imaging

KAREN E. LINDER, ADRIAN D. NUNN, and H. WILLIAM STRAUSS

Radionuclide imaging is useful to evaluate cardiac function, determine relative (and, with positron imaging, absolute) myocardial perfusion, detect acute necrosis, measure the regional and global utilization of substrates, and define the distribution of adrenergic innervation in the myocardium. This chapter provides an overview of the available radiopharmaceuticals for cardiac imaging, categorized by the physiologic parameters measured.

CARDIAC FUNCTION

Measurements of ventricular function utilize radiopharmaceuticals that meet two criteria: (a) Provide a sufficient photon flux for recording data during the time allocated, and (b) remain in the vascular compartment during the interval of measurement. To provide the photon flux with an acceptable absorbed dose, a radionuclide with a relatively short half-life and favorable biodistribution is required. For practical purposes, this limits the choice to ^{99m}Tc.

Data can be recorded either during the initial passage of the tracer through the central circulation, or after the tracer has equilibrated in the blood pool. Recording data during the first pass is technically demanding on the imaging device, hence the preference for equilibrium imaging.

FIRST PASS

First pass data can be recorded with any agent that traverses the chambers of interest and provides the necessary photon flux to record cardiac function during the 10–15 second interval that the tracer is present in the central circulation. Typically, doses of at least 15 mCi must be administered to provide about 100,000 cts/second with a state-of-the-art camera (representing about 5,000 cts/frame in a 50 msec/frame acquisition). Exceeding this count rate, particularly with older instruments, can result in distortions of the recorded information. Before recording first pass studies, it is helpful to perform phantom studies, with sources in petri dishes, to determine the behavior of the camera at high count rates. Most new instruments provide a linear response with activity up to ~125,000 cts/second. Table 15.1 summarizes agents that have been used for first pass studies. When the primary purpose of the study is to record data from the right heart only, either ^{99m}Tc-labeled agents, or ^{133}Xe dissolved in saline, or ^{81m}Kr dissolved in dextrose can be used. The dissolved gases are particularly useful if the patient's right ventricular function is measured several times in rapid succession, such as when testing agents that alter pulmonary vascular resistance.

To measure ejection fraction and ventricular volumes, the radiopharmaceutical must be administered in the smallest possible volume (preferably less than 0.5 ml) in a central vein (through a catheter placed in the vena cava if possible) to permit accurate delineation of the left and right heart chambers. Typically, a small volume bolus is not well-mixed as it traverses the right heart making quantitation of right heart function with this technique problematic. Passage of the compact bolus through the tricuspid and pulmonic valves, plus transit through the lung, provides sufficient mixing to delineate the entire left ventricle, except in cases of severe focal ventricular dysfunction, where mixing in the left heart blood pool may be impaired.

Radiopharmaceuticals employed for this study must not diffuse in the lungs. Pertechnetate and DTPA both lose about 10–15% of the dose in the lungs, which increases the lung background on the first pass examination. This is corrected by subtracting the lung background during quantitation, but the reduced contrast between the left heart and lungs may limit detection of subtle wall motion abnormalities. Lung extraction is less of a problem with ^{99m}Tc-sulfur colloid, unless patients have underlying systemic or pulmonary disease, when the lung extraction of sulfur colloid is increased.

EQUILIBRIUM IMAGING

Albumin

To maintain contrast between the cardiac chambers and the lungs, radiopharmaceuticals used for equilibrium imaging must have an effective vascular clearance half-time of at least several hours. This is accomplished by coupling the tracer to proteins or cells. In vivo labeling of proteins occurs with some radionuclides (e.g., gallium-67 or indium-111) which are carried by the β-globulin transferrin, but the photon flux of these tracers is insufficient for cardiac imaging with clinical doses. Because $^{99m}TcO_4^-$ is not protein bound in vivo, it must be coupled to protein in vitro prior to administration. ^{99m}Tc-albumin kits are available, which reduce ^{99m}Tc with stannous chloride and allow the reactive species to bind to albumin. Although this type of stannous-technetium-protein interaction produces multiple albumin species (6), the material remains in the blood pool long enough to provide acceptable data. The multidose vial permits reconstitution with sufficient activity that a single vial can be used to study several patients.

Albumin is not a perfect intravascular marker because the body albumin space is about 30% larger than the true plasma volume (7), but the 65-kd size of albumin (some of which may exist as a dimer) slows the rate of equilibration. Within an hour of administration, the tracer is largely confined to the vascular space, providing images of sufficient quality to evaluate both global and regional ventricular function. One of the major organs with a large albumin space is the liver. In some instances, the relatively high concentration of activity in the liver can obscure the inferior border of the heart, making it difficult to identify lesions in this area. An advantage of ^{99m}Tc-albumin is the reproducible, though suboptimal, image quality provided by the agent. This can be particularly important in patients with multisystem disease treated with multiple medications, when the systems used to label autologous red cells (the preferred equilibrium agent) may not work well. Table 15.2 summarizes agents that have been used for equilibrium imaging.

Labeled Red Cells

Red cells (8) can be radiolabeled by three different methods: (a) in vitro, (b) directly in vivo, or (c) a modified in vivo technique (Table 15.3). The techniques differ in the quality of the label, but not in the labeling reaction. When red cells are exposed to a small amount of stannous ion, subsequent exposure to pertechnetate allows the technetium ion to bind to the β-chain of hemoglobin with high affinity. Binding of pertechnetate to hemoglobin requires some time, typically several minutes, for a high degree of labeling (9). The modified in vivo and in vitro labeling techniques limit diffusion of pertechnetate into other compartments during this interval, resulting in higher contrast between the blood pool and background. Direct in vivo labeling has the greatest variability, with frequent visualization of the stomach and the lowest contrast between heart and lung background. The modified in vivo method produces a reliable label, with 90% red cell binding, and rare visualization of the stomach. By far, the highest quality labeling is accomplished by the in vitro labeling technique. When multiple measurements of cardiac function are recorded for in-

Table 15.1.
First Pass Radiopharmaceutics

Agent	Comments	Distribution
^{99m}Tc-DTPA	available in high specific activity; high photon flux	total body extracellular fluid (ECF) space; concentration in blood decreases to ~5% within 10 minutes of injection; excreted by glomerular filtration in the urine
Na^{99m}TcO$_4$	available in high specific activity (small volume); high photon flux	total body ECF space; although blood concentration decreases rapidly, pertechnetate is concentrated in the choroid plexus, gastric mucosa and thyroid gland; renal excretion is slow, with a clearance rate of ~3 ml/min
^{99m}Tc-Sulfur Colloid	available in high specific activity; high photon flux	concentrates in reticuloendothelial cells of the liver resulting in high hepatic dose difficult to see inferior wall on second injection in some patients
^{133}Xenon	dissolved in saline; 80 keV photon has slightly lower resolution than ^{99m}Tc; short effective half-life permits administration of 30–50 mCi/injection.	right heart data only; in the pulmonary capillaries dissolved xenon partitions into the pulmonary airspace providing information about pulmonary perfusion—within a few breaths the tracer clears in proportion to local ventilation
Research Generator Systems		
^{81m}Krypton	obtained by eluting the rubidium-krypton generator with dextrose in water in place of air.[1,2] This is not an FDA approved procedure	right heart data only; excreted by lungs
^{191m}Iridium	4.7 second half-life radionuclide; eluted directly from an Osmium generator into the patient.[3] The agent is of limited value in patients with heart failure, since their prolonged circulation times result in substantial tracer decay, and poor visualization of the left heart	Vascular space, since the agent decays before significant amounts can distribute extravascularly
^{178}Tantalum	10 minute half-life radionuclide, eluted directly from a Tungsten generator[4,5]	vascular space primarily due to protein binding

Table 15.2.
Radiopharmaceutics for Equilibrium Imaging

Agent	Application	Comments	Distribution
^{99m}Tc-Red Blood Cells	Equilibrium or first pass	requires labeling autologous cells either in vivo or in vitro	vascular space; concentrates in spleen
^{99m}Tc-Albumin	Equilibrium or first pass	available in multidose kits that can be labeled with high specific activity	vascular space; concentrates in liver

Table 15.3.
Red Cell Labeling

Technique	Labeling Procedure	Comments
in vivo	• administer stannous ion in the form of stannous pyrophosphate or stannous DTPA • wait 10–15 minutes • administer 20–30 mCi pertechnetate	red cell labeling may be impaired by prior administration of dipyridamole
modified in vivo	• administer stannous ion in the form of stannous pyrophosphate or stannous DTPA • wait 10–15 minutes • withdraw 3–5 ml of blood into a heparinized, shielded syringe containing 20–30 mCi pertechnetate • incubate at 20–30°C for 10 minutes • administer contents of syringe	red cell labeling may be impaired by: • reduced incubation temperature • low hematocrit (<20%) • prior administration of dipyridamole
in vitro red cell kit	• withdraw 1–3 ml of whole blood into a reaction vial containing an anticoagulant (either 0.5 ml acid citrate dextrose or heparin), mix for 5 minutes • add syringe 1 (sodium hypochlorite), mix; • add syringe 2 (sodium Citrate); mix; • add 10–100 mCi$^{99m}TcO_4^-$; incubate for 20 minutes; • inject	

tervals of several hours, the in vitro labeling approach should be employed.

In contrast to labeled albumin, where the liver is very prominent, labeled red cells concentrate in the spleen (probably due to the high splenic hematocrit). This high concentration of activity is rarely a problem for blood pool images because of the posterior location of the spleen.

Equilibrium imaging is usually performed 5–15 minutes after administration of the radiopharmaceutical, to permit adequate mixing in the blood pool. Although first pass data can be recorded with these agents, both albumin and red cells are usually administered in volumes 1 ml, making the bolus less compact during the left heart phase. Mixing is usually incomplete, even after 15 minutes, but the difference in blood pool activity concentration is typically $<10\%$ over the interval of multiview imaging (typically 15–30 minutes). This gradual "loss" of activity can be important when quantifying chamber volumes using one of the techniques that call for comparing region of interest counts (corrected for attenuation) to a blood sample in a petri dish. When these techniques are used, the blood sample should be obtained at the same time as the image to minimize errors.

ACUTE MYOCARDIAL NECROSIS

It is difficult to determine when a myocyte is injured to the point that recovery of function is impossible. In the early hours of injury), enzyme loss, electrocardiographic changes, loss of regional wall motion, or zones of decreased perfusion, can rarely identify sites of irreversible damage. A goal of imaging is to differentiate zones of irreversible injury from areas that can recover. At present, this can be accomplished by a combination of techniques, utilizing either perfusion imaging and a necrosis agent, or a metabolic agent and a perfusion agent. Agents that specifically localize in areas of acute myocyte necrosis include ^{99m}Tc-pyrophosphate (probably binding to regions of high calcium concentration in the dying cell), ^{111}In-antimyosin Fab (binding specifically to exposed segments of the heavy chain of cardiac myosin), and ^{99m}Tc-glucarate (mechanism unknown). The timing of earliest and peak uptake of the agents vis-à-vis the acute injury is summarized in Table 15.4.

Table 15.4.
Agents for Imaging Acute Necrosis

Agent	Time After Onset to Initial Uptake	Time After Onset to Peak Uptake	Interval Between Injection and Imaging
^{99m}Tc-Pyrophosphate	6–10 hours	24–72 hours	2–6 hours
^{111}In-Antimyosin	3—6 hours	24–72 hours	24–72 hours
^{99m}Tc-Glucarate	1–3 hours	<24 hours	0.5–1 hour

Pyrophosphate

^{99m}Tc-pyrophosphate uptake can occur in tissue that is severely, but not irreversibly, damaged (10). The clinical implications of this finding are that the technique is sensitive, but not specific for the detection of necrosis. As a result, it is not widely used for the detection of infarction.

Antimyosin

^{111}In-antimyosin is both specific and sensitive for the detection of acute myocyte necrosis (11). The antibody can only bind to the heavy chain of cardiac myosin if the sarcolemma is irreversibly disrupted. The radiolabeled antibody fragment, unfortunately, is relatively large (~50 kd) and has a blood clearance half-time of about 6 hours. Because uptake in most infarcted tissue is ~0.5–1% of the dose, it is usually necessary to wait for 24–48 hours to record diagnostic images (later imaging times may be required for the detection of very small subendocardial infarcts). As a result, this procedure is not often used clinically, because the diagnosis of infarction is available from serial enzyme and electrocardiographic studies.

Antimyosin imaging can be particularly useful in circumstances where diffuse necrosis is suspected, but difficult to verify using enzymes and electrocardiograms. Patients presenting with congestive heart failure without an apparent cause may have myocarditis. Acute myocarditis usually requires endocardial biopsy for diagnosis. Endocardial biopsies taken from multiple sites may fail to capture samples of tissue with the classic histopathologic findings, making the diagnosis problematic in about 25% of patients. Antimyosin imaging can effectively sample the entire heart for areas of necrosis, making this a valuable diagnostic technique in this setting.

Other situations where diffuse mecrosis may be difficult to detect include acute rejection in patients with cardiac transplantation, and cancer chemotherapy or radiation induced myocarditis. Antimyosin imaging can be useful in these circumstances.

Glucarate

^{99m}Tc-glucarate (12) is a radiopharmaceutical that recently entered human trials for the detection of tumors and acute tissue necrosis. Experimental studies demonstrated prompt uptake ($<$30 minutes) in areas of myocardial and cerebral infarction. In contrast to pyrophosphate, this agent appears to localize only in zones of irreversibly damaged tissue. The combination of rapid blood clearance, and uptake of $\sim$1% in zones of irreversible injury, permit diagnostic quality images to be recorded within 60 minutes of injection.

The clinical utility of this agent awaits large scale clinical trials. Should the promising preliminary data be borne out, this imaging technique may become the method of choice for evaluating patients presenting as "rule out infarct." Two major advantages of imaging the zones of acute necrosis instead of zones of decreased perfusion are that uptake will represent only areas of acute injury (independent of prior damage), and the localization produces a "hot spot," making the lesion easier to identify than an area of reduced uptake.

PERFUSION

Perfusion is defined as blood flow at the cellular level—the delivery of nutrients and removal of waste products to maintain cellular function. This parameter is different than the large vessel flow seen arteriographically, because an occluded vessel may have adequate collateralization to provide perfusion to large segments of tissue. Perfusion can be determined by any substance that meets the following criteria: (a) The agent must be *rapidly cleared* from the blood, and (b) the agent must be *concentrated* by an organ. Under these circumstances, the regional distribution in the tissues of that organ will be proportional to perfusion. Thus, organs or regions with high blood flow will have a proportionally higher concentration of the indicator than those with low blood flow. This principle, which was first described by Leon Saperstein (13), forms the basis for perfusion imaging in all organs, and applies to a wide variety of radiopharmaceuticals, including microspheres, radiolabeled fatty acids, monovalent cations such as thallium, and the technetium-based heart and brain perfusion imaging agents.

There are no absolute guidelines to define the limits of a Saperstein tracer. At one extreme are microspheres, which are totally extracted by all organs in a single pass and have no recirculation. At the other extreme are ions such as cesium, which, while a potassium analog, has a circulating half-time of over 5 minutes and low extraction. Long circulating half-lives lead to the problem of changing perfusion during the interval of measurement, similar to the problem of blurring due to motion during a time exposure in photography. Extraction fraction (the fraction of the agent entering the arterial circulation of an organ that is concentrated by that organ) of perfusion tracers should be over 50% and remain constant over a wide range of blood flows. At rest, myocardial blood flow is normally 60–80 ml/min/100 g tissue, but can increase to four or five times this value at peak exercise or with vasodilators (adenosine or dipyridamole). In many instances, the extraction of radiotracer falls off under high flow conditions, leading to an underestimation of perfusion (14). Higher extraction fractions are associated with higher concentrations of the indicator in the tissue, and hence provide a better signal-to-noise ratio in the image. In general, radiotracers that have an extraction fraction that is less than 50%, or that clear slowly from the blood (clearance $T_{1/2}$ 5 minutes), do not adhere to the Saperstein principle, and are not appropriate for perfusion imaging.

From a practical perspective, the agent must be retained in the myocardium for a sufficient period of time to allow imaging. This is especially important during SPECT studies. Clearance from the heart should be slow, relative to image acquisition time, to prevent generation of artifacts in SPECT reconstructions.

None of the myocardial perfusion agents adhere completely to the characteristics of an ideal agent. However, clinically useful images can be obtained with them all, as long as the deficiencies of each agent are compensated for.

OVERVIEW OF AGENTS USED FOR PERFUSION

Radiotracers used to image perfusion in the heart can be divided into four classes: inorganic cationic potassium analogs (e.g., ^{201}Tl), complex cations (e.g., sestamibi), highly extracted neutral molecules (e.g., teboroxime, $H_2{}^{15}O$), and fatty acids (e.g., paraiodophenylhexadecanoic acid or the branched chain fatty acid betamethyliodophenylpentadecanoic acid (BMIPP)).

Inorganic Cationic Potassium Analogs

Most of the small inorganic cations that have been used for myocardial perfusion imaging are analogs of the potassium ion. Transport of potassium (K^+) into myocardial cells involves the Na^+/K^+ ATPase pump that is present in viable myocardial membranes. This pump, which concentrates potassium intracellularly and expels sodium, appears to be relatively nonspecific, as several other monocations that have an ionic radius close to that of K^+ are also taken up by the Na^+/K^+ ATPase pump. A list of potassium analogs that have been used for myocardial perfusion imaging is given in Table 15.5. Of these, thallous ion is the most avidly extracted.

Table 15.5.
Inorganic Cations Used for Myocardial Imaging

Inorganic Cation	% Coronary Extraction[15]	Ionic Radius	Energy (keV)	Physical $T_{1/2}$
^{43} Potassium (K)	71	1.38	373,619	22.4 h
^{201} Thallium (Tl)	88	1.50	68,83	73 h
^{129} Cesium (Cs)	22	1.70	375,416	32.1 h
^{82} Rubidium (Rb)	70	1.49	511	~75 sec
^{13} N NH_4^+	90	1.48	511	10 min
^{38} Potassium (K)	71	1.38	511	7.6 min

Potassium

Investigations with ^{43}K began in 1971 (16). However, this radionuclide (physical $T_{1/2}$ = 22.4 hours) has γ-emissions that are too high in energy (373 and 619 keV) to be useful for imaging with a 1.25-cm thick NaI crystal gamma-camera (intrinsic photopeak efficiency <25%, versus 90% for 140 keV photons), but was very useful for imaging with a rectilinear scanner. ^{43}K was the first radionuclide employed for stress myocardial perfusion imaging (17). Another radioisotope of potassium, ^{38}K, decays by positron emission so its annihilation photons can be detected using positron emission tomography (PET). Its short half-life (~7 minutes) limits its use to institutions with on-site accelerators, but in vivo measurements of myocardial perfusion with this isotope were reported as early as 1978 (18).

Thallium-201

The thallous ion (Tl^+) mimics potassium and, as a result of its low energy photons, rapidly replaced potassium-43 as the preferred myocardial perfusion agent (19, 20). It is avidly concentrated by the myocardium, with an extraction 80% at resting blood flow, and ~70% at maximal myocardial blood flow. Once inside the myocyte, Tl^+ equilibrates with potassium ions in the cell, and exits slowly, over several hours. The regional distribution of thallium provides a reasonable estimate of perfusion. Although ^{201}Tl myocardial perfusion imaging is currently the most widely used procedure in nuclear cardiology, the characteristics of the isotope are suboptimal. The abundant x-ray photons of 68–83 keV usually used for imaging make changes in tissue thickness very apparent on the images—hence attenuation artifacts are seen to a greater degree with this radiopharmaceutical than with ^{99m}Tc-labeled agents. Additionally, the agent has a physical half-life of 73 hours and a biologic half-life of 10 days, which leads to a radiation dose to the kidneys of ~1 rad/mCi and limits the allowable cumulative dose of thallium to ~3–4 mCi (21). Despite these drawbacks, ^{201}Tl remains the most popular agent for myocardial perfusion imaging, with proven efficacy in the identification of myocardial ischemia.

At rest, about 3.5% of injected ^{201}Tl localizes in the myocardium and increases to ~4.4% during exercise (22). After initial localization, thallium activity levels in the heart do not remain constant. The average half-time for loss of ^{201}Tl from the heart is 4–6 hours (23). Several factors can affect the rate of loss. Faster clearance is seen in patients that achieve high levels of exercise than in those at submaximal exercise levels (24). Activity clears in a differential fashion from zones of ischemia and normal segments: ischemic zones clear at a slower rate than from well-perfused segments. Clearance is also affected by plasma insulin levels, with faster washout from both ischemic and normoxic segments in animals infused with a glucose-insulin-potassium solution (25).

Thallium in myocardial tissue is in equilibrium with the trace amount of thallium that remains in the blood, which is in turn, in equilibrium with the pool of activity that is sequestered in other tissues, such as the liver and skeletal muscle. Over time, ischemic but viable tissue that initially showed reduced thallium levels due to underperfusion by stenotic coronary arteries, may appear to "fill in," a phenomenon known as redistribution, due to the differential clearance (26). Areas of fibrosis will not do this, allowing discrimination between tissue that is ischemic and infarcted by imaging the patient both immediately after injection and several hours later. In severely ischemic myocardium, however, about one-third of the lesions which have viable myocardium will appear unchanged at 3–4 hours, but may show redistribution at 24 hours, or show uptake with reinjection of thallium at rest (27–29). In a limited number of studies, lesions that fill in with reinjection have shown good concordance with segments that accumulate ^{18}F-fluorodeoxyglucose, suggesting that such segments remain viable (30–32).

Tc Complex Cations

The suboptimal imaging properties of ^{201}Tl led to research aimed at development of ^{99m}Tc-based agents for myocardial perfusion imaging to permit administration of larger doses (producing higher photon fluxes) to record higher quality images in a shorter interval of time.

Initial efforts at the development of ^{99m}Tc-labeled myocardial imaging agents were focused on producing cationic complexes with the expectation (33) that Tc complexes with a positive charge would mimic the behavior of thallium and be taken up by the Na^+/K^+ ATPase pump. (This has not proved to be true (46).) However, the Tc(III) cationic compounds trans-$[^{99m}Tc(DMPE)_2Cl_2]^+$ (34, 35) (DMPE = 1,2-bis(dimethylphosphino)ethane) and trans-$[^{99m}Tc(DEPE)_2Cl_2]^+$ (DEPE = 1,2-bis(diethylphosphino)ethane) (36) failed to give satisfactory localization in human heart, despite good myocardial uptake in rats and dogs. Several Tc(I) cations were also evaluated in humans (37). Three of these agents, $[^{99m}Tc\text{-}DMPE)3]^+$, $^{99m}Tc[(TMP)_6]^+$ (TMP = trimethylphosphite and $^{99m}Tc(POM\text{-}POM)3]^+$ (POM-POM = 1,2-bis(dimethoxyphosphino)ethane) cleared from the blood in humans very slowly, obscuring myocardial activity.

The behavior of these Tc(III) cationic compounds highly is species dependent (38). It has been proposed that the washout of the Tc(III) species is due to reduction of these compounds to neutral Tc(II) compounds in the human heart (39). The resulting lipophilic Tc(II) species formed after reduction clears rapidly from the heart. Several groups have found that Tc(III) (40, 41) and Tc(V) (42, 51) complexes that have had their redox potential tuned so that reduction cannot take place, *can* be used for myocardial perfusion.

For example, the agent ^{99m}Tc-Q12 is a nonreducible cationic complex that has recently shown potential as a myocardial imaging agent in animal studies and early human trials (40, 41). Unlike earlier cations, this agent shows rapid blood clearance and heart uptake and does not appear to undergo significant washout over 5 hours postinjection. Another solution to this problem was to produce technetium agents in the oxidation state Tc(I), which is very stable. Sestamibi, one of the two ^{99m}Tc-labeled perfusion agents approved by the FDA in December of 1990, falls into this class.

Sestamibi

^{99m}Tc-sestamibi is an isonitrile complex of technetium (also known as MIBI (methoxy-isobutyl-isonitrile)). Two earlier isonitrile complexes (^{99m}Tc-t-butyl isonitrile (TBI) (43, 44) and ^{99m}Tc-carboxyisopropyl isonitrile (CPI) (45)) were also tested in humans, but were not pursued due to high hepatic uptake. Interestingly, it has been shown that, unlike thallium, uptake of ^{99m}Tc-sestamibi is not blocked by ouabain, so the uptake of the agent does not appear to be dependent on the Na^+/K^+ ATPase transport system (46). Thus, the initial premise on which research into Tc agents began led to a compound that is retained by different mechanisms than were originally proposed. The agent appears to bind to cellular elements, particularly in the mitochondrial membrane. Viable tissue is required for uptake and retention. In contrast to the kinetics of thallium, sestamibi has a half-time for clearance from the myocardium of about 6 hours and no definite evidence of differential washout from ischemic and normal tissue (47, 48). Therefore, images obtained at 1 hour reflect perfusion at the time of injection. To differentiate exercise induced ischemic tissue from scar, the patient must have a second injection of the radiopharmaceutical at rest.

Sestamibi clears from the blood less rapidly than thallium, and its overall extraction efficiency is lower (about 60% at resting myocardial blood flow). As is true for $^{201}Tl^+$, extraction efficiency of sestamibi appears to fall at high flow rates (49). Because of this, only about 2% of the dose is extracted by the heart, as opposed to ~4% for Tl. However, the much higher dose of ^{99m}Tc used more than compensates for lower extraction. Dosimetry of sestamibi is very favorable relative to Tl, permitting doses of 20–30 mCi with a radiation burden of 3–5 rads to the bowel. This greatly increases the number of photons available for imaging. The 140 keV γ-photons are also of higher energy, so soft tissue attenuation is much less of a problem than it is with ^{201}Tl. Good correlation between the results of ^{201}Tl and ^{99m}Tc-sestamibi studies has been shown in a number of clinical comparisons (50).

Sestamibi also localizes in other organs, including skeletal muscle, liver, and kidneys. Initial hepatic uptake is pronounced, so imaging studies are normally delayed for 30–60 minutes to allow clearance from the liver into the gall bladder and bowel. With exercise, a larger fraction of activity localizes in the heart and skeletal muscles, with significantly lower activity in the liver.

Tetrofosmin

^{99m}Tc-tetrofosmin (P53) is a lipophilic, cationic diphosphine ^{99m}Tc-[(tetrofosmin)$_2$O$_2$]$^+$ complex. Phase I trials on this complex (51) report that 1.2% of the dose localizes in the heart and is retained, whereas rapid clearance is seen from lung, blood and liver. Activity is excreted through both the GI and urinary tracts. Exercise lowered the activity in the liver, resulting in a clearer image of the heart. Early liver uptake at rest ranged from 5–10% of the dose, but fell rapidly to <1.6% at 2 hours, with heart:liver ratios reported as 0.75 at 30 minutes (52). With exercise, there was a dramatic increase in skeletal muscle uptake, as is seen with Tl, sestamibi, and teboroxime. The total body dose for a 30 mCi dose is estimated to be 0.4 rad. The agent does not redistribute, so two injections are required for rest/stress studies. The product also has the advantage of being prepared at room temperature, as opposed to the boiling required for sestamibi and teboroxime. The compound is reconstituted with Tc and allowed to stand at room temperature for 15 minutes. Phase III studies (53, 54) have been carried out, and the results indicate that the optimal imaging time is 30 minutes postinjection. This presents an advantage relative to sestamibi, where imaging is usually delayed for 60 minutes.

Teboroxime

Unlike sestamibi and tetrofosmin, which are charged compounds, teboroxime is neutral. This compound (55) is a member of the boronic acid adduct of technetium dioxime (BATO) class (56) of compounds. The drug is readily produced by template synthesis (57) by adding $^{99m}TcO_4^-$ to a lyophilized vial that contains the appropriate vicinal dioxime and boronic acid, followed by heating at 100°C for 15 minutes. Once prepared, teboroxime is stable for greater than 6 hours.

Teboroxime has initial myocardial uptake that is closest to the Saperstein ideal. Its clearance from the blood is extremely rapid, with an extraction fraction in the myocardium exceeding that of thallium at all flows (58). Unfortunately, unlike thallium, teboroxime clears from the heart very rapidly, with biexponential clearance half-times of 2 minutes (68%) and 78 minutes (32%). As a result, images must be obtained *immediately* after injection. Clinical investigations have demonstrated a high degree of concordance of teboroxime uptake with thallium scintigraphy and the agent is reported to give similar diagnostic accuracy to angiography in ischemic heart disease (59, 60). Once cleared from the heart, teboroxime does not relocalize. Like sestamibi, the dosimetry of teboroxime is such that 20–30 mCi of the agent may be injected (usually as 12–15 mCi for initial stress test, followed by 20–25 for rest study). The agent is excreted primarily through the GI tract. The radiation doses to the liver and upper large bowel are 1.9 and 3.7 rad, respectively, from 30 mCi of ^{99m}Tc-teboroxime (61).

There are reports that the clearance rates from ischemic and normoxic tissue are different, both in experimental (62, 63) and clinical settings. If washout does prove to be flow-related, then either sequential images or regional washout curves may give valuable information that will assist in clinical diagnosis (64). Table 15.6 compares the extraction, clearance half-time, cardiac and hepatic uptake, and differential clearance of these agents. Figure 15.1 shows their chemical structures.

Table 15.6.
Comparison of ^{99m}Tc-teboroxime, ^{99m}Tc-sestamibi, and ^{201}Tl

Class	^{99m}Tc-teboroxime Neutral Complex (BATO)	^{99m}Tc-sestamibi Complex Cation (Isonitrile)	^{201}Tl Inorganic Cation
Peak extraction fraction	~0.90	~0.65	~0.8
Clearance $T_{1/2}$			
Heart	~4 minutes	~6 hours	~4 hours
Liver	~1.5 hour	~0.5 hour	
Differential clearance from normal and ischemic tissue	Yes	Slight	Yes

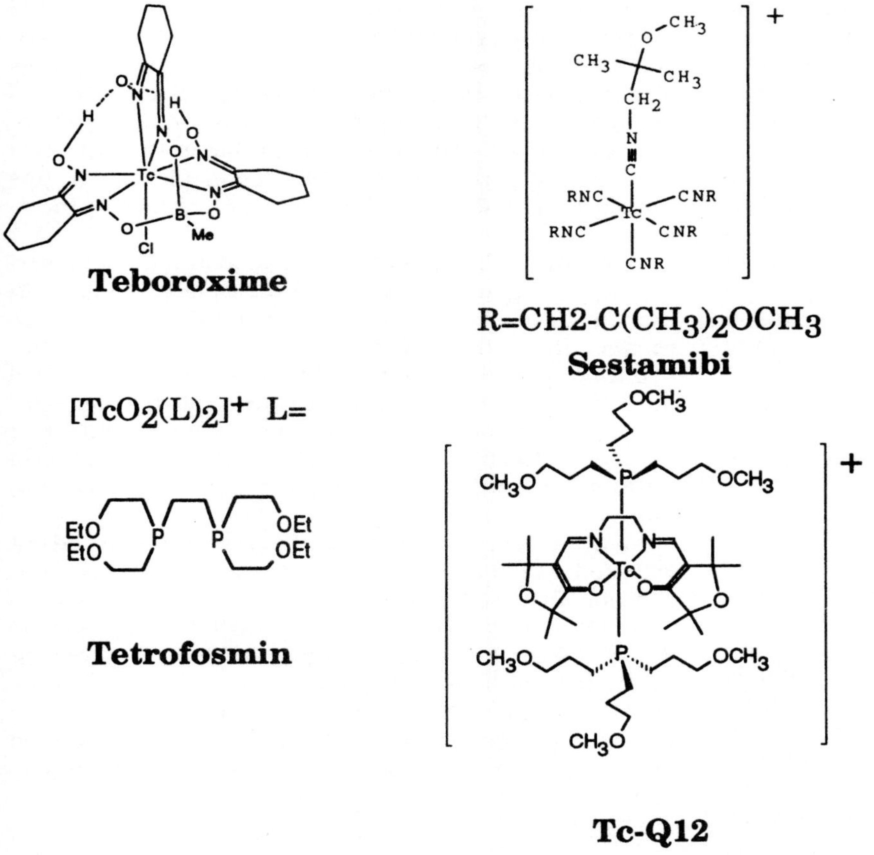

Figure 15.1. Chemical structures of teboroxime, sestamibi, tetrofosmin, and Tc-Q12.

Rubidium

Rubidium-82 is a short-lived ($T_{1/2}$ = 75 seconds), positron emitting, potassium analog produced by the decay of its parent strontium-82 ($T_{1/2}$ = 25 days). The parent-daughter relationship permits this agent to be sold as a generator system, allowing the short-lived agent to be used to make multiple measurements of myocardial perfusion with a modest radiation burden. One generator provides short-lived ^{82}Rb for about 1 month. Effective imaging of this agent is obtained with positron cameras with detectors optimized for its 511 keV emissions. Like potassium and thallium, cationic Rb is concentrated in the myocardium by the Na^+/K^+ ATPase pump, but because of the short half-life of ^{82}Rb, imaging protocols and pharmacokinetics are dominated by the physical characteristics of the nuclide. This agent is eluted directly from the strontium-82 generator (65) into the patient. Myocardial imaging with this isotope requires rapid acquisition of data, due to its short physical half-life, but this short half-life makes it very attractive for use in rapid repeat studies, such as stress/rest protocols and pre/postintervention studies (66). Images recorded within the first 1–2 minutes after intravenous injection show activity in the blood pool; images obtained after 2 minutes reflect myocardial perfusion. If gating is carried out during acquisition, ejection fraction and regional wall motion studies can also be performed. Good quality images can only be recorded for 4–6 half-lives after infusion.

N-13 Ammonia

In addition to generator produced ^{82}Rb, several small molecules labeled with short-lived cyclotron-produced positron-emitting isotopes have been used for myocardial per-

Table 15.7.
PET Radiopharmaceutics for Myocardial Perfusion

Agent	Physical Half-Life	Source
^{82}Rb	75 sec	strontium generator
$^{13}NH_3$	10 min	cyclotron
$H_2{}^{15}O$	122 sec	cyclotron

fusion imaging, including $^{13}NH_3$ and $H_2{}^{15}O$ (67). Like rubidium, $^{13}NH_3$ is taken up by the Na^+/K^+ ATPase pump, because it exists in solution as cationic NH_{4+}. ^{15}O-labeled water is a highly permeable, neutral, Saperstein tracer that shows strong correlation with blood flow as determined by microspheres over a wide range of flows (68). Despite this very desirable property, imaging the distribution of perfusion with water is difficult. To effectively image ^{15}O (with its short half-life) requires administration of 80–100 mCi/injection, with rapid data acquisition. This places marked constraints on the imaging device. Another major issue with ^{15}O water is the low contrast (about 1.5:1) between the heart and surrounding blood pool and lung tissue which makes the images difficult to interpret visually. In comparison, the typical contrast between myocardium and background is 2–3:1 for $^{13}NH_3$, ^{82}Rb, or ^{38}K. A comparison of PET agents used to measure myocardial perfusion is shown in Table 15.7.

Despite the major advantages of PET in terms of resolution and absolute quantitation, single photon imaging remains the technique of choice for the routine evaluation of myocardial perfusion because of cost and availability.

Metabolic Imaging

A major advantage of PET imaging is the ability to use positron-emitting ^{11}C in place of stable ^{12}C in metabolic substrates. When dynamic images are recorded following administration of a ^{11}C radiopharmaceutical, the dynamic changes in tracer distribution can be assessed using a metabolic model, to determine regional metabolic rates in an organ. In this fashion, the rate of oxidative metabolism can be determined from the kinetics of ^{11}C acetate. In some situations, particularly where metabolism is rapid and the end products are reutilized by several metabolic pathways, analogs such as 2-deoxyglucose, labeled with either ^{11}C or ^{18}F, are used. The analogs typically permit several key steps to take place before the catabolism cannot proceed. Then the concentration of tracer in the tissue is evaluated to determine its utilization up to the forbidden step.

In this text, Schwaiger and Bonow, in chapters 26 and 27, address the utilization of positron-labeled radiopharmaceuticals for evaluation of regional metabolism.

ADRENERGIC INNERVATION

Metaiodobenzylguanidine (mIBG) is an iodinated aromatic analog of the antihypertensive drug guanethidine (69). The compound is taken up by the postsynaptic sympathetic nerves in the heart that serve as a link between the brain and contracting heart muscles, and is stored in norepinephrine storage vesicles. It is also taken up by nonneuronal compartments, but efflux from these compartments is relatively rapid, so, by 3–4 hours after injection, images are thought to largely represent neuronal uptake (70). The primary use of mIBG is in studies of heart diseases that are characterized by alterations in sympathetic nerve function. Cardiac transplantation in humans (71, 72) (which destroys all sympathetic nerves), and chemical denervation of cardiac sympathetic nerves in dogs, abolishes mIBG localization in the heart at delayed times, although initial uptake in the dog, but not the human, is unaffected. Patients with severe diabetic autonomic neuropathy show decreased mIBG uptake that parallels sympathetic cardiac dysfunction (73). In humans with dilated (74–76) and hypertrophic (77) cardiomyopathy, mIBG has demonstrated altered cardiac sympathetic arterioatony. Metaiodobenzylguanidine can also be used as a means of identifying sites of arrhymogenesis in patients with right ventricular cardiomyopathy (78). In patients with myocardial infarction, the extent of denervation appears far larger than the area of decreased perfusion (79, 80). The significance of this finding, as an indication of potential arrhythmia, is uncertain.

Blocking studies in dogs have demonstrated that reserpine (1 mg/kg) will block 30% of the uptake of mIBG. In humans, it has been noted that the antidepressant imipramine, drugs which affect neuronal transport of norepinephrine such as labetolol (81), and calcium channel blockers can suppress mIBG uptake, and that the sympathomimetic phenylpropanolamine can increase the rate of loss of mIBG from the heart. Therefore, interpretation of mIBG studies should take drug treatment into consideration.

Metaiodobenzylguanidine studies have been carried out with both ^{131}I and ^{123}I labels. ^{123}I is the superior radionuclide for such studies as it has a $T_{1/2}$ of 13.3 hours and its 159 keV γ, with 83% abundance, provide a high photon flux at a desirable energy. Early sources of ^{123}I were contaminated with longer lived high energy isotopes that degraded images and contributed negatively to dosimetry. However, schemes for the production of ^{123}I have improved dramatically over the past several years, as has availability (82).

FATTY ACIDS

Under normal conditions 60–70% of myocardial energy is obtained from the metabolism of lipids (83). Nonesterified fatty acids are primarily carried in the blood pool bound to albumin. The albumin-bound pool is in equilibrium with a very small amount of free fatty acid, and with storage pools in the liver and muscles. The total plasma pool of long-chain fatty acids turns over very rapidly (half-life <2 minutes), and has high extraction by the heart and liver. As a result, fatty acid radiopharmaceuticals can be used as Saperstein tracers to measure perfusion (84). Information on metabolism can be determined by measuring the clearance of these agents from the myocardium (85). However, the rapid clearance of these agents makes their distribution very perfusion dependent. To understand metabolism, it is best to determine regional perfusion at the same time metabolic measurements are made.

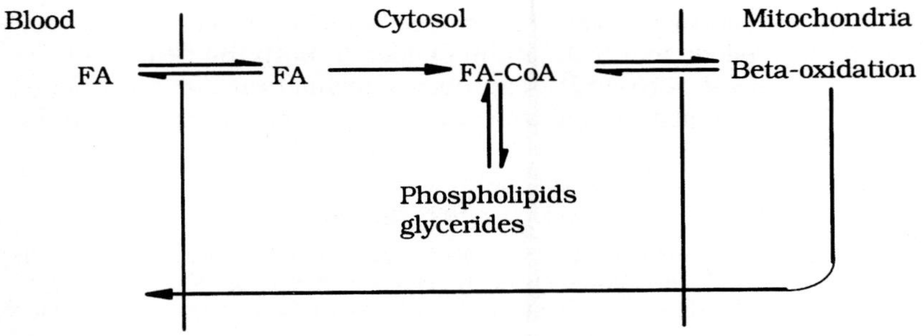

Figure 15.2. Fatty acid metabolism.

The metabolism and/or temporary storage of fatty acids in the cardiomyocyte is relatively well-understood (86). A simplified scheme is shown in Figure 15.2. It should be obvious from this scheme that there are various points within the cell at which differences in metabolism can influence retention of radioactivity in the cell.

The development of fatty acids labeled with SPECT radionuclides has taken two paths. A considerable amount of effort has been expended in attempts to incorporate a metal chelate into a fatty acid-like molecule so that ^{99m}Tc can be used as the radiolabel. All of these attempts have failed because the physicochemical characteristics of the metal chelate moiety—size, shape, lipophilicity, charge, etc.—are too different from the substitutions known now to be acceptable to the system. The difficulties have arisen not from rapid metabolism and egress of the radioactivity from the myocardium, but from an inability to synthesize a metal chelate-containing molecule that showed sufficient uptake by the heart together with the necessary clearance from the blood. The relatively recent documentation of a fatty acid transporter which facilitates the entry of fatty acids into the cell from the plasma (87, 88) may provide the tool that will allow success in these endeavors.

Radioiodinated fatty acids were initially utilized to determine regional perfusion (89, 90). The terminally iodinated compounds had excellent extraction, comparable to that of potassium, but their residence time in the myocardium was extremely short due to rapid metabolism and release of free iodide from the myocardium (91). Although these properties allowed one to obtain perfusion images of the myocardium, the short retention time of the radioactivity was prohibitive and the advent of routine thallium imaging reduced the value of these iodinated perfusion agents. It was recognized that methods for preventing deiodination and/or slowing down β-oxidation were needed to maintain the radioactivity in the myocardium (92), and that with these improvements it might be possible to assess metabolism rather than flow.

The problem of deiodination was solved by adding the iodine to a phenyl group at the ω position of the fatty acid chain to produce the 15-(p-^{123}I-iodophenyl-)-pentadecanoic acid (p-IPPA). The orthoisomer has been found to be retained longer than the paraisomer, apparently because the orthoisomer is bound to coenzyme A and is retained in the cytosolic pool, whereas the paraisomer progresses further to be metabolized by mitochondrial β-oxidation (93). Thus, it would seem that the orthoisomer contains both of the attributes necessary for metabolic imaging of the myocardium. Despite this, the orthoisomer has not been widely investigated and, instead, efforts have concentrated on improving the retention of the para isomer.

Table 15.8.
Adsorbed Doses in mGy/mBq for ^{123}I-BMIPP and ^{201}Thallium

Organ	^{123}I-BMIPP	^{201}TL
Heart	0.071	0.173
Liver	0.043	0.127
Spleen	0.013	0.108
Bladder Wall	0.038	0.122
Red Marrow	0.016	–
Ovaries	0.014	–
Testes	0.0098	0.192
Total Body	0.013	–

Prevention of β-oxidation has been addressed by placement of stearic blocks in the fatty acid chain. These have included the insertion of rings (94) or heteroatoms, but by far the most common method has been the addition of methyl groups to the chain (95, 96). Any branching of the fatty acid chain should lead to a reduction in metabolism, but the position and degree of substitution produce different effects (97). The 3- and the 9-methyl derivatives have been sponsored by commercial entities and have undergone clinical trials (98, 99). The 3-methyl derivative 15-(p-^{123}I-iodophenyl-)-3-*R,S*-methylpentadecanoic acid (BMIPP) is approved for use in Japan as Cardiodyne (Nihon Mediphysics).

The normal injected dose of BMIPP is about 3 mCi (111 mBq), which contains about 0.5 mg of stable fatty acid. The injection is performed at rest. There is rapid uptake of radioactivity by the myocardium which contains about 5% of the injected dose by 1.5 hours. Imaging of the myocardium can commence immediately after injection. There is little washout of radioactivity from the myocardium, so that by 24 hours the myocardium still contains about 4% of the injected dose. Radioactivity is taken up by the liver, but there is little hepatobiliary excretion.

The clinical utility of fatty acid imaging is uncertain. Cardiomyopathies have been shown to produce changes in fatty acid metabolism in animals (100, 101) and in man (102, 103), in addition to the changes produced by ischemia. However, it is unclear whether fatty acid imaging will play a role in clinical decisionmaking. Table 15.8 compares the radiation burden of ^{201}Tl and BMIPP in various organs.

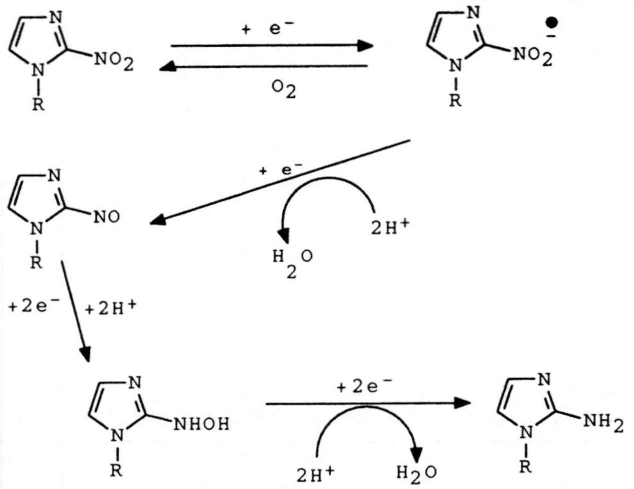

Figure 15.3. Proposed metabolic pathway for nitroimidazole based hypoxia agents.

HYPOXIA

Many compounds show differential activity between normoxic and hypoxic tissue, including antibiotics, such as metronidazole which shows activity against anaerobic infections, and sensitizers, such as misonidazole which has been used as a radiation or chemical sensitizer of hypoxic tissue during tumor therapy. Nitroimidazoles enter tissue and undergo reduction to a more reactive product. The formation of this derivative is initiated by the enzyme-mediated single electron reduction of the nitro group to a free radical which is an anion at neutral pH. The initial one electron reduction is catalyzed by some unidentified reductase(s) and is reversible in the presence of oxygen. Chemistry studies using model compounds show that the reduction pathway can proceed in successive steps past the hydroxylamine derivative to terminate at the relatively inactive amine derivative. These reactions are summarized in Figure 15.3.

The initial reduction occurs in all viable tissues. Selectivity is produced by reoxidation of the initial products by molecular oxygen. The rate of this reoxidation is dependent upon the local oxygen concentration, so that in normoxic tissue the unreduced species is predominant and leaves the tissues as blood levels drop. Thus, reduction occurs in all tissue with viable enzymatic processes, but trapping only occurs in those tissues with low oxygen tension where reoxidation and export of the original compound cannot occur.

The idea that nitroimidazoles might be adapted to allow the visualization of hypoxic tissue in vivo has been discussed for 10 years (104); however, it is only in the last 3 or 4 years that practical application of the idea has occurred using the positron emitting radionuclide ^{18}F to make ^{18}F-fluoromisonidazole (105, 106). Later, radioiodinated nitroimidazoles were developed (107). Successful in vivo imaging of hypoxic tissue using these compounds has been reported in animals and man, with most activity in the oncology field (108, 109). In the past few years, success has been reported in transferring the nitroimidazole technology to a technetium chelate in both the heart and the brain (110–112). A number of technetium complexes containing nitroimidazoles are due to enter clinical trials in the near future.

REFERENCES

1. Vanbilloen HP, Verbeke KA, DeRoo MJ, Verbruggen AM. Technetium-99m-labeled human serum albumin for ventriculography: a comparative evaluation of six labeling kits. Eur J Nucl Med 1993;20:465–472.
2. Verbeke KA, Vanbilloen HP, De Roo MJ, Verbruggen AM. Technetium-99m mercaptoalbumin as a potential substitute or technetium-99m-labeled red blood cells. Eur J Nucl Med 1993; 20:473–482.
3. Srivastava SC, Straub RP. Blood cell labeling with ^{99m}Tc: progress and perspectives. Sem Nucl Med 1990;20:41–51.
4. Callahan RJ, Froelich JW, McKusick KA, Leppo J, Strauss HW. A modified method for the in vivo labeling of red blood cells with ^{99m}Tc. J Nucl Med 1982;23:315–318.
5. Khaw BA, Scott J, Fallon JT, Cahill SL, Haber E, Homcy C. Myocardial injury quantitation by cell sorting initiated with antimyosin fluorescent spheres. Science 1982;217:1050–1053.
6. Khaw BA, Narula J, Strauss HW. Detection of adult myocardial infarction with antimyosin. Section 1. In: Khaw BA, Narula J, Strauss HW, eds. Monoclonal antibodies in cardiovascular diseases. Philadelphia PA: Lea & Febiger, 1993:1–66.
7. Yaoita H, Fischman AJ, Wilkinson R, Khaw BA, Juweid M, Strauss HW. Distribution of deoxyglucose and technetium-99m glucarate in the acutely ischemic myocardium. J Nucl Med 1993; 34:1303–1308.
8. Saperstein LA, Moses LE. Cerebral and cephalic blood flow in man: basic considerations of the indicator fractionation technique. In: Knisely RW, Tauxe WN, Anderson EB, eds. Dynamic clinical studies with radioisotopes. Vol. 3. Washington, DC: USAEC Division of Technical Information, 1964:135–152.
9. Weich HF, Strauss HW, Pitt B. The extraction of thallium-201 by the myocardium. Circulation 1977;56:188–191.
10. Hurley PJ, Cooper M, Reba RC, Poggenburg KJ, Wagner HN Jr. ^{43}KCl: a new radiopharmaceutical for imaging the heart. J Nucl Med 1971;12:516–519.
11. Zaret BL, Strauss HW, Martin ND, Wells HP Jr., Flamm MD Jr. Noninvasive regional myocardial perfusion with radioactive potassium. Study of patients at rest, with exercise and during angina pectoris. N Engl J Med 1973;288:809–812.
12. Lambrecht RM, Gallagher BM, Wolf AP, et al. Potassium-38 for myocardial perfusion in normal and acutely infarcted dogs. In: Abstracts of the Second International Congress World Federation of Nuclear Medicine and Biology, September 17–21, 1978. Washington, DC: 1978:6.
13. Lebowitz E, Greene MW, Fairchild R, et al. Thallium-201 for medical use. J Nucl Med 1975;16:151–155.
14. Strauss HW, Harrison K, Langan JK, Lebowitz E, Pitt B. Thallium-201 for myocardial imaging. Relation of thallium-201 to regional myocardial perfusion. Circulation 1975;51:641–645.
15. Miller DD, Elmaleh DR, McKusick KA, et al. Radiopharmaceuticals for cardiac imaging. Radiol Clin North Am 1985;23:765–781.
16. Palmer EL, Scott JA, Strauss HW. Practical Nuclear Medicine. Philadelphia: W.B. Saunders, 1992:77.
17. Pohost GM, Alpert NM, Ingwall JS, et al. Thallium redistribution: mechanisms and clinical utility. Semin Nucl Med 1980;10:76–93.
18. Kaul S, Chesler DA, Pohost GM, et al. Influence of peak exercise heart rate on normal thallium myocardial clearance. J Nucl Med 1986;27:26–30.

19. Wilson RA, Okada RD, Strauss HW, et al. Effect of glucose-insulin-potassium infusion on thallium clearance. Circulation 1983;68:203–209.
20. Pohost GM, Zir LM, Moore RH, et al. Differentiation of transiently ischemic from infarcted myocardium by serial imaging after a single dose of thallium-201. Circulation 1977;55:294–302.
21. Bonow RO, Dilsizian V. Thallium 201 for assessment of myocardial viability. Semin Nucl Med 1991;21(3):230–241.
22. Bonow RO, Dilsizian V, Cuocolo A, Bacharach SL. Identification of viable myocardium in patients with chronic coronary artery disease and left ventricular dysfunction. Comparison of thallium scintigraphy with reinjection and PET imaging with ^{18}F-fluorodeoxyglucose. Circulation 1991;83(1):26–37.
23. Rocco TP, Dilsizian V, McKusick KA, et al. Comparison of thallium redistribution with rest "reinjection" imaging for the detection of viable myocardium. Am J Cardiol 1990;66:158–163.
24. Marin Neto JA, Dilsiziam V, Arrighi JA, et al. Thallium reinjection demonstrates viable myocardium in regions with reverse redistribution. Circulation 1993;88(4:1):1736–1745.
25. Takami K, Ohtani H, Yonekura Y, et al. Viable myocardium identified by reinjection thallium-201 imaging: comparison with regional wall motion and metabolic activity on FDG-PET. J Cardiol 1992;22(2–3):283–293.
26. Dilsizian V, Freedman NM, Bacharach SL, et al. Regional thallium uptake in irreversible defects. Magnitude of change in thallium activity after reinjection distinguishes viable from nonviable myocardium. Circulation 1992;85(2):627–634.
27. Deutsch E, Bushong W, Glaven KA, et al. Heart imaging with cationic complexes of technetium. Science 1981;214:85–86.
28. Gerson MC, Deutsch EA, Nishiyama H, et al. Myocardial perfusion imaging with technetium-99m DMPE in man. Eur J Nucl Med 1983;8:371–374.
29. Dudczak R, Angelberger P, Homan R, Kletter K, Schmoliner R, Frischauf H. Evaluation of ^{99m}Tc-dichloro bis(1,2-dimethylphosphino)ethane (^{99m}Tc-DMPE) for myocardial scintigraphy in man. Eur J Nucl Med 1983;8:513–515.
30. Thakur ML, Park CH, Fazio F, et al. Preparation and evaluation of [^{99m}Tc]DEPE as a cardiac perfusion agent. Int J Appl Radiat Isot 1984;35:507–515.
31. Gerundini P, Savi A, Gilardi MC, et al. Evaluation in dogs and humans of three potential technetium-99m myocardial perfusion agents. J Nucl Med 1986;27:409–416.
32. Deutsch E, Ketring AR, Libson K, Vanderheyden J-L, Hirth WW. The Noah's ark experiment: species dependent biodistributions of cationic Tc complexes. Nucl Med Biol 1989;16:191–232.
33. Deutsch E, Bushong W, Glaven KA, et al. Heart imaging with cationic complexes of technetium. Science 1981;214:85–86.
34. Gerson MC, Deutsch EA, Nishiyama H, et al. Myocardial perfusion imaging with technetium-99m DMPE in man. Eur J Nucl Med 1983;8:371–374.
35. Dudczak R, Angelberger P, Homan R, Kletter K, Schmoliner R, Frischauf H. Evaluation of ^{99m}Tc-dichloro bis(1,2-dimethylphosphino)ethane (^{99m}Tc-DMPE) for myocardial scintigraphy in man. Eur J Nucl Med 1983;8:513–515.
36. Thakur ML, Park CH, Fazio F, et al. Preparation and evaluation of [^{99m}Tc]DEPE as a cardiac perfusion agent. Int J Appl Radiat Isot 1984;35:507–515.
37. Gerundini P, Savi A, Gilardi MC, et al. Evaluation in dogs and humans of three potential technetium-99m myocardial perfusion agents. J Nucl Med 1986;27:409–416.
38. Deutsch E, Ketring AR, Libson K, Vanderheyden J-L, Hirth WW. The Noah's ark experiment: species dependent biodistributions of cationic Tc complexes. Nucl Med Biol 1989;16:191–232.
39. Deutsch E, Hirth W. In vivo inorganic chemistry of technetium cations. J Nucl Med 1987;28:1491–1500.
40. Gerson MC, Millard RW, Roszell NJ, et al. Kinetic properties of ^{99m}Tc-Q12 in canine myocardium. Circulation 1994;89:1291–1300.
41. Rossetti C, Paganelli G, Vanoli G, Di Leo M, et al. Biodistribution in humans and preliminary clinical evaluation of a new tracer with optimized properties for myocardial perfusion imaging: [^{99m}Tc]Q12. J Nucl Biol Med 1992;36(Suppl 2):29–31.
42. Pasqualini R, Duatti A. Synthesis and characterization of the new neutral myocardial imaging agent [^{99m}TcN(noet)$_2$ (noet = N-ethyl-N-ethoxydithiocarbamato). J Chem Soc Chem Comm 1992;1354–1355.
43. Holman BL, Jones AG, Lister-James J, et al. A new Tc-99m labeled imaging agent, hexakis(t-butylisonitrile)-technetium(I) [Tc-99m TBI]: initial experience in the human. J Nucl Med 1984; 25:1350–1355.
44. Holman BL, Campbell CA, Lister-James J, Jones AG, Davison A, Kloner RA. Effect of reperfusion and hyperemia on the biodistribution of the myocardial imaging agent Tc-99m TBI. J Nucl Med 1986;27:1172–1177.
45. Holman BL, Sporn V, Jones AG, et al. Myocardial imaging with technetium-99m CPI: initial experience in the human. J Nucl Med 1987;28:13–18.
46. Mousa SA, Williams SJ, Sands H. Characterization of in vivo chemistry of cations in the heart. J Nucl Med 1987;28:1351–1357.
47. Okada R, Glover D, Gaffney T, Williams S. Myocardial kinetics of Tc-99m-hexakis-2-methoxy-2-methylpropylisonitrile. Circulation 1988;77:491–498.
48. Stirner H, Buell U, Kleinhans E, Bares R, Grosse W. Myocardial kinetics of ^{99m}Tc-hexakis-(2-methoxy-isobutyl-isonitrile)(HMIBI) in patients with coronary artery disease: a comparative study versus ^{201}Tl with SPECT. Nucl Med Commun 1988;9:15–23.
49. Glover DK, Okada RD. Myocardial kinetics of Tc-MIBI in canine myocardium after dipyridamole. Circulation 1990;81:628–637.
50. Berman DS, Kiat H, Maddahi J. The new ^{99m}Tc myocardial perfusion imaging agents: ^{99m}Tc-sestamibi and ^{99m}Tc-teboroxime. Circulation 1991;84(Suppl I):I-7–I-21.
51. Higley B, Smith FW, Smith T, et al. Technetium-99m-1,2-bis[(2-ethoxyethyl)phosphino]ethane: human biodistribution, dosimetry and safety of a new myocardial perfusion imaging agent. J Nucl Med 1993;34:30–38.
52. Lahiri A, Higley B, Smith T, et al. Myocardial perfusion imaging in man using new ^{99m}Tc-labeled diphosphine complexes. Nucl Med Commun 1987;28:721.
53. Sridhara B, Braat S, Rigo P, Itti R, Cload P, Lahiri A. Comparison of myocardial perfusion imaging with technetium-99m tetrophosmin vs. thallium-201 in coronary artery disease. Am J Cardiol 1993;72:1015–1019.
54. Rigo P, Leclercq B, Itti R, Lahiri A, Braat S. Tecnetium-99m-tetrofosmin myocardial imaging: a comparison with thallium-201 and angiography. J Nucl Med 1994;35(4):587–593.
55. Narra RK, Nunn AD, Kuczynski BL, Feld T, Wedeking P, Eckelman WC. A neutral technetium-99m complex for myocardial imaging. J Nucl Med 1989;30:1830–1837.
56. Treher EN, Gougoutas J, Malley M, Nunn AD. New technetium radiopharmaceuticals: boronic acid adducts of technetium dioximes. J Label Comp Radiopharm 1986;23:118–120.
57. Treher EN, Francesconi LC, Gougoutas JZ, Malley MF, Nunn AD. Mono-capped tris dioxime complexes of technetium(III): synthesis, and structural characterization of TcX(dioxime)$_3$B-R (X = Cl, Br; dioxime=dimethyl glyoxime, cyclohexane dione dioxime; R=CH_3, C_4H_9). Inorg Chem 1989;28:3411–3416.
58. Leppo JA, Meerdink DJ. Comparative myocardial extraction of two technetium-labeled BATO derivatives (SQ30217, SQ32014) and thallium. J Nucl Med 1990;31:67–74.
59. Johnson LL, Seldin DW Clinical experience with technetium-99m teboroxime, a neutral lipophilic myocardial perfusion agent. Am J Cardiol 1990;66:63E–67E.

60. Hendel RC, McSherry B, Karimeddini M, Leppo JA. Diagnostic value of a new myocardial perfusion agent, teboroxime (SQ30217), utilizing a rapid planar imaging protocol: preliminary results. J Am Coll Cardiol 1990;16:855–861.
61. Johnson L. Clinical experience with technetium-99m-teboroxime. Semin Nucl Med 1991;21(3):182–189.
62. Stewart RE, Heyl B, O'Rourke RA, Blumhardt R, Miller DD. Demonstration of differential post-stenotic myocardial technetium-99m-teboroxime clearance kinetics after experimental ischemia and hyperemic stress. J Nucl Med 1991;32:2000–2008.
63. Gray W, Gewirtz H Comparison of Tc-99m-teboroxime with thallium for myocardial imaging in the presence of a coronary artery stenosis. Circulation 1991;84:1796–1807.
64. Nunn AD. Is there additional useful information in the myocardial washout characteristics of teboroxime? J Nucl Med 1991; 32:1988–1991.
65. Waters SL, Coursey BM, eds. The strontium-82/rubidium-82 generator. Special issue. Appl Radiat and Isotopes 1987;38:171–239.
66. Selwyn AP, Allan RM, L'Abbate A, et al. Relation between regional myocardial uptake of rubidium-82 and perfusion: absolute reduction of cation uptake in ischemia. Am J Cardiol 1982;50:112–121.
67. Araujo LI, Lammertsma AA, Rhodes CG, et al. Noninvasive quantification of regional myocardial blood flow in coronary artery disease with oxygen-15-labeled carbon dioxide inhalation and positron emission tomography. Circulation 1991;83(3):875–885.
68. Bergmann SR, Herrero P, Markham J, et al. Noninvasive quantitation of myocardial blood flow in human subjects with oxygen-15-labeled water and positron emission tomography. J Am Coll Cardiol 1989;14(3):639–652.
69. Wieland DM, Brown LE, Rogers WL, et al. Myocardial imaging with a radioiodinated norepinephrine storage analog. J Nucl Med 1981;22:22–31.
70. Nakajo M, Shimabukuro K, Yoshimura K. Iodine-131 metaiodobenzylguanidine intra- and extravascular accumulation in the rat heart. J Nucl Med 1986;27:84–89.
71. Glowniak JV, Turner FE, Gray LL, et al. Iodine-123-metaiodobenzylguanidine imaging of the heart in idiopathic congestive cardiomyopathy and cardiac transplants. J Nucl Med 1989; 30:1182–1191.
72. Dae MW, De Marco T, Botvinick EH, et al. Scintigraphic assessment of MmIBG uptake in globally denervated human and canine hearts—implications for clinical studies. J Nucl Med 1992; 33:1444–1450.
73. Sisson JC, Shapiro B, Beyers L, et al. Metaiodobenzylguanidine to map scintigraphically the adrenergic nervous system in man. J Nucl Med 1987;28:1625–1636.
74. Henderson EB, Kahn JK, Corbett JR, et al. Abnormal I-123 metaiodobenzylguanidine myocardial washout and distribution may reflect myocardial adrenergic derangement in patients with congestive cardiomyopathy. Circulation 1988;78:1192–1199.
75. Yamakado K, Takeda K, Kitano T, et al. Serial change of iodine-123 metaiodobenzylguanidine (mIBG) myocardial concentration in patients with dilated cardiomyopathy. Eur J Nucl Med 1992; 19(4):265–270.
76. Schofer J, Spielman R, Schuchert A, Weber K, Schluter M. Iodine-123-metaiodobenzylguanidine scintigraphy: a noninvasive method to demonstrate myocardial adrenergic nervous system disintegrity in patients with idiopathic dilated cardiomyopathy. J Am Coll Cardiol 1988;12:1252–1258.
77. Nakajima K, Bunko H, Taki J, Shimizu M, Muramori A, Hisada K. Quantitative analysis of I-123 metaiodobenzyguanidine (MmIBG) uptake in hypertrophic cardiomyopathy. Am Heart J 1990;1329–1337.
78. Wichter T, Hindricks G, Lerch H, et al. Regional myocardial sympathetic dysinnervation in arrhythmogenic right ventricular cardiomyopathy. Circulation 1994;89:667–683.
79. Hirosawa K, Tanaka T, Hisada K, Bunko H. Clinical evaluation of ^{123}I-MmIBG for assessment of the sympathetic nervous system in the heart (multicenter clinical trial) (Japanese). Kaku-Igaku 1991;28:461–476.
80. Stanton MS, Tuli MM, Radtke NL, et al. Regional sympathetic denervation after myocardial infarction in humans detected noninvasively using I-123 metaiodobenzylguanidine. J Am Coll Cardiol 1989;14:1519–1529.
81. Fagret D, Wolf JE, Michel C. Myocardial uptake of meta-[^{123}I]-iodobenzylguanidine ([^{123}I]-MmIBG in patients with myocardial infarct. Eur J Nucl Med 1989;15:624–628.
82. Kulkarni PV, Corbett JR. Radioiodinated tracers for myocardial imaging. Semin Nucl Med 1990;20:119–129.
83. Brunken RC, Schelbert HR. Evaluation of myocardial substrate metabolism in ischemic heart disease. In: Marcus ML, Skorton DJ, Schelbert HR, Wolf GL, eds. Cardiac imaging. Chap. 67. Philadelphia: W.B. Saunders, 1991:1191–1240.
84. Miller DD, Gill JB, Livni E, et al. Fatty acid analogue accumulation: a marker of myocyte viability in ischemic-reperfused myocardium. Circ Res 1988;63:681–692.
85. Stanton MS, Tuli MM, Radtke NL, et al. Regional sympathetic denervation after myocardial infarction in humans detected noninvasively using I-123 metaiodobenzylguanidine. J Am Coll Cardiol 1989;14:1519–1529.
86. Tahiliani AG. Myocardial fatty acid metabolism. In: Fozzard HA, Haber E, Jennings RB, Katz AM, Morgan HE, eds. The heart and cardiovascular system. New York: Raven Press, 1991:1599–1620.
87. Stremmel W. Fatty acid uptake by isolated rat heart myocytes represents a carrier-mediated transport process. J Clin Invest 1988;81:844–852.
88. Vyska K, Machulla HJ, Stremmel W, et al. Regional myocardial free fatty acid extraction in normal and ischemic myocardium. Circulation 1988;78:1218–1233.
89. Evans JR, Gunton RW, Baker RG, et al. Use of radioiodinated fatty acids for photoscans of the heart. Circ Res 1965;16:1–10.
90. Poe ND, Robinson GD, Graham LS, et al. Experimental basis for myocardial imaging with ^{123}I-labeled hexadecanoic acid. J Nucl Med 1976;17:1077–1082.
91. Machulla HJ, Stocklin G, Kupfernagel C, et al. Comparative evaluation of fatty acids labeled with C-11, Cl-34m, Br-77 and I-123 for metabolic studies of the myocardium. J Nucl Med 1978; 19:298–302.
92. Machulla HJ, Marsmann M, Dutschka KP. Biochemical concept and synthesis of radioiodinated phenylfatty acid for in vivo metabolic studies of the myocardium. Eur J Nucl Med 1980;5:171–173.
93. Kaiser KP, Geuting B, Grossman K, et al. Tracer kinetics of 15-(ortho-123,^{131}I-phenyl)-pentadecanoic acid (oPPA) and 15-(para-123,^{131}I-phenyl)-pentadecanoic acid (pPPA) in animals and man. J Nucl Med 1990;31:1608–1616.
94. Eisenhut M, Liefhold J. Radioiodinated p-phenylene bridged fatty acids as new myocardial imaging agents: synthesis and biodistribution in rats. Int J Appl Radiat Isot 1988;39:639–649.
95. Livni E, Elmaleh DR, Levy S, Brownell GL, Strauss HW. β-methyl[1-^{11}C]-heptadecanoic acid: a new myocardial metabolic tracer for positron emission tomography. J Nucl Med 1982; 23:169–175.
96. Goodman MM, Kirsch G, Knapp FF. Synthesis of radioiodinated ω-p-(iodophenyl)-substituted methyl branched long-chain fatty acids. J Labeled Cpd Radiopharm 1992;19:1316–1318.
97. Otto CA, Brown LKE, Scott AM. Radioiodinated branched chain fatty acids: substrates for β oxidation? J Nucl Med 1985;25:75–80.

98. Torizuka K, Yonekura Y, Nishimura T, et al. The phase I study of β-methyl-p-(^{123}I)-iodophenyl-pentadecanoic acid (^{123}I-BMIPP). Jpn J Nucl Med 1991;28:681–690.
99. Chouraqui P, Maddahi J, Henkin R, Karesh SM, Galie E, Berman DS. Comparison of myocardial imaging with Iodine-123–Iodophenyl-9–methy pentadecanoic acid and Thallium-201-chloride for assessment of patients with exercised-induced myocardial ischemia. J Nucl Med 1991;32:447–452.
100. Kubota K, Som P, Oster ZH, et al. Detection of cardiomyopathy in an animal model using quantitative autoradiography. J Nucl Med 1988;29:1697–1703.
101. Wakasugi S, Fischman AJ, Babich JW, et al. Myocardial substrate utilization and left ventricular function in adriamycin cardiomyopathy. J Nucl Med 1993;34:1529–1535.
102. Takeishi Y, Chiba J, Abe S, Tonooka I, Komatani A, Tomoike H. Heterogeneous myocardial distribution of iodine-123 15-(p-iodophenyl-)-3-*R,S*-methylpentadecanoic acid (BMIPP) in patients with hypertrophic cardiomyopathy. Eur J Nucl Med 1992; 19:775–782.
103. 0taki J, Nakajima K, Bunko H, Shimizu M, Taniguchi M, Hisada K. ^{123}I-labeled BMIPP fatty acid myocardial scintigraphy in patients with hypertrophic cardiomyopathy: SPECT comparison with stress ^{201}Tl. Nucl Med Commun 1993;14:181–188.
104. Chapman JD, Franko AJ, Sharplin L. A marker for hypoxic cells in tumors with potential for clinical application. Br J Cancer 1981;4:546–550.
105. Rasey JS, Grumbaum Z, Magee S, et al. Characterization of radiolabeled fluoromisonidazole as a probe for hypoxic cells. Radiat Res 1987;111:292–304.
106. Shelton ME, Dence CS, Hwang DR, et al. Myocardial kinetics of fluorine-18 misonidazole: a marker of hypoxic myocardium. J Nucl Med 1989;30:351–358.
107. Mannan RH, Somayaji VV, Lee J, et al. Radioiodinated 1-(5-Iodo-5-deoxy-β-D-arabinofuranosyl)-2-nitroimidazole (iodoazomycin arabinoside: IAZA): a novel marker of tissue hypoxia. J Nucl Med 1991;32:1764–1770.
108. Rasey JS, Koh WJ, Grierson JR, et al. Radiolabeled fluoromisonidazole as an imaging agent for tumor hypoxia. Int J Radiation Oncology Biol Phys 1989;17:985–991.
109. Valk PE, Mathis CA, Prados MD, Gilbert JC, Budinger TF. Hypoxia in human gliomas: demonstration by PET with fluorine-18-fluoromisonidazole. J Nucl Med 1992;33:2133–2137.
110. Linder KE, Chan Y-W, Cyr JE, Malley MF, Nowotnik DP, Nunn AD. TcO(PnAO-1-(2-nitroimidazole)) [BMS-181321], a new technetium-containing nitroimidazole complex for imaging hypoxia: synthesis, characterization, and xanthine oxidase-catalyzed reduction. J Med Chem 1994;37:9–17.
111. Rumsey WL, Cyr JE, Raju N, Narra RK. A novel [^{99m}]technetium-labeled nitroheterocycle capable of identification of hypoxia in heart. Biochem Biophys Res Commun 1993;193:1239–1246.
112. DiRocco RJ, Kuczynski BL, Pirro JP, et al. Imaging ischemic tissue at risk of infarction during stroke. J Cereb Blood Flow Metab 1993;13:755–762.

16 Accelerators and Positron Emission Tomography Radiopharmaceuticals

BONNIE B. DUNN* and RONALD G. MANNING

There are more than 60 radiopharmaceuticals currently being used as positron emission tomography (PET) imaging agents; however, there are less than a dozen that are routinely employed (1, 2). These agents are typically distinguished by good radiochemical yields, acceptable specific activity, simple, easy, synthetic procedures, and, most importantly, good in vivo selectivity.

The only Food and Drug Administration (FDA) approved PET radiopharmaceutical is rubidium-82-labeled rubidium chloride ($[^{82}Rb]RbCl$) produced from generators (Table 16.1). Since the development and advance in technology of small medical cyclotrons, the most commonly used PET radiopharmaceuticals are those containing a fluorine-18 or carbon-11 radioisotope because (a) the replacement of a hydrogen atom by a fluorine atom often has little effect on a drug's behavior, (b) carbon is ubiquitous in nature, and (c) the relatively long half-lives allow sufficient time for preparation of complex molecules and enough radioactivity for the radiosynthesis of more than one dose per preparation. Other positron emitting radionuclides having short half-lives which have been incorporated into useful PET radiopharmaceuticals are $[^{13}N]$nitrogen and $[^{15}O]$oxygen (Table 16.1).

PARTICLE ACCELERATORS

PET radioisotopes can be produced by a variety of particle accelerators (1, 3–6). Traditionally, cyclotrons have been used to make the isotope of interest. In a cyclotron, charged particles are produced, accelerated, and then directed against a target material. The nuclear reaction between the accelerated particles and the target material gives the positron emitting radionuclide (Table 16.2). Charged particles or ions are produced in an ion source located in the center of the cyclotron, as shown in Figure 16.1. The ions gain energy due to a high-voltage alternating electric field. This electric field is induced on an electrode. Cyclotron electrodes are hollow metal structures whose charge can be switched rapidly. When the ions are inside the electrode, they are not affected by the electrode's charge. As the ions exit an electrode the charge on the electrode is changed so that it repels the ions (like charges repel). In a similar manner, the charge on the next electrode along the path of the ions is changed so that it attracts the ions. Thus the ions gain energy each time they are between electrodes. In the simplest configuration, two electrodes are used. To constrain the ions to a roughly circular orbit, a strong magnetic field is applied. As the ions gain in energy, the radius of their orbit increases. The ions gradually spiral outward as they are accelerated. Their distance from the center of the cyclotron is a measure of the kinetic energy they possess. At the appropriate radius they have acquired enough energy to induce the nuclear reaction of interest. Particle energies needed to induce the nuclear reactions shown in Table 16.2 are several million electron volts (MeV). After one packet of charged particles has been accelerated, the cyclotron is ready to start another group of ions on its journey from the center of the cyclotron. Although the cyclotron produces pulses of high energy-charged particles, the frequency of this event is very high so that the cyclotron appears to be continuously producing ions. The stream of high energy particles produced is referred to as a beam.

Cyclotrons themselves can be differentiated according to several features. Some of these features include the (a) types of particles accelerated, (b) particle beam current, and (c) particle energy. In theory, any charged particle can be accelerated by virtue of its net electrical charge. As a practical matter, only protons (p^+) and deuterons (d^+) are used routinely in medical cyclotrons. These particles are easy to produce from hydrogen or deuterium gas, respectively. Also, their nuclear interactions with selected target atoms give high yields of the radioisotopes of interest. Particle beam current refers to the amount of charged particles that a cyclotron can accelerate. It is possible to electrically isolate several parts of the cyclotron including the target. Thus an electrical current can be measured. Cyclotron beam currents are in the microampere (μA) range. The yield of the radioisotope as a function of the bombarding particle energy can be determined. This yield can be expressed in nuclear terms as a cross-section, or in radiopharmaceutic radiopharmaceutical terms as the saturation yield of the product. The saturation yield has units of mCi per μA (mCi/μA). It is the maximum yield of radioisotope that one would obtain if the irradiation were continued until a steady state occurred. At steady state, isotope production and radioactive decay are equal. The saturation yield differs for each nuclear reaction and is dependent on the energy of the bombarding particle. Table 16.3 lists saturation yields for several nuclear reactions that produce PET radioisotopes. In Table 16.3, the energy of the bombarding particle is 9.5–11 MeV. The saturation yields are different for different energy ranges. Over certain ranges, it is advantageous to have higher beam energies, since the saturation yield is still increasing. The larger cyclotrons needed to achieve higher beam energies are more expensive and more complex.

Until about 1980, all the cyclotrons that were available

*The views expressed in this chapter are those of the authors and do not necessarily reflect those of the Food and Drug Administration.

Table 16.1.
Properties of Some Common PET Radioisotopes

Radioisotope	Half-life (minutes)	Maximum β^+ Energy (keV)	Atoms/mCi	Comment
Fluorine-18	109.7	635	3.5×10^{11}	can ship short distances
Gallium-68	68.3	1880	2.2×10^{11}	generator daughter
Carbon-11	20.4	970	6.5×10^{10}	need accelerator
Nitrogen-13	9.96	1190	3.2×10^{10}	need accelerator
Oxygen-15	2.07	1700	6.6×10^{9}	need accelerator
Rubidium-82	1.25	3350	4.0×10^{9}	generator daughter

Table 16.2.
Common PET Radioisotopes and Their Production Methods in Small Particle Accelerators Using Protons and Deuterons

Nuclide	Halflife	Production Method	Target Material	Comment
^{18}F	109.7 min	$^{18}O(p,n)^{18}F$	^{18}O-water or ^{18}O-ice	enriched isotope
		$^{20}Ne(d,\alpha)^{18}F$	Ne gas	yields F_2
^{11}C	20.4 min	$^{11}B(p,n)^{11}C$	boric oxide	used in linacs
		$^{14}N(p,\alpha)^{11}C$	N_2 gas	used in cyclotrons
		$^{10}B(d,n)^{11}C$	boric oxide	not common
		$^{11}B(d,2n)^{11}C$	boric oxide	not common
		$^{14}N(d,\alpha n)^{11}C$	N_2 gas	not common
^{13}N	9.96 min	$^{16}O(p,\alpha)^{13}N$	water	used in cyclotrons
		$^{12}C(d,n)^{13}N$	graphite	used in linacs
		$^{13}C(d,n)^{13}N$	CO_2 gas	not common
^{15}O	2.07 min	$^{14}N(d,n)^{15}O$	N_2 gas	need deuterons
		$^{15}N(p,n)^{15}O$	$[^{15}N]N_2$ gas	enriched gas
		$^{16}O(p,pn)^{15}O$	O_2 gas	not common

for the routine production of medical radioisotopes were designed to circulate positive ions such as H^+ (15). The H^+ ions were easy to obtain and accelerate. The next step was to have the particle beam impact a target containing the materials to be bombarded. Targets can either be outside the vacuum chamber of the cyclotron (external targets) or inside the cyclotron (internal targets). If the target were external, the particle beam would have to be directed outside the cyclotron. Removing the ions from their outward spiraling orbit so that they could bombard a target required a sophisticated extraction apparatus. This extraction apparatus consisted of, for example, high current and high voltage assemblies that overcame the tendency of the particles to follow the roughly circular orbit induced by the large electromagnets above and below the plane of the particles' orbit. The extraction apparatus was vulnerable to being struck by the beam of accelerated particles if the beam deviated slightly from the correct path during an irradiation. If the extraction apparatus were struck by the beam it could become intensely radioactive or, on occasion, damaged. A damaged extraction apparatus could require extensive repairs resulting in high radiation exposures to the cyclotron staff. As an alternative to directing the beam to targets external to the cyclotron itself, an internal target can be used. An internal target can intersect the circulating beam without the need of an extraction apparatus. However, if an internal target were to malfunction, the cyclotron vacuum chamber would have to be entered in order to perform repairs. This could be a costly and time-consuming operation.

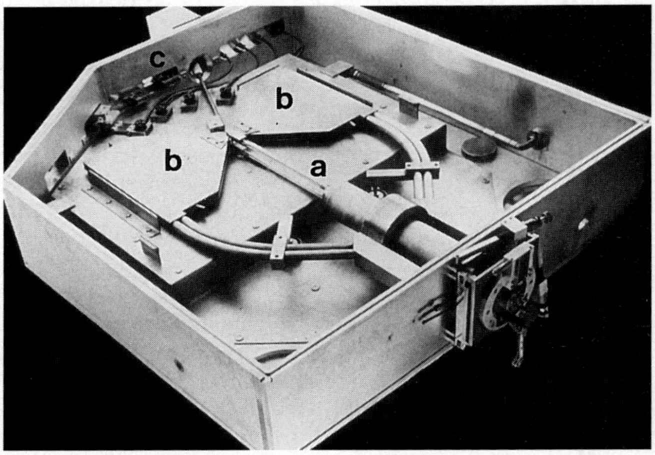

Figure 16.1. Vacuum chamber from the Siemens 11 MeV negative-ion cyclotron with the top removed. (**a**) Ion source; (**b**) radiofrequency electrodes; (**c**) carbon stripping foils.

Negative-ion cyclotrons accelerate particles such as H^- (see Fig. 16.2 for an example). The first negative-ion cyclotrons designed specifically for PET were built by Computer Technology and Imaging, Inc. (CTI). Negative ions can be easily produced. They are more prone to lose their charge than are positively charged ions. As a result, negative-ion cyclotrons require a vacuum about 10 times better than comparable positive-ion cyclotrons. Such vacuums are

Table 16.3.
Production of PET Radioisotopes at 9.5–11 MeV

Nuclear Reaction	Saturation Yield (mCi/μAmp)	Chemical Form of Precursor	Reference
$^{14}N(p,\alpha)^{11}C$	84	$^{11}CO_2$	7
$^{16}O(p,\alpha)^{13}N$	7	$^{13}NO_3^-$, $^{13}NO_2^-$, $^{13}NH_4^+$	8
$^{13}C(p,n)^{13}N$	110	$^{13}NH_4^+$	9
$^{15}N(p,n)^{15}O$	70	$^{15}O_2$	10,11
$^{14}N(d,n)^{15}O$	70	$^{15}O_2$	12
$^{18}O(p,n)^{18}F$	120	$^{18}F^-$(aq)	13
$^{20}Ne(d,\alpha)^{18}F$	76	$^{18}F_2$	14

achievable through the use of larger roughing and diffusion pumps and better vacuum seals. Negative-ion cyclotrons have the distinct advantage of not requiring a conventional extraction apparatus. Instead, the circulating ion beam can be directed against a thin carbon foil. This foil will remove two electrons from each of the accelerated particles. This changes the net charge on the circulating ions from −1 to +1 (e.g., from H^- to H^+). Since each particle is now oppositely charged, each ion will be induced by the magnetic field to curve in the opposite direction. That is, instead of curving in toward the center of the cyclotron, the ion will curve out toward the edge of the vacuum chamber. By properly situating the carbon foils, the newly formed positive-ion particle beam can then exit the cyclotron and impact a target.

Negative-ion cyclotrons have the additional advantage that the carbon foil can be moved radially so that it only partially intersects the packet of accelerated particles. In such a case, the portion of the packet of accelerated particles that does not strike the carbon foil remains negatively charged and continues to curve inward. A second carbon foil situated further around the perimeter of the vacuum chamber can intersect the beam and result in a second beam of positively charged particles. This second packet of particles can then be directed at a second target. Thus two targets can be irradiated simultaneously. This feature can be useful clinically. A long irradiation to produce ^{18}F does not preclude an irradiation to produce a shorter-lived radioisotope such as ^{15}O or ^{13}N.

Table 16.4 compares beam parameters of some commercially available cyclotrons. These cyclotrons can typically accelerate protons at energies ranging from about 10 MeV up to about 17 MeV. By comparison, the average kinetic energy of a gas molecule at room temperature is about 1/40 eV. The Ion Beam Applications (IBA) Cyclone 30 has a much higher energy. Although it has been used for PET, it is primarily sold for non-PET applications. Many of the cyclotrons listed in Table 16.4 also accelerate deuterons. The change from protons (hydrogen ions) to deuterons is accomplished by changing the gas in the ion source from hydrogen to deuterium. Table 16.2 lists several nuclear reactions to produce PET radioisotopes that require deuterons. Especially useful are $^{14}N(d,n)^{15}O$ and $^{20}Ne(d,\alpha)^{18}F$. The first produces oxygen-15 without the need for isotopically enriched $[^{15}N]N_2$ (Table 16.2). The reaction of deuterons with neon-20 produces ^{18}F as F_2 gas. This is a chemical form of fluorine that cannot be obtained from the fluoride ion (F^-). Fluorine gas is a useful chemical reactant for the synthesis of many fluorine-containing radiopharmaceuticals.

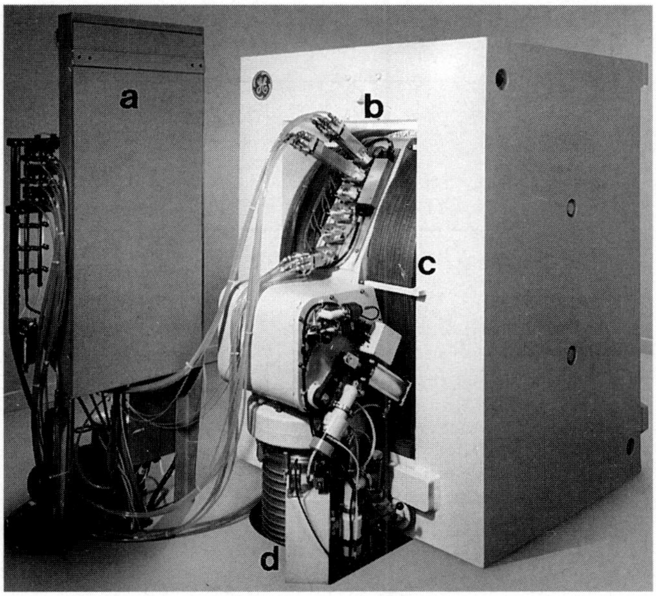

Figure 16.2. The General Electric PETtrace Cyclotron. The beam circulates in a vertical plane. (**a**) Electronics cabinet; (**b**) electromagnet; (**c**) vacuum chamber; and (**d**) vacuum diffusion pump.

The particle beam currents listed in Table 16.4 are the maximum that a given cyclotron model can produce during normal operating conditions. These beam currents have been shown experimentally to be sufficient to produce enough radioisotope for clinical PET. Table 16.5 shows the yields of the four short-lived PET radioisotopes for various cyclotrons.

By constraining the accelerated particles to travel in a circular orbit in a cyclotron, the same acceleration elements (the radiofrequency electrodes) can be used again and again. A cyclotron requires a strong magnetic field to maintain the accelerated particles in this roughly circular orbit. Linear accelerators, or linacs, accelerate particles in a straight line and therefore do not require strong magnets to bend the beam. In situations where very high energy particles (thousands of MeV) are needed, the linac can be a mile or more in length. The energies required to produce the PET radioisotopes are relatively low, and linacs of only a few feet in length suffice.

Several types of linacs are available. One such linac is

Table 16.4.
Beam Characteristics of Some Small Particle Accelerators for PET

Company & Model	Proton Energy (MeV)	Deuteron Energy (MeV)	Beam Current (μA)	Comment
AAI TCA	3.7	3.7	750 (p), 200 (d)	linear accelerator
AccSys PET Linac	7	none	150	linear accelerator
CGR-Sumitomo 370	17	10	50	positive-ion cyclotron
CTI RDS 112	11	none	50	negative-ion cyclotron
Ebco TR 13/8	13	8	50	negative-ion cyclotron
GE PETtrace	16	8	75 (p), 60 (d)	negative-ion cyclotron
IBA Cyclone 30	15–30	none	350	negative-ion cyclotron
IBA Cyclone 10/5	10	5	50	negative-ion cyclotron
JSW BC 126	12	6	50	positive-ion cyclotron
JSW BC 168	16	8	50	positive-ion cyclotron
JSW BC 1710	17	10	50	positive-ion cyclotron
Oxford	12	none	100	positive-ion cyclotron
PracSys NHVG	4.3	4.3	300	linear accelerator

Table 16.5.
Sample Performance Characteristics of Some Small Particle Accelerators for PET

	Radioisotope Yield in mCi at Specified Irradiation Time				
Company & Model	$[^{11}C]O_2$ 40 min	$[^{13}N]NH_3$ 10 min	$[^{15}O]O_2$ 10 min	$[^{18}F]F$ 60 min	$[^{18}F]F_2$ 60 min
AAI TCA	1000	670	1000	640	—
AccSys PET linac	1500	670	1190	1000	—
CGR-Sumitomo 370	2280	280	1700	660	—
CTI RDS 112	1250	80	2000	500	—
Ebco TR 13/8	2260	350	1000	1000	350
GE PETtrace	3490	250	1340	1000	300
IBA Cyclone 10/5	1500	250	500	500	150
JSW BC 1710	2300	150	1900	890	375
Oxford	650	25	280	750	—
PracSys NHVG	1500	750	1100	660	700

the Tandem Cascade Accelerator (TCA, Fig. 16.3). The TCA is a dual (or tandem) electrostatic accelerator. In an electrostatic accelerator a beam of particles gains energy from charged electrodes. In the TCA a beam of negative particles (H^- or D^-) is initially accelerated down an evacuated tube consisting of a series of high voltage electrodes. This first beam is then sent through a carbon foil so that the two electrons on each negatively charged ion are removed. The resulting positive-ion beam is then accelerated by the same amount in a second, connected electrostatic acceleration tube. Beam energies of up to a few MeV can be produced. Because this energy is much lower than the energies used in a small medical cyclotron, less of the nuclear reaction cross-section is accessed. The reaction cross-section is a measure of the intrinsic yield of radioisotope. To make about the same amount of radioisotope product and compensate for lower cross-sections, much higher beam currents are required. The TCA has a maximum design beam current of 750 μA.

The product of beam current and beam energy is the beam power. Specially designed targets are required to withstand the higher beam power of the TCA. The entire high voltage apparatus is housed in a pressure vessel electrically insulated with 100 psig of sulfur hexafluoride gas.

A second type of linear accelerator is the PracSys nested high voltage generator (NHVG). This linac is similar to the TCA in that it can be operated in a tandem acceleration mode. In the NHVG, power transmission is accomplished via transformer coupling and the insulation is plastic instead of gas.

AccSys Technology has also developed a linac for PET. The AccSys linac employs slightly different technology from the other two linacs.

Linacs are new to PET. The performance specifications and yields shown in Tables 16.4 and 16.5 are generally based on calculations and not on results from routine clinical practice. Linacs offer the promise of increased ease of use and lower cost. As such, they are an exciting development for clinical PET. Manufacturers of accelerators for PET are listed in Table 16.6.

QUALITY ASSURANCE AND QUALITY CONTROL

Cyclotron targets (Fig. 16.4) and the target materials used to produce these radionuclides are not generally manufactured in the PET facility. However, the quality of the target materials must be ensured by the PET center because, together with the nuclear reactions, these materials deter-

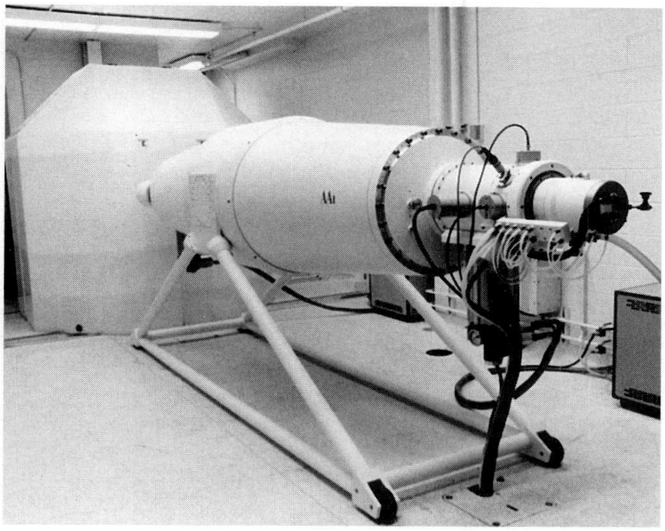

Figure 16.3. Accelerator Applications, Inc. Tandem Cascade Accelerator. The total length is 10 feet and the diameter is 3 feet.

mine the radionuclidic, radiochemical, and chemical purity of the radioisotope. The critical nuclear parameters include the beam current, particle energy, threshold energy, and the purity of the target substance. Multichannel analysis or pulse height γ-ray spectroscopy of radioisotopes other than positron emitters can be determined 3–4 half-lives after the end of the target bombardment with little interference from the main 511 keV photopeak of the positron emitters.

The manufacture and quality control of PET radiopharmaceuticals present some unique challenges because PET radiopharmaceuticals must be analyzed for purity and meet quality assurance specifications before administration to humans (16–20). Because of the short half-life of the PET imaging agents, it is essential that the quality assurance be completed as rapidly as possible and that it be fully documented. The quality control method for determining radiochemical purity is usually based on a chromatographic method with sensitive radioactivity detection. Chromatography is chosen because of its speed. High performance liquid chromatography (HPLC) is the most applicable because of high speed, sensitivity, resolution, and in-line measurement of both chemical and radiochemical purity. Routine HPLC analysis using analytical HPLC columns can be performed by comparison to a standard.

Low level impurities, separated by HPLC are generally easy to detect if they are ultra-violet (UV) absorbing. Poorly absorbing compounds can be detected by pulsed amperometric detectors. The mass quantities of radioactive active ingredients contained in a PET radiopharmaceutical can vary from nanogram to milligram amounts. The chemical purity requirement is to verify the chemical identity of the drug product, including stereoisomeric purity. The method for chemical purity analysis has the additional requirement to verify the absence of any chemical impurities or solvent residues in the final preparation. File samples are to be kept on every radiopharmaceutical prepared for human use. Although long-term stability studies are not usually required because the shelf-life of the PET radiopharmaceutical is limited by the physical half-life of the radionuclide, stability studies of the radiopharmaceutical must be determined experimentally for the time period from the end of synthesis to administration to the subject. The stability of the active ingredients should also be determined for a known container under set storage conditions. Stress stability tests may also need to be performed when the drug substance is known to be susceptible to degradation. Total mass and specific activity can usually be determined before injection to humans. Assuring compliance to specifications for those positron emitters with half-lives less than 10 minutes is an extremely difficult task. For quantitative PET receptor studies there must be high specific activity which make the procedures susceptible to trace interferences in reagents, solvents, glassware, etc. Many of these trace interferences will be seen in the UV chromatogram. The reagents and solvents must be high purity HPLC grade. The analyses also require an HPLC injection of a known standard each time before the quality analysis of the final radiopharmaceutical. In this way the accuracy of the system is determined each time.

It should be standard operating procedure to determine periodic radionuclidic purity of the PET radionuclides produced and in the final product. When no volatile compounds are present, radio-thin layer chromatography (TLC) is done as an additional purity test because of the advantage that all the radioactivity that is applied to the plate is detected. TLC is the most frequently used method for routine analysis of intermediates and end products during the developmental stages of radiopharmaceutical production. Purity limits and quality control specifications must indicate the final radiopharmaceutical to be at a specified chemical and radiochemical purity, with a limit on total mass and minimum specific activity at the end of synthesis.

There should be written procedures to ensure specified limits and controls for drug product quality. Tests should be done to ensure sterility, apyrogenicity, isotonicity and suitable acidity (pH) before administration to humans. The liquid injectable drug product should be formulated in an isotonic diluent and sterilized by terminal filtration through a 0.22 μm filter as a final step in the radiosynthesis procedure. The sterility test must be carried out retrospectively to assure the safety of the overall procedure. The pH and isotonicity are adjusted to physiologic values by the addition of sterile buffers or sterile saline. Sterility should be determined on each batch of every parenteral radiopharmaceutical using United States Pharmacopeia (USP) methods. Since an entire lot of a PET radiopharmaceutical may be administered to one or several subjects, depending upon the radioactivity remaining in the container at the time of administration, then the administration of the entire quantity of the lot to a single patient should be anticipated for every lot manufactured. This is an important consideration in establishing the maximum limit for endotoxins and impurities. Verification of a lack of pyrogenicity should be determined by the USP Limulus Amebocyte Lysate (LAL) test on each batch of every non-gaseous radiopharmaceutical prepared for human use.

Table 16.6.
Manufacturers of Accelerators for the Production of PET Radioisotopes

Manufacturer	Address
Accelerator Applications (AAI)	15 Ward St., Somerville, MA 02143, (617) 547–1019
AccSys Technology	1177 Quarry Lane, Pleasanton, CA 94566 (510) 462–6949
Sumitomo Heavy Industries (CGR-Sumitomo)	Suite 3669 One World Trade Center New York, NY 10048 (212) 432–0572
Computer Technology and Imaging (CTI/Siemens)	810 Innovation Drive, Knoxville, TN 37932 (615) 966–7539
Ebco Technologies	7851 Alderbridge Way, Richmond, B.C. Canada V6X 2A4 (604) 278–5578
General Electric Medical Systems (GE)	175 Anderson Drive, Marlborough, MA 01752 (508) 229–2620
Ion Beam Applications (IBA)	39 Hawthorne Avenue, San Anselmo, CA 94960 (415) 453–1499
Japan Steel Works America (JSW)	200 Park Avenue, New York, NY 10166 (212) 867–5600
Oxford Instruments	130A Baker Avenue, Concord, MA 01742 (800) 447–4717
PracSys Corporation	400 West Cummings Park, Suite 6650 Woburn, MA 01801 (617) 938–7144

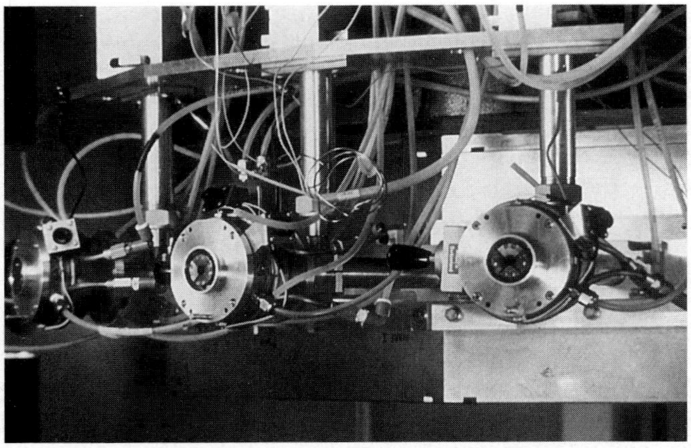

Figure 16.4. Cyclotron targets on the Siemens/CTI model T205 112 negative-ion cyclotron.

Each PET radiopharmaceutical intended for inhalation should incorporate a particulate filter (0.45 μm) as a component of the administration procedure. With every major change or initial production of a new radiopharmaceutical, three independent production runs should be performed to verify the drug product quality, strength, and purity.

It is an optimum condition when there is dedicated equipment and personnel for each synthesis and analysis for purity. Each PET center must provide for the assessment of scientific and technical quality of the manufacturing and quality control operations by a radiopharmacist and radiochemist. The dedicated equipment should include materials of a specified grade and standards of identity, and standard operation procedures for all raw materials. For critical components, a certificate of analysis should be obtained from the supplier, and at least one identity test be performed. Components, containers and closures, and supplies used in the radiosynthesis of PET radiopharmaceuticals should be stored in a controlled access area according to written procedures. These raw materials are logged in, assigned lot numbers and expiration dates based upon either the manufacturer's expiration date, or assigned an expiration date based on the physical and chemical properties of the component, material, or supply.

Documentation in the form of batch production records and quality control records is essential. The information contained in the label should include the date, name of the radiopharmaceutical, the total radioactivity, the time of the measurement, the expiration time, the volume, and the specific activity. The label should also state, "Caution: Radioactive Material." Chemical reactions with the radiopharmaceutical storage container should also be investigated since the container itself can be a potential source leading to impurities. Assurance must be provided that no extractables are leached from the container/closure system into the final PET radiopharmaceutical.

It is important that the analytical test be validated and the limits for all tests be specified. It is anticipated that all PET facilities will be required to prepare an application for the authorization to use PET radiopharmaceuticals. Generators and kits are the shared responsibility of an industrial manufacturer and the hospital pharmacy, while the short half-life of PET radionuclides requires that a cyclotron facility be within the vicinity of the clinical PET center, and therefore requires the PET facility to be responsible for the aseptic processing and to be in compliance with Federal regulations. PET has been used for many years for research purposes under the authority of the Institutional Review Board (IRB). However, with the advent of numerous clinical PET centers the FDA intends to regulate the production and use of these pharmaceuticals through revised drug provisions of the Federal Food, Drug and Cosmetic Act (21).

The most frequently used PET radiopharmaceutical is 2-deoxy-2-[^{18}F]fluoro-D-glucose (2-[^{18}F]FDG) (20), with many PET centers reporting the use of 6-[^{18}F]fluoro-3,4-dihydroxyphenylalanine (6-[^{18}F]FDopa), 6-[^{18}F]fluoro-3,4-dihydroxyphenethylamine (6-[^{18}F]fluorodopamine), sodium [^{18}F]fluoride, and fluorine-18- and carbon-11-labeled central nervous system receptor ligands. Carbon-11-labeled products are numerous and varied because of the ubiquitous nature of the carbon atom and have, therefore, been incorporated into many classes of compounds such as ligands for opiate receptors ([^{11}C]carfentanil), dopamine D_1 receptors ([^{11}C]SCH 23390), dopamine D_2 receptors ([^{11}C]raclopride), and benzodiazepine receptors ([^{11}C]flumazenil). Radioactive gases ([^{11}C]CO, [^{11}C]CO_2), fatty acids, and acetate have also been prepared. Carbon-11 has also been used to label serotonin receptor ligands (altanserin) and serotonin reuptake ligands (McN5652). Oxygen-15-labeled water and nitrogen-13 ammonia are used at many PET centers with a great deal of frequency.

The USP issued the first monograph for a PET radiopharmaceutical labeled with a cyclotron generated radionuclide in 1989 for 2-[^{18}F]FDG in the ninth supplement to the United States Pharmacopeia XXI, and was given the United States Adopted Name (USAN), Fludeoxyglucose F 18 (2). In 1990, the second PET radiopharmaceutical standard was published in the USP XXII for nitrogen-13-labeled ammonia, Ammonia N 13 Injection. Soon ^{18}F-labeled fluoromethane, and ^{18}F sodium fluoride were included. In 1991, 6-[^{18}F]fluorodopa (23) became an official monograph. ^{11}C-labeled carbon monoxide was listed with the USAN name carbon monoxide C 11 in 1992, as well as Water O 15, although neither is an official monograph in the USP at the time this publication goes to press. The use of PET radiopharmaceuticals continues to grow with increased interest and utility to provide a powerful tool for the evaluation of physiologic parameters and biochemical processes based on the in vivo distribution of the radioactivity.

2-DEOXY-2-[^{18}F]FLUORO-D-GLUCOSE

2-Deoxy-2-[^{18}F]fluoro-D-glucose (2-[^{18}F]FDG) is a metabolic tracer used for the quantitation of glucose metabolic rate, and has persisted since 1977, as the most frequently used and important fluorine-18-labeled radiopharmaceutical for studying local organ metabolism by PET (24, 25). This radiopharmaceutical is routinely employed for functional studies of brain (26), heart (27), psychiatry (28), oncology (29), neurology (30), and tumor growth (31, 32). Figure 16.5 shows the structures of D-glucose and of 2-FDG. D-Glucose is the natural metabolic substrate. In FDG, a fluorine has been substituted for a hydroxyl (-OH) at the second carbon. When the fluorine is radioactive ([^{18}F]), then the radiotracer 2-[^{18}F]FDG results. 2-[^{18}F]FDG is

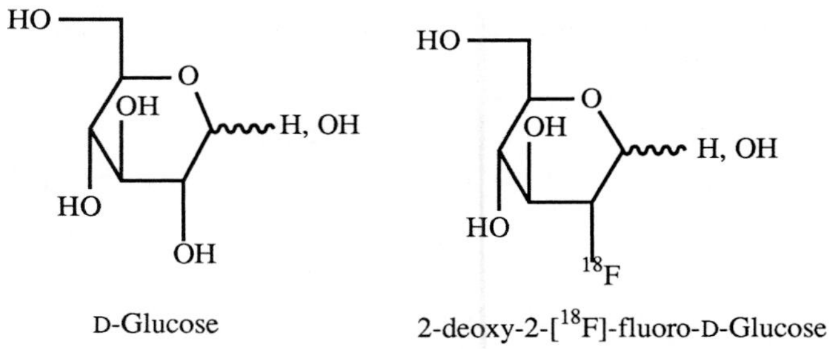

Figure 16.5. The structures of D-Glucose and 2-deoxy-2-[^{18}F]-fluoro-D-Glucose.

phosphorylated to 2-[^{18}F]FDG-6-phosphate by the enzyme hexokinase. Further metabolism does not occur in tissues that do not have phosphatase enzyme during the time required for imaging. In tissues with this enzyme (such as the liver, spleen, and kidneys), 2-[^{18}F]FDG is dephosphorylated and cleared from the tissue (24, 25).

Fluorine-18 can be produced by a number of nuclear reactions. The most common nuclear reactions utilized via cyclotron production are those using deuterons or protons: ^{20}Ne(d,α)^{18}F or ^{18}O(p,n)^{18}F (Table 16.2).

2-[^{18}F]FDG was first synthesized using [^{18}F]F_2 produced by the ^{20}Ne(d,α)^{18}F nuclear reaction. The yields were low (33). Fluorine-18 is produced from the bombardment of neon-20 with deuterons. The target is constructed of nickel, passivated with F_2, and filled with 0.1% F_2 in neon. The effect of the target gas purity on the chemical form of ^{18}F during F_2 production using fluorine in neon has been described (34). A regioselective synthesis using the electrophilic fluorinating agent [^{18}F]acetyl hypofluorite, CH_3COOF was developed (35). The stereoselectivity of the addition of acetyl hypofluorite to tri-O-acetyl glucal (compound **1** in Fig. 16.6) was found to be poor and resulted in poor isomeric purity (36–38). The [^{18}F]acetyl hypofluorite was reacted with tri-O-acetyl glucal in glacial acetic acid to yield compounds **2** and **3** in Figure 16.6. Hydrolysis with hydrochloric acid (HCl) of **2** gave the final product which was purified by passage through anion retention resin, neutral alumina, and activated charcoal. Reaction intermediate **3** resulted in the formation of the mannose isomer (2-deoxy-2-[^{18}F]fluoro-D-mannose, FDM) as a radioimpurity. Quality control included radiochemical purity by HPLC utilizing a carbohydrate HPLC analysis column and a sodium iodide (NaI) detector. A quality control method utilizing just HPLC could not detect free fluoride, therefore TLC is used to detect the free fluoride [^{18}F]. Additionally, the TLC technique can confirm the HPLC analysis for [^{18}F]acetylfluorodeoxyglucose. Alternative radiosyntheses were investigated (39), including cyclic sulfate (40). Electrophilic fluorination methods produced low radiochemical yields with low specific activities, and the formation of both epimeric forms. As a result, nucleophilic substitution reactions were investigated.

A currently popular alternative nucleophilic fluorination method has been developed by Hamacher, et al. (41), utilizing the [^{18}F]fluoride nucleophilic displacement reaction with 1,3,4,6-tetra-O-acetyl-2-trifluoromethansul-

Figure 16.6. The synthetic routes for the production of 2-FDG (* = [18]F or ^{18}F).

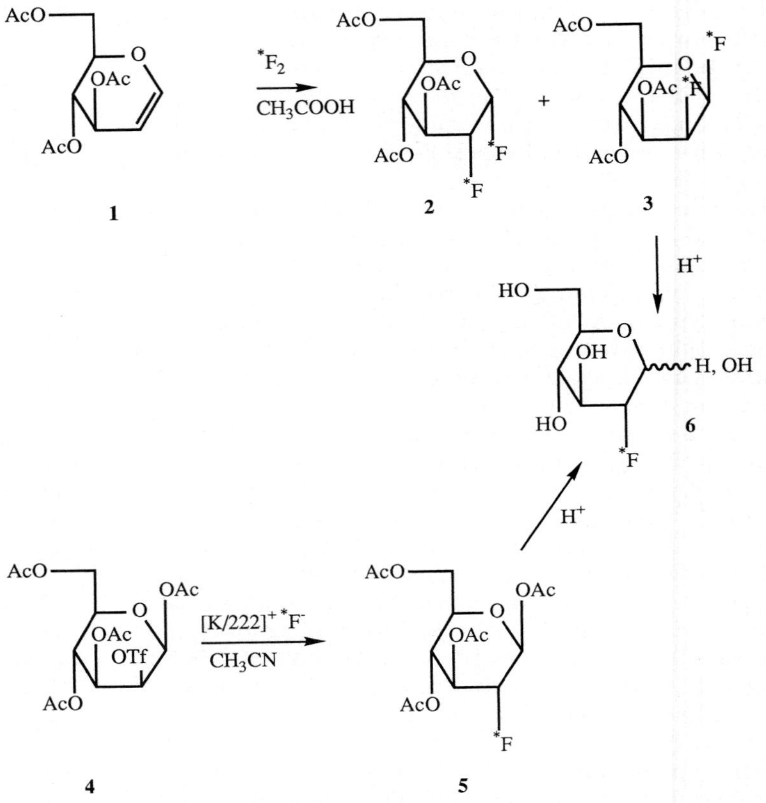

fonyl-β-D-mannopyranose (compound **4**, Fig. 16.6). After displacement, acid hydrolysis of the acetylated intermediate **5** gives 2-[^{18}F]FDG (compound **6**, Fig. 16.6) in good yield.

[^{18}F]Fluoride is produced by the ^{18}O(p,n)^{18}F reaction of protons on oxygen-18-enriched water (42–48). These targets are of varying design constructed of metals (silver, copper, titanium, nickel, and stainless steel) with oxygen-18-enriched water target cavities of 0.1–4 ml volumes. The high cost and lack of availability of the oxygen-18-enriched water has led to the development of anion exchange separation methods (49, 50), and quaternary ammonium resins for the separation of [^{18}F]fluoride from the isotopically enriched water (51, 52). The nucleophilic synthesis has improved the specific activity, stereospecificity, and yield. When the radiopharmaceutical is synthesized from ^{18}F prepared by the ^{18}O(p,n)^{18}F reaction in a target chamber constructed of titanium, the quality control analysis should include an investigation for the presence of vanadium-48 ($t_{1/2}$ = 16 days). Periodic radionuclidic purity assessment of the final product by multichannel analysis 10 half-lives later will ensure compliance with specifications.

The Hamacher, et al., synthesis utilizes Kryptofix 2.2.2 as a phase transfer catalyst to increase the reactivity of the fluoride ions (Fig. 16.6). A quality control analysis for any radiosynthesis using Kryptofix 2.2.2 must include a TLC method for investigation for possible minor contamination of the final radiopharmaceutical. Kryptofix 2.2.2 has an acute toxicity evidenced by ptosis, apnea, and convulsions. Recently, Moerlein, et al. (53), reported a quantitative TLC system for screening 2-[^{18}F]FDG radiopharmaceutical preparations for the possible impurities fluoride, Kryptofix 2.2.2 and glucose. These authors found that by increasing the volume of 0.1 N HCl in the initial solid-phase extraction to 10 ml, all the Kryptofix 2.2.2 was eliminated as an impurity.

Chaly and Dahl (54) have developed a rapid, simple, TLC quality control procedure where a silica gel 60 HPTLC plate is developed in a mixture of methanol/ammonium hydroxide (9:1). The developed plate is dried, and iodine vapor is used for visualization. A yellow spot (R_f 0.38) indicates the presence of Kryptofix 2.2.2. Radio-TLC quality control can be used to determine not only the percent radiochemical purity of 2-[^{18}F]FDG, but also the presence of both [^{18}F]fluoride and partially unhydrolyzed 2-[^{18}F]FDG by using silica gel 60 TLC plates developed in acetonitrile/water (95:5). HPLC (carbohydrate column with acetonitrile/water (93:7)) can serve as an independent confirmatory method. HPLC cannot determine the amount of [^{18}F]fluoride present in the final product because the fluoride does not elute off the column.

The use of ion chromatographic analysis has been reported (55). The method described by Alexoff uses a high pressure ion chromatograph with highly sensitive (10–100 pmol) pulsed amperometric detection. Radionuclidic purity should be determined by multichannel analysis from 40–2,000 keV with 99% 511 keV. Multichannel scaling should indicate a half-life of 110 ±5 minutes (22). The nucleophilic substitution has been found to be free of 2-fluoro-2-deoxymannose, and 99% radiochemically and radionuclidically pure. The possible impurities are Kryptofix 2.2.2, glucose, mannose, and 2-chloro-2-deoxyglucose

(55). Additional requirements are set for pH (within a 0.4 pH unit range between 4.5 and 8.5) isotonicity, specific activity (not less than 37×10^9 mBq (1 Ci) per mmol), bacterial endotoxin, and sterility (22). To assure sterility, the final product is filtered through a 0.22 μm filter prior to formulation. The stability of the drug product should be determined for the length of possible use of the product and the expiry date/time determined. Any possibility of an impurity which could be leached from the container-closure system should be investigated, and teflon or siliconized rubber stoppers employed.

[^{13}N]AMMONIA

[^{13}N]Ammonia has attracted interest as an imaging agent to study brain (56), liver (57, 58), and myocardial ischemia and/or altered myocardial perfusion (59–61), and has a history of use in biologic research (62) and nuclear medicine (63). Hundreds of healthy volunteers and patients have been evaluated for cerebral, hepatic, and myocardial perfusion using [^{13}N]ammonia in the United States (59, 60, 64, 65), Europe (66), and Japan (58, 67–69). These studies were performed with subjects both at rest and during exercise (70).

[^{13}N]Ammonia is a USP approved drug (71). When [^{13}N]ammonia is injected intravenously, [^{13}N]NH_3 rapidly clears from the circulation, 85% leaving the blood in the first minute (63) and only 1.4% remaining in the circulation after 200 seconds (56). It is taken up mainly by the myocardium, the brain, the liver, and the kidneys (72, 73). Cardiac imaging is based on myocardial tissue uptake of [^{13}N]NH_3 which is related to regional myocardial blood flow. Although myocardial uptake was once thought to be the result of ammonium competition with potassium transport, it is now accepted that myocardial localization is due to infusion across capillary and cellular membranes as [^{13}N]ammonia. Retention in myocardial cells is the result of metabolism to [^{13}N]glutamine by glutamine synthetase (56, 74, 75), and becomes trapped within the tissues by incorporation into the cellular pool of amino acids. The myocardial uptake of [^{13}N]ammonia has been demonstrated to be proportional to the coronary blood flow (76). In myocardial infarct patients, the slow blood pool clearance and prolonged lung retention is apparently the result of a large pulmonary distribution volume. Imaging studies of the distribution pattern allow for quantitation of regional myocardial perfusion in vivo with patients affected with coronary artery disease, hypertrophic cardiomyopathy, or chest pain syndrome with normal coronary arteries. In the blood more than 95% is in the form of ammonium ion ([^{13}N]$NH4^+$). The clinical feasibility of using PET for the assessment of myocardial perfusion has been established in studies involving [^{82}Rb]RbCl (77, 78), [^{15}O]H_2O (79, 80), and [^{13}N]NH_3 (60, 61). The advantages over thallium imaging include better resolution, the ability to quantitate flow, and the ability to perform multiple serial studies within a brief period of time under varied conditions (81). [^{13}N]Ammonia has also been used in conjunction with 2-[^{18}F]FDG for evaluation of myocardial ischemia (59).

The chemical name is nitrogen-13-labeled ammonia, chemical formula [^{13}N]NH_3, molecular weight 16, labeled with the short-lived positron emitter ^{13}N ($t_{1/2}$ = 9.97 minutes). The ^{13}N radioactive label allows for the distribution of the drug uptake in the myocardium which can be imaged with a PET scanner. The compound was first synthesized and used in animals and humans in the early 1970s (56, 72, 82). No adverse effects have been found. No pharmacologic effects should be elicited by [^{13}N]ammonia. The USP DI (75) states that there are no known drug interactions and/or related problems associated with the use of [^{13}N]ammonia, nor is there evidence of any diagnostic interference associated with the use of [^{13}N]ammonia. There is no information regarding medical problems that would present an increased risk or interfere with the use of [^{13}N]ammonia.

In the past, $^{13}NO_x$ species were chemically reduced with Devarda's alloy or some other reducing reagent and the [^{13}N]ammonia distilled prior to use. The recent synthetic method reported by Wieland, et al. (83), utilized in-target high yield production of [^{13}N]ammonia by proton irradiation of a pressurized aqueous mixture of ethanol (5 mM). The addition of ethanol as a hydroxy radical scavenger greatly enhances the yield of [^{13}N]ammonia (84). [^{13}N]Ammonia is produced on cyclotrons by the $^{16}O(p,\alpha)^{13}N$ nuclear reaction, employing protons on dilute aqueous ethanol. The ethyl alcohol is 190 proof diluted in sterile water for injection, USP. The target chamber can be constructed of titanium or silver. When [^{13}N]ammonia is transferred from the target through a strong anion-exchange resin membrane, all anionic interferences are removed. The aqueous ethanol mixture is convenient since it is suitable for human intravenous injection after sterilization by terminal filtration through the 0.22 μm vented filter into a sterile vial or syringe. To aid in the assurance of a lack of pyrogenicity, the target and product delivery lines are flushed with target water/ethanol mixture. Each batch should be tested for chemical and radiochemical purity, lack of pyrogenicity by the LAL test, pH, and sterility. The USP specification for specific activity is $\geq$100 Ci/mmol. The apparatus should be constructed of disposable tubing and needles in addition to the vial or syringe.

Cation exchange chromatography is the best choice for quality assurance because [^{13}N]NH_3 elutes with a definite retention time (85, 86) and a single HPLC column allows for a dedicated system for the routine quality assurance of [^{13}N]ammonia. The primary aqueous ^{13}N species after irradiation are nitrite and nitrate. Strong anion exchange (SAX) high performance ion chromatography (HPIC) can be performed with a Wescan Anion/R anion column, 100×4.6 mm (available through Alltech Associates, Deerfield, IL), or equivalent, using 4 mM p-hydroxybenzoic acid, pH 8.5 at a flow rate of 2.0 ml/min. The effluent can be monitored for conductivity and radioactivity. Strong cation exchange HPIC can be performed on a cation column (for example, a Wescan cation/S (50×4.6 mm, 3 μm) using 3 mM nitric acid as eluent at a flow of 2.0 ml/min. Specific activity can be determined by comparison of integrated area for the ammonia peak to that of a standard calibration. Radiochemical purity can be determined using an in-line, flow through NaI detector. The radiochromatographic peak which elutes with a retention time of 0.33 minutes (SAX HPIC) can be collected and the half-life determined within

3 minutes of end of bombardment (87). A quality control method should include a test for formaldehyde. A colorimetric test for formaldehyde using Fast Formalert (Baxter Healthcare, McGaw Park, IL), which has a limit of detection of 2 ppm, has been reported (87).

The radionuclidic product γ-ray spectrum should be used to routinely determine the radionuclidic purity. This can be accomplished by either multichannel pulse height analysis and/or multichannel scaling to ensure a lack of detectable radionuclidic impurities. Possible impurities using the titanium target could be vanadium-48 ($t_{1/2}$ = 16 d; 983 keV), scandium-44 ($t_{1/2}$ = 2.44 d; 1156 keV), fluorine-18 ($t_{1/2}$ = 109.7 minutes), and oxygen-15 ($t_{1/2}$ = 2.07 minutes). The primary radionuclidic impurity not removed by the SAX membrane filter is ^{15}O, most likely present as [^{15}O]water, produced by the ^{16}O(p,pn)^{15}O nuclear reaction. ^{48}V, ^{44}Sc, and ^{18}F will be completely retained by a SAX filter membrane and consequently not detected.

The USP monograph specifies the pH of the radiopharmaceutical be between 4.5 and 8.5. The injectate should be terminally filtered through a 0.22 μm filter prior to injection to assure sterility. Each batch should be tested for pyrogenicity using the USP LAL assay test prior to human administration.

[^{82}Rb]RUBIDIUM CHLORIDE

Rubidium-82 rubidium chloride (Table 16.1) has been found to be useful clinically as a blood flow agent, especially in the heart (88–94). The drug has also been used to evaluate blood-brain barrier changes in brain-tumor patients because there is little uptake by normal brain as ^{82}Rb does not cross an intact blood-brain barrier (95–99). Rubidium Rb 82 (USAN name) is currently the only FDA approved PET radiopharmaceutical. The accepted indication is for PET myocardial perfusion imaging. It is used in the diagnosis of myocardial infarction to distinguish normal from abnormal regions of myocardial perfusion in patients with suspected myocardial infarction. Indications not included in the U.S. product labeling include the diagnosis of coronary artery disease. [^{82}Rb]RbCl PET has been used in studies of myocardial perfusion before and after exercise with dipyridamole or adenosine stress.

Rubidium-82 decays with a half-life of 75 seconds (100). It has two decays modes: 95% positron emission and 5% electron capture (101). Besides the 511 keV photons resulting from positron annihilation, it also emits a 776 keV γ (15% abundance) and a 1395 keV γ (0.5% abundance). The isotope is the daughter of the radioisotope strontium-82 (^{82}Sr). Strontium-82 has a half-life of 25.3 days (102, 103). It decays by 100% electron capture with no γs. The ^{82}Sr radioisotope is produced in high-energy accelerators, such as the Los Alamos Meson Physics Facility (LAMPF), where a molybdenum target is irradiated with 700–800 MeV protons (104, 105). Strontium-85 is formed as a radioimpurity during the bombardment to produce ^{82}Sr (104). Strontium-85 has a half-life of 64.8 days. It is produced in amounts roughly equal to ^{82}Sr at the end of the bombardment. Strontium-85 decays exclusively by electron capture. It has a 514 keV γ-ray with 93% abundance.

Rubidium is a group 1A chemical element (an alkali metal). It forms ionic solids such as RbCl and yields +1 cations (Rb^+) in solution. This cationic character is the basis for its imaging applications as it emulates potassium ions physiologically (97). Rubidium accumulates in the cells of the myocardium as a function of blood flow. Areas of ischemia or infarction exhibit low [^{82}Rb]RbCl uptake because of diminished blood flow and/or viability.

A commercial ^{82}Rb infusion system is being sold by Squibb Diagnostics under the name CardioGen-82″ (106). The infusion system consists of two components: the ^{82}Sr-^{82}Rb generator and the semiautomated infusion apparatus. The infusion apparatus is a mobile cart with (a) a lead shield for the generator, (b) a waste bottle and shield, (c) a syringe pump, (d) a radioactivity detector, (e) an electronics control console, and (f) valves and tubing. The ^{82}Rb is obtained from the infusion system by eluting with sterile normal saline for direct injection into a patient.

The generator contains a ^{82}Sr/^{85}Sr mixture adsorbed on a hydrous stannic oxide column. (107). The activity on the column is typically 90–150 mCi ^{82}Sr at calibration time. The ratio of ^{85}Sr to ^{82}Sr on the column doubles each 40.6 days. The generator is replaced at roughly 30-day intervals. The expired generator is returned to Squibb Diagnostics in the original shipping container.

The ^{82}Rb is intravenously administered directly from the generator. The amount of radioactivity to be injected is assayed on-line by the self-contained positron (β-particle) probe which consists of a plastic scintillator and a photomultiplier tube. The quantity of ^{82}Rb to be delivered to the patient can be selected prior to beginning the administration. The automated infusion continues until the patient dose is achieved. A maximum volume can also be set as a backup safety control to avoid excessive radiation dose to the patient in the event of radioactivity detector failure during infusion (the cumulative volume is not to exceed 200 ml). The infusion rate is generally 50 ml/min. The maximum single dose to a patient is 60 mCi; the maximum cumulative dose is 120 mCi. The critical organs are the kidneys which receive 4.02 rads per 60 mCi dose (108). Myocardial radioactivity allows images to be obtained 2–7 minutes after injection.

During elution of ^{82}Rb from the generator some strontium is also removed. The strontium constitutes a radioimpurity that is of no benefit to the patient. The strontium that elutes off the column in the generator is referred to as breakthrough. The user of the CardioGen-82″ system is required to perform a daily quality control determination of the amount of ^{82}Sr and ^{85}Sr breakthrough. The allowable limit for ^{82}Sr breakthrough is 0.02 μCi ^{82}Sr/mCi ^{82}Rb. The limit for ^{85}Sr is 0.2 μCi/mCi ^{82}Rb. The ratio is determined by eluting the generator and measuring the ^{82}Rb activity. After the ^{82}Rb has decayed the total strontium activity is measured. Strontium ratios have been determined at the factory. The ^{82}Sr/^{85}Sr ratio can be determined at any later point using a chart supplied by Squibb Diagnostics with each generator.

The tubing used to deliver the ^{82}Rb to the patient is changed each time a new patient is imaged. This patient line contains its own sterilizing filter. There is another sterilizing filter located upstream between the syringe pump and the generator. The use of two filters in-line helps ensure sterility. The user of the CardioGen-82″ system is not required to check generator eluate for sterility or apyrogenicity. Aseptic technique should be observed in the assembly of the generator tubing, the handling of the eluate, and the installation of the patient line.

^{15}O-LABELED WATER

Oxygen-15-labeled water has been used for the investigation of blood flow in brain (109–111), heart (112–114), pancreas (115), and in breast tumors (116). The short half-life of ^{15}O (2.07 minutes) has been an advantage for in vivo investigations because it allows for rapid sequential administrations.

Oxygen delivery to the brain depends on cerebral blood flow. A number of studies have shown that regional cerebral blood flow (rCBF) (117, 118) and cerebral metabolism depend on regional functional activity (119, 120). Changes in rCBF can be useful indicators of changes in regional functional activation (121). Decreased hemispheric blood flow and oxygen metabolism have been reported in Parkinson's disease (122–125).

The composition of the formulated drug is tracer amounts of ^{15}O-labeled water in 0.9% sodium chloride solution. The most convenient method for the production of ^{15}O-labeled water is by the $^{14}N(d,n)^{15}O$ nuclear reaction (126–129) in a nitrogen gas target. The palladium catalyzed reaction of oxygen $[^{15}O]O_2$ with hydrogen was used for the radiosynthesis (127); however, the advantages of using platinum wire have been described (130). When the deuteron energy is not greater than 6 MeV no significant radionuclidic impurities are produced. When the nitrogen target gas contains some small percentage of oxygen (~1%) oxygen-15 is produced mainly as $[^{15}O]O_2$. It is also possible to produce some ammonia from the reaction of N_2 and H_2 over the catalyst. To ensure the purity of the final radiopharmaceutical, traps containing active carbon and soda lime can be used to remove nitrogen oxides and carbon dioxide. The $[^{15}O]H_2O$ vapor is trapped in sterile 0.9% sodium chloride for injection, USP, and is terminally sterilized by passage through a 0.22 μm filter into a sterile vial or syringe. The saline solution assures isotonicity. Flow rate, pressure, and radioactivity should be constantly monitored during the production. Rapid sequential dispensing of many doses of high level ^{15}O-labeled water is often required due to the short half-life of oxygen-15 and because the radiopharmaceutical is used multiple times each day. To lower the radiation exposure to the processing chemist, the quality control of each sample is to be avoided. It is customary to test the first and last lot of a continuous batch for compliance with quality control specifications. The optimum situation would be to have an ^{15}O gas production system which could monitor the gas delivery conditions and perform quality control by on-line, real time sampling and analysis of the continuous flow (130). Appropriate batch forms should ensure recording of patient administration. The ^{15}O-labeled water samples prepared for administration must be shown to be sterile and pyrogen free. To guarantee that the ^{15}O-labeled water samples are sterile and pyrogen free, components of the system can be rinsed and stored in bacteriostatic saline (USP) overnight and then flushed with sterile, normal saline prior to filling for production. Each batch of ^{15}O-labeled water should be tested for pyrogenicity levels using the USP LAL test. Other tests include pH, chemical, and radiochemical purity. The γ-ray spectrum of the final product should be periodically analyzed by multichannel pulse height analysis. The radionuclidic specification should be 99.0%.

^{11}C AND ^{15}O-LABELED GASES

Carbon-11- and ^{15}O-labeled gases are the most widely used cyclotron produced radioactive gases to date. Carbon-11 can be used as $[^{11}C]CO$ and $[^{11}C]CO_2$. Oxygen-15 may be produced as $[^{15}O]O_2$, $C^{15}O$, and $C^{15}O_2$. These short-lived radioactive gases are valuable tracers for the investigation of in vivo regional determination of many physiologic parameters, especially in the clinical investigation of pulmonary and cardiac malfunctions.

^{11}C-LABELED CARBON MONOXIDE

The use of ^{11}C-labeled carbon monoxide, $[^{11}C]CO$, has allowed dynamic measurements of carbon-11-labeled red blood cells for assessment of regional blood volume using PET. Inhalation of $[^{11}C]CO$ has been developed for noninvasive assessment of cerebral blood volume (CBV) in humans. This technique has been applied by several investigators (131–135). $[^{11}C]CO$ also has been used as a blood pool label in cardiac studies (56). Additionally, $[^{11}C]CO$ studies may be used in conjunction with other positron-emitting radiopharmaceuticals. In these cases, the $[^{11}C]CO$ image is used to correct for the effects of residual amounts of the other radiopharmaceuticals in the blood pool. Upon inhalation, labeled carbon monoxide is absorbed at the gas-tissue interface within the lung and enters the pulmonary blood circulation, where it is bound to hemoglobin and is assumed to be uniformly distributed throughout the total blood volume. Data obtained from these types of studies provide clinically important information about ventricular function in a variety of cardiac diseases. Typically, 5–15 mCi of $[^{11}C]CO$ is used in PET protocols for bolus inhalation. The critical organ is the spleen, which receives a higher radiation absorbed dose than the lungs. The spleen dose is 1.4 rad/15 mCi of administered $[^{11}C]CO$ (136).

^{11}C-labeled carbon monoxide is routinely prepared from the proton bombardment of a nitrogen gas target ($^{14}N(p,\alpha)^{11}C$) (137–139). The gaseous target produces $[^{11}C]CO_2$, which is subsequently converted via catalytic reduction to $[^{11}C]CO$. The catalytic conversion of $[^{11}C]CO_2$ to $[^{11}C]CO$ is carried out with both zinc and magnesium at high temperatures. Unreacted $[^{11}C]CO_2$ and NO_2 can be removed by the addition of a soda lime trap in the effluent line. The impurity $[^{11}C]CH_4$ could be formed when hydrogen and/or hydrocarbons are present in the target gas. The elimination or conversion of $[^{11}C]CH_4$ to $[^{11}C]CO$ can be achieved through proper adjustment of catalyst temperature and flow rate.

$[^{11}C]CO$ has also been prepared by the deuteron bombardment of a boric oxide target ($^{10}B(d,n)^{11}C$) (126, 140, 141). Possible radionuclidic impurities include ^{13}N (formed via the $^{14}N(p,pn)^{13}N$ process), ^{10}C (formed via the $^{14}N(p,\alpha n)^{10}C$ reaction), and ^{14}O (formed by the $^{14}N(p,n)^{14}O$ reaction). The target gas (99.9% nitrogen) should not contain more than 1 ppm oxygen (142). Oxygen concentrations greater than 1 ppm could result in the formation of both labeled and unlabeled nitrogen oxide impurities (138, 142).

Radiogas chromatography is the method of choice for the determination of the radiochemical purity of gaseous radiopharmaceuticals (17, 18, 127, 138). Routine quality control analysis is necessary and can be simplified by an on-line analysis of a gas stream, either directly from the target or after initial chemical processing. [^{11}C]CO can be introduced into an injection loop valve and split injected onto each of two columns. A radioactivity detector and a thermal conductivity detector (for mass determination of carbon monoxide) are used to determine both radiochemical purity and mass of carbon monoxide along with other gaseous impurities (143). The use of a molecular sieve column allows separation of CO from different air components (O_2, N_2, and CH_4). A Porapak-Q column (Waters Associates, Milford, MA) of sufficient length is used to separate CO_2 from N_2 and CO (which coelutes) and CO_2 from NO_2.

[^{11}C]CO poses no pharmacologic or toxic response in humans when prepared in the no carrier-added concentrations. Carbon monoxide impairs oxygen transport by blood. The affinity of human hemoglobin for carbon monoxide is 210 times greater than it is for oxygen (144). Excess exposure to this compound causes symptoms that include headache, dizziness, vomiting, nausea, tinnitus, perspiration, and systemic pain (144). A carbon monoxide concentration of 50 ppm would produce a carboxyhemoglobin level of 8–10% (145). When 8% of the hemoglobin exists as carboxyhemoglobin, approximately 1.23 mmol of carbon monoxide would be the threshold limit for a bolus inhalation. The proposed USP monograph sets the mass limit for use of [^{11}C]CO at 1.23 mmol in the dose to be administered (146). These calculations are based on the standard 70 kg man and should be adjusted dependent upon the weight of the subject.

^{15}O-LABELED GASES

Oxygen-15 has been used as a medical tracer for studying both the intake of oxygen and its rate of clearance into the blood in small regional volumes of lung (147) and to investigate rCBF, blood volume, and oxygen metabolism. Oxygen-15 has been used to label oxygen, carbon monoxide, and carbon dioxide. The short half-life of oxygen-15 (2.07 minutes) has proven to be an advantage for in vivo investigations allowing for rapid sequential injections.

Molecular [^{15}O]O_2 allows the study of cerebral oxygen metabolism following continuous inhalation (148–150) or brief inhalation (151). Oxygen-15-labeled CO_2 allows the measurement of the blood circulation and exchange of carbon dioxide in the lungs. [^{15}O]CO has been used for measurement of cerebral blood volume. Red cells can be labeled with [^{15}O]carbon monoxide (135, 152).

[^{15}O]CO is preferable to the use of ^{11}CO in that the rapid decay allows for the use of other PET agents in a single PET scanning session, and there is less radiation exposure (136).

Use of inhalation of [^{15}O]CO_2 has been investigated for measuring rCBF (149, 150) in which [^{15}O]CO_2 was continuously delivered in air at a constant rate. Inhalation of the [^{15}O]CO_2 results in the carbonic anhydrase in the red blood cells to transfer the ^{15}O label to water (149). The PET tracer most commonly used to measure rCBF is oxygen-15-labeled water, which is administered by intravenous injection and has the advantage of being biologically inert and chemically stable with no undesirable physiologic effects.

[^{11}C]ACETATE

^{11}C-acetate has attracted interest as an imaging agent to assess oxidative myocardial metabolism using PET (153–157). The use of ^{11}C-acetate and PET imaging has been proposed as a means of early noninvasive detection of myocardial metabolic abnormalities of diverse cardiac diseases. ^{11}C-acetate is converted to acetyl coenzyme A by the enzyme acetyl CoA synthetase after myocardial uptake. Acetyl coenzyme A enters the tricarboxylic acid cycle (TCA or Kreb's cycle) and is predominantly metabolized to the end product, $^{11}CO_2$, which is then cleared from the myocardium. Because the TCA cycle is tightly coupled to oxidative phosphorylation, assessment of ^{11}C-acetate kinetics in myocardium provides an index of oxidative metabolism.

The ^{11}C is a radioactive label so that the distribution of the drug's perfusion, metabolism, and clearance in the myocardium can be imaged with a PET scanner. The chemical formula is $CH_3$11COOH with a formula weight of 59.05. The positron emitting ^{11}C atom is located at the carboxylate carbon. ^{11}C-acetate is the radiolabeled isotope tracer of endogenous acetate. The chemical structure of ^{11}C-acetate differs from acetate only at the carboxylic carbon where a carbon-12 atom is replaced by a carbon-11 atom. Chemically the two compounds are alike.

The radiopharmaceutical is used as a diagnostic research tool for regional myocardial oxidative metabolism and in patients in conjunction with other imaging agents such as ^{15}O-labeled water. The use of PET scanning with ^{15}O-labeled water allows for the measurement of myocardial blood flow and its changes occurring in normal and pathologic states. Myocardial oxidative metabolism relative to blood flow can be used to evaluate the location, extent, and severity of myocardial cardiotoxicity. ^{11}C-acetate has been validated as a tracer of myocardial oxidative metabolism in both animals and humans. Henes, et al. (157), measured ^{11}C-acetate clearance with PET in seven normal patients at rest and during dobutamine infusion (employed to increase cardiac work). At rest, ^{11}C-acetate clearance was monoexponential and homogenous. During dobutamine infusion the rate pressure product increased 141% and the clearance of ^{11}C-acetate became biexponential. The k_1 at rest and during dobutamine infusion strongly correlated with the rate pressure product. This study suggested that this procedure would allow evaluation of regional myocardial oxidative metabolic reserve in patients with cardiac diseases and the assessment of the efficacy of interventions to enhance the recovery of metabolically comprised myocardium. Ambrecht, et al. (158), used normal volunteers engaged in supine bicycle exercise to show similar (as Henes, et al.) biexponential homogeneous time-activity curves. By splitting the resting studies into a fasting group and a group done after an oral glucose load, they confirmed independence of fast, first-phase ^{11}C-acetate kinetics from changes in myocardial substrate supply. Chan, et al. (159), studied 15 patients with chronic coronary artery disease and resting perfusion abnormalities. Regional myocardial uptake of ^{11}C-acetate was compared to regional myocardial perfusion measured by nitrogen-13 ammonia in 119 segments. These investigators found that the initial relative myocardial concentrations and segmental net extractions of the two tracers closely correlated. This study indicated that ^{11}C-acetate can be used exclusively to evaluate regional oxidative metabolism and regional myocardial perfusion. Walsh, et al. (160), utilized the tracers ^{11}C-acetate and ^{15}O-labeled water, and PET to demonstrate that in six patients with myocardial infarction, oxidative metabolism in the center of zones of infarction was markedly depressed. In four patients studied within 48 hours of the infarction and again more than 7 days after the acute event, regional myocardial oxidative metabolism did not change with time. Kotzerke, et al. (161), devised an analysis algorithm which generated polar coordinate maps of myocardial ^{11}C-acetate kinetics. It was observed, in 10 normal subjects, that left ventricle k_1 values, ^{11}C-acetate clearance rate, varied only 10.6 ±2.4%. There existed a small increase but a significant variation in septal, anterior, and basal regions. The ability to detect these small changes of variation permitted characterization of the location, extent, and severity of the myocardial disease. Miller, et al. (162), developed a methodology to construct quantitative accurate three-dimensional images of myocardial oxidative consumption from serial images of myocardial washout of ^{11}C-acetate. The three-dimensional functional displays permitted assessment of the inferoposterior wall and also permitted viewing of the myocardium from all angles. Four human subjects with acute myocardial infarction and one normal subject were injected via the antecubital vein with ^{11}C-acetate, and the rate of myocardial utilization was determined by monoexponential fitting of the clearance of ^{11}C-acetate at 2–3 minutes. Hicks, et al. (163), obtained results that showed that right ventricular ^{11}C-acetate clearance rate constants obtained by PET imaging provided a noninvasive evaluation of right ventricular oxidative metabolism. Twenty-one patients with aortic valve disease and 10 normal volunteers were shown to have right ventricular free wall ^{11}C-acetate clearance rate constants that positively correlated with the product of systolic pulmonary artery pressures and heart rate for all patients, whereas septal ^{11}C-acetate clearance rate constants did not. These data suggest that regional right ventricular clearance of ^{11}C-acetate reflects local oxygen demand. Hicks, et al. (164), studied myocardial regional substrate metabolism in nine healthy male volunteers under tightly controlled metabolic conditions of hyperinsulinemic-euglycemic clamping with and without a concurrent lipid emulsion infusion. There was found small, but significant, inhomogeneity of regional glucose metabolism. However, this was less than under fasting conditions. A 13% decrease was observed in glucose utilization in the septum versus the lateral wall with and without lipid infusion, which cannot be explained by a decrease in metabolic demand because $^{11}CO_2$ clearance was greater in the septum than in the lateral wall. This PET acquisition protocol consisted of simultaneous imaging of transaxial slices encompassing the entire heart which used a reorientation algorithm to generate short-axis cardiac planes from transaxial slices. The short-axis data was fed to semiautomated regional analysis programs to create polar coordinate maps of ^{11}C-acetate clearance rate constants and myocardial glucose utilization.

Synthetic methods have been developed by Pike, et al. (165), and Norenberg, et al. (166). ^{11}C-carbon dioxide is produced on a cyclotron by the $^{14}N(p,\alpha)^{11}C$ nuclear reaction by bombarding ultra-high purity nitrogen gas with protons. The $^{11}CO_2$ produced is trapped from the sweep gas in a hollow stainless steel spiral immersed in liquid nitrogen. The stainless steel trap is sealed and removed from the liquid nitrogen using a remote system. The stainless steel trap is then warmed and the $^{11}CO_2$ is released into freshly prepared methyl magnesium bromide in diethyl ether at ambient temperature. Hydrochloric acid is added to the reaction vessel and the phases allowed to separate and the aqueous layer withdrawn from the reaction vessel. Sodium bicarbonate in water for injection is added to the reaction vessel. The aqueous layer is again withdrawn, and the solution is heated at 60°C for 5 minutes under a stream of nitrogen. The product is terminally sterilized through a 0.22 μm filter. Pike, et al. (165), reported a radiosynthesis time of 20 minutes with production of [^{11}C]acetate in high radiochemical yield (73 ±12%; based on the initial activity of consumed ^{11}C-labeled carbon dioxide and corrected for radioactive decay).

Norenberg, et al. (166), report the use of a solid phase extraction which uses a remote production system employing reduced total volume solvents, which also removes trace amounts of labeled byproducts. Once $^{11}CO_2$ is produced the radioactivity is eluted from the target and trapped on a collection loop of Porapak-Q in nickel tubing cooled in liquid argon. The collection loop is removed from the liquid argon and the remote system apparatus directs the flow into a reaction vessel. A remote manipulator is used to submerge the input needle into an ice-cold Grignard solution of methyl magnesium bromide in ether (0.12 M, 2 ml). After the $^{11}CO_2$ is transferred, 0.2 ml of water is added via the remote switching of a six-way valve. The ether is evaporated with helium flow (about 100 ml/min) and heat (200°C). After dryness is attained, 0.5 ml of 1 N H_3PO_4 is added by switching another six-way valve and the ^{11}C-acetate is codistilled along with the water into a syringe containing 0.4 ml of water. When the distillation is complete, the distillate is pushed through a C-18 SepPak (available from Waters Associates, Milford, MA) and a 0.22 μm filter into a sterile serum vial. The distillation effectively removes the salts and the C-18 Sep-Pak retains ^{11}C-acetone, the major organic contaminant. The entire procedure requires approximately 15 minutes from end of bombardment. The trapping efficiency of the $^{11}CO_2$ is 50–75%.

Each batch of ^{11}C-acetate should be subjected to quality control and adjusted for isotonicity with saline prior to use. Aliquots of the product should be assayed for pH, specific activity, and chemical and radiochemical purity. The high performance liquid chromatography quality control procedure uses a reverse phase C-8, 10 μm (4.6×250 mm, available from Alltech, Deerfield, IL) column with a UV detector set at 210 nm for acetate (R_t = 2.12 minutes) and 260 nm for impurities (R_t = 4.15 minutes, acetone; 4.71

minutes, t-butyl-alcohol). The eluent is 7 mN H_3PO_4 at a flow rate of 2 ml/min. Radioactive determinations can be made using a radioisotope detector in-line with the flowing liquid sample in series following the UV detector (166). The mass determinations can be made using the UV detector and comparing the result to a standard curve. This method is sensitive enough to detect and quantify the TCA metabolite acetate, the chemical and radiochemical purity, and specific activity before injection into humans. The ^{11}C-acetate should be 95% chemically pure and 98% radiochemically pure with the impurities being acetone and t-butyl-alcohol. The radionuclidic purity should have been determined during development of the product and should be investigated by radionuclidic product γ-ray spectrum routinely, by either multichannel pulse height analysis to determine the absence of radiation other than a major photo peak at 0.511 MeV and a sum peak at 1.022 MeV, over a finite time period, or multichannel scaling to ensure a lack of detectable radionuclidic impurities. The proper proton bombardment energy incident on the target gas and the use of high-purity materials in the fabrication of the target chamber help ensure high radionuclidic purity. The pH of the radiopharmaceutical should be between 5 and 9. To assure sterility the injectate should be filtered through a 0.22 μm filter prior to injection. Every sample should be tested for sterility, and each batch should be tested for pyrogenicity by the LAL assay immediately upon end of synthesis (EOS). Each product formulated should be labeled with a lot number, compound name, volume, and activity at the end of synthesis.

A toxicologic concern is that trace amounts of magnesium and bromide ions may be injected along with ^{11}C-acetate. Quality control analysis should include a determination of the magnesium and bromide levels in the drug product during the development of the radiosynthetic method to assure the final drug product will consistently contain a lack of, or very low levels of, magnesium and bromide. A gas chromatographic procedure can be used to determine the absence of diethyl ether in the head space gases of the drug product container.

6-[^{18}F]FLUORODOPA

6-[^{18}F]Fluoro-L-3,4-dihydroxyphenylalanine (Fig. 16.7) is the positron-emitting fluorinated L-dopa analog which has attracted interest as an imaging agent for brain dopamine neurons using positron emission tomography (167–171). The cell bodies of the central dopaminergic neurons are located in the pars compacta of the substantia nigra and ventral tegmental area (172). 6-[^{18}F]fluorodopamine is actively stored in sympathetic synaptic vesicles and can be released by sympathetic nerve stimulation (169). It has been demonstrated in the rhesus monkey, that after peripheral intravenous administration of 6-[^{18}F]fluorodopa, 6-[^{18}F]fluorodopamine is synthesized and retained in that part of the brain having the highest density of dopaminergic nerve fibers, the striatum (173). In certain diseases, this neurotransmitter is deficient. 6-[^{18}F]fluorodopa is converted to 6-[^{18}F]fluorodopamine by decarboxylation and behaves similarly to endogenous dopamine, thus allowing investigation of regional brain metabolism and catecholamine biochemistry. Baboon studies using 6-[^{18}F]fluorodopa were performed to test the validity of 6-fluorodopa as an analog of L-dopa and of fluorodopamine as a false neurotransmitter. These studies (174) show that the radioactivity is released by reserpine most probably because of fluorodopamine release. This suggests that 6-[^{18}F]fluorodopa is decarboxylated and stored in vesicles as 6-[^{18}F]fluorodopamine (169). Dopamine receptor binding studies have confirmed that both 5- and 6-fluorodopamine have high affinities and properties similar to dopamine at D_2 sites (175). In an attempt to understand the role of the dopaminergic system in Parkinsonism and other neurologic disorders, studies of presynaptic dopaminergic function using 6-[^{18}F]fluorodopa in animals and in humans have been conducted (176–178) and in hemiparkinsonian patients a reduced accumulation of ^{18}F activity has been found in the contralateral striatum (179). The pharmacologic effects and the mechanism of action of 6-[^{18}F]fluorodopa will be similar to those of L-dopa. These effects are generally dose-dependent and reversible (180). The main effects are on the central nervous system, the cardiovascular system and the endocrine system. L-dopa can affect attention, arousal, mood, and have motor manifestations, most notably in patients with Parkinson's disease. Abnormal involuntary movements and encephalopathic states have been seen with chronic therapy. Orthostatic hypotension and cardiac arrhythmias have been described with high doses of L-dopa. L-dopa can affect the secretion of prolactin and growth hormone from the pituitary. Also, nausea and vomiting are well-known adverse effects of L-dopa therapy. Since dopamine cannot cross the blood-brain barrier, its precursor, 6-[^{18}F]fluorodopa, the analog of L-dopa which crosses the blood-brain barrier, is administered. Often carbidopa, a drug routinely used in combination with L-dopa in the treatment of Parkinson's disease, is given by oral admin-

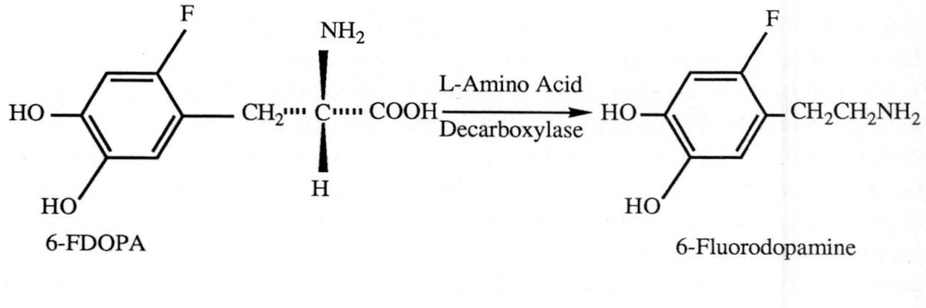

Figure 16.7. Enzymatic conversion of 6-fluorodopa to 6 fluorodopamine.

istration. Carbidopa does not cross the blood-brain barrier but acts only peripherally. It inhibits peripheral decarboxylation of L-dopa (as well as 6-[^{18}F]fluorodopa) by aromatic amino acid decarboxylase. By preventing the peripheral breakdown of 6-[^{18}F]fluorodopa, a greater amount of radiotracer reaches the brain. The only labeled compounds present in plasma of subjects pretreated with carbidopa as long as 120 minutes after 6-[^{18}F]fluorodopa injection are 6-[^{18}F]fluorodopa itself and 3-O-methyl-6-[^{18}F]fluorodopa (181).

6-[^{18}F]fluorodopa PET scanning has proven of value in characterizing aberrations of dopaminergic function in Parkinson's disease (182–184) and other movement disorders such as dystonia (185) and Huntington's disease (186).

The chemical structure of 6-[^{18}F]fluorodopa differs from L-dopa only at the 6 position of the catechol moiety where a fluorine atom replaces a hydrogen atom. The physical and chemical properties of the ring-fluorinated catechols are similar to the endogenous biogenic catechols. The first commonly used synthetic method was developed by Adam, et al. (187). ^{18}F-fluorine gas was produced by the nuclear reaction ^{20}Ne(d,α)^{18}F, employing deuterons on neon gas in a nickel target. The beam current was varied (usually 10–35 μA) for various durations of bombardment to adjust for yield. The target was filled with a small (<1%) percentage of fluorine. The synthesis starting material L-methyl-N-acetyl-[β-(3-methoxy-4-acetoxyphenyl)alaninate was prepared from the reaction of 3-O-methyl-L-dopa with gaseous HCl and anhydrous methanol followed by reaction with dry pyridine-acetic anhydride. This synthetic method produced 6-[^{18}F]fluorodopa in nearly equivalent amounts with the 2-[^{18}F]fluorodopa isomer. 6-[^{18}F]fluorodopa was then separated from the starting material and the 2-[^{18}F]fluorodopa isomer using an extensive high pressure liquid chromatography purification procedure. The presence of 2-[^{18}F]fluorodopa in the 6-[^{18}F]fluorodopa preparation decreases the signal-to-noise ratio of the images and compromises the PET data (188). Regioselectivity is important in the synthesis since the 6-[^{18}F]fluorodopa isomer is the most desirable, as substitution at that position has the least effect on the behavior of the parent dopa molecule (substitution at the 2 and 5 positions produces fluorodopa molecules with radically different rates of 3-O-methylation by catecholamine o-methyltransferase (COMT)).

Initially, half of the ^{18}F activity is unreactive fluoride and half of the [^{18}F]acetyl hypofluorite is labeled in the 2 position. Due to a lack of regioselectivity, 6-[^{18}F]fluorodopa was frequently produced in low yields. In 1990, Luxen, et al. (189), developed a regioselective radiofluorodemercuration procedure. The key radiosynthetic step involves the radiofluorodemercuration of N-(trifluoroacetyl)-3,4-dimethoxy-6-trifluoroacetoxymercurio-L-phenylalanine ethyl ester with [^{18}F]acetylhypofluorite, which, upon acid hydrolysis, provides only the 6-[^{18}F]fluorodopa isomer. In this synthesis, all the [^{18}F]acetylhypofluorite generated is utilizable activity for the production of 6-[^{18}F]fluorodopa. A 1992 publication by Luxen, et al. (190), reviews synthetic methods based on labeling by nonregioselective electrophilic fluorination, regioselective fluorodemetalation, and nucleophilic substitution. The use of a mercury intermediate proved to give higher yields while increasing the pressure in the neon target can increase the recovery of ^{18}F and increase the specific activity (191). The fluorine exchange for the mercury is highly selective and obviates the need for a chromatographic purification step. The fluorodemercuration route is the current preferred route. Nucleophilic labeling using imidazolidinone chiral agent to produce 6-[^{18}F]fluorodopa has not been optimized in terms of ease of preparation, synthesis time, and radiochemical yields at the present time. To obviate any potential pharmacologic effect, a high specific activity compound would be advantageous and may be the preferential route in the future. The product can be diluted with sterile saline for injection, USP, for a 0.9% final concentration to achieve isotonicity, and sterilized by terminal filtration through a 0.22 μm filter into an amber sterile vial with a teflon-faced stopper.

The following quality control procedures should be used: An aliquot of the product should be assayed for specific activity, radiochemical and chemical purity, radionuclidic purity, verification of a lack of pyrogenicity using the USP LAL test, pH, and isotonicity before human administration. For this reason, quality control must be based on rapid chromatographic procedures. Luxen, et al. (190), report on various quality control methods and discuss the advantages and disadvantages of each method.

The radionuclidic product γ-ray spectrum should be analyzed routinely by either multichannel pulse height analysis to determine the absence of radiation other than a major photopeak at 0.511 MeV and a sum peak at 1.022 MeV, over a finite time period, or by multichannel scaling to ensure a lack of detectable radionuclidic impurities. The acceptance specification in the USP monograph for the radionuclidic half-life determination is 110 ±5 minutes. Appropriate specifications should be set for the carbon and nitrogen impurity substances in the commercial neon gas. The high energy deuterons that initiate the nuclear reaction (^{20}Ne(d,α)^{18}F) may cause the formation of other possible nuclidic impurities via the reactions ^{10}B(d,n)^{11}C, ^{12}C(d,n)^{13}N, and ^{14}N(d,n)^{15}O. Analysis by MCA should indicate no other significant radionuclidic impurities in the range from 40–2,000 keV in the final radiopharmaceutical. To assure that the specifications are maintained from batch to batch the cyclotron parameters should be fixed and daily values recorded in a cyclotron log and verified by a cyclotron engineer. Proper deuteron energy incident on the target and use of the proper materials in the fabrication of the target chamber ensure high radionuclidic purity.

Even though preparative reverse phase HPLC (192–194) or ion pair chromatography (189, 195) provide good assurance of the chemical and radiochemical purity of 6-[^{18}F]fluorodopa, the USP monograph (23) states that appropriate tests should be performed to demonstrate this and specifically to show the absence of mercury-containing starting materials or reagents used in the synthesis. The USP specification (23) for mercury is <0.5 μg/ml. To determine the absence of mercury-containing starting materials or reagents an HPLC quality control procedure using a C-18 column eluting with 50 mM tetrabutylammonium iodide (TBAI) in 60% acetonitrile:40% water with

UV detection at 270 nm (196). This method is rapid (R_t 6.6 minutes) (197). Atomic absorption spectroscopy is the recognized method by the USP (23). This method is not always available to a PET radiopharmacy and may be time consuming. Radiochemical purity can be assured with HPLC analysis equipped with an in-line sodium iodide detector. Chemical purity can be determined using a C-18 column with absorbance detection at 280 nm (189, 192) or at 220 nm. At 220 nm the sensitivity is approximately twice that using absorbance at 280 nm (194). Electrochemical detection has also been used with good results (192). Possible impurities are L-dopa, 6-hydroxy-dopa, and 2- and 5-fluorodopa. The distribution of impurities is dependent upon the synthetic method used. Pike, et al. (193), recommend an upper acceptable limit of 50 μg for this compound, a potent neurotoxin when it is converted to the L-6-hydroxydopamine in vivo (198).

The USP value for the specific activity specification is ≥100 mCi/mmol (23). 6-[^{18}F]fluorodopa at this specific activity will behave as a true tracer at the blood-brain barrier. Currently, there are no requirements to produce 6-[^{18}F]fluorodopa at high specific activity.

Enantiomeric purity can be determined by injection onto an HPLC system equipped with a chiral ligand exchange HPLC column, as specified in the USP, to determine enantiomeric purity with each new batch of starting material, or by TLC (199).

Drug product stability has been addressed by Dunn and Kiesewetter (200) and Chen, et al. (192). Dunn and Kiesewetter found that 6-[^{18}F]fluorodopa samples had no decrease in chemical or radiochemical purity up to 4 hours without the needed addition of a preservative when the formulation was stored in an amber vial at room temperature at a pH between 6 and 7. These results are in concurrence with Pike, et al. (193), who report that their preparations of 6-[^{18}F]fluorodopa maintain radiochemical purity for at least 1 hour without the need for added stabilizers. Chen, et al. (192), found that the drug product as a dilute saline solution is nonenzymatically oxidized and sensitive to light exposure and high temperature. Chen, et al., also found that if exposed to light and allowed to sit at room temperature there is a progressive loss of 6-[^{18}F]fluorodopa over time with a 20% loss at 1 hour and 50% loss at 4 hours. For this reason, the USP monograph states that the drug product be dispensed into an amber, sterile vial and administered immediately after the quality control release. No color change or precipitate should be noted in the final radiopharmaceutical formulation. The pH of each formulated preparation should be in the range of 4–5 to avoid possible product oxidation. During the standardization and development of the synthetic procedure, the stability, isotonicity, and the sterility and apyrogenicity of the finished product should be established. The tonicity can be determined during the development stage by a commercial osmometer and then repeated at regular intervals to ensure compliance with the specifications. The sterility test method should be according to the USP method using the approved media, fluid thioglycollate medium, and soybean-casein digest medium. A quantitative bacterial endotoxin specification level for the LAL test would recommend ≤175 Endotoxin Units per dose.

6-[^{18}F]FLUORODOPAMINE

6-[^{18}F]fluoro-3,4-dihydroxyphenethylamine, abbreviated 6-[^{18}F]fluorodopamine, has been shown to be a promising PET imaging agent for the visualizing cardiac sympathetic innervation and function in humans. 6-[^{18}F]fluorodopamine can be obtained from 6-fluorodopa via the enzyme DOPA decarboxylase (Fig. 16.7). 6-[^{18}F]fluorodopamine has been utilized to study sympathetic innervation and function (201). 6-[^{18}F]fluorodopamine has been prepared by various methods. Dunn, et al. (194), report the preparation of 6-[^{18}F]fluorodopamine by in vitro enzymatic conversion from 6-[^{18}F]fluorodopa prepared by the direct fluorination of L-methyl-N-acetyl-[β-(3-methoxy-4-acetoxyphenyl)]alaninate and then incubated with the enzyme L-amino acid decarboxylase and pyridoxal phosphate cofactor at 37°C for 15 minutes. Besides low radiochemical yields, this synthetic method requires a quality control test that determines both fluorodopa isomers and fluorodopamine isomers. Ding, et al. (202), later reported an improved no-carrier-added synthesis of high specific activity 6-[^{18}F]fluorodopamine via a nucleophilic aromatic substitution reaction using [^{18}F]fluoride ion. In PET studies in baboons, rapid uptake and concentration of the tracer in myocardial tissue and rapid clearance from the blood with no change in vital signs at any time during the study was shown, indicating it was at true tracer levels (below the mass which would lead to pharmacologic effects). Recently another method of preparation of 6-[^{18}F]fluorodopamine has been reported (203) by the National Institutes of Health. The 6-[^{18}F]fluorodopamine was prepared in a fashion similar to that already described by Luxen, et al. (189). The key radiosynthetic step involves the radiofluorodemercuration of N-(trifluoroacetyl)-3,4-dimethoxy-6-trifluoroacetoxymercurio-β-phenethylamine with [^{18}F]acetyl hypofluorite. The final drug product should be sterilized by terminal filtration through a 0.22 μm filter into a sterile amber vial (teflon-faced septa). To the final sample may also be added sterile phosphate buffer and sterile saline for injection, 0.9%, USP, to adjust for pH and isotonicity.

Quality control procedures should include testing each batch of 6-[^{18}F]fluorodopamine for specific activity, radiochemical and chemical purity, pH, lack of pyrogenicity by LAL test, and for the presence of mercury immediately upon end of synthesis. The quality control procedures for this radiopharmaceutical have been reported (197), stating radionuclidic purity determination by γ-ray spectrum of the final product should be analyzed by multichannel pulse height analysis as described earlier for 6-[^{18}F]fluorodopa. The radionuclidic purity specification for the final drug product should be ≥99%. The radiochemical and chemical purity determination was done immediately at the end of synthesis by high performance liquid chromatography with isocratic elution with 10% acetonitrile/buffer for separation of L-dopa, dopamine, and other possible contaminants of the 6-[^{18}F]fluorodopamine synthesis. Even though preparative HPLC provides good assurance of the chemical and radiochemical purity, appropriate tests to demonstrate 90% radiochemical and chemical purity, and specifically to show the absence of mercury-containing starting materials or reagents used in the synthesis (≤0.5

ppm mercury) should be performed. An HPLC quality control procedure based on Tajima, et al. (204), using an Axxiom C-18 (Axxiom Chromatography, Calabas, CA) reversed phase column (4.6×100 mm, 3 μm) (eluent 50 mM tetrabutylammonium iodide (TBAI) in 60% acetonitrile:40% water, flow rate 2 ml/min, UV detection at 270 nm) has been developed for standard linear responses for mercury solutions between 1 ppm and 10 ppb.

AUTOMATED RADIOCHEMICAL SYNTHESIS DEVICES

The routine, repeated synthesis of radiopharmaceuticals can result in unnecessarily high exposure to ionizing radiation. The exposures can be especially high at facilities that prepare pharmaceutics labeled with short-lived positron-emitting radioactive isotopes such as carbon-11, nitrogen-13, oxygen-15, and fluorine-18. Partly to comply with the concept of "as low as is reasonably achievable" (ALARA) personnel exposures, automated radiochemical synthesis devices or chemical "synthesis modules" have been developed. Such synthesis modules can use prefilled chemical templates (Fig. 16.8) or user prepared reagent vials connected to the apparatus via tubing (Fig. 16.9). These automated synthesis devices can be more efficient and precise than existing manual methods. Such automated methods are especially useful when a radiopharmaceutical synthesis requires repetitive, uniform manipulations on a daily basis.

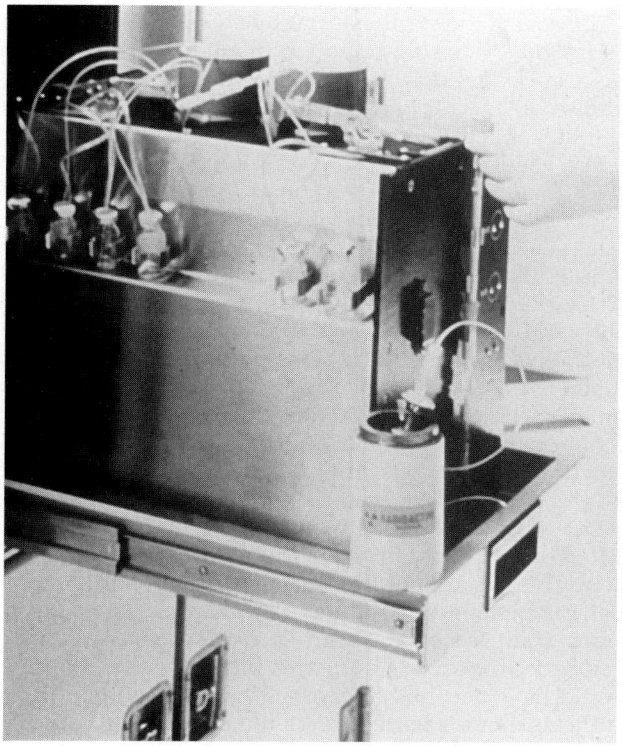

Figure 16.9. Automated synthesis device from the Siemens Medical Systems.

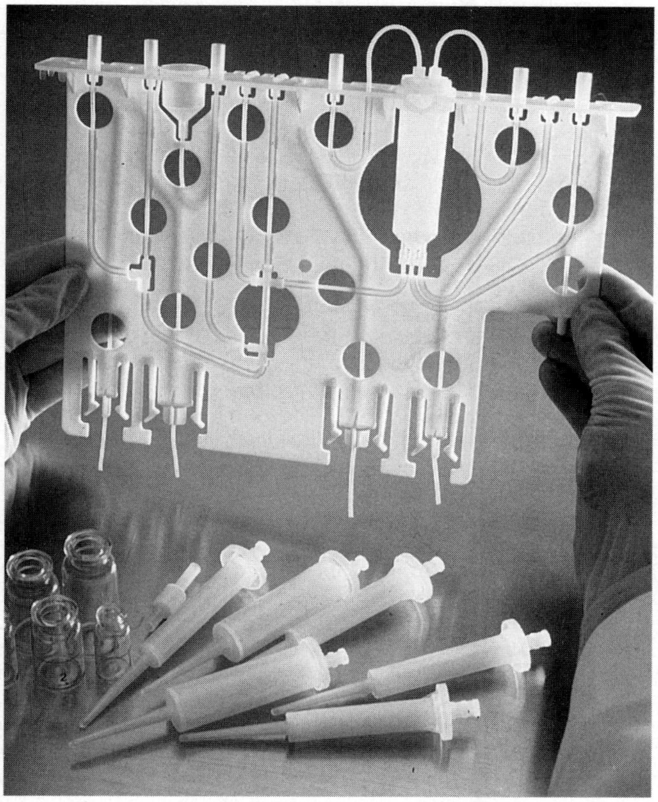

Figure 16.8. Template from the General Electric FDG Micro-lab System.

It is advisable to compare the drug products from automated radiosynthetic devices with the substances prepared by conventional manual syntheses. In the case of positron-emitting radiopharmaceuticals, this testing will include many of the same determinations as previously discussed and listed in the USP.

Manual methods described in the USP are amenable to control by synthesis modules. For example, the Fludeoxyglucose F 18 Injection can be readily adapted to automated synthesis. Of special concern is the methodology involved in validating that an automated apparatus is performing correctly. For a manual procedure, human intervention and correction by inspection can effectively nullify any procedural errors. However, in an automated system, effective feedback will generally only begin at the quality control step.

Synthesis modules are not limited to black boxes. The term encompasses any automated device used in the synthesis of radiochemicals. Robotics are thus explicitly included. The exact method of control is also variable. Both hard-wired and software controlled synthesis devices fall under this general designation. All synthesis modules consist of remotely-controlled devices for manipulating a chemical apparatus to effect the synthesis of a radiochemical. For each synthesis module there are devices for controlling parameters such as time, temperature, pressure, volume, sequencing, and other synthesis procedures. These parameters should be monitored and constrained to fall within certain bounds.

The goal of the synthesis module quality assurance is to ensure that the subsequent radiopharmaceutical meets preset specifications. Although medical device GMP regulations per 21 CFR Part 820 (Code of Federal Regulations) are not applicable, they may be helpful in developing a quality assurance program. As a practical matter, this involves documented measurement and control of all relevant physical parameters which are controlled by the synthesis module. Quality control testing of a synthesis module implies routine testing of all parameters initially certified during the qualification. Depending on the criticality and the stability of the parameter setting, testing may be as often as daily. This process performance assessment is best aided by the end-product testing. For example, variations in the temperature of an oil bath may be acceptable if the radiochemical (end-product) can be shown to meet all relevant testing criteria. The specification, testing, storage, and use of reagents for a synthesis module should follow a program similar to provisions in 21 CFR Parts 210 and 211. In this context, a reagent is defined as anything that contacts end-product precursors or the final radiochemical product. For example, in some processes compressed nitrogen is used to move liquid reagents. In this case, both the nitrogen and the tubing should have acceptable characteristics documented. Key synthesis module variables should be monitored and documented. These characteristics include all physical, chemical, electrical, and performance attributes. Especially important for microprocessor and computer-controlled devices is a method for specifying, testing, and documenting computer software and hardware. Such a program should include a periodic generalized testing of the computer hardware. Additionally, the software code should be examined to determine that it has not been modified and that it continues to result in a drug product meeting all specifications.

Some mechanical changes in the synthesis module can be considered trivial. This category often includes changes not affecting any of the monitored parameters. An example is replacing a length of tubing with an identical piece. However, care must be taken to ensure that seemingly innocuous changes do not have an unexpected impact. For example, changes in a comment line of a computer program may inadvertently result in a vital instruction being changed or deleted. Any changes to monitored parameters have the potential for changing the process output. If the resultant radiochemical does not meet specifications, then the change must be corrected and the process revalidated. All changes should be approved by a change control committee and recorded in a log book.

REFERENCES

1. JAMA Council on Scientific Affairs, Positron Emission Tomography Panel. Cyclotrons and radiopharmaceuticals in positron emission tomography. JAMA 1988;259:1854–1860.
2. Fowler JS, Wolf AP. New developments in radiotracers for positron emission tomography. NIDA Res Monograph 1991;112:146–167.
3. Birattari C, Bonardi M, Ferrari A, Milanesi L, Silari M. Biomedical applications of cyclotrons and review of commercially available models. J Med Eng Technol 1987;11:166–176.
4. Comar D, Crouzel C. Biomedical cyclotrons for radioisotope production. Int J Rad Appl Instrum B 1986;13:101–107.
5. Wolf AP. Cyclotrons, radionuclides, precursors, and demands for routine versus research compounds. Ann Neurol 1984; 15(Suppl):S19–24.
6. Salvadori PA, Bottigli U, Guzzardi R, Crouzel C, Comar D. Cyclotrons for medical use: characteristics and installation aspects. J Nucl Med Allied Sci 1982;26:41–54.
7. Bida GT, Ruth TJ, Wolf AP. Experimentally determined thick target yields for the $^{14}N(p,\alpha)^{11}C$ reaction. Radiochim Acta 1980; 27:181–185.
8. Daube ME. Development and comparison of myocardial tracers for positron emission tomography [Dissertation]. Madison, WI: University of Wisconsin, 1983.
9. Austin SM, Galonsky A, Bortins J, et al. A batch process for the production of ^{13}N-labeled nitrogen gas. Nucl Instr Meth 1975; 126:373–379.
10. Murphy K, Byrd RC, Guss PP, et al. The $^{15}N(p,n)^{15}O$ reaction below 9.3 MeV. Nucl Phys A 1981;355:1–12.
11. Wieland BW, Schmidt DG, Bida G, et al. Efficient, economical production of oxygen-15-labeled tracers with low energy protons. J Label Comp Radiopharm 1986;23:1214.
12. Vera-Ruiz H, Wolf AP. Excitation function for the ^{15}O production via the $^{14}N(d,n)^{15}O$ reaction. Radiochim Acta 1977;26:65–67.
13. Ruth TJ, Wolf AP. Absolute cross-sections for the production of ^{18}F via the $^{18}O(p,n)^{18}F$ reaction. Radiochim Acta 1979;26:21–24.
14. Nozaki T, Iwamoto M, Ido T. Yield of ^{18}F for various reactions from oxygen and neon. Int J Appl Rad Isot 1974;25:393–399.
15. Burgerjon JJ. H^- cyclotrons for radioisotope production. Invited paper at Conference on the Application of Accelerators in Research and Industry, Denton, TX, November 12–14, 1984.
16. Vera-Ruiz H, Marcus CS, Pike VW, et al. Quality control of cyclotron-produced radiopharmaceuticals. Int J Radiat Appl Instrum Part B 1990;17:445–456.
17. Krohn KA, Jansholt AL. Radiochemical quality control of short-lived radiopharmaceuticals. Int J Appl Radiat Isot 1977;28:213–227.
18. Meyer GJ. Some aspects of radioanalytical quality control of cyclotron-produced short-lived radiopharmaceuticals. Radiochim Acta 1982;30:175–184.
19. Manning RG, Wolfangel RG. Pharmacy involvement with positron-emitting radiopharmaceuticals. J Pharm Practice 1989; 2:185–190.
20. Kung HF. Overview of radiopharmaceuticals for diagnosis of central nervous disorders. Crit Rev Clin Lab Sci 1991;28:269–286.
21. U.S. Department of Health and Human Services, Public Health Service, Food and Drug Administration, 5600 Fishers Lane, Rockville, Maryland 20857, DHHS Publication No.(FDA) 93-1051, ISBN 0-16-041900-X, amended February 1993.
22. United States Pharmacopeia. Fludeoxyglucose F 18 Injection. USP 1989;22:579–580.
23. United States Pharmacopeia. 6–Fluorodopa F18 Injection. USP 1991;22(5th Suppl):2616–2617.
24. Ido T, Wan C-N, Fowler JS, et al. Fluorination with molecular fluorine. A convenient synthesis of 2-deoxy-2-fluoro-D-glucose. J Org Chem 1977;423:2341–2342.
25. Reivich M. Application of the deoxyglucose method to human cerebral dysfunction: the use of 2-[^{18}F]fluoro-2-deoxy-D-glucose in man. Neurosci Res Program Bull 1976;14:502–504.
26. Phelps ME, Mazziotta JC. Positron emission tomography: human brain function and biochemistry. Science 1985;228:799–809.
27. Phelps ME, Hoffman EJ, Selin C, et al. Investigation of [^{18}F]2-

fluoro-2-deoxyglucose for the measure of myocardial glucose metabolism. J Nucl Med 1978;19:1311–1319.

28. Ferris SH, DeLeon MJ, Wolf AP, et al. Positron emission tomography in the study of aging and senile dementia. Neurobiology of Aging 1980;1:127–131.
29. Hoh CK, Hawkins RA, Glaspy JA, et al. Cancer detection with whole-body PET using 2-[^{18}F]fluoro-2-deoxy-D-glucose. J Comput Asst Tomog 1993;17:582–589.
30. Zametkin AJ, Nordahl TE, Gross M, et al. Cerebral glucose metabolism in adults with hyperactivity of childhood onset. New Eng J Med 1990;323:1361–1366.
31. DiChiro G, Fulham MJ. Virchow's shackles: can PET-FDG challenge tumor histology? AJNR 1993;14:524–527.
32. DiChiro G, DeLaPaz RL, Brooks RA, et al. Glucose utilization of cerebral gliomas measured by [^{18}F]fluorodeoxyglucose and positron emission tomography. Neurology 1982;32:1323–1329.
33. Ido T, Wan C-N, Casella V, et al. Labeled 2-deoxy-D-glucose analogs ^{18}F-labeled 2-deoxy-2-fluoro-D-glucose, 2-deoxy-2-fluoro-D-mannose, and ^{14}C-2-deoxy-2-fluoro-D-glucose. J Labeled Cmpd Radiopharm 1978;14:175–182.
34. Bida GT, Ehrenkaufer RL, Wolf AP, Fowler JS, MacGregor RR, Ruth TJ. The effect of target gas purity on the chemical form of ^{18}F during [^{18}F]F_2 production using the neon/fluorine (Ne/F_2) target. J Nucl Med 1980;21:758–762.
35. Fowler JS, Shiue C-Y, Wolf AP, Salvador PA, MacGregor RR. Synthesis of ^{18}F-labeled acetyl hypofluorite for radiotracer synthesis. J Labeled Cmpd Radiopharm 1982;19:1634–1636.
36. Bida GT, Satyamurthy N, Barrio JR. The synthesis of 2-[^{18}F]F-fluoro-2-deoxy-D-glucose using glucals: a reexamination. J Nucl Med 1984;25:1327–1334.
37. Ishiwata K, Ido T, Nakanishi H, Iwata R. Contamination of 2-deoxy-2-[^{18}F]fluoro-D-glucose preparations synthesized from [^{18}F]acetyl hypofluorite and [^{18}F]F_2. Appl Radiat Isot 1987; 38:463–466.
38. Shiue C-Y, Fowler JS, Wolf AP, Alexoff D, MacGregor RR. Gas-liquid chromatographic determination of relative amounts of 2-deoxy-2-fluoro-D-glucose and 2-deoxy-2-fluoro-D-mannose synthesized from various methods. J Labeled Cmpd Radiopham 1985;22:503–508.
39. Dunn BB, Bennett J, Channing M, Kiesewetter DO, Finn R. Comparative evaluation of synthetic routes to 2-fluoro-[^{18}F]-2-deoxy-D-glucose. J Labeled Cmpd Radiopharm 1986;23:1094.
40. Tewson TJ. Synthesis of no-carrier added fluorine-18 2-fluoro-2-deoxy-D-glucose. J Nucl Med 1983;24:718–721.
41. Hamacher K, Coenen HH, Stocklin G. Efficient stereospecific synthesis of NCA 2-[^{18}F]fluoro-2-deoxy-D-glucose using aminopolyether supported nucleophilic substitution. J Nucl Med 1986; 27:235–238.
42. Berridge MS, Tewson TJ. Effects of target design on the production and utilization of [^{18}F] fluoride from [^{18}O]water. J Labeled Cmpd Radioparm 1986;23:1177–1178.
43. Huszan I, Weinreich R. Production of ^{18}F with an ^{18}O enriched water target. Radioanal Nucl Chem Lett 1985;93:349–354.
44. Iwata R, Ido T, Brady F, Takahashi T, Ujuie A. [^{18}F]fluoride production with a circulating [^{18}O]water target. Appl Radiat Isot 1987;38:979–984.
45. Keinonen J, Fontell A, Kairento A-L. Effective small volume [^{18}O]water target for the production of [^{18}F]fluoride. Appl Radiat Isot 1986;37:631–632.
46. Kilbourn MR, Hood JT, Welch MJ. A simple ^{18}O-water target for ^{18}F production. Int J Appl Radiat Isot 1984;35:599–602.
47. Vora MM, Boothe TE, Finn RD, et al. Multimillicurie preparation of 2-^{18}F-fluoro-2-deoxy-D-glucose via nucleophilic displacement with fluorine-18 labeled fluoride. J Labeled Cmpd Radiopharm 1985;22:953–970.
48. Wieland BW, Hendry GO, Schmidt DG, Bida G, Ruth TJ. Efficient small-volume ^{18}O-water targets for producing ^{18}F fluoride with low energy protons. J Labeled Cmpd Radiopharm 1986; 23:1205–1207.
49. Schlyer DJ, Bastos M, Wolf AP. A rapid quantitative separation of fluorine-18 fluoride from oxygen-18 water. J Nucl Med 1987; 28:764.
50. Jewett DM, Toorongian SA, Mulholland GK, Watkins GL, Kilbourn MR. Multiphase extraction: a rapid phase-transfer of [^{18}F]fluoride for nucleophilic radiolabeling reactions. Appl Radiat Isot 1988;39:1109–1111.
51. Mulholland GK, Mangner TJ, Jewett DM, Kilbourn MR. Polymer-supported nucleophillic radiolabeling reactions with [^{18}F]fluorine and [^{11}C]cyanide ion on quaternary ammonium resins. J Labeled Cmpd Radiopharm 1989;267:378–380.
52. Mulholland GK, Toorongian SA, Jewett DM, Kilbourn MR. Polymer supported NCA nucleophilic radiofluorination. Rapid new synthesis of [F-18]FDG with recovery of [O-18]water. J Nucl Med 1988;29:754.
53. Moerlein SM, Brodack JW, Siegel BA, Welch, MJ. Elimination of contaminant kryptofix 2.2.2 in the routine production of 2-[^{18}F]fluoro-2-deoxy-D-glucose. Appl Radiat Isot 1989;40:741–743.
54. Chaly T, Dahl JR. Thin layer chromatographic detection of kryptofix 2.2.2 in the routine synthesis of [^{18}F]-2-fluoro-deoxyglucose. Nucl Med Biol 1989;16:385–387.
55. Alexoff DL, Casati R, Fowler J, et al. Ion chromatographic analysis of high specific activity ^{18}FDG preparations and detection of the chemical impurity 2-deoxy-2-chloro-D-glucose. Appl Radiat Isot 1992;43:1313–1322.
56. Phelps ME, Hoffman EJ, Coleman RE, et al. Tomographic images of blood pool and perfusion in brain and heart. J Nucl Med 1976; 17:603–612.
57. Chen B, Huang SC, Germano G, et al. Noninvasive quantification of hepatic arterial blood flow with nitrogen-13 ammonia and dynamic positron emission tomography. J Nucl Med 1991; 32:2199–2206.
58. Hayashi N, Tamaki N, Yonekura Y, et al. Imaging of the hepatocellular carcinoma using dynamic positron emission tomography with nitrogen-13 ammonia. J Nucl Med 1985;26:254–257.
59. Marshall R, Tillisch JH, Phelps ME, et al. Identification and differentiation of resting myocardial ischemia and infarction in man with positron computed tomography, F-18 labelled fluorodeoxyglucose and N-13 labelled ammonia. Circulation 1983;67:766–778.
60. Krivokapich J, Smith GT, Huang SC, et al. ^{13}N ammonia myocardial imaging at rest and with exercise in normal volunteers. Circulation 1989;80:1328–1337.
61. Hutchins GD, Schwaiger M, Rosenspire KC, et al. Noninvasive quantification of regional blood flow in the human heart using N-13 ammonia and dynamic positron emission tomographic imaging. J Am Coll Cardiol 1990;15:1032–1042.
62. Cooper A, Gelbard A, Freed B. Nitrogen-13 as a biochemical tracer. In: Meister A, ed. Advances in enzymology and related areas of molecular biology. New York: Wiley and Sons, 1985; 57:251–356.
63. Harper PV, Lathrop KA, Krizek H, Lembares N, Stark V, Hoffer PB. Clinical feasibility of myocardial imaging with $^{13}NH_3$. J Nucl Med 1972;13;278–280.
64. Kuhl DE, Phelps ME, Kowell AP, Metter EJ, Selin C, Winter J. Effects of stroke on local cerebral metabolism and perfusion: mapping by emission computed tomography of ^{18}FDG and $^{13}NH_3$. Ann Neurol 1980;8:47–60.
65. Parodi O, Schelbert HR, Schwaiger M, Hansen H, Selin C, Hoffman EJ. Cardiac emission computed tomography: underestimation of regional tracer concentrations due to wall motion abnormalities. J Comput Assist Tomogr 1984;8:1083–1092.

66. Schelstraete K, Simons M, Deman J, et al. Uptake of ^{13}N-ammonia by human tumours as studied by positron emission tomography. British J Radiol 1982;55:797–804.
67. Yoshida K, Endo M, Himi T, et al. Measurement of regional myocardial blood flow in hypertrophic cardiomyopathy: application of the first-pass flow model using [^{13}N]ammonia and PET. Am J Physiol Imag 1989;4:97–104.
68. Tamaki N, Senda M, Yonekura Y, et al. Dynamic positron computed tomography of the heart with a high sensitivity positron camera and nitrogen-13 ammonia. J Nucl Med 1985;26:567–575.
69. Senda M, Yonekura Y, Tamaki N, et al. Interpolating scan and oblique-angle tomograms in myocardial PET using nitrogen-13 ammonia. J Nucl Med 1986;27:1830–1836.
70. Tamaki N, Yonekura Y, Yamashita K, et al. Value of rest-stress myocardial positron tomography using nitrogen-13 ammonia for the preoperative prediction of reversible asynergy. J Nucl Med 1989;30:1302–1310.
71. United States Pharmacopeia. Ammonia N 13 Injection. USP 1990;22(3rd Suppl):2367–2368.
72. Schelbert HR, Phelps ME, Huang SC, et al. N-13-ammonia as an indicator of myocardial blood flow. Circulation 1981;63:1259–1272.
73. Monahan WG, Tilbury RS, Laughlin RS, et al. Uptake of ^{13}N-labeled ammonia. J Nucl Med 1972;13:274–277.
74. Harper PV, Schwartz V, Beck RN, et al. Clinical myocardial imaging with Nitrogen-13 ammonia. Radiology 1973;108:613–617.
75. The United States Pharmacopeial Convention, Inc. Ammonia N 13 Systemic. Drug Information for the Health Care Professional (DI). Vol. 1. 14th ed. Rockville, MD: United States Pharmacopeial Convention, Inc., 1994:77–79.
76. Walsh W, Harper PV, Resnekov L, Fill H. Noninvasive evaluation of regional myocardial perfusion in 112 patients using a mobile scintillation camera and intravenous nitrogen-13-labeled ammonia. Circulation 1976;54:266–275.
77. Selwyn AP, Allan RM, L'Abbate AL, et al. Relation between regional myocardial uptake of rubidium-82 and perfusion: absolute reduction of cation uptake in ischemia. Am J Cardiol 1982; 50:112–121.
78. Gould KL, Goldstein RA, Mullani NA, et al. Noninvasive assessment of coronary stenoses by myocardial perfusion imaging during pharmacologic coronary vasodilation. VIII. Clinical feasibility of positron cardiac imaging without a cyclotron using generator-produced rubidium-82. Am J Cardiol 1986;7:775–789.
79. Bergmann SR, Herrero P, Markham J, et al. Noninvasive quantitation of myocardial blood flow in human subjects with oxygen-15-labeled water and positron emission tomography. J Am Coll Cardiol; 1989;14:639–652.
80. Walsh MN, Bergmann SR, Steele RL, et al. Delineation of impaired regional myocardial perfusion by positron emission tomography with O-15 water. Circulation 1988;78:612–620.
81. Niemeyer MG, Kuijper AF, Gerhards LJ, D'Haene EG, van der Wall EE. Nitrogen-13 ammonia perfusion imaging: relation to metabolic imaging. Am Heart J 1993;125:848–854.
82. Tilbury RS, Dahl JR, Monahan WG, Laughlin JS. The production of ^{13}N-labeled ammonia for medical use. Radiochem Radioanel Lett 19771;8:317–323.
83. Wieland B, Bida G, Padgett H, et al. In-target production of [^{13}N]ammonia via proton irradiation of dilute aqueous ethanol and acetic acid mixtures. Appl Radiat Isot 1991;42:1095–1098.
84. Ferrieri R, MacDonald K, Schlyer DJ, Wolf AP. Proton irradiation of dilute aqueous ethanol for in-target production of [^{13}N]ammonia: studies on the fate of ethanol. J Label Compds Radiopharm 1993;32:461–463.
85. Nieves E, Rosenspire KC, Filc-DeRicco S, Gelbard AS. High performance liquid chromatographic on-line flow-through radioactivity detection system for analyzing amino acids and metabolites labeled with Nitrogen-13. J Chromatogr 1986;383:325–327.
86. Welch MJ, Straatman MG. The reactions of recoil N-13 atoms with some organic compounds in the solid and liquid phases. Radiochim Acta 1973;20:124–129.
87. Channing MA, Dunn BB, Kiesewetter DO, Plascjak P, Eckelman W. The quality of [^{13}N]ammonia produced by using ethanol as a scavenger. Symposium proceeding of the Tenth International Symposium on Radiopharmaceutical Chemistry, Kyoto, Japan, October 25–28, 1993.
88. Jones T. Introduction—clinical uses of $^{82}Sr/^{82}Rb$ generators. Appl Radiat Isot 1987;38:171–174.
89. MacIntyre WJ, Go RT, King JL, et al. Clinical outcome of cardiac patients with negative thallium-201 SPECT and positive rubidium-82 PET myocardial perfusion imaging. J Nucl Med 1993; 34:400–404.
90. Marwick TH, Cook SA, Lafont A, Underwood DA, Salcedo EE. Influence of left ventricular mass on the diagnostic accuracy of myocardial perfusion imaging using positron emission tomography with dipyridamole stress. J Nucl Med 1991;32:2221–2226.
91. Grover-McKay M, Ratib O, Schwaiger M, et al. Detection of coronary artery disease with positron emission tomography and rubidium-82. Am Heart J 1992;123:646–652.
92. Gould KL. Clinical cardiac positron emission tomography: state of the art. Circulation 1991;84(Suppl):122–136.
93. Stewart RE, Schwaiger M, Molina E, et al. Comparison of rubidium-82 positron emission tomography and thallium-201 SPECT imaging for detection of coronary artery disease. Am J Cardiol 1991;67:1303–1310.
94. Tamaki N, Alpert NM, Rabito CA, Barlai-Kovach M, Correia JA, Strauss HW. The effect of captopril on renal blood flow in renal artery stenosis assessed by positron tomography with rubidium-82. Hypertension 1988;11:217–222.
95. Yen C-K, Yano Y, Budinger TF, et al. Brain tumor evaluation using Rb-82 and positron emission tomography. J Nucl Med 1982; 23:532–537.
96. Jarden JO, Dhawan V, Moeller JR, Strother SC, Rottenberg DA. The time course of steroid action on blood-to-brain and blood-to-tumor transport of ^{82}Rb: a positron emission tomographic study. Ann Neurol 1989;25:239–245.
97. Brooks DJ, Beany RP, Lammertsma AA, et al. Quantitative measurement of blood-brain barrier permeability using rubidium-82 and positron emission tomography. J Cerebral Blood Flow Metab 1984;4:535–545.
98. Yen CK, Budinger TF. Evaluatin of blood-brain barrier permeability changes in rhesus monkeys and man using ^{82}Rb and positron emission tomography. J Comp Asst Tomog 1981;5:792–799.
99. Lammertsma AA, Brooks DJ, Frackowiak RSJ, Heather JD, Jones T. A method to quantitate the fractional extraction of rubidium-82 across the blood-brain barrier using positron emission tomography. J Cerebral Blood Flow Metab 1984;4:523–534.
100. Woods MJ, Judge SM, Lucas SEM. The half-life of ^{82}Rb. Appl Radiat Isot 1987;38:191–192.
101. Judge SM, Woods MJ, Waters SL, Butler KR. A partial decay scheme study of ^{82}Rb and consequences for radiation dose measurements. Appl Radiat Isot 1987;38:185–190.
102. Judge SM, Privitera, Woods MJ. The half-life of ^{82}Sr. Appl Radiat Isot 1987;38:193–194.
103. Hoppes DD, Coursey BM, Schima FJ, Yang D. National Bureau of Standards decay-scheme investigations of strontium-82–rubidium-82. Appl Radiat Isot 1987;38:195–204.
104. Thomas KE. Strontium-82 production at Los Alamos National Laboratory. Appl Radiat Isot 1987;38:175–180.
105. Mausner LF, Prach T, Srivastava SC. Production of ^{82}Sr by proton irradiation of RbCl. Appl Radiat Isot 1987;38:181–184.

106. Squibb Diagnostics. CardioGen-82″ Rubidium Rb 82 Generator product brochure J4-263, January 1990.
107. Neirinckx RD, Cochavi S, Gennaro G, et al. Application of a commercial Sr-82/Rb-82 generator for heart and kidney imaging. Nucl Med Biol Adv 1982;1:613–616.
108. International Commission on Radiological Protection (ICRP). Publication 53: radiation dose to patients from radiopharmaceuticals. Oxford: Pergamon Press, 1987.
109. Matthew E, Andreason P, Carson RE, et al. Reproducibility of resting cerebral blood flow measurements with $H_2\,^{15}O$ positron emission tomography in humans. J Cereb Blood Flow Metab 1993;13:748–754.
110. Quarles RP, Mintun MA, Larson KB, Markham J, MacLeod AM, Raichle ME. Measurement of regional cerebral blood flow with positron emission tomography: a comparison of [^{15}O]water to [^{11}C]butanol with distributed-parameter and compartmental models. J Cereb Blood Flow Metab 1993;13:733–747.
111. Raichle ME, Martin WRW, Herscovitch P, Mintun MA, Markham J. Brain blood flow measured with intravenous $H_2\,^{15}O$. II Implementation and validation. J Nucl Med 1983;24:790–798.
112. Merlet P, Mazoyer B, Hittinger L, et al. Assessment of coronary reserve in man: comparison between positron emission tomography with oxygen-15–labeled water and intracoronary Doppler technique. J Nucl Med 1993;34:1899–1904.
113. Yamamoto Y, de Silva R, Rhodes CG, et al. A new strategy for the assessment of viable myocardium and regional myocardial blood flow using ^{15}O-water and dynamic positron emission tomography. Circulation 1992;86:167–178.
114. de Silva R, Yamamoto Y, Rhodes CG, et al. Preoperative prediction of the outcome of coronary revascularization using positron emission tomography. Circulation 1992;86:1738–1742.
115. Kubo S, Yamamoto K, Magata Y, et al. Assessment of pancreatic blood flow with positron emission tomography and oxygen-15 water. Ann Nucl Med 1991;5:133–138.
116. Wilson CB, Lammertsma AA, McKenzie CG, Sikora K, Jones T. Measurements of blood flow and exchanging water space in breast tumors using positron emission tomography: a rapid and noninvasive dynamic method. Cancer Res 1992;52:1592–1597.
117. Raichle ME, Grubb RL, Gado MH, Eichling JO, Ter-Pogossian NM. Correlation between regional cerebral blood flow and oxidative metabolism. Arch Neurol 1976;33:523–526.
118. Sokoloff L. Relationships among local functional activity, energy metabolism and blood flow in the central nervous system. Fed Proc 1981;40:2311–2316.
119. Yarowsky PJ, Ingvar DH. Neuronal activity and energy metabolism. Fed Proc 1981;40:2353–2362.
120. Cherry SR, Woods RP, Hoffman EJ, Mazziotta JC. Improved detection of focal cerebral blood flow changes using three-dimensional positron emission tomography. J Cereb Blood Flow Metab 1993;13:630–638.
121. Mintun MA, Fox PT, Raichle ME. A highly accurate method of localizing regions of neuronal activation in the human brain with positron emission tomography. J Cereb Blood Flow Metab 1989; 9:96–103.
122. Lavy S, Melamed E, Cooper G, Bentin S, Rinot Y. Regional cerebral blood flow in patients with Parkinson's disease. Arch Neurol 1979;36:344–348.
123. Lenzi GL, Jopnes T, Reid J, Moss S. Regional impairment of cerebral oxidative metabolism in Parkinson's disease. J Neurol Neurosurg Psychiatry 1979;42:59–62.
124. Leenders KL, Wolfson L, Jones T. Cerebral blood flow and oxygen metabolism measurement with positron emission tomography in Parkinson's disease. Monogr Neural Sci 1984;11:180–186.
125. Leenders KL, Wolfson L, Gibbs J, Wise R, Jones T, Legg N. Regional cerebral blood flow and oxygen metabolism in Parkinson's disease and their response to L-dopa. J Cereb Blood Flow Metab 1983;3:S448–489.
126. Welch MJ, Ter-Pogossian MM. Preparation of short half-lived radioactive gases for medical studies. Radiat Res 1968;36:580–587.
127. Clark JC, Buckingham PD. Short lived radioactive gases for clinical use. London: Butterworth & Co., 1975.
128. Welch MJ, Kilbourn MR. A remote system for the routine production of oxygen-15 radiopharmaceuticals. J Labeled Cmpd Radiopharm 1985;22:1193–1200.
129. Jackson JR, Dembowski BS, Ehrenkaufer RL, McIntyre E, Reivich M. [^{15}O]H_2O, [^{15}O]O_2 and [^{15}O]CO gas production, monitoring and quality control system. Appl Radiat Isot 1993;44:631–634.
130. Berridge MS, Terris AH, Cassidy EH. Low-carrier production of [^{15}O]oxygen, water and carbon monoxide. Int J Radiat Appl Instrum 1990;41:1173–1175.
131. Glass HI, Brant A, Clark JC, deGaretta AC, Day LG. Measurement of blood volume using red cells labeled with radioactive carbon monoxide. J Nucl Med 1968;9:571–575.
132. Glass HI, Edwards RHT, deGarreta AC, Clark JC. CO red cell labeling for blood volume and total hemoglobin in athletes: effect of training. J Appl Physiol 1969;26;131–134.
133. Weinreich R, Ritzl F, Feinendegen LE, Schnippering HG, Stocklin G. Fixation, retention and exhalation of carrier-free ^{11}C-labeled carbon monoxide by man. Rad and Environ Biophys 1975; 12:271–280.
134. Brownell GL, Cochavi S. Transverse section imaging with carbon-11 labeled carbon monoxide. J Comp Asst Tomog 1978; 2:533–538.
135. Grubb RL Jr, Raichle M, Higgins CS, Eichling JO. Measurement of regional cerebral blood volume by emission tomography. Ann Neurol 1978;4:322–328.
136. Kearfott KJ. Absorbed dose estimates for positron emission tomography (PET): $C^{15}O$, ^{11}CO, and $CO^{15}O$. J Nucl Med 1982; 23:1031–1037.
137. Del Fiore G, Depresseux JC, Bartsch P, Quaglia L, Peters JM: Production of oxygen-15, nitrogen-13 and carbon-11 and of their low molecular weight derivatives for biomedical applications. Int J Appl Radiat Isot 1979;30:543–549.
138. Christman DR, Finn RD, Karlstrom KI, Wolf AP. The production of ultra-high activity ^{11}C-labeled hydrogen cyanide, carbon dioxide, carbon monoxide and methane via the $^{14}N(p,\alpha)^{11}C$ reaction (XV). Int J Appl Radiat Isot 1975;26:435–442.
139. Shishido F, Tateno Y, Takashima T, Tamachi S, Yamaura A, Yamasaki T. Positron CT imaging using a high resolution PCT device (Positologica-I), ^{11}CO, $^{13}NH_3$, and ^{18}FDG in clinical evaluation of cerebrovascular diseases. Eur J Nucl Med 1984;9:265–271.
140. Buckingham PD, Forse GR. The preparation and processing of radioactive gases for clinical use. Int J Appl Radiat 1963;14:439–445.
141. Lederer CM. Shirley VS, eds. Table of isotopes. 7th ed. New York: John Wiley and Sons, 1978.
142. Wolf AP, Redvanly CS. Carbon-11 and radiopharmaceuticals. Int J Appl Radiat Isot 1977;28:29–48.
143. Clark JC, Buckingham PD. The preparation and storage of carbon-11-labeled gases for clinical use. Int J Appl Radiat Isot 1971; 22:639–646.
144. Goldsmith JR, Landaw SA. Carbon monoxide and human health. Science 1968;162:1352–1359.
145. Grut A, Astrup P, Challen JR, Gerhardsson G. Threshold limit values for carbon monoxide. Arch Environ Health 1970;21:542–544.
146. Dunn BB, Channing MA, Kiesewetter DO. USP standards for C 11 labeled carbon monoxide; stimuli to the revision process. Pharmacopeial Forum 1992;18(6):4414–4415.
147. Ter-Pogossian MM. Short-lived isotopes and positron emitters in medicine. In: Lawrence JH, ed. Progress in atomic medicine. Ch 1. New York: Grune & Stratton, 1965;107–126.

148. Jones SC, Chesler DA, Ter-Pogossian MM. The continuous inhalation of oxygen-15 for assessing regional oxygen extraction in the brain of man. Br J Radiol 1976;49:339–343.
149. Frackowiak RSJ, Lenzi G-L, Jones T, Heather JD. Quantitative measurement of regional cerebral blood flow and oxygen metabolism in man using ^{15}O and positron emission tomography: theory, procedure and normal values. J Comput Assist Tomog 1980; 4:727–736.
150. Subramanyam R, Albert NM, Hoop B Jr, Brownell GL, Taveras JM. A model for regional cerebral oxygen distribution during continuous inhalation of $^{15}O_2$, $C^{15}O$, and $C^{15}O_2$. J Nucl Med 1978;19:48–53.
151. Mintun MA, Raichle ME, Martin WRW, Herscovitch P. Brain oxygen utilization measured with O-15 radiotracers and positron emission tomography. J Nucl Med 1984;25:177–187.
152. Martin WRW, Powers WJ, Raichle ME. Cerebral blood volume measured with inhaled $C^{15}O$ and positron emission tomography. J Cereb Blood Flow Metab 1987;7:421–426.
153. Brown MA, Marshall DR, Sobel BE, Bergmann SR. Delineation of myocardial oxygen utilization with carbon-11-labeled acetate. Circulation 1987;76:687–696.
154. Brown MA, Myears DW, Bergmann SR. Validity of estimates of myocardial oxidative metabolism with carbon-11 acetate and positron emission tomography despite altered patterns of substrate utilization. J Nucl Med 1989;30:187–193.
155. Brown MA, Myears DW, Bergmann SR. Noninvasive assessment of canine myocardial oxidative metabolism with carbon-11 acetate and positron emission tomography. J Am Coll Cardiol 1988; 12:1054–1063.
156. Buxton DB, Schwaiger M, Nguyen A, Phelps ME, Schelbert HR. Radiolabeled acetate as a tracer of myocardial tricarboxylic acid cycle flux. Circ Res 1988;63:628–634.
157. Henes CG, Bergmann SR, Walsh MN, Sobel BE, Gletman EM. Assessment of myocardial oxidative metabolic reserve with positron emission tomography and carbon-11 acetate. J Nucl Med 1989;30:1489–1499.
158. Armbrecht JJ, Buxton DB, Brunken RC, Phelps ME, Schelbert HR. Regional myocardial oxygen consumption determined noninvasively in humans with 1-[^{11}C]acetate and dynamic positron tomography. Circulation 1989;80:863–872.
159. Chan SY, Brunken RC, Phelps ME, Schelbert HR. Use of the metabolic tracer ^{11}C-acetate for evaluation of regional myocardial perfusion. J Nucl Med 1991;32:665–672.
160. Walsh MN, Geltman EM, Brown MA, et al. Noninvasive estimation of regional myocardial oxygen consumption by positron emission tomography with carbon-11 acetate in patients with myocardial infarction. J Nucl Med 1989;30:1798–1808.
161. Kotzerke J, Hicks RJ, Wolfe E, et al. Three-dimensional assessment of myocardial oxidative metabolism: a new approach for regional determination of PET-derived ^{11}C-acetate kinetics. J Nucl Med 1990;31:1876–1893.
162. Miller TR, Wallis JW, Geltman EM, Bergmann SR. Three-dimensional functional images of myocardial oxygen consumption from positron tomography. J Nucl Med 1990;31:2064–2068.
163. Hicks RJ, Kalff V, Savas V, Starling MR, Schwaiger M. Assessment of right ventricular oxidative metabolism by positron emission tomography with C-11 acetate in aortic valve disease. Am J Cardiol 1991;67:753–757.
164. Hicks RJ, Herman WH, Kalff V, et al. Quantitative evaluation of regional substrate metabolism in the human heart by positron emission tomography. J Am Coll Cardiol 1991;18:101–111.
165. Pike VW, Eakins MN, Allan RM, Selwyn AP. Preparation of 1-[^{11}C]acetate—an agent for the study of myocardial metabolism by positron emission tomography. Appl Radiat Isot 1982; 33:505–512.
166. Norenberg JP, Simpson NR, Dunn BB, Kiesewetter DO. Remote synthesis of [^{11}C]acetate. Appl Radiat Isot 1992;43:943–945.
167. Firnau G, Garnett ES, Sourkes TL, Missala K. [^{18}F]-Fluorodopa: a unique γ-emitting substrate for dopa decarboxylase. Experimentia 1975:31:1254–1255.
168. Garnett ES, Firnau G, Nahmias C. Dopamine visualized in the basal ganglia of living man. Nature 1983;305:137–138.
169. Chiueh CC, Zukowska-Grojec Z, Kirk KL, Kopin IJ. 6-Fluorocatecholamines as false adrenergic neurotransmitters. J Pharmacol Exp Ther 1983;225:529–533.
170. Martin WRW, Adam MJ, Bergstom M, Ammann W. In vivo study of dopa metabolism in Parkinson's disease. In: Fahn S, Marsden CD, Jenner P, Teychenne P, eds. Recent developments in Parkinson's disease. New York: Raven Press, 1986:97–102.
171. Chiueh CC, Kirk KL, Channing MA, Kessler RM. Neurochemical basis of the use of 6–F-dopa for visualizing dopamine neurons in the brain by the positron emission tomography. Neurosci Abs 1984;10:883.
172. Anden NE, Carlsson A, Dahlstom A, Fuxe K, Hillarp NA, Larsson K. Demonstration and mapping out of nigro-neostriatal dopamine neurons. Life Sci 1964;3:523–530.
173. Firnau G, Sood S, Chiral R. Cerebral metabolism of 6-[^{18}F]fluoro-L-3,4-dihydroxyphenylalanine in the primate. J Neurochem 1987;48:1077–1082.
174. Firnau G, Garnett ES, Chan PKH, Belbeck KW. Intracerebral dopamine metabolism studies by a novel radioisotope technique. J Pharm Pharmacol 1976;28:584–585.
175. Firnau G, Garnett ES, Marshall AM, Seeman P, Tedesco J, Kirk KL. Effects of fluoro-dopamines on dopamine receptors (D1, D2, D3 sites). Biochem Pharmacol 1981;30:2927–2930.
176. Garnett ES, Firnau G, Nahmias C, Chirakal R. Striatal dopamine metabolism in living monkeys examined by positron emission tomography. Brain Res 1983;280:169–171.
177. Garnett ES, Firnau G, Nahmias C. Dopamine visualized in the basal ganglia of living man. Nature 1983;305:137–138.
178. Martin WRW, Palmer MR, Patlak CS, Calne DB. Nigrostriatal function in humans studies with positron emission tomography. Ann Neurol 1989:26:535–546.
179. Garnett ES, Nahmias C, Firnau G. Central dopaminergic pathways in hemiparkinsonism examined by positron emission tomography. Can J Neurol Sci 1984;11:174–179.
180. Bianchine JR. Drugs for Parkinson's disease centrally acting muscle relaxants. In: Gilman AG, ed. The pharmacological basis of therapeutics. New York: MacMillian Publishing Co., 1980:472–482.
181. Boyes BE, Cumming P, Martin WRW, McGeer EG. Determination of plasma [^{18}F]-6-fluorodopa during positron emission tomography; elimination and metabolism in carbidopa treated subjects. Life Sci 1986;39:2243–2252.
182. Martin WRW, Stoessl AJ, Adam MJ. Positron emission tomography in Parkinson's disease: glucose and dopa metabolism. In: Yahr MD, Bergmann KJ, eds. Advances in neuorology: Parkinson's disease. New York: Raven Press, 1986;45:95–98.
183. Leenders KL. Parkinson's disease and PET tracer studies. J Neural Transm 1988;27:219–225.
184. Leenders K, Palmer A, Turton D. DOPA uptake and dopamine receptor binding visualized in the human brain in vivo. In: Fahn S, Marsden CD, Jenner P, Teychenne P, eds. Recent developments in Parkinson's disease. New York: Raven Press 1986:103–114.
185. Lang, AE, Garnett ES, Firnau G, Nahmias C, Talalla A. Positron tomography in dystonia. Adv Neurol 1988;50:249–253.
186. Leenders KL, Frackowiak SJ, Quinn N, Marsden CD. Brain energy metabolism and dopaminergic function in Huntington's disease measured in vivo using positron emission tomography. Movement Disorders 1986;1:69–77.
187. Adam MJ, Ruth TJ, Grierson JR, Abeysekera B, Pate BD. Routine synthesis of L-[^{18}F]6-fluorodopa with fluorine-18 acetyl hypofluorite. J Nucl Med 1986;27:1462–1466.

188. Cumming P, Hausser M, Martin WRW, et al. Kinetics of in vitro decarboxylation and the in vivo metabolism of 2-[^{18}F] and 6-[^{18}F]fluorodopa in the hooded rat. Biochem Pharm 1988;37:247–250.
189. Luxen A, Perlmutter M, Bida G. Remote, semiautomated production of 6-[^{18}F]fluoro-L-dopa for human studies with PET. Appl Radiat Isot 1990;41:275–281.
190. Luxen A, Guillaume M, Melega WP, Pike VW, Solin O, Wagner R. Production of 6-[^{18}F]fluoro-L-dopa and its metabolism in vivo—a critical review. Nucl Med Biol 1992;19:149–158.
191. Casella V, Ido T, Wolf AP, Fowler JS, MacGregor RR, Ruth TJ. Anhydrous F-18-labeled elemental fluorine for radiopharmaceutical preparation. J Nucl Med 1980;21:750–757.
192. Chen J, Huang S, Finn R. Quality control procedure for 6-[^{18}F]fluoro-L-dopa: a presynaptic PET imaging ligand for brain dopamine neurons. J Nucl Med 1989;30:1249–1256.
193. Pike VW, Kensett MJ, Tuton DR, Waters SL, Silvester DJ. Labelled agents for PET studies of the dopaminergic system—some quality assurance methods, experience and issues. Appl Radiat Isot 1990;41:483–492.
194. Dunn B, Channing M, Adams H, Goldstein D, Kirk K, Kiesewetter D. A single column, rapid quality control procedure for 6-[^{18}F]fluoro-L-dopa and [^{18}F]fluorodopamine PET imaging agents. Nucl Med Biol 1991;18:209–213.
195. Coenen HH, Franken K, Kling P, Stocklin G. Direct electrophilic radiofluorination of phenylalanine, tyrosine and dopa. Appl Radiat Isot 1988;39:1243–1250.
196. Luxen A, Barrio JR, Van Moffaert G, Perlmutter M, Cook JC, Phelps ME. Remote, semiautomated production of 6–[^{18}F]fluoro-L-dopa for human studies with PET. Seventh International Symposium on Radiopharmaceutical Chemistry. Groningen, Netherlands, 4–8 July, 1988.
197. Dunn BB, Channing MA, Regdos S, Kiesewetter DO. Issues concerning quality control of five routinely used PET imaging compounds. Fourth European Symposium on Radiopharmacy and Radiopharmaceuticals. Baden, Switzerland, May 1991.
198. Sachs C, Jonsson G. Selective 6-hydroxy-dopa induced degeneration of central and peripheral noradrenalin neurons. Brain Res 1972;40:563–568.
199. Gunther K, Martens J, Schickedanz M. Resolution of optical isomers by thin layer chromatography (TLC). Enantiomeric purity of L-dopa. Z Anal Chem 1985;322:513–514.
200. Dunn BB, Kiesewetter DO. Stability of 6-[^{18}F]fluorodopa preparations [Letter; Comment]. J Nucl Med 1991;32:894.
201. Goldstein DS, Eisenhofer G, Dunn BB, et al. Positron emission tomographic imaging of cardiac sympathetic innervation using 6-[^{18}F]fluorodopamine: initial findings in humans. J Am Coll Cardiol 22;1993:1961–1971.
202. Ding YS, Fowler JS, Gately SJ, Dewey SL, Wolf AP, Schlyer DJ. Synthesis of high specific activity 6-[^{18}F]fluorodopamine for positron emission tomography studies of sympathetic nervous tissue. J Med Chem 1991;43:861–863.
203. Adams HR, Channing MA, Divel JJ, et al. Trend analysis of quality control data. American Chemical Society Symposium on "Chemists Views of Imaging Centers." Chicago, IL, August 22–27, 1993.
204. Tajima K, Nakamura M, Takagi S, Kai F, Osajima Y. Analysis of mercury (II) halides by reverse-phase ion-pair chromatography. J Liquid Chromatog 1986;9:1021–1032.

17 Receptor Site Imaging

WILLIAM C. ECKELMAN

The greatest strength of nuclear medicine lies in its ability to detect and quantitate biologic function rather than fixed anatomic properties. These functional studies can be divided into two categories: the determination of tissue blood flow and the determination of biochemistry. Many of the radiopharmaceuticals used in routine clinical diagnosis measure changes in blood flow to an organ as a function of disease. The gold standard for tissue blood flow measurements in experimental animals is usually radiolabeled microspheres that are extracted by the capillary vessels with an extraction fraction of 1. This extraction fraction is independent of flow. Many radiopharmaceuticals are compared to microspheres over a range of blood flows expected in normal and diseased tissues. For example, cationic salts of the Group 1 alkali metals potassium, rubidium, and cesium, and the group III element thallium are indicators of blood flow and correlate with microspheres in a linear fashion over a limited range (1). Certainly, ^{99m}Tc macroaggregated albumin, having an identical mechanism of localization as microspheres, is a measure of blood flow to the lung (2). Likewise, the extraction of colloid by the phagocytic cells in the liver is flow dependent (3). In the case of reduced flow (e.g., cirrhosis and hepatitis), the uptake of ^{99m}Tc sulfur colloid is decreased proportionally (4). ^{131}I *o*-iodohippurate (Hippuran) is also used to measure effective renal plasma flow because of its high extraction by the kidneys (5). Blood flow in two major target tissues, the myocardium and the cerebrum with a normal blood-brain barrier, can now be studied with ^{99m}Tc-labeled compounds. In the heart, ^{201}Tl is the thallous cation is most often used. However, ^{99m}Tc cations, such as hexakis (2-methoxy-2-methylpropyl) isonitrile (sestamibi) and neutral ^{99m}Tc complexes such as [bis[1,2-cyclohexanedionedioximato(1′)-O]-1,2-cyclohexane-dione-dioximato (2-O) methylborato(2)-N,N′,-N′′,N′′′,N′′′′,N′′′′′] chlorotechnetium (teboroxime) (6–8), are being used as myocardial perfusion agents. ^{133}Xe is approved by the United States Food and Drug Administration (FDA) for the measurement of cerebral perfusion. In 1989, ^{123}I-labeled N-isopropylamphetamine (9) (Spectamine) became the second commercially available agent that crosses the intact blood-brain barrier. The distribution immediately after injection is flow related, but the immediate uptake and later distribution are dependent on amine uptake processes. Several neutral ^{99m}Tc-labeled compounds are available for measuring cerebral blood flow in disease states in which the blood-brain barrier is intact. The series of propyleneamineoximes are interesting cerebral perfusion agents (10). Whereas ^{99m}Tc PNAO (propyleneamine oxime) is taken up efficiently and released from the cerebrum rapidly, a derivative, ^{99m}Tc, d,l hexamethylpropyleneamine oxime (HMPAO) is taken up and retained.

In recent years, research emphasis has been placed on tracers that predominately measure biochemistry. This emphasis has occurred for a number of reasons: the competition of other imaging modalities for anatomic definition, the success in measuring biochemical pathways using both positron emitting and single photon emitting radiopharmaceuticals, and the improvements in both positron emission tomography and single photon emission computed tomography. Many new imaging modalities, such as x-ray computed tomography, ultrasound, and nuclear magnetic resonance imaging, are better suited to analyze anatomic changes. On the other hand, the success with compounds such as ^{18}F-2-fluorodeoxyglucose (11) in measuring glucose metabolism demonstrates that in vivo biochemical tracers are possible.

DEFINITION OF RECEPTOR

Several classes of radiotracers can be studied. Of these classes, receptor-binding radiotracers are especially interesting in that changes in receptor concentration are thought to be related to certain disease states. Throughout the history of science, investigators have realized that there must be a substance that imparts specificity to a particular cell type. Ehrlich (12) realized this in his study of the interaction of antigens with specific, complementary, preformed "receptors."

Many important biologic functions are controlled by receptors, and many changes in receptor concentration as a function of disease have been noted. There are only a few structural determinations of receptors. As a result, the definition of a receptor is operational (13) and is determined by certain properties observed in vitro. The usual criteria are high ligand affinity, specificity, saturability, and distribution in relation to physiologic response. The determination of those properties has been made possible by the development of high specific activity radiotracers. In general, receptor protein is present in limited concentration, about 10^{-7}–10^{-10} mol/liter in homogenized tissue. Therefore, the receptor is easily saturated by the appropriate ligand. Specificity and high ligand affinity are closely related because, by the nature of the high affinity between the receptor and the ligand, specificity results. Often, ligands at high concentration can cause physiologic effects at numerous receptor sites, but are specific for only one receptor at low concentration. In vivo tests for saturability require the administration of a physiologically active amount of the biochemical or drug which would probably be unacceptable for a routine diagnostic procedure because of possible toxicity. The final criterion is that the binding of the ligand to the sites can be related to the biologic effect of the ligand. Experimentally, this is shown by comparing the affinity of various ligands with their in vivo biologic effect. If a correlation is obtained, then the receptor is defined. In the radiotracer context, the distribution of the receptor is determined in vivo and correlated with the known distribution of receptors from biologic studies in vivo or from in vitro assays of various organs and tissues. In general, receptor-binding radiotracers offer an area of research that allows the noninvasive monitoring of the change in receptor as a function of disease.

CHOICE OF A RECEPTOR SYSTEM

The choice of a receptor system must be made on both chemical and clinical grounds. There is no value in developing a receptor-binding radiotracer for a clinically important receptor disease if the radiotracer does not concentrate in the target tissue in an amount such that an external image can be obtained. Although this requirement may seem obvious, there were a number of cases in which low-affinity radiotracers were prepared, only to discover that the fraction of the radioligand binding to the target receptor is very low.

CHEMICAL BASIS: MATHEMATIC MODEL

The chemical basis of choosing a receptor system is made easier by using relatively simple equations, for example, the Scatchard transformation of the second-order binding equation (14):

$$B/F = KR_0 - KB;$$

when $R_0 > L$ then $B/F = KR_0$ = target/background (17)
In conditions of high specific activity, the bound-to-free ratio (B/F), which in vivo would be the maximal target-to-nontarget ratio, can be estimated by the product of the affinity constant (K) and the receptor concentration (R_0) when the radioligand concentration (L) is small compared to R_0. This equation is an easy rule of thumb that appears to hold for most of the receptor systems. Although this is an equilibrium equation, it appears that the kinetic expression reduces to a similar form under specific conditions (15).

Using this rule of thumb ($B/F = KR_0$), it becomes clear that agonists for biogenic amine receptors usually do not have large enough affinity constants to permit external imaging. Some antagonists do have affinity constants large enough to produce reasonable ratios. However, the balance in nature is such that most antagonists barely have high enough affinity to achieve a B/F ratio of 10 for receptor concentrations in the range of 10^{-7}–10^{-9} mol/liter. Nonspecific binding, or more precisely nonreceptor binding, also plays a major role in the target-to-nontarget ratio.

CLINICAL BASIS

An exponential increase has occurred in the number of publications relating a change in receptor concentration to a particular drug therapy or disease state. Many reviews on the clinical importance of receptor concentration have been written by Wagner (16), Gibson (17), Melnechuk (18), Blecher and Bar (19), Clayton (20), and others (21). From the reviews, one can easily recognize the vast clinical potential open to receptor binding radiotracers. In general, many hormones (insulin, growth hormone, luteinizing hormone-human chorionic gonadotropin, thyrotropin-releasing hormone, glucagon, vasopressin, catecholamines, and calcitonin) are able to decrease the number of receptors by a feedback mechanism often described as down regulation. Two receptor systems are being imaged routinely in nuclear medicine. Transferrin receptors are imaged using ^{67}Ga-citrate (see Chapter 67) and somatostatin receptors are imaged using ^{111}In octreotide (see Chapter 55). Two examples of other receptor systems are given here.

Steroid Hormone Receptors

Estrogen receptor-binding radiotracers have perhaps the greatest potential clinical utility, and, therefore, estrogen receptors are one of the most studied receptors. There have been numerous reports dating to 1896 that endocrine ablation induces breast tumor regression in certain patients (22). The development of high specific activity tritiated estradiol by Jensen and Jacobson (23) led to the routine determination of estrogen receptors in breast tumors prior to antiestrogen therapy (24). Nearly 60% of primary breast cancer and 55% of metastatic lesions contain estrogen receptors, and approximately 55–60% of patients exhibiting detectable estrogen receptors respond to ablative or hormone therapy. Conversely, if estrogen receptors are not present, then the response rate to ablative therapy is only 5–10%.

Muscarinic Acetylcholine Receptor

The muscarinic receptor appears to play an essential role in many physiologic or behavioral responses (25). For example, the muscarinic receptor has been implicated as a factor in Alzheimer's dementia. Analysis of postmortem brain shows a conservation of M1 subtype receptors, but a significant reduction in the quantity of M2 subtype in cortical regions (26).

RADIOTRACERS FOR THE DETERMINATION OF RECEPTOR DENSITY CHANGES

Comar, et al. (27), reviewed the positron-emitting, receptor-binding radiotracers. They list more than 25 radiotracers that have been synthesized. Additional receptor-binding radiotracers were added to this list in general reviews by Fowler and Wolf (28), Eckelman (29), Stocklin (30), and Eckelman (31). Many have been validated in animals as receptor-binding radiotracers. Some have been validated in animals as sensitive probes for a change in radioactivity as a function of a change in receptor concentration, but, at the time of this writing, few have been shown to be sensitive probes in humans.

There are four criteria for producing radioligands sensitive to changes in binding site concentration (32).

1. Find a binding site change as a function of a specific disease based on in vitro literature or surrogate measurements in vivo.
2. Develop a radiolabeled biochemical that binds preferentially to the chosen binding site.
3. Determine the sensitivity of the radiotracer to a change in the binding site concentration.

4. Determine if the sensitivity of the radiotracer matches the changes expected in the specific disease.

Many radiotracers bind to the target either by ionic or covalent interactions. In general, the pharmaceutical literature points to many compounds that have nM binding affinities. Although the binding site concentration is generally ignored in this search, the B/F ratio is usually sufficient if the affinity constant is subnanomolar. In fact, if the affinity is too strong, the radiopharmaceutical will measure flow or permeability surface area rather than biochemical changes. Targeting (criterion 2) is a necessary, but not sufficient, criterion for the development of a receptor binding radiopharmaceutical. To complete the development of the ideal radiotracer, the sensitivity of the radiotracer to a change in the binding site concentration must be determined (criterion 3).

SPECIFIC ACTIVITY

Because of the potential clinical application for receptor-binding radiotracers, much effort has been made in the synthesis and purification of these compounds. The synthetic procedure must be carried out with high specific activity radiotracer without added carrier. Additionally, the effective specific activity of the product must be high (about 1000 Ci (37,000 GBq)/mmol). Therefore, elaborate separation schemes must be developed to separate all nonradioactive receptor-active material from the product. Separation schemes are usually performed using reversed-phase high-performance liquid chromatography. If the starting material elutes before the desired product—the most likely order for halogenated radiotracers—then the relatively large amounts of starting material can contaminate the radiolabeled products even if the elution volumes differ by large amounts.

There have been reports that the specific activity of ^{11}C does not attain theoretic maximum when separated as CO or CO_2 because of contamination of solvents, gases, and pump oil with these oxides (33). Even for ^{11}C HCN, the ratio of ^{11}C to ^{12}C is 1:3000 and for ^{11}C HCHO 1:8000 (34). Few radioligands are actually produced at the theoretical specific activity of the no-carrier-added radionuclide (35).

IN VITRO ASSAYS

With ^{11}C compounds in which the ^{11}C replaces a stable carbon, there is no need to prove that the radiolabeled compound has the same properties as the parent compound. However, with halogenated derivatives or compounds labeled with ^{99m}Tc, the properties of the new derivative must be ascertained relative to the parent structure. Very few biochemicals and drugs used in clinical medicine actually concentrate exclusively in the target organ, that is, the dream of a "magic bullet" has not been realized. In fact, most drugs and biochemicals have low target-to-blood ratios, often less than 10. Therefore, any decrease in the localization caused by substitution, either by a halogen or a metallic radionuclide, can cause a decrease in specificity that makes the radioligand useless. The substitution of the halogen or metal must be made in a portion of the molecule that does not interact with the receptor. This is often a difficult task for two reasons. First, the sensitive and insensitive parts of the molecule must be determined. Much effort has gone into so-called structure-activity relationships, but their predictive value is continually questioned (36, 37). Second, the synthesis and purification of a derivative substituted in a part of the molecule that will not affect the receptor interaction is a difficult task. Much synthetic effort has gone into the development of the relatively few successful receptor-binding radiotracers. This is especially true for ^{99m}Tc.

The choice of radionuclide is based not only on the perturbation to the parent drug or biochemical and the ease of synthesis but also on the nuclear properties. ^{11}C and ^{18}F are positron-emitting radionuclides and have the advantage of using imaging systems that can quantify the amount of radioactivity in vivo. However, the half-life of ^{11}C might be too short for measuring biologic phenomena. Additionally, both radionuclides are only available from a cyclotron. The single photon-emitting radionuclides are more generally available, but with regard to regional quantitation the imaging devices for them are not as advanced.

In vitro studies using radioreceptor assays have been very helpful in determining the properties of the new radiolabeled derivative. Often, the in vitro test is carried out using the nonradioactive halogenated compound. The radioactive compound is usually much more difficult to prepare because of the special requirement of high specific activity that necessitates reactions at low molarity and extensive purification of the product.

ANIMAL DISTRIBUTION STUDIES

The distribution of radiolabeled compounds is usually determined in small animals. Similarities between the distribution of the radiolabeled derivative and the ^{3}H-labeled substrate are considered as proof that receptor binding is the major cause of the localization. Likewise, similarities between the distribution of the radiotracer and a theoretic model are also considered as proof. Both of these considerations must be accepted with caution because distribution is only one criterion in the operational definition of a receptor.

VALIDATION OF RECEPTOR BINDING

The other criteria that distinguish receptor binding from other types of binding are saturability and stereospecificity. For example, the binding of ^{3}H (*R*)-QNB to the muscarinic cholinergic receptor in heart and brain in vitro has been well-documented (38–40). The burden of proof for receptor binding is based on the pharmacologic profile whereby agonists and antagonists are used in the in vitro assay and the relative binding affinity is compared with physiologic response. To this can be added the criterion of stereoselectivity. For example, the *R* and *S* isomers of QNB were shown to have affinity constants in vitro that differ by a factor of 58 in caudate-putamen and by a factor of 153 in ventricular muscle preparations (40). The proof that ^{3}H (*R*)-QNB is binding to the muscarinic receptor in vivo is shown by the difference in displacement of ^{3}H (*R*)-QNB by the *R* and *S* isomer of QNB. Again, the competition appears to be stereoselective, with the more active isomer causing the greater displacement (40). From these experiments, one can conclude that the distribution of QNB both in vitro and in vivo is determined by the muscarinic receptor.

Another proof of receptor binding is to demonstrate the saturability of the binding either by a preinjection, a coinjection, or a postinjection of a saturating amount of receptor-binding ligand. These experiments are more difficult to perform and interpret because the injection of pharmacologic amounts can perturb various pharmacokinetic factors other than receptor binding. Coinjection of QNB with ^{125}I (*R*)-IQNB (40) or coinjection of estradiol with 11β-methoxy-17α (^{125}I) iodovinylestradiol (41) decreased the concentration of radioactivity in the receptor-containing organs by a significant factor compared to control animals. The use of a posttracer-injection of nonradioactive estradiol displaced only 50% of the ^{125}I localized in the uterus of immature rats (41). The interpretation of these data in terms of percentage receptor binding is not straightforward and further clarification is necessary to transfer techniques used in vitro to in vivo animal studies.

Qualitative and Quantitative Indicator of Receptor Concentration Change

Although there is some added information in being able to quantify the concentration of receptors in breast cancer, good correlation is still obtained using a straightforward positive or negative interpretation with 10 fmol/mg protein as the cutoff point (42). The estrogen receptor-binding radiotracer would fall into this category. One clinical study has been published using 16α-(^{77}Br)-bromoestradiol (43). Eight patients were studied following the intravenous administration of 4 mCi (148 MBq) ^{77}Br. In vitro estrogen assays of the primary tumor were performed for comparison. Two patients were on tamoxifen therapy and, therefore, the negative scan results were expected. But three of the four patients who had estrogen-dependent breast cancer also had positive scans. There is also preliminary evidence that ^{18}F-labeled 16α-fluoroestradiol can be used to detect estrogen receptors (44). The radiolabeled steroids demonstrate the general guideline of the B/F ratio. Katzenellenbogen's group (45) pursued such radiotracers for many years. They have correlated the affinity constant and both receptor binding and nonreceptor binding with the uptake in receptor containing organs. Aldosterone is considered to bind to Type I and Type II rat receptors with Kd values of 2.8–3.5 and 33–47 nM. Estrogens, progestins, and androgens have much higher in vitro, as well as in vivo, affinities for their receptors. For example, estradiol has a 0.1 nM affinity for rat uterine estrogen receptor, R5020 has a 0.41 nM affinity for the rat uterine progestin receptor, and R1881 has a 0.6 nM affinity for the rat prostate androgen receptor. The comparable receptor concentrations are 1000 fmol/mg for estrogen and 800 fmol/mg for progestins in the immature rat uterus, 120 fmol/mg for the androgen receptor, and 140–200 fmol/mg for Type II aldosterone receptors in the hippocampus. The B/F ratio is 10,000 for estradiol, 1,951 for R5020, 200 for androgen, and about the same for aldosterone.

These relationships predict the results obtained in the human studies. The most selective PET radiotracer for estrogen receptor is 16α-[^{18}F] fluoro-17β-estradiol (FES). Uptake in the tumor shows a good correlation with estrogen receptor concentration determined by in vitro assay (46). The same investigators later found that metastases of breast carcinoma can be detected with FES. A decrease in the tumor uptake of FES occurred after treatment with antiestrogen drugs. For progestin binding ligands, there was no correlation between tumor uptake and in vitro values (47). The affinity of the progestin (21-[^{18}F] fluoro-16α-ethyl-19-norprogesterone, FENP) is high but the binding potential is not as high as that for FES. Additionally, the nonreceptor binding is high as a result of its higher lipophilicity and perhaps its lower binding potential.

Vera, et al. (48), investigated a receptor system based on the recognition and binding of specific carbohydrate sequences. They chose hepatic binding protein and studied the interaction of iodine- and technetium-labeled glycoproteins. Their early studies were with ^{99m}Tc asialoceruloplasmin for hepatic imaging in rabbits (49). For human studies they used albumin substituted with galactose moieties, which they call neogalactoalbumin (NGA). The number of galactose moieties conjugated to the albumin determines the rate of clearance by altering the affinity constant and possibly various transport phenomena. They have developed a kinetic model to calculate the receptor concentration in the liver given the other system parameters. The model allows blood flow effects to be separated from binding parameters if the two are the same order of magnitude in units of reciprocal time. Because hepatic blood flow cannot easily be changed, this equality is brought about by altering the affinity constant of NGA. The pharmacokinetic model analyzes binding data to determine the receptor concentration. Second-order kinetics are established by using relatively large quantities of ^{99m}Tc NGA. This approach is most useful in those receptor systems that have relatively innocuous substrates.

A number of patients have been studied with this agent (48, 50–53). The amount of radioactivity in the liver as a function of time is analyzed. The first portion of the curve is related to blood flow, the second to excretory function/metabolism. A computer program to analyze these curves has been written (54). Of the patients studied, which include patients with hepatomas, metastatic ovarian cancer, breast metastases, and severe chronic hepatic dysfunction, those with normal parameters of flow and receptor concentration seemed to have the highest survival time.

The muscarinic acetylcholine receptor (m-AChR) is another receptor system that has been studied in a limited number of patients. Over 10 years ago, R-3-quinuclidinyl-4-iodobenzilate [(*R*)-4-IQNB] has been prepared using ^{123}I or ^{125}I (55). The product is a mixture of two stereoisomers because of the unresolved optically active center in the benzilate moiety. The distribution was studied in rats and validated as receptor mediated by coinjecting 50 nmol of QNB (56). ^{3}H-labeled (*R*)-QNB was used as a control. The distribution of the two radiotracers is qualitatively similar. More ^{125}I is detected in the lungs than ^{3}H. This site of loss for 4-IQNB is probably due to the increased lipophilicity caused by the addition of an iodine atom. As a result, the concentration of ^{125}I was lower in target organs, such as cerebrum and heart, when compared to ^{3}H. The experiments using 50 nmol of coinjected (*R, S*)-QNB support the hypothesis that the distribution is primarily receptor mediated by demonstrating the saturability of the binding sites. Previously, ^{3}H (*R*)-QNB binding in rat brain and heart was shown to decrease, compared to the control, when 50 nmol of the pharmacologically active isomer (*R*)-QNB was coinjected with ^{3}H (*R*)-QNB, but was not decreased when the inactive isomer (*S*)-QNB was used. This stereoselective competition adds support to a receptor-mediated mechanism of localization in vivo (40).

With ^{3}H (*R*)-QNB, the striatum-to-cerebellum ratio is approximately 1 in vivo, whereas in vitro it is 603:51 in units of picomoles per gram protein in homogenized rat brain (57). With ^{125}I (*R*)-4-IQNB, we observed an increased striatum-to-cerebellum ratio because of an increased offrate of ^{125}I (*R*)-4-IQNB in the cerebellum. The concentration of radioactivity in the striatum and cerebellum at each time point is a complex function of blood flow, rate constants, and receptor concentration. The receptor concentration can only be obtained by employing a pharmacokinetic model.

Conversely, in cat and dog studies using 4-IQNB we observed radioactivity in the cerebrum but not in the cerebellum. The concentration of m-AChR has not been determined in cats, but in dogs is 475 pmol/g protein in the caudate nucleus, 147 in the thalamus, 57 in the hypothalamus, and 36 in the cerebellar cortex (58). In humans, the concentration in the caudate is 950 pmol/g protein, 707 in the putamen, and 15 in the cerebellar hemisphere, as determined by Wastek and Yamamura (59). Enna, et al. (60), determined that the concentration of m-AChR was 480 pmol/g protein in the caudate and 472 pmol/g in the putamen, but could not find m-AChR in the cerebellum. Nordström, et al., determined that the cerebral cortex of untreated patients contained 500 pmol/g protein (61). The cerebrum was detected using ^{123}I (*R*)-4-IQNB in humans, but not the cerebellum. If the latter values of Enna, et al., are accurate, then the high caudate putamen-to-cerebellum ratio obtained in images of dogs, cats, and humans are understandable.

A comparison of the distribution of a flow-mediated agent, such as ^{123}I-labeled HIPDM, with ^{123}I (*R*)-4-IQNB (56) suggests that the uptake of ^{123}I (*R*)-4-IQNB is receptor mediated in humans. Single photon emission computed tomography using a ring system showed good definition of the caudate putamen area and the cerebral cortex in humans (56). These data indicate that receptor-binding radiotracers can be used to visualize m-AChR by external imaging.

One patient with Alzheimer's disease has been studied by Holman and colleagues (62). The control study using a cerebral perfusion agent showed a defect in the temporoparietal cortex, whereas the study using ^{123}I (*R*)-4-IQNB did not show the same defect. Because the kinetic sensitivity of IQNB has not been demonstrated yet, the small decrease that was detected could be due to relative insensitivity to change in receptor as a function of disease or to a relatively normal concentration of receptor despite a profound decrease in blood flow. The most interesting data are that of Weinberger, et al. (63), who have shown a very high sensitivity to the change in receptor concentration using the data from a single image collected 21 hours after injection of [^{123}I] 4-IQNB. In numerous studies in man, there are various cases of differences in distribution of radiotracers measuring perfusion, glucose metabolism, and mACh receptor concentration, which indicate, in a preliminary sense, that 4-IQNB is a sensitive probe of mAChR concentration and may be useful in detecting and monitoring diseases related to change in this receptor system. This biochemical probe, 4-IQNB, is presently being used in a number of clinical studies, mainly in patient populations with dementia.

The development of a receptor binding radiotracer is a two-part problem: (a) the development of a radioligand that has a high receptor-to-nonreceptor binding and fulfills the operational definition, and (b) the development of an analytic technique that shows a high sensitivity between the radioactivity in the target organ and the receptor concentration. Many experiments have been done to support the former, but few have been done to support the latter. The kinetic analysis has involved two approaches: (a) the use of a high specific activity radioligand, and (b) the use of a low specific activity ligand or the ligand at varying specific activities.

In a conference on receptor binding radiotracers, Krohn et al. (49), put forth the hypothesis that the maximum sensitivity to receptor concentration change will come at ligand-to-receptor ratios of between 0.2 and 0.8. The ability to separate mathematically the total receptor concentration from the rate of ligand-receptor binding was also related to the receptor saturation level, but in most cases investigators have treated the product of the receptor concentration and the binding rate constant as a single variable. The assumption that the binding rate constant has not changed in disease addresses the latter issue, but the former issue is still a major point of discussion. The sensitivity of determining receptor concentration change is best studied using simulations because there are few animal models in which the receptor concentration can be systematically changed. An elegant analysis was done by Vera, et al. (64), that shows the coefficient of variation in the measurement of receptor concentration as a function of the binding affinity and the fractional receptor saturation. The receptor concentration is more precisely determined at higher fractional receptor saturation. The precision of determining receptor concentration has a parabolic dependence on the binding rate constant. At low ligand-receptor binding rate constant, the fraction of receptor binding to nonreceptor binding is low. At a very high rate constant, the radioactivity determined in the target organ is independent of receptor concentration, and the rate-determining step becomes the flow or membrane transport rather than the ligand-receptor binding process.

Friedman, et al. (65), and Farde, et al. (66), both used thermodynamic equilibrium to describe the binding process. Their studies show the same results as obtained by, Vera et al. (64): the sensitivity to receptor change is maximal at about 50% saturation.

The use of high specific activity ligands to estimate the receptor concentrations was first developed on an empirical basis using ^{3}H ligands. Wagner, et al. (67), used the same approach and found that the slope of the tissue ratio versus time plot changed as a function of age. They used the D_2 receptor binding ligand ^{11}C-*N*-methylspiperone and postulated that the D_2 receptor decreases as a function of age (68). The analysis can be derived from basic principles, as was done by Patlak and Blasberg (69), for an irreversible binding ligand, and then applied to the three-compartment model.

The current trend in receptor binding radiotracer design is to choose compounds that are in steady state at some defined time after administration as a bolus or administration by an infusion to reach steady state (70). For some time, there were attempts to apply the equilibrium equations describing binding studies carried out in vitro to the distribution of radiopharmaceuticals in vivo. These relationships were used both to screen compounds before radiolabeling and to analyze the pharmacokinetics in vivo to determine the binding potential. In the first application, the Scatchard form of the law of mass action is used (71–75). At high specific activity, the Bound (B) to Free (F) ratio is equal to the product of the Equilibrium Constant (K_A) and the Binding Site Concentration (B_{max}).

$$\frac{B}{F} = K_A \times B_{\max} - K_A \times B \sim K_A \times B_{\max}$$

The higher the K_A and/or the B_{max}, then the better the chance of achieving a B/F ratio of ≥ 10 which is generally considered a reasonable goal for external planar imaging, whereas a lower ratio is required for tomography (76). Eckelman and Gibson (77) recently reviewed the applicability of this approach for nononcologic radiopharmaceuticals. In the second application, these equations are used to analyze the change in B_{max} or binding potential (78) from in vivo data. The equation describing in vitro binding applies to in vivo studies when the distribution is in steady state, i.e., the clearance (β) is smaller than the rate of return to the central compartment for a two-compartment model (79). For the two-compartment model as the time after injection approaches infinity, the equation is:

$$\frac{B}{F} = \frac{k_1}{k_2 - \beta}$$

where k_1 is the rate constant for transfer from the central compartment to the bound compartment and k_2 is the reverse process. β is the rate constant for the elimination process. In certain specific cases, the ratio appears to be constant from some time in the β-phase. If β is small compared to k_2, then the B/F ratio will approach the binding potential. The form of the three-compartment model is more complicated, although similar arguments can be made. At steady state, the B/F ratio is given by:

$$\frac{B}{F} = \frac{k_1}{k_2}\left(1 + \frac{k_3}{k_4}\right)$$

where k_3 is the rate of association with the receptor and k_4 is the rate of dissociation of the radioligand-receptor complex. These equations have been used for many radiopharmaceuticals, e.g., raclopride (80) and cyclofoxy (81) which approach steady state in vivo. Other more sophisticated equations that incorporate nonspecific binding and the vascular volume have been used (24).

The key to the agreement between the B/F ratio obtained in vitro and the ratio obtained in vivo by external imaging is the purity of the radiopharmaceutical in both blood (or another reference region) and the target organ, and the approach of the distribution in vivo toward steady state. Metabolite studies of the blood radioactivity can be used to correct the plasma input function, but it is difficult to obtain the same information in the target organ. Modeling of multiple species in the target organ, e.g., for ^{11}C-amino acids, is complicated. An incomplete list of radiopharmaceuticals that appear to give a change in radioactivity as a function of a change in receptor concentration was compiled by Eckelman (32) and Kilbourn (82).

SUMMARY

The success of any field depends on its ability to adapt to changing situations. The strength of nuclear medicine is the ability to measure functional changes. Its strength is not in measuring anatomic structures. Receptor-binding radiotracers are ideal candidates for the measurement of a specific process in humans using a noninvasive technique. Preliminary results using estrogen receptor-binding radiotracers are encouraging, and many receptor-binding radiotracers should be in clinical trials in the immediate future. The expectation is that we will be able to measure the change in concentration of receptor as a function of disease which will permit physicians to individualize therapy and to monitor the progress of that therapy by a noninvasive method.

REFERENCES

1. Budinger T. Physiology and physics in nuclear cardiology. In: Breast A, ed. Nuclear cardiology (Cardiovascular Clinic Series 10/2). Philadelphia: F.A. Davis, 1979:9.
2. Tow DE, Wagner HN Jr, Lopex-Majano V, Smith EM, Migita T. Validity of measuring regional pulmonary arterial blood with macroggregates of human serum albunim. Am J Roentgenol 1966; 96:664–676.
3. Shaldon S, Chiandussi L, Guevara L, Caesar J, Sherlock S. The estimation of hepatic blood flow and intrahepatic shunted blood flow by colloidal heat-denatured human serum albumin labeled with I-131. J Clin Invest 1961;10:1346–1354.
4. Sherlock S. Measurement of hepatic blood flow. In: Kniseley RM, Tampe WN, Anderson EB, eds. Dynamic clinical studies with radioisotopes. Oak Ridge, TN: USAEC Technical Information Center, 1964:359.
5. Tubis M, Posnick E, Nordyke RA. Preparation and use of I^{131} labeled sodium iodohippurate in kidney function tests. Proc Soc Exp Biol Med 1960;103:497–498.
6. Johnson LL, Seldin DW, Muschel MJ, et al. Comparison of planar SQ 30,217 and Tl-201 myocardial imaging with coronary anatomy [Abstract]. Circulation 1987;76(IV):217.
7. Seldin DW, Johnson LL, Blood DK, et al. Myocardial perfusion imaging with technetium-99m SQ 30,217: comparison with thallium-201 and coronary anatomy. 1989;30:312–319.
8. Meerdink DJ, Thuber M, Savage S, et al. Comparative myocardial extraction of two technetium labeled boron oxime derivatives (SQ 30,217, SQ 32014) and thallium. J Nucl Med 1988;29:972.
9. Winchell HS, Horst WD, Braun L, et al. N-isopropyl-[^{123}I]p-io-

doamphetamine: single pass brain uptake and washout, binding to brain synaptosomes, and localization in dog and monkey brain. J Nucl Med 1980;21:947–952.
10. Volkert WA, Hoffman TJ, Seger TM, et al. ^{99m}Tc-propylene amine oxime (Tc-99m-PnAO): a potential brain radiopharmaceutical. Eur J Nucl Med 1984;11:511–516.
11. Phelps ME, Mazziotta JC, Huang SC. Study of cerebral function with positron computed tomography. J Cerebral Blood Flow Metab 1982;2:113–162.
12. Ehrlich P. Collected studies in immunity. New York: Wiley, 1906. (See Himmelweit F, ed. The collected papers of Paul Ehrlich. Vol. II: Immunology and cancer research. New York: Pergamon Press, 1957.)
13. Kahn CR. Membrane receptors for hormones and neurotransmitters. J Cell Biol 1976;70:261–280.
14. Eckelman WC, Reba RC, Gibson RE, et al. Receptor binding radiotracers: a class of potential radiopharmaceuticals. J Nucl Med 1979;20:350–357.
15. Wagner JG. Fundamentals of clinical pharmacokinetics. Hamilton, IL: Drug Intelligence, 1981.
16. Wagner HN Jr. Introduction: The role of receptors in disease. In: Eckelman WC, ed. Receptor binding radiotracers. Vol. II. Boca Raton, FL: CRC Press, 1982:177.
17. Gibson RE. Quantitative changes in receptor-concentration as a function of disease. In: Eckelman WC, ed. Receptor binding radiotracers. Vol. II. Boca Raton, FL: CRC Press, 1982:185.
18. Melnechuk T. Cell receptor disorders. La Jolla, CA: Western Behavioral Sciences Institutes, 1978.
19. Blecher M, Bar RS. Receptors and human disease. Baltimore: Williams & Wilkins, 1981.
20. Receptors in health and disease. In: Clayton RN, ed. Clinics in endocrinology and metabolism. Vol. 12, no. 1. London: Saunders, 1983.
21. Parker, M, ed. Nuclear hormone receptors: molecular mechanisms, cellular functions, clinical abnormalities. London: Academic Press, 1991.
22. Beatson GT. On the treatment of inoperable cases of carcinoma of the mammae: suggestions for a new method of treatment, with illustrative cases. Lancet 1896;2:104, 162.
23. Jensen EV, Jacobson HI. Basic guides to the mechanism of estrogen action. Rec Prog Horm Res 1962;18:387–414.
24. Edwards DP, Chamness GC, McGuire WL. Estrogen and progesterone receptor proteins in breast cancer. Biochim Biophys Acta 1979;560:457–486.
25. Subtypes of muscarinic receptors V. Proceedings of the Fifth International Symposium on subtypes of muscarinic receptors. Life Sciences 1993;52:405–594.
26. Quirion R, Aubert I, Lapchak PA, et al. Muscarinic receptor subtypes in human neurodegenerative disorders: focus on Alzheimer's disease. TIPS (December 1989 Supplement) 1989;80–84.
27. Comar D, Berridge M, Maziere B, Crouzel C. Radiopharmaceuticals labeled with positron-emitting radioisotopes. In: Ell PJ, Holman BL, eds. Computer emission tomography. New York: Oxford University Press, 1982:42–90.
28. Fowler JS, Wolf AP. The synthesis of carbon-11, fluorine-18 and nitrogen-13 labeled radiotracers for biomedical applications (NAS-NS-3201). Washington, DC: Technical Information Center, US Department of Energy, 1982.
29. Eckelman WC. Clinical potential of receptor based radiopharmaceuticals. In: Fritzberg AR, ed. Radiopharmaceutical progress and clinical perspectives. Vol. II. Boca Raton, FL: CRC Press, 1986:89–114.
30. Stocklin G. Tracers for metabolic imaging of brain and heart. Radiochemistry and radiopharmacology. Eur J Nucl Med 1992; 19(7):527–551.
31. Eckelman WC. The testing of putative receptor binding radiotracers in vivo. In: Diksic M, Reba RC, eds. Radiopharmaceuticals and brain pathology studied with PET and SPECT. Ch. 4:. Boca Raton, FL: CRC Press, 1990:41–68.
32. Eckelman WC. The status of radiopharmaceutical research [Editorial]. Nucl Med Biol 1991;18(7):iii–vi.
33. Christman DR, Finn RD, Karlstrom KI, Wolf AP. The production of ultra high activity $^{14}N(p,\alpha)^{11}C$ reaction. Int J Appl Radiat Isot 1975; 26:435–442.
34. Fowler JS, Arnett CD, Wolf AP, MacGregor RR, Norton EF, Findley AM. [^{11}C] spioperidol: synthesis, specific activity determination, and biodistribution in mice. J Nucl Med 1982;23:437–445.
35. Welch MJ, McElvany K, Tewson TJ. Production of high specific activity compounds with short-lived radionuclides. In: Eckelman WC, ed. Receptor binding radiotracers. Vol. I. Boca Raton, FL: CRC Press, 1982:55.
36. Martin YC. A practitioner's perspective of the role of quantitative structure-activity analysis in medicinal chemistry. J Med Chem 1981;24:229–237.
37. Waldrop MM. The reign of trial and error draws to a close. Science 1990;247:28–29.
38. Rzeszotarski WJ, Gibson RE, Eckelman WC, et al. Analysis of R, S-3-quinuclidinyl benzilates. J Med Chem 1982;25:1103–1106.
39. Gibson RE, Weckstein DJ, Jagoda EM, Rzeszotarski WJ, Reba RC, Eckelman WC. The characteristics of I-125 QNB and H-3 QNB in vivo and in vitro. J Nucl Med 1984;25:214–222.
40. Eckelman WC, Grissom M, Conklin J, et al. In vivo competition studies with analogues of quinuclidinyl benzilate. J Pharm Sci 1984;73:529–533.
41. Jagoda EM, Gibson RE, Goodgold H, et al. I-125 17-α-iodovinyl 11-β-methoxyestradiol: in vivo and in vitro properties of a high affinity estrogen-receptor radiopharmaceutical. J Nucl Med 1984; 25:472–477.
42. Allegra JC, Lippman MC, Thompson EB, et al. Estrogen receptor status: an important variable in predicting response to endocrine therapy in metastatic breast cancer. Eur J Cancer 1980;16:323.
43. McElvaney KD, Katzenellenbogen JA, Shafer KE. 16α-^{77}Br] bromoestradiol: dosimetry and preliminary clinical studies. J Nucl Med 1982;23:425–430.
44. Mintun MA, Welch MJ, Mathias CJ, Brodack JA, Siegel BA, Katzenellenbogen JA. Application of 16α-[F-18]-fluoro-17β-estradiol (I) for the assessment of estrogen receptors in human breast carcinoma. J Nucl Med 1987;28:561.
45. Pomper MG, Kochanny MJ, Thieme AM, et al. Fluorine-substituted corticosteroids: synthesis and evaluation as potential receptor-based imaging agents for PET of the brain. Nucl Med Biol 1992; 19:461–480.
46. Mintun MA, Welch MJ, Siegel BA, et al. Breast cancer: PET imaging of estrogen receptors. Radiology 1988;69:45–48.
47. Dehdashti F, McGuire AH, VanBrocklin HF, et al. Assessment of 21-[18F]fluoro-16α-ethyl-19-norprogesterone as a positron-emitting radiopharmaceutical for the detection of progestin receptors in human breast carcinomas. J Nucl Med 1991;32(8):1532–1537.
48. Vera DR, Krohn KA, Stadalnik RC, Scheibe PO. [^{99m}Tc] galactosylneoglycoalbumin: in vivo characterization of receptor-mediated binding. Radiology 1984;151:191–196.
49. Krohn K, Vera DR, Stadalnik RC. A complementary radiopharmaceutical and mathematical model for quantitative hepatic-binding receptor. In: Eckelman WC, ed. Receptor binding radiotracers. Vol. II. Boca Raton, FL: CRC Press, 1982:41.
50. Stadalnik RC, Vera DR, Krohn KA. Receptor-binding radiopharmaceuticals: experimental and clinical aspects. In: Freeman LM, Weissman HE, eds. Nuclear medicine annual. New York: Raven Press, 1986:105–139.
51. Stadalnik RC, Vera DR, Woodle ES, et al. Technetium-99m-NGA functional hepatic imaging: preliminary clinical experience. J Nucl Med 1985;26:1233–1242.

52. Kudo M, Vera DR, Stadalnik RC, et al. Measurement of functioning hepatocyte mass via [^{99m}Tc]-galactosylneoglycoalbumin. Dig Dis Sci 1993;17:814–819.
53. Kudo M, Todo A, Ikekubo K, Yamamoto K, Vera DR, Stadalnik RC. Quantitative assessment of hepatocellular function via in vivo radioreceptor imaging: technetium-99m-galactosyl human serum albumin (Tc-GSA). Hepatology 1993;17:814–819.
54. Vera DR, Stadalnik RC, Trudeau WL, Schiebe PO, Krohn KA. Measurement of receptor quality and forward binding rate constant via radiopharmaceutical modeling of [^{99m}Tc]-galactosyl-neoglycoalbumin. J Nucl Med 1991;32:1169–1176.
55. Rzeszotarski WJ, Eckelman WC, Francis BE, et al. Synthesis and evaluation of radioiodinated derivatives of I-azabicyclo (2.2.2) oct-3–yl-α-hydroxy-α-(4-azabicyclo) phenylacetate as potential radiopharmaceuticals. J Med Chem 1984;27:156–159.
56. Eckelman WC, Reba RC, Gibson RE, et al. External imaging of cerebral muscarinic acetylcholine receptors. Science 1984; 223:291–293.
57. Kobayashi RM, Palkovits M, Hruska RE, Rothschild R, Yamamura HI. Regional distribution of muscarinic cholinergic receptors in rat brain. Brain Res 1978;154:13–23.
58. Hiley CR, Burgen ASV. The distribution of muscarinic receptor sites in the nervous system of the dog. J Neurol Chem 1974; 22:159–162.
59. Wastek GJ, Yamamura HI. Biochemical characterization of the muscarinic cholinergic receptor in human brain: alterations in Huntington's disease. Molec Pharmacol 1978;14:768–780.
60. Enna SJ, Bennett JP Jr, Bylund DB, et al. Neurotransmitter receptor binding: regional distribution in human brain. J Neurol Chem 1977;28:233.
61. Nordström O, Weslind A, Unden A, Meyerson B, Sachs C, Bartfai T. Pre- and postsynaptic muscarinic receptors in surgical samples from human cerebral cortex. Brain Res 1982;234:387–397.
62. Holman BL, Gibson RE, Hill TC, Eckelman WC, Albert M, Reba RC. Muscarinic acetylcholine receptors in Alzheimer's disease. JAMA 1985;254:3063–3066.
63. Weinberger DR, Gibson R, Coppola R, et al. The distribution of cerebral muscarinic acetylcholine receptors in vivo in patients with dementia. Arch Neurol 1991;48:169–176.
64. Vera DR, Krohn KA, Scheibe PO, Stadalnik RC. Identifiability analysis of an in vivo receptor-binding radiopharmacokinetic system. IEEE Trans Biomed Eng 1985;32:312–322.
65. Friedman AM, DeJesus OT, Revenaugh J, Dinerstein RJ. Measurements in vivo of parameters of the dopamine system. Ann Neurol 1984;15(Suppl):566–567.
66. Farde L, Erling E, Erikson L, et al. Substituted benzamides as ligands for visualization of dopamine receptor binding in the human brain by positron emission tomography. Proc Natl Acad Sci USA 1985;82:3863–3867.
67. Wagner HN Jr, Burns HD, Dannals RF, et al. Imaging dopamine receptors in the human brain by positron tomography. Science 1983;221:1264–1266.
68. Wong DF, Wagner HN Jr, Dannals RF, et al. Effects of age on dopamine an serotonin receptors measured by positron tomography in the living human brain. Science 1984;226:1393–1396.
69. Patlak CS, Blasberg RG. Graphical evaluation of blood-to-brain transfer constants from multiple-time uptake data. Generalization. J Cereb Blood Flow Metab 1985;5:584–590.
70. Lassen NA. Neuroreceptor quantitation in vivo by the steady state principle using constant infusion or bolus injection of radioactive tracers. J Cereb Blood Flow Metab 1992;12:709–716.
71. Eckelman WC, Reba RC, Gibson RE, et al. Receptor binding radiotracers: a class of potential radiopharmaceuticals. J Nuc Med 1979;20:350–357.
72. Eckelman WC. Radiolabeled adrenergic and muscarinic blockers for in vivo studies. In: Eckelman WC, ed. Receptor binding radiotracers. Vol. I. Boca Raton, FL: CRC Press, 1982:69–91.
73. Eckelman WC. The testing of putative receptor binding radiotracers in vivo. In: Diksic M, Reba RC, eds. Radiopharmaceuticals and brain pathology studied with PET and SPECT. Ch. 4. Boca Raton, FL: CRC Press, 1990:41–68.
74. Katzenellenbogen J. The development of gamma-emitting hormone analogs as imaging agents for receptor-positive tumors. In: The prostatic cell: structure and function. New York: Alan R. Liss, Inc., 1981:313–327.
75. Katzenellenbogen JA, Heiman DF, Carlson KE, Lloyd JE. In vitro and in vivo steroid receptor assays in the design of estrogen radiopharmaceuticals. In: Eckelman WC, ed. Receptor binding
radiotracers. Vol. I. Boca Raton, FL: CRC Press, 1982:93–126.
76. Goodenough DJ, Atkins FB. Theoretical limitations of tumor imaging. In: Srivastava S, ed. Radiolabeled monoclonal antibodies for imaging and therapy. New York: Plenum Press, 1988:495–512.
77. Eckelman WC, Gibson RE. The design of site directed radiopharmaceuticals for use in drug discovery. In: Burns HD, Gibson RE, Dannals RF, Siegl PKS, eds. Nuclear imaging in drug discovery, development and approval. Boston: Birkhauser Boston, Inc., 1992:113–134.
78. Mintun MA, Raichle ME, Kilbourn MR, Wooten GF, Welch MJ. A quantitative model for the in vivo assessment of drug binding sites with positron emission tomography. Ann Neurol 1984;15:217–227.
79. Wagner JG. Fundamentals of clinical pharmacokinetics. Hamilton, IL: Drug Intelligence, 1981.
80. Wienhard K, Herholz K, Coenen HH, et al. Increased amino acid transport into brain tumors measured by PET of L-2-[^{18}F] fluorotyrosine. J Nucl Med 1991;32:1338–1346.
81. Carson R, Channing MA, Blasberg RG, et al. Comparison of bolus and infusion methods for receptor quantitation: application to [^{18}F] cyclofoxy and positron emission tomography. J Cereb Blood Flow Metab 1993;13:24–42.
82. Kilbourn MR. Shades of grey: radiopharmaceuticals in the 90's and beyond. Nucl Med Biol 1991;412:109–117.

18 Radiation Protection

JERROLD T. BUSHBERG and EDWIN M. LEIDHOLDT, JR.

The use of ionizing radiation in nuclear medicine carries with it a responsibility to both patient and staff to maximize the diagnostic and therapeutic benefit while minimizing the potential for adverse health effects. Shortly after the discovery of the x-ray by Roentgen in 1895, the potential for acute health hazards of ionizing radiation became apparent. However, the risks of delayed effects from ionizing radiation were not known and many early users did not believe that anyone could be hurt by something that could not be detected by any of the human senses. Many experiments on the biologic effects of ionizing radiation began in the early 1900s, and the first radiation protection standards were proposed by the British Roentgen Society in 1915. We now realize that these pioneers had a very limited knowledge of the hazards of ionizing radiation and of the principles of radiation protection.

Some uncertainties remain regarding the risks to humans of certain health effects from ionizing radiation, particularly cancer and genetic effects from low dose and low dose rate radiation. Despite this, however, more scientific data are available today on the health effects of ionizing radiation than any other physical agent or chemical. Additionally, the use of most forms of ionizing radiation is heavily regulated at both the national and state levels.

QUANTITIES AND UNITS IN RADIATION DOSIMETRY

ABSORBED DOSE

The amount and rate of energy deposition in tissue are major determinants of biologic effects. The *absorbed dose* is defined as the amount of energy imparted to matter by ionizing radiation per unit mass (1–4). The Systeme Internationale (SI) unit of exposure is the gray (Gy). One gray is defined as 1 J/kg. The traditional unit of absorbed dose is the rad, originally an acronym for "*r*adiation *a*bsorbed *d*ose." One rad is defined as 0.01 J/kg; thus, 1 rad is equal to 0.01 gray. Absorbed dose is defined for all types of ionizing radiation and matter. Absorbed dose to soft tissue is most commonly encountered in radiation protection.

One disadvantage to the quantity absorbed dose is that it is difficult to directly measure, especially in radiation protection applications. Instead, it is usually inferred from measurements of other quantities, such as ionization per mass of air.

The x-rays and γ-rays used in nuclear medicine deposit their energy in matter by photoelectric absorption and Compton scattering. The absorbed dose can be calculated from the mass energy absorption coefficient of a material, if the fluence (number of photons per unit area) and the energies of the photons are known. The absorbed dose to an organ or tissue from a radiopharmaceutical includes energy deposition from both particulate radiations and photons.

Although 1 gray (100 rad) is a very large radiation dose to man, it represents an extremely small energy deposition per mass of matter. The energy in 1 gray, if deposited as heat, would raise the temperature of water by approximately 2.4×10^{-4}°C.

EXPOSURE

The intensity of x or γ radiation at a particular location can be expressed as the radiation's ability to ionize air at that location. *Exposure* is defined as the total amount of ionization (charge) produced per mass of air, when all the electrons produced in that mass of air are completely stopped in air (1, 2). The SI unit of exposure is the coulomb per kilogram (C/kg). The traditional unit of radiation exposure is the roentgen (R). One roentgen is defined as the amount of x or radiation that produces 2.58×10^{-4} coulombs of charge per kilogram of air.

Exposure is a useful quantity for several reasons. It is a direct measure of ionization, ionization being the initiating event in most biologic damage. Exposure can be easily measured by portable air-filled ionization chambers. Additionally, the atomic numbers of the elements constituting air are close to those of the elements comprising tissue and so exposure is nearly proportional to the absorbed dose to soft tissue over a considerable range of photon energies.

It is important to appreciate the limitations inherent in the use of exposure:

1. It is defined only for x- and γ-rays (i.e., not charged particles).
2. It is difficult to measure for photons with energies greater than a few MeV.
3. It is defined for ionization in air only.
4. An ambient air ionization chamber is affected by atmospheric pressure and temperature which determine the mass of air in the fixed volume of the chamber. Corrections for variations in atmospheric pressure and temperature are usually modest.
5. Exposure is a measure of integral (cumulative) ionization over a time interval and is independent of exposure rate.

The ratio of absorbed dose per unit of radiation exposure (i.e., rad/roentgen) is called the *f-factor* and has been determined for a number of tissues. Thus, if the exposure and the energy of the x- or γ-rays are known, the absorbed dose can be determined. The f-factors for water, muscle, and bone are shown in Figure 18.1. Notice that the exposure in roentgens is within approximately 10% of the absorbed dose to soft tissue in centigray (rad) over the range of photon energies encountered in nuclear medicine.

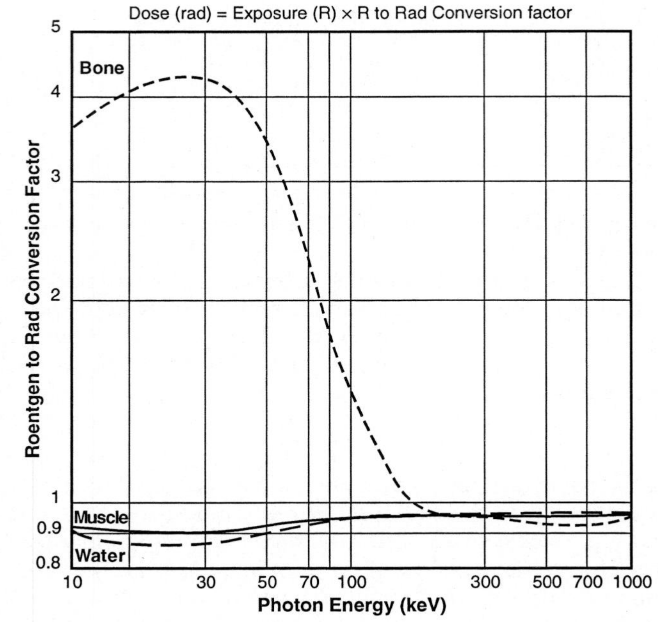

Figure 18.1. The roentgen-to-rad conversion factor versus photon energy for water, muscle, and bone.

EQUIVALENT DOSE AND DOSE EQUIVALENT

The absorbed dose and dose rate are not the only determinants of biologic damage. An additional factor is the microscopic energy deposition pattern. In interacting with an absorber, all forms of ionizing radiation liberate charged particles that, for the purpose of predicting their microscopic energy deposition patterns, can be described by mass, charge, and kinetic energy. The number of ion pairs formed by a particular radiation per unit path-length is referred to as its *specific ionization* and is expressed in units of ion pairs per micrometer. A related quantity is the *linear energy transfer* (LET), which is the energy deposited locally per unit path-length. LET is commonly expressed in keV/μM. Those forms of radiation that produce dense ionization patterns (i.e., high LET radiations) have been shown to produce greater amounts of irreparable damage in both cellular and complex biologic systems per unit dose than low LET radiations. Radiobiologists describe this difference in biologic response by comparing a particular "test" radiation to a standard radiation (often 250 kVp x-rays). A biologic end point is selected for observation (e.g., 37% cell survival in irradiated cell cultures) and the doses necessary to produce this end point for the test and standard radiations are determined experimentally. The ratio of the dose required for the standard radiation to the dose required for the test radiation is referred to as the *relative biologic effectiveness* (RBE) of the test radiation. The RBEs for various radiations typically range from 1 to 50 for both mammalian systems and cells in culture.

This information has been used to establish modifying *radiation weighting factors* (w_R) to the absorbed dose that express the relative biologic hazards of specified forms of radiation. These weighting factors have been established for both particulate and electromagnetic radiations of various energies and are listed in Table 18.1.

The absorbed dose (in gray or rad) can be modified to represent the biologic hazard of the radiation by multiplying the absorbed dose by the radiation weighting factor for that type of radiation. This product is referred to as the *equivalent dose*. If an individual is exposed to more than one type of radiation, the equivalent dose is the sum of the products of the absorbed doses from each type of radiation and the weighting factors:

$$H_T = \sum_R w_R \times D_{T,R} \quad (1)$$

where $D_{T,R}$ is the average absorbed dose to an organ or tissue T from radiation of type R (3, 4). The SI unit of equivalent dose is the sievert (Sv); thus 1 gray of a radiation with a radiation weighting factor of 1 will yield an equivalent dose of 1 Sv. The traditional unit of equivalent dose is the rem (originally an acronym for "roentgen-equivalent-man"); 1 rem is equal to 0.01 Sv.

For example, if a person were to accidentally ingest a mixture of radioactive materials from which the dose to the gastrointestinal tract is 50 mGy (5 rad) from α-particles, 30 mGy (3 rad) from β-particles, and 20 mGy (2 rad) from γ-rays, the absorbed dose would be:

$$D = 50\ mGy + 30\ mGy + 20\ mGy = 100\ mGy\ (10\ rad).$$

However, the equivalent dose to the gastrointestinal tract would be:

$$\begin{aligned} H &= (50\ mGy)(20) + (30\ mGy)(1) + (20\ mGy)(1) \\ &= 1.05\ Sv\ (105\ rem). \end{aligned}$$

The quantity equivalent dose coexists with an older but similar quantity, *dose equivalent*. The dose equivalent, similar to the equivalent dose, is intended to reflect the biologic harm from absorbed doses of different types of radiation. It is calculated as the sum of the products of the absorbed doses from each type of radiation and quality factors (Q), similar to the radiation weighting factors w_R, which reflect the relative harm from different types of radiation:

$$H = \sum_R Q_R \times D_R \quad (2)$$

where D_R is the absorbed dose from radiation R at a point and Q_R is the quality factor for that type of radiation (1–3).

Table 18.1.
Radiation Weighting Factors

Type and Energy of Radiation	Radiation Weighting Factor (w_T)
Photons (x- and γ-rays), all energies	1
Electrons and muons, all energies	1
Neutrons, energy < 10 keV	5
10 keV to 100 keV	10
> 100 keV to 2 MeV	20
> 2 MeV to 20 MeV	10
> 20 MeV	5
Protons, other than recoil protons, energy > 2 MeV	5
Particles, fission fragments, heavy nuclei	20

Adapted from International Commission on Radiological Protection. 1990 recommendations of the International Commission on Radiological Protection. ICRP publication 60, 21, 1991. Annals of the ICRP. Elmsford, NY: Pergamon Press, 1991.

Table 18.2.
Quality factors as a function of the linear energy transfer of the radiation. The quality factor is one for photons and electrons, because the linear energy transfer of electrons is less than 10 keV per μm.

Quality Factor	Linear Energy Transfer L (keV/μm)
1	$L \leq 10$
0.32 L–2.2	$10 < L < 100$
$300/\sqrt{L}$	$L \geq 100$

Adapted from International Commission on Radiation Units and Measurements. Quantities and units in radiation protection dosimetry. ICRU report 51. Bethesda, MD: International Commission on Radiation Units and Measurements, 1993.

The quality factors are listed as a function of LET in Table 18.2. The units of dose equivalent are the sievert (Sv) and the rem (traditional). The major distinction between the two quantities is that dose equivalent is computed from the absorbed dose at a point, whereas the equivalent dose is calculated from the average dose to a tissue or organ. The quantity dose equivalent is used in the current U.S. Nuclear Regulatory Commission (NRC) regulations.

EFFECTIVE DOSE

A common problem in personnel dosimetry occurs when the body is exposed to ionizing radiation in a nonuniform manner, either from external sources (e.g., the fluoroscopist who wears a lead apron) or internal sources (e.g., a person who inhales Iodine-131). In 1977, in an attempt to compare detriment from nonuniform exposure of the body with detriment from uniform exposure of the body, the International Commission on Radiological Protection (ICRP) proposed a new scheme for dose limitation (5). The scheme defined a weighted average of the dose equivalents to the various tissues or organs of the body:

$$E = \sum_T w_T H_T \quad (3)$$

where the H_T are the average dose equivalents to the various tissues or organs of the body and the weighting factors w_T, listed in column 2 of Table 18.3, reflect the relative risk of detrimental effects. The sum of the weighting factors w_T is 1:

$$\sum_T w_T = 1.0 \quad (4)$$

The weighted equivalent dose E became known as the *effective dose equivalent* (ede). In 1990, the ICRP revised the scheme, with new tissue weighting factors (Table 18.3, column 3) (4). The weighted equivalent dose was then given the name *effective dose* to distinguish it from the ede which was based upon the older tissue weighting factors. However, the system of dose limitation mandated by the U.S. Nuclear Regulatory Commission utilizes the older 1977 weighting factors. The quantities effective dose equivalent and effective dose are specified in the same units as equivalent dose, i.e., sievert (Sv) or rem (traditional).

To illustrate the concept of effective dose, let us compare the risk from 50 μSv (5 mrem) equivalent dose to the gonads with a similar exposure to the whole body. The effective dose from the gonadal exposure is:

Table 18.3.
Tissue weighting factors (w_T). The U.S. Nuclear Regulatory Commission's system of dose limitation (contained in Title 10, Part 20, of the Code of Federal Regulations) incorporates the ICRP 26 tissue weighting factors. ICRP Publications 26 and 60 describe how the remainder terms are to be applied to organs not assigned weighting factors.

Tissue	Tissue Weighting Factors (ICRP Publication 26, 1977)	Tissue Weighting Factors (ICRP Publication 60, 1990)
gonads	0.25	0.20
red bone marrow	0.12	0.12
colon		0.12
lung	0.12	0.12
stomach		0.12
bladder		0.05
breast	0.15	0.05
liver		0.05
esophagus		0.05
thyroid	0.03	0.05
skin		0.01
bone surfaces	0.03	0.01
remainder	0.30	0.05
Sum	1.00	1.00

$$\begin{aligned} E &= \text{(equivalent dose to the gonads)} \\ &\quad \text{(tissue weighting factor for the gonads)} \\ &= 50\ \mu Sv \times 0.20 = 10\ \mu Sv. \end{aligned}$$

In other words, the "detriment" from a gonadal dose of 50 μSv is similar to that from a uniform exposure of 10 μSv (1 mrem) to the entire body.

COMMITTED EQUIVALENT DOSE AND COMMITTED EFFECTIVE DOSE

Another facet of radiation dosimetry is the situation in which radioactive material is injected into, or inhaled, ingested, or absorbed through the skin. The exposure from incorporated radioactivity continues until the activity is eliminated from the body by biologic excretion and radioactive decay. If a radionuclide has a sufficiently long half-life and the biologic excretion is slow, the activity irradiates the individual over the remainder of his or her life. The *committed equivalent dose* is the equivalent dose to a particular tissue or organ over a specified length of time:

$$H_{c,T}(\tau) = \int_0^{\tau} \dot{H}_T(t)\, dt \quad (5)$$

where $\dot{H}_T(t)$ is the equivalent dose rate to the organ or tissue T from radioactivity throughout the body and τ is the specified time interval (4). The *committed effective dose* is the sum of committed equivalent doses to the various organs and tissues of the body, each weighted by the appropriate tissue weighting factor w_T:

$$E_c(\tau) = \sum_T w_T \times H_{c,T}(\tau) \quad (6)$$

The units of committed equivalent and effective dose are the sievert (Sv) and rem (traditional). If the length of time τ is not specified, it is assumed to be 50 years for adults and from intake to age 70 years for children (4).

DOSIMETRIC QUANTITIES FOR POPULATIONS

For a comparison of the possible effects of various sources of radiation on a population, the *collective effective dose* (S) is defined as the sum of the effective doses of each person in the population (4). The SI unit of collective effective dose is the man-sievert. For example, if 100 people were each exposed to 1 mSv (100 mrem), the collective effective dose would be 0.1 man-sievert (10 man-rem). This concept necessarily implies (a) linearity between radiation dose and detrimental effect and (b) that there is no threshold level for the detriment. The reliability of these assumptions are difficult to prove; however, most scientists believe that calculations made in this manner lead to a conservative estimate of detriment.

The *genetically significant dose* (GSD) is a measure of genetic detriment to a population. It is defined as the dose which, if given to every member of the population, would produce the same genetic detriment as the actual doses received by the various individuals.

SOURCES OF EXPOSURE

NATURAL SOURCES OF RADIATION EXPOSURE

Natural sources of radiation are particularly important because they are the largest contributor to the collective dose of the world's population. Natural irradiation is usually incurred at a relatively constant rate and has exposed all forms of life since the inception of life on the planet. Natural background radiation is from three sources: cosmic radiation, which includes both radiation from extraterrestrial sources and secondary radiation produced by the interactions of the primary cosmic rays with the atmosphere; cosmogenic radionuclides, which are radionuclides produced by the interaction of cosmic radiation; and primordial radionuclides, which are radionuclides that have existed on the earth since its creation and their radioactive decay products. The following information on population exposure from natural background radiation is from NCRP Report No. 94 (6), unless otherwise cited.

The vast majority of primary cosmic rays are charged particles, mostly protons and α-particles. Primary cosmic rays originate from galactic sources and the sun; however, the solar particles are of much lower average energy and contribute only slightly to cosmic ray dose at the earth's surface. The galactic particles are very energetic, with mean energies of $\sim 10^{10}$ eV, and interact with our atmosphere to produce a variety of secondary radiation (mainly photons, muons, electrons, and neutrons). The primary cosmic rays are substantially affected by the earth's magnetic field; the cosmic ray flux is much higher at the north and south poles of the earth than at the equator. At sea level, essentially all the primary particles have disappeared and the exposure is due to the secondary radiation. The atmosphere provides considerable attenuation; without the atmosphere, the cosmic ray dose rate at the earth's surface would be on the order of a 1000 times greater. At sea level in middle latitudes, the average annual dose equivalent is estimated as 240 μSv (24 mrem), taking into account shielding by buildings. At higher altitudes, there is less atmospheric shielding and the cosmic ray dose increases. In Denver (1600 meter altitude), for example, the cosmic ray dose equivalent is approximately 500 μSv (50 mrem) per year. The annual dose equivalent to the U.S. population from cosmic rays is estimated as 270 μSv (27 mrem), 10 μSv (1 mrem) of which is from exposure during air travel.

Cosmic rays also produce a number of cosmogenic radionuclides as a result of interaction with the atmosphere. Tritium (hydrogen-3), beryllium-7, carbon-14, and sodium-22 contribute the most to natural background exposure. The effective dose equivalent from cosmogenic radionuclides is estimated to be just over 10 μSv (1.0 mrem) per year, essentially all from carbon-14 incorporated in the body.

In addition to cosmogenic radionuclides, we are constantly exposed to primordial radionuclides that have existed in the earth's crust since its formation. These are the major source of terrestrial external whole body radiation exposure, producing an average γ dose equivalent rate of approximately 280 μSv/y (28 mrem/y) in the United States and Canada. There are some regions in the world where the terrestrial radiation exposure substantially exceeds the average. These include the monazite sands in Kerala, India; several areas in Brazil; and other areas in Italy, Egypt, Iran, Kenya, and Sweden (7). In Kerala, for example, the thorium concentration produces absorbed dose rates as high as 35 mGy/y (3.5 rad/y) (7).

Primordial radionuclides have half-lives that are comparable to the age of the earth (4.5×10^9 years). Primordial radionuclides may be classified into "series radionuclides," which decay to stable isotopes of lead through a series of radioactive decay products, and "nonseries" radionuclides, such as potassium-40, which decay directly to stable nuclides. The three decay chains are the uranium series, which originates with uranium-238; the thorium series, which originates with thorium-232; and the actinium series, which originates with uranium-235. The uranium series is the most significant of these as a source of natural radiation exposure. In this series, uranium-238 decays through a series of 13 radioactive daughters, ending as stable lead-206. The half-lives of the radioactive daughters range from 2.5×10^5 years (uranium-234) to 1.6×10^{-4} seconds (polonium-214).

Radon-222 is the sixth radioactive nuclide in the uranium-238 decay chain and is produced by the α decay of its parent, radium-226. Radon is a noble gas, behaving chemically and biologically like xenon and krypton. It decays by α-particle emission, with a 3.8-day half-life. Exposure to radon has long been associated with a higher incidence of lung cancer among uranium miners. The carcinogenic hazard is not posed by radon itself, but by its short-lived daughters, most notably polonium-218 and polonium-214, α-emitters with half-lives of 3.05 minutes and 1.64×10^{-4} seconds, respectively. Unlike radon, these daughters are quite reactive, combining readily with other chemicals and adhering to bronchial mucosa. There has recently been an increased interest in the exposure from radon, with investigations being undertaken at the state and federal levels to more accurately determine the extent of population radon exposure. The highest concentrations of radon and its daughters are found indoors, especially during winter months when buildings are more tightly sealed.

Exposure to radon is commonly described either in terms of the air concentration of radon alone or in terms of the concentration of its short-lived progeny. Exposure to the progeny of radon can be measured in terms of working level (WL). The WL is defined as any combination of short-lived daughter radionuclides in 1 liter of air that will result in the emission of 1.3×10^5 MeV of potential energy. One WL corresponds to 3.7 kBq/m^3 (100 pCi/liter), if the radon daughters are in equilibrium with radon. However, ventilation of occupied spaces usually prevents the radon daughters from achieving equilibrium and so a WL usually corresponds to a considerably higher radon concentration than 100 pCi/l. The exposure to an individual is the product of the number of working levels and the exposure time. For this purpose, the working level month (WLM) is defined as 170 hours of exposure to 1 WL of radon daughters.

The U.S. Environmental Protection Agency has established a radon concentration limit of 150 Bq/m^3 (4 pCi/liter) for members of the public, above which action is advised to reduce radon exposure (8). This action level is controversial, being lower than action levels recommended by internationally recognized radiation protection organizations. For example, the National Council on Radiation Protection and Measurements (NCRP) recommends, as the remedial action level, an annual exposure of 2 WLM; this corresponds to an average radon concentration of 300 Bq/m^3, if the radon decay products are in 50% equilibrium with radon (9).

Although there is some external whole body dose from radon daughters, it is very small compared to the α dose to the tracheobronchial region of the lung from inhalation. The absorbed dose is typically calculated to the bronchial epithelium, which is the radiobiologic target of interest. Radon and its progeny contribute more than 98% of the annual dose equivalent from inhaled radionuclides to the bronchial epithelium, 24.0 mSv (2.40 rem). They deposit relatively little energy in the remainder of the lungs. If the tissue weighting factor w_T of 0.08 recommended by the ICRP for bronchial epithelium is used, the resultant annual effective dose equivalent for inhaled radionuclides is approximately 2 mSv (200 mrem).

Radionuclides are found in the body as the result of ingestion of food and water that contain small amounts of naturally occurring radionuclides. These radionuclides generally follow the same chemical metabolism as that of their stable isotopes. The shorter-lived radionuclides tend to be maintained at equilibrium concentrations, disappearing by decay but continually replenished by intake. The long-lived radionuclides are usually maintained at equilibrium concentrations or increase slowly with age. The average annual effective dose equivalent from noncosmogenic radionuclides in the body is approximately 0.40 mSv (40 mrem). The most significant contributors to this dose are potassium-40, which is present in all body tissues, although with considerable variation, and polonium-210, an α-emitter delivering the majority of its dose to bone surfaces and bone marrow.

In summary, natural sources of radiation include cosmic rays and cosmogenic and primordial radionuclides. Cosmic rays are an external source of exposure, cosmogenic radionuclides are primarily an internal source, whereas primordial radionuclides contribute to both the external and internal exposure, as well as exposure to the bronchial epithelium from airborne activity. The exposures from radionuclides in the soil and cosmic rays vary significantly throughout the world. The average annual effective dose equivalent to the populations of the United States and Canada from all natural sources is estimated to be approximately 3 mSv (300 mrem) per year.

TECHNOLOGY BASED SOURCES

Human activities have significantly increased the radiation exposure to the population. Technology based sources can be classified into two categories—enhanced natural sources and artificial radiation sources. Enhancement of natural radiation sources occurs when man's activities increase the population exposure from naturally occurring radioactive materials. Artificial radiation sources include x-ray machines, particle accelerators, nuclear reactors, and fallout from tests of nuclear weapons.

Enhanced Natural Sources

Domestic water supplies release radon inside buildings; they are estimated to contribute 10–60 μSv (1–6 mrem) to the annual per capita effective dose equivalent (10). The burning of fossil fuels (natural gas, coal, and oil) increases radiation exposure by the dispersion of primordial radionuclides. The annual per capita effective dose equivalent from this source is estimated to be between 3.5 and 6.2 μSv (0.35–0.62 mrem) (10). Phosphate rock is mined and used mainly as a fertilizer, with the byproduct (gypsum) used as a building material in homes. Radiation exposure from this source is predominantly from the primordial radionuclides of the uranium decay series. The annual per capita effective dose equivalent from phosphate fertilizer is estimated to be less than 10 μSv (1 mrem) (10). Building materials such as rock, cement, and gypsum wallboard contain primordial radionuclides which cause an estimated annual per capita effective dose equivalent of 35 μSv (3.5 mrem) (10). Buildings also increase the concentration of radon. The average radon concentration indoors is approximately 10 times that of the outdoor environment (6); however, there are large variations in indoor concentration between different buildings and even between different locations in a particular building.

As was mentioned earlier, cosmic ray exposure increases with altitude. Thus, cosmic ray exposure is enhanced by air transportation or space travel. A typical round trip airplane flight from New York to Paris results in an additional cosmic ray dose of 30 μSv (3 mrem). The average annual effective dose equivalent for aircraft crew members is approximately 3.5 mSv (350 mrem) (7).

Tobacco contains natural radionuclides, most significantly ^{210}Pb and ^{210}Po. Thus, the smoking of tobacco causes the bronchial epithelium to be irradiated with α-particles. However, due to several uncertainties, the NCRP has not assigned a per capita effective dose equivalent for the smoking of tobacco (10). A number of manufactured products, including older instruments with radioluminous dials, some optical glass, tungsten welding rods, static eliminators, and fluorescent lamp starters, contain primordial radioactive material, but they contribute little to the per capita effective dose equivalent (10).

In summary, technologic enhancement of natural sources occurs under many circumstances, with the largest exposure being the result of energy conservation and exposure to radon in buildings.

Artificial Sources Other Than Those Used in Medicine

Artificial sources of radiation include fallout from nuclear weapons, nuclear power, occupational exposure, and medical uses of ionizing radiation. Approximately 360 atmospheric nuclear weapons tests were performed from 1945 through 1962; an additional 63 were conducted in the period from 1962 through 1980, when the atmospheric testing of these weapons was discontinued. Radionuclides released in these atmospheric explosions may enter the body as a result of inhalation or ingestion. The radionuclide that contributes the most (86%) to the dose from weapons testing is carbon-14. The annual per capita effective dose equivalent from fallout radionuclides is approximately 20 μSv (2 mrem) (7).

Nuclear power production increases population exposure during mining of the fuel, uranium fuel fabrication, reactor operation, and waste storage and disposal, collectively called the nuclear fuel cycle. Additionally, there is environmental dispersion of radionuclides. The annual per capita effective dose equivalent from the nuclear fuel cycle is estimated to be approximately 0.5 μSv (0.05 mrem) (11).

Occupational radiation exposure occurs in the nuclear fuel cycle, medicine, scientific research, the military, and various commercial industries. Although it is not possible to determine from the literature the total number of workers who are occupationally exposed, about 1.5 million workers are monitored for radiation exposure in the United States. The mean annual effective dose equivalent to them from occupational exposure is estimated to be approximately 1.5 mSv (150 mrem) (12). The frequency distribution of occupational doses is highly skewed for most radiation-related occupations, with few workers having doses approaching the annual limit (12). The contribution of occupational radiation exposure to the average per capita effective dose equivalent of the entire U.S. population is estimated to be approximately 10 μSv (1 mrem) (11).

Exposure to Patients from Medical Radiation

The exposure of patients to radiation for medical purposes provides the largest population exposure of any technologic-based source. Medical radiation exposure is normally divided into three categories: (a) diagnostic x-ray examinations, (b) administration of radiopharmaceuticals in nuclear medicine, and (c) therapeutic use of radiation. Medical radiation is difficult to compare to other sources because it is predominantly in the form of partial body exposures, the exposures are at higher rates than most other sources, the mean age of the irradiated population is much greater than that of the overall population, and much of the dose is to ill or injured persons.

For the year 1980, the estimated per capita effective dose equivalent from diagnostic x-ray procedures was 0.40 mSv (40 mrem) per year (13). For the year 1982, the estimated effective dose equivalent per capita from nuclear medicine in the United States was 140 μSv (14 mrem) per year (13). More recent data on medical exposures were unavailable at the time of writing; changes in medical practice and technology may have caused current doses to differ from these estimates.

Radiation therapy generally falls into three categories: (a) external beam therapy, (b) brachytherapy (the implantation of sealed radioactive sources), and (c) radiopharmaceutical therapy. The high absorbed doses utilized lead generally to effects such as cell killing rather than detriment in terms of long-term carcinogenesis. Many of the patients receiving treatment for malignancies have limited life expectancies and are usually beyond child-bearing age. Thus, one cannot easily calculate a reasonable collective effective dose or genetically significant dose for radiotherapy.

In summary, the major sources of radiation exposure to the population are natural background and medical exposure. Radon and tobacco predominantly affect the bronchial epithelium, and are important, and often overlooked, contributors to the population exposure. The components of the average annual effective dose equivalent to the population of the United States are listed in Table 18.4.

REGULATIONS PERTAINING TO THE USE OF RADIATION

ADVISORY BODIES

A number of advisory groups promulgate information and advice relevant to protection against ionizing radiation. Although the recommendations of these groups do not carry the force of law, they often become "standards of practice" and may be incorporated into regulations by regulatory agencies. The International Commission of Radiological Protection (ICRP), founded in 1928, is the most eminent of these bodies. It is composed of internationally-recognized experts in many fields relevant to radiation protection. It was founded to provide guidance relevant to the use of x-rays and radium in medicine, but has since broadened its interests to encompass other sources and uses of radiation and radioactive material. However, it retains a special relationship with the profession of radiology.

The National Council on Radiation Protection and Measurements (NCRP) is a prestigious nonprofit corporation chartered by Congress in 1964. Its members consist of experts in ionizing and nonionizing radiation and related disciplines. It has a role similar to that of the ICRP, but provides recommendations with a national rather than international perspective. The ICRP and NCRP have issued well over 160 monographs relevant to radiation protection.

REGULATORY AGENCIES

The U.S. Nuclear Regulatory Commission (NRC) is a federal agency charged with regulating the production and use of radioactive material created by nuclear reactors, called *by-product material*, or that can be used to fuel nuclear reac-

Table 18.4.
Contributions to the annual effective dose equivalent of the population of the United States circa 1980–1982[a]

Source	Number of People Exposed (thousands)	Average Annual Effective Dose Equivalent in the Exposed Population (mSv)	Average Annual Effective Dose Equivalent in the U.S. Population (mSv)	% of Total Average Annual Effective Dose Equivalent in the U.S. Population
Natural Sources				
Radon	230,000	2.0	2.0	55
Cosmic radiation	230,000	0.27	0.27	8
Cosmogenic radionuclides	230,000	0.01	0.01	< 1
External terrestrial	230,000	0.28	0.28	8
Internal radionuclides	230,000	0.39	0.39	11
Occupational	930	2.3	0.009	<< 1
Nuclear Fuel Cycle	—	—	0.0005	<< 1
Consumer Products				
Tobacco	50,000	—	—	
Other	120,000	0.05–0.3	0.05–0.13	3
Miscellaneous Environmental Sources	25,000	0.006	0.0006	<< 1
Medical				
Diagnostic x-rays	—*	—	0.39	11
Nuclear medicine	—*	—	0.14	4
Rounded Total	230,000		3.6	100

[a]Adapted from National Council on Radiation Protection and Measurements. Ionizing radiation exposure of the population of the United States. NCRP report no. 93. Bethesda, MD: National Council on Radiation Protection and Measurement, 1987.
*The number of examinations is known, but not the number of exposed persons.

tors. It was established by the Energy Reorganization Act of 1974, which abolished the Atomic Energy Commission and transferred its licensing and regulatory functions to the NRC. The NRC has no jurisdiction over radioactive materials produced by particle accelerators and many naturally-occurring radioactive materials.

The NRC's regulations are contained in Title 10 of the Code of Federal Regulations (CFR). Portions of these regulations relevant to the medical use of byproduct material include Part 19 (10 CFR 19), which requires the training of workers in radiation safety precautions and notification of workers of their radiation exposures; Part 20 (10 CFR 20), entitled *Standards for Protection Against Radiation*, which establishes a system for the limitation of radiation doses to workers and members of the public and contains regulations on many other topics, including the disposal of radioactive waste; and Part 35 (10 CFR 35), entitled *Medical Use of Byproduct Material*, which contains regulations regarding to the use of radioactive material in nuclear medicine and radiation oncology (14–16). Part 35, for example, requires the testing of dose calibrators, radiation surveys in the nuclear medicine department, and the use of syringe shields; specifies precautions to be followed in radiopharmaceutical therapies and precautions to prevent the misadministration of radiopharmaceuticals to patients; and requires the reporting to the NRC of misadministrations. In addition to promulgating regulations, the NRC issues advisory documents, called regulatory guides, containing suggested methods for complying with the regulations (19–26).

The NRC has an enforcement program to ensure compliance with their regulations. The NRC regularly inspects facilities it has licensed. Should violations be discovered, the NRC can levy fines, place additional restrictions on the use of byproduct material, and even withdraw permission to utilize byproduct material.

The NRC is permitted to transfer its responsibilities for regulating byproduct material to state governments, provided that the states establish and enforce regulations similar to those of the NRC. States granted these powers are called *agreement states*. Twenty-nine states are currently agreement states.

The shipping of radioactive material is jointly regulated by the NRC and the U.S. Department of Transportation (DOT). The regulations of the DOT are contained in Title 49 of the Code of Federal Regulations. The production of radiopharmaceuticals, the testing in humans of radiopharmaceuticals under development, and the administration of radioactive substances to humans for basic research are regulated by the U.S. Food and Drug Administration (FDA), whose regulations are contained in Title 21 of the Code of Federal Regulations. Releases to the atmosphere of radioactive material are jointly regulated by the NRC and the U.S. Environmental Protection Agency (EPA). The EPA's National Emission Standards for Hazardous Air Pollutants (NESHAPS) limit the effective dose equivalent to "members of the public" from airborne emissions of radioactivity to 100 μSv (10 mrem) per year, of which no more than 30 μSv (3 mrem) can be from isotopes of iodine (17). The term "members of the public" in NESHAPS refers to individuals who are off-site, unless there is a nursing home, dormitory, or other housing on-site.

STANDARDS FOR PROTECTION AGAINST RADIATION

As mentioned in the preceding section, the NRC has promulgated *Standards for Protection Against Radiation* (10 CFR 20) to protect members of the public and persons who are occupationally exposed to radiation. A major revision to *Standards for Protection Against Radiation* was approved by the NRC in 1991; institutions were required to be in compliance with the revised regulations by January 1, 1994. The revised regulations incorporate, with modifications, the system for dose limitation published in ICRP Publications 26 and 30 (5, 18). This system was intended to prevent deterministic effects (effects whose severities increase with increasing dose, such as cataracts, reduction in fertility, and hematologic consequences of bone marrow depletion) and limit the probability of stochastic effects (effects whose probabilities increase with increasing dose, but whose severities are unaffected by dose, such as cancer and hereditary defects).

The system of dose limitation imposes two requirements: (a) all exposures must be maintained as low as reasonably achievable (ALARA), social and economic factors being taken into account, and (b) the exposures to individuals must not exceed the limits provided in the regulations. These NRC regulations adopt, with modifications, the system proposed in ICRP Publications 26 and 30 for summing doses from radionuclides incorporated into the body and doses from sources external to the body and provide a set of limits for the sums.

Summing Internal and External Doses

External doses to an individual are usually determined by a body dosimeter worn by an exposed individual on the part of the body, other than the extremities, likely to receive the greatest dose. The body dosimeter indicates the deep dose equivalent and the shallow dose equivalent from external sources. The *deep dose equivalent* is the dose equivalent at a depth of 1 cm of tissue and the *shallow dose equivalent* is the dose equivalent at a depth of 0.007 cm of tissue. The NRC's main modification to the ICRP Publication 26 system is that, under the NRC scheme, all organs and tissues of the body (except the skin and the lenses of the eyes) are assumed to receive the deep dose equivalent from external sources.

The committed dose equivalent and committed effective dose equivalent are due only to exposure from radionuclides incorporated into the body. The *committed dose equivalent* ($H_{T,50}$) is the dose equivalent to a tissue or organ T over the 50 years following the ingestion or inhalation of radioactivity. The *committed effective dose equivalent* ($H_{E,50}$) is the weighted average of the committed dose equivalents to the various organs and tissues of the body:

$$H_{E,50} = \sum_{T} w_T \times H_{T,50} \qquad (7)$$

where the weighting factors w_T are those from ICRP Publication 26 (Table 18.3, Column 2).

The *total effective dose equivalent* is the sum of the deep dose equivalent and the committed effective dose equivalent.

Dose Limits

The dose limits for persons who are occupationally exposed are:

1. Total effective dose equivalent: 0.05 Sv (5 rem) per year
2. The sum of the deep dose equivalent and the committed dose equivalent to any individual organ or tissue: 0.5 Sv (50 rem) per year
3. Shallow dose equivalent to the skin or any extremity: 0.5 Sv (50 rem) per year
4. Eye dose equivalent (dose equivalent to the lens of the eye): 0.15 Sv (15 rem) per year

Occupational exposures to minors (persons under 18 years of age) may be no more than 10% of the above limits. The dose to an embryo or fetus, from the occupational exposure of a declared pregnant woman, may not exceed 0.005 Sv (0.5 rem) over the duration of the pregnancy. (A declared pregnant woman is a woman who has voluntarily chosen to declare her pregnancy in writing to her employer.) Efforts must be made to avoid substantial variation above a uniform monthly exposure rate.

The total effective dose equivalent to "individual members of the public" shall not exceed 1 mSv (100 mrem) per year. The dose of radiation in an unrestricted area may not exceed 0.02 mSv (2 mrem) in any one hour. "Individual members of the public" include employees who are not occupationally exposed. For example, a dietician whose office is adjacent to the radiopharmacy in nuclear medicine would probably be considered an "individual member of the public."

Based upon recent increases in the estimated risk of cancer per unit of effective dose and in an attempt to maintain the risk to radiation workers comparable to those of workers in industries deemed to be safe, both the ICRP and the NCRP have recently recommended occupational dose limits more stringent than those currently set by the NRC (Table 18.5). It is therefore likely that the NRC will reduce their occupational dose limits in the future.

Annual Limits on Intake and Derived Air Concentrations

In practice, the committed dose equivalent and committed effective dose equivalent are rarely used for demonstrating compliance with the dose limits. Instead, compliance is usually demonstrated by one of two methods. In the first method, an individual's intake of radioactive material is estimated and compared to an *annual limit on intake* (ALI). The ALI is the activity of a radionuclide that, if inhaled or ingested, would produce a committed dose equivalent of 0.5 Sv (50 rem) in any individual organ or tissue or a committed effective dose equivalent of 0.05 Sv (5 rem). ALIs for inhalation of airborne radioactive materials of interest in nuclear medicine are listed in Table 18.6. ALIs are not listed for noble gases because very little of the inhaled activity is retained in the body; most of the dose from them is due to external exposure from the cloud of gas surrounding the exposed individual. When the ALI is determined by the limit on the committed dose equivalent to an organ (0.5 Sv), as is the case for iodine-131, the name of the organ is listed after the ALI, followed in parentheses by the activity that would cause a committed effective dose equivalent of 5 rem.

Alternatively, the air concentration of a radionuclide may be measured and compared to its *derived air concentration* (DAC). The DAC is the concentration of a radionu-

Table 18.5.
Comparison of current U.S. Nuclear Regulatory Commission dose limits, which are largely based upon recommendations of the ICRP published in 1977 and 1979, with the current recommendations of the ICRP and NCRP. All limits are annual limits, unless otherwise specified.

	Recommendations		Regulations
	ICRP Publication 60 (1990)	NCRP Report No. 116 (1993)	U.S. NRC 10 CFR 20
Occupational Limits			
effective dose	50 mSv *and* 100 mSv in 5 years	50 mSv *and* 10 mSv × age (y)	50 mSv (effective dose equivalent*)
lens of eye	150 mSv	150 mSv	150 mSv
skin, hands, feet	500 mSv	500 mSv	500 mSv
any organ or tissue	—	—	500 mSv
embryo or fetus	2 mSv external dose to abdomen and limit intakes to 1/20 of an ALI for remainder of pregnancy**	equivalent dose to fetus 0.5 mSv per month**	dose to fetus 5 mSv during entire pregnancy
Public Dose Limits			
effective dose	1 mSv *and, if needed,* higher values provided 5 mSv not exceeded over 5 years	1 mSv for continuous exposures *and* 5 mSv for infrequent exposures	1 mSv (effective dose equivalent*)

*The effective dose equivalent is similar to the effective dose, but based upon tissue weighting factors published by the ICRP in 1977.
**After pregnancy is known.

Table 18.6.
Annual limits on intake (ALIs) and derived air concentrations (DACs) established by the NRC for radionuclides likely to become airborne in the nuclear medicine department. ALIs and DACs pertain to restricted areas, whereas airborne effluent concentrations apply to effluents released to unrestricted areas.

Radiochemical	ALI for Inhalation (μCi)	DAC (μCi/ml)	Airbone Effluent Concentration (μCi/ml)
^{99m}Tc aerosol	20,000	1×10^{-4}	3×10^{-7}
^{131}I	50 (thyroid)	2×10^{-8}	2×10^{-10}
(any form)	200*		
^{133}Xe	not defined**	1×10^{-4}	5×10^{-7}

*Whenever the concentration of a particular radionuclide is limited by the dose to a specific organ, the critical organ is listed after the ALI, followed by the activity that would cause an effective dose equivalent of 0.05 mSv (5 rem).
**ALI is not listed, because the vast majority of the dose is from photons emitted from the cloud of gas surrounding the worker and very little is from gas inhaled by the worker.

clide in air that, if breathed under conditions of light activity for 2000 hours, would result in the inhalation of the ALI. Table 18.6 also lists the DACs of airborne radioactive materials likely to be encountered in nuclear medicine.

If an individual is exposed to a single airborne radionuclide and his or her exposure from external sources is less than one-tenth of the dose limit (0.5 rem for a nonpregnant adult worker), it is sufficient to demonstrate that his or her intake is less than an ALI. However, if these conditions are not met, it must be demonstrated that the dose to each organ does not exceed 50 rem and the total effective dose equivalent does not exceed 5 rem.

Example Assume that a worker could receive a deep dose equivalent up to 2.5 rem in a year from external sources. What is the maximal activity of iodine-131 that could be inhaled by this worker without causing the worker to exceed the limits?

Solution To ensure the dose equivalent to the worker's thyroid does not exceed 50 rem:

$$\frac{2.5\ rem}{50\ rem} + \frac{\text{intake}}{50\ \mu Ci} \leq 1$$

$$\text{intake} \leq 47.5\ \mu Ci$$

To ensure the worker's total effective dose equivalent does not exceed 5 rem:

$$\frac{2.5\ rem}{5\ rem} + \frac{\text{intake}}{200\ \mu Ci} \leq 1$$

$$\text{intake} \leq 100\ \mu Ci$$

The maximal intake of ^{131}I is therefore the smaller of the two, or 47.5 μCi.

PERSONNEL DOSIMETRY

Personnel dosimetry is the measurement of the individual exposures of people to ionizing radiation. There are many devices available today that may serve as personnel dosimeters. One way to assess currently available devices is to compare them to an "ideal" dosimeter. An ideal dosimeter would have the following characteristics:

1. The response of the dosimeter would be independent of radiation energy (linear energy response).
2. The response of the dosimeter would be independent of its orientation relative to the incident radiation field. This is called "geometry independence."
3. The dosimeter would be sensitive enough to record exposure slightly over background (~20 μGy/week (2 mrad/week)) and have a range large enough to record serious overexposures (e.g., ~5 Gy (500 rad)).
4. The dosimeter would respond only to ionizing radiation, would not be affected by other environmental conditions (e.g., heat and humidity), and would not lose stored information with time.
5. The dosimeter would indicate separately the doses from α, β, γ, and neutron radiations of various energy ranges.
6. The radiation dose would be readable immediately but also permanently recorded for future analysis.
7. The dosimeter would be tissue equivalent so that the results can be expressed directly as absorbed dose to tissue.

8. The dosimeter would be small, lightweight, rugged, easy to use, and inexpensive.

No dosimeter available today meets all of the ideal requirements. In fact, some of the "ideal" characteristics are not satisfied by any currently available dosimeters.

The NRC requires all persons whose doses from external sources are likely to exceed 10% of the occupational limits listed above to wear dosimeters (15). The NRC requires dosimeters used to measure the dose to the body to indicate the deep, eye, and shallow dose equivalents and extremity dosimeters (wrist or finger dosimeters) to indicate shallow dose equivalents. The deep dose equivalent is the dose equivalent at a tissue depth of 1 cm, the eye dose equivalent is the dose equivalent at a tissue depth of 0.3 cm, and the shallow dose equivalent is the dose equivalent at a tissue depth of 0.007 cm. The NRC also requires personnel dosimeters other than pocket ion chambers and electronic dosimeters to be processed by a dosimetry processor accredited by the National Voluntary Laboratory Accreditation Program (NVLAP) of the National Institute of Standards and Technologies.

FILM BADGE DOSIMETERS

The film badge, despite its limitations, is still the most widely used personnel dosimeter. All film badges are constructed in a manner similar to that in Figure 18.2. A piece of x-ray film, contained in a light-tight and moisture-resistant envelope, is sandwiched between a series of plastic and metal filters in a plastic holder that also has an "open window" section in which there is no plastic or metal filter in front of the film. This open window permits a portion of the film to detect all radiation with the exception of α and weak β particles. The metal filters provide different attenuation factors for photons, and thus the relative darkening behind these filters, called the "filter pattern," helps to identify the energy of the x- and γ-rays. Additionally, the metal filters help to compensate for the over-response of the film to low-energy photons due to the high photoelectric cross-section of the silver halide (AgBr) crystals in the film.

These films are typically used for a 1-month period and then sent to a commercial dosimetry company where they are developed and read. The optical densities of all the areas of the film are read by a densitometer. The radiation dose is determined by comparing the optical densities to predetermined standards.

Advantages of Film Badges

1. Film has a broad dose range: 0.1 mGy–15 Gy (0.01–1500 rad) for x- and γ-rays and 0.5 mGy–10 Gy (0.05–1000 rad) for high energy β-particles.
2. Plastic and metal filters in the film badge permit it to distinguish between penetrating radiation (i.e., photons) and nonpenetrating radiation (β-particles and low-energy x-rays). The energy of the photons can be grossly evaluated as high, medium, or low energy.
3. The developed film provides a permanent record of the exposure that can be reanalyzed at a future date.
4. Film badges are small, lightweight, easy to use, and inexpensive.

Disadvantages of Film Badges

1. Film is sensitive to environmental effects such as heat and humidity. For example, a film badge left on the dash of a car on a hot summer day may be rendered unreadable by the heat.

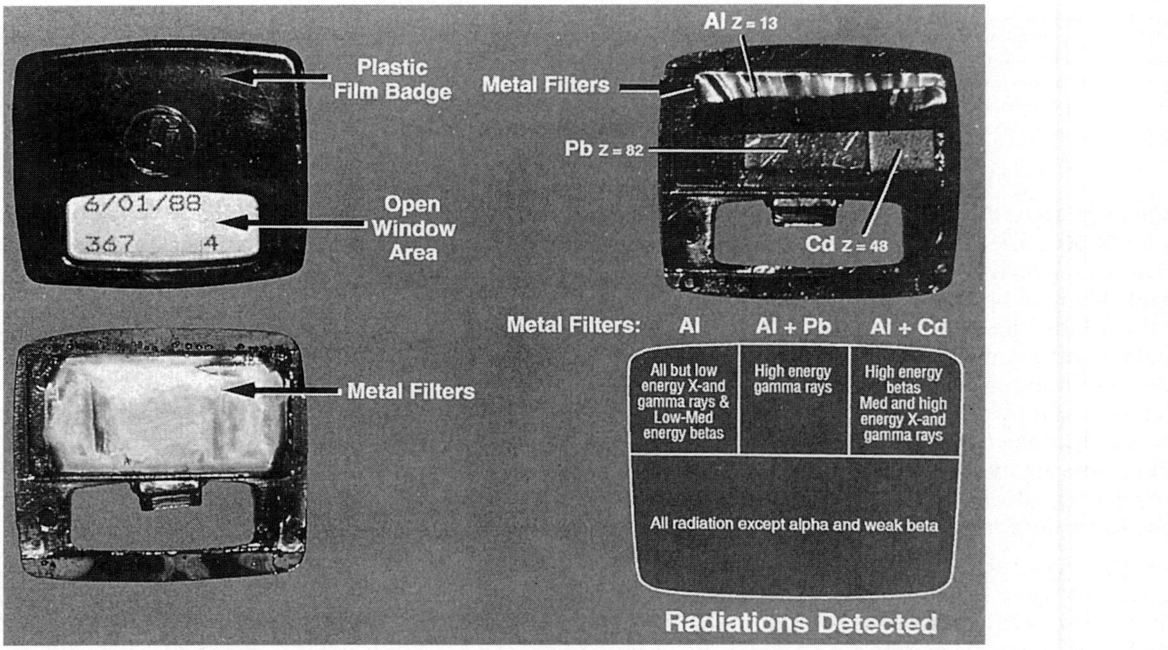

Figure 18.2. Film badge. The film is sandwiched between two sets of metal filters. The relative darkening on the developed film (filter patterns) provides a crude but useful assessment of the energy of the radiation exposure. The diagram shows the types of radiation that can penetrate and thus be recorded in each section of the film badge. (Reproduced by permission from Bushberg JT, Seibert JA, Leidholdt EM Jr., Boone JM. The essential physics of medical imaging. Baltimore: Williams & Wilkins, 1994.)

2. Film must be processed by the film badge supplier, and the evaluation of an exposure cannot be made immediately. In the event of a suspected serious overexposure, the film can be sent to the vendor and processed within approximately 48 hours.

THERMOLUMINESCENT DOSIMETERS

Thermoluminescent dosimeters (TLDs) have a wide range of applications in radiation dosimetry. They are typically small chips of inorganic crystalline materials in which excited electrons become trapped in metastable states. When ionizing radiation interacts with the TLD, the energy deposition raises electrons from the valence band into the higher-energy conduction band, where they settle into metastable electron traps. The electron vacancies left in the conduction band by the removal of the electrons are called *holes*. The more radiation received by the TLD, the more valence electrons will inhabit these electron traps. The TLD is "read" by heating it (300–400°C) in a light-tight enclosure in front of a photomultiplier tube (PMT). The heating causes the metastable electrons to reenter the conduction band, filling the holes, with the emission of visible and UV light photons. These visible and UV photons interact with the PMT, producing an electrical current in it. The PMT amplifies this current through a process of electron multiplication. The current from the PMT is integrated (accumulated) to produce a signal whose amplitude is proportional to the absorbed dose to the TLD.

Lithium fluoride (LiF) is the TLD material most commonly used for personnel dosimetry. Because its effective atomic number is similar to that of soft tissue, the absorbed dose to LiF is similar to that of soft tissue over a wide range of x- and γ-ray energies. Its electron traps are sufficiently "deep" that there is relatively little loss of trapped electrons at normal ambient temperatures, even over several months. Body dosimeters using LiF usually have two or more chips; single chips are used in finger rings to monitor extremity exposures (Fig. 18.3). The lower limit of detection of LiF is about 0.1 mGy (10 mrad). Other TLD materials, such as aluminum oxide activated with carbon, can be used if smaller doses must be assessed. However, measures must be taken to compensate for their nonlinear energy responses relative to soft tissue.

Advantages of TLDs

1. LiF TLDs have a very wide dose-response range: 0.1 mGy–1000 Gy (0.01–100,000 rad).
2. LiF TLDs are tissue equivalent ($Z \approx 7$), which means that the quantity of light emitted by a TLD is nearly proportional to dose to soft tissue over a wide range of x- and γ-ray energies.
3. They can be reused following heating at high temperature for about 24 hours. This process is referred to as *annealing*.
4. They are very small and so can be used on finger rings.
5. They are lightweight and as easy to use as film.

Disadvantages of TLDs

1. TLDs cannot be read without a TLD reader, which is expensive and requires repeated calibration. Most TLDs are returned to the vendor to be processed (read).

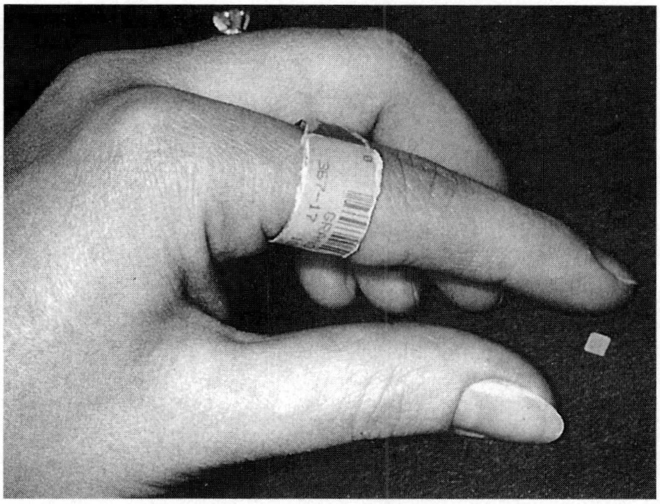

Figure 18.3. A small chip of LiF (shown above) is sealed in a ring (underneath the identification label) which is worn on the palmar surface such that the chip would be facing a radiation source held in the hand. (Reproduced by permission from Bushberg JT, Seibert JA, Leidholdt EM Jr., Boone JM. The essential physics of medical imaging. Baltimore: Williams & Wilkins, 1994.)

2. Once the TLD is processed, the radiation exposure information is lost from the TLD crystal; it cannot be reprocessed at a later date.
3. TLDs are also susceptible to environmental effects (heat and humidity) and the information stored on the TLD will eventually fade or degrade with time.

POCKET ION CHAMBERS

The pocket ion chamber is a simple electroscope. A central insulated electrode can be charged with respect to the outside case. A quartz fiber located on the end of the central electrode is deflected in proportion to the charge. This fiber can be viewed through a simple optical system in which it appears as a hairline cursor on a superimposed exposure scale. The dosimeter is charged before use so that the quartz fiber is deflected to indicate a reading of zero exposure. Radiation causes ionization of the air in the chamber. These ions partially neutralize the stored charge, causing the quartz fiber to experience less repulsion and therefore to move closer to its uncharged position. This movement is seen as a uprange deflection of the hairline on the exposure scale (Fig. 18.4).

Advantages of Pocket Ion Chambers

1. The most significant advantage of this instrument is that it can be read immediately by the user without a loss of information.
2. Pocket ion chambers are manufactured with several range scales (e.g., 0–200 mR, 0–5 R, or 0–500 R).
3. They are reusable, lightweight, and small.

Disadvantages of Pocket Ion Chambers

1. Many models are unable to detect low energy photons or any particulate radiation because of the thick chamber wall. However, special low energy models are available.

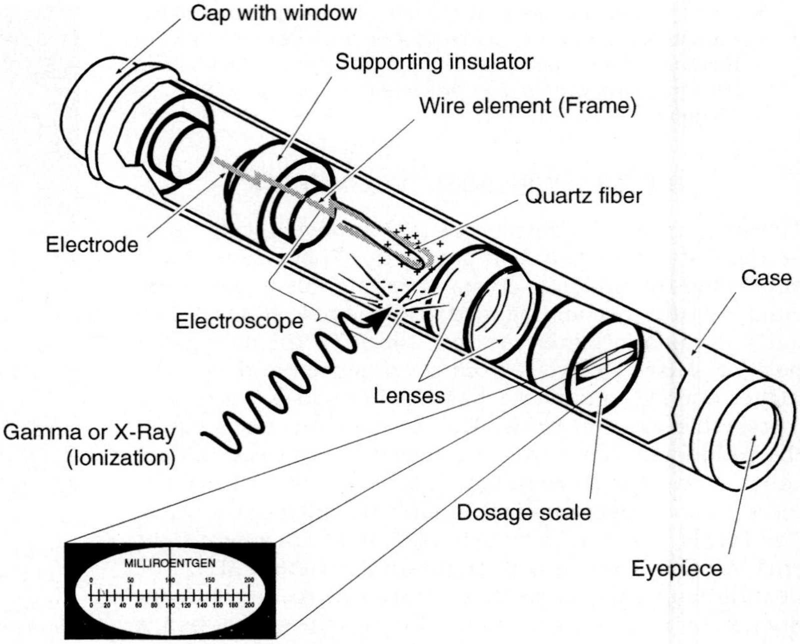

Figure 18.4. Cross-section of a analogue pocket ion chamber. (Reproduced by permission from Bushberg JT, Seibert JA, Leidholdt EM Jr., Boone JM. The essential physics of medical imaging. Baltimore: Williams & Wilkins, 1994.)

2. The dosimeter may spontaneously discharge if dropped on a hard surface, resulting in a spurious high exposure reading.
3. They are fragile and may break if dropped.
4. When they are recharged for reuse, the prior exposure information is lost; therefore, they provide no permanent record.

ELECTRONIC PERSONNEL DOSIMETERS

Electronic personnel dosimeters may use GM tubes or silicon solid-state diodes as detectors. Their major advantage is that, like pocket ion chambers, they provide the user a visible display of his or her current exposure. Older models were generally unreliable, fragile, bulky, and insensitive to low energy x- and γ-rays. Recent models have overcome many of these limitations and will no doubt become more commonly used in the future (Fig. 18.5). The better models use solid-state diodes.

Advantages of Electronic Personnel Dosimeters

1. They can be read immediately by the user without any loss of information.
2. They are reusable.
3. Some models can be programmed to sound an alarm at a preset dose-rate.
4. The best models have very high sensitivity, accurately measure doses over a very wide range (1 μGy–10 Gy (0.1 mrad–1,000 rad)), and have a linear energy response to photons over a wide energy range (±20% from 20 keV to 7 MeV).

Disadvantages of Electronic Personnel Dosimeters

1. They are relatively expensive compared to film and TLD badges.
2. They are bulky compared to film and TLD badges.

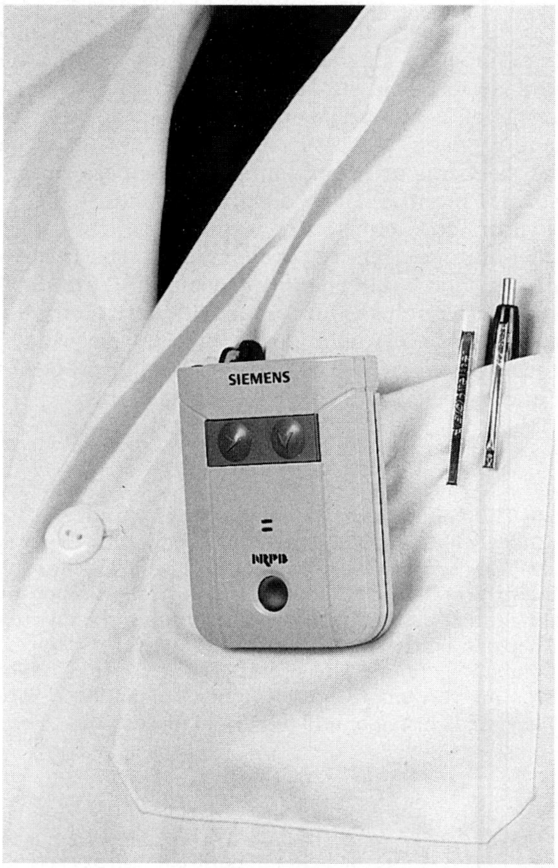

Figure 18.5. Electronic personnel dosimeter. Courtesy of Siemens Inc.

3. Less expensive models may be unable to detect low energy photons or any particulate radiation and may have a non-linear energy response.
4. They require periodic replacement of electrical batteries.

Common problems encountered with all personnel dosimeters include erroneous high exposures resulting from the dosimeter having been inadvertently left in a radiation field or having been contaminated with radioactive material and false low exposures from not being worn.

BIOASSAYS

Bioassays are measurements to assess the amount of radioactive material incorporated in the body. Assays of excreta, usually urine, are performed in many occupations utilizing radioactive material. However, the most common bioassay in nuclear medicine is the measurement of the activities of iodine-125 or 131 in the thyroid glands of staff handling large activities of these isotopes. This assay is usually performed using a thyroid uptake probe equipped with a sodium iodide scintillation detector. In all bioassays, the detector efficiency must be known. The efficiency of the thyroid probe is determined by counting a known activity of the isotope of interest in a thyroid phantom, such as the American National Standards Institute (ANSI) thyroid phantom which simulates the attenuation of the average adult neck. For any bioassay procedure, the *minimum detectable activity* must be determined to ensure that the procedure is capable of detecting a sufficiently small activity (27). The minimum detectable activity is reduced (the bioassay becomes more sensitive) as the detection efficiency and counting time are increased and as the background count-rate is reduced. Methods have been developed that permit the effective dose to the person to be estimated from the activity measured during the bioassay (19, 28–30).

RADIATION SURVEY INSTRUMENTS AND SURVEY PROCEDURES

Radiation surveys are performed in the nuclear medicine laboratory to evaluate external radiation fields from a variety of sources and to detect and measure contamination of facilities and personnel. These surveys are an important part of keeping occupational radiation exposures as low as reasonably achievable. External radiation fields can be measured with a portable ionization chamber (ion chamber) or, under the appropriate conditions, a Geiger-Mueller (G-M) survey instrument.

PORTABLE IONIZATION CHAMBER SURVEY METERS

Theory of Operation

An ion chamber survey meter for measuring exposure-rate consists of an air-filled chamber containing two electrodes, a battery to provide a voltage between the electrodes, and a sensitive electrometer to measure the current flowing between the electrodes (Fig. 18.6). Exposure to radiation causes partial ionization of the air in the chamber. Ionization of the air from x-rays and γ-rays results primarily from electrons released following photoelectric or Compton interactions in the chamber walls. The ions are attracted to the electrodes, producing an ionization current that is measured by the electrometer. The ion chamber can thus be considered a current generator whose output current is proportional to the rate of internal air ionization. When the radiation source is x- or γ-rays, the current is proportional to the exposure-rate (e.g., mR/hr). Most ion chambers have plastic or metal caps that must be placed over the thin entrance windows of the chambers for measurements of higher energy photons. The cap can also be used to determine if the indicated exposure-rate is partially caused by β-radiation.

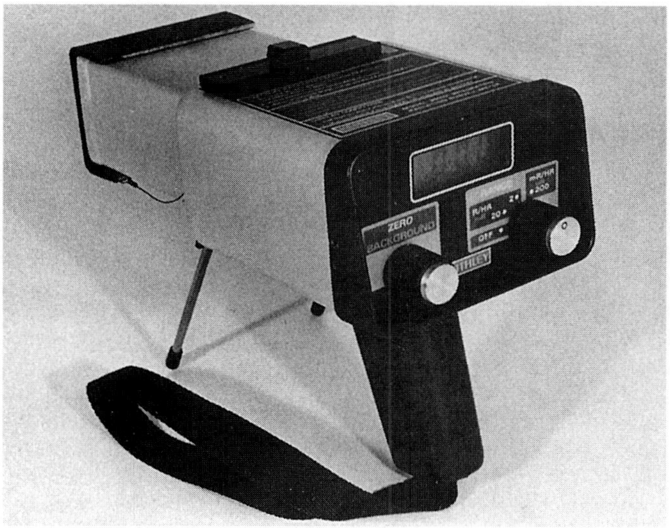

Figure 18.6. Portable air-filled ionization chamber survey meter. This particular instrument measures exposure-rates ranging from about 0.1 mR/hour to 20 R/hour. (Photograph courtesy Keithley Instruments, Inc.) (Reproduced by permission from Bushberg JT, Seibert JA, Leidholdt EM Jr., Boone JM. The essential physics of medical imaging. Baltimore: Williams & Wilkins, 1994.)

Advantages of the Ion Chamber

1. The exposure rate can be accurately measured over a wide range of photon energies. The measured exposure is typically within ±10% of the actual exposure between 40 keV and several MeV.
2. Ion chamber survey meters have a wide exposure range, typically 0.001–500 R/hr.
3. Ion chamber survey meters will not saturate in moderately high radiation fields and express minimal dose-rate effects (typically less than 10% error between 10 mR/hr and 10 R/hr).
4. Changes in atmospheric temperature and pressure do affect measurements from ambient air ion chambers; however, correction factors are typically minor.

Disadvantages of Ion Chambers

1. The response times of these instruments are moderately slow and thus careful observation is required to make accurate measurements.
2. The very small electrical charge produced by each interaction causes ion chambers to be relatively insensitive. An ion chamber would not be the instrument of choice to locate minor contamination or a low-activity source. A more suit-

able instrument for these applications would be a G-M survey meter.

GEIGER-MUELLER SURVEY INSTRUMENTS

Theory of Operation

The most common and versatile portable radiation survey instrument in the nuclear medicine laboratory is the G-M survey meter. These instruments are available from many vendors in a variety of designs. The typical instrument consists of a handheld probe housing the G-M tube, connected by a cable to a separate case containing the detector circuitry and display (Fig. 18.7).

A G-M detector consists of a thin, cylindrical metal shell with a wire mounted at the center of the cylinder. The detector is filled with a noble gas (e.g., neon or argon) and a small amount (~0.1%) of a halogen such as chlorine (quenching gas). A potential difference (voltage) of approximately 900 volts is maintained between the shell and the central wire, which is the positive electrode (anode). As in the ion chamber, radiation produces ion pairs in the sensitive volume. However, in the case of the G-M counter, the large potential difference across the tube accelerates the electrons toward the positively-charged anode, supplying them with sufficient kinetic energy to produce additional ionization. This "avalanche" continues as secondary ionizations trigger additional gas ionization, eventually resulting in a large number of electrons being collected on the anode. This cascade effect, resulting in approximately 10^9 electrons being collected per ionization event, produces, in a typical G-M instrument, a signal of about 1 volt, which is used to activate a counting circuit. The counting circuit registers each avalanche as a "count." The number of counts per minute (cpm) is proportional to the amount of radiation incident on the G-M tube.

Geiger-Mueller tubes contain "quenching" gases to prevent the positive ions, which slowly drift to the cathode, from triggering additional avalanches. The time between the initial avalanche and the neutralization is typically 100 msec. During this time interval, referred to as the *deadtime* of the detector, the detector is insensitive to additional interactions.

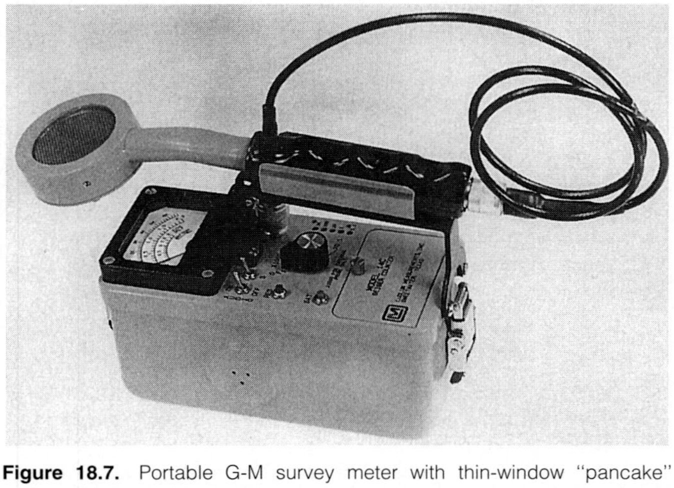

Figure 18.7. Portable G-M survey meter with thin-window "pancake" probe. (Photograph courtesy Ludlum Measurements, Inc.) (Reproduced by permission from Bushberg JT, Seibert JA, Leidholdt EM Jr., Boone JM. The essential physics of medical imaging. Baltimore: Williams & Wilkins, 1994.)

The magnitude of the multiplication effect, and thus the voltage pulse, is independent of the type or energy of the initial ionizing radiation. Therefore, the G-M counter cannot be used to determine radiation energies; however, discrimination between electrons (β-particles and conversion electrons) and photons is possible by sliding a metal or plastic window over a portion of the G-M tube. The thickness of the wall of the G-M tube determines the minimum electron energy detectable.

G-M detectors are extremely sensitive to charged particles of sufficient energy to penetrate the wall of the tube; almost every charged particle reaching the interior of the tube is registered as a count. Flat large-area thin-window probes, called "pancake probes," are especially useful for surveys for radioactive contamination (Fig. 18.7). The high sensitivity of these detectors to charged particles allows them to detect small amounts of activity.

G-M detectors are relatively insensitive to x- and γ-rays, relative to other detectors such as sodium iodide scintillators. Most x- and γ-rays pass through the gas without interaction. Those photons that are detected usually interact with the wall of the tube, with the resultant electrons entering the gas.

G-M survey meters may be calibrated to indicate either exposure-rate (mR/hr) or count-rate (cpm). Those calibrated to indicate exposure rate (mR/hr) usually exhibit a nonlinear energy response relative to an air-filled ion chamber. If calibrated with a high energy γ-ray source (typically ^{137}Cs, 662 keV γ-rays), they overrespond by a factor as much as 5 for photons in the range of 40–100 keV. An energy response curve supplied by the manufacturer can be used to correct the indicated exposure rate, if the energy of the incident photons is known. Some manufacturers offer "energy compensated" G-M probes in which the G-M tube is covered by a sleeve of higher Z metal; the increased photoelectric absorption of lower energy photons by the sleeve gives the detector a flat energy response, permitting accurate measurement of exposure-rate over a wide range of photon energies. However, the energy-compensated probe is not very useful for contamination surveys, because the metal sleeve attenuates most charged particles, and it is much less sensitive to low energy photons than an uncompensated probe.

Advantages of G-M Detectors

1. G-M detectors are extremely sensitive to charged particles of sufficient energy to penetrate the walls of the tubes. G-M instruments equipped with thin window "pancake" probes are very useful for locating radioactive contamination.
2. G-M survey meters are useful for locating areas of high exposure-rate, although for most meters, the indicated exposure-rate may be substantially in error.
3. G-M detectors are relatively inexpensive, portable, lightweight, and rugged, and thus are the instrument of choice for most surveys in the nuclear medicine laboratory.

Disadvantages and Limitations of G-M Detectors

1. Most probes exhibit considerable energy dependence, causing significant errors when exposure rates are measured for

photons of energies other than that for which the detector was calibrated. "Energy compensated" G-M probes have a response relatively independent of photon energy, but at the cost of reduced sensitivity to low energy photons and insensitivity to charged particles.

2. Deadtime count losses cause the G-M detector to indicate a falsely-low interaction rate at high interaction rates. In extremely high radiation fields, the interaction rate may be so high that the long deadtime inherent in G-M detectors results in complete saturation of the detector system. Depending on the design of the instrument, this will result in either a continuous full scale or a zero reading on the meter. The latter is obviously a serious and potentially dangerous limitation of the G-M detector; therefore, ion chambers should always be used to evaluate high radiation fields. The exposure range of G-M detectors is typically limited to ~200 mR/hr (~300,000 cpm).
3. G-M detectors, even with very thin windows, are relatively insensitive to contamination from certain radionuclides, such as ^{125}I and ^{51}Cr. The weak Auger electrons from these radionuclides are unable to penetrate the entrance window and most of their x- or γ-rays pass through the gas without interaction. Other types of instruments, such as portable scintillation survey meters, are preferable for these radionuclides.

USE OF PORTABLE SURVEY INSTRUMENTS

Portable survey instruments should be calibrated at least annually. Following calibration, a small check source (typically 1 μCi of ^{137}Cs for G-M instruments and 10 μCi of ^{137}Cs for ion chamber survey meters) is placed against the detector and the indicated reading recorded on the instrument. On each day of use of a meter, the same check source is placed against the meter at the same location; if the reading is not within ±20% of the reading when last calibrated, the instrument should be recalibrated. The instrument's battery should also be checked each day that the instrument is used.

Surveys with a G-M detector for radioactive contamination are usually performed with the instrument set to its most sensitive scale while the probe is moved slowly approximately 1 cm above the surface to be surveyed. Most G-M survey instruments have speakers that enable the operator to locate sites of contamination or excessive exposure without looking at the meter.

WIPE TESTS FOR REMOVABLE CONTAMINATION

Depending on the survey technique, portable radiation survey instruments may fail to detect contamination less than approximately 4 kBq (~0.1 μCi) of technetium-99m per 100 cm². Although this amount of activity does not constitute a serious personnel hazard, it is good practice to detect and eliminate all unnecessary sites of contamination.

Contamination is simply the presence of noncontained radioactive material in an amount and/or location that is undesirable. Contamination can be either fixed or removable (transportable). This distinction is important with regard to the potential for spread of the contamination to other facilities or personnel. Removable contamination is detected and measured by wipe tests. A piece of filter paper or similar material is wiped over a surface area of approximately 100 cm² (~4 × 4 inches) and counted in an appropriate detector.

The activity on a wipe sample can be assayed using a G-M survey instrument, a proportional counter, a liquid scintillation counter, or a NaI(Tl) well counter or probe system. The selection of one particular instrument over another will be a function of the radionuclide in question, availability of instrumentation, desired minimum detectable activity, accuracy of result, and speed of analysis. In most nuclear medicine laboratories, a NaI(Tl) well detector is the instrument of choice for assaying wipe test samples because of its high detection efficiency for x- and γ-ray emitting radionuclides. If the NaI(Tl) well detector is connected to a multichannel analyzer, the energy spectrum of an unknown radionuclide can be readily displayed and the radionuclide identified by matching its energy spectrum with previously collected spectra from radionuclides used in the laboratory. This information can be extremely useful in tracing a source of contamination.

Regulatory agencies commonly require contamination levels to be recorded in units of disintegrations per minute (dpm) /100 cm². The measured count-rate must be corrected for the background count-rate of the detector and the detection efficiency for the specific radionuclide. For most NaI(Tl) well counters, a conservative estimate of the detection efficiency for common radionuclides used in nuclear medicine is 50%. Thus, when the detector efficiency has not been determined, multiplying the observed counts per minute by 2, after subtracting background, should provide a reasonable estimate of the disintegrations per minute.

LOCATION, FREQUENCY, AND ACTION LEVELS FOR RADIATION SURVEYS

The NRC requires areas where radiopharmaceuticals are routinely prepared or administered to be surveyed at the end of each day of use and all areas where radiopharmaceuticals or radioactive waste are stored to be surveyed weekly with a portable radiation survey meter (16). The instrument used must be able to detect exposure rates of 0.1 mR/h. A Geiger-Mueller survey meter equipped with a large area thin-window detector is recommended for these surveys. NRC regulations also require surveys for removable contamination (wipe tests) to be performed weekly of all areas where radiopharmaceuticals are routinely prepared, administered, or stored (16). Action levels are required to be established for both the instrument surveys and the wipe tests; if the measured dose-rate or removable contamination exceeds its action level, the individual performing the survey must notify the Radiation Safety Officer.

It is common practice to remove any contamination found by either survey meter or wipe test. If proper precautions are taken, most contamination occurs on disposable plastic-backed paper which can be discarded into the radioactive waste. Typically, contaminated surfaces not protected by disposable coverings are cleaned until the removable contamination is less than 200 dpm per 100 cm².

The NRC also requires surveys to be performed of radiation levels in restricted and unrestricted areas and of radioactive material in effluents to demonstrate compliance with the dose limit for individual members of the public (1 mSv (100 mrem) per year) (15). Very sensitive dosimeters, such as those using aluminum oxide TLDs, may be placed in unrestricted areas to demonstrate compliance with respect to external sources of radiation.

PRINCIPLES AND APPLICATIONS OF RADIATION PROTECTION

SOURCES OF EXPOSURE IN NUCLEAR MEDICINE

The average whole body dose for a nuclear medicine technologist in a busy 500-bed hospital is approximately 2 mSv (200 mrem) per year. The exposure received by the individual technologist is determined by factors such as:

1. The activities and photon energies of the radionuclides used.
2. The radiopharmaceuticals' biodistribution and biologic half-life in the patients.
3. Lengths of the imaging procedures. Critically ill and uncooperative patients typically require more positioning time and may require retakes because of patient motion.
4. The distance from the patient to the technologist during imaging. The computer and camera console should be as far from the patient as is practical in an imaging room.

Although the nuclear medicine technologists' hands are exposed to large dose-rates for short periods of time during radiopharmaceutical preparation and injection, the majority of the effective dose to the technologists is from activity in the patient during imaging (31). Over the last 20 years, the replacement of older radiopharmaceuticals with ones labeled with short-lived non-β-particle emitting radionuclides has permitted the administration of much larger activities to patients. These large activities, while necessary for good image quality, produce much higher exposure-rates in the vicinity of the patient. Typical exposures to imaging personnel from various nuclear medicine procedures are listed in Table 18.7.

PROTECTION AGAINST EXTERNAL EXPOSURE

Three techniques can be used to reduce radiation exposure from sources external to the body: decreasing time, increasing distance, and using shielding. These radiation protection principles are ubiquitous in all aspects of health physics and have special applications in nuclear medicine.

Time

Limiting radiation exposure from high radiation fields occasionally encountered in nuclear medicine can be accomplished in many cases by simply reducing the time spent working with or near the source. Typically, the highest radiation fields encountered in the nuclear medicine laboratory are associated with the preparation of the radiopharmaceuticals. The amount of time spent preparing vials and syringes of radiopharmaceuticals in the radiopharmacy is usually directly proportional to one's experience in these tasks. Training technologists initially with nonradioactive solutions is a good way to provide the needed experience while preventing unnecessary radiation exposure.

Distance

Perhaps the most effective and commonly used radiation protection principle used in nuclear medicine is the use of distance to reduce exposure. With some exceptions, the dimensions of most radiation sources are small compared to the distance between the source and personnel. Under these conditions, the radiation field intensity can be assumed to decrease inversely with the square of the distance. The effect of this "inverse square law" can be seen in the example in Table 18.8 demonstrating the effectiveness of remote handling devices in reducing radiation exposure from unshielded radionuclides. Long tongs or forceps should always be used, when handling unshielded sources or vials, to reduce the radiation dose to the hands.

It is important to remember that the patient is a radiation source. Facilities should be designed so that, following patient positioning, personnel can adequately monitor both the patient and acquisition of the image while maintaining a large distance between themselves and the patient. In particular, imaging rooms should be as large as is reasonable and computer consoles in the imaging rooms should be placed as far as possible from the location of the patient being imaged.

The exposure rate at a particular distance from an un-

Table 18.7.
Typical exposure rate at 1 meter from adult nuclear medicine patient after radiopharmaceutic administration

Study	Radiopharmaceutic	Dose (mCi)[a]	Exposure Rate at 1 m (mR/hr)[b]
Thyroid cancer therapy	^{131}I (NaI)	200	~28
Cerebral perfusion scan	^{18}F (FDG)	10	~1.5
Cardiac gated imaging	^{99m}Tc RBC	20	~1.4
Bone scan	^{99m}Tc MDP	25	~1.2
Tumor imaging	^{67}Ga Citrate	3	~0.4
Liver-spleen scan	^{99m}Tc Sulfur colloid	4	~0.2
Myocardial perfusion imaging	^{201}Tl Chloride	3	~0.1

[a]Multiply by 37 to obtain MBq.
[b]Multiply by 258 to obtain nC/kg-hr.
Reprinted from Bushberg JT, Seibert JA, Leidholdt EM Jr., Boone JM. The essential physics of medical imaging. Baltimore: Williams & Wilkins, 1994:600.

Table 18.8.
Effect of Distance on Exposure with Common Radionuclides Used in Nuclear Medicine

Radionuclide (10 mCi)[a]	Exposure Rate (mR/hr)[b,c] at 1 cm	Exposure Rate (mR/hr)[b] at 10 cm (~4 inches)
^{67}Ga	10,870	109
^{99m}Tc	12,000	120
^{123}I	27,050	270
^{131}I	27,770	278
^{133}Xe	10,070	100
^{201}Tl	8,580	85

[a]Multiply by 37 to obtain MBq.
[b]Multiply by 258 to obtain nC/kg-hr.
[c]Source: Shleien, B. The health physics and radiological health handbook, Silver Spring, MD: Scinta, Inc., 1992:165–172. For photons ≥ 10 keV (i.e., Γ_{10}).

shielded radioactive source is a function of its decay scheme and is expressed as the *exposure rate constant* (Γ). Γ is the exposure rate from x- and γ-rays above a specified minimum energy (e.g., Γ_{10} is the exposure rate constant for all photons with energies above 10 keV) per unit activity and at a unit distance. Γ is commonly expressed as roentgens per hour from 1 mCi at 1 cm, which has the units: R • cm²/mCi • hr. The exposure rate from any activity and at any distance may be calculated as:

$$X = \Gamma A/r^2 \tag{8}$$

where Γ is the exposure rate constant, *A* is the activity of the source, and *r* is the distance from the source. The dramatic effect of distance on lowering the exposure rate is shown in Table 18.8 for radionuclides commonly used in nuclear medicine.

Shielding

In addition to time and distance, shielding of the radiation source is commonly used to reduce the exposure rate to personnel. The choice of shielding material is a function of the type of radiation and its energy. β-Radiation is best shielded with low atomic number (Z) materials, such as plastic or water, to minimize the production of bremsstrahlung x-rays, which are much more penetrating than the β-particles. When large activities of high-energy β-emitters are to be shielded, lead shielding outside the plastic shield will help attenuate the bremsstrahlung that is produced.

External radiation fields from radionuclides used in nuclear medicine consist primarily of x- and γ-rays. High-Z materials such as lead are very effective in attenuating these forms of radiation.

The half-value layer (HVL) is the thickness of a specified shielding material necessary to reduce the intensity of the incident radiation by one-half. Thus, two HVLs reduce the intensity by one-fourth, three HVLs reduce it by one-eighth, and so on. The general formula for the reduction factor is $1/2^n$ where *n* is equal to the number of HVLs. The HVL is a function of the radionuclide being shielded and the shielding material. The exposure rate constants and HVLs of lead for several radionuclides common to nuclear medicine are listed in Table 18.9.

Lead aprons (0.5 mm lead equivalent), which are commonly worn in diagnostic x-ray departments to shield personnel from low-energy scattered radiation, are not usually recommended for use in nuclear medicine departments because they do not provide very effective attenuation for the higher energy photons from radiopharmaceuticals (~65% attenuation for 140 keV γ-rays).

Considerations in Shield Construction

When erecting or relocating a shield, the following points should be considered:

1. All six sides adjacent to the shield should be considered in terms of affording adequate protection for both radiation workers and others. In particular, the bottoms of bench-top work areas should be sufficiently shielded to protect the lower part of the body.
2. The working surface must be able to support the weight of the shielding and both should be covered with plastic-backed absorbent paper or other material to aid in the removal of contamination.
3. Consideration must be given to the radiation exposure to the head of a person manipulating objects behind the shield. Leaded glass is commonly used for this purpose. Mirrors located over or in storage areas often permit sources to be manipulated without direct radiation exposure to the head.
4. After construction, the shield should be evaluated by placing a source behind the shield and measuring the exposure rates in surrounding areas.

Table 18.9.
γ-Exposure rate constants (Γ_{10}) and half value layers (HVL) of lead for radionuclides of interest to nuclear medicine

Radionuclide	Γ_{10} (R·cm²/mCi·hr)[a,c]	Half Value Layer in Pb (mm)[b,d]
^{57}Co	1.5	0.18
^{99m}Tc	1.2	0.25
^{111}In	5.0	0.67
^{123}I	2.7	0.36
^{131}I	2.8	2.88
^{67}Ga	1.1	1.45
^{201}Tl	0.8	0.26
^{133}Xe	1.0	0.17

[a]Multiply by 6.97 to obtain μC/kg·cm²/MBq-hr.
[b]The first HVL will be significantly greater than subsequent HVLs for those radionuclides with multiple photon emissions at significantly different energies (e.g., Ga-67) because the lower energy photons will be preferentially attenuated in the first HVL.
[c]Source: Shleien, B. The health physics and radiological health handbook, Silver Spring, MD: Scinta, Inc., 1992:165–192. For photons ≥ 10 keV (i.e., Γ_{10}).
[d]Adapted from Shleien, B. The health physics and radiological health handbook, p. 165–172.

Radiopharmaceutical Preparation Areas

Table-top lead shields with leaded glass windows are used to protect the heads and bodies of persons preparing doses of radiopharmaceuticals (Fig. 18.8). Most commercial table-top shields do not have lead in their bases; a separate sheet of lead should be placed on the table top beneath the table-top shield. Shielding is commonly placed against the wall behind the dose preparation area to protect personnel in the adjacent room.

Syringe and Vial Shields

All stock solutions of radioactive material should be stored in vial shields. Virtually all radionuclides shipped to nuclear medicine departments arrive in lead vial shields that are adequate for the purpose of radiation safety. Commercial vial shields with leaded glass windows are helpful in determining the fluid level in the vial when withdrawing an aliquot with a syringe.

Syringe shields made from lead or tungsten with lead-glass windows are commonly used to reduce exposures during radiopharmaceutical preparation and administration (Fig. 18.9). Syringe shields can reduce exposure to the technologists' hands by 50% during radiopharmaceutical preparation and as much as 80% during injection (31).

Shielding During Imaging

Techniques which minimize the exposure to technologists during imaging procedures will substantially reduce their

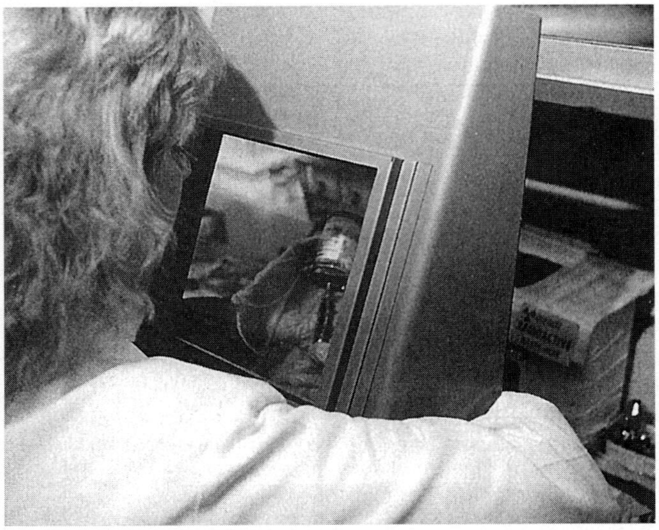

Figure 18.8. Dose preparation work station. The technologist is drawing the radiopharmaceutical from a vial shielded by a "lead pig" into a syringe contained in a syringe shield. Further protection from radiation exposure is afforded by working behind the lead "L-shield" with a leaded glass window. The technologist is wearing a lab coat and disposable gloves to prevent contamination. A film badge is worn on the lab coat to record whole body exposure and a TLD finger ring dosimeter is worn inside the glove to record the extremity exposure. (Reproduced by permission from Bushberg JT, Seibert JA, Leidholdt EM Jr., Boone JM. The essential physics of medical imaging. Baltimore: Williams & Wilkins, 1994.)

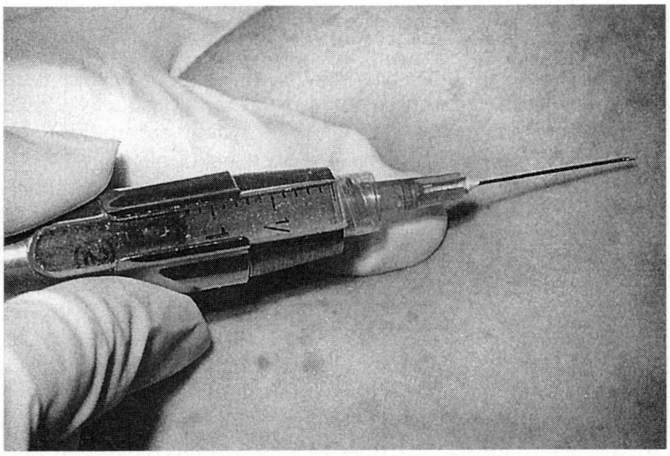

Figure 18.9. Syringe shield for a 3 cc syringe. The barrel is made from high Z material (e.g., lead or tungsten) in which a leaded glass window is inserted so that the syringe graduations and the dose can be seen. (Reproduced by permission from Bushberg JT, Seibert JA, Leidholdt EM Jr., Boone JM. The essential physics of medical imaging. Baltimore: Williams & Wilkins, 1994.)

annual effective doses. To that end, fixed or mobile leaded glass or acrylic shields between the computer terminal and the location of the patient being imaged are being increasingly used to protect the technologist. This is particularly important in situations in which the computer terminal and imaging equipment are in close proximity.

PROTECTION AGAINST PERSONNEL CONTAMINATION AND THE INCORPORATION OF RADIOACTIVITY INTO THE BODY

Small amounts of radioactivity on the skin or in the body can produce large radiation doses. For example, the intake of 37 kBq (1 μCi) of ^{131}I will produce a dose to the thyroid of approximately 0.01 Gy (1 rad). Additionally, it is often difficult or impossible to significantly hasten the elimination of radioactivity once it has been incorporated into the body. Incorporation of radioactivity into the body can occur by inhalation, ingestion, absorption through the skin, or through wounds. For these reasons, it is important to handle unsealed radioactive material in such a manner as to prevent it from coming into contact with the skin and to minimize the release of radioactivity into the air.

The degrees of hazard of radioactive materials as potential internal contaminants varies widely and is determined by the following factors: (a) the types and energies of the particles and photons emitted, (b) the physical half-life of the material, (c) the kinetics of the material in the body, and (d) the potential of the material to become airborne or absorbed through the skin. Radionuclides emitting α-particles are, in general, more hazardous than those emitting electrons and those emitting energetic electrons tend to be more hazardous that those mainly emitting photons. Radioactive materials of longer physical half-life tend to be more hazardous than those of shorter half-life. The kinetics of the radioactive material in the body is important; materials retained by the body tend to be more hazardous than those which are rapidly eliminated. Also, those which concentrate in or near radiosensitive tissues (e.g., the bone marrow) are, in general, more hazardous than those which are more uniformly distributed in the body or concentrate in less radiation sensitive tissues. The most hazardous radionuclides commonly used in nuclear medicine are ^{131}I, ^{125}I, ^{89}Sr, and ^{32}P.

Radiation Protection—Practical Considerations for the Nuclear Medicine Department

Provided the radioactive material is not likely to become airborne, the main precautions when handling unsealed radioactivity resemble the "universal precautions" used to protect staff from blood-borne pathogens. The following is a list of basic rules that should be observed when working with radioactive material:

1. Unsealed radioactive material should be handled in designated work areas posted with radioactive material warning signs and covered with plastic-backed absorbent paper or other suitable material that will absorb spills and prevent the spread of contamination. The paper should be replaced regularly.
2. Lab coats or other protective clothing must be worn when in rooms where unsealed radioactivity is used. Lab coats should be buttoned while handling radioactivity. This protective clothing should be changed if contaminated and should not be worn outside the work area.
3. Disposable impermeable gloves should be worn when handling unsealed radioactive material and replaced frequently.
4. Hands should be washed after removing the disposable gloves and surveyed with a suitable survey instrument.

The hands should also be washed and the hands and clothing surveyed before eating, drinking, or smoking, and at the end of the workday.

5. Body dosimeters should be worn in the department and finger dosimeters should be worn whenever eluting generators, handling radioactivity, or positioning patients.
6. All radioactive material should be kept in adequately shielded containers when not in use. Mirrors should be placed behind open storage areas to reduce exposure to the head.
7. All potentially volatile or gaseous radioactive materials (e.g., ^{131}I and ^{133}Xe) should be stored and used in a fume hood with adequate air flow (i.e., between 100 and 150 linear feet/minute).
8. No eating, drinking, or smoking should be allowed in rooms in which radionuclides are stored or used, nor should storage of food or beverages be permitted.
9. All containers of radioactive material should be clearly labeled with radionuclide name, chemical form, activity, and date and time of assay.
10. Pipetting should never be done by mouth. Instead, remote or mechanical pipetting devices should be used.
11. Work areas should be kept as clear and clutter free as possible.
12. All spills should be contained and cleaned up immediately in order to minimize the spread of contamination. Spills should be cleaned from the areas of low contamination toward the area of highest contamination.
13. Office, study, and reading areas should be located as far away from radionuclide storage areas as practical.
14. Syringe and vial shields should always be used for preparing and administering doses of radiopharmaceuticals to patients.
15. Long tongs or forceps should be used to reduce the radiation dose to the hands when handling unshielded vials and other sources.
16. All preparations of radiopharmaceutical stock solutions and patient doses should be performed behind a leaded glass drawing station.
17. Daily G-M meter surveys and weekly wipe tests of the laboratory area should be conducted to evaluate and document exposure and contamination.
18. The recapping of needles should be discouraged to reduce the hazards of blood-borne pathogens. However, when recapping a needle is necessary, the cap must not be held with the hands.

Radioactive Aerosols and Gases

A number of radioactive noble gases (e.g., ^{133}Xe and ^{81m}Kr) and ^{99m}Tc DTPA aerosol are used in nuclear medicine for lung ventilation studies. Additionally, radioiodine in the form of sodium iodide can evolve a radioactive gas. The risk to workers from airborne radioactivity depends upon the radionuclide, its chemical form, its concentration in the air, and the duration of time that persons are exposed to it. The dose from radioactive noble gases is usually due to external exposure from the cloud of gas, since little of the gas is absorbed from the lungs. For most other airborne radioactive material, there is significant uptake and retention of radioactivity by the body. The methods for protecting personnel from airborne radioactivity are to minimize the activity that is released, use dilution to minimize the concentration of radioactivity in the air, and limit the time that people are exposed to airborne radioactivity.

The primary method of protecting workers and the public from airborne radioactivity is to minimize the release of activity to the atmosphere. For example, vials of radioactive iodine should be kept tightly capped. Solutions of radioiodine in the form of sodium iodide should be maintained at a basic pH, because the volatility is enhanced at low pH.

Filters or traps are commonly used to minimize the release of activity to the atmosphere. In nuclear medicine, disposable filters are used to collect the technetium-99m aerosol and charcoal traps are commonly used to collect ^{133}Xe exhaled by patients during lung ventilation studies. A charcoal xenon trap consists of a charcoal filter cartridge, surrounded by lead shielding, to trap the xenon in the air expired by the patient and a blower to pull the air through the charcoal cartridge. Each xenon trap is equipped with a moisture trap to prevent moisture in the air expired by the patient from wetting the charcoal and reducing its trapping efficiency. The desiccant in the moisture trap should be checked frequently and replaced when it changes color. Some xenon traps, which permit the patients to rebreathe expired air, are also equipped with containers of soda lime to absorb carbon dioxide and prevent the patients from becoming acidotic during the recirculation phase of the studies. The soda lime must be replaced frequently. The effluent from charcoal traps must be monitored to ensure that the charcoal traps are functioning acceptably. Many traps are equipped with exhaust monitors which continuously measure the concentration of xenon in the exhaust from the traps. The charcoal cartridges should be replaced when indicated by the exhaust monitors. When a trap is not equipped with an exhaust monitor, the exhaust gas should be collected once a month and counted to ensure the trap is functioning acceptably.

Significant activities of volatile or gaseous radioactive materials should be stored and manipulated in fume hoods. The average air velocity at the face of the fume hood should be between 100 and 150 feet per minute with the sash of the hood at a reasonable working height (typically 45 cm). The fume hood should be free of clutter that might create areas of reduced air flow. The average face velocity should be measured at least annually, and the hood marked with the date of the inspection, the average face velocity, and the maximal acceptable sash height. The fan for the hood should be located at the exhaust (roof) end of the ducting and the ducting should terminate in a stack far from building air intakes.

Rooms in which ventilation studies are performed should be at a negative pressure with respect to surrounding rooms, so that the air flow at doors is into rather than out of the ventilation study rooms, thereby limiting the loss of radioactive gas or aerosol into surrounding rooms. Negative pressure is achieved by ensuring that the supply air flow into the room is substantially exceeded by the exhaust flow. The room exhaust should be entirely released to the exterior of the building away from intake vents; it should not be recirculated. Additionally, the exhaust flow must be sufficient to keep the average airborne concentration in the room substantially less than the less than the derived air concentration (DAC) specified by the U.S. Nuclear Regulatory Commission for that radionuclide. (DACs for certain radionuclides of interest to nuclear medicine are listed in

Table 18.6.) The average air activity concentration in the room is calculated from the equation:

$$C = \frac{A/T}{Q} \quad (9)$$

where C is the average air concentration, A is the average activity released in a specified time period (typically a month), T is the time period, and Q is the room's exhaust flow (typically in cubic feet per minute). NRC regulations require the measurement of ventilation rates in rooms in which radioactive gases are used every 6 months (16).

For example, assume that a room used for ^{133}Xe lung ventilation studies has an exhaust air flow of 400 cubic feet per minute, that an average of 10 ventilation studies are performed per month, and that an average activity of 10 mCi is used per study. If it assumed that 25% of the xenon-133 is lost to the room, the average air concentration is:

$$C = \frac{(0.25)(10\ pts)(10\ mCi/pt)/(1\ month)}{400\ cu.\ ft./min}$$

Converting millicuries to microcuries and cubic feet to milliliters, and recognizing that there are approximately 10,000 working minutes in a month, the average air concentration is:

$$C = 2.2 \times 10^{-7}\ \mu Ci/ml$$

which is much less than the DAC for ^{133}Xe listed in Table 18.6.

More detailed information on radiation protection principles can be found in several publications (32–34).

PROTECTION OF THE NUCLEAR MEDICINE PATIENT

ENSURING THE RADIOPHARMACEUTICAL IS ADMINISTERED AS INTENDED

Among the most important aspects to protecting the nuclear medicine patient are to ensure that appropriate studies are performed correctly on the intended patients and that female patients who may be pregnant or are breast-feeding children are identified prior to the administration of radiopharmaceuticals. Each nuclear medicine department should have written procedures regarding the administration of radiopharmaceuticals to patients; staff members must be trained in these procedures upon employment and regularly thereafter. The following procedures are recommended for routine diagnostic studies:

1. All requests for patient studies must be reviewed by a nuclear medicine staff physician for appropriateness. The request for a study should then be sent to the technologists in writing. It is the responsibility of the physician to ensure that the desired procedure is clearly described.
2. When a vial of a radiopharmaceutical is placed in a vial radiation shield, the shield must be conspicuously labeled with the name of the radiopharmaceutical.
3. The activity of each dosage of a photon-emitting radiopharmaceutical must be assayed using a dose calibrator prior to administration, even if it is a precalibrated unit dosage prepared by a commercial radiopharmacy.
4. The radiopharmaceutical and prescribed activity or activity range for each procedure should be posted near the dose calibrator and/or contained within the department's policy and procedure manual.
5. Whenever a syringe of a radiopharmaceutical is placed in a syringe radiation shield, the shield must be conspicuously labeled with the name of the radiopharmaceutical and the name of the patient, even if the syringe is to be immediately administered to a patient.
6. The patient must be identified by two independent means (e.g., requesting the patient to recite his or her name and social security number) at the time of radiopharmaceutical administration. The information received from the patient, the approved request for the procedure, and the label on the syringe shield must be compared. If more than one dosage is to be administered to a patient, the patient must be properly identified at the time of each administration.
7. All female patients of childbearing potential must be asked if they might be pregnant or are breast-feeding a child before the administration of a radiopharmaceutical. Adolescent female patients should not necessarily be assumed to be not sexually active.

REDUCTION OF THE RADIATION DOSE TO THE PATIENT

The radiopharmaceutical chosen for a procedure significantly affects the radiation dose to the patient. In particular, ^{123}I sodium iodide should be used instead of ^{131}I sodium iodide for routine thyroid uptake measurements and imaging. Also, ^{123}I-labeled radiopharmaceuticals should be used, whenever possible, instead of ones labeled with ^{131}I. Whenever ^{131}I-labeled radiopharmaceuticals, other than NaI, are used (e.g., ^{131}I hippuran), the patient's thyroid should be first blocked with nonradioactive iodine to limit the thyroidal uptake of unbound radioiodine.

The radiation doses to patients from radiopharmaceuticals that are excreted in the urine can be reduced significantly by encouraging the patients to drink fluids and void frequently. It is important, of course, to first screen for patients for whom this recommendation is contraindicated, such as patients suffering from congestive heart failure.

PATIENTS WHO ARE PREGNANT OR NURSING A CHILD

It is essential that female patients between the ages of 13 and 50 be asked if they might be pregnant or are breast-feeding infants. Also, patient waiting and reception areas should be posted with prominent signs requesting such patients to notify the staff. Patients who might be pregnant or are breast-feeding must be referred to a nuclear medicine staff physician who will determine whether the study should be performed and, if the study is to be performed, any modifications to the procedure and precautions to be followed by the patient. A pregnancy test can be performed if it is uncertain whether the patient is pregnant.

When the patient is pregnant, the physician should consider other diagnostic modalities and radiopharmaceuticals which might reduce or even avoid the irradiation of the fetus. The physician may wish to ask a medical physicist to estimate the radiation dose to the fetus from the intended procedure. Estimations of fetal dose are relatively simple when the radiopharmaceutical does not cross the placenta. Reducing the administered activity will reduce the fetal dose; however, it must first be ascertained whether the patient is capable of remaining immobile for the increased duration of the study. Because of the proximity of the bladder to the uterus, it is important to encourage the patient to drink fluids and void frequently to reduce the fetal dose from radiopharmaceuticals eliminated via the kidneys. The physician should discuss the potential risks, alternatives, and precautions with the patient. It is prudent to have the patient sign a statement acknowledging the discussion and consenting to the study.

Patients who are breast-feeding children must be counseled by the nuclear medicine physician to cease breast-feeding until the radionuclide in the milk has reached a sufficiently low concentration. As in the case of the pregnant patient, the physician should consider whether the study is necessary, alternate diagnostic modalities, and other radiopharmaceuticals which might reduce the length of time that cessation of nursing is required. Table 18.10 contains recommendations for the cessation of breast feeding following the administration of common radiopharmaceuticals. The patient should be instructed to manually express and discard her breast milk during this period to avoid discomfort and maintain lactation. The physician should discuss the potential risks, alternatives, and precautions with the patient, and have the patient sign a statement acknowledging the discussion and consenting to the study.

RADIOLABELED BLOOD PRODUCTS

Certain procedures, such as indium-111- and technetium-99m-labeled leukocyte scans and chromium-51 erythrocyte studies, require the in vitro labeling and reinjection into the patient of blood elements. Tragic consequences can occur if blood or blood components from a patient with blood-borne pathogens are mistakenly reinjected into the wrong patient. Each nuclear medicine department should have stringent procedures requiring the labeling of blood samples and identification of the patient at the time the blood is drawn and again prior to reinjection to avoid such accidents. All staff must be trained in such procedures upon employment and regularly thereafter.

MISADMINISTRATIONS

NRC regulations require that each dose of a photon-emitting radiopharmaceutical be assayed using a dose calibrator prior to administration to a patient (16). The NRC has defined a *misadministration* as the administration of:

1. An activity greater than 30 microcuries of ^{125}I or ^{131}I sodium iodide when
   a. it is administered to the wrong patient,
   b. the patient is administered the wrong radiopharmaceutical, or
   c. the administered activity differs from the prescribed activity by more than 20% of the prescribed activity and the difference exceeds 30 microcuries;
2. A therapeutic radiopharmaceutical dosage, other than ^{125}I or ^{131}I sodium iodide, when
   a. it is administered to the wrong patient or by the wrong route of administration,
   b. the patient is administered the wrong radiopharmaceutical, or
   c. the administered activity differs from the prescribed activity by more than 20% of the prescribed activity;
3. A diagnostic radiopharmaceutical dosage, other than activities greater than 30 μCi of either ^{125}I or ^{131}I sodium iodide, when both

Table 18.10.
Recommendations for Cessation of Breast Feeding after Administration of Radiopharmaceutic to Mothers[c]

Radiopharamceutic	Administered Activity[a]	Imaging Procedure	Safe Breast Milk Concentration (μCi/ml)	Cessation of Breast Feeding until Breast Milk is Safe
^{99m}Tc Sodium Pertechnetate	10 mCi	Thyroid scan and Meckel's scan	8.2×10^{-2}	24 hrs
^{99m}Tc kits (general rule)	5–25 mCi	All	8.2×10^{-2}	24 hrs
^{99m}Tc DTPA	10–15 mCi	Renal scan	1.2×10^{-1}	17 hrs
^{99m}Tc MAA	3–5 mCi	Lung perfusion scan	1.2×10^{-1}	10 hrs
^{99m}Tc Sulfur Colloid	5 mCi	Liver spleen scan	1.6×10^{-1}	15 hrs
^{99m}Tc MDP	15–25 mCi	Bone scan	2.1×10^{-1}	17 hrs
^{67}Ga Citrate	6–10 mCi	Infection and tumor scans	2.1×10^{-3}	4 wks
^{201}Tl Chloride	3 mCi	Myocardial perfusion	2.4×10^{-3}	3 wks
Sodium ^{123}I	30 μCi	Thyroid uptake	1.2×10^{-4}	3 days
	50–400 μCi	Thyroid scan	1.2×10^{-4}	5 days
Sodium ^{131}I	5 μCi	Thyroid uptake	4.1×10^{-7}	68 days
Sodium ^{131}I	10 mCi	Thyroid cancer Scan or Graves Therapy	4.1×10^{-7}	Discontinue[b]
Sodium ^{131}I	29.9 mCi	Outpatient therapy for Hyperfunctioning nodule	4.1×10^{-7}	Discontinue[b]
Sodium ^{131}I	100 mCi or more	Thyroid cancer treatment (ablation)	4.1×10^{-7}	Discontinue[b]

[a]Multiply by 37 to obtain MBq.
[b]Discontinuance is based not only on the excessive time recommended for cessation of breast feeding but also on the high dose the breasts themselves would receive during the radiopharmaceutical breast transit.
[c]Adapted from Conte AC, Bushberg JT. Essential science of nuclear medicine. In: Brant WE, Helms CA, eds. Fundamentals of diagnostic radiology. Baltimore: Williams & Wilkins, 1994.

a. it is administered to the wrong patient, by the wrong route of administration, or the administered activity differs from the prescribed activity, and
b. the effective dose equivalent to the patient exceeds 5 rem or the dose equivalent to any organ exceeds 50 rem.

When a misadministration is discovered, immediate action must be taken to minimize the radiation dose to the patient. Methods include the use of emetics or gastric lavage to remove orally administered radiopharmaceuticals and the use of blocking agents such as potassium iodide for ^{131}I sodium iodide and $KClO_4$ for ^{99m}Tc pertechnetate. NCRP Report No. 65 provides useful guidance (41). NRC regulations require the licensee to notify the NRC and the referring physician within 24 hours, followed by a written report to the NRC within 15 days (16). The patient, or patient's responsible relative or guardian, must also be notified within 24 hours, unless the referring physician informs the licensee either that he or she will inform the patient or that, based on medical judgment, notifying the patient would be harmful. The licensee is not required to notify the patient or the patient's responsible relative or guardian without first consulting the referring physician. A written report must be furnished to the patient or the patient's relative or guardian if either was notified verbally. The written report to the NRC must state whether the licensee informed the patient or the patient's relative or guardian and if not, why not. The report to the NRC must *not* include the patient's name or other identifying information. Whenever a misadministration is suspected, the current NRC regulations should be consulted to ensure all legal requirements are met.

QUALITY MANAGEMENT PROGRAM

The NRC requires each of its medical licensees to develop and implement a "quality management" (QM) program to ensure that certain higher-risk radiopharmaceuticals are administered to patients as directed by the nuclear medicine physician (16). A written directive must be prepared by the physician prior to the administration of activities of either ^{125}I or ^{131}I sodium iodide exceeding 30 μCi or any administration of a radiopharmaceutical for therapeutic purposes. Prior to each administration, the patient's identity must be verified by more than one method as the individual named in the written directive and the administration must be in accordance with the directive. Any unintended deviations from the directive must be identified and corrective action taken. The QM program must be reviewed at intervals not to exceed 12 months. Each licensee must prepare written procedures for its QM program and submit them to the NRC. The licensee must maintain all written directives, records of all administrations subject to the QM program, the reviews of the program, and records of the investigations of all recordable events for 3 years. It is recommended that a form be prepared for written directives. Figure 18.10 shows such a form.

RADIOPHARMACEUTICAL THERAPIES

Radiopharmaceuticals are used for therapy in a number of diseases. The most common is the use of activities of 111 mBq–1.1 Gbq (3–30 mCi) of ^{131}I sodium iodide for the treatment of hyperthyroidism and 1.85–7.4 GBq (50–200 mCi) of ^{131}I sodium iodide for the treatment of thyroid carcinoma. Activities up to 555 mBq (15 mCi) of phosphorus-32 as sodium phosphate are used for the treatment of diseases of the bone marrow such as polycythemia vera, thrombocythemia, and certain leukemias and for palliation of pain in patients with multiple skeletal metastases from cancer. Activities of approximately 148 mBq (4 mCi) of strontium-89 are administered for palliation of pain in patients with multiple skeletal metastases from cancer. A variety of monoclonal and polyclonal antibodies, the majority of which are labeled with ^{131}I, are under investigation for radioimmunotherapy of cancer. The properties of these radionuclides are summarized in Table 18.11.

All radionuclides used for therapy emit a significant fraction of their decay energy as charged particles. The properties that make these radionuclides useful in therapy also render them relatively hazardous to medical staff, the patients' families, and the public. In general, the primary precaution for radionuclides emitting only charged particles, such as ^{32}P and ^{89}Sr, is to control contamination from the patients. External exposure from x-rays (bremsstrahlung) is neglible. In the case of therapeutic radionuclides with significant photon emissions, such as ^{131}I, precautions must be taken against both contamination and external exposure.

THERAPY OF THE OUTPATIENT

Medical facilities licensed by the U.S. Nuclear Regulatory Commission are permitted to administer radiopharmaceuticals for therapeutic purposes to outpatients, provided that the administered activity is less than 1.11 Gbq (30 mCi) or the measured dose equivalent rate is less than 50 μSv/hr (5 mrem/hr) at 1 meter (16). Therefore, patients being treated with ^{32}P and ^{89}Sr and most patients being treated for hyperthyroidism with ^{131}I may be treated without being hospitalized, except when hospitalization is required for medical reasons. However, each patient should be interviewed regarding his or her home and work situation before administration of the radiopharmaceutical and instructed in radiation safety precautions to be followed after treatment. It may occasionally be necessary to hospitalize patients for radiation safety reasons, for example, if the patient lives with a pregnant woman or small children in a small apartment, or if it is believed that the patient is unlikely to follow radiation safety precautions. The precautions should be given both verbally and in writing. The following is an example of such precautions for ^{131}I:

Safety Precautions Following Administration of Radioactive Iodine-131: 370 mBq–1.11 GBq (10–30 mCi)

The dose of radioactive iodine that you have received is beneficial to you, but it is desirable that other persons not be unnecessarily exposed to radiation. The following precautions will help minimize the radiation exposure to other persons.

A. During the first 5 days

Much of the radioactivity in your body will be eliminated in your

CHECKLIST FOR RADIOPHARMACEUTICAL THERAPY OR ADMINISTRATION OF I-125 OR I-131 AS SODIUM IODIDE

Radiopharmaceutical Prescription
(completed by Nuclear Medicine Attending Physician)

Patient____
Social Security Number____________________ Date of Birth____________________
Procedure____

Radiopharmaceutical Prescribed______________ in the chemical form of______________
Route of administration____________________ Activity Prescribed__________ millicuries

Signature of Nuclear Medicine Attending Physician__________________ Date__________

Radiopharmaceutical Administration
(Two Nuclear Medicine staff members shall verify that the patient's identity, radionuclide, chemical form, activity, and route of administration match the above prescription.)

Patient identification: The patient's identity has been verified immediately prior to administration of the radiopharmaceutical and compared to the prescription above by at least two of the following methods:

_____1. Asking the patient to state and spell his/her full name and compare with the prescription above.
_____2. Comparing stated social security number with prescription above.
_____3. Comparing stated date of birth with prescription above.
_____4. Comparing stated address with patient's record and prescription above.
_____5. Comparing photographic identification (e.g., driver's license) with prescription above and patient's appearance.
_____6. Comparing in-patient identification wrist band with patient record and prescription above.
_____7. Relative or friend attests to patient's identify:
Name of attestor____________________ Relationship to patient____________________

Pregnant or breast-feeding: If patient is female and between 13 and 50, patient was asked if she might be pregnant or is breast-feeding a child.__________

Radiopharmaceutical dosage verification: (completed by person administering radiopharmaceutical)

Radiopharmaceutical being administered__________ in the chemical form of______________
Radiopharmaceutical lot number______________________________
Measured activity____________________ millicuries at____________________
Route of administration______________________________
Date and time of administration______________________________

Signature of person administering dose______________________________
Signature of person verifying patient's identity, radiopharmaceutical, activity, and route of administration______________________________

Review After Administration for Unintended Deviations

Deviations:____
____________________ Radiation Safety Officer______________ Date__________

Figure 18.10. Checklist for radiopharmaceutical therapy or administration of ^{125}I or ^{131}I as sodium iodide.

urine. Also, some radioactivity will be found in your saliva and perspiration. To minimize the spread of radioactivity:

1. Wash cups, plates, and eating utensils immediately after use or use disposables.
2. Do not kiss anyone.
3. Do not share towels and washcloths with others.
4. Sleep in a separate bed.
5. Wash any clothing you have worn (including pajamas, underwear, towels, and bed linens) separately from those used by other members of your family.
6. Do not touch or hold infants or pregnant women.
7. Stay at least 3 feet away from other people, except for very brief contact.
8. Flush the toilet twice after using it. If you spill any urine

Table 18.11.
Physical Properties of Radionuclides Commonly Used for Therapy

Nuclide	Half-life (days)	Maximum β Energy (keV)	Average β Energy (keV)	x- and γ-Ray Emissions (keV)
^{32}P	14.3	1710	695	none
^{89}Sr	50.6	1491	583	rare
^{131}I	8.04	807	182	364 (81%) others < 723

on the toilet or elsewhere, wash the area three times using toilet paper and flush it down the toilet.

9. Wash your hands frequently, especially before touching another person.

B. During the next 5 days

Your thyroid gland will contain significant radioactivity. To minimize the radiation exposure to others:

1. Sleep in a separate bed.
2. Avoid sitting close to others (within 2 feet) for hours at a time (for example, at a movie theater).
3. Do not hold infants or young children, except for short periods.

C. If you are breast-feeding an infant, you must discontinue breast-feeding. Your doctor will advise you when you may resume.

The precautions described in items A and C above are sufficient for patients administered ^{32}P or ^{89}Sr for therapeutic purposes or activities of ^{131}I sodium iodide between 37–370 mBq (1–10 mCi).

THERAPY OF THE HOSPITALIZED PATIENT

Institutions licensed by the NRC are required to hospitalize patients administered radiopharmaceuticals until the activity in the patient falls below 1.11 Gbq (30 mCi) or the dose equivalent rate at 1 meter falls below 50 μSv/hr (5 mrem/hr) (16). Although the patient is usually released from the hospital when the retained activity or dose equivalent rate fall below these limits, patients are sometimes hospitalized longer for radiation protection purposes. In some cases, it may be appropriate to release patients from the hospital before the conditions specified are met. If the patient is compliant and their home environment is unlikely to result in an effective dose to others in excess of 50 μSv (5 mrem), regulations should be consulted before the patient is discharged.

The following radiation safety precautions are recommended for hospitalized ^{131}I therapy patients:

1. Room selection: The patient must be confined to a private room selected to minimize the exposure to staff and other patients. Corner rooms are often used. Adjacent rooms, other than infrequently occupied rooms such as storage rooms, often must be placed off limits, unless shielding is used. The patient's room must have a private toilet.
2. Training of staff: The nursing staff on the ward and the ward team (medical students, residents, fellows, and staff physicians) must be trained in radiation safety precautions. Written nursing instructions should be placed in the patient's chart and a warning label indicating the patient contains radioactive material should be placed on the cover of the patient's chart. Housekeeping personnel must be instructed not to enter the room or remove anything from the room. Dietetics personnel must be instructed to provide disposable table service and not to enter the room when delivering meals. Personnel on all shifts must receive training.
3. Room preparation: The majority of the ^{131}I will be excreted in the urine in the first 24 hours; however, iodine-131 will also be found in perspiration and saliva. Surfaces likely to become contaminated should be covered with plastic or plastic-backed absorbent paper to aid in decontamination. These include the floor of the room and bathroom, the mattress, the pillows, toilet seat, rim of the toilet bowl, tops of all tables and night stands, and anything the patient is likely to touch (e.g., the phone, light switches, TV and bed controls).
4. The patient's door should be posted with a "Radioactive Materials" warning sign and instructions that the room not be released for general use without the approval of the Radiation Safety Officer and that visitors and ancillary personnel contact the nursing station or Radiation Safety Office before entering the room.
5. Radiation safety instructions for the patient: The patient should be instructed in radiation safety precautions. These include not leaving the room, keeping distance from and not touching visitors, flushing the toilet twice after use, and frequent hand washing. Male patients should be asked to sit when urinating into the toilet. Patients for whom it is not contraindicated for medical reasons should be encouraged to drink fluids and urinate frequently while confined.
6. Personnel dosimetry: Nursing staff providing care for the patient must be issued dosimeters.
7. Administration of the dose: The dose usually arrives precalibrated for the correct activity at the time of administration. The activity must be measured using a dose calibrator, preferably twice, before it is administered to the patient. The therapy dose should be transported to the patient's room on a cart and should be shielded to reduce the exposure rate at 1 meter to less than 2 mR/hr. Prior to administration of the dose, a written directive must be prepared by the nuclear medicine staff physician naming the patient and specifying the radionuclide, chemical form, and administered activity. The administration must be in accordance with the directive and the identity of the patient must be verified by at least two independent means. (See "Quality Management Program" under "Protection of the Patient" earlier in this chapter.) If the patient is female and between the ages of 13 and 50, she must be asked if she might be pregnant or is nursing a child. Although the technologist may administer therapeutic quantities of radioactive material, it is recommended that the nuclear medicine staff physician supervise the administration of the dose.
8. Survey of dose-rates in adjacent areas: Promptly after administration of the dose, the dose rates should be measured in all adjacent occupied areas, including rooms above and below (unless demonstrated not to be required by previous measurements), to verify that the dose rates in unrestricted areas (including hallways) do not exceed 20 μSv/hr (2 mrem/hr) and that no "member of the public" (which includes nearby patients, visitors, and office workers) will receive more than 1 mSv (100 mrem) in a year. Access must be restricted to any areas in which the dose rate exceeds 20 μSv/hr (2 mrem/hr).
9. Care of these patients is analogous to the treatment of isolation patients. All food should be served with disposable plates and utensils that will be discarded after use into a designated radioactive waste container. Used linens must not be sent to the laundry without a release by the radiation safety staff. Nursing staff must promptly notify nuclear medicine or radiation safety of spills of excreta in the room, medical emergencies, or the patient's death. Nurses and ward team members should wear their assigned radiation dosimeters and disposable shoe covers and gloves when entering the room. This protective clothing should be

removed and placed in radioactive waste containers when personnel leave the room. If the nurses' duties are likely to cause their clothing to become contaminated, they should wear aprons or isolation gowns. Used aprons or gowns should be placed in the contaminated linen container in the patient's room at the end of each shift. If the patient is medically stable, discontinuing the routine monitoring of the patient's vital signs can significantly reduce the exposure to nursing staff. If this monitoring is discontinued, the nursing staff should check on the patient as frequently as necessary from the doorway of the patient's room. If monitoring of vital signs is necessary, a sphygmomanometer should be left in the patient's room. The head of the stethoscope should be placed in a disposable glove before being placed against the patient.

10. Visitors should be informed of the contamination and exposure hazard and be instructed to remain outside the patient's room or wear protective clothing and remain at or beyond a safe distance (as determined by radiation safety) from the patient during the visit. No direct patient contact should be permitted. Pregnant women and children under 18 years of age should be discouraged from visiting the patient in the hospital.
11. Release of the patient: The NRC and most state regulatory agencies require that patients not be discharged from the hospital until the exposure rate from the patient is below 50 μSv/hr (5 mrem/hr) at 1 meter or their radioactivity content is less than 1.11 GBq (30 mCi). The activity remaining in the patient can be easily estimated from the exposure-rate at a fixed distance from the patient. The exposure-rate is initially measured with an ionization chamber at 1 meter from the patient's abdomen approximately 15 minutes after the dose has been administered. The exposure rate at 1 meter, when the activity in the patient had fallen to 30 mCi, will be approximately:

$$X_{30mCi} = \frac{(30mCi)X_o}{A_o} \qquad (10)$$

where X_o is the initial exposure rate (mR/hr) and A_o is the administered activity (mCi). For example, if the exposure rate at 1 meter from a patient shortly after the administration of a 100 mCi dose is 20 mR/hr, the patient may be discharged when the exposure rate is less than:

$$X_{30mCi} = \frac{(30\ mCi)(20\ mR/h)}{100\ mCi} = 6\ mR/h$$

Patients are usually discharged between 24 and 48 hours after administration of the radioiodine.

12. Discharge instructions to patients: The patient should be interviewed regarding his or her situation at home and at work. The patient should be given, both verbally and in writing, radiation safety precautions to be followed after discharge from the hospital. (The earlier "Safety Precautions Following Administration of Radioactive Iodine-131: 370 mBq–1.11 GBq (10–30 mCi)" are recommended.)
13. Decontamination of the patient's room: Once the patient is discharged, all protective coverings and trash should be removed and treated as radioactive trash. Linens may be stored for decay or treated as radioactive trash. The room must be decontaminated and surveyed before it is released for routine use. The room is surveyed with a sensitive survey instrument, such as a G-M survey meter with a thin window "pancake" probe, and with wipe tests. NRC regulations do not permit the room to be reassigned until the removable contamination on each wipe sample is less than 200 disintegrations per minute per 100 square centimeters wiped (16).

The recent introduction of radioimmunotherapy with ^{131}I-labeled monoclonal antibodies directed toward various tumors has increased the number of therapies with high activities of radioiodine. These patients are typically in much poorer health than thyroid cancer patients and often require longer hospitalization. This fact, together with an increased likelihood of acute medical intervention and life support, greatly enhances the possibility of radioiodine contamination of healthcare personnel and facilities. Special efforts should be made to adequately train these individuals in appropriate radiation safety practices. Pathology personnel should also be trained and prepared to deal with this complication. Health physics assistance may be necessary to evaluate and monitor radiation fields and help with contamination control if patients require surgery or autopsy within a few days following the radiotherapy dose.

The precautions for treatment of patients with ^{32}P or ^{89}Sr are identical to those listed above for therapy with ^{131}I, except that there is little external exposure from these patients. Dose rates need not be measured in adjacent rooms following administration, adjacent rooms are not placed off limits, and nursing staff need not be issued dosimeters. Additional recommendations and precautions for managing patients who have received therapeutic amounts of radionuclides may be found in NCRP Report No. 37 (36). A revision of this document is being prepared by the NCRP and is due to be published in 1995.

MISCELLANEOUS ASPECTS OF RADIATION SAFETY IN NUCLEAR MEDICINE

RECEIVING RADIOPHARMACEUTICAL PACKAGES

The NRC (15) and agreement states require institutions to establish procedures for the receipt of radioactive packages to minimize the potential for contamination and personnel exposure. If packages are received in a mailroom or warehouse rather than directly by the nuclear medicine department, the mailroom or warehouse staff must be instructed in radiation safety precautions, including the requirement to immediately report packages that are damaged or appear to be leaking. The packages should first be inspected visually to confirm the integrity of the containers. The external surfaces of most radioactive packages must be surveyed by wipe tests for removable contamination. Additionally, the radiation levels emitted by packages containing especially large activities must be measured. Most institutions monitor all radioactive packages for removable contamination and radiation levels to avoid accidentally failing to perform one of these tests of a package for which it is required. If removable contamination is found, personnel should take precautions to prevent its spread. If the removable contamination on the external surface exceeds 6600 disintegrations per minute (dpm) per 300 cm^2, the final delivery carrier and the NRC or the state radiologic health organization must be immediately notified. Although not required, some departments perform wipe tests of the innermost containers (the vials and syringes), using swabs or forceps to minimize exposure to the hands, to ensure that the inner containers are not leaking or badly contaminated. When the receipt of this material is properly recorded, it should be stored in a manner that minimizes radiation exposure to personnel. If the shipping package is not reusable, it is usually surveyed for contamination in a low background area, using a thin-window G-M survey meter, all radioactive warning labels are rendered unrecognizable, and it is discarded into the nonradioactive waste.

RADIOACTIVE WASTE

There are a number of methods for disposal of radioactive waste. These include: (a) decay in storage, followed by disposal as nonradioactive waste; (b) disposal into the sanitary sewer system; (c) shipment to a recipient licensed to receive the waste; (d) incineration; and (e) shipment to a licensed radioactive burial site. The NRC and agreements states permit patient excreta to be discarded into the sanitary sewer without regard for its radioactivity (15).

Because of significant increases in the cost of radioactive waste disposal and the loss of certain disposal options, minimization of radioactive waste is important. Items that are not radioactive should not be discarded into the radioactive waste. In particular, disposable shipping cartons from radioactive material shipments should be surveyed in a low-background area with a portable G-M survey meter and, if they are not contaminated, discarded into the normal trash once their warning labels have been removed or rendered unrecognizable.

Decay in storage is an attractive option for the nuclear medicine department, due to the short half-lives of most radionuclides used. The NRC permits its licensees to discard as ordinary trash radioactive waste containing radionuclides with half-lives less than 65 days, provided that the material is stored for at least 10 half-lives, any radiation warning labels are obliterated, and the material is surveyed with a sensitive survey meter in a low-background area to determine that its radioactivity cannot be distinguished from background. It is recommended that the radioactive waste be segregated by half-life into the categories of (a) ^{99m}Tc, (b) radionuclides with half-lives less than 6 days (i.e., ^{67}Ga, ^{111}In, ^{123}I, ^{133}Xe, and ^{201}Tl), and (c) others (e.g., ^{131}I), to minimize the volume of waste in storage.

Many commercial radiopharmacies will accept the return of used syringes and vials. However, this constitutes the shipping of radioactive materials and is subject to either NRC or agreement state and also DOT regulations. Many departments prefer to decay this material in storage to avoid the shipping requirements.

Radioactive materials may also be shipped to a licensed radioactive waste burial site. However, due to an organization of the states into regional compacts under the federal Low-Level Radioactive Waste Policy Act of 1980, many states no longer have access to any radioactive waste burial sites. Even when available, this option is very expensive and, as is the case when returning waste to a radiopharmacy, subject to complicated regulatory requirements.

The NRC (15) and agreement states permit the sewer disposal of radioactive material, provided that it is soluble or readily dispersible biologic material. The disposals must not exceed limits on the activity that may be released annually and monthly limits on the average concentration of activity in the sewage. In many areas, however, local agencies have established regulations regarding the sewer disposal of radioactive waste that are more restrictive than state and federal regulations.

An institution may request permission from the NRC or agreement state agency to permit the incineration of radioactive waste. The application must demonstrate that releases of airborne radioactivity from the stack will be within permissible limits. The ash must be monitored and, if it contains significant amounts of radioactivity, must be treated as radioactive waste.

SHIPPING RADIOACTIVE MATERIALS

The transportation of radioactive materials, including radioactive waste, is jointly regulated by the NRC and the U.S. Department of Transportation (DOT). DOT regulations (Title 49 of the Code of Federal Regulations) contain requirements for shipping papers, packaging, and package labeling. The DOT also requires training of workers who ship radioactive materials. Returning used syringes, used vials, and unused doses to a radiopharmacy constitutes shipping of radioactive materials and is subject to DOT regulations.

In general, limited quantities of radioactive material and low-specific activity radioactive material (as defined in DOT regulations) may be shipped in strong tight packages that will not leak radioactive materials under conditions normally incident to transportation. Other radioactive material must be shipped in containers certified to withstand accidents. In either case, shipping papers must be prepared describing the contents of the packages. The radiation levels at the surface of a package and at 1 meter, and the removable contamination on the outside of the package, must be measured and be within limits specified by DOT regulations. The labels on a package are determined by the measured radiation levels.

RADIATION ACCIDENTS

A radiation accident may be defined as inadvertent exposure to ionizing radiation or unintentional contamination with a radionuclide. Several texts and reviews of the preparation for and response to radiation accidents are available (37–41). Although clinically significant radiation accidents are rare, it is prudent for each hospital to have a written procedure to cope with such accidents. Emergency room and employee health staff should also have regular training in such accidents. The radiation accident victims most likely to be treated are hospital staff members who have contaminated themselves, splashed radioactivity into their eyes, or punctured themselves with contaminated sharps.

Radiation accidents may be classified into those caused by irradiation by external sources and those involving contamination of the victims by radioactive material. It should be noted that more than one "type" of accident may occur in a given circumstance. For example, an individual may be exposed and contaminated in the same accident.

IRRADIATION BY EXTERNAL SOURCES

Exposure to a source of radiation causes an individual to be *irradiated.* Under most circumstances, the exposure ends once the radiation source is turned off, removed, or shielded or the individual is removed from the area. Unless the exposure is massive, the clinical effects of the radiation injury are not immediately apparent. The actual symptoms and ultimate injury depend on the absorbed dose, tissues exposed, and penetrating capabilities of the radiation. Unless there has been a massive exposure to neutrons, the individual does not become radioactive and may be handled without special precautions. Medical management in such cases is initially symptomatic, with particular care being taken to assess the absorbed dose by using biologic criteria such as nausea, vomiting, diarrhea, skin erythema, lymphocyte count, and chromosomal aberration frequency.

CONTAMINATION

The second major type of radiation accident is *contamination* with a radionuclide. The contamination may be on the surface of the skin (external contamination), may be within the body (internal contamination), or may be in the form of an embedded object. Contamination usually refers to unsealed radionuclides rather than sealed sources.

External contamination rarely reaches levels that cause acute medical effects. There are a few instances in which there may be absorption of the radionuclide through the skin, such as contamination with tritium or radioiodine. α-Emitting radionuclides do not pose a hazard if the skin is intact since the particles are unable to penetrate to the viable layer of the dermis. Energetic β-particles can cause skin erythema and in some cases skin necrosis. As a practical matter, these effects are seen only in circumstances in which there is very high specific activity (such as fresh fallout from nuclear weapons). Skin contamination with γ-emitting radionuclides usually poses more hazard to the sensitive internal organs than to the skin itself. The major hazard associated with external contamination is that it may become internal, either through inhalation, through transdermal absorption, by absorption through wounds, or, more likely, through ingestion. The medical management of external contamination consists of removal of the contamination. Simply removing the outer clothing often removes 70–90% of external contamination, with the remainder usually being on the hands, face, and hair. After the clothing is removed, washing with soap and water usually removes 90–95% of surface contamination.

In instances in which there is a physical injury associated with external contamination, the transportation of such a patient into the emergency room area must be carefully controlled to prevent spread of the contamination to personnel, facilities, and equipment. Overall, emergency room management is a matter of having some form of protective clothing available (such as shoe covers, water-repellent gowns or coveralls, surgical masks, and gloves). If time permits, the floor should be covered and the area roped-off. Medical stabilization of the patient always takes priority. After the patient is stabilized, removal of external contamination can be performed.

Management of internal contamination is a much more difficult problem. Early diagnosis and treatment are necessary in order to have much effect in most cases. As an example, soluble transuranic radionuclides administered intravenously or absorbed through wounds are almost completely localized in the osseous tissues within 2 hours. The best early treatment is specific to the radionuclide and its chemical form. Unfortunately, this type of information is often difficult to obtain within the first 2 hours after an accident. Most early treatment of internal contamination is based on preplanning and educated guesses. NCRP Report No. 65 provides guidance for the management of internal contamination (41).

The major treatment methods for internal contamination utilize one or more of the following principles:

1. Blocking or isotopic dilution (e.g., oral administration of nonradioactive potassium iodide to prevent thyroidal uptake of radioactive iodine). Suspected or known exposure to radioactive iodine can be conveniently treated by having the patient drink a glass of water containing 5 drops of saturated solution of potassium iodide (SSKI) (41).
2. Limiting the uptake (e.g., administration of aluminum-containing antacids to reduce uptake from the gut).
3. Increasing the transit through the body (treatment with fluids in the case of tritium contamination or administration of cathartics in the case of ingestion).
4. Local removal (e.g., debridement of a contaminated wound).
5. Decorporation (e.g., administration of chelating agents such as calcium- or zinc-DTPA for treatment of transuranic internal contamination).

The amount of internal contamination from inhalation can be assessed if the concentrations in the atmosphere and the occupancy time are known. Lacking these, other facts about the accident are also useful. Accidents in which there was a grinding procedure suggest large particles, which are usually deposited in the anterior nose and pharynx. An accident involving a fire would suggest much smaller particles that may well be deposited much further down in the bronchial tree or in alveoli. To assess the possibility of internal contamination, nasal swabs may be useful; such samples should be obtained as early as possible following a contamination accident since the nose and nasopharynx clear relatively quickly. Swab samples should be obtained from both nostrils to assure that there is, in fact, inhalation rather than contamination of a nares by a finger.

Whole body counters are very sensitive devices that are utilized at many nuclear power plants to assess internal contamination. Unfortunately, they are cumbersome and their extreme sensitivities often render them useless when clinically significant amounts of radionuclides are present. In cases in which a whole body counter cannot be utilized, a γ-camera may provide useful information. A relatively crude photopeak analysis can be performed and localization of radionuclide within the body by imaging methods is often possible. There should always be follow-up of patients suspected of having internal contamination with analysis of serial urine and/or fecal samples. Follow-up thyroid counting is useful in those patients who have internal contamination with radioiodine.

RADIATION SAFETY PROGRAMS AT MEDICAL INSTITUTION

RADIOACTIVE MATERIALS LICENSE

Any individual or institution wishing to perform nuclear medicine or to use radioactive materials for research or radiation oncology must first apply to the NRC or pertinent agreement state agency for a license. A license application must be prepared describing the facilities where the radioactive material is to be used, the persons who are to supervise the use of the material and their qualifications, the uses of the material (i.e., uptake, dilution, and excretion studies; imaging studies; or therapies), and the possession limits for certain categories of material. The license application must also contain proposed procedures for such matters as receiving and opening packages of radioactive material, testing dose calibrators, handling radioactive material safely, surveys of use areas for exposure and contamination, personnel dosimetry, radiopharmaceutical therapies, and disposal of radioactive waste. The NRC (25) and agreement state agencies provide suggested procedures. When the license is issued, all commitments made by the applicant in the license application become legally binding. A common cause of violations noted during inspections by the NRC or agreement state agencies is unawareness of provisions of the license.

RADIATION SAFETY OFFICER

Each facility performing nuclear medicine must designate a radiation safety officer (RSO). In small departments, the RSO is usually the nuclear medicine physician. Hospitals with large nuclear medicine programs may have a full-time RSO. This person will usually hold a doctorate or masters degree in an appropriate discipline and may be certified by the American Board of Radiology, the American Board of Medical Physics, the American Board of Science in Nuclear Medicine, or the American Board of Health Physics. In very large programs, such as those at research and teaching hospitals, the RSO may be assisted by other health physicists, technicians, and clerical personnel. The duties of the RSO include investigating incidents, writing procedures, performing periodic radiation surveys, training personnel, monitoring personnel dosimetry, directing action during emergencies such as spills and personnel contamination, performing periodic audits of users of radioactive material, and preparing license applications and amendments.

RADIATION SAFETY COMMITTEE

Each medical institution licensed to use radioactive materials must have a radiation safety committee. The NRC requires each committee to consist of at least three individuals, including an authorized user for each type of use permitted by the license (e.g., if nuclear medicine is performed, a nuclear medicine physician must be a member of the committee), the radiation safety officer, a representative of nursing, and a representative of management (16). The committee must meet at least quarterly. The committee must review the qualifications of proposed authorized users and a proposed radiation safety officer prior to submitting license applications or license amendment requests to the NRC or an agreement state agency, review the doses to workers quarterly, review incidents and corrective action taken, and perform an annual review of the radiation safety program.

Some larger institutions, typically research and teaching hospitals, are issued *licenses of broad scope*. In a broad scope license, the radiation safety committee is delegated the authority to approve authorized users for clinical and research uses of radioactive material.

TRAINING PROGRAM

One of the most important aspects of a radiation safety program is the training of workers who enter restricted areas. These workers must be trained prior to assuming their duties and regularly thereafter and their training must be commensurate with the complexity of their duties and the magnitude of the risk. Workers who must be trained include nuclear medicine physicians and technologists, nurses who provide care for radiopharmaceutical therapy patients, and other staff who may routinely enter restricted areas. Housekeepers who clean the nuclear medicine department or who work on wards where radiopharmaceutical therapy patients are confined, maintenance personnel who enter restricted areas, and hospital security personnel also should receive limited training commensurate with the risks encountered. Additionally, all nursing staff should receive some general training because they encounter patients who have been administered radiopharmaceuticals for diagnostic purposes. NRC regulations require this training to describe the sources of radiation; the health risks associated with ionizing radiation; precautions to minimize exposure; applicable portions of regulations and license conditions; the requirement to report to the appropriate supervisor anything which might cause a violation of regulations or license conditions or unnecessary exposure of persons to radiation; and the workers' right to obtain their radiation exposure reports (14). Women must be notified of their right, should they become pregnant, to declare their pregnancies, thereby causing their embryos or fetuses to be subject to a more restrictive dose limit (see "Standards for Protection Against Radiation" under "Regulations Pertaining to the Use of Radiation" earlier in this chapter).

REFERENCES

1. International Commission on Radiation Units and Measurements. Radiation quantities and units. ICRU report 33. Bethesda, MD: International Commission on Radiation Units and Measurements, 1980.
2. National Council on Radiation Protection and Measurements. SI Units in radiation protection and measurements. NCRP report no. 82. Bethesda, MD: National Council on Radiation Protection and Measurement, 1985.

3. International Commission on Radiation Units and Measurements. Quantities and units in radiation protection dosimetry. ICRU report 51. Bethesda, MD: 1993.
4. International Commission on Radiological Protection. 1990 recommendations of the International Commission on Radiological Protection. ICRP publication 60, 21, 1991. Annals of the ICRP. Elmsford, NY: Pergamon Press, 1991.
5. International Commission on Radiological Protection. Recommendations of the International Commission on Radiological Protection. ICRP publication 26, 1, 1977. Annals of the ICRP. Elmsford, NY: Pergamon Press, 1977.
6. National Council on Radiation Protection and Measurements. Exposure of the population in the United States and Canada from natural background radiation. NCRP report no. 94, Bethesda, MD: National Council on Radiation Protection and Measurement, 1987.
7. United Nations Scientific Committee on the Effects of Atomic Radiation. Sources and effects of ionizing radiation, 1993. Report to the General Assembly. United Nations, New York: United Nations Scientific Committee on the Effects of Atomic Radiation, 1993.
8. National Technical Information Service. A citizen's guide to radon, what it is and what to do about it. OPA-86-004. Springfield, VA: National Technical Information Service, 1986.
9. National Council on Radiation Protection and Measurements. Limitation of exposure to ionizing radiation. NCRP report no. 116, Bethesda, MD: National Council on Radiation Protection and Measurement, 1993.
10. National Council on Radiation Protection and Measurements. Radiation exposure of the U.S. Population from consumer products and miscellaneous sources. NCRP report no. 95. Bethesda, MD: National Council on Radiation Protection and Measurement, 1987.
11. National Council on Radiation Protection and Measurements. Ionizing radiation exposure of the population of the United States. NCRP report no. 93. Bethesda, MD: National Council on Radiation Protection and Measurement, 1987.
12. National Council on Radiation Protection and Measurements. Exposure of the U.S. Population from occupational radiation. NCRP report no. 101. Bethesda, MD: National Council on Radiation Protection and Measurement, 1989.
13. National Council on Radiation Protection and Measurements. Exposure of the U.S. Population from diagnostic medical radiation. NCRP report no. 100. Bethesda, MD: National Council on Radiation Protection and Measurement, 1989.
14. U.S. Nuclear Regulatory Commission. Notices, instructions, and reports to workers: inspection and investigations. Title 10 of the Code of Federal Regulations, Part 19. Washington, DC: U.S. Government Printing Office, January 1, 1994.
15. U.S. Nuclear Regulatory Commission. Standards for protection against radiation. Title 10 of the Code of Federal Regulations, Part 20. Washington, DC: U.S. Government Printing Office, January 1, 1994.
16. U.S. Nuclear Regulatory Commission. Medical use of byproduct material. Title 10 of the Code of Federal Regulations, Part 35. Washington, DC: U.S. Government Printing Office, January 1, 1994.
17. U.S. Environmental Protection Agency. National emission standards for hazardous air pollutants. Title 40 of the Code of Federal Regulations, Part 61. Washington, DC: U.S. Government Printing Office, January 1, 1994.
18. International Commission on Radiological Protection. Limits for intakes of radionuclides by workers. ICRP publication 30 (four parts, including supplements). Annals of the ICRP. Elmsford, NY: Pergamon Press, 1979–1988.
19. U.S. Nuclear Regulatory Commission. Regulatory guide 8.9: acceptable concepts, models, equations, and assumptions for a bioassay program. Revision 1. Washington, DC: U.S. Government Printing Office, July, 1993.
20. U.S. Nuclear Regulatory Commission. Regulatory guide 8.10: operating philosophy for maintaining occupational radiation exposure as low as is reasonably achievable. Washington, DC: U.S. Government Printing Office, September, 1975.
21. U.S. Nuclear Regulatory Commission. Regulatory guide 8.13: instruction concerning prenatal radiation exposure. Revision 2. Washington, DC: U.S. Government Printing Office, December, 1987.
22. U.S. Nuclear Regulatory Commission. Regulatory guide 8.18: information relevant to ensuring that occupational radiation exposure at medical institutions will be as low as reasonably achievable. Revision 1. Washington, DC: U.S. Government Printing Office, October, 1982.
23. U.S. Nuclear Regulatory Commission. Regulatory guide 8.23: radiation safety surveys at medical institutions. Washington DC: U.S. Government Printing Office, January, 1981.
24. U.S. Nuclear Regulatory Commission. Regulatory guide 8.33: quality management program. Washington, DC: U.S. Government Printing Office, October, 1991.
25. U.S. Nuclear Regulatory Commission. Regulatory guide 10.8: guide for the preparation of applications for medical programs. Revision 2. Washington, DC: U.S. Government Printing Office, August, 1987.
26. U.S. Nuclear Regulatory Commission. Appendix X to regulatory guide 10.8: guidance on complying with new part 20 requirements. Washington DC: U.S. Government Printing Office, 1992.
27. National Council on Radiation Protection and Measurements. A handbook of radioactivity measurements procedures. NCRP report no. 58. 2nd ed. Bethesda, MD: National Council on Radiation Protection and Measurement, 1985.
28. International Commission on Radiological Protection. Individual monitoring for intake of radionuclides by workers: design and interpretation. ICRP publication 54. Elmsford, NY: Pergamon Press, 1988.
29. Lessard ET, Yihua X, Skrable KW, et al. Interpretation of bioassay measurements. U.S. Nuclear Regulatory Commission. NUREGCR-4884. Washington DC: U.S. Government Printing Office, July, 1987.
30. Eckerman KF, Wolbarst AB, Richardson AC. Limiting values of radionuclide intake and air concentration and dose conversion factors for inhalation, submersion, and ingestion. Federal guidance report No. 11. EPA-520/1-88-20. Washington DC: U.S. Government Printing Office, September, 1988.
31. Barrall RC, Smith SI. Personal radiation exposure and protection from Tc-99m radiation. In: Kereiakes JG, Corey KR, eds. Biophysical aspects of the medical use of technetium-99m. AAPM monograph no 1. Cincinnati: University of Cincinnati, 1976.
32. International Commission on Radiological Protection. The handling, storage, use and disposal of unsealed radionuclides in hospitals and medical research establishments. ICRP publication 25. Elmsford, NY: Pergamon Press, 1977.
33. U.S. Department of Health, Education and Welfare (USDHEW). Radiation safety in nuclear medicine: a practical guide. USDHEW Publ FDA-82 8180. Washington, DC: U.S. Government Printing Office, 1981.
34. National Council on Radiation Protection and Measurement (NCRP). Radiation protection for medical and allied health personnel. NCRP report no. 105. Washington, DC: National Council on Radiation Protection and Measurement, 1989.
35. Committee 3 of the International Commission on Radiological Protection. Summary of the current ICRP principles for protection of the patient in nuclear medicine, Oxford: Pergamon Press, 1993.
36. National Council on Radiation Protection and Measurements (NCRP). Precautions in the management of patients who have re-

ceived therapeutic amounts of radionuclides. NCRP report no. 37. Washington, DC: National Council on Radiation Protection and Measurements, 1970.

37. Hubner KF, Fry SA, eds. The medical basis for radiation accident preparedness. In: Proceedings of a Conference, Oak Ridge, TN. New York: Elsevier, 1980.
38. Shleien B. Preparedness and response in radiation accidents. U.S. Department of Health & Human Services publ. FDA-83 8211. Washington, DC: U.S. Government Printing Office, 1984.
39. Leonard RB, Ricks RC. Emergency department radiation accident protocol. Ann Emerg Med 1980;9:9.
40. Mettler FA, Kelsey CA, Ricks RC, eds. Medical management of radiation accidents. Boca Raton, FL: CRC Press, 1990.
41. National Council on Radiation Protection and Measurements (NCRP). Management of persons accidentally contaminated with radionuclides. NCRP report no. 65. Washington, DC: National Council on Radiation Protection and Measurements, 1980.

19 Radiopharmaceutical Dosimetry

JERROLD T. BUSHBERG and MICHAEL G. STABIN

The objective of internal radiation dosimetry calculations is to determine the absorbed energy (i.e., "dose") to various organs delivered from internally deposited radionuclides (radiopharmaceuticals). The first systematized formulation for determining the radiation absorbed dose from internally deposited radionuclides was developed by Marinelli, et al. (1), in 1948. This work was extended and standardized by Loevinger, et al. (2), in 1956, and later developed by Loevinger and Berman (3) into a generalized formalism for internal dose calculations applicable to all radionuclides. In 1968, this system was adopted by the Society of Nuclear Medicine's Medical Internal Radiation Dose Committee (MIRD). The MIRD schema (4), with subsequent revisions and additions, is currently the most widely accepted method for estimating the internal radiation dose from radionuclides of general interest in nuclear medicine.

As a practical matter, physicians engaged in the clinical practice of nuclear medicine are rarely called upon to perform dosimetry calculations. The organ doses for approved diagnostic radionuclides are determined by the radiopharmaceutical supplier and provided as part of the package insert. There are, however, circumstances when dosimetry must be performed. Examples include requests for use of new diagnostic agents, requests for use of an old agent by a new route of administration, and certain therapeutic administrations. Additionally, the original dosimetry provided by the manufacturer is rarely updated as new (often more accurate) information becomes available. It is also important that the clinician have at least some understanding of the most common method by which dosimetry data are calculated. Unfortunately it is impossible to present such material without resorting to algebraic formulas and use of relatively unfamiliar symbols. The level of presentation of material in this section is a compromise, allowing the reader actually to perform model calculations by the MIRD method while avoiding more complex dosimetry problems.

PARAMETERS AND UNITS

One way to think about calculating organ doses from internally administered radiopharmaceuticals is to organize and define those parameters or variables that are the necessary determinants of the absorbed dose in tissue. This process begins by identifying three major categories of parameters to be considered:

1. *Radionuclide parameters:* These are parameters related only to the physical and immutable properties of the radionuclide.
2. *Biologic parameters:* These are parameters related only to the biologic system and the pharmacokinetics of the radiopharmaceutical.
3. *Combined parameters*: These are parameters that are a function of both the radionuclide and the biologic system.

RADIONUCLIDE PARAMETERS

The term used to indicate the total average energy available from a given radionuclide per nuclear transformation is the *mean energy per disintegration* (δ), which is expressed in the unit gram-rad per microcurie-hour (g-rad/μCi-hr). Nuclear transformation is usually referred to as disintegration (dis). The unit of radiation quantity, or activity, is expressed in μCi, which is equal to 3.7×10^4 disintegrations/second or 1.33×10^8 disintegrations/hour. The unit for radiation dose is the *rad*, which is defined in terms of absorbed energy per gram of material (energy/g). If we choose the unit of time to be hours (i.e., dis/hr), the equivalent units of δ are energy/dis, as shown below:

$$\Delta_i = \frac{\text{g-rad}}{\mu\text{Ci-hr}} = \frac{\text{g}\cdot\left(\frac{\text{energy}}{\text{g}}\right)}{\left(\frac{\text{dis}}{\text{hr}}\right)\cdot\text{hr}} = \frac{\text{energy}}{\text{dis}} \qquad (1)$$

The expression δ_i is used to denote the energy per disintegration for a particular radiation emission. The *i* is used to denote the general equation as it applies to any value of *i* (i.e., δ_1 δ_2, δ_3, etc.). When the value *i* appears in any equation, it denotes the general form applicable to any discrete entity. Values of δ_i have been calculated for the principal particulate and electromagnetic (photon) emissions resulting from the nuclear transformation process. The photons include γ- and x-rays and the particulate radiations include α and β^- particles, positrons (β^+), internal conversion electrons (ICEs), and Auger electrons (AEs). One can appreciate the contribution of these various radiations to the overall energy emitted by considering, for example, the decay scheme and radiations from ^{99m}Tc (Fig. 19.1).

Although we usually think of ^{99m}Tc as a relatively simple monoenergetic 140-keV photon emitter, the actual decay scheme and spectrum of emissions is considerably more complex, consisting of three isomeric transitions (γ_1, γ_2, γ_3) and a number of particulate radiations, as well as low-energy characteristic x-rays. The δ_i for each type of radiation is calculated from the relationship:

$$1 = 2\ 3\ 4 \qquad (2)$$
$$\Delta_i \quad 2.13\ n_i\ E_i$$

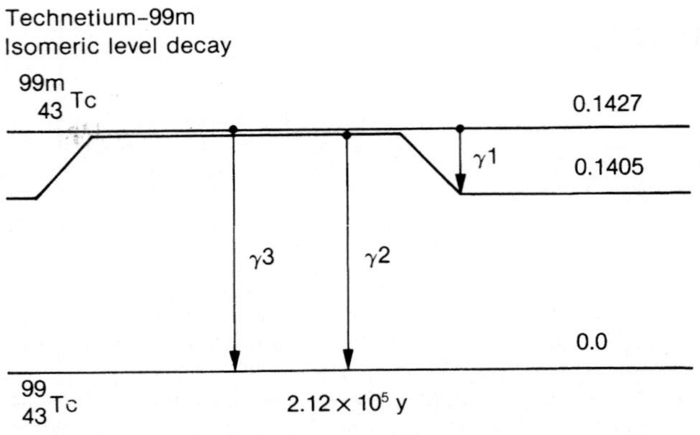

SIGNIFICANT RADIATION EMISSIONS OUTPUT DATA

Radiation	n_i (mean number/ dis)	E_i (mean energy/ particle or photon) (MeV)	Δ_i (mean energy/dis) (g-rad/μCi-hr)
γ 1	0.0000	0.0021	0.0000
M Int Con Elect	0.9860	0.0016	0.0035
γ 2	0.8787	0.1405	0.2630
K Int Con Elect	0.0913	0.1194	0.0232
L Int Con Elect	0.0118	0.1377	0.0034
M Int Con Elect	0.0039	0.1400	0.0011
γ 3	0.0003	0.1426	0.0001
K Int Con Elect	0.0088	0.1215	0.0022
L Int Con Elect	0.0035	0.1398	0.0010
M Int Con Elect	0.0011	0.1422	0.0003
K α-1 -ray	0.0441	0.0183	0.0017
K α-2 -ray	0.0221	0.0182	0.0008
K β-1 -ray	0.0105	0.0206	0.0004
KLL Auger Elect	0.0152	0.0154	0.0005
KLX Auger Elect	0.0055	0.0178	0.0002
LMM Auger Elect	0.1093	0.0019	0.0004
MXY Auger Elect	1.2359	0.0004	0.0011

Figure 19.1. Decay scheme and radiation emission information for ^{99m}Tc. *Top*: Decay scheme. *Bottom*: Radiation emission information. *K, L, M, X, Y* = orbital shells; *Int Con Elect* = internal conversion electron; *Auger Elect* = Auger electron.

Code	Symbol	Explanation
1.	Δ_i	Mean energy per disintegration for the *i*th emission.
2.	2.13	A conversion constant to convert MeV/disintegration to g-rad/μCi-hr.
3.	n_i	Mean number (average number) of *i*th-type radiation emitted per disintegration.
4.	E_i	Mean energy of the *i*th particle or photon emitted (in MeV).

Two other important parameters of the radionuclide are the quantity of radioactivity initially administered (A_o), expressed in μCi, and the characteristic physical half-life (T_p), expressed in hours. The physical half-life is an immutable property of the radionuclide and is defined as the time necessary to decrease a quantity of radioactivity from a specified radionuclide by one-half (e.g., T_p for ^{99m}Tc = approximately 6 hours).

A summary of these radiation-specific variables, their relationship, and units is shown in Table 19.1.

BIOLOGIC PARAMETERS

Biologic parameters identify the target organ for which the dose is being calculated (r_k), the various source organs in which the radiopharmaceutical is distributed (r_h), the fraction of the injected activity localized in each source organ (f_h), the mass of the target organ (m_k) in grams, and the biologic half-life of the radiopharmaceutical in a specified source organ (T_b). The biologic half-life expressed in hours is defined as the time necessary for the egress of one-half the initially deposited radiopharmaceutical from a specified source organ. This will, of course, depend only on the pharmacokinetics of the radiopharmaceutical in an individual patient and not on any of the decay characteristics of the radionuclide. For the majority of radiopharmaceuticals, or in the absence of more accurate kinetics data, the biologic elimination rate is assumed to follow a single exponential function (i.e., e^{-x}). These factors are summarized in Table 19.2.

Table 19.1.
Variables That Identify or Quantify Some Aspects of the Radiation Source (Radionuclide)

Symbol	Quanitty	Describes	Equivalent	Units
i		*i*th type of radiation photon or particle (i.e., γ, x-ray, ICE, AE)		
n_i		Mean number of the *i*th type of radiation emitted per disintegration		
E_i		Mean energy of radiation *i*		MeV/particle or photon
Δ_i	Mean energy per disintegration for radiation *i*	Total average energy emitted as radiation *i* per disintegration	$2.13\ n_i\bar{E}_i$	g-rad/μCi-hr
A_o	Activity	Quantity of radioactivity present at time = 0 expressed as the number of disintegrations per second (dps)	3.7×10^4 dps	μCi
T_p	Physical half-life	Time required to decrease a quantity of radioactivity by one-half		hours (hr)

Table 19.2.
Variables That Identify or Are a Function of the Biologic System

Symbol	Quantity	Describes	Units
r	region	A specific tissue or organ system	
r_t	target	Identity of the target tissue for which the dose is being calculated	
r_b	source	Identity of the source tissue in which some fraction of the activity is distributed	
f_n	fractional uptake	The fraction of the administered activity taken up by the source tissue (r_b)	
m_k	mass	Mass of the target tissue	grams (g)
T_b	biologic half-life	The time required by the source tissue (r_b) to biologically eliminate one-half of the deposited radiopharmaceutical from the source organ	hours (hr)

COMBINED PARAMETERS (PHYSICALLY AND BIOLOGICALLY DEPENDENT)

The final category of parameters includes quantities that are functions of both the physical characteristics of the radionuclide and the biologic system in which it is located. As we have seen, the quantity referred to as *half-life* is a generic term that represents the time required for activity to decrease by one-half of its original value. The effective half-life (T_e) represents the time required for the activity initially present in a specified source organ to decrease by one-half. The effective half-life is a function of the combined effects of physical decay and biologic elimination of the radiopharmaceutical from the source organ. The quantitative relationship between T_p, T_b, and T_e is

$$T_e = \frac{T_p \cdot T_b}{T_p + T_b} \tag{3}$$

If T_b is infinite (i.e., the material is not excreted) or very long compared to T_p (e.g., ^{99m}Tc sulfur colloid in the liver), T_p becomes controlling and the T_e is effectively equal to T_p. This can be proved by inserting a larger number for T_b relative to T_p in equation 3.

The fraction of each *i*th type of radiation emitted from a radionuclide in a source organ (r_h) that is absorbed in a specified target organ (r_k) is symbolized as $\phi_i(r_k \leftarrow r_h)$ and referred to as the *absorbed fraction* (i.e., energy emitted by r_h and absorbed by r_k for each $_i$). The value of the absorbed fraction (ϕ_i) depends on (a) the type and energy of the radiation emitted, and (b) the geometric relationships, elemental composition, and attenuation characteristics of the source, target, and interposing tissues.

The radiation emission data are known with a high degree of accuracy for most radionuclides; however, the complex interactions and energy deposition patterns represented in the absorbed fraction $\phi_i(r_k \rightarrow r_h)$ for a particular combination of radionuclide, source, and target are best estimated by computer algorithms that apply the Monte Carlo technique (5, 6). The Monte Carlo technique determines the energy deposited in tissue by tracing the randomly generated, but probabilistically determined, pathways and interactions of emissions from a large number of disintegrations, and averaging the results.

The anatomic model used for many years in these calculations was that of a 70-kg "standard" or "reference" hermaphrodite person. Various simplifications regarding elemental composition, organ size, position, contents, and geometry were made. Figures 19.2 and 19.3 show the dimensions of the reference hermaphrodite phantom and the geometric simplifications and relationships of the principal organs. Calculations of absorbed dose using this phantom are thus really estimates of doses to the organs of this phantom, and, hopefully, are somewhat representative of an average of the adult population. Significant improvements to this model have been made over the years. First in the category of improvements was the addition of certain improved organ systems, including the heart (7), brain (8), peritoneal cavity (9), prostate gland (10), esophagus (11), and subregions of the brain (12). A significant improvement in the ability to extend dose calculations to more individuals was realized in the pediatric phantom series of Cristy and Eckerman (13) and the pregnant woman phantom series of Stabin, et al. (14). The pediatric phantom series consisted of six phantoms, representing individuals of age 0 (newborn), 1 year, 5 years, 10 years, 15 years, and 18 years (adult). The Cristy and Eckerman adult phantom is slightly different than the original adult phantom described in MIRD Pamphlet No. 5, Revised (15).

The basic MIRD expression of mean absorbed dose in a particular target organ $\overline{D}(r_k)$ from all source organs is shown below in equation 4. This equation takes into account all of the physical and biologic variables discussed thus far.

$$\underbrace{\overline{(D)(r_k)}}_{①} = \frac{\overset{②}{\overline{\Sigma_h}}\ \overset{③}{\overline{A_o}} \bullet \overset{④}{\overline{f}} \bullet \overset{⑤}{\overline{1.44T_e}}}{\underset{⑥}{\underline{m_k}}}\ \overset{⑦}{\overline{\Sigma_i}}\underset{⑧}{\underline{\Delta_i}}\overset{⑨}{\overline{\Phi_i(rk \leftarrow r_h)}} \tag{4}$$

Code	Symbol	Quantity	Describes	Equivalence	Units
1.	$\bar{D}(r_k)$	absorbed dose	Energy deposited per unit mass of the target organ (r_k)	$\frac{100 \text{ erg}}{\text{g}}$	rad
2.	Σ_h		The sum of all the determinations from emissions originating within both the target organ and all other organs		
3.	A_o	activity	Activity at time 0	3.7×10^4 dps	μCi
4.	f	fractional	Fraction of the administered activity in a source organ		
5.	$1.44T_e$		The "average" life of the radioactivity in a source organ	$\frac{1.44T_p \cdot T_b}{T_p + T_b}$	hr
6.	m_k	mass	Mass of the target organ		g
7.	Σ_i		Sum of all the emissions		
8.	Δ_i	mean energy per disintegration for radiation i	Total average energy emitted as radiation i per disintegration	$2.13n_iE_i$	g-rad/μCi-hr
9.	ϕ_i $(r_k \leftarrow r_h)$	absorbed fraction	The fraction of the energy emitted by the radionuclide in the source organ (r_h) that is deposited in the target organ (r_k)		

Note that the summation sign [Σ_i, δi, $\phi_i(r_k \leftarrow r_h)$] indicates that one must sum the individual products of the amount of energy released by radiation ($_i$) per disintegration (δ_i) and the fraction of that energy absorbed by the designated target [$\phi_i(r_k \leftarrow r_h)$]. The symbol ($\Sigma_h$) reflects the need to calculate the target organ dose by adding together not only the individual doses from activity located within the target organ itself (i.e., $r_k = r_h$—the self-irradiating dose) but also the dose resulting from other source tissues irradiating the target tissue.

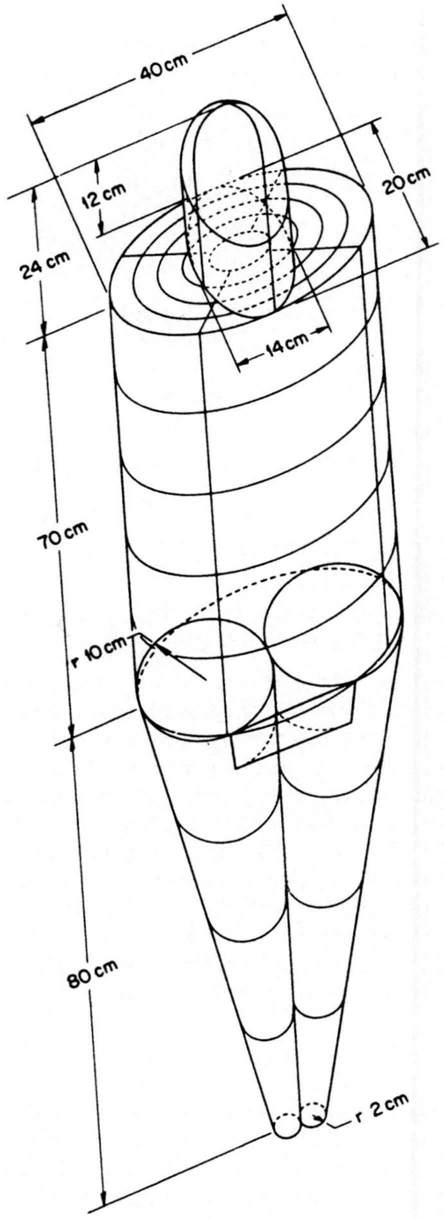

Figure 19.2. Exterior of the adult human phantom. Dimensions and coordinate system of adult human phantom. (Reproduced by permission from Snyder WJ, Ford MR, Warner GG. Estimates of absorbed fraction for photon sources uniformly distributed in various organs of the heterogeneous phantom. nm/MIRD Pamphlet #5 (Revised). New York: Society of Nuclear Medicine, 1978.)

SIMPLIFIED DOSE CALCULATION TECHNIQUE

The cumulated activity ($\tilde{A}_h$) represents the total number of disintegrations from the specified amount of activity in the source organ. This can be seen by a simple analysis of units (i.e., $\tilde{A}_h = A_o$ (dis/time) • T_e (time) = dis).

The cumulated activity in the source organ, expressed in μCi-hr, can be represented by a single term ($\tilde{A}_h$) incorporating the biodistribution and kinetics information as shown in equation 5:

$$A_h = A_o \bullet f_h \bullet 1.44\ T_e \tag{5}$$

The MIRD Committee has further simplified the dose calculation procedure by combining the appropriate values of δ_i, $\phi_i(r_k \leftarrow r_h)$, and m_k for each combination of source, target, and radionuclide into a so-called S factor as shown in equation 6:

$$S\ (r_k \leftarrow r_h) = \frac{\Sigma\Delta\phi_i(r_k \leftarrow r_h)}{m_k} \tag{6}$$

The S factor thus represents the mean absorbed dose in the target organ per unit cumulated activity in a designated

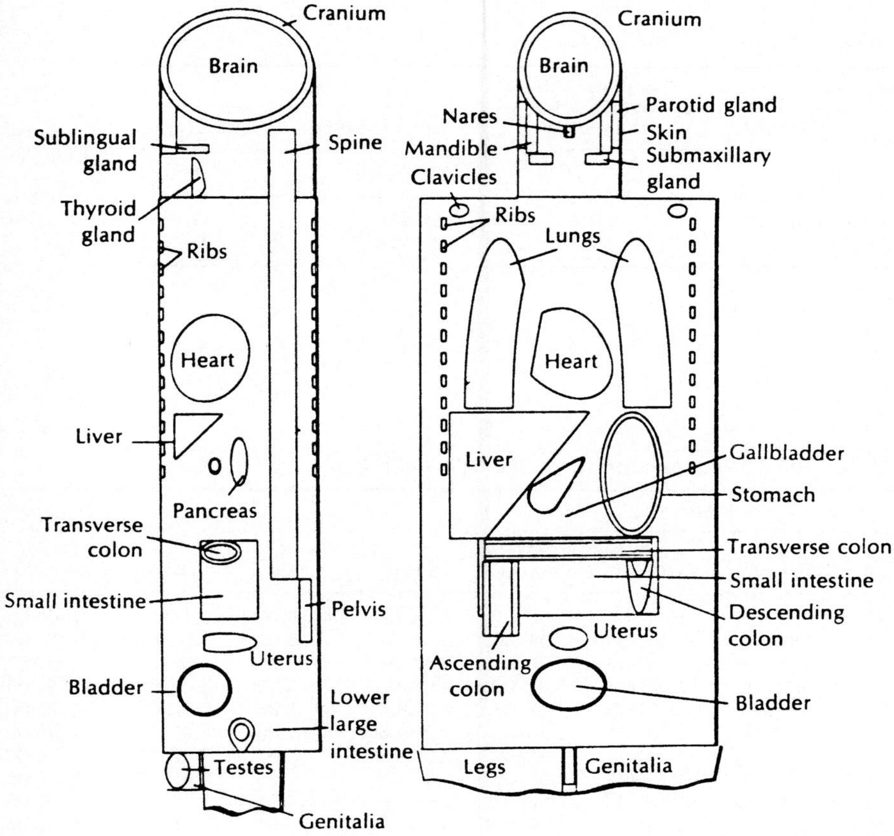

Figure 19.3. Computer plots of phantom sections. Computer plots of sections through adult hermaphrodite phantom illustrating the shape of the internal organs and their relative position. (Reproduced by permission from Smith EM, Warner GG. Estimates of radiation dose to the embryo from nuclear medicine procedures. J Nucl Med 1976;17:836–839.)

source organ in rad/μCi-hr. Thus the equation for calculating the absorbed dose to r_k reduces to

$$\underset{\bar{D}(r_k)}{\overset{\textcircled{1}}{|}} = \underset{\Sigma_h}{\overset{\textcircled{2}}{|}}\ \underset{\tilde{A}_h}{\overset{\textcircled{3}}{|}}\ \underset{S(r_k \leftarrow r_h)}{\overset{\textcircled{4}}{|}} \qquad (7)$$

The MIRD Committee has compiled S factors for more than 110 radionuclides and 20 source/target combinations (16).

Code	Symbol	Quantity	Equivalence	Units
1.	$\bar{D}(r_k)$	target organ dose	$\Sigma h A h s(r_k \leftarrow r_h)$	rad
2.	Σh	sum of the determinations from emissions originating within both the target organ and all other organs		
3.	$\tilde{A}_h$	cumulated activity	$A_o \cdot f \cdot 1.44T_e$	μCi-hr
4.	$S(r_k \leftarrow r_h)$	S factor	$\Sigma i \Delta i \phi_i(r_k \leftarrow r_h)$	rad/ μCi-hr

A WORD ABOUT UNITS

The traditional radiologic units of Ci, R, rad, and rem are maintained throughout this section rather than switching to the equivalent Systeme Internationale (SI) units (Bq, C/Kg, Gy, and Sv, respectively) because the former are still the most commonly used in nuclear medicine in the United States. The relationship between these two systems is given in Table 19.3. Other units are chosen for their utility in a given example or because of common usage. Although any variety of units may be employed in a radiation dose calculation, care must be taken to assure unit *consistency* throughout (i.e., not mixing seconds with hours or μCi with Ci) and some effort should be made to choose units that are either best suited to a particular problem or that follow some logical and/or established convention. One could express velocity in furlongs per fortnight, but this would hardly be a very useful term!

EXAMPLES OF DOSE CALCULATIONS

The simplest example of a MIRD calculation would be a situation in which the radiopharmaceutical *instantaneously* localized in a *single organ* and remained there with an *infinite* biologic *half-life*.

For the purpose of demonstrating the basic MIRD technique, a hypothetical situation is presented below in example 1.

EXAMPLE 1

A patient is injected with 3 mCi (111 mBq) of ^{99m}Tc sulfur colloid. Estimate the radiation absorbed dose to the:

(a) liver
(b) testes
(c) red bone marrow
(d) total body

Table 19.3.
Conventional and SI Radiologic Units and Conversion Factors

Quantity	Conventional Units: Name	Conventional Units: Symbol	Multiply by the Conventional Units to Obtain SI Units	SI Units: Name	SI Units: Symbol
Activity	Curie	Ci	3.7×10^{10}	Becquerel[a]	Bq
Exposure	Roentgen	R	2.58×10^{-4}	Coulomb per kilogram	C/kg
Absorbed dose	Radiation absorbed dose	rad	10^{-2}	Gray[b]	Gy
Dose equivalent	Roentgen-equivalent man	rem	10^{-2}	Sievert	Sv

[a]Bq = 1 disintegration/sec (dis sec^{-1}).
[b]Gray = 1 Joule/kg.

Table 19.4.
Absorbed Dose Per Unit Cumulated Activity (RAD/μCi-hr) Technetium-99m (Half life 6.02 hours)[a]

Target Organs (r_k)	Adrenals	Bladder Contents	Source Organs (r_b) Intestinal Tract: Stomach Contents	SI Contents	ULI Contents	LLI Contents	Kidneys	Liver	Lungs	Other Tissue (Muscle)
Adrenals	3.1E-03	1.5E-07	2.7E-06	1.0E-06	9.1E-07	3.6E-07	1.1E-05	4.5E-06	2.7E-06	1.4E-06
Bladder Wall	1.3E-07	1.6E-04	2.7E-07	2.6E-06	2.2E-06	6.9E-06	2.8E-07	1.6E-07	3.6E-08	1.8E-06
Bone (total)	2.0E-06	9.2E-07	9.0E-07	1.3E-06	1.1E-06	1.6E-06	1.4E-06	1.1E-06	1.5E-06	9.8E-07
GI (stom wall)	2.9E-06	2.7E-07	1.3E-04	3.7E-06	3.8E-06	1.8E-06	3.6E-06	1.9E-06	1.8E-06	1.3E-06
GI (SI)	8.3E-07	3.0E-06	2.7E-06	7.8E-05	1.7E-05	9.4E-06	2.9E-06	1.6E-06	1.9E-07	1.5E-06
GI (ULI wall)	9.3E-07	2.2E-06	3.5E-06	2.4E-05	1.3E-04	4.2E-06	2.9E-06	2.5E-06	2.2E-07	1.6E-06
GI (LLI wall)	2.2E-07	7.4E-06	1.2E-06	7.3E-06	3.2E-06	1.9E-04	7.2E-07	2.3E-07	7.1E-08	1.7E-06
Kidneys	1.1E-05	2.6E-07	3.5E-06	3.2E-06	2.8E-06	8.6E-07	1.9E-04	3.9E-06	8.4E-07	1.3E-06
Liver	4.9E-06	1.7E-07	2.0E-06	1.8E-06	2.6E-06	2.5E-07	3.9E-06	4.6E-05	2.5E-06	1.1E-06
Lungs	2.4E-06	2.4E-08	1.7E-06	2.2E-07	2.6E-07	7.9E-08	8.5E-07	2.5E-06	5.2E-05	1.3E-06
Marrow (red)	3.6E-06	2.2E-06	1.6E-06	4.3E-06	3.7E-06	5.1E-06	3.8E-06	1.6E-06	1.9E-06	2.0E-06
Oth Tiss (musc)	1.4E-06	1.8E-06	1.4E-06	1.5E-06	1.5E-06	1.7E-06	1.3E-06	1.1E-06	1.3E-06	2.7E-06
Ovaries	6.1E-07	7.3E-06	5.0E-07	1.1E-05	1.2E-05	1.8E-05	1.1E-06	4.5E-07	9.4E-08	2.0E-06
Pancreas	9.0E-06	2.3E-07	1.8E-05	2.1E-06	2.3E-06	7.4E-07	6.6E-06	4.2E-06	2.6E-06	1.8E-06
Skin	5.1E-07	5.5E-07	4.4E-07	4.1E-07	4.1E-07	4.8E-07	5.3E-07	4.9E-07	5.3E-07	7.2E-07
Spleen	6.3E-06	6.6E-07	1.0E-05	1.5E-06	1.4E-06	8.0E-07	8.6E-06	9.2E-07	2.3E-06	1.4E-06
Testes	3.2E-08	4.7E-06	5.1E-08	3.1E-07	2.7E-07	1.8E-06	8.8E-06	6.2E-08	7.9E-09	1.1E-06
Thyroid	1.3E-07	2.1E-09	8.7E-08	1.5E-08	1.6E-08	5.4E-09	4.8E-08	1.5E-07	9.2E-07	1.3E-06
Uterus (nongrvd)	1.1E-06	1.6E-05	7.7E-07	9.6E-06	5.4E-06	7.1E-06	9.4E-07	3.9E-07	8.2E-08	2.3E-06
Total body	2.2E-06	1.9E-06	1.9E-06	2.4E-06	2.2E-06	2.3E-06	2.2E-06	2.2E-06	2.0E-06	1.9E-06

Target Organs (r_b)	Ovaries	Pancreas	Source Organs (r_b) Skeleton: R Marrow	Cort Bone	Tra Bone	Skin	Spleen	Testes	Thyroid	Total body
Adrenals	3.3E-07	9.1E-06	2.3E-06	1.1E-06	1.1E-06	6.8E-07	6.3E-06	3.2E-08	1.3E-07	2.3E-06
Bladder Wall	7.2E-06	1.4E-07	9.9E-07	5.1E-07	5.1E-07	4.9E-07	1.2E-07	4.8E-06	2.1E-09	2.3E-06
Bone (total)	1.5E-06	1.5E-06	4.0E-06	1.2E-05	1.0E-05	9.9E-07	1.1E-06	9.2E-07	1.0E-06	2.5E-06
GI (stom wall)	8.1E-07	1.8E-05	9.5E-07	5.5E-07	5.5E-07	5.4E-07	1.0E-05	3.2E-08	4.5E-08	2.2E-06
GI (SI)	1.2E-05	1.8E-06	2.6E-06	7.3E-07	7.3E-07	4.5E-07	1.4E-06	3.6E-07	9.3E-09	2.5E-06
GI (ULI wall)	1.1E-05	2.1E-06	2.1E-06	6.9E-07	6.9E-07	4.6E-07	1.4E-06	3.1E-07	1.1E-08	2.4E-06
GI (LLI wall)	1.5E-06	5.7E-07	2.9E-06	1.0E-06	1.0E-06	4.8E-07	6.1E-07	2.7E-06	4.3E-09	2.3E-06
Kidneys	9.2E-07	6.6E-06	2.2E-06	8.2E-07	8.2E-07	5.7E-07	9.1E-06	4.0E-08	3.4E-08	2.2E-06
Liver	5.4E-07	4.4E-06	9.2E-07	6.6E-07	6.6E-07	5.3E-07	9.8E-07	3.1E-08	9.3E-08	2.2E-06
Lungs	6.0E-08	2.5E-06	1.2E-06	9.4E-07	9.4E-07	5.8E-07	2.3E-06	6.6E-09	9.4E-07	2.0E-06
Marrow (red)	5.5E-06	2.8E-06	3.1E-05	4.1E-06	9.1E-06	9.5E-07	1.7E-06	7.3E-07	1.1E-06	2.9E-06
Oth Tiss (musc)	2.0E-06	1.8E-06	1.2E-06	9.8E-07	9.8E-07	7.2E-07	1.4E-06	1.1E-06	1.3E-06	1.9E-06
Ovaries	4.2E-03	4.1E-07	3.2E-06	7.1E-07	7.1E-07	3.8E-07	4.0E-07	0.0	4.9E-09	2.4E-06
Pancreas	5.0E-07	5.8E-04	1.7E-06	8.5E-07	8.5E-07	4.4E-07	1.9E-05	5.5E-08	7.2E-08	2.4E-06
Skin	4.1E-07	4.0E-07	5.9E-07	6.5E-07	6.5E-07	1.6E-05	4.7E-07	1.4E-06	7.3E-07	1.3E-06
Spleen	4.9E-07	1.9E-05	9.2E-07	5.8E-07	5.8E-07	5.4E-07	3.3E-04	1.7E-08	1.1E-07	2.2E-06
Testes	0.0	5.5E-08	4.5E-07	6.4E-07	6.4E-07	9.1E-07	4.8E-08	1.4E-03	5.0E-10	1.7E-06
Thyroid	4.9E-09	1.2E-07	6.8E-07	7.9E-07	7.9E-07	6.9E-07	8.7E-08	5.0E-10	2.3E-03	1.5E-06
Uterus (nongrvd)	2.1E-05	5.3E-07	2.2E-06	5.7E-07	5.7E-07	4.0E-07	4.0E-07	0.0	4.6E-09	2.6E-06
Total body	2.6E-06	2.6E-06	2.2E-06	2.0E-06	2.0E-06	1.3E-06	2.2E-06	1.9E-06	1.8E-06	2.0E-06

[a]From Snyder WS, Ford MR, Warner GG, Watson SB: *Absorbed Dose Per Unit Accumulated Activity for Selected Radionuclides and Organs* (MIRD Pamphlet No. 11). New York, Society of Nuclear Medicine, 1975.

Assumptions

1. All of the injected activity is uniformly distributed in the liver.
2. The uptake of ^{99m}Tc sulfur colloid in the liver from the blood is essentially instantaneous.
3. There is no biologic removal of ^{99m}Tc sulfur colloid from the liver.

In this case the average dose ($\bar{D}$) to any target organ (r_k) can be estimated by applying the simplified MIRD formulation in equation 7:

$$\bar{D}(r_k) = \Sigma_h \tilde{A}_h \, S(r_k \rightarrow r_h) \qquad (7)$$

Step 1. Calculate the cumulated activity ($\tilde{A}_h$) in the source organ (i.e., liver). By inserting the appropriate values into equation 5 we have

$$\tilde{A}_h = (3000\ \mu\text{Ci})\ (1)\ (1.44)\ (6\ \text{hr}) = 2.60 \times 10^4\ \mu\text{Ci-hr}$$

Note that because $T_b = \infty$, $T_e = T_p$.

Step 2. Find the appropriate S factors for each target/source combination and the radionuclide of interest (i.e., ^{99m}Tc). A reproduction of the appropriate MIRD table for this calculation is shown in Table 19.4. The appropriate *S* factors are found at the intersection of the source organ (i.e., liver) column and the individual target organs (i.e., liver, testes, red marrow, or total body) row. (A complete listing of *S* factors is contained in MIRD Pamphlet #11 (16).)

Target (r_k)	Source (r_h)	*S* Factor
Liver	Liver	4.6×10^{-5}
Testes	Liver	6.2×10^{-8}
Red bone marrow	Liver	1.6×10^{-6}
Total body	Liver	2.2×10^{-6}

Step 3. Organize the assembled information in a table of organ doses.

Target organ (r_k)	$\tilde{A}_h$(μCi-hr)		$S(r_k r_h)$ (rad/ μCi-hr)		$\bar{D}(r_k)$(rad)
1. Liver	$2.60 \times 10_4$	×	4.6×10^{-5}	=	1.2
2. Testes	$2.60 \times 10_4$	×	6.2×10^{-8}	=	0.002
3. Red bone marrow	$2.60 \times 10_4$	×	1.6×10^{-6}	=	0.042
4. Total body	$2.60 \times 10_4$	×	2.2×10^{-6}	=	0.057

Note that the relatively small dose to target organs other than the liver is mostly due to:

1. Only a small fraction of the isotropically emitted penetrating radiation (i.e., γ-rays) being intercepted by the other organ systems (e.g., testes and red bone marrow), *or*
2. The relatively large mass over which the radiation is distributed (e.g., total body).

The first example is simplified by that fact that there was only one source organ (liver) and no biologic elimination of the radiopharmaceutical. The second example is a more complex but realistic dosimetry problem.

EXAMPLE 2

A patient receives 20 mCi of ^{99m}Tc methylene diphosphonate for a bone scan. Estimate the radiation absorbed dose to the

(a) Red bone marrow
(b) Bladder wall

Assumptions

1. Thirty-five percent of the activity is uniformly distributed in the bone where T_b = 18.6 days. (*Note*: 18.6 days × 24 hours/day = 446.4 hours.)
2. Sixty percent of the activity is in the bladder where T_b = 0.67 hours.
3. Five percent of the activity is uniformly distributed in the whole body where T_b = 0.43 hours.
4. The uptake in all of the source organs was essentially instantaneous.

We will still use the formalism in equation 7.

Step 1. Calculate A_h for each source organ, remembering

$$\tilde{A}_h = A_o \cdot f_h \cdot 1.44\ T_e \text{ and } T_e = \frac{T_p \cdot T_b}{T_p + T_b}$$

Source organ	A_o (μCi)		f_h		1.44		T_e(hr)		A_h(μCi-hr)
Bone	20,000	×	0.35	×	1.44	×	5.94	=	5.99×10^4
Bladder contents	20,000	×	0.60	×	1.44	×	0.603	=	1.04×10^4
Total body	20,000	×	0.05	×	1.44	×	0.40	=	5.78×10^2

Step 2. Find the appropriate S factors for each target/source combination. Note that because the injected activity is localized in multiple source organs, for every target organ (i.e., red bone marrow and bladder wall) there are three sources of radiation (i.e., bone, bladder contents, and total body). An additional complication is that *S* factors in Table 19.4 have been calculated separately for cortical (cort) and trabecular (tra) bone. Thus one must assume that the cumulated activity ($\tilde{A}_h$) in the bone is equally divided between the two bone tissues, and therefore consider each as an individual source organ. The permutations of target/source combinations and associated *S* factors are as follows:

Target (r_k)	Source (r_h)	S factor (rad.μCi-hr)
Red bone marrow	Cort bone	4.1×10^{-6}
Red bone marrow	Tra bone	9.1×10^{-6}
Red bone marrow	Bladder contents	2.2×10^{-6}
Red bone marrow	Total body	2.9×10^{-6}
Bladder wall	Cort bone	5.1×10^{-7}
Bladder wall	Tra bone	5.1×10^{-7}
Bladder wall	Bladder contents	1.6×10^{-4}
Bladder wall	Total body	2.3×10^{-6}

It is interesting to note that the dose per unit activity (*S* factor) for the trabecular bone irradiating the bone marrow (9.1×10^{-6}) is more than twice as large as the *S* factor for the cortical bone irradiating the bone marrow (4.1×10^{-6}), even though the activity is evenly distributed between the two bone tissues. This occurs because the marrow is exposed to a larger effective surface area in the trabecular bone than in cortical bone, providing a greater opportunity for the nonpenetrating radiation (i.e., ICEs, AEs, and low-energy γ- and x-ray photons) to interact with the marrow.

Yet another complication arises in that we have calculated an $\tilde{A}$ for the *remainder of the body* (in this problem total body minus bone and bladder contents), while we have available *S*-values for the *total body*. Cloutier, et al. (17), showed how to correct either the $\tilde{A}$ values or the S-values for this problem. Although the $\tilde{A}$ correction is technically easier (18), correction of the *S*-values is a more intuitive process. The S-value correction is performed as follows:

$$S(r_k \leftarrow RB) = S(r_k \leftarrow TB)\left(\frac{m_{TB}}{m_{RB}}\right) - \sum_h S(r_k \leftarrow r_h)\left(\frac{m_h}{m_{RB}}\right)$$

where

$S(r_k \leftarrow RB)$ is the S-value for "remainder of the body" irradiating target region r_k
$S(r_k \leftarrow TB)$ is the S-value for the total body irradiating target region r_k
$S(r_k \leftarrow r_h)$ is the S-value for source region h irradiating target region r_k
m_{TB} is the mass of the total body
m_{RB} is the mass of the remainder of the body, i.e., the total body minus all other source organs used in this problem, and
m_h is the mass of source region h.

For this problem the S-values for remainder of body irradiating the red marrow and the bladder wall are 2.7×10^{-6} and 1.9×10^{-6} rad/μCi-hr, respectively, instead of 2.9×10^{-6} and 2.3×10^{-6} rad/μCi-hr.

Step 3. Organize the assembled information into a table of organ doses for each target from each source.

Target (r_k) = Red bone marrow (RM)

Source organ	Ah(μCi-hr)		(rad/μCi-hr)		(rad)
Cort bone (CB)	½(5.99 × 10⁴)	×	4.1×10^{-6}	=	0.123
Tra bone (TrB)	½(5.99 × 10⁴)	×	9.1×10^{-6}	=	0.272
Bladder contents (BC)	1.04×10^4	×	2.2×10^{-6}	=	0.023
Total body (TB)	5.78×10^2	×	2.7×10^{-6}	=	0.002

The total dose to red bone marrow is the sum of the dose from each source: $\bar{D}(r_k) = \Sigma\, \bar{D}(r_k \leftarrow r_h) = \Sigma\, \bar{D}(RM \leftarrow CB) + \bar{D}(RM \leftarrow TrB) + \bar{D}(RM \leftarrow BC) + \bar{D}(RM \leftarrow TB)$ (i.e., $\bar{D}(r_k) = 0.123 + 0.272 + 0.023 + 0.002 = 0.42$ rad (420 mrad, 4.2 mGy)).

Target (r_k) = Bladder wall (BW)

Source organ	Ah(μCi-hr)		$S(r_k \leftarrow r_h)$ (rad/μCi-hr)		$(\bar{D} \leftarrow r_h)$ (rad)
Cort bone (CB)	½(5.99 × 10⁴)	×	5.1×10^{-7}	=	0.015
Tra bone (TrB)	½(5.99 × 10⁴)	×	5.1×10^{-7}	=	0.015
Bladder contents (BC)	1.04×10^4	×	1.6×10^{-4}	=	1.700
Total body (TB)	5.78×10^2	×	1.9×10^{-6}	=	0.001

As before, $\bar{D}(r_k) = \Sigma\, \bar{D}(r_k \leftarrow r_h) = 0.015 + 0.015 + 1.700 + 0.001 = 1.7$ rad (1700 mrad, or 17 mGy). Note that the dose to the bladder wall is almost entirely (98.2%) due to activity in the bladder. From these calculations one can appreciate how the effective half-life (T_e) of activity in an organ affects the dose to a target. In this situation, a recommendation to have the patient void 1–2 hours after the administration of the activity, not only improves the scintigram, but can reduce the dose to the bladder wall by as much as 75% (19).

EXAMPLE 3

This example employs a model with several source organs, in which the kinetics of an agent have been determined in a population of adult volunteers, but for which dose estimates are desired for children of all ages as well as adults. Very few investigators have the time or resources to study the kinetics of radiopharmaceuticals in children and adults, so it is typical to use a single set of $\tilde{A}$ values with S-values determined for several different age groups. A diagram of the model is shown in Figure 19.4. The $\tilde{A}$'s determined from the experimental studies with this ^{99m}Tc-labeled compound are:

Thyroid	35 μCi-hr
Lungs	200 μCi-hr
Liver	550 μCi-hr
Gallbladder	120 μCi-hr
Small Intestine	630 μCi-hr
Upper Large Intestine	850 μCi-hr
Lower Large Intestine	400 μCi-hr
Kidneys	520 μCi-hr
Spleen	210 μCi-hr
Urinary Bladder	2000 μCi-hr
Remainder of Body	450 μCi-hr

The dose estimates for this problem would be calculated exactly the same as for example 2, except that there are a lot more calculations to do. The easiest way to perform the calculation may be in a matrix format. If the set of dose estimates we want is a 1×14 matrix (dose estimates for 14 target organs—thyroid, lungs, liver, gallbladder, small intestine, upper large intestine, lower large intestine, kidneys, urinary bladder, spleen, ovaries, testes, red marrow, and total body), this can be found by multiplication of a 1×11 matrix of residence times (for the 11 source organs above) and a 11×14 matrix of S-values:

$$[\bar{\mathbf{D}}] = [\tilde{\mathbf{A}}] \times [\mathbf{S}]$$

Additionally, we can repeat this calculation six times to obtain dose estimates for each member of the Cristy-Eckerman phantom series, thus simulating a set of dose estimates for children of various ages and adults. Table 19.5 gives dose estimates for these six ages for the cumulated activities shown above.

Note how the dose estimates increase with decreasing age, as the organs get smaller and closer together. The overall increase for any organ going from an adult to a new-

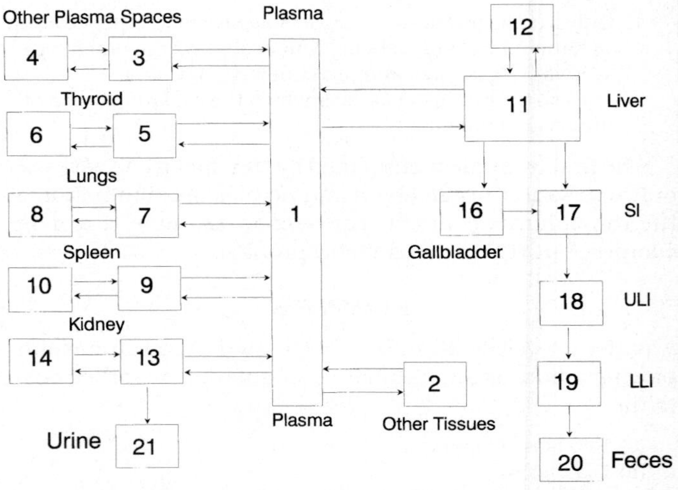

Figure 19.4. Compartmental model for ^{99m}Tc compound of example 3.

Table 19.5.
Radiation Dose Estimates for the Compound of Example 3

Organ	Estimated Radiation Dose (mGy/mBq)					
	Newborn	1-yr-old	5-yr-old	10-yr-old	15-yr-old	Adult
Adrenals	3.6E-02	1.9E-02	1.1E-02	7.4E-03	4.8E-03	3.7E-03
Brain	3.3E-03	1.4E-03	7.8E-04	4.8E-04	3.0E-04	2.5E-04
Breasts	9.6E-03	4.3E-03	2.4E-03	1.4E-03	7.7E-04	6.2E-04
Gallbladder Wall	3.6E-01	1.7E-01	5.7E-02	3.4E-02	2.5E-02	2.2E-02
LLI Wall	3.7E-01	1.5E-01	8.2E-02	5.2E-02	3.2E-02	2.5E-02
Small Intestine	2.3E-01	1.0E-01	5.7E-02	3.6E-02	2.2E-02	1.8E-02
Stomach	3.7E-02	1.8E-02	1.1E-02	7.1E-03	4.5E-03	3.5E-03
ULI Wall	4.8E-01	2.1E-01	1.1E-01	7.0E-02	4.2E-02	3.3E-02
Heart Wall	1.7E-02	8.3E-03	4.7E-03	3.1E-03	2.0E-03	1.5E-03
Kidneys	2.9E-01	1.2E-01	6.9E-02	4.8E-02	3.4E-02	2.8E-02
Liver	9.0E-02	4.3E-02	2.4E-02	1.7E-02	1.1E-02	8.7E-03
Lungs	5.4E-02	2.2E-02	1.1E-02	7.5E-03	5.3E-03	3.6E-03
Muscle	2.3E-02	1.2E-02	6.7E-03	4.4E-03	3.0E-03	2.5E-03
Ovaries	8.9E-02	4.7E-02	2.9E-02	2.0E-02	1.4E-02	1.1E-02
Pancreas	4.5E-02	2.2E-02	1.3E-02	8.9E-03	5.5E-03	4.4E-03
Red Marrow	1.4E-02	7.8E-03	5.7E-03	4.5E-03	3.2E-03	2.6E-03
Bone Surfaces	3.1E-02	1.5E-02	8.1E-03	5.5E-03	3.8E-03	3.0E-03
Skin	1.1E-02	4.9E-03	2.6E-03	1.7E-03	1.1E-03	8.8E-04
Spleen	2.9E-01	1.2E-01	6.5E-02	4.3E-02	2.8E-02	2.0E-02
Testes	4.5E-02	2.4E-02	1.3E-02	8.2E-03	4.7E-03	3.3E-03
Thymus	8.4E-03	3.9E-03	2.2E-03	1.4E-03	9.1E-04	7.1E-04
Thyroid	2.8E-01	2.1E-01	1.1E-01	5.0E-02	3.3E-02	2.0E-02
Urinary Bladder Wall	1.0E+00	4.4E-01	2.3E-01	1.6E-01	1.2E-01	9.7-02
Uterus	1.1E-01	6.0E-02	3.7E-02	2.5E-02	1.6E-02	1.3E-02
Effective Dose Equivalent (mSv/mBq)	1.9E-01	8.8E-02	4.7E-02	3.1E-02	2.1E-02	1.7E-02

born is typically about a factor of 10 for ^{99m}Tc. An adjustment which might reasonably be made to this set of dose estimates is to decrease cumulated activities for the urinary bladder and gastrointestinal tract organs to reflect more rapid clearance in young children. Note also the calculation of a new quantity, the effective dose equivalent, instead of the "total body" dose (the total energy absorbed in the body divided by the mass of the total body). The effective dose equivalent (EDE) is calculated by multiplying the dose estimates (after conversion to dose equivalent) for individual organs by a risk-related weighting factor (Table 19.6)(20) and adding up the individual weighted dose equivalents to a single value. For "Remainder of Body," choose the five organs with the highest doses which do not have a specifically assigned weighting factor and assign each a weighting factor of 0.06. For example, for the adult:

Organ	Dose Equivalent (mSv/mBq)	Weighting Factor	Weighted Dose Equivalent (mSv/mBq)
Ovaries	0.011	0.25	0.0028
Breasts	0.00062	0.15	0.000093
Lungs	0.0036	0.12	0.00043
Red marrow	0.0026	0.12	0.00031
Thyroid	0.020	0.03	0.00060
Bone surfaces	0.0030	0.03	0.000090
Urinary bladder	0.097	0.06	0.0058
ULI wall	0.033	0.06	0.0020
Kidneys	0.028	0.06	0.0017
LLI wall	0.025	0.06	0.0015
Gallbladder wall	0.022	0.06	0.0013
TOTAL (EDE)			0.017 mSv/mBq

Table 19.6.
Organ Weighting Factors Assigned in ICRP 30

Organ	Weighting Factor
Gonads	0.25
Breast	0.15
Red Marrow	0.12
Lung	0.12
Thyroid	0.03
Bone Surfaces	0.03
Remainder	0.30

Although originally derived for an adult working population (20), the ICRP has proposed the quantity as useful in nuclear medicine and applicable to all age groups (21). This quantity is thought by many to be better than "total body" dose in comparing radiopharmaceuticals, procedures, etc. It is important, however, not to attach too much significance to the number, as it is a derived quantity based on many assumptions, subject to change. Indeed, a new set of weighting factors has already been published by the ICRP (22). The MIRD Committee has strongly cautioned against the use of this quantity in nuclear medicine (23), and points out that the quantity is especially not to be applied to therapy situations or to evaluate the risk to an individual.

LIMITATIONS OF THE MIRD METHOD

The MIRD formulation is a significant improvement over other previously used methods, specifically the widely used formulation recommended by the International Committee on Radiological Protection (ICRP #2) in 1959 (24). However, the MIRD method as traditionally applied usually includes several assumptions, limitations, and simplifications, which include:

1. Activity is assumed to be uniformly distributed in the source organs.
2. Energy deposition is averaged over the entire mass of the target organ (i.e., no microdosimetric models are considered).
3. Simple geometric shapes and interorgan relationships are used to approximate human anatomy.
4. The phantoms used for a "reference" adult (i.e., 154 lbs and 5′8″), adolescent, and child are only an approximation of the physical dimensions of any particular individual.
5. Each organ is assumed to be of homogeneous density and composition.
6. Minor dose contributions from bremsstrahlung radiation and Coster-Kronig transitions are ignored.
7. With a few exceptions, low-energy photons and all particulate radiation are assumed to be absorbed locally (i.e., nonpenetrating).

The general MIRD dose equation (equation 4) does *not*, however, contain these assumptions. It is a generally applicable absorbed dose equation whose application is only limited by the assumptions inherent in the specific values for the parameters entered. If the absorbed fractions, for instance, are derived for tissue or cellular level geometries (instead of whole organ geometries), the absorbed doses will be accurate for this domain.

While it is beyond the scope of this section to delve into all of the potential ramifications of the MIRD assumptions, limitations, or simplifications, let us consider some of these factors in a little more detail.

SMALL SCALE AND MICRODOSIMETRY

When there is significant uptake of the radiopharmaceutical in a target organ of interest, the averaging of the dose over the entire organ system is an oversimplification of the actual energy deposition pattern. If dose estimation formulas are to be successfully used to provide a quantitative variable in a dose-response risk projection model, then the appropriate dose(s) to be considered may not only be the average organ system dose but also the detailed energy deposition pattern over short (i.e., macromolecular or cellular) ranges. This is especially important for nonpenetrating radiations (e.g., low-energy photons, ICE, AE, β^-, β^+) in radiobiologically critical targets.

For example, the work of Rao, et al. (25), with mouse testes demonstrated that intratesticular administration of thallous chloride resulted in a significant concentration of the thallium cation in the basal layer ($\leq$10 μm) of the seminiferous epithelium. This region is generally populated with spermatogonia, which are the stem cells for sperm. The authors demonstrated that ^{201}Tl, which emits predominantly low energy mercury x-rays, AEs, and ICEs, was 2–4 times more effective in reducing testis weight and sperm number than ^{204}Tl (an energetic β-emitter) per microcurie administered. However, this result is contrary to what one would expect by considering only the total testicular dose (rad) per microcurie of ^{201}Tl and ^{204}Tl in the organ as calculated by conventional dosimetry, or 8.3 and 54.0 rad, respectively. Thus it appears that the abundance of low-energy electrons emitted during ^{201}Tl decay, which deliver the majority of their energy over a very short range, have a more significant influence over the measured biologic effect than the average total energy deposited per gram would have predicted. Although it is likely that the intravenous route of administration of ^{201}Tl in the clinical setting and blood-testis barrier prevent the inorganic thallous ion from being in intimate contact with the germinal layer of the seminiferous tubules, it is important to note that the estimate of average dose to the testes would not have represented this biologically significant dose distribution pattern.

On the other hand, if one were to consider ^{111}In platelet scintigraphy, the situation may be reversed. A 5-rad organ dose to the spleen is predicted during radioplatelet imaging with modest amounts (<200 μCi) of injected activity. It is important to remember, however, that the 5-rad splenic dose calculation was made by dividing the energy from radiation absorbed in the spleen during decay by the organ's entire mass. This simplification ignores the fact that a significant fraction of the particulate radiation emitted by ^{111}In is in the form of low-energy (0.6–25.4 keV) Auger electrons, which undoubtedly deposit some of their energy within the platelet itself or in adjacent platelets that have formed small platelet aggregates. Thus, in this case, the estimated average dose may overestimate the actual energy deposition pattern realized by sensitive sites within cells of the spleen.

CALCULATIONAL TECHNIQUES

Calculating absorbed dose as a function of distance from point or extended photon or electron-emitting sources has been facilitated for many years by the formulas of Loevinger, et al. (26), and the point kernels of Berger (27). Through the use of the formulas of Loevinger, et al., or the point kernels of Berger, dose as a function of distance may be estimated for most source geometries. Development of the actual techniques and examples is beyond the scope of this chapter. More recently, similar efforts have been attempted by Cross, et al. (28), Werner, et al. (29), and Howell, et al. (30). Certain radiation transport codes are also available which can simulate the transport and absorption of photon and electron energy. Current examples include the EGS code series (31) and the MCNP code (32). The point kernels of Berger and Cross, et al., were generated by similar codes. Most of these authors have produced very similar results, differing only slightly at short distances or at high energies. Useful applications of these results have been published by a number of authors, including Howell, et al. (30), Faraggi, et al. (33), Hui, et al. (34), and Werner, et al. (29), usually for activity in and around tumors of various sizes.

The problems discussed (dose to the testes from thallium isotopes and dose to the spleen from ^{111}In platelets), however, can be addressed through use of these methods, to evaluate where the energy is actually deposited. One of the barriers encountered in this analysis is knowledge of the microscopic distributions of the radionuclides. This information is not accessible by current external imaging techniques, although some information may be gleaned from autoradiography studies.

INTRACELLULAR DOSIMETRY

Since the introduction of ^{111}In 8-hydroxyquinoline (In-Oxine) as a cellular radiolabel by McAfee and Thakur in 1976 (35), the use of this lipid-soluble chelate and its chemical analogs (e.g., tropolone) for cell labeling has rapidly expanded. The diagnostic utility of ^{111}In-labeled formed blood elements (specifically platelets and granulocytes) has been demonstrated by numerous investigators (36–44). Of more recent concern has been the intracellular dose to these circulating blood cells and its potential radiobiologic significance.

Basson and McAfee have calculated cellular radiation doses to neutrophils and platelets for a number of radionuclides of clinical interest (45). Table 19.7 shows the dose and dose rate estimates for ^{111}In based on this work, together with those of ^{99m}Tc and ^{51}Cr for comparison. Note that although the dose and dose rates shown here are considerably higher than those seen from commonly used radiopharmaceuticals and organ system dosimetry, this is mainly a result of the relatively small mass represented by these cells. Studies of structure, function, survival, and margination of these cells have not demonstrated any significant abnormalities (46, 47). While the fact that platelets are enucleated and both platelets and neutrophils are postmitotic may help explain their relative radioresistivity, such is not the case for lymphocytes, which have large nuclei, long mitotic futures, and variable mitotic rates. It has been known for some time that lymphocytes are among the most radiosensitive targets in the body, and several investigators have evaluated the effect of intracellular ^{111}In in lymphocytes (48, 49).

MICRODOSIMETRY

Dosimetry at the cellular level, DNA level, etc., is yet another level of dosimetry, called microdosimetry by some, and is distinguished from small scale dosimetry by its stochastic nature. Much of the work in this field, useful in radiation detection as well as tissue dosimetry, has been developed by Harold Rossi. A summary of some of the concepts of microdosimetry is given in an article by Rossi and Zaider (50). Some applications of these concepts have been attempted by Makrigiorgos, et al. (51, 52), Gardin, et al. (53), and Leichner (54). Although these calculations are possible, the interpretation of the results is uncertain at present, and more development is needed.

Table 19.7
Doses and Dose Rates for Cellular Radiolabels

Cells	Nuclide	Dose rate[a] (rad/hr)	T_c (hr)	Dose (rad)[a]
Neutrophils	Tc-99m	91	3	390
	In-111	187	5.5	1,480
	Cr-51	115	6	990
Platelets	Tc-99m	125	5.7	1,030
	In-111	213	42	12,900
	Cr-51	193	93	25,900

[a]Assumes 1 mCi uniformly distributed in 1.3×10^8 neutrophils or 7.5×10^9 platelets typically contained in 30 ml of whole blood. Modified from Bassano and McAfee (21).

ACCURACY OF DOSE CALCULATIONS

The time integral activity ($\tilde{A}_h$) used for each initial organ dose estimate generated during the IND phase of radiopharmaceutical development is usually based on laboratory animal data, which are only slowly adjusted by human investigation and quantitative evaluation of biodistribution and kinetics. The animal model assumption and biodistribution kinetics will always be associated with some error in attempting to predict the human dosimetry. In an analysis of data sets for several radiopharmaceuticals first using animal data and then human data gathered in clinical trials, the animal data typically predicted correctly the organ receiving the highest absorbed dose, and determined most estimates for most organs within a factor of 2 (55). One notable exception was for prediction of the dosimetry of ^{99m}Tc ECD using monkeys. The monkeys retained significantly more of the activity than did humans, thus overestimating the dose to many visceral organs, but badly underestimating the dose to the gallbladder wall and urinary bladder wall (the latter of which was the critical organ—this dose was underestimated by about a factor of 7). This was probably due to anesthetizing the animals for imaging. However, it shows that predictions of human dosimetry based on animal models are only approximate at best.

Another consideration is the applicability of human dosimetry data when they are available. If the data are based primarily on normal healthy adult volunteers, it is clear that biodistribution and kinetics for this group will be different from a patient population of dissimilar ages and in whom the normal metabolic process may be compromised by the presence of various pathophysiologic conditions. Additionally, our estimate of the impact on human health from a particular dose-response model may be off by an order of magnitude in either direction.

Considering this, one may ask, why bother to do these calculations at all if they are fraught with so many assumptions and potential errors? The answer is that this system and other dose estimate models give us at least a yardstick for comparison from which we can make some decisions regarding the safety or potential hazards of future radiopharmaceuticals. Additionally, the calculated dose estimates also serve as a guide to the safe and selective use of currently used radiopharmaceuticals in various patient populations. As more detailed information regarding the dose-response relationship becomes available the utility of our cumulative knowledge base of radiopharmaceutical dosimetry will have even greater significance.

MIRD PUBLICATIONS AND DOSE ESTIMATES

Since the publication of the first MIRD schema in 1968 (4), the Committee has published a number of pamphlets containing additional information, refinements, and simplifications of the technique. Additionally, various task groups of the Committee periodically publish dose estimate re-

Appendix 1[a]

Radiopharmaceutical	Typical Adult Dose		Organ Receiving Highest Dose	Organ Dose[b]		Effective Dose[c,d]		Gonadal Dose[b,e]			Early Pregnancy Dose[b,f]		
	mBq	mCi		mGy	rad	mSv	rem	mGy		rad	mGy	rad	
F-18 Fluorodeoxyglucose	370	10	Bladder Wall	69	6.9	11	1.1	6.3 4.8	ov ts	0.63 0.48	8.5	0.85	56,57
P-32 Sodium Phosphate	148	4	Red Marrow	2,100	210	390	39	100 100	ov ts	10 10	140	14	58
P-32 Chromic Phosphate	370	10	Pleural surface Peritoneal surface	115,000 90,000	11,500 9,000	NA[g,h]		NA[g]			NA[g]		59
Cr-51 Sodium Chromate RBC	5.6	0.15	Spleen	7	0.7	0.92	0.092	0.54 0.40	ov ts	0.054 0.040	0.54	0.054	60
Co-57 Sodium Cyanocobalamin (B-12)	0.037	0.001	Liver	0.85	0.085	0.11	0.011	0.031 0.017	ov ts	0.0031 0.0017	0.057	0.0057	60
Ga-67 Citrate	185	5	Bone surface	120	12	22.5	2.25	14 9.5	ov ts	1.4 0.95	14	1.4	61
In-111 White Blood Cells	18.5	0.5	Spleen	110	11	12.5	1.25	2.4 0.55	ov ts	0.24 0.055	1.9	0.19	62–66
I-123 Sodium Iodide	14.8	0.4	Thyroid	52	5.2	1.8	0.18	0.18 0.076	ov ts	0.018 0.0076	0.24	0.024	67
Kr-81m Gas	370	10	Lungs	0.074	0.0074	9.8×10^{-3}	9.8×10^{-4}	5×10^{-5} 3.8×10^{-6}	ov ts	5×10^{-6} 3.8×10^{-7}	3.7×10^{-5}	3.7×10^{-6}	66
I-125 Albumin	0.74	0.02	Heart Wall	0.44	0.044	2	0.2	0.15 0.12	ov ts	0.015 0.012	0.19	0.019	66
I-131 Sodium Iodide	3700	100	Thyroid	1.3×10^{6}	1.3×10^{5}	NA[g,h]		180 100	ov ts	18 10	220	22	67
I-131 Sodium Iodohippurate	13	0.35	Bladder wall (Thyroid blocked with Lugol's solution or SSKI)	18	1.8	1.3	0.13	0.30 0.22	ov ts	0.030 0.022	0.83	0.083	68
Xe-133 Gas (5-minute breathing and 10-liter spirometer volume	555	15	Lung	0.63	0.063	0.42	0.042	0.39 0.36	ov ts	0.039 0.036	0.39	0.039	69
TI-201 Chloride	Planar 74	 2	Testes Thyroid (female)	60 46	6.0 4.6	26	2.6	7.4 60	ov ts	0.74 6.0	6.2	0.62	70–71
Tc-99m Sodium Pertechnetate	Thyroid Imaging 370	 10	Bladder wall (5 h void)	13	1.3	3.9	0.39	3.2 1.2	ov ts	0.32 0.12	3.0 4.2	0.3 0.42	72
Tc-99m Red Blood Cells	740	20	Bladder wall (5 h void)	16	1.6	5.4	0.54	3.4 2.4	ov ts	0.34 0.24			73
Tc-99m Pyrophosphate	Planar 555 SPECT 925	 15 25	Bone Surfaces (5 h void)	36	3.6	4.1	0.41	2.1 1.4	ov ts	0.21 0.14	2.7	0.27	74
Tc-99m Medronate also known as Tc-99m Methyenediphosonate or MDP	Planar 740 SPECT 1,110	 20 30	Bone Surfaces	44	4.4	5.4	0.54	2.4 1.6	ov ts	0.24 0.16	3.8	0.38	74
Tc-99m Mertiatide also known as MAG_3 (Mallinckrodt)	370	10	Bladder wall (5 h void)	50	5.0	4.4	0.44	2.5 1.7	ov ts	0.25 0.17	5.5	0.55	75

Appendix 1—*continued*

Radiopharmaceutical	Typical Adult Dose		Organ Receiving Highest Dose	Organ Dose[b]		Effective Dose[c,d]		Gonadal Dose[b,e]			Early Pregnancy Dose[b,f]		
	mBq	mCi		mGy	rad	mSv	rem	mGy		rad	mGy	rad	
Tc-99m Pentetate also known as Tc-99m DTPA	370	10	Bladder wall (5 h void)	28	2.8	3	0.3	2.0 1.4	ov ts	0.20 0.14	3.7	0.37	76
Tc-99m Sulfur Colloid	296	8	Liver	26	2.6	4.1	0.41	0.47 0.07	ov ts	0.047 0.007	0.40	0.040	77
Tc-99m Disofenin also known as HIDA (iminodiacetic acid)	185	5	Gallbladder wall	20	2.0	4.7	0.47	3.6 0.32	ov ts	0.36 0.032	0.26	0.026	60
Tc-99m Sestamibi also known as Cardiolite	740	20	Upper large intestine wall	37 Rest 30 Stress	3.7 3.0	11.2 Rest 9.6 Stress	1.12 0.96	10 2.6	ov ts	1.0 0.26	8.9	0.89	66
Tc-99m Exametazime also known as Ceretec and HMPAO	740	20	Kidneys	26	2.6	10.2	1.02	5.2 1.7	ov ts	0.52 0.17	5.2	0.52	78
Tc-99m Macro aggregated albumin (MAA)	148	4	Lungs	10	1.0	1.9	0.19	0.27 0.16	ov ts	0.027 0.016	0.34	0.034	60

[a]Modified and reproduced by permission from Bushberg JT, et al. The Essential Physics of Medical Imaging. Baltimore: Williams and Wilkins, 1994: 650–652.

[b]Gray and rad per typical administered adult dose

[c]Sievert and rem per typical administered adult dose

[d]Although the effective dose was developed for (and thus incorporates assumptions relevant to) a healthy occupationally exposed population (as compared with an ill elderly population characteristic of medical imaging) its application in medicine has been recommended by the ICRP and, at the very least, offers a relative basis upon which doses may be compared between various diagnostic examinations (nuclear medicine; diagnostic x-rays) using ionizing radiation

[e]ov = ovaries; ts = testes

[f]Dose to the nongravid uterus of the adult female phantom. Some activity in the remainder of the body assumed to be in the uterus.

[g]NA = Not applicable.

[h]The effective dose is not a relevant quantity for therapeutic doses of radionuclides because it provides an estimate of effective stochastic risk (e.g., cancer and genetic detriment) and is not relevant to deterministic (i.e., nonstochastic) risks (e.g., acute radiation syndrome).

ports in the Journal of Nuclear Medicine that utilize the MIRD formalisms and the best available human and animal data to estimate organ doses in humans from radiopharmaceuticals, either in routine clinical use or under current clinical evaluation. Information on MIRD documents is available through the Society of Nuclear Medicine. Adult patient and early pregnancy doses from commonly used radiopharmaceuticals is provided in Appendix one together with their references.

REFERENCES

1. Marinelli LD, Quimby EH, Hine GJ. Dosage determination with radioactive isotopes; practical considerations in therapy and protection. Am J Roent Radium Ther 1948;59:260.
2. Loevinger R, Holt JG, Hine GJ. Internally administered radioisotopes. In: Hine GJ, Brownell GL, eds. Radiation dosimetry. Chap. 17. New York: Academic Press, 1956.
3. Loevinger R, Berman M. A formalism for calculation of absorbed dose from radionuclides. Phys Med Biol 1968;13:205.
4. Loevinger R, Berman M. A schema for absorbed dose calculations for biologically distributed radionuclides. J Nucl Med 1968;(Suppl 1, Pamphlet #1).
5. Ellett WH, Callahan AB, Brownell GL. Gamma-ray dosimetry of internal emitters. I. Monte Carlo calculations of absorbed dose from point sources. Br J Radiol 1964;37:45.
6. Ellett WH, Callahan AB, Brownell GL. Gamma-ray dosimetry of internal emitters. II. Monte Carlo calculations of absorbed dose from uniform sources. Br J Radiol 1965;38:541.
7. Coffey J, Cristy M, Warner G. MIRD Pamphlet No 13: Specific absorbed fractions for photon sources uniformly distributed in the heart chambers and heart wall of a heterogeneous phantom. J Nucl Med 1981;22:65–71.
8. Eckerman KF, Cristy M, Warner GG. Dosimetric evaluation of brain scanning agents. In: Watson EE, Schlafke-Stelson AT, Coffey JL, Cloutier RJ, eds. Third international radiopharmaceutical dosimetry symposium. HHS Publication FDA 81–8166. Rockville, MD: U.S. Dept. of Health and Human Services, Food and Drug Administration, 1981:527–540.
9. Watson EE, Stabin MG. A model of the peritoneal cavity for use in internal dosimetry [Abstract]. J Nucl Med 1986;27:979.
10. Stabin MG. A model of the prostate gland for use in internal dosimetry. J Nucl Med 1994;35(3):516.
11. Eckerman KF, Ryman JC. External exposure to radionuclides in air, water, and soil. Federal Guidance Report No. 12, EPA Report No. EPA 402-R-93–081. Washington, DC: Government Printing Office, 1993.
12. Crady DL, Bolch WE, Weber DA, Atkins HL. Specific absorbed fractions for photon sources in a revised dosimetric model of the

brain. Health Physics. Supplement to Vol. 64, No. 6. Baltimore: Williams and Wilkins, 1993:S17.

13. Cristy M, Eckerman K. Specific absorbed fractions of energy at various ages from internal photon sources. ORNL/TM-8381 V1-V7. Oak Ridge, TN: Oak Ridge National Laboratory, 1987.
14. Stabin MG, Watson EE, Cristy M, Ryman JC, Davis J, Marshall DA. Mathematical models and specific absorbed fractions of photon energy in the adult female at various stages of pregnancy. Oak Ridge, TN: Oak Ridge National Laboratory, 1994 (in press).
15. Snyder W, Ford M, Warner G. Estimates of specific absorbed fractions for photon sources uniformly distributed in various organs of a heterogeneous phantom. MIRD Pamphlet No. 5 (revised). New York: Society of Nuclear Medicine, 1978.
16. Snyder WS, Ford MR, Warner GG, Watson SB. "S" absorbed dose per unit cumulated activity for selected radionuclides and organs. nm/MIRD Pamphlet #11. New York: Society of Nuclear Medicine, 1975.
17. Cloutier R, Watson E, Rohrer R, Smith E. Calculating the radiation dose to an organ, J Nucl Med 1973;14(1):53–55.
18. Coffey J, Watson E. Calculating dose from remaining body activity: a comparison of two methods. Med Phys 1979;6(4):307–308.
19. Smith EM, Warner GG. Practical methods of dose reduction to the bladder wall. In: Cloutier RJ, Coffey JL, Snyder WS, Watson EE, eds. Radiopharmaceutical dosimetry, proceedings of a symposium at Oak Ridge, April 1976. Bureau of Radiological Health Publication (EDS)76–8044. Washington, DC: U.S. Government Printing Office, 1976.
20. International Commission on Radiological Protection. Limits for intakes of radionuclides by workers. ICRP Publication 30. New York: Pergamon Press, 1979.
21. International Commission on Radiological Protection. Protection of the patient in nuclear medicine. ICRP Publication 52. New York: Pergamon Press, 1987.
22. International Commission on Radiological Protection. 1990 recommendations of the International Commission on Radiological Protection. ICRP Publication 60. New York: Pergamon Press, 1991.
23. Poston J. Application of the effective dose equivalent to nuclear medicine patients. J Nucl Med 1993;34(4):714–716.
24. International Committee on Radiological Protection. Report of ICRP Committee II on permissible dose for internal radiation. Health Phys 1959;3:1.
25. Rao DV, Govelitz DF, Sastry KSR. Radiotoxicity of thallium-201 in mouse testes: inadequacy of conventional dosimetry. J Nucl Med 1983;24:145.
26. Loevinger R, Japha E, Brownell G. Discrete radiosotope processes. In: Hine G, Brownell G, eds. Radiation dosimetry. Chap. 16. New York: Academic Press, 1956:694–802.
27. Berger, M. MIRD Pamphlet No 7. Distribution of absorbed dose around point sources of electrons and beta particles in water and other media. J Nucl Med 1971;12(Suppl 5):5.
28. Cross W, Freedman N, Wong P. Tables of beta-ray dose distributions in water. AECL-10521. Chalk River, Ontario: Chalk River Nuclear Laboratories, 1992.
29. Werner B, Rahman M, Salk W. Dose distributions in regions containing beta sources: uniform spherical source regions in homogeneous media. Med Phys 1991;18(6):1181–1191.
30. Howell R, Rao D, Sastry K. Macroscopic dosimetry for radioimmunotherapy: nonuniform activity distributions in solid tumors. Med Phys 1989;16(1):66–74.
31. Bielajew A, Rogers D. PRESTA: the parameter reduced electron-step transport algorithm for electron monte carlo transport. Nucl Instrum Methods 1987;B18:165–181.
32. Briesmeister, JF. MCNP—a general Monte Carlo N-particle transport code. LA-12625-M. Los Alamos, NM: Los Alamos National Laboratory, 1993.
33. Farragi M, Gardin I, Labriolle-Vaylet C, et al. The influence of tracer localization on the electron dose rate delivered to the cell nucleus. J Nucl Med 1994;35:113–119.
34. Hui T, Fisher D, Press O, et al. Localized beta dosimetry of ^{131}I-labeled antibodies in follicular lymphoma. Med Phys 1992; 19(1):97–104.
35. McAfee JG, Thakur ML. Survey of radioactive agents for in vitro labeling of phagocytic leukocytes. I. Soluble agents. J Nucl Med 1976;17:480.
36. Goodwin DA, Bushberg JT, Doherty PW, et al. In-111 labeled autologous platelets for location of vascular thrombi in humans. J Nucl Med 1978;19:626.
37. Davis HH, Siegel BA, Joist JH, et al. Scintigraphic detection of atherosclerotic lesions and venous thrombi in man by indium-111-labeled autologous platelets. Lancet 1978;1:1185.
38. Smith N, Chandler S, Hawker RJ, et al. Indium-labeled autologous platelets as diagnostic aid after renal transplantation. Lancet 1979;1:1241.
39. Thakur ML, Lavender JP, Arnot RN, et al. Indium-111 labeled autologous leukocytes in man. J Nucl Med 1977;18:1014.
40. Doherty PW, Bushberg JT, Lipton MJ, Meares CF, Goodwin DA. The use of indium-111-labeled leukocytes for abscess detection. Clin Nucl Med 1978;3:108.
41. Ezekowitz MD, Burow RD, Heath PW, et al. The diagnostic accuracy of indium-111 platelet scintigraphy in the diagnosis of left ventricular thrombi. Am J Cardiol 1983;51:1563–1564.
42. Goss TP, Monahan JJ. Indium-111 white blood cell scan. Orthop Rev 1981;10:91.
43. Ezekowitz MD, Wilson DA, Smith EO, et al. The comparison of indium-111 platelet scintigraphy and two-dimensional echocardiography in the diagnosis of left ventricular thrombi. N Engl J Med 1982;306:1509–1513.
44. Thakur ML, Gottschalk AG, eds. In-111 labeled neutrophils, platelets and lymphocytes. New York: Trivirum Publishing Co., 1980.
45. Bassano DA, McAfee JG. Cellular doses of labeled neutrophils and platelets. J Nucl Med 1979;20:255.
46. Zakhireh B, Thakur ML, Malech HL, et al. Indium-111 labeled human polymorphonuclear leukocytes: viability, random migration, chemotaxis, bacterial capacity and ultrastructure. J Nucl Med 1979;20:741.
47. Welch MJ, Mathias CJ. Platelet viability following In-111 oxine labeling in electrolyte solutions. In: Thakur ML, Gottschalk AG, eds. In-111 labeled neutrophils, platelets and lymphocytes. New York: Trivirum Publishing Co., 1980:93–102.
48. Rannie GH, Thakur ML, Ford WL. Indium-111 labeled lymphocytes: preparation, evaluation and comparison with Cr-51 lymphocytes in rats. Clin Exp Immunol 1977;29:509.
49. Chisholm PM, Danpure HJ, Healey G, et al. Cell damage resulting from the labeling of rat lymphocytes and HeLa S3 cells with In-111 oxine. J Nucl Med 1979;20:1308.
50. Rossi H, Zaider M. Elements of microdosimetry. Med Phys 1991; 18(6):1085–1092.
51. Makrigiorgos G, Ito S, Baranowska-Kortylewicz J, et al. Inhomogeneous deposition of radiopharmaceuticals at the cellular level: experimental evidence and dosimetry implications. J Nucl Med 1990;31:1358–1363.
52. Makrigiorgos G, Adelstein S, Kassis A. Limitations of conventional internal dosimetry at the cellular level. J Nucl Med 1989;30:1856–1864.
53. Gardin I, Linhart N, Petiet A, Bok B. Dosimetry at the cellular level of Kupffer cells after technetium-99m-sulphur colloid injection. J Nucl Med 1992;33:380–384.
54. Leichner P. Macrodosimetry and microdosimetry in radioimmunotherapy. DOE/ER/61195. Omaha: University of Nebraska Medical Center, 1991.
55. Stabin M. Radiation dosimetry and the predictive value of preclinical models. Presentation, Drug Information Association, July 13, 1989.

56. Gallagher BM, Ansari A, Atkins H, et al. Radiopharmaceuticals XXVII. ^{18}F-labeled 2-deoxy-2-fluoro-D-glucose as a radiopharmaceutical for measuring regional myocardial glucose metabolism in vivo: tissue distribution and imaging studies in animals. J Nucl Med 1977;18(10):990–996.
57. Jones SC, Alavi A, Christman D, et al. The radiation dosimetry of 2-[F-18]fluoro-2-deoxy-D-glucose in man. J Nucl Med 1982; 23(7):613–617.
58. International Commission on Radiological Protection. Limits for intakes of radionuclides by workers. ICRP Publication 30. New York: Pergamon Press, 1979.
59. Watson EE, Stabin MG, Davis JL, Eckerman KF. A model of the peritoneal cavity for use in internal dosimetry. J Nucl Med 1989; 30:2002–2011.
60. International Commission on Radiological Protection. Radiation dose to patients from radiopharmaceuticals. ICRP Publication 53. Pergamon Press, New York, 1988.
61. Cloutier RJ, Watson EE, Hayes RL, et al. MIRD dose estimate report no. 2: gallium-66-, gallium-67-, gallium-68-, and gallium-72-citrate. J Nucl Med 1973;14:755–756.
62. Thakur ML, Seifert CL, Madsen MT, et al. Neutrophil labeling: problems and pitfalls. Sem Nucl Med 1984;14:107–117.
63. Weiblen BJ, Forstrom L, McCullough J. Studies of the kinetics of indium-111-labeled granulocytes. J Lab Clin Med 1979;94:246–255.
64. Goodwin, DA, Finston, RA, Smith, SI. The distribution and dosimetry of In-111-labeled leukocytes and platelets in humans. Third International Radiopharmaceutical Dosimetry Symposium, Oak Ridge, TN. HHS publication FDA-81-8166. Washington, DC: Bureau of Radiological Health (Government Printing Office), 1980: 88–101.
65. Marcus C, Stabin M, Watson E. Dosimetry of leukocytes labeled with ^{99m}Tc-albumin colliod. Nucl Med Comm 1988;9:249–254.
66. Stabin M. Personal communication. Oak Ridge, TN: Radiation Internal Dose Information Center, 1992.
67. Berman M, Braverman L, Burke J, et al. MIRD dose estimate report no. 5: radiation absorbed dose estimates for I-123, I-124, I-125, I-126, I-130, I-131, and I-132 as sodium iodide. J Nucl Med 1975;16:857–860.
68. Lindmo T, Skretting A, Nakken KF. An examination of different mathematical models for renal function as measured by ^{131}I-hippuran renography. Med Phys 1974;1(4):193–197.
69. Atkins HL, Robertson JS, Croft BY, et al. Estimates of radiation absorbed doses from radioxenons in lung imaging. MIRD dose estimate report no. 9. J Nucl Med 1980;21:459–465.
70. Krahwinkel W, Herzog H, Feinendegen L. Pharmacokinetics of thallium-201 in normal individuals after routine myocardial scintigraphy. J Nucl Med 1988;29(9):1582–1586.
71. Gupta SM, Herrera N, Spencer RP, et al. Testicular-scrotal content of ^{201}Tl and ^{67}Ga after intravenous administration. Int J Nucl Med and Biol 1981;8:211–213.
72. Lathrop K, Atkins H, Berman M, et al. MIRD dose estimate report no. 8: radiation absorbed dose estimates for technetium-99m as sodium pertechnetate. J Nucl Med 1976;17:74–77.
73. Atkins H, Thomas SR, Buddemeyer U, Chervu LR. MIRD dose estimate report no. 14: radiation absorbed dose from ^{99m}Tc-labeled red blood cells. J Nucl Med 1990;31:378–380.
74. Weber D, Makler PT Jr., Watson EE, et al. MIRD dose estimate report no 13: radiation absorbed dose from ^{99m}Tc-labeled bone agents. J Nucl Med 1989;30:1117–1122.
75. Stabin M, Taylor A, Eshima D, et al. Radiation dosimetry for technetium-99m-MAG_3, technetium-99m-DTPA, and iodine-131-OIH based on human biodistribution studies. J Nucl Med 1992;33:33–40.
76. Thomas SR, Atkins HL, McAfee JG, et al. MIRD dose estimate no. 12: radiation absorbed dose from ^{99m}Tc diethylenetriaminepentaacetic acid (DTPA). J Nucl Med 1984;25:503–505.
77. Atkins HL, Cloutier RJ, Lathrop KA, et al. MIRD dose estimate report no. 3: summary of current radiation dose estimates to humans with various liver conditions from ^{99m}Tc sulfur colloid. J Nucl Med 1975;16:108A–108B.
78. Soundy RG, Tyrrell DA, Pickett RD, Stabin MG. The radiation dosimetry of ^{99}Tc^{m}-exametazime. Nucl Med Comm 1990;11:791–799.

20 Radiobiology

S. JULIAN GIBBS

It has been recognized for almost a century that ionizing radiation, in sufficient doses, produces damage in living systems (1). However, despite decades of intensive research worldwide, it has not been established conclusively that small doses, such as those encountered by staff and patients in diagnostic procedures in the healing arts, are harmful. Neither has it been demonstrated that such doses are safe, i.e., devoid of injurious effects. This dilemma led the scientific community, on grounds of prudence, to establish the no-threshold model, which states that any dose of radiation, however small, *may* carry a small probability of biologic damage. Estimates of risk in this chapter are based on this model. It must be emphasized at the outset that there is a large uncertainty in these risk estimates, not only in their magnitudes, but also in whether these risks exist at all. There are no confirmed data demonstrating that any patient has ever been harmed by current techniques of the diagnostic use of ionizing radiation in the healing arts.

The public, the media, and even some scientists have confused the no-threshold model with established fact. The model fits available data, but not to the exclusion of other models. Some data support the concept of beneficial effects of small doses of radiation, called radiation hormesis (2). It seems clear that the facts lie somewhere between the two extremes, but their precise location in this space is unknown. We must proceed, however, with the information we have to estimate risks to patients and staff from diagnostic radiation in the healing arts, and to determine that those risks are within the range that society considers acceptable (Table 20.1). To do otherwise could ignore a radiation dose that might be avoided or prevent a patient from receiving a clinically indicated procedure.

Table 20.1.
One in a Million Risks[a]

Risk	Quantity
Existence, male, age 60	20 min
Living in New York	2 days
Living in Denver	2 months
Living in stone building	2 months
Drinking Miami water	1 year
Living near PVC plant	10 years
Travel by canoe	6 min
Travel by bicycle	10 miles
Travel by automobile	300 miles
Travel by commercial air	1000 miles
Working in coal mine	1 hour
Typical factory work	10 days
Smoking	1.4 cigarettes
Drinking wine	500 cc

[a]Data from Pochin (3) and Wilson (4)

It is first necessary to provide basic information dealing with radiation effects at the cellular level to create rational understanding of effects in intact organisms, especially humans.

CELLULAR RADIOBIOLOGY

Radiation effects result from the chemical events that follow ionization within a cell. Ion pairs are created randomly, either in biologically important molecules (direct action) or through damage to these molecules as a result of free radicals formed by radiolysis of water (indirect action). Overwhelming experimental evidence points to DNA as the target molecule. Numerous alterations in DNA have been described, including alteration or deletion of bases; strand breaks, or disruption of the sugar-phosphate backbone of either one (single-strand break) or both (double-strand break) of the double helix; and cross-linking, or production of covalent bonds between the two chains.

TRANSFORMATION AND MUTATION

Relatively modest DNA damage involving only one or a few molecules per cell, resulting from small radiation doses, is thought to be associated with subtle changes in cell chemistry. These apparently minor chemical changes, however, can lead to serious alterations in cell function. In vitro transformation has been demonstrated in mammalian cells exposed to doses as small as 10 mGy. Frequency of transformation is relatively low, of the order of 10^{-2} per Gy. Transformed cells are characterized by loss of contact inhibition in culture, and the generation of malignant tumors when injected in sufficient numbers into susceptible animals (5). In other cases, rather severe damage, such as deletion of large numbers of base pairs, may result in cells that are not perceptibly altered (6). Some relatively large regions of DNA contain no genetic information essential for cell survival or function. Specific locus mutations in vitro have been studied by a number of investigators. Frequency is much lower than that of transformation, typically of the order of 10^{-4}–10^{-6} per Gy (7).

CELL DEATH

More severe DNA damage, especially strand breaks, has been associated with cell death. Three modes of radiation-induced cell death have been described. *Reproductive cell death*, or loss of clonogenicity, has been extensively studied in cultured mammalian cells. Classically, cell survival curves have been generated using the target theory model (8) shown in Figure 20.1**A**. With high-LET radiation (e.g., heavy charged particles), the survival curve is exponential,

$$S = e^{-D/D_0}$$

where S is the surviving fraction, D is radiation dose, and D_0 is a parameter, the reciprocal of the slope. This is known as the single-target model. With low-LET radiation (e.g., x-ray) the curve is exponential with a shoulder,

$$S = 1 - (1 - e^{-D/D_0})^n$$

where n is the extrapolation number, the intercept on the ordinate of the extrapolation of the linear portion of the curve. This is the multihit or multitarget model. A cell survival curve can be characterized using this model by specifying D_0 and, with low-LET radiation, n. In general, D_0 is smaller, i.e., the curve is steeper, with high LET radiation.

An alternative to target theory is the theory of dual radiation action, which models survival curves as

$$S = e^{-(\alpha D + \beta D^2)}$$

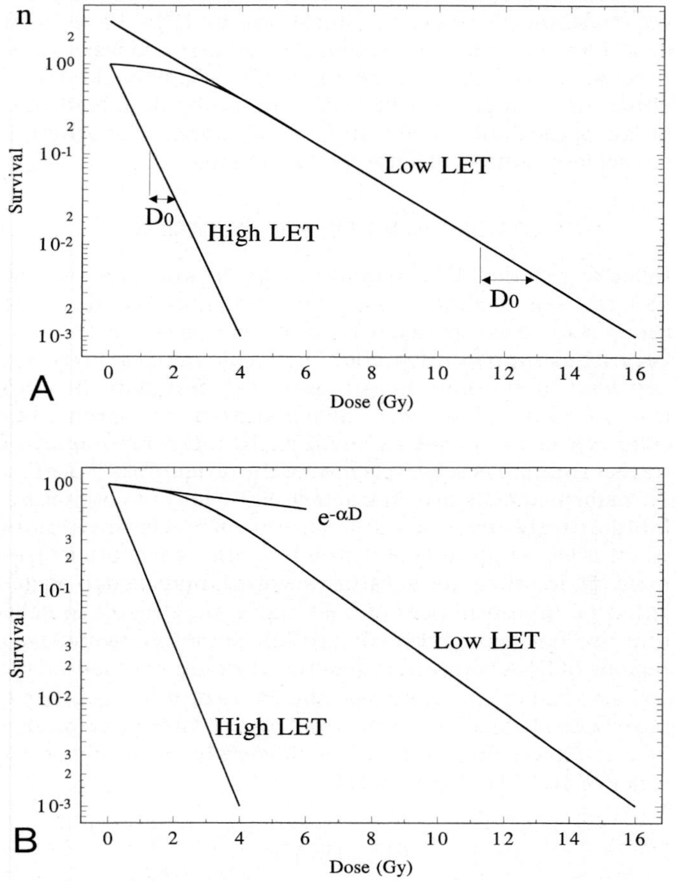

Figure 20.1. Cell survival curves, hypothetical. **A.** Target theory. The curve following exposure to neutrons or charged particles (*high LET*) is exponential, characterized by D_0, the reciprocal of the slope. From exposure to x-rays, γ-rays, or electrons (*low LET*), there is a shoulder resulting from repair of sublethal damage at low doses. The curve is characterized by D_0 and n, the intercept of the linear portion of the curve extrapolated to zero dose. **B.** Theory of dual radiation action. The curve following exposure to *high-LET* radiation is exponential, characterized by α, the reciprocal of D_0. The initial slope in the curve from low-LET radiation, characterized by $e^{-\alpha D}$, estimates effects from small doses. Downward concavity comes from the βD^2 term.

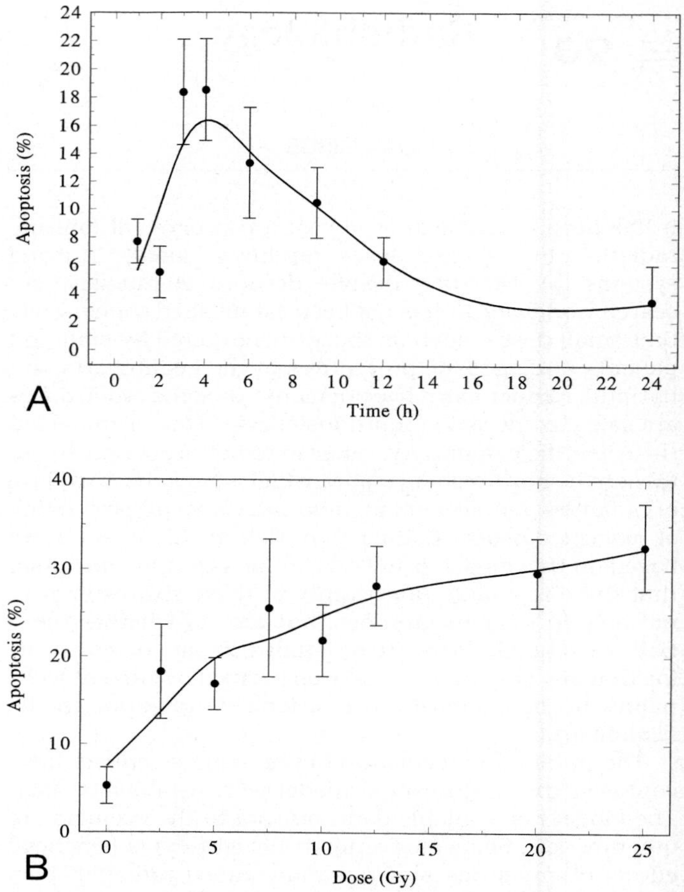

Figure 20.2. Apoptosis, or programmed cell death, in mouse ovarian tumors irradiated in vivo. **A.** Time course. A brief wave of apoptosis occurs after single exposure of 2.5 Gy, peaking at 4–6 hours postexposure, and returning to control levels at 24 hours. **B.** Dose-response curve at 4 hours after single exposure. The response appears to saturate at about 10 Gy, with little further increase at doses above 12.5 Gy. Error bars in both plots represent standard deviations. (Data from Stephens LC, Hunter NR, Ang KK, Milas L, Meyn RE. Development of apoptosis in irradiated murine tumors as a function of time and dose. Radiat Res 1993;135:75–80.)

where α and β are parameters, as shown in Figure 20.1**B** (9). In general, $\alpha > \beta$. Thus, with low LET radiation at low doses or low dose rates, the βD^2 term is negligible. At higher doses, the curve remains concave downward. At high LET $\beta \approx 0$. The model is broadly applicable to a number of radiation effects, including carcinogenesis.

For most mammalian cells in culture exposed to low LET radiation, D_0 is about 1–2 Gy, and n is 2–3. Several investigators have shown by ingenious techniques that most mammalian cells in vivo exhibit similar radiosensitivity. The major exceptions are lymphocytes and bone marrow colony forming cells, for which the D_0 is about 0.7 Gy (10).

Programmed cell death, or apoptosis, is a mode of cell death whose first visible sign is chromatin condensation. The dying cell then disintegrates to form a cluster of apoptotic bodies that are membrane bound and which are soon phagocytosed. Since membranes remain intact until phagocytosis, no cellular contents are released, and no inflammatory response occurs. In irradiated radioresponsive tumors, brief waves of apoptotic bodies are seen (Fig. 20.2), peaking about 4 hours postexposure, with a D_0 of about 4 Gy (11). Apoptosis is an active, genetically programmed process. Presence of p53 tumor suppressor gene is required for radiation-induced apoptosis in mouse thymocytes (12). It plays a role in a number of physiologic processes, e.g., embryonic development (10). Its overall importance in radiobiology is not yet fully understood or appreciated.

Interphase cell death, not genetically programmed, requires very large doses that disrupt cellular membranes and organization or, in extreme cases, molecules, such as denaturation of proteins. This is the classically-described mode of death of nondividing cell populations. It is of limited importance in radiobiology. The doses required to produce it occur only in such things as nuclear explosions, and then only when the exposed individuals are close enough to the detonation to be killed by blast or heat.

MODIFYING FACTORS

A number of factors and conditions may either increase or decrease the magnitude of the effect of a given dose. In general, these factors must be present at the time of exposure.

Physical factors generally interact at the level of ionization. *Linear energy transfer* (LET), or the spatial density of ion pairs produced along the track of an ionizing particle, affects not only the shape but also the slope of the cell survival curve (Fig. 20.1). Densely-ionizing particles, such as neutrons or heavy charged particles, will deposit a lethal dose in any cell they traverse. Conversely, sparsely-ionizing particles, such as photons, may deposit only a single interaction in a cell, resulting in sublethal damage. Only when a second particle deposits an independent second event in the same cell will the cell be killed—the origin of the D^2 term in the theory of dual radiation action (13). *Dose rate* directly affects damage. If a dose is protracted over time by either low dose rate or fractionation, injury is less than that caused by the same dose delivered in a single brief exposure (13). *Heat* sensitizes cells to lethal effects of low LET radiation (10).

Chemical factors generally interact at the level of the initial physical chemical event, promptly after the physical event of ionization. *Oxygen* sensitizes cells to lethal effects of radiation. Cells exposed in total absence of oxygen are much more resistant. The oxygen enhancement ratio measured as change in D_0 is usually about 2–3. The mechanism is thought to be interaction of molecular oxygen with radicals produced by radiolysis of water, yielding more reactive hydroperoxyl radicals (10, 13). *Radioprotectors*, generally chemicals containing sulfhydryl groups, protect cells and organisms from lethal radiation effects, presumably acting as free radical scavengers (14). *Radiosensitizers* have the opposite effect, especially on hypoxic cells (10). These factors are effective only with low LET radiation.

Biologic factors are intrinsic to the cell population at the time of exposure. *Repair* of sublethal damage occurs between dose fractions or during exposure at low dose rate (15). Radiation injury may be regarded as an equilibrium between damage and repair—at high dose rates, the equilibrium shifts toward damage, while at lower dose rates it may shift toward survival. *Cell cycle* stage is a major player. Cells in M and G_2 are the most sensitive, while those in late S are most resistant, with early S and G_1 intermediate (10). The difference in sensitivity, measured as D_0, between the most sensitive and most resistant phases is generally a factor of 2–3. Nondividing cells—those not in the cell division cycle—are among the most resistant.

MAMMALIAN RADIOBIOLOGY

Biologic effects of radiation in mammals fall into two categories. *Stochastic* effects are those in which the probability of occurrence is a function of dose, the effect being all or nothing. They are the result of subtle alterations in cell chemistry, such as transformation or mutation. *Deterministic* effects are those in which the severity is a function of dose. They are generally the result of cell killing—the more cells killed, the more severe the effect.

STOCHASTIC EFFECTS

Available data are consistent with the widely-held hypothesis of the absence of a threshold dose for these effects, the major examples of which are cancer and genetic effects. As the dose approaches zero, the probability of occurrence approaches zero—but is not zero for the smallest doses for which conclusive data are available, about 50–100 mSv. Thus, if a threshold dose exists, it is quite small.

The problem with extending the database to smaller doses is that radiation mimics nature. Radiation-induced cancer or mutation cannot be distinguished by any known method from spontaneous cancer or mutation. The only observable event in an irradiated population is increased incidence of the stochastic effect. A tiny increment on a substantial spontaneous incidence is undetectable unless the study population is quite large. For example, Land estimated that a prospective study to examine the risk of screening mammography in asymptomatic women would require enrolling 60 million subjects at age 35, half of whom get screening mammography, with all followed for life (16). Even this large study population would yield a statistical power of only 0.5

Data from studies of stochastic effects in a number of exposed populations have been extensively reviewed by the Committee on the Biological Effects of Ionizing Radiation (BEIR) of the U.S. National Research Council (17) and the United Nations Scientific Committee on the Effects of Atomic Radiation (UNSCEAR) (18). Two alternative models are used to estimate risk. The additive model results in absolute risk, for example cancer deaths per million person years per sievert. The multiplicative model produces relative risk, essentially the incidence of the effect in the exposed population divided by incidence in controls. It is sometimes expressed as excess relative risk, or relative risk minus one. That is, a relative risk of 1.5 and excess relative risk of 0.5 both project a 50% increase in the event in the exposed population. The multiplicative model is generally more conservative and fits most data better; it is, therefore, used for risk estimation in this chapter.

Cancer

Radiation-induced cancer was observed as early as 1904 (19). However, despite the accumulation of anecdotal evidence, cancer was not widely recognized as a risk of low-dose radiation until excess leukemia appeared in the Japanese atomic bomb survivors (Fig. 20.3) beginning shortly after World War II (20).

Japanese Atomic Bomb Survivors. The Hiroshima and Nagasaki populations of more than 75,000 survivors have been intensively studied. Although deaths from solid tumors greatly outnumber those from leukemia, the relative risk of leukemia has been greater than that of solid tumors. Relative risk is normalized to spontaneous incidence, which for leukemia is quite low in the Japanese population. The temporal increase in deaths from solid tumors (Fig. 20.3**A**) reflects both the increase in spontaneous cancer in the aging population and the long latent period for radiation-induced solid tumors, now thought to be the remainder of the lifespan of exposed subjects. However, it appears that virtually all excess leukemia deaths occurred within 25 years of exposure (Fig. 20.3**B**). Although there has been an increase in cancer death rate in most organs and tissues in the Japanese atomic bomb survivors, only leukemia, esophagus, stomach, colon, lung, female breast, ovary, bladder, and multiple myeloma are clearly statistically significant (Fig. 20.4). Lack of significance for many organs relates to small numbers of cases (e.g., 52 deaths in the study population from prostate cancer).

Most earlier studies of cancer risk in the Japanese survivors have utilized death as the end point. Death is sharply defined and cause of death can be determined retrospectively from death certificates. However, recent studies have used cancer incidence as the end point, so nonfatal cancer can be included in the calculation of detriment (21–23). As shown in Table 20.2, risk of cancer incidence is generally greater than that for cancer death, reflecting either curative treatment or intercurrent death from other causes.

The dose response (Fig. 20.5) for radiation-induced can-

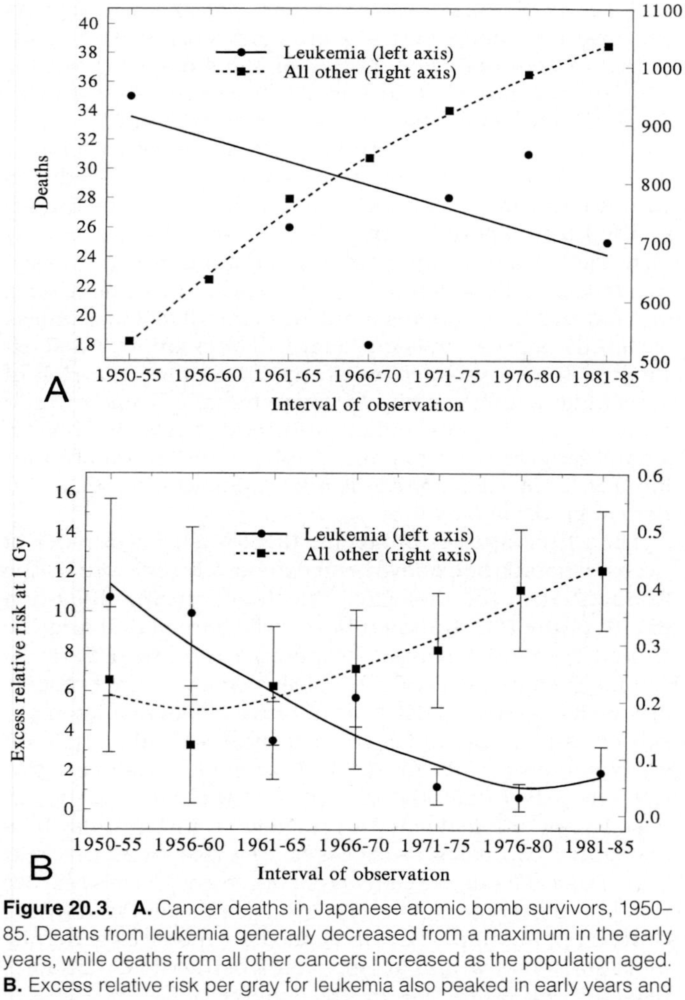

Figure 20.3. **A.** Cancer deaths in Japanese atomic bomb survivors, 1950–85. Deaths from leukemia generally decreased from a maximum in the early years, while deaths from all other cancers increased as the population aged. **B.** Excess relative risk per gray for leukemia also peaked in early years and has declined, while risk of other tumors has increased. Error bars represent standard errors. (Data from Shimizu Y, Kato H, Schull WJ. Life span study report 11. Part 2. Cancer mortality in the years 1950–85 based on the recently revised doses (DS86). Technical Report RERF TR 5–88. Hiroshima: Radiation Effects Research Foundation, 1988.)

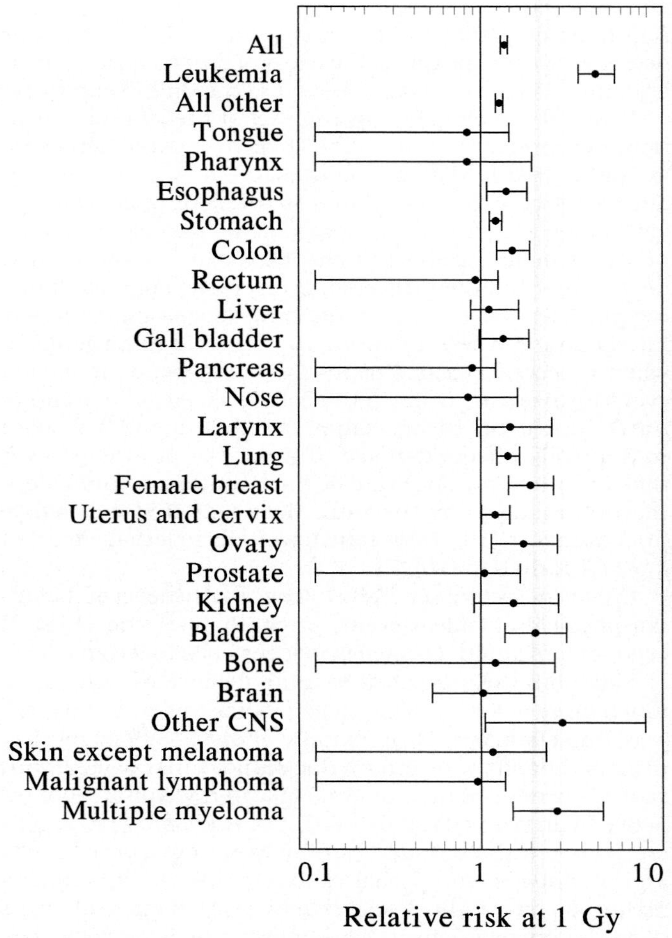

Figure 20.4. Relative risk of cancer death, by organ or tissue, in Japanese atomic bomb survivors. Excess (relative risk > 1) has been found in nearly all organs, but in many cases is not statistically significant because of the small numbers involved. Error bars represent 90% confidence limits. (Data from Shimizu Y, Kato H, Schull WJ. Life span study report 11. Part 2. Cancer mortality in the years 1950–85 based on the recently revised doses (DS86). Technical Report RERF TR 5–88. Hiroshima: Radiation Effects Research Foundation, 1988.)

Table 20.2.
Cancer in Japanese Atomic Bomb Survivors

	Incidence 1958–87[a]			Mortality 1950–85[b]		
Organ or Tissue	ERR[c] at 1 Sv	EAR[d] per 10^4 PY Sv	AR[e] %	ERR[c] at 1 Sv	EAR[d] per 10^4 PY Sv	AR[e] %
Digestive system	0.38	10.4	7.8	0.24	3.39	6.6
Esophagus	0.28	0.30	6.5	0.43	0.34	12.7
Stomach	0.32	4.8	6.5	0.23	2.07	6.3
Colon	0.72	1.8	14.2	0.56	0.56	15.1
Liver	0.49	1.6	10.9	0.12	0.05	3.9
Gallbladder	0.12	0.18	2.2	0.37	0.22	8.2
Respiratory system	0.80	4.4	16.3	0.40	1.29	10.1
Lung	0.95	4.4	18.9	0.46	1.25	11.4
Female breast	1.6	6.7	31.9	1.00	1.02	22.1
Uterus	−0.15	−1.1	−3.3	0.22	0.60	5.3
Ovary	0.99	1.1	17.7	0.81	0.45	18.7
Prostate	0.29	0.61	7.0	0.05	0.03	1.9
Urinary tract	1.2	2.1	22.3	1.02	0.55	22.7
Thyroid	1.2	1.6	25.9			
Total solid tumors	0.63	29.7	11.6	0.29	7.41	7.9
Lymphoma	0.62	0.56	14	−0.05	−0.02	−1.8
Multiple myeloma	0.25	0.08		1.86	0.21	32.5
Leukemia	3.9	2.7	50	3.92	2.29	55.4
ALL	9.1	0.62	70			
AML	3.3	1.1	46			
CML	6.2	0.9	62			
Other	3.6	0.21	51			

[a]Except lymphoma, myeloma, and leukemia, 1950–1987. Data from Thompson, et al. (21), and Preston, et al. (22)
[b]Data from Shimizu, Kato, and Schull (20)
[c]Excess relative risk
[d]Excess absolute risk
[e]Attributable risk

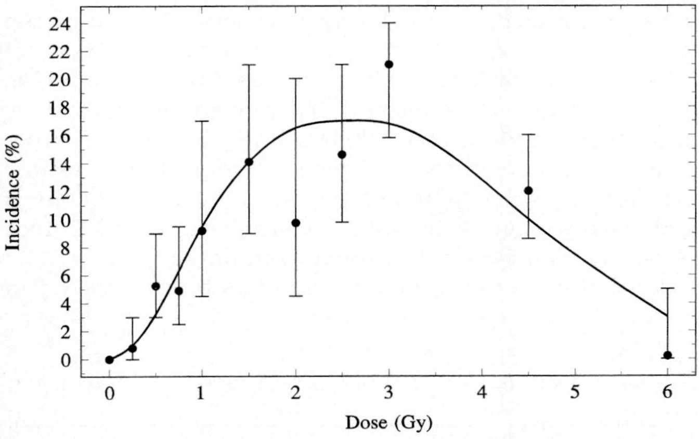

Figure 20.5. Dose response curve for radiation-induced myeoid leukemia in mice. In carefully controlled animal experiments, the curve typically extrapolates to spontaneous incidence at zero dose, is initially concave upward, reaches a maximum, and then declines at high doses. Transformed cells are killed by large doses, accounting for the reduced effectiveness. (Data from Mole RH, Papworth DG, Corp MJ. The dose response for x-ray induction of myeloid leukemia in male CBA.H mice. Br J Cancer 1983; 47:285–291.)

cer in carefully controlled animal experiments can be fit by a curve from the theory of dual radiation action,

$$I = (\alpha D + \beta D^2)e^{-(\alpha D + \beta D^2)}$$

where I is incidence and D is dose. The initial $\alpha D + \beta D^2$ expression defines the carcinogenic process, with the βD^2 term accounting for the upward concavity. The exponential term includes cell killing at higher doses. However, for solid tumors in the Japanese atomic bomb survivors, there are no significant deviations from linearity at doses below 2 Sv. Exclusion of cases with doses greater than 2 Sv eliminates only 55 cases from a total of 8613 cases in a study population of 79,972 (21). For leukemia in this population, the data were consistent with linear nonthreshold models except for acute myelogenous leukemia, which showed statistically significant upward concavity (22). Radiation can interact with other factors in the carcinogenic process. Risk of cancer in the Japanese survivors depended not only on dose, but also on age at exposure, interval since exposure, and sex.

Other Irradiated Populations. Studies of the Japanese atomic bomb survivors have provided the most extensive, quantitative data dealing with radiation carcinogenesis. However, excess cancer has been identified in a large number of other populations. Most have followed exposure from medical sources; a few instances of nonmedical exposure are important.

Excess leukemia was identified in several studies, including patients receiving therapeutic radiation for ankylosing spondylitis (25) and for carcinoma of the uterine cervix (26, 27). Statistically significant association between diagnostic x-ray exposure and adult-onset leukemia was detected in some (28, 29), but not all (30), case-control studies.

Excess breast cancer was first seen in women who had undergone repeated fluoroscopy to the chest (31). Numerous other populations with excess breast cancer were subsequently identified, including, in both Canada (32) and Massachusetts (33), women who had been treated for tuberculosis by repeated pneumothorax under fluoroscopic control and women who had been treated with small therapeutic doses of radiation for acute postpartum mastitis (34). The BEIR V committee concluded from these and other data that breast cancer risk was greater in women irradiated before age 20 than in those irradiated later in life, is influenced by hormonal status, and that there was little effect of dose protraction (17).

Lung cancer was extensively studied in uranium miners (Fig. 20.6) who worked in an atmosphere contaminated with radon and its radioactive progeny (35). The interaction of radiation with smoking appears to be multiplicative rather than additive. Excess lung cancer has also been detected in the ankylosing spondylitis patients (26).

Elevated stomach cancer was detected in patients treated with therapeutic irradiation for peptic ulcer between 1937 and 1955, with a relative risk of 3.7 from the fractionated dose of 16–17 Gy (36).

Radiogenic thyroid cancer was studied in a number of populations, of which the most extensive were young people who were epilated for tinea capitis upon arrival in the new state of Israel (37) and infants irradiated for thymic enlargement (38). Effects of internally-deposited ^{131}I are difficult to interpret because of problems of dosimetry. Older studies suggested that the relative effectiveness per unit dose of internal emitters was less than one-half that of external radiation (39). Patients treated with ^{131}I for thyrotoxicosis were studied. Doses were generally very large (50–100 Gy), resulting in extensive death of cells that might have been transformed. Further, the incidence of thyroid cancer among thyrotoxicosis patients is quite high, making control groups difficult to identify (40). Relative risks varied from 1.01 to 9.1, depending on control group selected (17). Follow-up of more than 10,000 subjects who had undergone diagnostic procedures using ^{131}I in Sweden (average thyroid dose 0.5 Gy) yielded a relative risk of thyroid cancer of 1.27 (95% confidence interval 0.94–1.67). However, many of these studies were ordered because of suspected thyroid tumors and many subsequent tumors were either medullary or poorly differentiated, and one was a sarcoma—none of which have been seen in excess numbers in other irradiated populations (41). Thyroid cancer was extensively investigated in Marshall Islanders exposed from nuclear weapons testing in 1954 to both external γ-radiation from fallout and ingested radioiodides (Table 20.3) (42). Children living in portions of Nevada and Utah were exposed to radioactive fallout from weapons testing in 1952–1955, resulting in thyroid doses up to 1 Gy. The relative risk of thyroid cancer was found to be 1.9, which was not statistically significant (43). Finally, a large and detailed animal study found essentially no difference in the effectiveness per unit dose of external versus internal radiation in thyroid carcinogenesis (44). The BEIR V committee estimated the effectiveness ratio for ^{131}I compared to x-rays as 0.66, but with a 95% confidence interval of 0.14–3.15. It now seems clear that the juvenile thyroid is more sensitive than the adult, females are more sensitive than males to both spontaneous and radiogenic thyroid cancer by a factor of about 3, and radiogenic thyroid cancer is commonly accompanied or preceded by benign nodules and its histology is usually low-grade papillary. Tumor growth is promoted by hormonal stimulation (17).

Excess cancer of the esophagus has been observed in

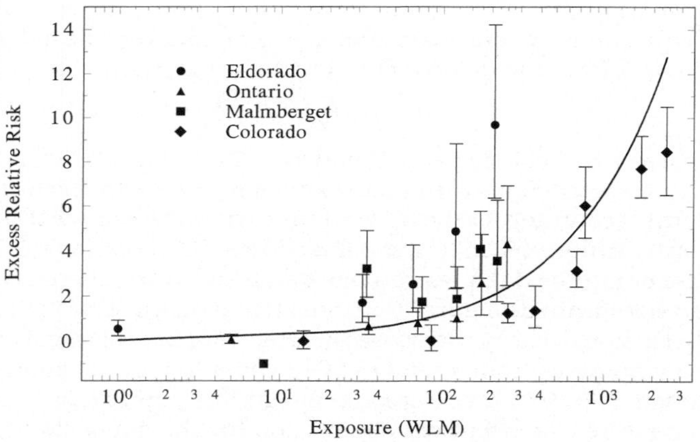

Figure 20.6. Lung cancer in four cohorts of uranium miners as a function of occupational exposure in working level months (WLM). The four groups were miners at Eldorado and Ontario in Canada, Malmberget in Sweden, and the Colorado Plateau in the U.S. One WLM represents 1 typical month (22 working days) in an atmosphere containing radioactive particulates (radon and its progeny) in a concentration equivalent to a "working level," which has a complicated definition depending on ventilation, etc. Curve represents fitted power function. Risk, expressed as excess relative risk, is increased at higher exposures. There is considerable discordance in the data amongst the four cohorts, probably the result of cofactors such as smoking. Conversion of exposure in WLM to dose equivalent to bronchial epithelium requires a number of assumptions, leading to considerable uncertainty in the results. Current data suggest a range of 60–200 mSv/WLM. (Data from BEIR IV (31).)

Table 20.3.
Thyroid Tumors in Marshall Islanders Exposed to Radioactive Fallout[a]

Atoll	Age at exposure (y)	Dose (Gy)	Nodules (%)	Cancer (%)
Rongelap	1	≥15	66.7	0
	2–9	8–15	81.2	6.2
	≥10	3.4–8	13.3	6.7
Alingnae	<10	2.8–4.5	28.6	0
	≥10	1.4–1.9	33.3	0
Utirik	<10	0.6–1.0	7.8	1.6
	≥10	0.3–0.6	12.0	2.0
Controls	<10		2.6	0.9
	≥10		7.8	0.8

[a]Data from Conard (42)

the ankylosing spondylitics. In fact, esophageal cancer is the major tumor seen to continue in excess more than 25 years postexposure (25).

Colon cancer in excess incidence has been unequivocally identified in the Japanese atomic bomb survivors. Other studies, however, are not so convincing. Statistically significant associations between colon cancer and therapeutic radiation for benign gynecologic conditions were established in some (45, 46), but not all (47, 48), studies. No excess colon cancer deaths were seen in a 30-year follow-up of a large series of patients irradiated for carcinoma of the uterine cervix (27). Excess colon cancer was detected in the ankylosing spondylitics (25). However, these results have been excluded from risk estimations because of the well-known associations between ankylosing spondylitis and ulcerative colitis and between ulcerative colitis and colon cancer (17). Radiogenic cancer of the small intestine has been detected in experimental animals but not in humans.

In the liver, excess cancer has been seen mainly in human and animal populations with intrahepatic concentrations of radionuclides. Thorotrast, containing 25% colloidal $^{232}ThO_2$, was used extensively as a radiologic contrast agent until about 1955. Three major epidemiologic studies of its association with liver cancer were summarized by the BEIR IV committee, showing, for example, 413 excess liver cancers in a population of 2334 in the largest study (34). No excess liver cancers were detected in the ankylosing spondylitics (25) or patients irradiated for carcinoma of the uterine cervix (27).

The recognition in the mid-1920s of "radium jaw" in watch-dial painters (49), the result of ingestion of minute quantities of ^{226}Ra, and sometimes ^{228}Ra, from "tipping" their artists' brushes on their tongues, led to abandonment of the technique and to the first standards for occupational radiation protection (50). Osteogenic sarcoma is the common result of the high-LET radiation of radium (35). Additionally, low-LET radiation is associated with bone cancer in the ankylosing spondylitis patients (25) and the long-term follow-up for occurrence of second caners following radiotherapy (27), but not from low-LET occupational exposure in British radiologists (51).

Radiation was noted to increase the incidence of tumors of the nervous system in several populations, including the previously-mentioned Israeli tinea capitis subjects (52) and the ankylosing spondylitics (25). Mortality from brain cancer was about three times greater in early American radiologists than in other medical specialists (53), suggesting an effect of occupational exposure. Associations between intracranial meningiomas and diagnostic exposure were reported (54–56). Although the dose response curve remains unknown, available data clearly indicate that the brain is relatively sensitive to radiation carcinogenesis.

Organs of the genital system, except the ovary, appear relatively insensitive to radiogenic cancer (17). The urinary tract, especially the bladder, is somewhat sensitive, as seen in the ankylosing spondylitics (25) and in women therapeutically irradiated for benign uterine bleeding (46).

Both animal and human studies have detected excess parathyroid disease, including hyperparathyroidism, hyperplasia, adenomas, and, occasionally, cancer (17). The paranasal sinuses were found sensitive to the carcinogenic influence of high-LET radiation in the radium-dial painters and Thorotrast subjects (35). No associations with low-LET exposure were identified (17).

Death from radiogenic skin cancer, occurring in an area of radiodermatitis, was observed as early as 1904 (19). In the Israeli tinea capitis studies, excess basal cell carcinoma was noticed on the skin of the head, face, and neck in white, but not nonwhite, subjects (57), suggesting an interaction of ionizing radiation with ultraviolet exposure.

Excess multiple myeloma was seen in 12 of 17 irradiated populations, with the greatest risk occurring in those exposed to internal emitters (58). No excess Hodgkin's disease was identified in irradiated populations; non-Hodgkin's lymphomas were shown to be elevated in some populations, but not in others (17).

Radiogenic cancers of the pharynx and larynx were observed as a late complication of high-dose therapeutic radiation (17). Salivary gland tumors were noted in excess incidence in patients treated with external radiation (52) and ^{131}I (59), and associated with diagnostic exposure (60). Data on pancreatic cancer following radiation exposure are sparse and inconsistent, perhaps related to the well-known difficulty of detection of the disease (17).

Prenatal Exposure. A great deal of attention has been devoted to study of the relationship of prenatal diagnostic radiation exposure to childhood cancer since the first report by Stewart and associates in 1956 (61). Numerous studies soon followed, with conflicting results. A prospective study, which is less sensitive but more specific than retrospective case-control studies, found a significant association between prenatal exposure and childhood leukemia, but not other cancers, in white children—but no such association in blacks. Furthermore, there was a similar level of association with childhood accidental death (62). If one accepts the results of this study as showing that prenatal radiation is carcinogenic, then one must also accept its role in the etiology of accident proneness. In all of these studies, it is presumed that the prenatal diagnostic exposure was rational—that is, the attending physician had a valid reason for prescribing the exposure. One large scale study investigated the effects of routine pelvimetry at term, finding no significant association with childhood cancer (63). Early reports in the Japanese survivors exposed in utero showed no increase in childhood cancer; however, as this population has reached middle age, excess cancer has been detected (64).

Risk of Radiation-Induced Cancer. The BEIR V committee estimated that the risk of radiogenic cancer, averaged over both sexes and all ages, following acute whole-body exposure to low-LET radiation at high dose rate, is 8% per sievert (17). They further estimated that this risk estimate should be reduced by a factor of 2 or more for small doses or low dose rate. The UNSCEAR committee concluded that this dose and dose-rate effectiveness factor (DDREF) is close to 1 for solid tumors and 2 for leukemia, or about 1.7 overall, with a 90% confidence interval of 1.1–3.1 (18).

Genetic Effects

There are obvious uncertainties in estimation of risk of radiogenic cancer because of inconsistencies in the human data. However, there are no directly confirmed data dealing with human genetic effects of radiation. Thus, genetic risk estimation depends on a general knowledge of human genetics and extrapolation from animal studies.

In 1955, Macht and Lawrence reported increased likelihood of congenital anomalies in offspring of radiologists as compared to children of other physicians (65). Gardner, et al., reported, in 1990, the increased incidence of leukemia and lymphoma among children in and around the Sellafield nuclear plant in the United Kingdom, associated with occupational exposure of the fathers (66). However, extensive analysis of eight indicators of genetic effect in offspring of the Japanese atomic bomb survivors (stillbirths, congenital anomalies, childhood death, childhood cancer, chromosomal rearrangements, protein electrophoretic behavior and enzyme activity, sex ratio, and childhood physical development) failed to demonstrate any statistically significant genetic effect (67). The average dose to the parents was 0.4 Sv, in the range of the doubling dose estimated from early animal experiments.

Animal data, on the other hand, have been so convincing as to make certain the existence of a genetic effect of radiation. Data from Muller's studies in the 1920s using the geneticist's favorite organism, *drosophila* (68), were used for decades for the estimation of genetic risk. The "megamouse studies" at Oak Ridge National Laboratory in the 1950s and early 1960s (Fig. 20.7), named for the size of the study population, examined specific-locus recessive mutations in mice (69). They were major contributors to early BEIR and UNSCEAR estimates of the doubling dose, in the range of 0.5–2.5 Sv. The doubling dose is the dose required to double the spontaneous mutation rate. Usual early calculations used the human spontaneous mutation rate and the radiation response of mice, generally half the radiation response of the male mouse at low dose rates, since the female was much less sensitive. Thus, the doubling dose was for a mythical creature with the spontaneous mutation rate of humans and half the radiation response of a male mouse. The direct method of risk estimation avoided these complications by examining the frequency of dominant mutants in first generation offspring. For example, if the frequency of skeletal defects in mice was 4×10^{-4} per Gy per gamete, and in humans about 20% of serious dominant disorders involve the skeleton, then the frequency of serious first-generation dominant disorders in humans should be about 2000 per million live births per sievert (70).

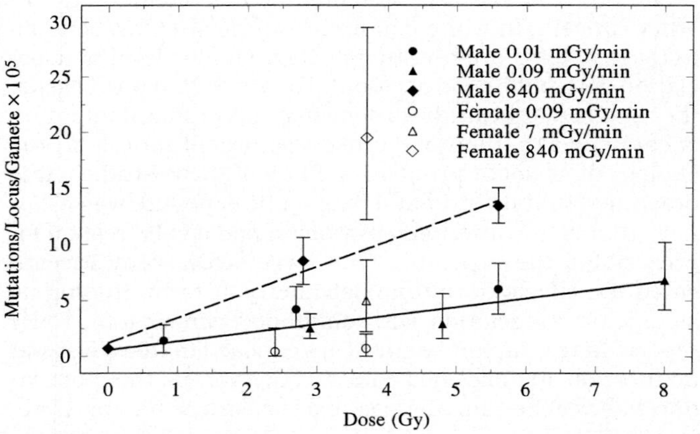

Figure 20.7. The "megamouse studies": specific locus mutations in mice exposed to x-rays, showing effects of sex and dose rate. Error bars represent 90% confidence intervals. *Solid line* is linear regression of low dose rate data for males (0.01 and 0.09 mGy/min combined) and *dashed line* is linear regression for high dose rate (840 mGy/min) data for males. No regression is possible for females because the spontaneous mutation rate was so low as to be statistically unacceptable, even in a population of hundreds of thousands. The dose rate effect is as expected in both sexes; damage is proportional to dose and dose rate. At low dose rates, the mutation rate in females given up to 4 Gy was no greater than the spontaneous rate in males, but at high dose rates females were more sensitive than males. (Data from Russell WL. The nature of the dose-rate effect of radiation on mutation in mice. Japan J Genet 1964;40(Suppl):128–140.)

Genetic Risk. The BEIR V Committee concluded that the human doubling dose is not likely to be less than the value of approximately 1 Sv from animal studies (17). Indeed, reappraisal of data from the first-generation offspring of Japanese atomic bomb survivors indicated that this value probably overestimated the risk (71). The UNSCEAR 1993 report concluded that the doubling dose is not likely to be less than 2 Sv. Their best estimate of the doubling dose for low dose rate exposure was 4 Sv (18).

The National Council on Radiation Protection and Measurements has estimated that the genetically significant dose to the average U.S. citizen is approximately 1.3 mSv per year. About 1 mSv comes from natural sources in the environment, and about 0.3 mSv is from manmade radiation, including medical, consumer products (tobacco, luminous watch dials, smoke detectors, etc.), occupational, and miscellaneous sources (72). Thus, the total genetic radiation burden of the population is approximately 40 mSv per generation. The estimated increased incidence of genetic disease is so small as to be nearly impossible to detect in a study population of finite size, as shown in Table 20.4, especially since about 75% is from unavoidable natural sources that have been with us since the beginning of time.

DETERMINISTIC EFFECTS

Deterministic effects occur in all exposed individuals, provided doses exceed thresholds. Thus, the statistical problems obvious in estimation of risk of stochastic effect do not exist for deterministic effects. These effects are a concern in radiation oncology and some interventional radiologic procedures, but are never encountered in patients from the doses employed in diagnostic medicine.

Acute Radiation Syndromes

The best known deterministic effects are the acute radiation syndromes. They are a serious concern in the event of radiation accidents or nuclear war, but are not a consideration in the analysis of risks of diagnostic or occupa-

Table 20.4.
Estimated Incidence of Genetic Disease from Environmental Exposure (40 mSv per generation)

	Incidence (per Million Live Births)		Effects of 40 mSv per Generation (per Million Live Births)			
			UNSCEAR[a]		BEIR[b]	
Genetic Disease	UNSCEAR[a]	BEIR[b]	First Generation	Equilibrium	First Generation	Equilibrium
Autosomal dominant	10,000		60	400		
Clinically severe		2500			20–80	100
Clinically mild		7500			4–60	300
X-linked		400			<4	<20
Autosomal recessive	2500	2500	0.2	60	<4	Very slow ↑
Chromosomal anomalies						
Structural	400	600	10	16	<20	Very little ↑
Numeric	3400	3800	Very small	Very small	<4	<4
Congenital anomalies	60,000	20,000–30,000	Not estimated		40	40–400
Multifactorial diseases	600,000		Not estimated			
Heart disease		600,000			Not estimated	
Cancer		300,000			Not estimated	
Other		300,000			Not estimated	
Total			70	480		

[a]Data from UNSCEAR (18)
[b]Data from BEIR V (17)

tional exposure. The dose levels given in relation to these effects are for acute whole-body exposures. The acute radiation syndromes were recently reviewed by Hall (73).

The *hematopoietic* or *bone marrow syndrome* is the result of killing of proliferating cells of the hematopoietic series in the bone marrow, resulting in depression of circulating leukocytes and platelets and the possibility of death within 60 days. The threshold dose is about 250 mSv for detectable suppression of white count, 1 Sv for symptoms, and 3 Sv for death within 60 days. Individuals receiving doses in this range go first into prodromal phase, characterized by nausea and vomiting within hours of exposure. Recovery usually follows within about 24 hours, and there may be several symptom-free days. White cells in circulation at the time of exposure are relatively unaffected, and continue to function through their normal lifespan. However, they are not replaced by the failing bone marrow. Symptoms of the hematopoietic syndrome begin as white and platelet counts fall, and consist of chills, fever, fatigue, petechial hemorrhages in the skin, ulceration of the oral mucosa, and epilation. The $LD_{50/60}$ (the dose that kills half the population within 60 days) has been estimated as about 3–4 Sv. However, several Chernobyl workers survived doses up to about 8 Sv with only supportive care. The $LD_{50/60}$ with treatment may be as great as 7 Sv. Bone marrow transplantation was used for 13 Chernobyl victims; only two survived, one of whom showed signs of autologous marrow repopulation. Apparently only one transplant was successful. The dose window for effective marrow transplantation is quite narrow. Below 8 Sv it should be unnecessary and above 10 Sv it is ineffective because of the results of the gastrointestinal syndrome.

At doses above 10 Sv, the *gastrointestinal syndrome* results in death within about 10 days from denudation of the epithelial lining of the small intestine, the result of killing of proliferating cells in the crypts of Lieberkuhn. Characteristic symptoms are nausea, vomiting, and extended diarrhea. Several Chernobyl victims, in whom bone marrow transplants failed, died of this syndrome 7–10 days postexposure.

The *cerebrovascular* or *CNS syndrome* occurs following doses above about 100 Gy. All systems are severely damaged at this dose. However, the CNS syndrome evolves so rapidly that death occurs within 48 hours, before the other syndromes have a chance to develop. Symptoms usually begin in minutes, and consist of severe nausea and vomiting followed by disorientation, loss of muscular coordination, respiratory distress, seizures, coma, and death. The precise cause of death is not fully known. The most widely held view is a direct effect on the microvasculature, resulting in massive intracranial edema. However, animal studies showed that the dose required to produce this syndrome is greater if the head alone is irradiated, rather than the whole body.

Cataract

A great deal of attention in the medical literature has been devoted to risk of radiogenic cataract from small radiation doses, such as diagnostic or occupational. Most early studies of patient dosimetry from diagnostic procedures included determination of dose to the optic lens. However, human data from a number of exposed populations indicate a clear threshold (Fig. 20.8)—0.6–1.5 Gy in Japanese atomic bomb survivors and about 2 Gy in patients receiving fractionated radiotherapy (74). The International Commission on Radiological Protection has concluded that the threshold for progressive, vision-impairing cataract in the general population from highly protracted exposure is not likely to be less than 8 Sv. This is well beyond the levels encountered by virtually all individuals from environmental, occupational, or medical diagnostic sources.

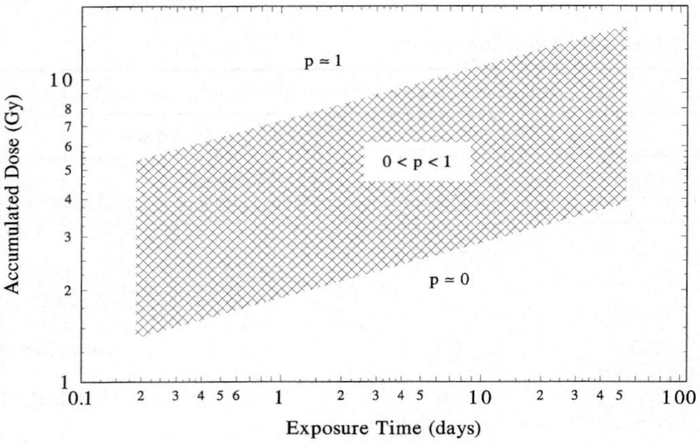

Figure 20.8. Time-dose isoeffect plot for radiogenic cataract. Any point (combination of time over which radiation is administered and total accumulated dose) falling below the shaded area is virtually certain to be below the threshold for clinically significant cataract. Any point above the shaded area is virtually certain to produce such a cataract. Any point within the shaded area falls in the range of biologic variation, and may or may not produce a progressive cataract in a given individual. (Data from Merriam GR, Szechter A, Focht EF. The effects of ionizing radiation on the eye. Front Radiat Ther Oncol 1972;6:346–385.)

Table 20.5.
Threshold Doses for Sterility[a]

Tissue/Effect	Acute Dose (Sv)	Protracted Dose (Sv)	Protracted Dose Rate (Sv/y)
Testes			
Temporary sterility	0.15	Not applicable[b]	0.4
Permanent sterility	3.5	Not applicable	2
Ovaries			
Sterility	2.5–6	6	>0.2

[a]Data from ICRP (74)
[b]Threshold depends on dose rate rather than total dose

Sterility

The germinal cells of testes and ovaries, especially at certain stages of their production and maturation, are highly radiosensitive. Threshold doses for temporary sterility are rather small (Table 20.5). Permanent sterilization, however, requires large doses or protracted doses delivered at rather high dose rates (74).

Other Organs and Tissues

Threshold doses for production of deterministic effects in adults are much greater than those employed in diagnostic medicine. Table 20.6 lists the doses required to produce such effects in 5% (ED_5, an effective threshold) and 50% (ED_{50}, the median effective dose) of exposed subjects in 5 years. In growing children, the required doses are much smaller, but still beyond diagnostic levels (Table 20.7). The data in Tables 20.6 and 20.7 are for conventionally fractionated therapeutic doses. For smaller fields, the required doses are somewhat greater; conversely, for larger fields, they are smaller. Acute doses to produce the effect will be smaller. Growth retardation, measured as decreased adult height, was seen in Japanese atomic bomb survivors less than 5 years old at exposure and whose dose equivalent was greater than 1 Sv (18).

Effects on Embryo and Fetus

Just as the growing child is more sensitive than the adult, the embryo is even more sensitive to deterministic effects. Gestational age at exposure determines the nature of the effect, as shown in Figure 20.9 (77, 78). The only effect observed from preimplantation exposure in mice is early prenatal death. A large portion of medical exposure of the unrecognized pregnancy occurs during this period. If the

Table 20.6.
Estimated Total Accumulated Dose for Deterministic Effects in Adults 5 Years After Fractionated Radiotherapy[a]

Organ	Treated Field	Injury	ED_5 (Gy)	ED_{50} (Gy)
Bone marrow	Whole	Hypoplasia	2	5
Ovary	Whole	Permanent sterility	2–3	6–12
Testis	Whole	Permanent sterility	5–15	20
Lens	Whole	Cataract	5	12
Kidney	Whole	Nephrosclerosis	23	28
Liver	Whole	Liver failure	35	45
Lung	Lobe	Fibrosis	40	60
Heart	Whole	Pericarditis	40	>100
Thyroid	Whole	Hypothyroidism	45	150
Pituitary	Whole	Hypopituitarism	45	200–300
Brain	Whole	Necrosis	50	>60
Spinal cord	5 cm²	Necrosis	50	>60
Breast	Whole	Atrophy, necrosis	>50	>100
Skin	100 cm²	Ulcer, fibrosis	55	70
Eye	Whole	Panophthalmitis	55	100
Esophagus	75 cm²	Ulcer, stricture	60	75
Bladder	Whole	Ulcer, contracture	60	80
Bone	10 cm²	Necrosis, fracture	60	150
Ureter	5–10 cm	Stricture	75	100
Muscle	Whole	Atrophy	>100	

[a]Data from UNSCEAR (18), ICRP (74), and Rubin and Casarett (76)

Table 20.7.
Estimated Total Accumulated Dose for Deterministic Effects in Growing Children 5 Years After Fractionated Radiotherapy[a]

Organ	Field	Injury	ED_5 (Gy)	ED_{50} (Gy)
Breast	5 cm^2	No development	10	15
Cartilage	5 cm^2	Arrested growth	10	30
Bone	10 cm^2	Arrested growth	20	30
Muscle	10 cm^2	Hypoplasia	20–30	40–50

[a]Data from UNSCEAR (18), ICRP (74), and Rubin and Casarett (76).

mouse data could be extrapolated directly to humans, then the continuing pregnancy could be taken as evidence that there was no effect from that exposure. There were no survivors in the Hiroshima and Nagasaki populations who were exposed during the first 2 weeks of gestation. Thus, human and animal data are consistent, but do not provide conclusive proof that conclusions drawn from the mouse studies may be applied directly to humans.

Exposure of the pregnant mouse during the period of major organogenesis leads to congenital anomalies and neonatal death. The sensitive period for induction of a specific anomaly is brief; exposure must occur at a critical stage of development or differentiation of the involved tissues. An exception is the central nervous system, which is rapidly developing throughout organogenesis. Thus, the spectrum of anomalies in irradiated populations is weighted toward CNS anomalies, which was also seen in pregnant patients treated in the early days of radiotherapy (79).

The major effects seen in Japanese survivors irradiated in utero were growth retardation, especially microcephaly (80) and mental retardation (78). Survivors exposed within 3000 m of the hypocenter were shorter in stature, lighter in weight, and had smaller head circumference than those exposed at distances greater than 3000 m (81). Microcephaly (head smaller than 2 standard deviations below the mean for age) was seen after exposures in the first 25 weeks of pregnancy, with maximum sensitivity in the first 16 weeks (Fig. 20.10). Mental retardation was not seen from exposure before 8 weeks or after 25 weeks. Maximum sensitivity occurred at 8–15 weeks; at 16–25 weeks, sensitivity was about half of the maximum (Fig. 20.11). These effects were reflected in IQ scores and school performance.

Most data, both from human studies and animal experiments, are consistent with a threshold of approximately 100 mSv for early prenatal death and for teratogenic effects (82). The NCRP has concluded that statistically significant increase in these effects is not likely below about 150 mSv (83). However, a few studies have shown effects, including human microcephaly down to about 50 mSv (81). Although there is agreement that these effects are deterministic, the magnitude of the threshold dose remains uncertain. The ICRP has concluded that the threshold for radiation protection purposes should be taken as 100 mSv (84). Early mouse studies indicated that the incidence of prenatal death was well above 50% and that of congenital anomalies approached 100% at 2 Sv delivered at the times of peak sensitivities (77). The shape of the dose response curve between 0.1 and 2 Sv remains unclear.

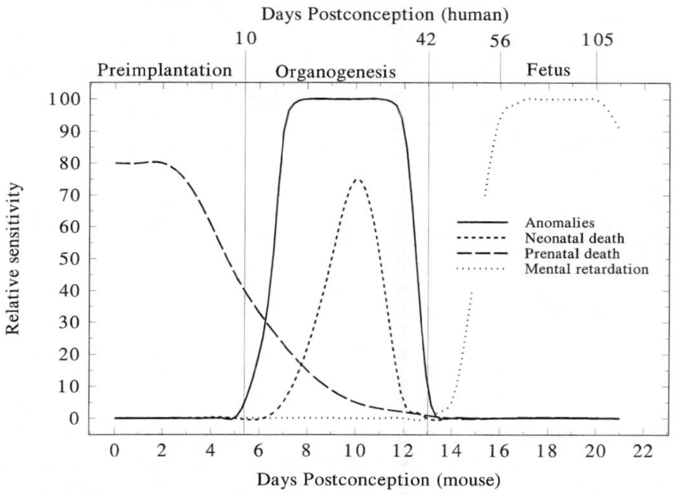

Figure 20.9. Influence of gestational age on deterministic effects in mice and mental retardation in humans. Prenatal death is the overwhelming probability from preimplantation exposure, while congenital anomalies and neonatal death are most likely from exposure during major organogenesis in mice. In the Japanese atomic bomb survivors, maximum sensitivity to mental retardation occurred from exposure between 8th and 15th weeks of gestation. Note that human development does not map linearly to mouse development. In humans, the fetal period occupies most of pregnancy; in mice it is a minor component. (Data from Russell LB, Russell WL. An analysis of the changing radiation response of the developing mouse embryo. J Cell Physiol 1954;43(Suppl 1):103–149; Otake M, Schull WJ. In utero exposure to A-bomb radiation and mental retardation: a reassessment. Br J Radiol 1984;57:409–414.)

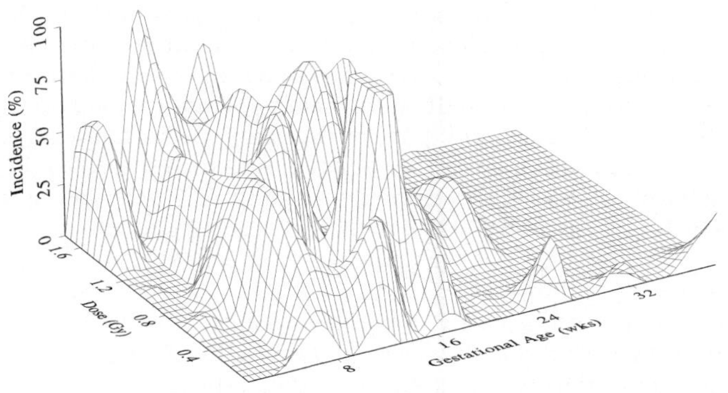

Figure 20.10. Influence of gestational age and dose on incidence of microcephaly in Hiroshima atomic bomb survivors irradiated in utero. There was a general dependence on dose. There were a total of 8 cases in the 115 individuals exposed to doses less than 100 mGy. These followed exposure at all gestational ages. Virtually all cases that were exposed to more than 100 mGy followed exposure in the first 25 weeks of pregnancy. (Data from Miller RW, Mulvihill JJ. Small head size after atomic irradiation. In: Sever JL, Brent RL, eds. Teratogen update: environmentally induced birth defect risks. New York: Alan R. Liss, 1986:141–143.)

Assessment of risk of human mental retardation from exposure in utero is a bit clearer. Maximum likelihood analysis of data from the Japanese indicated an incidence of severe retardation of 43% at 1 Sv and a threshold of 200–400 mSv, with a lower 95% confidence limit of about 100 mSv, delivered during the period of maximum sensitivity, gestational age 8–15 weeks (85). IQ scores declined by

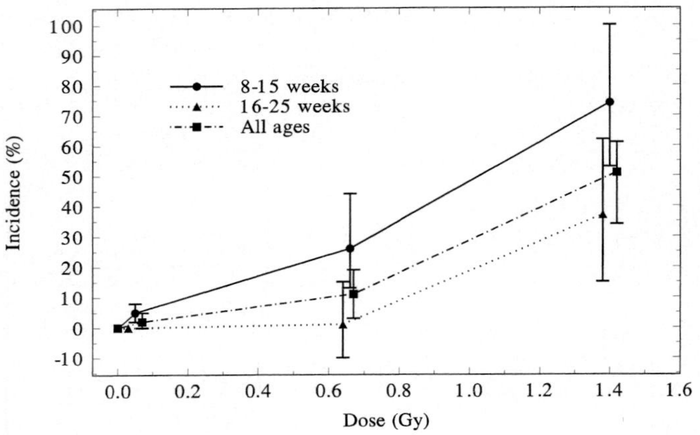

Figure 20.11. Dose response for mental retardation in Japanese atomic bomb survivors exposed in utero. No cases were seen from exposure prior to 8 weeks gestational age. Maximum sensitivity occurred from exposure 8–15 weeks gestational age. Sensitivity at 16–25 weeks was about half that at 8–15 weeks. (Data from Otake M, Schull WJ. In utero exposure to A-bomb radiation and mental retardation: a reassessment. Br J Radiol 1984;57:409–414.)

Table 20.8.
Detriment[a] (Percent per Sv)

Tissue or Organ	Adult Workers	Entire Population
Bladder	0.24	0.29
Bone marrow	0.83	1.04
Bone surface	0.06	0.07
Breast	0.29	0.36
Colon	0.82	1.03
Esophagus	0.19	0.24
Liver	0.13	0.16
Lung	0.64	0.80
Ovary (cancer)	0.12	0.15
Gonads (genetic)	0.80	1.33
Skin	0.03	0.04
Stomach	0.80	1.00
Thyroid	0.12	0.15
Remainder	0.47	0.59
Subtotals (rounded)		
Fatal cancer	4.0	5.0
Nonfatal cancer	0.8	1.0
Severe hereditary effects	0.8	1.3
Total (rounded)	5.6	7.3

[a]Data from ICRP (84).

about 30 per Sv from exposure during this interval (86). Response was significantly less (about half) at 16–25 weeks, and near zero at other times.

RISK ASSESSMENT

A number of indicators of risk, e.g., whole-body and critical organ doses, have been used in older publications. More recently, the effective dose has become the standard. The effective dose provides an estimate of the uniform whole-body dose that would carry the same risk of stochastic effect as the dose actually administered nonuniformly over the body, or over only part of the body, as in medical or occupational exposure. The concept was introduced by Jacobi in 1975 (87). He defined detriment, the probability of stochastic effect weighted by severity of that effect,

$$G = \sum s_i \, \alpha_i \, d_i.$$

where s is the severity, α the probability of the effect per unit dose, and d is the average dose to the ith organ. If the dose is uniform to the total body (D_{TB}), then

$$G = \sum s_i \, \alpha_i \, D_{TB} = D_{TB} \sum s_i \, \alpha_i.$$

The effective dose, for the total body, is then

$$D_E = D_{TB} = \frac{\sum s_i \, \alpha_i \, d_i}{\sum s_i \, d_i}.$$

Defining a weight factor for each organ as the fraction of total body stochastic effect attributable to that organ,

$$w_i = \frac{s_i \, \alpha_i}{\sum s_i \, \alpha_i},$$

then simplifies the effective dose to

$$D_E = \sum w_i \, d_i.$$

The ICRP adopted a simplified version of the Jacobi effective dose, which they called effective dose equivalent, in Publication 26 in 1977 (88). They eliminated the severity factors and used only lethal cancer or genetic effect expressed in the first two postirradiation generations as end points. Laws and Rosenstein adapted the effective dose to apply to somatic effects only (89). In 1990, the ICRP returned to the effective dose concept, defining the product $s_i\alpha_i$ as detriment (84). They concluded that detriment, which is a weighted probability of stochastic effect, is 5.6% per Sv for the adult working population, and 7.3% per Sv for the entire population (Table 20.8). Risk is greater in the entire population because of inclusion of children, whose radiosensitivity is greater. Inclusion of older retired adults, whose genetic risk is zero and whose cancer risk substantially lower, in the entire population mitigates but does not completely counteract the effect of the children.

The ICRP has provided organ weight factors for calculation of effective dose, shown in Figure 20.12 (84). The same set of factors is used for either the working or the entire population. Differences are beyond the precision of the method. The effective dose, calculated for a given set of exposure circumstances, e.g., occupational or a given diagnostic procedure or set of procedures, can then be compared with environmental exposure (Fig. 20.13). The NCRP has calculated this average exposure to the American population, from all sources, as effective dose equivalent (72). That is, they used the 1977 ICRP method (88). In general, 1990 effective doses are less than 1977 effective dose equivalents. The ratio ranges from about 0.6 for ^{99m}Tc gluconate to very nearly 1.0 for ^{99m}Tc MAA (18). The major factor in this difference was the large weight for remainder in the 1977 method (Fig. 20.12**A**), which was required by the paucity of data on specific organ risks at the time. The Commission recommended that the remainder be estimated by the five organs (excluding those with specific weights), each assigned a weight of 0.06, which overestimated the influence of the remainder on effective dose equivalent in many cases (92). For thyroid studies the effective dose is greater than effective dose equivalent by a

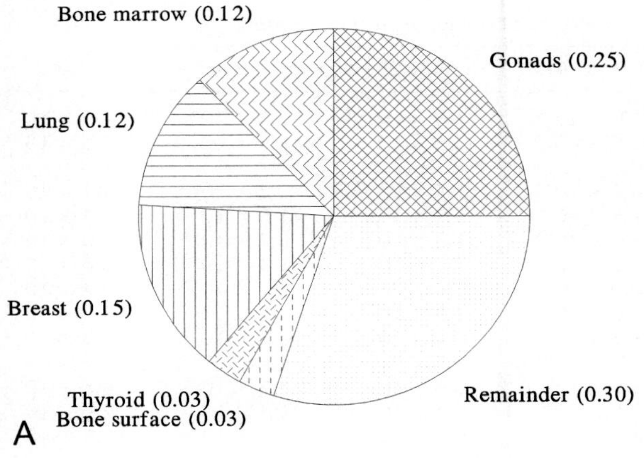

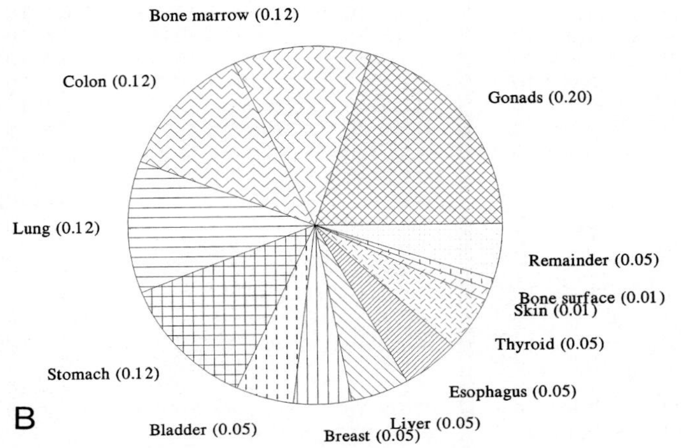

Figure 20.12. Organ weight factors for calculation of ICRP 1977 effective dose equivalent (**A**) and 1990 effective dose (**B**). The effective dose equivalent or effective dose is calculated from organ doses. It is an estimate of the uniform whole-body dose carrying the same risk of stochastic effect as the dose administered nonuniformly. In general, the 1990 effective dose is less than the 1977 effective dose equivalent, calculated from the same organ dose data. (Data from International Commission on Radiological Protection. 1990 Recommendations of the International Commission on Radiological Protection. ICRP Publication 60. Ann ICRP 1991;21(1–3); International Commission on Radiological Protection. Recommendations of the International Commission on Radiological Protection. ICRP Publication 26. Ann ICRP 1977;1(3).)

factor of up to 1.6 for radioiodide uptake. The weight factor for the thyroid was reduced for the 1990 effective dose, in accord with new data. Thus, the 1990 effective dose and 1977 effective dose equivalent may be used interchangeably only for crude first order approximations.

Effective dose equivalents in children and adults are presented for most radiopharmaceuticals in Table 20.9 (90, 91). Similar data for exposure in utero are presented in Tables 20.10 and 20.11, and for exposure during lactation in Table 20.12. These data have replaced specific organ doses, critical organ doses, etc., as indices of patient dose in most recent publications. The data in Tables 20.9 through 20.12 apply to healthy individuals. Isotope distribution may vary with disease states, possibly producing differences in radiation dose distribution and effective dose equivalent or effective dose. ICRP Publication 53 and its supplement (90, 91) provide some examples of alteration of effective dose equivalent in certain diseases. They also provide doses to specific organs used in calculation of effective dose equivalent.

The major advantage of effective dose equivalent or effective dose calculated for a diagnostic procedure is that it can be compared with environmental radiation as an estimate of the radiation burden to the patient. For example, the effective dose equivalent of a typical study using 500 mBq (about 15 mCi) of ^{99m}Tc pertechnetate with blocking is about 2.8 mSv (Table 20.9), the equivalent of about 11 months of natural background (Fig. 20.13). It may be tempting to calculate detriment from the patient effective dose equivalent, but this tacitly assumes that the linear nonthreshold model is established fact. Such is definitely not the case. Results of the calculation could be worse than worthless—they could be misleading.

RECOMMENDATIONS

Diagnostic nuclear medicine procedures deliver small radiation doses to the patient. The effective dose equivalent or effective dose is the best estimate of the radiation burden to the patient from that dose. The linear nonthreshold model suggests that these doses carry small risks of stochastic effects. It is not certain, however, that this model is really the best fit to available data in this dose range. Therefore, all recognized authorities recommend that med-

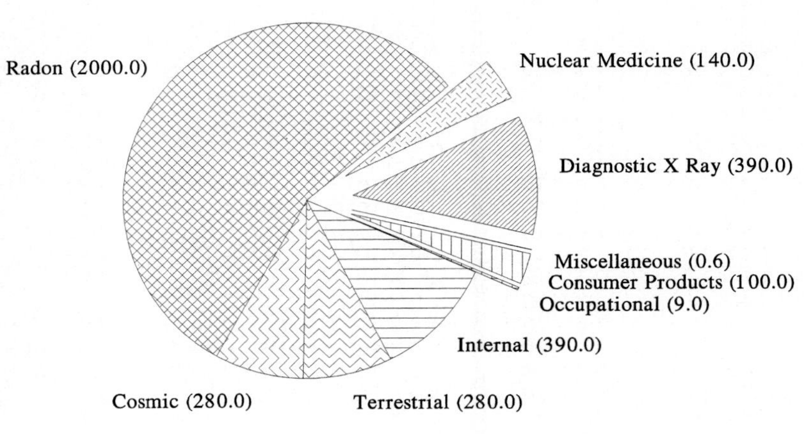

Figure 20.13. Annual radiation dose, average, 3600 μSv/y to U.S. population, from all sources. Natural sources, radon and progeny, cosmic, terrestrial, and internal, account for 3000 μSv/y, while manmade sources (diagnostic x-ray, nuclear medicine, consumer products, occupational, and miscellaneous) contribute only 600 μSv/y. The healing arts account for the majority of manmade radiation exposure. (Data from National Council on Radiation Protection and Measurements. Ionizing radiation exposure of the population of the United States. NCRP Report No. 93. Bethesda, MD: National Council on Radiation Protection and Measurements, 1987.)

Table 20.9.
Effective Dose Equivalents from Diagnostic Nuclear Medicine Procedures[a]

Isotope	Pharmaceutical	Conditions of Administration[b]	Effective Dose Equivalent (mSv/mBq)[c] Adult	Age 15	Age 10	Age 5	Age 1
^{3}H	Water		1.6×10^{-2}	1.6×10^{-2}	1.8×10^{-2}	2.4×10^{-2}	4.5×10^{-2}
	Inulin		1.2×10^{-3}	1.5×10^{-3}	2.4×10^{-3}	3.8×10^{-3}	7.5×10^{-3}
	Neutral fat and free fatty acids		2.2×10^{-1}				
^{11}C	Erythrocytes		6.9×10^{-3}	8.4×10^{-3}	1.4×10^{-2}	2.2×10^{-2}	4.2×10^{-2}
	Spiperone		5.9×10^{-3}	7.8×10^{-3}	1.2×10^{-2}	1.8×10^{-2}	3.4×10^{-2}
^{14}C	CO	20 s inhalation	6.6×10^{-3}	8.0×10^{-3}	1.3×10^{-2}	2.1×10^{-2}	4.0×10^{-2}
		1 h continuous	4.3×10^{-3}	5.3×10^{-3}	5.3×10^{-3}	1.4×10^{-2}	2.6×10^{-2}
	CO_2	20 s inhalation	1.7×10^{-3}	2.0×10^{-3}	3.1×10^{-3}	4.9×10^{-3}	9.4×10^{-3}
		1 h continuous	1.1×10^{-3}	1.3×10^{-3}	2.0×10^{-3}	3.1×10^{-3}	6.0×10^{-3}
	Inulin		1.1×10^{-2}	1.3×10^{-2}	2.1×10^{-2}	3.3×10^{-2}	6.5×10^{-2}
	Neutral fat and free fatty acids		2.1				
^{13}N	N_2 gas	20 s inhalation	3.7×10^{-4}	5.8×10^{-4}	8.4×10^{-4}	1.3×10^{-3}	2.5×10^{-3}
		1 h continuous	4.2×10^{-4}	6.5×10^{-4}	9.4×10^{-4}	1.4×10^{-3}	2.9×10^{-3}
	N_2 solution		4.0×10^{-4}	6.2×10^{-4}	8.9×10^{-4}	1.4×10^{-3}	2.7×10^{-3}
	NH_3		2.7×10^{-3}	3.2×10^{-3}	4.9×10^{-3}	7.7×10^{-3}	1.5×10^{-2}
	L-Glutamate		1.3×10^{-2}	1.7×10^{-2}	2.9×10^{-2}	3.9×10^{-2}	7.7×10^{-2}
^{15}O	CO	20 s inhalation	1.1×10^{-3}	1.5×10^{-3}	2.4×10^{-3}	3.9×10^{-3}	7.6×10^{-3}
		1 h continuous	7.6×10^{-4}	1.0×10^{-3}	1.6×10^{-3}	2.6×10^{-3}	5.1×10^{-3}
	CO_2	20 s inhalation	5.4×10^{-4}	6.8×10^{-4}	1.1×10^{-3}	1.7×10^{-3}	3.3×10^{-3}
		1 h continuous	4.0×10^{-4}	5.0×10^{-4}	7.8×10^{-4}	1.2×10^{-3}	2.4×10^{-3}
	O_2 gas	20 s inhalation	3.9×10^{-4}	5.7×10^{-4}	8.5×10^{-4}	1.3×10^{-3}	2.7×10^{-3}
		1 h continuous	4.3×10^{-4}	6.4×10^{-4}	9.5×10^{-4}	1.5×10^{-3}	3.0×10^{-3}
^{18}F	F^-		2.7×10^{-2}	3.4×10^{-2}	5.2×10^{-2}	8.6×10^{-2}	1.7×10^{-1}
	FDG		2.7×10^{-2}	3.2×10^{-2}	4.7×10^{-2}	7.3×10^{-2}	1.3×10^{-1}
^{22}Na	Na^+		2.8	3.3	4.9	8.0	1.5×10^{1}
^{24}Na	Na^+		3.4×10^{-1}	3.9×10^{-1}	6.1×10^{-1}	1.0	1.9
^{28}Mg	Mg^{2+}		8.3×10^{-1}	9.8×10^{-1}	1.6	3.0	6.4
^{32}P	PO_4^{3-}		2.2	3.0	5.1	1.0×10^{1}	2.2×10^{1}
^{33}P	PO_4^{3-}		3.3×10^{-1}	4.4×10^{-1}	7.5×10^{-1}	1.5	3.2
^{35}S	S_4^{2-}		9.8×10^{-2}	1.2×10^{-1}	2.0×10^{-1}	3.4×10^{-1}	6.8×10^{-1}
^{34m}Cl	Cl^-		8.6×10^{-3}	1.8×10^{-2}	2.9×10^{-2}	4.6×10^{-2}	9.0×10^{-2}
^{36}Cl	Cl^-		8.0×10^{-1}	9.6×10^{-1}	1.6	2.8	5.6
^{38}Cl	Cl^-		1.6×10^{-2}	1.8×10^{-2}	3.0×10^{-2}	4.9×10^{-2}	9.7×10^{-2}
^{38}K	K^+		2.7×10^{-2}	3.6×10^{-2}	5.5×10^{-2}	9.4×10^{-2}	1.7×10^{-1}
^{42}K	K^+		1.9×10^{-1}	2.3×10^{-1}	3.8×10^{-1}	6.4×10^{-1}	1.3
^{43}K	K^+		1.7×10^{-1}	2.0×10^{-1}	3.0×10^{-1}	4.8×10^{-1}	9.0×10^{-1}
^{45}Ca	Ca^{2+}		2.1	2.8	4.8	8.9	1.9×10^{1}
^{47}Ca	Ca^{2+}		1.4	1.8	2.9	5.0	1.1×10^{1}
^{46}Sc	Nonabsorbable	Oral fluid	1.4	1.8	2.8	4.4	7.8
	marker	Oral solid	1.5	1.8	2.9	4.4	8.0
^{47}Sc	Nonabsorbable	Oral fluid	5.6×10^{-1}	7.3×10^{-1}	1.3	2.1	4.2
	marker	Oral solid	5.7×10^{-1}	7.4×10^{-1}	1.3	2.2	4.3
^{51}Cr	$CrCl_3$		1.1×10^{-1}	1.4×10^{-1}	2.1×10^{-1}	3.1×10^{-1}	5.5×10^{-1}
	EDTA		2.3×10^{-3}	3.1×10^{-3}	4.6×10^{-3}	7.0×10^{-3}	1.3×10^{-2}
	Platelets		2.4×10^{-1}	3.5×10^{-1}	5.3×10^{-1}	8.2×10^{-1}	1.5
	Erythrocytes		2.6×10^{-1}	3.3×10^{-1}	5.2×10^{-1}	8.0×10^{-1}	1.5
		Denatured	4.0×10^{-1}	5.4×10^{-1}	8.3×10^{-1}	1.3	2.3
	Leukocytes		1.9×10^{-1}	2.8×10^{-1}	4.3×10^{-1}	6.7×10^{-1}	1.3
	Nonabsorbable	Oral fluid	3.4×10^{-2}	4.7×10^{-2}	7.7×10^{-2}	1.2×10^{-1}	2.3×10^{-1}
	marker	Oral solid	3.4×10^{-2}	4.8×10^{-2}	7.8×10^{-2}	1.2×10^{-1}	2.3×10^{-1}
^{52}Fe	$Fe^{2+,3+}$	Oral	1.0	1.1	1.9	3.4	7.0
^{55}Fe	$Fe^{2+,3+}$	Parenteral	5.9	8.0	1.3×10^{1}	2.3×10^{1}	4.6×10^{1}
		Oral	5.9×10^{-1}	8.1×10^{-1}	1.3	2.3	4.6
^{59}Fe	$Fe^{2+,3+}$	Parenteral	1.3×10^{1}	1.5×10^{1}	2.4×10^{1}	3.7×10^{1}	6.8×10^{1}
		Oral	2.0	2.5	4.0	6.2	1.1×10^{1}
^{57}Co	Bleomycin		5.6×10^{-2}	7.1×10^{-2}	1.0×10^{-1}	1.6×10^{-1}	2.8×10^{-1}
	Vitamin B_{12}	IV, Carrier free	5.8	7.3	1.1×10^{1}	1.6×10^{1}	2.8×10^{1}
		IV, Carrier	5.8×10^{-1}	7.3×10^{-1}	1.1	1.6	2.9
^{58}Co	Vitamin B_{12}	IV, Carrier free	1.1×10^{1}	1.3×10^{1}	2.0×10^{1}	2.9×10^{1}	4.9×10^{1}
		IV, Carrier	1.1	1.3	2.0	2.9	5.0
^{64}Cu	$Cu^{+,2+}$		5.3×10^{-2}	6.6×10^{-2}	1.0×10^{-1}	1.5×10^{-1}	2.8×10^{-1}
^{67}Cu	$Cu^{+,2+}$		2.2×10^{-1}	2.7×10^{-1}	4.1×10^{-1}	6.1×10^{-1}	1.2
^{62}Zn	Zn^{2+}		4.9×10^{-1}	6.6×10^{-1}	1.0	1.6	3.1
^{65}Zn	Zn^{2+}		1.1×10^{1}	1.3×10^{1}	1.9×10^{1}	2.8×10^{1}	4.8×10^{1}
^{69m}Zn	Zn^{2+}		2.1×10^{-1}	2.5×10^{-1}	3.9×10^{-1}	6.1×10^{-1}	1.2
^{66}Ga	Citrate		3.4×10^{-1}	4.3×10^{-1}	7.0×10^{-1}	1.2	2.3
^{67}Ga	Citrate		1.2×10^{-1}	1.6×10^{-1}	2.5×10^{-1}	4.0×10^{-1}	7.9×10^{-1}
^{68}Ga	Citrate		2.7×10^{-2}	3.4×10^{-2}	5.6×10^{-2}	9.5×10^{-2}	1.9×10^{-1}
	EDTA		4.0×10^{-2}	5.2×10^{-2}	7.5×10^{-2}	9.5×10^{-2}	1.8×10^{-1}
^{72}Ga	Citrate		3.5×10^{-1}	4.4×10^{-1}	7.0×10^{-1}	1.1	2.1
^{72}As	AsO_3^{3-}, AsO_4^{3-}		4.8×10^{-1}	5.9×10^{-1}	9.2×10^{-1}	1.4	2.7
^{74}As	AsO_3^{3-}, AsO_4^{3-}		6.3×10^{-1}	7.6×10^{-1}	1.2	1.8	3.4

Table 20.9—continued

Isotope	Pharmaceutical	Conditions of Administration[b]	Effective Dose Equivalent (mSv/mBq)[c] Adult	Age 15	Age 10	Age 5	Age 1
^{76}As	AsO_3^{3-}, AsO_4^{3-}		3.9×10^{-1}	4.8×10^{-1}	7.6×10^{-1}	1.2	2.4
^{75}Se	SeO_3^{2-}		3.5	4.4	6.8	9.6	1.6×10^{1}
	Methionine		3.0	3.8	6.5	9.2	1.5×10^{1}
	Methylcholesterol		1.7	2.1	3.1	4.5	7.7
	Bile acid		1.1	1.3	1.8	2.9	6.2
^{76}Br	Br^-		3.0×10^{-1}	3.5×10^{-1}	5.5×10^{-1}	8.6×10^{-1}	1.6
^{77}Br	Br^-		7.8×10^{-2}	9.1×10^{-2}	1.3×10^{-1}	2.0×10^{-1}	3.5×10^{-1}
	Spiperone		8.7×10^{-2}	1.1×10^{-1}	1.6×10^{-1}	2.4×10^{-1}	4.2×10^{-1}
^{82}Br	Br^-		4.3×10^{-1}	4.9×10^{-1}	7.3×10^{-1}	1.1	1.9
^{81m}Kr	Kr		2.7×10^{-5}	4.0×10^{-5}	5.7×10^{-5}	8.8×10^{-5}	1.7×10^{-4}
^{82}Rb	Rb^+		4.8×10^{-3}	6.7×10^{-3}	1.0×10^{-2}	1.8×10^{-2}	3.3×10^{-2}
^{81}Rb	Rb^+		3.1×10^{-2}	3.7×10^{-2}	5.7×10^{-2}	1.1×10^{-1}	2.2×10^{-1}
	Erythrocytes	Denatured	2.7×10^{-1}	3.8×10^{-1}	5.8×10^{-1}	9.1×10^{-1}	1.7
^{84}Rb	Rb^+		3.6	4.4	6.6	1.1×10^{1}	2.0×10^{1}
^{86}Rb	Rb^+		3.9	4.8	7.7	1.4×10^{1}	2.9×10^{1}
^{85}Sr	Sr^{2+}		8.5×10^{-1}	1.0	1.5	2.3	4.3
^{87m}Sr	Sr^{2+}		6.7×10^{-3}	8.1×10^{-3}	1.3×10^{-2}	2.1×10^{-2}	4.1×10^{-2}
^{89}Sr	Sr^{2+}		2.9	3.8	6.5	1.2×10^{1}	2.5×10^{1}
^{99m}Tc	Albumin	IV	7.9×10^{-3}	9.7×10^{-3}	1.5×10^{-2}	2.3×10^{-2}	4.2×10^{-2}
		Intrathecal lumbar	1.1×10^{-2}				
		Intrathecal cisternal	6.8×10^{-3}				
	Citrate		8.3×10^{-3}	1.0×10^{-2}	1.5×10^{-2}	2.2×10^{-2}	3.9×10^{-2}
	Colloid, large		1.4×10^{-2}	1.8×10^{-2}	2.8×10^{-2}	4.1×10^{-2}	7.3×10^{-2}
	Colloid, small		1.4×10^{-2}	1.9×10^{-2}	2.9×10^{-2}	4.3×10^{-2}	7.6×10^{-2}
	DMSA		1.6×10^{-2}	1.9×10^{-2}	2.7×10^{-2}	4.0×10^{-2}	6.9×10^{-2}
	DTPA	IV	6.3×10^{-3}	7.8×10^{-3}	1.1×10^{-2}	1.7×10^{-2}	3.0×10^{-2}
		Intrathecal lumbar	1.1×10^{-2}				
		Intrathecal cisternal	6.6×10^{-3}				
	HM-PAO		9.3×10^{-3}	1.1×10^{-2}	1.7×10^{-2}	2.6×10^{-2}	4.8×10^{-2}
	MAG3		7.3×10^{-3}	9.3×10^{-3}	1.2×10^{-2}	1.2×10^{-2}	2.2×10^{-2}
	MIBI	Resting	8.5×10^{-3}	1.1×10^{-2}	1.7×10^{-2}	2.6×10^{-2}	5.0×10^{-2}
		Exercise	8.5×10^{-3}	9.7×10^{-3}	1.5×10^{-2}	2.2×10^{-2}	4.3×10^{-2}
	Plasmin		1.1×10^{-2}	1.5×10^{-2}	2.2×10^{-2}	3.4×10^{-2}	6.0×10^{-2}
	Gluconate, glucoheptonate		9.0×10^{-3}	1.1×10^{-2}	1.6×10^{-2}	2.4×10^{-2}	4.2×10^{-2}
	Penicillamine		1.3×10^{-2}	1.6×10^{-2}	2.3×10^{-2}	3.4×10^{-2}	5.9×10^{-2}
	Pertechnetate	IV, no blocking	1.3×10^{-2}	1.6×10^{-2}	2.5×10^{-2}	4.0×10^{-2}	7.3×10^{-2}
		IV, blocking	5.5×10^{-3}	6.6×10^{-3}	9.8×10^{-3}	1.5×10^{-2}	2.6×10^{-2}
		Oral, no blocking	1.5×10^{-2}	1.9×10^{-2}	2.9×10^{-2}	4.6×10^{-2}	8.4×10^{-2}
	IDA derivatives		2.4×10^{-2}	2.9×10^{-2}	4.4×10^{-2}	7.0×10^{-2}	1.5×10^{-1}
	Fibrinogen		8.1×10^{-3}	9.9×10^{-3}	1.5×10^{-2}	2.4×10^{-2}	4.3×10^{-2}
	Erythrocytes		8.5×10^{-3}	1.1×10^{-2}	1.6×10^{-2}	2.5×10^{-2}	4.6×10^{-2}
	Denatured erythrocytes		4.1×10^{-2}	5.6×10^{-2}	8.4×10^{-2}	1.3×10^{-1}	2.2×10^{-1}
	Phosphates, phosphonates		8.0×10^{-3}	1.0×10^{-2}	1.5×10^{-2}	2.5×10^{-2}	5.0×10^{-2}
	Aerosols	Fast clearance	7.0×10^{-3}	9.1×10^{-3}	1.3×10^{-2}	2.0×10^{-2}	3.6×10^{-2}
		Slow clearance	1.5×10^{-2}	2.2×10^{-2}	3.1×10^{-2}	4.6×10^{-2}	8.5×10^{-2}
	Heparin		7.3×10^{-3}	9.3×10^{-3}	1.4×10^{-2}	2.1×10^{-2}	3.8×10^{-2}
	Macroaggregated albumin		1.2×10^{-2}	1.8×10^{-2}	2.5×10^{-2}	3.8×10^{-2}	6.9×10^{-2}
^{99m}Tc	Nonabsorbable markers	Oral fluids	2.4×10^{-2}	2.9×10^{-2}	4.7×10^{-2}	7.3×10^{-2}	1.3×10^{-1}
		Oral solids	2.4×10^{-2}	2.9×10^{-2}	4.6×10^{-2}	7.1×10^{-2}	1.3×10^{-1}
	Albumin microspheres		1.1×10^{-2}	1.6×10^{-2}	2.2×10^{-2}	3.3×10^{-2}	6.2×10^{-2}
	Platelets		2.2×10^{-2}	2.9×10^{-2}	4.4×10^{-2}	6.7×10^{-2}	1.2×10^{-1}
	Leukocytes		1.7×10^{-2}	2.3×10^{-2}	3.5×10^{-2}	5.4×10^{-2}	9.8×10^{-2}
^{111}In	In^{3+}		2.6×10^{-1}	3.3×10^{-1}	4.9×10^{-1}	7.5×10^{-1}	1.4
	DTPA	IV	2.5×10^{-2}	3.1×10^{-2}	4.5×10^{-2}	6.7×10^{-2}	1.2×10^{-1}
		Intrathecal lumbar	1.4×10^{-1}				
		Intrathecal cisternal	1.2×10^{-1}				
	Aerosols	Fast clearance	2.8×10^{-2}	3.6×10^{-2}	5.3×10^{-2}	7.9×10^{-2}	1.4×10^{-1}
		Slow clearance	2.9×10^{-1}	3.9×10^{-1}	5.6×10^{-1}	8.4×10^{-1}	1.5
	Nonabsorbable markers	Oral fluids	3.0×10^{-1}	3.7×10^{-1}	6.0×10^{-1}	9.3×10^{-1}	1.7
		Oral solids	3.1×10^{-1}	3.8×10^{-1}	6.1×10^{-1}	9.4×10^{-1}	1.7
	Platelets		7.0×10^{-1}	9.3×10^{-1}	1.4	2.1	3.7
	Leukocytes		5.9×10^{-1}	7.9×10^{-1}	1.2	1.8	3.2
	Bleomycin		1.6×10^{-1}	2.0×10^{-1}	2.9×10^{-1}	4.4×10^{-1}	7.7×10^{-1}
^{113m}In	In^{3+}		1.3×10^{-2}	1.7×10^{-2}	2.8×10^{-2}	4.6×10^{-2}	9.2×10^{-2}
	Hydroxide, colloidal		1.7×10^{-2}	2.3×10^{-2}	3.6×10^{-2}	5.7×10^{-2}	1.1×10^{-1}
	DTPA		1.4×10^{-2}	1.8×10^{-2}	2.7×10^{-2}	4.2×10^{-2}	7.9×10^{-2}
	Aerosols	Fast clearance	1.8×10^{-2}	2.5×10^{-2}	3.6×10^{-2}	5.6×10^{-2}	1.1×10^{-1}
		Slow clearance	2.6×10^{-2}	3.8×10^{-2}	5.5×10^{-2}	8.5×10^{-2}	1.7×10^{-1}
	Nonabsorbable markers	Oral fluids	2.7×10^{-2}	3.3×10^{-2}	5.6×10^{-2}	9.1×10^{-2}	1.8×10^{-1}
		Oral solids	2.8×10^{-2}	3.4×10^{-2}	5.5×10^{-2}	9.1×10^{-2}	1.8×10^{-1}

Table 20.9—continued

Isotope	Pharmaceutical	Conditions of Administration[b]	Effective Dose Equivalent (mSv/mBq)[c]				
			Adult	Age 15	Age 10	Age 5	Age 1
^{123}I	I^-	Thyroid uptake 0%	1.3×10^{-2}	1.6×10^{-2}	2.4×10^{-2}	3.7×10^{-2}	6.7×10^{-2}
		Uptake 25%	1.1×10^{-1}	1.7×10^{-1}	2.6×10^{-1}	5.4×10^{-1}	1.0
	Amphetamine		3.2×10^{-2}	4.3×10^{-2}	6.2×10^{-2}	9.4×10^{-2}	1.7×10^{-1}
	Fibrinogen		2.7×10^{-2}	3.3×10^{-2}	5.3×10^{-2}	8.3×10^{-2}	1.6×10^{-1}
	Albumin	IV	2.6×10^{-2}	3.2×10^{-2}	5.0×10^{-2}	8.0×10^{-2}	1.5×10^{-1}
		Intrathecal lumbar	3.9×10^{-2}				
		Intrathecal cisternal	2.8×10^{-2}				
	Microaggregated albumin		2.4×10^{-2}	3.1×10^{-2}	4.7×10^{-2}	7.2×10^{-2}	1.3×10^{-1}
	Hippuran		1.5×10^{-2}	1.9×10^{-2}	2.8×10^{-2}	4.3×10^{-2}	7.8×10^{-2}
	MIBG		1.8×10^{-2}	2.3×10^{-2}	3.4×10^{-2}	5.0×10^{-2}	9.0×10^{-2}
^{123}I	Rose bengal		7.6×10^{-2}	9.4×10^{-2}	1.5×10^{-1}	2.4×10^{-1}	4.7×10^{-1}
^{124}I	I^-	Thyroid uptake 0%	1.1×10^{-1}	1.3×10^{-1}	2.0×10^{-1}	3.1×10^{-1}	5.6×10^{-1}
		Uptake 25%	6.5	1.0×10^{1}	1.5×10^{1}	3.3×10^{1}	6.1×10^{1}
^{125}I	I^-	Thyroid uptake 0%	1.2×10^{-2}	1.5×10^{-2}	2.3×10^{-2}	3.7×10^{-2}	7.3×10^{-2}
		Uptake 25%	7.1	1.0×10^{1}	1.3×10^{1}	2.5×10^{1}	4.0×10^{1}
	Fibrinogen		1.2×10^{-1}	1.5×10^{-1}	2.4×10^{-1}	3.9×10^{-1}	7.7×10^{-1}
	Albumin		3.4×10^{-1}	4.1×10^{-1}	6.8×10^{-1}	1.1	2.2
	Nonabsorbable	Oral fluids	1.5×10^{-1}	1.9×10^{-1}	3.3×10^{-1}	5.4×10^{-1}	1.0
	markers	Oral solids	1.6×10^{-1}	2.0×10^{-1}	3.4×10^{-1}	5.6×10^{-1}	1.1
	Hippuran		1.0×10^{-2}	1.3×10^{-2}	2.0×10^{-2}	3.1×10^{-2}	6.0×10^{-2}
	Antipyrene		1.3×10^{-2}	1.6×10^{-2}	2.6×10^{-2}	4.1×10^{-2}	8.0×10^{-2}
	Thalamate		9.7×10^{-3}	1.2×10^{-2}	1.9×10^{-2}	3.0×10^{-2}	5.7×10^{-2}
	PVP		1.2	1.5	2.3	3.5	6.6
	T4		1.2×10^{-1}	1.4×10^{-1}	2.3×10^{-1}	3.8×10^{-1}	7.6×10^{-1}
	T3		4.9×10^{-2}	6.1×10^{-2}	1.0×10^{-1}	1.7×10^{-1}	3.3×10^{-1}
	rT3		3.6×10^{-2}	4.6×10^{-2}	7.7×10^{-2}	1.2×10^{-1}	2.4×10^{-1}
	Diiodothyronine		3.6×10^{-2}	4.5×10^{-2}	7.6×10^{-2}	1.2×10^{-1}	2.4×10^{-1}
^{131}I	I^-	Thyroid uptake 0%	7.2×10^{-2}	8.8×10^{-2}	1.4×10^{-1}	2.1×10^{-1}	4.0×10^{-1}
		Uptake 25%	1.1×10^{1}	1.7×10^{1}	2.5×10^{1}	5.6×10^{1}	1.0×10^{2}
	Fibrinogen		5.6×10^{-1}	6.9×10^{-1}	1.1	1.8	3.6
	Albumin	IV	8.6×10^{-1}	1.1	1.7	2.8	5.4
		Intrathecal lumbar	9.0×10^{-1}				
		Intrathecal cisternal	8.4×10^{-1}				
	Macroaggregated albumin		5.0×10^{-1}	7.0×10^{-1}	1.0	1.6	3.1
	Nonabsorbable	Oral fluids	9.3×10^{-1}	1.1	2.0	3.2	6.3
	markers	Oral solids	9.5×10^{-1}	1.2	2.0	3.3	6.5
	Microaggregated albumin		2.4×10^{-2}	3.1×10^{-2}	4.7×10^{-2}	7.2×10^{-2}	1.3×10^{-1}
	Hippuran		6.6×10^{-2}	8.3×10^{-2}	1.3×10^{-1}	1.9×10^{-1}	3.7×10^{-1}
	Antipyrine		7.8×10^{-2}	9.5×10^{-2}	1.5×10^{-1}	2.3×10^{-1}	4.4×10^{-1}
^{131}I	Norcholesterol		1.5	2.2	3.4	6.8	1.3×10^{1}
	PVP		9.7×10^{-1}	1.2	1.8	2.7	5.1
	T4		4.4×10^{-1}	5.2×10^{-1}	8.5×10^{-1}	1.4	2.6
	T3		2.7×10^{-1}	3.3×10^{-1}	5.4×10^{-1}	8.7×10^{-1}	1.7
	rT3		2.2×10^{-1}	2.7×10^{-1}	4.5×10^{-1}	7.3×10^{-1}	1.4
	Diiodothyronine		2.2×10^{-1}	2.7×10^{-1}	4.4×10^{-1}	7.2×10^{-1}	1.4
	MIBG		2.0×10^{-1}	2.6×10^{-1}	4.0×10^{-1}	6.1×10^{-1}	1.1
	Rose bengal		9.1×10^{-1}	1.1	1.9	3.2	6.3
^{127}Xe	Gas	30 s inhalation	1.4×10^{-4}	1.8×10^{-4}	2.7×10^{-4}	4.1×10^{-4}	7.5×10^{-4}
		10 m rebreathe	1.2×10^{-3}	1.5×10^{-3}	2.2×10^{-3}	3.5×10^{-3}	6.3×10^{-3}
^{133}Xe	Gas	30 s inhalation	1.9×10^{-4}	2.6×10^{-4}	4.0×10^{-4}	6.4×10^{-4}	1.3×10^{-3}
		10 m rebreathe	1.3×10^{-3}	1.5×10^{-3}	2.5×10^{-3}	4.1×10^{-3}	8.3×10^{-3}
^{129}Cs	Cs^+		4.7×10^{-2}	5.4×10^{-2}	8.1×10^{-2}	1.2×10^{-1}	2.2×10^{-1}
^{130}Cs	Cs^+		2.4×10^{-3}	2.6×10^{-3}	3.9×10^{-3}	5.9×10^{-3}	1.1×10^{-2}
^{131}Cs	Cs^+		4.9×10^{-2}	5.4×10^{-2}	7.8×10^{-2}	1.2×10^{-1}	2.1×10^{-1}
^{134m}Cs	Cs^+		5.1×10^{-3}	4.9×10^{-3}	6.6×10^{-3}	8.7×10^{-3}	1.5×10^{-2}
^{131}Ba	Ba^{2+}		5.0×10^{-1}	7.0×10^{-1}	1.1	1.8	3.4
	Nonabsorbable	Oral fluids	4.5×10^{-1}	6.6×10^{-1}	1.1	1.7	3.1
	markers	Oral solids	4.6×10^{-1}	6.7×10^{-1}	1.1	1.7	3.2
^{133m}Ba	Ba^{2+}		4.1×10^{-1}	6.4×10^{-1}	1.1	1.9	3.8
^{135m}Ba	Ba^{2+}		3.1×10^{-1}	3.8×10^{-1}	6.7×10^{-1}	1.1	2.3
^{140}La	DTPA		1.9×10^{-1}	2.3×10^{-1}	3.5×10^{-1}	5.3×10^{-1}	9.9×10^{-1}
^{169}Yb	DTPA	IV	4.6×10^{-2}	5.8×10^{-2}	8.9×10^{-2}	1.4×10^{-1}	2.5×10^{-1}
		Intrathecal lumbar	2.3×10^{-1}				
		Intrathecal cisternal	2.2×10^{-1}				
^{198}Au	Colloid		1.5	2.1	3.3	5.3	1.0×10^{1}
^{197}Hg	$HgCl_2$		3.2×10^{-1}	4.0×10^{-1}	5.8×10^{-1}	8.7×10^{-1}	8.8×10^{-1}
	BMHP		3.9×10^{-1}	5.0×10^{-1}	7.5×10^{-1}	1.1	1.4
	Chlormerodrin		1.8×10^{-1}	2.3×10^{-1}	3.4×10^{-1}	5.2×10^{-1}	9.8×10^{-1}
^{203}Hg	Chlormerodrin		1.7	2.2	3.3	4.9	8.8
^{201}Tl	$Tl^{+,3+}$		2.3×10^{-1}	3.6×10^{-1}	1.5	2.0	3.0

[a]Data from ICP (90, 91)

[b]IV unless otherwise specified

[c]Multiply numbers in table by 3.7 to convert to rem/mCi

Table 20.10.
Estimated Dose to Embryo from Maternal Diagnostic Nuclear Medicine Procedures[a]

Isotope	Pharmaceutical	Embryo Dose (mGy/ mBq to Mother)
^{99m}Tc	Albumin	4.9×10^{-3}
	Lung aggregate	9.5×10^{-3}
	Polyphosphate	9.7×10^{-3}
	Pertechnetate	1.0×10^{-2}
	Stannous glucoheptonate	1.1×10^{-2}
	Sulfur colloid	8.6×10^{-3}
^{123}I	Nal (15% uptake)	8.6×10^{-3}
	Rose bengal	3.5×10^{-2}
^{131}I	Nal (15% uptake)	2.7×10^{-2}
	Rose bengal	1.8×10^{-1}

[a]Data from Kereiakes and Rosenstein (93).

Table 20.11.
Estimated Fetal Thyroid Dose from Maternal Radioiodine

Gestation Period	Fetal/Maternal Ratio (Thyroid Gland)	Dose to Fetal Thyroid (mGy/mBq)
10–12 weeks	—	2.7×10^{-7} (precursors)
12–13 weeks	1.2	1.9×10^{-4}
Second trimester	1.8	1.6×10^{-3}
Third trimester	7.5	—
Term	—	2.2×10^{-3}

Table 20.12.
Estimated Dose to Mother and Breast-Feeding Child from Diagnostic Nuclear Medicine Procedures During Lactation[a]

Radiopharmaceutical	Effective Dose Equivalent (mSv/mBq)	
	Mother	Child
^{99m}Tc pertechnetate	1.1×10^{-2}	3.0×10^{-2}
^{131}I iodohippurate	5.0×10^{-2}	7.0
^{51}Cr EDTA	2.5×10^{-3}	1.5×10^{-3}
^{125}I fibrinogen	1.1×10^{-1}	3.2

[a]Data from UNSCEAR (18).

ical needs of the patient take precedence over potential radiation risk. That is, radiation exposure for a procedure that is clinically justified should not be an overriding concern. All effort should obviously be made to optimize the procedure so as to minimize exposure to both patients and staff. On the other hand, procedures whose purposes are nonmedical, such as mass screening, occupational, medicolegal, insurance, or research, should be carefully weighed as to what benefit is received by whom versus the radiation burden to the subject.

The most frequent source of radiation exposure problems in diagnostic medicine is the unwitting exposure of an early, unrecognized pregnancy. The question is at what dose level should consideration be given to termination of the pregnancy on grounds of radiation effect to the embryo. Although there are no clear data, there is reason to believe that the embryo/fetus is more sensitive to stochastic effects, in particular cancer, than the adult or even the child. However, the problem of the applicability of the linear nonthreshold model again enters. In any event, even by the most conservative models, the probability of a stochastic effect from such an exposure is very small and therefore difficult to deal with. However, thresholds for deterministic effects in the early embryo are in the range of 50–150 mGy. It is possible to deliver doses in this range in diagnostic medicine, especially from a complicated workup. In years past, several authors recommended specific dose levels for recommending therapeutic abortion (94, 95). Now it seems more reasonable to consider an action range rather than an action level. Doses to the embryo below about 50 mGy should carry little or no risk of deterministic effect. Doses in the range of 50–150 mGy may be associated with small, perhaps statistically insignificant, risk, and the patient should be so counseled. Above 150 mGy, however, the risk is likely to be statistically significant, and pregnancy termination should be considered.

These recommendations are not intended for blind application to any specific case. They should be tempered with judgement. The patient still comes first.

REFERENCES

1. Rollins WH. Notes on x-light. Boston: Privately published, 1904.
2. Sagan LS, ed. Radiation hormesis. Proceedings of a conference held at Oakland CA, Aug. 14–16, 1985. Health Phys 1987;52:519–680.
3. Pochin EE. Why be quantitative about radiation risk estimates? L.S. Taylor Lecture Series, no. 2. Washington, DC: NCRP Publications, 1978.
4. Wilson R. Risks caused by low levels of pollution. Yale J Biol Med 1978;51:37–51.
5. Borek C. In vitro cell transformation by low doses of x-irradiation and neutrons. In: Yuhas JW, Tennant RW, Regan JD, eds. Biology of radiation carcinogenesis. New York: Raven Press, 1976:309–326.
6. Rinchik EM, Stoye JP, Frankel WN, et al. Molecular analysis of viable spontaneous and radiation-induced albino (c)-locus mutations in the mouse. Mutat Res 1993;286:199–207.
7. Thacker J. Radiation-induced mutation in mammalian cells at low doses and dose rates. In: Nygaard OF, Sinclair WK, Lett JT, eds. Effects of low dose and low dose rate radiation. New York: Academic Press, 1992:77–124.
8. Lea DE. Actions of radiations on living cells. 2d ed. Cambridge, UK: Cambridge University Press, 1955.
9. Kellerer AM, Rossi HH. A generalized formulation of the theory of dual radiation action. Radiat Res 1978;75:471–488.
10. Hall EJ. Radiobiology for the radiologist. 4th ed. Philadelphia: J.B. Lippincott, 1994.
11. Stephens LC, Hunter NR, Ang KK, Milas L, Meyn RE. Development of apoptosis in irradiated murine tumors as a function of time and dose. Radiat Res 1993;135:75–80.
12. Lowe SW, Schmitt EM, Smith SW, Osborne BA, Jacks T. p53 is required for radiation-induced apoptosis in mouse thymocytes. Nature 1993;362:847–849.
13. Kollmorgen GM, Bedford JS. Cellular radiation biology. In: Darymple GV, Gaulden ME, Kollmorgen GM, Vogel HH, eds. Medical radiation biology. Philadelphia: W.B. Saunders, 1973:100–127.
14. Bacq ZM, Alexander P. Fundamentals of radiobiology. New York: MacMillan, 1961.
15. Elkind MM, Sutton H. Radiation response of mammalian cells grown in culture. I. Repair of x-ray damage in surviving Chinese hamster cells. Radiat Res 1960;13:556–593.

16. Land CE. Estimating cancer risks from low doses of ionizing radiation. Science 1980;209:1197–1203.
17. Committee on the Biological Effects of Ionizing Radiation. Health effects of exposure to low levels of ionizing radiation (BEIR V). Washington, DC: National Academy Press, 1990.
18. United Nations Scientific Committee on the Efects of Atomic Radiation. Sources and effects of ionizing radiation. New York: United Nations, 1993.
19. Upton AC. Cancer research 1964: thoughts on the contributions of radiation biology. Cancer Res 1964;24:1861–1868.
20. Shimizu Y, Kato H, Schull WJ. Life span study report 11. Part 2. Cancer mortality in the years 1950–85 based on the recently revised doses (DS86). Technical Report RERF TR 5–88. Hiroshima: Radiation Effects Research Foundation, 1988.
21. Thompson DE, Mabuchi K, Ron E, et al. Cancer incidence in atomic bomb survivors. Part II: Solid tumors, 1958–1987. Radiat Res 1994;137(Suppl):S17–S67.
22. Preston DL, Kusumi S, Tomonaga M, et al. Cancer incidence in atomic bomb survivors. Part III: Leukemia, lymphoma and multiple myeloma, 1950–1987. Radiat Res 1994;137(Suppl):S68–S97.
23. Ron E, Preston DL, Mabuchi K, Thompson DE, Soda M. Cancer incidence in atomic bomb survivors. Part IV. Comparison of cancer incidence and mortality. Radiat Res 1994;137(Suppl):S98–S112.
24. Mole RH, Papworth DG, Corp MJ. The dose response for x-ray induction of myeloid leukemia in male CBA.H mice. Br J Cancer 1983;47:285–291.
25. Darby SC, Doll R, Gill SK, Smith PG. Long-term mortality after a single treatment course with x-rays in patients treated for ankylosing spondylitis. Br J Cancer 1987;55:179–190.
26. Boice JD Jr, Blettner M, Kleinerman RA, et al. Radiation dose and leukemia risk in patients treated for cancer of the cervix. J US National Cancer Inst 1987;79:1295–1311.
27. Boice JD Jr, Enghohm G, Kleinerman RA, et al. Radiation dose and second cancer risk in patients treated for cancer of the cervix. Radiat Res 1988;116:3–55.
28. Stewart A, Pennypacker W, Barber R. Adult leukemia and diagnostic x-rays. Br Med J 1962;2:882–890.
29. Gibson R, Graham S, Lilienfeld A, et al. Irradiation in the epidemiology of leukemia among adults. J US National Cancer Inst 1972;48:301–311.
30. Linos A, Gray J, Orvis A. Low dose radiation and leukemia. N Engl J Med 1980;302:1101.
31. MacKenzie I. Breast cancer following multiple fluoroscopies. Br J Cancer 1965;19:1–9.
32. Miller AB, Howe GR, Sherman GJ, et al. Breast cancer mortality following irradiation in a cohort of Canadian tuberculosis patients. N Engl J Med 1989;321:1285–1289.
33. Hrubec Z, Boice J, Monson R, Rosenstein M. Breast cancer after multiple chest fluoroscopies: second follow-up of Massachusetts women with tuberculosis. Cancer Res 1989;49:229–234.
34. Shore R, Hildreth N, Woodward E, Dvoretsky P, Hempelmann L, Pasternack B. Breast cancer among women given x-ray therapy for acute postpartum mastitis. J US Natl Cancer Inst 1986; 77:689–696.
35. Committee on the Biological Effects of Ionizing Radiation. Health risks of radon and other internally deposited alpha-emitters (BEIR IV). Washington, DC: National Academy Press, 1988.
36. Griem ML, Justman J, Weiss L. The neoplastic potential of gastric irradiation. Am J Clin Oncol 1984;7:675–677.
37. Ron E, Modan B. Thyroid and other neoplasms following childhood scalp irradiation. In: Boice JD Jr, Fraumeni JF Jr, eds. Radiation carcinogenesis: epidemiology and biological significance. New York: Raven Press, 1984:139–151.
38. Shore RE, Woodward ED, Hempelmann LH. Radiation-induced thyroid cancer. In: Boice JD Jr, Fraumeni JF Jr, eds. Radiation carcinogenesis: epidemiology and biological significance. New York: Raven Press, 1984:131–138.
39. National Council on Radiation Protection and Measurement. Induction of thyroid cancer by ionizing radiation. NCRP Report No. 80. Bethesda, MD: National Council on Radiation Protection and Measurement, 1985.
40. Hoffman DA. Late effects of I-131 therapy in the United States. In: Boice JD Jr, Fraumeni JF Jr, eds. Radiation carcinogenesis: epidemiology and biological significance. New York: Raven Press, 1984:273–280.
41. Holm L-E, Wicklund KE, Lundell GE, et al. Thyroid cancer after diagnostic doses of iodine-131: a retrospective study. J US Natl Cancer Inst 1988;80:1132–1136.
42. Conard RA. Late radiation effects in Marshall Islanders exposed to fallout 28 years ago. In: Boice JD Jr, Fraumeni JF Jr, eds. Radiation carcinogenesis: epidemiology and biological significance. New York: Raven Press, 1984:57–71.
43. Rothman RJ. Significance of studies of low-dose radiation fallout in the western United States. In: Boice JD Jr, Fraumeni JF Jr, eds. Radiation carcinogenesis: epidemiology and biological significance. New York: Raven Press, 1984:73–82.
44. Lee WR, Chiacchierini RP, Shlein B, Telles NC. Thyroid tumors following I-131 or localized x-irradiation to the thyroid and the pituitary glands in rats. Radiat Res 1982;92:307–319.
45. Brinkley D, Haybittle JL. The late effects of artificial menopause by x-radiation. Br J Radiol 1969;42:519–521.
46. Smith PG, Doll R. Late effects of x-irradiation in patients treated for metropathia haemorrhagica. Br J Radiol 1976;49:224–232.
47. Dickson RJ. The late results of radium treatment for benign uterine hemorrhage. Br J Radiol 1969;42:582–594.
48. Wagoner JK. Leukemia and other malignancies following radiation therapy for gynecological disorders. In: Boice JD Jr, Fraumeni JF Jr, eds. Radiation carcinogenesis: epidemiology and biological significance. New York: Raven Press, 1984:153–159.
49. Blum T. Osteomyelitis of the mandible and maxilla. J Am Dent Assoc 1924;11:802–805.
50. Taylor LS. Radiation protection standards. Cleveland: CRC Press, 1971.
51. Smith PG, Doll R. Mortality from cancer and all causes among British radiologists. Br J Radiol 1981;54:187–194.
52. Shore RE, Albert RE, Pasternack BS. Follow-up study of patients treated by x-ray epilation for tinea capitis: resurvey of posttreatment illness and mortality experience. Arch Environ Health 1976; 31:17–24.
53. Matanoski GM. The current mortality rates of radiologists and other physician specialists: specific causes of death. Am J Epidemiol 1975;101:199–210.
54. Preston-Martin S, Paganini-Hill A, Henderson BE, Pike M, Wood C. Case control study of intracranial meningiomas in women in Los Angeles County, California. J US Natl Cancer Inst 1980; 65:67–73.
55. Soffer D, Pittalura S, Feiner M, Beller AJ. Intracranial meningiomas following low-dose irradiation to the head. J Neurosurg 1983; 59:1048–1053.
56. Rubinstein AB, Shalit MN, Cohen ML, Zandbank U, Reichenthal E. Radiation-induced cerebral meningioma: a recognizable entity. J Neurosurg 1984;61:966–971.
57. Harley N, Kolber AB, Shore RE, Albert RE, Altman SM, Pasternack B. The skin dose and response for the head and neck in patients irradiated with x ray for tinea capitis: implications for environmental radioactivity. In: Proceedings of the 16th Midyear Topical Meeting of the Health Physics Society. Springfield, VA: National Technical Information Service, 1983:125–142.
58. Cuzick J. Radiation-induced myelomatosis. N Engl J Med 1981; 304:204–210.
59. Land CE. Carcinogenic effects of radiation on the human digestive tract and other organs. In: Upton AC, Albert RE, Burns FJ, Shore

RE, eds. Radiation carcinogenesis. New York: Elsevier, 1986:347–378.
60. Preston-Martin S, Thomas DC, White SC, Cohen D. Prior exposure to medical and dental x-rays related to tumors of the parotid gland. J US Natl Cancer Inst 1988;80:943–949.
61. Stewart A, Webb J, Giles D, Hewitt D. Malignant disease in childhood and diagnostic irradiation in utero. Lancet 1956;1:447.
62. Diamond EL, Schmerler H, Lilienfeld AM. The relationship of intra-uterine radiation to subsequent mortality and development of leukemia in children. Am J Epidemiol 1973;97:283–313.
63. Oppenheim BE, Griem ML, Meier P. Effects of low-dose prenatal irradiation in humans: analysis of Chicago Lying-In data and comparison with other studies. Radiat Res 1974;57:508–544.
64. Yoshimoto Y, Kato H, Schull WJ. Risk of cancer among in utero children exposed to A-bomb radiation: 1950–84. RERF Technical Report 4–88. Hiroshima: Radiation Effects Research Foundation, 1988.
65. Macht SH, Lawrence PS. National survey of congenital malformation, resulting from exposure to roentgen radiation. Am J Roentgenol 1955;73:442–466.
66. Gardner MJ, Snee MP, Hall AJ, et al. Results of case-control study of leukaemia and lymphoma among young people near Sellafield nuclear plant in West Cumbria. Br Med J 1990;300:423–428.
67. Neel JV. Update on the genetic effects of ionizing radiation. JAMA 1991;66:698–701.
68. Muller HJ. Artificial transmutation of the gene. Science 1927; 66:84–87.
69. Russell WL. The nature of the dose-rate effect of radiation on mutation in mice. Japan J Genet 1964;40(Suppl):128–140.
70. Selby PB, Selby PR. Gamma-ray-induced dominant mutations that cause skeletal abnormalities in mice. I. Plan, summary of results and discussion. Mutat Res 1977;43:357–375.
71. Schull WJ, Otake M, Neel JV. Genetic effects of the atomic bombs: a reappraisal. Science 1981;213:1220–1227.
72. National Council on Radiation Protection and Measurements. Ionizing radiation exposure of the population of the United States. NCRP Report No. 93. Bethesda, MD: National Council on Radiation Protection and Measurements, 1987.
73. Hall EJ. Radiobiology for the radiologist. 4th ed. Philadelphia: J.B. Lippincott, 1994.
74. International Commission on Radiological Protection. Nonstochastic effects of ionizing radiation. ICRP Publication 41. Ann ICRP 1984;14(3).
75. Merriam GR, Szechter A, Focht EF. The effects of ionizing radiation on the eye. Front Radiat Ther Oncol 1972;6:346–385.
76. Rubin P, Casarett GW. A direction for clinical radiation pathology. The tolerance dose. Front Radiat Ther Oncol 1972;6:1–16.
77. Russell LB, Russell WL. An analysis of the changing radiation response of the developing mouse embryo. J Cell Physiol 1954; 43(Suppl 1):103–149.
78. Otake M, Schull WJ. In utero exposure to A-bomb radiation and mental retardation: a reassessment. Br J Radiol 1984;57:409–414.
79. Goldstein L, Murphy DP. Microcephalic idiocy following radium therapy for uterine cancer during pregnancy. Am J Obstet Gynecol 1929;18:1890–195.
80. Miller RW, Mulvihill JJ. Small head size after atomic irradiation. In: Sever JL, Brent RL, eds. Teratogen update: environmentally induced birth defect risks. New York: Alan R. Liss, 1986:141–143.
81. Committee on the Biological Effects of Ionizing Radiations. The effects on populations of exposure to low levels of ionizing radiation (BEIR III). Washington, DC: National Academy of Sciences, 1980.
82. Brent RL, Gorson RO. Radiation exposure in pregnancy. Curr Probl Radiol 1972;2:1–48.
83. National Council on Radiation Protection and Measurements. Medical exposure of pregnant and potentially pregnant women. NCRP Report No. 54. Bethesda, MD: National Council on Radiation Protection and Measurement, 1977.
84. International Commission on Radiological Protection. 1990 Recommendations of the International Commission on Radiological Protection. ICRP Publication 60. Ann ICRP 1991;21(1–3).
85. Otake M, Yashimaru H, Schull WJ. Severe mental retardation among the prenatally exposed survivors of the atomic bombing of Hiroshima and Nagasaki: a comparison of the old and new dosimetry systems. RERF Technical Report 16–87. Hiroshima: Radiation Effects Research Foundation, 1987.
86. Schull WJ, Otake M. Effects on intelligence of prenatal exposure to ionizing radiation. RERF Technical Report 7–86. Hiroshima: Radiation Effects Research Foundation, 1986.
87. Jacobi W. The concept of effective dose—a proposal for the combination of organ doses. Radiat Environ Biophys 1975;12:101–109.
88. International Commission on Radiological Protection. Recommendations of the International Commission on Radiological Protection. ICRP Publication 26. Ann ICRP 1977;1(3).
89. Laws PW, Rosenstein M. A somatic dose index for diagnostic radiology. Health Phys 1978;35:629–642.
90. International Commission on Radiological Protection. Radiation dose to patients from radiopharmaceuticals. ICRP Publication 53. Ann ICRP 1987;18(1–4).
91. International Commission on Radiological Protection. Addendum 1 to radiation dose to patients from radiopharmaceuticals. Ann ICRP 1991;22(3):1–28.
92. Gibbs SJ. Influence of organs in the ICRP's remainder on effective dose equivalent computed for diagnostic radiation exposures. Health Phys 1989;56:515–520.
93. Kereiakes JG, Rosenstein M. Handbook of radiation doses in nuclear medicine and diagnostic radiology. Boca Raton, FL: CRC Press, 1980.
94. Hammer-Jacobsen E. Therapeutic abortion on account of x-ray examination during pregnancy. Dan Med Bull 1959;6:113–121.
95. Dekaban AS. Abnormalities in children exposed to x-radiation during various stages of gestation: tentative timetable of radiation to the human fetus. J Nucl Med 1968;9:471–477.

21 Cardiac Pathology and Morphology Relevant to Cardiovascular Imaging

HENRY S. CABIN and K. SONI CLUBB

The potential of cardiovascular imaging to define cardiac structure and function has expanded dramatically during the past several years. Crucial to the interpretation of these images is an understanding of cardiac structure in the normal and diseased heart. In this chapter, an overview of cardiac pathology is provided, emphasizing three areas: coronary artery disease and myocardial infarction (MI), valvular heart disease, and cardiomyopathy.

CORONARY HEART DISEASE

CORONARY ARTERY DISEASE

Coronary artery atherosclerosis is the structural abnormality underlying the three major clinical manifestations of coronary artery disease: angina pectoris, MI, and sudden coronary death. Atherosclerotic plaque consists predominately of fibrous tissue with areas of fat. Atherosclerotic lesions involve the intimal layer of the artery, but may also extend into the media with replacement of portions of smooth muscle by fibrous and elastic tissue. The intimal plaque may contain calcium. Although atherosclerosis may be focally severe, the atherosclerotic process is almost always diffuse, with involvement of virtually every portion of the epicardial coronary arteries (Fig. 21.1). Quantitative autopsy studies have found no difference in the extent or severity of atherosclerotic narrowing among patients with angina pectoris, acute MI, or sudden coronary death (1–5). The clinical outcome of the atherosclerotic process must, therefore, be influenced by other factors such as coronary artery thrombus or spasm.

The role of coronary artery thrombus in the production of MI has been debated for years. Although most necropsy investigators reported the frequent presence of thrombus

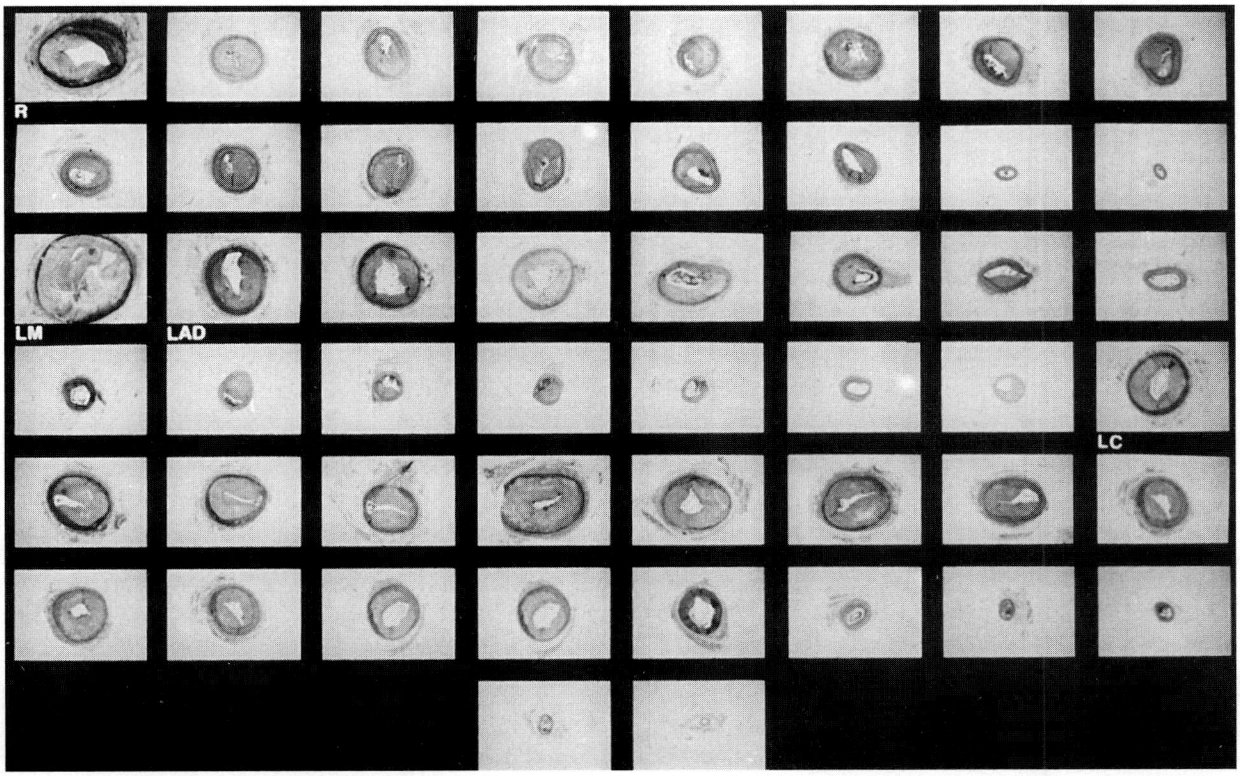

Figure 21.1. The atherosclerotic process. Histologic sections from the entire length of the right (*R*), left main (*LM*), left anterior descending (*LAD*), and left circumflex (*LC*) coronary arteries, from a 58-year-old man with angina pectoris and death during cardiac catheterization. There is diffuse atherosclerotic narrowing of all four coronary arteries.

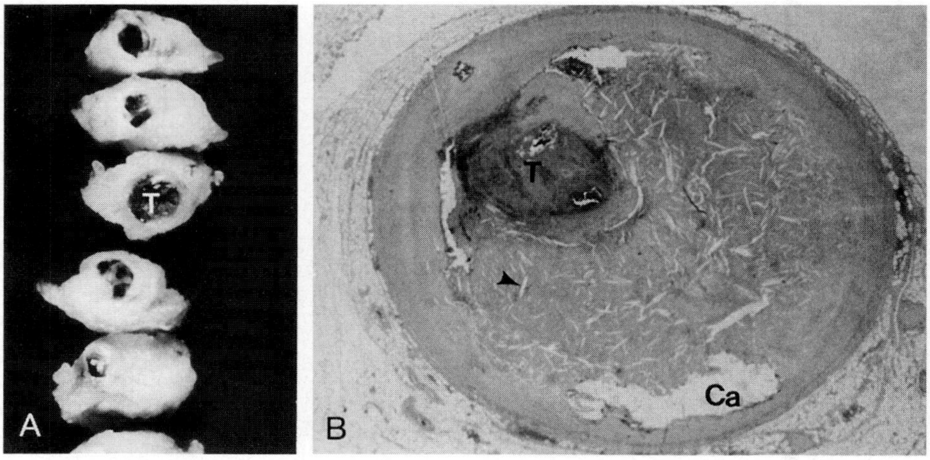

Figure 21.2. Thrombus at site of atherosclerotic narrowing. **A:** Gross photograph of the left anterior descending (*LAD*) coronary artery cut transversely into 5 mm segments. Each segment is surrounded by epicardial fat. A thrombus (*T*) occluded the lumen of the artery. **B:** A histologic section of the LAD (×20, hematoxylin and eosin) reveals 90% cross-sectional area narrowing by atherosclerotic plaque. The plaque consists of fibrous tissue with areas of calcium (*Ca*) and cholesterol clefts (*arrowhead*) and the residual lumen is occluded by thrombus (*T*).

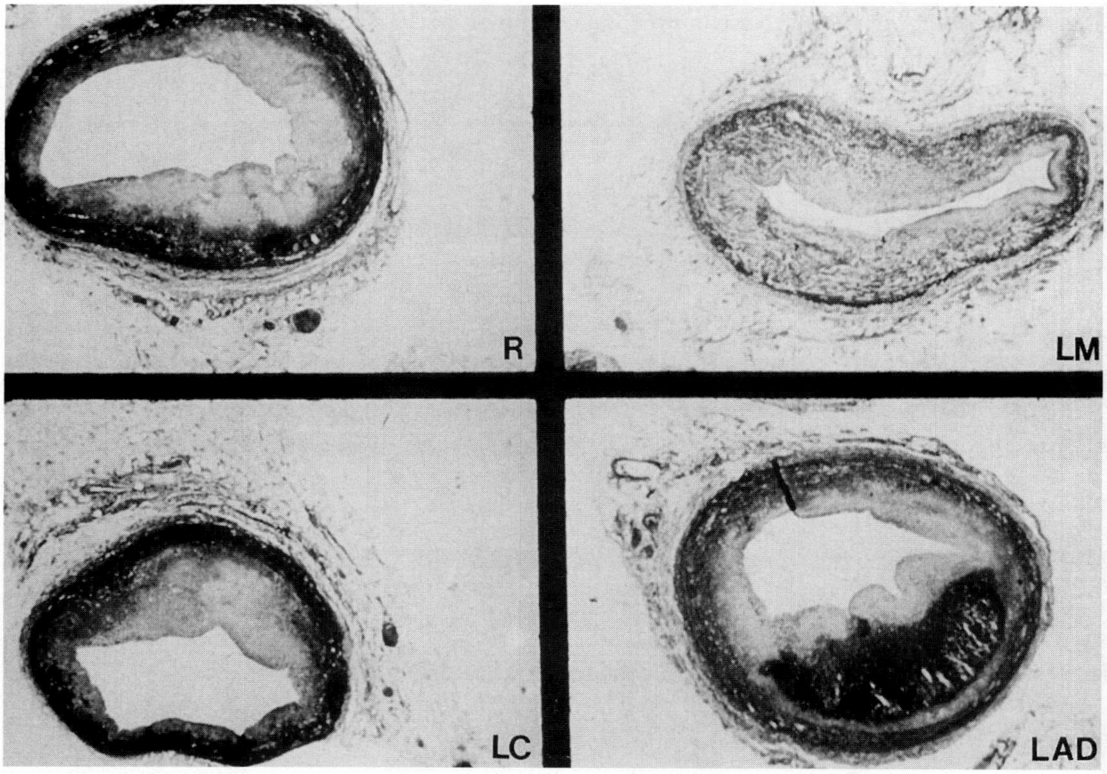

Figure 21.3. Hemorrhage into atherosclerotic plaque. Photomicrographs of transverse histologic sections (×10, hematoxylin and eosin) of the proximal right (*R*), left main (*LM*), left circumflex (*LC*), and left anterior descending (*LAD*) coronary arteries from a 43-year-old woman with mitral regurgitation who died of an acute anterior wall myocardial infarction. At autopsy, each coronary artery was narrowed less than 50% in cross-sectional area by atherosclerotic plaque. Hemorrhage was present in a proximal LAD plaque, producing significant stenosis of that vessel.

at a site of severe atherosclerotic narrowing in patients with fatal acute MI (Fig. 21.2), others did not confirm this finding (1, 6). Recently, the use of thrombolytic agents for the treatment of acute MI has resulted in an extensive experience with cardiac catheterization performed early in acute transmural MI. Coronary angiography performed within hours of the onset of chest pain often reveals occlusion of major coronary artery by thrombus at a site of severe atherosclerotic narrowing (7–9). Although thrombus may be important in the initiation of acute MI, there is little evidence that it plays a role in sudden coronary death. Thrombus is rarely found in autopsy patients who die suddenly and have coronary artery narrowing by atherosclerotic plaque (3). There is increasing angiographic (10, 11) and angioscopic (12) evidence that thrombus is often present in patients with unstable, but not stable, angina pectoris. This information suggests that thrombus may be important in converting stable to unstable pectoris. Support for this concept is provided by studies suggesting that anticoagulation (13) and thrombolytic therapy (14) are effective in the treatment of unstable angina pectoris.

Coronary artery spasm, like thrombus, occurs most often at a site of atherosclerotic narrowing. It has been reported most frequently in patients with variant or Prinzmetal's angina, in whom chest pain is usually unrelated to exertion and is associated with ST segment elevation (15). Angiographic studies using ergonovine to induce coronary spasm have also reported spasm in patients with typical exertional angina pectoris (16), as well as in the patient with nonexertional angina without ST segment elevation. Other less important coronary artery abnormalities resulting in clinical cardiac disease are hemorrhage into an atherosclerotic plaque (Fig. 21.3), which is found occasionally at necropsy in a patient with a fatal coronary event, and coronary artery dissection. Hemorrhage into atherosclerotic plaque has been reported in patients receiving thrombolytic therapy in association with coronary artery angioplasty (17).

MYOCARDIAL INFARCTION

The major structural consequence of coronary artery disease is myocardial infarction. Neither recurrent reversible ischemia nor sudden coronary death result in gross structural abnormalities of the myocardium in the absence of MI.

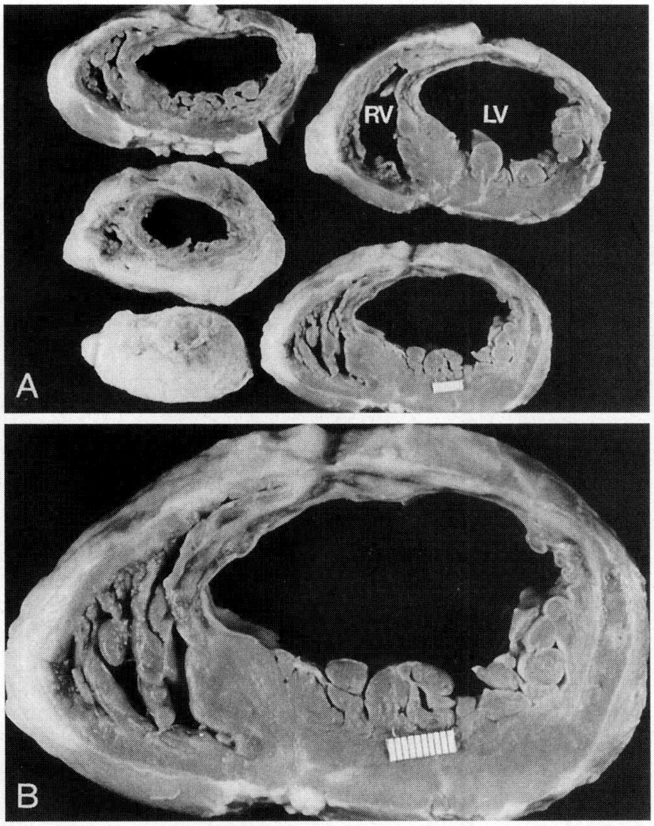

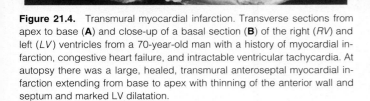

Figure 21.4. Transmural myocardial infarction. Transverse sections from apex to base (**A**) and close-up of a basal section (**B**) of the right (*RV*) and left (*LV*) ventricles from a 70-year-old man with a history of myocardial infarction, congestive heart failure, and intractable ventricular tachycardia. At autopsy there was a large, healed, transmural anteroseptal myocardial infarction extending from base to apex with thinning of the anterior wall and septum and marked LV dilatation.

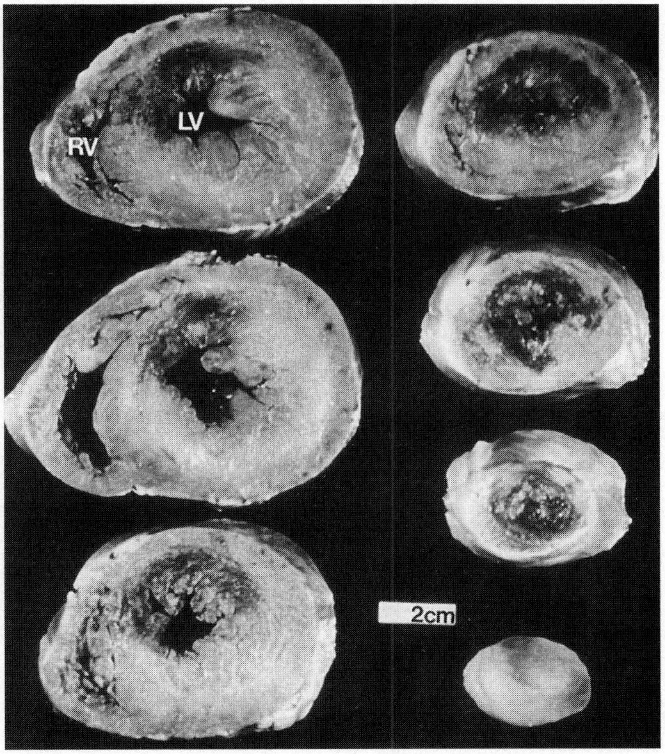

Figure 21.5. Nontransmural myocardial infarction. Transverse sections, from apex to base of the right ventricle (*RV*) and left ventricle (*LV*) from a 64-year-old man with long-standing hypertension who died 6 days after his first MI. At autopsy there is a hemorrhagic anteroseptal infarct, which is nontransmural in the basal and mid-left ventricle but becomes circumferential and transmural at the apex. There is also left ventricular hypertrophy.

Although the terms subendocardial and transmural are often used, these terms do not adequately define the anatomic features of MI. The term *subendocardial* implies a limitation of the infarct to the inner half of the myocardium. At autopsy, however, there is always extension of the necrosis or scar into the epicardial half of the muscle wall. More useful terms to describe the extent of an MI are *transmural* and *nontransmural*. Transmural suggests involvement of the entire thickness of the wall and, in patients who survive the first few days of the infarct, is often associated with thinning (Fig. 21.4). In nontransmural MI, significant areas of normal myocardium are present in the same region as infarcted myocardium, and there is rarely thinning of the wall (Fig. 21.5). In addition to these general terms, an adequate anatomic description of an MI includes regional location. A number of schemata have been proposed for the localization of MI and there is no general accepted terminology. A useful system for localizing an infarct at autopsy as well as by imaging during life is to divide the ventricle into basal, medial, and apical thirds. Within each third, the wall can be divided into anterior, lateral, posterior, and septal portions (18).

The size of an MI has been related both clinically and at autopsy to the clinical consequence of the infarct. Although determining infarct size is relatively easy and accurate at autopsy, it is considerably more difficult during life. Infarct size has been estimated from cardiac enzymes, electrocardiogram (ECG) abnormalities, and extent of regional wall motion abnormality by echocardiography, radionuclide angiography, and contrast angiography. In general, an infarct involving more than 40–50% of the left ventricular wall is associated with cardiogenic shock and death. An infarct involving from 20–40% of the left ventricular wall can lead to congestive heart failure and a shortened survival when compared to infarct involving less than 20% of the left ventricular wall (19). In addition to length of survival, MI size may also correlate with the frequency and type of post-MI symptoms; congestive heart failure usually suggests a larger infarct and angina pectoris is often associated with a smaller infarct (20).

ISCHEMIC CARDIOMYOPATHY

When MI involves more than 20% of the left ventricular wall, ischemic cardiomyopathy may develop. The morphologic features of this condition include left ventricular chamber dilatation and hypertrophy of the noninfarcted myocardium (Fig. 21.6). Additionally, associated right

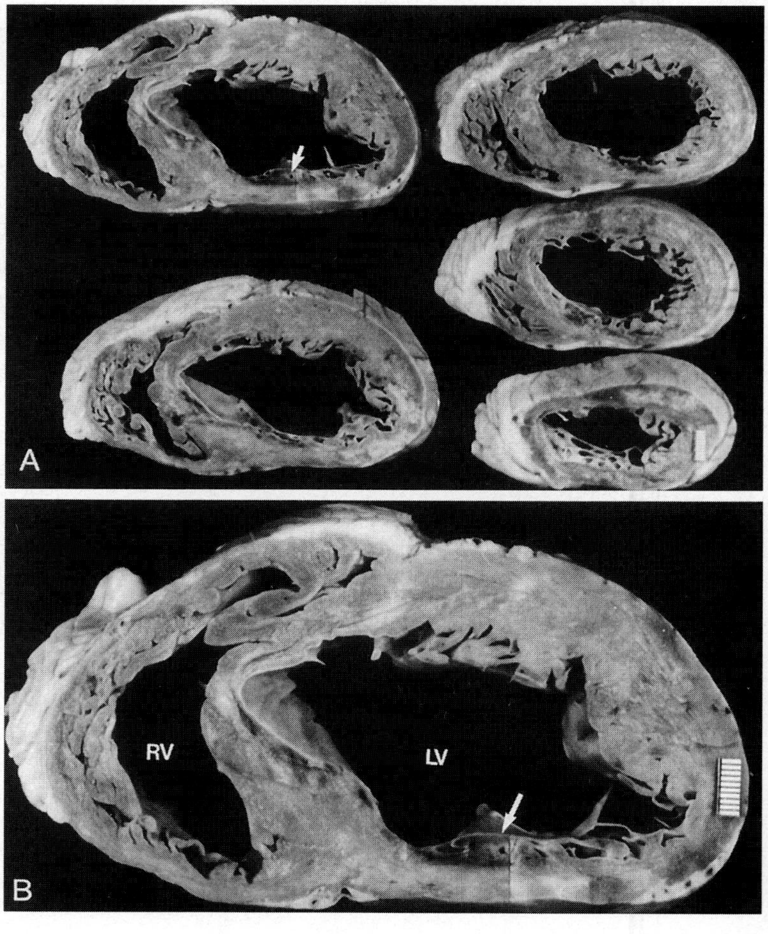

Figure 21.6. Ischemic cardiomyopathy. Transverse sections from apex to base of the right (*RV*) and left (*LV*) ventricles (**A**), and close-up of the basal-most section (**B**), from an 86-year-old man with a history of MI and congestive heart failure. Autopsy revealed ischemic cardiomyopathy with biventricular dilation and healed anteroseptal and posterolateral transmural MI. Note associated infarction and thinning of the posteromedial papillary muscle (*arrow*).

atrial, right ventricular, and left atrial chamber dilatation are often seen. The clinical features of ischemic cardiomyopathy include systolic dysfunction with congestive heart failure, systemic emboli from left ventricular thrombus, ventricular arrhythmias, and shortened survival when compared to patients with smaller MI with ischemic cardiomyopathy.

LEFT VENTRICULAR ANEURYSM

A subgroup of patients with ischemic cardiomyopathy are those with left ventricular aneurysm (Fig. 21.7). A left ventricular aneurysm is a wide-mouthed, convex, cavitary protrusion of the left ventricular free wall during both systole and diastole (21, 22). The aneurysm wall is thin and consists of fibrous tissue with or without residual myocardial fibers. Left ventricular aneurysms are associated with large MIs in all locations, but are most frequent with anterior MI. The noninfarcted portion of the left ventricle dilates and hypertrophies, and the left atrium and right-sided chambers often dilate. The usual clinical consequences of left ventricular aneurysm are congestive heart failure and ventricular arrhythmias. Although older studies also reported frequent peripheral emboli, more recent reports have suggested that patients with left ventricular aneurysm rarely have clinically apparent systemic emboli (21) despite the high frequency (50%) of the intra-aneurysmal thrombus (Fig. 21.8). This has been attributed to the noncontractile nature of the aneurysm wall (scar) and relative protection of the thrombus from left ventricular turbulent blood flow because of its intra-aneurysmal location. If a clinical embolic event occurs, it usually does so during the first several weeks after MI (23). Recent clinical and autopsy studies have suggested that the development of a left ventricular aneurysm after MI is associated with a high 1-year mortality rate (22, 24). Although left ventricular aneurysmectomy may result in symptomatic improvement (congestive heart failure and ventricular arrhythmias), there is no evidence that surgery improves long-term survival.

RIGHT VENTRICULAR MYOCARDIAL INFARCTION

Right ventricular MI has been recognized at autopsy for several decades (25–29). Although there have been reports of isolated right ventricular infarction, it is virtually always associated with infarction of the left ventricular wall and septum. Although most recent autopsy studies have re-

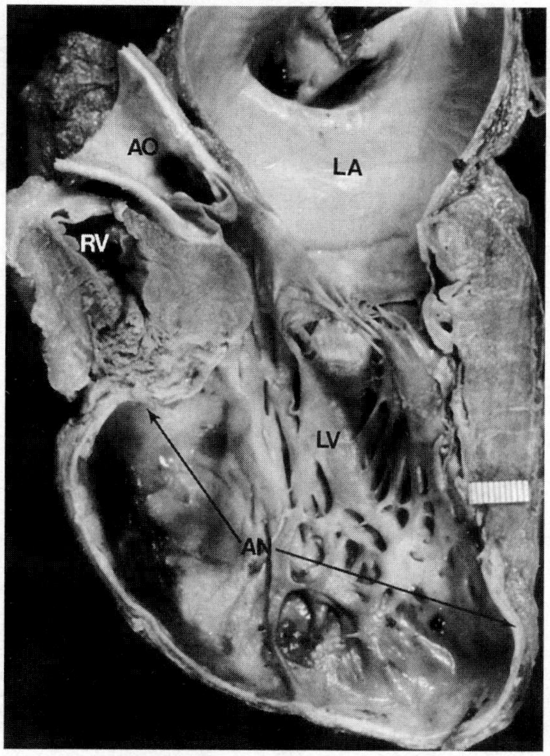

Figure 21.7. Left ventricular aneurysm. Longitudinal section through the left atrium (*LA*), left ventricle (*LV*), aorta (*AO*), and right ventricular outflow tract (*RV*) of a 72-year-old woman with a history of myocardial infarction and subsequent congestive heart failure who died of intractable ventricular arrhythmias. At autopsy a large, anteroapical aneurysm (*AN*) was seen.

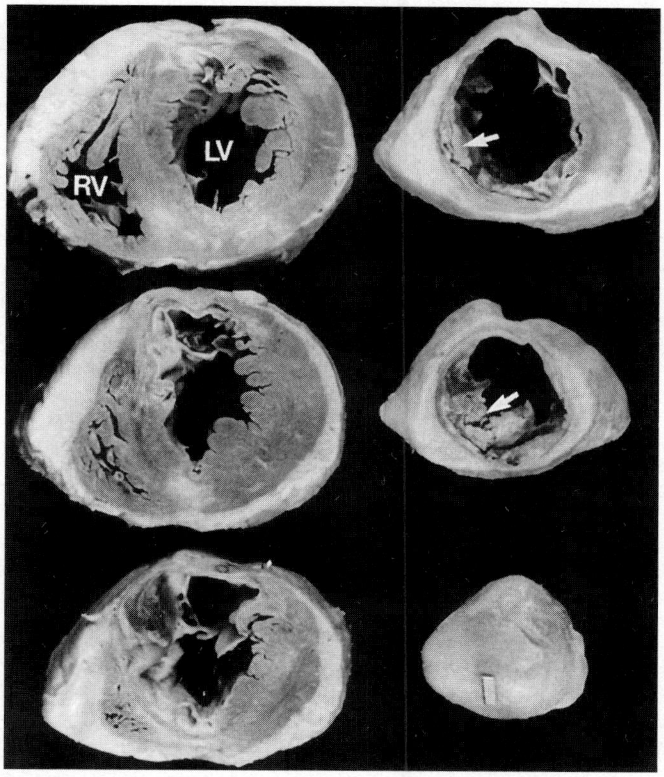

Figure 21.8. Intra-aneurysmal thrombus. Transverse 1-cm thick sections from apex to base of the right (*RV*) and left (*LV*) ventricles from an 86-year-old woman with a history of hypertension, congestive heart failure, and MI. At autopsy there was a transmural anteroseptal MI extending from base to apex with an anteroapical left ventricular aneurysm containing thrombus (*arrow*).

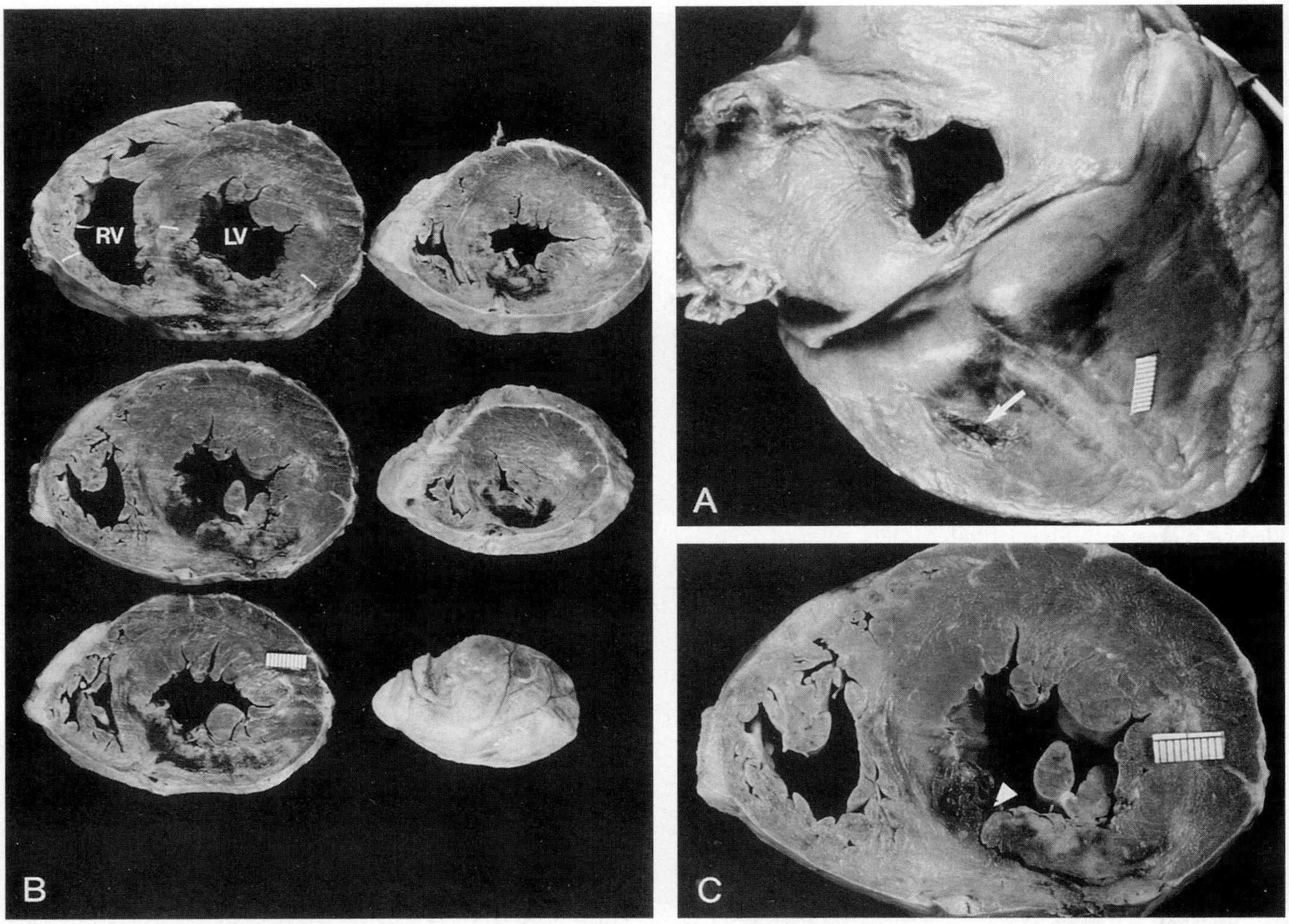

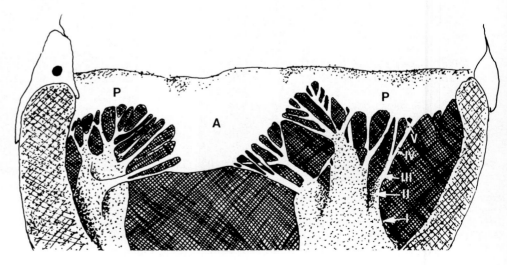

Figure 21.9. Right ventricular myocardial infarction. The heart from a 61-year-old man who died suddenly 3 days after his first myocardial infarction. Two hundred milliliters of blood filled the pericardial space. **A:** A rupture site was identified on the posterior surface of the left ventricle before it was opened (*arrow*). **B:** Transverse section of the ventricles revealed an acute posterior and septal infarct that extended from base to apex, and involved the posterior right ventricle (*RV*) with consequent dilatation of that chamber. The extent of the MI in the basal slice is delineated by brackets. *LV* = left ventricle. **C:** A close-up of a single slice shows the entry site of the rupture at the junction of the free wall and septum (*arrowhead*).

Figure 21.10. Mitral valve apparatus. The anterolateral and posteromedial papillary muscles each provide support for both the anterior (*A*) and posterior (*P*) leaflets. The branching structure of the support system is demonstrated: *I* = papillary muscle base; *II* = papillary muscle head; *III* = primary cord; *IV* = secondary chord; and *V* = tertiary chord. The hemodynamic significance of rupture in the support system is determined by the level of the rupture. Rupture of a papillary muscle head or primary chord can produce severe regurgitation, whereas rupture of a tertiary chord may have no clinical consequence.

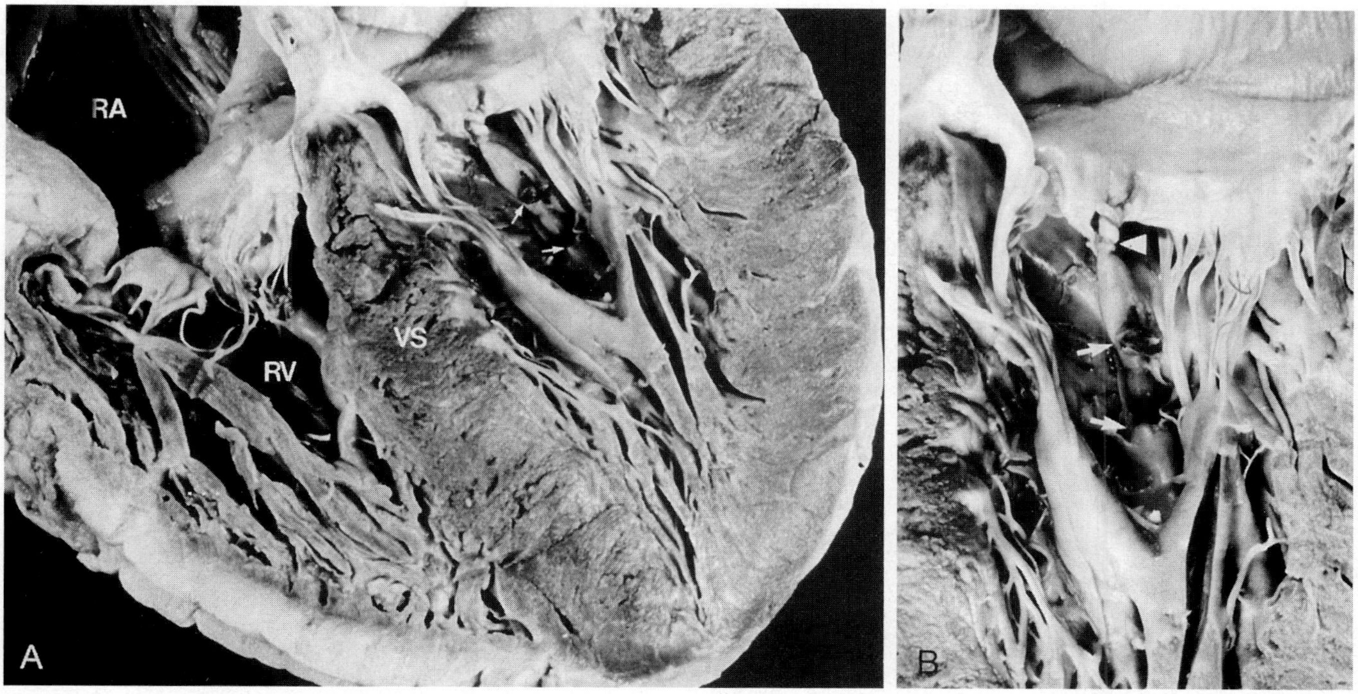

Figure 21.11. Rupture of papillary muscle head. Longitudinal section of the heart (**A**) and close-up of the mitral valve apparatus (**B**) from a 94-year-old woman with no prior cardiac history who developed acute pulmonary edema and died 3 days after MI. At the time of acute hemodynamic deterioration a new murmur of mitral regurgitation was noted and echocardiography revealed an echogenic mass attached to the posterior leaflet of the mitral valve that prolapsed into the left atrium during ventricular systole. At autopsy, an acute posteroseptal infarction was complicated by rupture of one head of the posteromedial papillary muscle (*arrows*), which was attached to the posterior leaflet of the mitral valve. Note coiling of the chordal attachments (*arrowhead*), which is often seen with papillary muscle rupture and presumably results from vigorous movements of the ruptured head. *RA* = right atrium; *RV* = right ventricle; and *VS* = ventricular septum.

ported right ventricular infarction occurring exclusively in association with inferior (posterior) wall left ventricular MI (27, 28) (Fig. 21.9), older studies and a recent autopsy study have described a similar frequency of anterior and posterior right ventricular infarction (29, 30). Right ventricular infarction can produce right ventricular and right atrial dilation. This can be seen on radionuclide and echocardiographic images, and is often seen at autopsy (Fig. 21.9). A recent report suggested that right ventricular MI can be diagnosed with a high degree of certainty if regional right ventricular dysfunction is present on equilibrium radionuclide angiography (31). Right ventricular MI may cause predominant right-sided congestive heart failure and may present as significant systemic hypotension because of inadequate left ventricular filling. Right heart catheterization of patients with right ventricular infarction may demonstrate high right atrial and right ventricular end-diastolic pressures that approach or exceed mean pulmonary capillary wedge pressure (32). It is important to recognize right ventricular MI as a cause of hypotension in the peri-MI period because appropriate treatment (volume expansion) may significantly improve short-term prognosis. Although clinical features of right ventricular MI are well-described, clinicopathologic studies have reported many patients with right ventricular infarction at autopsy without signs of right ventricular dysfunction during life (27).

PAPILLARY MUSCLE INFARCTION

Myocardial infarction can involve the anterolateral or posteromedial papillary muscle and produce dysfunction and consequent mitral regurgitation. Occasionally, infarction of a papillary muscle results in papillary muscle rupture. Since each papillary muscle provides support for both the anterior and posterior mitral valve leaflets (Fig. 21.10), rupture of either papillary muscle can undermine support of both leaflets. Rupture through the base of the papillary muscle (usually posteromedial) is associated with acute onset of severe mitral regurgitation and congestive heart failure. It is rare for a patient to survive this type of papillary muscle rupture long enough to undergo corrective surgery. Each papillary muscle divides into two or three heads, and rupture of one of the heads (Fig. 21.11) produces less severe hemodynamic compromise than rupture of the entire papillary muscle and may allow surgical repair.

LEFT VENTRICULAR RUPTURE

Rupture of the left ventricular free wall is a complication of anterior (Fig. 21.12) or posterior (inferior) (Fig. 21.9) MI and causes pericardial tamponade and sudden death. Rare

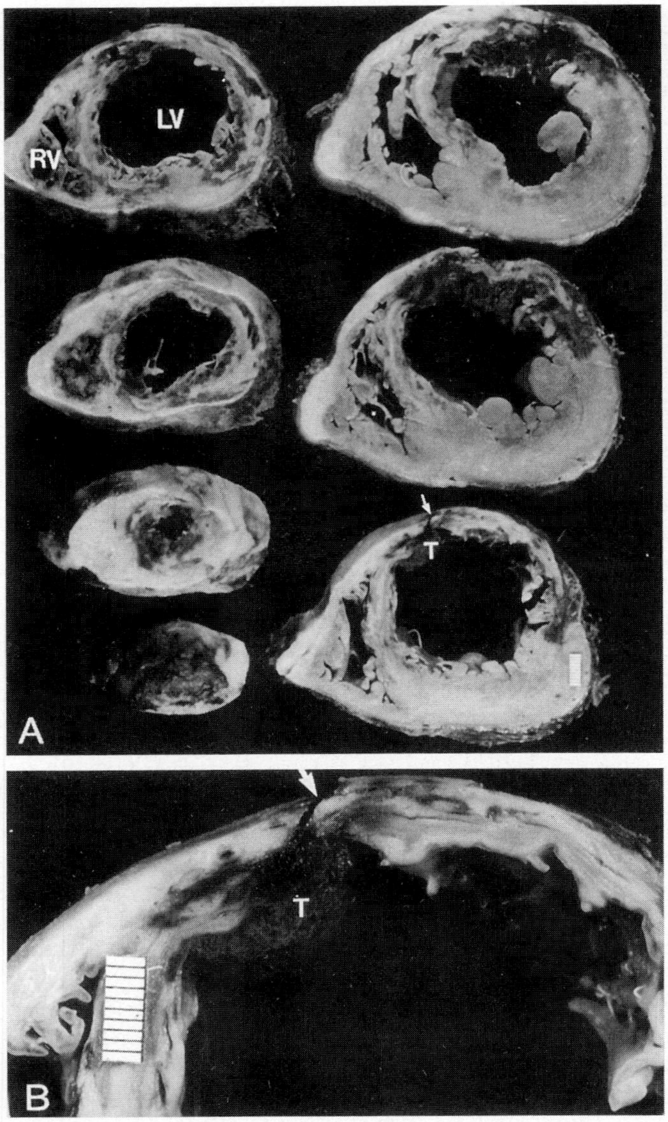

Figure 21.12. Rupture of left ventricular free wall. Transverse sections from apex to base of the right (*RV*) and left (*LV*) ventricles (**A**), and close-up of the anterior wall (**B**) from the heart of a 36-year-old man with a history of hypertension who developed electromechanical dissociation and died suddenly 13 days after his first MI. At autopsy 300 ml of blood filled the pericardial space. There was transmural necrosis of the anterior wall and the anterior septum from base to apex, becoming circumferential at the apex. An anterior mural thrombus (*T*) was adjacent to the rupture site (*arrow*) at the junction of the anterior left ventricular wall and the interventricular septum.

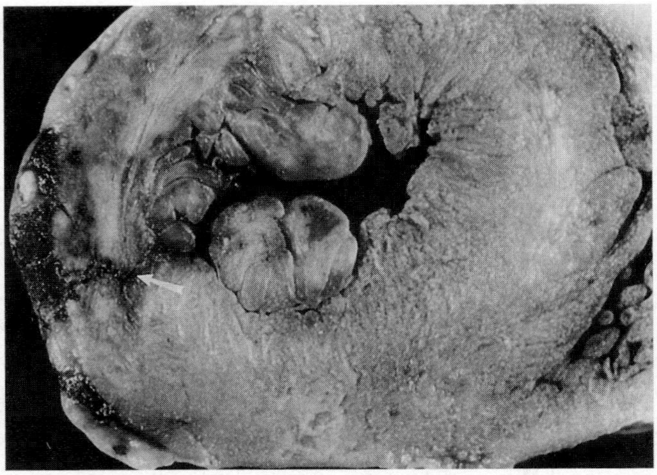

Figure 21.13. Rupture at normal-necrotic myocardium junction. Transverse section through the mid-left ventricle of a 68-year-old woman with a history of systemic hypertension and angina pectoris who died in electromechanical dissociation 4 days after her first MI. At autopsy 300 ml of blood filled the pericardial space, with rupture through the lateral wall of the left ventricle at the junction of the normal and necrotic myocardium (*arrow*). The infarct involves the anterolateral wall of the left ventricle from base to apex and there is significant left ventricular hypertrophy. The MI is relatively small and consequently there is no left ventricular chamber dilation.

cases of subacute rupture with surgical repair have been reported (33, 34). Rupture usually occurs 2–5 days after MI, but can occur up to 2 weeks after MI. It most commonly occurs with first MI and in patients with a history of systemic hypertension (35, 36). Thinning of the wall and dilatation in the area of infarction (expansion) is often seen (37). The most likely sites for rupture are the junction of the normal and necrotic myocardium (Fig. 21.13) (36) and the junction of the free wall and septum in the area of infarction (Figs. 21.9 and 21.12). Rarely, if extensive visceral and parietal pericardial adhesions overlie the area of infarction, rupture may result in formation of a false aneurysm (38). The rupture in that case is usually clinically silent and the false aneurysm is detected by noninvasive (39) or invasive imaging or at autopsy. A false aneurysm is distinguished during life from a true aneurysm by its narrow mouth, which is usually apparent on echocardiographic, radionuclide, or angiographic images. A false aneurysm, in contrast to a true aneurysm, is likely to rupture, and, therefore, documentation of its presence is an indication for resection.

Rupture of the ventricular septum (Fig. 21.14) may occur with anterior or posterior infarction and is marked by the acute onset of congestive heart failure, hypotension, and a new systolic murmur. Like free wall rupture, septal rupture usually occurs 2–5 days after MI and is commonly associated with a history of systemic hypertension (40). In contrast to free wall rupture, septal rupture may be compatible with survival and subsequent surgical repair.

CORONARY ARTERY BYPASS SURGERY

It is increasingly common to study hearts at autopsy from patients who have undergone previous coronary artery bypass surgery. Intimal thickening occurs in all saphenous vein grafts within a few months of insertion (41). Occlusion of vein grafts can be due to thrombus formation or atherosclerotic plaque. Patients who develop graft occlusion

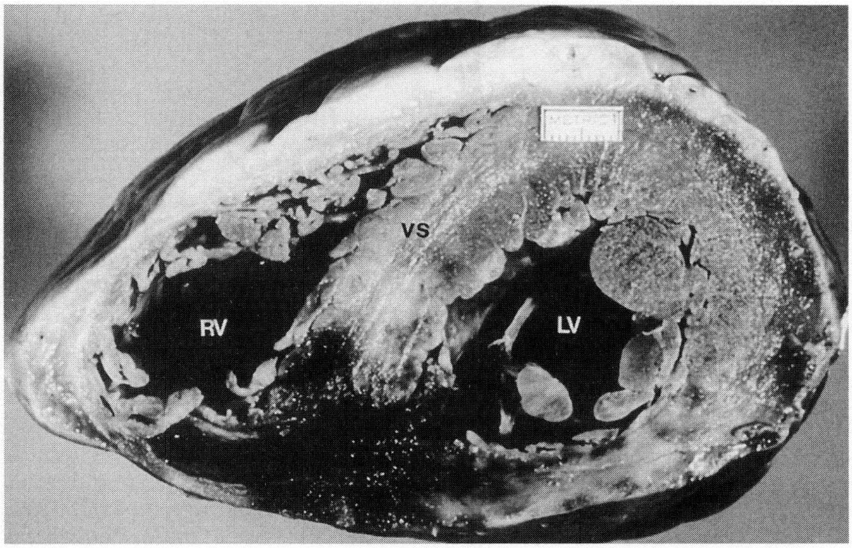

Figure 21.14. Rupture of the ventricular septum. Transverse section of both ventricles at the level of the papillary muscles from a 59-year-old woman who suddenly developed cariogenic shock 4 days after inferior wall myocardial infarction. At autopsy there was transmural necrosis of the posterior left ventricle (*LV*), right ventricle (*RV*), and interventricular septum (*VS*). Rupture at the junction of the posterior wall of the LV and VS caused a ventricular septal defect. Note the increased epicardial fat often found in patients with ventricular septal or free wall rupture.

within a few months of surgery generally have occlusion by thrombus and almost always have severe atherosclerosis in the native coronary artery at, or distal to, the anastomotic site (42). In patients with late graft occlusion, the appearance of the grafts is similar to that of native atherosclerotic coronary arteries, with intimal fibrous proliferation and occasional lipid deposition. It is unclear whether development of atherosclerosis in vein grafts is caused by an underlying systemic propensity for atherosclerosis (i.e., hypercholesterolemia) or by mechanical factors.

VALVULAR HEART DISEASE

MITRAL VALVE

Mitral Stenosis

Although (rarely) infective endocarditis (Fig. 21.15) or intracardiac tumor can cause mitral stenosis, mitral stenosis in the adult is usually a consequence of rheumatic heart disease. Rheumatic disease may cause functional abnormalities of any of the four cardiac valves, but is most commonly associated with abnormalities of the mitral valve with or without involvement of the aortic, tricuspid, or pulmonic valves. The most common functional consequence of rheumatic mitral valve disease is stenosis with or without regurgitation (43). The mitral valve abnormality can range from mild thickening or retraction of the leaflets to extensive thickening and calcification with fusion of one or both commissures and fusion of the chordae tendineae (Fig. 21.16). The basal part of the leaflets, particularly the anterior leaflet, are usually less thickened and maintain some degree of flexibility. Thickening of the free edges produces a funnel-like appearance with narrowing of the orifice. Functional narrowing may be exacerbated by subvalvular obstruction from severe chordal fusion. Because of elevated left atrial pressure in mitral stenosis, the left atrium dilates, and there may also be associated right atrial and ventricular dilatation. Although thrombus in the left atrial appendage occurs in a variety of cardiac diseases (Fig. 21.17), thrombus in the body of the left atrium is virtually only seen with mitral stenosis. Clinical consequences of mitral stenosis include congestive heart failure from elevated pulmonary venous pressure and systemic embolization from left atrial thrombus. When elevated right-sided pressures develop, signs and symptoms of right heart failure may predominate.

Mitral Regurgitation

Pure mitral regurgitation of the basis of rheumatic disease occurs, but is unusual (44). Mitral regurgitation is usually caused by an abnormality in the support system of an otherwise normal mitral valve. Such abnormalities include myocardial infarction with papillary muscle dysfunction or rupture, dilated cardiomyopathy (ischemic or nonischemic) with displacement of the papillary muscles, and elongation or spontaneous rupture of a chord. The clinical outcome of chordal rupture is determined by the level at which rupture occurs (Fig. 21.10). The other common etiology of pure mitral regurgitation is mitral valve prolapse (45). With prolapse, the valve leaflets are hooded, thickened, and have an increased surface area relative to the annular size (Fig. 21.18). The chordae may be lengthened and can rupture. It has not been determined whether the "click-murmur syndrome" without severe mitral regurgitation is usually associated with this typical morphologic appearance. Mitral valve prolapse is usually an isolated phenomenon, but has been reported in association with a variety of disorders, including atrial septal defect, Ebsteins's anomaly, and Marfan's syndrome. Other causes of pure mitral regurgitation include infective endocarditis with destruction or perforation of a valve leaflet and mitral "annular" calcification (Fig. 21.19).

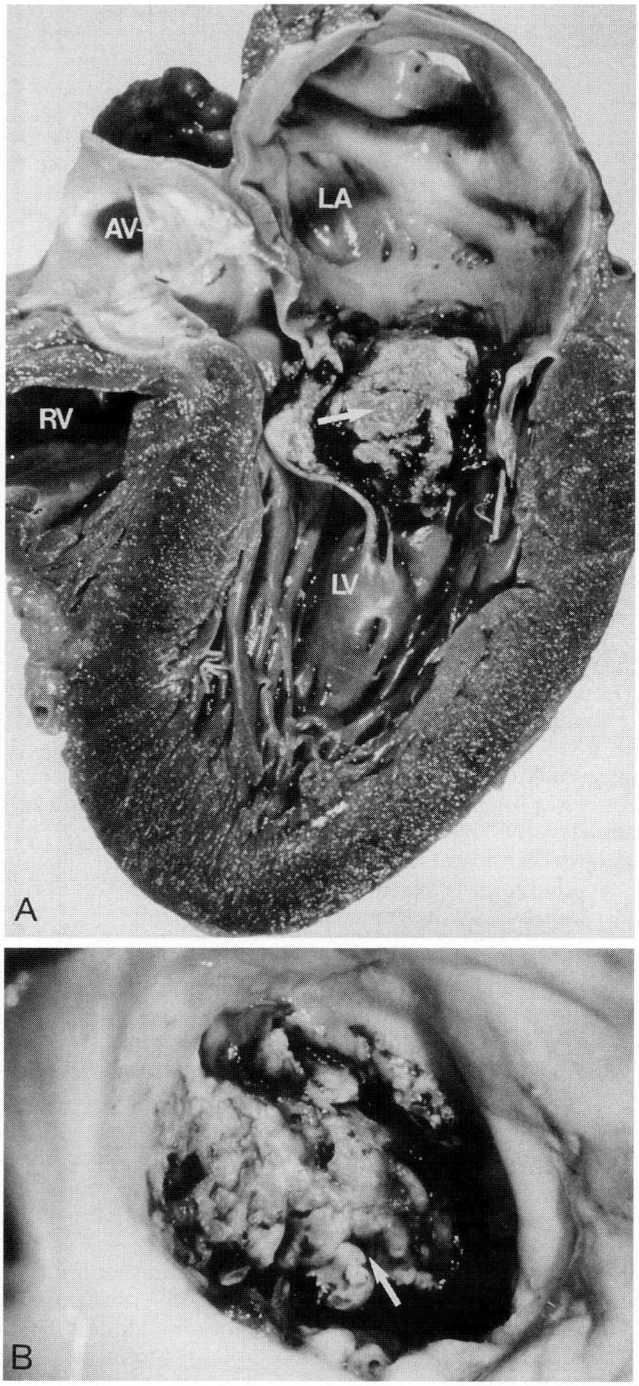

Figure 21.15. Mitral stenosis with infective endocarditis. Longitudinal section of the heart (**A**), and view of the mitral valve through the left atrium (**B**) of 71-year-old man who died 8 weeks after *Staphylococcus aureus* infective endocarditis was diagnosed. At autopsy, a massive infected vegetation (*arrow*) wad adherent to the anterior mitral valve leaflet, causing significant mitral stenosis. The usual functional consequence of infective endocarditis is valvular regurgitation, but rarely, as in this case, a massive vegetation may obstruct the valve orifice. *AV* = aortic valve; *LA* = left atrium; *RV* = right ventricle; and *LV* = left ventricular.

AORTIC VALVE DISORDERS

Aortic Stenosis

Aortic stenosis may be congenital or acquired. The age of the patient at the time aortic stenosis presents is strongly related to the etiology (45). Within the first 15 years of life, aortic stenosis is usually caused by a congenitally stenotic, unicommisural (unicuspid) valve. Aortic stenosis developing between the ages of 15 and 65 years is most commonly associated with a bicuspid aortic valve. A bicuspid valve is rarely congenitally stenotic but, because of its abnormal structure, may become stenotic through acceleration of degenerative changes. The valve leaflets become thickened and may become calcified, with fusion of one or both commissures. Occasionally a bicuspid aortic valve does not develop any functional abnormalities and is an incidental finding at autopsy (Fig. 21.20). The incidence of bicuspid aortic valve has been reported to be as high as 2% (45) of the population. Ninety percent or more of patients over the age of 65 with aortic stenosis have a tricuspid valve with fibrous thickening and calcification of each of the cusps. Calcification generally occurs on the aortic aspects of the cusps and severe commissural fusion is rare (Fig. 21.21). This type of aortic stenosis may be confused morphologically with rheumatic aortic stenosis. The latter is rare and is always associated with anatomic abnormalities of the mitral valve. Additionally, rheumatic stenosis is usually associated with severe fusion of one or more of the commissures. Critical aortic stenosis produces left ventricular hypertrophy, with thickening of the free wall and septum, but usually without dilatation of the left ventricular cavity (Fig. 21.21). The impaired diastolic function of the thick-walled, noncompliant left ventricle may combine with outflow obstruction by the stenotic valve to elevate left ventricular end-diastolic and stolic and left atrial pressures, causing left atrial dilatation and congestive heart failure.

Aortic Regurgitation

Aortic regurgitation usually occurs in association with aortic stenosis. Pure aortic regurgitation is caused by abnormalities of the valve leaflets or aortic root. Rarely, thickening and retraction of a bicuspid aortic valve (46) or rheumatic involvement of a tricuspid valve produces pure aortic regurgitation. Infective endocarditis can also cause aortic regurgitation by damaging one or more of the valve leaflets (Fig. 21.22). Dilatation of the aortic root can occur with Marfan's syndrome, syphilitic aortitis, systemic hypertension (47), or atherosclerotic aneurysm, and can produce aortic regurgitation by preventing coaptation of the normal valve leaflets. Aortic root dissection may also produce acute aortic regurgitation by undermining the support of one or more cusps.

PROSTHETIC VALVE DISORDERS

Bioprostheses (most commonly porcine) can become stenotic or regurgitant. Stenosis is caused by thickening, cal-

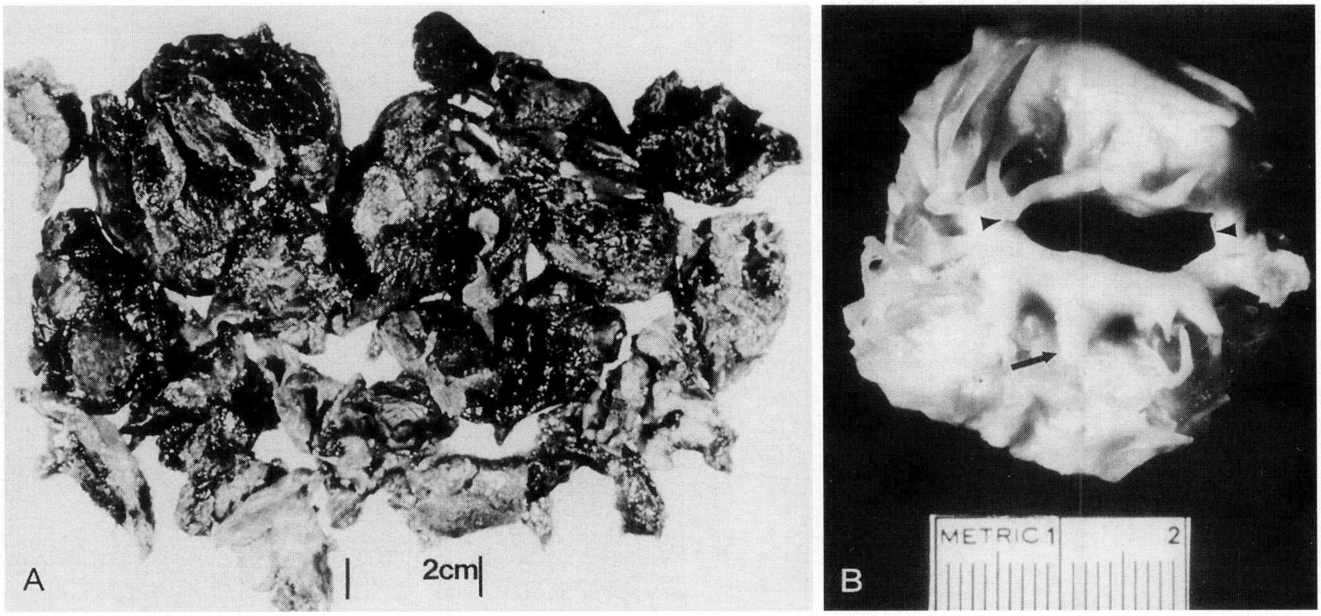

Figure 21.16. Rheumatic mitral stenosis. Left atrial thrombus (**A**) and ventricular side of the excised mitral valve (**B**) from a 44-year-old woman with a history of mitral stenosis, atrial fibrillation, and a brainstem stroke 6 months prior to mitral valve replacement. At surgery, a massive thrombus filled the left atrium. The valve shows the typical "fishmouth" appearance of rheumatic mitral stenosis, with fibrous thickening of both leaflets, commissural fusion (*arrowheads*), and thickening and fusion of the chordae tendineae (*arrow*).

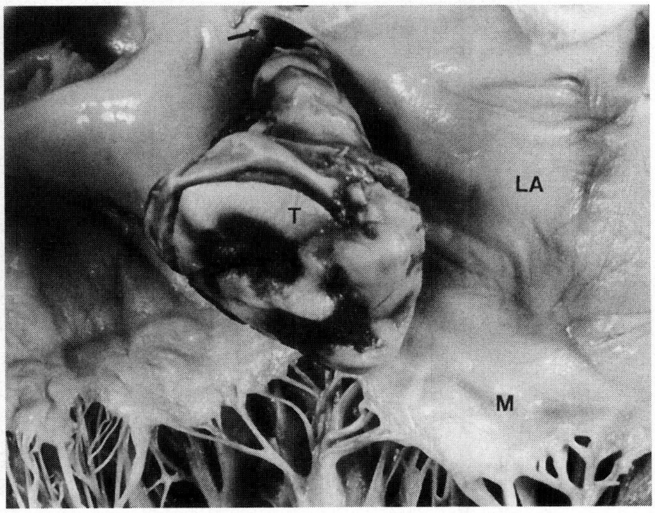

Figure 21.17. Thrombus in left atrial appendage. Opened left atrium from 70-year-old woman with a history of chronic atrial fibrillation and multiple strokes who died of congestive heart failure. At autopsy, a large pedunculated thrombus (*T*) originated in the left atrial appendage (*arrow*) and protruded into the left atrium (*LA*). The mitral valve (*M*) was normal.

cification, and immobilization of the leaflets (Fig. 21.23) and regurgitation by disruption of the leaflets from degenerative changes of infective endocarditis. Mechanical prostheses are of two general types: caged ball and tilting disc (Fig. 21.24). Caged ball valves always have an intrinsic pressure gradient. The gradient may produce hemodynamically significant stenosis if a large prosthesis is placed in a small orifice (Fig. 21.24). A caged ball prosthesis can become regurgitant from ingrowth of fibrous tissue or thrombus formation at the base of the cage, preventing adequate seating of the ball. Thrombus formation or fibrous ingrowth can also impede disc motion in the tilting disc valves, causing stenosis or regurgitation. The valve disc can become "frozen" in a partially open position, producing a mixture of stenosis and regurgitation. Rarely, suture overhang can cause regurgitation by preventing closure (48). Regurgitation through a paravalvular leak can occur with any type of prosthesis and can be due to inadequate suturing or infection at the suture line.

CARDIOMYOPATHY

Dilated Cardiomyopathy

Dilated cardiomyopathy is associated with left ventricular systolic dysfunction. It is frequently a consequence of a previous large MI (ischemic cardiomyopathy) (Fig. 21.6), but may also be idiopathic or secondary to an infiltrative process or to long-standing valvular dysfunction (9). Alcoholic and peripathum cardiomyopathies are included in the category of idiopathic dilated cardiomyopathy. Idiopathic dilated cardiomyopathy is characterized by dilatation of all four cardiac chambers with a markedly increased heart weight and normal or increased wall thickness (Fig. 21.25). The left ventricle contains mural thrombus in approximately 50% of cases and the frequency of clinically apparent systemic emboli may be as high as 25–30%. Histologically, there are no distinguishing features of idio-

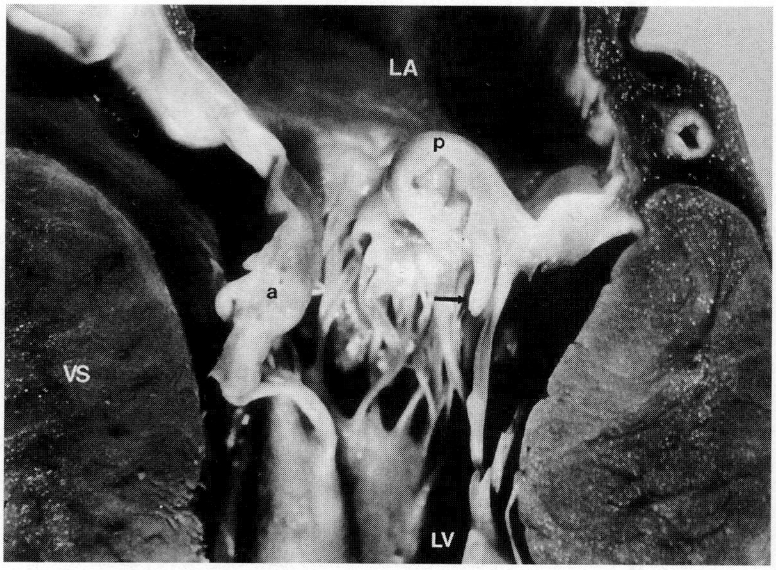

Figure 21.18. Mitral valve prolapse. Longitudinal section through the left atrium (*LA*), anterior (*a*) and posterior (*P*) mitral valve leaflets, interventricular septum (*VS*), and left ventricle (*LV*) from a patient with sudden death. At autopsy a redundant, "floppy," posterior leaflet of the mitral valve prolapsed into the left atrium and was associated with a ruptured chord (*arrow*).

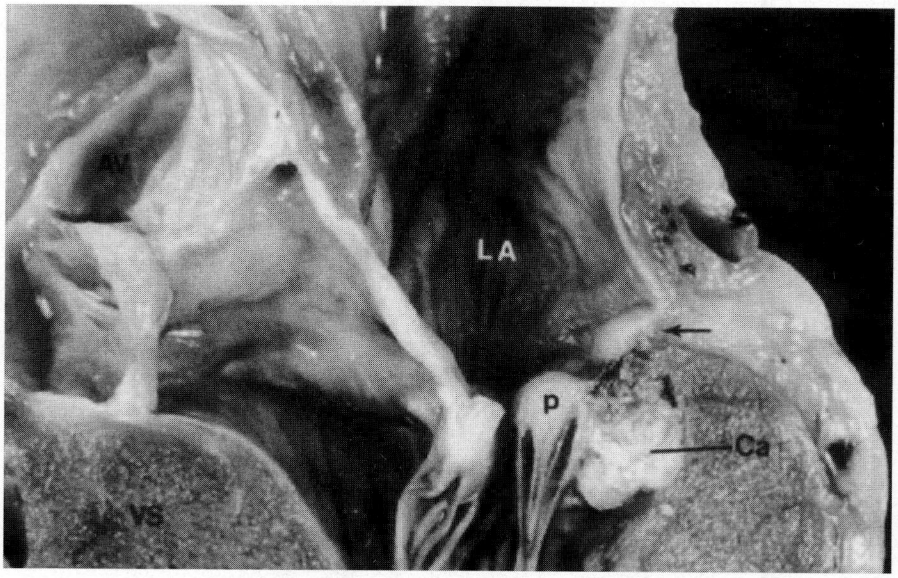

Figure 21.19. Mitral "annular" calcification. Left atrium (*LA*), mitral valve, and aortic valve (*AV*), in a longitudinal section of the heart from a 68-year-old woman with a history of angina pectoris, MI, and cardiac rupture. A large deposit of mitral "annular" calcium (*Ca*) is seen behind the posterior mitral valve leaflet (*p*) and below the anulus (*arrow*). Mitral "annular" calcium can be detected by cardiac ultrasound and is often found at autopsy in elderly patients. The term annular is inaccurate because the calcium is usually within the myocardium behind the valve leaflet and below the anulus. Although "annular" calcium rarely compromises valve function, it has been reported in association with mitral regurgitation.

pathic dilated cardiomyopathy, although increased interstitial myocardial fibrosis is sometimes seen. Some investigators have postulated that idiopathic dilated cardiomyopathy results from a previously undiagnosed episode of myocarditis. This has not been substantiated either clinically or pathologically. Dilated cardiomyopathy may develop as a consequence of left ventricular volume overload associated with aortic or mitral regurgitation. Although initially ventricular function is preserved, longstanding volume overload of the left ventricle may produce an irreversible cardiomyopathy. Such patients may have progressive congestive heart failure despite valve replacement.

Nondilated Cardiomyopathy

Nondilated cardiomyopathy is generally associated with normal systolic function and abnormal diastolic function

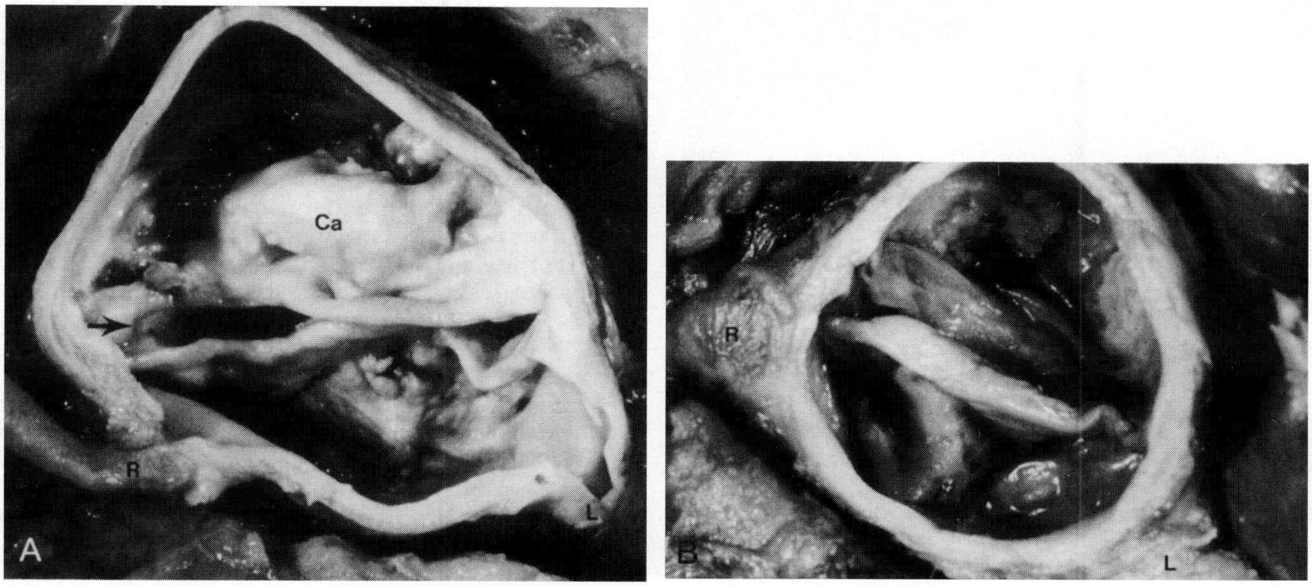

Figure 21.20. Bicuspid aortic valve. Stenotic (**A**) and nonstenotic (**B**) bicuspid aortic valves. The stenotic valve is from a 50-year-old man who died in congestive heart failure. It is thickened and calcified (*Ca*) and there is partial fusion of one commissure (*arrow*). The nonstenotic valve was an incidental finding at autopsy in a 61-year-old man who died of cardiac rupture as a complication of MI. The leaflets are mildly thickened but freely mobile. The cusps of a bicuspid aortic valve may be oriented to the right and left, with each coronary artery originating from its own coronary sinus, or anteriorly and posteriorly, as pictured here, with both the right (*R*) and left (*L*) coronary artery arising from the anterior sinus.

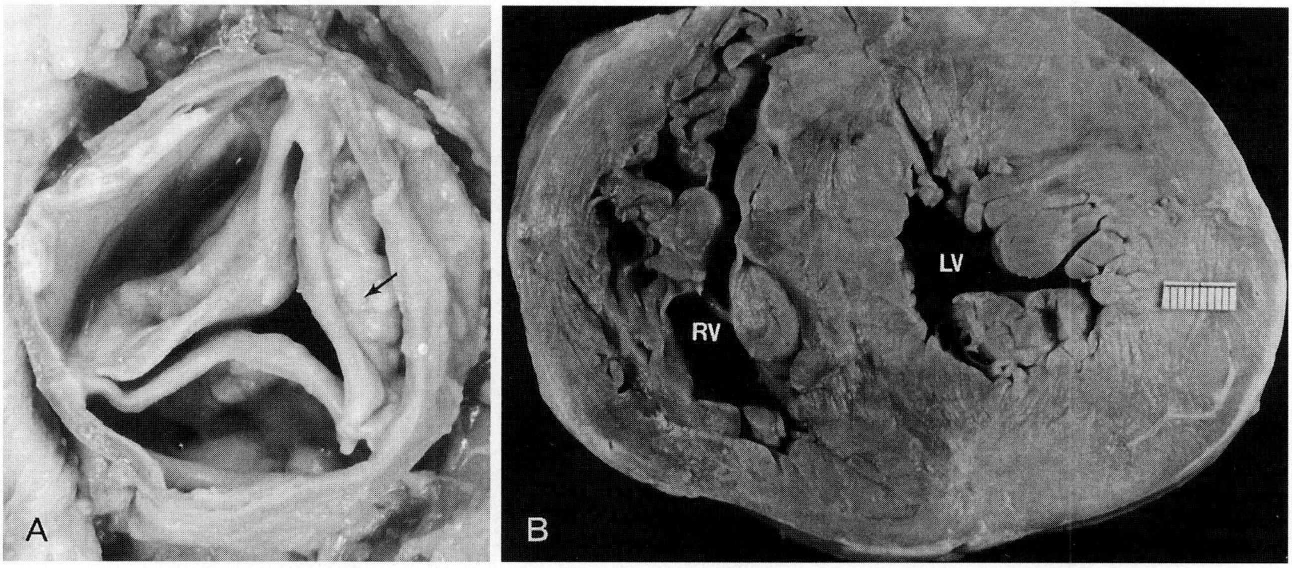

Figure 21.21. Degenerative aortic stenosis. Aortic valve (**A**) and left ventricle (**B**) from an 83-year-old man with a history of syncope who died in congestive heart failure. At autopsy, the left ventricle was hypertrophied and nondilated. The aortic valve was severely stenotic with fibrous thickening of all three cusps and extensive calcium deposition (*arrow*) on the aortic side of the valve leaflets. In contrast to the findings in rheumatic aortic stenosis, there was little commissural fusion and the mitral valve was normal. *LV* = left ventricle; *RV* = right ventricle.

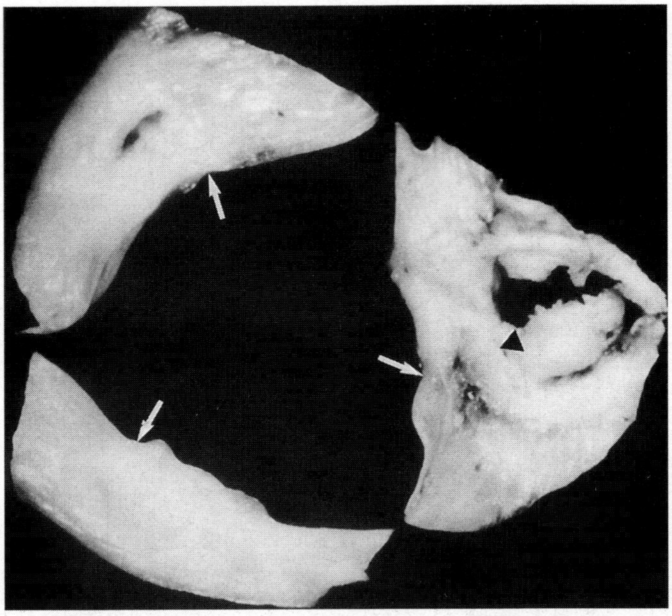

Figure 21.22. Aortic regurgitation with infective endocarditis. Surgically excised tricuspid aortic valve from a 28-year-old intravenous drug abuser with a history of infective endocarditis and subsequent aortic regurgitation. A large perforation of one cusp (*arrowhead*) and retraction and indentations (*arrows*) of all three cusps are hallmarks of healed infective endocarditis.

(the left ventricle empties normally but fills abnormally because of abnormal myocardial compliance). As a result, left atrial pressure and pulmonary venous pressure become elevated and congestive heart failure develops. Nondilated cardiomyopathy may be caused by severe long-standing hypertension with thickening of the left ventricular wall (Fig. 21.26).

Hypertrophic cardiomyopathy (also referred to as idiopathic hypertrophic subaortic stenosis, asymmetric septal hypertrophy, etc.) is defined as hypertrophy of the left ventricle without left ventricular dilatation and the absence of other causes of left ventricular hypertrophy (i.e., hypertension, aortic stenosis) (49). It is generally associated with asymmetric septal hypertrophy, and in approximately 50% of cases left ventricular outflow tract obstruction is present (Fig. 21.27). Rarely, significant hypertrophy of the right ventricle is associated with right ventricular outflow obstruction. Extensive myocardial fiber disarray can be seen on microscopic examination of the left ventricular free wall or ventricular septum. The left atrium is dilated in most patients with hypertrophic cardiomyopathy and the right atrium and right ventricle may also be dilated. Hypertrophic cardiomyopathy may be inherited and is associated with an increased risk of sudden death, particularly in young people.

Nondilated cardiomyopathy may also result from extensive myocardial amyloid deposition. Amyloidosis of the heart is rarely an isolated finding and one usually sees extensive amyloid infiltration of other tissues.

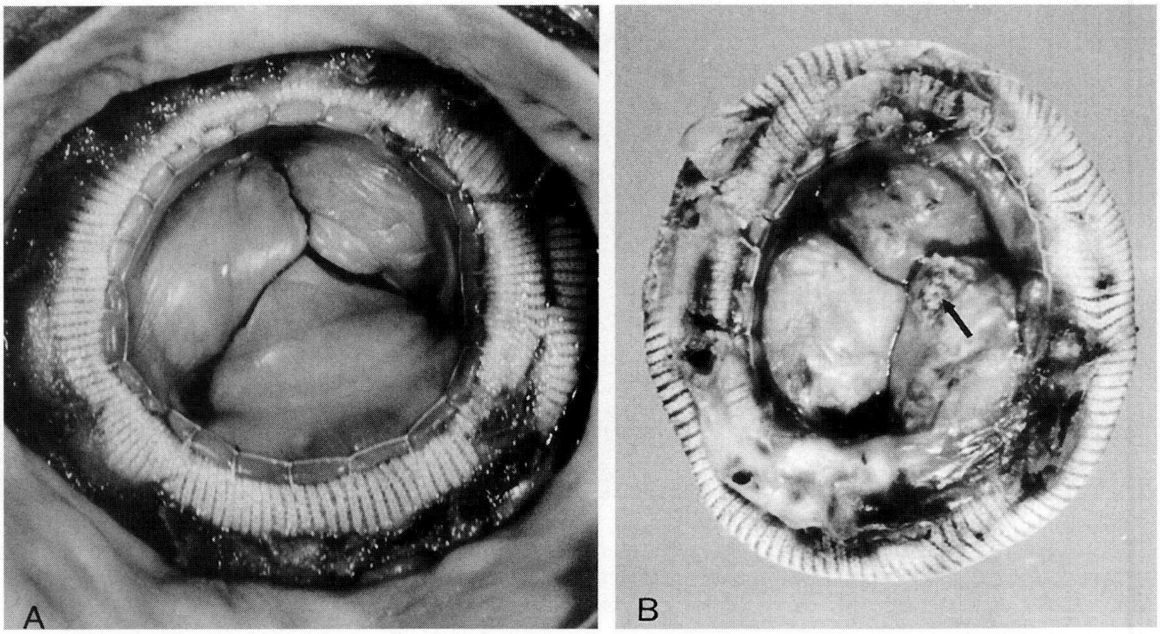

Figure 21.23. Stenosis of prosthetic valve. Normal in situ (**A**) and stenotic excised (**B**) porcine bioprostheses. There is calcification (*arrow*) and fibrous thickening of the stenotic valve.

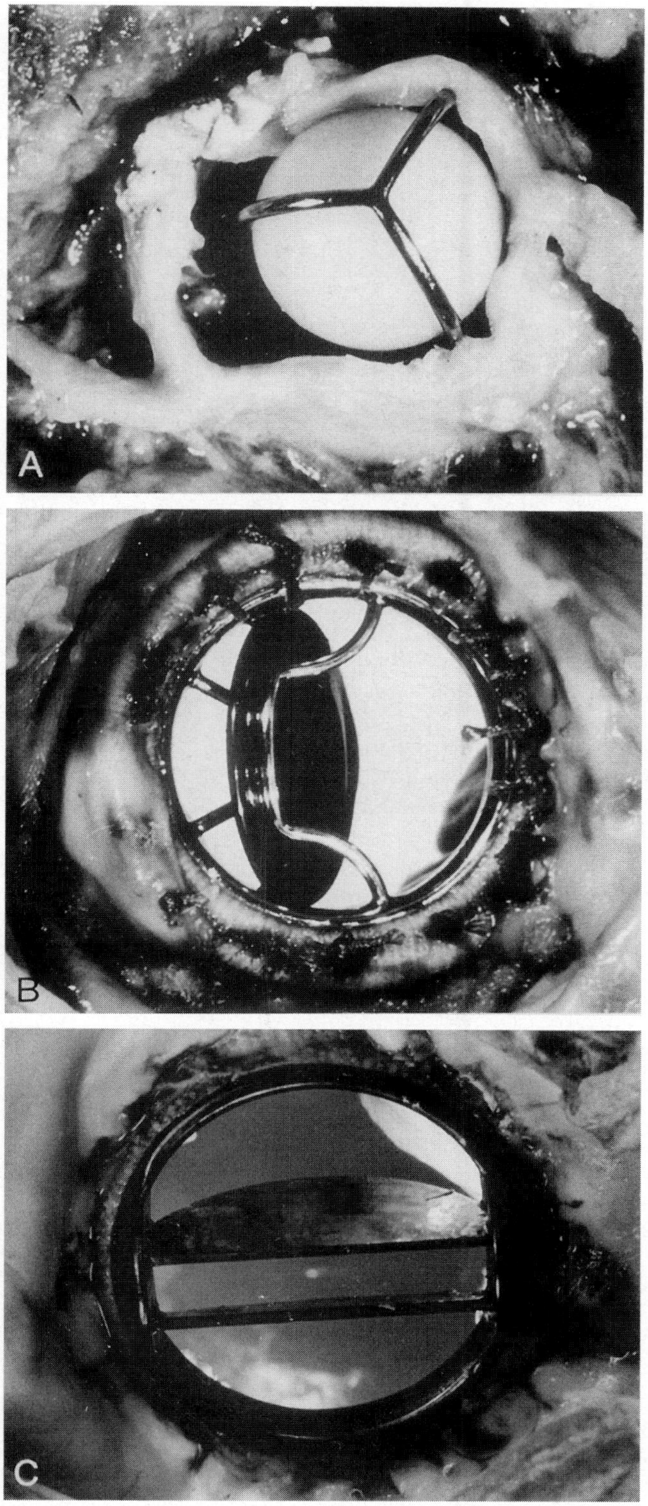

Figure 21.24. Types of mechanical prostheses. St. Judes mitral (**C**), Bjork-Shiley mitral (**B**), and Starr Edwards aortic (**A**) prosthetic valves are shown in the open position. The ball of the Starr Edwards prosthesis fills a major portion of the aorta and may be associated with a significant pressure gradient between the left ventricle and aorta.

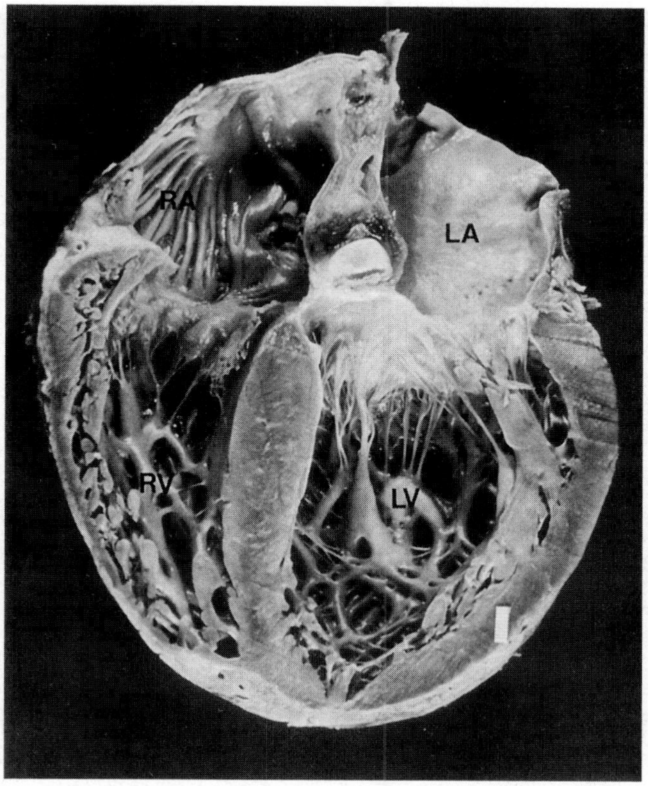

Figure 21.25. Idiopathic dilated cardiomyopathy. Longitudinal section of the heart from a 29-year-old man with idiopathic dilated cardiomyopathy (IDC) and congestive heart failure. Characteristic morphologic features of IDC are present and include four-chamber dilatation and marked hypertrophy (1100 g with normal <400 g) without wall thickening. This contrasts with the type of left ventricular hypertrophy seen with aortic stenosis or systemic hypertension (wall thickening without left ventricular dilation). Although approximately 50% of patients with IDC have left ventricular mural thrombus at autopsy, none is seen here. *RA* = right atrium; *RV* = right ventricle; *LA* = left atrium; and *LV* = left ventricle.

Myocardial tumor infiltration, either primary or metastatic, has also been reported as a cause of nondilated cardiomyopathy (50).

SUMMARY

In this brief overview of coronary, valvular, and myocardial heart disease, the structural abnormalities associated with these disorders are described. Cardiac imaging attempts to portray the structural and functional abnormalities of the heart that cause symptomatic cardiac disease. Appreciation of the pathologic anatomy of this disorder will allow a better understanding of the images generated by the various nuclear medicine modalities that are discussed in the next several chapters.

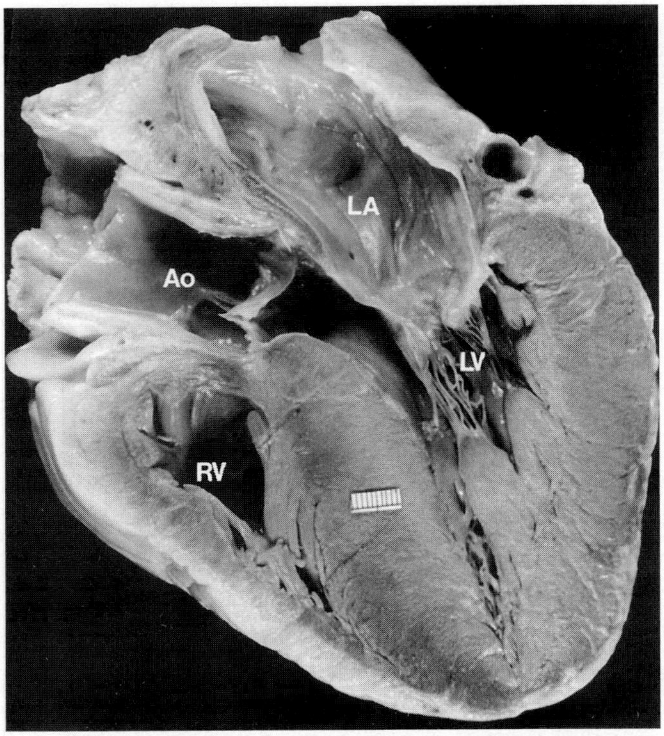

Figure 21.26. Nondilated cardiomyopathy. Longitudinal section through the right ventricular outflow tract (*RV*), left atrium (*LA*), left ventricle (*LV*), and aorta (*Ao*) of a 56-year-old hypertensive man. Left ventricular hypertrophy with wall thickening, a nondilated LV, and a dilated LA are the characteristic morphologic features of the hypertensive heart.

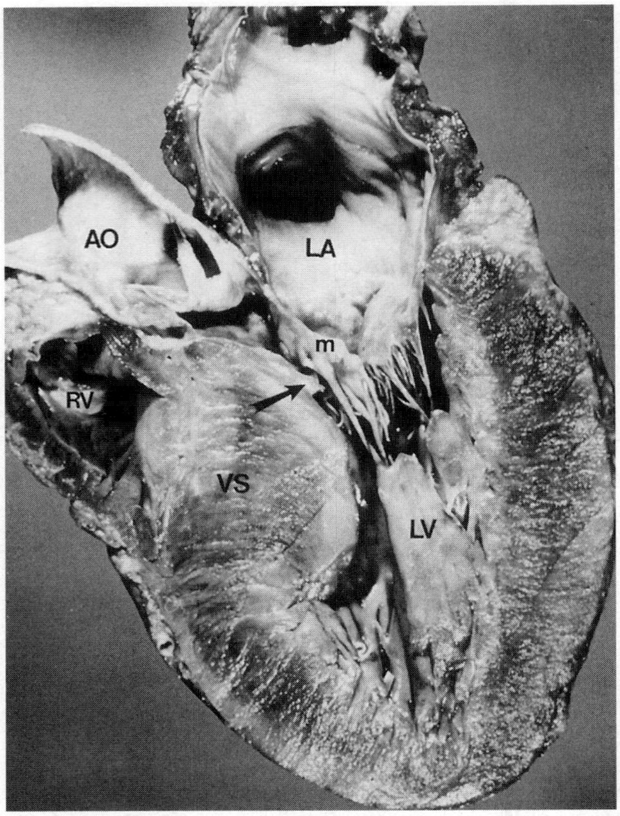

Figure 21.27. Hypertrophic cardiomyopathy. Longitudinal section through the right ventricular outflow tract (*RV*), left atrium (*LA*), and ventricular septum (*VS*), left ventricle (*LV*), and aorta (*Ao*) of a 23-year-old man with hypertrophic cardiomyopathy. There is asymmetric septal hypertrophy with LA but with LV dilation. Thickening of the endocardium overlying the basal septum (*arrow*) and of the anterior leaflet of the mitral valve (*m*) were present and are the anatomic markers of systolic anterior motion of the mitral valve with secondary LV outflow tract obstruction.

REFERENCES

1. Brosius FC, Roberts WC. Comparison of degree and extent of coronary narrowing by atherosclerotic plaque in anterior and posterior transmural acute myocardial infarction. Circulation 1981; 64:715.
2. Cabin HS, Roberts WC. Comparison of amount and extent of coronary narrowing by atherosclerotic plaque and of myocardial scarring at necropsy in anterior and posterior healed transmural myocardial infarction. Circulation 1982;66:93.
3. Jones AA, Roberts WC. Quantitation of coronary arterial narrowing at necropsy in sudden coronary death. Am J Cardiol 1979; 44:39.
4. Cabin HS, Roberts WC. Quantitative comparison of extent of coronary narrowing and size of healed myocardial infarct in 33 necropsy patients with clinically recognized and in 28 with clinically unrecognized ("silent") previous acute myocardial infarction. Am J Cardiol 1982;50:677.
5. Cabin HS, Roberts WC. Fatal cardiac arrest during cardiac catheterization for angina pectoris: an analysis of 10 necropsy patients. Am J Cardiol 1981;48:1.
6. Roberts WC, Buka LM. The frequency and significance of coronary arterial thrombi and other observations in fatal acute myocardial infarction: a study of 107 necropsy patients. Am J Med 1972; 52:425.
7. Wood MA, Spores J, Notske R, et al. Prevalence of total coronary occlusion during the early hours of transmural myocardial infarction. N Engl J Med 1980;303:897.
8. Anderson JL, Marshall HW, Bray BE, et al. A randomized trial of intracoronary streptokinase in the treatment of acute myocardial infarction. N Engl J Med 1983;308:1312.
9. Kennedy JW, Ritchie JL, Davis KB, Fritz JK. Western Washington randomized trial of intracoronary streptokinase in acute myocardial infarction. N Engl J Med 1983;309:1477.
10. Bresnahan DR, Davis JL, Holmes DRJ, Smith HC. Angiographic occurrence and clinical correlates of intraluminal coronary artery thrombus—role of unstable angina. J Am Coll Cardiol 1985; 6:285.
11. Capone G, Wolf NM, Meyer B, Meister SG. Frequency of intracoronary filling defects by angiography in angina pectoris at rest. Am J Cardiol 1985;56:403.
12. Sherman CT, Litvack F, Grundfest W, et al. Coronary angioscopy in patients with unstable angina pectoris. N Engl J Med 1986; 315:913.
13. Telford AM, Wilson C. Trial of heparin vs. atenolol in prevention of myocardial infarction in intermediate coronary syndrome. Lancet 1981;1:1225.
14. Gold HK, Johns JA, Leinback RC, et al. A randomized, blinded, placebo-controlled trial of recombinant human tissue-type plasminogen activator in patients with unstable angina pectoris. Circulation 1987;75:1192.
15. Prinzmetal M, Kennamer R, Merliss R, Wada T, Bor N. Angina Pectoris I: a variant form of angina pectoris. Am J Med 1959;27:375.
16. Bertrand ME, LaBlanche JM, Tilmant PY, et al. Frequency of pro-

voked coronary arterial spasm in 1089 consecutive patients undergoing coronary arteriography. Circulation 1982;65:1299.
17. Waller BF, Rothbaum DA, Pinkerton CA, et al. Status of the myocardium and infarct-related coronary artery in 19 necropsy patients with acute recanalization using pharmacologic (streptokinase, r-tissue plasminogen activator), mechanical (percutaneous transluminal coronary angioplasty) or combined types of reperfusion therapy. J Am Coll Cardiol 1987;9:785.
18. Roberts WC, Gardin JM. Location of myocardial infarcts: a confusion of terms and definitions. Am J Cardiol 1978;42:868.
19. Cabin HS, Roberts WC. Relation of healed transmural myocardial infarct size to length of survival after acute myocardial infarction, age at death, and amount and extent of coronary atrial narrowing by atherosclerotic plaques: analysis of 70 necropsy patients. Am Heart J 1982;104:216.
20. Cabin HS, Roberts WC. Angina pectoris after healing of acute myocardial infarction: an indicator of small posteriorly located left ventricular infarcts[Abstract]. Lab Invests 1981;44:7A.
21. Cabin HS, Roberts WC. Left ventricular aneurysm, intraneurysmal thrombus and systemic embolus in coronary heart disease. Chest 1980;77:586.
22. Cabin HS, Roberts WC. True left ventricular aneurysm and healed myocardial infarction, clinical and necropsy observations including quantification of degrees of coronary arterial narrowing. Am J Cardiol 1980;46:754.
23. Reeder GS, Lengyel M, Tajik AJ, Seward JB, Smith HC, Danielson GK. Mural thrombus in the left ventricular aneurysm; incidence, role of angiography, and relation between anticoagulation and embolization. Mayo Clin Proc 1981;56:77.
24. Meizlish JL, Berger HJ, Plankey M, Errico D, Levy W, Zaret BL. Functional left ventricular aneurysm formation after acute anterior transmural myocardial infarction; incidence, natural history, and prognostic implications. N Engl J Med 1984;311:1001.
25. Wartman WB, Hellerstein HK. The incidence of heart disease in 2000 consecutive autopsies. Ann Intern Med 1948;28:41.
26. Yater WM, Traum AH, Brown WG, Fitzgerald RP, Grisler MA, Wilcox BB. Coronary artery disease in men 18–39 years of age: report of 860 cases, 450 with necropsy examination. Am Heart J 1948; 36:683.
27. Isner JM, Roberts WC. Right ventricular infarction complicating left ventricular infarction secondary to coronary heart disease: frequency, location, associated findings and significance from analysis of 236 necropsy patients with acute or healed myocardial infarction. Am J Cardiol 1978;42:885.
28. Ratliff NB, Hackel DB. Combined right and left ventricular infarction: pathogenies and clinicopathologic correlations. Am J Cardiol 1980;45:217.
29. Wade WG. The pathogenesis of infarction of the right ventricle. Br Heart J 1959;21:545.
30. Cabin HS, Clubb KS, Wackers FJ, Zaret BL. Right ventricle myocardial infarction with anterior wall left ventricular infarction: an autopsy study. Am Heart J 1987;113:16.
31. Cabin HS, Clubb KS, Wackers FJ. Regional right ventricular dysfunction: an excellent predictor of right ventricular necrosis with anterior as well as inferior myocardial infarction. Circulation 1985;72:413.
32. Cohn JN, Guiha NH, Broder MI, Limas CJ. Right ventricular infarction: clinical and hemodynamic features. Am J Cardiol 1974; 33:209.
33. Eisenmann B, Bareiss P, Pacifico AD, et al. Anatomic, clinical and therapeutic features of acute cardiac rupture. J Thorac Cardiovasc Surg 1978;76:78–82.
34. Nunex L, de la Llana R, Lopez Sendon J, Coma I, Gil Aguado M, Larrea JL. Diagnosis and treatment of subacute free wall ventricular rupture after infarction. Ann Thorac Surg 1983;35:525–529.
35. Edmonson HA, Hoxie HJ. Hypertension and cardiac rupture: clinical and pathological study of 72 cases, in 13 of which rupture of the interventricular septum occurred. Am Heart J 1942;24:719.
36. Alpert JS, Braunwald E. Acute myocardial infarction: pathological, pathophysiological, and clinical manifestations. In: Braunwald E, ed. Heart disease: a textbook of cardiovascular medicine. Vol. II. Philadelphia: WB Saunders, 1984:1262.
37. Schuster EH, Bulkley BH. Expansion of transmural myocardial infarction: pathophysiologic factor in cardiac rupture. Circulation 1979;60:1532–1538.
38. Roberts WC, Morrow AG. Pseudonaneurysm of the left ventricle. An unusual sequel of myocardial infarction and rupture of the heart. Am J Med 1967;43:639.
39. Gatewood RP Jr, Nanda NC. Differentiation of left ventricular pseudoaneurysm from true aneurysm with two dimensional echocardiography. Am J Cardiol 1980;46:869.
40. Edwards BS, Edwards WD, Edwards JE. Ventricular septal rupture complicating acute myocardial infarction: identification of simple and complex types in 53 autopsied hearts. Am J Cardiol 1984;54:1201.
41. Silver MD, Wilson GJ. Pathology of cardiovascular prostheses including coronary artery bypass and other vascular grafts. In: Silver MD, ed. Cardiovascular pathology. New York: Churchill Livingstone, 1983:1225–1296.
42. Waller BF, Roberts WC. Amount of narrowing by atherosclerotic plaque in 44 non-bypassed and 52 bypassed major epicardial coronary arteries in 32 necropsy patients who died within 1 month of aortocoronary bypass grafting. Am J Cardiol 1983;46:956.
43. Roberts WC. Morphologic features of the normal and abnormal mitral valve. Am J Cardiol 1983;51:1005.
44. Waller BF, Morrow AG, Maron BJ, et al. Etiology of clinically isolated, severe, chronic, pure mitral regurgitation: analysis of 97 patients over 30 years of age having mitral valve replacement. Am Heart J 1982;104:276.
45. Roberts WC. Congenital cardiovascular abnormalities usually "silent" until adulthood: morphologic features of the floppy mitral valve, valvular aortic stenosis, hypertrophic cardiomyopathy, sinus of Valsalva aneurysm, and the Marfan syndrome. In: Roberts WC, ed. Congenital heart disease in adults. Philadelphia: FA Davis, 1979:407–453.
46. Roberts WC, Morrow AG, McIntosh CL, Jones M, Epstein SE. Congenitally bicuspid aortic valve causing severe, pure aortic regurgitation without superimposed infective endocarditis. Analysis of 13 patients requiring aortic valve replacement. Am J Cardiol 1981;47:206.
47. Waller BF, Zoltick JM, Rosen JH, et al. Severe aortic regurgitation from systemic hypertension (without aortic dissection) requiring aortic valve replacement: analysis of four patients. Am J Cardiol 1982;49:473.
48. Roberts WC. Complications of cardiac valve replacement: characteristic abnormalities of prostheses pertaining to any or a specific site. Am Heart J 1982;103:113.
49. Roberts WC, Ferrans VJ. Pathologic anatomy of the cardiomyopathies. Idiopathic dilated and hypertrophic types, infiltrative types, and endomyocardial disease with and without eosinophilia. Hum Pathol 1975;6:287.
50. Cabin HS, Costello RM, Vasudevan G, Maron BM, Roberts WC. Cardiac lymphoma mimicking hypertrophic cardiomyopathy. Am Heart J 1981;102:466.

22 Digital Techniques for the Acquisition, Processing, and Analysis of Nuclear Cardiology Images

GUIDO GERMANO, KENNETH VAN TRAIN, HOSEN KIAT, and DANIEL S. BERMAN

Computers are an integral and irrenounceable part of the way nuclear medicine is practiced today. Not only do computers control the acquisition of nuclear data, but the data is also made available in digital form for further computer processing, display, and storage. Nuclear medicine images can be examined in conjunction with, and displayed merged with, images from other modalities (MRI, CT, etc), electronically transferred to and from remote sites, and integrated with other image and text information in a departmental or hospital-wide information system. Quantification of nuclear medicine images is gaining wide acceptance, and artificial intelligence techniques and algorithms are increasingly being used to help physicians diagnose and characterize coronary artery disease.

This chapter provides a comprehensive review of the way computers are used in nuclear cardiology today, as well as identifying future directions towards which hardware and software development is proceeding. In the first section, various acquisition strategies employed in nuclear cardiology are reviewed and discussed. The second section deals with the processing necessary to pass from the collected raw data to the final images on which visual or quantitative analysis is performed. The third section describes methods of quantitative analysis of the cardiac images aimed at extracting global and regional information on myocardial perfusion and function. Finally, the fourth section examines the future of computers in nuclear cardiology.

The reader of this chapter should be familiar with the basic principles of computer operation explained in Chapter 8, as well as with the principles of single photon emission computed tomography (SPECT) outlined in Chapter 9. SPECT imaging is used in the vast majority of all cardiac nuclear procedures performed in the United States, and, consequently, is given special prominence in this chapter. For clinical performance, interpretation, and rationale of cardiac nuclear medicine studies, both planar and SPECT, the reader is referred to Chapters 23 through 27.

ACQUISITION

There are a large number of acquisition protocols and techniques used in nuclear cardiology today. Most of them are based on the Anger scintillation camera, or a variation of this camera, described in Chapter 7. To recall some basic concepts, a scintillation camera (or gamma-camera) consists of one or more scintillation detectors, typically made of high-density materials such as thallium activated NaI. When radiation impinges on and penetrates the scintillation detector, it dissipates its energy by conversion into light photons, which are in turn converted into electrons and amplified into an electric current by a set of photomultiplier tubes (PMTs) directly coupled to the scintillation crystal. The amount of energy dissipated in the detector is proportional to the energy of the original γ-ray, and the point of impact is derived by analysis of the fraction of light photons collected by different PMTs (1).

PLANAR VERSUS TOMOGRAPHIC ACQUISITION

The first major distinction in nuclear cardiology acquisitions is between planar and tomographic (SPECT) techniques. In planar imaging, the camera is fixed relative to the patient, so one obtains a two-dimensional image that reflects the projection of the three-dimensional distribution of activity in the patient. This is why planar images are also called projection images or "projections." Since planar images cannot differentiate between overlapping structures, image contrast suffers. It is often necessary to acquire more than one projection image. The planar projections most commonly used for myocardial perfusion imaging are the anterior, the 45° left anterior oblique (LAO), and a left lateral view. In SPECT imaging, the camera's detector rotates around the patient, collecting a projection image at every few degrees. The key to SPECT imaging is the fact that the three-dimensional distribution of activity can be "reconstructed" from a set of two-dimensional projection images, provided that the latter are adequately spaced and cover a large enough arc (180° or more). This process was first described by Bracewell for astronomic applications (2), and subsequently applied to medical tomography by Shepp and Logan (3).

The most popular form of tomographic reconstruction from projections in nuclear medicine is backprojection. Figure 22.1 shows a graphic explanation of backprojection, with the two-dimensional projection images (perpendicular to the plane of the page) simplified into one-dimensional profiles, and the three-dimensional activity distribution simplified into a two-dimensional "point" source. Each profile represents the integrated sum of the activity distribution along that particular angle. In standard backprojection (linear superimposition of backprojections or LSBP), the counts in each profile are uniformly "smeared" back onto the tomographic image matrix, with consequent loss of resolution, contrast, and creation of the characteristic "star" artifact. In filtered backprojection (linear superimposition of filtered backprojections or LSFBP), each profile is filtered with a damped oscillating function before backprojection, so as to eliminate the star artifact and recover image contrast and resolution. The canonic filter

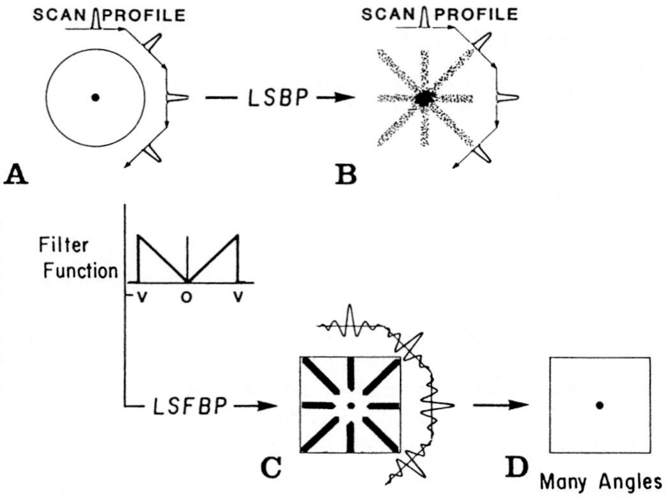

Figure 22.1. Reconstruction of tomographic images via backprojection. The counts in scan profiles collected at different angles around a point source (**A**) can be uniformly "backprojected" onto an image matrix (linear superimposition of backprojections or LSBP), The original point source distribution is recreated, but at the cost of blurring and loss of contrast; moreover, the characteristic "star artifact" results (**B**). Alternatively, the profile counts can be first processed by a filter function shaped like a ramp in the Fourier domain and an oscillating damped curve in the space domain, and then backprojected onto the image matrix (linear superimposition of filtered back projections or LSFBP) **C.** The curve sections below zero cancel the star artifact, the cancellation being closer to perfect the more profiles that are used for reconstruction (**D**). In modern tomography, LSFBP is universally preferred to LSBP. (Reproduced by permission from Phelps ME, Hoffman EJ, Gado M, et al. Computerized transaxial reconstruction. In: DeBlanc H, Sorenson J, eds. Noninvasive brain imaging, computerized tomography and radionuclides. New York: Society of Nuclear Medicine, 1975:111–145.)

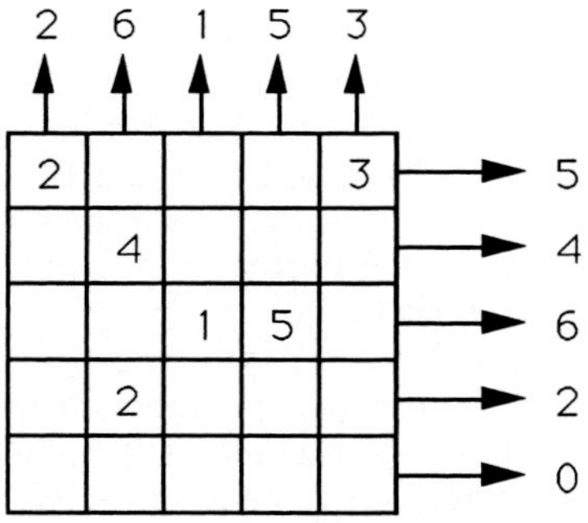

Figure 22.2. Algebraic reconstruction (ART) of tomographic images. Each point in the profiles of Figure 22.1 is the sum of a row, a column, or a diagonal distribution of image matrix pixels. A system of equations can then be constructed and solved for those pixels. The concept is exemplified in this Figure by showing the numeric components of two discretized profiles along the horizontal and vertical directions. For other angles, the sum of fractional pixels must be considered.

function used corresponds to a ramp in the frequency or Fourier domain. As we shall see, filters are usually described in terms of their shape in this domain.

Filtered backprojection is not the only reconstruction method used in nuclear cardiology, although it is by far the most widely used. Algebraic reconstruction techniques (ART) also utilize the projection images as input, but aim at finding the exact mathematic solution to the problem of activity distribution in the field of view (FOV) by considering the value in each pixel of the reconstructed image as an unknown, and each point in a profile (projection image) as an equation. The basic concept of ART is shown in Figure 22.2, again applied to a simple two-dimensional activity distribution and two representative profiles.

SPECT ACQUISITION ISSUES

Issues of much debate in cardiac SPECT imaging include 180° vs. 360° acquisition, and circular vs. noncircular (patient-contoured) orbit. The rationale for 180° acquisition of data (usually from 45° RAO to LPO) is that myocardial counts in the remaining projections are overwhelmingly attenuated or scattered by the patient's body, and consequently do not contribute much additional information to the final images. Overall, 180° SPECT acquisition is generally preferred today for both ^{201}Tl and ^{99m}Tc studies because of the higher contrast and resolution of the reconstructed images (4–9), although the use of 360° acquisition has been advocated based on its superior image uniformity and the lesser distortion it causes (10–14). It should be noted that with modern triple-detector cameras the concept of 180° acquisition and 180° reconstruction are not synonymous, because the three detectors completely surround the patient and one always acquires data corresponding to the full 360° arc when 180° data are acquired. Concerning noncircular acquisition, the rationale for its use is that the rotating detector can be made to follow the patient's contour, reducing the distance between collimator and heart and increasing image resolution and uniformity on a projection-by-projection basis (15–18). However, it has been shown that noncircular acquisition may introduce artifacts by pooling together projection images reflecting widely varying heart-detector distances, and possessing widely different spatial resolution characteristics (19). Of interest, the same problem may present itself (although to a lesser degree) in circular acquisition, because the heart is not positioned exactly at the center of rotation of the detector(s). Currently there is no clear consensus on whether circular or elliptical orbiting is preferred for cardiac SPECT.

Another important issue in SPECT acquisition is step-and-shoot vs. continuous rotation. In step-and-shoot, the camera collects data at a discrete number of angles around the patient, and temporarily stops collection as it "steps" from one angle to the adjacent one. We have observed that the stepping "dead time" varies from 3–7 seconds/projection for various systems in our laboratory.

In continuous acquisition, the detector rotates continuously and at constant speed around the patient. The acquisition arc is temporally divided in a number of segments equal to the number of projections desired, and data collected along each segment is assigned to the corresponding projection image. Pseudocontinuous (or modified step-and-shoot) is a hybrid of the previous two methods: the detector still moves as in step-and-shoot acquisition, but data collection is enabled during the stepping and "settle-down" period. The advantage of continuous or pseudocontinuous acquisition is the time savings derived from elim-

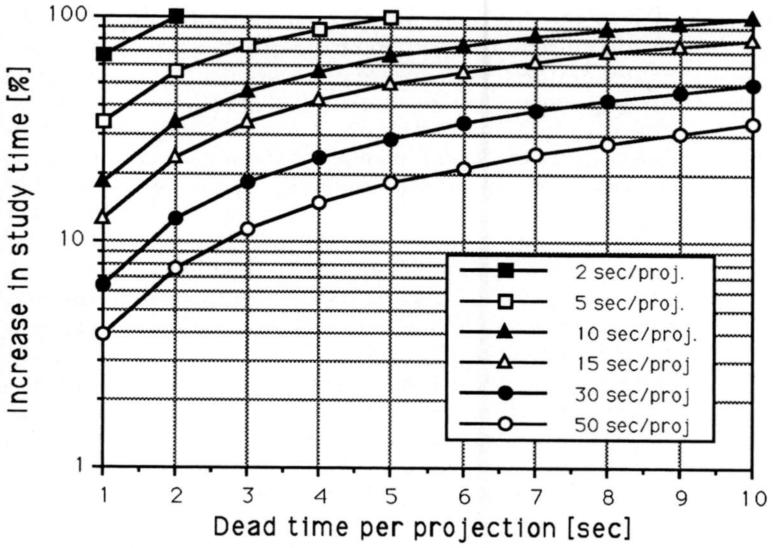

Figure 22.3. Increase in study duration due to dead time in step-and-shoot acquisition. For standard ^{201}Tl or ^{99m}Tc-sestamibi acquisitions at 15 sec/projection, a typical dead time of 4 seconds results in a 40% increase in study duration compared to continuous or pseudocontinuous acquisition.

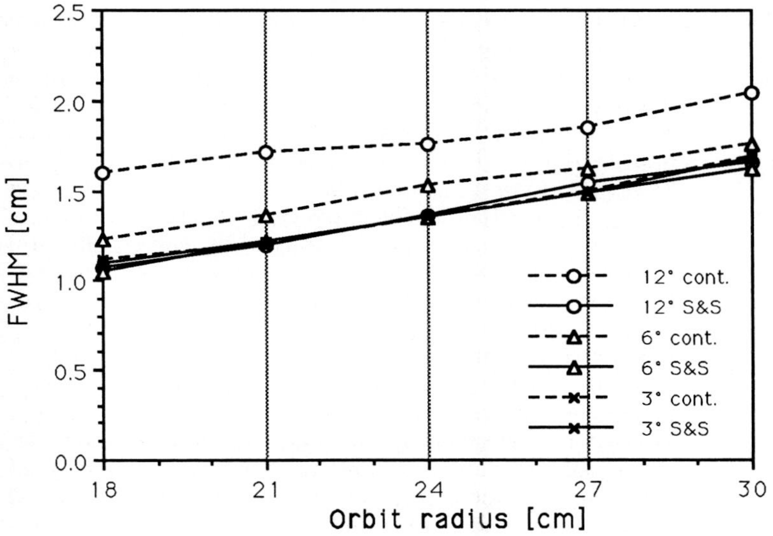

Figure 22.4. Line source resolution (FWHM) as a function of type of acquisition (continuous vs. step-and-shoot), orbit radius, and angular length of the arc assigned to one projection. As expected, resolution is progressively worse as the orbit radius increases. The use of continuous acquisition protocols yields virtually identical resolution to that of step-and-shoot protocols, as long as projection images are acquired at an angular spacing of 3°.

inating dead time. The savings are proportional to the dead time, to the number of projections acquired, and inversely proportional to the total duration of the acquisition (Fig. 22.3). The potential disadvantage of non step-and-shoot approaches is the loss of resolution associated with assigning to a given angle data which has really been acquired along an arc. However, line source experiments show that the loss of resolution with continuous acquisition is negligible as long as projection data are collected at least every 3° (Fig. 22.4). Continuous or pseudocontinuous acquisition is virtually indispensable in dynamic SPECT protocols to image agents with rapid uptake and washout (20–25), or when temporal image fractionation is employed to reduce motion artifacts in static SPECT (26, 27).

DYNAMIC, FIRST PASS AND ECG-GATED ACQUISITION

Dynamic acquisitions are used to better follow a dynamic process, such as the change in myocardial radionuclide distribution with time. In principle, a dynamic study can be seen as a collection of N static studies, where N is the number of time intervals at which we take a "snapshot" of the activity distribution in the field of view. Each image (planar) or set of images (SPECT) corresponding to a time interval is termed a "frame" or "temporal frame," with notation similar to cinematography. Dynamic planar or dynamic SPECT acquisitions have been effectively employed to image ^{99m}Tc-teboroxime, a myocardial perfusion agent with rapid uptake and washout (20–44), with frame duration ranging from 15 seconds to 1–2 minutes.

The first pass technique is a type of dynamic acquisition which uses very fine temporal sampling (20–100 frames per second (fps)) to look at the initial transit of a radionuclide bolus through the central circulation (Fig. 22.5). For SPECT, this very rapid acquisition requires a ring detector, and such systems are not currently available for nuclear cardiology. Thus, this form of imaging for purposes of nuclear cardiology is limited to the planar approach. In principle, the radionuclide should remain in the vascular space for the duration of the study. In practice, since the duration

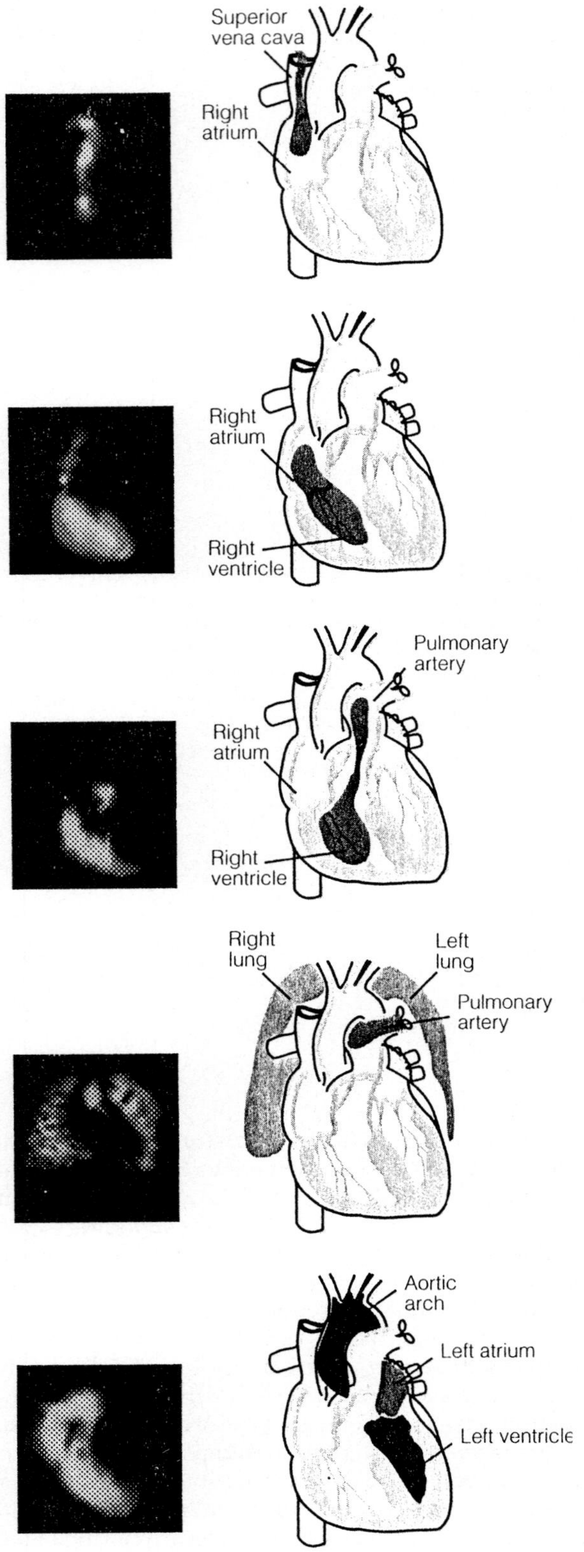

Figure 22.5. First pass acquisition. Serial anatomic (*right column*) and nuclear (*left column*) temporal display of the initial transit of the radionuclide bolus through the heart. (Reproduced by permission from English CA, English RJ, Gierink CP, Manspeaker H, Murphy JU, Wise PA. Introduction to nuclear cardiology. 3rd ed. Boston: Du Pont Pharma, 1993:217.)

of first pass studies is so short, virtually all nonparticulate technetium-labeled radiopharmaceuticals are appropriate for this study. With technetium-labeled myocardial perfusion agents, a minor error in first pass studies is introduced by the small fraction of the injected dose that is taken up in the initial transit by the myocardium. Nonetheless, since the amount taken up by the myocardium is only a small fraction of the initial amount in the cardiac blood pool, these errors are minimal. Thus, the perfusion agents ^{99m}Tc-sestamibi and ^{99m}Tc-teboroxime have also been used with success in first pass studies (25, 45). Key to the successful application of the first pass technique is the administration of the bolus, which should be extremely compact (less than 1 ml in volume). Acquisition is completed in less than 1 minute, and can be performed in any desired view, since distinct temporal relationships in the arrival and disappearance of radioactivity from the various cardiac chambers allow their separation with first pass studies.

Electrocardiographic (ECG)-gated acquisitions can also be seen as a form of dynamic acquisition, in which each frame corresponds to a specific portion (interval or gate) of the cardiac cycle, identified relative to the R wave on the patient's ECG. Because the cardiac cycle is divided in as many as 8–64 intervals, data from many different cycles (up to several hundreds) must be averaged to ensure adequate count statistics. Although this form of imaging can be applied to first pass data (46, 47), it is commonly used for equilibrium blood pool or myocardial perfusion imaging methods. Unlike first pass scintigraphy, for equilibrium gated blood pool scintigraphy the imaged radiopharmaceutical must stay within the vascular compartment for a prolonged period. Although labeled proteins such as technetium-99m albumin could be employed for blood pool imaging, labeled red blood cells are most commonly employed, labeled either through in vivo or in vitro methods. The latter provides the highest target to background ratio. Figure 22.6 explains the way cycles are averaged in gated planar acquisition: counts collected during the nth interval from the occurrence of each R wave trigger are accumulated in the same projection image (frame n). Acquisition stops when a preset number of counts has been collected, or when a predetermined period of time has elapsed. In gated SPECT, the same sorting process is repeated projection after projection.

In the standard gating approach, also referred to as the "fixed temporal" (FT) resolution with "forward-gating" (48–50), all gating intervals have the same length (generally, between 10–20 and 50–100 msec), and this length is fixed and based on the number of intervals and the average duration of the cardiac cycle. In clinical medicine, all cardiac cycles do not have exactly the same length. Therefore, in some cases the time between two consecutive R wave triggers will be longer than average, and once the time corresponding to the last interval has elapsed, all additional data would be discarded. Perhaps more troublingly, in other cases an R wave will occur sooner than average, so that at the end of the acquisition the last few intervals will consistently contain lower counts than the initial ones. Because one or the other situation will nearly always present itself to some degree, methods have been developed to com-

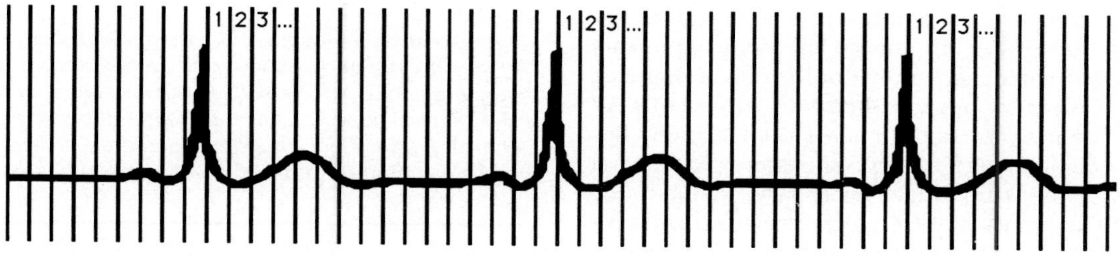

Figure 22.6. Electrocardiographic (ECG) gating. Each cardiac cycle (defined by two successive R wave peaks) is divided into a number of fixed-length temporal intervals or frames (gates). Data collected during homologous frames in different cycles are summed together, as they refer to the same dynamic cardiac state.

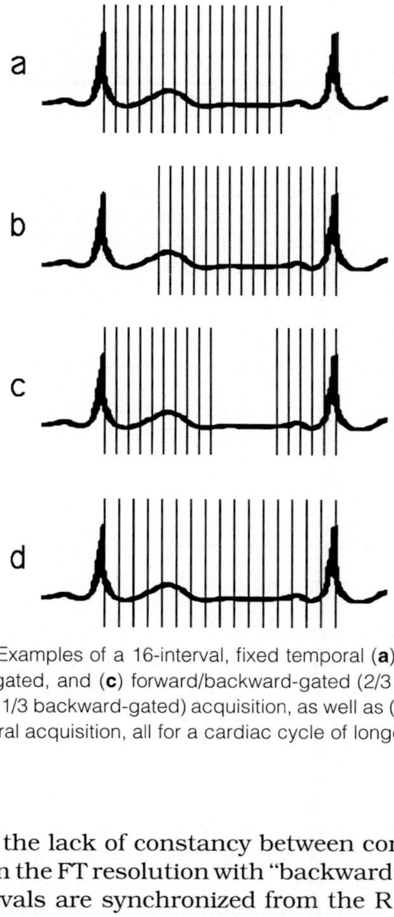

Figure 22.7. Examples of a 16-interval, fixed temporal (**a**) forward-gated, (**b**) backward-gated, and (**c**) forward/backward-gated (2/3 of the intervals forward-gated, 1/3 backward-gated) acquisition, as well as (**d**) a 16-interval, variable temporal acquisition, all for a cardiac cycle of longer than average duration.

pensate for the lack of constancy between consecutive R-R triggers. In the FT resolution with "backward-gating," the gating intervals are synchronized from the R wave backward, and applied to the latest heartbeat's data stored in a memory buffer. As this method causes similar problems to those encountered in forward-gating, a combination of forward and backward gating is often used (Fig. 22.7) (51). In a totally different approach, called the "variable temporal" (VT) resolution method, the R-R duration is dynamically adjusted to match the average length of the latest few heart cycles, and the length of the gating intervals (which remain constant in number) changes accordingly (Fig. 22.7). This method is computationally more intensive, requiring the alteration of the intervals' length on a beat-by-beat basis (48, 52). ECG-gated planar studies are commonly performed using blood pool agents (53, 54), but can also be used with myocardial perfusion agents. ECG-gated SPECT studies may use either blood pool agents (55, 56) or perfusion agents (57, 58). Of note, first pass studies utilize data averaged over a few heart cycles (generally 4–10), and can, therefore, also benefit from ECG gating (46, 59).

FRAME MODE VERSUS LIST MODE ACQUISITION

Most acquisition protocols operate in frame mode. Simply put, this means that the individual events are sorted or "framed" into projection images at the camera electronics level, and part of the information associated with such events is lost to the user. In other words, when a projection image is produced as the result of a planar acquisition, we know the number of events associated with every pixel of that image. However, we do not know *at what time* each individual event accumulated in that pixel (we only know it was during acquisition, or, at best, during a specific gating interval), nor do we know *what energy* did that particular event have (we only know that its energy was within a range specified by the energy acquisition window).

The concept of list mode has been introduced in nuclear cardiology mainly to answer the problem of nonconstancy of the R-R interval in gated first pass studies (60, 61), and, consequently, the term list mode is traditionally employed in lieu of the more correct "temporal list mode." In temporal list mode, each individual event is stored in a memory bin, which contains information on the event's location in the XY detector plane, and the exact time of its arrival (as determined by the camera's internal clock). In gated applications, the ECG curve is also stored as timed by the same clock. When the acquisition is completed, the cardiac cycle lengths (R-R interval) can be histogrammed, an acceptance window selected which straddles the histogram's peak, and events occurring during cycles of acceptable length sorted into frames based on either the FT resolution or VT resolution method. It is obvious that list mode acquisition requires substantially more memory and more postacquisition processing than standard acquisition. For instance, 200,000 counts accumulated in a projection image in frame mode would occupy 64^2 (i.e., 4096) memory locations if a 64×64 pixel^2 matrix is used, as opposed to 200,000 memory locations in temporal list mode. Moreover, the individual memory location in list mode would have to be more expansive, as it must contain the additional timing information. To obviate memory and processing problems, it has been recently proposed that the processing of list mode data should occur concurrently with its acquisition, i.e., in real-time (62).

In addition to temporal list mode, it is possible to acquire data in "energy list mode." In energy list mode, the exact energy associated with each individual event is digitized and stored in a memory bin together with the event's XY location (63). The main attraction of energy list mode lies in the fact that commitment to a specific energy window at the acquisition stage is no longer necessary. Instead, one can acquire all the events in the energy spectrum, and process them at a later time to purge the data set of undesired events. One class of undesirable events is represented by scattered events, a fraction of which is always found in the photopeak window when conventional acquisition is used. Although dual-window acquisition in conjunction with subtraction techniques has been used to estimate the scatter fraction (64–69), it has long been recognized that optimal scatter correction would require knowledge of the full spectral distribution of Compton photons (70, 71), information that only energy list mode acquisition can provide (72, 73).

As a particularly interesting case, the problem of correcting for isotope crosstalk in dual isotope myocardial perfusion SPECT may be best approached using this form of acquisition. As the phenomenon of isotope crosstalk in simultaneous dual isotope acquisition is closely related to scatter, energy list mode may be the key to making simultaneous ^{99m}Tc stress/^{201}Tl rest myocardial perfusion studies a clinical reality, thus taking advantage of the substantial improvements in patient throughput and quantitative accuracy possible with this technique (26, 74–76).

Of course, it is conceivable that an event might be acquired in "energy/temporal list mode," i.e., digitizing and preserving information relative to its XY location, its energy, and the time of its arrival. This approach is not yet implemented, but it may become practical as totally digital gamma-cameras (77), super-fast processors, and lower-cost computer memory become widely available.

DIMENSIONALITY OF ACQUISITION

It is helpful to look at all acquisition techniques and group them based on the "dimensionality" of the acquisition (Table 22.1). In this respect, a static planar study requires a two-dimensional acquisition, because events are collected in two dimensions (X and Y in the image). A dynamic, first pass or gated planar study requires a three-dimensional acquisition (X, Y, and time), as does a static SPECT study (X, Y, and angle of rotation). Gated and dynamic SPECT require a four-dimensional acquisition (X, Y, angle of rotation, and time).

It is important to understand that, all other factors being equal, one wants to employ the highest dimensionality acquisition technique available. Additional information is gathered from additional dimensions, and, in fact, lower dimension studies are contained in higher dimension ones. By definition, a SPECT study contains a number of planar studies equal to the number of projection angles, while a gated SPECT study contains a number of standard SPECT studies equal to the number of gating intervals used. What prevents us from using high-dimensionality acquisition is, of course, count statistics. It is clearly seen from Table 22.1 that higher dimension acquisitions produce greater numbers of images. Since the isotope dose administered is limited by dosimetry considerations and can be considered a constant for all studies utilizing the same isotope, and since the acquisition time is limited by patients' tolerance and capability of mantaining a still position, a higher-dimension study must distribute approximately the same number of counts amongst more images. (First pass studies, which collect the largest number of images over only three dimensions, are no exception. They derive their counts from radioactivity in the bloodstream immediately after injection, which is several tenfolds higher in concentration than radioactivity taken up by the myocardium).

Table 22.1.
Dimensionality of acquisition in nuclear cardiology studies. Higher-dimension acquisition protocols produce a larger number of images, which consequently have lower statistical quality if the injected dose and the total acquisition time do not change. Generally, statistical considerations are addressed by increasing the acquisition time or making heavier use of smoothing filters.

Study	Dimensionality	Variables	# images
Standard planar	2	X, Y	1–4
Dynamic planar (^{99m}Tc-teboroxime)	3	X, Y, time	40–60
First pass	3	X, Y, time	500–5000
Gated planar	3	X, Y, time	14–100
Standard SPECT	3	X, Y, angle	30–120
Dynamic SPECT	4	X, Y, angle, time	180–3000
Gated SPECT	4	X, Y, angle, time	240–1920

Table 22.2.
Duration of SPECT studies acquired with single- and multidetector cameras. All cameras rotate at the same speed, continuous or pseudocontinuous rotation is assumed, and the time T *employed by a single-detector camera for a 180° acquisition is taken as reference. Note that triple-detector cameras are excellent for 360° acquisition, but 90° dual-detector cameras are the best choice for 180° acquisition.*

	180° acquisition	360° acquisition
1 detector	T	2T
2 detectors 180° apart	T	T
3 detectors 120° apart	2/3 T	2/3 T
2 detectors 90° apart	T/2	T

MULTIDETECTOR CAMERAS AND SPECIALIZED COLLIMATORS

The need for higher statistics has led to the introduction of multidetector cameras. The three-detector configuration, with the detectors arranged in a equilateral triangle, and the two-detector configuration, with the detectors at 90° forming an L, are the most popular for cardiac use. In planar studies, multidetector cameras allow collection of multiple views simultaneously. In SPECT studies, they make it possible to acquire studies of higher statistical content without increase in the acquisition time or, conversely, to reduce the time necessary to acquire a study of a given statistical content. The benefits of this latter approach (generally preferred for efficiency reasons) are exemplified in Table 22.2, where three-detector and two-detector (90°) cameras are compared to one-detector and two-detector (180°) cameras for 180° and 360° acquisition.

Since physical collimation (as opposed to electronic collimation in positron emission tomography) reduces the photonic flux in nuclear cardiology, collimator design has been another way to try and improve count statistics. Standard collimators have parallel holes which offer the benefit of no spatial distortion and uniform counting efficiency. To increase count statistics, high sensitivity parallel hole collimators may be used which are shallower than standard all-purpose collimators. To increase resolution, high resolution collimators may be employed which are deeper than all-purpose collimators. There is a direct trade off between sensitivity and resolution with parallel hole collimators. Fan beam collimators were designed to increase volume sensitivity by magnifying the principal activity distribution and mapping it to a larger portion of the camera's detector (78). This is achieved by focusing to a line parallel to the axis of rotation of the camera and beyond the patient. Extension of this concept led to the current development of astigmatic collimators, which focus to two orthogonal lines, and cone-beam collimators, which focus to a point (79, 80). The main problem to be addressed with this type of collimator is that projection data are not completely sampled, and distortions may result from reconstruction (4). Effective use of these new collimators in myocardial SPECT will require developing software and algorithms to solve these problems.

IMAGE PROCESSING AND DISPLAY

IMAGE RESTORATION

Even in a well-functioning gamma-camera system, there are known inaccuracies of the hardware acquisition chain which need to be compensated in software before the data is analyzed. For instance, the nonlinearity of the X and Y positioning signals across the face of the detector would typically result in "pincushion" or "barrel" distortion of the image, easily detectable with the use of straight-line test patterns (15). The common approach to correcting these and other "image nonuniformities" is that of acquiring a very high-count image of a uniform radiation field or "flood."

For multidetector cameras, an image per detector is acquired. Each pixel in this test image would have the same value (within statistical precision) if uniformity were perfect. Therefore, the differences in counts between pixels in the image can be used to generate a correction matrix to be applied to all subsequent clinical studies. Correction generally occurs "on the fly" during acquisition, so that any projection data available for processing will have been already corrected for nonuniformities.

Another image restoration technique important for SPECT acquisitions is the center of rotation (COR) correction, which ensures perfect alignment of the mechanical axis of rotation of the camera detector(s) with the electronic axis of rotation of the image reconstruction matrix (81). Without this correction, "tuning fork" artifacts and general image degradation may appear in the reconstructed images (82). The usual way to perform the COR correction is to acquire a 360° SPECT study of a point source, then plot the X-Y position of the point source's centroid on the projection images as a function of the projection angle. If alignment were perfect, the Y (axial) coordinate of the point source would be constant, while the X (transaxial) coordinate would describe a sinusoid of amplitude proportional to the source's distance from the physical axis of rotation (83). Deviations from this ideal behavior are used to compute correction matrices to be stored on the computer hard disk and applied to all subsequent studies.

On multidetector cameras, COR correction also allows for checking the registration of the different detectors. Figure 22.8 shows a three-detector camera with detector 3 misaligned by over 0.1 pixels in the axial dimension, relative to detectors 1 and 2. COR correction can be performed less often than nonuniformity correction (weekly vs. daily).

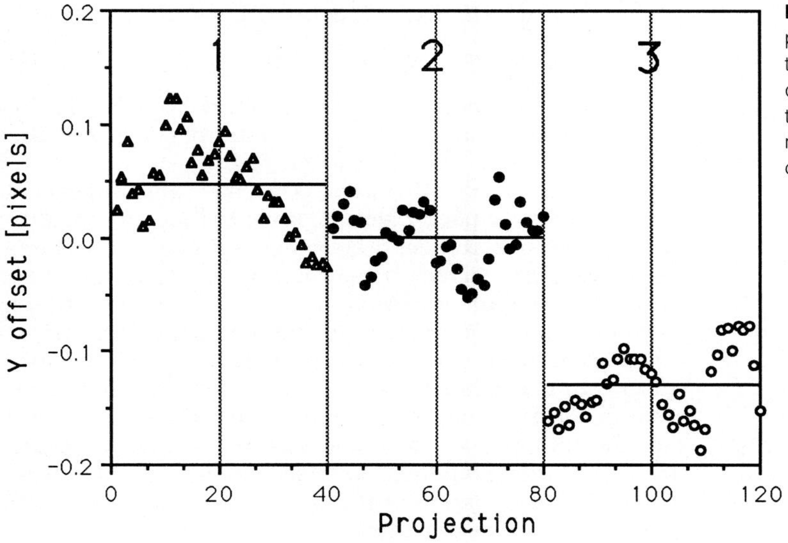

Figure 22.8. Detector misalignment in a three-detector camera. A point source was imaged over 360° and 120 projections (1–40 = detector 1, 41–80 = detector 2, 81–120 = detector 3), and its centroid determined in the 120 projection images. For each individual detector, the axial (*y*) components of the centroid are clustered around the mean y (*solid segments*), but the means are noticeably different from one another, especially for detector 3.

IMAGE ENHANCEMENT

Image enhancement is the process of altering the acquired image or set of images so as to make them ready for visual or quantitative analysis. "Enhancing" an image may consist of changing its temporal or spatial resolution, contrast, and uniformity. Since these parameters are interrelated, maximizing one can only be done at the expense of others. A tradeoff, depending on the particular study or type of analysis desired, is usually sought. Most types of image enhancement involve the use of filters. Images are generally thought of and represented in the conventional two-dimensional or three-dimensional space, that is, in the "space domain." However, filters are just as frequently defined in the "frequency or Fourier domain." It will now be necessary to briefly explain the relationship between these two concepts.

Space and Frequency Domain

The often misunderstood concept of "frequency domain" is easier to appreciate if one thinks of it as of a different way to express size and distance relationship between physical objects in an image. In Figure 22.9, three rectangular objects regularly repeat themselves along the horizontal direction, spaced by a distance equal to their horizontal dimension. In "spatial domain" terms, one would say that the first object repeats itself every 20 pixels, the second every 10 pixels, and the third every 2 pixels. In "frequency domain" terms, one could equivalently say that the frequency of occurrence of the three objects is 0.05 times per pixel (or, in common parlance, 0.05 cycles/pixel), 0.1 cycles/pixel, and 0.5 cycles/pixel, respectively. This reasoning can be extended to a two- or three-dimensional situation, the basic concept remaining the following: distance or size in the spatial domain corresponds (with inverse relationship) to frequency in the frequency domain. Consequently, small structures in an image are said to have high frequency, and the resolution capability of a camera system is often expressed by means of the Nyquist frequency (Ny), i.e., the highest frequency that the system can recover (15). To be accurate, what we refer to as frequency is more correctly termed "spatial frequency," because an analogous relationship to the one between space and spatial frequency exists between time and frequency. An example of the latter relationship is the "phase analysis" technique, which is examined in detail in the Image Processing section of this chapter.

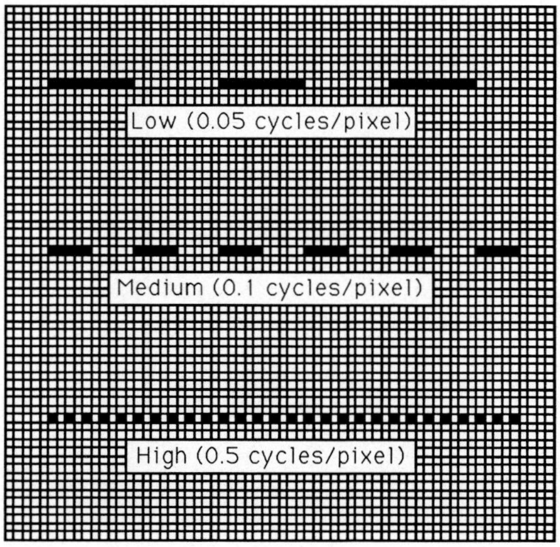

Figure 22.9. Frequency or Fourier domain. The "frequency" of occurrence of the long, medium, or short segments can be expressed as the inverse of the number of pixels between two consecutive segments. The frequency of 0.5 cycles/pixels is the highest achievable, since the unit of image resolution is the pixel. As a general rule, high frequencies are associated with small objects, and low frequencies with large, uniform objects.

The mathematic operators that allow us to pass from the space to the frequency domain are the Fourier transform and the Fourier series. The Fourier transform translates a continuous function in the space domain into a continuous function in the frequency domain, while the Fourier series translates a continuous function in the space domain into a discrete function in the frequency domain. A complete discussion of this topic is available in (84); for the purposes of this chapter, it suffices to refer to either one as the Fourier transform. In intuitive terms, the Fourier transform of a spatial function $f(x)$ expresses that function as a sum of sine and cosine functions of different frequencies. The reason why the Fourier transform and the frequency or Fourier domain are so extensively used in image processing is because the relatively complex operation of "convolution" of two functions in the physical space is equivalent to the simple multiplication of their Fourier transforms in the frequency domain.

Convolution as a Smoothing or Sharpening Tool

Convolution is represented by the symbol, and can be thought of as a "shift and multiply" operation. The well-known "three-point smoothing" used with one-dimensional discrete curves is a typical example of convolution. In this technique, the value at each point of the curve is replaced by the sum (or the average) of itself, the previous value, and the following value, thus reducing sudden variations between adjacent points. In other words, as shown in Figure 22.10, three-point smoothing of a function $f(x)$ is achieved by dragging or "shifting" a three-point "kernel" k containing the weights $k_1 = 1$, $k_2 = 1$, and $k_3 = 1$ across $f(x)$, and computing at each point x_i the sum:

$$g(x_i) = k_1\, f(x_{i-1}) + k_2\, f(xi) + k_3\, f(x_{i+1}) \qquad (1)$$

The resulting function $g(x)$, often normalized to $f(x)$ by transforming it into $g(x)/3$, is the result of convolving the kernel k with the original function $f(x)$.

It is intuitive that other kernels will have different effects on $f(x)$. A three-point "kernel" k containing the weights $k_1 = -1$, $k_2 = 2$, and $k_3 = -1$ convolved with $f(x)$ will enhance its edges. In fact, the kernel −1, 2, −1, also referred to as the one-dimensional Laplacian operator, performs a second derivative operation on $f(x)$. While the first derivative of a curve has value zero in correspondence of the function's minima and maxima, the second derivative has value zero in correspondence of the function's inflection points, i.e., the minima and maxima of the function's slope. Figure 22.11 shows a simplified example where $f(x)$ is piecewise constant: its second derivative $g(x)$ is zero (a) in the trivial case where $f(x)$ is constant and (b) at the "zero crossings"

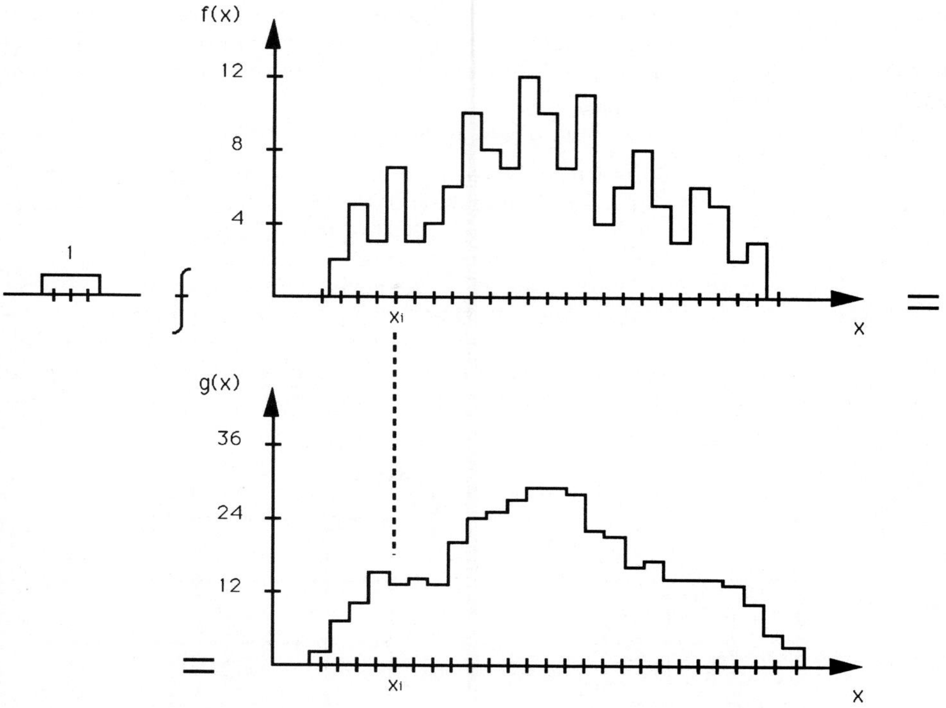

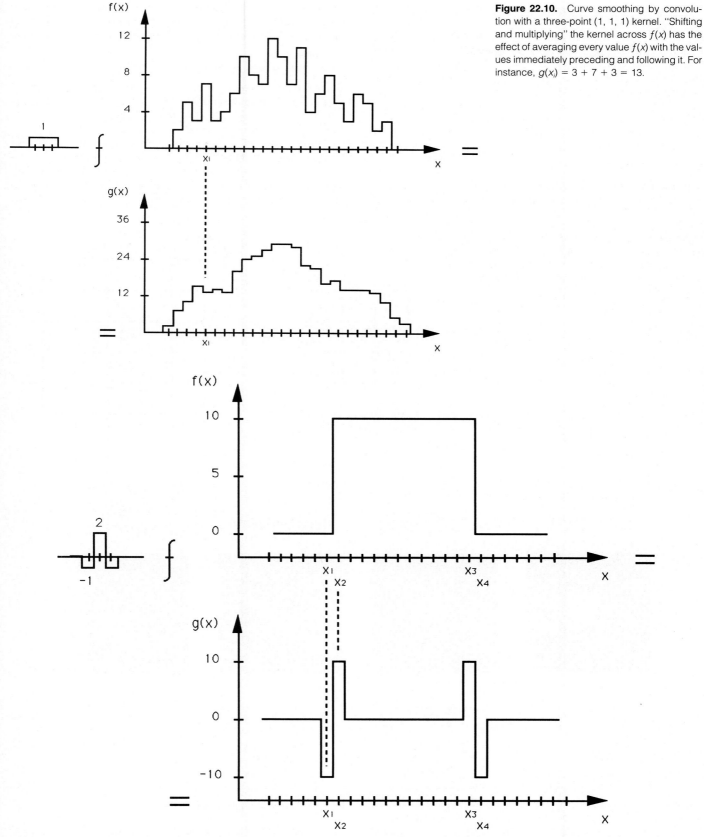

Figure 22.10. Curve smoothing by convolution with a three-point (1, 1, 1) kernel. "Shifting and multiplying" the kernel across $f(x)$ has the effect of averaging every value $f(x)$ with the values immediately preceding and following it. For instance, $g(x_i) = 3 + 7 + 3 = 13$.

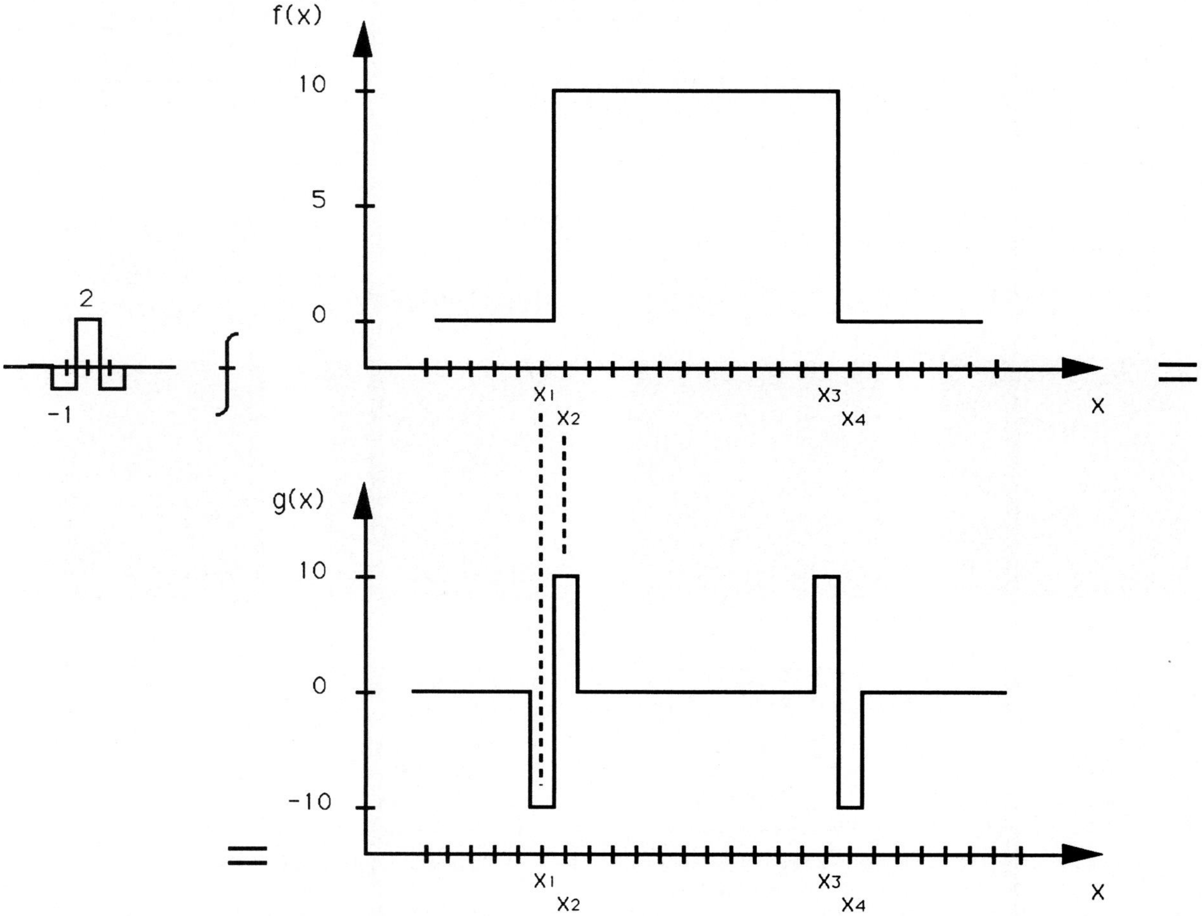

Figure 22.11. Edge enhancement by convolution with a three-point (−1, 2, −1) kernel. Shifting and multiplying the kernel across $f(x)$ has the effect of highlighting points where sudden transitions in value (discontinuities) of $f(x)$ occur. For instance, $g(x_1) = 0 + 0 - 10 = -10$ and $g(x_2) = 0 + 20 - 10 = +10$. The "zero-crossing" transition of $g(x)$ in passing from x_1 to x_2 (as well as from x_3 to x_4) is used as a marker of the edge location.

between x_1 and x_2, and between x_3 and x_4, corresponding to the "edges" of $f(x)$.

These concepts can be extended to two-dimensional functions, i.e., images. The kernel k will be two-dimensional, and can be shifted across the image both horizontally and vertically. At each pixel P, also identified by its coordinates (x_i, y_i), it will be:

$$\begin{aligned} g(x_i,y_i) = {} & k_1\, f(x_{i-1},y_{i-1}) + k_2\, f(x_{i-1},y_i) + k_3\, f(x_{i-1},y_{i+1}) \\ & + k_4\, f(x_i,y_{i-1}) + k_5\, f(x_i,y_i) + k_6\, f(x_i,y_{i+1}) \\ & + k_7\, f(x_{i+1},y_{i-1}) + k_8\, f(x_{i+1},y_i) \\ & + k_9\, f(x_{i+1},y_{i+1}) \end{aligned} \tag{2}$$

if the kernel used has dimensions 3×3, as is the case in Figure 22.12. Just as in the one-dimensional case, the values of $k_1 \ldots k_9$ shall determine the type of operation performed. Figure 22.13 shows a smoothing and a sharpening kernel, and their effect on a planar ^{201}Tl myocardial image.

Smoothing and Sharpening in the Frequency Domain

Convolution kernels in the one-, two-, or three-dimensional space achieve the desired effect of blurring, sharpening, or otherwise altering the original curve or image. However, the process is not intuitive, as it is often difficult to relate a kernel to the result of its convolution with an image. Since image filtering is always performed to enhance certain characteristics, or to better visualize certain structures in the image, it would be desirable to design a filter based on the "frequency content" of those structures.

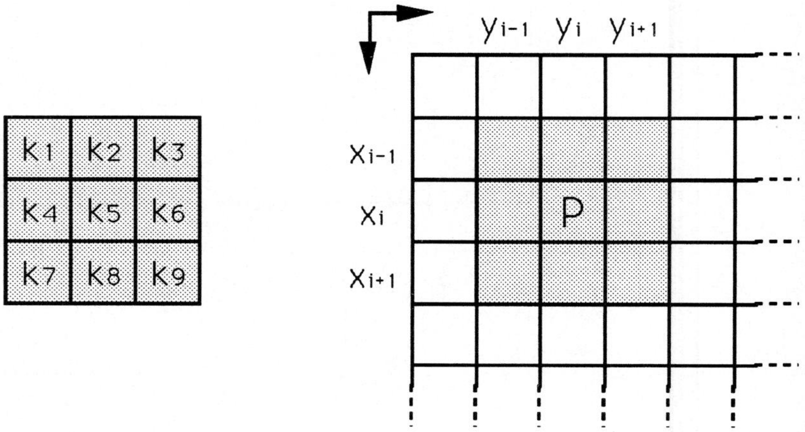

Figure 22.12. Convolution of an image with a two-dimensional, 9-point kernel. The kernel is shifted across the image horizontally and vertically, and modifies the value of each image pixel *P* based on the values of P's nearest eight neighbors, as well as on the nine kernel "weights" $k_1 \ldots k_9$.

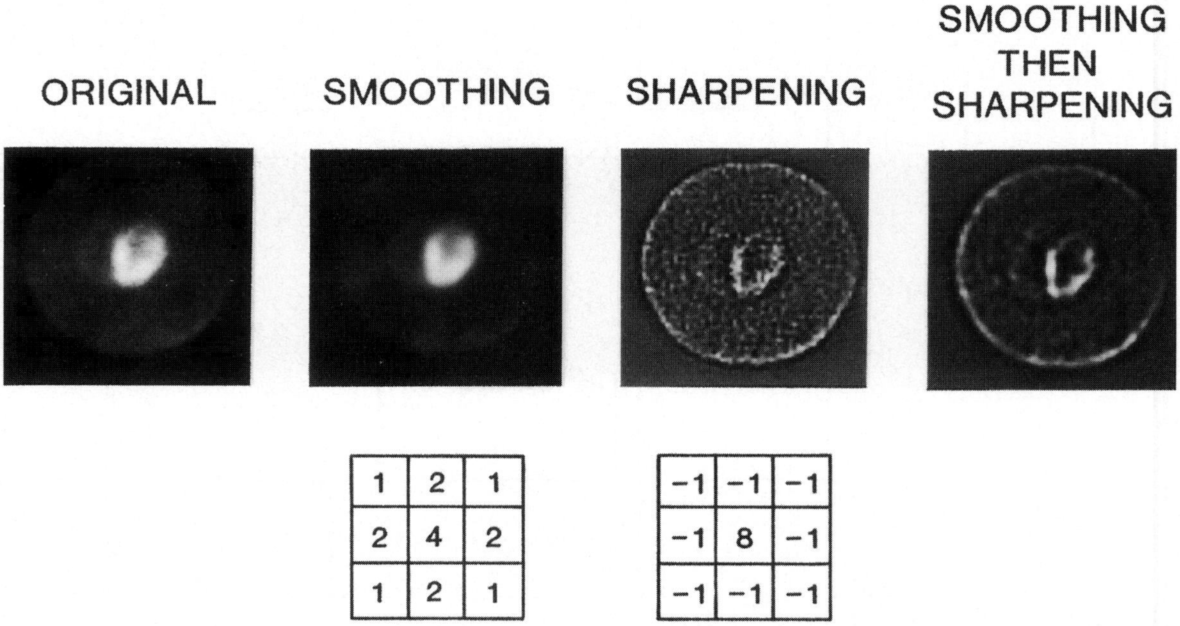

Figure 22.13. Convolution of a ^{201}Tl planar image with two different two-dimensional, 9-point kernels. The smoothing kernel (with weights 1, 2, and 4) blurs the image, while the sharpening kernel (with weights −1 and 8) enhances the myocardial edges as well as the statistical noise present in the image. Sequential application of the kernels reduces noise in the sharpened image while preserving the edge information. (Reproduced by permission from Garcia EV, Bateman TM, Berman DS, et al. Computer techniques for optimal radionuclide assessment of the heart. In: Gottschalk A, Hoffer PB, Potchen EJ, eds. Diagnostic nuclear medicine. Vol. I. 2d ed. Baltimore: Williams and Wilkins, 1988:259–290.)

Here is where the Fourier transform comes to our help. As stated earlier, a spatial function $f(x)$ can be expressed as a summation of sine and cosine functions of different frequencies. Without probing the mathematics of the process, suffice it to say that it is also possible to represent an image $f(x,y)$ through its frequency components by "transforming" it into an image $F(u,v)$, where u and v are the image's coordinates in a new domain, the frequency or Fourier do-

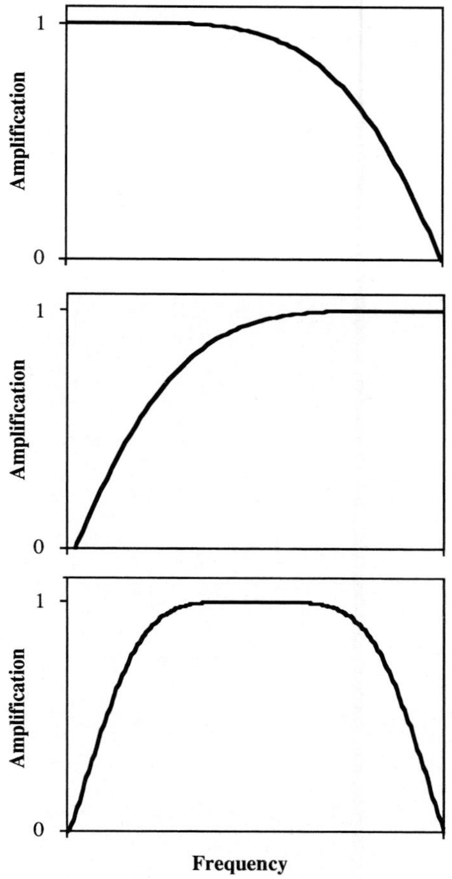

Figure 22.14. Low-pass (*top*), high-pass (*center*), and band-pass (*bottom*) filters shown in the frequency or Fourier domain. Image smoothing is accomplished by attenuating the higher frequencies, and image sharpening by attenuating the lower frequencies in the image. Consequently, a low-pass filter smooths, and a high-pass filter sharpens the image.

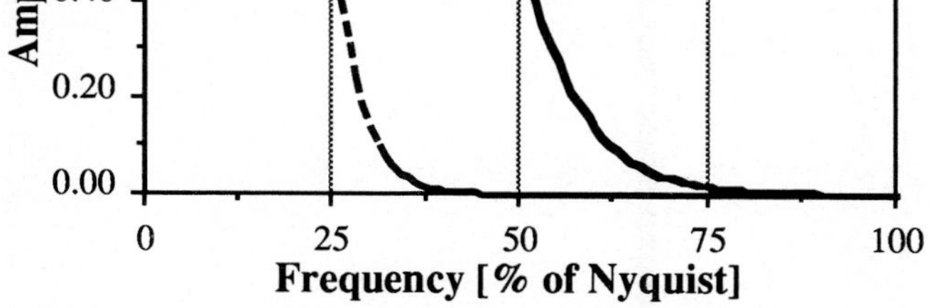

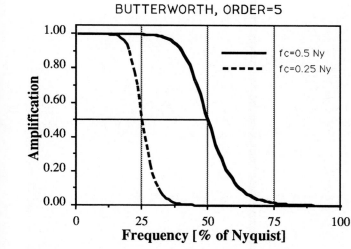

Figure 22.15. Frequency-domain curves for two Butterworth filters with the same order but different critical frequencies. The slope of the curves is identical, being determined by filter order. The critical frequencies (at which filter amplification is 0.5) and all spatial frequencies are expressed as percentages of the Nyquist frequency, which depends on the specific camera system used.

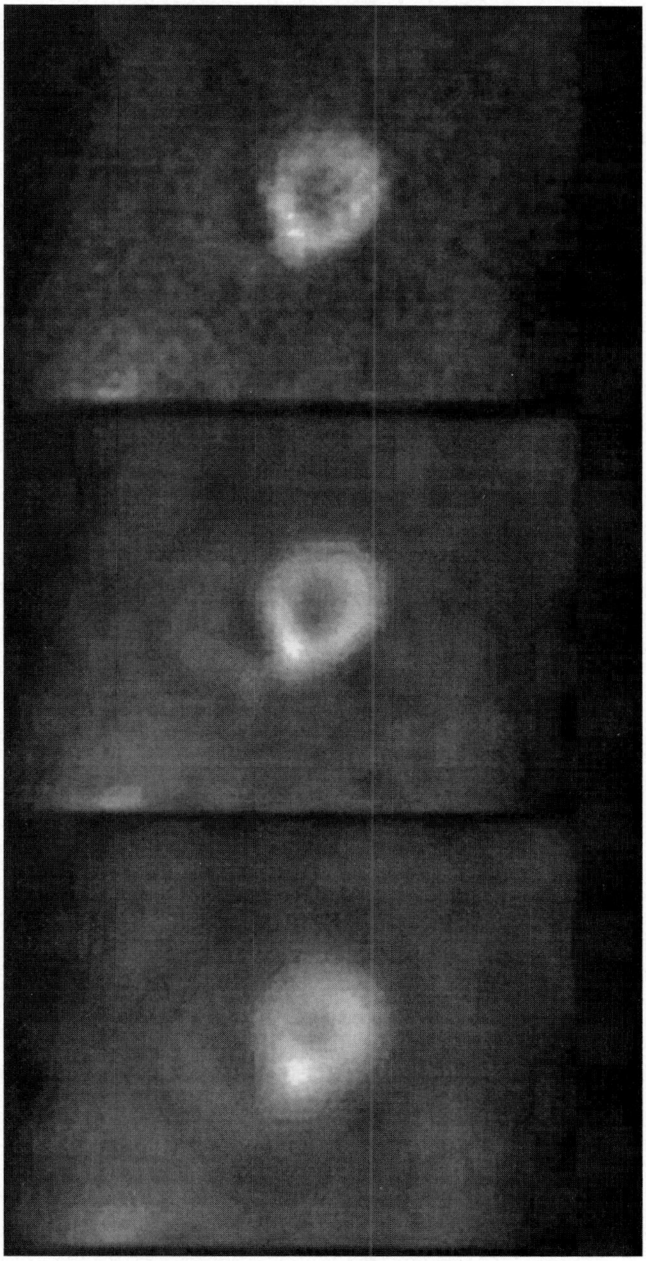

Figure 22.16. Application of the two filters in Figure 22.15 to a planar ^{99m}Tc-sestamibi image (*top*). The Butterworth filter, with order 5 and critical frequency equalling 50% of Nyquist, blurs the image enough to eliminate "salt-and-pepper" noise (*center*). However, further decreasing the critical frequency to 25% of Nyquist artificially results in "filling" of the LV cavity (*bottom*).

main. It is not critical to expand on what this new image looks like, because (a) it is not generally displayed and (b) even if it were, it would be obvious that it bears no visual resemblance to the original image. In the new domain, high frequencies correspond to small structures or areas of sharp changes in image intensity (i.e., bone edges in an x-ray of the hand, brain circumvolutions in a SPECT, PET, or MR study of the head, small tumors in whole body planar or tomographic studies, a small defect in a SPECT or PET myocardial perfusion study), while low frequencies correspond to relatively large and uniform image areas. If we want to increase the resolution of an image, we amplify its high frequencies, or attenuate its low frequencies; if we want to blur the image, we do the opposite. These requirements can be expressed in a straightforward way by specifying a one-dimensional filter function that will be multiplied by $F(u,v)$—in fact, multiplication in the frequency domain is mathematically equivalent to convolution in the space domain. The resulting image is then "inverse-Fourier transformed," giving back the filtered image $g(x,y)$ in the space domain, in a way totally transparent to the user.

The entire concept becomes clear once it is understood that the filter function in the frequency domain is exactly the same as the frequency response curve of a stereo amplifier. The filter's values at the various abscissae specify by how much the corresponding spacial frequencies must be attenuated. In Figure 22.14 we show examples of a low-pass, a high-pass, and a band-pass filter, appropriately named after the type of spacial frequencies that they "let pass" unattenuated when applied to an image. Making reference to Figure 22.13, a low-pass filter has the same effect as a smoothing kernel, and a high-pass filter the same as a sharpening kernel.

Common Types of Filters

Nuclear cardiac images are relatively count-poor, due to limitations in the injected dose, the use of physical collimation, and the attenuation properties of the thorax. The planar projections in a tomographic study are usually stored in 64×64 pixels^2 matrices (as opposed to 128×128 for PET studies or up to 2048×2048 for chest x-rays), so as to avoid distributing the collected counts over too many pixels. Even so, planar images are affected by random noise, i.e., the "salt-and-pepper" pattern caused by statistical variations in the counting rate. Salt-and-pepper

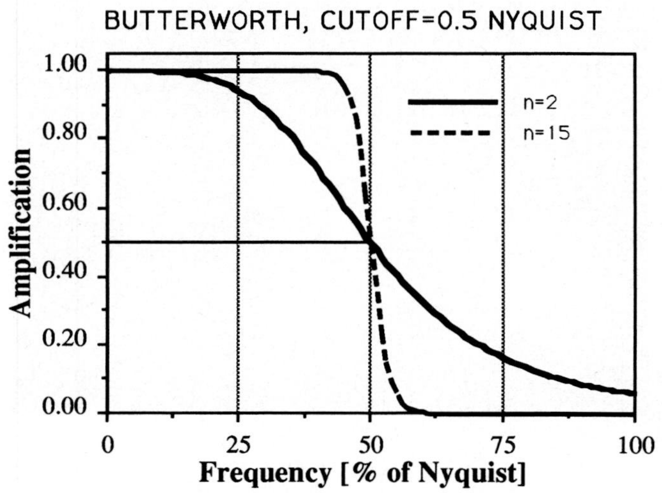

Figure 22.17. Frequency-domain curves for two Butterworth filters with the same critical frequency but different orders. The slopes of the curves are proportional to filter order.

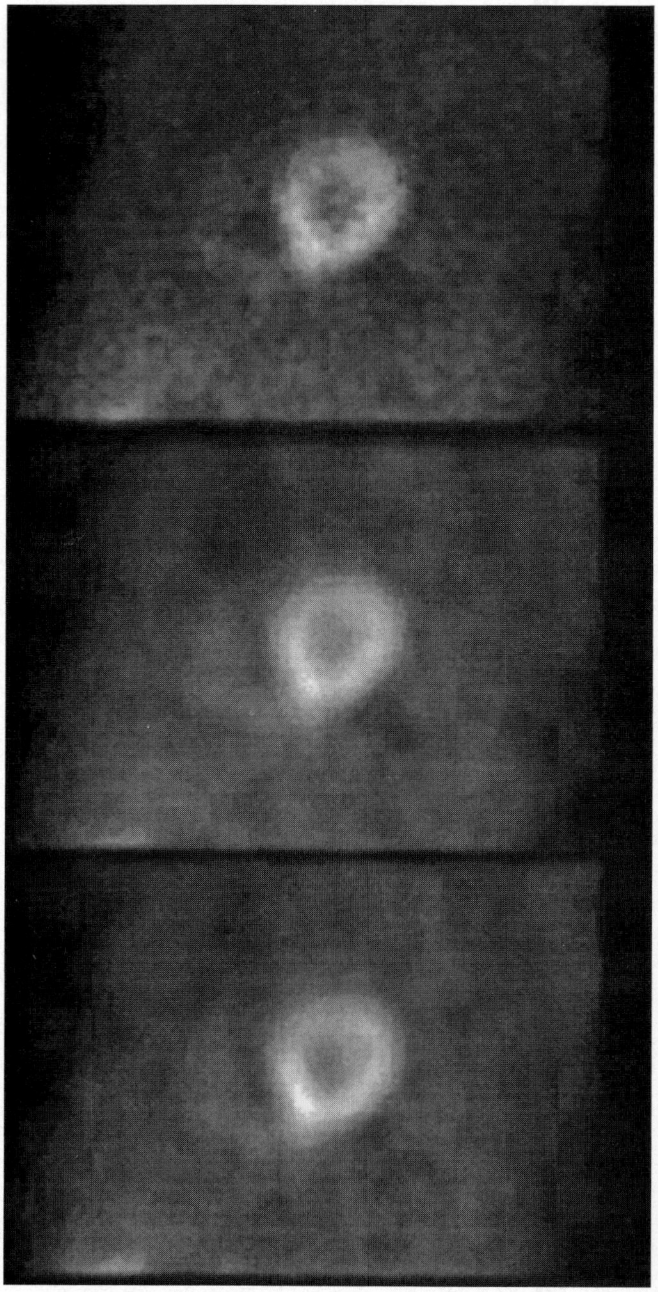

Figure 22.18. Application of the two filters in Figure 22.17 to the same planar ^{99m}Tc-sestamibi image (*top*) as in Figure 22.16. The Butterworth filters with order 2 (*center*) and order 15 (*bottom*) do not yield dramatically different images, suggesting that varying the order of this type of filter is a fine-tuning operation compared to varying its critical frequency.

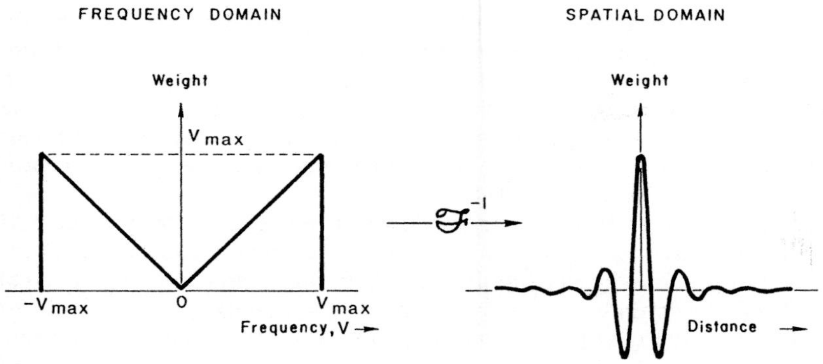

Figure 22.19. Frequency domain (*left*) and spatial domain (*right*) representation of the ramp filter used in the filtered backprojection reconstruction of tomographic images. V_{max} is the Nyquist frequency, while the operator F^{-1} expresses the "inverse Fourier transform" operation necessary to pass from the Fourier to the spatial domain. Since Fourier transforms are defined for symmetrical functions, the ramp has been mirrored about the y-axis in the frequency plot. However, negative spatial frequencies have no physical meaning, and filter curves in the frequency domain are essentially always shown from the zero frequency up. (Reproduced by permission from Phelps ME, Hoffman EJ, Gado M, et al. Computerized transaxial reconstruction. In: DeBlanc H, Sorenson J, eds. Noninvasive brain imaging, computerized tomography and radionuclides. New York: Society of Nuclear Medicine, 1975:111–145.)

("mottle") noise by definition involves high frequencies, or sudden changes from dark to light in adjacent pixels, and as such it can be reduced by low-pass filtering (smoothing). This operation is best performed on the projection images before reconstruction, to avoid propagating that noise. The most popular low-pass filters used in nuclear cardiology belong to the Hanning and Butterworth families. The former has been traditionally employed to process ^{201}Tl images; the latter was initially preferred for ^{99m}Tc images, but its flexibility and ease of design have made it the filter of choice in many nuclear medicine procedures. The Butterworth filter family is described in the frequency domain by the class of functions:

$$B(f) = \frac{1}{1 + \frac{f^{2n}}{f_c}} \quad (3)$$

where f_c is the critical or "cutoff" frequency, and n the order of the filter. From simple mathematic considerations it descends that any Butterworth filter has amplitude 1 when f is small (low frequencies), amplitude 0 when f is large (high frequencies), and amplitude 0.5 at $f = f_c$. However, the mode of transition from 1 to 0 can be profoundly altered by acting on the filter's parameters n and f_c. Essentially, n controls the slope of that transition, while f_c controls the location of the slope's middle point. Figure 22.15 shows two Butterworth filters of the same order but with different critical frequencies, and Figure 22.16 demonstrates that their application to a reference planar image produces images whose smoothness is strongly and inversely proportional to f_c. On the other hand, Figure 22.17 shows two Butterworth filters of different order but with the same critical frequency. Although the curves are different, Figure 22.18 demonstrates that their application to a reference planar image results in images that are smoother than the original, but not strikingly different from one another. This happens because each filter has a frequency range where it attenuates more than the other, and, therefore, varying the order of a Butterworth achieves a tradeoff between higher and lower frequencies. It should be noted that the frequency f in Figures 22.15 and 22.17 is not expressed in cycles/cm, but as a percentage of the Nyquist (Ny) frequency (the highest frequency that the camera system can "see" with its resolution capabilities). This is appropriate because frequencies that are not "seen" by the camera and yet are present in the image must represent noise, and as such should always be completely attenuated by the filter. Ny is generally lower than 1 cycle/cm in current systems.

Having introduced the concepts of space and frequency domains, it is now easier to understand why a ramp filter is used in filtered backprojection (LSFBP). As seen in Figure 22.1, the process of backprojection (LSBP) inherently creates large and uniform (i.e., low frequency) structures, as it smears the measured count profile activities uniformly across the image matrix. The ramp filter, shown in Figure 22.19 together with its inverse Fourier transform or spatial representation, progressively amplifies higher frequencies (attenuates lower frequencies), thus compensating for that phenomenon and minimizing the star artifact. The ramp filter is a high-pass filter, and as such it amplifies noise; it is, therefore, often necessary that the individual projection images be smoothed before filtered backprojection. In principle, a smoothing Butterworth filter could be combined with the ramp filter, creating a hybrid filter to be applied to the unprocessed projection data during backprojection and thus avoiding two separate filtering operations. In practice, however, this approach is rarely used.

Background Subtraction in Planar Images

SPECT does not require background subtraction, as it maps a three-dimensional radioisotopic activity distribution onto a three-dimensional image volume. On the other hand, background subtraction is a form of image enhancement usually needed in planar imaging. As was explained, a two-dimensional projection image reflects the distribution of activity in the three-dimensional patient volume, and as such it will contain contributions from structures underlying and overlying the heart. These spurious contributions, cumulatively termed background, reduce the contrast of potential perfusion defects in the myocardium, possibly resulting in a normal diagnosis in the presence of perfusion abnormalities. A processing approach that minimizes background contributions is the bilinear interpolative background subtraction technique developed by Goris, et al. (85), and later modified by Watson, et al. (86). In this approach, a human operator defines the heart's location by sizing and positioning a rectangular boundary region tightly around the heart in the planar image. The region serves as a mask in that all pixels outside it are zeroed. The value of each pixel $P(x,y)$ inside the mask is modified by subtracting from it an estimated, spatially-variant background value based on the shortest distance of $P(x,y)$ from the four sides of the mask and the pixel values at the mask's boundary. In different implementations of interpolative background subtraction, the boundary region is irregular (87), polygonal (88), or elliptical (89), no one method being clearly superior to the others (90). Of note, positioning a boundary region around the left ventricle in static planar images effectively segments the left ventricle and isolates it from other structures (see Image Analysis section).

Background subtraction should be applied on a frame-by-frame basis in dynamic planar studies, such as ECG-gated blood pool studies (87, 88, 91). Although the uncorrected images may be just as effective as the background-corrected ones for ejection fraction determination (92, 93), the improvement in the corrected image's contrast facilitates LV edge detection, as well as the assessment of wall motion abnormalities. In some approaches, it is necessary that the edges of the left ventricle be detected before background estimation and subtraction (94).

Scatter Correction

At the present time, no scatter correction is routinely used with either planar or SPECT myocardial imaging. Both in planar and in SPECT imaging, the great majority of the radiation emitted from the heart is scattered by the surrounding tissue through Compton-type interactions (1). Scattered γ-rays typically carry incorrect positional information (95), and, if imaged, result in reduced lesion contrast (much as background activity in planar images). Most scattered radiation can be prevented from reaching the camera's detector by using a collimator; however, some scatter is always present because collimators must be efficient enough to yield images of good counting statistics (15). Rejection of scattered radiation that reaches the detector is performed at the time of data acquisition by using a "tight" energy discrimination window centered on the isotope's photopeak; but once again, the window cannot be too tight for statistical reasons. Consequently, scatter correction methods have been introduced which can be applied to the projection data at the image enhancement step. Most scatter correction methods rely on modern cameras' capability to acquire data in multiple energy windows. One popular approach uses a standard window centered on the isotope's photopeak and another at lower energy, in the Compton region of the spectrum (1). The scatter image is scaled and subtracted from the photopeak image (66, 69), yielding, in first approximation, a scatter-purged image. Since scatter in the photopeak region is different from scatter at lower energies, alternative approaches have used two windows adjacent to each other and positioned on the photopeak so as to "split" it (67, 96), a window centered on the photopeak and two small subwindows on both sides of the main window (97), or as many as 5–30 separate windows variously distributed on the spectrum (73). Another class of software methods for scatter correction is based on the principle that scatter can be expressed as the convolution of the unscattered projection data with a "scatter function." If the scatter function can then be estimated from Monte Carlo simulations or line source measurements, the inverse operation (in the space or frequency domain) can be applied to deconvolve the scatter kernel from the projection data (98–101).

Even a cursory review of the literature on scatter correction algorithms will reveal that no one algorithm is universally accepted. This probably stems from the lack of comparative data on their relative efficacy, especially in clinical patient images. This limitation may be overcome through the acquisition of data in energy list mode and their successive sorting and processing as required by the various windowing or deconvolution algorithms. Since scatter correction in single-isotope studies and isotope crosstalk correction in dual- or multiple-isotope studies are two aspects of the same problem, it is reasonable to assume that progress toward their solution will be parallel.

Attenuation Correction

Photon attenuation is a concept that applies to SPECT or planar imaging. Its correction, however, is, for practical purposes, limited to SPECT. Photon attenuation is perhaps the single most serious impediment to absolute quantitation in myocardial SPECT. Unlike PET, attenuation in SPECT is dependent on the length of travel of the photons, and on the thickness and types of materials they traverse before impinging on the detector. The traditional way to address this problem has been to acquire projection data over 360°, and then to average data from opposing projections using the arithmetic or geometric mean, before reconstruction. This approach is easy to implement and results in attenuation that is reasonably depth independent and uniform in the field of view. However, the acquisition time for 360° data sets is generally longer than for 180°, the reconstructed images are less sharp and contrasty, and the algorithm itself is accurate for brain studies, but not for myocardial studies.

Another, more computationally demanding class of techniques to correct for attenuation is based on modifications of the backprojection process. In these approaches, each pixel in each projection image is divided by an attenuation factor estimated from the distance between that pixel and the x-axis of a rotating coordinate system (102). The normalized set of projection images is termed the exponential Radon transform, and from that set transaxial images can be reconstructed by applying a modified backprojection algorithm (103–105).

A simple, widely adopted correction method that is applied directly to the reconstructed data is Chang's method (106). In this approach, an image reconstructed without attenuation correction provides an estimate of the outline of the patient's section. The average distance D from the outline is calculated for each pixel within that section, and the counts at the pixel are assumed to have been attenuated by $e^{-\mu D}$, where μ is an uniform attenuation coefficient at the energy of interest. Unfortunately, μ is far from uniform in the human thorax. Thus, this attenuation correction method is not routinely used in myocardial SPECT studies. Chang's algorithm can be modified to include spatially varying attenuation coefficients, but the attenuation maps must be somehow determined from additional measurements. A way to do this is by acquiring transmission images in addition to emission images. Transmission images can be acquired using computerized tomography (107, 108), or a radioactive flood source positioned opposite the detector and on the other side of the patient. If the flood source contains a different isotope from that within the patient, emission and transmission images can be acquired simultaneously (109), otherwise two separate imaging sessions are required (110–112). In more recent developments, flood sources have been replaced by one or more line sources, and same-isotope transmission and emission images are acquired simultaneously. This is achieved by either committing one detector of a multidetector camera exclusively to transmission imaging (113), or by electronically mapping the position of a moving line source onto an opposing detector (114). Finally, hybrid approaches have used transmission images to isolate a small number of structures of markedly different density characteristics (i.e., lungs vs. muscle tissue in myocardial imaging) assigning to each of them a constant attenuation coefficient (115–117).

As with scatter correction, no single attenuation correction method has proved able to completely solve the problem (118), and the goal of absolute quantitation in myocardial SPECT remains elusive. Absolute quantitation links the count value in an image pixel to the concentration of radionuclide activity in the myocardial region corresponding to that pixel, so that region of interest (ROI) analysis of a portion of the myocardium would yield the perfusion of that area in ml/min/g. Nevertheless, application of some of the attenuation correction algorithms described has been reported to achieve quantitation accuracy of better than $\pm 10\%$ in phantoms, as well as dramatic changes in the visual appearance of perfusion patterns in clinical patients. It is likely that within the near future several different approaches for routine attenuation correction will be commercially available.

IMAGE ANALYSIS

The ultimate goal of a nuclear cardiac study is to gain information on the state of the heart, and computerized image analysis allows us to extract that information automatically from the reconstructed and enhanced images. The first image analysis step usually involves image segmentation to isolate the heart from neighboring structures (in myocardial perfusion imaging, the "heart" refers to the left ventricular myocardium). Application of edge detection or pattern recognition algorithms can further outline the boundaries of the LV cavity or the myocardium, both in planar and in SPECT studies. ROI analysis of dynamic studies results in the generation of one-dimensional time-activity curves, which can then be fitted to a variety of mathematic functions. Parametric imaging is used to extract information concerning a specific parameter from a set of images, and to represent it in a visually meaningful way.

Image Segmentation

The simplest form of image segmentation is thresholding. If the heart is the "hottest" structure in an image, setting to zero all the pixels below a certain fraction of the image's maximal pixel count will reduce or eliminate extracardiac activity. Unfortunately, simple thresholding is often inadequate to isolate the left ventricle. In myocardial perfusion studies, hepatic activity may be well above that of the heart (21), and pulmonary, splenic, and intestinal uptake is often of concern. Additionally, the relatively poor image resolution (further worsened by smoothing or reorientation) causes "smearing" of activity (119), so that organs containing radioactivity and in close proximity of one another may appear connected in an image. In planar studies, it is especially problematic to separate the ventricles from the atria.

More sophisticated approaches to segmentation have been devised which use adaptive thresholding. In one such approach, a set of two-dimensional tomographic images are filtered with a kernel reflecting the expected shape of the myocardium, then a threshold is applied and the pixels above the threshold are grouped in various clusters based on adjacency criteria (120, 121). In a more advanced algorithm, segmentation of the myocardium in SPECT studies is performed in the three-dimensional space and makes use of the expected location, size, and shape of the heart, together with iterative "erosion" and "dilatation" of voxel clusters (122, 123). In particular, an initial threshold is applied to the three-dimensional image volume, and the relative clusters determined by depth-first search from seed voxels (124). A candidate left ventricle cluster is selected. If its volume is greater than the physiologic range, erosion of the cluster is performed by raising the threshold in small steps until the cluster is broken down into two or more subclusters. Once the left ventricle cluster is identified, the effect of the previous thresholding is relieved by dilatation, i.e., by adding 1-voxel-wide layers to the cluster while making sure that no one pixel reconnects the Left ventricle to other clusters. An example of the application of this method to a ^{99m}Tc-sestamibi myocardial SPECT study with prominent intestinal uptake is shown in Figure 22.20.

In ECG-gated studies, isolation of the left ventriculear cavity or myocardium can also be effected by identifying and clustering pixels whose count value changes the most during the cardiac cycle. In fact, count variations in an image region are a consequence of motion of the corresponding body region imaged (left ventricle myocardium in myocardial gated SPECT, or radioactive blood in planar- or SPECT-gated blood pool studies). This analysis can be implemented in the space, as well as in the frequency, domain (125). Motion-based segmentation was applied to gated blood pool planar studies by Nelson, et al. (126), who determined the minimum count value throughout the cardiac cycle for each image pixel, then pooled those values together into a "minimum image" and subtracted it from each dynamic frame. Since the minimum image represented, in first approximation, structures that did not move, the result was "stroke images" with the isolated ventricles at end-diastole and the isolated atria at end-systole.

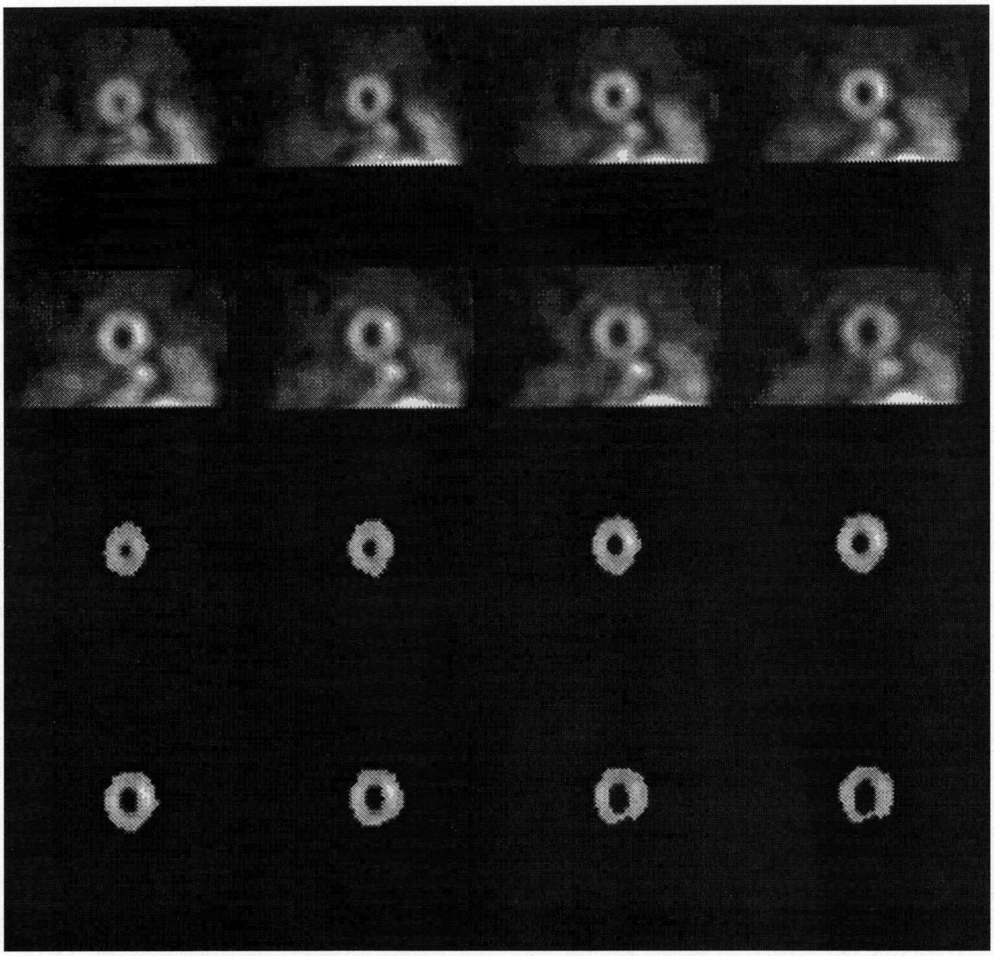

Figure 22.20. Image segmentation. *Top two rows:* Eight consecutive short axis slices (left to right = apex to base) of a ^{99m}Tc-sestamibi patient study with considerable hepatic and intestinal uptake. *Bottom two rows:* Application of the segmentation algorithm described by Germano, et al. (123), identifies the LV myocardium and isolates it for further processing.

Edge Detection

In addition to isolating the heart from other structures in the image set, image segmentation can be used to define heart edges or boundaries, such as the left ventricular endocardial and epicardial surfaces in SPECT studies. The attractiveness of this approach is that it leads to the determination of myocardial and left ventricular cavity volumes, whose knowledge is critical in a number of applications. For example, transient ischemic dilatation of the left ventricular cavity (a marker of severe and extensive coronary artery disease (127, 128)) as a result of exercise or pharmacologic stressing can be measured from static rest/stress SPECT studies. Also, quantities such as stroke volume, ejection fraction, myocardial motion, and thickening can be derived from volume measurements in gated SPECT studies, adding functional information to the conventional perfusion pattern analysis (129–131). Endocardial surfaces have been estimated in gated blood pool SPECT studies by operator-guided thresholding, combined with constraints that the surfaces be smooth, continuous, and convex (132). In gated myocardial SPECT studies, endocardial and epicardial surfaces have been estimated by computing image intensity gradients along radials originating from the left ventricle's long axis (133). Note that the gradient of a count distribution is equivalent to the first derivative of that distribution's profile, and that the endocardial and epicardial surfaces are the loci of the gradients' local maxima and minima, respectively. Since the maximum and minimum of the first derivative of a function are located at the zero-crossing points of the second derivative, this method is equivalent to application of the Laplacian operator described earlier. As we saw, a sharpening kernel like the Laplacian enhances the edges of a structure, but also increases high-frequency noise in the image; consequently, the myocardial surfaces estimated by this process exhibit sharp discontinuities and artifacts, and require the use of relaxation algorithms (133, 134). A similar application of gradient analysis to a set of two-dimensional, reformatted long axis images studies was described to permit delineation of endocardial and epicardial surfaces in ungated myocardial SPECT studies (135), although successive versions of the same algorithm use the simpler assumption of fixed myocardial thickness (136, 137).

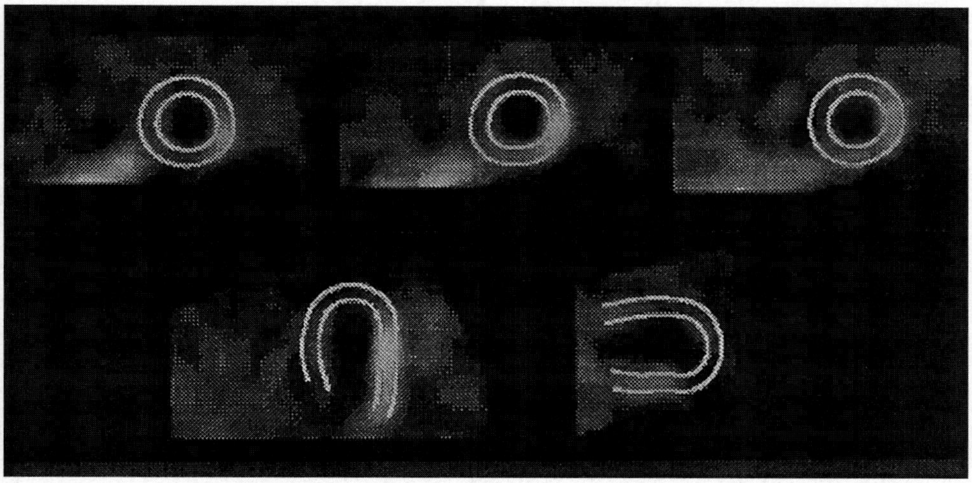

Figure 22.21. Three-dimensional edge detection in a ^{99m}Tc-sestamibi patient study with extensive perfusion defects. The algorithm described by Germano, et al. (123), determines and displays LV endocardial and epicardial contours overlayed to the perfusion images. Edges in correspondence of perfusion defects are estimated based on the artificial intelligence constraints of smoothness, continuity and expected shape of the LV. *Top three images:* Short axis (left to right = apex to base). *Bottom two images:* Horizontal (*left*) and vertical (*right*) long axis.

A different technique for the detection of left ventricular endocardial and epicardial surfaces from gated and ungated myocardial SPECT studies uses the count profiles drawn from the long axis perpendicularly to the mid-myocardial surface of the left ventricle. These profiles are fitted to asymmetric gaussian distributions, the standard deviations of those gaussians calculated and the myocardial surfaces estimated by "straddling" the mid-myocardial surface with appropriate fractions of the standard deviations. (123, 138). Surface discontinuities representing perfusion defects, identified by subthreshold profiles, are iteratively filled in the three-dimensional space using smoothness, the isocontours of the coordinate system, and the geometry of the defect boundaries as constraints. In other words, the algorithm uses the artificial intelligence concepts of smoothness, myocardial shape, and connectivity to find edges even in the absence of perfusion. An example of the application of this method to the end-diastolic frame of an ECG-gated myocardial SPECT study with considerable hepatic uptake and large perfusion defects is shown in Figure 22.21.

In planar first pass and gated equilibrium blood pool studies, the edge of the left ventriclear cavity has been determined in various ways (139–145). The most widespread approach uses a combination of the Laplacian operator and thresholding: the Laplacian operator is applied to the image(s) horizontally and vertically (125), and possibly along the image diagonals (144). Statistical noise is a major hindrance with this method, and it leads to the creation of spurious edges. The edges themselves are often discontinuous and/or more than 1 pixel wide, so that further processing is required to achieve "edge thinning" and edge continuity (52). Recently proposed edge detection algorithms make extensive use of artificial intelligence concepts such as knowledge (a) of the expected shape and location of the left venticle and (b) of the structure and complexity of the entire image domain (146, 147).

Image Reorientation (SPECT)

Figure 22.20 shows a series of tomographic short-axis (also termed "oblique") images of the myocardium. Most visual and quantitative analysis is performed on the short-axis images, as opposed to the tomographic transaxial images. Transaxial images resulting from tomographic reconstruction represent planes (slices) perpendicular to the long axis of the patient, and, therefore, usually not perpendicular to the long axis of the left venticle. A plane cutting obliquely through the myocardium sees an apparent myocardial thickness that depends on the angle of intersection, and artifactual inhomogeneities in the regional count densities may result (119). Also, the heart's orientation in a patient's chest varies amongst different individuals. Thus, the orientation of the transaxial images is not standardized, and visual interpretation in these conditions has been reported to cause lower sensitivity and specificity for the detection of perfusion defects (148, 149). By contrast, short-axis images, which are perpendicular to the long axis of the left ventricle, standardize both display and interpretation of myocardial SPECT studies. Additionally, they make it possible to present three-dimensional information in two-dimensional polar maps, a standard tool for quantification of myocardial parameters (150).

The transformation of transaxial into short-axis image sets is realized via the reorientation process. Reorientation typically consists of two operator-guided steps. First, a transaxial image containing a good-sized cavity is selected, and the long axis in that transaxial plane is manually drawn and overlayed onto the image (Fig. 22.22, *left*). The image volume is then reformatted along planes perpendicular to the transaxial plane and parallel to the long axis. Again, the operator selects a sagittal slice and draws the long axis projection in that plane (Fig. 22.22, *center*). The orientation of the long axis in the transaxial and the sagittal plane uniquely defines its orientation in the three-dimensional space, and the image volume is finally reformatted along planes perpendicular to that direction, generating a set of short-axis images (Fig. 22.22, *right*) (151). It was demonstrated that incorrectly performed reorientation results in serious artifacts (152, 153), yet the operator-guided process is fraught with subjective judgment and prone to inter- and intraobserver variability.

Several algorithms have been proposed to automate the reorientation process. In one approach, the myocardial

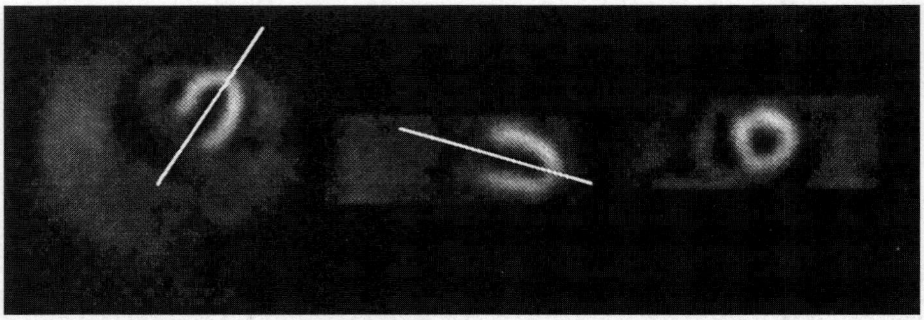

Figure 22.22. Reorientation of transaxial into short axis images. The LV long axis is determined in a transaxial image (*left*) and a vertical long axis image (*center*). Then the image volume is resliced perpendicularly to the LV, resulting in "doughnut-like" images (*right*).

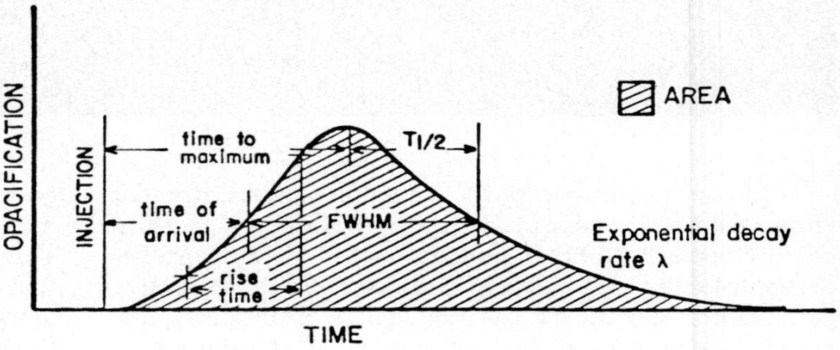

Figure 22.23. Time-activity curve from an ROI centered on the LV cavity, describing the first passage of a bolus of radioactivity through the LV. (Reproduced by permission from Garcia EV, Bateman TM, Berman DS, et al. Computer techniques for optimal radionuclide assessment of the heart. In: Gottschalk A, Hoffer PB, Potchen EJ, eds. Diagnostic nuclear medicine. Vol. I. 2d ed. Baltimore: Williams and Wilkins, 1988:259–290.)

apex is identified as the point of maximum count gradient along the myocardial midline in a two-dimensional transaxial image. The long axis is assumed to lie along the line passing through the apex, and encountering the least amount of activity in its path (154). A similar approach requires the initial manual drawing of the long axis in two tomographic images, and then iteratively improves on that estimate by comparing it to the locus of the minimal count pixels, calculated along profiles perpendicular to the long axis itself (155). More sophisticated algorithms exploit the fact that the left ventricle has roughly ellipsoidal shape, and therefore its midsurface or "skeleton" can be fitted to a quadratic function in the three-dimensional space, with the major axis of the ellipsoid coinciding with that of the long axis (156). Extraction of the mid-myocardial surface is achieved either by computing the locus of the centers of the maximal spheres included in a binarized mask of the myocardium (157), or more simply by pooling together the maxima along count profiles originating from the center of mass of the segmented left ventricle (122).

Regions of Interest, Time-Activity Curves and Phase Analysis

All dynamic acquisition protocols produce images that can be used to generate time-activity curves. A time-activity curve is a discrete, one-dimensional function displaying the average count activity in a fixed ROI of the image as a function of the temporal frames at which imaging takes place. In planar first pass imaging, the ROI can be positioned on the left ventricular cavity so that the initial transit of a bolus of radioactivity through the ventricle can be followed. Because frames in first pass studies are very tightly spaced (each lasting on the order of 10 msec), the "temporal sampling" or "temporal resolution" of the related time-activity curve is excellent, resulting in an almost continuous function (Fig. 22.23). This, in turn, allows the extraction of a good number of information items, amongst which the time of arrival, the rise time, and the time to maximum.

In dynamic myocardial SPECT imaging with ^{99m}Tc-teboroxime, it is possible to place an ROI on a myocardial wall and derive a time-activity curve showing the uptake and washout from the myocardium for this agent (20, 22, 24). At 1 minute per frame as a minimum, the temporal resolution of this curve is much lower than in first pass imaging, due to count statistics constraints. However, preliminary results from animal studies and computer simulations (41, 158) show that, if a temporal sampling of $\leq$15 sec per frame could be achieved, compartmental modeling analysis could be implemented in SPECT as done in ^{13}N-ammonia and ^{18}FDG myocardial PET (159). Linear compartmental models are used to estimate parameters that characterize biologic processes from the kinetics of a tracer participating in those processes. A compartment is defined as a space (not necessarily a physical space) into which the tracer is uniformly distributed. The amount of tracer (per unit time) that leaves a compartment for another is defined by a rate constant, and is graphically represented as an arrow connecting the two compartments. A simple compartmental model for the delivery (extraction) of a tracer from blood vessels to tissue is shown in Figure 22.24. Several compartments can be grouped into a larger, global compartment, or a compartment can be broken down into subcompartments. With terminology borrowed from the theory of linear systems, each compartment is a black box with one or more inputs and outputs. The relationship between an input $i(t)$ and an output $o(t)$ is

$$o(t) = I(t) \otimes h(t) \quad (4)$$

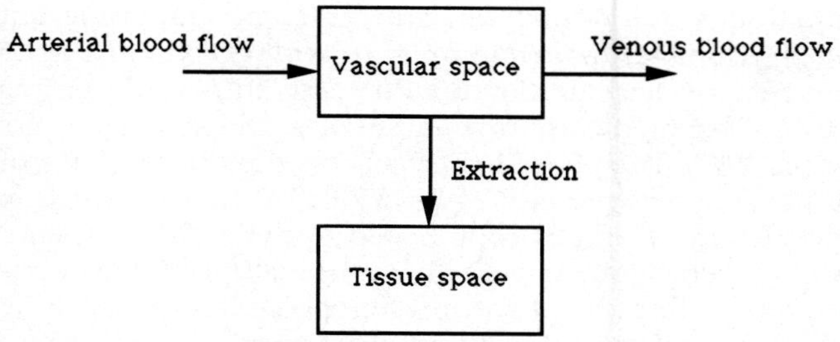

Figure 22.24. A simple two-compartment model for blood supply to tissue. In compartmental modeling analysis, a biologic process can be defined and measured in terms of a radioactive tracer's transfer between "compartments" characterized by input and output rate constants.

where $h(t)$ is the transfer function of the compartment for that specific I/O pair. An extensive description of tracer kinetic modeling, compartmental analysis and its application to nuclear medicine has been reported by Huang (160).

A time-activity curve is a discrete sequence of data points, but it can be approximated by, or "fitted" to, a continuous mathematic function of time. Fitting consists in (a) selecting a type of function whose general shape matches that of the time-activity curve, then (b) iteratively varying the function's parameters to improve the match. In the least-squares fitting method, the optimal match is obtained by minimizing the squared distances of the data points from the fitting function (161, 162). The fitting process reduces the statistical variability intrinsic to the data, thus representing a form of smoothing. With reference to Figure 22.23, the rightmost portion of the curve could be fitted by an exponential function of the type $k\,e^{-\lambda t}$, where λ is the decay rate of activity in the left ventricle.

ROIs are used to generate time-activity curves, but also to measure average activities (as well as ratios of activities) in various regions of static images. Regrettably, an issue not often addressed in the literature is the appropriate size and location of ROIs. The ROI should be large enough (contain enough pixels) to average out statistical noise, but small enough with respect to the structure on which it is placed to minimize the count loss from partial volume effects. Partial volume penalizes objects of dimensions smaller than twice the resolution of the camera system, making the apparent concentration of activity in those objects lower than the true concentration (119). Figure 22.25 explains the partial volume effect in one-dimensional objects: A "large" object containing a uniform activity concentration of 100 (*dashed line, top*) is seen by the camera system as containing a smoother, gaussian-like activity distribution with maximum value of 100 (*solid line, top*), while a "small" object with the same activity concentration (*dashed line, bottom*) appears as containing a gaussian activity distribution of maximal value $C_m < 100$. It should be easily understood, then, that an ROI centered on the apparent maximal-count pixel of a large object will yield measurements fairly independent of the ROI's size. By contrast, an ROI centered on the maximal-count pixel of a small object will yield measurements of value inversely proportional to the ROI's size. Based on the reconstructed resolution (10–20 mm full width at half maximum (FWHM))

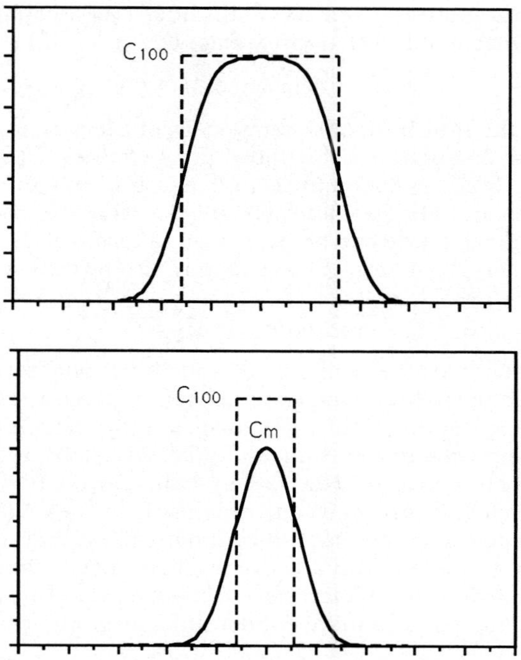

Figure 22.25. Partial volume effect. When an object containing an uniform concentration of radioactivity (*dashed line, top*) is larger than twice the resolution of the nuclear camera system, the imaged distribution is somewhat blurred but its maximum value coincides with the original concentration C_{100} (*solid line, top*). If, however, the object is smaller (*dashed line, bottom*), the maximum value of the imaged distribution C_m is lower than C_{100} (*solid line, bottom*). In other words, the "recovery coefficient" of the activity distribution in the bottom graph is <1 (119).

of current camera systems, the LV cavity can be considered a large object, but the myocardial wall cannot. Therefore, extreme caution should be used when collecting data from myocardial ROIs, a possible rule of thumb being that of using ROIs of a diameter lower than half the apparent myocardial thickness (163). A complete discussion of the effect of the ROI size and shape on the measured myocardial activity can be found in the work of Gambhir (164).

An interesting generalization of the ROI concept is to consider each pixel in the image as an ROI; in other words, time-activity curves can be generated for every pixel in the image. The main application of this technique is phase analysis of gated planar first pass or blood pool studies (165), although the same analysis can be performed for each voxel in gated SPECT blood pool studies (166). Phase analysis is a particular case of Fourier analysis. As explained earlier for a spatial function $f(x)$, the Fourier transform (rigorously, the Fourier series) of a temporal function $f(t)$ expresses that function as a sum of sine and/or cosine functions of different frequencies and amplitudes. It descends that each time activity curve $f_{i,j}(t)$ corresponding to the image pixel (i,j) can be expressed as

$$f_{i,j}(t) = A_0 + A_1\cos(ft+f_1) + A_2\cos(2ft+f_2) + A_3\cos(3ft+f_3) + \ldots \quad (5)$$

where $A_0, A_1, A_2, A_3, f_1, f_2, f_3 \ldots$ are, of course, functions of the specific pixel considered (167). Since time-activity curves for a gated blood pool study are always periodic functions without major discontinuities (168), equation 5 can be reasonably well approximated by

$$f_{i,j}(t) = A_0 + A_1\cos(ft+f_1) \quad (6)$$

i.e., by the first harmonic component of the series. A distribution histogram of the pixel phase values $f_1(i,j)$ can then be built, and examined to detect wall motion asynchronies and abnormalities (169–171). Moreover, the entire dynamic study can be expressed in terms of the three parameters A_0, A_1, and f_1, as explained in the next section.

Parametric Images

The terms "parametric imaging" and "functional imaging" are often used interchangeably. Based on the observation that most nuclear medicine images are, by their very nature, functional rather than anatomic, Goris (52, 172) distinguished between descriptive, true parametric, true functional or physiologic, and diagnostic images. What all these types of images have in common is that they are derived or extracted from a set of original images, and that they provide a particular piece of information present in the original set in a more condensed, easily interpretable form.

Examples of true parametric images are the phase and the amplitude images from gated planar first pass or blood pool studies (165, 167, 168, 170, 173). Figure 22.26 shows two cosinusoidal curves with the same phase but different amplitudes (*top graph*), or with the same amplitude but different phases (*bottom graph*). In both graphs, the solid curve expresses equation 6 with $f_1=0$, thus representing the first harmonic approximation of a time-activity curve for pixel (i,j). The phase image collects the phases $f_1(i,j)$ of all the time-activity curves for pixels in the left ventricle, and displays them in color-coded format. If the LV contracts synchronously or "in phase," the $f_1(i,j)$ will have similar values, and the phase image representation of the LV will have uniform color. Similarly, two amplitude images can be built by collecting all the $A_0(i,j)$ and the $A_1(i,j)$. The reason why phase and amplitude images are called true parametric images is that they contain full information on the study from which they originate. To the extent that the first harmonic approximation of time-activity curves is valid, the entire gated planar first pass or blood pool study can be reconstituted from the knowledge of the three pixel-dependent "parameters" A_0, A_1, and f_1. An example of phase and amplitude images for a gated planar first pass study performed on a normal patient is shown in Figure 22.27.

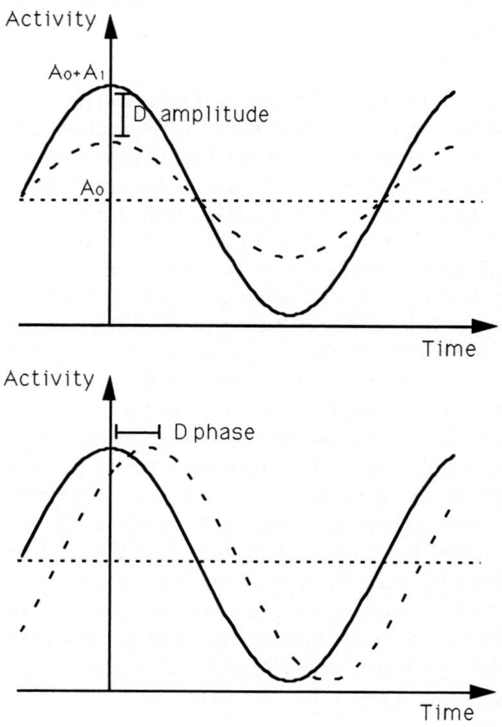

Figure 22.26. Phase analysis of time-activity curves. The two cosinusoidal curves in the *top* graph are "in phase" but have different amplitudes, while the two in the *bottom* graph have the same amplitude but are "out of phase," or shifted relative to each other. All curves are described by modifications of equation 6, in particular: $f(t) = A_0+A_1 \cos(ft)$ (*solid curves*), $f(t) = A_0+(A_1-\text{D amplitude}) \cos(ft)$ (*dashed curve, top*), and $f(t) = A_0+A_1 \cos(ft+\text{D phase})$ (*dashed curve, bottom*).

True functional or physiologic images do not contain enough information to allow mathematic reconstruction of the original data; however, they are important because of their immediate physiologic meaning. Examples of physiologic images are the ejection fraction image and the stroke volume image. The stroke volume (SV) and the ejection fraction (EF) images, proposed by Maddox, et al., for gated blood pool studies (174), are built from the background-corrected end-systolic (ES) and end-diastolic (ED) images in the study. For each pixel (i,j) within the left ventricular cavity, it is simply

$$SV_{(i,j)} = ED_{(i,j)} - ES_{(i,j)} \quad (7)$$

$$EF_{(i,j)} = \frac{ED_{(i,j)} - ES_{(i,j)}}{ED_{(i,j)}} \quad (8)$$

The ejection fraction image permits visual evaluation of regional left ventricuallar wall motion by highlighting the decrease in counts in the outer peel (ejection shell) of the left ventricular cavity from ED to ES. This change in counts is related to the volume difference between ED and ES (175, 176). The stroke volume image (which is not normalized to the patient's ED configuration) is more difficult to interpret, as it shows substantial variability in normal patients. Therefore, it is more often used for delineation of the left ventricular perimeter (174).

Diagnostic images combine the information extraction, synthesis and display capabilities of true parametric and true functional images with the incorporation of one or several diagnostic criteria. For example, one could estimate the range of values ("normal range") for the regional ejection fraction in a population of healthy patients, then zeroing the pixels whose values are outside that range in the ejection fraction image. This would provide immediate visual identification of areas of abnormal contraction in the left ventricle. Similarly, one could estimate the normal range of values for regional myocardial perfusion in a healthy population, and use that information to modify the abnormal patient's perfusion polar map, another type of parametric image to be defined in the quantification sec-

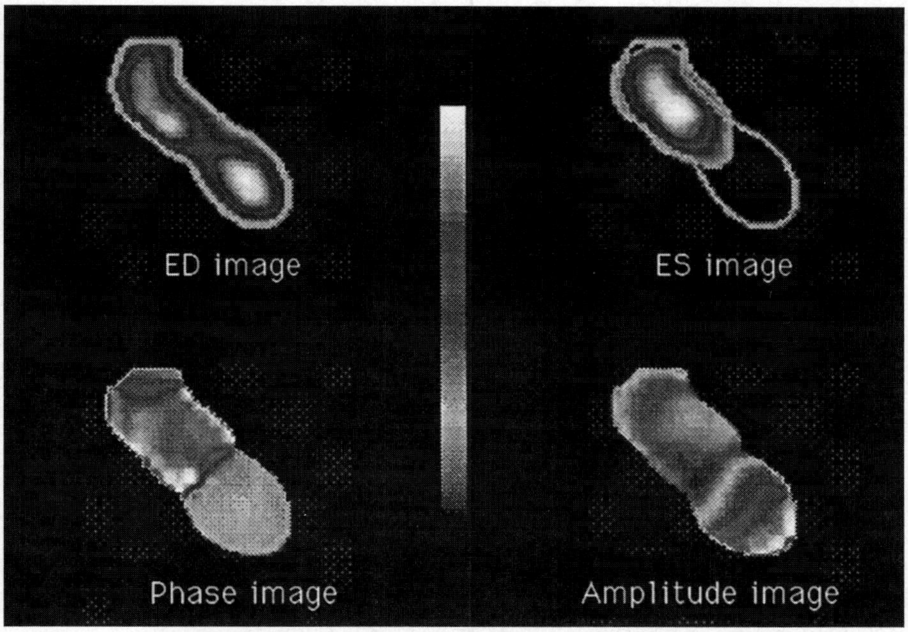

Figure 22.27. ^{99m}Tc-sestamibi first pass study of a normal patient. *Top:* End-systolic and end-diastolic images with superimposed ED contour. *Bottom:* Phase and amplitude images. Note the uniformity of color in the LV portion of the phase image, indicating uniform contraction of the LV myocardium. The amplitude image has a wider range of colors in the same area, reflecting the fact that different parts of the myocardium move by different amounts, albeit in phase.

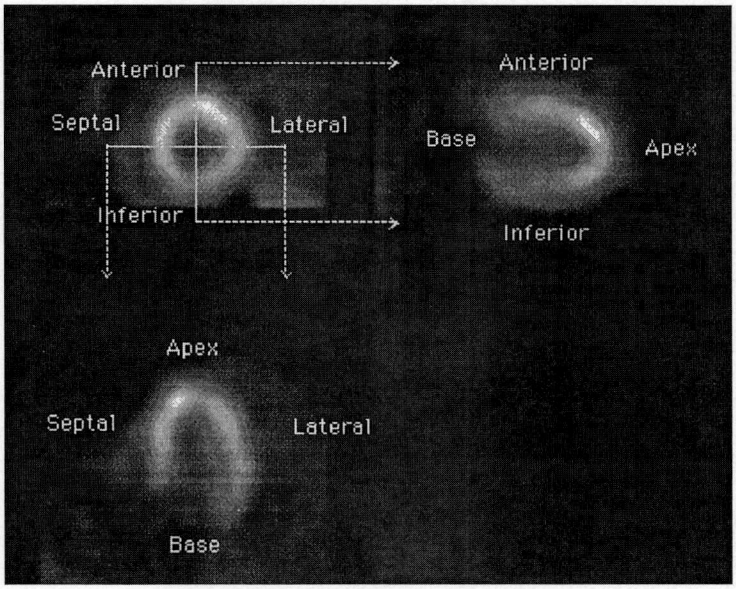

Figure 22.28. Standardized display of myocardial perfusion images. A midventricular short axis image (*top left*), vertical long axis image (*top right*), and horizontal long axis image (*bottom*) are shown.

tion of this chapter. Zeroing all pixels in the map with values outside the normal range allows for immediate visual assessment of the extent of perfusion abnormalities, while color-coding pixels in the abnormal area in a manner consistent with their degree of abnormality allows for clear assessment of the severity of perfusion abnormalities.

Image Display

As explained in the Acquisition section of this chapter, two-dimensional acquisition protocols produce two-dimensional images. Three-dimensional acquisition protocols may produce (a) a temporal sequence of two-dimensional images (dynamic, first pass, or gated planar studies), or (b) a three-dimensional set of stacked two-dimensional images (static SPECT studies). Display of studies of the first type is straightforward, being usually implemented by "endless loop" cineing of the sequential images. By contrast, the display of static SPECT studies requires some standardization (177). It is not generally preferred to display static SPECT studies as three-dimensional volumes; rather, the two-dimensional images constituting the volume are presented side-by-side for immediate visualization of the entire myocardium. In addition to the short axis images, vertical (horizontal) long axis images are generated by slicing the image volume along vertical (horizontal) planes perpendicular to the short axis planes. By convention, the myocardial apex will point upward in the horizontal long axis images, rightward in the vertical long axis images (Fig. 22.28). The number of images displayed for a myocardial SPECT study is 32 (16 short axis, 8 vertical long axis, and 8 horizontal long axis) in the Cedars-Sinai display. The images are arranged in 4 rows of 8: left-to-right, the short axis images progress from apex to base, the vertical long axis images from the septal to the lateral wall, and the horizontal long axis from the inferior to the anterior wall of the LV. When two studies (i.e., rest and stress perfusion) are displayed together, their rows are interlaced to permit easier comparison of homologous images (Fig. 22.29).

Three-dimensional displays are implemented through surface or volume rendering techniques. "Rendering" can be considered a form of parametric imaging, in that it condenses the three-dimensional data set into a two-dimensional picture containing depth cues (178). Surface rendering is essentially equivalent to threshold-based segmentation plus surface extraction. The extracted surface is approximated by a wire mesh tiled with a mosaic of polygons (179), or by the outward faces of the voxels (cuberilles) belonging to the surface itself (180). In either case, the main depth cue is derived from simulated "illumination" of the surface (181).

Surface rendering is the least computationally demanding form of rendering, because it discards all nonsurface information about the rendered object. Nevertheless, interactive rotation of surface-rendered images requires real-time redrawing of all the polygons in the wire mesh, a taxing task for computers not employing specialized hardware. Display of interactively rotated, temporally varying surface-rendered images (as in gated blood pool SPECT studies of the heart (132, 182)) compounds the problem.

Volume rendering visualizes data from the entire image volume, as opposed to from just a surface (183, 184). This is accomplished by tracing rays from each pixel in the rendered image plane to the sampled image volume (backward mapping), or by directly mapping the sampled image volume onto the rendered image plane (forward mapping). The advantages of volume rendering are that the final image

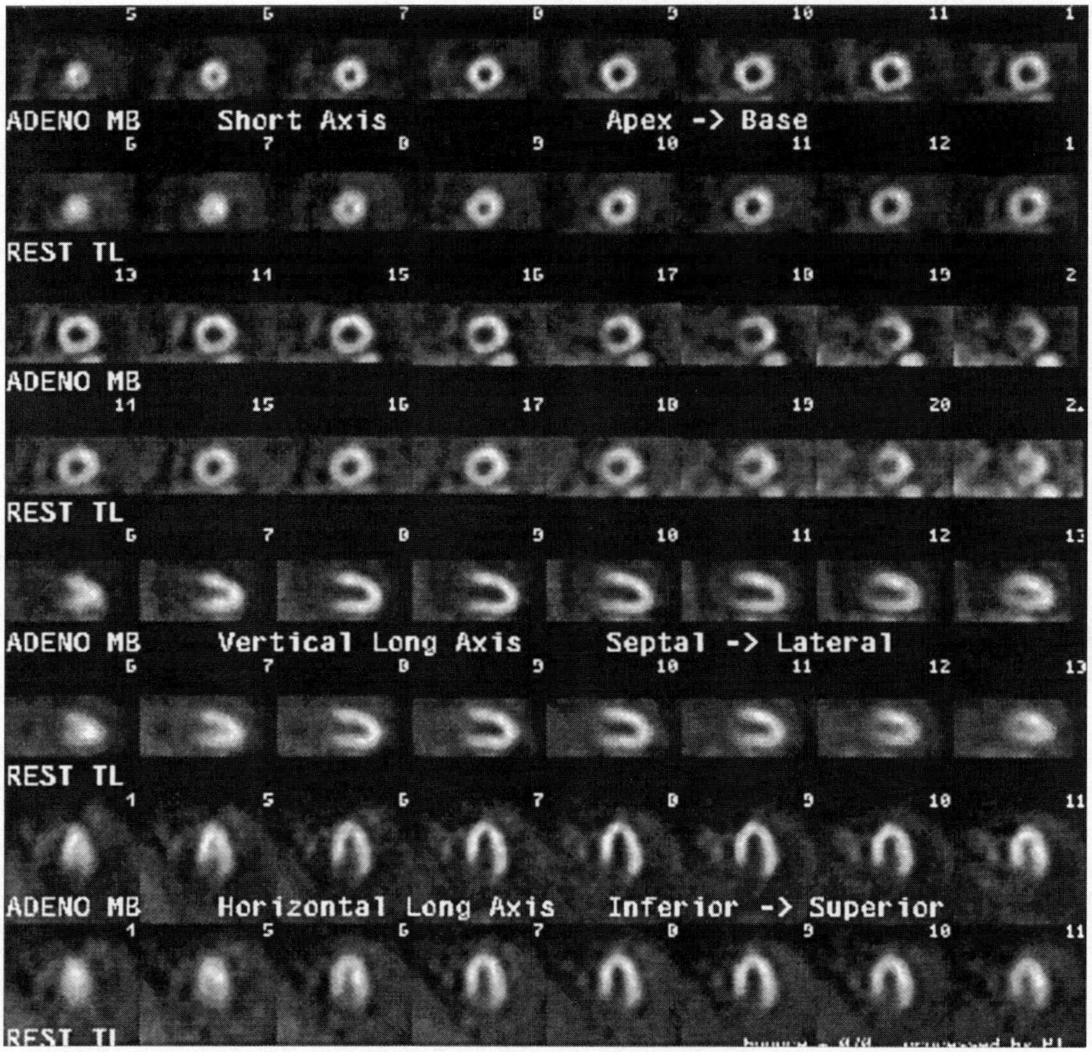

Figure 22.29. Cedars-Sinai standardized display of rest/stress myocardial perfusion studies. Short axis, vertical long axis, and horizontal long axis images for the rest and stress study are displayed in interlaced rows for ease of comparison. In this normal patient example, the rest ^{201}Tl/adenosine stress ^{99m}Tc-sestamibi separate dual isotope protocol described by Berman, et al. (74), was used.

retains more information and does not suffer from artifacts consequent to incorrect surface determination (178); however, every voxel in the image volume must be processed, and the algorithm is more computationally expensive.

Nuclear cardiology planar and SPECT images should be displayed in a gray or monochrome scale, although a 10- or 20-step color scale may be occasionally used to gauge the relative activity of different organs or structures in the image. On the other hand, parametric images make wide use of color scales to accentuate the information they present. Finally, it should be noted that three-dimensional color display requires 24-bit display capabilities; most nuclear medicine workstations have an 8-bit display and need additional graphic boards, at an increase in cost and a decrease in the portability of the display software.

QUANTIFICATION OF CARDIAC PERFUSION AND FUNCTION

The interpretation of nuclear cardiology myocardial perfusion and function is more accurately performed by integrating quantitative with qualitative analysis. While visual interpretation is subjective and more prone to observer variability, quantitative analysis offers an objective approach, providing a more accurate means of assessing the extent, severity, and reversibility of perfusion defects or estimating their functional significance. Quantitative techniques are well-suited to objectively analyzing a patients study over a period of time or following medical or surgical intervention. This section examines quantitative techniques developed at Cedars-Sinai for analyzing myocardial perfusion ^{201}Tl planar (9, 185, 186) and tomographic (150, 187, 188) studies, as well as Tc-sestamibi quantitative tomographic studies (189–191) which were developed at Cedars-Sinai and Emory University, followed by a discussion of quantitative techniques for the analysis of myocardial function.

The type of software developed at Cedars-Sinai over the past 15 years for analysis of relative myocardial perfusion is referred to as semiautomatic interpretative software. This software quantitatively compares a patient's results to a database of normal values, producing a report indicating the normal and abnormal areas of the patient's study. The physician reviews these results and integrates them with the other information related to the patient's study to make the final interpretation.

The development of this type of software follows various labor intensive stages of evolution. Initially, the software is designed, written, and tested. The optimal acquisition, reconstruction, and processing protocols are determined and sample sizes for patient populations are calculated. There are four patient populations utilized in the evaluation: normal, pilot, prospective, and multicenter trial. The gender-matched normal population is used to determine the mean and variance of the normal perfusion distribution of the tracer (150, 185, 190). The pilot population consists of both normal and abnormal patients, and it is used to determine the optimal criteria for detection of disease (186, 187, 190). The prospective population is used to validate the final normal limits and criteria for disease detection (186, 187, 190). The final multicenter trial validation consists of determining the accuracy of the program in a population from different geographic locations (9, 188, 190). The myocardial perfusion programs developed utilizing this technique are described later.

QUANTITATION OF PLANAR ^{201}Tl PERFUSION

The quantitative analysis of planar ^{201}Tl images is divided into three major steps: (a) image processing, (b) extraction of the ^{201}Tl myocardial distribution and washout characteristics, and (c) comparison of the patient's myocardial ^{201}Tl distribution and washout characteristics to those of a normal population. Image processing involves compensation for tissue crosstalk via bilinear interpolative background subtraction (85). The image is then spatially smoothed using a 3×3 filter with weight factors of 4-2-1. The ^{201}Tl myocardial distribution is extracted from the processed image utilizing a maximum count circumferential profile sampling method. A profile consists of 60 points, representing the maximum count values along 60 rays spaced by 6° and originating at the center of the patient's LV cavity. The stress profile is normalized so that its maximum value is 100%, and the corresponding delayed profile is normalized by the same factor. The stress and delayed circumferential profiles are then aligned so that the 90° point in each profile corresponds to the scintigraphic left ventricular apex. This step was implemented to correct for slight differences in patient positioning and to align all curves to a standard frame of reference.

The stress distribution profile is used to represent how the relative ^{201}Tl concentration in one segment of the myocardium compares to another segment during the same period of time. Washout circumferential profiles are also calculated using the following formula:

$$\% \text{ Washout} = \frac{\text{Stress-delayed}}{\times\ 100 \text{ Stress}} \tag{9}$$

These washout profiles are used to determine how the ^{201}Tl concentration in a segment of the myocardium compares to itself at a later time.

The stress and washout profiles are then compared to the corresponding normal limit profiles to identify normal and abnormal myocardial segments. The normal limits are determined from the pooled profiles of male and female "low-likelihood normals," who are classified as normal by having a less than a 1% likelihood of coronary artery disease based on Bayesian analysis of age, sex, symptom classification, coronary risk factors, and the results of an electrocardiographic stress test (192, 193). All "low likelihood" subjects must have a normal resting ECG, as well as achieve more than 85% of their age-predicted maximum heart rate without chest pain or electrocardiographic changes during exercise. The mean and standard deviation are computed for each of the 60 angular segments represented in the stress and washout normal profiles, the threshold for abnormality being 2.5 standard deviations below the mean. Following comparison of the patient's profiles to these normal limits, the normal and abnormal areas are calculated and a quantitative report is generated. An example of the quantitative output of a patients study is demonstrated in Figure 22.30. The multicenter trial vali-

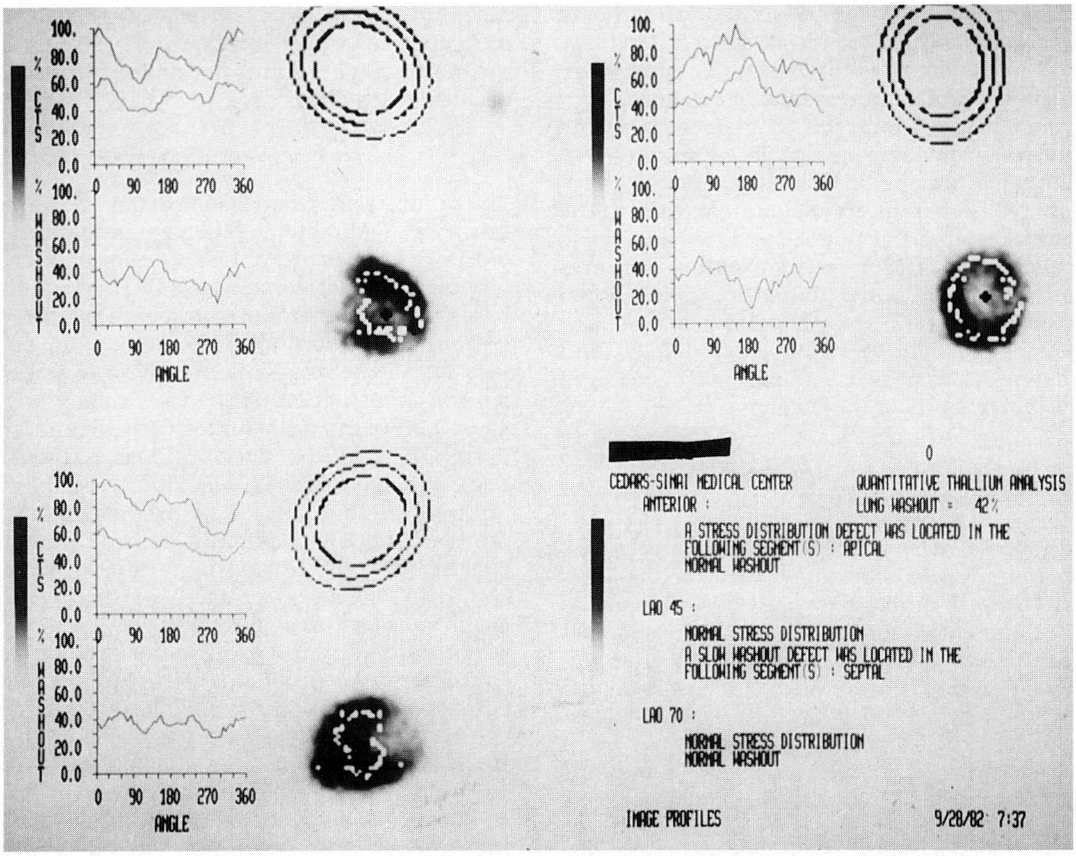

Figure 22.30. Quantitative results for a planar ^{201}Tl study, including stress and rest circumferential profiles, washout profile, abnormality ellipses, and stress quality control image for the anterior (*upper left*), LAO 45 (*upper right*), and LAO 70 (*lower right*) views. The inner ellipse is used as a reference, while breaks in the center ellipse indicate the location of stress defects, and breaks in the outer ellipse indicate washout abnormalities. The English report is also presented (*lower right*).

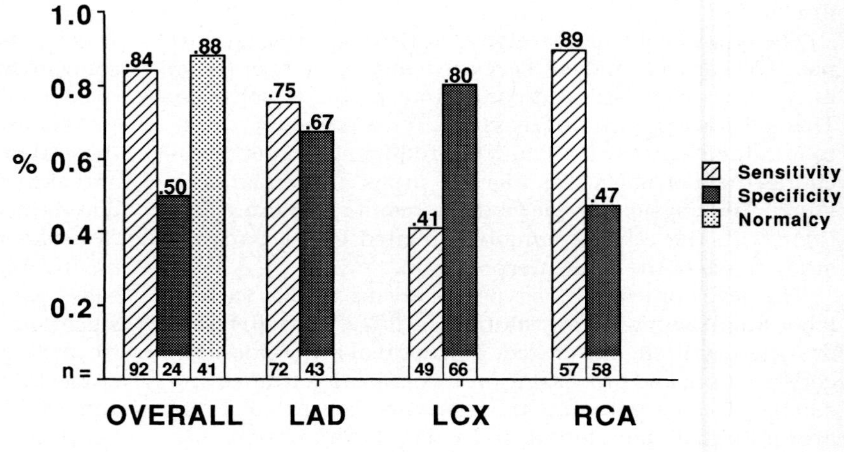

Figure 22.31. Multicenter trial validation results for overall detection and localization of coronary artery disease by the Cedars-Sinai quantitative ^{201}Tl planar analysis program. The trials included four centers contributing a total of 157 patients.

dation results for this approach (9) are shown in Figure 22.31.

There have been other methods utilized for quantitating the myocardial activity distribution (86, 194, 195). While these approaches differ in the way they sample and align the images, the basic processing steps, i.e., smoothing, background subtraction, and myocardial sampling, are employed by all of the techniques.

QUANTITATION OF SPECT ^{201}Tl PERFUSION

SPECT myocardial perfusion imaging is technically more exacting than planar imaging, requiring more expertise and stricter quality control. Several investigators have shown that the tomographic approach offers improved accuracy for the evaluation of coronary artery disease (196–198). Additionally, successful implementation of the technique has been shown to allow objective and accurate analysis of myocardial perfusion (150, 187, 199). The SPECT quantitative program developed by Cedars-Sinai for ^{201}Tl (150, 187, 188) is reviewed, along with comparisons to other approaches.

Analysis of ^{201}Tl SPECT images involves three steps: (a) selection of the myocardial image volume, (b) selection of the LV cavity center and radius, and (c) generation and alignment of the circumferential profiles. The short axis tomograms selected are those extending from the subendocardial portion of the apex to the base of the heart (Fig. 22.32**A**). The last three basal tomograms are not considered for quantitation, due to the variability in drop-off of activity in the inferior and septal regions. The vertical long axis tomograms selected are those extending from the subendocardial portion of the septum to the subendocardial portion of the lateral wall (Fig. 22.32**A**). In the Cedars-Sinai program, vertical long axis slices are used to assess the myocardial perfusion distribution at the apex. The LV cavity center and radius (Fig. 22.32**B**) are then manually selected and used as references for sampling the myocardium and generating the maximum count circumferential profiles. Finally, the profiles are aligned to a common anatomic landmark, i.e., the inferior junction of the right ventricle with the left ventricle for the short axis, and the apex for the vertical long axis tomograms. Alignment is performed to account for differences in heart orientation, and to improve the ability to localize disease (Fig. 22.32**C**). The program generates maximum count circumferential profiles for each of the selected short and vertical long axis tomograms. These profiles are mapped onto a two-dimensional polar map representing the left ventricular myocardium.

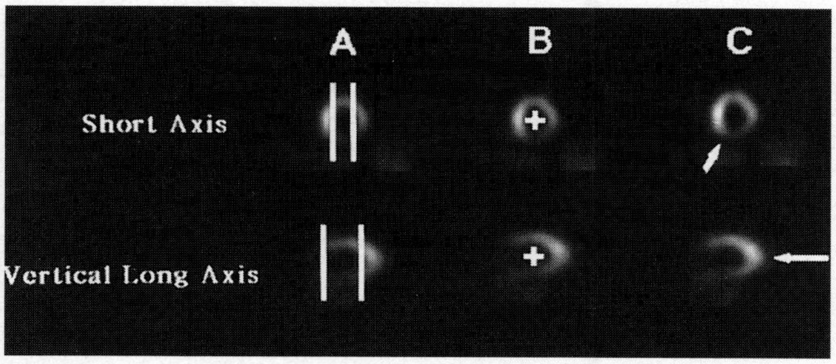

Figure 22.32. Three operator-interactive steps are required when using the Cedars-Sinai quantitative ^{201}Tl tomographic program for processing. The operator selects the slices to be quantitated (**A**), then the LV cavity center (**B**), and the most apical point for alignment purposes (**C**).

Polar maps are a form of parametric imaging, since information regarding the three-dimensional SPECT image volume is extracted and condensed into a two-dimensional representation. They are the two-dimensional equivalent of the one-dimensional circumferential profile curve used in planar imaging. Indeed, a polar map consists of a number of circumferential profiles, which are represented as concentric annuli or rings having the same thickness. Since the size of the polar map is fixed, the thickness of the annuli depends on how many profiles there are, i.e., on the size of the patient's LV. In ^{201}Tl polar maps, the apical portion of the LV myocardium is mapped to the innermost rings in the map, while the circumferential profiles from the short axis images are mapped to the outer rings (Fig. 22.33). The tomograms and quantitative polar map report for a patient are shown in Figures 22.34 and 22.35.

The gender-matched normal limits are derived from patients with a <5% likelihood of having coronary artery disease (low likelihood patients). Given the variable number of annuli in a polar map, annuli corresponding to the short axis profiles are further mapped to five superannuli of greater thickness. Similarly, five superannuli represent the volume displayed by the apex (150). It is with reference to these superannuli that normal limits are generated, so as to ensure standardization. Due to the non-Gaussian distribution of normal circumferential profile points around the mean in the anterolateral and inferoseptal regions, it was determined that profiles constructed by connecting the lowest observed points in the individual normal patient profiles (range approach) represent the best estimate of the limits of normality (187). To account for the different distribution patterns between male and females (200, 201), gender-matched normal limits are utilized. The analysis program determines the values for total defect size and localizes disease to individual coronary territories. These ter-

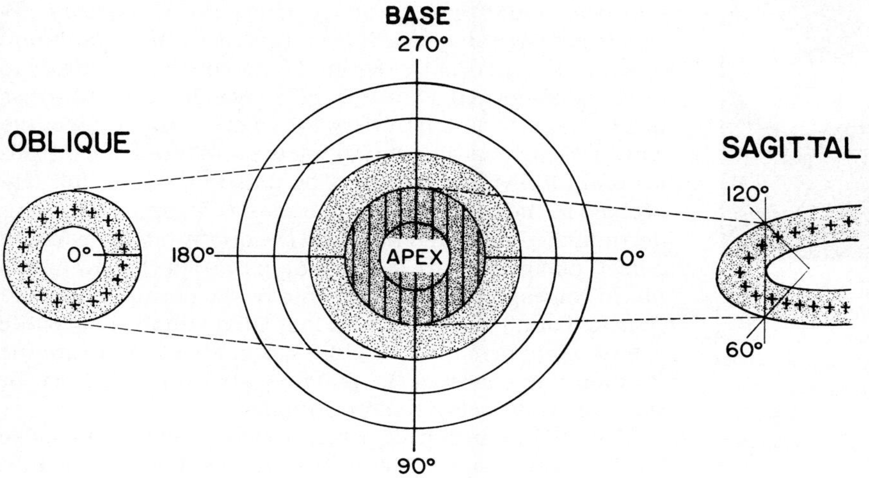

Figure 22.33. Polar map generation for ^{201}Tl SPECT studies. By reducing the information contained in the tomographic image volume to (a) the maximal-count circumferential profiles for the short axis (oblique) images and (b) the apical portion of the maximal-count profiles for the vertical long axis (sagittal) images, one can map a three-dimensional volume onto a two-dimensional plane. (Reproduced by permission from Garcia EV, Bateman TM, Berman DS, et al. Computer techniques for optimal radionuclide assessment of the heart. In: Gottschalk A, Hoffer PB, Potchen EJ, eds. Diagnostic nuclear medicine. Vol. I. 2d ed. Baltimore: Williams and Wilkins, 1988:259–290.)

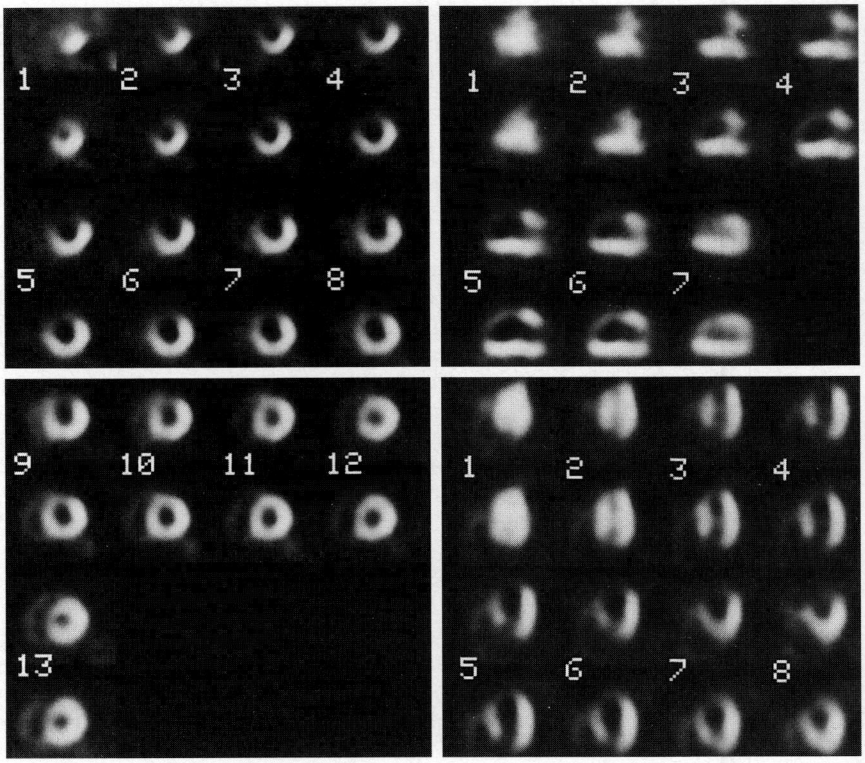

Figure 22.34. ^{201}Tl stress (*odd rows*) and rest (*even rows*) tomographic study. The short axis (*left*), vertical long axis (*upper right*), and horizontal long axis (*lower right*) are displayed. The quantitative results for this study are shown in Figure 22.35.

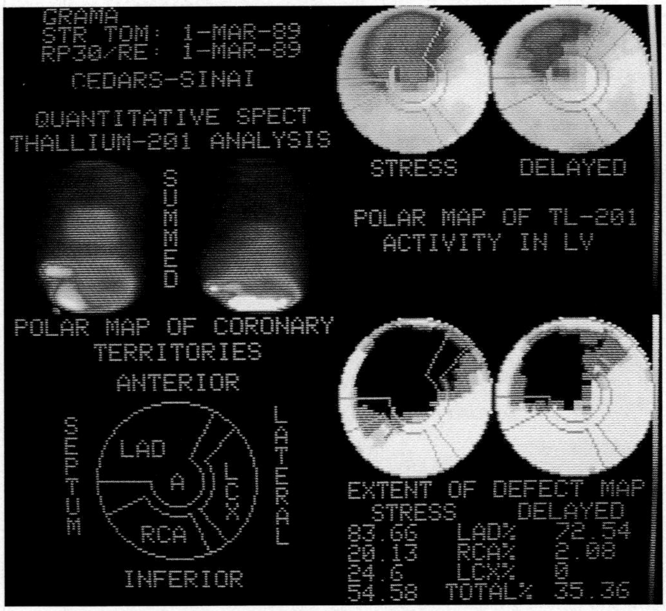

Figure 22.35. An example of the Cedars-Sinai SPECT ^{201}Tl quantitative output for a patient with left anterior descending disease. The report consists of patient information with summed projection images used for quality control (*upper left*), a diagram of vascular territories (*lower left*), raw data stress and rest polar maps (*upper right*), and defect polar maps with quantitative results (*lower right*). In the defect polar maps, pixels corresponding to segments below normal limits are "blacked out," so as to give an immediate impression of the extent of abnormality.

ritories are defined by examining patients with single vessel coronary artery disease (187, 202). The territory borders are visible in the patient example shown in Figure 22.35.

The criteria for disease detection were determined using receiver operating characteristics (ROC) curve analysis to assess what percentage of the polar map should be below normal limits for the relative coronary territory to considered abnormal. Various percentages of abnormality were compared to determine those which provided the optimum tradeoff of sensitivity and specificity for identification of disease in each of the three coronary vascular territories. The optimum threshold was determined to be 12% for the left anterior descending (LAD) and left circumflex (LCX), and 8% for the right coronary artery (RCA) territory, respectively. These percentages represent the minimum amount of abnormality required for a coronary territory to be called abnormal. Figure 22.35 shows the rest and stress polar maps, demonstrating the distribution of counts within the myocardium for the stress and the delayed studies of an individual patient. The patient's stress and rest profiles in the maps are compared to the appropriate gender-matched normal limits, and the quantitative "extent of defect" polar maps are generated. In the defect polar maps, pixels corresponding to segments below normal limits are "blacked out," so as to give an immediate impression of the extent of abnormality. The blacked out areas indicate the location and extent of the patients' abnormal territory for the stress and delayed distribution.

The ^{201}Tl quantitative program was validated in-house (187) and in a multicenter trial study (188). Since the pub-

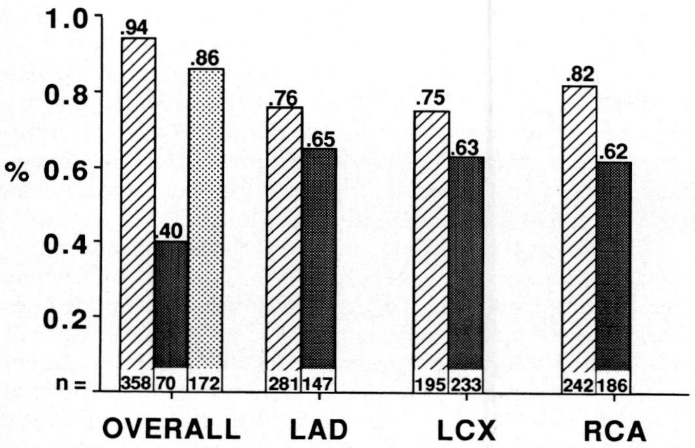

Figure 22.36. Multicenter trial validation results for overall detection and localization of coronary artery disease for the Cedars-Sinai quantitative tomographic Tl-201 program. The trials comprised 22 sites, nine different computer systems, and a total of 600 patients.

lication of the multicenter trial results, which included studies acquired with ADAC, Siemens, and MDS camera systems, there were further multicenter trial studies with six additional systems (Elscint, Picker, Summit, Medasys, Toshiba, and Sophy). The global multicenter trial results for the nine camera/computer systems are listed in Figure 22.36.

Another approach for quantitating ^{201}Tl tomograms is the General Electric Bullseye method (199). The technique is similar to the Cedars-Sinai method, except that it utilizes different filters, analyzes only the short axis slices, samples the myocardium using circumferential profiles consisting of 40 points, and normalizes the profiles to the most normal region of the myocardium. Additionally, normal limits are derived based on a standard deviation approach and offer analysis of washout and reversibility (203–205). Despite these differences, the results of the Bullseye method's multicenter trial validation were very similar to the Cedars-Sinai results. Tamaki, et al. (206), and Caldwell, et al. (207), also developed programs for the quantitative analysis of ^{201}Tl myocardial perfusion. There are slight variations between these approaches and the two previously described.

QUANTITATION OF SPECT ^{99m}Tc-SESTAMIBI PERFUSION

In 1989, investigators at Cedars-Sinai Medical Center and Emory University undertook a research project to develop a program to quantitatively analyze ^{99m}Tc-sestamibi myocardial perfusion SPECT. This effort included the development of optimized imaging, acquisition, and processing protocols (208, 209). Once those protocols were established, a quantitative algorithm was developed for the analysis of the ^{99m}Tc-sestamibi images (189, 190). This quantitative algorithm incorporated many of the features previously described for the Cedars-Sinai quantitative ^{201}Tl and Emory bullseye programs, along with some new features.

The algorithm substantially reduces operator interaction at the LV segmentation stage by performing automatic selection of the processing parameters, i.e., the images to quantitate, the LV cavity center, and the radius of search (121). This enhancement improves the reproducibility and objectivity of the quantitative analysis compared to previous ^{201}Tl approaches. Once the automatically determined parameters are verified or (if erroneous) manually corrected by the operator, the program quantitatively analyzes the data. Sampling of the myocardium uses a hybrid approach, where the apical portion of the myocardium is sampled using spheric coordinates, and the remainder of the myocardium is sampled using cylindric coordinates (Fig. 22.37). This technique results in radial sampling which is mostly perpendicular to the myocardial wall at all

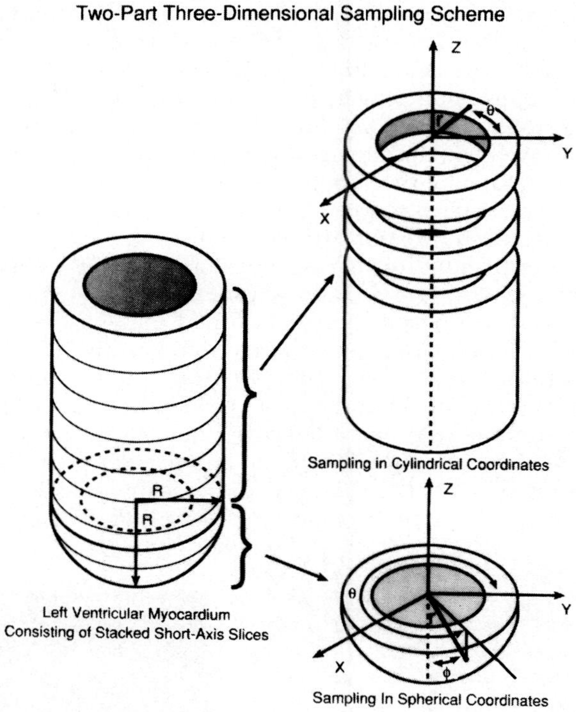

Figure 22.37. Three-dimensional sampling for circumferential profiles extraction and polar map generation in ^{99m}Tc SPECT studies (CEqual). Modeling the apical portion of the LV myocardium as a sphere and sampling along the sphere's radii promotes perpendicularity to the myocardium at the apex. (Reproduced by permission from Garcia EV, Bateman TM, Berman DS, et al. Computer techniques for optimal radionuclide assessment of the heart.In: Gottschalk A, Hoffer PB, Potchen EJ, eds. Diagnostic nuclear medicine. Vol. I. 2d ed. Baltimore: Williams and Wilkins, 1988:259–290.)

points, and thus yields a more accurate representation of the perfusion distribution (203). Using this two-part sampling scheme, maximum count circumferential profiles (each comprised of 40 points) are generated from all of the short axis tomograms.

Gender-matched normal limits have been derived for a rest/stress, low dose/high dose imaging protocol (210) using studies obtained in men and women who have a low likelihood of disease and acquired at Cedars-Sinai Medical Center and Emory University on different commercial camera systems. The two normal populations were combined after it was determined that no significant differences existed between them, and the mean and standard deviation for both the men and women circumferential profiles were generated. The normal limits consist of a set of 12 different profiles, containing a total of 480 points. Normal limits are calculated for each of the measurements of interest, i.e., stress, rest, and reversibility. Since the actual number of patient profiles varies with the size of the person's heart and the pixel size (zoom) of the acquired images, the algorithm maps each patient profile to one of the 12 normal limit profiles (190). The patient's rest profiles are normalized to the most normal area of the patient's stress profiles for calculation of reversibility. Severity assessment is performed by determining the number of standard deviations by which each pixel falls below the mean normal value.

The threshold for disease detection, expressed as the number of standard deviations from the mean which would best separate normal from abnormal patients, is determined by comparing an expert visual reading of the tomographic slices to the output of the quantitative program. Multiple standard deviations were evaluated for each territory, and receiver operating curve analysis was employed to determine the optimal threshold for each area. In the evaluation of a patients' study, the patient's profile points are compared to their respective normal limit values and are considered abnormal if they fall below the normal limit threshold. Localization of disease is determined based on the territories previously defined for ^{201}Tl, which were verified in a subsequent investigation. This investigation further determined that the minimal percentage of abnormal points required for the ^{99m}Tc-sestamibi study to be considered as having a defect in a given vascular territory was 10% for the LAD and LCX, and 12% for the RCA territory.

The severity polar map indicates the number of standard deviations by which each pixel in the defect falls below the mean normal limit. Different numbers of standard deviations are coded in different colors, since the purpose of this map is to give an impression of the degree of abnormality. Conversely, only points above the mean normal limit are considered in the reversibility map. Reversibility is calculated by scaling the rest and stress polar maps to a common value (the most normal region of the stress distribution), subtracting the stress from the rest, and evaluating the difference map for areas of significant change. The stress blackout map forms the basis for the reversibility map, which is created from the stress blackout map by highlighting all abnormal areas with a statistically significant reversibility. Highlighting is performed by coding blacked-out pixels into white.

Quantitative polar maps generated from the profile data represent information related to the defect extent, severity and reversibility. The raw data contained in the profiles are represented in two polar map configurations—distance and volume weighted. The distance-weighted polar map is the basic map described in the ^{201}Tl SPECT quantitation section, and is constructed by mapping sequential maximal-count profiles (from apex to base) onto successive rings in the polar map. Each ring within the polar map is assigned the same width in pixels. The volume-weighted polar map is constructed in much the same way as the distance-weighted polar map, except that the width of each

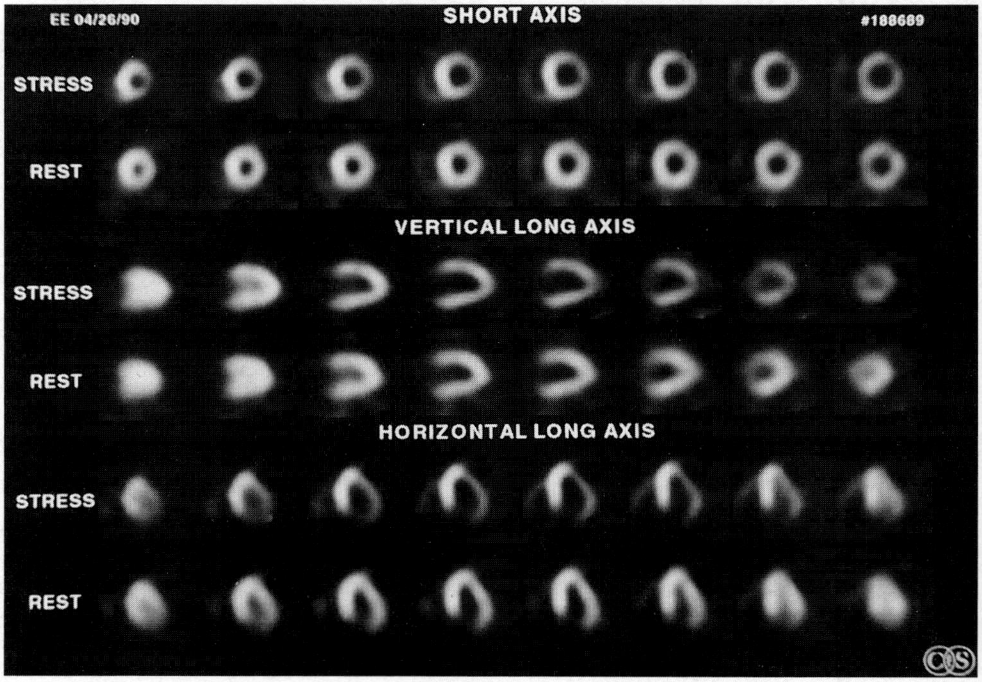

Figure 22.38. Same day rest-stress ^{99m}Tc-sestamibi tomographic study of a patient with prior myocardial infarction. The homologous stress and rest tomograms of the short, vertical long, and horizontal long axis are shown.

ring is decreased from the apex to the base. To determine the width of each ring, the total volume of the myocardium is estimated. The volume of the apical hemisphere is then estimated, and its percentage of the total volume calculated. The apical hemisphere is mapped so that the area it occupies is the same percentage of the total area of the polar map as the volume of the apical hemisphere is of the total volume of the myocardium. Each ring in the apical hemisphere has equal width. For those slices outside the apical hemisphere, the percentage of area that each slice occupies in the polar map is proportional to its percentage of the total volume of the myocardium.

The tomograms and quantitative polar maps of a patient acquired using the same day rest-stress ^{99m}Tc-sestamibi protocol are shown in Figures 22.38 and 22.39. This study is from a 60-year-old male with chronic typical angina and a history of prior myocardial infarction. The study was conducted to assess the extent of ischemia in the area of infarction and to determine if remote ischemia was present. Visual interpretation demonstrated moderately extensive reversible defects in the lateral and midanterior wall of the left ventricle. Quantitative analysis (Fig. 22.39) demonstrated a 22% defect in the LAD territory and a 74% defect in the LCX territory, both reversible. Coronary angiographic findings demonstrated a totally occluded circumflex artery with collaterals from RCA and 80% stenosis of the diagonal. The cardiac catheterization findings correlated with both the visual and quantitative interpretations.

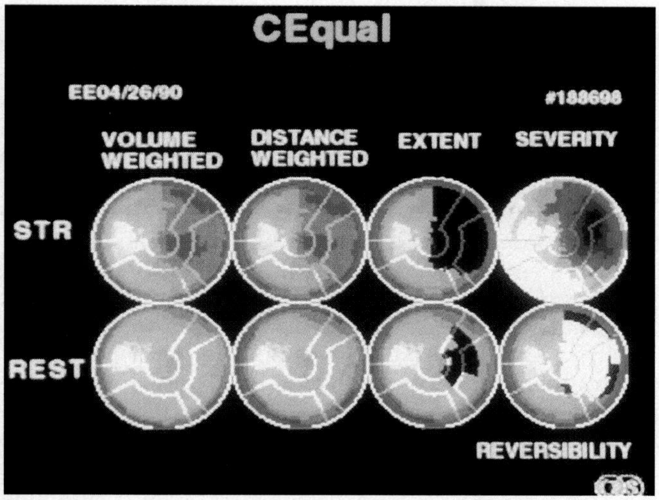

Figure 22.39. CEqual quantitative report for the patients study shown in Figure 22.38. *Top row:* Stress polar maps. *Bottom row:* Rest polar maps. Volume- and distance-weighted, as well as extent, severity (*top right*), and reversibility (*lower right*) polar maps are shown.

The SPECT ^{99m}Tc-sestamibi quantitation program has been validated in a multicenter trial comprising 161 patients from seven different clinical sites utilizing various camera/computer systems (191). The results of this study are shown in Figure 22.40. To summarize, the quantitative approach for ^{99m}Tc-sestamibi SPECT offers improvements over the previous ^{201}Tl approaches (150, 199). Improvements include automatic processing, spherical coordinate sampling of the apex, and the generation of volume-weighted polar maps. Additionally, normal limits include variable standard deviations and profile normalization is accomplished using eight, rather than four, segments (199), which results in improved accuracy for detection of disease. Of note, with all of the quantitative approaches to image interpretation, it is imperative that the acquisition and reconstruction protocols be standardized. The need for standardization in quantitative analysis may help further the whole area of standardization in nuclear cardiology.

Further research is underway to develop normal databases pertaining to the following acquisition protocols: 2-day ^{99m}Tc-sestamibi, separate and simultaneous acquisition dual isotope rest ^{201}Tl/stress ^{99m}Tc-sestamibi, pharmacologic studies, ^{201}Tl, other ^{99m}Tc-based myocardial perfusion agents, as well as protocols incorporating attenuation and scatter correction. Additional SPECT ^{99m}Tc-sestamibi perfusion (CEqual) developments will include prognostic evaluation involving indexes related to severity and reversibility, and defect sizing before and after medical or surgical intervention.

QUANTIFICATION OF MYOCARDIAL FUNCTION

Myocardial function is evaluated in terms of how well the heart pumps blood (ejection fraction, stroke volume), and how much it contracts (myocardial motion) and thickens (myocardial thickening) during the cardiac cycle. Since subsecond temporal resolution is needed to study these phenomena, myocardial function studies utilize dynamic

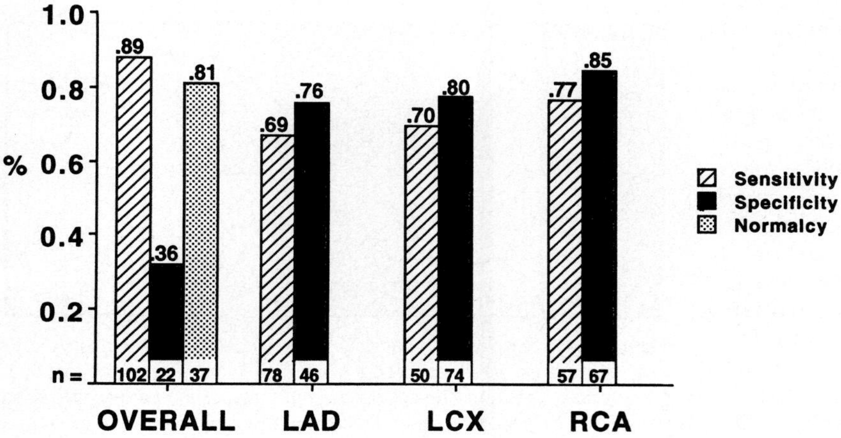

Figure 22.40. CEqual multicenter trial validation results for the overall sensitivity, specificity, normalcy rate, and sensitivity and specificity for localization of disease in individual coronary arteries.

acquisition, either gated or first pass. Quantitative measurements of cardiac function can be global (if they relate to the entire left ventricle or right ventricle) or regional.

The global stroke volume SV and the global ejection fraction EF for the left ventricle are measured from the end-systolic (ESV) and end-diastolic (EDV) left ventricular cavity volumes, as follows:

$$SV = EDV - ESV \tag{10}$$

$$EF = \frac{EDV - ESV}{EDV} \tag{11}$$

The techniques to estimate ESV and EDV can be essentially divided in geometric and count-based techniques. Geometric methods can be applied to three-dimensional (gated blood pool SPECT, myocardial SPECT) or two-dimensional images (planar-gated blood pool, first pass). In the first case, the three-dimensionality of the data makes it possible to simply add up all the voxels bound by the endocardial surface of the left ventricle and the valve plane, then multiply that number by the unit volume that each voxel represents (132). The problem is then reduced to one of edge detection, and the accuracy of the estimated volume is directly proportional to the accuracy with which one can estimate the left ventricular cavity boundaries. When geometric methods are applied to planar first pass or gated blood pool studies, some assumptions must be made to derive a volume estimate from the two-dimensional images. Usually, the left ventricular cavity is assumed to have the shape of an ellipsoid or a prolate spheroid, and its volume is estimated from its area and long axis in the specific projection acquired (53, 211, 212). To the extent that the left ventricle deviates from the postulated model, the results will be incorrect (213). The error in determining EDV and ESV is propagated in the computation of SV and EF, resulting in larger errors for these derived quantities.

Count-based methods for the calculation of left ventricular volumes can be applied to three-dimensional (214) or two-dimensional data and rely on the measurement of counts in an ROI traced over the left ventriucular cavity boundary. The total amount of counts C_{tot} in the ROI is proportional to the cavity volume, and, in the absence of tissue attenuation, that volume can be calculated as C_{tot}/C, where C is a normalization factor expressing the number of counts per unit volume and can be measured from a reference blood sample. Corrections for tissue attenuation have been proposed (215, 216), although these approaches have been reported to be error prone (52). Massardo, et al. (217, 218), suggested that one can eliminate the effect of attenuation by ratioing attenuated counts. In their approach, applied to gated blood pool (217) and first pass data (218), the ratio between the total counts and the maximal pixel counts in the left ventricular cavity is calculated and multiplied by a camera-specific constant to obtain the left ventricualrlar cavity volume. The relative accuracy of count-based ratio methods and other count-based methods for volume estimation has been investigated (219, 220). Count attenuation is not a major problem in EF calculations, because the counts in EDV and ESV (equally affected by attenuation) are ratioed in equations 10 and 11.

Identification of the ES and ED frames, from which EDV and ESV are derived, is done on the time-activity curve generated from an ROI encompassing the left ventricular cavity. Figure 22.41 shows one such curve for a gated blood-pool study: ED corresponds to the curve's maximum (conventionally plotted as the first point in the curve), while ES occurs at the curve's minimum. Temporal smoothing of the curve prior to calculation of EF should be avoided, as it artificially decreases the EF value. There is additional information to be derived from the time-activity curve, if the temporal sampling is fine enough. For example, the left ventricular systolic function can be examined in terms of the ejection rate (ER), i.e., the derivative or slope of the time-activity curve during systole. Similarly, the left ventricular diastolic function can be investigated by examining the peak-filling rate (the maximum slope of the curve after ES) and the time-to-peak-filling rate (the time interval between ES and the point of peak-filling rate). Finally, time-activity curves can be derived for the right ventricle, and the right ventricleular ejection fraction calculated as for the left ventricle (170). The assessment of diastolic function requires some form of bad-beat rejection, which is not required for the assessment of systolic function. In fact, variations in beat length predominantly affect the diastolic phase of the cardiac cycle.

The calculation of regional functional cardiac parameters is somewhat more complex than that of global parameters. The calculation of regional EFs and SVs, for example, requires the definition of regional volumes and their measurement at ES and ED. In planar-gated blood pool or first pass studies, this is done by taking the ROI used to generate the global time-activity curve, dividing it into a number of angular sectors, and generating as many time-activity curves as there are sectors, proceeding then as in the global parameters calculation. The origin of the sectors is the geometric center of the ROI (221), and the statistical quality of the curves is proportional to the sectors' size, which ranges from 6° (222) to 45° (221). In three-dimensional gated blood pool SPECT images, wedge-shaped regional volumes can be defined by connecting the vertexes of endocardial surface "patches" to the left ventricle's long axis (132).

Regional wall motion is closely related to regional EFs. In planar imaging, the same ROI subdivision in sectors used for regional EF determination has been applied to wall motion analysis (91). The change in the sectors' areas be-

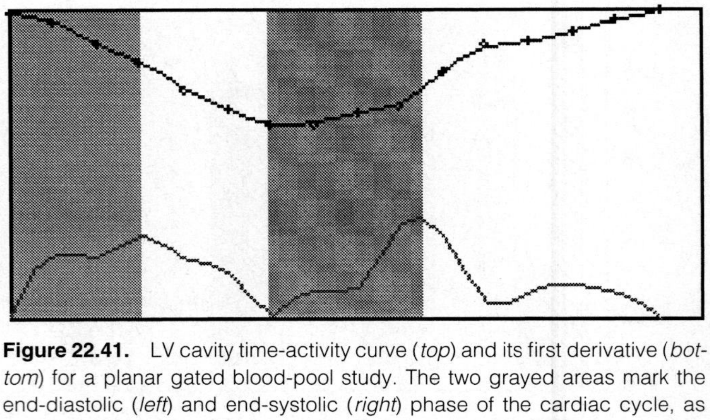

Figure 22.41. LV cavity time-activity curve (*top*) and its first derivative (*bottom*) for a planar gated blood-pool study. The two grayed areas mark the end-diastolic (*left*) and end-systolic (*right*) phase of the cardiac cycle, as determined from the maxima and minima of the derivative curve.

tween ED and ES is a first-order measure of the regional "contraction fraction," as long as motion was not perpendicular to the image plane. Other geometric methods use radial or chord shortening as a measure of wall motion, but the area method has been reported to yield superior results (223). As with regional function, regional wall motion is better estimated from tomographic images, as planar images suffer from the overlapping of different portions of the heart with different motion. In gated blood pool SPECT, regional wall motion has been measured by creating a midsurface as the locus of the points equidistant from the location of the endocardial surface at ES and ED. The lengths of the segments perpendicular to the midsurface and connecting the ED and ES surfaces are taken as a measure of regional wall motion (131).

Myocardial wall thickening cannot be determined from planar- or SPECT-gated blood pool studies, since in those studies essentially no activity is present in the myocardium. In perfusion studies, the thickness of the myocardial wall is generally smaller than twice the resolution of the camera system, and, consequently, it cannot be accurately measured due to the partial volume effect (119). However, the partial volume effect can be exploited to assess the *variation* in myocardial thickness between systole and diastole. The apparent concentration of activity in the myocardium is proportional to the myocardial thickness, as visually confirmed by the "brightening" of the myocardium at ES when gated images are displayed in cine mode. Therefore, the difference between the regionally measured counts at ES and ED (usually normalized to the counts measured at ED) is a good estimate of myocardial thickening. This approach has been used with planar (224) and SPECT (225, 226) perfusion studies.

Of course, normal limits can be generated for regional ejection fractions, wall motion, and thickening by measuring these parameters in normal volunteers or low-likelihood patients. Circumferential profiles and polar maps can also be built, much in the same way as for perfusion quantification. Gated myocardial SPECT using ^{99m}Tc-sestamibi has made it possible for perfusion, wall motion, and thickening to be assessed simultaneously through one injection and one 20-minute SPECT study (129), and it can be considered one of the fastest and more complete nuclear cardiology procedures of the future.

FUTURE DIRECTIONS

DATA EXCHANGE AND REGISTRATION

In nuclear cardiology, as in other branches of medical imaging, it is important to develop easy-to-implement, standardized protocols for the exchange of image data amongst systems and computers produced by different manufacturers. There are several reasons why this is desirable. The rest and stress cardiac perfusion studies for a specific patient may have been acquired on different cameras, while the quantification algorithm calls for the studies to be analyzed on the same platform. One may want to display dynamic first pass or gated SPECT images alongside static perfusion images, or to pool together for analysis patient populations studied on different cameras. In short, the ideal goal is that of processing, analyzing, and displaying image data on "off-the-shelf," low-cost workstations, regardless of where the data was acquired. This objective is attainable because cameras and computers in the nuclear medicine division are often part of a local area network, and because the transfer speeds associated with standard local area network configurations are generally adequate for the transmission of nuclear images.

On a departmental scale, one may want to display SPECT and angiographic or MRI images simultaneously. In fact, patient information, images, and text data describing the results of the individual tests performed, should be integrated and presented on-screen to the inquiring radiologist or nuclear cardiologist. The issues involved with setting up this environment (termed the Radiology Information System or RIS) are similar to those encountered when nuclear data alone are considered. However, radiologic images are typically larger than nuclear images, and image compression is needed for transmission and storage (227). Furthermore, the operation of the various divisional databases (nuclear, MRI, CT, etc.) must be tightly coordinated. The RIS will eventually be integrated with the Hospital Information System (HIS), for hospital-wide transmission and display of images and other data.

Image data can also be exchanged between different institutions, or locations separated by large distances. This approach goes under the name of telemedicine, and has been traditionally used for field hospitals in war zones (228) or for small hospitals in rural areas of the country. A much larger role for telemedicine is being advocated in the current debate on the containment of medical care costs. In one such scenario, smaller community hospitals, where not all medical specialties are represented, would transmit images to specialists at larger institutions for expert interpretation (229, 230). Standard telephone lines, optical fiber lines, or commercial communications satellites can be used for data transmission in telemedicine. The coarser matrixes of nuclear medicine data (generally 64×64 or 128×128) result in much lower throughput requirements for nuclear medicine than for standard radiography, ultrasound, CT, or MRI. Thus, for most of nuclear medicine, telemedicine can be accomplished through standard phone lines.

In nuclear medicine, as in other fields, manufacturers are reluctant to disclose their proprietary image formats, therefore the most straightforward way to ensure data exchange compatibility is to use an "open" format to which all images are converted. The nuclear medicine image format most used in Europe (and rapidly emerging as the de facto standard in the United States) is the INTERFILE format (231). Another approach, DICOM (also referred to as ACR-NEMA), involves defining not just the file format, but the entire data communication protocol (232). Camera users must request and verify that their system provide output image data in conformance with accepted "open" image formats, or at least that translators from proprietary to standardized formats be available.

Once image data sets from the same or from different modalities are available in a common format and on the same computer platform, it is often desirable to have them "registered." Registration or "correlation" of image data sets consists of identifying and matching homologous points, curves, or planes, so that the data sets can be aligned to one another by a combination of scaling, translations, and rotations. The most immediate example of correlation in cardiac SPECT is the registration of rest and stress image volumes in individual patients. Rather than trying to position the patient on the bed in exactly the same way in the two studies, it is more practical (and accurate) to start with roughly equivalent positioning, perform the acquisition, and electronically match the data at the time of analysis/processing. A more challenging correlation is that between image sets from modalities with somewhat different characteristics, such as PET and SPECT (233, 234). Even more problematic is the correlation between anatomic (MRI, CT, Ultrasound) and functional or nonanatomic modalities (PET, SPECT). Correlation of three-dimensional MRI/PET image sets has been successfully accomplished for brain studies (235–237), and needs to be extended to myocardial MRI/SPECT studies. In this respect, simultaneous emission/transmission protocols being investigated for attenuation correction in SPECT may prove useful in outlining the physical anatomy of the heart, playing the same role as transmission PET scans in MRI/PET correlation.

AUTOMATION OF DATA PROCESSING

With the advent of higher-dimensionality acquisition techniques, the size of nuclear cardiology data sets has increased, and so has the time necessary for their processing. For instance, the prefiltering and reconstruction of a 16-interval gated SPECT study requires about 10–20 minutes on most current machines, and operator interaction is required for the selection of various parameters. Faster computers and algorithms will no doubt be increasingly available, but the complexity of the operations they are expected to perform will also likely increase (an example might be iterative reconstruction of tomographic images, a very computationally intensive approach). In future perspective, the solution consists in eliminating as much of the operator interaction as possible, so that the entire processing can be performed in the background and transparently to the user, either concurrently with acquisition or after hours, in batch mode. This push-button operation would also improve speed, reproducibility, and accuracy of the processing.

The challenge in totally automated processing is that the success rate of the processing chain is the product of the success rates for the individual modules in the chain. Let us assume that the processing of a SPECT study consists of the following steps: (a) filtering and reconstruction, (b) reorientation, and (c) quantification, and that each of these steps can be performed by a totally automated software module. Even if each individual module were successful in 90% of the cases, the chain would have a success rate of $0.9 \times 0.9 \times 0.9 = 73\%$, which means that more than one in four studies would have to be reprocessed with some form of operator interaction. Also, it will be important to equip the algorithms with the built-in capability of evaluating the results they produce. If the results are "unlikely" (based on what the algorithm has been trained to expect or "knows" from previous experience), the results should be flagged as dubious and operator action should be automatically requested. This bring us to the concepts of artificial intelligence and "expert systems."

EXPERT SYSTEMS AND NEURAL NETWORKS

Artificial intelligence can be loosely defined as "the study of the computations that make it possible to perceive, reason and act" (124). The ambitious goal of artificial intelligence is that of "emulating" the behavior of the human brain as it performs specific tasks. Two tasks of special importance to nuclear cardiology are the identification or segmentation of the LV in image data sets, and the diagnostic interpretation of myocardial perfusion studies. Software modules that perform those tasks are often referred to as "expert systems."

An expert system (or, more appropriately, a rule-based system) uses rules to express knowledge, and "rule chaining" to apply that knowledge to solving problems. A rule is generally expressed by "if-then" patterns: *if* a specific condition is verified, *then* a specific action should be taken. In the Image Analysis section of this chapter, we described the automatic segmentation of the LV through clusterification. In that context, two segmentation rules reflecting knowledge of the expected size of the LV could be "if the cluster size is lower than 5 ml, then discard the cluster because it cannot represent the LV," or "if the cluster size is greater than 500 ml, then erode the cluster because the liver is probably connected to the LV's inferior wall" (122, 123, 146). Rules must be prioritized to avoid conflicts, and this can be visually expressed by arranging them in a "decision tree." In artificial intelligence terms, key to the solution of a problem is the description of the problem using an appropriate representation. In other words, if the appropriate rules are chosen, the expert system is usually able to solve the problem. The complexity of the overall task is apparent when one considers the problem of interpreting myocardial perfusion studies by determining the existence, location, and characteristics of perfusion defects based on the quantitative polar maps outputs (238). In building this expert system's decision tree, the rules are specified by experienced clinicians (239). However, some investigators argue that lack of agreement between clinicians may make it difficult to model the diagnostic decision making process, and therefore advocate decision rules derived statistically from patient populations (240). While expert systems cannot replace physicians, they can assist them in the diagnosis of cardiac disease much in the same way as quantitative analysis does, eliminating inter- and intraobserver variability (241).

In addition to expert systems, where decision rules are clearly expressed, artificial intelligence techniques include the use of simulated neural networks (242). In a simulated neural network, neurons and dendrites are modeled with electronic nodes and connections. There may be several layers of neurons, each of which "fires" whenever the sum of its inputs exceeds a threshold (238). The appeal of this approach is that networks can be "trained" to recognize data patterns and regularities, which might not be easy to formalize in rules. With reference to the interpretation of myocardial perfusion studies, an experienced clinician could present a number of polar maps (inputs) to the network, together with the relative diagnoses (outputs). The nodes would then automatically assign higher or lower weights to their interconnections so as to produce a global system transfer function consistent with the training input-output sets (243), and the "tuned" configuration could be used on successive sets. Replicating a real neural network is impossible—the human brain consists of more than 10^{11} neurons, each of them with 10^5 connections, and its supermassive parallelization would not be achievable by any computer. Electronic emulations consist of only a few layers of nodes. Success has been reported as to their application to various nuclear cardiology problems (243–247), although their design is still widely regarded as a form of art (124).

BAYESIAN IMAGE ALTERATION

Images of the heart acquired with two different modalities can be correlated and analyzed together. However, it should also be possible to incorporate information of typically nonimage format into nuclear cardiology images. Examples of this information are the epidemiologic knowledge of the prevalence of disease in the patient population studied, the symptoms, family, and personal medical history of each individual patient, and the results of tests such as treadmill ECG (192, 193). Research performed at Cedars-Sinai Medical Center aims at developing a Bayesian algorithm that transforms the three-dimensional tomographic image set, voxel by voxel, modifying image contrast as a function of the pretest likelihood of coronary artery disease. The relationship between normalized voxel intensity before (raw) and after (adjusted) enhancement is of the type

$$\text{Adjusted density} = 1 - \frac{1}{\dfrac{\text{Raw density}}{1 - \text{raw density}} \, \dfrac{\text{Pretest probability}}{1 - \text{pretest probability}} + 1} \qquad (12)$$

Key to this approach is the correct identification of the LV's endocardial and epicardial boundaries, so that the Bayesian algorithm can be applied only to voxels corresponding to the myocardium, leaving the LV cavity and the background unchanged. An example of patient study before and after Bayesian enhancement is shown in Figure 22.42. Much refinement and validation is still needed for this algorithm; in particular, images should be interpreted before and after enhancement by experienced clinicians, and improvements in accuracy obtained by the algorithm should be compared to those provided by multiple logistic regression.

FINAL CONSIDERATIONS

Nuclear medicine and nuclear cardiology are relatively recent disciplines and are rapidly and continually evolving. The fact that electronic computers and nuclear medicine were born within a short time of each other has naturally led to the extensive use of digital equipment and techniques in nuclear medicine. As a result, nuclear medicine is today more heavily computerized than older disciplines like conventional radiography or ultrasonography, and its technologic content is very high. This chapter addressed issues connected with the digital nature of nuclear cardiology, particularly the acquisition, processing, display, and analysis of the digital cardiac data. In many instances, the same or similar issues are to be found in computer science, electrical and electronic engineering, and mathematics, attesting to the increasing interdisciplinarity of modern medicine.

The future of nuclear cardiology will depend on software and computer advances, but is also dependent on developments in other areas—isotopes, study protocols, hardware and instrumentation, and the economics of nuclear cardiology and medicine. It is essential to understand that these areas are not independent, but rather very tightly connected. In fact, initial advances in one area often justify and inspire research and progress in others. A typical example of this process can be seen in gated myocardial SPECT imaging. The concept of electrocardiographically gated cardiac imaging was introduced as early as 1971 (53), but it is the recent advent of ^{99m}Tc-based myocardial agents, multidetector cameras, and fast, 32- and 64-bit microprocessors which are making routine gating of clinical myocardial SPECT studies practical and effective. At the same time, the possibility of gaining information on both myocardial perfusion *and* function with one injection and one gated acquisition sequence (129) is extremely attractive in the era of healthcare reform. The issues of instrumentation, radiopharmaceuticals, and diagnostic protocols for nuclear cardiology and nuclear medicine are presented in other chapters of this book, to which the reader is referred.

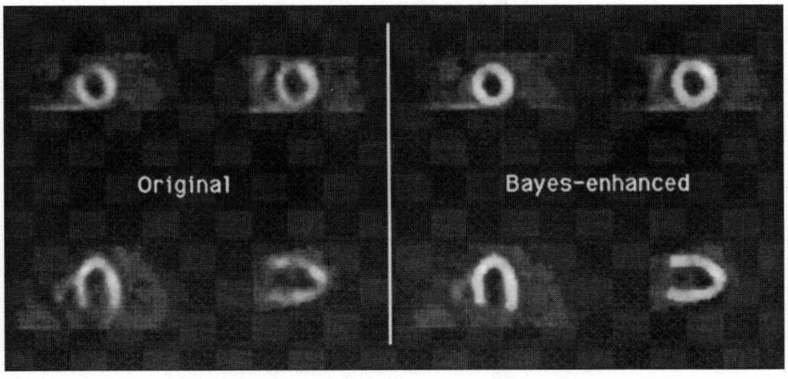

Figure 22.42. Bayesian image enhancement. Two short axis (*top row*), a horizontal and a vertical long axis image (*bottom row*) are shown for a patient with apparent anterior and inferior perfusion defects but only a 15% pretest likelihood of disease (*left*). The same images after Bayesian modification of the myocardial voxels (*right*) show no defects. Note that the background and the extramyocardial activity have not been affected by the Bayesian algorithm.

ACKNOWLEDGMENTS

The authors would like to acknowledge the collaboration of Joseph Areeda, John Friedman, Paul Kavanagh, and Hsiao-Te Su in the development of some of the algorithms described, as well as the technical assistance of Mark Hyun and Ponce Tapnio.

REFERENCES

1. Knoll G. Radiation detection and measurement. New York: John Wiley and Sons, 1979.
2. Bracewell R, Riddle A. Inversion of fan-beam scans in radioastronomy. Astrophys J 1967;150:427–434.
3. Shepp L, Logan B. The Fourier reconstruction of a head section. IEEE Trans Nucl Sci 1974;21:21–43.
4. Gullberg G, Zeng G, Christian P, Datz F, Morgan H. Cone beam tomography of the heart using SPECT. Invest Radiol 1991; 26(1):681–688.
5. Inoue Y, Machida K, Honda N, et al. Comparison between 180 degree and 360 degree data collection in ^{99m}Tc-tetrofosmin SPECT of the myocardium. Kaku Igaku (Japan J Nucl Med) 1993;30(1):85–88.
6. Eisner R, Martin S, Leon A, et al. Inhomogeneity of gated and ungated SPECT technetium-99m-sestamibi bull's-eyes in normal dogs: comparison with thallium-201. J Nucl Med 1993; 34(2):281–287.
7. Maublant J, Peycelon P, Kwiatkowski F, et al. Comparison between 180 and 360 data collection in technetium-99m MIBI SPECT of the myocardium. J Nucl Med 1989;30(3):295–300.
8. Eisner R, Nowak D, Pettigrew R, Fajman W. Fundamentals of 180 degree acquisition and reconstruction in SPECT imaging. J Nucl Med 1986;27(11):1717–1728.
9. Van Train K, Berman D, Garcia E, et al. Quantitative analysis of stress Tl-201 myocardial scintigrams: a multicenter trial. J Nucl Med 1986;31(7):1168–1180.
10. Knesaurek K. Comparison of 360 degree and 180 degree data collection in SPECT imaging. Phys Med Biol 1987;32(11):1445–1456.
11. Knesaurek K, King M, Glick S, Penney B. Investigation of causes of geometric distortion in 180 degree and 360 degree angular sampling in SPECT. J Nucl Med 1989;30(10):1666–1675.
12. Go R, MacIntyre W, Houser T, et al. Clinical evaluation of 360 degree and 180 degree data sampling techniques for transaxial SPECT thallium-201 myocardial perfusion imaging. J Nucl Med 1985;26(7):695–706.
13. Bice A, Clausen M, Loncaric S, Wagner H. Comparison of transaxial resolution in 180 degree and 360 degree SPECT with a rotating scintillation camera. Eur J Nucl Med 1987;13(1):7–11.
14. Hoffman E. 180 compared with 360 sampling in SPECT. J Nucl Med 1982;23:745–746.
15. Sorenson J, Phelps M. Physics in nuclear medicine. 2d ed. Orlando, Florida: Grune & Stratton, 1987.
16. Esser P, Jakimcius A, Foley L. The peanut orbit: a modified elliptical orbit for single-photon emission computed tomography imaging. Med Phys 1989;16(1):114–118.
17. Gottschalk S, Salem D, Lim C, Wake R. SPECT resolution and uniformity improvements by noncircular orbit. J Nucl Med 1983; 24(9):822–828.
18. Todd-Pokropek A. Noncircular orbits for the reduction of uniformity artefacts in SPECT. Phys Med Biol 1983;28(3):309–313.
19. Maniawski P, Morgan H, Wackers F. Orbit-related variation in spatial resolution as a source of artifactual defects in thallium-201 SPECT. J Nucl Med 1991;32(5):871–875.
20. Chua T, Kiat H, Germano G, et al. Tc-99m teboroxime regional myocardial washout in subjects with and without coronary artery disease. Am J Cardiol 1993;72:728–734.
21. Chua T, Kiat H, Germano G, et al. Rapid back-to-back adenosine stress/rest technetium-99m teboroxime myocardial perfusion SPECT using a triple-detector camera. J Nucl Med 1993; 34(9):1485–1493.
22. Gewirtz H. Differential myocardial washout of technetium-99m-teboroxime: mechanism and significance. J Nucl Med 1991; 32(10):2009–2011.
23. Johnson L, Seldin D. Clinical experience with technetium-99m teboroxime, a neutral, lipophilic myocardial perfusion imaging agent. Am J Cardiol 1990;66(13):63E–67E.
24. Nunn A. Is there additional useful information in the myocardial washout characteristics of teboroxime? J Nucl Med 1991; 32(10):1988–1991.
25. Berman D, Kiat H, Maddahi J. The new ^{99m}Tc myocardial perfusion imaging agents: ^{99m}Tc-sestamibi and ^{99m}Tc-teboroxime. Circulation 1991;84(3):I7–I21.
26. Germano G, Van Train K, Garcia E, et al. Quantitation of myocardial perfusion with SPECT: current issues and future trends. Nuclear cardiology: the state of the art and future directions. St Louis: Mosby Year Book, 1992:77–88.
27. Germano G, Kavanagh P, Kiat H, Van Train K, Berman D. Temporal image fractionation: rejection of motion artifacts in myocardial SPECT. J Nucl Med 1994 35;7:1193–1197.
28. Dahlberg S, Weinstein H, Hendel R, McSherry B, Leppo J. Planar myocardial perfusion imaging with technetium-99m-teboroxime: comparison by vascular territory with thallium-201 and coronary angiography. J Nucl Med 1992;33(10):1783–1788.
29. Drane W, Keim S, Strickland P, Tineo A, Nicole M. Preliminary report of SPECT imaging with Tc-99m teboroxime in ischemic heart disease. Clin Nucl Med 1992;17(3):215–225.
30. Fleming R, Kirkeeide R, Taegtmeyer H, et al. Comparison of technetium-99m teboroxime tomography with automated quantitative coronary arteriography and thallium-201 tomographic imaging. J Am Coll Cardiol 1991;17(6):1297–1302.
31. Gray W, Gewirtz H. Comparison of 99m-Technetium-teboroxime with thallium for myocardial imaging in the presence of a coronary artery stenosis. Circulation 1991;84:1796–1807.
32. Iskandrian A, Heo J, Nguyen T, Mercuro J. Myocardial imaging with Tc-99m teboroxime: technique and initial results. Am Heart J 1991;121(3):889–894.
33. Johnson L. Myocardial perfusion imaging of a flow tracer: clinical experience with teboroxime. Nuclear cardiology: the state of the art and future directions. St Louis: Mosby Year Book, 1992:209–215.
34. Leppo J, DePuey E, Johnson L. A review of cardiac imaging with sestamibi and teboroxime. J Nucl Med 1991;32(10):2012–2022.
35. Iskandrian A, Heo J, Nguyen T, et al. Tomographic myocardial perfusion imaging with technetium-99m teboroxime during adenosine-induced coronary hyperemia: correlation with thallium-201 imaging. J Am Coll Cardiol 1992;19(2):307–312.
36. Li Q, Solot G, Frank T, Wagner H, Becker L. Tomographic myocardial perfusion imaging with technetium-99m-teboroxime at rest and after dypiridamole. J Nucl Med 1991;32(10):1968–1976.
37. Marshall R, Leidholdt E, Zhang D, Barnett C. The effect of flow on technetium-99m-teboroxime (SQ30217) and thallium-201 extraction and retention in rabbit heart. J Nucl Med 1991; 32(10):1979–1988.
38. Oshima M, Ishihara M, Sano H, et al. Comparison of thallium-201 and technetium-99m teboroxime myocardial single photon emission tomography with coronary arteriography. Eur J Nucl Med 1992;19(7):522–526.
39. Pieri P, Yasuda T, Fischman A, et al. Myocardial accumulation and clearance of technetium 99m Teboroxime at 100%, 75%, 50% and zero coronary blood flow in dogs. Eur J Nucl Med 1991; 18:725–731.
40. Serafini A, Topchik S, Jimenez H, et al. Clinical comparison of technetium-99m-teboroxime and thallium-201 utilizing a con-

tinuous SPECT imaging protocol. J Nucl Med 1992;33(7):1304–1311.
41. Smith A, Gullberg G, Christian P, Datz F. Using teboroxime kinetics as an indicator of myocardial blood flow [Abstract]. J Nucl Med 1993;34(5):91P.
42. Stewart R, Heyl B, O'Rourke R, Blumhardt R, Miller D. Demonstration of differential poststenotic myocardial technetium-99m-teboroxime clearance kinetics after experimental ischemia and hyperemic stress. J Nucl Med 1991;32(10):2000–2008.
43. Taillefer R, Lambert R, Essiambre R, Phaneuf D, Leveille J. Comparison between thallium-201, technetium-99m-sestamibi and technetium-99m-teboroxime planar myocardial perfusion imaging in detection of coronary artery disease. J Nucl Med 1992; 33(6):1091–1098.
44. Weinstein H, Reinhardt C, Leppo J. Teboroxime, sestamibi and thallium-201 as markers of myocardial hypoperfusion: comparison by quantitative dual-isotope autoradiography in rabbits. J Nucl Med 1993;34(9):1510–1517.
45. Bisi G, Sciagra R, Bull U, et al. Assessment of ventricular function with first-pass radionuclide angiography using technetium-99m hexakis-2-methoxyisobutylisonitrile: a European multicentre study. Eur J Nucl Med 1991;18(3):178–183.
46. Myers R, Drasin E. EKG gated first-transit radionuclide angiocardiography. Clin Nucl Med 1980;5(4):143–148.
47. Maddahi J, Berman D, Matsuoka D, et al. A new technique for assessing right ventricular ejection fraction using rapid multiple-gated equilibrium cardiac blood pool scintigraphy. Description, validation and findings in chronic coronary artery disease. Circulation 1979;60(3):581–589.
48. Bacharach S, Bonow R, Green M. Comparison of fixed and variable temporal resolution methods for creating gated cardiac blood-pool image sequences. J Nucl Med 1990;31:38–42.
49. Green M, Ostrow H, Douglas M, et al. High temporal resolution ECG-gated scintigraphic angiocardiography. J Nucl Med 1975; 16(1):95–98.
50. Bacharach S, Green M, Borer J, et al. A real-time system for multi-image gated cardiac studies. J Nucl Med 1977;18:79–84.
51. Juni J, Chen C. Effects of gating modes on the analysis of left ventricular function in the presence of heart rate variation. J Nucl Med 1988;29(7):1272–1278.
52. Garcia E, Bateman T, Berman D, Maddahi J. Computer techniques for optimal radionuclide assessment of the heart. In: Gottschalk HAP, ed. Diagnostic nuclear medicine 2d ed. Baltimore: Williams and Wilkins, 1988:259–290.
53. Strauss H, Zaret B, Hurley P, Natarajan T, Pitt B. A scintiphotographic method for measuring left ventricular ejection fraction in man without cardiac catheterization. Am J Cardiol 1971; 28:575–580.
54. Wackers F, Berger H, Johnstone D, et al. Multiple gated cardiac blood pool imaging for left ventricular ejection fraction: validation of the technique and assessment of variability. Am J Cardiol 1979;43:1159–1166.
55. Maublant J, Bailly P, Mestas D, et al. Feasibility of gated single-photon emission transaxial tomography of the cardiac blood pool. Radiology 1983;146:837–839.
56. Fischman A, Moore R, Gill J, Strauss H. Gated blood pool tomography: a technology whose time has come. Semin Nucl Med 1989;19(1):13–21.
57. Berman D, Kiat H, Van Train K, et al. Technetium-99m sestamibi in the assessment of chronic coronary artery disease. Semin Nucl Med 1991;21(3):190–212.
58. Mannting F, Morgan-Mannting M. Gated SPECT with technetium-99m sestamibi for assessment of myocardial perfusion abnormalities. J Nucl Med 1993;34(4):601–608.
59. Morrison D, Turgeon J, Kotler J, Henry R. Gated first pass radionuclide ventriculography. Methods, validation, and applications. Clin Nucl Med 1984;9(9):506–512.
60. Bacharach S, Green M, Borer J. Instrumentation and data processing in cardiovascular nuclear medicine: evaluation of ventricular function. Semin Nucl Med 1979;9:257–274.
61. Jengo J, Mena I, Blaufuss A, Criley J. Evaluation of left ventricular function (ejection fraction and segmental wall motion) by single pass radioisotope angiography. Circulation 1979;57(2): 326–332.
62. Lear J, Pratt J. Real-time list-mode processing of gated cardiac blood pool examinations with forward-backward framing. Eur J Nucl Med 1992;19(3):177–180.
63. Lewellen T, Miyaoka R, Kohlmyer S, Pollard K. An XYE acquisition interface for General Electric Starcam anger cameras. Proc IEEE Med Imag Conf 1991;3:1861–1865.
64. Harrison R, Haynor D, Lewellen T. Dual energy window scatter corrections for positron emission tomography. Proc IEEE Med Imag Conf 1991;3:1700–1704.
65. Jaszczak R, Floyd C, Coleman R. Scatter compensation techniques for SPECT. IEEE Trans Nucl Sci 1985;32:786–793.
66. Jaszczak R, Greer K, Floyd C, Coleman R. Improved SPECT quantification using compensation for scattered photons. J Nucl Med 1984;25:893–900.
67. King M, Hadamenos G, Glick S. A dual-photopeak window method for scatter correction. J Nucl Med 1992;33(4):605–612.
68. Yanch J, Flower M, Webb S. A comparison of deconvolution and windowed subtraction techniques for scatter compensation in SPECT. IEEE Trans Med Imag 1988;7:13–20.
69. Oppenheim B. Scatter correction for SPECT. J Nucl Med 1984; 25:928–929.
70. Beck R, Zimmer L, Charleston D, Hoffer P. Aspects of imaging and counting in nuclear medicine using scintillation and semiconductor detectors. IEEE Trans Nucl Sci 1972;19:173–178.
71. Beck R, Zimmer L, Charleston D, Harper P, Hoffer P. Advances in fundamental aspects of imaging systems and techniques. Medical radioisotope scintigraphy. Vienna: IAEA, 1973:3–45.
72. Gagnon D, Todd-Pokropek A, Arsenualt A, Dupras G. A method for the correction of scatter using energy information: holospectral imaging. J Nucl Med 1988;29:864.
73. Haynor D, Harrison R, Lewellen T. SPECT scatter correction algorithms using position and energy information: preliminary simulation studies [Abstract]. Proc IEEE Med Imag Conf 1991; 3:1803.
74. Berman D, Kiat H, Friedman J, et al. Separate acquisition rest thallium-201/stress technetium-99m sestamibi dual isotope myocardial perfusion SPECT: a clinical validation study. J Am Coll Cardiol 1993;22(5):1455–1464.
75. Kiat H, Germano G, Friedman J, et al. Comparative feasibility of separate or simultaneous rest thallium-201/stress technetium-99m sestamibi dual isotope myocardial perfusion SPECT. J Nucl Med 1994;35(4):542–548.
76. DePuey E. Simultaneous thallium-201/technetium-99m dual-isotope cardiac SPECT: ready for prime time [Editorial]? J Nucl Med 1993;34(11):2006–2008.
77. Stark I. Scintillation camera detector head: technical observations, comments and comparison of the Anger principle with a new arithmetic digital detector system. Personal Communication 1992.
78. Jaszczak R, Chang L, Murphy P. Single photon emission computed tomography using multi-slice fan beam collimators. IEEE Trans Nucl Sci 1979;26:610–618.
79. Jaszczak R, Floyd C, Manglos S, Greer K, Coleman R. Cone-beam collimation for single-photon emission computed tomography: analysis simulation and image reconstruction using filtered backprojection. Med Phys 1986;13:484–489.
80. Moore S, Kouris K, Cullum I. Collimator design for single photon emission tomography. Eur J Nucl Med 1992;19(2):138–150.
81. Greer K, Jaszczak R, Coleman R. An overview of a camera-based SPECT system. Med Phys 1982;9(4):455–463.

82. Jaszczak R, Greer K, Coleman R. SPECT system misalignment: comparison of phantom and patient images. In: Esser PD, ed. Emission computed tomography current trends. New York: Society of Nuclear Medicine, 1983:81–90.
83. Germano G, Chua T, Kavanagh P, Kiat H, Berman D. Detection and correction of patient motion in dynamic and static myocardial SPECT using a multidetector camera. J Nucl Med 1993; 34(8):1349–1355.
84. Parker J. Image reconstruction in radiology. Boca Raton: CRC Press, 1990.
85. Goris M, Daspit S, McLaughlin P, Kriss J. Interpolative background subtraction. J Nucl Med 1976;17:744–747.
86. Watson D, Campbell N, Read E, et al. Spatial and temporal quantitation of plane thallium myocardial images. J Nucl Med 1981; 22(7):577–584.
87. Nichols K. Interpolative background corrections for gated bloodpool studies of low signal-to-noise ratios. In: Esser P, ed. Digital imaging: clinical advances in nuclear medicine. New York: Society of Nuclear Medicine, 1982:227–240.
88. Leidholdt E, Watson D, Read M, Croft B, Teates C. Interpolative background subtraction using polygonal boundary regions for gated blood pool imaging. Functional mapping of organ systems and other computer topics. New York: Society of Nuclear Medicine, 1981:91–101.
89. Okada R, Lim Y, Boucher C, et al. Clinical, angiographic, hemodynamic, perfusional and functional changes after one-vessel left anterior descending coronary angioplasty. Am J Cardiol 1985;55:347–356.
90. Douglass K, Links J, Gedra T, Wagner H. A comparison of interpolative background subtraction algorithms using analytical surfaces. Functional mapping of organ systems and other computer topics. New York: Society of Nuclear Medicine, 1981:83–90.
91. Areeda J, Garcia E, Van Train K, et al. Comprehensive analysis of rest/exercise segmental left ventricular function from radionuclide ventriculograms. Computers in cardiology. Long Beach, CA: IEEE Computer Society, 1982:109–112.
92. Gandsman E, Shulman R, Tyson I, Bough E. Calculation of the left ventricular ejection fraction by gated radionuclide angiography without direct background correction. Radiology 1982; 144(2):377–381.
93. Karsch K, Schicha H, Rentrop P, Kreuzer H, Emrich D. Validity of different gated equilibrium blood pool methods for determination of left ventricular ejection fraction. Eur J Nucl Med 1980; 5(5):439–445.
94. Burow R, Strauss H, Singleton R, et al. Analysis of left ventricular function from multiple gated acquisition cardiac blood pool imaging. Comparison to contrast angiography. Circulation 1977; 56(6):1024–1028.
95. Gagnon D, Pouliot N, Laperriere L. Statistical and physical content of low-energy photons in holospectral imaging. IEEE Trans Med Imag 1991;10(3):284–289.
96. Hademenos G, Ljungberg M, King M, Glick S. A Monte Carlo investigation of the dual photopeak window scatter correction method. Proc IEEE Med Imag Conf 1991;3:1814–1821.
97. Ogawa K, Harata Y, Ichihara T, Kubo A, Hashimoto S. A practical method for position-dependent compton-scatter correction in single photon emission CT. IEEE Trans Med Imag 1991; 10(3):408–412.
98. Axelsson B, Msaki P, Israelsson A. Subtraction of compton-scattered photons in single-photon emission computerized tomography. J Nucl Med 1984;25:490–494.
99. Egbert S, May R. An integral-transport method for Compton-scatter correction in emission computed tomography. IEEE Trans Nucl Sci 1980;27:543–548.
100. Floyd C, Jaszczak R, Greer K, Coleman R. Deconvolution of compton scatter in SPECT. J Nucl Med 1985;26:403–408.
101. Msaki P, Axelsson B, Dahl C, Larsson S. A generalized scatter correction technique in SPECT using point scatter distribution functions. J Nucl Med 1987;28:1861–1869.
102. Blockland K, Reiber H, Pauwels E. Quantitative analysis in single photon emission tomography (SPECT). Eur J Nucl Med 1992; 19(1):47–61.
103. Tretiak O, Metz C. The exponential radon transform. SIAM J Appl Math 1980;39:341–354.
104. Gullberg G, Budinger T. The use of filtering methods to compensate for constant attenuation in single-photon emission computed tomography. IEEE Trans Biomed Eng 1981;28:142–157.
105. Tanaka E. Quantitative image reconstruction with weighted backprojection for single photon emission computed tomography. J Comput Assist Tomogr 1983;7:692.
106. Chang L. A method for attenuation correction in radionuclide computed tomography. IEEE Trans Nucl Sci 1978;-25:638–643.
107. Moore S. Attenuation compensation. In: Ell PJ, Holman BL, eds. Computed emission tomography. New York: Oxford University Press, 1982:339–360.
108. Hasegawa B, Lang T, Brown J, et al. Object-specific attenuation correction of SPECT with correlated dual-energy x-ray CT. IEEE Trans Nucl Sci 1993;40(4):1242–1252.
109. Bailey D, Hutton B, Walker P. Improved SPECT using simultaneous emission and transmission tomography. J Nucl Med 1987;28(5):844–851.
110. Almquist H, Palmer J, Ljundberg M, et al. Quantitative SPECT by attenuation correction of the projection set using transmission data: evaluation of a method. Eur J Nucl med 1990;16(8–10):587–594.
111. Ljundberg M, Strand S. Scatter and attenuation correction in SPECT using density maps and Monte Carlo simulated scatter functions. J Nucl Med 1990;31(9):1560–1567.
112. Ljundberg M, Strand S. Attenuation correction in SPECT based on transmission studies and Monte Carlo simulations of buildup functions. J Nucl Med 1990;31(4):493–500.
113. Tung C, Gullberg G, Zeng G, et al. Nonuniform attenuation correction using simultaneous transmission and emission converging tomography. IEEE Trans Med Imag 1992;39(4):1134–1143.
114. Tan P, Bailey D, Meikle S, et al. A scanning line source for simultaneous emission and transmission measurements in SPECT. J Nucl Med 1993;34(10):1752–1760.
115. Huang S, Carson R, Phelps M, et al. A boundary method for attenuation correction in positron emission tomography. J Nucl Med 1981;22:627–637.
116. Faber T, Lewis M, Corbett J, Stokely E. Attenuation correction for SPECT: an evaluation of hybrid approaches. IEEE Trans Med Imag 1984;3:101–107.
117. Digby W, Hoffman E, Dahlbom M, Bidaut L. Application of measured/calculated attenuation correction for high-resolution PET imaging of the heart. J Nucl Med 1987;28(4):696.
118. Manglos S, Jaszczac R, Floyd C, et al. A quantitative comparison of attenuation-weighted backprojection with multiplicative and iterative post-processing attenuation correction in SPECT. IEEE Trans Med Imag 1988;7:127–134.
119. Hoffman E, Huang S, Phelps M. Quantitation in positron emission tomography: 1. Effect of object size. J Comput Assist Tomogr 1979;3(3):299–308.
120. Marr D, Hildreth E. Theory of edge detection. Royal Soc London Proc B 1980;187–217
121. Ezekiel A, Van Train K, Berman D, et al. Automatic determination of quantitation parameters from Tc-sestamibi myocardial tomograms. Proc IEEE Comput in Cardiol 1991;237–240.
122. Germano G, Kavanagh P, Su H, et al. Automatic reorientation of 3-dimensional transaxial myocardial perfusion SPECT images. J Nucl Med 1995J Nucl Med (In press).
123. Germano G, Kiat H, Moriel M, et al. Quantitative, automatic measurement of left ventricular ejection fraction by gated SPECT:

development and preliminary validation [Abstract]. Clin Nucl Med 1993;18(10):924.
124. Winston P. Artificial intelligence. 3rd ed. Reading, MA: Addison-Wesley, 1992.
125. Gonzalez R, Wintz P. Digital image processing. 2d ed. Reading, MA: Addison-Wesley, 1987.
126. Nelson T, Verba J, Bhargava V, Shabetai R, Slutski R. Automatic analysis of left ventricular ejection fraction using stroke volume images. Invest Radiol 1983;18(2):130–137.
127. Weiss A, Berman D, Lew A, et al. Transient ischemic dilation of the left ventricle on stress thallium-201 scintigraphy: a marker of severe and extensive coronary artery disease. J Am Coll Cardiol 1987;9(4):752–759.
128. Chouraqui P, Rodrigues E, Berman D, Maddahi J. Significance of dipyridamole-induced transient dilation of the left ventricle during thallium-201 scintigraphy in suspected coronary artery disease. Am J Cardiol 1988;66(7):689–694.
129. Chua T, Kiat H, Germano G, et al. Gated technetium-99m sestamibi for simultaneous assessment of stress myocardial perfusion, postexercise regional ventricular function and myocardial viability: correlation with echocardiography and rest thallium-201 scintigraphy. J Am Coll Cardiol 1994;23(5):1107–1114.
130. DePuey E, Nichols K, Dobrinsky C. Left ventricular ejection fraction assessed from gated technetium-99m-sestamibi SPECT. J Nucl Med 1993;34(11):1871–1876.
131. Faber T, Akers M, Pesnock R, Corbett J. Three-dimensional motion and perfusion quantification in gated single photon emission computed tomograms. J Nucl Med 1991;32(12):2311–2317.
132. Faber T, Stokely E, Templeton G, et al. Quantification of three-dimensional left ventricular segmental wall motion and volumes from gated tomographic radionuclide ventriculograms. J Nucl Med 1989;30(5):638–649.
133. Faber T, Stokely E, Peshock R, Corbett J. A model-based four-dimensional left ventricular surface detector. IEEE Trans Med Imag 1991;10(3):321–329.
134. Kittler J, Illingworth J. Relaxation labeling algorithms—a review. Image Vision Comput 1985;8:206–216.
135. Nuyts J, Mortelmans L, Suetens P, Oosterlinck A, de Rou M. Model-based quantification of myocardial perfusion images from SPECT. J Nucl Med 1989;30(12):1992–2001.
136. Nuyts J, Suetens P, Oosterlinck A, De Roo M, Mortelmans L. Delineation of ECT images using global constraints and dynamic programming. IEEE Trans Med Imag 1991;10:489–498.
137. Mortelmans L, Nuyts J, Scheys I, et al. A new quantitative method for the analysis of cardiac perfusion tomography (SPECT): validation in postinfarct patients treated with trombolytic therapy. Eur J Nucl Med 1993;20(12):1193–1200.
138. Ratib O, Huang H. CALIPSO: an interactive software package for multimodality medical image analysis on a personal computer. J Med Imag 1989;3:205–216.
139. DePuey E. Gated cardiac imaging: automated blood pool studies. Diagn Imag 1985;4:24–29.
140. Jackson P, Wilde P, Watt I, Davies E. An edge detection algorithm for use in radionuclide imaging. Eur J Nucl Med 1981;6:33–38.
141. Todd-Pokropek A. Edge detection and wall motion: an intercomparison of different algorithms in nuclear cardiology. Physical techniques in cardiological imaging. Bristol, England: Adam Hilger, 1982:125–141.
142. Federman J, Brown M, Tancredi R, et al. Multiple-gated acquisition cardiac blood-pool isotope imaging. Evaluation of left ventricular function correlated with contrast angiography. Mayo Clinic Proc 1978;10:625–633.
143. Hecht H, Mirell S, Rolett E, Blahd W. Left-ventricular ejection fraction and segmental wall motion by peripheral first-pass radionuclide angiography. J Nucl Med 1978;19(1):17–23.
144. Goris M, McKillop J, Briandet P. A fully automated determination of the left ventricular region of interest in nuclear angiocardiography. Cardiov Interv Radiol 1981;4(2):117–123.
145. Yang K, Thompson C, Mena I. Automatic ventricular edge detection for determination of left ventricular volumes, ejection fraction and regional ejection fractions from first pass radioisotope angiography. Compu Med Imag Graph 1988;12(3):147–158.
146. Duncan J. Knowledge-directed left ventricular boundary detection in equilibrium radionuclide angiocardiography. IEEE Trans Med Imag 1987;6:325–336.
147. Lilly P, Jenkins J, Bourdillon P. Automatic contour definition on left ventriculograms by image evidence and a multiple template-based model. IEEE Trans Med Imag 1989;8:173–185.
148. Senda M, Yonekura Y, Tamaki N, et al. Interpolating scan and oblique-angle tomograms in myocardial PET using nitrogen-13 ammonia. J Nucl Med 1986;27(12):1830–1836.
149. Kuhle W, Porenta G, Huang S, Phelps M, Schelbert H. Issues in the quantitation of reoriented cardiac PET images. J Nucl Med 1992;33(6):1235–1242.
150. Garcia E, Van Train K, Maddahi J, et al. Quantification of rotational thallium-201 myocardial tomography. J Nucl Med 1985; 26:17–26.
151. Borrello J, Clinthorne N, Rogers W, Thrall J, Keyes J. Oblique-angle tomography: a reconstructing algorithm from transaxial tomographic data. J Nucl Med 1981;22:471–473.
152. Lancaster J, Starling M, Kopp D, Lasher J, Blumhardt R. Effect of errors in reangulation on planar and tomographic thallium-201 washout profile curves. J Nucl Med 1985;26(12):1445–1455.
153. DePuey E, Garcia E. Optimal specificity of thallium-201 SPECT through recognition of imaging artifacts. J Nucl Med 1989; 30:441–449.
154. Cooke C, Folks R, Jones M, Ezquerra N, Garcia E. Automatic program for determining the long axis of the left ventricular myocardium used for thallium-201 tomographic reconstruction [Abstract]. J Nucl Med 1989;30:806.
155. He Z, Maublant J, Cauvin J, Veyre A. Reorientation of the left ventricular long axis on myocardial transaxial tomography by a linear fitting method. J Nucl Med 1991;32:1794–1800.
156. Cauvin J, Boire J, Maublant J, et al. Automatic detection of the left ventricular myocardium long axis and center in thallium-201 single photon emission computed tomography. Eur J Nucl Med 1992;19(12):1032–1037.
157. Serra J. Image analysis and mathematical morphology. London: Academic, 1984.
158. Smith A, Gullberg G, Datz F, Christian P. Kinetic modeling of teboroxime using dynamic SPECT imaging [Abstract]. J Nucl Med 1992;33(5):878–879.
159. Schelbert H, Schwaiger M. PET studies of the heart. In: Phelps M, Mazziotta J, Schelbert H, eds. Positron emission tomography and autoradiography. Principles and applications for the brain and heart. New York: Raven Press, 1986:581–661.
160. Huang S, Phelps M. Principles of tracer kinetic modeling in positron emission tomography and autoradiography.In: Phelps M, Mazziotta J, Schelbert H, eds. Positron emission tomography and autoradiography. Principles and applications for the brain and heart. New York: Raven Press, 1986:287–346.
161. Bevington P. Data reduction and error analysis for the physical sciences. New York: McGraw-Hill, 1969.
162. Dell R, Sciacca R, Lieberman K, Case D, Cannon P. A weighted least-squares technique for the analysis of kinetic data. Circ Res 1973;32:71–84.
163. Germano G, Chen B, Huang S, et al. Use of the abdominal aorta for arterial input function determination in hepatic and renal PET studies. J Nucl Med 1992;33(4):613–620.
164. Gambhir S. Quantitation of the physical factors affecting the tracer kinetic modeling of cardiac positron emission tomography data [Dissertation]. Los Angeles: University of California, 1990.
165. Adam W, Tarkowska A, Bitter F, Stauch M, Geffers H. Equilib-

rium (gated) radionuclide ventriculography. Cardiovasc Radiol 1979;2:161–173.
166. Neumann D, Go R, Myers B, et al. Parametric phase display for biventricular function from gated cardiac blood pool single-photon emission tomography. Eur J Nucl Med 1993;20(11):1108–1111.
167. Barnes W, Gose E. Functional image data acquisition and processing. Semin Nucl Med 1987;17(1):58–71.
168. Pavel D, Briandet P. Quo vadis phase analysis. Clin Nucl Med 1983;8(11):564–575.
169. Links J, Douglass K, Wagner H. Patterns of ventricular emptying by Fourier analysis of gated blood-pool studies. J Nucl Med 1980; 21(10):978–982.
170. Gregoire J, Parker J, Holman B. Quantitative radionuclide angiocardiography. Cardiovasc Intervent Radiol 1987;10:384–399.
171. Van Dyke D, Anger H, Sullivan R, et al. Cardiac evaluation from radioisotope dynamics. J Nucl Med 1972;13(8):585–592.
172. Goris M. Functional or parametric images. J Nucl Med 1982; 23(4):360–362.
173. Boudreau R, Loken M. Functional imaging of the heart. Semin Nucl Med 1987;17(1):28–38.
174. Maddox D, Holman B, Wynne J, et al. Ejection fraction image: a noninvasive index of regional left ventricular wall motion. Am J Cardiol 1978;41:1230–1238.
175. Parker J, Secker-Walker R, Hill R, Siegel B, Potchen E. A new technique for the calculation of left ventricular ejection fraction. J Nucl Med 1972;13(8):649–651.
176. Secker-Walker R, Resnick L, Kunz H, et al. Measurement of left ventricular ejection fraction. J Nucl Med 1973;14(11):798–802.
177. Committee on Advanced Cardiac Imaging and Technology, et al. Standardization of cardiac tomographic imaging. Circulation 1992;86(1):338–339.
178. Wallis J, Miller T. Three-dimensional display in nuclear medicine and radiology. J Nucl Med 1990;32(3):534–546.
179. Mazziotta J, Huang H. THREAD: Three-dimensional reconstruction and display with biomedical applications in neuron ultrastructure and display. Am Fed Inform Proc Soc 1976;45:241–250.
180. Herman G, Liu H. Three-dimensional display of human organs from computed tomograms. Comput Graph Image Proc 1979; 9:1–21.
181. Phong B. Illumination for computer generated pictures. Communications of the ACM 1975;18(6):311–317.
182. Miller T, Wallis J, Sampathkumaran K. Three-dimensional display of gated cardiac blood-pool studies. J Nucl Med 1989; 30(12):2036–2041.
183. Kajiya J, Von Herzen B. Ray tracing volume densities. Comput Graph 1984;18(3):165–174.
184. Drebin R, Carpenter L, Hanrahan P. Volume rendering. Computer Graphics 1988;22(4):65–74.
185. Garcia E, Maddahi J, Berman D, Waxman A. Space-time quantitation of Tl-201 myocardial scintigraphy. J Nucl Med 1981; 22:309–317.
186. Maddahi J, Garcia E, Berman D, et al. Improved noninvasive assessment of CAD by quantitative analysis of regional stress myocardial distribution and washout of thallium-201. Circulation 1981;64:924–935.
187. Maddahi J, Van Train K, Prigent F, et al. Quantitative single photon emission computerized thallium-201 tomography for detecting and localization of coronary artery disease: optimization and prospective validation of a new technique. J Am Coll Cardiol 1989;14:1689–1699.
188. Van Train K, Maddahi J, Berman D, et al. Quantitative analysis of tomographic stress thallium-201 myocardial scintigrams: a multicenter trial. J Nucl Med 1990;31:1168–1179.
189. Garcia E, Cooke C, Van Train K, et al. Technical aspects of myocardial SPECT imaging with technetium-99m sestamibi. Am J Cardiol 1990;66(13):23E–31E.
190. Van Train K, Areeda J, Garcia E, et al. Quantitative same-day rest-stress technetium-99m-sestamibi SPECT: definition and validation of stress normal limits and criteria for abnormality. J Nucl Med 1993;34(9):1494–1502.
191. Van Train K, Garcia E, Maddahi J, et al. Multicenter trial validation for quantitative analysis of same-day rest-stress technetium-99m-sestamibi myocardial tomograms. J Nucl Med 1994; 35(4):609–618.
192. Diamond G, Forrester J. Analysis of probability as an aid in the clinical diagnosis of coronary artery disease. N Engl J Med 1979; 300:1350–1358.
193. Diamond G, Forrester J, Hirsch M, et al. Application of conditional probability analysis to the clinical diagnosis of coronary artery disease. J Clin Invest 1980;65:1210–1221.
194. Wackers F, Fetterman R, Mattera J, Clements J. Quantitative planar thallium-201 stress scintigraphy: a critical evaluation of the method. Semin Nucl Med 1985;15(1):46–66.
195. Lim Y, Okada R, Chesler D, et al. A new approach to quantitation of exercise thallium-201 before and after an intervention: application to define the impct of coronary angioplasty on regional myocardial perfusion. Am Heart J 1984;108:917–925.
196. Maddahi J, Van Train K, Wong C, et al. Comparison of Tl-201 single photon emission computerized tomography (SPECT) and planar imaging for evaluation of coronary artery disease [Abstract]. J Nucl Med 1986;27(6):999.
197. Tamaki S, Nakajima H, Murakami T, et al. Estimation of infarct size by myocardial emission computed tomography with thallium-201 and its relation to creatine kinase-MB release after myocardial infarction in man. Circulation 1982;66:994–1001.
198. Vogel R, Kirch D, LeFree M, et al. Thallium-201 myocardial perfusion scintigraphy: results of standard and multi-pinhole tomographic techniques. Am J Cardiol 1979;43:787–793.
199. De Pasquale E, Nody A, De Puey E, et al. Quantitative rotational thallium-201 tomography for identifying and localizing coronary artery disease. Circulation 1988;77:316–327.
200. Eisner R, Tamas M, Cloninger K, et al. Normal SPECT thallium-201 bull's-eye display: gender differences. J Nucl Med 1988; 29:1901–1909.
201. Van Train K, Maddahi J, Wng C, et al. Definition of normal limits in stress Tl-201 myocardial rotational tomography [Abstract]. J Nucl Med 1986;27(6):899.
202. Prigent F, Maddahi J, Berman D. Quantitative stress-redistribution Tl-201 single-photon emission tomography (SPECT): development of a scheme for localization of coronary artery disease [Abstract]. J Nucl Med 1986;27(6):997–998.
203. Garcia E, DePuey E, Sonnemaker R, et al. Quantification of the reversibility of stress-induced thallium-201 myocardial perfusion defects: a multicenter trial using bull's-eye polar maps and standard normal limits. J Nucl Med 1990;31(11):1761–1765.
204. Klein J, Garcia E, DePuey E, et al. Reversibility bull's eye: a new polar bull's eye map to quantify reversibility of stress-induced SPECT thallium-201 myocardial perfusion defects. J Nucl Med 1990;31(7):1240–1246.
205. Luna E, Klein L, Garcia E, Robbins W, DePuey E. Reversibility bullseye polar map: accuracy in detecting myocardial ischemia [Abstract]. J Nucl Med 1988;29(5):951.
206. Tamaki N, Yonekura Y, Mukai F, et al. Stress thallium-201 transaxial emission computed tomography: quantitative vs. qualitative analysis for evaluation of coronary artery disease. J Am Coll Cardiol 1984;4:1213–1221.
207. Caldwell J, Williams D, Harp G, Stratton J, Ritchie J. Quantitation of size of relative myocardial perfusion by single-photon emission computed tomography. Circulation 1984;70(6):1048–1056.

208. Van Train K, Folks R, Wong C, et al. Optimization of Tc-mibi SPECT acquisition and processing parameters: collimator, matrix size and filter evaluation [Abstract]. J Nucl Med 1989; 30(5):757–758.
209. Folks R, Van Train K, Wong C, et al. Evaluation of Tc-mibi SPECT acquisition parameters: circular vs. elliptical and 180° vs. 360° orbits [Abstract]. J Nucl Med 1989;30(5):795–796.
210. Taillefer R, Gagnon A, Laflamme L. Same day injections of Tc-99m methoxy isobutyl isonitrile (hexamibi) for myocardial tomographic imaging: comparison between rest-stress and stress-rest injection sequences. Eur J Nucl Med 1989;15:113–117.
211. Uren R, Newman H, Hutton B, et al. Geometric determination of left ventricular volume from gated blood-pool studies using a slant-hole collimator. Radiology 1983;147:541–545.
212. DePuey E. Evaluation of cardiac function with radionuclides. In: Gottschalk HAP, ed. Diagnostic nuclear medicine. 2d ed. Baltimore: Williams and Wilkins, 1988:355–398.
213. Slutsky R, Karliner J, Ricci D, et al. Left ventricular volumes by gated equilibrium radionuclide angiography: a new method. Circulation 1979;60(3):556–564.
214. Graham M, Caputo G. Measurement of left ventricular volume using emission computed tomography. In: Esser P, ed. Emission computed tomography. New York: Society of Nuclear Medicine, 1983:147–153.
215. Links J, Becker L, Shindledecker J, et al. Measurement of absolute left ventricular volume from gated blood pool studies. Circulation 1982;65:82–90.
216. Schweiger M, Ratib O, Henze E, et al. Left ventricular stroke volume determinations from radionuclide ventriculograms: the effects of photon attenuation. Radiology 1984;153(1):235–240.
217. Massardo T, Gal R, Grenier R, Schmidt D, Port S. Left ventricular volume calculation using a count-based ratio method applied to multigated radionuclide angiography. J Nucl Med 1990; 31(4):450–456.
218. Gal R, Grenier R, Port S, Dymond D, Schmidt D. Left ventricular volume calculation using a count-based ratio method applied to first-pass radionuclide angiography. J Nucl Med 1992; 33(12):2124–2132.
219. Levy W, Cerqueira M, Matsuoka D, et al. Four radionuclide methods for left ventricular volume determination: comparison of a manual and an automated technique. J Nucl Med 1992; 33(5):763–770.
220. Levy W, Jacobson A, Cerqueira M, et al. Radionuclide cardiac volumes: effects of region of interest selection and correction for Compton scatter using a buildup factor. J Nucl Med 1992; 33(9):1642–1647.
221. Douglass K, Tibbits P, Kasecamp W, et al. Performance of a fully automated program for measurement of left ventricular ejection fraction. Eur J Nucl Med 1982;7(12):564–566.
222. Freeman M, Garcia E, Berman D, et al. An objective and quantitative method for assessment of regional left ventricular wall motion using multiple-gated equilibrium scintigraphy [Abstract]. J Nucl Med 1980;21:P62.
223. Gelberg H, Brundage B, Glantz S, Parmley W. Quantitative left ventricular wall motion analysis: a comparison of area, chord and radial methods. Circulation 1979;59:991–1000.
224. Marcassa C, Marzullo P, Parodi O, Sambuceti G, L'Abbate A. A new method for noninvasive quantification of segmental myocardial wall thickening using technetium-99m 2–methoxy-isobutyl-isonitrile scintigraphy—results in normal subjects. J Nucl Med 1990;31:173–177.
225. Mochizuki T, Murase K, Fujiwara Y, et al. Assessment of systolic thickening with thallium-201 ECG-gated single-photon emission computed tomography: a parameter for local left ventricular function. J Nucl Med 1991;32(8):1496–1500.
226. Galt J, Garcia E, Robbins W. Effects of myocardial wall thickness on SPECT quantification. IEEE Trans Med Imag 1990;9:144–150.
227. Huang H. Elements of digital radiology: a professional handbook and guide. Englewood Cliffs, NJ: Prentice-Hall, 1987.
228. Crowter J, Fernandez M. Telemedicine in Somalia. Advanced Imaging October 1993:28–31.
229. Brauer G. Telehealth: the delayed revolution in health care. Med Progress Technol 1992;18:151–163.
230. Brunner B. Healthcare-oriented telecommunications: the wave of the future. Topics Health Inform Manag 1993;14(1):54–61.
231. Todd-Pokropek A, Cradduck T, Deconinck F. A file format for the exchange of nuclear medicine data: a specification of Interfile version 3.3. Nucl Med Comm 1992;13:673–699.
232. Bidgood W, Horii S. Introduction to the ACR-NEMA DICOM standard. Radiographics 1992;12(2):345–355.
233. Altehoefer C, Kaiser H, Dorr R, et al. Fluorine-18 deoxyglucose PET for assessment of viable myocardium in perfusion defects in ^{99m}Tc-MIBI SPECT: a comparative study in patients with coronary artery disease. Eur J Nucl Med 1992;19(5):334–342.
234. Lucignani G, Paolini G, Landoni C, et al. Presurgical identification of hibernating myocardium by combined use of techetium-99m hexakis 2-methoxyisobutylisonitrile single photon emission tomography and fluorine-18 fluoro-2-deoxy-D-glucose positron emission tomography in patients with coronary artery disease. Eur J Nucl Med 1992;19(10):874–881.
235. Pelizzari C, Chen G, Spelbring D, Weichselbaum R, Chen C. Accurate three-dimensional registration of CT, PET and/or MR images of the brain. J Comput Assist Tomogr 1989;13(1):20–26.
236. Evans A, Marrett S, Torrescorzo J, Ku S, Collins L. MRI-PET correlation in three dimensions using a volume-of-interest (VOI) atlas. J Cerebr B 1991;11(2):A69–A78.
237. Valentino D. Mapping human brain structure-function relationships [Dissertation]. Los Angeles: University of California, 1991.
238. Garcia E, Cooke D. Computer methods in nuclear cardiology. Nuclear cardiology: the state of the art and future directions. St Louis: Mosby Year Book, 1992:97–108.
239. Houston A, Craig A. The role of expert system shell induction in the analysis of phase and amplitude images obtained from nuclear cardiology. Medical Informatics 1991;16(2):109–113.
240. Gilpin E, Olshen R, Chatterjee K, et al. Predicting 1-year outcome following acute myocardial infarction: physicians versus computers. Comput Biomed Res 1990;23(1):46–63.
241. Horino M, Hosoba M, Wani H, et al. Development and clinical application of an expert system for supporting diagnosis of ^{201}Tl stress myocardial SPECT. Kaku Igaku (Japan J Nucl Med) 1990; 27(2):93–106.
242. McClelland J, Rumelhart D. Parallel distributed processing. Cambridge, MA: MIT Press, 1986.
243. Wang D, Juni J. Artificial neural network interpretation of cardiac stress thallium studies [Abstract]. Radiology 1992; 185(P):283.
244. Fujita H, Katafuchi T, Uehara T, Nishimura T. Application of artificial neural network to computer-aided diagnosis of coronary artery disease in myocardial SPECT bull's-eye images. J Nucl Med 1992;33(2):272–276.
245. Fukuda H, Usuki N, Saiwai S, et al. Usefulness of an artificial neural network for assessing the ventricular size [Abstract]. Radiology 1992;185(P):156.
246. Tourassi G, Floyd C, Coleman R. Detection and localization of cold lesions on SPECT images with artificial neural networks [Abstract]. Radiology 1992;185(P):156.
247. Tsai C, Sun Y, Chung P, Lee J. Endocardial boundary detection using a neural network. Pattern Recognition 1993;26(7):1057–1068.

23 General Concepts of Ventricular Function, Myocardial Perfusion, and Exercise Physiology Relevant to Nuclear Cardiology

MARVIN W. KRONENBERG and LEWIS C. BECKER

Knowledge of ventricular mechanics, the physiology of the coronary circulation, and exercise physiology is necessary for the accurate interpretation of radionuclide ventriculographic and myocardial perfusion images. This chapter outlines these important basic concepts as applied to the heart. For further elaboration, and for subcellular and cellular mechanisms, the reader is referred to the texts in the list of suggested readings.

VENTRICULAR FUNCTION

BASIC CONCEPTS

Ventricular function is controlled by four major factors: preload, afterload, heart rate and rhythm, and contractility (Fig. 23.1). *Left ventricular performance* can be measured in several ways, some of which include cardiac output (blood flow per minute) and stroke volume (blood flow per beat). *Preload* is defined as the myocardial tension at end-diastole. It is estimated by myocardial segment length in the isolated muscle and by end-diastolic volume in the intact heart. *Afterload* is defined as the resistance to myocardial fiber shortening or to chamber contraction. It is estimated by the systolic load in papillary muscle experiments and by the systolic blood pressure or calculated wall stress in the intact heart. *Contractility* is defined as the intensity or quality of myocardial contraction. Each of these factors has multiple determinants. In addition to the properties of the veins and the arteries, neural and humoral factors greatly influence cardiac performance by affecting preload, afterload, heart rate, and contractility. Also, the contiguous adjacent structures—the lungs, pericardium, and pleura—affect cardiac function by influencing the filling and emptying of the heart. In conditions of heart failure, hypertrophy and dilatation are important modifying, compensatory mechanisms.

The *cardiac cycle* illustrates a sequence of electrical events that trigger mechanical events, producing pressure and flow. Figure 23.2 demonstrates these events for the left heart. In response to atrial depolarization, the atria contract, increasing the atrial and left ventricular diastolic pressure (a wave). In response to ventricular electrical depolarization, the left ventricle contracts. "Isovolumic contraction" is analogous to isometric contraction, in which the myocardial force or pressure increases, but no external work is performed. When the intraventricular pressure rises to a level sufficient to open the aortic valve, forward flow begins. The greatest flow occurs in early systole. The aortic pressure rises and then falls as ejection subsides. At the end of ventricular ejection, ventricular pressure falls to a level below the aortic diastolic pressure, and the aortic valve closes. The aortic pressure tracing shows a "dicrotic notch" resulting from elastic rebound of the aorta. Left ventricular pressure then falls (isovolumic relaxation) to a level low enough to allow the mitral valve to reopen, and the process of rapid ventricular filling ensues. The heart sounds correspond to atrial contraction (S4), mitral valve closure (S1), aortic valve closure (S2), and rapid ventricular filling (S3), respectively.

The ventricular volume increases during atrial contraction and decreases during the rapid ejection of blood (stroke volume) after aortic valve opening. These events are followed by rapid ventricular filling in early diastole, then a period of slow ventricular filling. The same electrical and mechanical events and the same pressure-volume relations apply to the right ventricle. Rapid heart rates reduce the ejection time somewhat, and reduce the slow ventricular filling period markedly.

A useful method for depicting ventricular function is the relationship between pressure and volume. Figure 23.3 shows such a *pressure-volume loop*. In the isolated papillary muscle, this can be portrayed as a force-length relationship. Since left ventricular pressure and volume are more easily measured in the intact heart than myocardial force and segment length, these are the more common modes for expression. The curve AB depicts the diastolic filling of the left ventricle. The curve BC demonstrates isometric contraction before reaching the level of pressure sufficient to open the aortic valve at point C. The curve CD represents isotonic contraction (ejection at relatively constant pressure after the aortic valve has opened). At the end of ejection, when ventricular pressure falls below the aortic diastolic pressure, the aortic valve closes. The curve DA represents isometric or isovolumic relaxation, an active process of relaxation of the left ventricular muscle, allowing pressure to diminish to levels sufficient to open the mi-

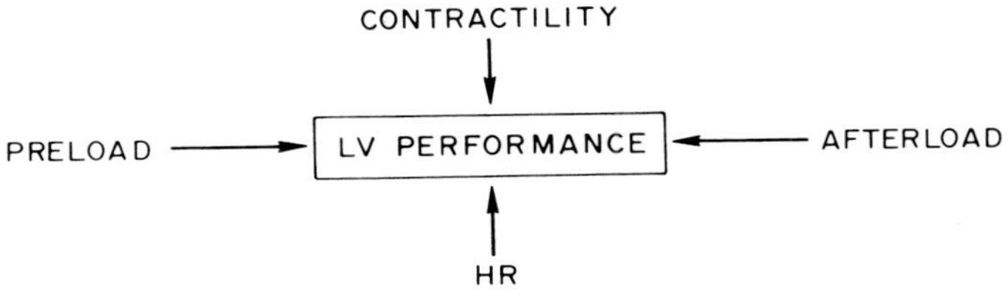

Figure 23.1. Determinants of left ventricular performance. *LV* = left ventricular, *HR* = heart rate.

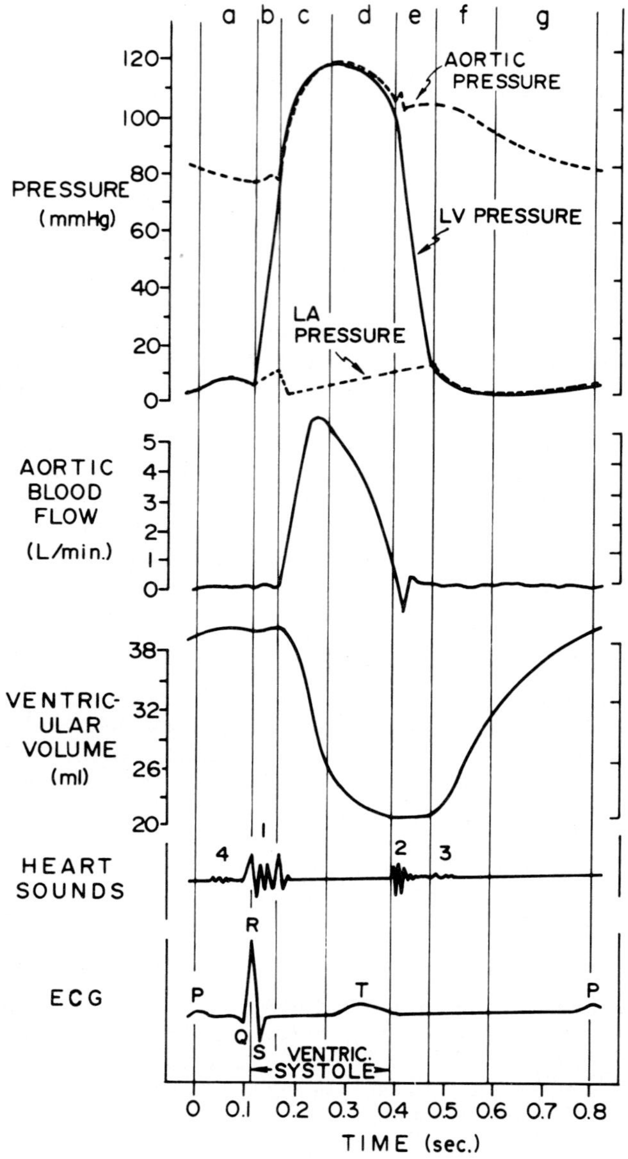

Figure 23.2. The cardiac cycle. Electrical events, followed by left heart flow and pressure, are illustrated. *a* = atrial contraction, *b* = isovolumic ventricular contraction; *c* = rapid ventricular ejection; *d* = slow ventricular ejection; *e* = isovolumic ventricular relaxation; *f* = rapid ventricular filling; and *g* = slow ventricular filling. *LV* = left ventricular; *LA* = left atrial; *ECG* = electrocardiogram. (Reproduced by permission and modified from Berne RM, Levy M. Cardiovascular physiology. 6th ed. St. Louis: CV Mosby, 1992.)

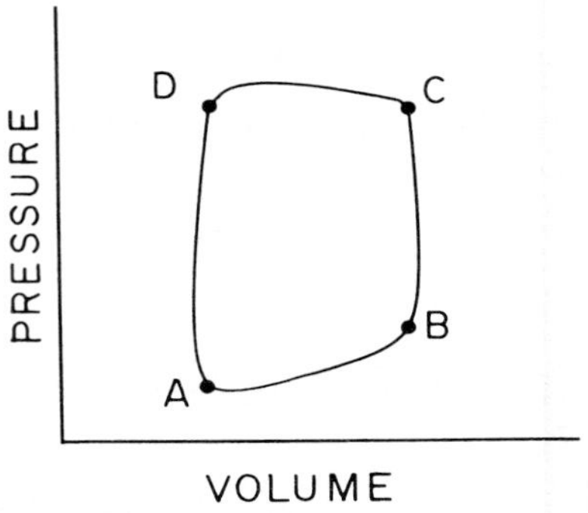

Figure 23.3. The ventricular pressure-volume relationship. See text for details.

tral valve and restart ventricular filling at point A. The diastolic pressure-volume relationship AB represents ventricular "compliance" (dV/dP), which is a measure of ventricular distensibility. The systolic pressure-volume relationship measured by BCD is a measure of ventricular systolic function, stiffening or "elastance," as stored power is turned into kinetic energy.

There are several "ejection-phase indices" of cardiac performance. The stroke volume (ml/beat) is represented by the distance on the volume axis between C and D. The "ejection fraction" is calculated as (EDV−ESV)/EDV, where EDV = end-diastolic volume (B), and ESV = end-systolic volume (D). Normal values for the left ventricle range from 0.50–0.70, and this index of global left ventricular performance is frequently calculated from radionuclide ventriculograms. An "isovolumic index" of contractility is the rate of rise of pressure (dP/dt).

Preload

The early studies of Frank, Starling, and Wiggers demonstrated that increasing myocardial stretch (length) produced stronger contractions (force). Studies in the frog ventricle by Frank in the late 1800s led to studies in the intact dog on right heart bypass (to control left ventricular filling characteristics) and also to elegant studies in the papillary muscle. Each of these emphasized the relationship between preload (ventricular stretch or volume) and a measure of cardiac performance (stroke volume, stroke work, cardiac output, etc.). As noted in Figure 23.4, the normal relationship between the end-diastolic volume (or pressure) and performance is curvilinear. Thus, as the ventricle is filled (stretched), ventricular performance (as measured by an ejection-phase index) increased, but asymptotically, so that beyond certain limits further stretch does not increase stroke volume, but merely raises the level of end-diastolic ventricular pressure and volume. Under steady state conditions, this relationship is a reflection of myocardial contractility. Conditions or agents that enhance contractility are termed *positive inotropic stimuli*. Under these conditions, stroke volume can be increased for any given level of pressure or volume, such that the ventricle contracts to a greater degree for the same end-diastolic volume. Conversely, ventricular function can be depressed by so-called *negative inotropic factors*, and, thus, there will be a lower stroke volume for the same level of diastolic volume.

The "operating point" for the intact heart is a more narrow range of diastolic pressure and volume. In practice, the description of ventricular function as normal, enhanced, or depressed is often based on single observations of ventricular contraction, stroke volume, or cardiac output. However, the care of patients with congestive cardiac failure is based on optimizing cardiac output while avoiding the excessively high end-diastolic pressures and volumes that produce pulmonary and systemic venous pressure elevation and congestion. Conversely, inadequate ventricular filling leads to low cardiac output syndromes, which

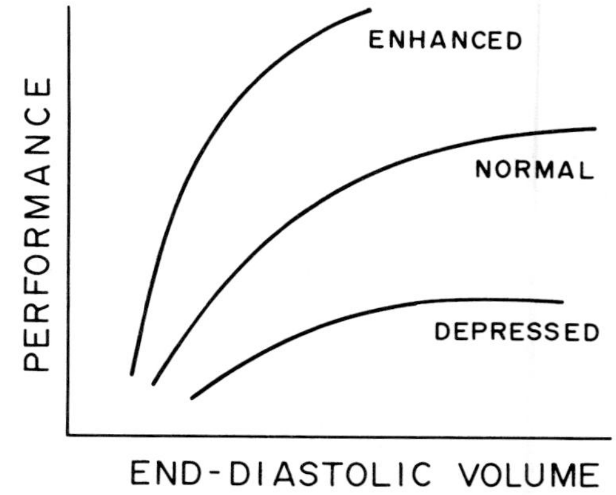

Figure 23.4. The Frank-Starling mechanism. Greater end-diastolic volume produces greater ventricular performance. Curves for normal, enhanced, and depressed contractility are shown.

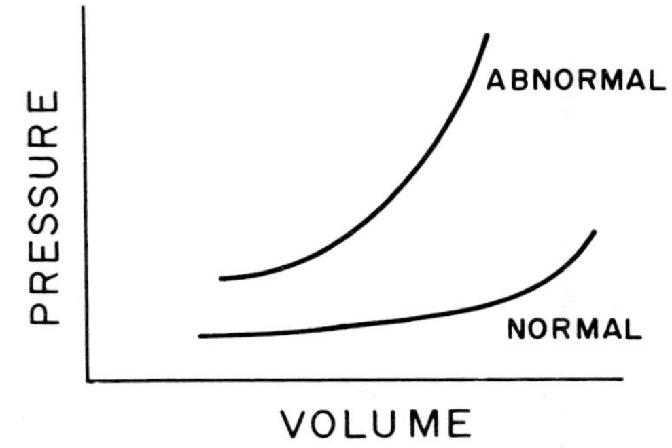

Figure 23.5. Ventricular compliance. Normal and abnormal curves are shown. In the normal state, there is a large change in volume for a small change in pressure (*dV/dP*), thus compliance is high.

may be reversed by appropriate volume loading. Clinical examples associated with increased ventricular preload include valvular regurgitant lesions, intracardiac shunts (congenial or acquired), and pulmonary or systemic arteriovenous fistulas. Such alterations in preload can produce abnormalities of diastolic pressure and volume, even though myocardial contractility is normal.

Ventricular filling is determined by the degree of active (energy requiring) relaxation of the myocardium (active calcium removal from the cytoplasm surrounding actin and myosin), venous return of blood, atrial contraction, the duration of diastole, and importantly, ventricular compliance (1), and perhaps diastolic "suction" (2). The term *compliance* (dV/dP) defines the relationship between diastolic pressure and volume (Fig. 23.5). The normal curve is nonlinear and demonstrates a large change in volume with a minimal increase in diastolic pressure, which remains low. The abnormal curve shows that small changes in volume are accompanied by large increases is diastolic pressure, and the diastolic pressures are higher at similar volumes. Chamber compliance itself is multifactorial. The ventricular size, its wall thickness, the completeness of active myocardial relaxation, the material properties of the ventricular wall (fibrous tissue versus normal), external compressive forces, and internal restriction to filling (such as endocardial fibroelastosis) all determine compliance. The pericardium itself has a pressure-volume relationship. Normally, the pericardium is a thin, compliant structure, and progressive increments of fluid added to the pericardial space cause minimal increases in pressure until a threshold level at which further increments in volume cause marked increases in the intrapericardial pressure. This condition of decompensated pericardial tamponade limits ventricular preload, and cardiac output can fall in spite of normal myocardial muscle characteristics. Similarly, a thickened pericardium can limit ventricular filling and cause the syndrome of chronic constrictive pericarditis. Removal of pericardial fluid or the pericardium itself produces a more normal ventricular diastolic pressure-volume relationship. Chronic disorders of the myocardium, such as hypertrophy, fibrosis after infarction, and infiltrative disorders, such as amyloidosis, reduce compliance. Transient myocardial ischemia causes stiffening and reduced compliance also (discussed later). Also, right ventricular dilatation affects left ventricular filling (see Ventricular interaction later in this chapter).

Afterload

Afterload is the resistance to fiber shortening or ventricular systolic emptying. A combination of inertial forces, aortic impedance and arteriolar tone constitute the ventricular afterload. Valvular aortic stenosis is an example of excess afterload due to high outflow impedance, whereas systemic hypertension can cause increased vascular resistance. The systolic arterial pressure and left ventricular wall "stress" (discussed later) are related to ventricular afterload. Figure 23.6 demonstrates the concept of the inverse, curvilinear relationship between ventricular performance and afterload (outflow resistance). Curves from ventricles with normal, moderately depressed, and severely depressed contractility are shown. For each curve, performance diminishes as the afterload increases. Conversely, reducing afterload increases performance. At low levels of afterload, the performance of each ventricle is roughly similar, but at greater levels of afterload, ventricles with reduced contractility, which operate on depressed curves, have lower stroke volume (3, 4).

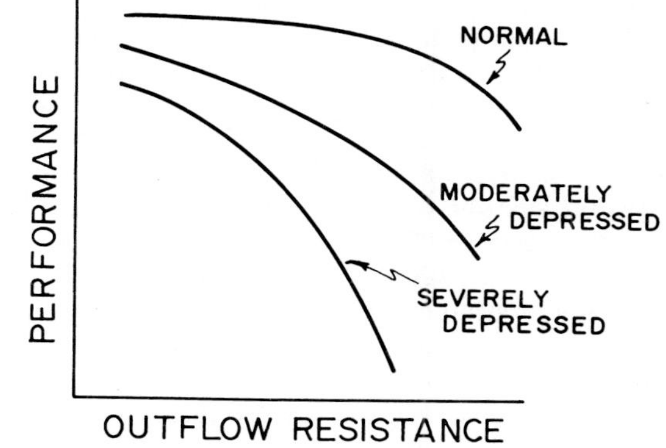

Figure 23.6. Concept of afterload regulation of ventricular performance. Ventricular performance (e.g., stroke volume) decreases as outflow resistance increases. The role of afterload is greatest when ventricular function is severely depressed. (Abstracted by permission of The New England Journal of Medicine and redrawn after Cohn JN, Franciosa JA. Vasodilator therapy of cardiac failure. N Engl J Med 1977;297:27.)

Contractility

Contractility is a broad term that describes the quality or intensity of myocardial contraction or fiber shortening. It may be influenced by diverse stimuli, such as ischemia, hypoxia, acidosis, drugs (both positive and negative inotropic agents), and intrinsic disorders of the myocardium.

The cellular mechanisms underlying contractility have been studied intensely, but estimation of contractility in the intact state has been difficult because cardiac performance (as an estimate of contractility) is also influenced by preload, afterload, and heart rate (Fig. 23.1). Such "ejection phase" indices as cardiac output, ejection fraction, stroke volume, stroke work, and V_{cf} (the velocity of circumferential fiber shortening) are each interdependent and dependent upon loading conditions and heart rate. Thus, they are inadequate estimates of contractility, although they may reflect the contractile state in certain situations. Other nonejection phase indices, such as isovolumic *dP/dt* (the rate of rise of pressure during isovolumic systole), estimate contractility better because they are less influenced by loading conditions. Maximal *dP/dt* is affected by loading conditions and is generally inadequate for estimating contractility if loading conditions change (5).

To circumvent these problems there has been extensive study of the contractile state in the isolated supported heart, intact animal models and in human subjects (6–13). The end-systolic pressure-volume relationship (ESPVR) and modifications have received extensive attention as indices of contractility that are relatively independent of loading conditions. The ESPVR incorporates pressure afterload into the estimate of contractility whereas other estimates of contractility such as the ejection fraction and *dP/dt* at maximal pressure do not account for loading conditions. Figure 23.7 demonstrates the concept of the generally linear relationship of end-systolic pressure and volume in the isolated supported heart. Several manipulations of ventricular pressure and volume are shown. Using the ESPVR concept, the myocardium is considered to have systolic behavior somewhat analogous to a spring. In a spring, there is a linear relationship between force and length such that greater stretch produces greater tension, and, similarly, in the heart there is a linear relationship between the afterload (as end-systolic pressure) and the end-systolic volume. Figure 23.7**A** demonstrates that preload may vary widely (*solid lines*) and when the ventricle is allowed to eject after reaching the same systolic pressure, in each case the ventricle ejects to the same end-systolic volume. Thus, under such conditions, regardless of preload, the end-systolic volume is determined by the level of end-systolic pressure. The pressure-volume loops depicted by the *dashed lines* show that end-systolic volume may become larger or smaller depending upon the systolic pressure afterload against which the ventricle ejects. When the end-systolic pressure-volume points are connected, the relationship is linear. Figure 23.7**B** illustrates that the ESPVR is relatively independent of end-diastolic volume. Here, with end-diastolic volume set constant, the ventricle is allowed to eject at low, medium, and high levels of systolic pressure. Under such conditions the end-systolic pressure determines the level of end-systolic volume, and

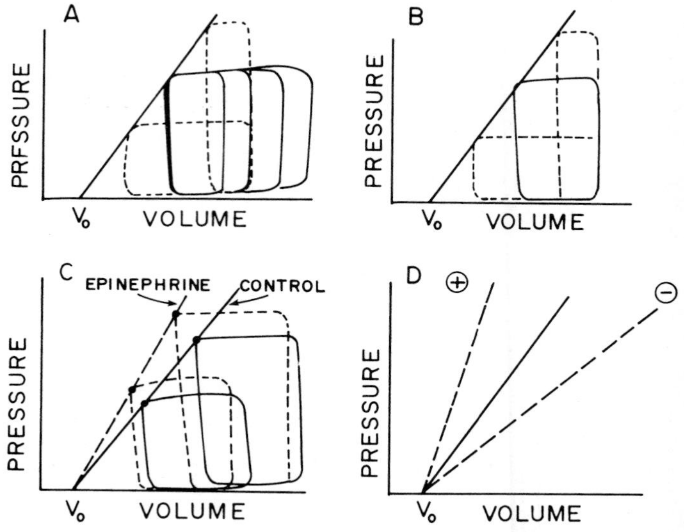

Figure 23.7. Ventricular end-systolic pressure-volume relationship (ESPVR) in the isolated, supported heart. **A.** *Solid lines* represent cardiac cycles at four levels of end-diastolic volume and demonstrate that the ventricle contracts to similar end-systolic volume, dependent on the systolic pressure and relatively independent of the end-diastolic pressure or volume. *Dashed lines* represent cardiac cycles at two other levels of end-systolic pressure. The curve connecting the end-systolic pressure-volume points is linear. V_0 represents ventricular volume when P = 0. **B.** Pressure-volume loops from similar end-diastolic volumes. The end-systolic pressure determines the end-systolic volume. **C.** The ESPVR is shifted leftward by the positive inotropic drug epinephrine. **D.** Positive inotropic drugs shift the ESPVR leftward, and negative inotropic drugs shift the ESPVR rightward. V_0 is relatively constant in the isolated heart, in spite of changes in contractility. (Reproduced by permission, redrawn and modified after Suga H, Sagawa K, Shoukas AA. Load independence of the instantaneous pressure-volume ratio of the canine left ventricle and effects of epinephrine and heart rate on the ratio. Circ Res 1974;32:314.)

the linearity is apparent. Thus, under constant contractile conditions, the ESPVR is an index of contractility, which is expressed in terms of ventricular "elastance" (*E*) and described by the equation $E_{es} = P_{es}/(V_{es} - V_o)$, where *P* and *V* are end-systolic (es) pressure and volume, and V_o represents the volume when $P = 0$. In Figure 23.7**C**, the pressure-volume relationship defined under control conditions in one contractile state is shifted leftward when an infusion of epinephrine produces a new steady state of increased contractility. In Figure 23.7**D**, to summarize, the pressure-volume relationship shifts leftward under positive inotropic states and shifts rightward with negative inotropic conditions.

There are some modifiers to the general concept. First, in acute experiments performed in the isolated heart, V_o is relatively constant. In the intact animal and in humans, V_o is more variable, partly due to acute changes in contractility and partly because of chronic adaptation by ventricular dilatation to conditions such as congestive cardiac failure. Second, in contrast to the engineering model of the spring, myocardial elastance increases with time during the cardiac cycle and is maximal at end-systole. This is termed "time-varying elastance" and is probably due to the interaction of calcium and the contractile apparatus, fiber properties, chamber geometry, and the sequence of activation. Third, further careful work has shown that the ESPVR is somewhat curvilinear (9), especially at high contractile states, and that all indices of contractility may have this property because of the time-varying enhancement of contractility during systole. Further enhancements to the measurement of contractility have included the linearity of preload recruitable stroke work (10) and preload adjusted maximal power (12), a measurement of the maximum rate of ventricular work (instantaneous ventricular pressure × rate of volume change) adjusted for end-diastolic volume. This latter index holds promise for future noninvasive study because the rate of rise of the arterial pressure and the decrease in ventricular volume may be estimated noninvasively (13). However, further study is necessary before embarking on clinical application. This further work has strengthened our knowledge of left ventricular chamber function and allows use of the ESPVR concept with appropriate caveats.

The ESPVR concept has been applied in clinical studies, with volume or dimension estimates by contrast ventriculography, echocardiography, or radionuclide ventriculography. Pressure afterload may be estimated by direct intra-arterial recording or by indirect sphygmomanometer measurements, sometimes extrapolated to end-systolic pressure by using the so-called calibrated carotid pulse tracing (13, 14). Ventricular wall stress is an important measure of afterload. Within the ventricle, tension, or force per unit area (Fig. 23.8), is compensated by wall thickness and yields the term "stress." Stress-shortening relations

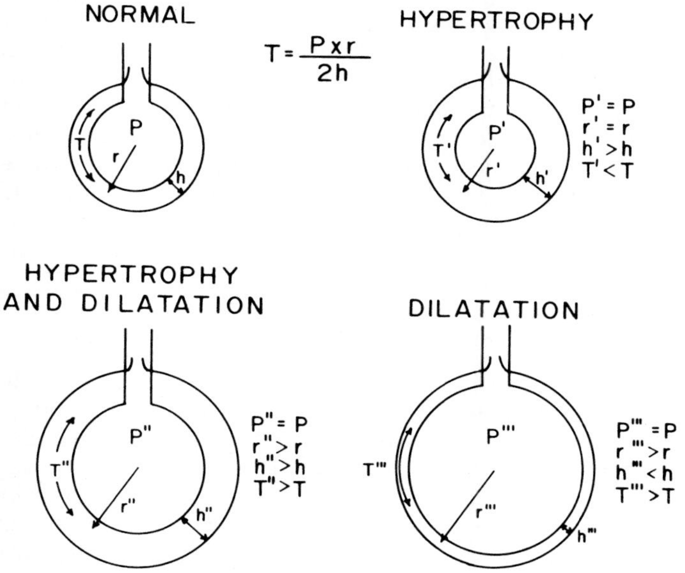

Figure 23.8. Compensatory mechanisms. As a consequence of heart failure, the left ventricle may dilate to produce an adequate stroke volume. Hypertrophy may accompany dilation or may occur alone as a response to systemic hypertension. The Laplace equation demonstrates the effects of hypertrophy, dilation, and the combination on wall tension (*T*). Increasing wall thickness (*h*) reduces tension and myocardial oxygen demand. However, increasing systolic pressure (*P*) or the ventricular end-diastolic radius (*r*) increases wall tension above normal and increases myocardial oxygen consumption. (Reproduced by permission and redrawn after Shepherd JT, Vanhoutte PM. The human cardiovascular system. New York: Raven Press, 1979:73.)

(stress-V_{cf}) usefully incorporate compensatory mechanisms such as hypertrophy into the afterload estimate (15, 16). This index of contractility also allows easier comparison between ventricles of different sizes. However, the assumptions in all such calculations may be compromised in the frequent case of regional ventricular dyssynergy following myocardial infarction.

Rhythm and Conduction Abnormalities

Cardiac conduction normally proceeds from the sinoatrial node through the atrioventricular node and His bundle to ramify into the left and right bundle branch systems and Purkinje fibers. This rapid electrical depolarization produces an orderly sequence of atrial contraction followed by ventricular contraction. Well-timed atrial systole may increase the stroke volume by 10–20%. Conversely, atrial arrhythmias such as atrial fibrillation reduce the end-diastolic volume and stroke volume, other factors remaining equal. The contributions of sinus rhythm and atrial systole to end-diastolic volume may be especially important in low cardiac output syndromes (i.e., reduced systolic performance) or in hearts with poor compliance.

Given a normal sequence of atrial and ventricular activation (normal sinus rhythm), the heart rate has obvious importance in generating the cardiac output (stroke volume × heart rate). Thus, bradycardia must reduce cardiac output, if stroke volume remains constant. Also, there are rate-dependent changes in contractility. Faster rates increase the strength of contraction through calcium mechanisms. This effect is most pronounced at rates in the 60–100 range.

Ventricular premature contractions have several deleterious effects. Early in diastole, the ventricular volume may be small. By itself, this would reduce stroke volume. Also there is reduced contraction based on a lower than normal amount of calcium available for transport to the active sites on actin and myosin. Postpremature beats tend to be more forceful contractions, probably as a result of greater calcium available to the contractile apparatus and a larger end-diastolic volume. Frequent premature ventricular contractions and salvos of such beats may severely reduce the cardiac output. Conduction disorders, such as right or left bundle branch block, disrupt the normal sequence of ventricular depolarization and contraction. This out-of-phase contraction sequence produces unusual motion of the interventricular septum, which can be observed on echocardiography and radionuclide ventriculography. This sequence also reduces septal perfusion. The combination of dyssynchrony and hypoperfusion reduces contractility (17).

Regional Left Ventricular Performance

All of the foregoing discussion relates to measurements of global (overall) ventricular performance. Such concepts are applicable to the normal heart or to the heart that is affected uniformly by generalized disorders of contractility. Coronary artery disease produces regional functional abnormalities that are acute or chronic. For example, a myocardial infarction in the distribution of the left anterior descending coronary artery may cause septal, anterior, and apical akinesis. Such regional disorders modify regional function. Their effect on global left ventricular performance depends on the extent of the regional abnormality and secondary compensatory events, such as increased contraction and hypertrophy of the remaining normal myocardium.

COMPENSATORY ADJUSTMENTS

Left Ventricular Factors

The left ventricle responds to a chronic, pathologic increase in afterload or preload by myocardial hypertrophy, dilatation, or both. This process is termed ventricular remodeling. The Laplace equation describes the relationship between wall tension, pressure, radius, and wall thickness (Fig. 23.8). Wall tension increases with dilation. It is reduced when there is adequate compensatory hypertrophy. When pressure and volume increase beyond the ability of hypertrophy to compensate, tension (or wall stress) rises to inappropriately high levels. Eventually left ventricular dysfunction occurs. This results in inadequate ventricular performance and is characterized by reduced forward output, unusually high filling pressures with their congestive consequences, or both. If the adjustment is inadequate, further dilatation may occur. Such dilatation further stretches the myofibrils, and the actin and myosin subunits. Theoretically, when dilatation is extreme, cardiac output may decline. Secondary pulmonary hypertension and right ventricular dysfunction may occur. Systemic hypertension and myocardial infarction are the two commonest causes of ventricular dilatation and hypertrophy. After myocardial infarction these compensatory processes are termed remodeling and involve both the infarct regions (expansion) and the noninfarcted regions which also dilate and hypertrophy (18). The right ventricle is anatomically thinner and less well-suited for compensating for this pressure and volume stress. Thus, right ventricular dilatation occurs and leads to right atrial hypertension, volume overload, or both, plus annular dilatation and possible tricuspid valvular regurgitation as well. The right ventricle is quite sensitive to pressure or volume overload and its contractility declines under such stress (19).

Neurohormonal Factors

The systemic arterial blood pressure is determined by the blood volume, the characteristics of the arteries and veins, and the characteristics of the heart as a pump. In the presence of inadequate pump performance, high-pressure and low-pressure mechanoreceptors (baroreceptors) form the afferent limb for central sympathetic and vagal compensatory activity. Consequently, the heart rate increases. Norepinephrine is released from adrenergic fibers in the heart in an attempt to increase contractility, and in the arterioles for regional vasoconstriction. Such vasoconstriction occurs in the skin, the splanchnic circulation, and the renal afferent arterioles. The systemic capacitance vessels constrict to increase right heart venous return, which increases preload in an attempt to increase cardiac performance. Hormonal adjustments are proportional to the degree of left ventricular dysfunction (20) and include elevated levels of circulating norepinephrine, renin, angiotensin II, aldosterone, and arginine vasopressin, the latter two being related to increasing the circulating blood volume. Additionally, the circulating concentration of endothelin is elevated in heart failure. Arteriolar vasoconstriction helps normalize the blood pressure, but at a higher level of peripheral resistance. Volume adjustments increase preload, but sometimes at the cost of pulmonary or peripheral edema. The chronically elevated levels of circulating catecholamines and the excess sympathetic activation are associated with downregulation of β-adrenergic receptors (21). This leads to less myocardial responsiveness to these positive inotropic factors plus chronotropic downregulation such that the heart rate is relatively lower than normal for the amount of circulating norepinephrine. Such chronotropic downregulation of the sinoatrial node is especially pronounced during exercise. Lastly, inadequate cardiac output leads to changes in oxyhemoglobin dissociation which favor oxygen unloading. Gradually, the heart, arteries, and veins come to a new operating point based on these circulatory adjustments. These adjustments may be sufficient to produce a normal cardiac output without circulatory congestion (asymptomatic left ventricular dysfunction), but may be inadequate to compensate for progressive myocardial dysfunction and lead to symptomatic dysfunction (congestive heart failure).

Ventricular Interaction

The right ventricle responds to the same mechanisms for altering performance as the left. Right and left ventricular interaction can be important. When examined in series, left heart failure can cause right heart failure. However, when examined in parallel, they interact through the interventricular septum, through common muscle fibers, and through the pericardium, which surrounds both chambers. For example, pulmonary hypertension can produce right ventricular hypertrophy and dilatation, eventually bowing the interventricular septum toward the left ventricle, adversely changing both the systolic and diastolic left ventricular pressure-volume relations.

Cardiopulmonary Interaction

Cardiopulmonary interactions have been incompletely characterized. However, several obvious models of interaction have been described. For instance, marked decreases in the intrapleural pressure on inspiration can reduce left ventricular performance by sequestering blood in the pulmonary circuit, thereby reducing left ventricular filling. Also, positive end-expiratory ventilatory pressure can reduce venous return to the right heart and limit cardiac output. Hypoxia has complex effects, with a primary depressant effect on the myocardium and a secondary stimulatory effect produced by adrenergic norepinephrine release. Local pulmonary reflexes may alter the heart rate.

Pharmacologic Effects on Cardiovascular Homeostasis

Positive inotropic agents increase the stroke volume for the same level of preload (Fig. 23.4) and reduce the end-systolic volume for the same level of afterload. (Fig. 23.7**C** and **D**). They increase the cardiac output and arterial blood pressure, thereby reducing the secondary vascular volume shifts and neurohormonal compensations for hypotension, hypovolemia, and reduced perfusion. Negative inotropic agents act conversely. Afterload-reducing drugs act by reducing vascular resistance and the arterial blood pressure. These changes improve stroke volume (Fig. 23.6) and sometimes the left ventricular developed pressure.

In recent years, there has been intense investigation of positive inotropic drugs to treat heart failure. Both β-adrenergic agonists and phosphodiesterase inhibitors can increase left ventricular performance sharply (as judged by the cardiac output and the ejection fraction). However, these short-term effects lead to β-adrenergic receptor downregulation and, in several studies of the phosphodiesterase mechanism, to excess mortality. Paradoxically, β-adrenergic receptor blockade has improved exercise capacity and the left ventricular ejection fraction in some patients with systolic dysfunction and heart failure. Angiotensin converting enzyme inhibitors have produced the most striking improvements in the drug therapy of left ventricular dysfunction, have lessened ventricular remodeling (22), and have decreased the morbidity and mortality of heart failure.

From a diagnostic nuclear medicine standpoint, both positive inotropic drugs and vasodilators such as dipyridamole have been employed as agents for pharmacologic stress testing and the evaluation of myocardial viability (23). Dobutamine stimulates β_1-, β_2- and α-adrenergic receptors. Predominantly, it exerts a positive inotropic effect on the heart with little net effect on the peripheral arterial tree. At low doses this drug may increase the contractility of viable "hibernating" or "stunned" myocardium. The improved performance may presage improvement after revascularization. At higher doses the net effect may be to produce ischemia. Such pharmacologic stress is useful for diagnosing ischemia when exercise is impractical or contraindicated.

Dipyridamole prevents the reuptake of adenosine, potentiates its effects on its receptors, and produces both coronary and systemic vasodilatation. Because of systemic vasodilatation ventricular afterload is reduced. In normal subjects, the left ventricular ejection fraction increases and wall motion remains normal or is enhanced. However, in patients with "significant" coronary atherosclerosis the drug may induce myocardial ischemia and the ejection fraction fails to increase or may decrease, and there may be new wall motion abnormalities. This is the basis for the dipyridamole echo test (24) and also for studies of dipyridamole radionuclide ventriculography (25). Adenosine infusion may also be employed with similar effects. The effects of dipyridamole on myocardial blood flow and perfusion are discussed in a later section (Myocardial Perfusion, Pharmacologic Alteration).

MYOCARDIAL PERFUSION

NORMAL REGULATION OF CORONARY BLOOD FLOW

Anatomic Factors

The left and right coronary arteries provide the major conduits for blood flow to the left and right ventricles and atria. A much smaller contribution, more important for the atria and right ventricle than the left ventricle, is provided by channels originating directly from the heart's cavities and running into the inner layers of the wall. Although the epicardial arteries usually provide only a minor portion of the total coronary vascular resistance, their contribution may be considerable under circumstances of atherosclerotic narrowing or spasm.

The major site of coronary vascular resistance normally resides in small intramural arteries and arterioles 10–40 μm in diameter, which exhibit important degrees of vasomotive constriction and dilation in response to various metabolic, humoral, and/or neural stimuli. Many of these small intramural arteries arise as perforating vessels from the epicardial arteries and course directly through the ventricular wall to the subendocardium, where they branch profusely to form a subendocardial vascular plexus or network. This network provides the major source of intercoronary collateral flow in the event of a coronary artery occlusion, although large epicardial artery-to-epicardial artery connections also play an important role.

As in other organs, the myocardial capillaries serve as semipermeable membranes for delivery of oxygen and nutrients and removal of metabolic waste products. The transport of molecules occurs between the capillary lumen and interstitial space via passive diffusion, pinocytosis, or passage through interendothelial pores. Capillary density is normally high ($2–5 \times 10^5$ capillaries per mm^2, with one capillary per muscle fiber), although the density can be reduced by disease processes, such as left ventricular hypertrophy. Whether a given capillary bed is perfused or not at any given moment is controlled by arteriolar precapillary sphincters. During hypoxia the sphincters relax, resulting in an increase in effective capillary density and a reduction in effective intercapillary distance.

Perfusion Pressure

Coronary blood flow is determined by the interaction between perfusion pressure and coronary vascular resistance (flow = perfusion pressure divided by resistance). Since the major portion of coronary blood flow occurs in diastole, perfusion pressure is frequently assumed to be equal to aortic diastolic pressure. However, in the presence of atherosclerotic stenoses of the coronary arteries, very significant pressure drops may occur along the course of the major epicardial arteries, reducing effective perfusion pressure markedly. Depending on the distribution of coronary stenoses, perfusion pressure may be significantly lower in one coronary bed than an adjacent one, encouraging the growth and development of intercoronary collaterals from the high- to the low-pressure bed.

The concept of perfusion pressure must also take into account the presence of "backpressure," that is, pressure at the level of the myocardial capillaries. The effective coronary "driving pressure" is actually equal to the perfusion pressure minus the backpressure. In most cases, the backpressure is equal to tissue pressure and is determined by the level of the left ventricular diastolic pressure. This is especially true for the subendocardial layer of the left ventricle, which is directly compressed when left ventricular cavity pressure rises. However, coronary sinus pressure may determine backpressure if it exceeds left ventricular diastolic pressure, as in some patients with right ventricular infarction or severe pulmonary hypertension.

Coronary Resistance

Extrinsic Compressive Forces. One of the most remarkable things about the heart is that during systolic contraction the intramural coronary vessels are compressed and coronary blood flow is effectively throttled. Blood is squeezed into the coronary veins and also backward into the epicardial arteries, which store the blood until the next beat ("capacitive" function). Systolic compressive forces are believed normally to be higher in the inner than the outer portion of the left ventricular wall, causing a greater reduction in systolic flow in the deeper layers. This "deficit" in myocardial perfusion must be made up for in diastole, and, in fact, about 85% of total coronary flow is diastolic under normal conditions. Because of greater inhibition of subendocardial perfusion in systole, diastolic perfusion of this region is higher in order to keep flow uniform across the wall. This compensation is mediated by greater dilatation of resistance vessels in the subendocardium, leading to some loss of total subendocardial vascular reserve. These concepts explain the critical dependence of subendocardial perfusion on diastolic hemodynamics. Subendocardial blood flow is affected out of proportion to subepicardial flow by decreases in effective diastolic perfusion pressure. Reduced diastolic pressure, in turn, could be due to a generalized drop in arterial pressure, a localized coronary artery stenosis, a rise in left ventricular filling pressure, or a shortening of diastolic time per beat as a result of an increase in heart rate. Because the subendocardium must normally utilize some of its vasodilatory reserve to maintain baseline perfusion, the subendocardium is especially vulnerable to ischemia and to ischemic damage during stress. The adequacy of subendocardial flow has been assessed experimentally using the diastolic pressure-time index (DPTI) divided by the systolic pressure-time index (SPTI), essentially an estimate of the "supply/demand balance" of the subendocardium (27).

Ordinarily, extravascular compressive forces represent only about 20% of the total (systolic plus diastolic) coronary resistance. However, the contribution of extravascular forces is exaggerated when the coronary vessels are greatly dilated, for example, during ischemia or severe exercise. For this reason, an increase in left ventricular filling pressure, leading to further compression of subendocardial vessels, could have a major adverse effect on perfusion in the setting of severe coronary atherosclerosis.

Metabolic Regulation. The most potent factor regulating coronary blood flow is the tight coupling that exists between coronary blood flow and myocardial oxygen demand, necessitated by the almost complete dependence of the myocardium on aerobic metabolism. In theory, myocardial oxygen delivery could be increased by either an increase in coronary blood flow or an increase in oxygen extraction, although the latter mechanism is limited by the high degree of extraction that exists under normal conditions. In practice, however, myocardial blood flow increases and decreases *pari passu* with changes in oxygen requirements, while increased extraction is generally found only when vasodilator reserve is exhausted. The close coupling between myocardial oxygen consumption and flow is adjusted on a second-by-second basis and represents the dominant mechanism for regulation of coronary blood flow.

The major determinants of myocardial oxygen consumption are heart rate, myocardial contractility, and wall stress (Fig. 23.8). Maximal exercise, associated with increases in all three major determinants of myocardial oxygen consumption, may cause as much as a fourfold increase in coronary blood flow with an opposite reduction in coronary vascular resistance. This increase is impressive, but it does not represent the full maximal vasodilating capacity of the coronary bed, which can be elicited by administration of potent arteriolar vasodilating agents, such as adenosine or dipyridamole. Under these conditions, as much as a sixfold increase in flow may occur.

Tight coupling of myocardial oxygen demands and flow results in the phenomenon of coronary autoregulation. Over a wide range of perfusion pressure, from about 50 to 150 mm Hg, coronary flow stays relatively constant as coronary vascular resistance adjusts to balance the change in pressure. Below 50 mm Hg, however, the vasodilating capacity of at least a portion of the ventricular wall is exceeded, autoregulation is no longer possible, and coronary flow falls abruptly. Above 150 mm Hg, the coronary vessels cannot or do not constrict further, and coronary flow increases rapidly. The concept of coronary autoregulation explains why relatively large changes in hemodynamics, above and below the normal level, may have little effect on the level of coronary blood flow.

A related phenomenon is *coronary reactive hyperemia* (Fig. 23.9). Following release of a brief coronary occlusion, flow increases above the previous baseline value (hyperemia) and the excess flow delivered to the myocardium ("repayment") equals or exceeds the amount of flow "debt" incurred during the occlusion. The amount and duration of hyperemia depend on the duration of occlusion, but the peak flow response is maximal after 15–30 seconds of occlusion. Reactive hyperemia has been measured in patients undergoing cardiac surgery using a Doppler flow meter placed over an epicardial coronary artery (28). It has

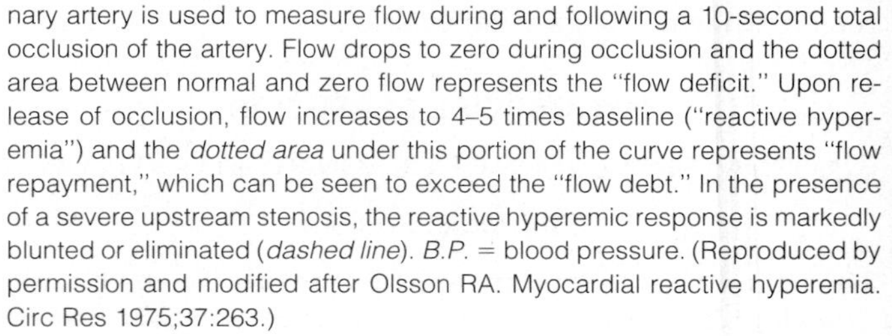

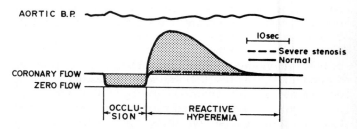

Figure 23.9. Reactive hyperemia. A flow meter implanted around a coronary artery is used to measure flow during and following a 10-second total occlusion of the artery. Flow drops to zero during occlusion and the dotted area between normal and zero flow represents the "flow deficit." Upon release of occlusion, flow increases to 4–5 times baseline ("reactive hyperemia") and the *dotted area* under this portion of the curve represents "flow repayment," which can be seen to exceed the "flow debt." In the presence of a severe upstream stenosis, the reactive hyperemic response is markedly blunted or eliminated (*dashed line*). *B.P.* = blood pressure. (Reproduced by permission and modified after Olsson RA. Myocardial reactive hyperemia. Circ Res 1975;37:263.)

also been identified in patients undergoing angioplasty following balloon deflation, using an intracoronary Doppler flow velocity catheter (29), and after reversal of transient coronary spasm using thallium perfusion imaging (30).

Despite its importance, the precise mechanism responsible for the metabolic regulation of coronary flow is uncertain. A number of chemical mediators have been proposed, including oxygen, potassium, and calcium, but the most likely mediators are one or more of these: adenosine, other nucleotides, prostaglandins, carbon dioxide, and/or hydrogen ion. These substances are all produced rapidly during ischemia and can cause relaxation of arterial smooth muscle. For example, adenosine is produced during metabolism of high-energy adenine nucleotides, diffuses across the myocardial cell membrane into the interstitial space, and is thought to interact with adenosine receptors to relax arteriolar smooth muscle and cause a decrease in coronary vascular resistance. ATP-sensitive potassium channels also contribute to reactive hyperemia by opening during ischemia, resulting in hyperpolarization and relaxation of vascular smooth muscle. Blockade of these channels by glibenclamide reduces reactive hyperemia by nearly 50% (31). It is likely that no single mediator exists, but rather that the tight coupling of metabolic needs and flow is a complex process that can be modulated by a number of compounds.

Neural and Humoral Regulation. The large and small coronary vessels and myocardial conduction tissue receive an abundant supply of autonomic nerves. Cardiac sympathetic nerves arise from the sympathetic ganglia, including the stellate ganglion, and densely innervate the epicardial coronary arteries and veins, as well as the intramural arteries, venules, and capillaries. Efferent parasympathetic cholinergic innervation arrives via the vagal nerves and supplies the coronary vessels and conduction system.

Sympathetic stimulation causes an increase in heart rate and myocardial contractility, resulting in an increase in myocardial metabolism and a compensatory rise in coronary blood flow via metabolic autoregulation. Vagal stimulation, in contrast, causes a striking bradycardia, modest decrease in myocardial contractility, and a resultant decrease in myocardial metabolism. The coronary arteries constrict in response to these effects on the myocardium, although the "direct" effect of vagal stimulation is to produce mild coronary dilation.

Infusions of adrenergic or cholinergic agonist drugs produce a much greater effect than can be elicited by more physiologic neural stimulation. For example, infusion of phenylephrine or methoxamine, both α-adrenergic agonists, can produce a twofold coronary constrictor response, compared to a 10–25% increase produced by selective sympathetic stimulation. Dobutamine, a synthetic sympathomimetic amine that stimulates β-adrenergic receptors, produces an increase in myocardial contractility and a secondary increase in myocardial blood flow. It is used in conjunction with echocardiography or perfusion imaging to diagnose coronary artery disease in patients who are unable to exercise (32). During dobutamine infusion, the presence of a coronary stenosis limits the flow increase that can occur through that vessel, leading to a maldistribution of perfusion and/or the appearance of a left ventricular wall motion abnormality (resulting from an imbalance between myocardial oxygen supply and demand).

A number of endogenous and exogenous humoral substances can produce significant coronary vasoconstriction. Among these are angiotensin, vasopressin, serotonin and the prostaglandins thromboxane A_2 and leukotriene D. Humoral coronary vasodilators include adenosine, acetylcholine, histamine, and the prostaglandins (PG) PGE_1 and prostacyclin (PGI_2). Infusion of these humoral agents can produce several-fold changes in coronary vascular resistance.

Pharmacologic Alteration. Potent coronary vasoactive substances have been developed for experimental, as well as therapeutic, manipulation of the coronary circulation. The most familiar of these are the nitrate preparations, including nitroglycerin and the longer acting isosorbide dinitrate. Nitrates cause a relaxation of arterial smooth muscle, particularly in the large epicardial coronary arteries, resulting in an increase in vessel caliber and a reversal of coronary spasm. Nitric oxide (NO) is believed to represent the direct mediator of these effects by increasing cellular levels of cyclic guanosine monophosphate (cGMP), which in turn inhibits calcium release from internal stores and calcium influx through membrane channels. NO is derived from organic nitrates following their conversion to inorganic nitrite in the presence of intracellular thiols such as cysteine. Nitroprusside, another nitrovasodilator, releases NO directly.

Administration of nitroglycerin sublingually causes a transient increase in coronary blood flow lasting 1–2 minutes, related to a dilation of arteriolar resistance vessels, combined with a longer lasting (up to 30 minutes) increase in epicardial vessel diameter, which is not associated with altered flow unless a significant coronary stenosis is present. Prolonged intravenous infusion of nitroglycerin similarly results in coronary dilation, usually without an increase in coronary blood flow, unless atherosclerotic narrowings are present and cause the epicardial arteries to become an important site of vascular resistance. If nitroglycerin is given within a few minutes of thallium injection during an exercise perfusion study, perfusion defects are often obliterated because of an increase in flow to the ischemic region at a time when significant amounts of thallium are still circulating in the blood.

Nonnitrate vasodilators, such as adenosine and dipyridamole, exert potent dilatory effects on resistance arterioles, resulting in large increases in coronary blood flow. In contrast to nitrates, the effects on epicardial conductance arteries are minimal. Dipyridamole has been used in conjunction with thallium perfusion imaging to increase coronary blood flow and uncover occult coronary stenoses, as with exercise (24, 33). This drug works by blocking the cellular uptake and metabolism of adenosine, thereby increasing its concentration at vascular smooth muscle receptors. Its effects can be reversed by aminophylline. In contrast to exercise, there is generally little change in heart rate or blood pressure following dipyridamole, and therefore little change in myocardial oxygen demands. Thallium is injected following a 4-minute intravenous infusion of the drug, and imaging is performed several minutes later. A thallium defect signifies the presence of a flow limiting coronary artery stenosis (usually reducing arterial diameter by ≥50%). Whereas flow increases several fold in response to dipyridamole in myocardium perfused by nonstenotic coronary arteries, the flow increase is blunted in areas fed by stenotic vessels; this is the basis of the maldistribution of thallium uptake that occurs in patients with coronary artery disease. There is also evidence that collateral-dependent regions of myocardium may experience an actual decrease in flow below baseline ("coronary steal") because of a decrease in collateral driving pressure (discussed later). Recently, adenosine itself has also been used to increase myocardial blood flow in conjunction with radionuclide perfusion imaging (34). Because of its very short half-life, adenosine must be continued for several minutes after the tracer is injected to ensure that its uptake is completed while flow is increased. Calcium-blocking drugs, such as nifedipine, verapamil, and diltiazem, are also coronary vasodilators. These drugs inhibit the transsarcolemmal passage of calcium through voltage-gated calcium channels, and have potent effects on both arteriolar resistance vessels and epicardial conductance arteries. They represent an important class of agents for reversal of coronary spasm and treatment of myocardial ischemia.

Coronary constrictor agents, such as ergonovine, are used clinically to provoke coronary artery spasm (35). In certain patients with rest angina, spontaneous coronary spasm may be responsible for attacks of episodic ischemia. Ergonovine is believed to induce spasm only in those susceptible individuals in whom spontaneous spasm is already occurring. Frequently spasm occurs at the site of an atherosclerotic plaque, but sometimes the coronary arteries appear normal. Ergonovine has been used in conjunction with thallium imaging to noninvasively detect spasm-induced perfusion defects, but because of the risk of inducing complete heart block, ventricular fibrillation, or difficult-to-reverse coronary spasm, ergonovine testing should probably only be done in the cardiac catheterization laboratory. Emergency intracoronary administration of vasodilators can then be performed if necessary.

Endothelium Dependent Vasomotion. Normal regulation of vasomotor tone in vivo is critically dependent on a normally functioning vascular endothelium. The endothelium participates in the metabolism of circulating vasoactive compounds such as angiotensin, bradykinin, and serotonin, and synthesizes vasodilator substances such as prostacyclin and NO, as well as constrictor substances such as endothelin. Many vasodilating substances (e.g., acetylcholine and bradykinin) produce their effect in vivo by stimulating specific endothelial cell receptors, leading to production of NO from L-arginine by the enzyme nitric oxide synthase. NO is then released from the endothelium and diffuses to overlying smooth muscle, where it produces relaxation through an increase in cGMP (36). The dilatation of an epicardial coronary artery that occurs during an increase in flow (i.e., during exercise or during an infusion of adenosine) is endothelium-dependent (37). Coronary atherosclerosis, as well as the presence of coronary risk factors such as hypertension and hypercholesterolemia, are associated with endothelial dysfunction and impaired endothelium-dependent vasodilation. Nitroglycerin and nitroprusside release NO directly and are considered *endothelium-independent* vasodilators (see earlier discussion).

MYOCARDIAL ISCHEMIA

Coronary Stenoses

Obstruction to coronary blood flow is usually caused by atherosclerotic narrowing in the epicardial coronary arteries, most often proximally at sites of turbulence, bending, or vessel bifurcations. Much less commonly, coronary obstruction may be related to embolization, vasculitis, dissection, or myocardial muscle bridging.

When hemodynamically significant, a coronary stenosis produces a pressure gradient within the artery, with downstream pressure falling below upstream pressure. The severity of stenosis is most related to the minimum luminal area available for passage of blood, but is also affected by the length and the shape of the narrowing. Eccentric stenoses may cause greater turbulence and loss of kinetic energy, resulting in larger pressure gradients. Stenosis severity is most often assessed by coronary angiography and is usually expressed as a percentage diameter stenosis relative to the diameter of an adjacent normal arterial segment. Experimentally, it has been determined that at least 50% diameter narrowing is required to reduce the maximal coronary flow response and that a stenosis must exceed 90% before resting flow is reduced. It is important to note that a 50% diameter stenosis is equivalent to a 75% reduction in cross-sectional area and a 70% diameter stenosis to a 90% reduction in area.

The severity of coronary artery disease in a patient is frequently described in terms of the most severe diameter stenosis in the three major arteries: anterior descending, circumflex, and right. Although convenient, this approach ignores the length of narrowings, the presence of lesions in series, and the diffuseness of arterial involvement. The narrowings are frequently estimated visually without actual measurements, resulting in reports that appear more quantitative than they really are. Furthermore, measurements of percentage diameter narrowing assume that the adjacent comparison segments are truly normal and are not themselves narrowed by disease, which is only infrequently the case. Studies by Marcus and associates (28), comparing coronary angiographic data with physiologic measurements of coronary flow obstruction, showed that the angiographic estimates of severity correlate poorly with true obstruction except when the stenosis is judged very severe (>90%) or very slight (<10%).

An additional problem in relating anatomic narrowings to physiologic effects is that the degree of stenosis is probably not fixed in most cases, but rather is dynamic and changing in response to a wide variety of factors. Decreases in distending pressure appear to increase stenosis severity by partial collapse of the stenotic segment. The opposite occurs with increases in distending pressure. Increased flow through a stenotic segment results in increased turbulence and energy loss, a fall in downstream pressure, and a possible increase in stenosis severity as a result of collapse of the distal end of the stenosis. Various humoral and neural stimuli could also have important effects on stenosis severity by constriction of arterial smooth muscle in the stenotic segment.

As a stenosis increases in severity, compensatory arteriolar dilatation must occur to maintain normal flow, utilizing in the process a portion of the vasodilator reserve of the involved myocardium. Experimentally, this loss of reserve is detected by a decrease in the reactive hyperemic response, the peak flow following a brief coronary occlusion. As discussed earlier, vasodilator reserve is lost quickly from the subendocardium because of the need to compensate for extravascular compressive forces, which are highest in this region.

Increasing stenosis severity also leads to a progressive reduction in distal coronary pressure and increasing vulnerability to subendocardial ischemia, since perfusion of the endocardial layers of the left ventricle is critically dependent on distal coronary pressure. Paradoxically, even though exercise increases epicardial coronary *flow* through a severe stenosis, subendocardial *perfusion* may actually decrease, because ischemia can increase the left ventricular filling pressure and increase the subendocardial diastolic compressive forces.

Coronary Collaterals

Coronary collateral vessels are vascular channels that connect large coronary arteries to one another. Native coronary collaterals are small, thin-walled structures with an endothelial lining and a sparse smooth muscle layer. Ischemia, however, can induce these primitive collaterals to develop into a major vascular network that can substantially modify the effects of coronary artery occlusion. Thus, following the onset of occlusion or the development of a severe stenosis (>80% diameter), a pressure gradient develops between occluded and nonoccluded vascular beds that stretches the collaterals, leading to rupture of the internal elastic lamina and migration of monocytes into the vessel wall. Over the next 1–2 weeks vascular growth occurs by mitotic division of endothelial cells, smooth muscle cells, and fibroblasts, resulting in larger, relatively thin-walled channels. Subsequently, over a period of months, the vessel wall becomes thicker and more organized by continued cellular proliferation and synthesis of elastin and collagen, so that the collateral vessel ultimately resembles a normal coronary artery. Experimentally, the functional capacity of collateral channels is near maximal by 4 weeks after coronary occlusion. Although effective resistance through immature native collaterals may be 60–80 times greater than minimal resistance through normal coronary vessels, the resistance falls to only 2–3 times normal in well-developed mature collaterals. Myocardium totally dependent on collaterals may have completely normal flow under resting conditions and may also possess substantial vascular reserve, with maximal flow as much as 50% of normal. Exercise perfusion imaging in patients may fail to detect a total coronary artery occlusion if collateralization of the occluded region is extensive, particularly if exercise heart rate is less than maximal (38).

Flow through collaterals is primarily dependent on the pressure gradient existing between the myocardial region perfused by the occluded or stenosed artery and the adjacent myocardial regions. Native immature collaterals may exhibit some vasomotion to neural, humoral, or pharmacologic stimuli, but the response is minimal because of the sparse numbers of smooth muscle cells present. Fully developed collaterals, however, have thick muscle coats and substantial neural connections are therefore capable of significant vasomotor activity. Nitroglycerin may be effective in angina in part because of a dilatation of the collaterals as well as the nonoccluded arteries supplying the collateral flow.

"Coronary steal" is a vasodilator-induced decrease in collateral flow to a collateral-dependent region (39). This response is seen with small vessel arteriolar-type dilators, such as dipyridamole or adenosine, and is most likely to occur in the setting of multivessel disease, where the arteries supplying collateral flow are themselves narrowed by coronary stenoses. An increase in flow through these stenosed arteries leads to a decrease in downstream pressure (see earlier discussion), which reduces the pressure head across the collaterals and causes a decrease in collateral perfusion. This mechanism is believed to account for the high prevalence of myocardial ischemia (chest pain or electrocardiographic changes) seen in patients with severe coronary artery disease given dipyridamole during thallium perfusion imaging.

Relation between Perfusion, Function, and Other Manifestations of Ischemia

A decrease in blood flow to a region of myocardium is associated with metabolic, functional, and electrocardiographic abnormalities, usually accompanied by the symptom of angina pectoris. Decreased oxygen delivery results in a cessation of aerobic metabolism, switchover to anaerobic glycolysis, buildup of lactic acid with tissue acidosis, and depletion of tissue high-energy phosphates. There is an almost immediate decrease in regional mechanical function, apparently related to an inability to cycle calcium normally to the myofilaments. Alterations in membrane function cause cell depolarization and relative inexcitability of the ischemic tissue, resulting in electrocardiographic ST segment abnormalities and QRS changes. All of these alterations are completely reversible if flow is restored within 15–20 minutes, although mechanical dysfunction may persist for hours to days before returning to normal ("stunned myocardium") (Fig. 23.10) (40). Stunning is caused in part by oxygen-free radicals generated during reperfusion (41), and the dysfunction associated with stunning can be transiently reversed by catecholamines or calcium. Longer ischemic durations result in progressive cellular necrosis, beginning with the most vulnerable subendocardial layers and proceeding in wave-like fashion toward the epicardium (42).

Of the various clinical manifestations of ischemia, regional mechanical dysfunction appears first, followed by electrocardiographic abnormalities, and finally by the symptom of chest pain. When monitoring patients with unstable angina in the coronary care unit, it is common to see electrocardiographic changes without chest pain as a manifestation of early ischemia. Chest pain may occur seconds to minutes later, or not at all ("silent ischemia"). Rest thallium imaging under these circumstances may demonstrate perfusion defects, despite the absence of chest pain or electrocardiographic abnormalities, which disappear after successful coronary bypass surgery (Fig. 23.11). Reduced blood flow can be associated with a proportional down-regulation of contractility and oxygen demands, resulting in myocardial dysfunction without the usual signs of ischemia (i.e., no chest pain or electrocardiographic or metabolic abnormalities). This phenomenon is known as "hibernating myocardium" (43). Function can be promptly restored to normal by increasing blood flow, commonly by means of percutaneous transluminal coronary angioplasty or bypass surgery. Hibernating myocardium can be detected by a rest-injected thallium study that demonstrates an initial perfusion defect filling in over 3–4 hours (indicative of regional myocardial viability). Positron emission tomography (PET) may also be used to detect hibernating myocardium. A perfusion defect accompanied by evidence of metabolic activity in a region with reduced contractile function ("perfusion-metabolism mismatch") identifies myocardium that is viable but ischemic at rest and, therefore, "hibernating."

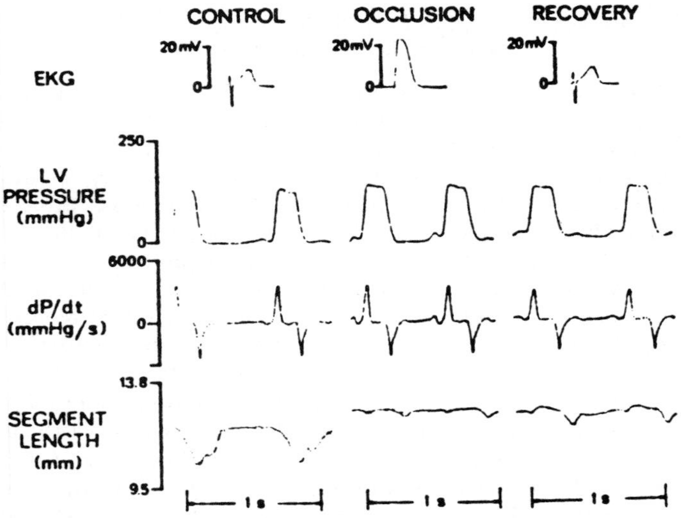

Figure 23.10. "Stunned myocardium." Myocardium remains dysfunctional after a brief (5-minute) occlusion of the coronary artery, despite normalization of the surface electrocardiogram (ECG). Residual dysfunction is denoted by increased myocardial segment length and markedly depressed shortening in the previously ischemic zone 5 minutes after release of the occlusion, and dysfunction may persist for up to 2 hours after such a brief occlusion. *LV* = left ventricle, *dP/dt* = rate of rise of ventricular pressure. (Reproduced by copyright permission of The American Society for Clinical Investigation from Heyndrickx GR, Millard RW, McRitchie RJ, Maroko PR, Vatner SF. Regional myocardial function and electrophysiological alterations after brief coronary occlusions in conscious dogs. J Clin Invest 1975;56:978.)

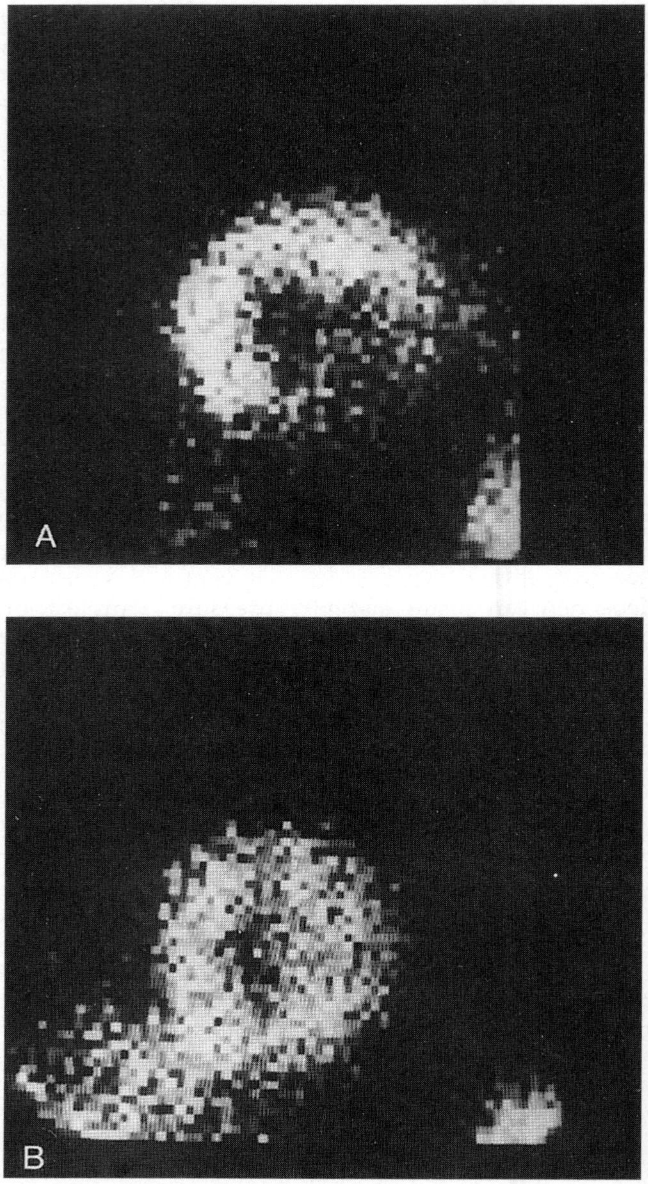

Figure 23.11. Rest thallium scintigrams before and after coronary artery bypass surgery. The 40° left anterior oblique view is shown. **A.** Preoperative demonstrating a moderately severe inferolateral perfusion defect unassociated with clinical signs of ischemia at the time of injection. **B**. After multivessel bypass surgery showing disappearance of the resting defect. (Reproduced by permission from Becker LC. Myocardial perfusion. In: Harbert JC, da Rocha AFG, eds. Textbook on nuclear medicine: Clinical applications. 2nd ed. Philadelphia: Lea & Febiger, 1984.)

EXERCISE PHYSIOLOGY

NORMAL MECHANISMS AND TYPES OF CARDIAC STRESS

Ventricular function can be examined more effectively and minor dysfunction may be exposed more easily if a "stress" is applied to the heart. Electrical pacing or handgrip (isometric exercise) may be used, but rhythmic ("isotonic," dynamic) exercise is most frequently employed.

Three major adjustments occur during *rhythmic exercise.* First, in response to the metabolic demands of the exercising muscles, those arterioles dilate, and the muscular blood flow increases. Second, to prevent systemic hypotension, the central nervous system produces arteriolar constriction in the nonexercising beds, such as the renal and splanchnic circulations. Also, the splanchnic venous capacitance vessels constrict. These changes help maintain the arterial pressure, in spite of vasodilation in the exercising muscular beds, and they increase the venous return to the right heart. The mechanical pumping effects of exercising muscles help to return blood to the right heart as well. The splanchnic and renal circulations are capable of withstanding such vasoconstriction, because their resting flow is considerably greater than their metabolic demands.

The third compensation is thermal. The excess heat produced by the exercising muscles is dissipated by cutaneous vasodilation, mediated by temperature-sensitive cells in the hypothalamus. The greater the degree of muscular and skin vasodilation, the greater the splanchnic and renal vasoconstriction. These homeostatic mechanisms help preserve cardiac and cerebral perfusion.

The heart and lungs are the limiting factors in maintaining adequate tissue perfusion and oxygenation. The heart rate, stroke volume, blood pressure and the inotropic state of the myocardium increase during exercise. An increase in heart rate is the primary means for increasing the cardiac output. Although the stroke volume increases slightly during the initial phases of rhythmic exercise, it may decrease slightly during prolonged exercise, apparently as a result of dilation of the cutaneous veins with a reduction in venous return and end-diastolic volume. However, with increased sympathetic stimulation of the myocardium, contractility is enhanced and the end-systolic volume decreases. Through these mechanisms the stroke volume increases by 10–20% during supine exercise. The stroke volume decreases when standing, but it increases during upright exercise to levels equal to supine resting stroke volume. By the combination of slightly improved stroke volume and tachycardia, the cardiac output rises three- to sixfold during moderately severe rhythmic exercise. The arterial systolic blood pressure increases usually by 50%, based on the level of resting vasoconstriction, the character of the arterial walls, and the cardiac performance. The increased contractile state is also evident by tachycardia, shorter systolic ejection time, smaller end-systolic volume, increased dP/dt, and an increase in the ratio of peak systolic pressure to end-systolic volume.

All of these mechanisms cause an increase in myocardial oxygen consumption. However, in the face of such increased demand, the increase in the heart rate reduces the coronary diastolic filling time, and coronary atherosclerosis may limit coronary blood flow, causing myocardial ischemia in the susceptible heart. The rate-pressure product, heart rate multiplied by the systolic arterial blood pressure, correlates roughly with myocardial oxygen consumption and is an index of the severity of the exercise stress.

Isometric exercise has been employed in some instances for the evaluation of ischemic heart disease. The major effects of static exercise are an increase in the arterial blood pressure and moderate increase in heart rate. Under extreme conditions, the arterial blood pressure may increase more than during rhythmic exercise, but conventional rhythmic exercise testing produces greater heart rate responses and greater oxygen demands. It is difficult to maintain and quantitate the effects of isometric exercise, and this limits its usefulness for testing cardiac reserve, whether by conventional electrocardiography or by imaging methods.

Atrial pacing has been used to increase myocardial oxygen demands and coronary blood flow, particularly in patients who are unable to perform rhythmic exercise. However, pacing causes little increase in contractility or coronary flow compared to dynamic exercise.

Cold pressor testing has been used in the clinical laboratory as a type of stress in conjunction with blood pool or perfusion imaging. The cold pressor response is obtained by immersing one hand in ice water for 1–2 minutes. Systolic blood pressure usually increases 10%, but heart rate is unchanged. Coronary artery diameter decreases and focal coronary spasm may be elicited in patients with variant angina or coronary atherosclerosis. This response is probably mediated by α-adrenergic receptors in the coronary arteries stimulated through neural reflexes. Sufficient coronary constriction or spasm may be associated with thallium perfusion defects, but this test is much less efficient than dynamic exercise for uncovering occult coronary artery disease.

EFFECTS OF ISCHEMIA ON VENTRICULAR PERFORMANCE

Myocardial ischemia is usually a localized phenomenon, due to excess myocardial oxygen demands compared to supply (e.g., myocardial blood flow). Transient myocardial ischemia may be produced by primary reduction in supply, such as by coronary ligation in the experimental animal or by coronary spasm in humans. More commonly, coronary stenoses limit supply, and demand is increased by physical activity, excess endogenous circulating catecholamines, or positive inotropic agents.

Regional ischemia, as noted earlier, reduces contraction (Fig. 23.10). Ischemia also hampers the active process of diastolic relaxation. The remaining, normally perfused myocardium attempts to compensate for ischemic regional dysfunction by enhanced contraction, probably the result of ventricular dilation and the Frank-Starling mechanism.

These important local effects may be accompanied by global hemodynamic derangements, if the area of ischemia is sufficiently large. The inadequate regional contraction may cause an increase in end-systolic volume. The end-diastolic volume may increase subsequent to the increase in end-systolic volume. The myocardium "stiffens" as a consequence of ischemia, and compliance thus becomes abnormal (Fig. 23.5). Incomplete relaxation can cause further elevation of the diastolic ventricular pressures, both early and late in diastole. These global changes in systole and in diastole can resolve after ischemia is relieved or may become chronic, as after infarction when fibrous scar replaces the normally compliant myocardium.

Both contrast and radionuclide ventriculography can

detect and quantitate these abnormalities in systolic performance. Compliance abnormalities can only be measured by a combination of pressure and volume, but abnormal left ventricular filling rates due to reduced compliance may be seen using radionuclide ventriculography in some patients.

CORONARY BLOOD FLOW DURING DYNAMIC EXERCISE

Because of the tight coupling of myocardial blood flow and myocardial oxygen demands, coronary flow increases during exercise. Total myocardial oxygen consumption per beat increases about 60%. Myocardial oxygen demands are often approximated by the rate-pressure product but are also influenced by the inotropic state of the heart, left ventricular volume, and left ventricular wall thickness.

Left ventricular function during exercise is ordinarily not limited by coronary blood flow except in the presence of coronary artery disease. An exception may be during vigorous sprint exercise without a gradual warm-up, when systolic blood pressure increases rapidly, possibly leading to a transient subendocardial supply/demand imbalance.

In the presence of coronary stenoses, the normal increase in coronary flow during exercise is prevented. It is believed that flow increases in myocardium perfused by narrowed arteries, but not to the extent necessary to keep up with increased oxygen demands. However, some evidence suggests that flow may actually fall below baseline levels in ischemic regions during stress. Maseri and associates (44) have shown that the washout of xenon-133 gas from an ischemic region slows markedly during pacing-induced ischemia after the region has been preloaded with the radioactive xenon. Similarly, Selwyn and coworkers (45) have demonstrated that the uptake of rubidium-82, a very short half-life cationic flow tracer, is reduced below baseline during ischemic episodes.

An absolute reduction in regional myocardial perfusion could occur during exercise if distal coronary pressure were to fall sufficiently, left ventricular diastolic pressure were to rise to inhibit subendocardial perfusion, or both were to occur together, which may often be the case. Additionally, exercise-induced coronary spasm may sometimes occur, recognizable by the appearance of ST segment elevation during or following exercise.

The appearance of a perfusion defect during exercise signifies only that the perfusion of the area with the defect is less than that of the surrounding myocardium. Flow to the ischemic region could be increased or decreased in an absolute sense and the images would look the same. Similarly, flow to the apparently "normal" area may actually be normal or abnormal: one can only determine that the "normal" areas have the highest flow within the left ventricle.

ACKNOWLEDGMENT

The authors appreciate the suggestions of Gottlieb C. Friesinger, M.D.

REFERENCES

1. Gaasch WH, Levine HJ, Quinones MA, Alexander JK. Left ventricular compliance: mechanisms and clinical implications. Am J Cardiol 1976;38:645–653.
2. Udelson JE, Bacharach SL, Cannon RO III, Bonow RO. Minimum left ventricular pressure during β-adrenergic stimulation in human subjects. Evidence for elastic recoil and diastolic "suction" in the normal heart. Circulation 1990;82:1174–1182.
3. Weber KT, Janicki JS, Hefner LL, Reeves RC. Determinants of stroke volume in the isolated canine heart. J Appl Physiol 1974; 37:742–747.
4. Cohn JN, Franciosa JA. Vasodilator therapy of heart failure. N Engl J Med 1977;297:27–31.
5. Wallace AG, Skinner NS Jr, Mitchell JH. Hemodynamic determinants of the maximal rate of rise of left ventricular pressure. Am J Physiol 1963;205:30–36.
6. Suga H, Sagwa K. Instantaneous pressure-volume relationships and their ratio in the excised, supported canine left ventricle. Circ Res 1974;35:117–126.
7. Grossman W, Braunwald E, Mann T, McLaurin LP, Green LH. Contractile state of the left ventricle in man as evaluated from end-systolic pressure-volume relations. Circulation 1977;56:845–852.
8. Carabello BA, Spann JF. The uses and limitations of end-systolic indices of left ventricular function. Circulation 1984;69:1058–1064.
9. Burkhoff D, Sugiura S, Yue DT, Sagawa K. Contractility-dependent curvlinearity of end-systolic pressure-volume relations. Am J Physiol 1987;252(Heart Circ Physiol 21):H1218–H1227.
10. Glower DD, Spratt JA, Snow ND, et al. Linearity of the Frank-Starling relationship in the intact heart: the concept of preload recruitable stroke work. Circulation 1985;71:994–1009.
11. Little WC, Cheng C-P, Mumma M, Igarashi Y, Vinten-Johansen J, Johnston WE. Comparison of measures of left ventricular contractile performance derived from pressure-volume loops in conscious dogs. Circulation 1989;80:1378–1387.
12. Kass DA, Beyar R. Evaluation of contractile state by maximal ventricular power divided by the square of end-diastolic volume. Circulation 1991;84:1698–1708.
13. Marmor A, Sharir T, Shlomo IB, Beyar R, Frenkel A, Front D. Radionuclide ventriculography and central aorta pressure change in noninvasive assessment of myocardial performance. J Nucl Med 1989;30:1657–1665.
14. Borow KM, Green LH, Grossman W, Braunwald E. Left ventricular end-systolic stress-shortening and stress-length relations in humans. Am J Cardiol 1982;50:1301–1308.
15. Colan SD, Borow KM, Neumann A. Left ventricular end-systolic wall-stress velocity of fiber shortening relation: a load independent index of myocardial contractility. J Am Coll Cardiol 1984; 4:715–724.
16. Ross J Jr. Cardiac function and myocardial contractility: a perspective. J Am Coll Cardiol 1983;1:52–62.
17. Park RC, Little WC, O'Rourke RA. Effect of alteration of left ventricular activation sequence on the left ventricular end-systolic pressure-volume relation in closed-chest dogs. Circ Res 1985; 57:706–717.
18. McKay RG, Pfeffer MA, Pasternak RC, et al. Left ventricular remodeling after myocardial infarction: a corollary to infarct expansion. Circulation 1986;74:693–702.
19. Konstam MA, Cohen SR, Salem DN, et al. Comparison of left and right ventricular end-systolic pressure-volume relations in congestive heart failure. J Am Coll Cardiol 1985;6:1326–1334.
20. Francis GS, Benedict C, Johnstone DE, et al. Comparison of neuroendocrine activation in patients with left ventricular dysfunction with and without congestive heart failure. A substudy of the Studies of Left Ventricular Dysfunction (SOLVD). Circulation 1990;82:1724–1729.
21. Colucci WS, Ribeiro JP, Rocco MB, et al. Impaired chronotropic response to exercise in patients with congestive heart failure. Role of postsynaptic β-adrenergic desensitization. Circulation 1989; 80:314–323.
22. Konstam MA, Rousseau MF, Kronenberg MW, et al. Effects of the

angiotensin converting enzyme inhibitor enalapril on the long-term progression of left ventricular dysfunction in patients with heart failure. Circulation 1992;86:431–438.
23. Dilsizian V, Bonow RO. Current diagnostic techniques of assessing myocardial viability in patients with hibernating and stunned myocardium. Circulation 1993;87:1–20.
24. Gould KL. Noninvasive assessment of coronary stenoses by myocardial perfusion imaging during pharmacologic coronary vasodilatation. I. Physiologic basis and experimental validation. Am J Cardiol 1978;41:267–278.
25. Picano E, Lattanzi F. Dipyridamole echocardiography. A new diagnostic window on coronary artery disease. Circulation 1991; 83(Suppl III):III-19–III-26.
26. Cates CU, Kronenberg MW, Collins HW, Sandler MP. Dipyridamole radionuclide ventriculography: a test with high specificity for severe coronary artery disease. J Am Coll Cardiol 1989;13:841–851.
27. Buckberg GB, Fixler DE, Archie JP, Hoffman JIE. Experimental subendocardial ischemia in dogs with normal coronary arteries. Circ Res 1972;30:67–81.
28. White CW, Wright CB, Doty DB, et al. Does visual interpretation of the coronary arteriogram predict the physiologic importance of a coronary stenosis? N Engl J Med 1984;310:819–824.
29. Doucette JW, Corl PD, Payne HM, et al. Validation of a Doppler guide-wire for intravascular measurement of coronary artery flow velocity. Circulation 1992;85:1899–1911.
30. Kronenberg MW, Robertson RM, Born ML, Steckley RA, Robertson D, Friesinger GC. Thallium-201 uptake in variant angina: probable demonstration of myocardial reactive hyperemia in man. Circulation 1982;66:1332–1338.
31. Aversano T, Ouyang P, Silverman H. Blockade of the ATP-sensitive potassium channel modulates reactive hyperemia in the canine coronary circulation. Circ Res 1991;69:618–622.
32. Pennell DJ, Underwood SR, Swanton RH, Walker JM, Ell PJ. Dobutamine thallium myocardial perfusion tomography. J Am Coll Cardiol 1991;18:1471–1479.
33. Albro PC, Gould KL, Westcott RJ, Hamilton GW, Ritchie JL, Williams DL. Noninvasive assessment of coronary stenoses by myocardial imaging during pharmacologic coronary vasodilation. III. Clinical trial. Am J Cardiol 1978;42:751–760.
34. Verani MS, Mahmarian JJ, Hixson JB, Boyce TM, Staudacher RA. Diagnosis of coronary artery disease by controlled coronary vasodilation with adenosine and thallium-201 scintigraphy in patients unable to exercise. Circulation 1990;82:80–87.
35. Schroeder JS, Bolen JL, Quint RA, et al. Provocation of coronary spasm with ergonovine maleate. New test with results in 57 patients undergoing coronary arteriography. Am J Cardiol 1977; 40:487–491.
36. Griffith TM, Lewis MJ, Newby AC, Henderson AH. Endothelium-derived relaxing factor. J Am Coll Cardiol 1988;12:797–806.
37. Inoue T, Tomoike H, Hisano K, Nakamura M. Endothelium determines flow-dependent dilation of the epicardial coronary artery in dogs. J Am Coll Cardiol 1988;11:187–191.
38. Rigo P, Becker LC, Griffith LSC, et al. The influence of coronary collaterals on the results of thallium-201 myocardial stress imaging. Am J Cardiol 1979;44:452–458.
39. Becker LC. Conditions for vasodilator-induced coronary steal in experimental myocardial ischemia. Circulation 1978;57:1103–1110.
40. Heyndrickx GR, Millard RW, McRitchie RJ, Maroko PR, Vatner SF. Regional myocardial functional and electrophysiological alterations after brief coronary occlusion in conscious dogs. J Clin Invest 1975;56:978–985.
41. Bolli R, Jeroudi MO, Patel BS, et al. Marked reduction of free radical generation and contractile dysfunction by antioxidant therapy begun at the time of reperfusion. Evidence that myocardial "stunning" is a manifestation of reperfusion injury. Circ Res 1989; 65:607–622.
42. Reimer KA, Lowe JE, Rasmussen MM, Jennings RB. The wavefront phenomenon of ischemic cell death. I. Myocardial infarct size vs. duration of coronary occlusion in dogs. Circulation 1977; 56:786–794.
43. Rahimtoola SH. Coronary bypass surgery for chronic angina—1981: a perspective. Circulation 1982;65:225–241.
44. Maseri A, L'Abbate A, Pesola A, Michelassi C, Marzilli M, De Nes M. Regional Myocardial perfusion in patients with atherosclerotic coronary artery disease at rest and during angina pectoris induced by tachycardia. Circulation 1977;55:423–433.
45. Selwyn AP, Forse G, Fox K, Jonathan A, Steiner R. Patterns of disturbed myocardial perfusion in patients with coronary artery disease. Regional myocardial perfusion in angina pectoris. Circulation 1981;64:83–90.

SUGGESTED READING

Becker LC. Increasing coronary blood flow. In: Wagner GS, ed. Myocardial infarction: measurement and intervention. The Hague: Martinus Nijhoff Publishers, 1982:415–456.

Berne RM, Rubio R. Coronary circulation. In: Berne RM, ed. Handbook of physiology. Section 2: The cardiovascular system. Volume I. The heart. Bethesda: American Physiological Society, 1979:873–952.

Braunwald E. Pathophysiology of heart failure and assessment of cardiac function. In: Braunwald E, ed. Heart disease. 4th ed. Philadelphia: WB Saunders, 1992:393–418, 419–443.

Braunwald E, Sonnenblick EH, Ross J Jr. Mechanisms of cardiac contraction and relaxation. In: Braunwald E, ed. Heart disease. 4th ed. Philadelphia: WB Saunders, 1992:351–392.

Braunwald E, Sonnenblick EH, Ross J Jr. Mechanisms of contraction of the normal and failing heart. 2nd ed. Boston: Little, Brown & Co., 1976.

Hoffman JIE. Key references: coronary blood flow. Circulation 1980; 62:187–198.

Marcus ML. The coronary circulation in health and disease. New York: McGraw-Hill, 1983.

Olsson RA, Bunger R, Spann JAE. Coronary circulation. In: Fozzard HA, Haber E, Jennings RB, Katz AM, Morgan HE, eds. The heart and cardiovascular system. Scientific foundations. 2nd ed. New York: Raven Press, 1986:1390–1425.

Schlant RC, Sonnenblick EH. Normal physiology of the cardiovascular system. In: Schlant RC, Alexander RW, eds. Hurst's the heart: arteries and veins. 8th ed. New York: McGraw-Hill, 1994:113–151.

Schaper W, Bernotat-Danielowski S, Nienaber C, Schaper J. Collateral circulation. In: Fozzard HA, Haber E, Jennings RB, Katz AM, Morgan HE, eds. The heart and cardiovascular system. Scientific Foundations. 2nd ed. New York: Raven Press, 1991:1427–1464.

Shepherd JT, Vanhoutte PM. The human cardiovascular system. Facts and concepts. New York: Raven Press, 1979.

24 Radionuclide Evaluation of Left Ventricular Function

PATRICK B. MURPHY and STEVEN C. PORT

There are many techniques available to the clinician for the assessment of ventricular function. All the commonly used clinical imaging modalities, including conventional x-ray, CT x-ray, MRI, ultrasound, and γ-ray, can provide useful information about ventricular function. Because of its excellent spatial resolution and freedom from contamination by surrounding structures, contrast angiography has been the standard to which all of those have been compared. Of the noninvasive methods, the radionuclide techniques are unique because the radioactivity that is injected for the purpose of imaging the heart temporarily remains in the cardiac chambers in a concentration that is directly proportional to the volume of blood in those chambers, making the technique inherently quantitative. All the other noninvasive and invasive techniques require mathematical assumptions about the geometry of a ventricle to quantitate ventricular function. Such assumptions work well some of the time, but when the shape of a ventricle is distorted by localized infarction, severe hypertrophy, or marked dilatation, the accuracy of geometric approaches is questionable. One could argue that the radionuclide methods should be the standard to which others, including contrast angiography, are compared.

Although many different names have been used for the radionuclide methods of evaluating ventricular function, the term radionuclide angiography (RNA) is used here. It is a generic term which is appropriate because it acknowledges that it is not only the ventricles that are imaged but the great vessels, the atria, and other blood-filled organs as well. Radionuclide angiography is performed in two distinctly different ways, the gated equilibrium method (EqRNA) and the first-pass method (FPRNA). Each technique has its own particular strengths and weaknesses and the student or practitioner of radionuclide cardiac imaging should be thoroughly familiar with the unique attributes and technical requirements of each technique. In this chapter, the two techniques are described separately and then compared.

EQUILIBRIUM RADIONUCLIDE ANGIOGRAPHY

Equilibrium radionuclide imaging is known by other names: gated blood pool imaging (GBP), radionuclide ventriculography (RNV), or simply MUGA (multigated acquisition). The first clinical applications of the technology were reported by Strauss and Zaret who showed its use for measuring left ventricular ejection fraction and detecting regional ventricular dysfunction (1, 2). In the relatively short time since, there have been major enhancements in radiopharmaceuticals and in the hardware and software necessary for data acquisition and processing, but the fundamental concept of creating and imaging a stable blood pool tag has not changed. Blood pools in the body consist mainly of the cardiac chambers, great vessels, and spleen. Those organs contain large amounts of free blood as opposed to blood intermixed with tissue such as in the liver or kidney. The relatively large blood pools of those organs make them easy to identify once the circulating blood pool is labeled with an appropriate γ emitter. Spatial resolution of the photons can be maximized so that anatomically correct representations of the cardiac chambers and great vessels may be produced. With the use of a physiologic trigger, such as an ECG gate that links the acquisition to the cardiac cycle, elegant cinematic displays of the change in radioactivity within the cardiac chambers and great vessels can be generated. If the radionuclide has long enough biologic and physical half-lives, then images may be acquired in multiple views or during multiple physiologic conditions such as the sequential stages of an exercise test.

IMAGING AGENTS

The only radionuclide that has been used clinically for EqRNA is ^{99m}Tc. Initially, ^{99}Tc-human serum albumin was used to create an intravascular tag. Human albumin was the initial agent of choice for several reasons. Albumin was easily obtained in a purified form by electrophoresis. It was considered safe from transmission of hepatitis, and both the chemical and physical activity of the albumin were well-studied. However, image quality was, by present standards, relatively poor and acquisition times were prolonged because the large amount of albumin sequestered in the pulmonary arterial tree caused a low signal-to-background ratio (3). The use of labeled albumin was virtually replaced in the late 1970s by the more efficient method of labeling red blood cells (RBCs) in vivo (4, 5). The RBC tag had a much more favorable target-to-background ratio compared to labeled albumin. This initial work and subsequent technical advances made RBC labeling the technique of choice for EqRNA.

RBC LABELING TECHNIQUES

Technetium labeling of red blood cells requires that the technetium be reduced so that it will bind with intracellular protein. The reduced form of technetium binds to the globin chain of the hemoglobin molecule. That binding lowers the intracellular concentration of free technetium, promoting further influx of technetium and further eventual binding. The initial reducing agent used was the iron ion found in iron ascorbate. Although that was effective, separation by column chromatography was necessary and labeling efficiency was not high. A higher binding efficiency was found with the use of the stannous ion (6). Standardized kit formulations using stannous pyrophosphate were subsequently developed and have greatly facilitated the clinical application of this type of RBC labeling. The optimal dose of tin will maximize the percentage of technetium bound inside the RBC and minimize the extravascular and circulating free technetium. An inadequate amount of stannous ion will result in free technetium remaining outside the RBC, thus increasing background contamination of the images. An excess amount of stannous ion results in the reduction of technetium prior to its entrance into the cell, thereby preventing its binding to intracellular protein and again increasing background activity. There are currently three RBC labeling protocols in use: in vivo, in vitro, and modified in vivo (in "vivtro") techniques.

In Vivo Technique

The in vivo labeling technique, as the name describes, takes place within the bloodstream. Pretreatment of the RBC is performed with an intravenous injection of stannous pyrophosphate provided in a kit formulation. The optimal dosage of stannous pyrophosphate is between 10 and 20 micrograms per kilogram of body weight (7, 8). The stannous ion is allowed to circulate for 30 minutes, which results in maximum uptake by the RBCs. A dose of 15–30 mCi (550–1100 MBq) of ^{99m}Tc pertechnetate is then injected intravenously. The RBCs will be labeled over the succeeding 5–10 minutes. Some of the free circulating pertechnetate will be taken up by the thyroid, the kidneys, and the gastric mucosa. A large percentage of the unbound pertechnetate will be excreted by the kidneys. Uptake of free technetium by the gastric mucosa will create some background noise near the heart. The labeling efficiency of this method ranges from 85–95%. Injection of either of these components into a heparinized line is not recommended as heparin will oxidize the stannous ion and complex with the ^{99m}Tc pertechnetate. The in vivo technique is considered the easiest to perform because it is the least labor intensive and it results in the lowest radiation exposure to personnel. It also has the benefit of the injection of a small bolus of ^{99m}Tc pertechnetate which facilitates adjunctive first-pass imaging.

In Vitro Technique

In contrast, the in vitro method is the most technically complex and time consuming approach. A small amount (10–20 cc) of the patient's blood is withdrawn into a syringe. Stannous citrate is then added to provide approximately 1.5 μg of stannous ion and additionally help to prevent coagulation of the blood. After 5 minutes of gentle agitation, the syringe is centrifuged. The supernatant which contains any excess stannous ions is then discarded. The resultant packed RBCs are then mixed with 15–30 mCi (550–1110 MBq) of ^{99m}Tc pertechnetate. After another 5 minutes of gentle agitation, the mixture is considered properly incubated and is reinjected into the patient. Five to 10 minutes after this, the tagged RBCs are considered to be in equilibrium throughout the blood volume. The labeling efficiency of the in vitro technique is routinely above 95% (9). However, the more time, blood handling, and radiation exposure for the technologists required, and the need for a centrifuge, as well as the clinical adequacy of the alternate labeling methods, have precluded clinical acceptance of the in vitro technique.

Modified In Vivo Technique

The modified in vivo or in "vivtro" technique represents a compromise between the two previous methods. Increased labeling efficiency, compared to the in vivo technique, is achieved by tagging the RBCs with ^{99m}Tc pertechnetate outside the body, while less labor and exposure for the technologist is achieved by in vivo RBC preparation with stannous ion. In this technique, stannous pyrophosphate is injected intravenously. After 30 minutes, 5 ml of blood are withdrawn into a shielded syringe containing 15–30 mCi (550–1110 MBq) of ^{99m}Tc pertechnetate and 1 ml of ACD (acid-citrate-dextrose) solution. A closed system is often employed that uses a steel butterfly needle, attached via a three-way stopcock to a shielded syringe. A closed system lowers the chance of contamination. A shielded syringe is absolutely necessary in this situation because of the close proximity of the radioactivity to both the patient and the technologist. After 10 minutes of incubation, the red blood cells are reinjected. Five to 10 minutes are then adequate for equilibrium throughout the total blood volume.

Compared to the in vitro method, this technique is less time consuming, but the tagging efficiency of 90–93% is lower (10). In general, image quality will be better than that achieved with the in vivo technique. As a result, the in "vivtro" technique has become the method of choice in many clinical facilities (Fig. 24.1).

Factors That May Modify RBC Labeling

There are several drugs, intravenous solutions, and clinical conditions that may theoretically interfere with RBC labeling (11, 12). Heparin, because of its clinical ubiquity, is probably of most concern. Heparin may reduce the labeling efficiency by oxidizing the stannous ion and complexing

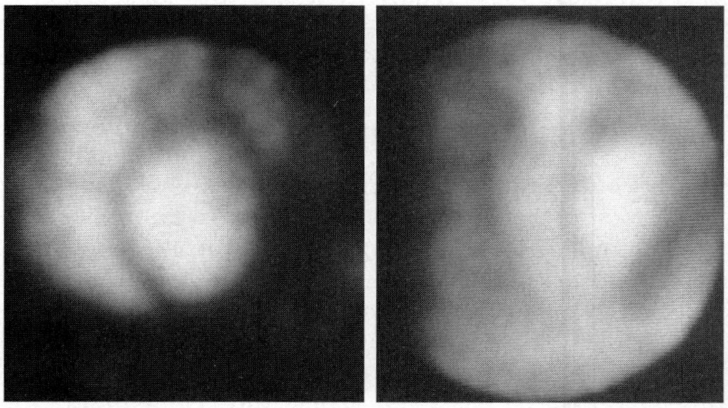

Figure 24.1. RBC Labeling. On the *left* is an example of a good quality RBC tag performed using the modified in vivo technique. The cardiac chambers are clearly delineated and the background activity is low. On the *right* is an example of a poor quality tag that was performed using the in vivo technique. Note the poor target-to-background ratio.

with the pertechnetate. One cannot avoid studying patients receiving heparin, but direct injection of the tin or the pertechnetate into intravenous lines that contain heparin should be avoided. Solutions of dextrose, mannitol, and sorbitol, and the presence of antibodies to the RBCs, as can occur in certain autoimmune diseases or after treatment with methyldopa or quinidine, may also reduce labeling efficiency.

INSTRUMENTATION

Camera

The goal of EqRNA is to obtain images of the cardiac chambers and great vessels with as high spatial a resolution as possible. The best quality images are obtained by positioning the detector as close to the subject's chest as possible. The small field-of-view (SFOV) cameras provide higher resolution images than do the large field-of-view (LFOV) systems. SFOV cameras are most adaptable to EqRNA since they can be more easily manipulated into the appropriate positions and can typically touch the chest during the acquisition of all views. The LFOV systems can certainly provide diagnostic quality images and are used frequently. Most SFOV systems are portable which allows imaging in hospital rooms. Multicrystal gamma-cameras have been used but are not recommended because of their lower spatial resolution.

Collimation

The collimator should be selected to meet the demands of the particular type of study to be acquired. For most resting EqRNA studies where the clinical question is the evaluation of ventricular function, a standard parallel hole, low energy, all-purpose collimator is adequate. With LFOV detectors, a slant hole collimator may be useful since it requires less angulation of the large head making oblique views easier and more comfortable to acquire (13). High resolution collimators do improve image quality, but the gain in resolution is not usually worth the prolonged imaging time for the average clinical study. For certain clinical questions such as the detection of right ventricular dysplasia or a ventricular thrombus or congenital anomalies of the great vessels, high resolution collimation can be quite useful.

For exercise studies, there is a premium on the count rate since time is limited. Some laboratories have used high sensitivity collimators during exercise, but the degradation in resolution may not be worth the higher count flux. In general, the all-purpose collimator is most often used for exercise acquisitions.

Computer/Software

All commercially available computers designed for nuclear imaging systems are capable of acquiring EqRNA data. Where systems differ is in the software. Ideally, the software should allow a variety of frame rates and pixel matrixes for both acquisition and processing. The system should permit both 64×64 and 128×128 acquisitions at frame rates of 8 to at least 32 frames per cycle. Arrhythmia detection and editing are essential. It is particularly helpful to be able to perform a time correction of the data as it is being acquired. With that approach, each accepted beat is interpolated to match the duration of other accepted beats so that a uniform time-activity curve can be generated. Standard temporal and spatial filters as well as Fourier filtering are necessary and available on most, if not all systems. Fourier filtering is particularly important for the assessment of diastolic ventricular function. Both frame mode and list mode acquisition protocols should be available. The software for data processing should allow manual, automatic, and semiautomatic approaches. One serious limitation of many commercial systems is the lack of validation of processing schemes. When that is the case, it is incumbent upon the operator to perform a validation study of the particular processing protocol chosen.

Most systems are capable of displaying multiple, synchronized cine displays of EqRNA images so that different views or previous and current studies can be viewed side-by-side. A wide assortment of color schemes is available for data display and are necessary for interpreting parametric images such as phase and amplitude images, but the contrast resolution of black and white images remains the standard for the cinematic assessment of wall motion.

DATA ACQUISITION

Imaging Angles

Most facilities employ three standard views for routine diagnostic work. As each of these views may require 10–15 minutes of scanning time, the patient must be positioned comfortably to prevent motion during scanning. The ability to view a study cinematically as it is progressing allows the technologist to reposition a patient or the detector to achieve an optimal image.

The primary view for quantitative analysis in EqRNA is the so-called "best septal" view. This view is typically obtained with the detector in a 40–50° LAO position. A slight caudal tilt is needed in most patients to enhance separation of the left atrium and the left ventricle. Ideally, the "best septal" view provides a true short axis view in which the LV appears spherical and there is clear separation of the two ventricles. Since this is the view that will be used for almost all the quantitative analyses applied to the study, several angles should be tested until the best possible angle is identified. Furthermore, this is the only view that can isolate that part of the LV perfused by the circumflex coronary artery. Either too shallow or too steep an angle will compromise that ability (Fig. 24.2).

Two additional views are obtained to visualize the remaining walls of the left ventricle and other cardiac structures. An anterior view is obtained by simply positioning the detector parallel to the chest or by rotating the detector approximately 45° anteriorly from the "best septal" view. The third view is the left lateral view which can be acquired by placing the patient in a right decubitus position with the detector parallel to the left chest or by rotating the detector 45° more laterally than the "best septal" view.

In some laboratories, a fourth view that is intermediate between the "best septal" and the left lateral views is acquired. Most important is that the technologist under-

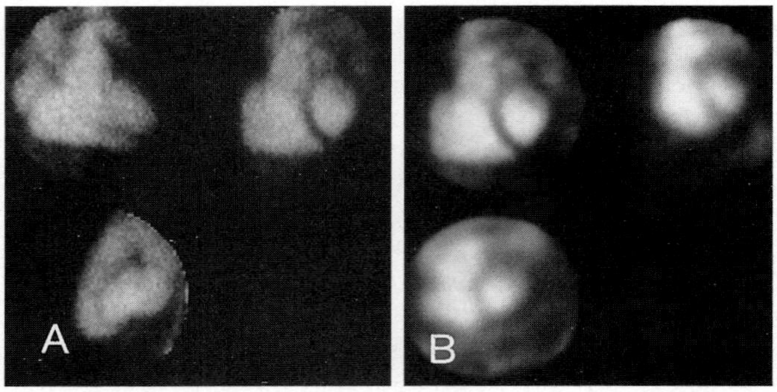

Figure 24.2. **A.** Examples of correctly positioned anterior, best septal and lateral views of a resting EqRNA examination. **B.** Three examples of septal views. The *upper left* image shows a true best septal view. The image at the *upper right* is an example of too shallow a septal view and the *lower* image is that of too steep a view. Note that the LV and RV can be separated in all three examples but only the upper left image is the correct one.

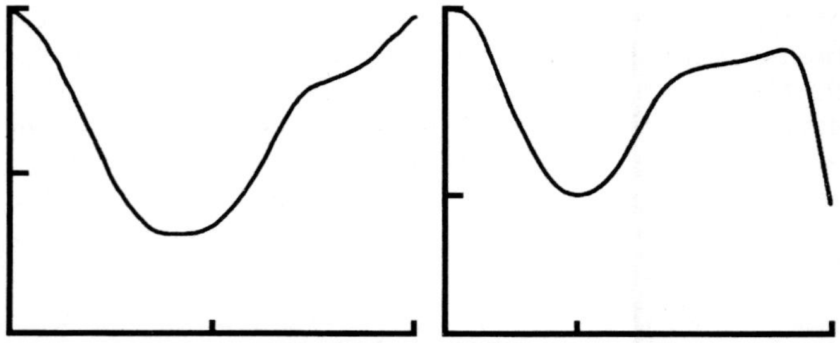

Figure 24.3. The left ventricular time-activity curve on the *left* was acquired in frame mode with software that allowed analysis and time correction of each accepted beat prior to storing the beat in memory. As a result there is preservation of the integrity of the diastolic portion of the curve. Studies acquired in such a fashion will always have the last frame return to end-diastole. On the right is an example of a similar curve acquired with a standard frame mode acquisition. Minor changes in heart rate within the beat acceptance window result in the last frame occurring at different times in the diastolic portion of the cardiac cycle. The shape of the curve is typical of this common problem.

stands the anatomy of the cardiac chambers so that the appropriate anatomic views are acquired even if the angles do not conform to what one would predict. For example, for some patients whose ventricles are rotated, a left posterior oblique view may be necessary to obtain a true left lateral image of the LV while in others, an RAO view may be necessary to obtain a true anterior image of the LV.

Gating

Gating is the technique that links the acquisition of the image data to the cardiac cycle. Most EqRNA studies are acquired in the so-called frame mode. In a frame mode acquisition, the cardiac cycle is arbitrarily divided up into a fixed number of frames and the data from each cycle are divided up and stored as individual frame memory bins. Individual beat information is lost once that beat has been added to the data. Theoretically, any physiologic event that varies with the cardiac cycle could be used to gate an acquisition. The ECG is the most convenient and is universally used for EqRNA. The accuracy of the gate depends upon the QRS recognition scheme used by the computer and the quality of the ECG signal. The QRS complex of the ECG identifies electrical depolarization of the ventricles. There is usually a small time lag between the onset of electrical depolarization and the onset of systolic contraction, so the peak (R wave) or the nadir (S wave) of the QRS complex actually corresponds fairly closely to end-diastole. However, the lag between the QRS and the onset of contraction varies from subject to subject and can be prolonged if there is a conduction delay such as left bundle branch block so that end-diastole may actually occur in frame 2 or 3 of the study.

There are a number of gating schemes for EqRNA. The standard method is the forward gating technique. In this case, the ECG signal is used to identify the beginning of frame 1 of the acquisition. Frame time is calculated as the average RR interval divided by the number of assigned frames. In the example of a 16-frame study, the events recorded during the first 16th of the RR cycle will be stored in frame 1, the information from the second 16th time interval of the cardiac cycle in the second frame, and so on until the last frame is acquired. The accuracy of this approach depends heavily upon the constancy of the RR interval during the acquisition. If a beat is longer than the previous beats, then the last frame acquired will not correspond to the end of the cycle. If a beat is shorter than the previous beats, then the last frame acquired will contain data from the beginning of the beat following the short beat. Variable beat length most significantly affects the diastolic portion of the cardiac cycle so that the end of the LV time activity curve may appear quite distorted (Fig. 24.3). One approach to avoiding beat variability is to use an RR interval screening method whereby the computer analyzes the beat length of each cycle and accepts or rejects the beat based on predetermined criteria. When a beat is rejected, the succeeding beats, usually beats 3 to 5, are often not collected. In fact, in many systems, acquisition is not reinitiated until an appropriate RR interval is sensed. Unfortunately, in some systems, the cycle that is outside the desired window, which initiates the rejection sequence, is admitted to the compiling data so variable beat length will still alter the final time-activity curve. Fortunately, the systolic portion of the cardiac cycle is insignificantly affected by most minor variations in cycle length. Difficulties with forward gating notwithstanding, with appropriate attention to RR window selection, accurate representations of both the systolic and diastolic portions of the left ventricular time activity curve could routinely be obtained (14).

Reverse Gating

Instead of assigning frame number 1 to the R wave, with reverse gating, the last frame is assigned to end on the R wave. As a result, the end-diastolic portion of the time-activity curve is protected and any distortions tend to occur in early systole. A compromise is the use of a combined forward-reverse gating technique. The first two-thirds of the cycle are gated in a forward direction and the end of the cycle in a reverse direction, and the two portions of the curve are joined. The forward gating improves the accuracy of the information obtained early in systole, while the backward gating portion preserves the end-diastolic data (15). Reverse gating and forward-reverse gating can be performed using either a list-mode acquisition or a frame mode acquisition that uses a memory buffer to screen and format beats.

Alternate R Wave Gating

Another approach is alternate R wave gating (16, 17). With this technique, frame 1 of the study is identified by every other R wave. Once a cycle is initiated, it is continued through the next R wave and ends with third R wave. The resultant time-activity curve encompasses two complete cardiac cycles and the diastolic portion of the first of the two cycles contains less distortion than would be seen in standard forward gating. Application of the alternate R wave gate is appropriate when evaluation of diastolic function is the clinical question at hand.

R-R Window and Arrhythmia Rejection

All commercially available systems have beat length acceptance criteria as part of the standard EqRNA acquisition protocol. Setting an RR interval acceptance window allows exclusion of ectopic beats from the data. The appropriate RR window for a given study depends upon the subjects rhythm, the type of study and the desired level of physiologic accuracy. Obviously, the narrower the RR window, the more homogeneous the beat lengths and the more physiologic the resultant time-activity curve. The tradeoff is always accuracy versus time since the narrower the window the longer the acquisition. For most routine clinical applications, a 10–15% window is appropriate. Virtually all premature beats will fall outside such a window. However, a number of sinus beats will also be rejected if there is any significant sinus arrhythmia which is common. Increasing the window will decrease acquisition time but at the expense of the diastolic portion of the time-activity curve. Since there is rarely any urgency during acquisition of a resting EqRNA, the added time with a narrow window is not a significant issue but if a subject cannot maintain a certain position for the requisite time period or if the time of acquisition is critical, then a wider window may be necessary. During an exercise study, the time available for imaging is very brief but the heart rate during exercise is usually so regular that the RR window is usually not important.

List Mode

List mode acquisition is the most memory intensive method. The scintigraphic data are stored continuously without any preset framing criteria. Time markers and the ECG signal are also stored. After the acquisition is terminated, the operator has the ability to screen all the cycles stored during the acquisition. The data can then be reformatted into a cycle that contains as many beats of whatever length is desired. With this approach the operator can set a very narrow RR window and then screen the resultant cycle to see if there are enough beats in the window to provide accurate statistics. If not, the window can be adjusted to accept more beats until the optimum combination of window length and statistics are produced. List mode allows formatting of multiple beat lengths for the study of the effects of cycle length or arrhythmia on ventricular function. Time-activity curves with very high temporal resolution can be generated with this technique since the timing markers are usually stored at 10 msec intervals. As a result, the list mode acquisition is particularly appropriate for studies of diastolic function (17).

Frame Rate and Frame Counts

Selection of the number of frames for an EqRNA study depends upon the clinical question being asked, the software capabilities, and the time available for acquisition. The greater the number of frames obtained during the cardiac cycle, the better the temporal resolution of the ventricular time-activity curve and, therefore, the more representative of the true cyclic variations in chamber volume. The influence of the frame rate on the measurements of systolic and diastolic function has been examined. It has been shown that the systolic phase of the cycle could be adequately assessed with as few as 16 frames per cycle, whereas the diastolic variables were best measured using 32–48 frames per cycle (15). For most clinical work, 32 frames per cycle is adequate temporal resolution. Practically, it is advisable to acquire all LAO views at 32 frames per cycle so that both systole and diastole can be adequately evaluated in all clinical studies. The other views of the acquisition can be acquired at 24 or even 16 frames per cycle. For exercise studies, where the scanning time is at a premium and where the interest is usually in systolic function, a frame rate of 16 frames per cycle is a good compromise between temporal resolution and statistics per frame.

To maintain image quality and statistical reliability for quantitation, a minimum number of counts must be contained in each frame. Most authorities believe that the absolute minimum number of counts per frame is 125,000, but would also agree that a more typically acceptable number would be 250,000 counts per frame (18). Whichever minimum number is selected, an increase in the number of frames will proportionally increase the scanning time to maintain the same count rate per frame.

STRESS PROTOCOLS

Exercise

The evaluation of ventricular function during exercise is helpful diagnostically and, in particular, prognostically. EqRNA can be applied to bicycle exercise in both the upright and supine positions. Treadmill exercise is unsuitable for equilibrium studies because of chest motion. Several commercially available exercise tables equipped with cycle ergometers have been specifically designed for simultaneous radionuclide imaging. The tables are narrow which facilitates approximation of the detector and are typically capable of being raised to a 30–60° head-up angle for semisupine exercise. Some tables are capable of being raised to the full upright position; however, the detector may not easily reach the chest in that configuration. Supine bicycle exercise places maximum strain on the legs and many patients will stop exercising with leg fatigue prior to achieving an adequate cardiovascular stress. That is especially true in older or deconditioned subjects. Semisupine or upright exercise is better tolerated. Supine cycling is accompanied by higher left ventricular end-diastolic pressure but lower peak heart rates than is upright cycling, but the overall stress on the heart is fairly similar at any given workload (19).

There is no absolutely correct imaging sequence for acquisition of an exercise EqRNA. Most protocols acquire the standard three-view resting study first. The resting LAO study should be performed in the same position as the exercise study so that the change in volumes and/or function will reflect the cardiac status rather than any change in position. Graded exercise should be performed allowing enough time at each workload for the heart rate to stabilize and for enough image statistics for reliable quantitation. Three-minute stages work reasonably well since the heart rate usually reaches a plateau in about 1 minute and 2 minutes remain for acquisition. Since it is difficult to predict when a subject will stop exercising, it is wise to acquire each stage of the study although it is not necessary to process all stages. The peak exercise stage should be extended as long as the patient can safely continue to insure image quality. However, the workload should never be lowered during the acquisition to prolong the exercise. Decreases in workload of as little as 25% are accompanied by immediate improvement in regional and global ventricular function which could result in underestimation of the magnitude of ischemia (20).

The primary view for an exercise study is, of course, the best septal view which allows generation of the quantitative data to be analyzed and reported. Wall motion abnormalities may be assessed in the septal, inferior, lateral, or posterior walls in the best septal view. If there is a specific clinical question regarding the anterolateral wall or apex, or if one wants to obtain maximum sensitivity for left anterior descending coronary artery disease, it may be useful to quickly rotate the detector to the anterior view once the septal view has enough statistics. Although not necessary in most cases, an immediate postexercise image may be of value in predicting recovery of function after revascularization in ventricular segments with severe motion abnormalities at rest (21, 22).

Alternatives to Exercise: Pacing, Cold Pressor and Pharmacologic Stress

Several options are available to challenge the coronary circulation and ventricular function in subjects who are unable to exercise. They include atrial pacing, cold pressor testing, catecholamine infusions, and coronary vasodilators. Prior to the widespread application of pharmacologic testing, atrial pacing was proposed as a mechanism of increasing myocardial oxygen demand, thereby provoking ischemia (23). Atrial pacing is well-suited to EqRNA since the heart rate at every increment is constant. It requires fluoroscopy and placement of an atrial electrode. Consequently, this type of stress is rarely, if ever, used at this point in time. Cold pressor testing stresses the heart by peripheral vasoconstriction induced during immersion of an extremity in ice water. That results in elevation of systolic and diastolic blood pressure as well as changes in the distribution of coronary blood flow. In patients with significant coronary artery disease, regional ventricular ischemia can be produced (24). Both normal subjects and subjects with coronary disease will show a drop in ejection fraction with cold pressor testing. In normal subjects, the LVEF quickly rebounds while in the subject with coronary disease there is a more prolonged depression of ventricular function (25). The overlap between normal subjects and patients and the intense discomfort of the procedure precluded widespread acceptance of this technique.

Catecholamine infusion is another approach to increasing myocardial oxygen demand in an effort to induce ischemia. Isoproterenol, dopamine, and dobutamine have all been tested, but only intravenous dobutamine has received significant clinical acceptance. Unlike atrial pacing, cold pressor stimulation, or the use of coronary vasodilators such as dipyridamole or adenosine, catecholamine infusions carry a significantly higher risk of tachyarrhythmia, both supraventricular and ventricular. Dobutamine is usually started at 5 μg/kg/min and the infusion rate is progressively increased every 5 minutes to 10, 20, 30, 40, and up to 50 μg/kg/min or until a target heart rate is reached or symptoms preclude continuation of the test (26, 27). As with an exercise test, each stage of the infusion should be imaged. Ischemic or arrhythmic effects can be reversed by either discontinuing the infusion or by intravenous administration of a rapidly acting beta blocker. Dobutamine produces a fairly consistent increase in heart rate and typically a modest elevation in blood pressure. Occasionally, the blood pressure and heart rate may suddenly drop during the infusion (27).

STANDARD DATA PROCESSING

There are as many approaches to processing of EqRNA data as there are vendors of gamma-cameras and software. It is beyond the scope of this chapter to review every nuance of data processing. However, the basic routines necessary to the processing of all studies are discussed. The operator is advised to view a cinematic display of the best septal view prior to beginning processing. That will provide a good visual sense of the spatial relationships between the two ventricles and between the ventricles and the atria, which becomes important during the creation of the regions-of-interest for the ventricular time-activity curve.

Left Ventricular Time-Activity Curve: Creating the Regions-of-Interest

Since all the quantitative data that will be used to describe the function of the LV are derived from the LV time-activity curve, every effort should be made to generate a curve that, as accurately as possible, reflects the changes in volume throughout the cardiac cycle. Most important to that process, of course, is the information density or counts within each frame and the sharpness of separation between the ventricle and surrounding chambers throughout the cardiac cycle, both of which are determined before processing begins. Despite all the temporal and spatial filters available

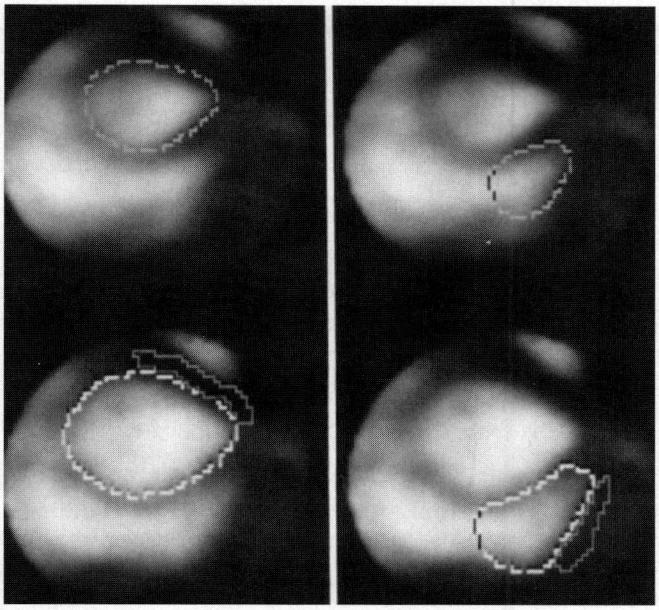

Figure 24.4. To calculate the left (*top*) or right (*bottom*) ventricular ejection fraction manually, ROIs are hand drawn around the chamber at end-diastole (*left*) and at end-systole (*right*) taking care to avoid nonventricular activity. A crescent-shaped background ROI is placed near the lateral border of the ventricle at end-diastole. For LV processing the background ROI avoids the activity from the adjacent spleen.

to the operator, technically inadequate raw data cannot be resurrected during processing. Given whatever raw data is available, the subsequent accuracy of the time-activity curve is highly dependent upon the accuracy of the regions-of-interest (ROI). There are three ways to generate the ROI; manual, semiautomatic, and automatic.

As its name implies, the manual method requires the operator to draw all the ROI to be used for the time-activity curve (Fig. 24.4). Since this is a labor intensive approach, it is usually restricted to drawing only the end-diastolic (ED) and end-systolic (ES) ROI. The ED ROI is usually drawn on frame 1 of the study. That ROI can then be used to generate a preliminary curve whose nadir identifies the ES frame. The operator can then draw the ES ROI. Two curves now exist, one from the ED ROI and the other from the ES ROI. The two curves can be interpolated to create the final LV time-activity curve.

The semiautomatic method requires the operator to identify the LV by manually drawing an initial ROI at ED. The program will then use an automated edge-detection algorithm to identify the LV perimeter in every frame of the study including the ED frame. There are two basic schemes for automated edge detection. The first is the threshold method in which the program tracks the counts from the center of the LV out to the periphery. The point at which counts drop precipitously is considered the edge of the LV. The second approach refines the threshold method by using the second derivative of the gradient in counts as one approaches the edge of the LV from the center. The maximum gradient is identified and considered the edge. All the computer generated ROI should be visually inspected in a large enough format to be easily checked for accuracy. In

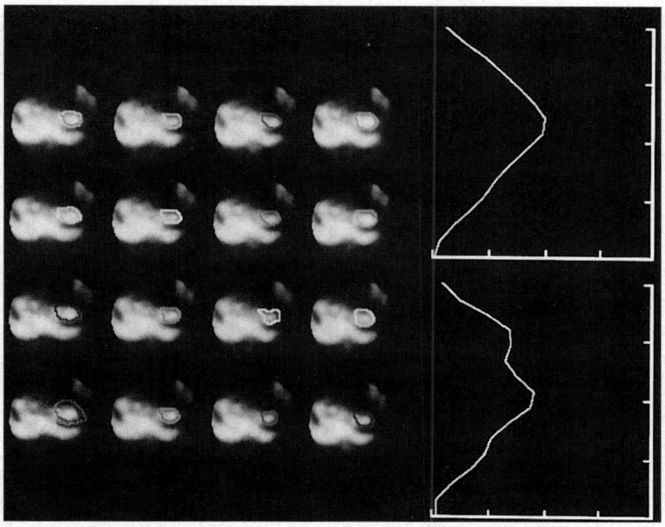

Figure 24.5. The computer can automatically generate regions-of-interest on each frame of the study once an initial, manual ROI is drawn to orient the computer to the borders of the chamber (*top*, *left*). As the time-activity curve on the *left middle* illustrates, the computer-generated ROIs not infrequently include noncardiac activity. A semiautomatic program allows the operator to selectively override the computer to correct any errant ROIs which then corrects the time-activity curve (*right*).

the semiautomated or interactive approach, the operator can then reject and recreate any ROI which either excludes ventricular activity or includes nonventricular activity.

In the fully automated method, the operator does not get the opportunity to review and adjust the computer determined ROI (Fig. 24.5). Operators should not be lulled into accepting automated ROI without visual inspection of each ROI. No algorithm is infallible. The automated approaches are not supplied for their accuracy, but rather for their speed and consistency. In direct comparisons of results obtained with manual and automated ROI, the manual method actually had the smallest intra- and interobserver variabilities (28). As a routine quality control technique, it is advisable to process each clinical study using both a manual and either an automated or semiautomated method.

Background Correction

For accurate quantitative analysis of EqRNA data, the time-activity curve must be corrected for the contribution of adjacent, noncardiac activity. When viewed in the LAO position, the left ventricle is adjacent to the lung and descending aorta. Occasionally, splenic or gastric activity is superimposed on the LV chamber. There will be some activity contained in the pulmonary vasculature, especially in patients with high pulmonary pressures, and some activity in the myocardium, itself. There is also a variable contribution from the left atrium which is difficult, if not impossible, to quantify. Background activity is estimated by drawing a ROI lateral to the left ventricle in the best septal view. Typically, a 2–3 pixel-wide crescent-shaped ROI, placed 1–3 pixels away from the LV ROI, is used to quantify the background (Fig. 24.4). The average count per pixel in that ROI is assumed to be representative of the entire background and is subtracted from each pixel count within the LV ROI. Care must be taken that "hot" noncardiac sites are not incorporated into the background ROI, e.g., liver or spleen. If that occurs, an artificially high ejection fraction would be calculated.

Temporal and Fourier Filtering

Once the background correction has been applied, the time-activity curve should be reviewed using a display of each data point. The operator should identify any points that do not appear to belong to the curve of that subjects data and then re-examine the ROI that produced those values. If necessary, the ROI should be redrawn. Even after the ROI are reviewed, the unfiltered time-activity curve may show fluctuations in counts that are not physiologic but due, instead, to the randomness of γ-photon emissions and unavoidable admixture of nonventricular activity in a ROI. To eliminate such random noise in the data, the time activity curve is typically subjected to a temporal filter which in its simplest form might be a 1–2–1 frame smoothing. That type of filtering helps to create a smooth curve for further analysis. There are multiple mathematical models for generating a "best fit" curve. Some of them take into account the slopes of the various line segments that connect adjacent data points, while others use the slopes of line segments between lines that are two or more points apart on the curve. Fourier filtering is somewhat more complex. It analyzes the data in the frequency domain and fits a curve that contains one or more frequencies (harmonics). Figure 24.6 shows the effects of applying Fourier filtering using progressively more harmonics in the filter. The optimum number of harmonics depends, to some degree, on the segment of the time-activity curve that is of interest but four or five harmonics seems to be quite sufficient (29).

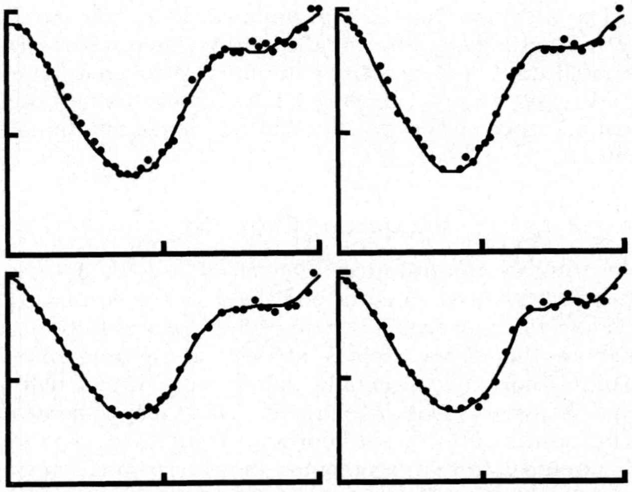

Figure 24.6. Applying a Fourier transform to the raw data eliminates noise. The figure shows the effects of increasing the number of harmonics used in the filtering process. With 3 harmonics (*top left*), the fitted curve appears to inadequately represent the true physiologic details of the actual data curve while 6 harmonics (*lower right*) appear to introduce variability that was not present in the raw data. Four (*top right*) or 5 (*bottom left*) harmonics appear to be adequate at average resting heart rates.

Left Ventricular Ejection Fraction

Once the data processing is completed, the left ventricular ejection fraction (LVEF) can be calculated as:

$$\frac{[\text{ED counts}-\text{Bkgd counts}] - [\text{ES counts}-\text{Bkgd counts}]}{\text{ED counts}-\text{Bkgd counts}}$$

Since background counts cancel out of the numerator, the term simplifies to:

$$\frac{\text{ED counts}-\text{ES counts}}{\text{ED counts}-\text{Bkgd counts}}$$

Consequently, LVEF varies directly with the background activity. An inappropriately high background would spuriously increase LVEF and insufficient background would lower the LVEF. The normal range for the LVEF at rest is approximately 0.50–0.80.

Another index of the systolic performance of the LV is the systolic ejection rate, expressed as the peak or the mean (30, 31). It is calculated using the first derivative of the time-activity curve. There has been no clinical demonstration that application of the ejection rate is diagnostically or prognostically more useful than LVEF.

Right Ventricular Ejection Fraction

A right ventricular time-activity curve may also be generated from EqRNA data. Again, the "best septal" view must be used to ensure separation of the left and right ventricles (32). In that projection, however, there is incomplete separation of the right atrium from the right ventricle. No matter what angulation is used, there is always some overlap of atrial and ventricular counts and since the atrial activity is maximal at ventricular end systole, the incorporation of atrial counts into the right ventricular end-systolic ROI frequently results in a spuriously low right ventricular ejection fraction. Correct identification of the pulmonary valve may also be problematic in an EqRNA study which creates more difficulty in drawing an accurate RV ROI. Phase images, which are useful in localizing valve planes, may be particularly helpful during RV processing. The range of normal values for the RVEF as measured from standard EqRNA data is 0.46–0.70 (33). When the RVEF is the main clinical question, then standard EqRNA is not the procedure of choice. Alternative methods such as the "gated first-pass" technique or traditional first-pass RNA may be used in that setting.

Left Ventricular Diastolic Filling

Several indices of diastolic filling of the LV can be calculated from the LV time-activity curve. Because of the complexity of the diastolic portion of the LV time-activity curve, it is important to acquire the data with sufficient temporal resolution. A minimum of 32 frames per cardiac cycle is necessary and, as indicated earlier, a 4th- or 5th-order

Fourier filter or other polynomial filter should be applied to the data before calculating any filling parameters. The most often cited indexes of diastolic function are the peak filling rate (PFR) and the time from end systole to the time at which the peak filling rate occurs (tPFR). The PFR is calculated by taking the first derivative of the time-activity curve (Fig. 24.7).

The first major positive peak in the first derivative curve corresponds to the point in the time-activity curve where counts are increasing at their fastest rate. The PFR is typically measured in counts/sec and normalized to end-diastolic counts to yield end-diastolic volumes/sec (EDV/sec). The tPFR should be expressed in milliseconds.

The second major positive peak in the first derivative curve corresponds to the most rapidly increasing count rate during atrial systole and has been referred to as the atrial filling rate, a somewhat misleading term since it is the ventricle that is filling. Calculation of the ratio of the PFR to the AFR or vice versa is useful as a quantitative descriptor of the relative contributions of early rapid filling and late (atrial) filling of the LV. The PFR and the AFR have been shown to correspond to the E and A waves of the Doppler echocardiographic mitral velocity waveform (34).

Normal values for the PFR and tPFR have been reported from many laboratories (35). The ranges are fairly wide and are dependent upon the temporal resolution, the type of gating, and the computer system used. As a general rule, at rest, the normal PFR should exceed 2.5 EDV/sec and the tPFR should be less than 180 msec. The AFR is typically 1.0 EDV/sec and the PFR/AFR ratio is usually greater than 2.5.

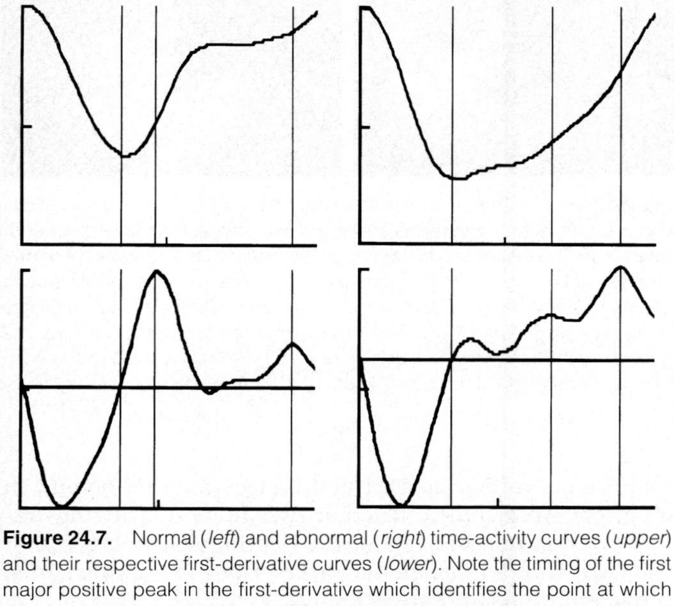

Figure 24.7. Normal (*left*) and abnormal (*right*) time-activity curves (*upper*) and their respective first-derivative curves (*lower*). Note the timing of the first major positive peak in the first-derivative which identifies the point at which counts are increasing in the ventricle at their most rapid rate, i.e., the peak filling rate (*PFR*). The time from end-systole (the nadir of the time-activity curve) to the PFR is the *tPFR*. The second positive peak in the first-derivative curve reflects the peak atrial contribution to LV filling (*AFR*). Note the relative heights of the early and late filling peaks of the first-derivative curve on the left compared to that on the right where the atrial contribution to filling is abnormally large and the early peak filling rate is both delayed and reduced.

Measurement of Left Ventricular Volume

Left ventricular volume has been measured with EqRNA using either geometric or count proportional approaches. The geometric method uses the same mathematical assumptions that are applied to contrast angiographic data (36–38). In that method, the area (A) of the LV in the LAO view and the longest length (L) of the LV in any view are used to calculate LV volume as $V = 8A^2/3L$. Although a significant correlation between the geometrically derived volumes from EqRNA and contrast angiographic data has been demonstrated (1), the geometric approach to EqRNA data suffers from its reliance on spatial resolution which cannot compare to contrast angiographic or other high resolution imaging modalities.

Count Proportional Methods with Blood Sampling

By definition, at equilibrium, the counts recorded from any chamber are directly proportional to the volume of that chamber. The relationship between counts and volume for any subject can be determined by withdrawing a known sample of blood and recording its activity. That relationship can then be used to calculate the volume of any chamber whose count rate can be measured. In practice, a small amount of labeled blood is withdrawn and counted in vitro using the gamma camera. Then, the background corrected, end-diastolic counts from the LV ROI are used to generate an approximate LV EDV as:

$$\frac{\text{ED counts corrected for the time per frame}}{\text{counts/ml of the reference blood sample}}$$

The EDV calculated in that manner is not, however, the actual EDV since the counts recorded from the LV are subject to attenuation, and the accuracy of the ROI, neither of which influences the counts recorded in vitro from the reference blood sample. In lieu of measuring the attenuation, the EDV calculated above has been correlated with the results of contrast angiography in the same subjects, so a regression equation could be used to calculate the absolute LV EDV from the attenuated radionuclide EDV (39). Other investigators have used chest wall markers to measure the distance from the detector to the center of the LV chamber. That distance and an assumed coefficient of attenuation are then used to correct the ED counts for attenuation (40). Still others have actually measured attenuation directly by counting a sealed source in air and then again in vivo (41, 42). Standard errors of the estimate for EDV and ESV using blood sampling methods have been ±36 ml and ±33 ml respectively.

Count Proportional Methods Without Blood Sampling

An alternative count-proportional method for calculating chamber volume is based on the idea of defining a reference volume within the image itself. One group suggested calculating the geometric volume of a cylindrically shaped segment of the aorta and then determining the counts in the same cylinder to establish the relationship of counts to volume for a given subject. Any chamber volume could then be determined from that relationship and the counts within the chamber (43). Another approach assumes the reference volume to be a rectangular solid whose dimensions are the depth of the LV and the sides of a pixel. It is assumed that the counts in the hottest pixel in the image are proportional to the volume of that rectangular solid. Assuming the LV to be spherical in shape, then the depth of the rectangular solid is equal to the diameter of the sphere. Ventricular volume (the volume of the sphere) can then be expressed in terms of the counts in the hottest pixel, the size of the pixel matrix, and the total counts recorded from the LV. (44, 45). Others have confirmed and refined that approach by including a term for eccentricity which is a measure of the deviation of an object from a true sphere (46). The advantages of this approach are its applicability to any system, its freedom from blood sampling, and its suitability to automation. Standard errors of the estimate for ED and ES volumes of the LV range from 23–34 ml and 10–36 ml, respectively, when using these methods.

Phase and Amplitude Images

Phase images derive their name from the fact that they are graphic representations of the timing of events in the cardiac cycle. The change in counts in each pixel in the image is analyzed in the frequency domain and a single harmonic Fourier filter, i.e., a cosine curve is fit to the data. Each pixel's cosine curve can be characterized by its amplitude and its relationship to the time of onset of the cardiac cycle, i.e., the R wave of the ECG signal. The beginning of the first frame is typically assigned a phase angle of 0° which results in a value of 180° for end systole and 360° for the end of diastole (the next R wave). In the normal situation, most, if not all, pixels in the two ventricles are filling and emptying at virtually the same time and atrial pixels are all filling and emptying together, but are 180° out of phase with the ventricular pixels. By assigning colors to each phase angle, a color coded, graphic display of the timing of events can be generated (Fig. 24.8). Phase images may be particularly helpful in identifying ventricular asynchrony as occurs in disturbances of conduction, in preexcitation syndromes, and in arrhythmias (47). They are routinely used in automated processing algorithms for identification of ROI borders.

Amplitude images derive their name from their relationship to the height of the fitted cosine curve described earlier. They represent the maximum change in counts between the peak and nadir of the fitted cosine curve. They are analogous to a stroke volume image. In the stroke volume image, end-systolic counts are subtracted from end-diastolic counts and the resultant difference is color coded. If end-systolic counts exceed end-diastolic counts, as occurs routinely in the atria and the aorta or in a dyskinetic ventricular segment, the negative value is set to zero so that such pixels drop out of the image. Hence, the atria, the aorta, and dyskinetic segments would not appear on a stroke volume image, but do appear in the amplitude image which does not recognize positive and negative values. Usually, the pixel with the largest change in counts during the cycle is assigned the brightest color and all other pixels are scaled appropriately. It is then relatively straightforward to identify groups of pixels whose colors indicate smaller amplitudes and, therefore, reduced systolic function (Fig. 24.9). Such images may be helpful in identifying regional ventricular dysfunction. Their advantage over visual analysis of the beating ventricles is that they are three-dimensional rather than two-dimensional representations and are objective.

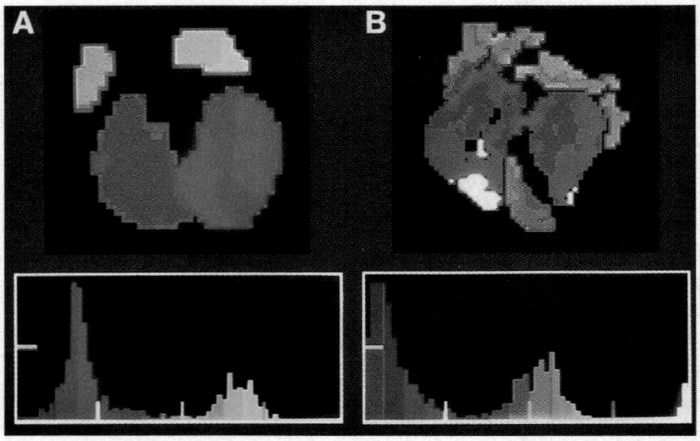

Figure 24.8. Normal (**A**) and abnormal (**B**) phase images (*upper*) and their respective phase angle histograms (*lower*). In the normal example, the pixels in both ventricles are of a fairly uniform color and the histogram shows a narrow distribution of phase angles consistent with synchronous contraction throughout both chambers. The phase angles of the atrial pixels are 180° out of phase with the ventricular pixels as one would expect since the atria fill while the ventricles empty. In the abnormal case, the pixels within the ventricles show several different phase angles. The septal and apical pixels in the LV have phase angles that are similar to those of the atrial pixels indicating that this part of the LV is 180° out of phase with the rest of the chamber which is typical of a dyskinetic segment. There is a band of black pixels in the LV indicating that there is no change in counts throughout the cardiac cycle in this area which is typical of an akinetic segment.

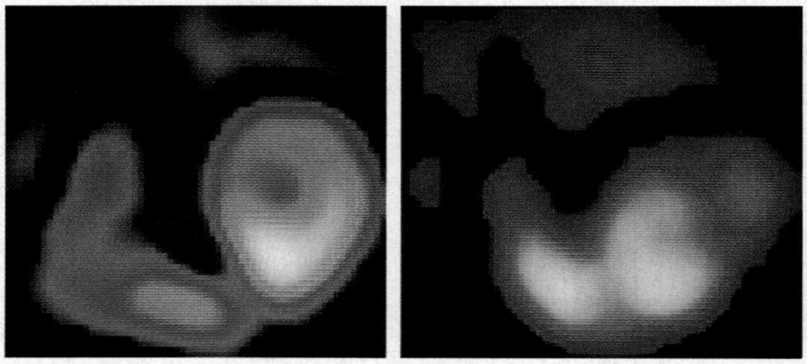

Figure 24.9. Normal (*left*) and abnormal (*right*) amplitude images. Pixels are color coded in direct relationship to the change in counts from end-diastole to end-systole. In these figures, the bright colors represent higher stroke counts. In the normal example, there is a shell of bright pixels around the periphery of the left ventricle which is where most of the change in counts during systole occurs. Near the aortic valve, the darker color occurs because the end-systolic volume is located there which results in a smaller change in counts. On the right, is an example of a patient with posterolateral dysfunction.

Both phase and amplitude images are influenced by the shape of the time-activity curve in each pixel. The shape will influence the cosine fit. For example, a distorted diastolic portion of the curve would change the shape of the cosine fit and influence the systolic measurements even though conduction and contraction may be completely normal. Because of that, some laboratories recommend truncating the time activity curve to eliminate the end of the cycle prior to applying the Fourier filter. When on-the-fly beat correction is used, or if the data are acquired in list mode, that issue is obviated.

DATA ANALYSIS AND INTERPRETATION

When reviewing EqRNA data, care should be taken to review each study in a systematic manner so that errors of omission do not occur. When looking at the views provided, they should be assessed for the spatial relationships, temporal relationships, and size and function of the cardiac chambers. To do that, the images should be reviewed in cinematic display, preferably simultaneously. Once the interpreting physician has assessed the data qualitatively, the clinical impression should be compared to the quantitative results. Discordance between qualitative and quantitative results should be resolved by either reprocessing or reevaluation of the cinematic displays.

Chamber Orientation

In the anterior view, the right ventricle is seen in the foreground with the left ventricle slightly posterior and to the right (Fig. 24.10). Although there is overlap between the RV and the inferior wall of the LV in this view, the higher count density of the LV allows clear visualization of the inferior wall. The other segments of the LV that are well seen in this view are the anterolateral wall and the apex. The body, apex, and outflow tract of the RV are typically seen in this projection. The right atrium is usually easily identified and occasionally the superior and inferior vena cavae are seen. The left atrium is usually hidden behind the great vessels and the LV. The pulmonary artery extends from the RV outflow tract upwards and toward the left lung crossing the ascending aorta. Part of the ascending aorta is almost always visible. The separation between the liver and the RV should be noted in the anterior view.

In the "best septal" view, the two most prominent features are the two ventricles separated by a very well delineated interventricular septum. It is probably the best view for assessing LV and RV chamber enlargement and is the best view to assess septal hypertrophy. The septum, true posterior, and inferoapical walls of the LV are seen in this view. The more horizontal the heart, the more inferior wall is seen; the more vertical the heart, the more the apex is seen.

Above the left ventricle, the left atrium, especially the left atrial appendage is usually well-delineated and left atrial enlargement is usually obvious in this projection. The right atrium is largely obscured by the RV in the best septal view, but may be seen at RV end systole and may include both vena cavae. Both the pulmonary artery and aorta are also seen. The size of the spleen should be noted in this view.

The lateral view offers the only totally unobstructed view of the inferior wall of the LV and is, therefore, an important view to acquire. No EqRNA, other than one being done for LVEF alone, is complete without a left lateral or at least a very steep LAO view. It may be the only view in which an inferior wall motion abnormality is detected. There is considerable overlap between the LV apex and the RV in this view, and it is occasionally impossible to assess apical wall motion. The anteroseptal wall of the LV is well seen. The left atrium and mitral valve plane are usually well seen in the lateral view. The right atrium is not visible.

Chamber Size

The evaluation of chamber or great vessel size is largely subjective and relative. With enough clinical experience on a given gamma-camera-computer system, the interpreter can fairly accurately identify varying degrees of chamber enlargement. Surrounding structures or other chambers in the same view are often the best references for assessing chamber size and are independent of the zoom factor used for acquisition or the distance of the chambers from the detector. For the LV, calculation of an absolute volume and comparison to normal limits for a given laboratory is the ideal way of defining LV chamber enlargement. The RV is typically smaller in its AP dimension than is the LV in the LAO view. When the AP dimension of the RV exceeds that of the LV, the RV may be enlarged, but when the LV chamber is small due to hypertrophy, the RV may appear relatively large even though it is normal in size. Moreover, the size of the RV inflow tract is quite variable and mild increases in RV size are difficult to distinguish from normal variants. The RV apex may extend beyond the LV apex in one or more views when the RV is dilated. The atria are the most difficult to evaluate. Depending on the imaging angle and cardiac orientation, the right atrium has a variable profile, appearing considerably larger in some normal subjects than in others. The left atrial appendage is visible in the best septal view, and if it is clearly identifiable through-

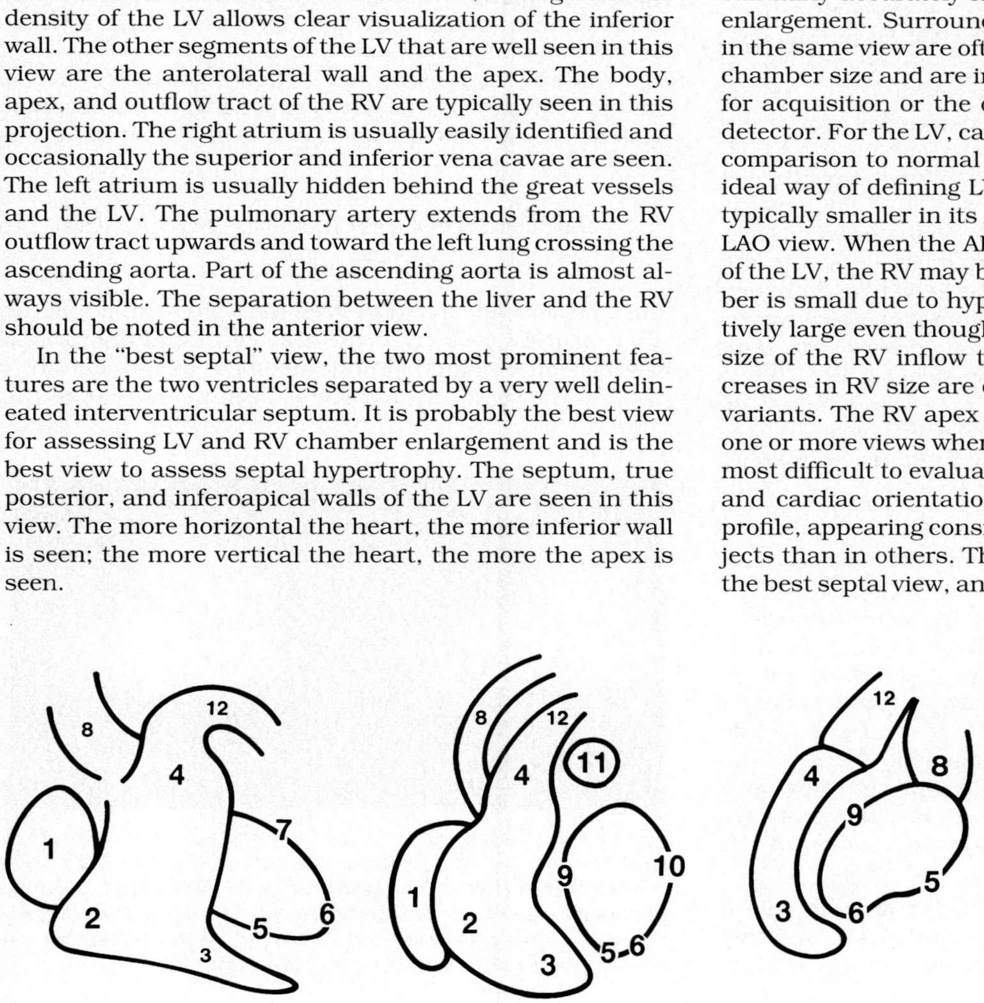

Figure 24.10. The commonly visualized chambers, vessels and ventricular segments in the anterior (*left*), best septal (*middle*) and lateral (*right*) views of a standard EqRNA. *1* = Right atrium; *2* = RV inflow; *3* = RV apex; *4* = RV outflow; *5* = LV-inferior wall; *6* = LV apex; *7* = LV anterolateral wall; *8* = Ascending aorta; *9* = LV septum; *10* = LV lateral or True posterior wall; *11* = Left atrium; *12* = Pulmonary artery.

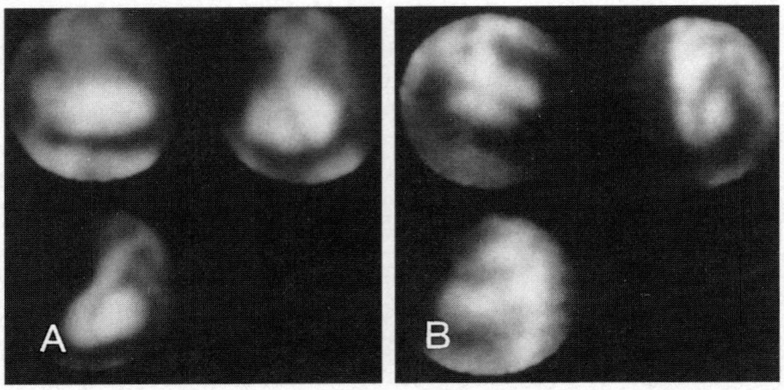

Figure 24.11. A percardial effusion is characterized by an increase in the silhouette surrounding the cardiac chambers, in particular the ventricles. In the anterior view, the space between the liver and the RV chamber is typically wider. Panel **A** shows a study from a subject with a moderate sized effusion and Panel **B** shows a large effusion.

out the cardiac cycle, it usually signifies left atrial enlargement. Usually the left atrial appendage becomes very small or frankly invisible during atrial systole.

Pulmonary Artery. The pulmonary artery is best assessed in the anterior and the best septal views. The pulmonary artery is usually comparable in size to the ascending aorta. The size of the pulmonary artery, when enlarged, may indicate increased pulmonary artery pressures, either secondary to lung disease, such as COPD, left ventricular dysfunction, or mitral valve disease. Careful examination of the left atrium and left ventricle may yield or a least exclude a particular cause of pulmonary hypertension. For example, a small left ventricle and a dilated left atrium would suggest mitral stenosis or diastolic dysfunction of the left ventricle as possible causes of the dilated pulmonary artery. Associated signs that need to be evaluated when looking at the size of a pulmonary artery include the size and function of the right ventricle and the activity in both lung fields. When there is significant pulmonary artery hypertension leading to a large pulmonary artery, the right ventricle is often dilated and hypocontractile. When pulmonary activity is increased it may signify left-sided failure as the cause of pulmonary hypertension. A rare cause of a large pulmonary artery would be a pulmonary embolus.

Aorta. Both the ascending and proximal descending aorta and occasionally the entire descending thoracic aorta may be evaluated qualitatively for size and tortuosity. In the best septal view, the ascending aorta may be seen and evaluated for significant dilatation. Mild dilatation is often missed on EqRNA studies, and this is certainly not the study of choice for that diagnosis. Tortuosity and aneurysmal dilatation of the descending aorta may be seen on this view as well. Both of those may be diagnostic of long-standing hypertension, or, in the case of a significantly tortuous descending aorta, advanced age. The EqRNA does not have the resolution necessary to identify a dissection of the aorta.

Pericardial Space. Surrounding the ventricular blood pools are the myocardium, the pericardial fat, and any pericardial fluid. The tracer-free space surrounding the ventricular cavities are enlarged when a pericardial effusion is present. However, because the thicknesses of the myocardium and pericardial fat vary, small pericardial effusions may be quite difficult to detect with certainty. When a pericardial effusion is large, there will be a proportionately large "halo" or darkened area around the heart (Fig. 24.11). In the anterior view, the space between the liver and the RV blood pool should be routinely examined. Enhanced separation of those two structures usually signifies the presence of a pericardial effusion. If the silhouette surrounding the LV blood pool appears enlarged in the LAO view but there is normal separation between the RV and the liver, then the increased silhouette is typically not due to a pericardial effusion.

Left Ventricular and Left Atrial Thrombi

Ventricular thrombi can be directly visualized in gated equilibrium studies (Fig. 24.12). They are typically found in association with ventricular segments that are akinetic, dyskinetic, or aneurysmal. The clots have been visualized and described as either an irregularity along the myocardium (3) or as a space-occupying lesion and, thus, an area of decreased count activity in the left ventricle (47). The exact role that EqRNA plays in the detection of ventricular thrombi is unknown. The minimum size of a thrombus that can be visualized is unknown and the relative sensitivities of EqRNA and echocardiography for detection of ventricular thrombi remains unstudied.

Left atrial thrombi are not typically visualized directly but the absence of the left atrial appendage in the best septal or steep LAO views is consistent with a left atrial thrombus (48).

ASSESSMENT OF RHYTHM AND CONDUCTION

Normal Sinus Rhythm

The anterior view, in which both the right atrium and the two ventricles are seen, is the best view for assessment of rhythm and conduction abnormalities. In normal sinus rhythm, the right atrium may be seen to contract at the

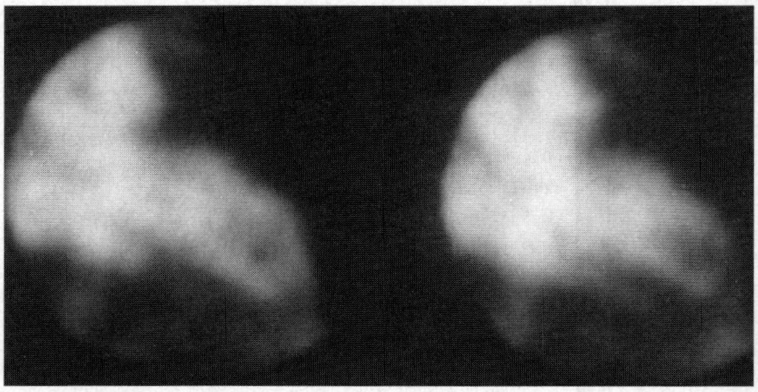

Figure 24.12. Patients with anterior and especially apical infarcts may have mural thrombi at the site of akinetic or dyskinetic myocardium. In this case, the anterior view shows a large space occupying mass in an anteroapical LV aneurysm at end-diastole (*left*) and end-systole (*right*). Given the appearance of this mass and its location within an aneurysmal segment, the overwhelming likelihood is that it represents a thrombus.

end of ventricular filling just prior to contraction of the ventricles. Visual inspection of the cine display in sinus rhythm will show a one-to-one correlation of atrial to ventricular contraction with the aforementioned timing sequence. Atrial contraction must be distinguished from the change in atrial size due to filling which can occur during any rhythm. Unequivocal contraction of the atria occurs virtually exclusively in sinus rhythm. Only the very rare patient with a slow atrial or AV nodal tachycardia will show organized atrial contraction and a one-to-one relationship to the ventricles.

Atrial Flutter—Fibrillation. Atrial fibrillation results in a loss of organized atrial activity and the atria do not appear to contract. The atria are usually dilated unless the fibrillation is of recent origin. The same is true of atrial flutter, although on occasion, in a well-organized and not too rapid flutter, a two-to-one or larger atrial to ventricular contraction ratio can be observed in the cine display. An extremely rare and typically transient cause of the atria failing to contract is atrial standstill from an atrial infarction.

Pacemaker Rhythm. There are two basic types of pacing, atrial or AV sequential pacing, which reproduce the normal hemodynamics of synchronized atrial and ventricular systole that are present in sinus rhythm and ventricular pacing, in which case, ventricular and atrial contractions may be completely asynchronous. Scintigraphically, atrial pacing cannot be distinguished from sinus rhythm. With AV sequential pacing, the timing of atrial and ventricular contractions appears normal but the ventricle is stimulated from the apex which creates an apical to basal wave of contraction through the ventricle that is easily distinguished from the normal pattern of ventricular depolarization. With ventricular pacing, both AV synchrony and the normal ventricular contraction pattern are lost.

Bundle Branch Block. There are two major types of bundle branch block that may be encountered clinically, left and right bundle branch block. With the three-lead configuration normally used for gating EqRNA studies, the widened QRS interval may be appreciated, but the type of bundle branch block may not be discernible. Careful visual interpretation of movement of the septum may be helpful in this regard.

In right bundle branch block, the septum is activated via the left Purkinje system, as is normally the case, and the ventricular contraction pattern appears normal. A phase image, however, may disclose the delayed onset of contraction in the right ventricle (49). With left bundle branch, the septum is initially depolarized from the right Purkinje system. The right ventricle actually is depolarized first and begins its systole prior to that of the left ventricle. It was shown that with left bundle branch block, the pressure inside the right ventricle during its systole causes a shift of the septum into the left ventricle prior to the beginning of left ventricular systole. With the delayed onset of left ventricular systole, the intraventricular pressures are equalized and the septum moves back towards the right ventricle as opposed to moving towards the center of the left ventricle (50). This paradoxical septal motion (moving towards the right ventricle during left ventricular systole) may be well seen in the "best septal" view. The phase image may be helpful in identifying or confirming the presence of left bundle branch block (Figs. 24.13 and 24.14). Paradoxical motion of the septum toward the RV during LV systole may be distinguished from septal dyskinesia due to infarction by the absence of the early motion of the septum toward the LV cavity in the setting of septal infarction.

Preexcitation and Ventricular Tachycardia. In a normally conducted ventricular beat, there is almost simultaneous contraction throughout both ventricles. This includes the septum and both free walls as seen in the "best septal" view. Using high resolution phase imaging, the timing of electrical-mechanical coupling may be viewed directly. Accessory pathways and circus movement tachycardias can be visually assessed using EqRNA study (51, 52) (Fig. 24.15).

ASSESSMENT OF SYSTOLIC FUNCTION

The evaluation of regional and global ventricular systolic function is probably the most important clinical role for EqRNA. As such, the interpreting physician should be methodic and diligent in analyzing the cinematic display of the data in all views acquired. The ventricular segments in the three typical views of an EqRNA study are indicated in Figure 24.11. An assessment should be recorded and reported for each of the segments. It is extremely helpful for students of radionuclide angiography to spend sufficient time studying contrast angiography to appreciate the variability of normal ventricular contraction patterns and the spectrum of LV and RV dysfunction. Regional dysfunction of the right ventricle is distinctly less common than global dysfunction, and typically results from right ventricular infarction in association with inferior infarction of the left ventricle (53). Regional dysfunction may also be seen in the right ventricular dysplasia, although even here the most

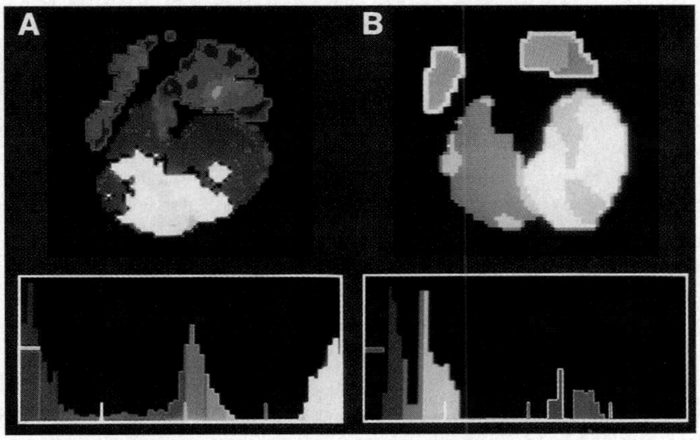

Figure 24.13. Phase images are particularly helpful in recognizing conduction abnormalities. In Panel **A,** systolic contraction begins at the apex of the RV and LV and spreads upward toward the base of the heart, a sequence that is distinctly different from normal (see Figure 24.8**A**) and which is typical of pacemaker rhythm. In **B,** the LV contracts considerably later than the RV (note the distinctly separate ventricular peaks on the phase histogram). This pattern is typical of left bundle branch block where depolarization and hence contraction are delayed in the left ventricular myocardium.

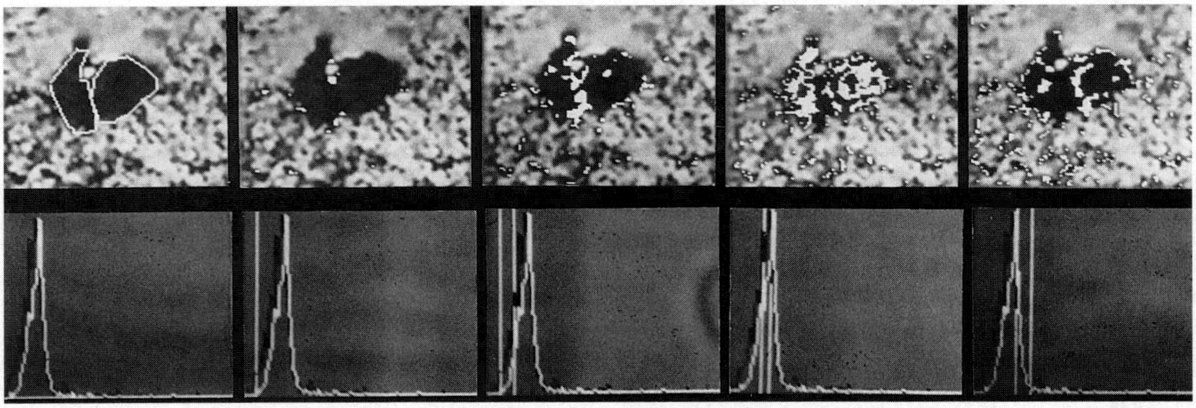

Figure 24.14. Phase image—normal study. *Top row:* Shown is the phase image in a normal patient in the best septal left anterior oblique projection. Ventricular regions of interest have been outlined and appear in homogeneous dark gray, indicating an early phase angle characteristic of normal ventricles. Above on the ventricular regions, the homogeneous light gray areas represent the atrial regions, out of phase with the ventricles. The background, lacking any relation to the cardiac cycle, appears as a random "salt and pepper" distribution of shades of gray. *Bottom row:* Shown are the normalized right (*black*) and left (*white*) ventricular phase histograms plotting phase angle on the abscissa and its frequency on the ordinate. In sequential panels, individual pixels in the phase image, which correspond to the serial windows marked on the phase histograms, are enhanced in white. The sequence, from left to right, indicates early septal phase angle with relatively symmetric subsequent involvement of both ventricles, the normal excitation (contraction) sequence. (Reproduced by permission from Frais M, Botvinick E, Shosa D, et al. Phase image characterization of localized and generalized left ventricular contraction abnormalities. J Am Coll Cardiol 1984;4:987.)

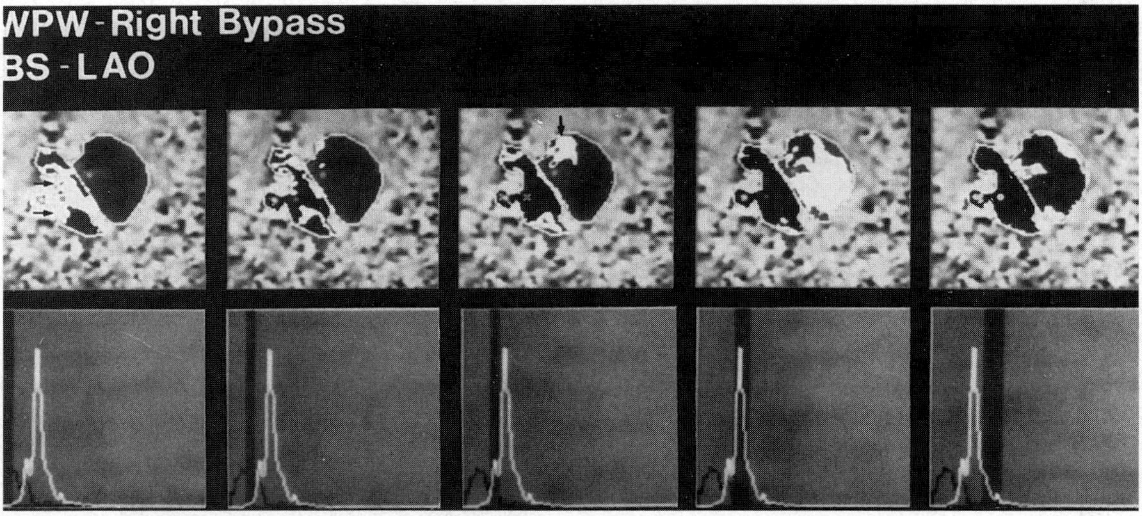

Figure 24.15. Right bypass pathway. Shown according to the format of the previous figure are the phase image and ventricular histograms, in a patient with a right-sided bypass pathway, Wolff Parkinson White Syndrome, imaged during preexcitation. Note the earlier occurrence of the right (*black*) histogram and the site of earliest phase angle in the right ventricle wall in this best septal left anterior oblique projection. A frame preceding those illustrated, would specifically localize the preexcitation pathway to the lateral base of the right ventricle.

common finding is a dilated and diffusely abnormal right ventricle (54). Many different types of parametric images are available to help the physician assess regional LV function including, stroke volume, regional LVEF, amplitude, and phase images. However, one should never be lulled into trusting such images without an independent evaluation of the cinematic display. Parametric images are arithmetic constructs whose validity depend upon the statistical strength of the raw data and the confounding influence of adjacent or overlying structures.

Regional LV Function

Regional systolic contraction or regional wall motion can be described in terms of synergy and synchrony. Synergy refers to the force of contraction and synchrony to the timing of contraction. The conventional terms for describing the severity of abnormal synergy (asynergy) are hypokinesia, akinesia, and dyskinesia. Abnormal synchrony is referred to as asynchrony. While the degrees of asynchrony have no special designations, the phase angle generated from a phase image can be used to quantify the degree of asynchrony. The extent of a regional wall motion abnormality is defined by the amount of the ventricular perimeter involved and should also be assessed and recorded routinely.

Normal. Normal wall motion is relatively simple to identify when all ventricular segments appear to contract at the same time, at the same rate, and to the same extent. Differentiating normal contraction from a synchronously contracting chamber, whose segments move somewhat less vigorously than normal, can be a very subjective decision and one which can only be made confidently with a lot of experience. In such a situation, quantitative information such as the regional LVEF or regional shortening statistics may be helpful. Altering the speed of the cinematic display can alter the subjective appreciation of the vigor of contraction and, therefore, the display speed should be kept within a narrow range for the sake of consistency.

Hypokinesia. The term signifies a reduction in the extent of contraction. Contraction is still present. Regional hypokinesia is best detected by comparison to other, more vigorously contracting segments in the same ventricle. As indicated earlier, when normally contracting segments are not present in the same ventricle, it may be difficult to recognize mild degrees of diffuse hypokinesia. The terms mild, moderate, and severe are used to characterize the spectrum of reduced wall motion between normal and akinesia. Contrast angiographers have used chord shortening to quantify regional systolic motion and a similar approach has been applied to radionuclide data even though the resolution of the typical RNA is not ideally suited to such an approach (55).

Akinesia. Akinesia signifies the absence of detectable contraction. In general, akinetic segments are fibrotic and devoid of viable myocardium (56). However, both stunned and hibernating myocardium may appear akinetic and, by inference, nonviable, yet may recover function with time or after revascularization.

Dyskinesia. A dyskinetic wall segment is one which passively bulges outward while the surrounding ventricular segments contract inward toward the center of the chamber. The pathologic substrate for dyskinetic myocardium is typically a thinned, fibrotic tissue devoid of any viable myocardial cells (56). Dyskinesia is typical of an aneurysm although some aneurysms appear akinetic rather than dyskinetic. As mentioned for akinesia, even dyskinesia may occasionally be seen in viable but stunned or hibernating myocardium.

Paradoxical Movement. The term paradoxical is used to characterize the motion of the ventricular septum that occurs in the presence of left bundle branch block or in certain right ventricular overload states. The septum appears to move inward early in systole and then bulge toward the right ventricular chamber as the rest of the left ventricle contracts. Although out of phase with the rest of the left ventricle, the paradoxically moving segment does contract. This is in contrast to a dyskinetic segment which does not contract at all. Dyskinesia can occur anywhere in the ventricle, whereas paradoxical movement is restricted to the septum.

Aneurysm. An aneurysm of the ventricle can be described angiographically, surgically, or pathologically, each definition containing the unique information from that particular approach. For the radionuclide diagnosis of an aneurysm, the angiographic definition is most appropriate. Simply stated, an aneurysm is a noncontractile part of the ventricle whose margins are clearly separable from the surrounding viable myocardium and where there is frequently a neck or waist formed by the contraction of the surrounding viable muscle (Fig. 24.16). One can think of an aneurysmal ventricle as consisting of two chambers, one of contracting muscle and the other of noncontracting scar tissue. Since an aneurysm is typically formed by a thin wall of fibrous tissue, it is typically dyskinetic but it may be akinetic. The most common locations for an aneurysm are the apex and anterior wall. Inferior and posterior aneurysms occur less frequently. Identification of an aneurysm may be important in a patient's clinical course. They are associated with an increased incidence of ventricular arrhythmias, congestive heart failure, and ventricular thrombi, the latter with the potential for systemic embolization.

Regional Ejection Fraction. The term regional ejection fraction has been applied to represent the ejection fraction of a varying number of subdivisions of the ventricle ranging in size from 1 pixel to one-third of the chamber. It may be of assistance in helping the interpreting physician detect regional dysfunction (57). Advantages of the regional EF over standard wall motion analysis include the facts that it is objective and that it represents three-dimensional data rather than two-dimensional data. Because of the latter, it

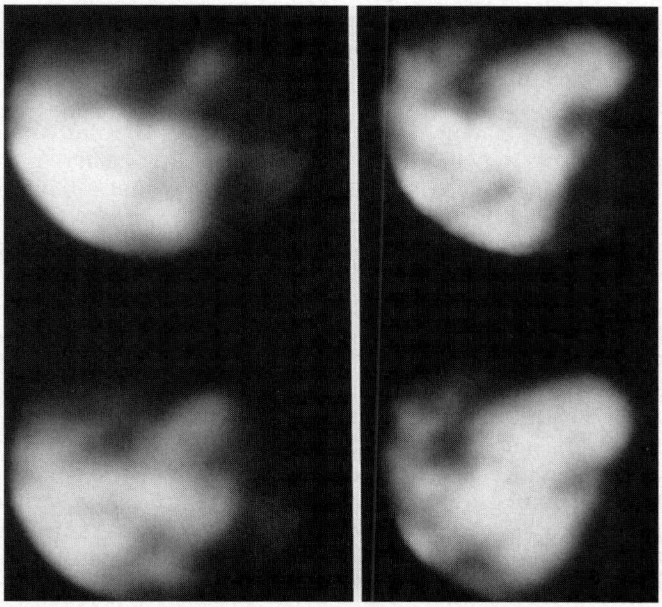

Figure 24.16. A small apical aneurysm is shown in the *top* panel with end-diastole on the *left* and end-systole on the *right*. The normal contraction of the base of the left ventricle makes the apical aneurysm appear very discrete and creates the narrow neck at end-systole. *Below*, the aneurysm is large and not as discrete because the myocardium outside the aneurysm does not contract normally.

should be clear that regional wall motion and regional EF are not equivalent. Comparisons of regional ejection fractions from one study to the next, or from one patient to another, presupposes that the alignment of the ventricles is identical and that the center of the ventricle remains in the same place, assumptions that are not always true.

Quantitative Regional Wall Motion

As in contrast angiography, regional wall motion may be quantified by calculating regional shortening fractions of a number of radii drawn from the center of the ventricle to the perimeter of the chamber at both ED and ES (58, 59). Rotation of the chamber during systole challenges the assumption that the center of the chamber remains constant, but the technique is fairly reproducible and is certainly valid for comparisons between interventions in the same individual. It is the latter application that is most suited to the use of this type of analysis (55). Quantification of regional wall motion is desirable because the qualitative analysis of wall motion is very subjective and interobserver variability is substantial. However, any geometric analysis of standard blood pool data is dependent upon the variable resolution of the images, resolution being dependent upon not just the intrinsic resolution of the imaging system, but also upon the quality of the red cell tag and the separation of the LV from surrounding structures.

Global Systolic Function: Left Ventricular Ejection Fraction

The performance of the entire ventricular chamber can be called global systolic function. The ejection fraction is used to quantify global ventricular function and typically ranges from 0.50–0.80 at rest and approximately 0.56–0.86 during exercise. Those values will vary somewhat among laboratories. Reductions in LVEF at rest are usually characterized as mild (0.40–0.49), moderate (0.25–0.40), and severe (<0.25).

The three major determinants of left ventricular function are preload, afterload, and the intrinsic contractility of the left ventricle itself. Preload refers to the amount of initial loading of the ventricle just prior to its contraction, i.e., the degree to which the muscle fibers are stretched from their resting state. It is typically expressed as the end-diastolic volume since it is clinically impossible to measure fiber stretch. Starling's law states that the greater the initial loading of the ventricle the greater the force of the subsequent contraction. Once a certain preload is exceeded, however, the ventricle becomes less efficient. Afterload refers to those forces which resist the ejection of blood from the left ventricle, i.e., peripheral resistance. The systolic blood pressure is a relative measure of peripheral vascular resistance. In general, increasing afterload results in less complete emptying of the ventricle. Myocardial contractility refers to the intrinsic inotropic state of the muscle and clinically can be thought of as the contractile performance of the ventricle at any given preload and afterload. An increase in contractility as might occur with an increase in catecholamines will result in the ventricle contracting to a smaller end-systolic volume, thus increasing the ejection fraction. A decrease in contractility will result in a decrease in ejection fraction. Because of that direct relationship, the ejection fraction is used clinically as a surrogate for contractility and works quite well as long as the loading conditions on the ventricle are within a physiologic range. The power of the ejection fraction as a clinical predictor of outcome in various cardiac diseases is testimony to its relationship to the intrinsic state of the myocardium. However, when loading conditions are changed, as occurs with the increased afterload of sudden hypertension, or severe aortic stenosis, or the decreased afterload of mitral insufficiency, ejection fraction may not reflect the contractility of the myocardium. Ejection fraction, unlike contractility, varies with loading conditions. As a result, investigators have looked for measurements other than ejection fraction that might more accurately reflect myocardial contractility regardless of loading conditions.

Peak-Systolic Pressure-End-Systolic Volume Relationship

It has been shown that the end-systolic volume is dependent almost exclusively upon afterload and not on preload. If contractility is held constant and afterload is varied, then a plot of end-systolic volume versus end-systolic pressure will be a straight line (60, 61). The slope of that line has been referred to as E_{max} (60). Increasing contractility increases the slope of the line and decreasing contractility lowers the slope. Clinically, end-systolic pressure can only be measured with a left ventricular catheter, but some authors have suggested the use of peak systolic pressure which can be measured with a cuff. Using the radionuclide end-systolic volume and cuff blood pressure, the slope of the peak systolic pressure end-systolic volume relationship has been described (62, 63). Potential applications of that approach include the assessment of patients with hypertrophic cardiomyopathies, aortic stenosis with depressed LVEF, aortic insufficiency, and mitral insufficiency. In particular, the timing of valve replacement might be facilitated by detecting changes in contractility before changes in ejection fraction occur.

DIASTOLIC LEFT VENTRICULAR FUNCTION

The filling of the left ventricle can be divided into active and passive phases. The active phase is an energy dependent phase that depends on the rate, synchrony, and extent of the breaking of the cross bridges between actin and myosin. This phase is referred to as a ventricular relaxation. During this phase, LV pressure falls below left atrial pressure, allowing the ventricle to fill. The pressure gradient between the left atrium and the left ventricle will then determine the flow across the mitral valve. For the most part, then, early rapid filling of the ventricle is dependent upon the rate and extent of myocardial relaxation and the LA-LV pressure gradient. Once rapid filling is over, passive filling continues. Passive filling is most dependent upon the compliance of the ventricle and can only be characterized by the relationship of pressure and volume throughout this portion of diastole. Unlike the end-systolic pressure volume relationship which is linear and can be defined by three data points, the diastolic pressure-volume relationship is curvilinear. Consequently, many more data points are required to define that relationship. Some investigators have coupled frame-by-frame radionuclide measurements of diastolic volume with high fidelity intraventricular pressure recordings to elegantly analyze compliance and its alteration with medication (64–66).

The interpretation of the diastolic filling portion of the left ventricular time-activity curve depends upon both the qualitative and quantitative assessment of the data. The qualitative assessment may be the most invaluable of the two because there are certain characteristic patterns of abnormal filling that recur frequently in clinical practice and because quantitation varies so much from laboratory to laboratory (16). Figure 24.17 shows several LV time-activity curves that are representative of the common patterns of abnormal diastolic filling. Prolongation of isovolumic relaxation, delayed and/or decreased early rapid filling, and exaggeration of the atrial contribution to filling are the typical disturbances of the normal filling pattern. They may occur alone or in combination. An exaggeration of the atrial contribution to filling associated with a variable decrease in the early peak filling rate is typical of both normal aging (17, 67, 68) and hypertension (69, 70). Prolongation of isovolumic relaxation is typical of hypertrophic myopathy (71) and delayed and decreased rapid filling is typical of coronary artery disease (72).

The isovolumic relaxation period may be measured, but is typically short and may only occupy the time between two frames of a standard EqRNA acquisition. Delayed early rapid filling may be quantified by prolongation of the tPFR. Decreased early rapid filling can be measured as a reduced PFR. The contribution of the atrium may be expressed as the absolute atrial filling rate (AFR), or the ratio of the atrial to early rapid filling rates (AFR/PFR), or its inverse PFR/AFR. Normal values for PFR, tPFR, and AFR vary substantially depending on the type of acquisition, frame rate, and, in the case of the EqRNA, the gating technique (16, 73).

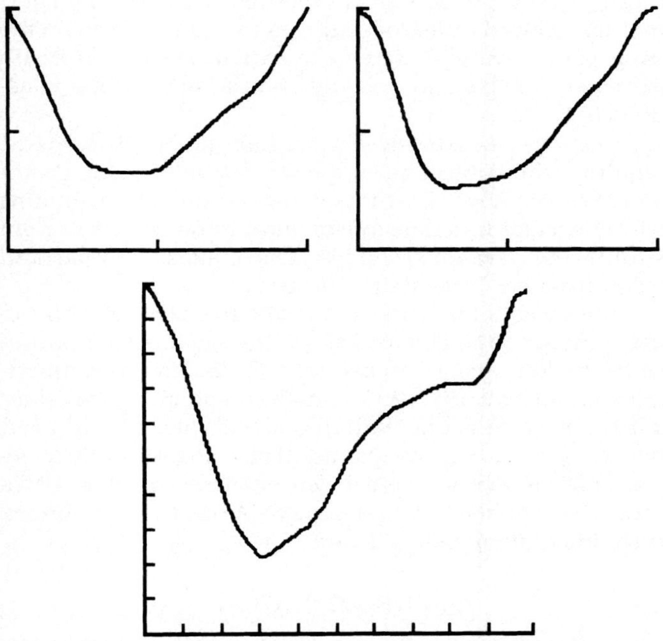

Figure 24.17. Typical clinical examples of abnormal diastolic filling patterns. In the curve on the *upper left*, the tPFR is prolonged due largely to a prolongation of the isovolumic relaxation phase. The atrial contribution to filling is increased. At the *top right*, the tPFR is prolonged largely because of decreased early rapid filling resulting in a reduced PFR. In the lower curve, the only abnormality is as exaggerated atrial contribution to filling.

It must be understood that the analysis of filling patterns and the timing of filling events represent the changes in volume during diastole, but obviously do not reflect the changes in intraventricular pressure. It is possible, therefore, to encounter normal filling times and a normal appearing filling pattern and still have abnormal diastolic pressure.

REGURGITANT FRACTION AND LEFT-TO-RIGHT SHUNTS

In an intact cardiac system, blood flows from one chamber to the next in one direction only, and so the amount of blood pumped per beat from one ventricle must equal that pumped from the other ventricle. Therefore, the stroke counts of the two ventricles must be equal. Any abnormality of structure or valve function that results in blood flow deviating from that unidirectional pattern will alter that fundamental relationship of stroke counts between the two ventricles.

In the case of mitral insufficiency or aortic insufficiency, left ventricular stroke counts will be higher than right ventricular stroke counts because each stroke of the LV contains both the counts destined to go forward in the circulation as well as the counts that will travel backward across the insufficient valve. The RV stroke counts represent only those counts going forward in the circulation. Hence the ratio of LV to RV stroke counts will exceed 1 by a fraction related to the magnitude of the insufficiency (74–76). The same concept applies to left-to-right shunts at the ventricular level, although, in that case, RV stroke counts are also increased above normal since the RV participates in the shunt (77). In contrast, right ventricular stroke counts will exceed left ventricular stroke counts in the presence of tricuspid or pulmonary insufficiency or with a left-to-right shunt at the atrial level.

Stroke count ratios derived from EqRNA have been found to be similar to the flow ratios measured at cardiac catheterization. Some authors believe that the RV/LV ratio may be compared directly to the Qp/Qs ratio derived from angiography. But because these numbers are derived during an equilibrium study, the exact location of a shunt or regurgitant lesion cannot be ascertained. Furthermore, the radionuclide data are highly dependent upon the accuracy of the ventricular ROI which are particularly problematic for the RV due to right atrial overlap and difficulty identifying the pulmonary valve. The right atrial overlap becomes even more of a problem when the right atrium is enlarged. As a result, reported LV to RV stroke count ratios usually exceed 1 in normal individuals. Other noninvasive techniques, such as Doppler echocardiography or first-pass RNA, are probably more accurate in detecting and quantifying both left-to-right shunts and valvular insufficiency.

TOMOGRAPHIC (SPECT) EqRNA

EqRNA may be acquired using a tomographic technique. When initially described, only the end-diastolic and end-systolic frames were stored for reconstruction (78–80) but with the expanded memory and increased speed of newer computers, all frames may be reconstructed. After routine RBC labeling, the subject may be imaged with standard tomographic equipment using a step and shoot protocol for 16–32 stops. At each stop, the acquisition is gated as is done in routine EqRNA, except that the number of frames per cardiac cycle is usually limited to approximately 8–12 because of time and memory constraints. Each stop is imaged for approximately 1 minute so that the entire acquisition takes no longer than an average three-view planar EqRNA study. The raw data then consist of 16 or 32 separate 8–12 frame EqRNA acquisitions. Tomographic reconstruction of each of the 8 frames of the study can then be performed to create axial and standard short axis, and vertical and horizontal long axis, images. Regional wall motion may then be interrogated tomographically. The advantages of tomographic EqRNA include the ability to examine regional wall motion throughout the entire depth of the ventricles, the freedom of the reconstructed data from background activity, and the fact that the acquisition does not require the technologist to identify specific imaging angles. At this point in time, however, it is not clear what real clinical benefit is achieved by acquiring an EqRNA study tomographically. In very specific situations, such as a large LV aneurysm where it may be difficult to accurately assess the margins of the aneurysm and the contraction pattern of the myocardium that may be hidden from view in a planar study, a tomographic acquisition would be helpful (79). The tomographic study may also be useful for measurement of chamber volume by calculation of the total number of three-dimensional pixels, i.e., voxels in the chamber of interest (80).

FIRST-PASS IMAGING

First-pass RNA is distinguished from EqRNA in two fundamental ways. First, no labeling of red blood cells is performed and second, all usable data are acquired during the initial transit of a radionuclide bolus through the central circulation. The first-pass study relies upon the temporal separation of chambers to generate chamber specific data as opposed to the requisite spatial separation in an EqRNA study. Inherent in the first-pass study is the ability to track the transit of the radionuclide through the heart and great vessels which makes it possible to detect abnormalities of tracer transit as is found in congenital heart disease, shunts and valvular insufficiency. Although the concept of first-pass RNA was first employed in 1927 (81) to measure the circulation time in man, it was not until 1969 that a ^{99m}Tc injection was used to sequentially visualize the heart and great vessels in patients (82). At that time, the technology was considered to be an improvement over contrast angiography as it was less invasive, less hazardous to the patient, and did not disturb their circulatory function.

IMAGING AGENTS

The requirements of a radionuclide for first-pass imaging are basically twofold: First, it must remain intravascular for the duration of the initial transit through the central circulation. Second, it must be safe for injection in a sufficiently large dose to generate the count rates necessary for this type of imaging.

^{99m}Tc Agents

Because of its high specific activity, ^{99m}Tc has been used for many years in nuclear medicine procedures. As we have seen previously, ^{99m}Tc pertechnetate is presently used in EqRNA studies. This agent may also be given as a bolus and is a very adequate agent for first-pass RNA. This agent may be used solely for a first-pass study or in conjunction with RBC labeling for an EqRNA study. An alternate technetium agent, DTPA (diethylenetriamine penta-acetic acid) is more commonly used because it is more rapidly cleared from the circulation by the kidneys. Of the technetium based myocardial perfusion imaging agents, sestamibi has been satisfactorily used for first-pass RNA (83, 84), as have teboroxime (85, 86) and tetrofosmin (87).

Ultra-Short-Lived Radionuclides

Although the 6-hour half-life of ^{99m}Tc is relatively short, the agents to which it is complexed have varying biologic clearance times. Therefore, radiation exposure limits the number of first-pass acquisitions that can be performed at a given time. Agents with extremely short half-lives (in the order of seconds to minutes) reduce the radiation exposure and allow more studies to be performed in a short period of time.

^{195m}Au has a half-life of 30.5 seconds. It is easily produced from a portable mercury generator. The correlation between first-pass ejection fractions using ^{195m}Au and those using ^{99m}Tc products exceeded 0.9 (88). The short half-life allowed numerous studies to be performed on the same patient without extreme radiation exposure and with extremely low background radiation from previous injections (89).

^{191m}Ir has an extremely short half-life of 4.9 seconds, requiring the subject be connected to the portable generator. Studies have shown its clinical utility for evaluating left ventricular function and for quantitation of left-to-right shunts (90). The 4.9 second half-life makes ^{191m}Ir particularly attractive for pediatric imaging.

^{178m}Ta was initially used to evaluate global left ventricular function (91). The half-life of this agent is 9.3 minutes which makes it easier to use than ^{191m}Ir. However, its primary photopeak of 55–65 keV make it suboptimal for standard gamma-cameras. With the clinical validation of a new type of gamma-camera, the multiwire proportional detector, and the development of an efficient portable ^{178m}Ta generator, satisfactory first-pass RNA has been performed with this radionuclide (92–94).

INSTRUMENTATION

Since all usable data are acquired during the initial transit of the radionuclide bolus, not many beats are available for processing. At rest, there are, on average, 6–10 beats, and at peak exercise 4–6 beats, during a typical study. As such, first-pass studies must have very high count rates to ensure the necessary count density for both image quality and statistical reliability of ejection fractions and volumes. Although first-pass ejection fractions may be generated with lower count rates, at least 150,000 counts/sec, and preferably ≥200,000 counts/sec, are necessary for adequate image quality, especially at end-systole.

Multicrystal Gamma-Camera

Historically, multicrystal gamma-camera systems were the first and only devices that could reliably record the count rates necessary for first-pass imaging. The initial multicrystal systems were able to record counts in excess of 250,000–300,000 counts/sec while maintaining enough spatial resolution for regional wall motion analysis. The latest generation of multicrystal gamma-cameras continues to deliver count rates in the same range but with enhanced energy and spatial resolution. To deliver such high count rates, the early multicrystal systems did sacrifice spatial resolution to the point that they were not particularly useful for other types of imaging. That may not be true of the newer generation of multicrystal cameras. Early systems were very large, very heavy, and not portable. Newer systems are substantially smaller and portable (Fig. 24.18).

Single-Crystal Gamma-Cameras

Conventional single-crystal gamma-cameras could count fairly linearly up to 60,000 counts/sec, but at higher rates there was substantial data loss and peak count rates with a clinical dose of technetium rarely exceeded 100,000 counts/sec with a collimator. As such, single-crystal cameras could not be used for high count rate first-pass RNA. More recent developments in camera-computer systems, specifically, all digital front end technology, allow single-crystal systems to achieve count rates up to 200,000 counts/sec. Clinically accurate, high count rate first-pass RNA has been performed with these newer single-crystal systems (95, 96).

Collimation

To achieve adequate count rates, high sensitivity and ultra-high sensitivity collimators are appropriate for first-pass studies. Some tradeoff between sensitivity and resolution is necessary and will depend upon the system in use. Collimators whose holes are aligned with the acquisition matrix offer the best combination of sensitivity and resolution.

Computer/Software

All current generation computer systems have enough speed and storage capacity for acquisition and processing of first-pass data. However, appropriate software is not universally available. First-pass acquisitions may be performed with either 64×64 or smaller matrixes. The 32×32 matrix has been used for some single-crystal systems (95), while the multicrystal systems now use a 20×20 matrix. The smaller matrixes increase the counts/pixel and are especially helpful in maintaining the integrity of the end-systolic image where the count density often becomes very marginal with a 64×64 matrix.

DATA ACQUISITION

Injection Techniques

Unlike the equilibrium study, the first-pass study requires bolus injection of a small volume with a high, specific activity. The quality of the first-pass study is very dependent upon the discreteness of the bolus. Consequently, the radionuclide must be injected into as large a bore vein as close to the central circulation as possible. In practice, there are only two sites that work well for that purpose, the medial antecubital and the external jugular veins. Lateral antecubital veins are reasonable alternatives. No other peripheral veins are acceptable. For the arm veins, an 18-gauge cannula is preferred while a 20-gauge cannula is adequate for the external jugular vein. When the right ventricular ejection fraction is of primary interest, it is helpful to prolong the radionuclide injection so that more right ventricular beats are available for data processing.

Radionuclide Dose

The appropriate radionuclide dose depends upon the sensitivity of the gamma-camera, the number of injections to

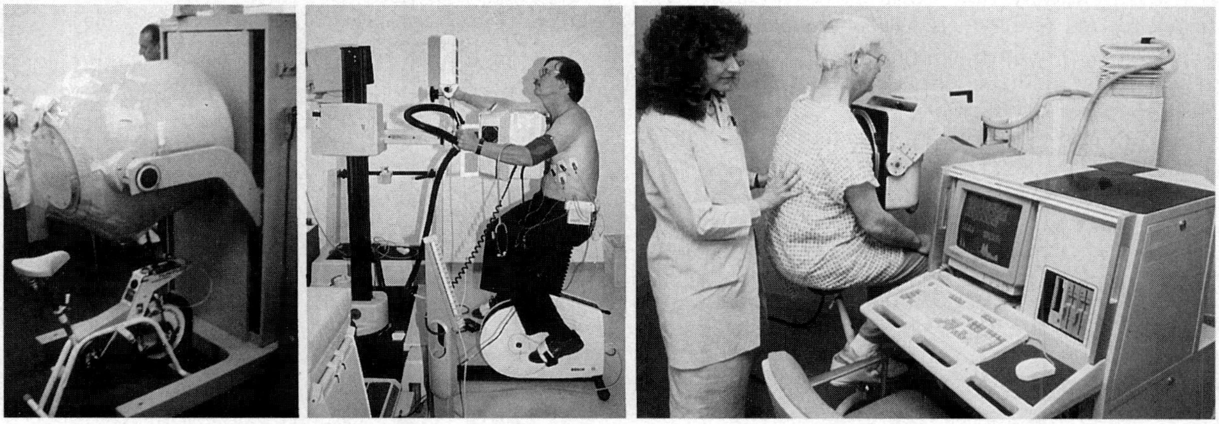

Figure 24.18. The evolution of cameras dedicated to first-pass imaging: (*left*) Baird Atomic System 77; (*middle*) Scinticor SIM400; (*right*) proportional-wire camera. (Courtesy of Dr. Jeffrey Lacy.)

be made, the size of the individual, and the specific radionuclide being used. With a multicrystal camera, doses as low as 8–10 mCi (296–370 MBq) may be used although 20–25 mCi (740–925 MBq) are recommended because lower doses may yield suboptimal statistics in large individuals or in cases where there are few beats available for processing. For single-crystal gamma-cameras, the dose should not be lower than 15 mCi (555 MBq) and should preferably be ±25 mCi (925 MBq) in the average adult. For the ultra-short-lived radionuclides, the doses can be substantially higher and doses of 50 mCi (1850 MBq) have been reported.

Imaging Angles

Because of the temporal separation of cardiac chambers, first-pass radionuclide studies can theoretically be acquired in any view. Typically, however, studies are acquired in either a shallow right anterior oblique view or a straight anterior projection. The shallow RAO view works well because it helps separate the atria from the ventricles and projects the LV away from the descending aorta. It is also a convenient view for direct comparison to contrast angiography. When the right ventricle is the chamber of primary concern, the 30° RAO view enhances right atrial-right ventricular separation. The anterior view works best for exercise studies because it is much easier to stabilize the chest against the detector. When the circumflex coronary artery is in question, an LAO view is useful. It should be noted that the count density in the left atrium is larger in first-pass studies than in equilibrium studies because of the activity in the bolus. As a result, a standard LAO view results in considerable left atrial-left ventricular overlap and an underestimation of LVEF. For shunt studies, as much of the lung fields as possible, particularly the right lung field, should be in the field of view, even to the exclusion of part or all of the left ventricle if necessary.

ECG Recording

For high count rate first-pass acquisitions using a multicrystal camera, no ECG signal is necessary. The counts within the time activity curve from a ventricular ROI are sufficient for the manual or automated identification of end-diastolic and end-systolic frames. When count rates may be lower, as frequently occurs with single crystal camera acquisitions, it is helpful to store an ECG signal which can then be used to facilitate data processing. Whether or not an ECG signal is stored, it is helpful to verify the cardiac rhythm prior to injection. Occasionally, the rhythm may be so irregular as to preclude a good quality first-pass study.

Frame Rates

The optimum frame rate depends upon the heart rate—the higher the heart rate, the faster the frame rate. At resting, heart rates of 50–100 beats/min, 20 frames/sec (50 msec/frame) is adequate. At heart rates of 150–200, frame rates of 40–100 frames/sec are necessary (97). Rather than constantly adjusting the frame rate, most laboratories compromise on 40–50 frames/sec for both rest and exercise studies. Data are usually acquired for 30 seconds from the time of injection to ensure that the entire transit is acquired.

Patient Positioning

First-pass studies cannot be repeated if an error in positioning is made. Therefore, it is important to verify that the chambers of interest will be in the field of view prior to study acquisition. Placing a uniform flood source or an exposed dose syringe behind the patient provides an image of the chest that allows identification of the lungs and mediastinum. Alternatively, a 1 mCi test dose can be injected for positioning. When more than one study is performed, the background activity from a preceding injection can be used for positioning.

STRESS PROTOCOLS

Bicycle Exercise Studies

First-pass RNA is particularly well-suited to the evaluation of ventricular function during exercise. The only caveat in acquiring such studies is that the chest must be relatively motionless with regard to the detector. Historically, that led to the use of bicycle ergometry as the method of choice for exercise first-pass studies. Although initial studies used supine bicycle exercise for correlation with data obtained in the cardiac catheterization laboratory, upright bicycle ergometry proved better for stabilizing the chest and was better tolerated (98, 99) (Fig. 24.19). Any graded exercise protocol is acceptable and because the acquisition time at peak exercise is so short, no time is required for stabilization of the heart rate. However, care should be taken to stabilize the patient's chest against the detector to minimize motion. Exercise should be continued until the bolus is seen to clear the LV. If technetium is used, a maximum of two injections may be made during the exercise study unless a resting study is not performed on the same day. For most clinical studies, rest and peak exercise acquisitions are sufficient.

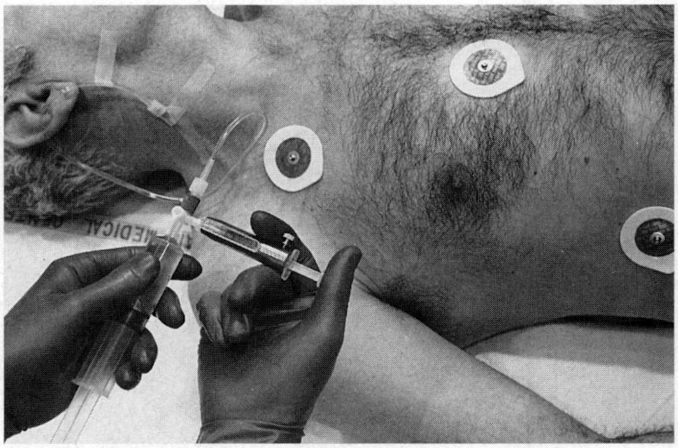

Figure 24.19. A typical setup for an external jugular vein approach to first-pass studies. The technique is well-tolerated, carries no additional risk compared to the antecubital approach, and leaves the patient's arms free for holding on to a handrail and for blood pressure recordings.

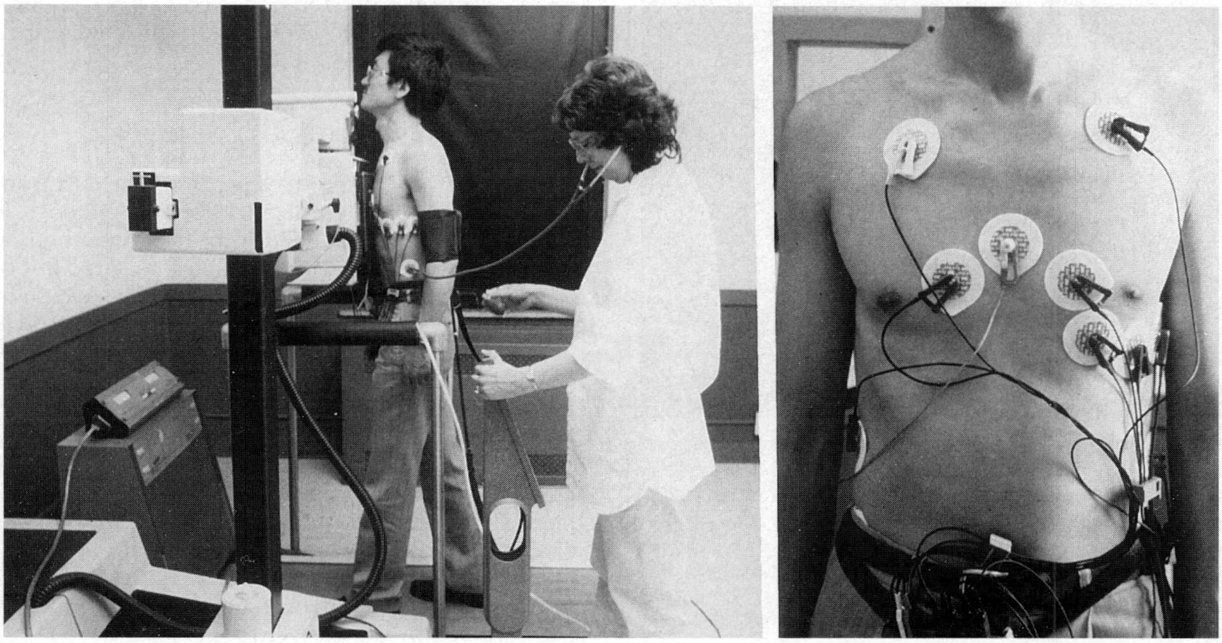

Figure 24.20. First-pass radionuclide angiography can be performed during treadmill exercise (*left*); however, a scheme for motion detection and correction is mandatory. In this case, an external sealed source containing ^{241}Am is affixed to the chest (what appears to be an electrode right over the middle of the sternum) so that a dual energy acquisition (using the 140 keV peak of ^{99m}Tc and the 50 keV of the americium) can be performed. (Courtesy of Dr. Jeffrey Lacy.)

Treadmill Exercise

During treadmill exercise, there is considerably more motion of the chest than during bicycle exercise. In fact, there is frequently so much motion that, until recently, first-pass RNA was never performed during treadmill exercise. With the introduction of a motion detection scheme that uses an external radioactive source attached to the chest, the image distortion due to chest motion has been considerably reduced. Clinically satisfactory first-pass RNA can now be routinely performed during treadmill exercise (84, 85, 100, 101). The external marker affixed to the chest is used to track chest wall and presumably cardiac motion. It must have a principal photopeak that lies outside the spectrum of the ^{99m}Tc so that both the marker photopeak and the technetium photopeak may be acquired simultaneously. Both ^{241}Am and ^{125}I have been used for that purpose. (Fig. 24.20)

STANDARD DATA PROCESSING

Analysis of Ventricular Function

First-pass data processing can be divided into four major steps. The first step is the creation of the time-activity curve from a ROI surrounding the ventricle of interest. Second is the selection of the beats to be included in the final analysis. Third is background subtraction and fourth is the creation of the final representative cycle from which all quantitative data are obtained. For details of data processing, the reader is referred to previously published articles describing those routines (98–104). Some of the more important aspects of processing are discussed here.

Region-of-interest Selection

An initial ventricular ROI is usually drawn manually on images generated by adding 20–40 frames of raw data together. That ROI is used to generate a time-activity curve from which an initial representative cycle is created. For both the left and right ventricles, the improved ventricular images from that initial representative cycle should then be used to draw separate end-diastolic and end-systolic ROI (Fig. 24.21). Both the RVEF and LVEF should be generated using two ROIs. The major pitfalls in creating accurate ROIs are the careful avoidance of left atrial activity and the identification of the aortic or pulmonary valve. Various parametric images such as stroke volume and phase images may be helpful in drawing the ROI. As in the processing of equilibrium data, the LV and RV ROI may be manually, semiautomatically, or automatically drawn.

Beat Selection

Once the final left ventricular region-of-interest has been identified, the operator has the opportunity to select those beats from the ventricular time-activity curve to be included in the final analysis. It is at this point that analysis or exclusion of individual beats may be performed. Premature ventricular beats will have a decreased ejection fraction when compared to sinus beats while postextrasystolic beats will have higher ejection fractions than sinus beats. For routine processing, ventricular premature beats, and, whenever possible, postextrasystolic beats should be excluded (Fig. 24.22). In ventricular bigeminy, when there are frequent PVCs, or when there is extremely irregular atrial fibrillation, data processing becomes ex-

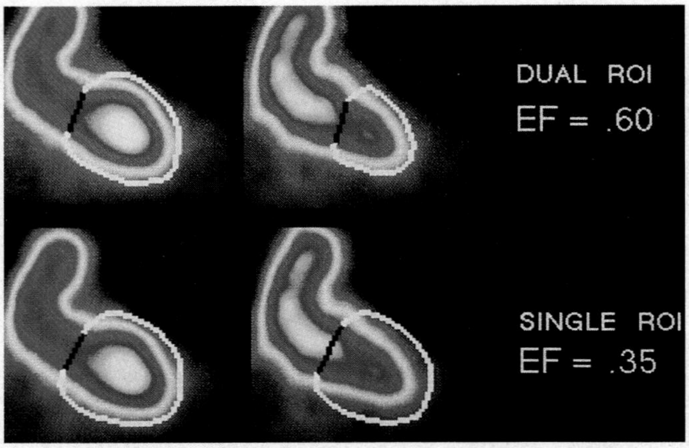

Figure 24.21. Although first-pass processing may be performed with a single ROI around the LV at end-diastole (*bottom left*), movement of the aortic valve toward the apex and filling of the left atrium during LV systole bring a variable, but sometimes significant, amount of nonventricular activity into the single ROI at end-systole (*bottom right*). Using a separate end-systolic ROI (*top right*) avoids that problem. In this case, because of a dilated left atrium, the dual ROI LVEF is much higher than the single ROI LVEF. In general, dual ROI ejection fractions are 5–10 EF units higher than their single ROI counterparts.

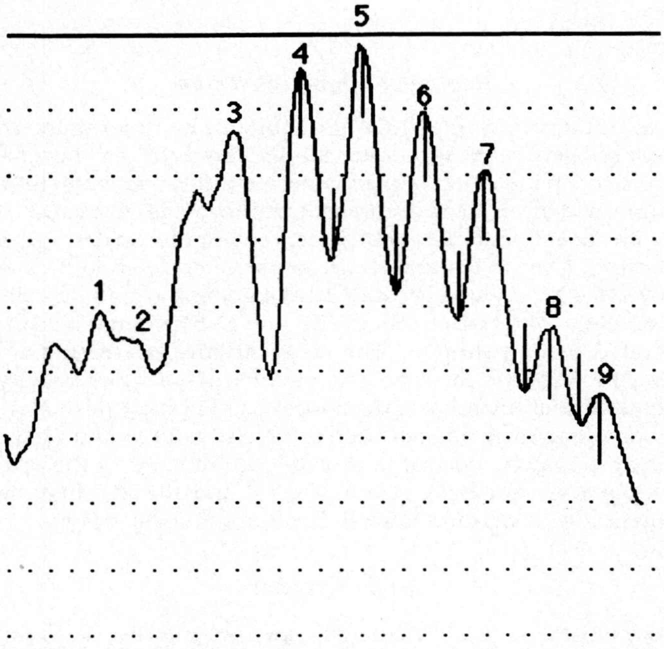

Figure 24.22. Beat selection is important during first-pass processing. In this example, beats numbered 3, 4, 5, and 6 are sinus beats, beat number 2 is a PVC, and beat number 3 is a post-PVC beat. The inclusion of PVC beats and post-PVC beats would spuriously lower or raise the ejection fraction respectively.

tremely difficult and often impossible. When such rhythms are present, the study should be postponed or an EqRNA acquisition performed.

Background Correction-LV

There are several different approaches to background correction in first-pass studies. However, the most accurate appears to be the so-called lung frame method (104). In this method, the distribution of counts in an image taken from the late pulmonary phase, just prior to appearance of the radionuclide in the LV, is used to correct the left ventricular phase. An adjustment for pulmonary washout is made. Background correction is crucial in the calculation of left ventricular ejection fraction and, unlike the background correction in EqRNA, changes in the background frame can cause large changes in the calculated LVEF. Occasionally, studies are encountered which cannot be appropriately corrected using the lung frame method because of persistent right ventricular activity throughout the pulmonary phase. In such situations, application of a regression equation to the uncorrected data may be the only way to generate an accurate LVEF.

Representative Cycle

After final beat selection and background correction, the individual beats are added together, frame by frame, to create the final representative cycle which may be displayed in a cine loop for analysis of regional wall motion. As in EqRNA, a host of parametric images may be created from the representative cycle. The most commonly used parametric images are the regional ejection fraction and stroke volume images (Fig. 24.23). Unlike those two images which are derived from the counts at end diastole and end systole, the mean transit time images, advocated by some authors (105), is more representative of the change in counts throughout systole or diastole. However, all parametric images are very count dependent for accuracy and very high count rate first-pass data are necessary for their routine clinical application.

The end-diastolic and end-systolic counts of the repre-

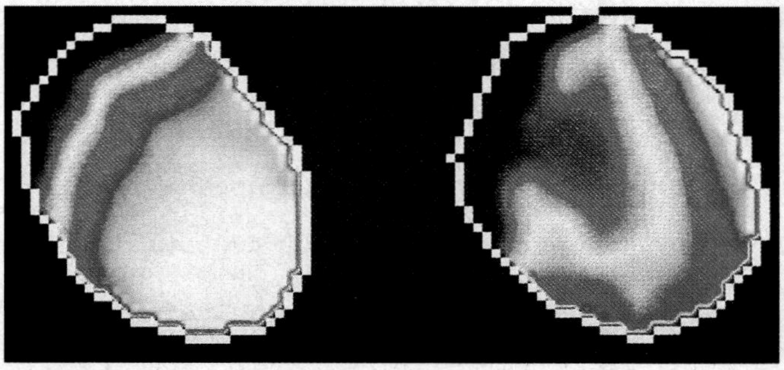

Figure 24.23. Parametric images may be helpful in defining localized abnormalities of contraction as indicated previously (see Figure 24.9). One of the most commonly used images is the regional ejection fraction image (REFI) generated by color coding the ejection fraction of each pixel in the LV image. A normal, homogeneous pattern is shown on the *left* and an example with clear regional dysfunction is shown on the *right*.

sentative cycle are used to calculate the LVEF using the same formula as that described previously for EqRNA. Left ventricular ejection fractions calculated by this measurement technique have correlated closely with ejection fractions measured during cardiac catheterization (103, 106, 107). Systolic ejection rates and diastolic filling parameters are also calculated from the representative cycle.

The accuracy of the first-pass LVEF is directly related to the statistical content of the data. The error in the measurement increases as the end-diastolic counts in the representative cycle decreases (108).

Although most exercise studies performed using bicycle exercise are free of major cardiac motion, mild degrees of motion occur frequently. A motion correction scheme can be applied to the representative cycle that uses a center of mass algorithm to identify the location of the ventricle throughout the LV phase and which then corrects each frame of the representative cycle accordingly.

Right Ventricular Function

The first-pass technique is the method of choice for measurement of right ventricular ejection fraction because of the ability to acquire the study in the RAO view, which maximizes right atrial-right ventricular separation (109). Despite that advantage, early studies using FPRNA reported RV ejection fractions that were as low as those reported using EqRNA (110). The cause of the low first-pass RV ejection fractions was the use of a single ROI drawn at end-diastole. Although the bolus does provide temporal separation of chambers, there is still a large quantity of activity in the right atrium during the majority of the RV phase. At RV end systole, the tricuspid valve moves toward the ventricle and a substantial portion of the right atrium, which is at its largest volume at that point, lies within an end-diastolic ROI drawn around the RV. Attempts to correct for atrial background by drawing a variable sized background ROI over the right atrium do not completely solve the problem. The solution is to calculate the RVEF using both end-diastolic and end-systolic ROI (109) (Fig. 24.24).

Right Ventricular Time-Activity Curve

In a typical FPRNA study performed for evaluation of the LV, the bolus is injected rapidly and the RV time-activity curve frequently contains 3 or 4 beats at most. Furthermore, there may be an inadequate amount of time for sufficient mixing to have taken place such that the concentration of the radionuclide in the RV is grossly different from beat to beat. The problem is compounded by exercise when tracer transit is very rapid, and by external jugular vein injections which result in rapid radionuclide delivery into the RV. As a result, it is occasionally impossible to generate statistically adequate RV data when the study was not acquired specifically for right ventricular analysis. Intentionally prolonging the injection will usually provide an adequate number of well-mixed beats for processing. Such prolongation of the bolus injection, however, may preclude a satisfactory LV study.

MEASUREMENT OF LEFT VENTRICULAR VOLUME

Geometric Method

As in EqRNA, left ventricular volume may be calculated by measuring the area of the LV and the length of the major axis in pixels. The pixel measurements can be converted to centimeters and the modified Sandler-Dodge equation (discussed earlier) can then be used to calculate LV volume. This approach has been validated (111). It is very dependent, however, on the criteria used for definition of the LV borders and upon the accuracy of the LV ROI.

Count-Proportional Methods

The reference volume approach described for EqRNA data has been successfully applied to first-pass data as well. The variables that must be measured include the total counts in the LV (T) and the counts in the hottest pixel in the LV (Nmax). With the size of a pixel (m) as a given, the volume of the LV is calculated as

$$\tfrac{1}{3}\,(T/Nmax-3.5)^{3/2}m^3$$

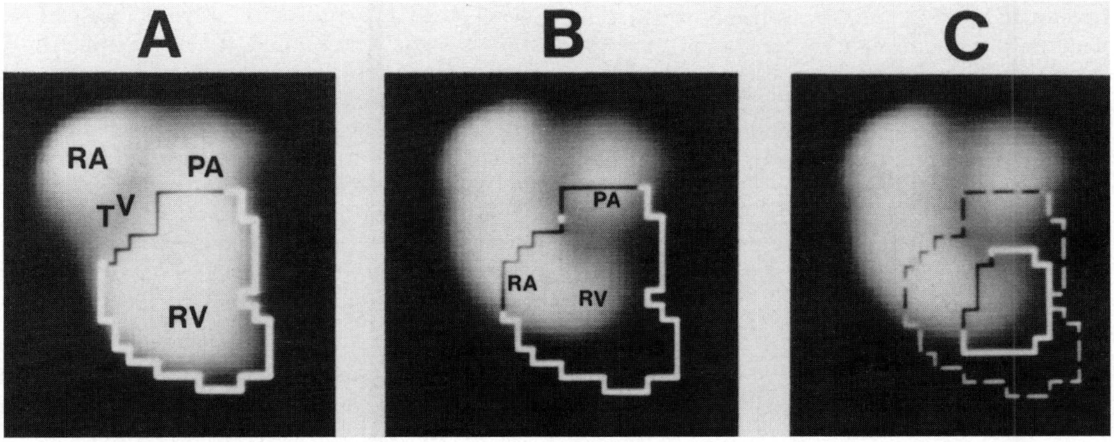

Figure 24.24. As indicated in Figure 24.21 for the LV, RV processing is best accomplished by using separate end-diastolic and end-systolic ROI. In panel **A,** a ROI is drawn around the RV at end-diastole. In panel **B,** the end-systolic frame is shown with the ROI from panel A. Note the inclusion of right atrial (*RA*) and pulmonary arterial (*PA*) activity within the ROI. Inclusion of that much nonventricular activity in a single end-diastolic ROI would underestimate the true RVEF. In panel **C,** a separate end-systolic ROI is drawn which excludes the atrial and pulmonary atrial activity.

The correlation coefficient between end-diastolic volume measured with that approach and the end-diastolic volume measured at cardiac catheterization exceeded 0.93 for both multi- and single-crystal systems (112). The standard error of the estimate for end-diastolic volume is ±35 ml. The stroke volume may then be calculated as the product of end-diastolic volume and ejection fraction and cardiac output as the product of the stroke volume and the heart rate.

Measurement of Pulmonary Transit Time and Pulmonary Blood Volume

The transit time between any two chambers may be calculated by generating a time-activity curve from the chambers of interest and measuring the time between the peaks of the curves (113). The mean transit time through the pulmonary circulation is calculated as the difference between the mean transit times of the pulmonary artery and the left atrium.

The product of the pulmonary mean transit time and the cardiac output is the pulmonary blood volume. Although, the pulmonary blood volume has not received widespread clinical application, it has been shown that an increase in pulmonary blood volume from rest to exercise may be used as a criterion for the diagnosis of coronary artery disease (114). In one study, an increase of more than 1.06 in the ratio of pulmonary blood volumes from exercise to rest had a sensitivity of 79% and a specificity of 100% in the detection of coronary artery disease involving the left ventricle (115). Other studies, though, have failed to confirm that clinical correlation.

DATA ANALYSIS AND INTERPRETATION

Normal Anatomy and Tracer Transit

The analysis of tracer transit through the central circulation is unique to first-pass RNA. The expected sequential appearance of the radionuclide in the superior vena cava, right atrium, right ventricle, pulmonary circulation, left side of the heart, and then the aorta should be confirmed in every study. Deviations from that sequence may indicate a congenital abnormality (Fig. 24.25). In the absence of a prolonged injection, prolongation of tracer transit through the right heart suggests pulmonary hypertension, tricuspid or pulmonary valve insufficiency, or a left-to-right intracardiac shunt. With a good bolus injection and normal tracer transit through the right heart and lungs, prolonged tracer transit through the left heart suggests mitral or aortic insufficiency or a left-to-right shunt. Left side valvular insufficiency can be quantified from first-pass data using a stroke count approach or a curve analysis technique.

Left Ventricular Systolic Function

The evaluation of both systolic and diastolic ventricular function begins with the inspection of the time-activity curve of the left ventricular ROI. Review of the beat selection, the background frame selection, and, in the case of the exercise study, the presence of cardiac motion, is important for the quality control of each study. Otherwise, the definitions and principles presented for the analysis of systolic function using EqRNA apply to first-pass data as well.

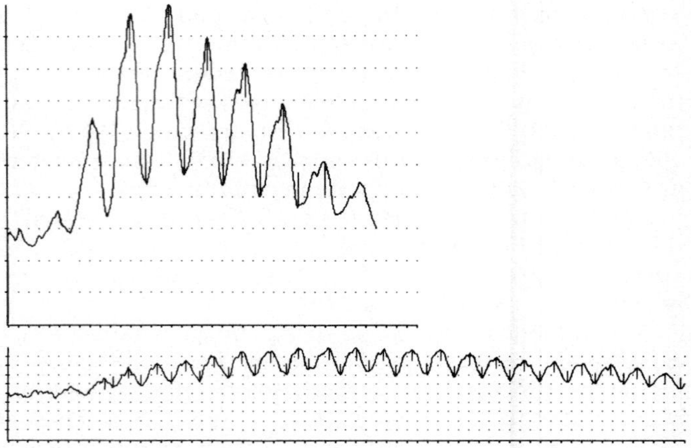

Figure 24.25. Visualizing tracer transit is helpful in detecting valvular insufficiency. Normal tracer transit through the left ventricle is shown *above* and markedly prolonged left ventricular tracer transit due to left sided valvular insufficiency is shown *below*. Correlation with the images may permit the Interpreter to distinguish between mitral and aortic insufficiency based on an enlarged left atrium or ascending aorta, respectively.

In the anterior first-pass left ventriculogram, the anterolateral, apical, and inferoseptal walls are visible. In an RAO first-pass left ventriculogram, the anterior, apical, and inferior walls are visible. The correlation between regional wall motion in the RAO first-pass study and wall motion in contrast ventriculography has been shown to be clinically acceptable (95). The weakest correlation occurred in the inferior wall which is probably due to the not uncommon oversubtraction of inferior wall activity when frames that contain right ventricular activity are chosen for the background correction. When background activity is very high, as occurs when there is considerable RV activity persisting through the LV phase, it may be impossible to accurately background correct the data without seriously oversubtracting LV activity causing LVEF to rise spuriously, volume to decrease, and wall motion to appear better than it may be. In such cases, it is advisable to view the cinematic display of the representative cycle without any background subtraction to assess regional wall motion. Since the first pass study is acquired in only one projection, and resolution is somewhat limited, it may be difficult to separate regional wall motion abnormalities in contiguous or overlapping segments. One typical example of that shortcoming is the appearance of anterior hypokinesia on a study acquired in the anterior view in a subject whose pathology actually involves the circumflex coronary artery. In this case, the three-dimensional effect of the posterior wall motion is interpreted in two-dimensional analysis as a problem with the anterior wall.

Parametric Images

As described earlier for EqRNA, a variety of parametric images can be generated to assist in the analysis of regional ventricular function. Phase and amplitude, stroke volume, regional ejection fraction, and mean transit time images may be helpful in certain clinical situations. They have the advantage of being more representative of the three-dimensional changes in counts throughout the ventricle than the cinematic display of the representative cycle. However, parametric images require very high count rates for accuracy. The potential diagnostic benefits of high count density parametric images have been thoroughly described (116).

Left Ventricular Diastolic Function

The same approach used for evaluating diastolic function in EqRNA studies may be applied to first-pass data as well. First-pass studies are usually acquired at frame rates fast enough for the evaluation of diastole. A frame time of 25 msec is roughly equivalent to a 32 frames/cycle gated acquisition at a heart rate of 60 beats/min (frame time 31 msec). The peak diastolic filling rate (PFR), the time to peak filling rate (tPFR), and filling fractions may all be calculated (117, 118). Because of the potential sensitivity of those measurements to the changing concentration of the radionuclide during the LV phase, it is considered important to select beats from both the ascending and descending limbs of the left ventricular time-activity curve.

Assessment of Valvular Insufficiency

As indicated earlier, prolongation of tracer transit through the left heart is typical of mitral or aortic insufficiency. Using the pulmonary time-activity curve as a monoexponential input function, the left ventricular time-activity curve may be deconvoluted so that the primary LV curve and the contribution from the regurgitation may be quantified. The degree of insufficiency calculated in that fashion has been correlated with standard invasive data (119). Others have taken a similar approach to that used in EqRNA and compared the total stroke count outputs of the left and right ventricles. The correlation between regurgitant fractions measured in that way and those measured at catheterization was 0.86 (120). Others have attempted to quantify tricuspid insufficiency (121).

Left-to-Right Shunts

The application of radionuclides to the detection and quantitation of intra- and extracardiac shunts is an extension of indicator dilution theory. Any measurable, nondiffusible indicator injected into the central circulation has a finite circulation time and a typical monoexponential appearance and disappearance when sampled downstream from the injection site. The agent classically used in the catheterization laboratory was indocyanine green whose concentration could be measured with a densitometer (122). In the case of an intracardiac left-to-right shunt as occurs with atrial and ventricular septal defects, injection of an indicator proximal to the shunt with sampling distal to the shunt yields a curve that is not monoexponential due to the early reappearance of the indicator that is shunted through the defect. The FPRNA can be used to create such a curve after injection of the indicator, in this case a radionuclide, into a peripheral vein with sampling downstream represented by the externally recorded appearance and clearance of the tracer in the lungs. Standard curve analysis techniques, such as the exponential and γ variate mathematical fits, can then be performed on a pulmonary time activity curve to separate that curve into a primary component and a shunt component. The areas of those two components are proportional to systemic and shunt flows and allow calculation of the ratio of pulmonary to systemic flow, or Qp/Qs, which is an index of the severity of the shunt (Figs. 24.26 and 24.27). With that type of analysis, shunts with a Qp/Qs as small as 1.2/1 have been accurately detected. The early reports using this technique showed excellent correlations with invasive oximetry readings (123, 124).

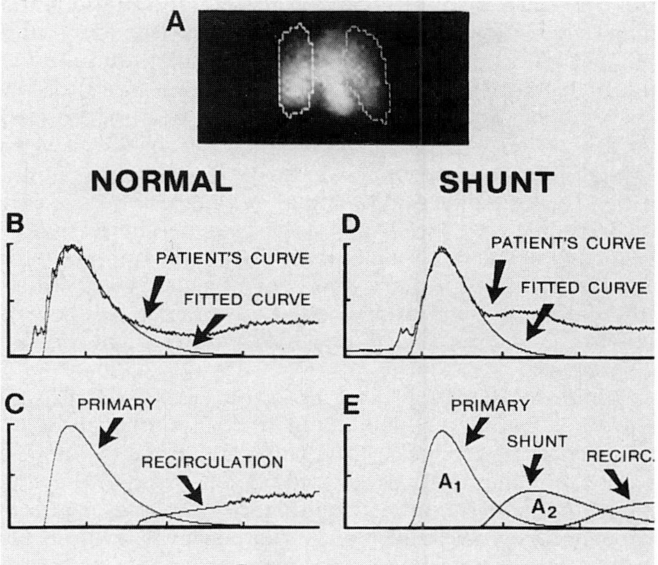

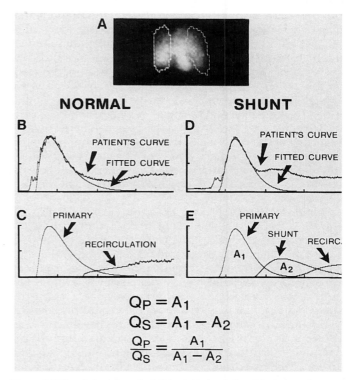

$$Q_P = A_1$$
$$Q_S = A_1 - A_2$$
$$\frac{Q_P}{Q_S} = \frac{A_1}{A_1 - A_2}$$

Figure 24.26. Calculation of a left-to-right shunt. Panel **A** shows a frame of the first-pass study selected because of the clear definition of the pulmonary activity. Manually drawn ROI are placed around each lung. The time-activity curve from the pulmonary ROI is indicated in panels **B** and **D** as the patient's curve. The superimposed mathematical fit is also shown. Panels **C** and **E** show the fitted curves alone. The areas *A1* and *A2* are used to calculate the Qp/Qs.

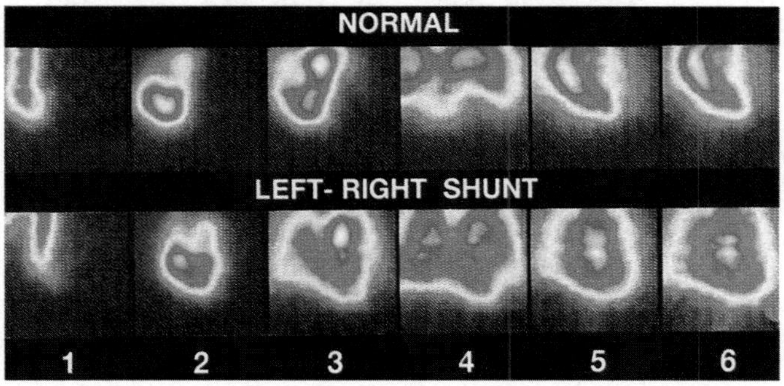

Figure 24.27. Serial images of a normal patient and a patient with a left-to-right intracardiac shunt are shown. Images 1–4 show the tracer appearing in the SVC, RA, RV, and lungs in both patients. In images 5 and 6, the normal patient shows a clearly identifiable LV chamber whereas the patient with the shunt shows activity in both ventricles because the tracer crosses from left to right at the same time it appears in the LV. No clear LV chamber can be identified. When the serial images show an LV phase as clearly as it is shown in the normal example here, a significant left-to-right intracardiac shunt is excluded.

For detection and quantitation of left-to-right shunts, pulmonary time-activity curves from the right lung, left lung, and, if necessary for adequate statistics, both lungs, may be analyzed. The right lung will usually provide the best time-activity curve for shunt analysis because it is most removed from the LV and thoracic aorta whose cyclic changes in activity can confound monoexponential curve analysis. Variability is to be expected since the curves from the two lungs frequently have statistical fluctuations that may be interpreted as breaks in the curve due to a shunt. The patient's curve should be time-smoothed to minimize the high frequency statistical noise that causes incorrect curve fitting. The mathematical fit must be superimposed on the patient's curve so that the quality of the fit is assessed. It is not uncommon to have to adjust the point at which the fit begins and the point at which it ends to avoid incorrect results. The output of the analysis should include hardcopy of the patient's curves, the superimposed mathematically fitted primary and secondary curves, and the calculation of the pulmonary (Q_p) to systemic (Q_s) flow ratios for each lung and, if necessary, both lungs together (Fig. 24.26).

Accurate detection and quantitation of left-to-right shunts is completely dependent upon the integrity of the bolus entering the lung. If the bolus is delayed by virtue of a poor injection or by prolonged transit through the right heart as might occur with significant tricuspid or pulmonary insufficiency, then the pulmonary curve will deviate from a true monoexponential even without a shunt. In such a situation, it may be impossible to quantify a left-to-right shunt. However, it is almost always possible to visually confirm the presence of a left-to-right shunt. The sequential appearance of the radionuclide bolus in the right atrium, right ventricle, pulmonary circulation, and left ventricle is obvious on a normal study, and the left ventricular phase is typically free of any right ventricular activity. In the case of an intracardiac left-to-right shunt, activity appears in the right and left ventricles simultaneously so that a clear left ventricular phase cannot be identified (Fig. 24.28). Therefore, the presence of a clearly identifiable left ventricular image during the first-pass virtually excludes a significant intracardiac left-to-right shunt. A patent ductus arteriosus, however, does not involve the right ventricle and cannot be excluded by that visual method.

First-pass RNA has also been used to detect right-to-left shunts. By placing a ROI over a systemic artery that is uncontaminated by pulmonary activity, early appearance of a radionuclide bolus in the systemic circulation following intravenous injection is consistent with a right-to-left shunt (125). Right-to-left shunts are most often seen in congenital heart disease in children, and the preferred method for detection and quantitation remains the intravenous injection of macroaggregated albumin. A ratio is generated from the activity that bypasses the lung through the shunt to arrive in organs such as the brain and kidney and the activity in the lung (126).

CLINICAL APPLICATIONS OF VENTRICULAR FUNCTION IMAGING

Screening for Coronary Artery Disease

There are several conditions that must be met by a diagnostic test to warrant its application to screening for a particular condition. First, the test must have an adequate sensitivity for detection of the disease. Second, it must have a very high specificity for the absence of the condition.

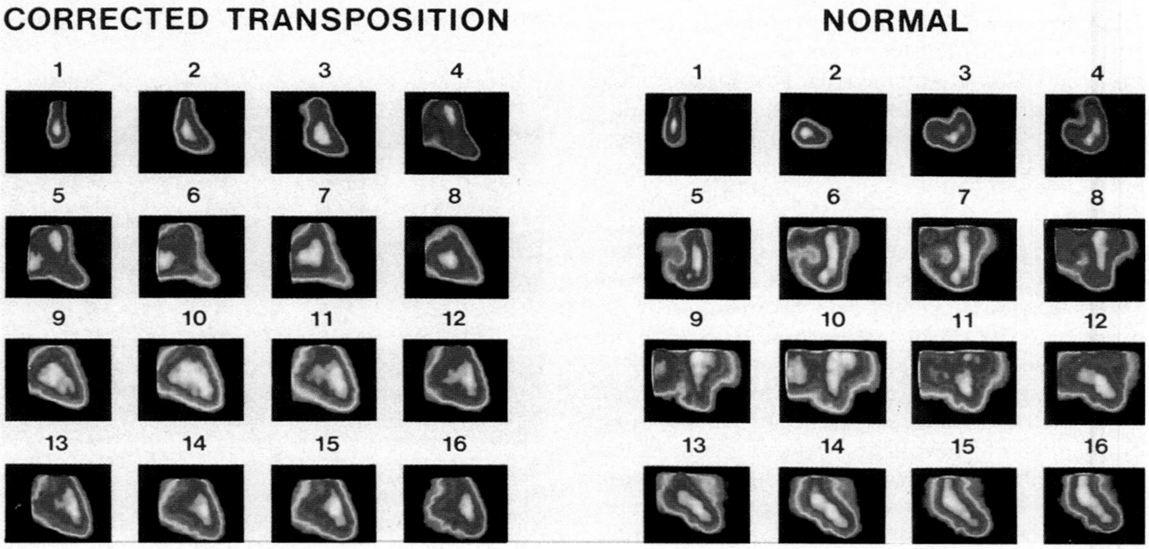

Figure 24.28. First-pass imaging enables one to examine the transit of a radionuclide bolus through the heart and great vessels. On the *right* is the normal sequence of superior vena cava, right atrium, right ventricle, lungs, left ventricle, and aorta. On the *left* is an example of corrected transposition where the venous ventricle has the morphologic appearance of a left ventricle and the systemic ventricle has the morphologic appearance of a right ventricle.

Third, one must have some idea of the disease prevalence in the population to be screened, because in the absence of 100% specificity, the lower the disease prevalence, the greater the number of false-positive test results. Fourth, since coronary disease has a wide range of potential severity, one must determine how severe the disease should be to be worth detecting. Fifth, the benefit of detecting the disease must outweigh any hazards that might occur during the testing for, or treatment of, the disease. Both EqRNA and FPRNA during stress fall far short of being an ideal screening test in all but populations in which the disease prevalence is very high. Consequently, screening for coronary artery disease with stress radionuclide ventricular function studies in an average population cannot be recommended.

Diagnosis of Coronary Artery Disease

When coronary blood flow is lower than the demand for flow, the ischemic cascade is initiated. Regional metabolic dysfunction ensues which leads to regional mechanical dysfunction which may then, if enough myocardium is involved, lead to global ventricular dysfunction. Electrocardiographic changes and symptoms tend to occur last. Since radionuclide ventriculography is an excellent test for the detection of regional and global ventricular dysfunction, it has been applied to the diagnosis of coronary artery disease. The typical ischemic response includes a new or worsened regional wall motion abnormality, an increase in end-systolic volume, a decrease in ejection fraction, a variable increase in end-diastolic volume, and alterations of diastolic filling. However, all or none of those responses may occur depending on the amount of myocardium rendered ischemic.

Left Ventricular Ejection Fraction Response to Exercise

Early experience with exercise RNA suggested that normal subjects increase their LVEF by at least 0.05 during dynamic exercise. Failure to increase the LVEF by at least 0.05 became a criterion for the diagnosis of coronary artery disease and reports appeared suggesting that use of that criterion had an extremely high sensitivity for the diagnosis of coronary disease. (127–130). However, as indicated earlier, localized ischemia may occur without any change in ejection fraction or end-diastolic volume if the overwhelming majority of the ventricle is not ischemic and contracting vigorously. Furthermore, after much more experience with exercise RNA, it is clear that there are many reasons for the ejection fraction failing to increase by at least 0.05 during exercise. Men and women appear to respond differently to exercise with men relying more upon a decrease in end-systolic volume and a concomitant increase in ejection fraction, and women relying more on an increase in end-diastolic volume and less on increasing ejection fraction (131, 132). Healthy older volunteers appear to have blunted ejection fraction responses to exercise (133). Isometric exercise results in an acute drop in ejection fraction (134) and the type of exercise protocol may have a dramatic effect on the ejection fraction response to exercise (135). Additionally, the resting ejection fraction appears to influence the ejection fraction response to exercise (136). The ejection fraction response may be altered by severe hypertension or by valvular heart disease. An inadequate exercise effort, defined as a rate-pressure product of 25,000, may also decrease the sensitivity for coronary disease (137). As a result of the numerous factors that can affect the left ventricular ejection fraction other than coronary artery disease, the use of ejection fraction criteria for the diagnosis of coronary artery disease has poor specificity (114, 138). In the largest study on the subject, the specificity for diagnosis of coronary artery disease of a failure to increase the LVEF during exercise by at least 0.05 had a specificity of 79%. Sensitivity was fairly high at 89% (138). As a result, some investigators have used regression equations to predict the ejection fraction response in a given subject based upon age, sex, and other criteria, including the end-diastolic volume. The diagnosis of coronary disease could then be made when the actual LVEF response was lower than that predicted (139). Another criterion for diagnosis is an exercise ejection fraction that is lower than the lowest exercise ejection fraction of a normal age-matched reference population. As indicated previously, however, any ejection fraction criterion is bound to have poor specificity.

Although ejection fraction criteria do not perform well for the diagnosis of any coronary involvement, exercise RNA has been used successfully to distinguish severe coronary disease from mild or no disease. In general, exercise LVEF varies inversely with the extent and severity of the coronary disease (138, 140). As a result, exercise LVEF can be used to identify patients with a large ischemic burden, those most likely to have multivessel or left main disease (141–143), and those most likely to benefit from revascularization procedures (144).

Regional Wall Motion

In direct contrast to abnormalities of the global ejection fraction during exercise, the detection of a regional abnormality of ventricular function either at rest or during exercise is highly specific for coronary artery disease. Regional dysfunction may be seen in certain cardiomyopathies but that is exceptionally rare. The specificity of a new or worsened regional wall motion abnormality during exercise has been reported to be as high as 93% (138). Unfortunately, the sensitivity of an exercise-induced wall motion abnormality is quite low in part due to the fact that exercise RNA is usually performed in only one view and in part due to the spatial resolution of the exercise RNA which is limited by statistics in the case of the EqRNA and by the lower intrinsic resolution in the case of the FPRNA. As indicated previously, various parametric images may be used to assist in detecting regional ventricular dysfunction. However, no large prospective studies have been performed to rigorously test their performance in the diagnosis of coronary artery disease.

Although not typically applied as diagnostic criteria, abnormalities of diastolic function are common in patients with coronary artery disease due to the impairment in ventricular relaxation seen with ischemia. Reduced and delayed peak filling rates, as well as decreased first-third filling fractions, have been described in patients with coronary disease, including those with normal systolic function (73, 145, 146). When blood flow is normalized, diastolic function may improve (147).

Pharmacologic Interventions

A large body of evidence exists that supports the diagnostic sensitivity and specificity of myocardial perfusion imaging in conjunction with the use of the coronary vasodilators dipyridamole (148, 149) and adenosine (150). There is also evidence to suggest that catecholamine administration coupled with myocardial perfusion imaging is useful for detecting coronary disease (151). There is considerably less evidence that ventricular function imaging during pharmacologic stimulation is useful diagnostically. Some investigators have found fairly high sensitivity for detection of disease by performing echocardiography during coronary vasodilation (152, 153) or during dobutamine infusion (154, 155). EqRNA has been found to be modestly sensitive but quite specific for the diagnosis of coronary disease when performed after a dipyridamole infusion (156), and was recently performed with some success during dobutamine infusion (157).

Combined Function-Perfusion Imaging

Early attempts at combined function-perfusion imaging used the simultaneous injection of ultra-short-lived radionuclides, such as ^{195m}Au (158) and ^{191}Ir (159), along with ^{201}Tl. With that approach, a first-pass study could be acquired during the injection and a perfusion image could be acquired soon thereafter when the gold or iridium had decayed to background levels. Difficulties with the generators for gold and iridium prevented widespread application of those techniques.

The advent of the technetium perfusion imaging agents makes it possible to perform combined ventricular function and myocardial perfusion imaging with a single radionuclide injection. At the time of injection of the radionuclide, a first-pass study can be acquired and perfusion imaging can be performed subsequently (83–87). The combined study can provide all the regional and global functional information and quantitative SPECT perfusion data. The functional impact of any given perfusion abnormality can be directly and quantitatively assessed. Preliminary evidence suggests that diagnostic sensitivity is enhanced using the combined approach (84). Routine addition of function to perfusion imaging appears to improve the detection of multivessel disease compared to the perfusion data alone (160). Additionally, diagnostic confidence is enhanced with the availability of both function and perfusion data. Perhaps most importantly, the addition of functional data adds the rest and/or exercise LVEF, two prognostically powerful variables in patients with coronary disease.

Another approach to combining function and perfusion data is to gate the SPECT perfusion acquisition. Because of the generally low statistics in SPECT studies using ^{201}Tl, gated SPECT for analysis of ventricular function has been performed exclusively with technetium perfusion agents. However, given the potentially high count rates obtainable with multiheaded detectors, gating SPECT thallium images may become more viable. Gating the SPECT acquisition allows a tomographic display of the changes in regional wall motion and wall thickening throughout the cardiac cycle. Qualitative assessment of regional wall motion and thickening from gated SPECT studies compares favorably to a similar assessment using echocardiography (161, 162). There has been some indication that LVEF can be measured using gated SPECT (163).

ASSESSMENT OF PROGNOSIS IN CHRONIC STABLE CORONARY ARTERY DISEASE

It has long been appreciated that the prognosis of patients with stable coronary artery disease is directly related to the contractile state of the left ventricle. Large series of both medically and surgically treated patients have been followed for several years, and the data from different investigators confirm that the resting left ventricular ejection fraction measured either invasively or noninvasively is a powerful predictor of subsequent outcome (164, 165). After the introduction of rest and exercise radionuclide angiography, a large series of patients with stable coronary artery disease was followed during medical management after baseline catheterization and rest and exercise RNA were obtained. As noted in previous studies, the resting radionuclide LVEF was a powerful predictor of subsequent outcome. However, the peak exercise LVEF proved to be even more powerful in predicting subsequent mortality (166, 167). The change in ejection fraction from rest to exercise was of no prognostic significance when a multivariable analysis was performed. Furthermore, when the radionuclide data were compared to the clinical and catheterization-derived variables, it was shown that the combination

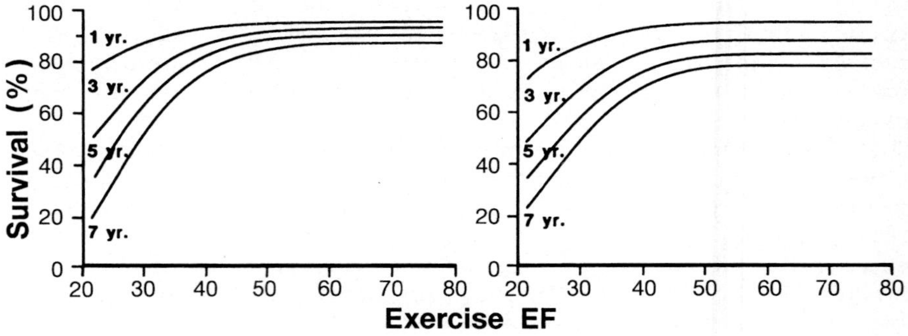

Figure 24.29. Overall survival (*left*) and infarct-free survival (*right*) are shown plotted against the exercise first-pass LVEF. Survival rates decrease rapidly once the exercise LVEF drops below 0.35. (Courtesy of Dr. Robert Jones.)

of the exercise ejection fraction and the clinical data contained almost all the prognostic information available from a catheterization. Figure 24.29 shows mortality plotted against the exercise ejection fraction. Patients with an exercise LVEF 0.50 have an excellent long-term outlook. Mortality begins to increase sharply once LVEF drops below 0.35. In a much smaller patient group, and using EqRNA, the resting LVEF proved to be a more important predictor of outcome than the exercise LVEF (168).

Other investigators have suggested that the change in the ejection fraction from rest to exercise is prognostically important. In a study of patients with three-vessel CAD who were mildly symptomatic, those subjects whose LVEF fell during exercise had more subsequent events than those subjects whose LVEF did not fall during exercise (169). In that study, all patients who died showed a decrease in LVEF and at least 1 mm of ST segment depression during exercise. Although there is some controversy about which of the three variables, resting LVEF, exercise LVEF, and the exercise-rest LVEF is most important in differing patient populations, there is certainly universal agreement that the LVEF can be used to stratify patients into high, low, and intermediate probabilities for subsequent cardiac events.

As yet, no prospective study has been performed that used the results of exercise radionuclide angiography to assign patients to medical or revascularization treatment strategies. In a nonprospective, nonrandomized study of subjects with normal resting LV function, it was shown that those subjects with the greatest fall in LVEF during exercise preoperatively showed the most benefit in terms of pain relief and longevity following bypass surgery (144). That type of data suggests that the exercise RNA can be used for segregating patients into those who should be treated medically and those who should receive some interventional strategy. Of note is the fact that there are no data on the clinical value of routine exercise RNA following coronary bypass surgery, especially in asymptomatic subjects, even though the prognostic power of the rest and exercise LVEF appears to be the same postoperatively as it is in patients with medically treated coronary disease.

ASSESSMENT OF ACUTE MYOCARDIAL INFARCTION

Diagnosis

The diagnosis of an acute MI is made by the history, the electrocardiogram, and the serum isoenzyme levels. Radionuclide angiography is not typically indicated for the diagnosis of acute MI, but in cases where there is diagnostic uncertainty, an assessment of ventricular function, specifically to detect any regional wall motion abnormality, can be very helpful. Of course, prior infarction cannot be distinguished from acutely infarcted myocardium.

Radionuclide angiography performed in patients who have sustained an acute myocardial infarction can be used to localize and size the infarct, diagnose coexistent complications such as right ventricular infarction or a ruptured interventricular septum, and predict both the short-term, in-hospital event rate and subsequent posthospital event rate. For a resting study during an acute MI, an EqRNA is preferred since it allows one to assess all the segments of both ventricles. During inferior wall infarction, it is advisable to acquire a first pass study during the injection of the labeled red cells or the technetium pertechnetate (in the case of in vivo labeling). The first-pass portion of the study provides the best measurement of RVEF and the gated portion of the study provides the high resolution wall motion assessment of the right and left ventricles and the LVEF. Having the first-pass study available also allows detection and quantitation of any shunt due to a ruptured septum.

Right Ventricular Infarction

It has been shown that over 30% of inferior wall infarctions are accompanied by right ventricular infarction (170). There is a broad spectrum of right ventricular involvement in acute inferior infarction. There may be mild, clinically silent, incidental RV dysfunction detected with an RNA or an echocardiographic study, or severe global RV dysfunction and minimal LV dysfunction. The entire gamut of findings between those two extremes may be encountered (171). The clinical criteria for RV infarction include ST segment elevation in right-sided precordial ECG leads and an elevated right atrial or RV end-diastolic pressure, which may exceed the LV pulmonary capillary wedge pressure (172). Scintigraphic methods for the detection of RV infarction include RV uptake of technetium pyrophosphate and regional and global RV dysfunction on RNA. The advantage of the RNA is that it not only identifies the RV infarct but defines its extent and severity. However, even apparently severe RV dysfunction during inferior infarction may not be accompanied by any hemodynamic derangement (173). It has been shown repeatedly that RV dysfunction associated with an acute inferior infarction frequently improves over time even without revascularization. Even severe RV dysfunction may improve in a matter of days (174), although usually, the more severe, the longer the time to recovery, and, on occasion, the RV dysfunction will never resolve. The fact that severe RV dysfunction may improve with time suggests that what has traditionally been called RV infarction may frequently represent stunning rather than infarction (Fig. 24.30).

Ruptured Septum and Acute Mitral Regurgitation

A ruptured interventricular septum is an uncommon but catastrophic complication of acute infarction, more often inferior infarction. The diagnosis may be established at the bedside by detecting an oxygen step-up in the RV or pulmonary artery, by demonstration of flow across the septum using Doppler echocardiography or by detection of a left-to-right shunt using RNA. Because of its widespread availability and increasing clinical experience, echocardiography is probably the test of choice in this setting. The same is true for mitral regurgitation due to papillary muscle dysfunction or frank rupture.

Assessment of Prognosis

The resting radionuclide left ventricular ejection fraction acquired at bedside early in the course of acute myocardial

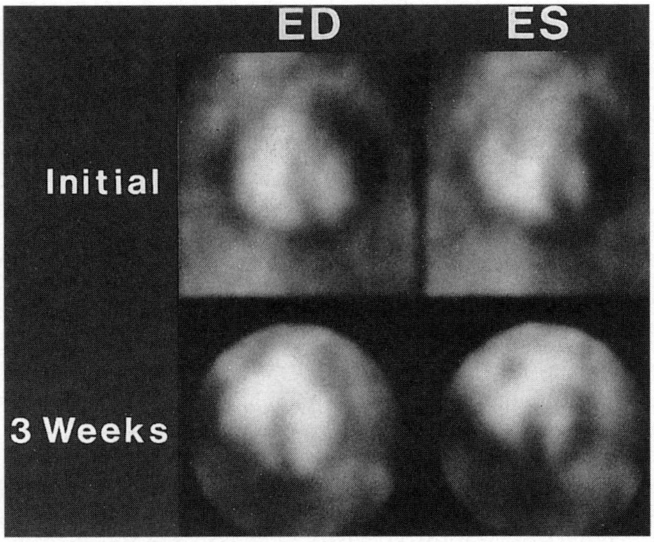

Figure 24.30. The EqRNA at the *top* was acquired soon after the patient presented with what appeared to be an inferior wall MI. The study suggested that the MI was primarily right ventricular in location. In this case, in which a thrombolytic was not administered, there is spontaneous improvement in RV function 3 weeks after the initial event.

infarction has been used to risk stratify patients into groups with varying probabilities of death or ventricular fibrillation during their hospitalization (175). The identification of coexisting RV infarction recently was shown to carry a worse short- and long-term prognosis compared to those patients without RV infarction (176). For those patients that survive their infarcts, RNA has been used to predict subsequent outcome. As in patients with stable coronary artery disease, both the resting (177) and the exercise LVEF (178, 179) have been shown to be highly predictive of subsequent event rates. Predischarge stress RNA has also been used to discriminate between subjects with low and high risks for future events and performs better than stress ECG in that capacity (180–183). There is, however, little data that addresses the role of stress RNA after infarction in the thrombolytic era. Considerably more focus has been given to the use of perfusion imaging for assessment of residual myocardial viability in the infarct area and detection of ischemia in segments remote from the infarct very soon after successful thrombolysis so that rapid decisions can be made regarding the need for catheterization and possible revascularization.

Assessment of Patients after PTCA

It is not surprising that those subjects who demonstrated an abnormal response to exercise pre-PTCA, would show improved left ventricular function following successful PTCA (184). Additionally, it has been shown that those patients whose LVEF or regional wall motion was abnormal during exercise soon after PTCA has a higher subsequent restenosis rate (185). Despite those findings, most post-PTCA patients have been followed with SPECT myocardial perfusion imaging because that type of imaging lends itself to more exact identification of the vascular territory involved.

Assessment of Myocardial Viability

The assessment of myocardial viability plays an important role in patients with coronary artery disease. In either stunned or hibernating myocardium, severe ventricular dysfunction that is typical of infarcted, nonviable myocardium may be present even though the myocardium is still viable. Identification of such tissue has become increasingly important since contractile function may be improved by restoration of blood flow. Despite, the profoundly depressed baseline function of stunned or hibernating myocardium, the viability of such muscle can be confirmed by demonstrating transiently improved function following acute afterload reduction, ventricular extrasystoles, inotropic stimulation, and immediately following cessation of exercise.

Systolic function of severely hypokinetic segments may improve after administration of nitroglycerin. Originally described during contrast ventriculography, the technique has been has also been performed using radionuclide angiography (186, 187). Improved function following nitroglycerin administration is a marker for improvement after revascularization. Catecholamines were also initially used in the catheterization lab to demonstrate inotropic reserve in severely depressed myocardial segments (188). More recently, low dose dobutamine infusions have been performed during echocardiographic examination to detect viable muscle. Radionuclide angiography could be used in place of echocardiography although some would argue that the ability to visualize wall thickening is an important part of the assessment of the catecholamine response (189–191). Immediately following cessation of exercise, there is an increase in ejection fraction and an improvement in the systolic function of myocardial segments that were severely abnormal at rest and which remained so during exercise (20, 21, 135). Furthermore, identification of that response proved to be a marker for improvement in resting function following revascularization (22). The radionuclide assessment of myocardial viability using ventricular function analysis has been largely replaced by perfusion imaging protocols using either single photon or positron techniques. Whether perfusion and function should both be evaluated or whether one assessment should follow the other if the result is not conclusive has never been tested.

EVALUATION OF THE PATIENT WITH DYSPNEA OR CONGESTIVE HEART FAILURE

There are many causes of dyspnea, both cardiac and noncardiac, but when a cardiac cause of dyspnea is being considered and the physical examination does not suggest any significant valvular heart disease, then a resting and, if necessary, an exercise RNA can frequently provide a diagnosis. If resting LV and RV function are normal in a patient being evaluated for dyspnea, especially dyspnea on exertion, then an exercise study should be performed. It may be useful to combine RNA, spirometry, and respiratory gas exchange measurements as a so-called cardiopulmonary stress test so that both cardiac and pulmonary causes, as well as the relative contribution of each, may be assessed (192).

In recent years, increasing attention has been paid to diastolic LV function as a cause of shortness of breath or congestive heart failure (CHF). It has been estimated that isolated diastolic dysfunction may be the cause of 30% of cases diagnosed with CHF (193, 194). RNA is the procedure of choice for distinguishing systolic from diastolic causes of CHF. As indicated previously, diastolic dysfunction may be recognized visually by inspection of the left ventricular volume curve and may be quantified by measurement of the peak filling rate (PFR), the time-to-peak (tPFR) and the atrial contribution to filling (AFR).

CARDIOMYOPATHY

Idiopathic Dilated

As its name implies, the sine qua non of the idiopathic dilated cardiomyopathy is the finding of a dilated and diffusely hypocontractile left ventricle. Radionuclide angiography is an ideal method for establishing the diagnosis. No absolute threshold of LVEF has been identified below which the diagnosis of cardiomyopathy is unequivocal, but for practical purposes, given the range of variability in the resting LVEF measurement in normal subjects, an LVEF of ≤0.40, when accompanied by a visual impression of LV enlargement and diffuse hypokinesia, should be considered evidence of a dilated cardiomyopathy. The etiology of diffuse LV dysfunction may not be apparent from a radionuclide, or for that matter, any type of ventriculogram. Findings that may be helpful in distinguishing idiopathic from so-called ischemic cardiomyopathies include the status of the right ventricle and the presence of akinetic or dyskinetic segments. There tends to be more involvement of the right ventricle in idiopathic dilated myopathies than in ischemic myopathies. In fact, the ratio of left ventricular to right ventricular end-diastolic volume has been used to discriminate ischemic from nonischemic myopathies (195). However, one should recognize that right ventricular dysfunction is a frequent finding with any long-standing LV dysfunction regardless of the etiology. The presence of akinetic or dyskinetic LV segments is very suggestive of an ischemic rather than an idiopathic cardiomyopathy. Occasionally, infiltrative myopathies, such as ventricular dysplasia, or inflammatory myocardial disease, such as sarcoid, may cause localized akinesia or dyskinesia. Associated findings in dilated cardiomyopathies are dilatation of the left and right atria and enlargement of the pulmonary artery, the latter a sign of pulmonary hypertension and atrial fibrillation.

The exercise response may be helpful in distinguishing ischemic from nonischemic causes of diffuse LV dysfunction. When due to coronary disease, the diffusely hypokinetic ventricle typically results from three-vessel disease. During exercise, such ventricles fail to increase the ejection fraction and typically show a drop in LVEF. In contrast, it is quite typical for patients with idiopathic dilated myopathies to show substantial increases in LVEF during exercise (196). Our own clinical findings support that concept. We have seen a severely depressed LVEF at rest increase to an almost normal EF during exercise.

Hypertrophic Cardiomyopathy

The hypertrophic cardiomyopathies are characterized by abnormal thickening of all or part of the left ventricular myocardium in the absence of an identifiable cause. The two most common types are the asymmetric and symmetric varieties. The asymmetric type is much more commonly seen. There are various types of asymmetric hypertrophy, specifically apical, midventricular, and septal. The ventricular septal variety is commonly referred to as asymmetric septal hypertrophy (ASH), or previously as idiopathic hypertrophic subaortic stenosis in the presence of a subvalvular pressure gradient (197).

Subjects with hypertrophic cardiomyopathy typically have small end-diastolic volumes due to the thickened myocardium and their ejection fractions are, therefore, typically quite high. Consequently, their left ventricles appear to be hyperdynamic but there is no evidence that such ventricles have any intrinsically greater contractility than normal. In the left anterior oblique view, septal hypertrophy may be recognized on an EqRNA. On the basis of radionuclide data, it has been demonstrated that diastolic dysfunction is present in the majority of patients with hypertrophic cardiomyopathy. In fact, it is the diastolic dysfunction that accounts for most of the clinical symptomatology in these patients. Radionuclide ventriculography has been used to demonstrate improvement in diastolic function when patients with hypotrophic myopathy are treated with drugs such as calcium blockers which appear to have a direct effect on diastolic filling (198).

Restrictive Cardiomyopathy

In restrictive cardiomyopathy, the primary pathologic disturbance is the impairment of left ventricular diastolic filling. As such, radionuclide ventriculography may be used to assist in the diagnosis. A recent study suggested that radionuclide ventriculography could be helpful in distinguishing restrictive cardiomyopathy from constrictive pericardial disease (199). In restrictive disease, early diastolic filling is typically delayed and/or reduced whereas in constrictive disease, early diastolic filling tends to be more rapid than normal.

Doxorubicin (Adriamycin) Cardiotoxicity

In patients undergoing chemotherapy with adriamycin, there is a significant risk of developing cardiotoxicity which is characterized by a decrease in left ventricular systolic function. The cardiotoxicity is dose-related and is rarely seen at cumulative doses of under 400 mg/m^2, but may be seen at doses under 300 mg/m^2. Once the dose exceeds 500 mg/m^2, the probability of cardiotoxicity increases dramatically (200). Radionuclide ventriculography has become the procedure of choice for serial evaluation of patients during adriamycin therapy (201–203). The primary measurement is the LVEF at rest. A study should be performed prior to any therapy so that baseline LV function is known. Thereafter, studies may be repeated at the discretion of the oncologist, but once the cumulative dose exceeds 250 mg/m^2, more frequent follow-up is recommended. Once the dose reaches 450–500 mg/m^2, LVEF should be checked prior to each dose. A decrease in LVEF 10–15 EF units or a decrease to below 0.45 is considered significant. If a significant decrease in LVEF is documented and the clinical decision is to proceed with further therapy, then the LVEF should be measured prior to each dose.

When the radionuclide data are equivocal or when the cumulative dose exceeds 500 mg/m^2 without radionuclide evidence of toxicity, myocardial biopsy may be useful (204).

VALVULAR HEART DISEASE

The primary role of radionuclide angiography in valvular heart disease is the serial evaluation of left ventricular size and ejection fraction. As indicated previously, both FPRNA and EqRNA have been used to quantify valvular insufficiency using stroke count and curve analysis techniques but in practice, the simplicity and accuracy of Doppler echocardiography make it the test of choice for that purpose. In stenotic valvular lesions, the only established role of RNA is to evaluate LV and RV function.

Aortic and Mitral Insufficiency

Patients with aortic insufficiency should be followed with serial measurements of LVEF and LV volumes. There is sufficient evidence to indicate that when the resting LVEF drops below 0.50, the prognosis for recovery of LV function after valve replacement decreases. Furthermore, once the LVEF drops below 0.50, there is a significantly greater risk of patients becoming symptomatic or even developing heart failure (205) and once the LVEF drops below 0.40, there is a higher long-term mortality even after valve replacement (206). Echocardiographic measurements of the end-diastolic and end-systolic volumes are also predictive of subsequent outcome. Radionuclide volumes have not yet been used for that purpose. It has been shown that the LVEF may decrease during exercise in asymptomatic patients with aortic insufficiency (207, 208), but there is no convincing evidence that the exercise LVEF is of any prognostic significance.

In patients with mitral insufficiency, the LVEF has also been shown to be of prognostic value. The clinical outcome and postoperative mortality of patients undergoing mitral valve replacement for mitral insufficiency were related to the preoperative LVEF. As in aortic insufficiency, when the LVEF dropped below 0.50, the clinical outcome was poorer (209). Since mitral insufficiency causes ventricular unloading compared to aortic insufficiency, the measured LVEF may be less reflective of actual ventricular contractility. Following mitral valve replacement, it is common to see the LVEF fall since the ventricle must now contract solely against systemic resistance (210). As a result, a method of evaluating left ventricular contractile function that is independent of the loading conditions would be useful in patients with mitral insufficiency.

ASSESSMENT OF PATIENTS WITH CHRONIC OBSTRUCTIVE PULMONARY DISEASE

The major determinant of right ventricular function is its afterload, the pulmonary artery pressure or resistance. Elevated pulmonary artery pressures, either transient or chronic, will result in a decrease in right ventricular systolic function.

Right ventricular systolic function tends to be reduced in patients with pulmonary hypertension. The relationship is not, however, linear, since many subjects with pulmonary hypertension may maintain normal RV systolic function for some time. In the setting of chronic obstructive pulmonary disease (COPD), RVEF does tend to be lower than normal and is inversely related to the pulmonary hypertension (211). An abnormal resting RVEF in a patient with COPD may be predictive of subsequent cor pulmonale (212). Patients with COPD and normal RV function at rest may show abnormal responses of the RVEF to exercise (213, 214).

TRANSPLANTATION

Currently, the primary modality for the detection of rejection in the cardiac transplant recipient is the serial evaluation of transvenous endomyocardial biopsy samples. There may, however, be an adjunctive role for RNA. It recently was demonstrated that left ventricular systolic dysfunction may be apparent on a radionuclide study when the biopsy shows only mild rejection or no rejection. Discordance between the RNA and the biopsy only occurred in 6 of 95 cases (215, 216). Since there are other potential causes of systolic LV dysfunction, such as coronary disease or hypertension, it is unlikely that the RNA would be useful routinely.

CONGENITAL HEART DISEASE

Congenital heart disease may be detected and characterized with FPRNA in children (217, 218) and in adults (219). However, given the spatial resolution of echocardiography, magnetic resonance imaging, and fast-CT, there is little, if any, primary role for radionuclide studies in the anatomic description of congenital heart lesions. However, FPRNA may still play a significant role in the detection and quantitation of left-to-right shunts. Left-to-right shunts are reliably detected on a FPRNA study. As indicated previously, any significant intracardiac left-to-right shunt can be detected visually by the absence of a clear LV phase (Fig. 24.24). Quantitatively, shunts with a Qp/Qs of $<1.2/1$ cannot be reliably distinguished from normal.

Serial Evaluation of LV Function: Reproducibility of Radionuclide LVEF

As indicated earlier, the serial measurement of ejection fraction may be important for the longitudinal evaluation of disease progression or regression, the response to specific therapy, or the toxicity of agents like doxorubicin. Since it is noninvasive, accurate, and quantitative, radionuclide angiography is the technique of choice for this purpose. However, the serial application of RNA presupposes that the reproducibility of the study has been demonstrated. One must know how much change in LVEF is acceptable on the basis of technical and biologic variability before one can conclude that there has been a real change in ventricular function. Variability data are available for both first pass RNA and EqRNA (220–222). At rest, the first-pass LVEF showed a mean difference of 0.04 ± 0.04 between measurements in the same subjects on different days (207). For EqRNA, the mean differences for same day studies and separate day studies were 0.03 ± 0.03 and 0.04 ± 0.03 respectively (207). Of note is the finding that the variability was greater in subjects with normal ventricles (0.05 ± 0.04) than in those with reduced LV function (0.02 ± 0.02). Intraobserver and interobserver variability for processing the same data are inconsequential.

FPRNA VERSUS EqRNA

Historically, the choice of performing a first-pass or a gated study depended upon the type of gamma-camera and the particular software available. Currently, both FPRNA and EqRNA can be adequately performed with several different gamma-cameras, and most current computers are fast enough and have sufficient storage capacity to handle either type of data. Virtually all clinical applications have been performed with both techniques. The selection of a procedure should be dictated by the clinical question at hand. Laboratories should have both modalities available and should be familiar with the acquisition of both types of studies. In general, EqRNA offers a higher spatial resolution but a relatively prolonged acquisition time and can only provide quantitative data in the "best septal" view. The FPRNA trades spatial resolution for speed.

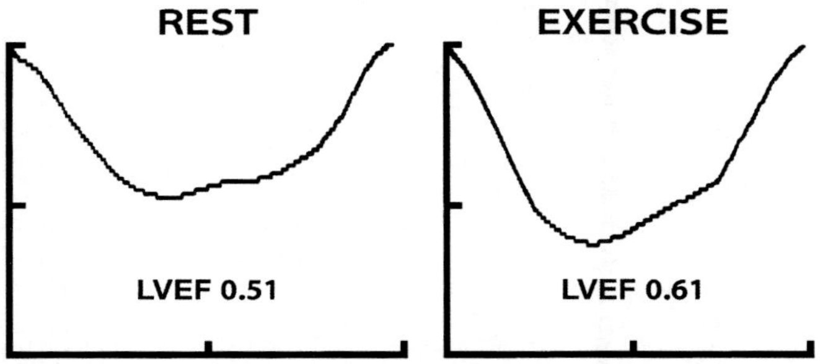

Figure 24.31. These curves were obtained in a man complaining of dyspnea on exertion. Regional wall motion and left ventricular ejection fractions were normal at rest and during exercise but diastolic dysfunction was obvious on both studies. When pulmonary causes of dyspnea are not apparent, rest and exercise ventricular function studies may be particularly helpful in identifying the cause. They may be combined with spirometry and blood gas measurements as a so-called cardiopulmonary stress test to quantify the relative contributions of the heart and lungs to the patient's dyspnea.

For most studies of left ventricular function at rest, the equilibrium method is preferred. At rest, time is not a significant factor, so the acquisition can be prolonged as much as necessary to achieve high count rates and maximum spatial resolution. Multiple views of the heart may be obtained. For the evaluation of RV function at rest, a combined FPRNA and EqRNA is recommended. The first-pass method remains the procedure of choice for measurement of RVEF while the EqRNA data offer better resolution of regional wall motion and multiple views.

During exercise, the speed of the first-pass study is a major advantage and FPRNA is, therefore, the procedure of choice for evaluation of LV function during exercise. When there is a specific question about ischemia in the circumflex distribution, an exercise EqRNA may be more appropriate than an exercise FPRNA because of the difficulty with left atrial-left ventricular overlap in LAO first-pass studies. The presence of arrhythmia such as very irregular atrial fibrillation, frequent premature beats or bigeminy is problematic for both techniques. FPRNA, however, is more susceptible to compromise by arrhythmia because of the paucity of beats available for analysis.

For the evaluation of diastolic LV function at rest, the EqRNA is preferred because of the ability to accumulate a large number of counts per frame throughout the cycle which decreases the percent error in the calculation of diastolic filling parameters (Figs. 24.31 and 24.32). FPRNA is certainly the preferred method of detecting and quantifying left-to-right shunts.

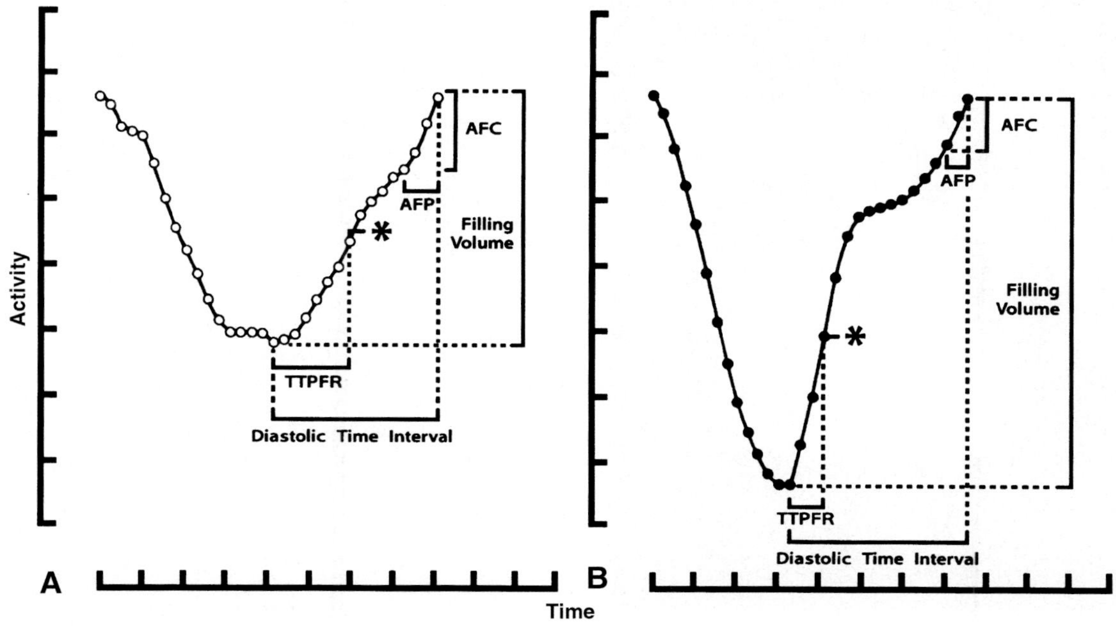

Figure 24.32. It has been suggested that radionuclide ventricular function imaging may be useful in distinguishing constrictive from restrictive heart disease. In restriction (panel **A**), early filling tends to be delayed thus prolonging the tPFR. In constriction (panel **B**), early filling is more rapid than usual thus shortening the tPFR. (With permission from Aroney CN, Ruddy TD, Dighero H, et al. Differentiation of restrictive cardiomyopathy from pericardial constriction: assessment of diastolic function by radionuclide angiography. J Am Coll Cardiol 1989;13:1007–1014.)

NONIMAGING PROBES

As yet, nonimaging probes have not assumed a significant role in clinical practice. They have been used successfully for research to evaluate changes in LV function in ambulatory subjects or to assess serial changes in LV function during spontaneous ischemic episodes in unstable patients. They have the benefit of displaying real-time variations in LV function, and have excellent temporal resolution. There are portable, freestanding units to assess the stationary patient, and there are miniaturized detectors that can be strapped to the patients chest for ambulatory monitoring.

Measurement of LVEF with the stationary probe correlates fairly well with values obtained with a standard gamma-camera. Correlations between 0.79 and 0.91 have been observed (223). Discordance is more common when there are regional wall motion abnormalities.

The miniaturized probes may be secured to the chest with a vest-like garment. Initial positioning of the probe is established with a standard gamma-camera and positioning is usually confirmed again when the acquisition is terminated. The LVEF measured with this type of probe has correlated well with the LVEF from a standard gamma-camera (224, 225). Reproducibility has been good with a correlation coefficient of 0.93 for sequential measurements in the same patients (226). With the aid of a patient recorder diary, changes in LV function may be correlated with normal activities in much the same manner as is done with a ambulatory ECG recordings. Silent ischemia may be readily detected with these particular probes (227), as well as changes in LV function during fluctuations in systolic pressure in hypertensives (228) (Fig. 24.33).

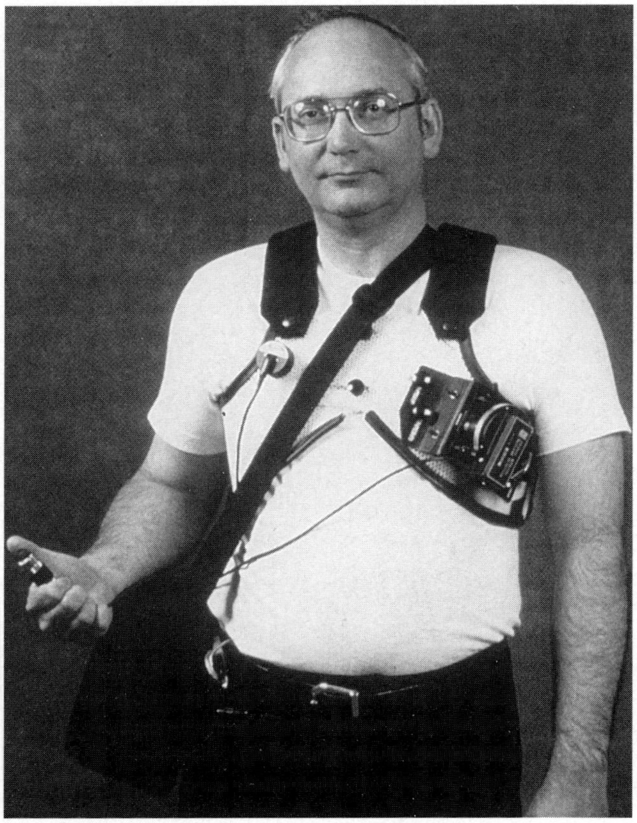

Figure 24.33. The "Vest" is a miniaturized nonimaging probe that has been used to evaluate changes in LVEF during routine daily activities and mental stress. (Courtesy of Capintec, Inc.)

REFERENCES

1. Strauss HW, Zaret BL, Hurley PJ, et al. A scintigraphic method for measuring left ventricular ejection fraction in man without cardiac catheterization. Am J Cardiol 1971;28:575–580.
2. Zaret BL, Strauss HW, Hurley PJ, et al. A noninvasive scintiphotographic method of detecting regional ventricular dysfunction in man. N Engl J Med 1971;284:1174–1180.
3. Strauss HW, McKusick KA, Boucher CA, et al. Of linens and laces—the eighth anniversary of the gated blood pool scan. Sem Nucl Med 1979;9:296–308.
4. Pavel DG, Zimmer AM, Patterson VN, et al. In vivo labeling of red blood cells with Tc-99m: a new approach to blood pool visualization. J Nucl Med 1979;18:308.
5. Thrall SH, Freitas JE, Swanson D, et al. Clinical comparison of cardiac blood pool visualization with technetium-99m red blood cells labeled in vivo and with technetium-99m human serum albumin. J Nucl Med 1978;19:796–803.
6. Lin M, Winchell HS, Shipley BA. Use of FE (II) or SN (II) alone for technetium labeling of albumin. J Nucl Med 1971;12:204–211.
7. Hamilton RG, Alderson PO. A comparative evaluation of techniques for rapid and efficient in vivo labeling of red blood cells with Tc-99m pertechnetate. J Nucl Med 1971;18:1010.
8. Kato M. In vivo labeling of red blood cells with Tc-99m with stannous pyridoxylideneamines. J Nucl Med 1979;20:1071.
9. Hegge FN, Hamiton GW, Larson SM, et al. Cardiac chamber imaging: a comparison of red blood cells labeled with Tc-99m invitro and in vivo. J Nucl Med 1978;19:129–134.
10. Callahan RG, Froelich JW, McKusick KA, et al. A modified method for the in vivo labeling of red blood cells with Tc-99m: concise communication. J Nucl Med 1982;23:315–318.
11. Parker DA, Karvelis KC, Thral JH, Froelich JW. Radionuclide ventriculography: methods. In: Gerson MC, ed. Cardiac nuclear medicine. New York: McGraw-Hill, 1991:84.
12. Hladik III WB, Nigg KK, Rhodes BA. Drug-induced changes in the biologic distribution of radiopharmaceuticals. Sem Nucl Med 1982;12:184–211.
13. Berthout P, Cardot JC, Faivre R, et al. Comparison between vertical parallel hole collimator and 30° rotating slant hole collimator for assessing global and regional left ventricular function by radionuclide angiography. Eur J Nucl Med 1988;14(3):120–124.
14. Juni JR, Chen CC. Effects of gating modes on the analysis of left ventricular function in the presence of heart rate variation. J Nucl Med 1988;29:1272–1278.
15. Bacharach SL, Green MV, Borer JS. Instrumentation in data processing in cardiovascular medicine: evaluation of ventricular function. Sem Nucl Med 1979;9:257–272.
16. Clements IP, Sinak LJ, Gibbons RG, et al. Determination of diastolic function by radionuclide ventriculography. Mayo Clin Proc 1990;65:1007–1019.
17. Sugrue DD, McKenny WJ, Dickie S, et al. Equilibrium radionuclide assessment of left ventricular ejection and filling. Comparison of list-mode and multi-gated frame mode measurements. Nucl Med Commun 1984;4:323–334.
18. Parker DA, Karvelis KC, Thral JH, Froelich AW. Radionuclide ventriculography: methods. In: Gerson MC, ed. Cardiac nuclear medicine. New York: McGraw-Hill, 1991:88–89.
19. Freeman MR, Berman DS, Staniloff H, et al. Comparison of up-

right supine bicycle exercise in the detection and evaluation of extent coronary artery disease by equilibrium radionuclide ventriculography. Am Heart J 1981;102:182–189.

20. Seaworth JF, Higginbotham MB, Coleman RE, Cobb FR. Effect of partial decreases in exercise work load on radionuclide indexes of ischemia. JACC 1983;2:522–529.
21. Rozanski A, Elkayam U, Berman DS, et al. Improvement of resting myocardial asynergy with cessation of upright bicycle exercise. Circulation 1983;67:529–535.
22. Rozanski A, Berman D, Gray R, Diamond G. Preoperative prediction of reversible myocardial asynergy by postexercise radionuclide ventriculography. N Engl J Med 1982;307:212–216.
23. Stratman HG, Kennedy HL. Evaluation of coronary artery disease in the patient unable to exercise: alternatives to exercise stress testing. Am Heart J 1989;117:1344–1365.
24. Stratton JR, Halter JB, Hallstrom AP, et al. Comparative plasma catecholamine and hemodynamic responses to hand grasp, cold pressor, and supine bicycle exercise testing in normal subjects. J Am Coll Cardiol 1983;2:93–104.
25. Vojacek J, Hannan WJ, Muir AL. Ventricular response to dynamic exercise and the cold pressor test. Eur Heart J 1982; 3:212–222.
26. McGillen MJ, DeBoe SF, Friedman HZ, Mancini GBJ. The effects of dopamine and dobutamine on regional function in the presence of rigid coronary stenoses and subclinical impairments of reactive hyperemia. Am Heart J 1988;115:970–977.
27. Iskandrian AS, Verani MS, Heo J. Pharmacologic stress testing: mechanism of action, hemodynamic responses, and results in detection of coronary artery disease. J Nucl Cardiol 1994;1:94–111.
28. Jensen FT, Lund O, Erlandsen M. Reliability of three computer methods in the analysis of ECG gated radionuclide left ventriculography: interrecording, interobserver, and intraobserver variability. Angiology 1991;42:866–877.
29. Bacharach SL, Green MV, Vitale D, et al. Optimum Fourier filtering of cardiac data: a minimum-error method: concise communication. J Nucl Med 1983;24:1176–1183.
30. Johnson LL, Marshall M, Johnson YE, et al. Radionuclide angiographic evaluation of left ventricular function by resting ejection rate during the first third of systole in patients with chronic aortic regurgitation. Am Heart J 1982;104:92–100.
31. Bacharach SL, Green MV, Borer JS, et al. Left ventricular peak ejection rate, filling rate, and ejection fraction—frame rate requirements at rest and exercise: concise communication. J Nucl Med 1979;20:189–193.
32. Maddahi J, Berman DS, Matsuoka DT, et al. A new technique for assessing right ventricular ejection fraction using rapid multiple-gated equilibrium blood pool scintigraphy: description, validation and findings in chronic coronary artery disease. Circulation 1979;60:581–589.
33. Winzelberg GG, Boucher CA, Prohous GM, et al. Right ventricular function in the aortic and mitral disease. Chest 1981; 79:520.
34. Spirito P, Maron BJ, Bonow RO. Noninvasive assessment of left ventricular diastolic function: comparative analysis of Doppler echocardiographic and radionuclide angiographic techniques. J Am Coll Cardiol 1986;7:518–526.
35. Bonow RO, Bacharach SL, Green MV, Kent KM. Impaired left ventricular diastolic filling in patients with coronary artery disease: assessment with radionuclide angiography. Circulation 1981;64:315–322.
36. Dodge HT, Sandler H, Baxley WA, Hawley RR. Usefulness and limitations of radiographic methods for determining left ventricular volume. Am J Cardiol 1966;18:10–24.
37. Sandler H, Dodge HT. The use of single plane angiocardiograms for the calculation of left ventricular volume in man. Am Heart J 1968;75:325–334.
38. Kennedy JW, Trenholme SE, Kasser IS. Left ventricular volume and mass from single-plane cineangiocardiogram. A comparison of anteroposterior and right anterior oblique methods. Am Heart J 1970;80:343–352.
39. Dehmer GJ, Lewis SE, Hillis LD, Twieg D. Nongeometric determination of left ventricular volumes from equilibrium blood pool scans. Am J Cardiol 1980;45:293–300.
40. Links JM, Becker LC, Shindledecker JG, Guzman P. Measurement of absolute left ventricular volume from gated blood pool studies. Circulation 1982;65:82–91.
41. Mauer AH, Siegel JA, Denenberg BS, Carabello BA. Absolute left ventricular volume from gated blood pool imaging with use of esophageal transmission measurement. Am J Cardiol 1983; 51:853–858.
42. Fearnow EC, Jaszczak RJ, Harris CC, Stanfield JA. Esophageal source measurement of Tc-99m attenuation coefficients for use in left ventricular volume determinations. Radiology 1985; 157:517–520.
43. Bourguignon MH, Douglas KH, Links JM, et al. Fully automated data acquisition processing and display in equilibrium radioventriculography. Eur J Nucl Med 1981;6:343.
44. Nickel O, Schad N, Andrews EJ, et al. Scintigraphic measurement of left ventricular volumes from the count-density distribution. J Nucl Med 1982;23:404–410.
45. Massardo T, Gal RA, Grenier RP, et al. Left ventricular volume calculations using a count based ratio method applied to multigated radionuclide angiography. J Nucl Med 1990;31:450–456.
46. Levy WC, Cerqueira MD, Matsuoka DT, et al. Four radionuclide methods for left ventricular volume determination: comparison of a manual and an automated technique. J Nucl Med 1992; 33:763–770.
47. Botvinick EH, Dae MW, O'Connell JW, et al. First harmonic Fourier (phase) analysis of blood pool scintigrams for the analysis of cardiac contraction and conduction. In: Gerson MC, ed. Cardiac nuclear medicine. New York: McGraw Hill, 1987:109.
48. Gerwitz H, Wilner A, Garriepy S. Diagnosis of left-ventricular mural thrombus by means of radionuclide ventriculography. J Nucl Med 1981;22:610–612.
49. Frais MA, Botvinick EH, Shosa DW, et al. Phase image characterization of ventricular contraction in left and right bundle branch block. Am J Cardiol 1982;50:95.
50. Grines CL, Bashore TM, Boudoulas H, Olson S, et al. Functional abnormalities in isolated left bundle branch block. Circulation 1989;79:845–853.
51. Botvinick EH, Frais M, O'Connell W, et al. Phase image evaluation of patients with ventricular pre-excitation syndromes. J Am Coll Cardiol 1984;3:799.
52. Swiryn S, Pavel D, Byrom E, et al. Sequential phase mapping of radionuclide gated biventriculograms in patients with sustained ventricular tachycardia: close correlation with electrophysiologic characteristics. Am Heart J 1982;103:319.
53. Starling MR, Dell'Italia LJ, Chaudhuri TK, et al. First transit and equilibrium radionuclide angiography in patients with inferior transmural myocardial infarction. Criteria for the diagnosis of associated hemodynamically significant right ventricular infarction. J Am Coll Cardiol 1984;4:923.
54. Hrooka Y, Urabe Y, Imaizumi T, et al. The usefulness of equilibrium radionuclide ventriculography in the diagnosis of arrhythmogenic right ventricular dysplasia and a report of cases of a familial occurrence. Jpn Circ J 1988;52:511–517.
55. Zaret BL, Wackers FJ. Radionuclide methods for evaluating the results of thrombolytic therapy. Circulation 1987;76(II):8–17.
56. Hackel DB, Wagner G, Ratliff NB, Cies A, Estes EH Jr. Anatomic studies of the cardiac conducting system in acute myocardial infarction. Am Heart J 1972;83(1):77–81.
57. Bodenheimer MM, Banka VS, Fooshee CM, et al. Comparative sensitivity of the exercise electrocardiogram, thallium im-

aging and stress radionuclide angiography to detect the presence and severity of coronary heart disease. Circulation 1979; 60:1270.
58. Sheehan FH, Dodge HT, Mathey DG, et al. Application of the centerline method: analysis of change in regional left ventricular wall motion in serial studies. In: Computers in Cardiology. Long Beach, CA: IEEE Computer Society, 1982:9–12.
59. Sheehan FH, Mathey DG, Schofer J, et al. Effect of interventions in salvaging left ventricular function in acute myocardial infarction: a study of intracoronary streptokinase. Am J Cardiol 1983; 52:431–438.
60. Sagawa K, Suga H, Shoukas AA, Bakalar KM. End-systolic pressure/volume ratio: a new index of ventricular contractility. Am J Cardiol 1977;40:748–753.
61. Kass DA, Maughan WL, Guo AM, et al. Comparative influence of load versus inotropic states on indexes of ventricular contractility: experimental and theoretical analysis based on pressure-volume relationships. Circulation 1988;76:1422.
62. Ramanathan KB, Erwin SW, Sullivan JM. Relationship of peak systolic pressure/end systolic volume ratio to standard ejection phase indices and ventricular function curves in coronary disease. Am J Med Sciences 1984;288:162–168.
63. Watkins J, Slutsky R, Tubau J, et al. A scintigraphic study of the relationship between left ventricular peak-systolic pressure and end-systolic volume in normal subjects and patients with coronary artery disease. Br Heart J 1982;48:39.
64. Magorien DJ, Shaffer P, Bush CA, et al. Assessment of left ventricular pressure-volume relations using gated radionuclide angiography, echocardiography and micromanometer pressure recordings. Circulation 1983;67:844.
65. Magorien DJ, Shaffer P, Bush C, Magorien RD. Hemodynamic correlates for timing intervals, ejection rate and filling rate derived from the radionuclide angiographic volume curve. Am J Cardiol 1984;53:567–571.
66. Monrad ES, McKay RG, Baim DS, et al. Improvement in indexes of diastolic performance in patients with congestive heart failure treated with milrinone. Circulation 1984;70:1030–1037.
67. Miyatake K, Okamoto M, Kinoshita N, et al. Augmentation of atrial contribution to left ventricular inflow with aging as assessed by intracardiac Doppler flowmetry. Am J Cardiol 1984; 53:586–589.
68. Bonow RO, Vitale DF, Bachararch SL, et al. Effects of aging on asynchronous left ventricular regional function and global ventricular filling in normal human subjects. JACC 1988;11:50–58.
69. Inouye I, Massie B, Loge D, et al. Abnormal left ventricular filling: an early finding in mild to moderate systemic hypertension. Am J Cardiol 1984;53:120–126.
70. Fouad FM, Slominski M, Tarazi RC. Left ventricular diastolic function in hypertension: relation to left ventricular mass and systolic function. JACC 1984;3:1500–1506.
71. Betocchi S, Bonow RO, Bacharach SL, et al. Isovolumic relaxation period in hypertrophic myopathy: assessment by radionuclide angiography. J Am Coll Cardiol 1986;7:74–81.
72. Bonow RO, Bacharach SL, Green MV, Kent KM. Impaired left ventricular diastolic filling in patients with coronary artery disease: assessment with radionuclide angiography. Circulation 1981;64:315–323.
73. Bonow RO. Radionuclide angiographic evaluation of left ventricular diastolic function. Circulation 1991;84(Suppl I):208–215.
74. Rigo P, Alderson DO, Robertson RM, et al. Measruement of aortic and mitral regurgitation by gated cardiac blood pool scans. Circulation 1979;60:306.
75. Urquhart J, Patterson RE, Packer M, et al. Quantification of valve regurgitation by radionuclide angiography before and after valve replacement surgery. Am J Cardiol 1981;47:287.
76. Henze E, Schelbert HR, Wisenberg G, et al. Assessment of regurgitant fraction and right and left ventricular function at rest and during exercise: a new technique for determination of right ventricular stroke counts from gated equilibrium blood pool studies. Am Heart J 1982;953–962.
77. Rigo P, Chevigne M. Measurement of left to right shunts by gated radionuclide angiography: concise communication. J Nucl Med 1982;23:1070.
78. Maublant J, Bailly P, Mestas D, et al. Feasibility of gated single-photon emission transaxial tomography of the cardiac blood pool. Radiology 1983;146:837–839.
79. Tamaki N, Mukai T, Ishii Y, et al. Multiaxial tomography of heart chambers by gated blood-pool emission computed tomography using a rotating gamma-camera. Radiology 1983;547–554.
80. Underwood SR, Walton S, Laming PJ, et al. Left ventricular volume and ejection fraction determined by gated blood pool emission tomography. Br Heart J 1985;53:216–222.
81. Blumgart HL, Weiss S. Studies on the velocity of blood flow. VII. The pulmonary circulation time in normal resting individuals. J Clin Investigation 1927;4:399–425.
82. Mason DT, Ashburn WL, Harbert JC, et al. Rapid sequential visualization of the heart and great vessels in man using the wide-field anger scintillation camera. Circulation 1969;39:19–28.
83. Jones RH, Borges-Neto S, Potts JM. Simultaneous measurement of myocardial perfusion and ventricular function during exercise from a single injection of technetium-99m sestamibi in coronary artery disease. Am J Cardiol 1990;66:68E–71E.
84. Borges-Neto S, Coleman RE, Potts JM, Jones RH. Combined exercise radionuclide angiocardiography and single photon emission computed tomography perfusion studies for assessment of coronary disease. Sem Nucl Med 1991;21:223.
85. Johnson LL, Rodney RA, Vaccarino RA, et al. Left ventricular perfusion and performance from a single radiopharmaceutical and one camera. J Nucl Med 1992;33:1411–1416.
86. Williams KA, Taillon LA, Draho JM, Foisy MF. First-pass radionuclide angiographic studies of left ventricular function with technetium-99m-teboroxime, technetium-99m sestamibi and technetium-99m-DTPA. J Nucl Med 1993;34:394–399.
87. Takahashi N, Tamaki N, Tadamura E, et al. Combined assessment of regional perfusion and wall motion in patients with coronary artery disease with technetium-99m-tetrofosmin. J Nucl Cardiol 1994;1:29–38.
88. Mena I, Narahara KA, de Jong R, Maublant J. Gold-195m, an ultra-short-lived generator-produced radionuclide: clinical application in sequential first pass ventriculography. J Nucl Med 1983;24:139–144.
89. Dymond DS, Elliott AT, Flatman W, Stone D. The clinical validation of gold-195m: a new short half-life radiopharmaceutical for rapid, sequential, first pass angiocardiography in patients. JACC 1983;2:85–92.
90. Treves S, Cheng C, Samuel A, et al. Iridium-191 angiocardiography for the detection and quantitation of left-to-right shunting. J Nucl Med 1980;21:1151–1157.
91. Holman BL, Neirinckx RD, Treves S, Tow DE. Cardiac imaging with tantalum-178. Radiology 1979;131:525–526.
92. Adams R, Lacy JL, Ball ME, Martin LJ. The count rate performance of a multiwire gamma camera measured by a decaying source method with 9.3-minute tantalum-178. J Nucl Med 1990; 31:1723–1726.
93. Lacy JL, Layne WW, Guidry GW, Verani MS, et al. Development and clinical performance of an automated, portable tungsten-178/tantalum-178 generator. J Nucl Med 1991;32:2158–2161.
94. Verani MS, Lacy JL, Guidry GW, et al. Quantification of left ventricular performance during transient coronary occlusion at various anatomic sites in humans: a study using tantalum-178 and a multiwire gamma-camera. J Am Coll Cardiol 1992;19:297–306.

95. Gal R, Grenier RP, Carpenter J, et al. High count rate first-pass radionuclide angiography using a digital gamma-camera. J Nucl Med 1986;27:198–206.
96. Nichols K, DePuey EG, Gooneratne N, et al. First-pass ventricular ejection fraction using a single-crystal nuclear camera. J Nucl Med 1994;35:1292–1300.
97. Bowyer KW, Konstantinow G, Rerych SK, Jones RH. Optimum counting intervals in radionuclide cardiac studies: In: Nuclear cardiology: selected computer aspects. New York: Society of Nuclear Medicine, 1978:85.
98. Rerych SK, Scholz PM, Newman GE, Sabiston DC Jr. Cardiac function at rest and during exercise in normals and in patients with coronary heart disease. Evaluation by radionuclide angiocardiography. Ann Surg 1978;187:449.
99. Berger HI, Reduto LA, Johnstone DE, et al. Global and regional left ventricular response to bicycle exercise in coronary artery disease. Am J Med 1979;66:13–21.
100. Potts JM, Borges-Neto S, Smith LR, Jones RH. Comparison of bicycle and treadmill radionuclide angiocardiography. J Nucl Med 1991;32:1918–1922.
101. Friedman JD, Berman DS, Kiat H, et al. Rest and treadmill exercise first-pass radionuclide ventriculography: validation of left ventricular ejection fraction measurements. J Nucl Cardiol 1994;4:382–388.
102. Jengo MA, Mena I, Blaufuss A, Criley JM. Evaluation of left ventricular function (ejection fraction and segmental wall motion) by single pass radioisotope aniography. Circulation 1978; 57:326.
103. Marshall RC, Berger HJ, Costin JC, Freedman GS. Assessment of cardiac performance with quantitative radionuclide angiocardiography. Circulation 1977;56:820–829.
104. Gal R, Grenier RP, Schmidt DH, Port SC. Background correction in first-pass radionuclide angiography: comparison of several approaches. J Nucl Med 1986;27:1480–1486.
105. Schad N, Nickel O. Radionuclide angiography of the heart in coronary artery disease: where do we stand? Cardiovasc Radiol 1978;1:27–35.
106. Scholz PM, Rerych SK, Moran JF, et al. Quantitative radionuclide angiocardiography. Cathet Cardiovasc Diagn 1980;6:265–283.
107. Bodenheimer MM, Banka VS, Fooshee CM, et al. Quantitative radionuclide angiography in the right anterior oblique view: comparison with contrast ventriculography. Am J Cardiol 1978; 41:718–725.
108. Wackers FJT. First-pass radionuclide angiocardiography. In: Gerson MC, ed. Cardiac nuclear medicine. New York: McGraw-Hill, 1991:67–80.
109. Morrison DA, Turgeon J, Ouitt T. Right ventricular ejection fraction measurements: contrast ventriculography versus gated blood pool and gated first-pass method. Am J Cardiol 1984; 54:651–653.
110. Berger HJ, Matthay RA, Loke J, et al. Assessment of cardiac performance with quantitative radionuclide angiocardiography: right ventricular ejection fraction with reference to findings in chronic obstructive pulmonary disease. Am J Cardiol 1978; 41:897–905.
111. Anderson PAW, Rerych SK, Moore TE, Jones RH. Accuracy of left ventricular end-diastolic dimension determinations obtained by radionuclide angiocardiography. J Nucl Med 1981;22:500.
112. Gal R, Grenier RP, Port SC, Dymond DS. Left ventricular volume calculation using a count-based ratio method applied to first-pass radionuclide angiography. J Nucl Med 1992;33:2124–2132.
113. Jones RH, Sabiston DC Jr, Bates BB, et al. Quantitative radionuclide angiocardiography for determination of chamber to chamber cardiac transit times. Am J Cardiol 1972;30:855–864.
114. Osbakken MD, Boucher CA, Okada RD, et al. Spectrum of global left ventricular responses to supine exercise: limitation in the use of ejection fraction in identifying patients with coronary artery disease. Am J Cardiol 1983;51:28.
115. Hanley PC, Gibbons RJ. Value of radionuclide-determined changes in pulmonary blood volume for the detection of coronary artery disease. Chest 1990;97:7–11.
116. Schad N, Andrews ES, Fleming JW. Colour atlas of first-pass functional imaging of the heart. Hingham: MTP Press Ltd., 1985.
117. Reduto LA, Wickemeyer WJ, Young JB, et al. Left ventricular diastolic performance at rest and during exercise in patients with coronary artery disease. Circulation 1981;63:1228–1237.
118. Polak JF, Kemper AJ, Bianco JA, et al. Resting early peak diastolic filling rate: a sensitive index of myocardial dysfunction in patients with coronary artery disease. J Nucl Med 1982;23:471–478.
119. Philippe L, Mena I, Darcourt J, French WJ. Evaluation of valvular regurgitation by factor analysis of first-pass angiography. J Nucl Med 1988;29:159–167.
120. Janowitz WR, Fester A. Quantitation of left ventricular regurgitant fraction by first pass radionuclide angiocardiography. Am J Cardiol 1982;49:85–92.
121. Kanishi Y, Tatsuta N, Hikasa Y, et al. Assessment of tricuspid regurgitation by analog computer analysis of dilution curves recorded by scintillation camera. Jpn Circulation 1982; J46:1147.
122. Braunwald E, Tannenbaum HL, Morrow AG. Localization of left-to-right cardiac shunts by dye-dilution curves following injection into the left side of the heart and into the aorta. Am J Med 1958; 24:203.
123. Maltz DL, Treves S. Quantitative radionuclide angiocardiography: determination of Qp:Qs in children. Circulation 1973; 47:1048–1056.
124. Askenazi J, Ahnberg DS, Korngold E, et al. Quantitative radionuclide angiocardiography: detection and quantitation of left-to-right shunts. Am J Cardiol 1976;37:382–387.
125. Peter CA, Armstrong BE, Jones RH. Radionuclide quantitation of right-to-left intracardiac shunts in children. Circulation 1981; 64:572.
126. Dogan AS, Rezai K, Kirchner PT, Stuhlmuller JE. A scintigraphic sign for detection of right-to-left shunts. J Nucl Med 1993; 34:1607–1611.
127. Rerych SK, Scholz PM, Newman GE, Sabiston DC Jr. Cardiac function at rest and during exercise in normals and patients with coronary artery disease. Ann Surg 1978;187:449.
128. Borer JS, Kent KM, Bacharach SL, et al. Sensitivity, specificity and predictive accuracy of radionuclide cineangiography during exercise in patients with coronary artery disease. Circulation 1979;60:572.
129. Berger H, Reduto L, Johnstone D, et al. Global and regional left ventricular response to bicycle exercise in coronary artery disease: assessment by quantitative radionuclide angiocardiography. Am J Med 1979;66:13.
130. Jengo JA, Oren V, Conant R, et al. Effects of maximal exercise stress on left ventricular function in patients with coronary artery disease using first pass radionuclide angiocardiography. A rapid noninvasive technique for determining ejection fraction and segmented wall motion. Circulation 1979;59:60–65.
131. Gibbons RJ, Lee KL, Cobb F, Jones RH. Ejection fraction response to exercise in patients with chest pain and normal coronary arteriograms. Circulation 1981;64:952–957.
132. Higginbotham MB, Morris KB, Coleman RE, Cobb FR. Sex-related differences in the normal cardiac response to upright exercise. Circulation 1984;70:357.
133. Port SC, Cobb FR, Coleman E, Jones RH. Effect of age on the

response of the left ventricular ejection fraction to exercise. N Engl J Med 1980;303:1133–1137.
134. Peter CA, Jones RH. Effects of isometric handgrip and dynamic exercise on left ventricular function. J Nucl Med 1980;21:1131.
135. Foster C, Dymond DS, Anholm JD, et al. Effect of exercise protocol on the left ventricular response to exercise. Am J Cardiol 1983;51:859–864.
136. Port SC, McEwan P, Cobb FR, Jones RH. Influence of resting left ventricular function on the left ventricular response to exercise in patients with coronary artery disease. Circulation 1981; 63:856.
137. Brady TJ, Thrall JH, Lo K, et al. The importance of adequate exercise in the detection of coronary heart disease by radionuclide ventriculography. J Nucl Med 1980;21:1125.
138. Jones RH, McEwen P, Newman GE, et al. Accuracy of diagnosis of coronary artery disease by radionuclide measurement of left ventricular function during rest and exercise. Circulation 1981; 64:586–601.
139. 'Gibbons RJ, Lee KL, Cobb FR, Jones RH. Ejection fraction response to exercise in patients with chest pain and normal coronary arteriograms. Circulation 1981;64:952–957.
140. DePace NL, Iskandrian AS, Hakki A, et al. Value of left ventricular ejection fraction during exercise in predicting the extent of coronary artery disease. J Am Coll Cardiol 1983;1:1002.
141. Johnson SH, Bigelow C, Lee KL, et al. Prediction of death and myocardial infarction by radionuclide angiocardiography in patients with suspected coronary artery disease. Am J Cardiol 1991;67:919–926.
142. Weintraub WS, Schneider RM, Seelaus PA, et al. Prospective evaluation of the severity of coronary artery disease with exercise radionuclide angiography and electrocardiography. Am Heart J 1986;111:537.
143. Gibbons RJ, Fyke FE III, Clements IP, et al. Noninvasive identification of severe coronary artery disease using exercise radionuclide angiography. J Am Coll Cardiol 1988;11:28–34.
144. Jones RH, Floyd RD, Austin EH, et al. The role of radionuclide angiocardiography in the preoperative prediction of pain relief and prolonged survival following coronary artery bypass grafting. Ann Surg 1983;197:743.
145. Austin EH, Jones RH. Radionuclide left ventricular volume curves in angiographically proved normal subjects and patients with three-vessel coronary disease. Am Heart J 1983;106:1357.
146. Miller TR, Goldman KJ, Sampathkumaran KS, et al. Analysis of cardiac diastolic function: application in coronary artery disease. J Nucl Med 1983;24:2–7.
147. Bonow RO, Kent KM, Rosing DR, et al. Improved left ventricular diastolic filling in patients with coronary artery disease after percutaneous transluminal angioplasty. Circulation 1982; 66:1159–1167.
148. Leppo J, Boucher CA, Okada RD, et al. Serial thallium-201, myocardial imaging after dipyridamole infusion: diagnostic utility in detecting coronary stenoses and relationship to regional wall motion. Circulation 1982;66:649–657.
149. Leppo JA. Dipyridamole-thallium imaging: the lazy man's stress test. J Nucl Med 1989;30:281–287.
150. Verani MS, Mahmarian JJ, Hixson JB, et al. Diagnosis of coronary artery disease by controlled coronary vasodilation with adenosine and thallium-201 scintigraphy in patients unable to exercise. Circulation 1990;82:80–87.
151. Pennell DJ, Underwood SR, Swanton RH, et al. Dobutamine thallium myocardial perfusion tomography. J Am Coll Cardiol 1991;18:1471–1479.
152. Picano E, Lattanzi F, Masini M, et al. Usefulness of the dipyridamole-exercise echocardiography test for diagnosis of coronary artery disease. Am J Cardiol 1988;62(1):67–70.
153. Masini M, Picano E, Lattanzi F, et al. High dose dipyridamole-echocardiography test in women: correlation with exercise-electrocardiography test and coronary arteriography. JACC 1988; 12:682.
154. Cohen JL, Greene TO, Ottenweller J, et al. Dobutamine digital echocardiography for detecting coronary artery disease. Am J Cardiol 1991;67:1311–1318.
155. Baudhuin T, Marwick T, Melin J, et al. Diagnosis of coronary artery disease in elderly patients: safety and efficacy of dobutamine echocardiography. Eur Heart J 1993;14:799–803.
156. Cates CU, Kronenberg MW, Collins HW, Sandler MP. Dipyridamole radionuclide ventriculography: a test with high specificity for severe coronary artery disease. J Am Coll Cardiol 1989;13:841–851.
157. Bahl VK, Vasan RS, Malhotra A, Wasir HS. A comparison of dobutamine infusion and exercise during radionuclide ventriculography in the evaluation of coronary arterial disease. Int J Cardiol 1992;35:49–55.
158. Narahara KA, Mena I, Maublaut JC, et al. Simultaneous maximum exercise radionuclide angiography and thallium stress perfusion imaging. Am J Cardiol 1984;53:812.
159. Verani MS, Lacy JL, Ball ME, et al. Simultaneous assessment of regional ventricular function and perfusion utilizing iridium-191m and thallium-201 during a single exercise test. Am J Cardiol Imaging 1988;2:206.
160. Palmas W, Friedman JD, Kiat H, et al. Improved identification of multiple-vessel coronary artery disease by addition of exercise wall motion analysis to Tc-99m-sestamibi myocardial perfusion SPECT [Abstract]. J Nucl Med 1993;34:1308.
161. Marcassa C, Marzulla P, Parod O, et al. A new method for noninvasive quantitation of segmental myocardial wall thickening using technetium-99m 2-methoxy-isobutyl-isonitrile scintigraphy: results in normal subjects. J Nucl Med 1990;31:173–177.
162. Mannting F, Morgan-Mannting MG. Gated SPECT with technetium-99m-sestamibi for assessment of myocardial perfusion abnormalities. J Nucl Med 1993;34:601–608.
163. DePuey EG, Nichols K, Dobrinsky C. Left ventricular ejection fraction assessed from gated technetium-99m-sestamibi SPECT. J Nucl Med 1993;34:1871–1876.
164. Harris PJ, Harrell FE Jr, Lee KL, Rosati RA. Nonfatal myocardial infarct in medically treated patients with coronary artery disease. Circulation 1980;62:240–248.
165. CASS Principal Investigators. Coronary artery surgery study (CASS): a randomized trial of coronary bypass surgery. Survival data. Circulation 1983;68:989.
166. Pryor DB, Harrel FE, Lee KL, et al. Prognostic indicators from radionuclide angiography in medically treated patients with coronary artery disease. Am J Cardiol 1984;53:18.
167. Lee KL, Pryor DB, Pieper KS, Harrell FE Jr. Prognostic value of radionuclide angiography in medically treated patients with coronary artery disease. Circulation 1990;82:1705–1717.
168. Talierao CP, Clements IP, Zingmeister AR, Gibbons RG. Prognostic value and limitations of exercise angiography in medically treated coronary artery disease. Mayo Clinc Proc 1988;63:573–582.
169. Bonow RO, Kent KM, Rosing DR, et al. Exercise-induced ischemia in mildly symptomatic patients with coronary artery disease and preseved left ventricular function: identification of subgroups at risk of death during medical therapy. N Engl J Med 1984;311:1339.
170. Isner JM, Roberts WC. Right ventricular infarction complicating left ventricular infarction secondary to coronary artery disease. Am J Cardiol 1978;42:885.
171. Baigrie RS, Haq A, Morgan CD, et al. The spectrum of right ventricular involvement in inferior myocardial infarction: a clinical, hemodynamic and noninvasive study. J Am Coll Cardiol 1983; 1:1396.

172. Cohn JN, Guiha NH, Broder MI, et al. Right ventricular infarction. Clinical and hemodynamic features. Am J Cardiol 1974; 33:209.
173. Rigo P, Murray M, Taylor DR, et al. Right ventricular dysfunction detected by gated scintiphotography in patients with acute inferior myocardial infarction. Circulation 1975;52:268.
174. Steele P, Kirch D, Ellis J, et al. Prompt return to normal of depressed right ventricular ejection fraction in acute inferior infarction. Br Heart J 1977;39:1319.
175. Ony L, Green S, Reiser P, et al. Early prediction of mortality in patients with acute myocardial infarction: a prospective study of clinical and radionuclide risk factors. Am J Cardiol 1986;57:33.
176. Zehender M, Kasper W, Kauder E, et al. Right ventricular infarction as an independent predictor of prognosis after acute inferior myocardial infarction. N Engl J Med 1993;328:81–88.
177. The Multicenter Post-Infarction Research Group. Risk stratification and survival after myocardial infarction. N Engl J Med 1983;309:331.
178. Morris KG, Palmieri ST, Califf RM, et al. Value of radionuclide aniography for predicting specific cardiac events after acute myocardial infarction. Am J Cardiol 1985;55:318.
179. Mazzotta G, Camerini A, Scopinaro G, et al. Predicting cardiac mortality after uncomplicated myocardial infarction by exercise radionuclide ventriculography and exercise-induced ST-segment elevation. Eur Heart J 1992;13:330–337.
180. Corbett JR, Dehmer GJ, Lewis SE, Woodward W. The prognostic value of submaximal exercise testing with radionuclide ventriculography before hospital discharge in patients with recent myocardial infarction. Circulation 1981;64:535–544.
181. Wasserman AG, Katz RJ, Cleary P, et al. Noninvasive detection of multivessel disease after myocardial infarction by exercise radionuclide ventriculography Am J Cardiol 1982;50:1242.
182. Hung J, Goris ML, Nash E, et al. Comparative value of maximal treadmill testing, exercise thallium myocardial perfusion imaging and exercise radionuclide ventriculography for distinguishing high- and low-risk patients soon after acute myocardial infarction. Am J Cardiol 1984;53:1221.
183. Kuchar DL, Freund J, Yeates M, Sammel N. Enhanced prediction of major cardiac events after myocardial infarction using exercise radionuclide ventriculography. Aust NZ J Med 1987;17:228–233.
184. Kent KM, Bonow RO, Rosing DR, et al. Improved myocardial function during exercise after successful percutaneous transluminal coronary angioplasty. N Engl J Med 1982;306:441.
185. DePuey EG, Leatherman LL, Leachman RO, et al. Restenosis after transluminal coronary angioplasty detected with exercise-gated radionuclide ventriculography. J Am Coll Cardiol 1984; 4:1103.
186. Helfrant RH, Pine R, Meister SG, et al. Nitroglycerin to unmask reversible asynergy. Circulation 1974;50:108–113.
187. Salel AF, Berman DS, DeNardo GL, Mason DT. Radionuclide assessment of nitroglycerin influence on abnormal left ventricular segmental contraction in patients with coronary heart disease. Circulation 1976;53:975–981.
188. Horn HR, Teichholz LE, Cohn PF, et al. Augmentation of left ventricular contraction pattern in coronary artery disease by an inotropic catecholamine. Circulation 1974;49:1063–1070.
189. McGillem MJ, DeBoe SF, Friedman HZ, Mancini GBJ. The effects of dopamine and dobutamine on regional function in the presence of rigid coronary stenoses and subcritical impairments of reactive hyperemia. Am Heart J 1988;115:970.
190. Bavilla F, Gheorghiade M, Alam M, et al. Low-dose dobutamine in patients with acute myocardial infarction identifies viable but not contractile myocardium and predicts the magnitude of improvement in wall motion abnormalities in response to coronary revascularization. Am Heart J 1991;122:1522–1531.
191. Smart S, Sawada S, Segar D, et al. Low-dose dobutamine echocardiography to assess prognosis after thrombolyses formyocardial infarction [Abstract]. Circulation 1991;84(Suppl II):478.
192. Boucher CA, Anderson MD, Schneider MS, et al. Left ventricular function before and after reaching the anaerobic threshold. Chest 1985;87:145–150.
193. Soufer R, Wohlgelernter D, Vita NA, et al. Intact systolic left ventricular function in clinical congestive heart failure. Am J Cardiol 1985;55:1032–1036.
194. Cohn JN, Johnson G, VA Cooperative Study Group. Heart failure with normal ejection fraction. Circulation 1990;81(Suppl III):4A.
195. Iskandrian AS, Helfeld H, Lemlek J, et al. Differentiation between primary dilated cardiomyopathy and ischemic cardiomyopathy based on right ventricular performance. Am Heart J 1992; 123:768–773.
196. Schoolmeester WL, Simpson AG, Saverbrunn BJ, et al. Radionuclide angiographic assessment of left ventricular function during exercise in patients with a severely reduced ejection fraction. Am J Cardiol 1981;47:804.
197. Wigle ED, Sasson Z, Henderson MA, et al. Hypertrophic cardiomyopathy. The importance of the site and the extent of hypertrophy. A review. Prog Cardiovasc Dis 1985;28:1–83.
198. Bonow RO, Rosing DR, Bacharach SL, et al. Effects of verapamil on left ventricular systolic function and diastolic filling in patients with hypertrophic cardiomyopathy. Circulation 1981; 64:787–796.
199. Aroney CN, Ruddy TD, Dighero H, et al. Differentiation of restrictive cardiomyopathy from pericardial constriction: assessment of diastolic function by radionuclide angiography. J Am Coll Cardiol 1989;13:1007–1014.
200. VonHoff DD, Layard MW, Basa P, et al. Risk factors for doxorubicin-induced congestive heart failure. Ann Intern Med 1979; 91:710.
201. Alexander J, Dainiak N, Berger HJ, et al. Serial assessment of doxorubicin cardiotoxicity with quantitative radionuclide angiocardiography. N Engl J Med 1979;300:278.
202. Gottdiener JS, Mathisen DJ, Borer JS, et al. Doxorubicin cardiotoxicity: assessment of late left ventricular dysfunction by radionuclide cineangiography. Ann Intern Med 1981;94:430.
203. Choi BW, Berger HJ, Schwartz PE, et al. Serial radionuclide assessment of doxorubicin cardiotoxicity in cancer patients with abnormal baseline resting left ventricular performance. Am Heart J 1983;106:638.
204. Mason JW, Bristow MR, Billingham ME, Daniels JR. Invasive and noninvasive methods of assessing adriamycin cardiotoxic effects in man: superiority of histopathologic assessment using endomyocardial biopsy. Cancer Treat Rep 1978;62:857.
205. Bonow RO. Radionuclide angiography in the management of asymptomatic aortic regurgitation. Circulation 1991;84(Suppl I):296–302.
206. Cohn LH. Timing of surgery in chronic mitral and aortic valve regurgitation. J Am Coll Cardiol Current J Review 1993uly/August:49–51.
207. Borer JS, Bacharach SL, Green MV, et al. Exercise-induced left ventricular dysfunction in symptomatic and asymptomatic patients with aortic regurgitation: assessment with radionuclide cineangiography. Am J Cardiol 1978;42:351–357.
208. Huxley RL, Gaffney FA, Corbett JR, et al. Early detection of left ventricular dysfunction in chronic aortic regurgitation as assessed by contrast angiography, echocardiography, and rest and exercise scintigraphy. Am J Cardiol 1983;51:1542–1550.
209. Crawford MH, Souchek J, Oprian CA. Determinants of survival and left ventricular performance after mitral valve replacement. Circulation 1990;81:1173–1181.
210. Levine HJ, Gaasch WH. Ratio of regurgitant volume to end-diastolic volume: a major determinant of ventricular response to

surgical correction of chronic volume overload. Am J Cardiol 1983;52:406–410.
211. Brent BN, Mahler D, Matthay RA, et al. Noninvasive diagnosis of pulmonary arterial hypertension in chronic obstructive pulmonary disease: right ventricular ejection fraction at rest. Am J Cardiol 1984;53:1349–1353.
212. Berger HJ, Matthay RA, Loke J, et al. Assessment of cardiac performance with quantitative radionuclide angiocardiography: right ventricular ejection fraction with reference to findings in chronic obstructive pulmonary disease. Am J Cardiol 1978; 41:897–905.
213. Matthay RA, Berger HJ, Davies RA, et al. Right and left ventricular exercise performance in chronic obstructive pulmonary disease: radionuclide assessment. Ann Intern Med 1980; 93:234.
214. Oliver RM, Fleming JS, Waller DG. Right ventricular function at rest and during exercise in chronic obstructive pulmonary disease. Chest 1993;103:74–80.
215. Olson LJ, Rodeheffer RJ. Management of patients after cardiac transplantation. Mayo Clin Proc 1992;67:775–784.
216. Lee KJ, Wallis JW, Miller TR, et al. The clinical utility of radionuclide ventriculography in cardiac transplantation. J Nucl Med 1990;31:1933–1939.
217. Hurley PJ, Wesselhoeft H, James AE Jr. Use of nuclear imaging in the evaluation of pediatric cardiac disease. Sem Nucl Med 1972;2:353.
218. Kriss JP, Enright LP, Hayden WG, et al. Radioisotopic angiocardiography: findings in congenital heart disease. J Nucl Med 1972;13:31.
219. Gal R, Port SC. Radionuclide angiography in congenitally corrected transposition of the great vessels in an adult. J Nucl Med 1987;28:116–118.
220. Marshall RC, Berger HJ, Reduto LA, et al. Variability in sequential measures of left ventricular performance assessed with radionuclide angiocardiography. Am J Cardiol 1978;41:531.
221. Upton MT, Rerych SK, Newman GE, et al. The reproducibility of radionuclide angiographic measurements of LV function in normal subjects at rest and during exercise. Circulation 1980; 62:126–132.
222. Wackers FJT, Berger HJ, Johnstone DE, et al. Multiple gated cardiac blood pool imaging for left ventricular ejection fraction: validation of the technique and assessment of variability. Am J Cardiol 1979;43:1159.
223. Wexler JP, Blaufox MD. Radionuclide evaluation of left ventricular function with nonimaging probes. Sem Nucl Med 1979; 9:310–319.
224. Tamaki N, Gill JB, Moore RH, et al. Cardiac response to daily activities and exercise in normal subjects assessed by an ambulatory ventricular function monitor. Am J Cardiol 1987; 59:1164–69.
225. Broadhurst P, Cashman P, Crawley J, et al. Clinical validation of a miniature nuclear probe system for continuous on-line monitoring of cardiac function and ST-segment. J Nucl Med 1991; 32:37–43.
226. Pfisterer M, Regenass S, Muller-Brand J, Burkart F. Ambulatory scintigraphic assessment of transient changes in left ventricular function: a new method for detection of silent myocardial ischaemia. Eur Heart J 1988;9(Suppl N):98–103.
227. Breisblatt WM, Weiland FL, McLain JR, et al. Usefulness of ambulatory radionuclide monitoring of left ventricular function early after acute myocardial infarction for predicting residual myocardial ischemia. Am J Cardiol 1988;62:1005–1010.
228. Breisblatt WM, Wolf CJ, McElhinny B, et al. Comparison of ambulatory left ventricular ejection fraction and blood pressure in systemic hypertension in patients with and without increased left ventricular mass. Am J Cardiol 1991;67:597–603.

25 Myocardial Perfusion Imaging

FRANS J. Th. WACKERS

Since 1975 Thallium-201 (^{201}Tl) has been widely employed as a radiopharmaceutical for imaging of the heart and assessment of regional myocardial perfusion (1, 2). Because of the less than optimal physical characteristics of ^{201}Tl for imaging, substantial research efforts have been directed towards the development of new ^{99m}Tc-labeled myocardial perfusion imaging agents. In 1990, ^{99m}Tc-sestamibi and ^{99m}Tc-teboroxime were approved for routine clinical imaging (3–6). ^{99m}Tc-tetrofosmin (7) and ^{99m}Tc-furifosmin (8) are presently in the phase of clinical evaluation and may be approved in the near future.

At the writing of this chapter, approximately 30% of all myocardial perfusion studies in the United States are performed using ^{99m}Tc-sestamibi. ^{99m}Tc-teboroxime has, because of its rapid clearance from the heart, found less acceptance for clinical imaging. In spite of the development of new imaging agents, the extensive experience accumulated in clinical imaging with ^{201}Tl remains relevant and is applicable to these newer imaging agents as well.

Myocardial perfusion imaging can be performed using either planar technique or single photon emission computerized tomography (SPECT). Although, at the present time, in many laboratories, SPECT is the most commonly performed imaging modality, the ability to perform good quality planar imaging is the cornerstone of optimal quality SPECT imaging. In fact, SPECT imaging consists of the acquisition of multiple *planar* projection images. Accordingly, the principles of planar imaging and the interpretation of planar images are discussed in detail as a preamble to SPECT imaging.

IMAGE ACQUISITION

Details of acquisition of planar and SPECT images have been discussed extensively in Chapter 22. Specific aspects of image acquisition using various radiopharmaceuticals are summarized in Table 25.1. For planar imaging, images are acquired in three views—the anterior, left anterior oblique (LAO), and the left lateral. For SPECT imaging, a series of 32 or more planar projection images is acquired in a 180–360° arc around the patient.

NORMAL PLANAR MYOCARDIAL PERFUSION IMAGE

Myocardial perfusion imaging agents accumulate in the heart proportional to the regional distribution of myocardial blood flow and of myocardial mass (9, 10). On planar gamma-camera images, the normal left ventricle displays a horseshoe, ovoid, or doughnut configuration (Fig. 25.1). Accumulation of myocardial perfusion tracers in the normal left ventricle is approximately homogeneous. However, some areas with apparent diminished uptake of radiotracer may occur in normal subjects. These variations of the normal image are discussed more extensively later in this chapter.

The right ventricle, because of its smaller myocardial mass and relatively less accumulation of radiotracer per

Table 25.1.
Summary of Acquisition Parameters for Planar and SPECT Myocardial Perfusion Imaging with ^{201}Tl and ^{99m}Tc-sestamibi

			^{99m}Tc-sestamibi			
	^{201}Tl		Planar		SPECT	
Dose	Planar	SPECT	Low	High	Low	High
mCi	2.5–3	3.5–4	10–15	20–25	10–15	20–25
Start imaging						
Post EX	5 min	15 min	15 min	15 min	15 min	15 min
Post pharm	5 min	5 min	60 min	60 min	60 min	60 min
Redist	3–4 h	3–4 h	n.a.	n.a.	n.a.	n.a.
Rest	45 min	45 min	60 min	60 min	60 min	60 min
Collimator	Hi Res/GAP	GAP	Hi Res/GAP	Hi Res/GAP	Hi Res	Hi Res
Peak	80 keV	80 keV	140 keV	140 keV	140 keV	140 keV
	167 keV	167 keV				
Matrix	128 × 128	64 × 64	128 × 128	128 × 128	64 × 64	64 × 64
Views	LAO	RAO-LPO	LAO	LAO	RAO-LPO	RAO-LPO
	ANT	180	ANT	ANT	180	180
	LLAT	32–64 st	LLAT	LLAT	32–64 st	32–64 st
Imaging time	8–10 min	40 s/st	5 min	5 min	40 s/st	25 s/st

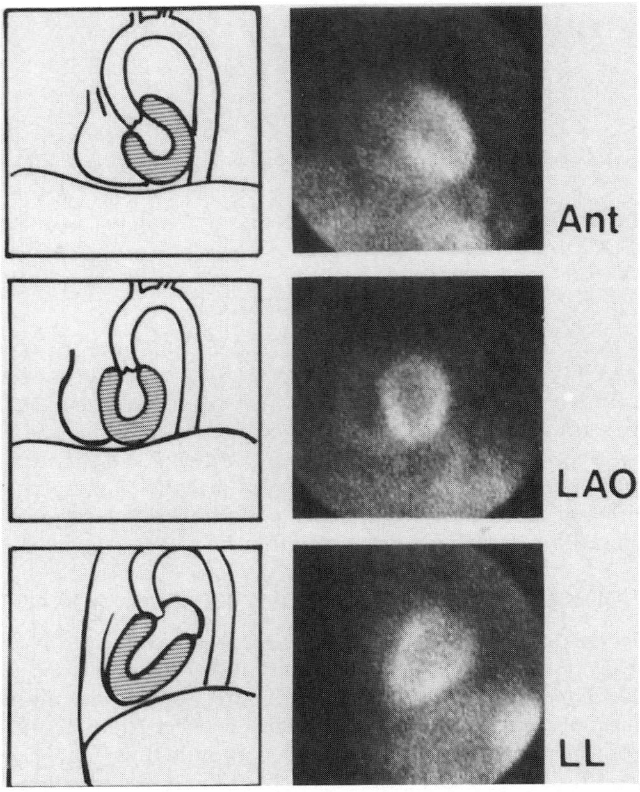

Figure 25.1. ^{201}Tl images in three planar projections of a normal subject. On the left, schematic representations of cardiac anatomy. The left ventricle is well-visualized; the right ventricle is only faintly visible. Accumulation of ^{201}Tl in the left ventricle is almost homogeneous. The central area of decreased activity is the left ventricular cavity. *Ant* = anterior, *LAO* = left anterior oblique, *LL* = left lateral.

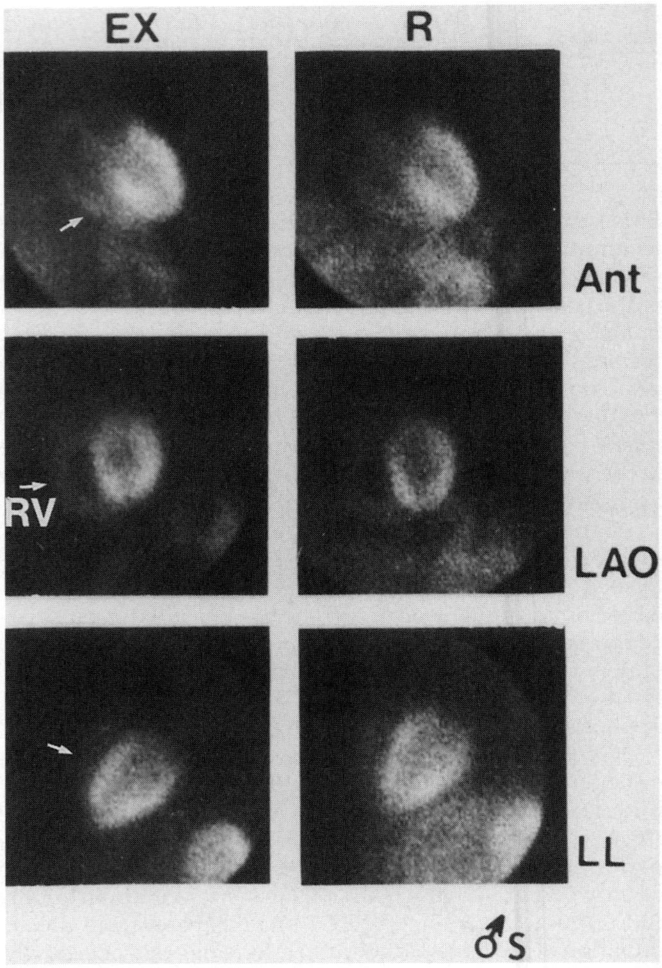

Figure 25.2. Planar ^{201}Tl images after injection during exercise (*EX*) and at rest (*R*) of a normal subject. In addition to the left ventricle, the right ventricle (*RV*) is also visualized after exercise (*arrows*). *Ant* = anterior, *LAO* = left anterior oblique, *LL* = left lateral.

gram of tissue, is usually only faintly visualized at rest. However, following exercise, the right ventricle is clearly visible (Fig. 25.2). Using ^{99m}Tc-sestamibi, the right ventricle is usually well-visualized, both at rest and after exercise (Fig. 25.3).

PROJECTION OF MYOCARDIAL RADIOTRACER ACTIVITY ON PLANAR IMAGES

In planar myocardial perfusion, imaging the anatomy of the heart is projected on images obtained from various angles. The configuration of the heart on the images is dependent on the amount of myocardial mass perpendicular to the crystal surface of the gamma-camera, regional radiopharmaceutical accumulation, and the effect of tissue attenuation. Figures 25.4**A** and **B** illustrate this for the left anterior oblique view. The familiar horseshoe appearance of the left ventricle on myocardial perfusion images is the result of (a) attenuation of radiation from the distant myocardial wall by the ventricular blood pool, and (b) the relatively greater myocardial mass of the walls perpendicular to the plane of view. Thus, the "left ventricular cavity" that appears to be visualized on planar images is an optical illusion caused by relatively lesser photons emanating from the facing left ventricular wall. The gamma-camera appears to look "through" this wall into the left ventricular cavity.

CARDIAC ANATOMY ON PLANAR MYOCARDIAL PERFUSION IMAGES

To visualize all left ventricular myocardial segments in planar imaging, it is necessary to obtain multiple images from different angles. Most laboratories routinely acquire three images (anterior, left anterior obliques, and left lateral views). Occasionally, additional images may be needed in individual patients.

The projection of myocardial activity in the three standard planar images can be understood by comparing myocardial perfusion images with sections through a normal human heart in comparable orientation (11).

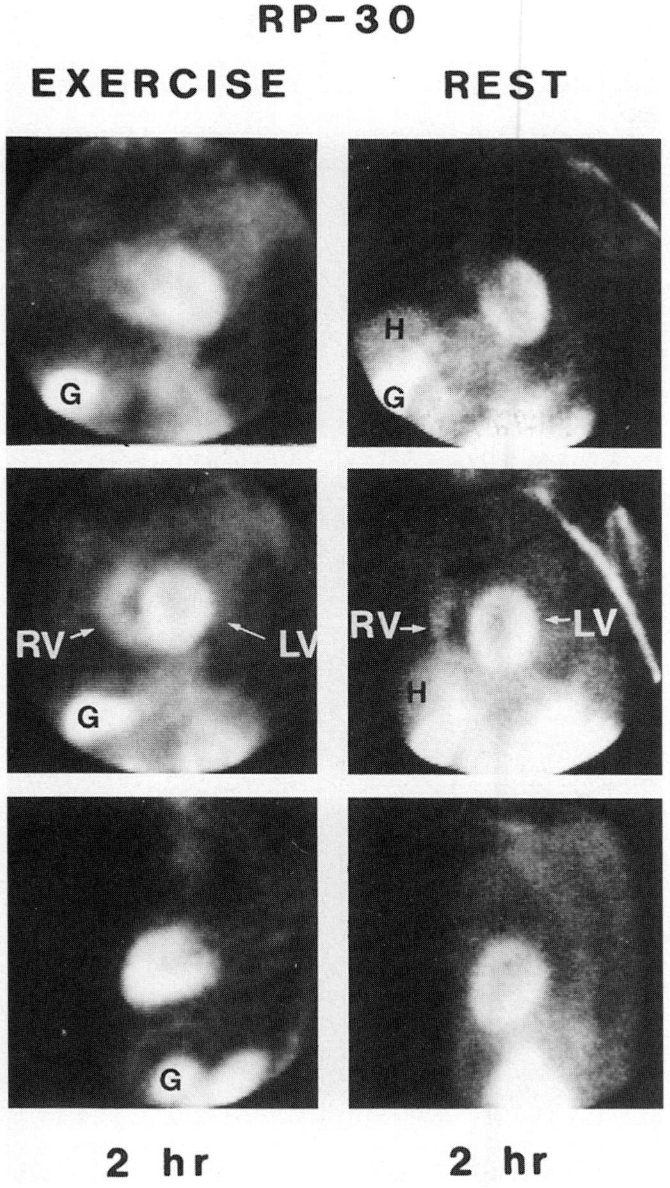

Figure 25.3. Planar myocardial perfusion images with ^{99m}Tc-sestamibi. Images of normal volunteer after exercise (*left*) and at rest (*right*). The images are taken with a large-field-of-view camera. The imaging agent is cleared into the gallbladder (*G*). After exercise, both the right (*RV*) and left (*LV*) ventricles are well-visualized. There is no significant liver accumulation. At rest, in contrast to resting ^{201}Tl imaging, both the right and left ventricles are still visible. The liver (*H*) shows significant accumulation of the radiopharmaceutical on the resting image.

Anterior View

Figure 25.5 shows a schematic drawing of the heart as it is projected on the surface of the crystal of the gamma-camera in the anterior position. It can be appreciated that in the anterior view the anterior wall overlies the ventricular cavity and blood pool. The border-forming walls of the left ventricle are the septum and the anterolateral wall. The anterolateral wall is projected as the cranial part of the "horseshoe." The interventricular septum is at an angle to the plane of section on the anterior image and contributes to the caudal part of the horseshoe image of the heart. However, activity from the inferoposterior wall is projected in this same area and therefore superimposed on that from the septum (Fig. 25.6).

Left Anterior Oblique View

In the left anterior oblique (LAO) projection, the interventricular septum is approximately perpendicular to the crystal surface and free of superimposed structures (Fig. 25.7). Septal activity is projected as the medial part of the "doughnut" or "horseshoe." The lateral part of the doughnut represents activity from the inferolateral and posterolateral left ventricular free wall. The anteroapical wall is viewed "en face," and is superimposed on the cardiac blood pool, therefore contributing relatively less to the image. The configuration of the left ventricle in the LAO projection may differ in individual patients depending upon the position of the heart in the chest (Fig. 25.8). The (typical) doughnut pattern is seen in approximately 65% of patients. In the remainder of patients, a horseshoe configuration is present. In 30% of patients, the left ventricle displays the shape of a vertical horseshoe with the open end (aortic orifice) facing up (11). In 5% of patients, the horseshoe is slanted and points toward the lower left corner of the image. The high-lateral area of lesser activity is the mitral valve area and is not a perfusion defect. The latter situation may be encountered in an occasional patient whose heart is rotated counterclockwise. Consequently, the resulting image is similar to the one seen on the regular left lateral view. The image can be converted into a normal doughnut pattern by changing the angle of obliquity from, for example, 45° to 30° (Fig. 25.9). It must be emphasized that the LAO image should not be acquired in a fixed angulation (e.g., 45°), but individualized so that the best possible separation between right and left ventricles is achieved. In such a view, the septum is vertical and straight. A curved septum usually indicates incorrect angulation.

Left Lateral View

For acquisition of a left lateral image of optimal diagnostic quality, imaging technique and patient positioning are of critical importance (see later). In the left lateral projection, the right ventricular outflow tract is anterior to the left ventricle (Fig. 25.10). The cranial portion of the horseshoe represents projected activity from the septum, but also from a part of the anterior wall perpendicular to the plane of view, and is superimposed on activity from the septum. Because of tissue attenuation, the contribution of the septum

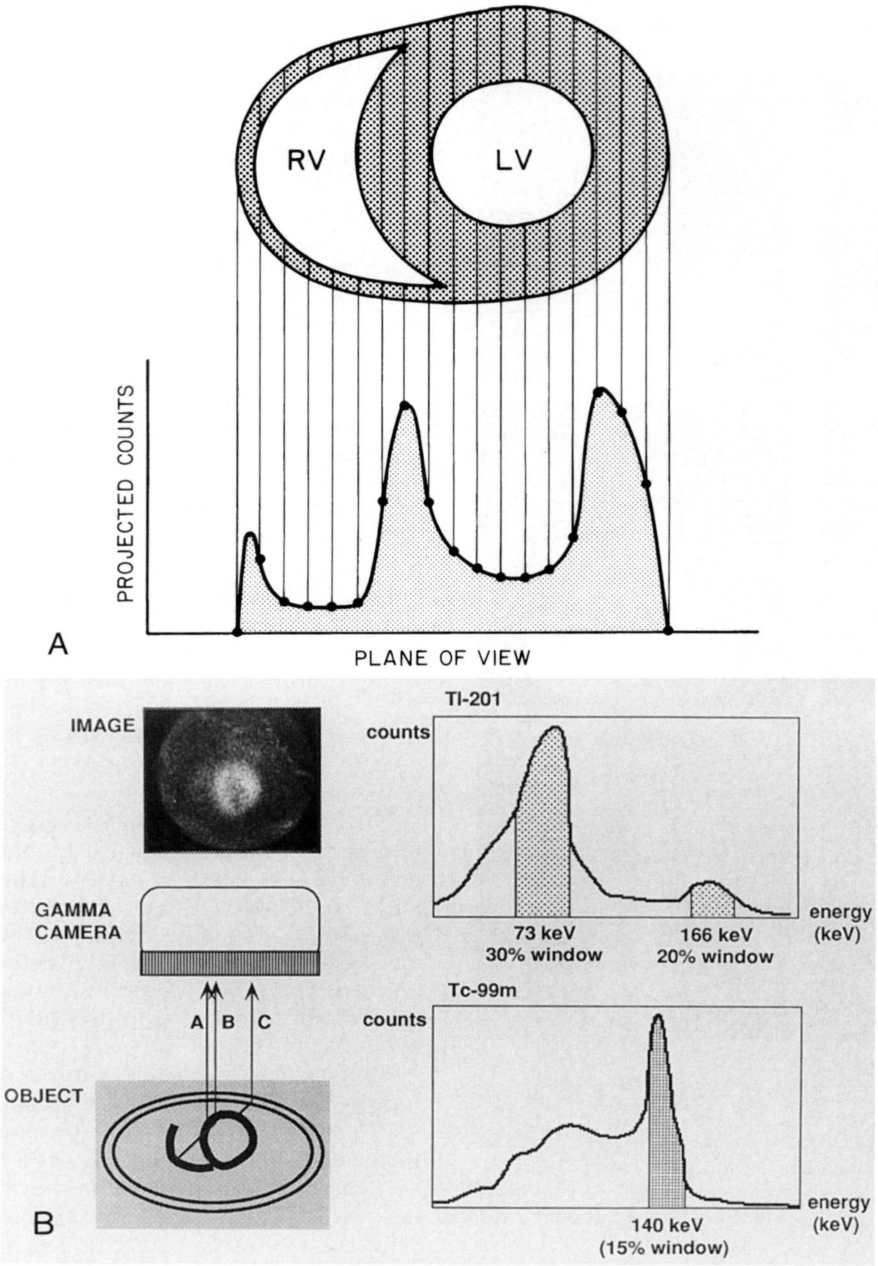

Figure 25.4. **A**. Schematic representation of the generation of a planar image. The projection of radioactivity on the planar view is demonstrated for the left anterior oblique projection (see text). (Reproduced by permission from Wackers FJTh. Thallium-201 myocardial imaging. In: Wackers FJTh, ed. Thallium-201 and technetium-99m pyrophosphate myocardial imaging in the coronary care unit. The Hague: Martinus Nijhoff Publishers, 1980:70–104.) **B.** Generation of myocardial perfusion images. *Left:* Schematic representation of image generation. The gamma-camera is equipped with a parallel-hole collimator. Only photons that travel through the parallel holes will generate scintillations in the gamma-camera crystal. *A, B,* and *C* are photons, but only *A* is a "good" photon, i.e., one that emanates from the septum and travels straight to the camera. *B* is originally from the right ventricle but, because of scatter, appears to come from the left ventricle. *C* originates from the middle of the anterior wall but, after scatter, appears to emanate from the lateral wall of the left ventricle. *Right:* Schematic representation of the energy spectra of ^{201}Tl and ^{99m}Tc. ^{201}Tl has two energy peaks: 73 keV x-rays and 166 keV γ-rays. As a result of scattered photons losing energy in the patient's body, the peaks are diffuse and confluent, not sharp. For ^{201}Tl imaging, two relatively wide windows (30% and 20%) are set symmetrically over both peaks, allowing scatter photons to contribute to the images. ^{99m}Tc has a single, better-defined peak at 140 keV. A relatively narrow window of 15% allows only a small number of scattered photons in the image. (Reproduced by permission from Wackers FJTh. Diagnostic pitfalls of myocardial perfusion in women. J Myocard Ischemia 1992;4:23–37.)

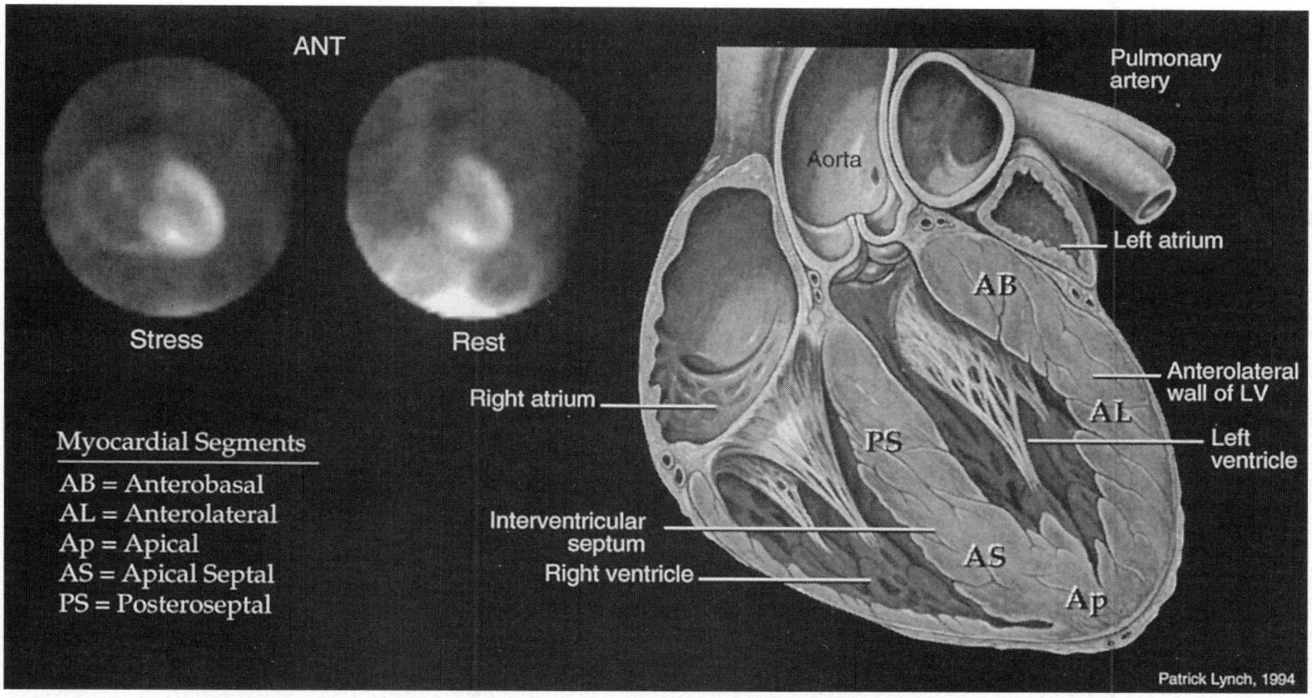

Figure 25.5. Anatomy of the left ventricle on planar anterior (ANT) images. Schematic anatomic drawing of the heart as projected in the planar anterior view (see text). Anterior stress/rest myocardial perfusion images are shown in the upper left.

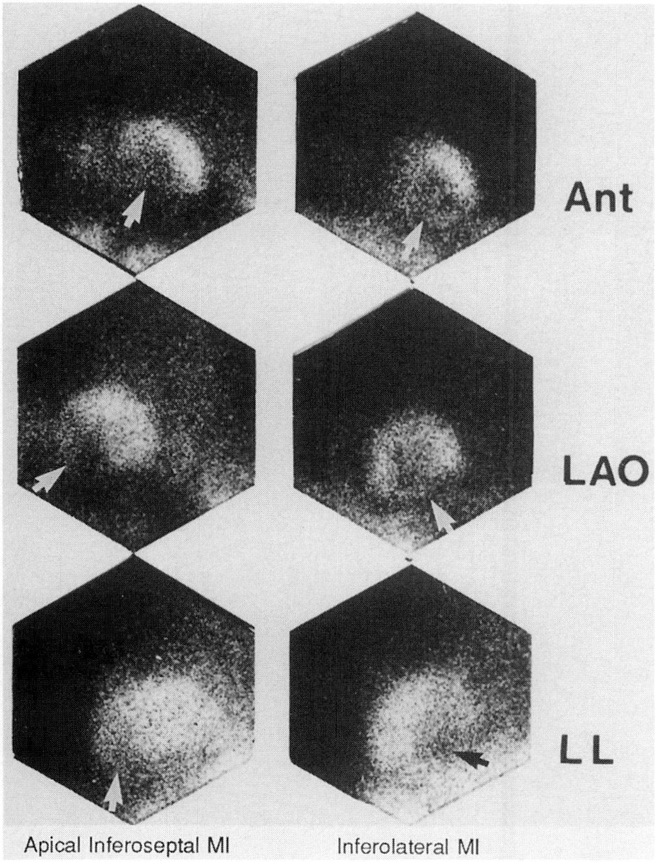

Figure 25.6. Planar ^{201}Tl images of myocardial infarction (MI). Planar ^{201}Tl myocardial images of a patient with an apical inferoseptal myocardial infarction (*left*) and a patient with an inferolateral and posterior infarction (*right*). Note that the anterior (*Ant*) view in both patients has a similar appearance. On the left anterior oblique (*LAO*) images, the location of the defect (*arrows*) is clearly shown to be septal in one patient (*left*), and inferolateral in the other patient (*right*). *LL* = left lateral. This demonstrates the necessity of multiple views in planar imaging for precise anatomic localization of a perfusion abnormality. (Reproduced by permission from Wackers FJTh, Busemann Sokole E, Samson G, van der Schoot JB. Atlas of Tl-201 myocardial scintigraphy. Clin Nucl Med 1977;2:64.)

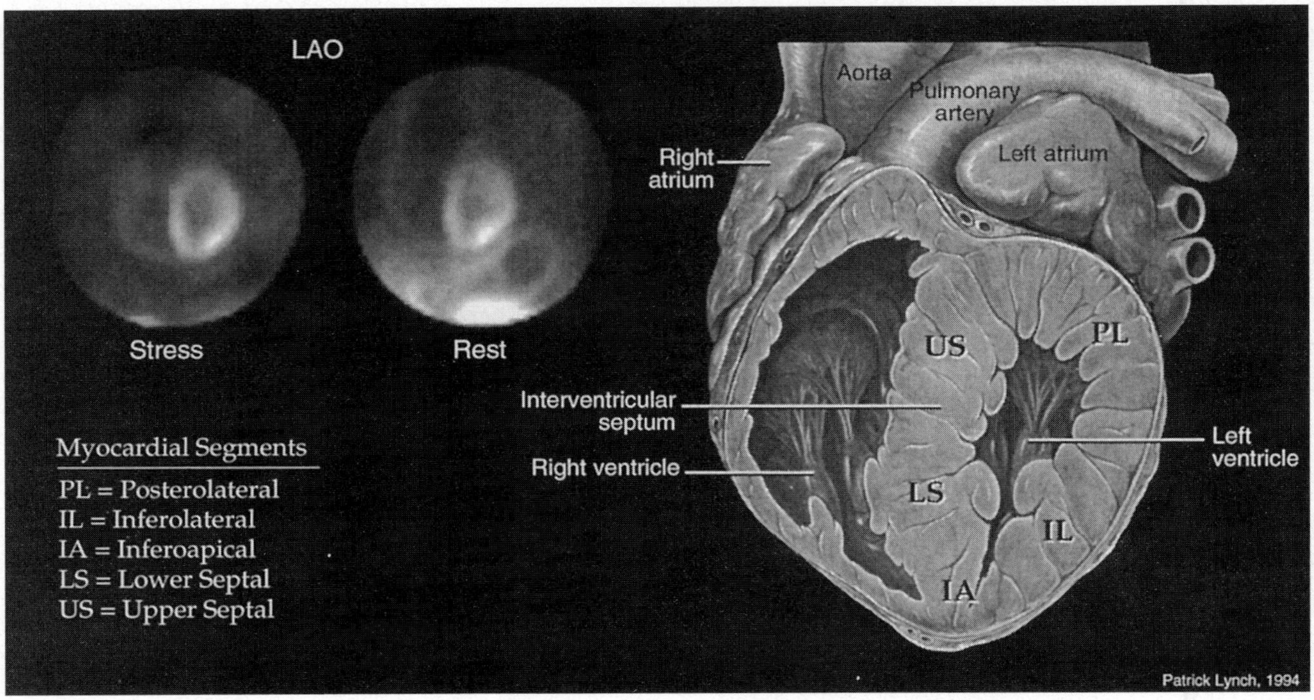

Figure 25.7. Anatomy of left ventricle on planar left anterior oblique (*LAO*) image. Schematic anatomic drawing on the heart as projected on a planar left anterior oblique image (see text). Stress/rest myocardial perfusion images are shown in the upper left.

Figure 25.8. Varying image pattern of the normal left ventricle in left anterior oblique (*LAO*) images. The percentages indicate the prevalence of each pattern in 500 unselected ^{201}Tl studies. The *arrows* indicate the area of diminished activity due to the aorta (*AO*) and the mitral orifice (*M*).

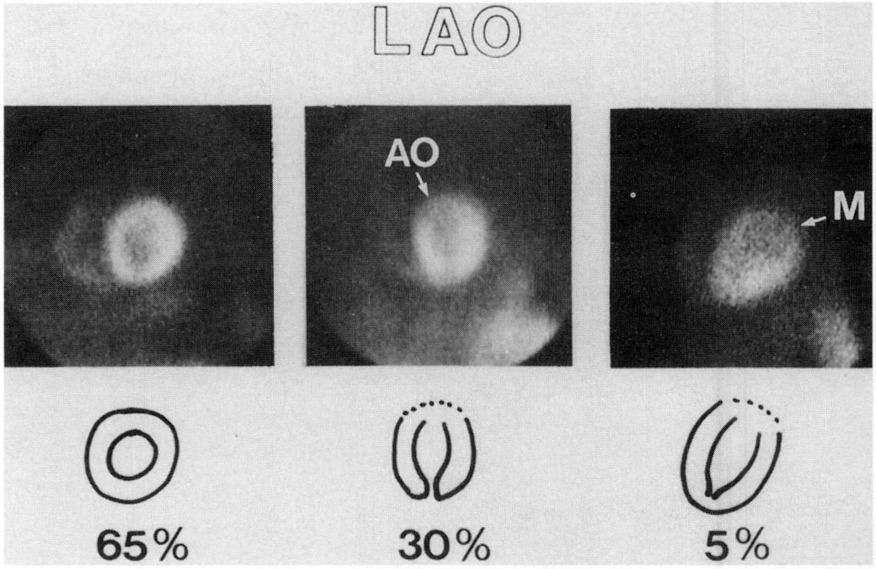

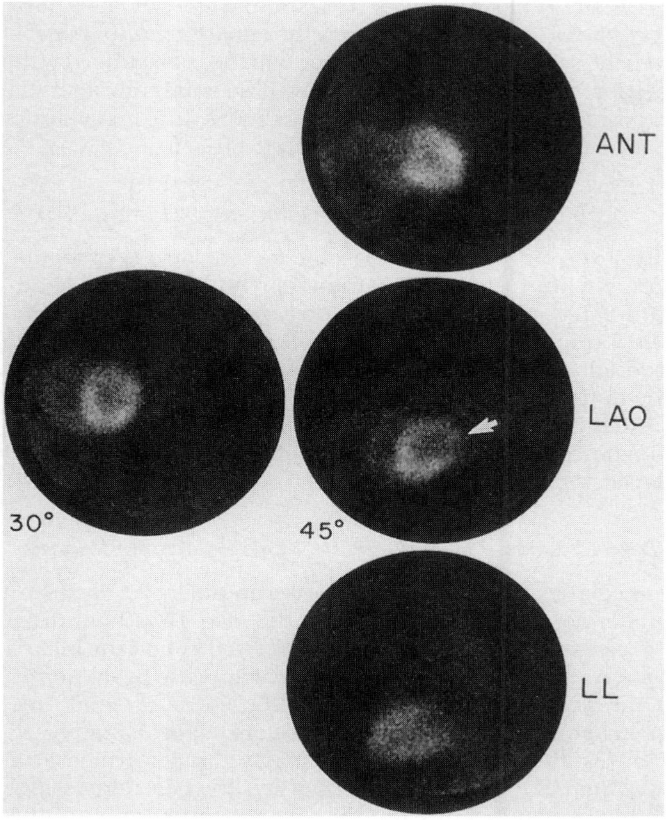

Figure 25.9. Postexercise planar ^{201}Tl images of a patient with counterclockwise-rotation of the heart. The standard planar 45° left anterior oblique (*LAO*) projection shows an apparent lateral wall myocardial perfusion defect (*arrow*). However, note that the septum is curved instead of straight. This indicates that the lateral aspect of the heart is viewed (compare the left lateral (*LL*) view in the same patient). By reimaging with rotating the position of the camera to 30°, a normal LAO projection is seen—the septum is straight and there is maximal separation of right and left ventricle. The "defect" with 45° obliquity is due to the mitral orifice. *ANT* = anterior. (Reproduced by permission from Wackers FJTh. Thallium-201 myocardial imaging. In: Wackers FJTh, ed. Thallium-201 and technetium-99m pyrophosphate myocardial imaging in the coronary care unit. The Hague: Martinus Nijhoff Publishers, 1980:70–104.)

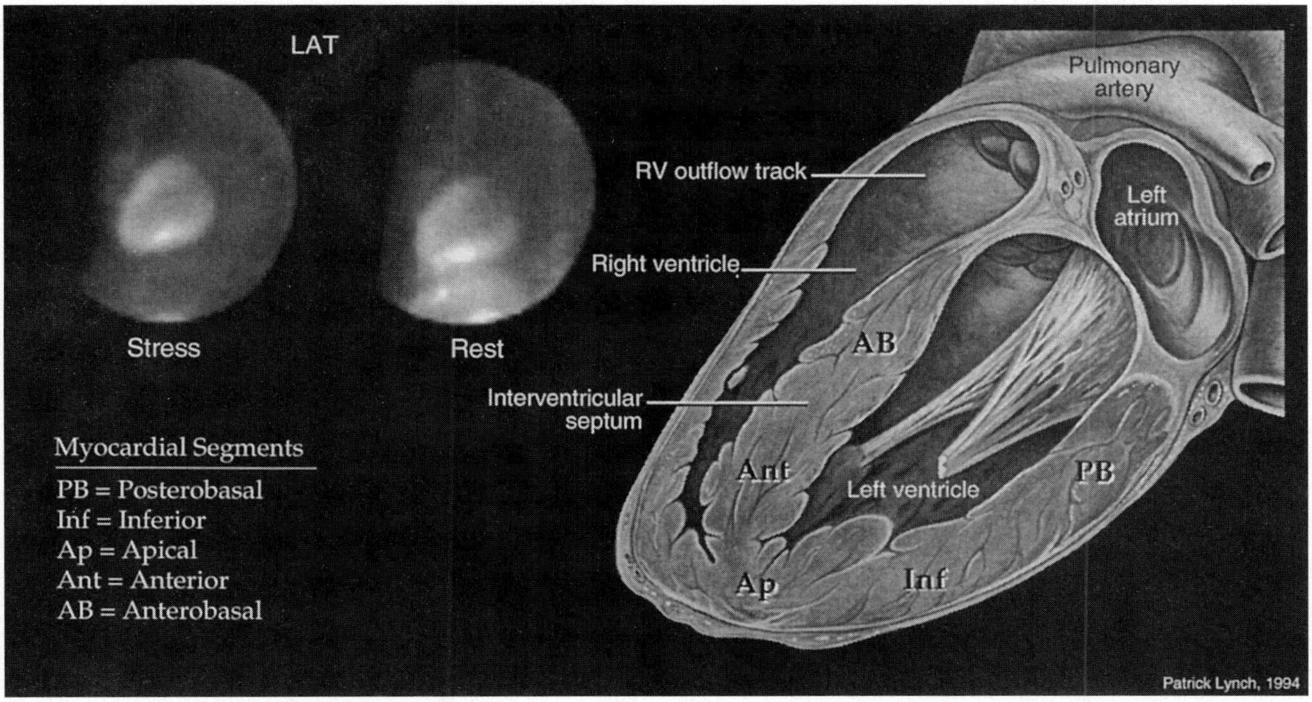

Figure 25.10. Anatomy of a left ventricle on planar left lateral (*LAT*) image. Schematic anatomic drawing of the heart as projected on a planar left lateral image (see text). Stress/rest myocardial perfusion images are shown in the upper left.

to the left lateral image may be less important. The inferoposterior wall is projected as the caudal part of the horseshoe.

The anatomy of the left ventricle, as projected onto the various planar scintigraphic views, is schematically shown in Figure 25.11.

CHARACTERISTICS OF NORMAL PLANAR IMAGES WITH VARIOUS MYOCARDIAL IMAGING AGENTS

The newly developed ^{99m}Tc-labeled agents, such as ^{99m}Tc-sestamibi, are promising in overcoming some of the limitations of imaging with ^{201}Tl. The low dose of 2.5–3.5 mCi of ^{201}Tl that is allowed to be administered, results in relatively count-poor images. Moreover, the low-energy emissions of ^{201}Tl result in substantial background scatter. The relatively high dose (25–30 mCi) and more favorable energy (140 keV) of ^{99m}Tc-sestamibi results in images of better count density, improved image resolution, and less low-energy background scatter (Fig. 25.12). Because of significantly improved image quality, interpretation of ^{99m}Tc-labeled tracer images is generally easier, and can be performed with greater confidence, than that of ^{201}Tl images.

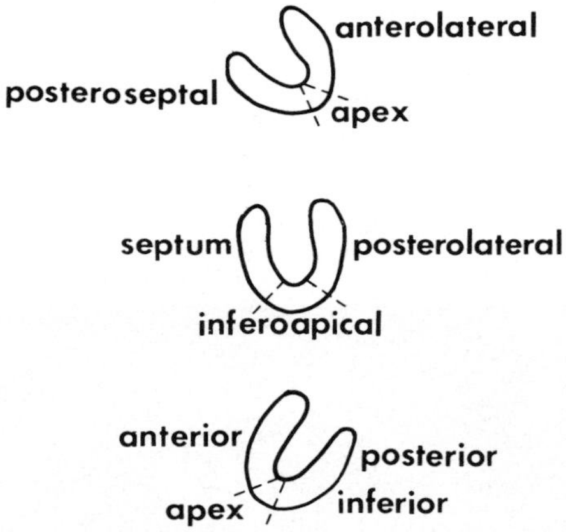

Figure 25.11. Anatomy of left ventricle. Schematic representation of left ventricular anatomy as projected on standard planar views (see text).

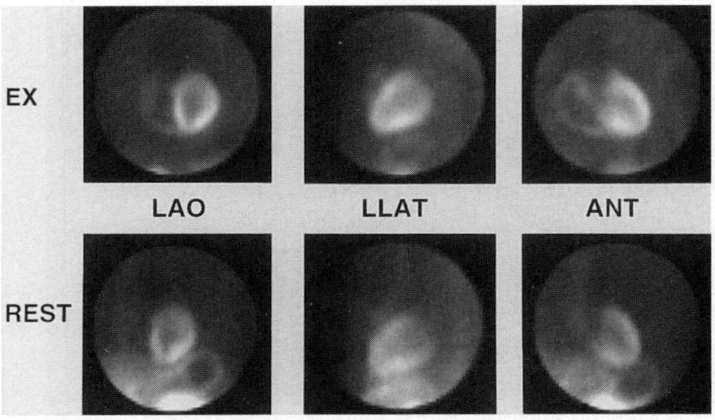

Figure 25.12. Normal sestamibi images after exercise and at rest. Note the considerable improved image quality compared to that with ^{201}Tl (Fig. 25.2).

On the other hand, ^{99m}Tc-sestamibi images also have drawbacks. Substantial subdiaphragmatic activity may be present, which at times interferes with interpretation of the inferior wall of the left ventricle. Marked subdiaphragmatic radiotracer uptake is characteristic for resting images and images obtained after pharmacologic stress.

Typical Normal Exercise-Delayed ^{201}Tl Images

After exercise, ^{201}Tl uptake in the field of view is predominantly within the heart. Minimal or no radiotracer is accumulated in subdiaphragmatic organs. At delayed or redistribution imaging, uptake of ^{201}Tl in the liver has gradually increased, whereas the heart has become fainter due to myocardial washout of ^{201}Tl (Fig. 25.2).

After a resting injection, or after pharmacologic stress, substantial subdiaphragmatic uptake of ^{201}Tl can be observed, which may degrade image quality.

Typical Normal Exercise-Rest ^{99m}Tc-Sestamibi Images

Immediately after exercise, intense uptake of ^{99m}Tc-sestamibi is noted in the liver. Within the next 15–30 minutes, ^{99m}Tc-sestamibi liver uptake is excreted through the biliary system and the radiopharmaceutical appears prominently in the gastrointestinal tract (Fig. 25.3). The optimal time for imaging after exercise is, therefore, approximately 15 minutes after injection. When imaging is performed at a later time, ^{99m}Tc-sestamibi activity in the gastrointestinal tract may significantly interfere with interpretation of the left ventricular inferior wall, in particular on left lateral pla-

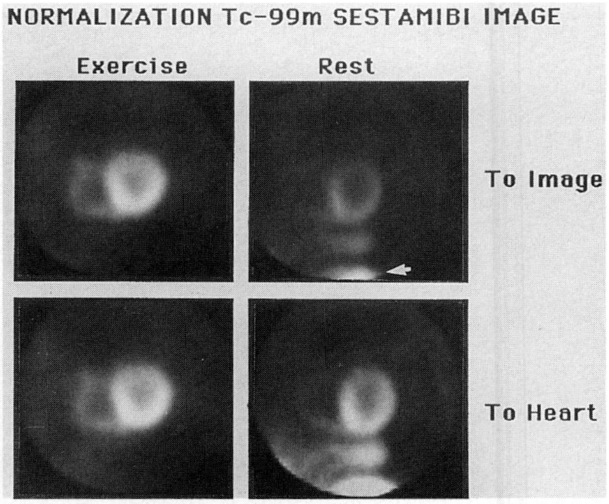

Figure 25.13. Normalization of exercise/rest ^{99m}Tc-sestamibi images. At times, intense subdiaphragmatic activity (*arrow*) may cause problems with adequate display of image of the heart at rest. On exercise images, the heart is the "hottest" organ. On the rest image, the "hottest" area is in the gastrointestinal tract. If the images are normalized to the hottest area in the field of view (i.e., subdiaphragmatic), the heart is only faintly visualized on the rest image (*top*). Using ^{99m}Tc-labeled myocardial perfusion imaging agents, images should be normalized to the heart, as shown in the *bottom panel*, for adequate visualization of the heart.

nar images. After a resting injection of ^{99m}Tc-sestamibi, intense uptake in the liver is again noted, but compared to following exercise, clearance from the liver is substantially slower and optimal timing of imaging is approximately 1–1 1/2 hours after resting injection. In contrast to general belief, digestion of a fatty meal with the purpose to enhance emptying of the gallbladder, has no appreciable favorable effect on image quality. In fact, undesirable subdiaphragmatic tracer accumulation may increase after a meal. Because of significant extracardiac activity, ^{99m}Tc-sestamibi images should be displayed with a gray scale normalized to the "hottest" pixel in the heart (Fig. 25.13).

VARYING SPECTRUM OF NORMAL PLANAR IMAGES

An important reason why the interpretation of planar images may be difficult is that on the *normal image* regionally decreased myocardial accumulation of the radiopharmaceutical may occur (11, 12). Familiarity with the spectrum of normal variations is necessary to avoid typical pitfalls in reading planar myocardial perfusion images (Table 25.2). These patterns are discussed later in detail.

Apex

A well-known and recognized area of normally decreased radiotracer activity is the apex of the left ventricle. This is caused by normal thinning of the myocardium at the apex. The apical defect is frequently noted in patients with a vertical position of the heart. It typically appears as a narrow slit or cleft-like area, aligned with the long axis of the ventricle, which usually can be appreciated on two or three views (Fig. 25.14). In patients with abnormal dilatation of the left ventricle (Fig. 25.15), this apical defect may be considerably larger, and at times is difficult to differentiate from apical infarction. A helpful guideline to distinguish a normal apical variant from an apical infarct is to recognize that the normal apical variant is *invariably* located symmetrically along the long axis of the left ventricle, whereas an apical infarct is asymmetric and usually extends into either the anterior or inferior wall.

Aortic Valve Area

Although the left ventricle on the planar LAO projection is visualized as a doughnut in most patients, occasionally a horseshoe configuration may be seen. The open end of the horseshoe, or apparent "high septal defect," in fact represents the membranous septum and aortic valve area (Fig. 25.8). This particular pattern is common and seldom poses a problem. However, in patients with a horizontally positioned heart and/or a tortuous ascending aorta, the base of the heart is in a near-vertical plane. The area of de-

Table 25.2.
Pitfalls in Interpretation of ^{201}Tl Images

Normal Variants	Characteristics
Apical defect	Narrow cleft aligned with left ventrical long axis; on multiple projections
Aortic valve defect	High septum; on LAO projection
Mitral valve defect	Open end horseshoe; on ANT and LL projections
Posterobasal defect	Inferior part horseshoe, caused by foreshortening; on LL and ANT projections
Typical Artifacts[a]	**Caused By**
ANT: inferoseptal defect	Attenuation by dilated right ventricle
LAO	
Septal defect	Clockwise rotation of dilated left ventricle
Lateral defect	Counterclockwise rotation of left ventricle
LL: posterobasal defect	Attenuation by hemidiaphragm when patient is imaged in supine position
Pendulous breasts	
Defect	Attenuation by breast tissue
Hot spot	Small-angle scatter by breast skinfold

[a]ANT = anterior, LAO = left anterior oblique view, LL = left lateral view.

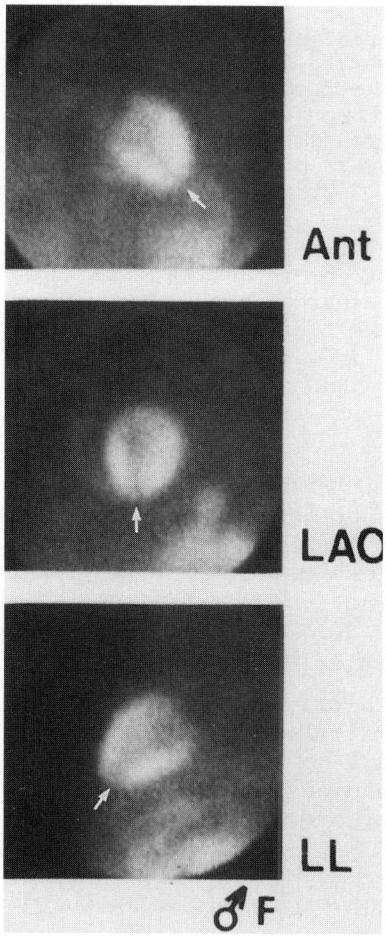

Figure 25.14. Apical thinning. Planar ^{201}Tl image of a normal subject with normal apical thinning (*arrows*). Apical thinning can be especially appreciated in the left anterior oblique (*LAO*) and left lateral (*LL*) projections, although it is also present in the anterior (*Ant*) projection. Note that this cleft-like defect is aligned with the long axis of the heart.

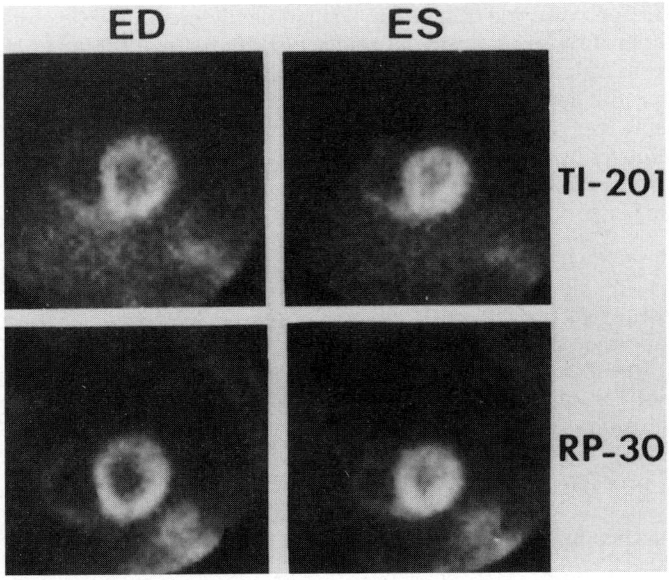

Figure 25.15. ^{201}Tl imaging in patient with dilated left ventricle. Planar ^{201}Tl images of a patient with long-standing hypertension. The left ventricle is enlarged and dilated. The apical defect (*arrows*) is due to partial volume effect and the enlargement and dilatation of the left ventricle. The apparent defect is not an infarct. The visualization of the right ventricle on this resting study is abnormal and is caused by moderate right ventricular hypertrophy in this patient, who also had associated chronic obstructive lung disease. *Ant* = anterior, *LAO* = left anterior oblique, *LL* = left lateral.

creased activity representing the aortic orifice then may be relatively large and can be mistaken for a septal perfusion defect. The clue to the proper interpretation of such an image usually is found on the anterior image, where the horizontal position of the heart can be readily recognized (Fig. 25.16).

Mitral Valve

At times the mitral valve plane may be responsible for artifactual defects on the LAO projection when the heart is rotated counterclockwise (Fig. 25.9). This situation can be recognized by the "curved" appearance of the septum.

Base of the Heart

On the anterior or left lateral view, high posterobasal defects (Fig. 25.17) always should be interpreted with caution. They may be caused by foreshortening of the inferior wall, which may be the case when the heart is in a horizontal position and points at a sharp angle toward the plane of view.

ARTIFACTS ON PLANAR IMAGES

Myocardial perfusion defects appearing on only one planar view are potentially artifactual. True myocardial infarction or ischemia usually presents as defects on more than one planar view (12–14). "Single-view" artifacts can be unmasked by repositioning the patient or by obtaining additional views. Typical artifacts can be described for each planar view (Table 25.2).

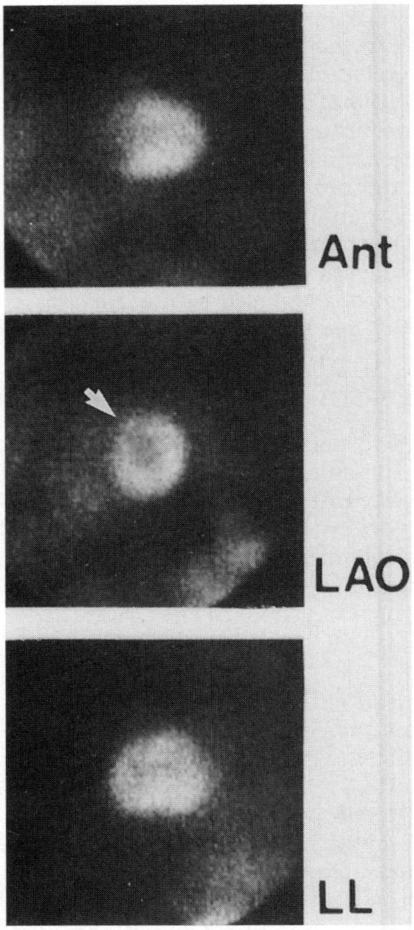

Figure 25.16. Horizontal position of the heart. Normal planar ^{201}Tl images of patient with a horizontal position of the heart and a tortuous ascending aorta. The heart is in a horizontal position, as can be seen on the anterior (*Ant*) and left lateral (*LL*) projections. The left anterior oblique (*LAO*) projection demonstrates an apparent perfusion defect high in the septum (*arrow*) that represents the aortic orifice. This is a normal variant.

Anterior View

In normal subjects, radiopharmaceutical uptake on planar images in the anterolateral wall is approximately equal to that in the inferoseptal region. Occasionally the inferoseptal region may have slightly less activity than the anterolateral wall. This is a normal variant. In patients with enlargement of the right ventricle (e.g., patients with chronic obstructive pulmonary disease) a typical artifact may be seen in the anterior view. The overlying enlarged right ventricle may attenuate radiation sufficiently to produce an artifactual defect in the inferoseptal wall (Fig. 25.18). Such an artifact can be unmasked by imaging the patient in the upright position. The possible explanation for this disappearance of the artifact is that by moving the patient from the standard supine position into the upright position the

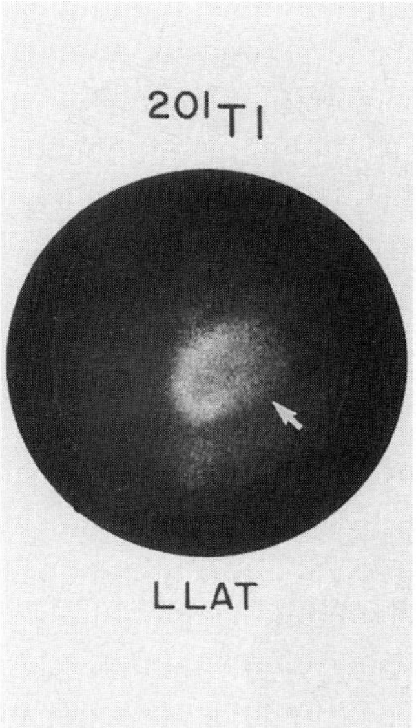

Figure 25.17. Planar ^{201}Tl image in left lateral projection of a normal subject. The anterior and the left anterior oblique views (not shown) are normal. A posterobasal perfusion defect appears to be present on the planar left lateral view, which was obtained with the patient supine. The apparent posterobasal myocardial perfusion defect (*arrow*) is caused by a foreshortening of the inferoposterior wall. Such an artifact can be avoided by acquiring left lateral images with the patient lying on the right side (see also Figs. 25.20–25.23).

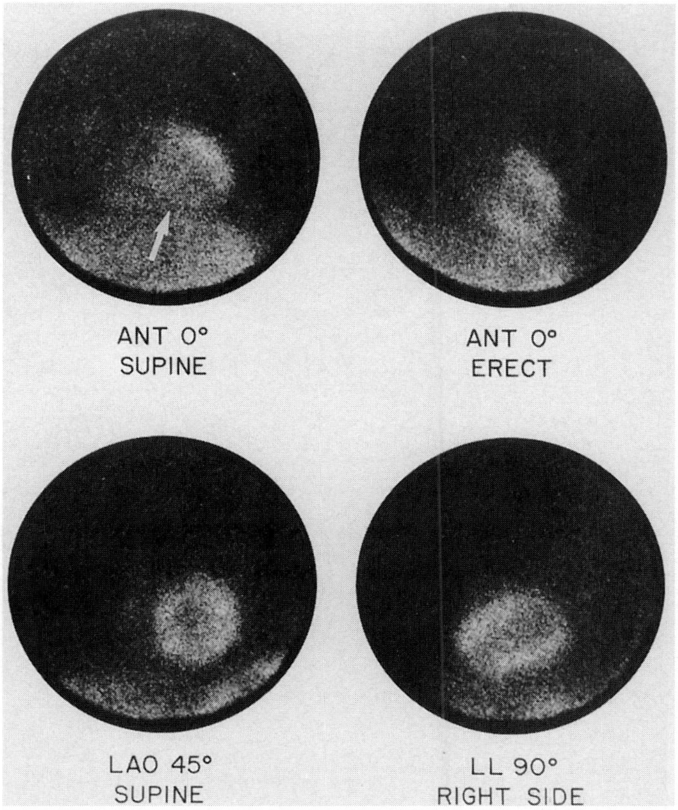

Figure 25.18. Planar ^{201}Tl imaging in chronic obstructive lung disease. Planar ^{201}Tl images at rest of a patient with chronic obstructive lung disease. In supine position, the anterior (*ANT*) projection shows an apparent defect in the inferior wall (*arrow*). When the anterior view is repeated with the patient sitting upright (erect) perfusion of the inferior wall is normal. This artifactual defect is most likely due to attenuation by the blood pool in the overlying enlarged right ventricle. The left anterior oblique (*LAO*) and left lateral (*LL*) projections are normal.

heart shifts into a more vertical position and at the same time the right ventricle rotates to the right. In the upright position there is less overlap of the right ventricle, and, consequently, a normal image of the left ventricle is seen.

Left Anterior Oblique View

On the LAO view, the position of the heart in the chest is often responsible for artifactual defects. One is an apparent lesion in the lateral wall. This is seen when the heart is rotated more medially than usual (Fig. 25.8). Another, as discussed earlier, is an apparent high septal defect, caused by horizontal position of the heart, usually representing the aortic orifice (Fig. 25.16).

In patients with enlargement and dilatation of the left ventricle, the long axis is frequently deviated to the left. In these cases, a routine 45° LAO view may display an image similar to that usually seen on the anterior projection (Fig. 25.19). The normal open end of the horseshoe could be misinterpreted as a septal defect. A steeper (60°) LAO angle may project the left ventricle correctly along the long axis and thereby restore the typical doughnut-shaped configuration. This phenomenon may in part explain previous reports of septal defects in patients with left bundle branch block (15). Many patients with complete left bundle branch block have an enlarged, dilated left ventricle with clockwise rotation. When the rotation is taken into consideration and the angulation of individual views is adjusted, the septum often is well-visualized, although it may appear thinner than usual (see also the discussion of the left bundle branch block later in this chapter).

Left Lateral View

On a left lateral view, inadequate acquisition technique may cause an apparent artifactual inferior defect. This important artifact is caused by attenuation of photons by structures superimposed on the inferior wall of the heart. The position of the patient during the acquisition of the left lateral view is crucial to avoid this problem (14, 16, 17). The left lateral image should be acquired with the patient *lying on his or her right side* (Fig. 25.20). Acquiring the left lateral view with the patient supine results in false-positive defects of the inferoposterior wall in 18% of patients (Fig. 25.21).

Furthermore, left lateral *supine* images are often technically inferior to those obtained with the patient lying on his or her *right side*. Explanations for this false-positive

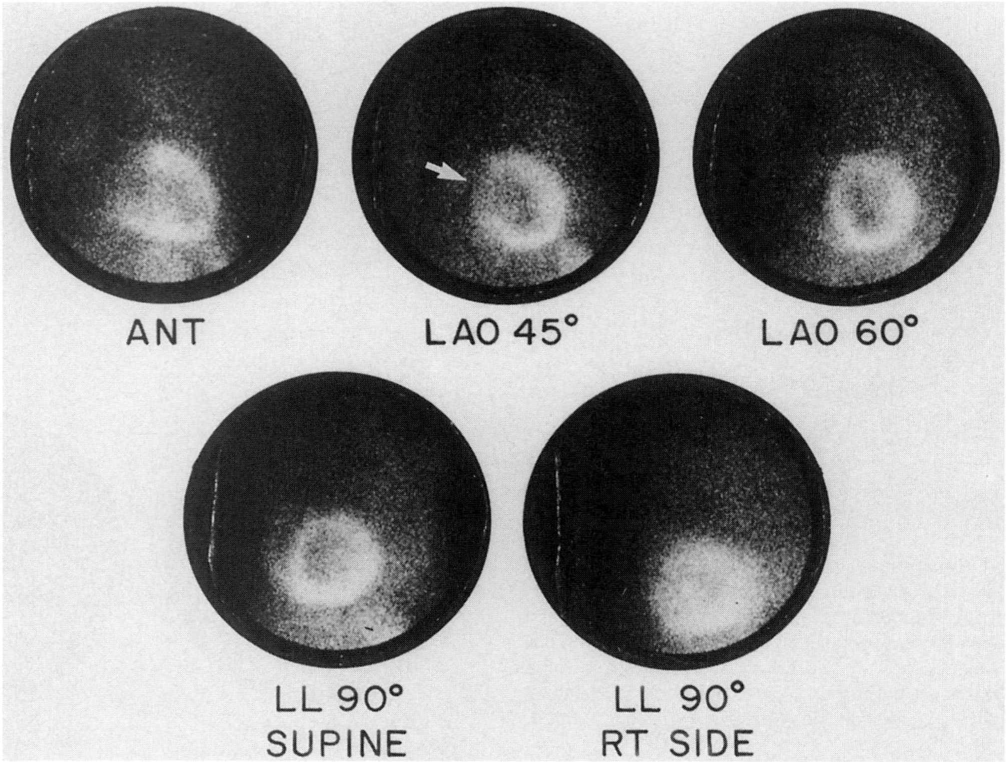

Figure 25.19. Planar ^{201}Tl images of a patient with complete left bundle branch block on the electrocardiogram. The left ventricle is enlarged, dilated, and rotated clockwise. On the standard planar 45° left anterior oblique (*LAO*) projection, a septal myocardial perfusion defect (*arrow*) appears to be present. However, the configuration of the left ventricle in this LAO projection is similar to that on the anterior (*ANT*) projection, indicating clockwise rotation. The LAO view at 60° and the left lateral (*LL*) views at 90° clearly visualize the septum. Although the septum is thinner than usual, no myocardial perfusion defect is present. (Reproduced by permission from Wackers FJTh. Thallium-201 myocardial imaging. In: Wackers FJTh, ed. Thallium-201 and technetium-99m pyrophosphate myocardial imaging in the coronary care unit. The Hague: Martinus Nijhoff Publishers, 1980:70–104.)

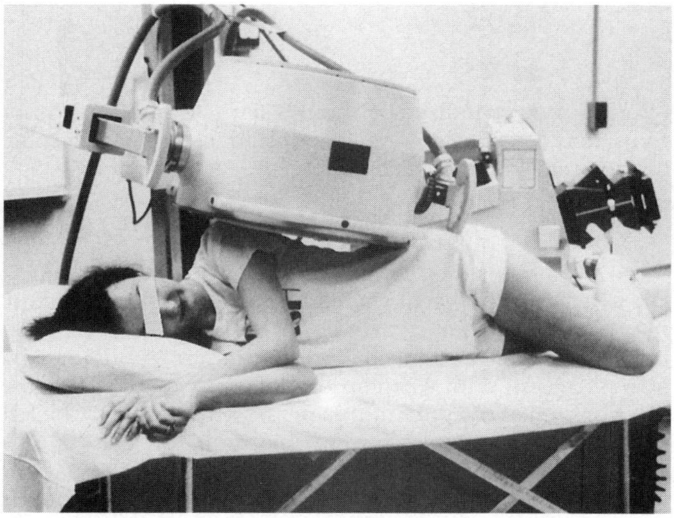

Figure 25.20. Correct patient positioning for acquisition of left lateral image. The patient should be lying on his or her right side with the camera detector above the table. The camera detector should be placed as close as possible to the chest wall.

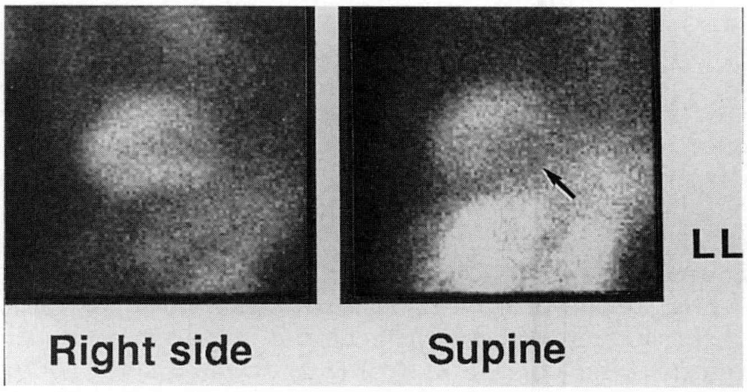

Figure 25.21. Artifactual inferoposterior defect in supine position. ^{201}Tl images following exercise in a patient with angiographic normal coronary arteries. A definite inferoposterior myocardial perfusion defect (*arrow*) is seen on the left lateral (*LL*) supine projection. A LL view obtained with the patient lying on his right side demonstrates a normal inferoposterior wall. The two left lateral images were obtained immediately after each other.

defect include geometric considerations and radiation attenuation by adjacent structures. Figure 25.22 demonstrates the change in alignment of the heart as the patient moves from the supine position to the right-side-down position: the long axis of the heart shifts from horizontal toward vertical. When the patient is on his or her right side, the inferoposterior segments are parallel to the detector, providing an *en face* image of this region. However, with the patient supine, the inferoposterior wall can be almost perpendicular to the detector, which results in a foreshortened projection of the inferoposterior segments (Fig. 25.17). Although false-positive defects in the left lateral supine position could potentially be the result of distorted projection of these segments, a more likely explanation is attenuation of radiation by the left hemidiaphragm (Fig. 25.23). SPECT imaging is usually performed with the patient lying supine. Not surprisingly, inferior wall attenuation is a frequently occurring problem in SPECT imaging.

The planar left-lateral view is an important projection for visualization of the inferoposterior wall without overlying radioactivity from other cardiac structures. If obtained with the right side down, the anterior and inferoposterior walls are spatially well-separated. In many laboratories, the left lateral view is not routinely obtained with the patient on the right side. Instead, a steep (70°) supine left anterior oblique projection is substituted. The latter view is often *not comparable* to the true left lateral image, especially in patients with enlarged left ventricles and/or clockwise rotation. On the supine steep oblique projection, the posterior wall is occasionally not visualized and therefore imaging is incomplete (Fig. 25.24).

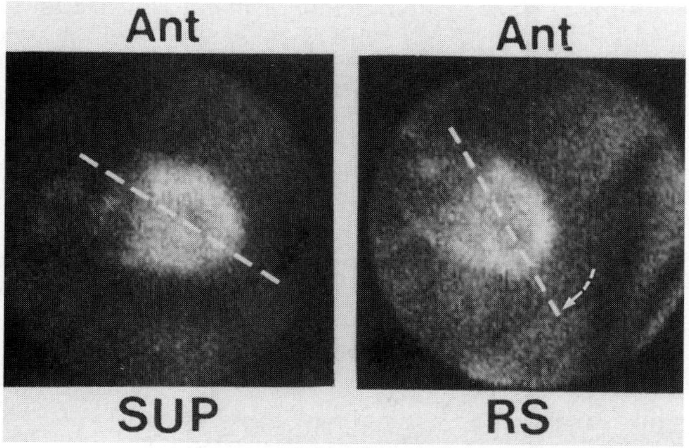

Figure 25.22. Patient positioning and inferoposterior wall visualization. Planar anterior ^{201}Tl images with the patient in supine position (*SUP*), and with the patient lying on his right side (*RS*). When the patient turns from supine position to the right-side-down position, the long axis of the heart (*broken line*) shifts to a more vertical position. This change in position of the heart is partly responsible for better visualization of the inferoposterior wall.

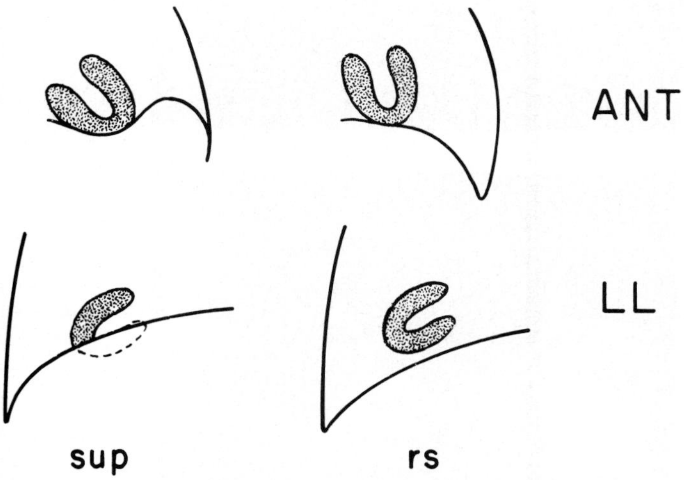

Figure 25.23. Patient positioning and hemidiaphragm/inferior wall. Schematic illustration of the relationship between left hemidiaphragm and inferior wall of the heart in supine (*sup*) position and with the patient on his or her right side (*rs*). The top panel shows the anterior (*ANT*) projection and the bottom panel shows the left lateral (*LL*) projection. In the supine position, the left hemidiaphragm is higher than in the right-side-down position and attenuates radiotracer in the inferoposterior myocardial segment. (Reproduced by permission from Johnstone DE, Wackers FJTh, Berger HJ, et al. Effect of patient positioning on left lateral thallium-201 myocardial images. J Nucl Med 1979;20:183.)

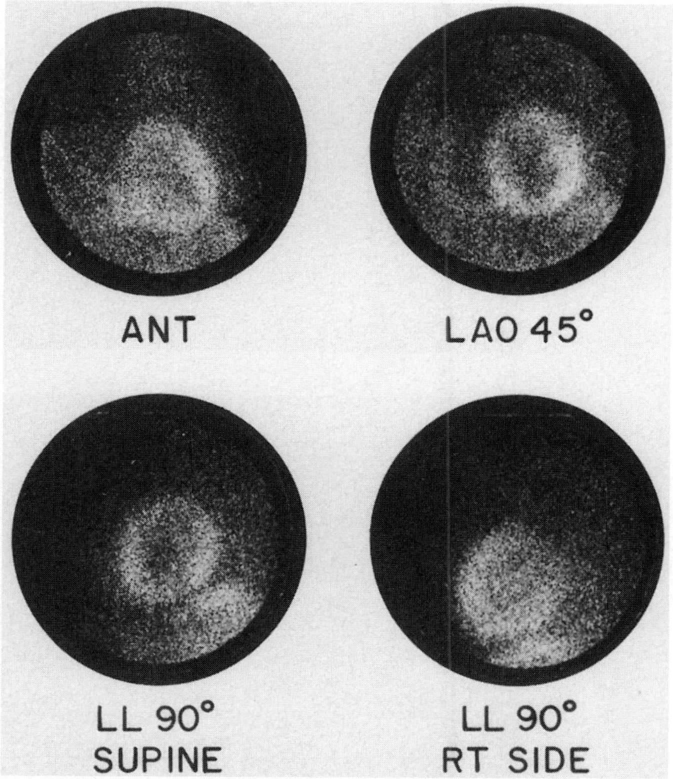

Figure 25.24. Myocardial perfusion image in dilated cardiomyopathy. Planar ^{201}Tl images of a patient with dilated cardiomyopathy. The left ventricle is enlarged. The left lateral (*LL*) supine projection shows the heart in a left anterior oblique (*LAO*)-like configuration because of cardiac enlargement. The inferoposterior wall is, consequently, not well-visualized. The LL view with the patient turned on his right side shows better projection of the long axis of the heart and visualizes the inferoposterior wall. *ANT* = anterior.

Obese Patients, Large Breasts

In extremely obese patients and/or in patients with large breasts, inhomogeneous attenuation of radiation may cause apparent diminished uptake of radiotracer in the heart. These areas often appear as anteroapical defects on the anterior and left lateral view, whereas the location may vary on the LAO view (Fig. 25.25). In addition to causing areas of diminished activity on myocardial perfusion images, the breast can also produce linear areas of increased activity. These areas of increased activity, which are caused by small-angle scatter of photons at the contour of the breast (Fig. 25.26), may further complicate the interpretation of breast artifacts. In some patients, inhomogeneous attenuation of photons by breast tissue may mimic an image of increased lung uptake. This may occur when the attenuation over the heart (by the full thickness of the breast) is greater than over the upper-lung fields. We have found it useful to employ radioactive string markers to outline the contour of the breast and define the relationship of the breast to the left ventricle and the apparent defects. Although the energy of ^{99m}Tc-labeled agents is higher than that of ^{201}Tl, tissue attenuation with ^{99m}Tc is decreased by only one-seventh. Therefore, breast attenuation artifacts can be expected to occur with ^{99m}Tc-labeled agents as well. However, in our experience, the artifacts associated with these newer agents are less marked than with ^{201}Tl. The most likely explanation is that less low-energy scatter photons are attenuated, as well as the use of high-resolution collimation and narrower (20%) energy window.

Typical ^{99m}Tc-Sestamibi Planar Imaging Artifacts

Because of substantial subdiaphragmatic accumulation of the radiopharmaceutical, planar images with ^{99m}Tc-sestamibi and other ^{99m}Tc-labeled agents may, at times, be significantly degraded. In particular, on the left lateral view the inferior wall of the left ventricle may be superimposed on subdiaphragmatic radioactivity, and interpretation of inferior wall abnormalities may be impossible or difficult. However, even without significant subdiaphragmatic ^{99m}Tc-labeled tracer uptake, the anterior wall-to-inferior wall count ratio on the planar left lateral view may be re-

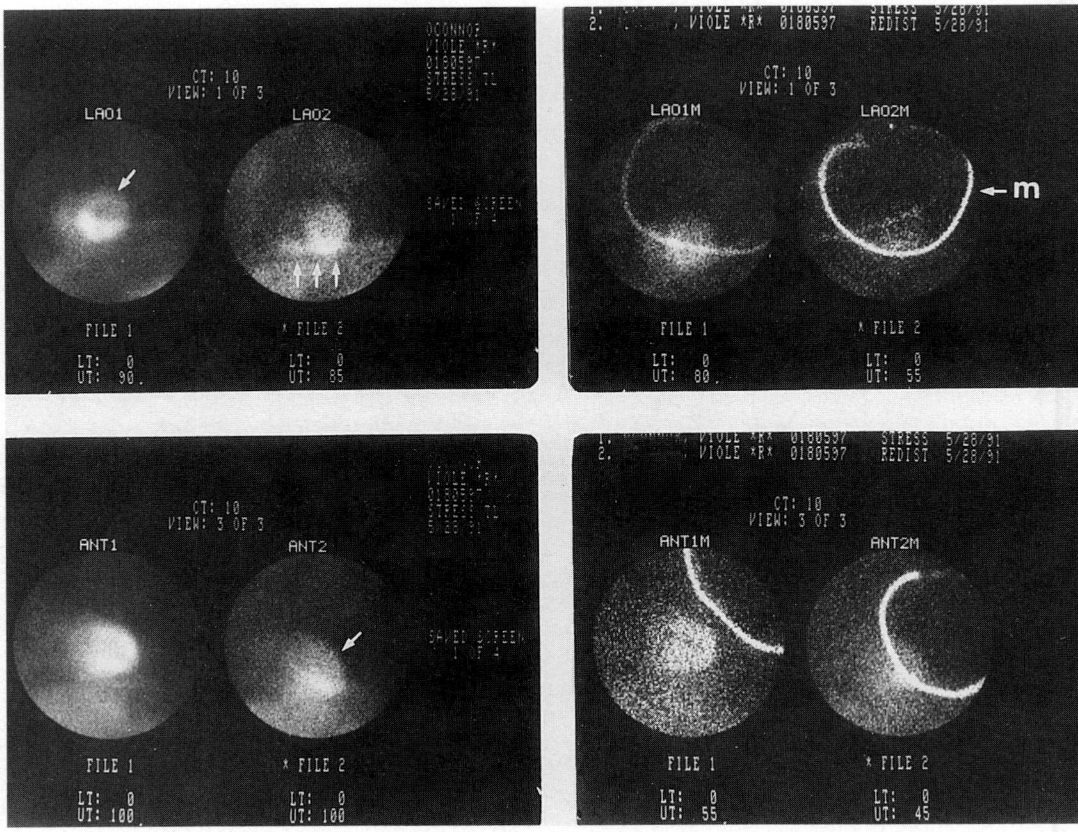

Figure 25.25. Planar ^{201}Tl left anterior oblique (*LAO*) and anterior (*ANT*) images in a woman with large breasts (*LAO, ANTI* = imaging during exercise; LAO2, *ANT2* = delayed imaging). Breast markers (*m*) are shown in the images on the right. On the LAO exercise images (*top*), a definite attenuation artifact is present (*arrow*). At delayed imaging, the breast contour is lower and is visualized as a linear area (*arrow*) with increased activity caused by small-angle scatter (see Fig. 25.26). The exercise anterior view (*bottom*) is normal, because the breast did not cover the heart. However, at delayed imaging, the contour of the breast is cross the heart, causing an attenuation artifact (*arrow*). This is an example of how breast attenuation artifacts can vary in the same view due to different breast positions. Note that on the delayed LAO image, unequal attenuation mimics an image with increased lung uptake of ^{201}Tl. (Reproduced by permission from Wackers FJTh. Diagnostic pitfalls of myocardial perfusion in women. J Myocard Ischemia 1992; 4:23–37.)

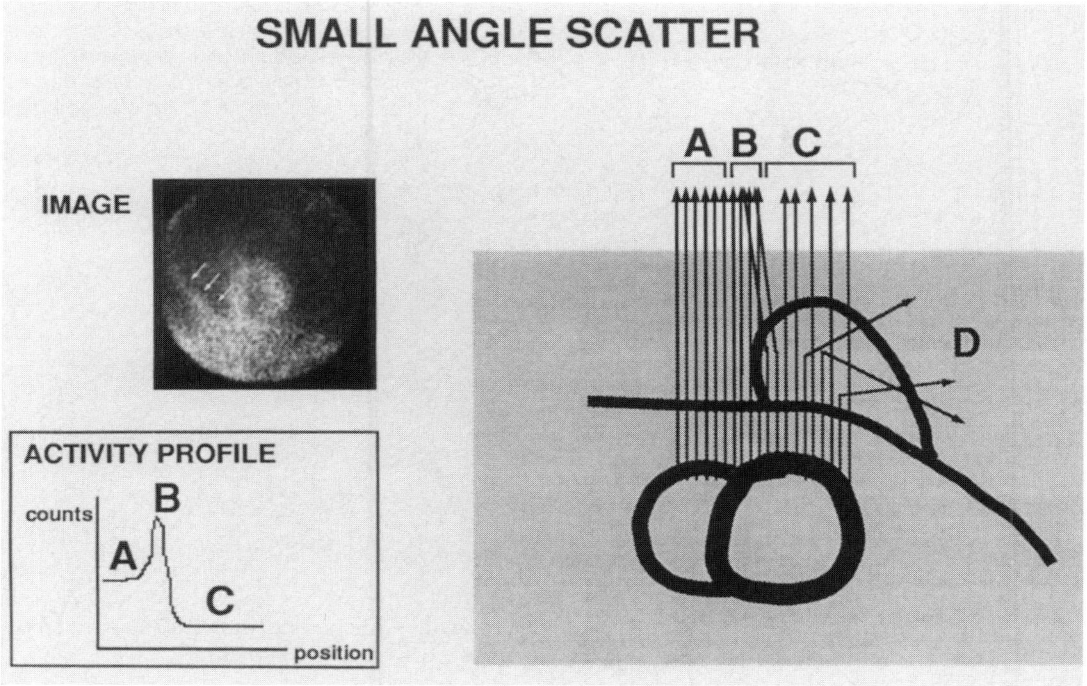

Figure 25.26. Attenuation and small-angle scatter. On the right is a schematic representation of the heart, chest wall, and left breast. Photons of *A* travel directly to the gamma-camera unattenuated, whereas photons at *D* are scattered in the breast and do not reach the gamma-camera (photon attenuation). Some photons (*C*) travel through the breast before they reach the gamma-camera, producing an image that suggests an area with apparently less activity. Other photons (*B*) travel through the border of the breast and scatter at a small angle (small-angle scatter). These are not attenuated photons, but rather, result in a linear area of increased activity (*arrows* on image), representing the contour of the breast. (Reproduced by permission from Wackers FJTh. Diagnostic pitfalls of myocardial perfusion in women. J Myocard Ischemia 1992;4:23–37.)

versed compared to that usually seen on a ^{201}Tl image: the inferior wall is more intense than the anterior wall. Thus, using ^{99m}Tc-labeled agents, because of increased intensity of the inferior wall, mild anterior wall defects may be mimicked. This is a normal and typical variant on planar imaging of ^{99m}Tc-labeled agents (Fig. 25.27).

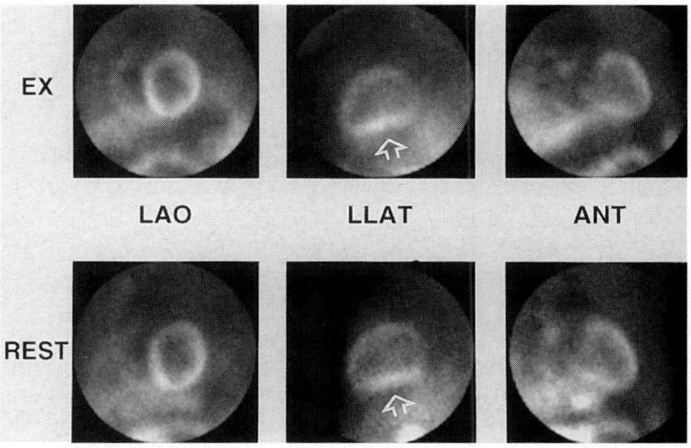

Figure 25.27. Typical normal variant on planar ^{99m}Tc-sestamibi imaging. Shown are exercise/rest ^{99m}Tc-sestamibi images. The left ventricle is slightly enlarged, but no myocardial perfusion defects are present. The left lateral images show a typical sestamibi normal variant; the inferior wall (*open arrow*) appears to be relatively "hotter" than to the anterior wall. This is due to superimposition of subdiaphragmatic activity over the inferior wall of the left ventricle. This typical ^{99m}Tc-sestamibi pattern should not be interpreted as a an anterior wall myocardial perfusion defect.

NORMAL SPECT MYOCARDIAL PERFUSION IMAGE

In SPECT myocardial perfusion imaging, the heart is displayed in short axis, horizontal long axis, and vertical long axis slices.

The short axis slices should be analyzed in three groups: apical slices, midventricular slices, and basal slices. To avoid artifacts by partial volume effect, only apical slices that clearly show the ventricular cavity should be analyzed. Figure 25.28 shows the standardized display of SPECT images. The anatomy of SPECT images and coronary territories are shown in Figures 25.29–25.32.

VARYING SPECTRUM OF NORMAL SPECT IMAGING

On the *short axis* slices, slightly less uptake of radiotracer can be appreciated in the septal wall, compared to the lateral wall (Fig. 25.33). Furthermore, there may be slightly less inferoseptal uptake in male patients as a normal variant, whereas radiotracer distribution in females is more homogeneous. The most apical short axis slices (without

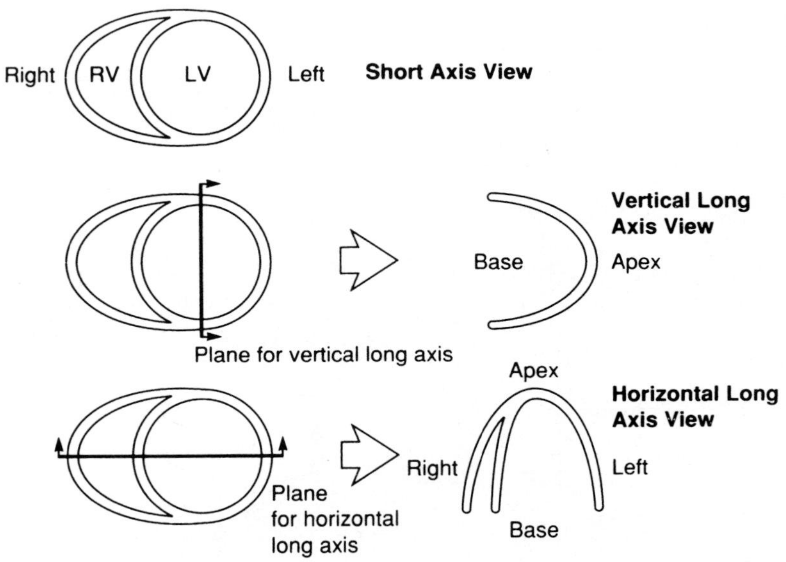

Figure 25.28. Standardized display of SPECT myocardial perfusion images. The short axis slices are displayed with the right ventricle left and the left ventricle right. The short axis slices are displayed as a horizontal row of images, starting with the apical slice on the left and the basal slices on the right. The vertical long axis slices are cut from the septum toward the lateral wall, displaying the septal slices on the left and the lateral slices on the right. The horizontal long axis slices are cut from the inferior wall towards the anterior wall, displaying the inferior wall slices on the left and the anterior wall slices on the right.

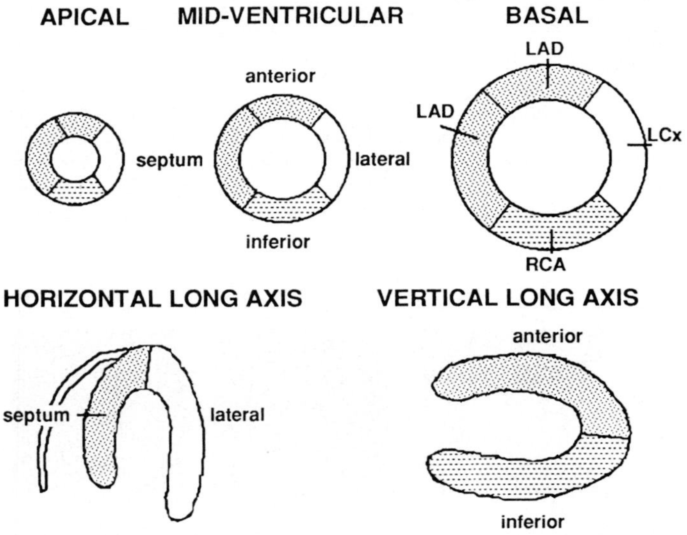

Figure 25.29. Anatomic segments and coronary artery territories on SPECT myocardial perfusion imaging.

ventricular cavity) often show somewhat inhomogeneous radiotracer distribution due to partial volume effect and due to the relative excentric location of the apex in the detector orbit (see later). The most basal slices of the short axis slices usually show an apparent septal defect. This is a normal finding that represents the *membranous portion of* the upper septum.

In contrast to planar imaging, where each view is an independently acquired and unique image, the *vertical long axis* slices and the *horizontal long axis* slices are reconstructed from the same raw data as the short axis slices. The main purpose for analyzing long axis slices is to inspect the apex and base of the heart without significant partial volume artifacts. Only slices that clearly show left ventricular cavity should be analyzed. On the horizontal long axis slices the septum is usually shorter than the lateral wall—this is a normal finding caused by the membranous portion of the septum.

ARTIFACTS ON SPECT IMAGES

Artifacts are particularly troublesome and may be difficult to recognize on reconstructed SPECT slices (14). When on planar imaging one view is of suboptimal quality, the remaining two views may be still acceptable for diagnostic interpretation. For SPECT imaging, the entire set of 32 or more projection images has to be of optimal quality. The basic concept of tomographic backprojection assumes that the object to be reconstructed remains unchanged during image acquisition from multiple angles. However, in reality, changes may occur during the time of SPECT acquisition.

Diaphragmatic Attenuation

The significant artifacts that can be caused by diaphragmatic attenuation have already been discussed for planar imaging. SPECT imaging is performed with the patient lying in a supine position. We have shown that in this position the left ventricular inferior wall frequently is attenuated (Fig. 25.21). Not surprisingly false-positive inferior wall defects are frequently seen on SPECT images (Fig. 25.34). Because such attenuation artifacts occur only in approximately 25% of patients, and since they are unpredictable, this variation is not readily incorporated in a normal SPECT database without decreasing sensitivity for detection of inferior wall perfusion defects. To recognize this potential SPECT artifact, we recommend completion of SPECT imaging with the additional *acquisition of two planar views:* one left lateral view with the patient lying *supine,* and another left lateral view with the patient lying on his/her *right side* (Fig. 25.20). This additional set of images will alert the interpreter to the possibility of inferior wall attenuation on SPECT. Other investigators recommend a different patient position for SPECT imaging to avoid artifacts—either in the prone (18) or the upright position (19).

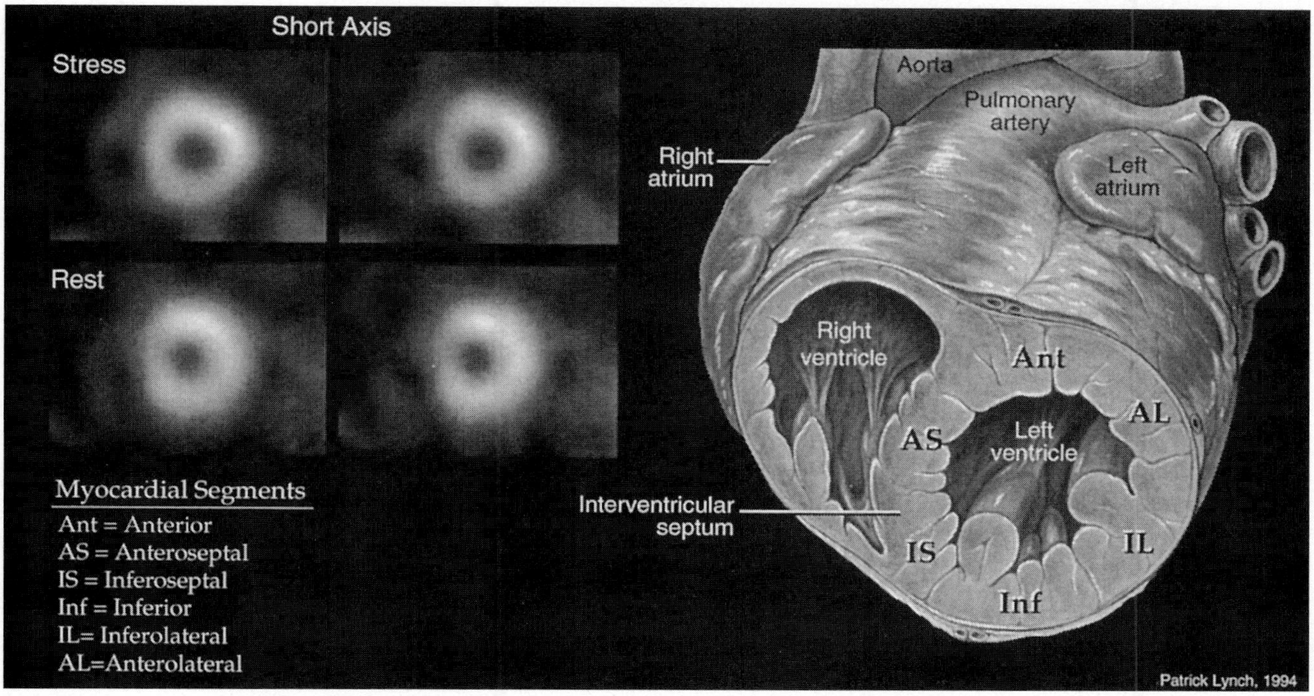

Figure 25.30. Anatomy of the left ventricle on short axis SPECT slices. Schematic anatomic drawing of the left ventricle as displayed in reconstructed short axis slices. Stress/rest scintigraphic short axis slices are shown in the left upper corner.

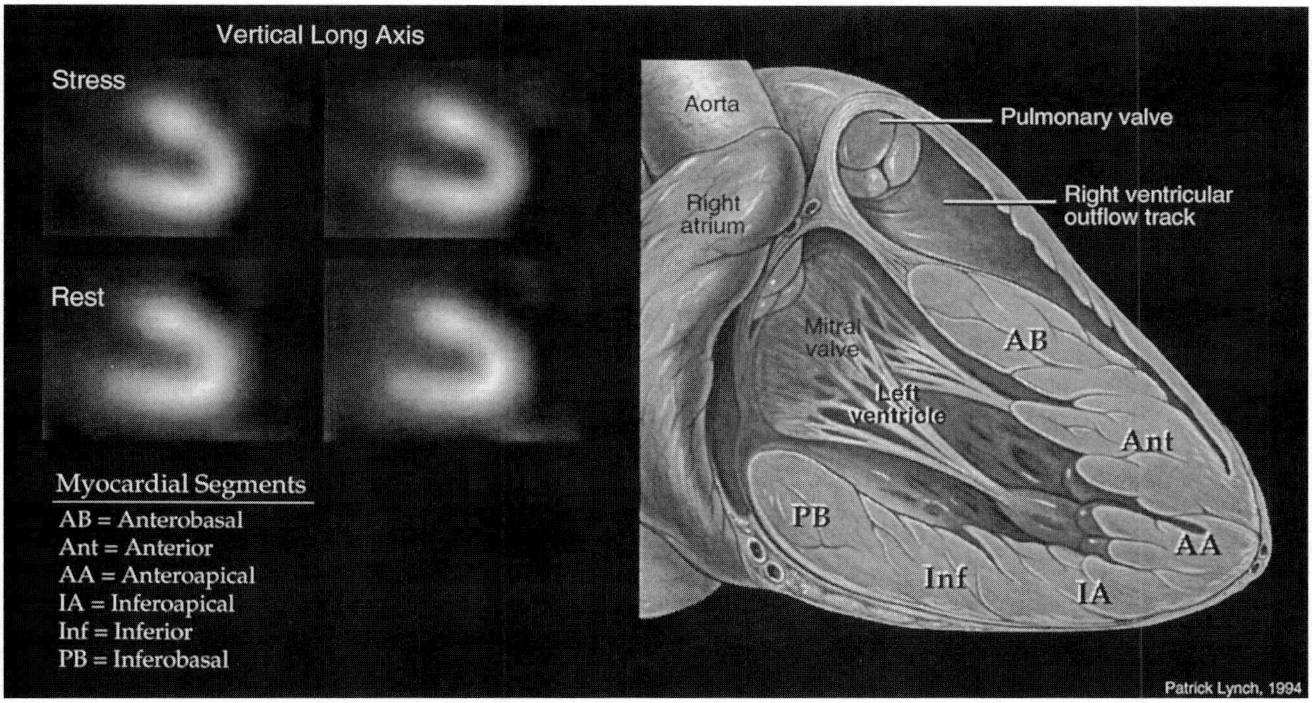

Figure 25.31. Anatomy on the left ventricle on vertical long axis SPECT slices. Schematic anatomic drawing of the left ventricle displayed in reconstructed vertical long axis SPECT slice is shown. Stress/rest scintigraphic vertical long axis slices shown in the left upper corner.

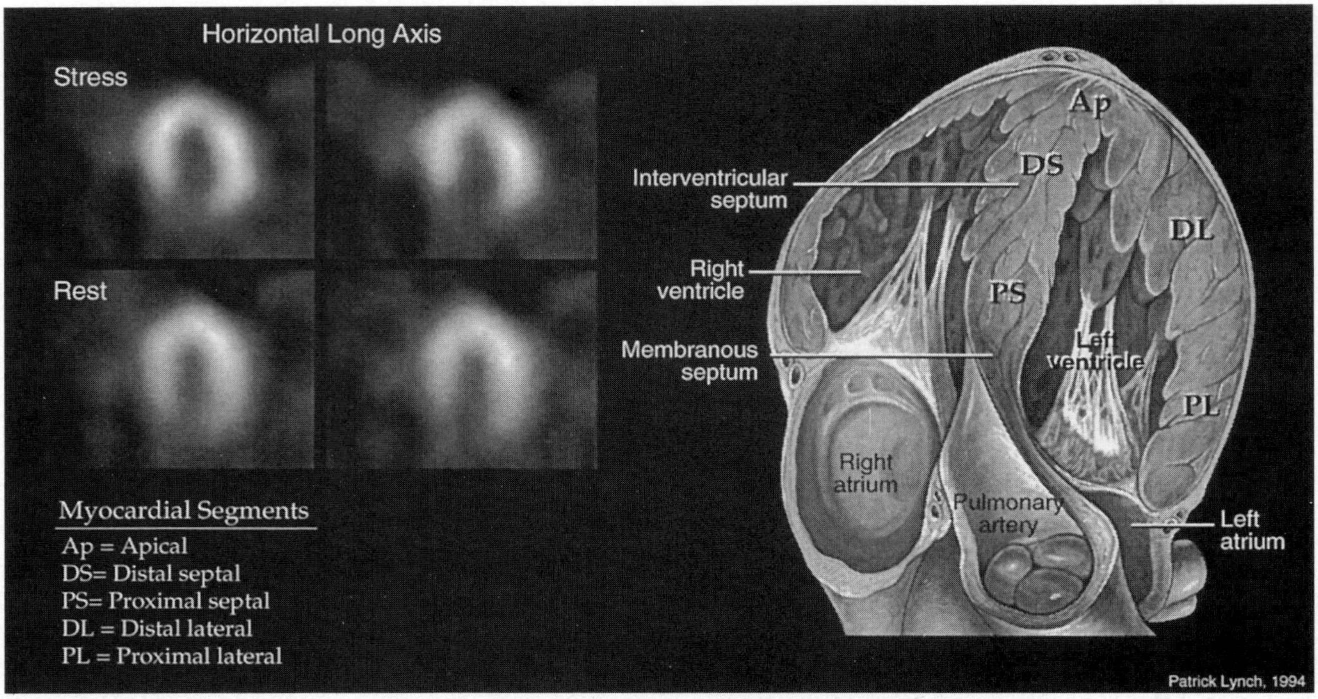

Figure 25.32. Anatomy of the left ventricle on horizontal long axis SPECT slices. Schematic anatomic drawing of the left ventricle as displayed in reconstructed horizontal long axis slices. Stress/rest scintigraphic horizontal long axis slices are shown in the upper left corner.

Visual analysis of ECG-gated SPECT images may also be helpful to recognize inferior wall attenuation artifacts. Normal wall motion of an apparent rest defect is suggestive of attenuation artifact. Until validated attenuation correction software can be applied routinely to SPECT images, attenuation artifacts may continue to limit specificity of SPECT imaging.

Breast Artifacts

On SPECT imaging, breast attenuation artifacts are less extensive than on planar imaging. However, on reconstructed slices they are difficult to distinguish from true myocardial perfusion defects (Fig. 25.35). Thus, recognition of breast artifacts on SPECT is even more difficult than on planar imaging. These artifacts remain a diagnostic dilemma. To detect the potential of breast artifacts on SPECT imaging, inspection of the "rotating projection images" prior to interpretation is an essential part of quality control. On cine display of the projection images (Fig. 25.36), one can observe the "breast shadow" moving over the heart, a sign that one should be alert for breast artifacts. Visual analysis of ECG-gated SPECT images may also be helpful to recognize breast attenuation artifacts. Normal wall motion of an apparent rest defect is suggestive of artifact. Attenuation correction software may in the future solve the problem of breast artifacts.

Upward Creep

During SPECT acquisition, the heart may change from a vertical position immediately postexercise, to a more horizontal position towards the end of image acquisition when the patient is rested. This change in position of the heart was observed to occur especially in subjects who exercised well and long. The explanation for the observation is that during SPECT acquisition the patient's breathing pattern changes from deep after exercise, to more shallow during recovery, with flattening of the diaphragm. This change in position is called "upward creep" of the heart and has been shown to cause artifactual inferior wall defects (20). To avoid these artifacts, it has been recommended that image acquisition not be started immediately postexercise, but be delayed for approximately 10 minutes to allow the patient to recover from the exercise effort. For ^{201}Tl imaging, this delay has been turned into an advantage, as this time allows for acquisition of a planar image for assessment of exercise-induced increased lung uptake, prior to starting SPECT imaging. Upward creep is less of a problem using ^{99m}Tc-sestamibi, since imaging is started, at the earliest, 15 minutes after injection at peak exercise.

Patient Motion

Many patients find it difficult to lie still for 20–30 minutes on a table with the arms extended over the head. Motion artifacts may seriously degrade the quality of SPECT images and may cause artifacts on reconstructed slices. Typical motion artifacts show the heart as if it is "broken up" and may mimic myocardial perfusion defects (Figs. 25.37**A** and **B**). Improved table design and different imaging positions could minimize this problem. Several investigators have noted that patients generally tolerate the prone or upright position better than the supine position, and have

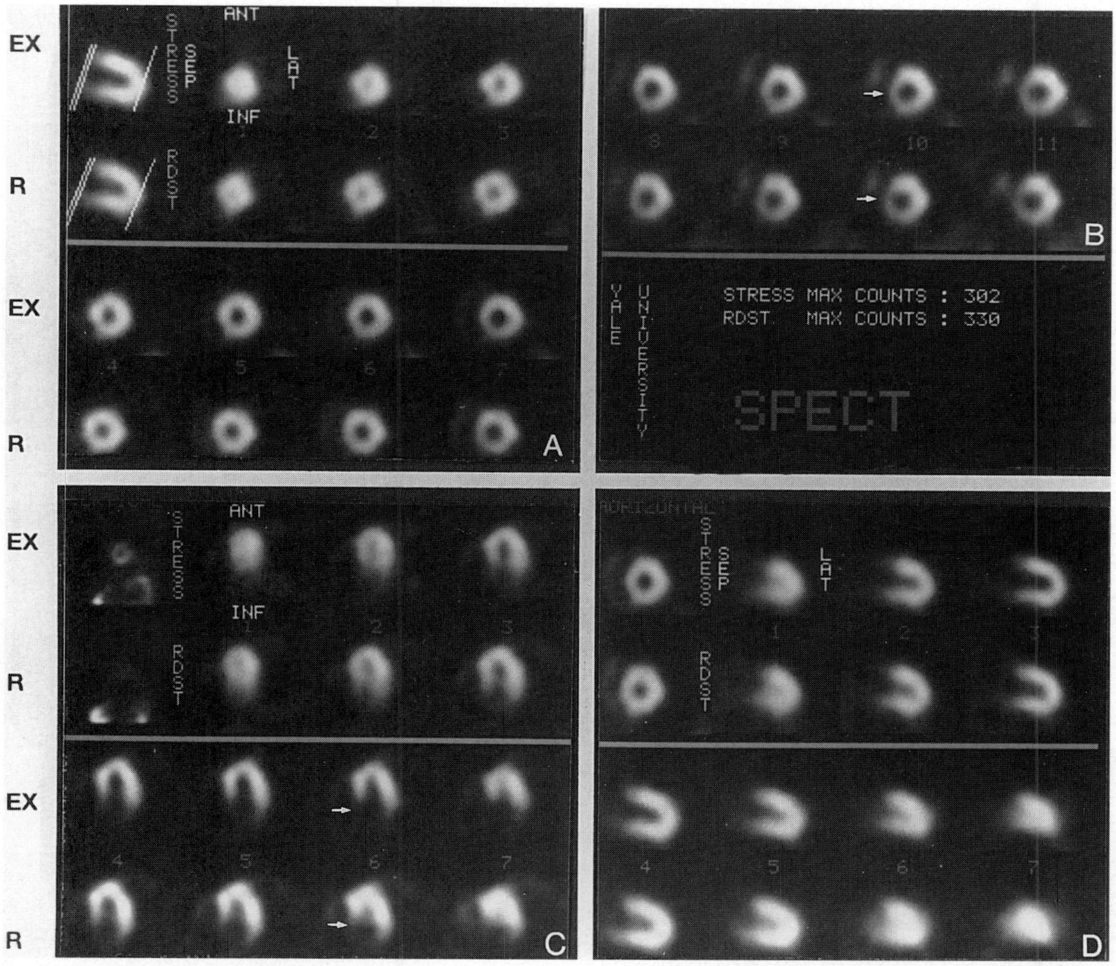

Figure 25.33. SPECT ^{99m}Tc-sestamibi myocardial images after exercise and at rest in a normal subject showing normal variation of radiopharmaceutic distribution. On the midventricular short axis slices (*A*), the inferior septal areas have slightly less activity than the lateral wall. On the basal slices (*B*), an apparent septal defect is present (*arrow*). This is the membranous portion of the septum. This is also seen in the horizontal long axis slices (*C*) where the septum is shorter (*arrow*) than the lateral wall. Vertical long axis slices are shown in *D*. (Reproduced by permission from Wackers FJTh. Artifacts in planar and SPECT myocardial perfusion imaging. Am J Cardiac Imaging 1992;6:42–58.)

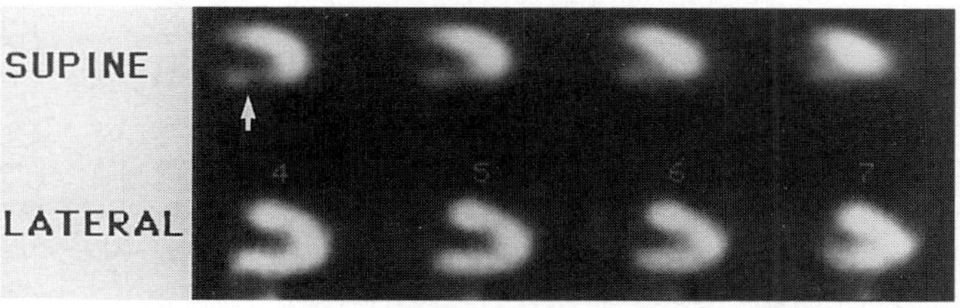

Figure 25.34. Vertical long axis ^{201}Tl SPECT images of the patient shown in Figure 25.21. Images acquired with the patient lying on his back (supine) are shown in the *top* panel. An inferior wall myocardial perfusion defect in present (*arrow*). The patient was turned on the right side (lateral) and SPECT imaging was repeated. This time the vertical long axis images are normal. The erroneous inferior wall defect on supine imaging is caused by attenuation by the left hemidiaphragm. Turning the patient onto her right side diminishes diaphragmatic attenuation. (Reproduced by permission from Wackers FJTh. Artifacts in planar and SPECT myocardial perfusion imaging. Am J Cardiac Imaging 1992;6:42–58.)

less motion artifacts when imaging is performed in those unconventional positions. Patient motion is best detected on the "rotating projection images," i.e., cine display of all planar projection images. This is an essential part of quality assurance before interpretation of the reconstructed slices. Unless well-validated motion correction software is used routinely, motion artifact will remain one of the most important technical problems with SPECT imaging.

Center of Rotation and Field Uniformity

Other artifacts typical for SPECT imaging, but usually less of a problem with improved technology and routine quality assurance of equipment, are those of the center-of-rotation offset and flood field nonuniformity. Offset of the center-of-rotation can produce apical artifacts. These artifacts are best observed on the horizontal long axis slices as defects and "smearing" near the apex (Fig. 25.38). Furthermore, center-of-rotation offset can cause a severe degradation of image resolution. Field nonuniformity causes typical ring artifacts. The latter artifacts are related to the mechanics of the SPECT gamma-camera and can be avoided by routine gamma-camera quality control. Center-of-rotation and uniformity are usually not a major source of problems in a well-run nuclear cardiology laboratory.

Orbit Related Artifacts

Another potential artifact is related to the orbit of the SPECT camera and the use of general-all-purpose collimation. Because of the relatively low count density of ^{201}Tl images, a general-all-purpose collimator is used to optimize count density. Some manufacturers have made it possible to preset an orbit that follows the body contour, i.e., during acquisition the camera head rotates as close as possible to the patient's chest wall at all 32 positions. However, because the heart is eccentric in the chest, such an orbit brings the camera head to varying distances from the target organ. With varying distance the resolution of the gamma-camera varies at each stop. Varying resolution may create typical artifacts—180° diametrically opposed defects on the short axis slices (21) (Fig. 25.39). These artifacts can be avoided by using a circular orbit. However, one should realize that even using a circular orbit, depending on the patient's body habitus, the heart may be eccentric and still be at varying distance from the camera head. The problem of variable resolution may be substantially lessened with the use of high resolution collimation, as is presently routinely used for imaging with ^{99m}Tc-labeled imaging agents and multihead gamma-cameras.

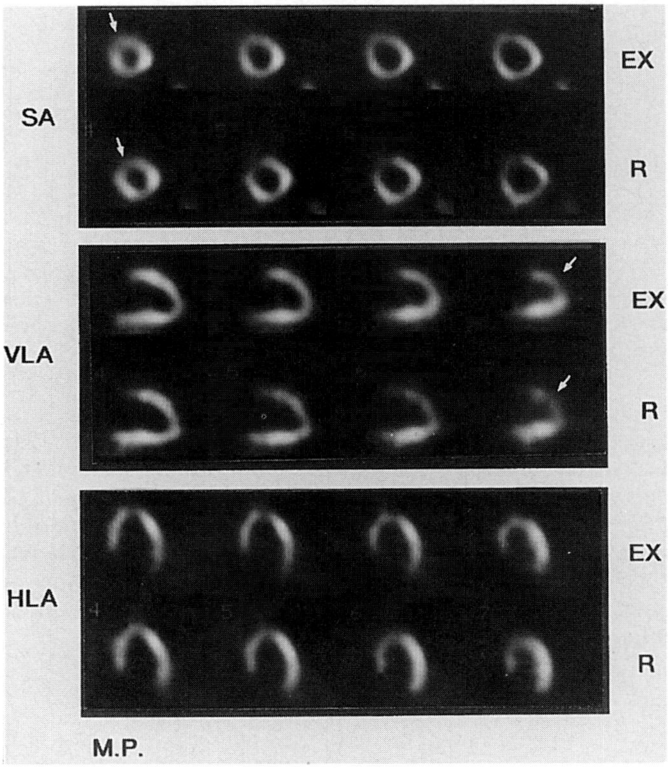

Figure 25.35. ^{201}Tl SPECT images with breast artifacts. On exercise (*EX*), short axis slices show that an anterior apical myocardial perfusion defect (*arrows*) is present. On the delayed redistribution (*R*) images, the anterior wall defect appears to be larger. The inconsistency of location of the defects is caused by change in position of the breast during repeat imaging. On the horizontal or vertical long axis slices anterior defects can be appreciated as well. (Reproduced by permission from Wackers FJTh. Artifacts in planar and SPECT myocardial perfusion imaging. Am J Cardiac Imaging 1992;6:42–58.)

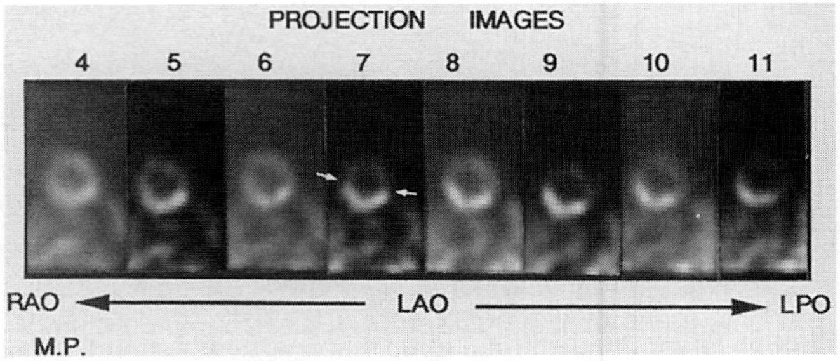

Figure 25.36. Serial consecutive planar projection images of the patient in Figure 25.35 with breast artifact. The breast shadow can be seen to be moving over the heart on frames 5–11 (*arrows*).

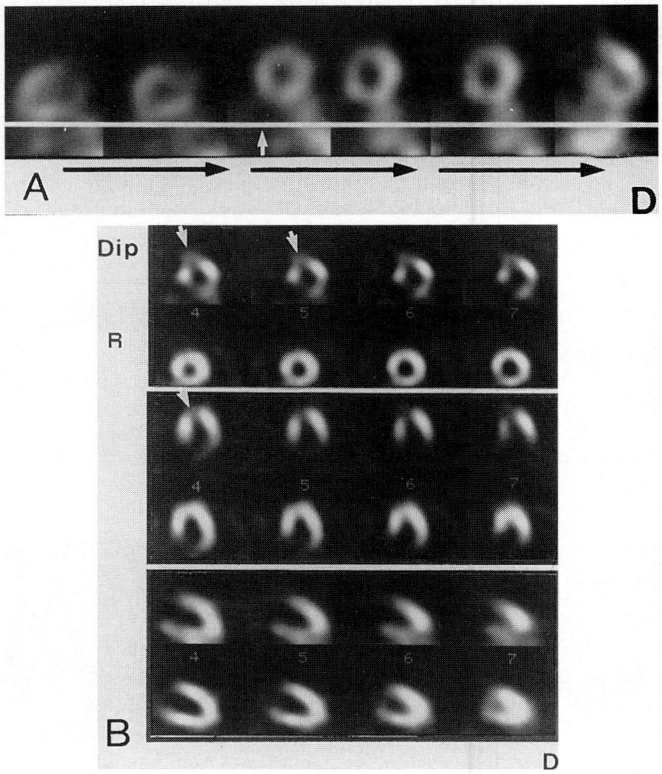

Figure 25.37. A. Selected planar projection images from LPO (*left*) to RAO position, before SPECT reconstruction. During acquisition of the LAO planar projection image position the patient moved upwards on the table (*arrow*). The *white bar* is a reference for initial position of the inferior wall. **B.** ^{201}Tl SPECT myocardial perfusion images of the same patient as in A. The initial images after infusion of dipyridamole (*Dip*) demonstrate apparent anteroapical defects (*arrows*). The redistribution (*R*) images are entirely normal. This is an example of marked distortion of image due to patient motion. Inspection of the planar projection images is essential for quality assurance and recognition of motion. (Reproduced by permission from Wackers FJTh. Artifacts in planar and SPECT myocardial perfusion imaging. Am J Cardiac Imaging 1992;6:42–58.)

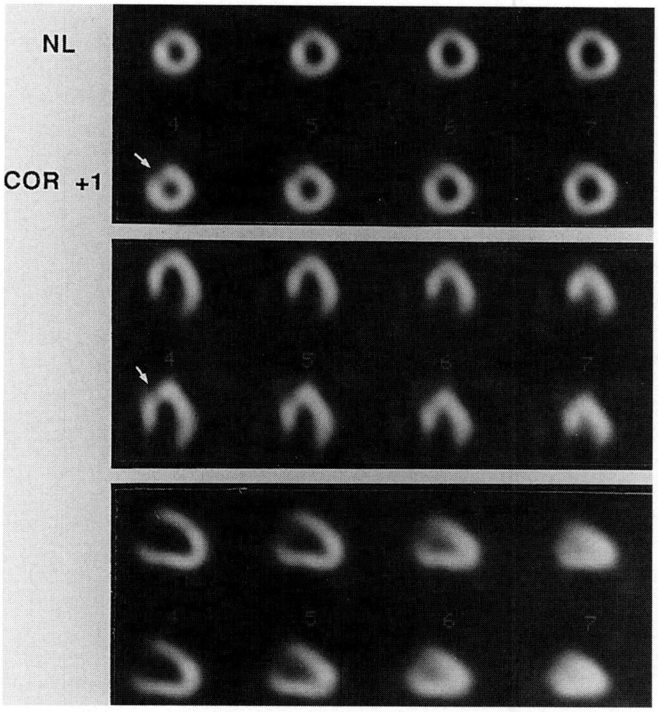

Figure 25.38. Offset of center rotation. ^{99m}Tc-sestamibi images of a normal subject. The original SPECT slices are shown on top (*NL*). One pixel center of rotation offset was introduced (*bottom*). Small artifactual defects are present on the short axis slices and long-axis slices (*arrow*). (Reproduced by permission from Wackers FJTh. Artifacts in planar and SPECT myocardial perfusion imaging. Am J Cardiac Imaging 1992;6:42–58.)

Artifacts Caused by Reconstruction and Display

During processing of a SPECT perfusion study, incorrect assignment of the left ventricular long axis on either the midtransaxial or midventricular long axis slices, may result in reconstructed slices that are distorted and not comparable. Furthermore, the "lineup" of stress-rest slices depends on subjective selection of comparable slices by the computer operator. "Pseudoreversibility" can be created by incorrect selection of slices (Fig. 25.40). Careful inspection of long axis selection and of all reconstructed slices is an important aspect of quality control.

Black Hole Sign

Dense cavity photopenia is occasionally noted in patients with large myocardial perfusion defects on both planar and SPECT imaging. This finding has been correlated with the presence of left ventricular aneurysm (22). The black hole sign is most likely caused by dyskinetic wall motion and partial volume effect.

Artifactual Defects Due to Intense Hepatic Activity

Intense hepatic or bowel activity adjacent to the heart may occur with ^{99m}Tc-labeled imaging agents. This may create artifactual myocardial perfusion defects after filtered back-

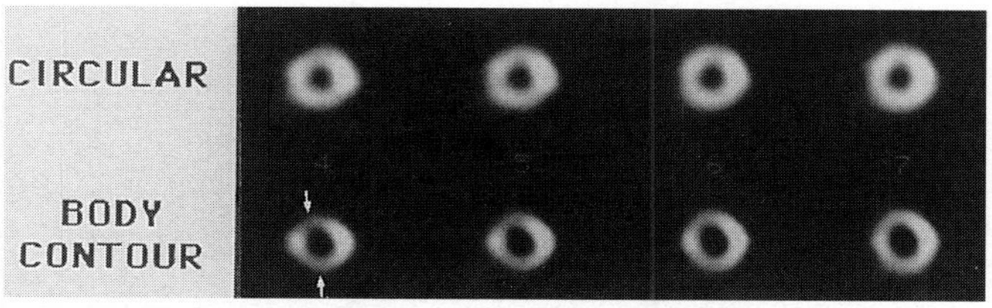

Figure 25.39. Effect of gamma-camera orbit. Short axis SPECT slices using a circular orbit (i.e., the heart is in the center of rotation of the camera head) are shown (*top*). The images are normal. Short axis SPECT slices using a body contour orbit are shown in *bottom* panel. Varying spatial resolution causes a typical artifact of 180° diametrical defects (*arrow*). (Reproduced by permission from Wackers FJTh. Artifacts in planar and SPECT myocardial perfusion imaging. Am J Cardiac Imaging 1992;6:42–58.)

projection (Fig. 25.41). Germano, et al. (23), showed that adjustment of appropriate prereconstruction filters may minimize such artifacts (see also Chapter 22).

Artifacts on Polar Map

Although the concept of creating a polar map or bull's-eye plot is attractive from the point of view of data reduction, it should be realized that this display is not a true image of the heart. Artifacts are extremely difficult to recognize once a polar map image has been created. An excellent discussion of the appearance of artifacts on tomographic bull's-eye plot can be found in the publication by DePuey and Garcia (24).

It follows that artifacts are plentiful with both planar and SPECT ^{201}Tl imaging (14). Artifacts are somewhat easier to recognize on planar imaging than on reconstructed SPECT slices. To deal with the potential problems of diaphragmatic attenuation, we routinely acquire additional planar images. Not only are planar images helpful for the recognition of artifacts, they also serve as backup studies when a SPECT study is invalid because of excessive patient motion.

Although SPECT imaging with ^{99m}Tc-labeled agents is consistently of better quality than SPECT imaging with ^{201}Tl (Fig. 25.42), these artifacts continue to be problem. It is important that the interpreter be always alert to the possibility of artifacts. Table 25.3 lists step-by-step quality assurance for planar and SPECT imaging.

RELATIVE ACCUMULATION OF RADIOPHARMACEUTICALS

Myocardial perfusion images are analyzed for *differences* in radiotracer accumulation. In patients suspected of ischemic heart disease, an area with relatively less activity usually is considered to be the abnormal area and to represent either exercise-induced myocardial ischemia or infarction. However, since myocardial perfusion images demonstrate *relative uptake* of radiotracer, occasionally the area with relatively *greater* uptake may be abnormal. For instance, this may occur on resting images of patients with idiopathic hypertrophic subaortic stenosis, in whom

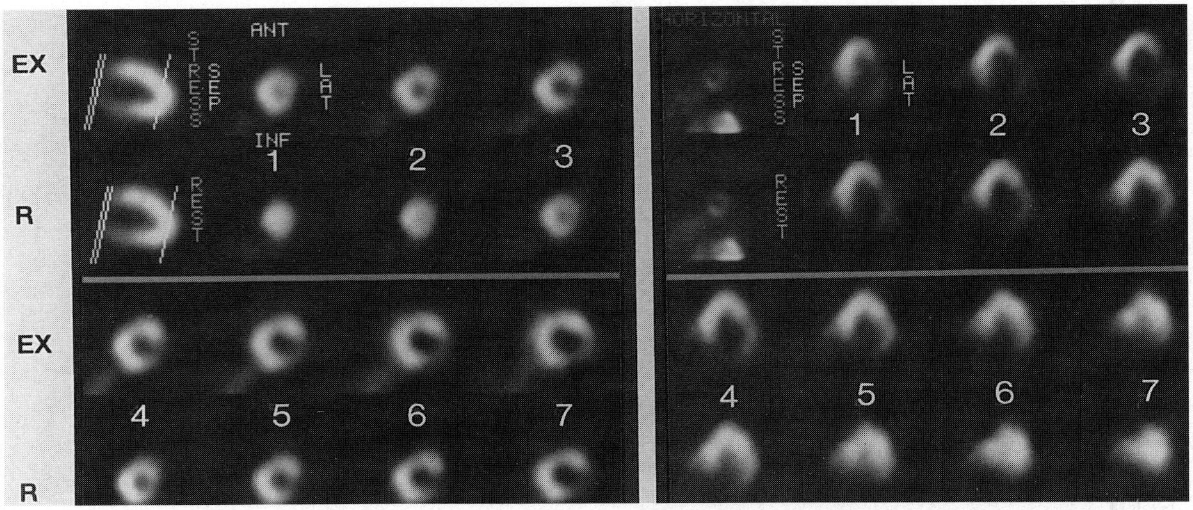

Figure 25.40. Pseudoreversibilty caused by misalignment of exercise (*EX*) and redistribution (*R*) slices in a patient with a fixed inferior wall defect. During processing the short-axis and horizontal long axis slices were not lined up correctly. Stress short axis slice no. 1 corresponds to rest slice no. 3. Without paying attention to the selection of slices, one could erroneously interpret these images as showing a reversible inferior wall defect. (Reproduced by permission from Wackers FJTh. Artifacts in planar and SPECT myocardial perfusion imaging. Am J Cardiac Imaging 1992;6:42–58.)

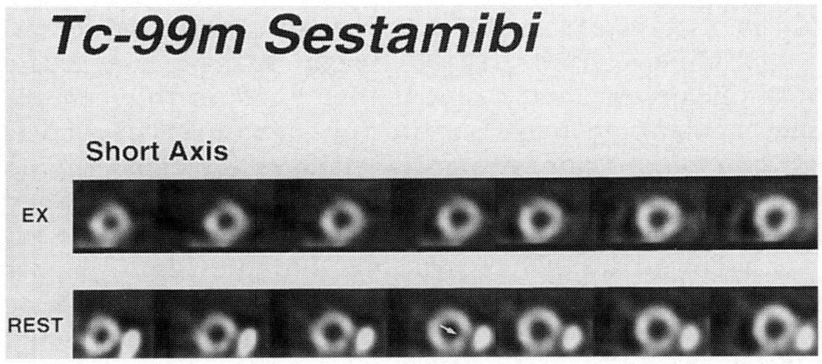

Figure 25.41. SPECT reconstruction artifact due to intense hepatic and intestinal activity. Exercise/rest short axis ^{99m}Tc-sestamibi SPECT images in patient with intense bowel activity at rest. The exercise (*EX*) image is normal. The septum on the EX image is relatively "hot" due to hypertrophy in this patient with hypertension. The resting images show intense uptake adjacent to the inferior lateral wall. Filtered backprojection using a standard Butterworth filter causes an artifactual defect in the inferior lateral wall (*arrow*). In patients with intense activity adjacent to the heart, the filter should be adjusted.

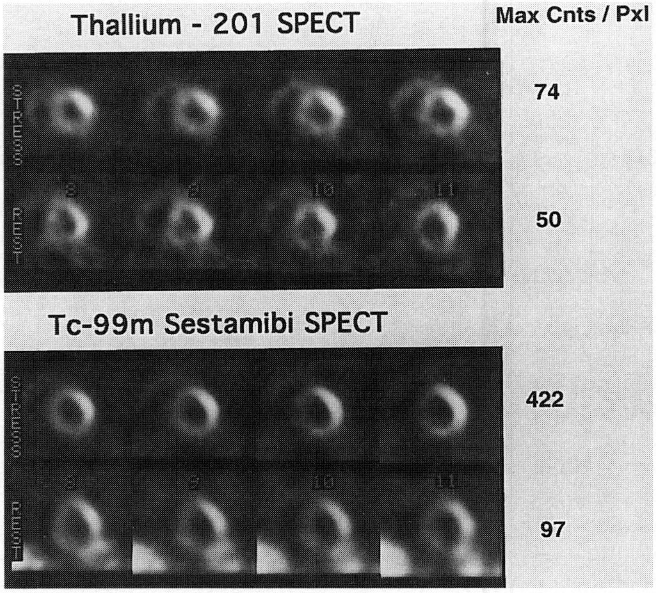

Figure 25.42. Comparison of ^{201}Tl SPECT imaging with ^{99m}Tc-sestamibi SPECT imaging in the same patient. Interval between the two studies was 5 days. The difference in quality of SPECT imaging using different radiopharmaceutics can be appreciated. Count density per pixel in projection images is substantially higher with ^{99m}Tc-sestamibi than with ^{201}Tl. ^{99m}Tc-sestamibi SPECT images are of better quality than the ^{201}Tl images. Nevertheless, both images show the presence of a fixed septal defect.

at rest the increased septal muscle mass accumulates a considerably greater amount of radiotracer than the remaining normal myocardium (25) (Fig. 21.43). After exercise, abnormally low ^{201}Tl uptake in the cardiomyopathic myocardium can be seen in some cases (26). In patients with hypertension and left ventricular hypertrophy, the septum has been noted to have increased tracer uptake in comparison to the lateral wall.

Another example can be encountered in patients with coronary spasm and postischemic reactive hyperemia (Fig. 21.44). If a perfusion imaging agent is injected shortly after relief of the pain, e.g., by sublingual nitroglycerin (27), a relatively greater amount of radiotracer may be accumulated in the abnormal, *now hyperemic,* myocardium than in the normal myocardium. Thus, the perfusion defect, or more appropriately, the area with relatively less uptake, appears to be at an erroneous anatomic location.

In patients with large perfusion defects, the display of relative activity of ^{201}Tl may lead to distortion of the images. Figure 25.45 shows three left lateral views in a normal subject, in a patient with a moderate-sized defect, and a pa-

Table 25.3.
Location of Acute Myocardial Infarction by Electrocardiography and by ^{201}Tl Myocardial Perfusion Imaging (200 Patients)[a]

	^{201}Tl Myocardial Perfusion Imaging			
Electrocardiogram	AS	A	I	IP
AS	59	1		
A	11	35	2	
I		1	14	35
IP			3	39

[a]AS = anteroseptal, A = anterior, I = inferior, IP = inferoposterior.

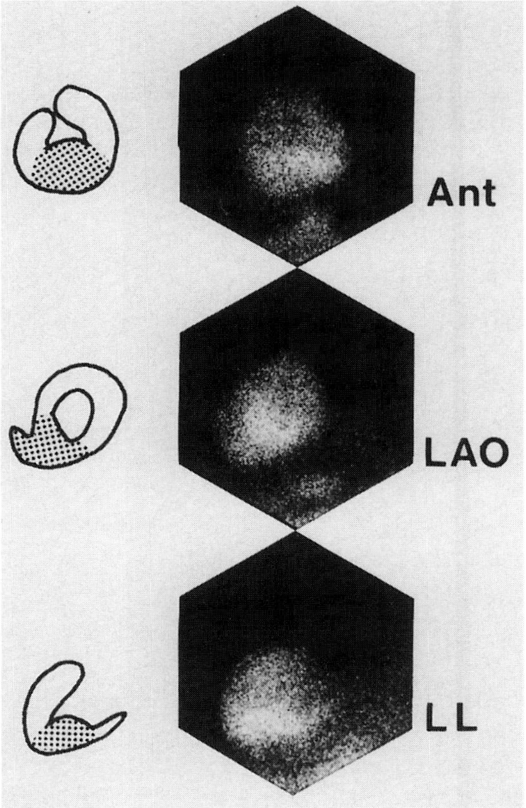

Figure 25.43. Planar ^{201}Tl images at rest of patient with idiopathic hypertrophic subaortic stenosis. Myocardial accumulation of ^{201}Tl is inhomogeneous and is higher in the pathologic hypertrophic septal muscle mass. At *left*, a schematic representation. (Reproduced by permission from Wackers FJTh. Thallium-201 myocardial imaging. In: Wackers FJTh, ed. Thallium-201 and technetium-99m pyrophosphate myocardial imaging in the coronary care unit. The Hague: Martinus Nijhoff Publishers, 1980:70–104.)

tient with a large perfusion defect. A normal horseshoe pattern is present in the normal subject. This normal pattern is still recognizable in the patient with a relatively small anterior wall defect. In contrast, in the patient with a large anterior wall defect the image is distorted; the base of the heart, which normally is the photopenic open end of the horseshoe is now intensely visualized, resulting in "closure" of the open end of the horseshoe.

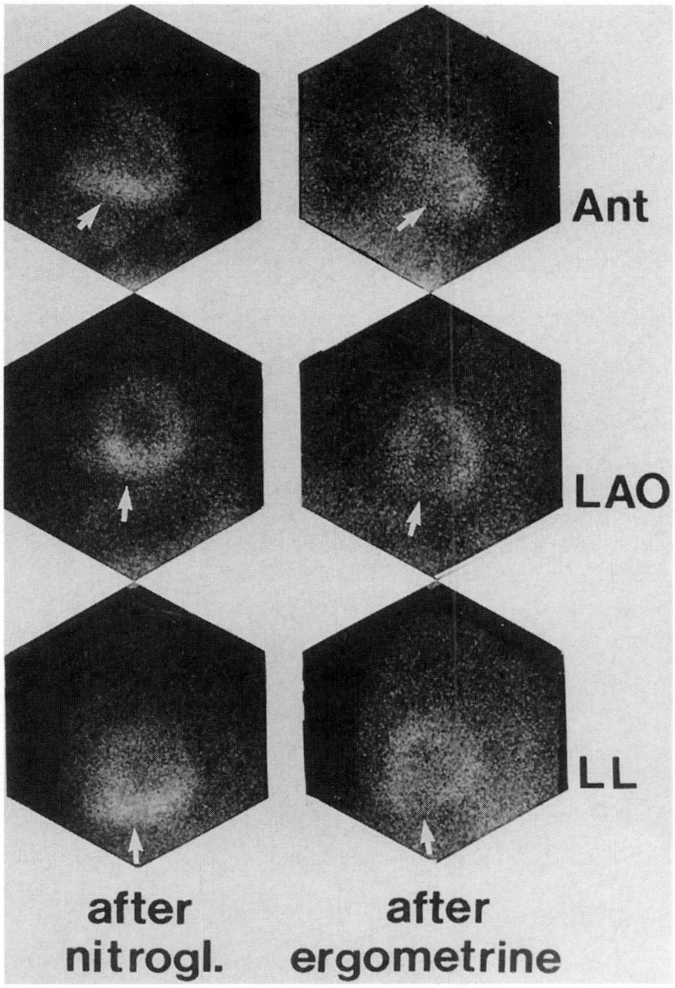

Figure 25.44. Planar ^{201}Tl imaging in patients with coronary artery spasm. ^{201}Tl images of a patient with angiographically normal coronary arteries and documented spasm of the right coronary artery. *Right*, ^{201}Tl images after provocation of coronary spasm by intravenous ergonovine. A myocardial perfusion defect is present in the inferior wall (*arrows*). *Left*, ^{201}Tl images of the same patient. The patient had a spontaneous attack of coronary spasm. ^{201}Tl was administered shortly after relief of pain by sublingual nitroglycerin. An area of diminished activity seems to be present in the anterolateral wall. However, the abnormal region is the area with *increased* ^{201}Tl activity (*arrows*), due to reactive hyperemia. (Reproduced by permission from Wackers FJTh. Thallium-201 myocardial imaging. In: Wackers FJTh, ed. Thallium-201 and technetium-99m pyrophosphate myocardial imaging in the coronary care unit. The Hague: Martinus Nijhoff Publishers, 1980:70–104.)

VISUALIZATION OF THE RIGHT VENTRICLE

Whether or not the right ventricle is visualized on myocardial perfusion images is determined by right ventricular myocardial blood flow and right ventricular myocardial mass (10). Under normal conditions the right ventricle has approximately 25% less myocardial mass and correspondingly less total myocardial blood flow than the left ventricle. Therefore, the right ventricle is usually faintly visualized at rest but almost always clearly visible after exercise (Fig. 25.2). Employing ^{99m}Tc-labeled agents, the right ventricle

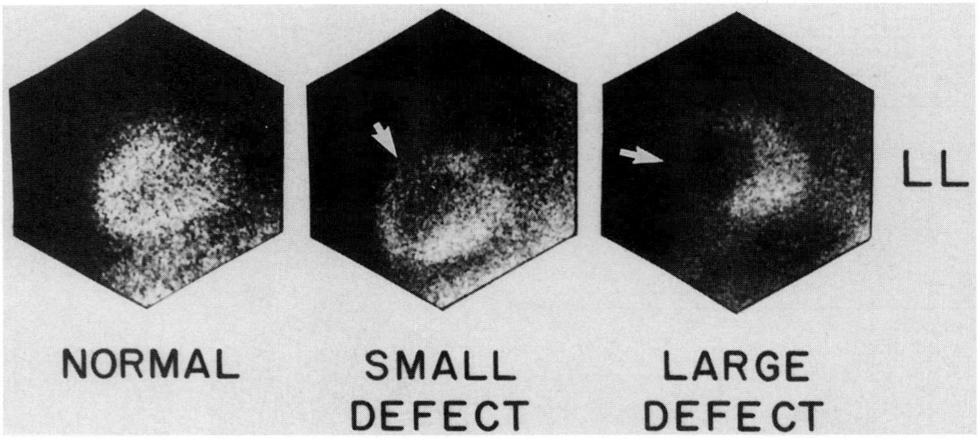

Figure 25.45. Distortion of image by large defect. *Left*, normal planar image displaying the usual horseshoe configuration. *Middle*, a small anterolateral myocardial perfusion defect. The horseshoe pattern is preserved. *Right*, a large anterior wall myocardial perfusion defect. The relative contribution of radioactivity from the base of the left ventricle is greater because of loss of emanating photons from the anterior wall. This results in a distorted image and "closure" of the open end of the horseshoe. (Reproduced by permission from Wackers FJTh. Thallium-201 myocardial imaging. In: Wackers FJTh, ed. Thallium-201 and technetium-99m pyrophosphate myocardial imaging in the coronary care unit. The Hague: Martinus Nijhoff Publishers, 1980:70–104.)

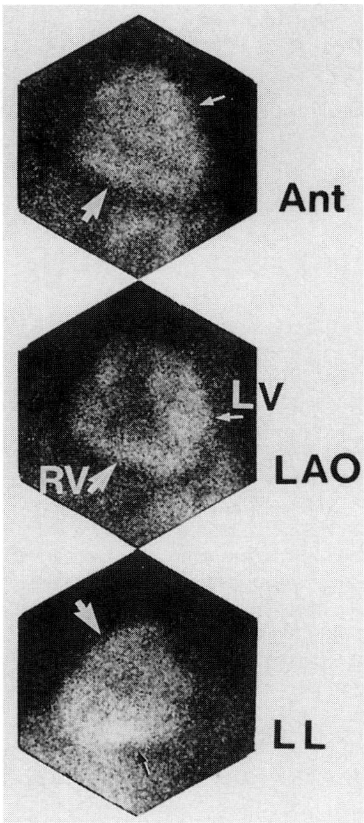

Figure 25.46. Planar ^{201}Tl images at rest in patient with severe pulmonary hypertension. Massive right ventricular enlargement and hypertrophy is present in three projections (*arrows*). The left ventricle (*LV*) is small compared to the right ventricle (*RV*) (*small arrows*). This image is diagnostic for massive right ventricular hypertrophy. *Ant* = anterior, *LAO* = left anterior oblique, *LL* = left lateral.

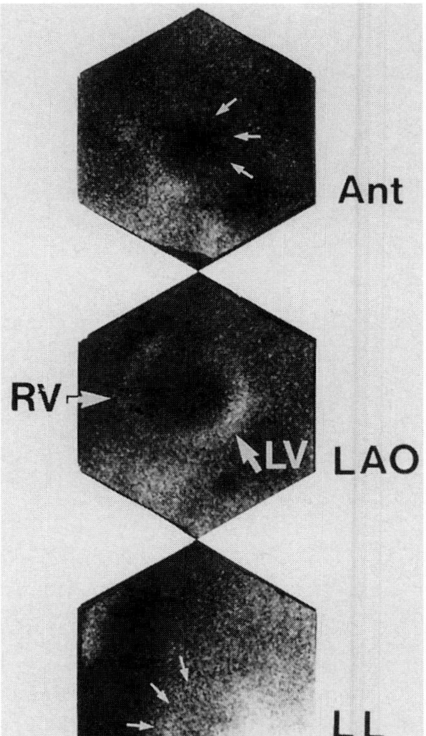

Figure 25.47. Planar ^{201}Tl images at rest in patient with extensive anteroseptal myocardial infarction. The left ventricle (*LV*) is hardly visible. A large anteroseptal myocardial perfusion defect is present (*small arrows*). On the left anterior oblique (*LAO*) view, the septum is completely absent. The right ventricle (*RV*) is clearly visualized. *Ant* = anterior, *LL* = left lateral. (Reproduced by permission from Wackers FJTh. Thallium-201 myocardial imaging. In: Wackers FJTh, ed. Thallium-201 and technetium-99m pyrophosphate myocardial imaging in the coronary care unit. The Hague: Martinus Nijhoff Publishers, 1980:70–104.)

is frequently well-visualized at rest (Fig. 25.12), probably because of less low-energy scatter.

Marked visualization of the right ventricle at rest is abnormal and indicates increased right ventricular workload and/or right ventricular hypertrophy (Fig. 25.46). This may be either pressure or volume overload (10). In patients with a variety of congenital heart diseases, acquired heart disease, or pulmonary disease (Fig. 25.15), the right ventricle may be visualized at rest (28–30).

In occasional patients with acute myocardial infarction, the right ventricle may be prominently visualized. This may be due to tachycardia, a relatively low contribution of photons emanating from the left ventricle because of an extensive perfusion defect (Fig. 25.47), increased right ventricular workload as a result of increased pulmonary wedge pressure, or a combination of these factors.

The right atrial appendix may also be visualized on planar images. It is frequently seen after exercise; however, visualization at rest is distinctly abnormal and is associated with anterior rotation and enlargement of the right heart in the same pathologic conditions that may cause right ventricular visualization (31).

On SPECT reconstructed slices, the right ventricular is usually poorly visualized in comparison to the left ventricle. However, using ^{99m}Tc-labeled agents, by masking the left ventricle, right ventricular polar maps can be generated that allow assessment of right ventricular perfusion (32).

ECG-GATED MYOCARDIAL PERFUSION IMAGING

The relatively short half-life of ^{99m}Tc allows the injection of a 10–50 times higher dose of a ^{99m}Tc-labeled imaging agent than of ^{201}Tl. Myocardial perfusion images with ^{99m}Tc-sestamibi, ^{99m}Tc-tetrofosmin, or ^{99m}Tc-furifosmin have sufficient count density in each image to allow *ECG-gated acquisition* for assessment of global and segmental myocardial contraction, in addition to myocardial perfusion. ECG-gating of myocardial perfusion imaging was initially attempted with ^{201}Tl (33–36). However, the relatively long acquisition time (20–30 minutes) required to obtain a single planar image with sufficient count density made this approach impractical. Using ^{99m}Tc-sestamibi, adequate quality ECG-gated planar and SPECT myocardial perfusion imaging has become feasible (Fig. 25.48). As with any new technique, one has to learn how to interpret these images. On inspection of planar gated myocardial perfusion images, not only motion of the walls can be recognized, but also changes in count density. This is due to partial volume effect of the walls in diastole (37–40). However, the interpretation of ECG-gated *planar* images is complicated by contraction of the overlapping facing myocardium, which erroneously exaggerates apparent *endocardial* motion. On the other hand, normal excursion of the *epicardial edges* is relatively small. These two confounding factors render the interpretation of ECG-gated planar imaging difficult and, at times, confusing (40). Nevertheless, several investigators found that resting, global, and segmental left ventricular systolic function can be assessed reproducibly and accurately from ECG-gated images in comparison two-dimensional echocardiography (41, 42). Various methods have been applied to ECG-gated planar imaging to quantify regional wall motion (37–40). The independent additive diagnostic value of planar ECG-gated perfusion imaging is, at the present time, still uncertain.

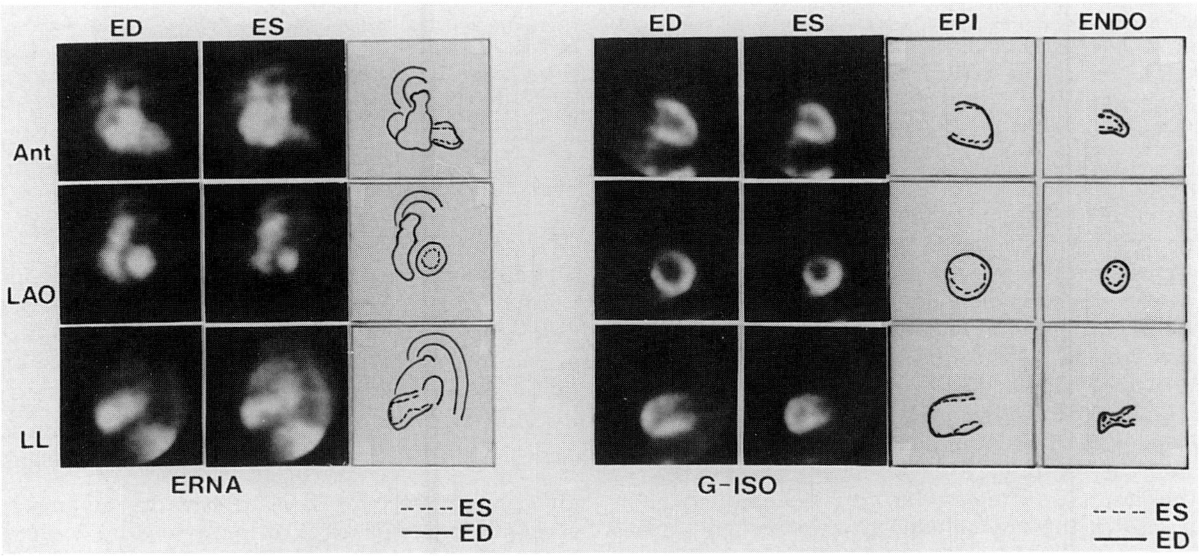

Figure 25.48. Equilibrium radionuclide angiocardiography (*ERNA*) and ECG-gated sestamibi images (*G-ISO*) of patient with nontransmural anterior wall myocardial infarction. End-diastolic (*ED*) and end-systolic (*ES*) images and schematic drawings of end-diastolic and end-systolic edges, are shown. *ERNA:* Endocardial anterolateral akinesis (*arrows*) is noted on anterior (*ANT*) and left lateral (*LL*) views. Regional wall motion is normal on left anterior oblique view (*LAO*). *G-ISO:* Although, no myocardial perfusion defect is present, regional wall motion is abnormal. Anterolateral akinesis (*arrows*) of epicardial (*EPI*) border is noted, whereas regional wall motion of endocardial (*ENDO*) portion appears normal. This patient had successful thrombolytic therapy for infarction. Although myocardial perfusion is restored, myocardial function has not yet recovered from ischemic insult (myocardial stunning). (Reproduced by permission from Wackers FJTh, Maniawski P, Sinusas AJ. Evaluation of left ventricular wall function by ECG-gated Tc-99m-sestamibi imaging. In: Beller GA, Zaret BL, eds. Nuclear cardiology: state of the art and future direction. St. Louis: Mosby, 1993:85–100.)

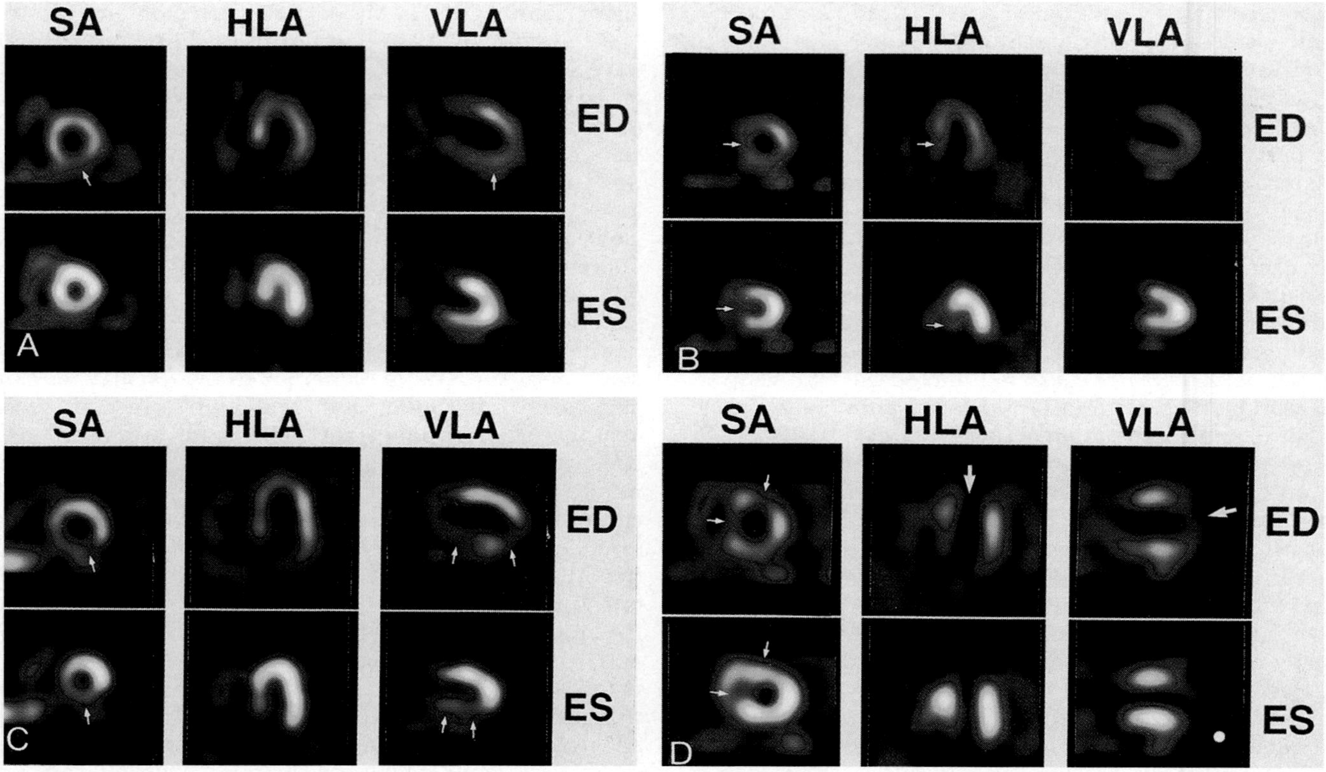

Figure 25.49. ECG-gated ^{99m}Tc-sestamibi SPECT images. The end-diastolic (*ED*) and end-systolic (*ES*) frames are shown in short axis (*SA*), horizontal long axis (*HLA*), and vertical long axis (*VLA*) slices. **A.** Normal image: During systole, homogenous thickening of the myocardium can be appreciated. The ED images show somewhat less uptake (*arrow*) in the inferior wall on the SA and VLA images. Because of the normal contraction shown in the ES images, this mild apparent defect is mostly likely caused by subdiaphragmatic attenuation. **B.** Patient with a septal infarct: The ED images show a septal defusion defect on the SA and HLA slices (*arrows*). During systole, this area does not show contraction, and the presence of akinesis confirms scarred myocardium. **C.** Inferior wall ischemia: The ED images show an inferoseptal myocardial perfusion defect (*arrow*). During ES the intensity of color increases, indicating myocardial thickening. This patient had reversible ischemia of the inferior wall on SPECT slices. **D.** Patient with infarction and ischemia: The ED postexercise images show a large anteroapical and septal myocardial perfusion defect on the horizontal and vertical long axis slices. The anteroapical segment (*long arrow*) does not contract during systole. However, the anterior and septal wall (*small arrow*) show increased color intensity during systole, indicating myocardial viability (*arrows*). (Reproduced by permission from Wackers FJTh, Maniawski P, Sinusas AJ. Evaluation of left ventricular wall function by ECG-gated Tc-99m-sestamibi imaging. In: Beller GA, Zaret BL, eds. Nuclear cardiology: state of the art and future direction. St. Louis: Mosby, 1993:85–100.)

ECG-gated *SPECT myocardial perfusion imaging* appears to be more promising (Fig. 25.49**A**, **B**, **C**, **D**). Again, good correlation with echocardiographic assessment of regional function has been demonstrated using visual analysis of regional wall motion on SPECT images (43, 44). In particular, inspection of the end-diastolic frame has been suggested to improve diagnostic accuracy (45). Promising preliminary results have been reported for quantification of myocardial wall thickening using count-based Fourier analysis (46–48). Although ECG-gated SPECT imaging is feasible, the clinical usefulness is still not well-defined. The technique appears to be most helpful for the recognition of artifactual defects due to attenuation (breast and diaphragm). ECG-gated SPECT images are useful to improve confidence of interpretation of "still" slices. Other investigators utilized ECG-gated SPECT perfusion images to calculate resting left ventricular ejection fraction from traced endocardial borders using Simpson's rule method (49–50).

ACUTE MYOCARDIAL INFARCTION

With the increasing clinical use of thrombolytic therapy during the early hours of acute myocardial infarction (51), radionuclide visualization of myocardial area at risk and of salvage myocardium has gained practical importance (52).

CHARACTERISTIC IMAGES OF MYOCARDIAL INFARCTION

Myocardial infarction is visualized on radionuclide myocardial perfusion images as an area with decreased tracer accumulation. The anatomic location and extent of myocardial infarction can be assessed reliably using either planar or SPECT imaging (53–56). Myocardial infarctions at various anatomic locations display characteristic myocardial perfusion images. Examples of planar and SPECT images in patients with acute myocardial infarction are shown in Figures 25.50, 25.51, and 25.52.

RIGHT VENTRICULAR INFARCTION

Since the right ventricle usually is not well-visualized on resting myocardial perfusion images, the diagnosis of right ventricular infarction can not be made directly. Right ventricular infarction occurs almost always in patients with inferior infarcts (57), and frequently involves the lower portion of the left ventricular septum. A septal defect can be easily appreciated on planar or SPECT myocardial perfusion images. Certainly, right ventricular infarction should be suspected in patients with electrocardiographic inferior infarction in cardiogenic shock and who have a normal-sized left ventricle on the myocardial perfusion image and a relatively small inferior wall perfusion defect (Fig. 25.53) If cardiogenic shock were due to extensive left ventricular damage, one would expect a left dilated ventricle. Occasionally, a negative (photopenic) image of a dilated and enlarged right ventricle provides a further clue for right ventricular infarction (58). Regional perfusion of the right ventricle can be assessed on SPECT images by masking left ventricular activity and displaying normalized reconstructed right ventricular slices or polar map. Right ventricular infarction can be visualized in this way. Combined imaging with ^{99m}Tc-stannous pyrophosphate infarct imaging and/or equilibrium radionuclide angiocardiography usually provides additional imaging modalities that aid in making the diagnosis of right ventricular infarction (58–60). Mahmarian, et al. (61), suggested that discordance between left ventricular inferior infarct size by SPECT imaging and enzymatic estimate may provide a means to assess the extent of right ventricular infarction.

Electrocardiographic and Postmortem Correlation of Location of Myocardial Infarction

Accurate location of acute myocardial infarction by noninvasive methods has clinical relevance, since the location of infarction is of prognostic importance. For instance, it is well-known that patients with anterior wall infarction have a poorer prognosis than patients with inferior wall infarc-

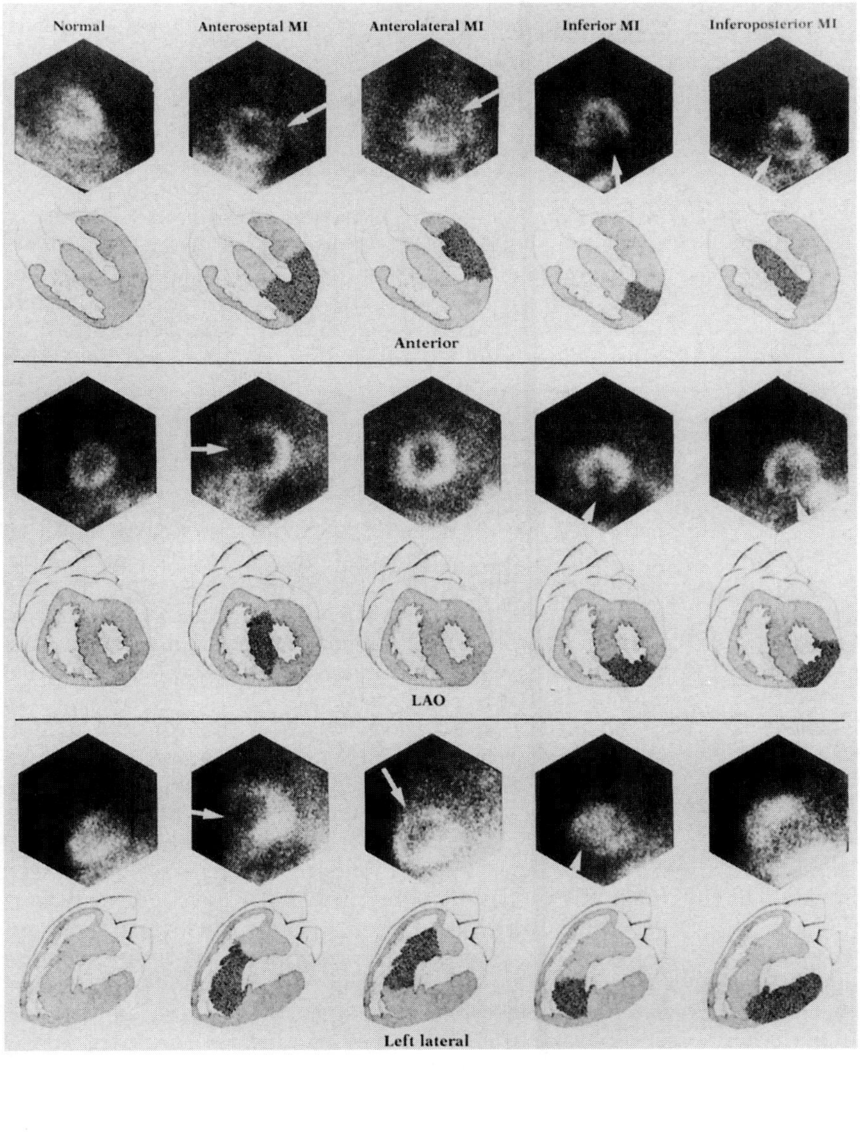

Figure 25.50. Planar ^{201}Tl images of acute myocardial infarction. Typical planar ^{201}Tl images of acute myocardial infarction in three projections: anterior (*top panel*), left anterior oblique (*LAO*) (*middle panel*), and left lateral (*lower panel*). The first column shows normal planar ^{201}Tl images. The second to fourth columns show abnormal planar ^{201}Tl images with defects (*arrows*) caused by acute myocardial infarction. Shown are examples of acute anteroseptal, anterolateral, inferior, and inferoposterior myocardial infarctions. Schematic representations of the infarcted area are shown on the diagrams below each ^{201}Tl image. (Modified by permission from Wackers FJTh, Busemann Sokole E, Samson G, et al. Value and limitations of thallium-201 scintigraphy in the acute phase of myocardial infarction. N Engl J Med 1976; 295:1.)

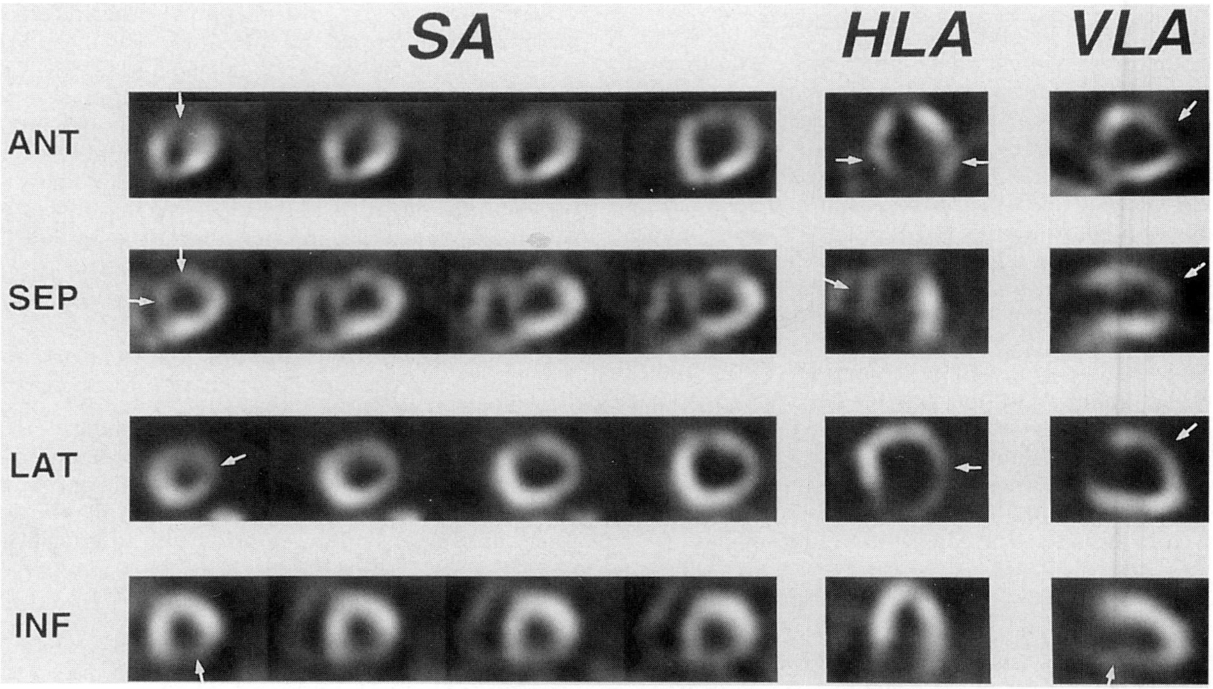

Figure 25.51. SPECT ^{99m}Tc-sestamibi images of acute myocardial infarction. Typical ^{99m}Tc-sestamibi SPECT images of acute myocardial infarction, in short axis (*SA*) horizontal long axis (*HLA*), and vertical long axis (*VLA*) slices. From top to bottom: anterior (*ANT*), anteroseptal (*SEP*), lateral (*LAT*), and inferior (*INF*) infarctions. Defects are indicated by *arrows*.

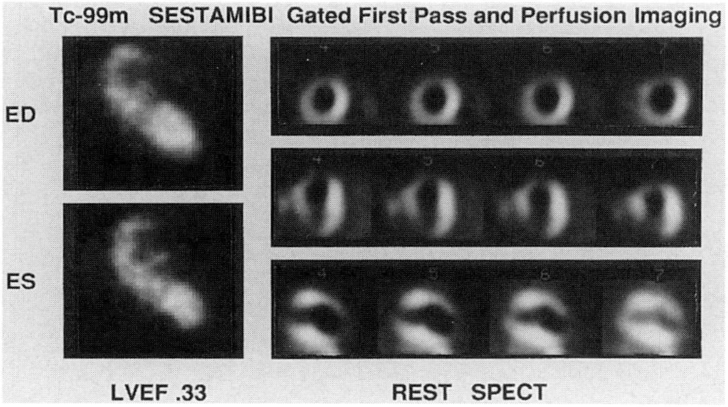

Figure 25.52. Simultaneous assessment of myocardial perfusion and function. ^{99m}Tc-sestamibi imaging in acute myocardial infarction allows assessment of both function and perfusion. In this patient with large anteroseptal infarction, the injection of sestamibi was utilized for first-pass radionuclide angiography (*left*). The end-diastolic and systolic frames are shown. Global left ventricular ejection fraction was severely depressed at 0.33. On the right are resting SPECT images in short axis, and vertical and horizontal long axis slices. A larged anteroseptal myocardial perfusion defect is present.

tion (62, 63). Moreover, involvement of the septum in anterior wall infarction indicates a large infarction and is associated with a mortality rate three times higher than in infarction at other locations (64). Since with radionuclide myocardial perfusion imaging the normally perfused and viable myocardium is visualized, precise anatomic location of the infarction is feasible (65, 66). Myocardial perfusion imaging may be helpful in patients with acute myocardial infarction to identify the infarct-related artery in patients with equivocal or nondiagnostic electrocardiograms. The correlation between scintigraphic location of infarction and the 12-lead electrocardiogram, as well as postmortem location of acute myocardial infarction, is shown in Tables 25.3 and 25.4.

Importance of Myocardial Infarction Size

The prognosis of a patient with acute myocardial infarction is directly related to the total amount of infarcted and necrotic myocardium (67). Since the earliest application of radionuclide imaging in patients with acute myocardial infarction, the potential value of this methodology to assess noninvasively and quantitatively the extent of myocardial damage has been recognized.

Since the normal and/or viable myocardium is visualized with a myocardial perfusion imaging agent, a perfusion defect can be expressed as a *percentage of the total visualized left ventricle* (56, 61, 65, 68–71). Moreover, since myocardial perfusion images demonstrate both acute and old infarction, the total amount of irreversibly damaged myocardium can be quantified. Early after acute myocardial infarction left ventricular ejection fraction or the extent of abnormal regional wall motion may not be an accurate measurement of the total amount of irreversible damage since stunned (but viable) myocardium may be present. Thus, myocardial perfusion imaging appears particularly

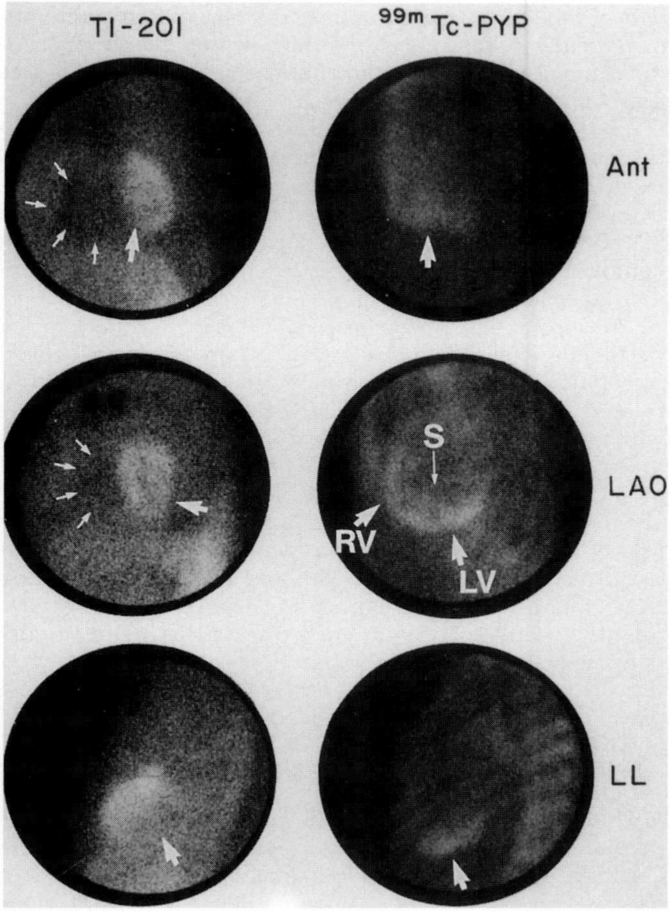

Figure 25.53. Inferior infarction with right ventricular involvement. Planar myocardial images with ^{201}Tl and ^{99m}Tc-pyrophosphate (*PYP*) in a patient with acute inferior wall myocardial infarction and right ventricular involvement. At the time of study, the patient was hypotensive with disproportionately elevated right ventricular pressure as compared to pulmonary wedge pressure. The ^{201}Tl image shows a normal size left ventricle (*LV*) with an inferoposterior myocardial perfusion defect (*large arrows*). In a patient in cardiogenic shock, dilatation of the left ventricle is expected. The absence of left ventricular dilatation suggests right ventricular involvement. The ^{99m}Tc-pyrophosphate image shows intense accumulation of the radiopharmaceutic in the heart (*arrows*). Although ^{99m}Tc-pyrophosphate has accumulated in the inferior wall of the left ventricle, substantial uptake is also present in the inferolateral wall of the *right* ventricle (*RV*), indicating right ventricular infarction. On the anterior (*Ant*) ^{201}Tl image, a negative image of the (dilated) right ventricle also can be appreciated (*small arrows*). *S* = interventricular septum. (Reproduced by permission from Wackers FJTh, Lie KI, Busemann Sokole E, Res J, van der Schoot JB, Durrer D. Prevalence of right ventricular involvement in inferior wall infarction assessed with myocardial imaging with thallium-201 and technetium-99m pyrophosphate. Am J Cardiol 1978;42:358.)

suited for early quantitative assessment of infarct size (see later for quantification). Indeed, in patients who had conventional (nonthrombolytic) treatment of myocardial infarction, planimetric size of planar ^{201}Tl myocardial perfusion defects correlated well with postmortem size of infarction (65) (Fig. 25.54). Furthermore, in patients with old infarction, an inverse relationship exists between the size of planar or SPECT myocardial perfusion defects and the left ventricular ejection fraction (72, 73).

Table 25.4.
Location of Myocardial Infarction by ^{201}Tl Myocardial Perfusion Imaging and Postmortem Findings (23 Patients)[a]

	^{201}Tl Myocardial Perfusion Imaging			
Postmortem	AS	A	I	IP
AS	11			1
A		2		
I				1
IP				8

[a]AS = anteroseptal, A = anterior, I = inferior, IP = inferoposterior.

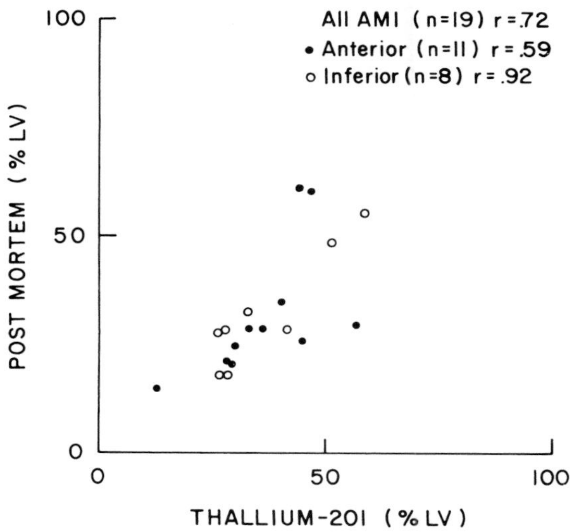

Figure 25.54. Postmortem infarction size and quantitative planar ^{201}Tl defect size. Correlations between measured size of myocardial infarction at postmortem and quantitative size of planar ^{201}Tl myocardial perfusion defects in 19 patients with acute myocardial infarction (*AMI*) is shown. *LV* = left ventricle.

DETECTION OF ACUTE MYOCARDIAL INFARCTION

Resting myocardial perfusion imaging with either ^{201}Tl or ^{99m}Tc-labeled agents is an extremely sensitive and reliable means of detecting acute myocardial infarction in the early stage. This was first demonstrated using ^{201}Tl (54) and more recently confirmed using ^{99m}Tc-sestamibi (52, 55).

Time of Imaging

There exists a clear relationship between diagnostic yield of myocardial perfusion imaging in acute myocardial infarction and the timing of myocardial imaging after onset of acute chest pain (Figs. 25.55 and 25.56). Wackers, et al. (54), showed that patients studied within 6 hours of onset of chest pain all had abnormal planar ^{201}Tl images. Of patients studied between 6 and 24 hours after chest pain, 88% had perfusion defects, whereas only 72% of patients studied later than 24 hours after onset of symptoms had myocardial perfusion defects. The overall sensitivity of planar ^{201}Tl myocardial imaging for detection of acute infarction was 82%. Boucher, et al. (55), confirmed similar excellent sensitivity (94%) and specificity (92%) for overall detection of myocardial infarction using planar ^{99m}Tc-sestamibi imaging.

Serial ^{201}Tl Imaging Following Acute Infarction

The characteristic relationship between results of ^{201}Tl imaging and the interval between onset of symptoms and time of imaging was elucidated by serial imaging (after repeat injection of ^{201}Tl) in the same patients (54). In approximately 25% of patients with acute myocardial infarction, serial imaging revealed changes in size of ^{201}Tl myocardial perfusion defects over time. Although in some patients an increase in size of defects could be demonstrated, in the majority of patients myocardial defects tended to become smaller with time. Moreover, changes in size of imaging defects occurred significantly more frequently within 24 hours of infarction than later. Furthermore, decrease in defect size tended to occur more often in patients with enzymatically small infarctions than in those with large infarctions. Examples of such changes are shown in Figures 25.57 and 25.58.

Smitherman, et al. (74), performed serial rest-redistribution myocardial imaging after a single dose of ^{201}Tl and reported results similar to those for serial imaging with repeat injections of ^{201}Tl. These temporal changes in size of ^{201}Tl defect following acute myocardial infarction have been confirmed by several investigators in clinical and experimental studies (75–77).

The earlier described changes in size of ^{201}Tl myocardial perfusion defects in acute infarction presently can be explained by spontaneous thrombolysis of clot in the infarct-related artery. DeWood, et al. (78), reported that in patients with acute myocardial infarction thrombosis of the infarct artery was demonstrable in 87% of patients when coronary angiography was performed within the first 4 hours after chest pain, whereas the prevalence of thrombosis in the infarct artery decreased when coronary angiography was performed later (Fig. 25.59). This and other studies suggest that spontaneous thrombolysis occurs relatively frequently (in 10–20% of patients) during the first 24 hours of infarction (51, 79).

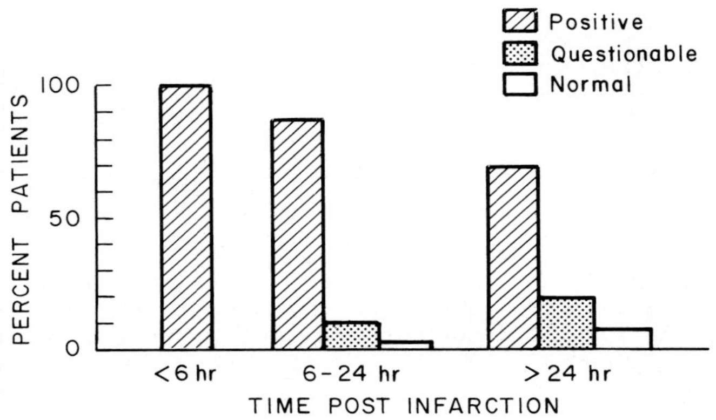

Figure 25.55. ^{201}Tl imaging results and time after infarction. Results of ^{201}Tl myocardial imaging in 200 patients with acute myocardial infarction in relation to time interval after onset of chest pain. (Reproduced by permission from Wackers FJTh. Thallium-201 myocardial imaging. In: Wackers FJTh, ed. Thallium-201 and technetium-99m pyrophosphate myocardial imaging in the coronary care unit. The Hague: Martinus Nijhoff Publishers, 1980:70–104.)

MYOCARDIAL PERFUSION IMAGING AND THROMBOLYTIC THERAPY FOR ACUTE MYOCARDIAL INFARCTION

Early thrombolytic treatment in patients with acute myocardial infarction can potentially salvage jeopardized myocardium. Myocardial perfusion imaging has been proposed as an objective means to document restoration of blood flow to the infarct region, as well as to visualize the extent of salvaged viable myocardium (80–90). Since marked changes in myocardial blood flow may occur during and after successful thrombolysis, various modes and times of administration of myocardial perfusion imaging agents have been investigated. Granato, et al. (91), demonstrated that the rate of reperfusion (rapidly or slowly) and *timing* of intravenous administration (before or immediately after reperfusion) have an effect on ^{201}Tl myocardial images. When, for example, ^{201}Tl is administered during or imme-

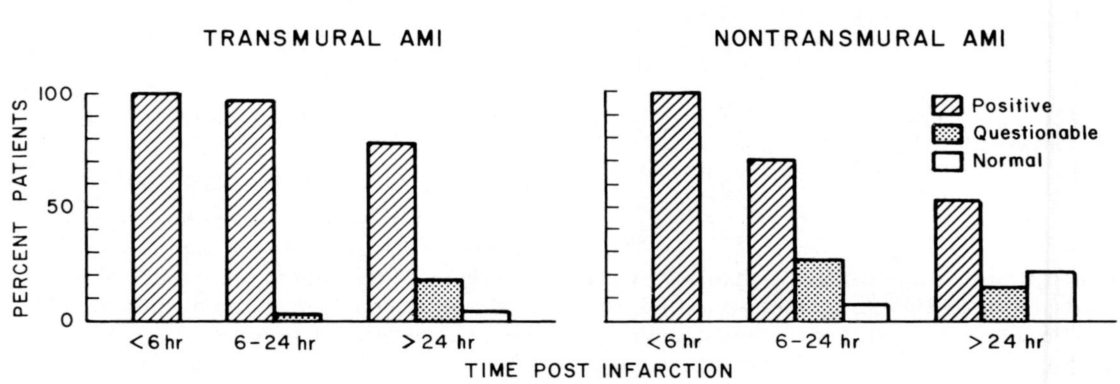

Figure 25.56. Transmural versus nontransmural infarction and time after infarction. Results of planar ^{201}Tl myocardial imaging in patients with transmural and nontransmural acute myocardial infarction (*AMI*) in relation to time interval after onset of chest pain. (Reproduced by permission from Wackers FJTh. Thallium-201 myocardial imaging. In: Wackers FJTh, ed. Thallium-201 and technetium-99m pyrophosphate myocardial imaging in the coronary care unit. The Hague: Martinus Nijhoff Publishers, 1980:70–104.)

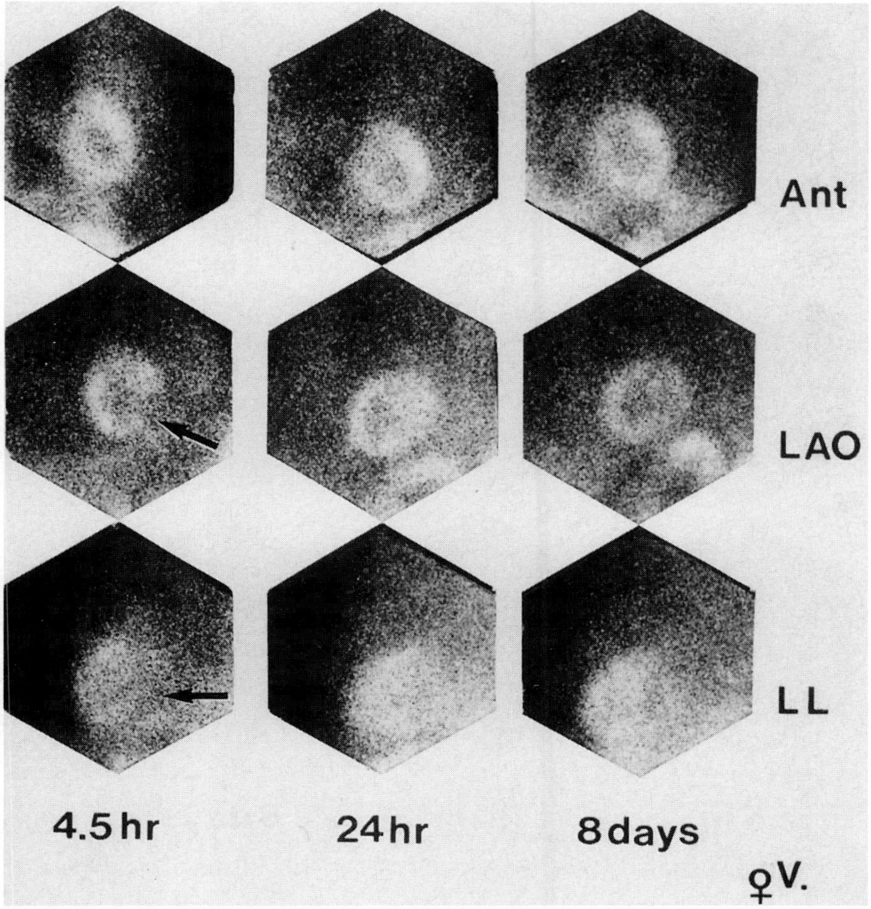

Figure 25.57. Serial planar ^{201}Tl myocardial imaging in a patient with acute inferoposterior myocardial infarction. At 4.5 hours after onset of chest pain, a definite myocardial perfusion defect is present at the inferolateral and posterior wall (*arrows*). Repeat imaging at 24 hours and at 8 days shows considerable reduction in size of the myocardial perfusion defect on the left anterior oblique (*LAO*) view and also on the left lateral (*LL*) view, although a posterior myocardial perfusion defect is still present at 8 days after myocardial infarction. *Ant* = anterior. (Reproduced by permission from Wackers FJTh, Busemann Sokole E, Samson G, et al. Value and limitations of thallium-201 scintigraphy in the acute phase of myocardial infarction. N Engl J Med 1976;295:1.)

diately after reflow to an infarct region, ^{201}Tl uptake may overestimate the degree of myocardial salvage because of reactive hyperemia in potential areas of necrosis. Nonviable necrotic myocardium may be masked by adjacent or superimposed hyperemia (91, 92). Consequently, a myocardial perfusion imaging agent is preferably administered *before* thrombolytic therapy is initiated to demonstrate the total area at risk. Using ^{201}Tl the interplay between initial myocardial uptake and redistribution and changes in infarct artery coronary blood flow is complex and variable in individual patients, and interpretation of serial ^{201}Tl images after a single intravenous injection may be uncertain.

On the other hand, ^{99m}Tc-sestamibi and ^{99m}Tc-tetrofosmin have characteristics that are well-suited for application in patients who undergo thrombolytic therapy for acute myocardial infarction (3, 7). Because of slow myocardial clearance, it is feasible to administer either agent immediately before or at the moment of initiation of thrombolytic therapy in the emergency department (93). Imaging can then be performed later at a convenient time. Extensive clinical experience has been accumulated using ^{99m}Tc-sestamibi for this clinical application (52, 94–98). When ^{99m}Tc-sestamibi is administered *before* thrombolytic therapy, the perfusion defect visualizes the *myocardium at risk*. When ^{99m}Tc-sestamibi is injected *after* thrombolytic therapy, the hypoperfused area reflects the *ultimate infarction* (Figs. 25.60 and 25.61). This basic concept has been validated in experimental animal models of coronary artery occlusion and reperfusion (56, 99). Thus, if the perfusion defect on the second image is smaller than on the first image, myocardial salvage and patency of the infarct artery is most likely achieved by thrombolytic therapy. Wackers, et al. (52, 93), and Gibbons, et al. (94), published the initial reports on the usefulness of ^{99m}Tc-sestamibi in the setting of thrombolytic therapy to assess the efficacy of therapy (Fig. 25.62). Their initial findings using planar and SPECT ^{99m}Tc-sestamibi imaging have been confirmed in numerous subsequent publications and in studies of hundreds of patients (95–98). The experience with ^{99m}Tc-sestamibi in acute myocardial infarction can be summarized as follows:

Serial myocardial perfusion imaging is feasible even in seriously ill patients. In the coronary care unit, planar imaging can be performed at the patient's bedside. However, several investigators have shown that SPECT imaging is feasible and can be performed safely in a nuclear medicine department, under supervision of a physician.

The myocardial area at risk varies greatly in individual patients with acute myocardial infarction (52, 94). There is no good correlation between the risk area as demonstrated with ^{99m}Tc-sestamibi imaging and the anatomic site of the occlusion of the infarct artery, i.e., distal or proximal (94). The area at risk in an acute anterior infarction is larger

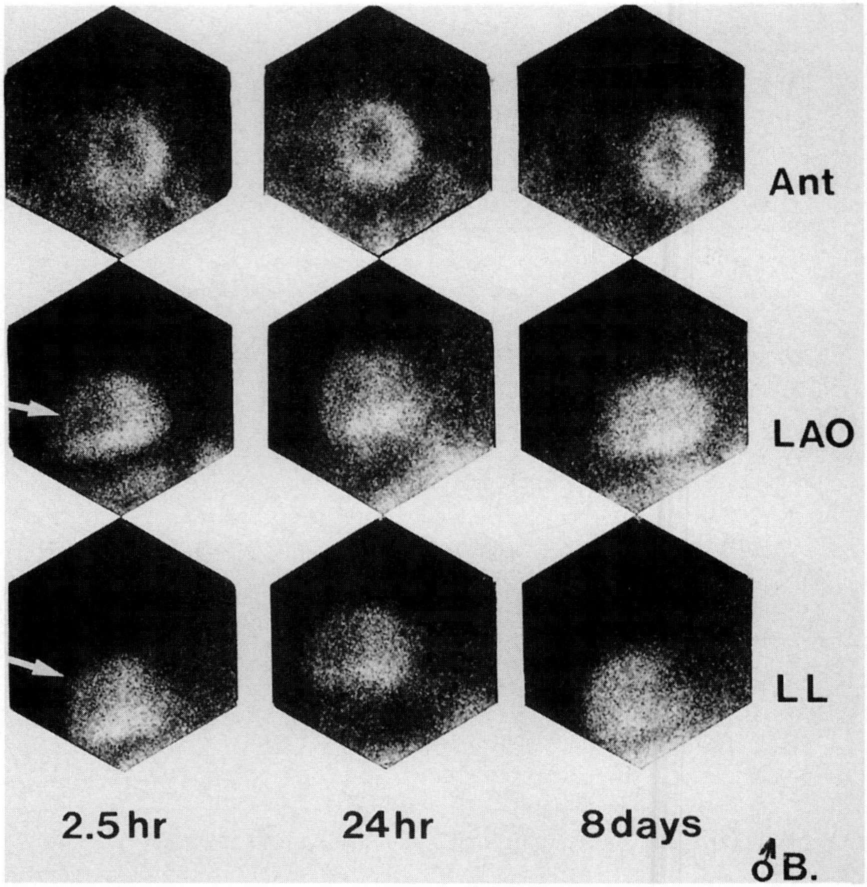

Figure 25.58. Serial planar ^{201}Tl myocardial perfusion images in patient with acute anteroseptal myocardial infarction. At 2.5 hours after onset of chest pain a definite anteroseptal myocardial perfusion defect is present (*arrows*). At 24 hours after onset of chest pain the area of diminished activity is still present. At 8 days after onset of symptoms the size of the myocardial perfusion defect has decreased significantly and the images are nearly normal. *Ant* = anterior, *LAO* = left anterior oblique, *LL* = left lateral. (Reproduced by permission from Wackers FJTh, Busemann Sokole E, Samson G, et al. Value and limitations of thallium-201 scintigraphy in the acute phase of myocardial infarction. N Engl J Med 1976; 295:1.)

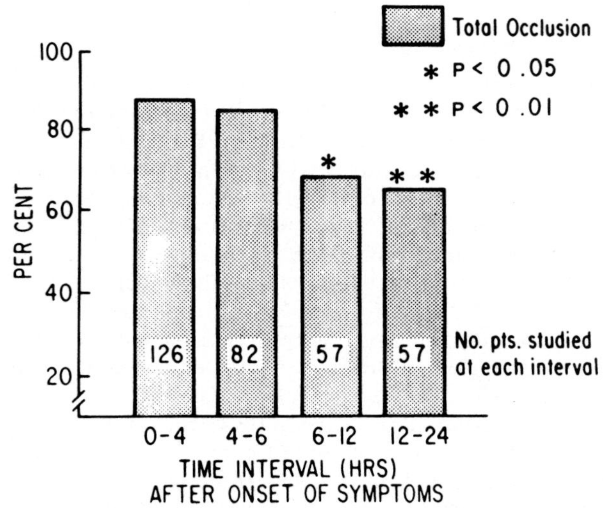

Figure 25.59. Frequency of infarct artery occlusion and time after infarction. Frequency of total occlusion of the infarct artery by thrombus on coronary angiography in relation to the time interval after onset of acute infarction. Eighty-eight percent of patients evaluated within 4 hours after onset of symptoms had total occlusion of the infarct artery. With increasing time interval there is a significant decrease in the number of patients with total occlusion, suggesting spontaneous thrombolysis. This observation most likely explains the decreasing sensitivity over time of perfusion imaging to visualize acute infarction. (Reproduced by permission from DeWood MA, Spores J, Notske R, et al. Prevalence of total coronary occlusion during the early hours of transmural myocardial infarction. N Engl J Med 1980;303:897.)

than that in acute inferior infarction (98). A decrease in size of myocardial perfusion defect (i.e., defect size before thrombolytic therapy compared to after thrombolytic therapy) is predictive of reperfusion of the infarct artery and subsequent improvement of left ventricular regional wall motion (73, 96). Serial myocardial perfusion imaging showed that in many patients (approximately 40%) defect size *continues to decrease* days after thrombolytic therapy was administered. Although this observation has been confirmed by others, the pathophysiologic basis of this phenomenon remains unclear. The size of a myocardial perfusion defect correlates well with left ventricular ejection fraction at hospital discharge (73, 100). Patients with collateral circulation to the infarct artery have smaller ultimate infarct size than in patients without collateral circulation (101).

Serial ^{99m}Tc-sestamibi imaging is now recognized as a potentially useful tool to assess the clinical efficacy of various thrombolytic strategies in acute myocardial infarction (102–106). The patient serves as his or her own control and, consequently, smaller numbers of patients need to be recruited for a clinical trial. Noninvasive assessment of reperfusion is important as the patient's prognosis is related to patency of the infarct artery. Assessment of myocardial perfusion after thrombolytic therapy may be particularly useful since global and regional left ventricular function may be initially depressed due to ischemic myocardial stunning.

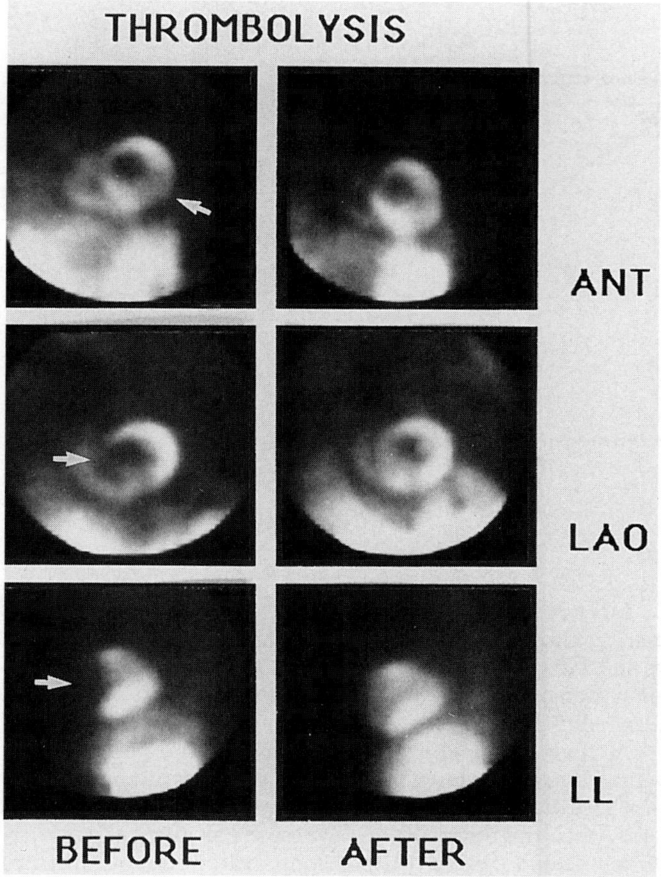

Figure 25.60. Planar myocardial perfusion imaging with ^{99m}Tc-sestamibi before and after thrombolytic therapy in a patient with an acute anteroseptal myocardial infarct. ^{99m}Tc-sestamibi was injected immediately before initiation of thrombolytic therapy and imaging was performed 2 hours later. Because of the lack of significant redistribution of ^{99m}Tc-sestamibi, the distribution of myocardial blood flow at the time of injection is "frozen" in time. The images before thrombolytic therapy show an anteroseptal myocardial perfusion defect (*arrows*) that was quantified as 53. The patient was reinjected with ^{99m}Tc-sestamibi after thrombolytic therapy was completed. These images show improved perfusion of the anteroseptal segments, indicating successful reperfusion of the infarct artery. The perfusion defect size after thrombolytic therapy was 35, consequently 33% of myocardium has been salvaged by thrombolytic therapy. (Reproduced by permission from Wackers FJTh, Gibbons RJ, Verani MS, et al. Serial quantitative planar technetium-99m-isonitrile imaging in acute myocardial infarction: efficacy for noninvasive assessment of thrombolytic therapy. J Am Coll Cardiol 1989;14:861–873.)

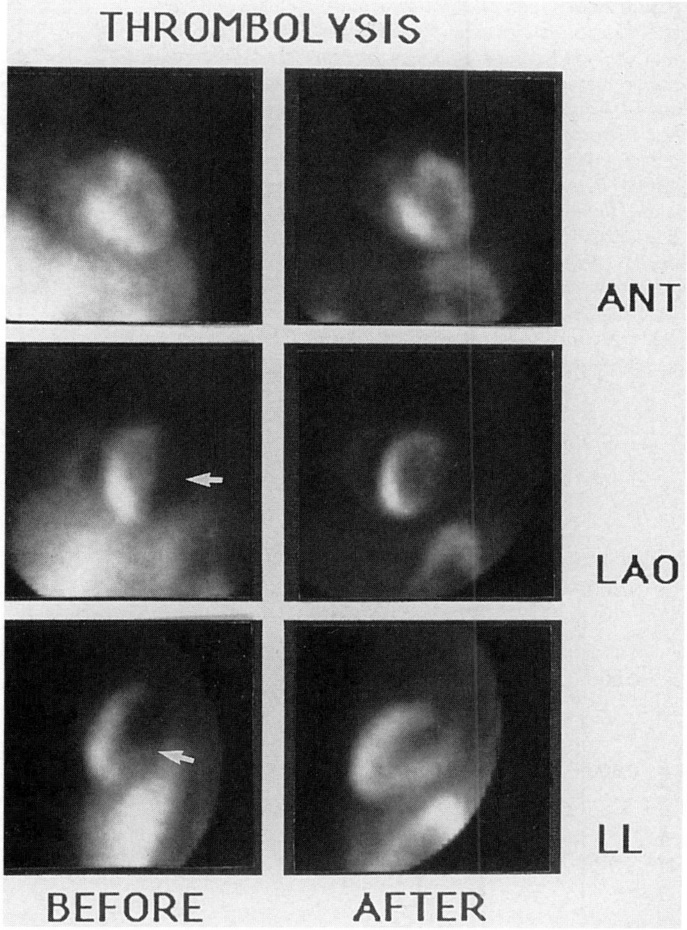

Figure 25.61. Planar myocardial perfusion imaging with ^{99m}Tc-sestamibi before and after thrombolytic therapy in a patient with a large posterior and lateral infarct. The images obtained with injection prior to thrombolytic therapy show a large inferoposterior myocardial perfusion defect (*arrow*), quantified as 49. After thrombolytic therapy there is evidence of successful reperfusion of the infarct artery. The inferoposterior wall is now visualized, although the posterolateral wall still shows a defect. The defect after thrombolytic therapy was 28 indicating 42% of myocardial salvage. (Reproduced by permission from Wackers FJTh, Gibbons RJ, Verani MS, et al. Serial quantitative planar technetium-99m-isonitrile imaging in acute myocardial infarction: efficacy for noninvasive assessment of thrombolytic therapy. J Am Coll Cardiol 1989;14:861–873.)

MYOCARDIAL PERFUSION IMAGING FOR THE ASSESSMENT OF PROGNOSIS AFTER ACUTE MYOCARDIAL INFARCTION

Myocardial perfusion imaging during the acute and subacute phase of infarction may provide prognostic information in two ways: (a) the size of myocardial perfusion defect and (b) detection of jeopardized myocardium.

As described earlier, the size of myocardial perfusion defects in acute infarction has important prognostic significance. This is not unexpected since an inverse relationship can be demonstrated between size of myocardial perfusion defect and left ventricular ejection fraction. Silverman, et al. (107), showed, using planar ^{201}Tl imaging, that patients with large perfusion defects had a poorer prognosis than patients with small defects, in spite of the fact that patients were clinically and hemodynamically comparable at the time of imaging. Patients with large defects had a mortality of 92%, compared to a mortality of 7% in patients with small defects, at an average follow-up of 9 months (Fig. 25.63). Other investigators have confirmed the prognostic value of determining the size of myocardial perfusion defects in acute myocardial infarction (72, 108, 109).

The demonstration of a decrease in size of myocardial perfusion defects during the course of acute myocardial infarction by serial imaging, suggests the presence of residual jeopardized myocardium within the infarct area (54, 74). Patients who have such a decrease in size of perfusion defect during their first admission for acute myocardial in-

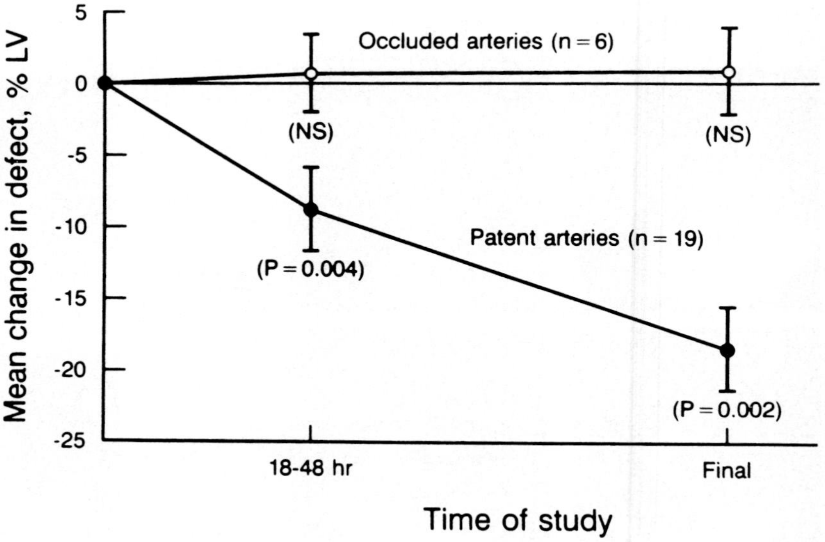

Figure 25.62. Serial SPECT myocardial perfusion imaging after thrombolysis for acute myocardial infarction. In patients with occluded coronary arteries and unsuccessful thrombolytic therapy, no change in myocardial defect size occurred. In contrast, patients who had successful thrombolytic therapy with reperfusion of the infarct artery (patent arteries) had a significant decrease in perfusion defect at 18–48 hours after onset of chest pain. Interestingly, there was a further decrease in defect size during subsequent days (Reproduced by permission from Pellikka PA, Behrenbeck R, Verani MS, Mahmarian JJ, Wackers FJTh, Gibbons RJ. Serial changes in myocardial perfusion using tomographic technetium-99m-hexakis-2-methoxy-2-methylpropyl-isonitrile imaging following reperfusion therapy of myocardial infarction. J Nucl Med 1990;31:1269–1275.)

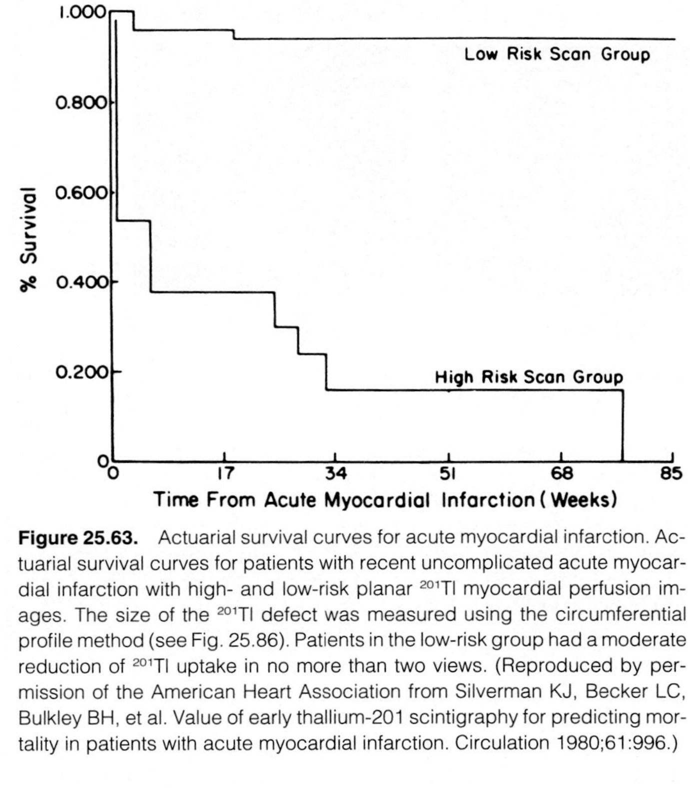

Figure 25.63. Actuarial survival curves for acute myocardial infarction. Actuarial survival curves for patients with recent uncomplicated acute myocardial infarction with high- and low-risk planar ^{201}Tl myocardial perfusion images. The size of the ^{201}Tl defect was measured using the circumferential profile method (see Fig. 25.86). Patients in the low-risk group had a moderate reduction of ^{201}Tl uptake in no more than two views. (Reproduced by permission of the American Heart Association from Silverman KJ, Becker LC, Bulkley BH, et al. Value of early thallium-201 scintigraphy for predicting mortality in patients with acute myocardial infarction. Circulation 1980;61:996.)

farction, may come back for a second admission with an acute extension of infarction in the same area. This suggests that the infarction was completed in two stages.

Nestico, et al. (110), noted that prominent visualization of the right ventricle at rest after acute myocardial infarction was a poor prognostic sign. These patients had a lower mean left ventricular ejection fraction, larger left ventricular ^{201}Tl defects, and more complex ventricular arrhythmias. It is conceivable that visualization of the right ventricle in these cases is caused by increased right ventricular afterload.

More recently Cerquiera, et al. (111), showed that in patients who had thrombolytic therapy for acute infarction, a similar relationship between SPECT myocardial perfusion defect size and long-term survival can be demonstrated (Fig. 25.64).

At hospital discharge, stress myocardial perfusion imaging has important prognostic value by demonstrating stress-induced myocardial ischemia within the infarct area and/or in the distribution of remote coronary artery territories. Gibson, et al. (112), demonstrated that quantitative analysis of predischarge ^{201}Tl stress images was superior to the stress ECG in identifying patients with multivessel disease and predicting subsequent cardiac events (Fig. 25.65). These investigators included only patients with an uncomplicated and natural course of their acute myocardial infarction in the study. Predischarge exercise tests after acute myocardial infarction are *submaximal* exercise tests. To improve diagnostic yield of myocardial perfusion imaging in this patient population, alternative modes of stress have been investigated. Leppo, et al. (113), reported that dipyridamole ^{201}Tl scintigraphy was a more sensitive predictor of subsequent cardiac events than a submaximal stress test in patients with a recent acute myocardial infarction. Brown, et al. (114), showed that dipyridamole myocardial perfusion imaging early (days 3–5) after acute infarction can be successfully employed to identify patients at increased risk for in-hospital complications.

Stress Myocardial Perfusion Imaging in Patients After Thrombolytic Therapy

In patients who received thrombolytic therapy for acute myocardial infarction, several investigators reported lower sensitivity and predictive values for subsequent cardiac events than those published previously in patients who had conventional treatment of infarction (115, 116). Plausible explanations for the apparent diminished sensitivity are several (117). Patients who are eligible for thrombolytic therapy constitute a selected group. They are usually

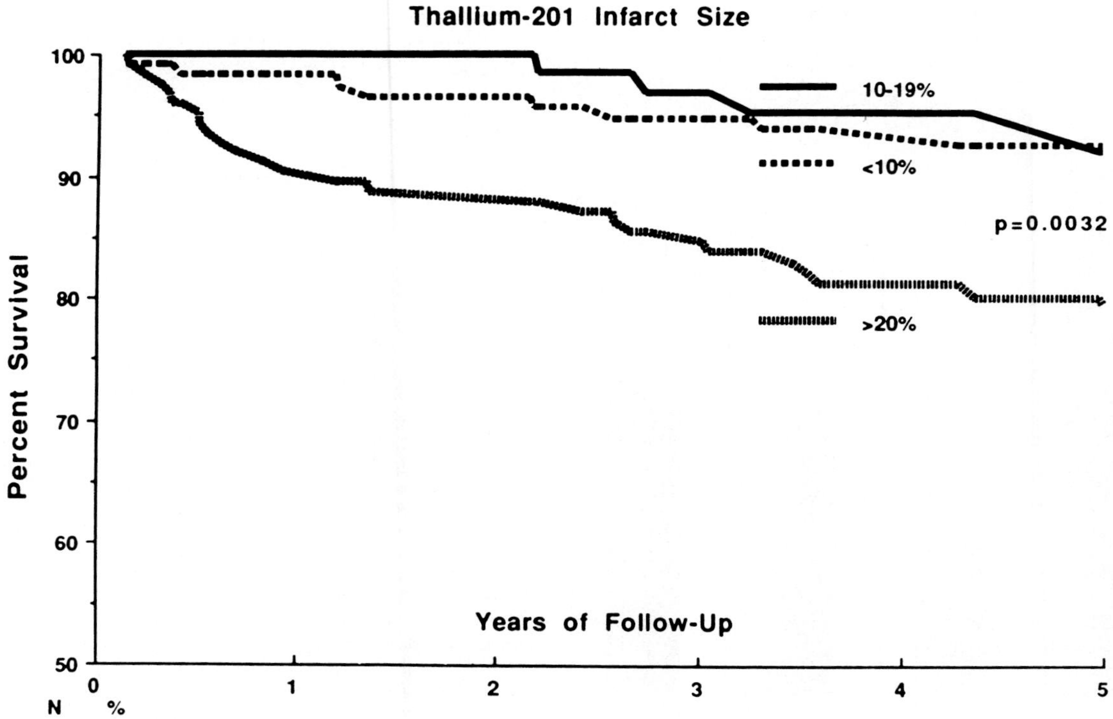

	N (0)	% (0)	N (1)	% (1)	N (3)	% (3)	N (5)	% (5)
<10%	117	100%	112	98%	104	95%	52	93%
10-19%	65	100%	64	100%	60	97%	28	92%
>20%	125	100%	111	90%	103	85%	57	79%

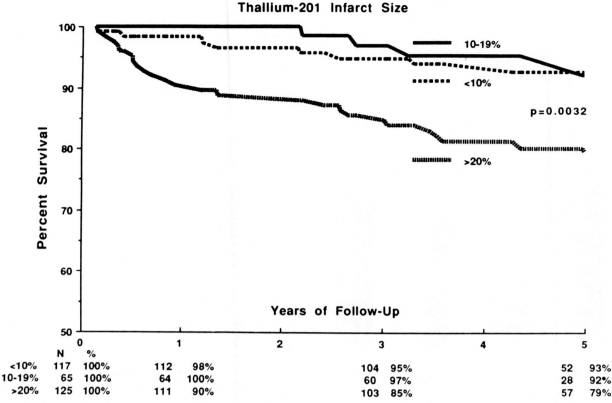

Figure 25.64. ^{201}Tl SPECT infarct size and percent survival during follow-up after thrombolytic therapy for acute myocardial infarction. Patients with large (≥20%) myocardial perfusion defects after thrombolytic therapy for myocardial infarction, had significantly poorer prognosis then patients with a small or moderate sized myocardial perfusion defects (Reproduced by permission from Cerqueira MD, Maynard C, Ritchie JL, Davis KB, Kennedy JW. Long-term survival in 618 patients from the western Washington streptokinase in myocardial infarction trials. J Am Coll Cardiol 1992;20:1452–1459.)

younger, have less prior myocardial infarction, have less non-Q wave infarctions, and have less severe multivessel coronary artery disease. Zaret, et al. (118), observed in the Thrombolysis in Myocardial Infarction (TIMI) Phase II trial, that although a relationship existed between left ventricular ejection fraction and 1-year mortality, the prognosis for any given level of ejection fraction was better for patients who received thrombolytic therapy than for those treated in the prethrombolytic era. McCallister, et al. (119), found that patients who had open infarct arteries after thrombolytic therapy and large infarcts (greater than 40% of the left ventricle measured by ^{99m}Tc-sestamibi imaging), nevertheless had a favorable outcome without heart failure. Since the cardiac event rate after thrombolytic therapy is extremely low, Bayesian principles would predict diminished predictive value for stress myocardial perfusion imaging. The excellent outcome is at least in part due to noninvasive risk stratification. Patients with abnormal stress tests are now routinely sent for angiography. Thus, since myocardial perfusion imaging can identify quantitatively size and reversibility of myocardial perfusion defects and the presence of remote ischemia, in individual patients, stress myocardial perfusion imaging still appears to be a valid approach to identify high risk patients.

MYOCARDIAL IMAGING FOR TRIAGE OF PATIENTS IN THE EMERGENCY DEPARTMENT

The preceding paragraphs addressed the clinical usefulness of myocardial perfusion imaging in patients with proven acute myocardial infarction. However, a relatively large number of patients are seen in the emergency department with atypical chest pain and nondiagnostic electrocardiograms. Their clinical diagnosis is uncertain. These patients are frequently admitted to "rule out myocardial infarction." After clinical observation and costly hospital admission, more than half of these patients are discharged with the "diagnosis" of noncardiac chest pain. Wackers, et al. (120), and others (121) demonstrated that resting myocardial perfusion imaging can be used to better triage these patients. Abnormal planar rest ^{201}Tl images had a sensitivity of 88%, a specificity of 88%, and a positive predictive value of 61% for the detection of acute infarction (Fig. 25.66). More recently, ^{99m}Tc-sestamibi has been used for triaging patients in the emergency department. Vareto, et al. (122), and Hilton, et al. (123), administered ^{99m}Tc-sestamibi in patients with acute chest pain but nondiagnostic electrocardiograms. Both studies showed that normal rest ^{99m}Tc-sestamibi SPECT imaging was associated with an excellent long- and short-term outcome, whereas patients who had abnormal ^{99m}Tc-sestamibi im-

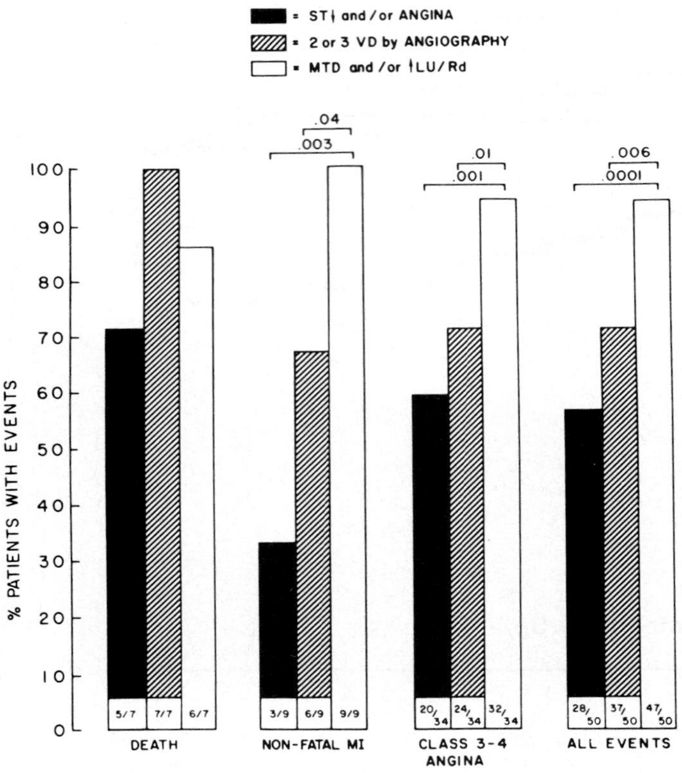

Figure 25.65. Sensitivity stress myocardial perfusion imaging for prediction of cardiac events after uncomplicated infarction. Sensitivity of stress electrocardiography (*black bar*), coronary angiography (*shaded bar*), and planar ^{201}Tl stress imaging (*white bar*) for identifying postinfarction patients who died, experienced reinfarction, or developed New York Heart Association class III or IV angina pectoris. The presence of multiple ^{201}Tl defects (*MTD*) and/or increased lung uptake and redistribution (↑ *LU/Rd*) identified significantly more patients at high risk for nonfatal myocardial infarction and class III and IV angina than did electrocardiographic ST segment depression (*ST* ⇌), stress-induced angina, or double- or triple-vessel disease (*VD*) by angiography. (Reproduced by permission of the American Heart Association from Gibson RS, Watson DD, Craddock GB, et al. Prediction of cardiac events after uncomplicated myocardial infarction: a prospective study comparing predischarge exercise thallium-201 scintigraphy and coronary angiography. Circulation 1983;68:321.)

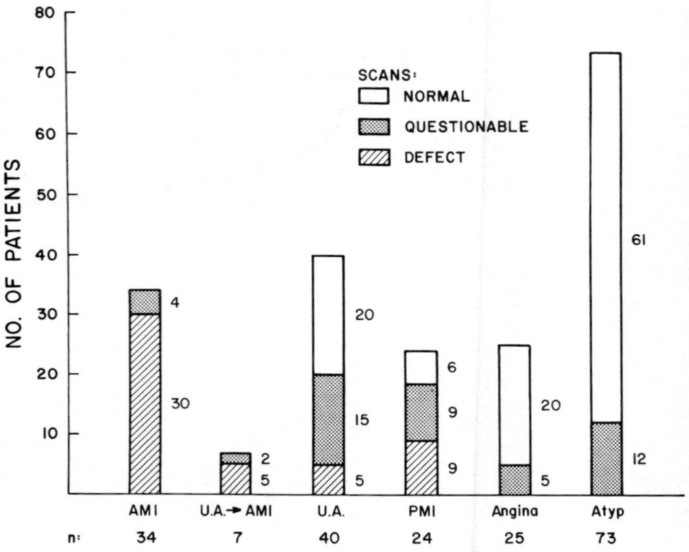

Figure 25.66. Planar ^{201}Tl imaging in emergency room and final diagnosis. Final diagnosis in 203 patients with chest pain and nondiagnostic ECG, admitted to rule out acute myocardial infarction, and the results of planar ^{201}Tl myocardial perfusion imaging on admission. The final diagnosis was based on results of enzyme level determinations, the development of electrocardiographic changes, and reevaluation of the patient's history. *AMI* = acute myocardial infarction, *PMI* = previous myocardial infarction, *U.A.* = unstable angina, *U.A.→AMI* = unstable angina progressing to acute myocardial infarction, *Atyp* = atypical complaints. (Reproduced by permission from Wackers FJTh, Lie KI, Liem KL, et al. Potential value of thallium-201 scintigraphy as a means of selecting patients for the coronary care unit. Br Heart J 1979;41:111.)

ages at the time of presentation in the emergency department, had a high incidence of cardiac events (Fig. 25.67). Although further studies are required to confirm these observations, these data suggest that this novel clinical application may be cost effective in patient management (124).

UNSTABLE ANGINA

Myocardial perfusion defects on resting myocardial perfusion images may represent either acute or old myocardial infarction, or a region of transient myocardial ischemia. Initial ^{201}Tl uptake and ^{99m}Tc-sestamibi uptake are primarily determined by regional myocardial blood flow (9, 125–132). Although intramyocyte sequestration is an active process, myocardial ischemia has minimal effect on cellular transmembrane transport of ^{201}Tl, and on mitochondrial membrane binding of ^{99m}Tc-sestamibi. Thus, myocardial ischemia *per se* does not cause image defects with either ^{201}Tl or ^{99m}Tc-sestamibi. Heterogeneity of radiotracer uptake reflects predominantly heterogeneity of regional myocardial blood flow.

An important portion of coronary care unit admissions consists of patients suspected to have the clinical syndrome of unstable angina. Often this diagnosis is tentative. Objective evidence of myocardial ischemia can be extremely helpful in patient management.

Wackers, et al. (133), evaluated the value of ^{201}Tl myocardial imaging in patients with unstable angina who were studied *during a pain-free period* (<18 hours) after an anginal attack. Forty percent of patients had abnormal resting myocardial perfusion images with ^{201}Tl, 27% had questionable images, and 33% had normal images. A definite relationship existed between the time of imaging after last anginal attack and the results of imaging (Fig. 25.68). Fifty percent of patients studied within 6 hours after the last anginal attack had abnormal ^{201}Tl images, compared to only 27% of patients studied later. Patients who had perfusion defects, showed filling-in of the defects on delayed redistribution imaging, indicating viable myocardium (Fig. 25.69). Others (134–136) have confirmed these observations in patients with unstable angina. These findings suggest that in patients with unstable angina, regional hypoperfusion exists and persists longer than can be judged from the patient's clinical status or electrocardiographic ST segment changes. Gewirtz, et al. (137), demonstrated

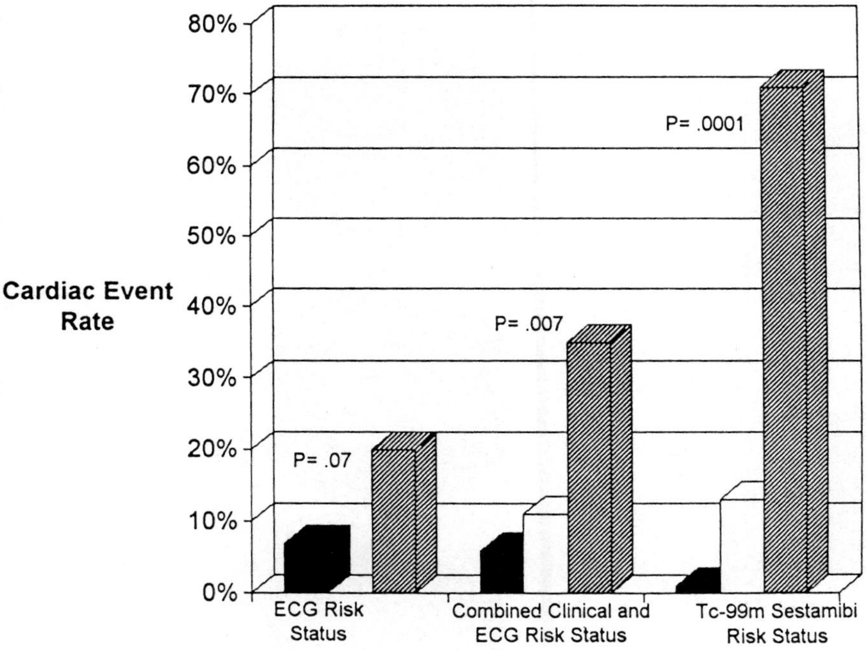

Figure 25.67. Cardiac event rate in patients with nondiagnostic electrocardiogram presenting with chest pain in the emergency room. There was no difference in cardiac event rate when only information on the electrocardiogram in the emergency room was considered. (*Black:* normal electrocardiogram; *shaded:* nondiagnostic electrocardiogram). When clinical risk factors were combined with ECG status, patients with more than three risk factors and nondiagnostic electrocardiogram had significantly higher cardiac event rate. When normal (*black*), equivocal (*white*), or abnormal (*shaded*) sestamibi images were compared, abnormal sestamibi images in the emergency room were highly predictive of future cardiac events. (Reproduced by permission from Hilton TC, Thompson RC, Williams HJ, et al. Technetium-99m-sestamibi myocardial perfusion imaging in the emergency room evaluation of chest pain. J Am Coll Cardiol 1994;23:1016–1022.)

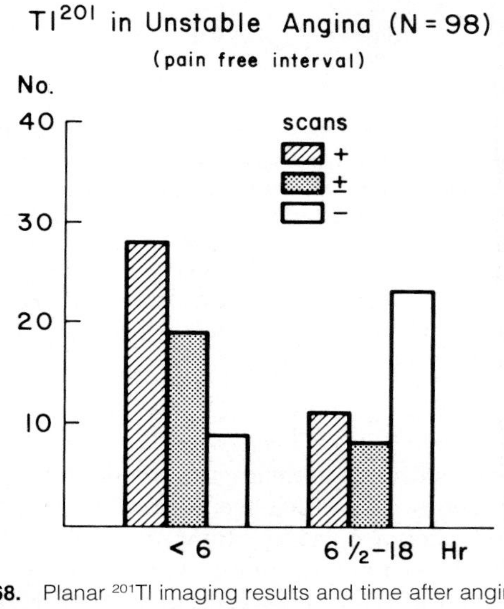

Figure 25.68. Planar ^{201}Tl imaging results and time after angina. Relationship between results of ^{201}Tl myocardial perfusion imaging in patients with unstable angina and the time of imaging after the last anginal episode. Symbols: + = abnormal ^{201}Tl image, ± = questionable ^{201}Tl images, − = normal ^{201}Tl image. (Reproduced by permission of the American Heart Association from Wackers FJTh, Lie KI, Liem KL, et al. Thallium-201 scintigraphy in unstable angina pectoris. Circulation 1978;57:738.)

that transient myocardial perfusion defects on resting ^{201}Tl scans can also be obtained in selected patients with severe but *stable* angina pectoris. In general, patients with coronary artery disease without history of infarction who demonstrate reversible resting defects have more severe coronary artery disease and a poorer prognosis than patients with chest pain syndromes and normal ^{201}Tl images.

Libodeau, et al. (138), recently confirmed and extended this observation using ^{99m}Tc-sestamibi imaging. When a patient is injected *during pain* with ^{99m}Tc-sestamibi, the presence of a myocardial perfusion defect, particularly if not present at rest, was highly sensitive and specific for severe coronary artery disease.

Frequently, reversible resting defects in patients with unstable angina are associated with abnormal wall motion on ventriculography. Coronary bypass surgery results in normalization of regional contractility and disappearance of the resting defects in these patients with ischemic cardiomyopathy (134). This condition is now recognized as being relatively common in patients with severe chronic coronary artery disease and is referred to as "hibernating myocardium." Resting reinjection myocardial perfusion imaging with ^{201}Tl has an unique role to identify this condition. The important subject of identification of myocardial viability using myocardial perfusion and metabolic imaging is discussed in detail in Chapter 27.

SUMMARY OF CLINICAL APPLICATION OF RESTING MYOCARDIAL PERFUSION IMAGING IN THE CORONARY CARE UNIT

In many patients admitted to the coronary care unit, the history and initial ECG will provide sufficient information to make the diagnosis of acute myocardial infarction at the time of presentation. In these patients, there is no need for resting myocardial perfusion imaging. However, in patients with complete left bundle branch block (Fig. 25.70), Wolff-Parkinson-White syndrome, or pacemaker rhythm, the ECG diagnosis of myocardial infarction may be difficult or impossible. In these patients, myocardial perfusion imaging may be helpful (139).

A most practical application of resting myocardial perfusion imaging is in patients with atypical history of chest pain and nondiagnostic ECG in whom acute myocardial

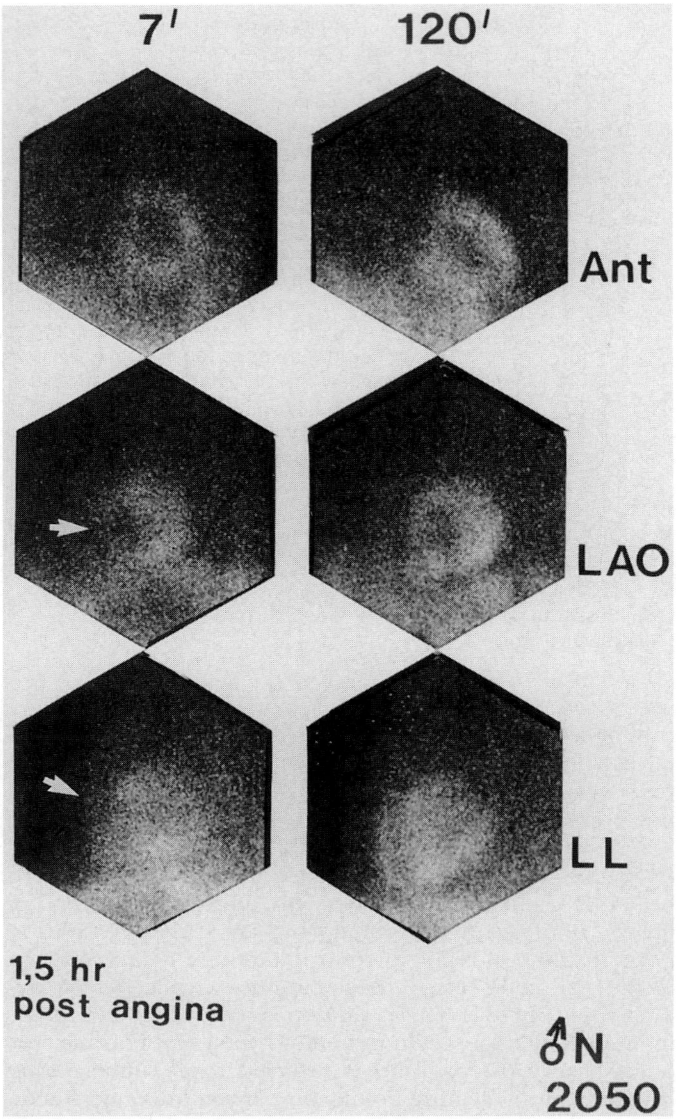

Figure 25.69. ^{201}Tl imaging in unstable angina. Initial and delayed planar imaging after a single dose of ^{201}Tl in a patient with unstable angina. *Left,* myocardial images obtained 1/2 hour after last anginal attack, 7 minutes after injection. The myocardial images show an anteroseptal myocardial perfusion defect (*arrows*). *Right,* myocardial images obtained 120 minutes after injection. The myocardial images show a nearly normal image as a result of filling in of the defect, indicating the presence of ischemic viable myocardium. *Ant* = anterior, *LAO* = left anterior oblique, *LL* = left lateral. (Reproduced by permission of the American Heart Association from Wackers FJTh, Lie KI, Liem KL, et al. Thallium-201 scintigraphy in unstable angina pectoris. Circulation 1978;57:738.)

infarction is to be ruled out. ^{99m}Tc-labeled myocardial perfusion imaging agents are preferred and more practical for this application. In this situation, it is important that imaging is performed as soon as possible, and not later than 6 hours after the last episode of chest pain. Furthermore, myocardial perfusion imaging provides means to quantify the area at risk, ultimate infarct size, and to evaluate the efficacy of thrombolytic therapy.

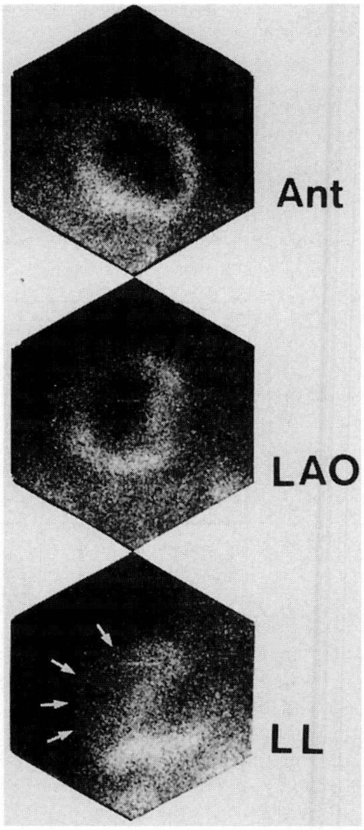

Figure 25.70. Planar ^{201}Tl images in patient with electrocardiographic complete left bundle branch block and acute myocardial infarction. The left ventricle is markedly enlarged and dilated. The left lateral (*LL*) view shows a large anterior wall defect (*small arrows*). The anterior (*Ant*) and left anterior oblique (*LAO*) views show no definite defect. However, the cavity is extremely photopenic since the anterior wall is viewed *en face* ("look-through" defect). The electrocardiogram in this patient did not provide information with respect to location of the myocardial infarction. Equilibrium radionuclide angiocardiography revealed an anterseptal aneurysm.

In patients with unstable angina, myocardial perfusion imaging provides a noninvasive method to objectively visualize the presence of resting hypoperfusion.

Myocardial perfusion imaging with pharmacologic vasodilation early after acute infarction allows for early identification of patients with increase risk for complicated in hospital course. At the time of hospital discharge, myocardial perfusion imaging using either ^{201}Tl or ^{99m}Tc-sestamibi and either planar or SPECT techniques, allows identification of high risk patients.

CHRONIC CORONARY ARTERY DISEASE

PATHOPHYSIOLOGIC BASIS FOR STRESS MYOCARDIAL PERFUSION IMAGING

Patients with chronic stable coronary artery disease usually are asymptomatic at rest. However, during exercise they may develop symptoms of angina pectoris. The pathophysiologic basis of this clinical syndrome is that at rest (even in the presence of a significant coronary stenosis) regional myocardial blood flow is adequate to meet myocar-

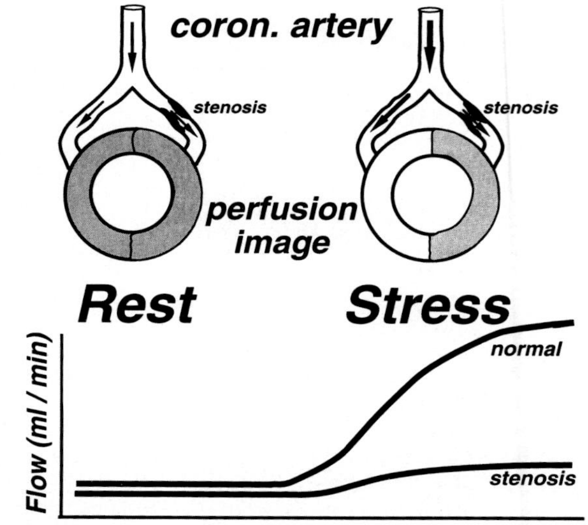

Figure 25.71. Schematic representation of the principle of rest/stress myocardial perfusion imaging. *Top:* Two branches of a coronary artery are schematically shown, one is normal (*left*), and one has a significant stenosis (*right*). *Middle:* Myocardial perfusion images of the territories supplied by the two branches. *Bottom:* Schematic representation of coronary blood flow in the branches at rest and during stress. At rest, myocardial blood flow is equal in both coronary artery branches. When a myocardial radiotracer is injected at rest, uptake is homogenous (normal image). During stress, coronary blood flow increases 2.0–2.5 times in the normal branch, but not to the same extent in the stenosed branch, resulting in heterogenous distribution of blood flow. This heterogeneity of blood flow can be visualized with ^{201}Tl or ^{201}Tl-sestamibi as an area with relatively decreased uptake (abnormal image with a myocardial perfusion defect). (Reproduced by permission from Wackers FJTh. Exercise myocardial perfusion imaging. J Nucl Med 1994;35:726–729.)

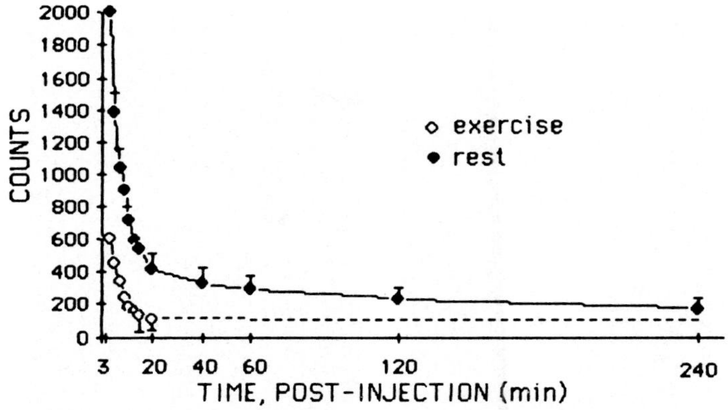

Figure 25.72. ^{201}Tl blood disappearance curves after intravenous injection during exercise and at rest. Blood activity declines exponentially after injection in both conditions. The $t_{1/2}$ of blood activity after exercise is 8 minutes, and at rest it is 7.2 minutes. However, despite initial similar clearances, absolute ^{201}Tl blood activity level is at all times 2.5–3 times higher after a rest injection than after exercise injection.

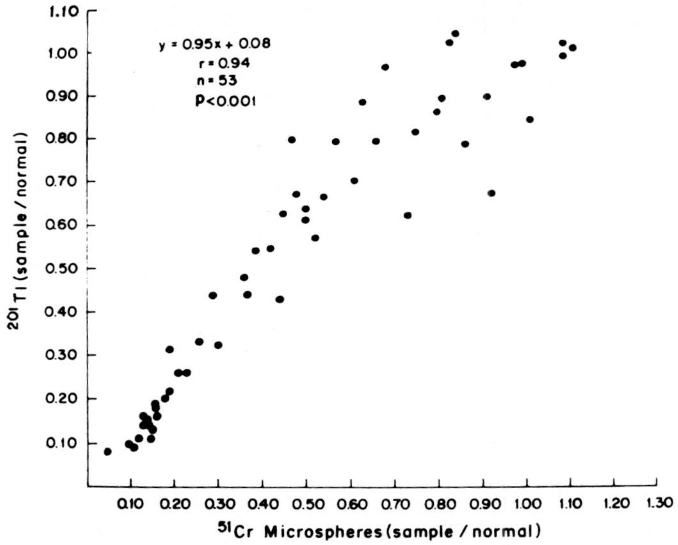

Figure 25.73. Transmural myocardial ^{201}Tl uptake and regional myocardial blood flow. Relationship between transmural myocardial ^{201}Tl uptake and relative regional myocardial blood flow as estimated by radioisotope microsphere technique in experimental animals. Activities are expressed as ratios between infarct sample and the mean of normal samples obtained in each individual study. The microsphere estimate of transmural regional myocardial blood flow correlates well with transmural ^{201}Tl uptake. (Reproduced by permission from DiCola VC, Downing SE, Donabedian RK, Zaret BL. Pathophysiological correlates of thallium-201 myocardial uptake in experimental infarction. Cardiovasc Res 1977;11:141.)

dial oxygen demands. However, during exercise, the same coronary artery stenosis limits appropriate augmentation of myocardial blood flow (coronary reserve) to meet increased metabolic demands (Fig. 25.71). Thus, insufficient regional oxygen supply to the myocardium supplied by a diseased coronary artery leads to local myocardial ischemia and clinical angina pectoris. Under these circumstances regional inhomogeneity of myocardial blood flow exists, which is relevant for myocardial perfusion imaging. After intravenous injection of a radiolabeled myocardial perfusion imaging agent (either at exercise or at rest), the radiotracer clears rapidly from the blood (Fig. 25.72) (140–143) and accumulates within the heart and body according to regional distribution of blood flow (Figs. 25.73 and 25.74). Although myocardial perfusion imaging agents are extracted relatively rapidly from the blood (94), an "ischemic steady state" of 1–2 minutes after tracer injection is required for sufficient tracer accumulation and visualization of perfusion defects (144, 145).

EXERCISE PROTOCOL

In most U.S. laboratories, treadmill exercise is the preferred method of stress in conjunction with myocardial perfusion imaging. Many American patients exercise better and feel more comfortable walking or running on a treadmill than exercising on an upright bicycle. The speed and grade of the motor driven treadmill can easily be adjusted to the physical condition and agility of the patient. In many other countries, the upright bicycle is the preferred exercise modality. The upright bicycle is preferred over the supine bicycle, since peak exercise heart rate (and, therefore, the increase of myocardial blood flow) usually is higher on upright bicycle (146). In preparation for the exercise test, the patient should be in a fasting state. Diabetic patients

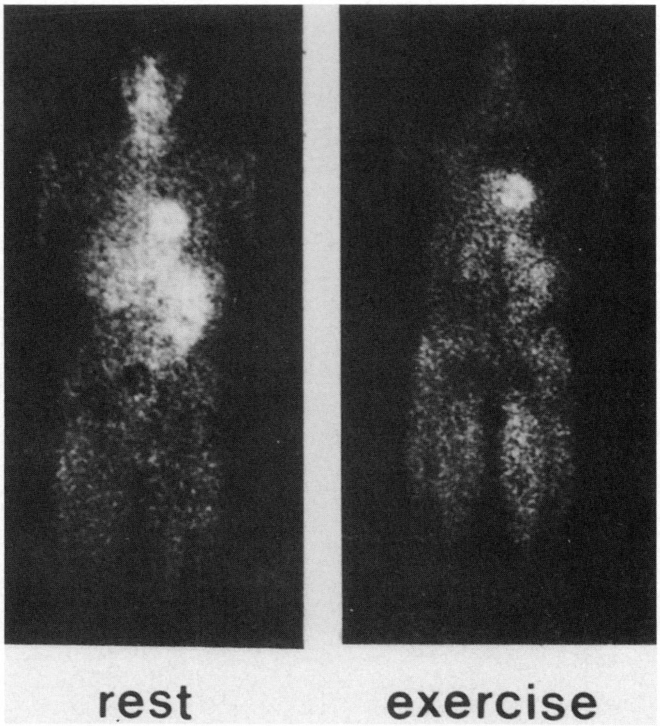

Figure 25.74. Whole body distribution of ^{201}Tl at rest and following exercise. At rest, ^{201}Tl accumulates in the heart, liver, spleen, kidneys, and gastrointestinal tract, proportional to the relative distribution of cardiac output. Following exercise, ^{201}Tl activity in the heart is prominent. Most of the remaining ^{201}Tl activity is accumulated in the exercising muscles of the thighs. Note the almost absent activity in the splanchnic region. (Reproduced by permission from Wackers FJTh, Busemann Sokole E, Samson G, van der Schoot JB. Atlas of Tl-201 myocardial scintigraphy. Clin Nucl Med 1977;2:64.)

should take their regular dose of insulin and have a light breakfast at least 1 hour prior to the test.

Several standardized exercise protocols exist. The most widely used protocol is that designed by Bruce (147). According to this protocol the subject starts out at 1.7 mph on a 10% grade (Table 25.5). Subsequently, every 3 minutes the speed and grade of the treadmill are increased until the patient reaches a predefined end point of exercise.

Generally accepted end points for exercise are: (a) angina pectoris or reproduction of the patient's symptoms, (b) severe fatigue, (c) hypotension, (d) ventricular arrhythmias, or (e) severe electrocardiographic ST segment depression (e.g., 3 mm or more) at 0.08 msec after the J-point. The age-predicted target heart rate should be considered a guideline for adequate exercise, but is in itself *not* a good end point, since maximal heart rate may vary importantly among individuals of the same age. A knowledgeable and experienced physician should supervise each stress test and monitor heart rate, blood pressure, electrocardiographic changes, and symptoms each 2–3 minutes. Serious complications as the direct result of stress testing are rare (approximately 1:10,000). The physician who administers the stress test should be trained in advanced cardiac life support.

Table 25.5.
Bruce Graded Treadmill Exercise Protocol

Stage	Speed (mph)	Grade (%)	Time (min)	METS[a]
1	1.7	10	3	5
2	2.5	12	3	7
3	3.4	14	3	10
4	4.2	16	3	13
5	5.0	18	3	16

[a]METS = metabolic equivalents.

An intravenous line should be in place in an antecubital vein for injection of radiopharmaceutical. When an end point of exercise is reached, the radiopharmaceutical is rapidly injected in the intravenous line and flushed with a bolus of 10 ml of saline. The patient is then encouraged to exercise for another 1–2 minutes at the same level of exercise. This continuation of exercise after the injection of the radionuclide is important for successful myocardial perfusion imaging as it takes at least 2–3 minutes for 80% of the injected radiopharmaceutical to be cleared from the blood (109) (Fig. 25.72). Consequently, it is crucial that during myocardial radiotracer uptake, heart rate and, presumably, myocardial blood flow are maintained at a "steady state." If the patient cannot continue to exercise at the same level, speed and grade of the treadmill can be decreased to a lower level. However, the patient should not be allowed to stop before 1–2 minutes after injection of the radiotracer. Obviously, clinical judgment must be employed at this time and patient safety is a first concern.

IMAGING AFTER EXERCISE

The timing of imaging after injection at exercise and at rest is different for different radiopharmaceuticals. Table 25.1 summarizes the details of imaging.

The image acquisition protocol should be strictly standardized in each laboratory for timing of imaging, sequence of imaging, and duration of imaging. In our laboratory, the technologists keep a detailed record of all aspects of image acquisition. This is an important aspect of quality control.

Before the patient is positioned under the gamma-camera, the injection site in the arm should be imaged just to identify any extravasation injection of the radiopharmaceutical.

Imaging Protocols

Myocardial perfusion imaging protocols have undergone substantial changes over the past few years. These changes have been implemented because of a better understanding of myocardial kinetics of ^{201}Tl and because of different requirements for imaging with the newly developed ^{99m}Tc-labeled imaging agents. An extensive review of various imaging protocols (148) in the mid-1990's is beyond the scope of this chapter. The most commonly used imaging protocols are the following:

Thallium-201. The patient is injected with ^{201}Tl (3.5 mCi) at peak exercise. Imaging is performed within 5 minutes of termination of exercise and delayed redistribution imaging is performed 3–4 hours later. In selected patients (see chapter 27), ^{201}Tl may be reinjected at rest either the same day (1 mCi) or on a different day (3.5 mCi). Rest imaging is started approximately 45 minutes after injection.

^{99m}Tc-Sestamibi. Two basic protocols are employed for ^{99m}Tc-sestamibi imaging, a 1-day protocol and a 2-day "split-dose" protocol. Using the 2-day protocol, 25–30 mCi of ^{99m}Tc-sestamibi is administered on one day at rest, and the same dose is administered on the other day at peak exercise. After exercise, imaging can be started approximately 15 minutes after injection of ^{99m}Tc-sestamibi. After injection of ^{99m}Tc-sestamibi at rest, imaging is delayed at least 1–1 1/2 hours to allow sufficient clearance of radiotracer from the liver. Using the 1-day protocol, the total dose administered to the patient per day is split in two: a low dose of 10–15 mCi is administered first, followed 3 hours later by the high dose of 20–25 mCi of ^{99m}Tc-sestamibi. Although there is a preference to perform the rest study first and the exercise study second, this sequence can be reversed without significant effect on the detection of coronary artery disease (149).

^{99m}Tc-Tetrofosmin. A 1-day "split-dose" imaging protocol has been proposed for ^{99m}Tc-tetrofosmin imaging (7). Similar doses of radiopharmaceutical as for ^{99m}Tc-sestamibi are administered. Because of relatively fast clearance of subdiaphragmatic uptake, imaging usually can be started at 15 minutes after injection, either at rest or exercise (Fig. 25.75).

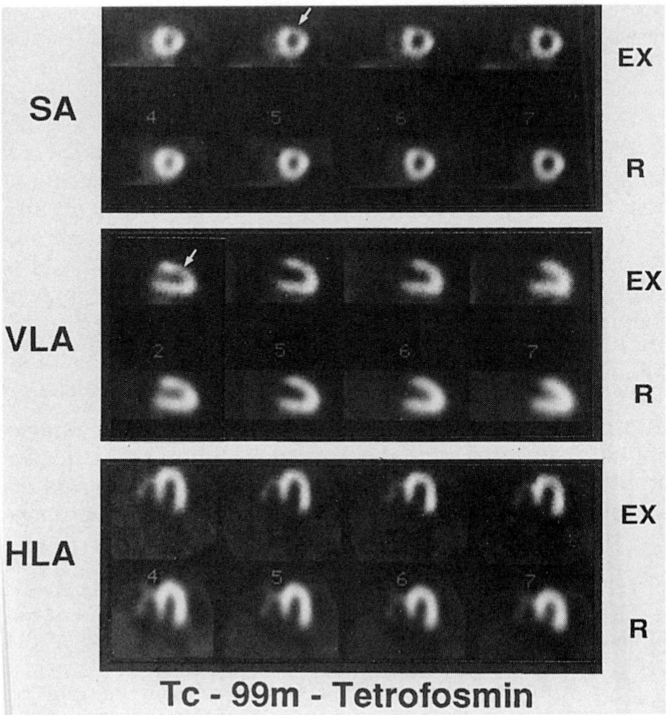

Figure 25.75. Exercise/rest SPECT myocardial perfusion imaging with ^{99m}Tc-tetrofosmin. The SPECT images were acquired 15 minutes after injection, both during exercise and rest. The images show a relatively small reversible anterior wall defect.

^{99m}Tc-Teboroxime. Because of the rapid clearance of ^{99m}Tc-teboroxime from the myocardium, imaging should be completed within the first 5–10 minutes after injection either at exercise or at rest. Rest and exercise imaging can be performed on one day using two 20–30 mCi doses of ^{99m}Tc-teboroxime. Rapid serial imaging by either planar or SPECT technique have been proposed (6, 150) (Fig. 25.76). For routine clinical use, these protocols are too demanding and not widely used at the present time.

Dual Isotope Imaging. According to this novel protocol, rest imaging is performed first with ^{201}Tl (3.5 mCi). As soon as rest ^{201}Tl-imaging is completed, the patient is stressed and 25 mCi of ^{99m}Tc-sestamibi is injected at peak stress. Stress imaging is then performed 15 minutes after completion of exercise. The advantage of this protocol is the relatively short time in which rest and stress imaging can be completed (151). Figure 25.77 shows an example of dual isotope images.

OPTIMAL PLANAR IMAGING

Planar stress myocardial perfusion imaging is started with the LAO projection. We prefer to start with the left anterior oblique (LAO) view since myocardial territories of the left anterior descending coronary artery (LAD) and of the left circumflex artery (LCx)/right coronary artery (RCA) are well-separated spatially in this image (Fig. 25.78). Next, a left lateral view is obtained, which again separates the territories of the LAD and LCx/RCA. Subsequently, an anterior view is obtained. On the anterior projection, the territories of the septal branches of the LAD and of the RCA are superimposed, and only the anterolateral wall is supplied by a single artery, the LAD (diagonal branches). Delayed or rest imaging is performed in the same sequence for the identical time as for exercise imaging.

Good quality planar images can be obtained relatively easily by paying attention to details of image acquisition (152). The most frequent reasons for poor quality images are (a) insufficient count density within the heart, (b) inconsistent patient positioning and repositioning, and (c) use of too large a zoom factor.

Adequate Count Density. One should aim for at least 600,000 counts in the field of view. When extracardiac activity is present, e.g., in lungs or subdiaphragmatic organs, greater count density in the field of view is needed (Fig. 25.79**A** and **B**).

Because of the relatively low dose of ^{201}Tl, imaging can be optimized in several ways:

1. Administration of adequate dose—at least 2.5 mCi for planar imaging. In obese patients, a larger dose is required.
2. Imaging on both energy peaks of ^{201}Tl.
3. Use general all-purpose collimator.
4. Imaging for a preset time rather than for counts, e.g., 8–10 minutes per view. This is of particular importance when substantial extracardiac activity is present, e.g., after dipyridamole infusion, or in patients with increased pulmonary uptake (see later).

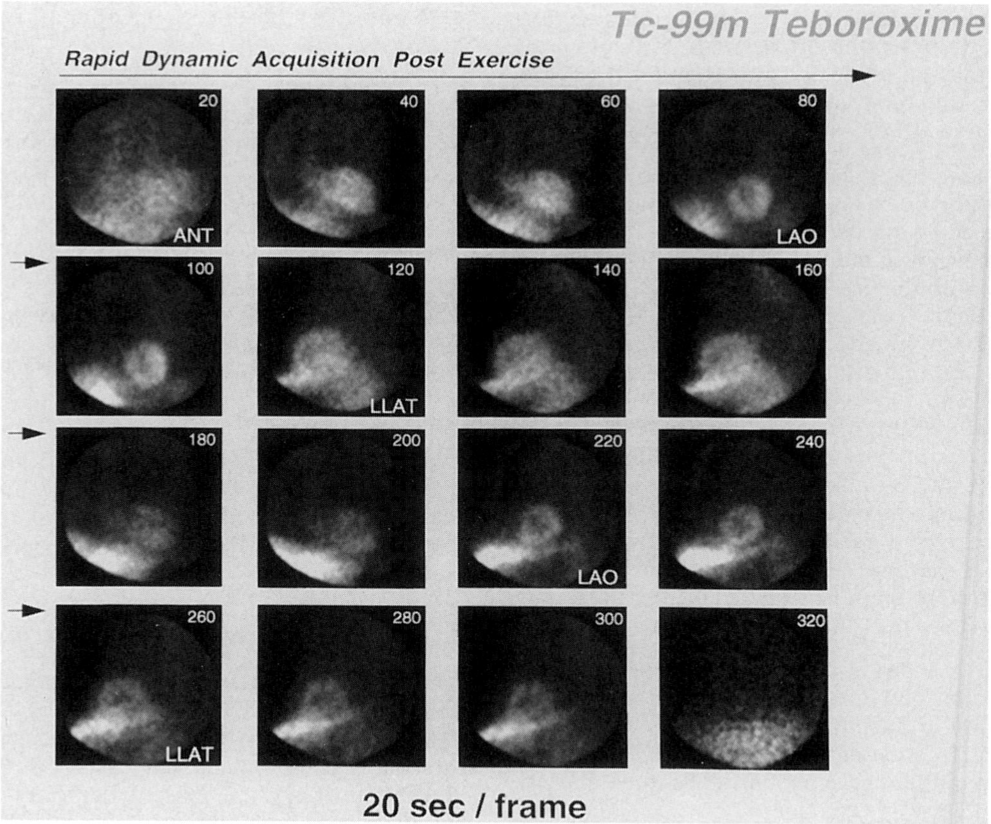

Figure 25.76. Rapid serial planar imaging with ^{99m}Tc-teboroxime. Each planar image is taken for 20 seconds, starting in the anterior (*ANT*) position immediately after termination of exercise. The patient was seated upright on a rotating chair and rotated from the anterior to the left anterior oblique (*LAO*) and left lateral (*LLAT*) position and again ANT, LAO, and LLAT. Note the rapid disappearance of ^{99m}Tc-teboroxime from the heart in 260 seconds and intensive liver uptake.

With the use of ^{99m}Tc-labeled imaging agents, adequate count density is readily achieved, since 20–30 mCi is administered. With the latter agents, one should aim for 1.5–2 million counts/field of view. This can usually be achieved with 5 minutes per view (3).

Patient Positioning. Imaging is routinely performed in three projections. The LAO view usually is obtained with the patient lying supine. This angulation should be used as a reference angle for the other views. The anterior view is obtained with the patient lying supine, with the camera 45° to the right of the LAO view. For the left lateral view, the patient should be decubitus and turned on the *right side*, with the camera head in the same position as for the anterior view. The detector head should be angled in such a way that it is as close as possible to the patient's chest wall. On all views, the heart should be in the center of the field of view. Repositioning of the patient at delayed imaging should be done with great care. The position of the heart on the exercise images should be reproduced as close as possible to that at rest.

Zoom Factor. It is a misconception to believe that the larger the heart in the field of view, the better the image. Too large a zoom factor creates a coarse image with poor resolution. Additionally, since the heart is displayed over a larger number of pixels, *greater* count density is required compared to without zoom. When a large field of view camera is used, the zoom factor (magnification) should not exceed 1.2 times. On an optimal planar image, the heart is approximately one-third to one-fourth of the diameter of the field of view (Figs. 25.1, 25.12, and 25.79).

Quality Assurance of Planar Image Interpretation

Interpretation of planar myocardial perfusion images should follow a systematic approach. Initial steps involve quality assurance. Next, images and computer graphics are analyzed using a step-by-step approach. We propose the following routine:

1. Did the patient continue to exercise for at least 1–2 minutes after administration of the radiotracer? If the patient terminated exercise too early (before 1 minute), false-negative images may occur.
2. Was initial imaging started at the appropriate time after injection of radiopharmaceutical? The technologist should keep precise records of actual timing of imaging. If, for example, ^{201}Tl imaging is delayed too much after exercise, false-negative images may be obtained because of early redistribution. Using ^{99m}Tc-labeled imaging agents, appro-

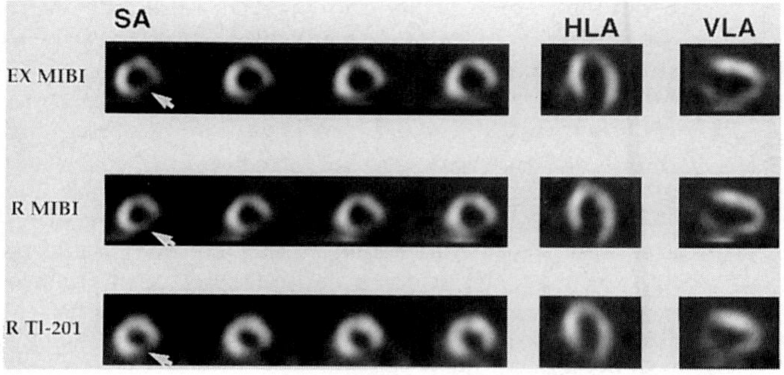

Figure 25.77. Dual isotope SPECT myocardial perfusion imaging. Dual isotope imaging employs ^{201}Tl for rest (*R*) imaging and ^{99m}Tc-sestamibi (*MIBI*) for exercise (*EX*) imaging. This figure illustrates the comparability of rest MIBI and rest ^{201}Tl SPECT imaging. The EX MIBI and R MIBI images show a fixed inferolateral defect (*arrow*) without evidence of ischemia. The R ^{201}Tl image similarly shows a inferolateral defect consistent with inferolateral infarction. However, compared to the EX MIBI image, the ^{201}Tl defect is slightly smaller. This is most likely due to the difference in physical characteristics of the two radiotracers. Such a small difference in defect size should not be misinterpreted as evidence for peri-infarction ischemia.

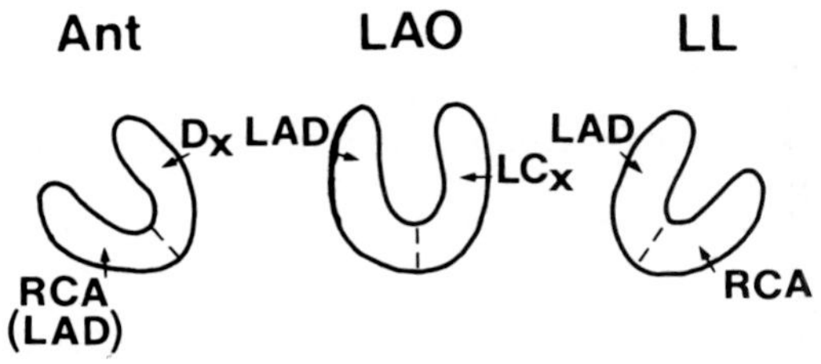

Figure 25.78. Diagrammatic representation of territories of various coronary arteries on three standard planar Tl-201 projections. *DX* = diagonal branch, *LAD* = left anterior descending coronary artery, *LCx* = left circumflex coronary artery, *RCA* = right coronary artery, *Ant* = anterior, *LAO* = left anterior oblique, *LL* = left lateral.

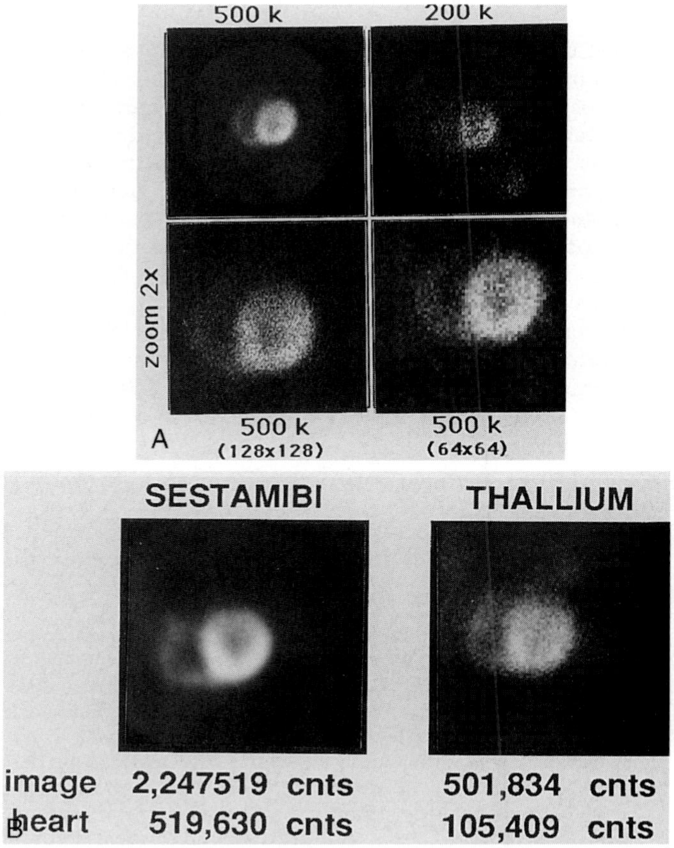

Figure 25.79. A. Effect of varying count density and zoom factor on image quality. LAO image of the same patient acquired in four different ways. *A:* Optimal image: 600,000 counts were acquired over 8 minutes using a 128 × 128 matrix. Maximal count per pixel in the heart is 191. The heart occupies approximately 1/3 of the field of view. *B:* Suboptimal image: because of the shorter acquisition time, only 200,000 counts are obtained in the field of view. The maximal count per pixel in the heart is only 65. *C:* Acquisition with a 2× zoom factor: 128 × 128 matrix. Although the image was acquired over the same time as image A was, a lower count was obtained in the field of view. The maximal count per pixel in the heart was only 52. This image is of suboptimal quality. *D:* Acquisition with a 2× zoom factor: 64 × 64 matrix. Although the count per pixel is higher (159), the resulting coarse and "boxy" image is of unsatisfactory quality. **B.** Comparative count density in ^{201}Tl and ^{99m}Tc-sestamibi images. Two planar images of the same patient are shown. The planar ^{99m}Tc-sestamibi images were acquired within 5 minutes after injection of 25 mCi, and the planar ^{201}Tl images were acquired within 8 minutes after injection of 2.5 mCi. ^{99m}Tc-sestamibi images are of considerably better quality and of higher count density than those with ^{201}Tl.

priate timing is important to allow for clearance of subdiaphragmatic activity.

3. Was the appropriate dose of radiopharmaceutical administered? Was there extravasation of radiopharmaceutical at the injection site? This would cause low count density in the heart. In our laboratory, the injection site is imaged and counted for 15 seconds immediately prior to imaging. Significant extravasation of radiopharmaceutical can be readily detected in this way.
4. Is there adequate count density in the image? For planar ^{201}Tl-imaging, at least 400,000 counts should be obtained in the whole field of view, or at least 35,000 counts in the background corrected left ventricle. This target count density is usually easily obtained with ^{99m}Tc-labeled radiotracers.
5. Particular attention should be paid to positioning and repositioning of the patient for rest or delayed imaging. Furthermore, the images should be inspected for potential artifacts caused by soft tissue attenuation (i.e., breast tissue). Breast markers (see earlier) are helpful in recognizing artifacts (Fig. 25.25).
6. The unprocessed images are displayed side-by-side, normalized to the "hottest" counts within the heart on the computer screen using a linear gray scale for visual analysis (Fig. 25.13).
7. Quantitative computer processing is displayed and reviewed. In general, quantitative data *should agree with the visual analysis*. Computer quantification has the advantage of confirming *the presence* of myocardial perfusion abnormality *and* providing a measure for *the degree* of abnormality.
8. Ascertain that the patient's exercise performance was adequate. Short duration of exercise and only a modest increase in heart rate may result in false-negative images, even if the patient has clinical symptoms of ischemia.

OPTIMAL SPECT IMAGING

For SPECT imaging careful attention to technical details is even more important than for planar imaging (153). Because of the potential movement during imaging, the patient should be immobilized using straps or devices that make it more comfortable for the patient to remain still. The arms should be above the head of the patient. The technologist should be attentive to potential patient motion. Motion may involve movement of the patient body, but may also involve a change in position of the heart within the chest (upward creep). The timing of SPECT acquisition after exercise and at rest or delayed imaging is identical to that for planar imaging. For SPECT imaging the rotation of the camera head may start either in the left posterior oblique (LPO) or right anterior oblique (RAO) position.

Quality Assurance of SPECT Image Interpretation

As for planar imaging, the interpretation of SPECT images should follow a systematic approach (14). We propose the following routine:

1. Inspection of cine display of rotating planar projection images (Fig. 25.80). This should always be the first step before interpretation of SPECT images. The rotating images allow assessment of overall study quality: (a) Is the left ventricle well-visualized? (b) Is there excessive extracardiac activity? Is this activity immediately adjacent to the heart? (c) Is there patient motion or upward creep of the heart? (d) Is there a breast shadow obscuring the heart in certain projections? (e) Is the orbit of the detector head around the heart circular (the heart "pivots" in the center of the screen) or elliptical (the heart "runs" across the screen from one side to the other) (Fig. 25.81).
2. Did the patient continue to exercise after injection of the radiotracer for 1–2 minutes?
3. Was timing of imaging appropriate after injection of radiotracer?
4. Was an appropriate dose of the radiopharmaceutical administered? What is the count density in the left ventricle? Software developed in our laboratory displays automatically the maximal number of counts in the "hottest" pixel in the heart in one of the anterior projection images.
5. Are displayed reconstructed tomographic slices appropriately chosen? Are stress and rest slices paired correctly (Fig. 25.40)?
6. Are there artifacts that are potentially due to motion (Fig. 25.37**A** and **B**), breast (Fig. 25.35), or diaphragmatic attenuation (Figs. 25.21 and 25.34)? If needed, one should inspect the cine of the rotating planar images again. Inspection of cine display of ECG-gated slices may be helpful.
7. Quantification (polar map or circumferential profiles) is compared with visual analysis.

IMAGE INTERPRETATION

Planar and SPECT images are interpreted by visual analysis, often aided by computer quantification, as follows (Fig. 25.82):

Normal. Homogeneous uptake of the radiopharmaceutical throughout the myocardium.

Defect. A localized myocardial area with a relative decrease in radiotracer uptake. Defects may vary in intensity, from slightly reduced activity to almost total absence of activity. Quantitative analysis allows severity of defects to be defined as "percent of normal activity" (140, 154).

Reversible Defect. A defect that is present on the initial stress images and no longer present or present to a lesser degree, on the resting or delayed images. This pattern indicates myocardial ischemia. Using ^{201}Tl, this change over time is referred to as "redistribution" (140, 155, 156).

Fixed Defect. A defect that is unchanged and present on both exercise and rest (delayed) images. This pattern generally indicates infarction and scar tissue. However, in some patients with fixed ^{201}Tl defects at 2–4-hour delayed imaging, improved uptake can be noted on 24-hour redistribution imaging or after a new resting injection (see later) (23, 24).

Reverse Redistribution. The initial images are either normal or show a defect, whereas the delayed or rest images show a more severe defect (Fig. 25.83). This pattern is frequently observed in patients who have undergone thrombolytic therapy

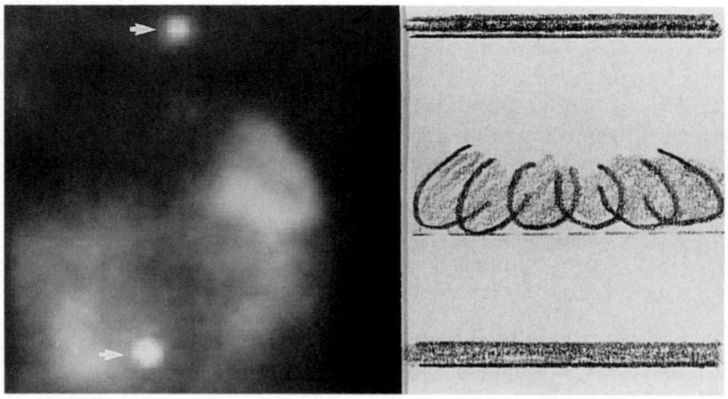

Figure 25.80. Cine display of projection images. Inspection of cine display of all 32 images acquired for SPECT reconstruction is an important step in quality control prior to image interpretation. Upward creep and/or body motion can be readily recognized in this display. Two point sources on the patient's chest in the field of view (*arrows*) can also be used as fixed reference marks. They should move on the cine display in a straight line. Presently, we use a white reference bar that can be positioned at the inferior wall (*LV*) (see Figs. 25.36 and 25.37).

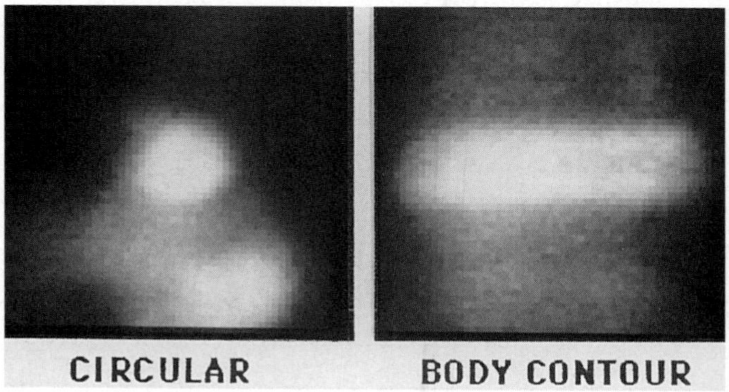

Figure 25.81. Inspection of cine display of 32 planar projection images for quality control of SPECT imaging. When the heart is excentric in the camera orbit, as for example, when the gamma-camera follows the *body contour*, the heart will move from the left of the screen to the right of the screen. When the heart is in the center of the orbit, as with a *circular* orbit with the imaging table moved laterally to position the heart in the center, the heart pivots in the center on the rotating image. The more the heart is off-center, the more likely artifacts occur (see Fig. 25.39).

or percutaneous coronary angioplasty (157). This phenomenon is thought to be caused by initial excess of tracer uptake in a reperfused area with a mixture of scar tissue and viable myocytes. Initial accumulation is thus followed by rapid clearance form scar tissue. Although the significance of this finding is controversial, it does not represent evidence of exercise-induced ischemia.

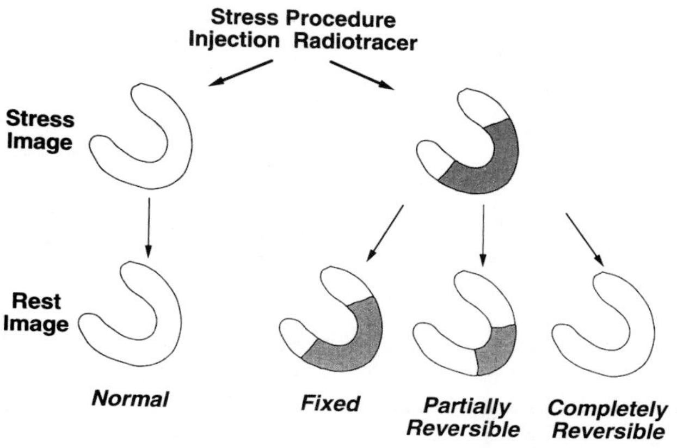

Figure 25.82. Schematic representation of interpretation of myocardial perfusion images. The *shaded* areas indicate myocardial perfusion defects. Not shown on this figure is reverse redistribution (see Fig. 25.83).

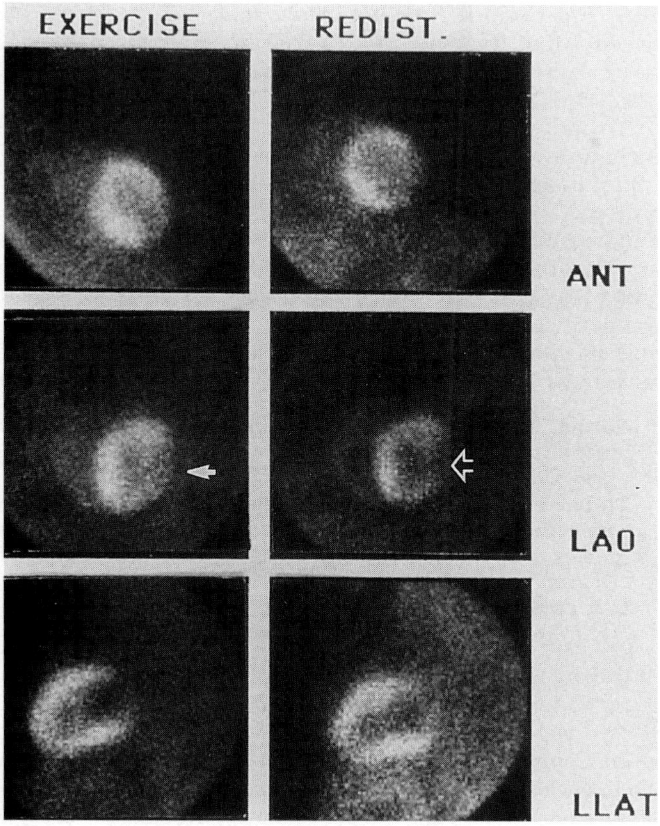

Figure 25.83. Example of reverse redistribution on planar ^{201}Tl imaging after exercise and redistribution. The exercise images show a relatively mild posterior lateral defect (*arrows*). This defect in more severe on redistribution imaging (*open arrow*). This pattern is referred to as reverse redistribution.

Lung Uptake. Normally no, or very little, ^{201}Tl is noted in the lung fields on postexercise images. Increased lung uptake can be quantitated as lung:heart ratio (normal <0.5) or as lung washout (normal <42%). This abnormality indicates exercise-induced ischemic left ventricular dysfunction (158).

Transient Left Ventricular Dilation. Occasionally, the left ventricle is noted to be larger following exercise than on the rest or delayed image. This pattern indicates exercise-induced left ventricular dysfunction (159).

Myocardial Kinetics of Radiopharmaceuticalals after Exercise

Thallium-201. After intravenous injection of ^{201}Tl during peak exercise, the radioisotope is rapidly distributed throughout the body proportional to the distribution of cardiac output (Fig. 25.74), and in the heart according to regional distribution of coronary blood flow (Fig. 25.73) (140–143). The first-pass extraction fraction of ^{201}Tl by the myocardial cells is 85–88% (125). During the first 7 minutes after exercise, ^{201}Tl clears rapidly from the blood pool, followed by a slower decrease over subsequent hours (Figs. 25.84 and 25.85) (140). In normal myocardium, ^{201}Tl uptake is maximal within 1–2 minutes of injection at peak exercise. As soon as initial uptake occurs, there is a continuous exchange between ^{201}Tl in the myocardium and

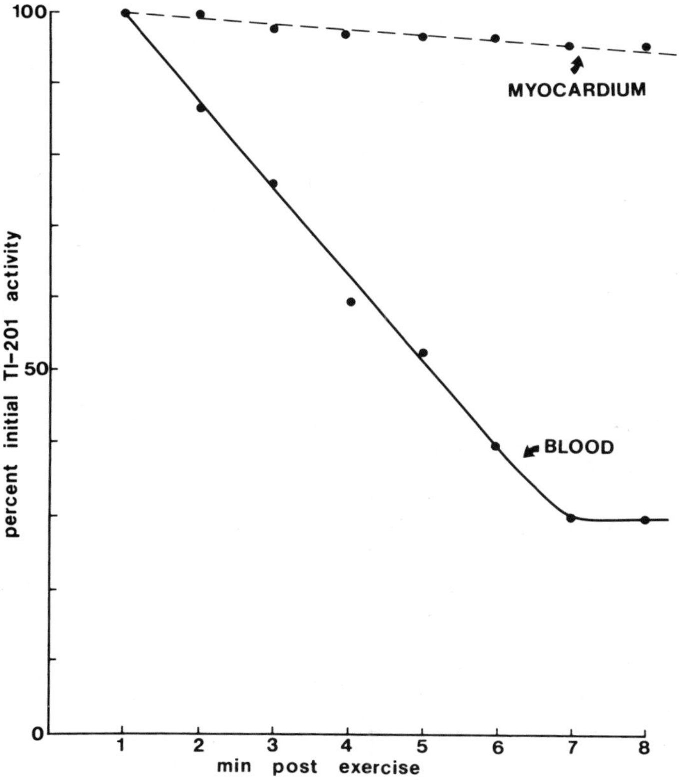

Figure 25.84. ^{201}Tl time-activity curve after exercise. Normal ^{201}Tl time-activity curve in blood and myocardium (total left ventricle in the left anterior oblique projection) during the first 8 minutes after termination of exercise. The data were obtained from a normal subject. (Reproduced by permission from Wackers FJTh, Fetterman RC, Mattera JA, Clements JP. Quantitative planar thallium-201 stress scintigraphy: a critical evaluation of the method. Semin Nucl Med 1985;15:46.)

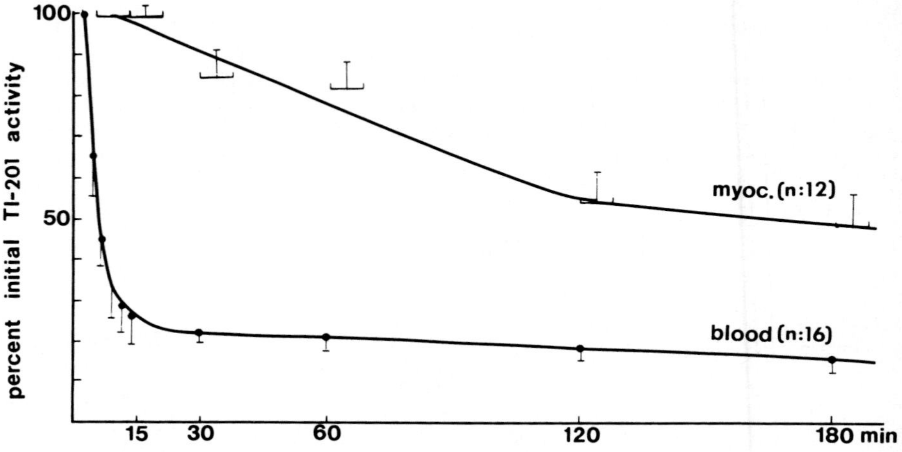

Figure 25.85. ^{201}Tl time-activity curve after exercise. Normal ^{201}Tl time-activity curve in blood and myocardium (total left ventricle in the left anterior oblique projection) up to 3 hours after termination of exercise. Data (mean ± standard deviation) were obtained in subjects with a low probability (less than 3%) of coronary artery disease. (Reproduced by permission from Wackers FJTh, Fetterman RC, Mattera JA, Clements JP. Quantitative planar thallium-201 stress scintigraphy: a critical evaluation of the method. Semin Nucl Med 1985;15:46.)

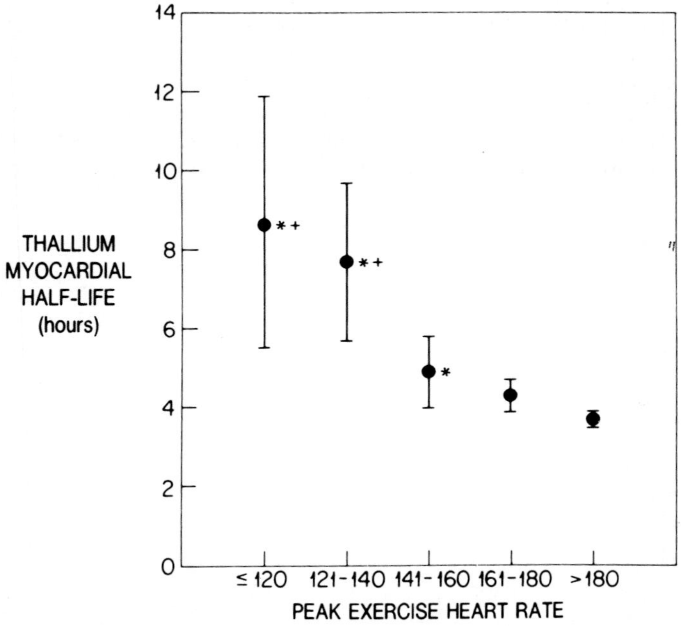

Figure 25.86. Relationship between ^{201}Tl myocardial clearance and peak heart rate achieved during exercise. ^{201}Tl clearance is expressed as $t_{1/2}$ of ^{201}Tl in the myocardium in hours. An inverse relationship exists between peak exercise heart rate and myocardial clearance ($t_{1/2}$). (Reproduced by permission from Kaul S, Chesler DA, Pohost GM, Strauss HW, Okada RD, Boucher CA. Influence of peak exercise heart rate on normal thallium-201 myocardial clearance. J Nucl Med 1986;27:26.)

^{201}Tl in the blood pool (155, 156). ^{201}Tl is continually clearing from the myocardial cells and being replaced by ^{201}Tl from the extracardiac pool. This continuous exchange explains the filling in or redistribution of defects after transient exercise-induced ischemia.

Normal myocardial ^{201}Tl kinetics are characterized by early peaking after injection, followed by gradual decrease over time (155, 160, 161). The half-time of ^{201}Tl net washout from normal myocardium is 4–8 hours. In normal patients, the lower limit (mean ±2 SD) of normal washout at 2 hours after exercise is approximately 30%, and at 4 hours 35%. The rate of ^{201}Tl washout is directly related to peak exercise heart rate (Fig. 25.86). When peak hart rate is lower than approximately 120 bpm (beats per minute) (inadequate exercise), abnormally low washout does not necessarily indicate ischemia (162, 163).

Myocardial ^{201}Tl kinetics in ischemic myocardium is variable. When significant coronary artery stenosis is present, the initial absolute level of ^{201}Tl *uptake* is lower than in the normal myocardium, creating a "defect" (156, 164–166). Furthermore, the *net washout* of ^{201}Tl measured between initial imaging and delayed imaging is, in general, lower in ischemic myocardial than in normal myocardium (Fig. 25.87) (166).

The differences in rate and direction of ^{201}Tl kinetics are most pronounced during the first 1–2 hours after exercise. Initial imaging should begin as soon as possible after exercise. A modest delay in obtaining the first set of images may result in false-negative images (140, 167). There are arguments in favor of delayed imaging at 2 hours after exercise, instead of at 4 hours after exercise, for detection of washout abnormalities (Fig. 25.88). Thallium-201 myocardial washout after adequate exercise can be summarized as follows (Fig. 25.87):

Normal Myocardium. Gradual clearance of ^{201}Tl over time. At 2 hours after exercise, at least 30% of initial ^{201}Tl activity has washed out.

Transiently Ischemic Myocardium. Net washout is *lower* than the normal limit. In more severe ischemia, *no change* in net myocardial ^{201}Tl content, or even an absolute *accumulation* of ^{201}Tl, may occur.

Infarcted Myocardium. Normal ^{201}Tl washout (probably partially due to overlying normal myocardium).

At the present time, detailed clinical analysis of ^{201}Tl *washout* is considered an art of the past. Reliable measurement of ^{201}Tl washout requires meticulous adherence to timing of the imaging protocol. Washout analysis was particularly useful, when done well, to enhance the diagnostic yield of *planar imaging.* With the increasing clinical use of ^{201}Tl SPECT imaging, it became clear that SPECT washout analysis was not as valuable as for planar imaging. This is most likely due to alteration of data during backprojection, image filtering, and lack of attenuation correction. More-

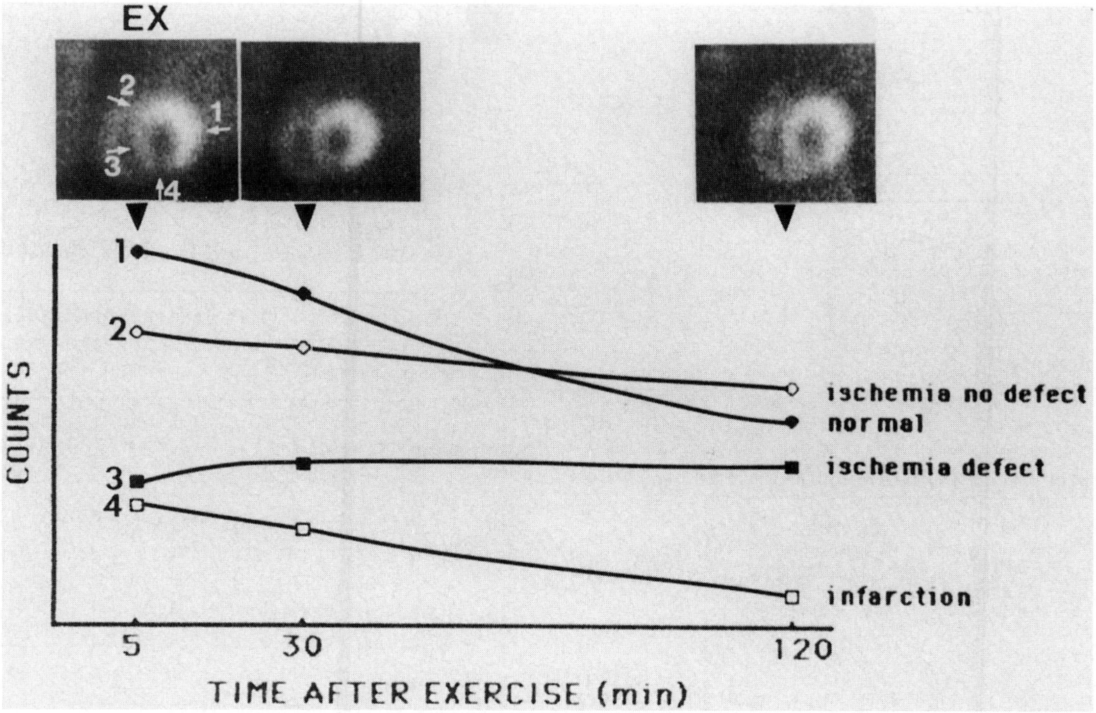

Figure 25.87. Comparative postexercise ^{201}Tl time-activity curves on planar imaging. ^{201}Tl time-activity curves after exercise in normal myocardium (*1*), transiently ischemic myocardium without visual defect (*2*), transiently ischemic myocardium with a visible defect (*3*), and old myocardial infarction (*4*). Normal myocardium (*1*) shows a gradual decrease of ^{201}Tl activity over time. After transient ischemia, ^{201}Tl activity may clear slower than normal (*2*) or actually increase (*3*) in the myocardium over time. An old infarct are (*4*) without exercise-induced myocardial ischemia shows gradual decrease in ^{201}Tl activity over time similar to normal myocardium. The images at the top show an example of a septal defect that gradually fills in over time, except at the apex where an old scar is present (*4*).

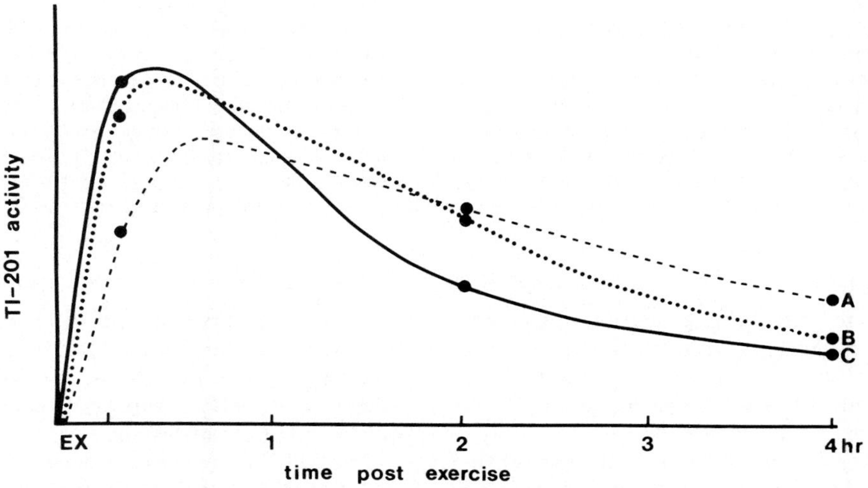

Figure 25.88. Schematic representation of myocardial ^{201}Tl time-activity curves after exercise, illustrating optimal timing of delayed imaging. *Curve A*, Severe ischemia: abnormal accumulation (defect) and abnormal washout. *Curve B*, Mild ischemia: normal accumulation (no defect) and abnormal washout. *Curve C*, Normal: normal accumulation and normal washout. Compared to myocardial ^{201}Tl activity immediately after exercise, ^{201}Tl washout is abnormal at any time of delayed imaging for *A* (exercise-induced myocardial ischemia with ^{201}Tl defect). However, for *B*, although ^{201}Tl washout initially is distinctly different from normal myocardium, at 4 hours after exercise no difference in overall washout is measured between *B* and *C*. The differences in direction and rate of ^{201}Tl kinetics are most prominent during the first 2 hours after exercise, which is the optimal time for delayed imaging and detection of washout abnormalities. (Reproduced by permission from Wackers FJTh, Fetterman RC, Mattera JA, Clements JP. Quantitative planar thallium-201 stress scintigraphy: a critical evaluation of the method. Semin Nucl Med 1985;15:46.)

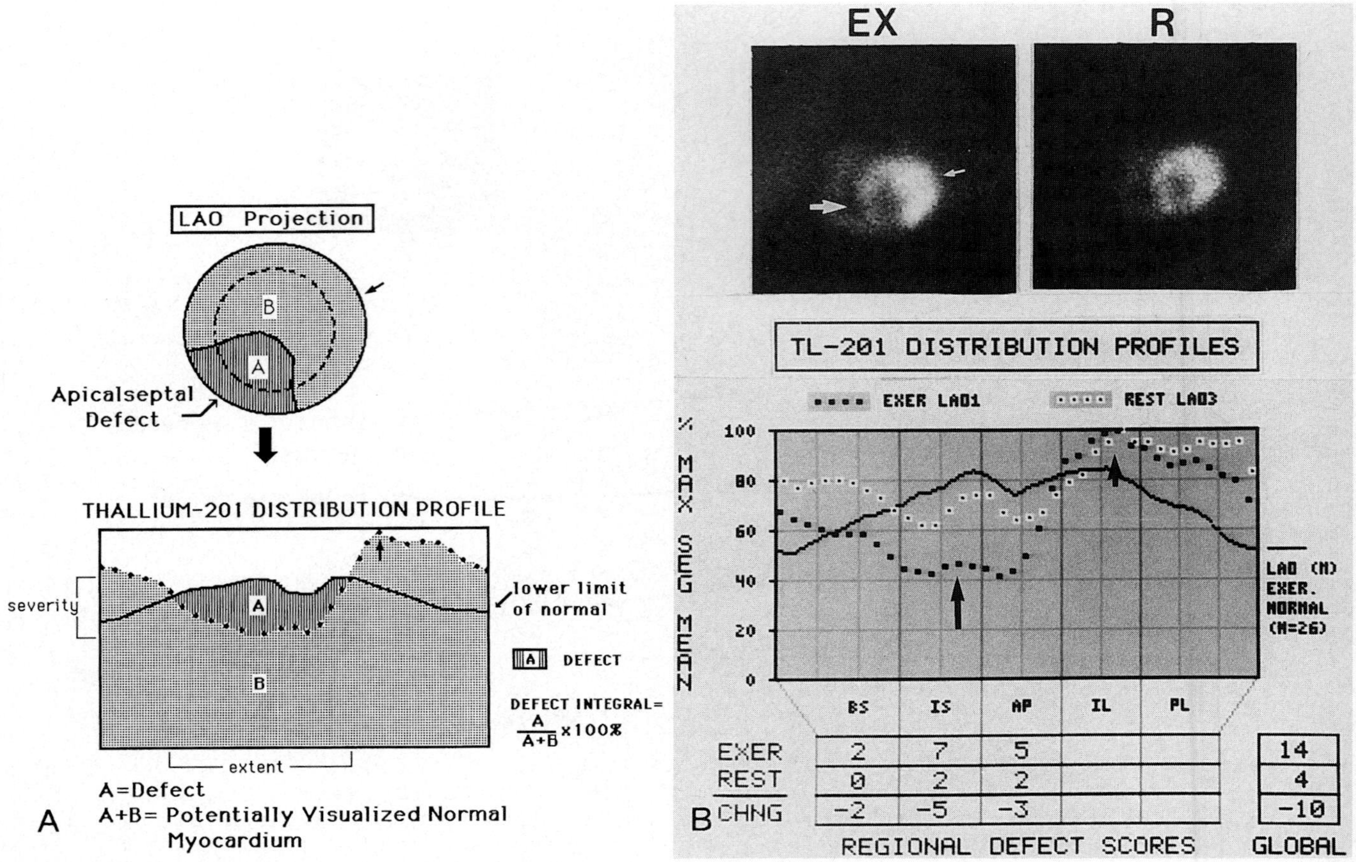

Figure 25.89. A. Generation of circumferential count distribution profile. *Top panel* shows a schematic LAO image with a apical septal perfusion defect (*A*). *B* is the normal myocardium. The *lower panel* displays the relative distribution of radiopharmaceutic in the myocardium graphically as a circumferential profile. The uptake of the radiopharmaceutic in the heart, even without perfusion defects, is usually not homogenous. The area in maximal count density (*small arrows*) is assigned the value of 100%. The activity within the heart is displayed as a percentage of maximal counts. The circumferential profile (*small dots, lower graph*) is displayed superimposed on a curve describing a lower limit of normal distribution. The defect is represented as the area below the lower limit of normal (*A*) and can be expressed as a defect integral relative to the total potentially visualized normal myocardium (*A* + *B*). **B.** Quantitative analysis of planar LAO ^{201}Tl exercise (*EX*) and redistribution (*R*) images using circumferential count profiles. Images in the *top panel* show a partially reversible inferoseptal defect (*arrow*). The *bottom panel* shows circumferential count distribution profiles, normalized to the area with the highest counts (i.e., inferolateral (*IL*) wall, *small arrow*). The continuous black curve indicates the lower limit (mean −2 sd) of normal radiotracer distribution. The exercise profile is below the lower limit of normal in the basal septal (*BS*), inferoseptal (*IS*), and apical (*AP*) segments in concordance with the visual impression. The redistribution profiles show significant improvement toward normal. The exercise defect is quantified as the integral below the normal curve 1.4. The remaining redistribution defect is small; 4 reversibility of the defect is 71%.

over, for most of the new ^{99m}Tc-labeled agents, myocardial clearance is slow (3, 128) and requires two separate radiotracer injections at rest and during stress. Therefore, radiopharmaceutical washout is *not* assessed using ^{99m}Tc-labeled imaging agents.

At present, quantitative measurement of stress and rest perfusion defects and of defect reversibility is the preferred approach to clinical myocardial perfusion imaging (154, 169).

Computer Processing and Analysis

Computer processing of planar and SPECT myocardial perfusion images is discussed in detail in Chapter 22. For planar myocardial perfusion imaging, circumferential count profiles with a normal reference database are widely accepted (Fig. 25.89**A** and **B**) (170). Although several different approaches and software have been published, the basic principles are the same (140, 171, 172). Figures 25.90–25.92 show representative clinical examples of quantitative planar imaging.

For SPECT myocardial perfusion imaging, two quantitative approaches have been published. The most widely used SPECT quantification software is that developed by the Cedars-Sinai/Emory group (154, 179). This software (CEQUAL) was discussed in Chapter 22. Another method, used in our laboratory, involves the generation of circumferential count distribution profiles, similar to that used for planar imaging (71, 169). Circumferential count profiles with display of the lower of the normal curve are generated for each of the short axis slices and displayed with a curve representing the lower limit of normal myocardial count

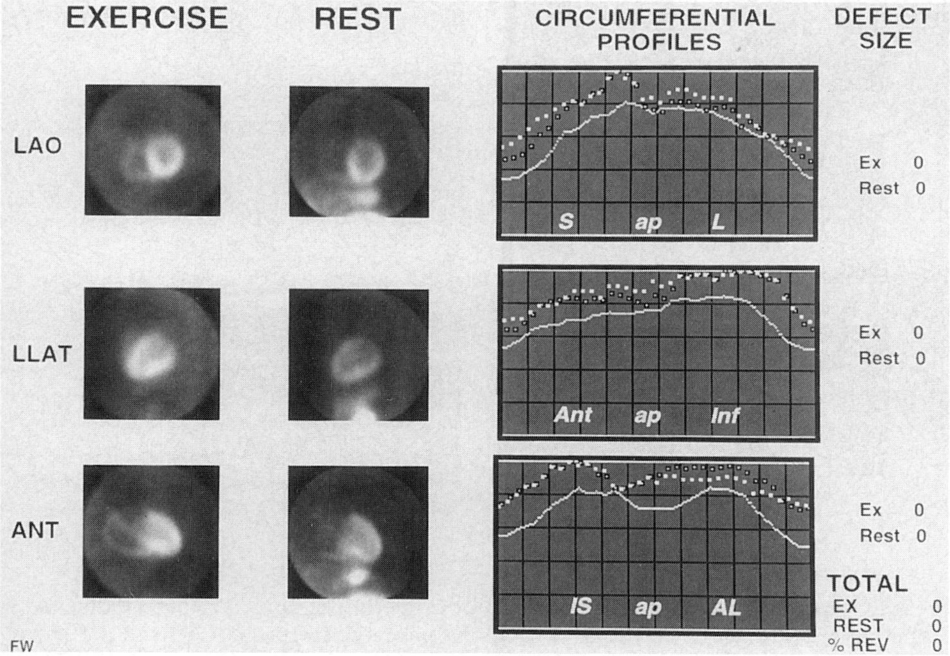

Figure 25.90. Normal planar quantitative myocardial perfusion imaging with ^{99m}Tc-sestamibi. The images on the *left* are normal: no myocardial perfusion defects on exercise or rest images. The relative distribution of counts is quantified as circumferential profiles on the *right*. The *large white dots* represent the exercise image. The *small white dots* represent the resting image. On all three views, all data points are above the lower-limit-of normal (*white line*).

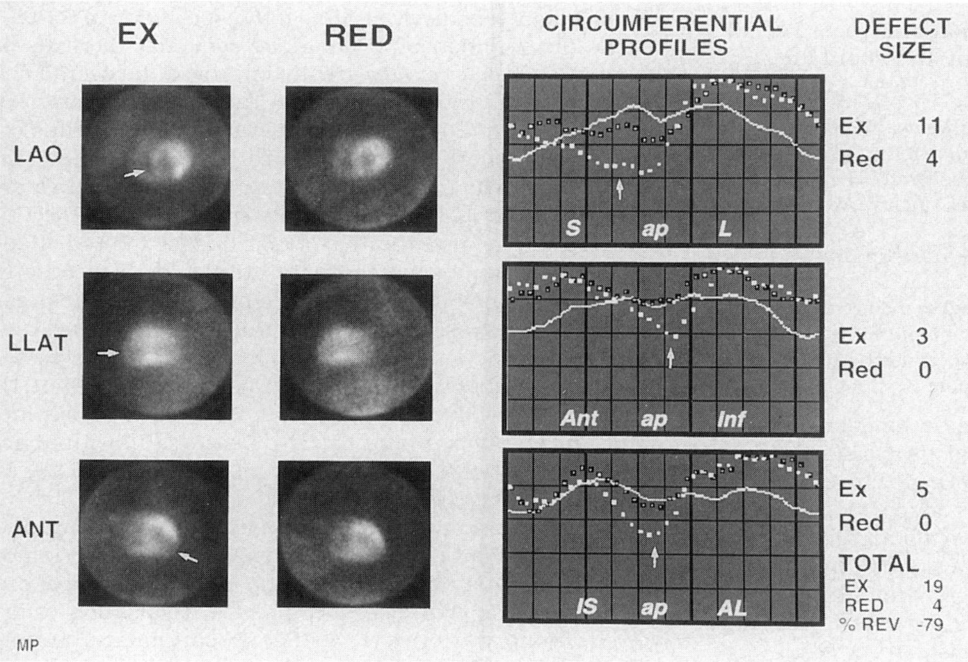

Figure 25.91. Planar quantitative myocardial perfusion imaging with ^{201}Tl in the patient with a reversible anteroseptal myocardial perfusion defect. The image on the *left* shows a myocardial perfusion defect in the inferoseptal and anteroapical and apical area (*arrows*) with substantial improvement on the redistribution images. Circumferential profiles at the *right* show the graphic display of a almost completely reversible defect. The patient is the same as in Figure 25.86B.

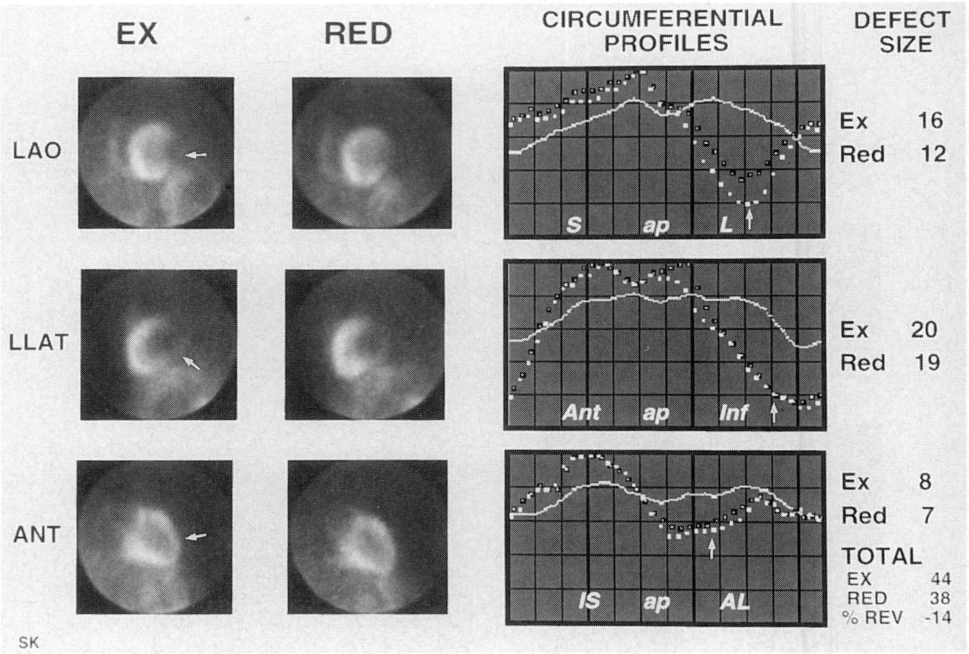

Figure 25.92. Planar quantitative myocardial perfusion imaging with ^{201}Tl in a patient with an infarction. The images of the left show a large posterolateral and inferoposterior perfusion defect (*arrow*) that is largely fixed. The graphic display of relative count distribution as circumferential profiles confirms this impression. The defect is fixed on the left lateral view, and the anterior view and shows only minimal reversibility on the LAO view.

distribution (174). This provides a readily appreciable quantitative measure of how abnormal the patient's image is compared to a normal database. Figures 25.93–25.97 show representative clinical examples of quantitative SPECT imaging.

Diagnostic Gain of Quantitative Image Analysis

We believe that reliable quantification of myocardial perfusion images is extremely important and should be used routinely for these reasons:

1. Quantification provides *greater confidence* in interpretation. Graphic display of relative count distribution serves as an objective and consistent "second observer." The normal database serves as a fixed "benchmark" against which images are compared.
2. Quantification provides *enhanced intra-* and *interobserver reproducibility* (175, 176).
3. Quantification provides a reproducible measure for the *degree of abnormality*. This is important since it is well-established that the more abnormal a myocardial perfusion image is, the poorer is the patient's outcome.

Quantitative analysis should always be *complementary* to visual analysis. Interpretation should always start with visual inspection of images, i.e., unprocessed planar images and SPECT slices. Images should be inspected for overall quality and the presence of possible artifacts. Quantitative display then serves to confirm the visual impression. Quantitative analysis should not, and cannot be expected to, provide entirely new information. We refer to this process as *"quantitative analysis with visual overread."*

DETECTION OF CORONARY ARTERY DISEASE

Since its introduction in the mid-1970s, numerous clinical studies have reported the clinical usefulness of planar ^{201}Tl stress imaging for detection of coronary artery disease in patients with chest pain syndromes (177–184). A 1981 review of the literature showed that the overall sensitivity and specificity of ^{201}Tl exercise imaging by *visual analysis* for coronary artery disease in a total of 2084 patients were 83% and 90% respectively (184). This compared favorably with that of the traditional stress ECG, which in this same review had a sensitivity of 58% and a specificity of 82%.

The introduction of *quantitative computer analysis* of planar ^{201}Tl stress images greatly improved the overall detection of coronary artery disease. Table 25.6 summarizes results of *quantitative* planar stress myocardial perfusion imaging as reported the literature (140, 184–189). The overall sensitivity to detect coronary artery disease in a total of 839 patients was 89%, with a specificity of 89%. The limited ability of quantitative planar images to predict accurately the number of coronary arteries with disease is shown in Table 25.7. Although the prediction of the presence of single-vessel disease and multivessel disease was good, the distinction between double-vessel or triple-vessel disease was suboptimal for planar imaging (140, 189–191). The predictive value of quantitative analysis of planar imaging to identify coronary artery disease in individual arteries using the schematic diagram in Figure 25.29, is shown in Table 25.8.

The limited accuracy of planar imaging to predict disease in individual coronary arteries is due to superimposition of various vascular beds on a planar projection. SPECT imaging provides more precise localization of involved coronary arteries (173, 192). In particular, the ability to predict left circumflex coronary artery disease and multivessel disease is improved using SPECT imaging (193). The overall detection of disease, however, is similar to that of planar imaging. Although sensitivity is improved, specificity and normalcy rate is lower than that of planar

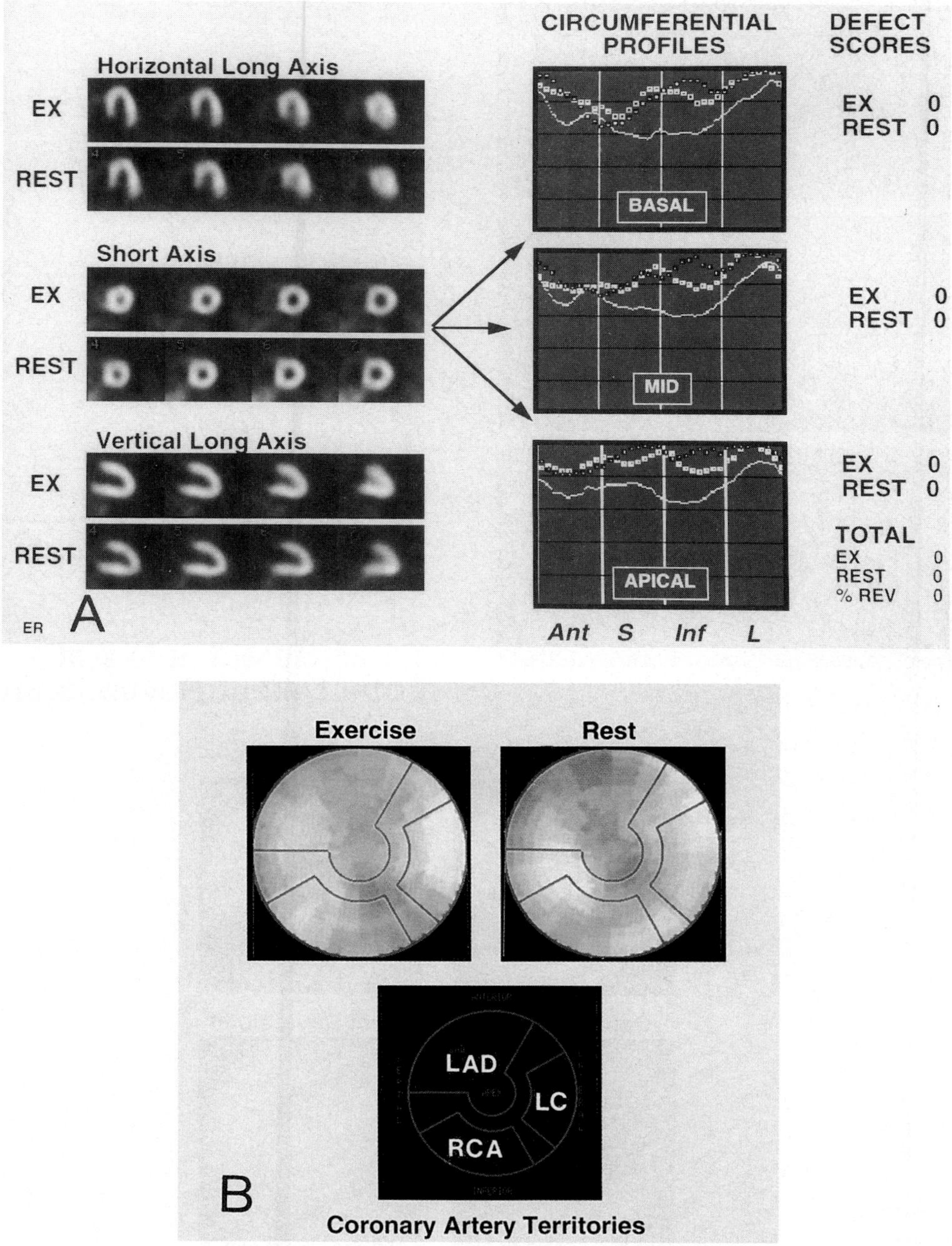

Figure 25.93. Quantitative SPECT myocardial perfusion imaging with ^{99m}Tc-sestamibi in a normal subject. **A.** The images (*left*) are normal. All short axis slices are quantified using circumferential profile analysis. Quantification of three representative apical, midventricular, and basal slices is shown (*right*). The exercise profile (*large white dots*) and rest profile (*small dots*) are displayed normalized to the area with maximal activity and compared to lower limit of normal distribution (*white curve*). In this example of a normal subject, all data points are above the lower limit of normal. Defect scores are tabulated at the far right. **B.** Bull's-eye or polar map display of normal SPECT images in A. The coronary artery territories are shown.

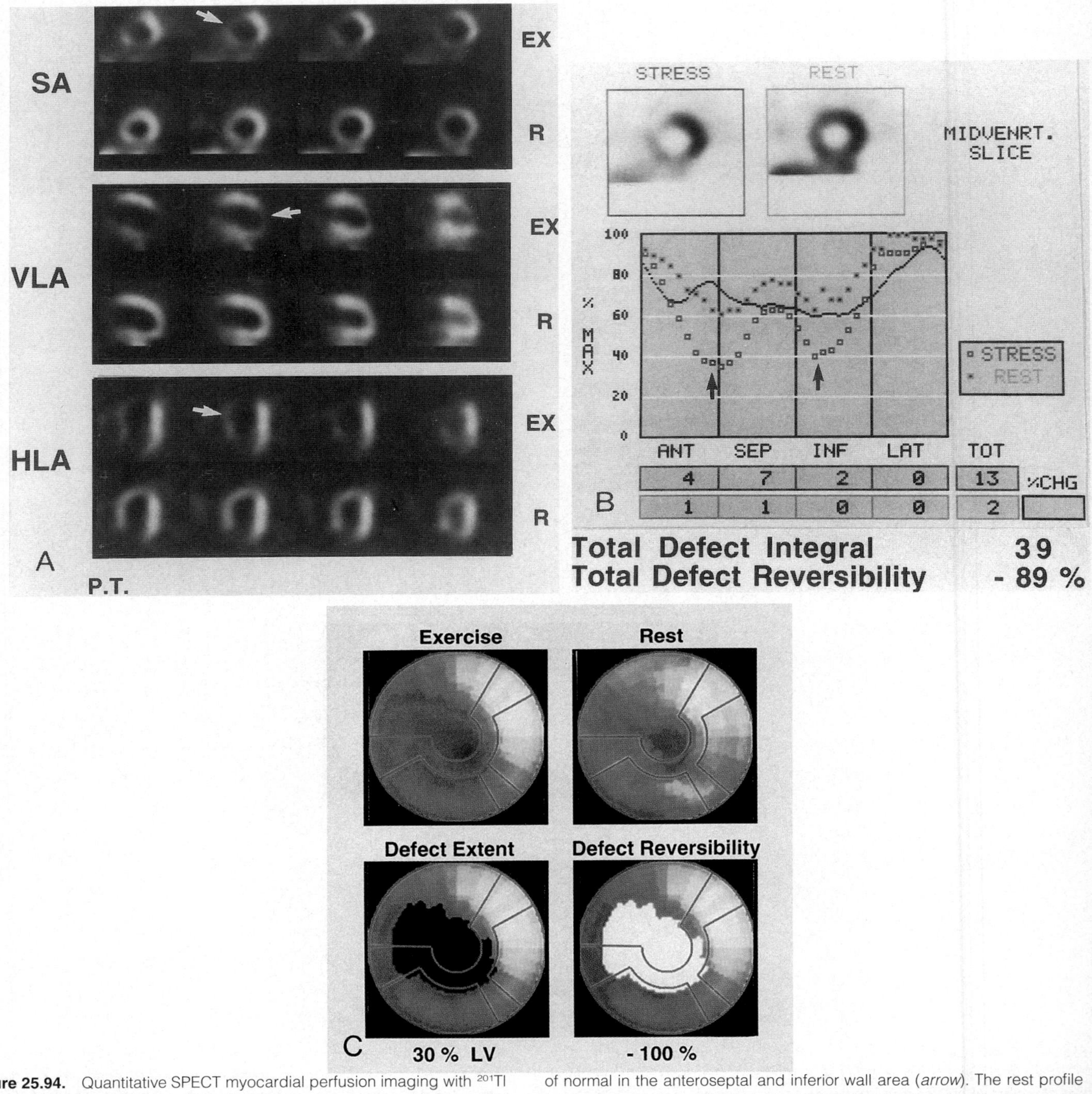

Figure 25.94. Quantitative SPECT myocardial perfusion imaging with ^{201}Tl in a patient with extensive exercise-induced anteroseptal and inferoseptal ischemia. **A.** The images (*left*) show an almost completely reversible anteroseptal and inferoseptal defect (*arrows*). **B.** Quantification of a representative midventricular short axis slice using circumferential profiles confirms the visual impression. The exercise circumferential profile is below the lower limit of normal in the anteroseptal and inferior wall area (*arrow*). The rest profile is near normal. Quantification of all short axis slices revealed a large exercise-induced total defect (total integral: 39) with near complete (89%) defect reversibility. **C.** Quantification using the CEQUAL polar map display. Using this method, total exercise defect size is 30% of left ventricle with complete defect reversibility.

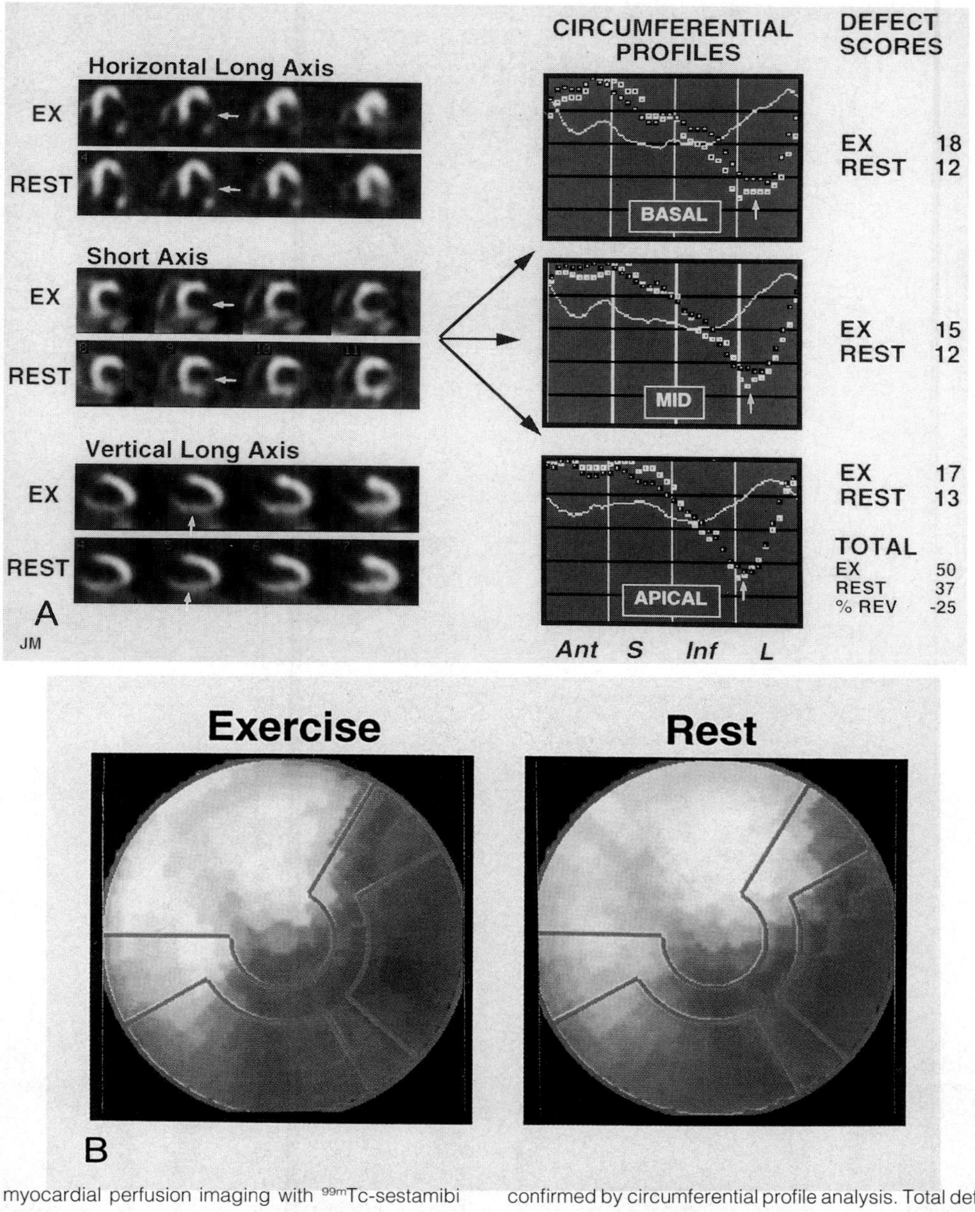

Figure 25.95. SPECT myocardial perfusion imaging with ^{99m}Tc-sestamibi in patient with inferior infarction. **A.** Exercise (*EX*) and rest images (*left*) show a fixed inferolateral (*arrows*) myocardial perfusion defect is present. This is confirmed by circumferential profile analysis. Total defect score is large (total integral: 50). There is some (25%) reversibility in the basal slices. **B.** Polar map display of images in A. The defect is in shades of *blue*.

Figure 25.96. Quantitative SPECT myocardial perfusion imaging with ^{99m}Tc-sestamibi in a patient with large anterior infarction. The images (*left*) show an extensive fixed anteroseptal myocardial perfusion defect (*arrows*). This is confirmed by circumferential profile analysis (*right*). Total defect score is large (total integral: 48) without reversibility.

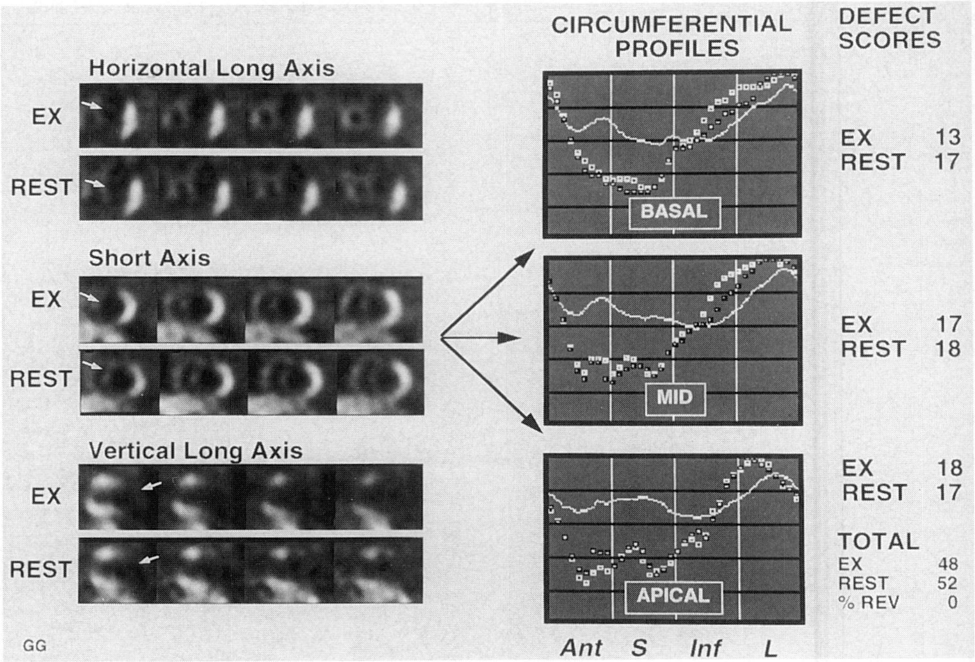

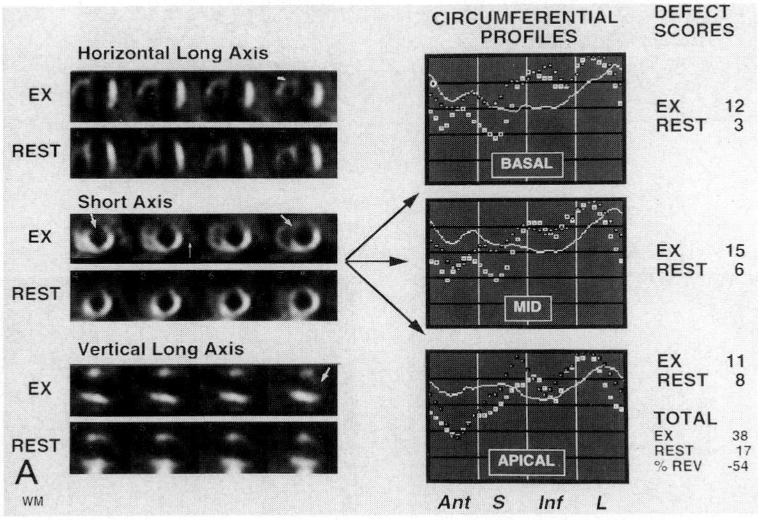

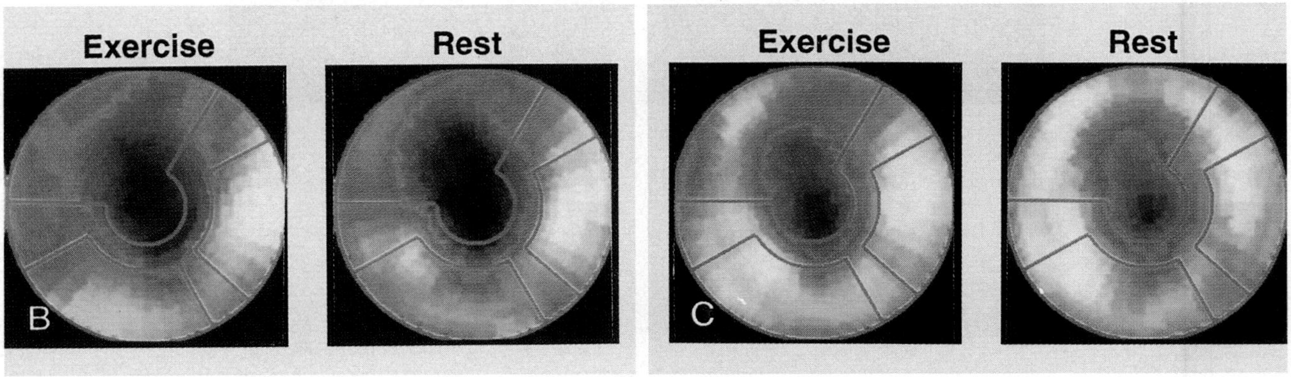

Figure 25.97. High-risk quantitative SPECT myocardial perfusion imaging with ^{99m}Tc-sestamibi. **A.** The images (*left*) show postexercise dilatation on short axis slices and increased lung uptake (*small arrow*). There is a partially reversible (basal and midventricular) anteroseptal myocardial perfusion defect (*arrow*). This is confirmed by quantitative circumferential profile analysis. The defect is large (total integral: 38), with 54% defect reversibility. ECG-gated images of this patient are shown in Figure 25.49D. **B.** Polar map display of images in A. The defect is in shades of *blue* and *red*. **C.** Polar map of the same patient after coronary bypass surgery. Note improvement of exercise defect, although some ischemia is still present in the anterior wall.

Table 25.6.
Sensitivity and Specificity to Detect Coronary Using Quantitative Planar Imaging

Author	Year	# Pts	Sens (%)	Spec (%)
Berger[185]	1981	140	91	90
Maddahi[184]	1981	67	93	91
Wackers[140]	1985	150	89	95
Kaul[186]	1986	325	90	80
Van Train[187]	1986	157	84	88
Total		839	89.4	88.8

Table 25.7.
Prediction of Number of Diseased Coronary Arteries by Quantitative Analysis of ^{201}Tl Stress Images (N = 131)[a]

Angiographic Coronary Artery Disease (*n*)[b]	Predictive Value (Positive)	Sensitivity
One vessel (65)	47/68 (69%)	47/65 (72%)
Two vessels (32)	9/26 (34%)	9/32 (28%)
Three vessels (20)	6/23 (26%)	6/20 (30%)
Multivessel (52)	31/49 (63%)	31/52 (60%)

[a]From Wackers FJTh, Fetterman RC, Mattera JA, Clements JP. Quantitative planar thallium-201 stress scintigraphy: a critical evaluation of the method. Semin Nucl Med. 1985; 15:46.

[b]Fourteen patients with false-negative studies were excluded.

Table 25.8.
Sensitivity, Specificity, and Predictive Value (Positive) of Quantitative Analysis in Patients with Single-Vessel Coronary Artery Disease (N = 77)[a]

Angiographic Coronary Artery Disease (*n*)[b]		Sensitivity	Specificity	Predictive Value
LAD	(41)	36/41 (99%)	28/36 (78%)	36/44 (82%)
RCA	(22)	15/22 (68%)	45/55 (82%)	15/25 (60%)
LCx	(14)	8/14 (57%)	49/63 (78%)	8/22 (36%)
RCA or LCx	(36)	28/36 (78%)	31/41 (76%)	28/38 (74%)

[a]From Wackers RJTh, Fetterman RC, Mattera JA, Clements JP. Quantitative planar thallium-201 stress scintigraphy: a critical evaluation of the method. Semin Nucl Med. 1985; 15:46.

[b]*AD* = left anterior descending artery, *LCx* = left circumflex artery, *RCA* = coronary artery.

imaging. Table 25.9 summarizes the results of ^{201}Tl SPECT stress myocardial perfusion imaging for detection of coronary artery disease as reported the literature (192–200). Overall, the sensitivity to detect coronary artery disease in a total of 1901 patients was 91%, with a specificity of 73%.

The relatively low specificity of SPECT imaging indicates that artifacts due to attenuation and motion are not always recognized. "*Referral bias*" has been proposed as another potential explanation for the limited specificity of SPECT imaging (201). With the increasing clinical acceptance of stress myocardial perfusion imaging in patients suspected of having coronary artery disease, patients with abnormal myocardial perfusion studies are preferentially referred for cardiac catheterization, whereas patients with normal myocardial perfusion images are generally not referred.

Table 25.9.
Sensitivity and Specificity to Detect Coronary Artery Disease Using SPECT Imaging

Author	Year	# Pts	Sens (%)	Spec (%)
Tamaki[197]	1984	104	91	92
DePasquale[193]	1988	210	95	71
Borges-Neto[200]	1988	100	92	69
Maddahi[192]	1989	110	96	56
Fintel[194]	1989	112	91	90
Iskandrian[198]	1989	461	88	60
Go[196]	1990	202	76	80
Mahmarian[195]	1990	360	93	87
Van Train[199]	1990	242	95	56
Total		1901	91	73

This practice limits angiographic confirmation of true negative patients. Patients with angiographic normal coronary arteries are likely to be referred because of abnormal perfusion (false-positive) images. To circumvent this problem, it is preferred to assess the "normalcy rate" of myocardial perfusion imaging in normal subjects as a surrogate for specificity.

^{99m}Tc-Labeled Myocardial Perfusion Agents

In recent trials, the new ^{99m}Tc imaging agents have been compared to ^{201}Tl as the gold standard. Only in limited subgroups of patients was the concordance with coronary angiography evaluated as well. For both planar and SPECT imaging, the reported average sensitivity and specificity of ^{99m}Tc-sestamibi (3, 4, 202–204), ^{99m}Tc-teboroxime (5, 6, 205, 206), ^{99m}Tc-tetrofosmin (207–209), and ^{99m}Tc-furifosmin (210) were similar to those obtained with ^{201}Tl.

An important advantage of the ^{99m}Tc-labeled agents is that, with the exception of ^{99m}Tc-teboroxime, SPECT imaging is of consistently better quality compared to ^{201}Tl SPECT imaging.

HIGH-RISK CORONARY ARTERY DISEASE

The more severe the patient's coronary artery disease, the more likely it is that abnormalities are present on stress myocardial perfusion imaging. For this reason it is important that myocardial perfusion abnormalities are quantified. Most patients (approximately 95%) with left main coronary artery disease have abnormal stress myocardial perfusion images. However, the expected typical left main pattern—defects in the distribution of the LAD and LCx, that is, anteroseptal and posterolateral myocardial perfusion defects—is found in only a minority (approximately 14%) of patients with left main disease (188–191). The majority (approximately 75%) of these patients have multiple defects and frequently increased ^{201}Tl lung uptake (Figs. 25.97–25.99).

Although almost all patients with triple-vessel disease have abnormal stress myocardial perfusion images, only approximately 60% have multiple defects in two or more vascular regions. Frequently, disease in the LCx is not detected, particularly when using planar ^{201}Tl imaging.

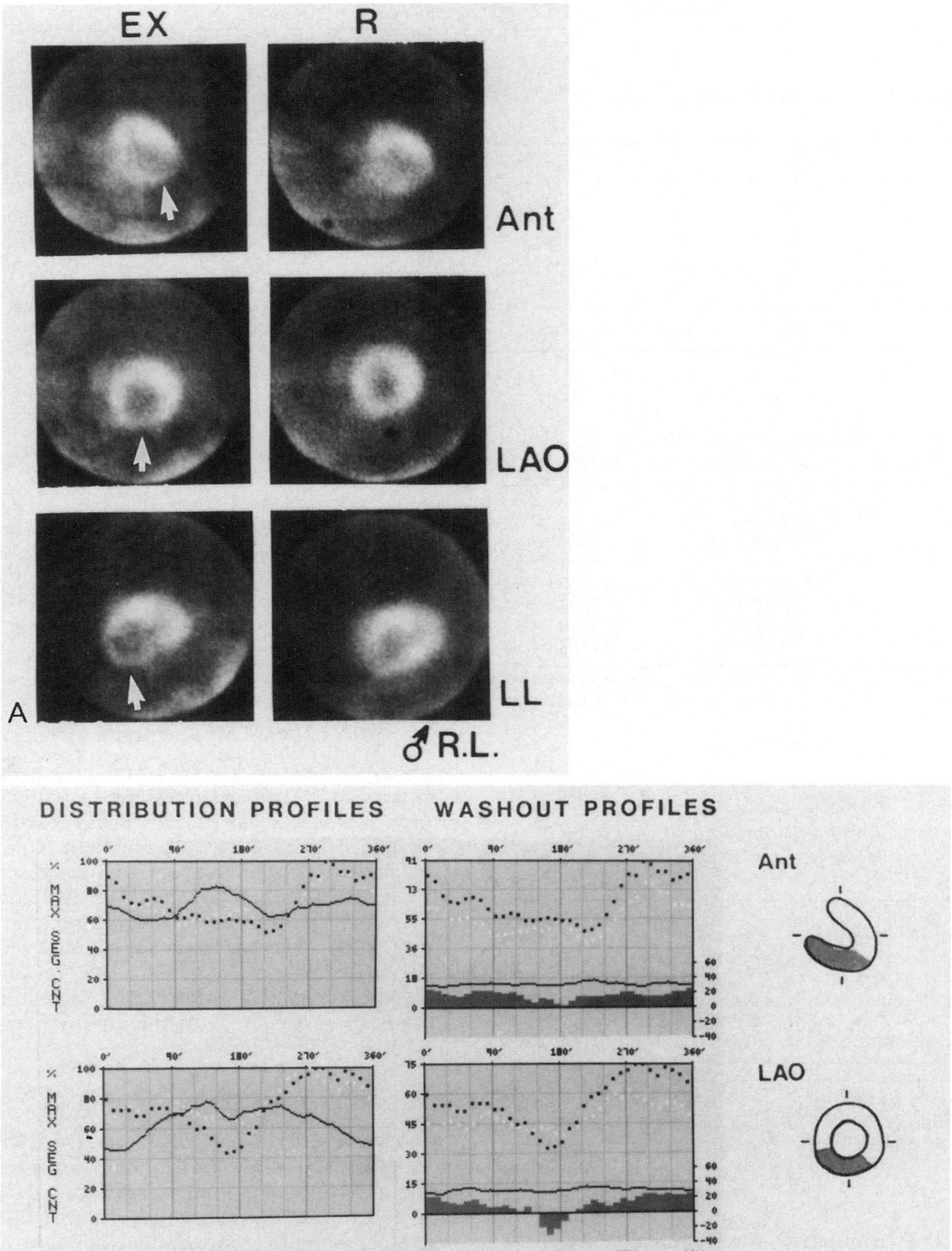

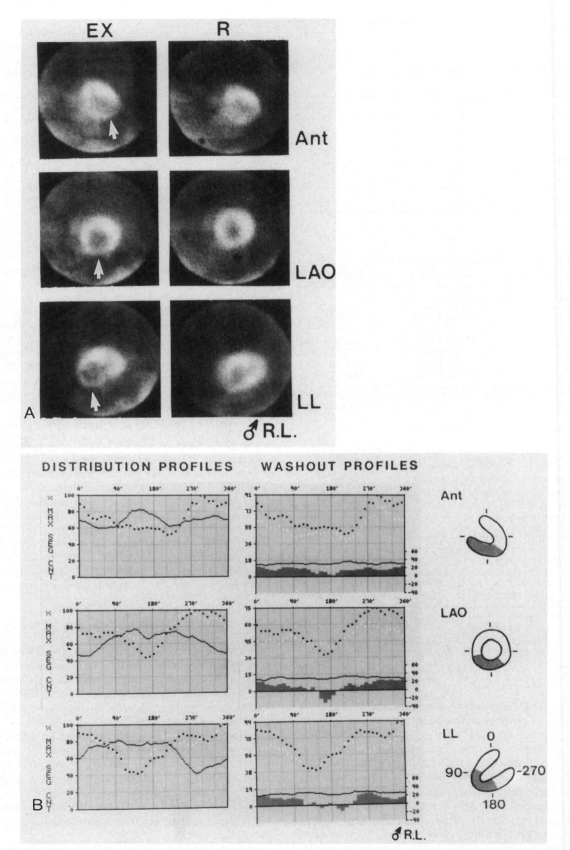

Figure 25.98. Prevalence of high-risk images with significant stenosis. Prevalence of high-risk ^{201}Tl stress images in 43 patients with significant (50%) stenosis of left main coronary artery. *LMCA* = left main coronary artery disease pattern (defect of mid- and upper septum and mid- and upper posterolateral walls); *MVD* = multivessel disease pattern (defects in two or more different vascular areas); ↑ *LU* = increased lung ^{201}Tl uptake. (Reproduced by permission from Nygaard TW, Gibson RS, Ryan JM, Gascho JA, Watson DD, Beller GA. Prevalence of high-risk thallium-201 scintigraphic findings in left main coronary artery stenosis: comparison with patients with multiple- and single-vessel coronary artery disease. Am J Cardiol 1984;53:462.)

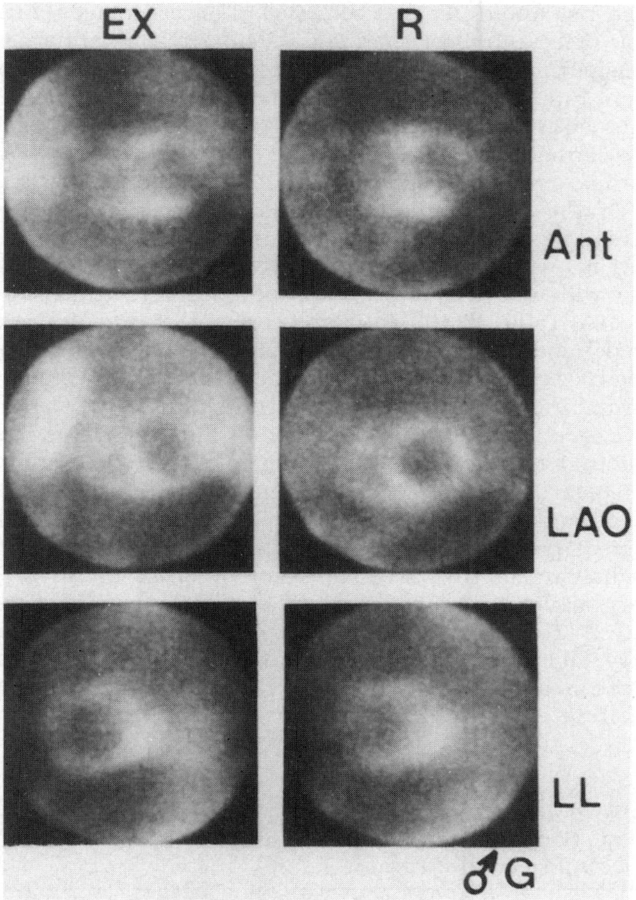

Figure 25.99. Typical example of high-risk planar ^{201}Tl stress images. On the postexercise planar images (*EX*), increased lung uptake of radiotracer can be noted on all three views, particularly on the left anterior oblique (*LAO*) view, which was the first view acquired after discontinuation of exercise. Furthermore, the heart is enlarged and shows a large anteroseptal myocardial perfusion defect. Additionally, there is an abnormal area in the inferolateral wall. The patient had severe triple-vessel coronary artery disease on coronary angiography. The images indicate multiple areas of exercise-induced myocardial ischemia and evidence of exercise-induced left ventricular dysfunction. *Ant* = anterior, *LL* = left lateral.

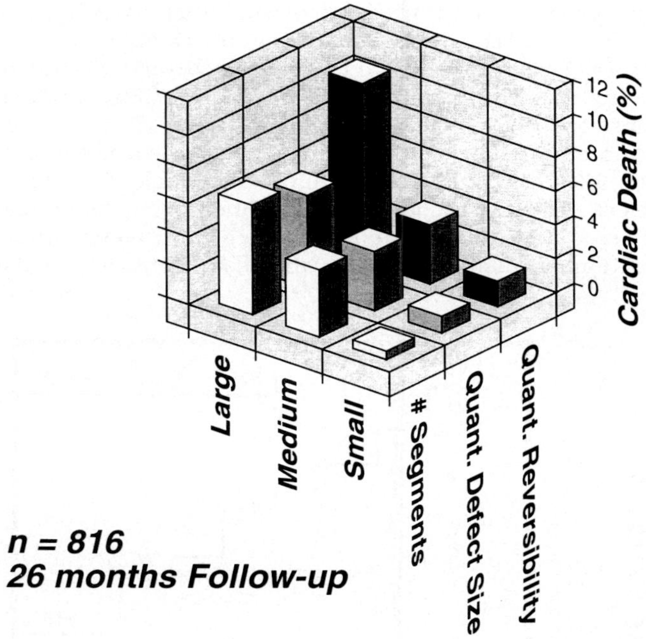

Figure 25.100. Prognostic importance of size and type in of myocardial perfusion abnormality. Data are from 816 patients with stable coronary artery disease enrolled in the Multicenter Study on Silent Myocardial Ischemia (MSSMI). The patients had 26 months follow-up. All patients had quantitative planar ^{201}Tl stress imaging. The graph relates the size of exercise defects, defect reversibility, and number of abnormal segments to cardiac death rate during follow-up. The highest cardiac death rate occurred in patients with the most abnormal images. In particular, patients with greatest defect reversibility had the highest cardiac death rate.

High-risk stress myocardial perfusion images (Figs. 25.97 and 25.99) can be characterized as follows:

1. Multiple defects in two or more coronary artery territories (112);
2. Increased pulmonary ^{201}Tl uptake after exercise (211, 212); and
3. Significant transient dilatation of the left ventricle immediately after exercise (159).

This high-risk pattern on either planar or SPECT imaging is highly specific (approximately 95%) for multivessel coronary disease; however, the sensitivity is only about 70%. Therefore, the absence of the foregoing scintigraphic characteristics should not be used to rule out the presence of high-risk disease.

The pattern of increased ^{201}Tl lung uptake indicates stress-induced left ventricular dysfunction and is associated with severe coronary artery disease. This pattern has been shown to be a very potent prediction of adverse outcome (213). Although there is some controversy among investigators, it is generally believed that by using ^{99m}Tc-labeled agents this important image pattern does not occur (214). However, we have occasionally observed increased lung uptake in patients with severe ischemia using ^{99m}Tc-sestamibi SPECT (Fig. 25.100). With the present tendency to image early after exercise, this pattern may be observed more frequently in the future. On the other hand, ^{99m}Tc-labeled agents can be used for first-pass radionuclide angiocardiography at rest and exercise, and thus provide direct measure of ventricular function (Fig. 25.52) (see Chapter 24).

STRESS MYOCARDIAL PERFUSION IMAGING AND PROGNOSIS

An extensive literature documents the important functional and prognostic information provided by stress myocardial perfusion imaging.

The literature of the 1980s was almost exclusively based upon planar ^{201}Tl imaging. Only in the early 1990s, did similar data obtained with SPECT imaging (using both ^{201}Tl and ^{99m}Tc-sestamibi) start appearing in the literature.

In patients without prior myocardial infarction, Brown, et al. (215), demonstrated that the number of reversible ^{201}Tl defects was the most important statistically significant predictor of future cardiac events. Similarly, Ladenheim, et al. (216), demonstrated that the extent and severity of ^{201}Tl defects correlated with the occurrence of cardiac events. We have confirmed these findings (Fig. 25.100). Gibson, et al. (112), evaluated quantitative ^{201}Tl stress imaging in patients after uncomplicated myocardial infarction (Fig. 25.65). Patients with a fixed, single ^{201}Tl stress defect without washout abnormalities at hospital discharge had a 6% cardiac event rate (death, recurrent infarction, or unstable angina), whereas patients who had a high-risk finding on predischarge ^{201}Tl stress images (multiple defects in more than one vascular region, abnormal washout, or increased lung uptake) had a 51% cardiac event rate. Several investigators have reported similar results on the prognostic value of ^{201}Tl stress imaging after myocardial infarction (218–220) and in patients with chronic coronary artery disease (221–226) (Fig. 25.101).

On the other hand, the presence of *normal* stress myocardial perfusion images by quantitative analysis, even in patients with known coronary artery disease, was associated with an extremely favorable prognosis (227–232) (Fig. 25.102; Table 25.10). The (rare) coronary events occurred predominantly in patients with a high likelihood of, or known, coronary artery disease (227–232). Interestingly, cardiac events occurred particularly in patients with a positive exercise electrocardiogram (232), and in patients who had undergone prior coronary angioplasty (233).

These data on abnormal and normal test results indicate that the extent of myocardial perfusion defects, or lack thereof, provides significant functional and prognostic information that surpasses anatomic information of coronary angiograms. Haronian, et al. (234), demonstrated with ^{99m}Tc-sestamibi imaging during PTCA that the coronary angiogram is of limited value in predicting the extent of the area at risk for a given coronary artery stenosis (Fig. 25.103).

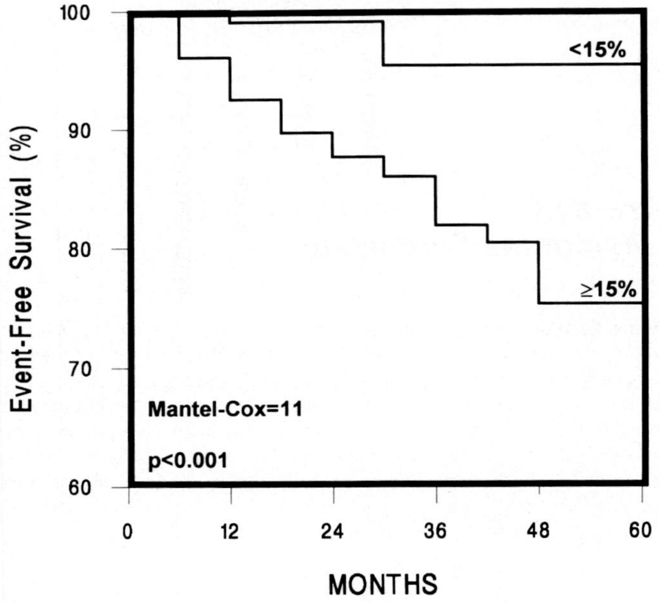

Figure 25.101. Actuarial event-free survival curves in patients with coronary artery disease. Patients were stratified according to size of exercise-induced myocardial perfusion defect on ^{201}Tl SPECT imaging. Patients with large perfusion defects (15% of left ventricle) had significantly poorer outcome than patients with smaller defects. (Reproduced by permission from Iskandrian AS, Chae SC, Heo J, Stanberry CD, Wasserleben V, Cave V. Independent and incremental prognostic value of exercise single-photon emission computed tomographic (SPECT) thallium imaging in coronary artery disease. J Am Coll Cardiol 1993;22:665–670.)

Table 25.10.
Yearly Cardiac Event Rate in Patients with Normal Myocardial Perfusion Images

	n:	Cardiac Death	Nonfatal MI
^{201}Tl			
Pamelia[228]	349	0.5%	0.6%
Wackers[227]	95	0%	1.0%
Wahl[229]	455	0.2%	0.6%
Staniloff[230]	372	0%	0.5%
Sestamibi			
Brown[231]	234	0%	0.5%
Raiker[232]	208	0%	0.5%

Figure 25.102. Distribution of pretest likelihood of coronary artery disease in 208 normal patients with quantitatively normal ^{99m}Tc-sestamibi exercise images. Occurrence of cardiac events during follow-up is indicated by *MI* (myocardial infarction). Reproduced by permission from Raiker K, Sinusas AJ, Zaret BL, Wackers FJTh. One-year prognosis of patients with normal Tc-99m-sestamibi stress imaging. Circulation 1993;88(Suppl):1486.)

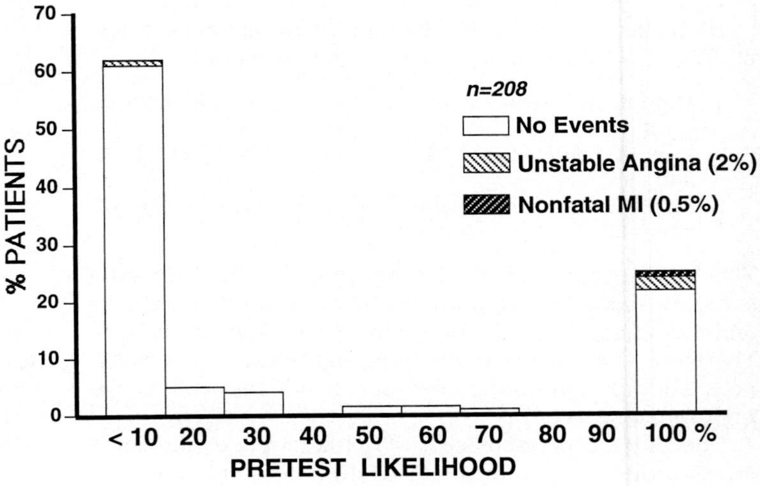

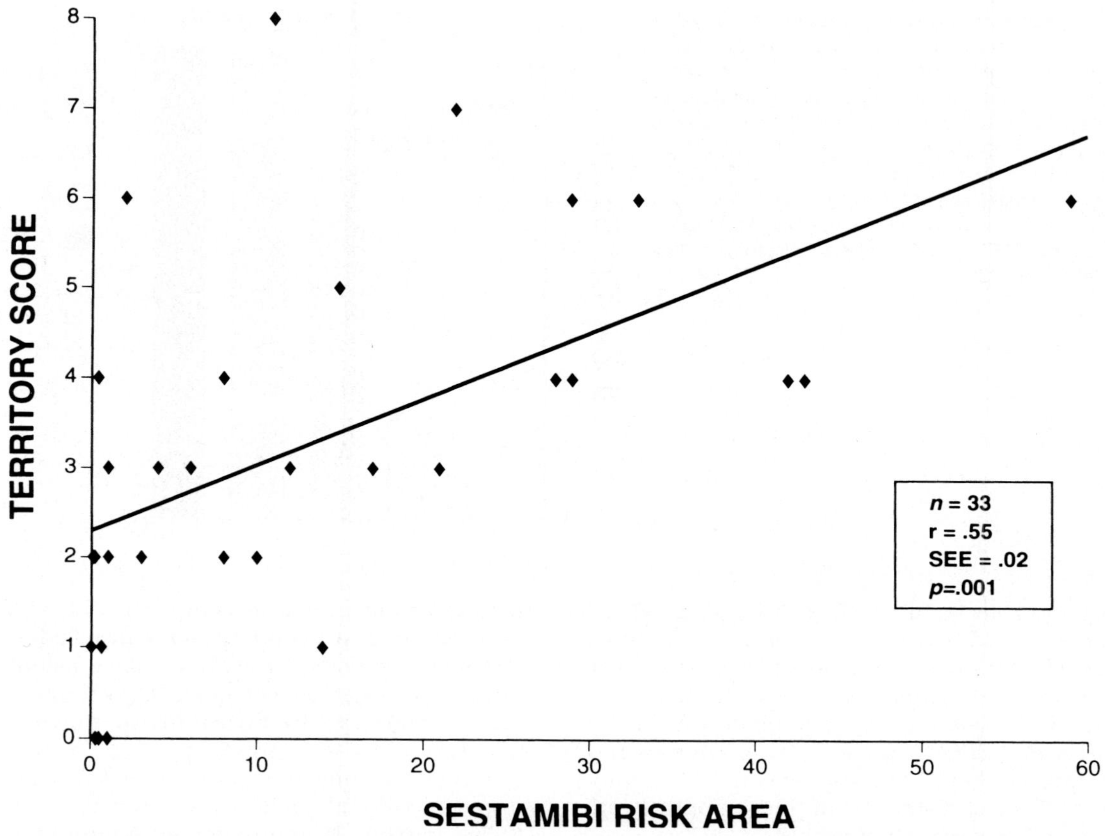

Figure 25.103. Correlation between ^{99m}Tc-sestamibi risk area and myocardial territory angiographic risk area. Note, again, a wide range of ^{99m}Tc-sestamibi defect sizes for similar angiographic scores. (Reproduced by permission from Haronian HL, Remetz MS, Sinusas AJ, et al. Myocardial risk area defined by technetium-99m sestamibi imaging during percutaneous transluminal coronary angioplasty: comparison with coronary angiography. J Am Coll Cardiol 1993;22:1033–1043.)

INDEPENDENT AND INCREMENTAL PROGNOSTIC VALUE OF STRESS MYOCARDIAL PERFUSION IMAGING

In clinical practice, a diagnostic test is not used in isolation. Other clinical and diagnostic data are usually available. The prognostic value of myocardial perfusion imaging, as demonstrated earlier, is important and supports the validity and accuracy of the test. However, if similar information can be derived from other less costly and readily available tests, it may not be cost effective to perform radionuclide myocardial perfusion imaging. Pollock, et al. (235), and Melin, et al. (236), assessed the incremental prognostic value of data obtained in succession (clinical, exercise ECG, planar ^{201}Tl stress imaging, and coronary angiography) in patients with suspected coronary artery disease. The combination of clinical and exercise ^{201}Tl variables provided greater prognostic information than the combination of clinical and angiographic data. Iskandrian, et al. (237), observed similar independent and incremental prognostic information using SPECT ^{201}Tl imaging, even when catheterization data are available. The extent of the perfusion abnormality on quantitative SPECT was the single most important prognostic predictor (Fig. 25.104). Petretta, et al. (238), and others (224) noted that the exercise ECG should be taken into consideration, when the exercise ECG is negative, the additive prognostic value of ^{201}Tl imaging is less than when the ECG is abnormal or nondiagnostic.

Although most of the published data were obtained using ^{201}Tl imaging, similar data are emerging for ^{99m}Tc-sestamibi (239).

STRESS MYOCARDIAL PERFUSION IMAGING BEFORE AND AFTER REVASCULARIZATION

In most instances, markedly abnormal stress myocardial perfusion images will lead to revascularization by either coronary bypass surgery (CABG) or percutaneous transluminal coronary angioplasty (PTCA). Myocardial perfusion imaging is not routinely performed after CABG and is only indicated when symptoms reoccur. Since many patients have abnormal ST-T segments on the electrocardiogram after CABG, these patients are better evaluated by myocardial perfusion imaging than by electrocardiographic treadmill testing.

Stress myocardial perfusion imaging is considered particularly useful after PTCA, since often only the culprit lesion is dilated. Optimal timing of imaging after PTCA is controversial. Although some investigators (240) have reported a high incidence of false-positive perfusion abnormalities early after PTCA, this is not a general experience.

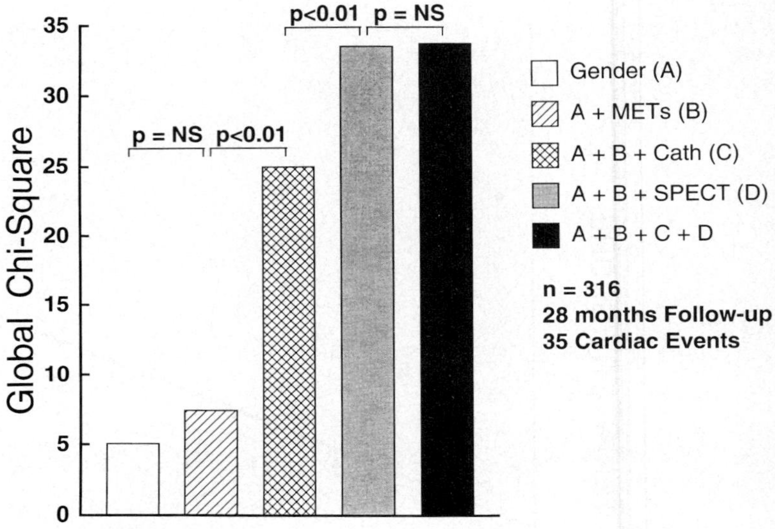

Figure 25.104. Independent and incremental prognostic power of clinical, exercise, catheterization, and quantitative ^{201}Tl SPECT variables. Data shown represent the global χ-square statistics of various clinical and diagnostic variables. SPECT imaging provides independent and incremental information to identify high risk patients. Note that angiography (*Cath*) has less incremental value than SPECT. (Reproduced by permission from Iskandrian AS, Chae SC, Heo J, Stanberry CD, Wasserleben V, Cave V. Independent and incremental prognostic value of exercise single-photon emission computed tomographic (SPECT) thallium imaging in coronary artery disease. J Am Coll Cardiol 1993;22:665–670.)

At approximately 4 weeks after PTCA, a close correlation has been demonstrated between stress-induced perfusion abnormalities and the presence or absence of restenosis, independent of clinical symptoms (241–243). SPECT imaging is particularly useful in these patients with known coronary anatomy. SPECT allows a determination of whether clinical ischemia is likely to be caused by saphenous vein graft closure, restenosis of the angioplasty site, or progression of disease in other vessels.

PHARMACOLOGIC STRESS AND MYOCARDIAL PERFUSION IMAGING

A considerable number (30–50%) of patients referred for stress testing are unable to perform adequate exercise on a motor-driven treadmill. This is particularly the case in patients with neurologic or orthopedic problems, patients with claudication because of severe peripheral vessel disease, patients with severe lung disease, or patients on β-blockers. In these patients, several alternative methods to evaluate the presence of significant coronary artery disease are available—vasodilatation with dipyridamole or adenosine, or β-adrenergic stress with dobutamine.

PHARMACOLOGIC VASODILATATION

Intravenous infusion of dipyridamole or adenosine is a practical and clinically proven useful alternative to physical exercise for provoking myocardial perfusion abnormalities (244–247). Adenosine is a direct potent dilator of the coronary resistance vasculature, and markedly increases coronary blood flow (248, 249). Dipyridamole achieves the same result in an indirect way: dipyridamole inhibits reabsorption of adenosine back into the myocytes, thus increasing blood and tissue adenosine level (Fig. 25.105) Adenosine is activated at adenosine receptor sites. These receptors can be blocked with aminophylline or xanthine derivatives.

Infusion of dipyridamole or adenosine results in a three- to fourfold increase of coronary artery blood flow. However, no such increase occurs in zones supplied by coronary arteries with hemodynamically significant stenosis. This produces *inhomogeneity of regional myocardial blood flow* that can be visualized by myocardial perfusion imaging (Fig. 25.71).

Extensive clinical experience exists with dipyridamole infusion. Dipyridamole is infused over a 4-minute period (0.568 mg/kg). At approximately 4 minutes after the completion of infusion, maximal coronary dilatory effect is achieved. This usually is associated with a modest (~10 bpm) increase in heart rate and approximately 10 mmHg decrease in systolic blood pressure. At this time of maximal vasodilatory effect, a myocardial perfusion imaging agent is injected intravenously. In many centers, dipyridamole infusion is combined, if at all feasible, with simultaneous low level treadmill exercise. Even minimal exercise decreases the incidence of subjective side effects, and decreases subdiaphragmatic tracer uptake, which can be a considerable problem with ^{99m}Tc-labeled agents.

The adenosine infusion protocol is as follows: Adenosine is infused intravenously starting with a dose of 50 μg/kg/min. The dose is increased every 3 minutes, if tolerated, to a maximal dose of 140 μg/kg/min. The radiopharmaceutical is injected at maximal dose and its infusion continued for 2–3 minutes. Myocardial perfusion imaging is performed as described earlier.

Using ^{99m}Tc-labeled agents, SPECT imaging is preferred after pharmacologic stress. On planar images, superimposition of intense subdiaphragmatic activity on the left ventricular inferior wall may degrade the quality of images substantially.

In patients with significant coronary artery disease, transient myocardial perfusion defects can be observed after pharmacologic vasodilation (Figs. 25.106 and 25.107**A** and **B**). During the infusion of vasodilators, most patients with abnormal myocardial perfusion images do have *heterogeneity of blood flow but no true myocardial ischemia.* Only occasional patients may clinically manifest ischemia with angina and ECG changes. The underlying pathophys-

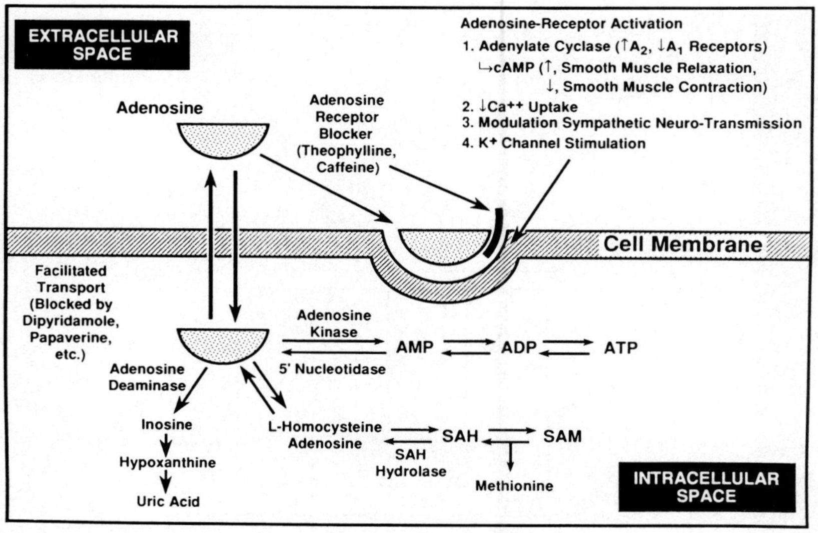

Figure 25.105. Mechanism of adenosine pharmacologic vasodilation. Adenosine is synthesized intracellularly from ATP or S-adenosyl homocysteine (SAM). Adenosine leaves the cell to act on surface membrane receptors, and then reenters the cell to be metabolized to ATP, S-adenosyl homocysteine, or uric acid. Theophylline and caffeine are competitive blockers at the receptor sites. *AMP* = Adenosine monophosphate; *SAH* = S-adenosyl-L-homocysteine. (Reproduced by permission from Verani MS. Adenosine thallium-201 myocardial perfusion scintigraphy. Am Heart J 1991;122:269–278.)

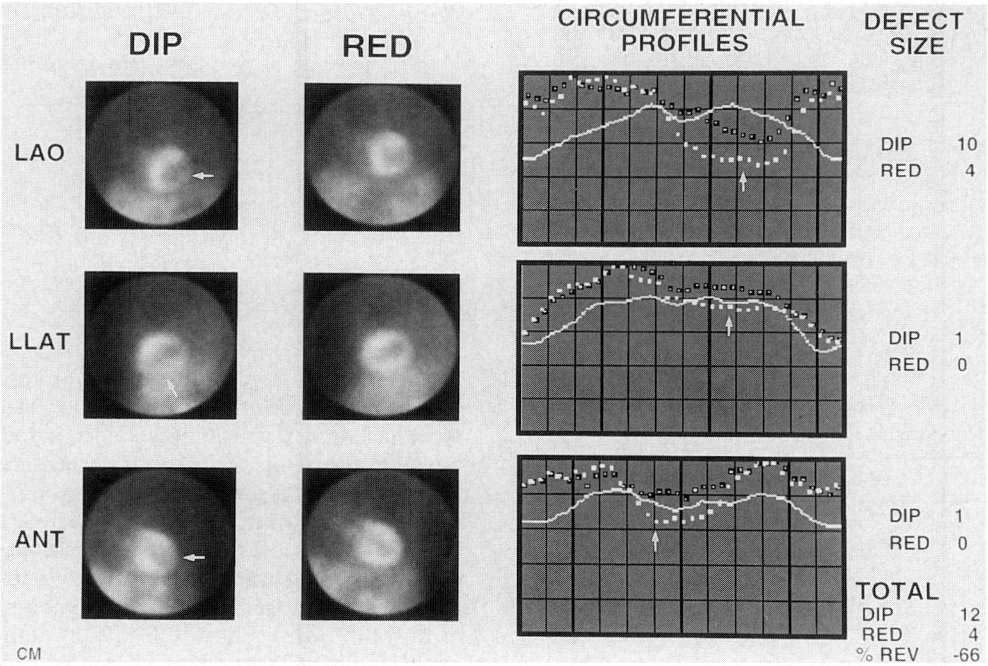

Figure 25.106. Planar dipyridamole ^{201}Tl imaging. Quantitative planar ^{201}Tl dipyridamole imaging in patient with chest pain and nondiagnostic treadmill test due to orthopedic problem. Note the substantial uptake in the region of the liver, which is typical for dipyridamole imaging. The images show a relative large reversible inferolateral myocardial perfusion defect (*arrow*). This is confirmed by quantitative circumferential profile analysis. Total defect integral is 12 with 66% defect reversibility.

iology of vasodilation-induced ischemia is "coronary steal." In this situation, the markedly increased coronary blood flow in the normal myocardial zones steals blood, via collaterals, away from the vascular bed supplied by a critical stenosis (245, 250). This undesirable effect of dipyridamole can be reversed relatively quickly by intravenous administration of aminophylline (249). Because of the short half-life of adenosine, termination of adenosine infusion is usually sufficient to relieve symptoms. Adenosine causes significantly more side effects than dipyridamole (251, 252). The most worrisome side effect of adenosine is that of high degree A-V block. However, this will revert quickly by discontinuing the infusion. The half-life of dipyridamole is considerably longer (20–45 minutes) and aminophylline is frequently needed to control side effects.

Myocardial perfusion imaging after dipyridamole vasodilatation with either ^{201}Tl or ^{99m}Tc-sestamibi has been reported to yield a sensitivity and specificity for the detection of coronary artery disease similar to that of exercise imaging (246, 247, 253, 254). Table 25.11 summarizes re-

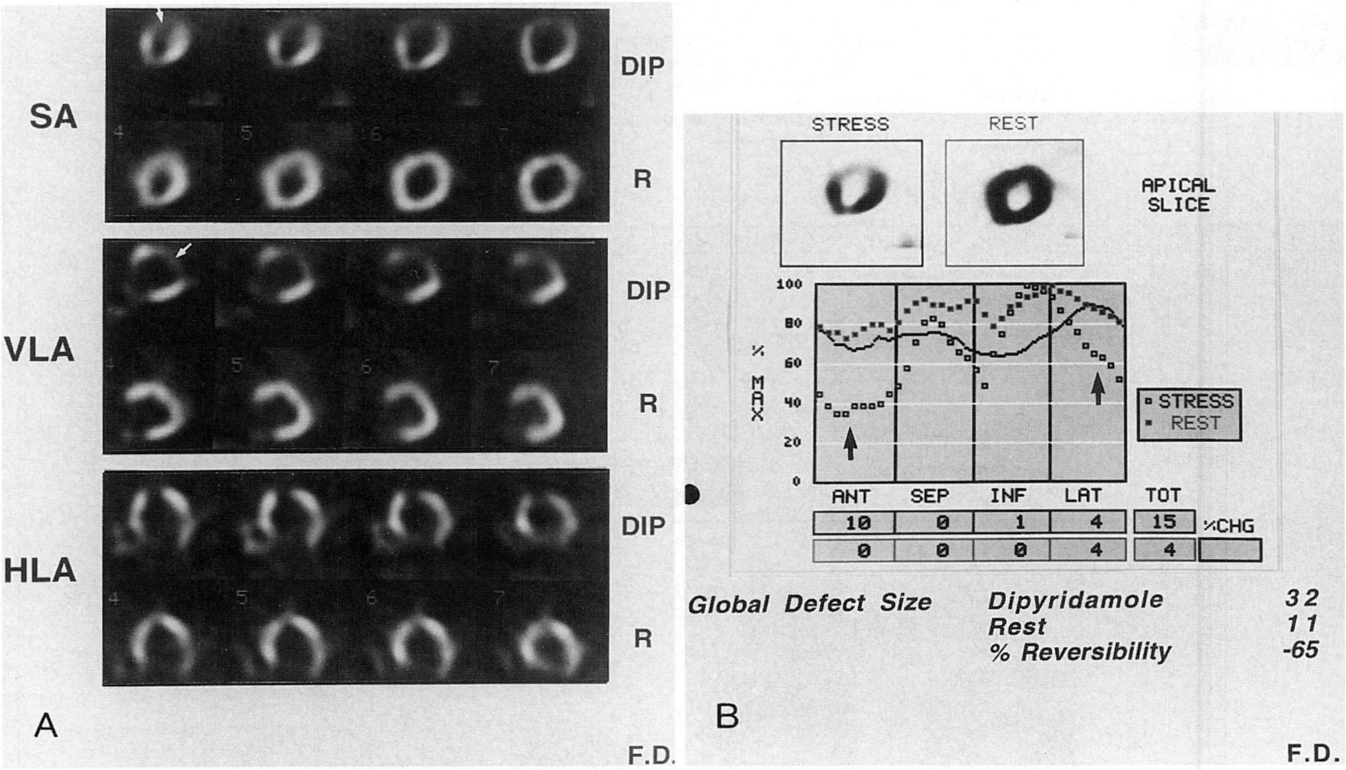

Figure 25.107. SPECT dipyridamole imaging. Quantitative ^{201}Tl SPECT imaging after infusion of dipyridamole (*DIP*) in a patient scheduled to undergo major abdominal surgery. **A.** The reconstructed slices show a marked reversible anterior myocardial perfusion defect (*arrows*). **B.** Representative circumferential profile of an apical short axis slice. The profile after dipyridamole infusion is below the lower limit of normal in the anterolateral wall (*arrow*) and is near normal at rest. Total defect size after dipyridamole is large (total integral: 32) with 65% defect reversibility at rest. The patient subsequently underwent coronary angiography and was found to have significant stenosis of the left anterior descending coronary artery.

Table 25.11.
Detection Coronary Artery Disease Using Pharmacologic Vasodilation and Myocardial Perfusion Imaging

	Methods	# Pts	Sens (%)	Spec (%)
Dipyridamole				
Francisco 1982[255]	Planar	420	81	66
Lam 1988[256]	SPECT	258	92	85
Huikuri 1988[257]				
Mendelson 1992[258]				
Kong 1992[259]				
Adenosine				
Verani 1990[260]				
Ngyen 1990[261]	SPECT	1053	87	89
Iskandrian 1991[262]				
Coyne 1991[263]				
Nishimura 1991[264]				
Gupta 1992[265]				

ported results in the literature for planar and SPECT dipyridamole and adenosine stress imaging (255–265).

RISK STRATIFICATION WITH VASODILATOR MYOCARDIAL PERFUSION IMAGING

Leppo, et al. (113), and Brown, et al. (114), reported that pharmacologic vasodilatation myocardial perfusion imaging has significant value for identifying high-risk patients after acute myocardial infarction.

Intravenous dipyridamole ^{201}Tl imaging has found a major clinical application in evaluating risk for perioperative cardiac events in patients scheduled for major noncardiac surgery. It is well-known that patients with severe peripheral vascular disease often have associated coronary artery disease which may, or may not, be clinically apparent. In these patients, perioperative morbidity and mortality is mostly due to underlying coronary artery disease. In patients who required peripheral vascular surgery, Boucher, et al. (266), and others (267, 268) demonstrated that dipyridamole ^{201}Tl imaging correctly predicted the occurrence of subsequent cardiac events. However, the predictive value of myocardial perfusion imaging was only 15–30%. Eagle, et al. (269), demonstrated that clinical variables, such as age, prior myocardial infarction, diabetes mellitus, history of angina, or congestive heart failure should be taken into consideration. If a patient has two or more of these variables, the patient is at high risk, whereas the patient having none of the clinical variables is at low risk. Pharmacologic vasodilatation myocardial perfusion imaging is most appropriately used for risk stratification in patients with an intermediate risk based on clinical variables. Additionally, it is important to consider the type of surgery that the patients are scheduled to undergo. For minor surgery, risk stratification with dipyridamole perfusion imaging is usually not indicated, whereas for major surgery, e.g., abdominal aortic aneurysm repair, risk stratification is appropriate.

As expected, the incidence of future cardiac events is related to *the extent* of perfusion abnormalities (270, 271). Short-term prognosis is determined by the presence of evidence of ischemia, i.e., reversible myocardial perfusion defects, whereas long-term prognosis is determined by the presence of fixed defects (272). In the latter situation, a fixed defect (i.e., scar) can be considered a surrogate for left ventricular ejection fraction.

Dobutamine Pharmacologic Stress

Dobutamine infusion is employed in patients who cannot perform physical exercise and who have contraindications for dipyridamole or adenosine infusion due to bronchospastic pulmonary disease, or patients who are on xanthine derivatives or had caffeine (273–275).

The dobutamine infusion protocol is as follows: Starting with intravenous infusion of 5 μg/kg/min, the dose is increased every 3 minutes, if tolerated, to a maximal dose of 40 μg/kg/min. The radiopharmaceutical is injected during infusion of the maximal dose, and infusion is continued for 2–3 minutes. Myocardial perfusion imaging is performed as described earlier.

Dobutamine increases myocardial oxygen demand by increasing myocardial contractility, heart rate, and systolic blood pressure. The increase in coronary blood flow is similar to that during physical exercise (two- to threefold) and less than that with adenosine or dipyridamole. The reported experience with dobutamine stress myocardial perfusion imaging shows that overall sensitivity and specificity to detect coronary artery disease is similar to that with physical exercise or pharmacologic vasodilatation (273–275) (Fig. 25.108).

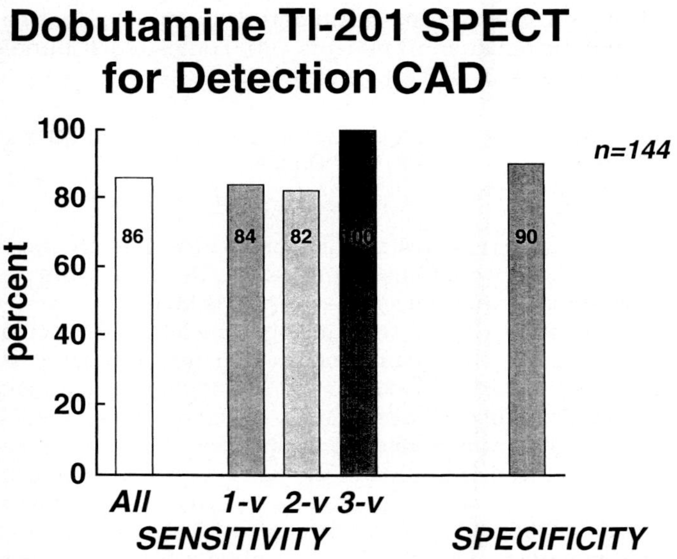

Figure 25.108. Detection of coronary artery disease by dobutamine stress imaging in 144 patients. *1-V, 2-V, 3-V* = single-vessel, double-vessel, and triple-vessel coronary artery disease. (Graph based on data from Hays JT, Mahmarian JJ, Cochran AJ, Verani MS. Dobutamine thallium-201 tomography for evaluating patients with suspected coronary artery disease unable to undergo exercise or vasodilator pharmacologic stress testing. J Am Coll Cardiol 1993;21:1583–1590.)

SELECTION OF PATIENTS FOR STRESS MYOCARDIAL PERFUSION IMAGING

Although the sensitivity and specificity of myocardial perfusion imaging is better than that of routine ECG exercise testing, stress myocardial perfusion imaging is a not a perfect diagnostic test. Some false-negative results can be expected in patients with angiographic coronary artery disease, and false-positive results may also occur. According to Bayes' theorem, the significance of a test result relates not only to the sensitivity and specificity of the test, but also to the prevalence of disease in the population under study (276–280). Assuming that myocardial perfusion stress imaging has an approximate sensitivity of 90% and a specificity of 95%, a positive result obtained in a population with a very low prevalence of coronary artery disease (e.g., $<3\%$) will have a low predictive value of only 36%, since, compared with expected true-positive results, a relatively large absolute number of false-positives can be anticipated. However, in a patient population with a high prevalence of coronary artery disease (e.g., 90%), a positive result has a predictive value of 99%. In this setting, relative to true-positive results, only a few false-positives are obtained. On the other hand, in a population with a high

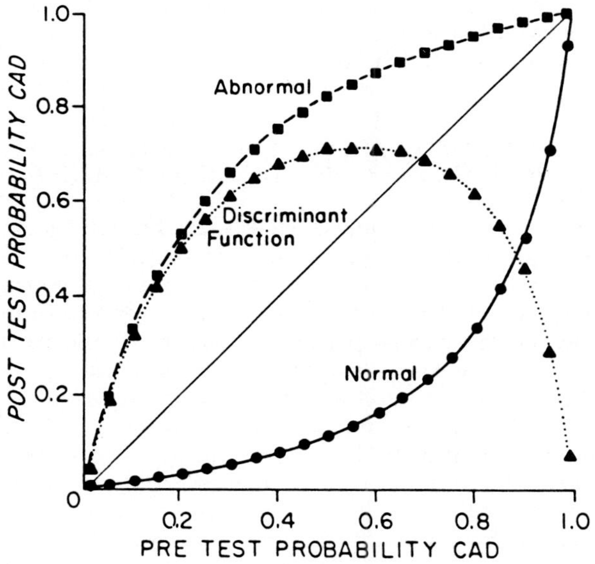

Figure 25.109. Probability of coronary artery disease. Pre- and posttest probability of coronary artery disease (*CAD*) for abnormal and normal results of quantitative ^{201}Tl stress imaging (sensitivity 90%, specificity 95%). The curve describes the difference between posttest probability of a normal and an abnormal test result, indicating the range of disease prevalence for which ^{201}Tl stress imaging discriminates most effectively between the presence or absence of disease. ^{201}Tl stress imaging is most useful when the pretest prevalence of coronary artery disease is 40–70%. Example: In a patient with a pretest probability of coronary artery disease of 60%, a positive ^{201}Tl stress test increases the probability of coronary artery disease to approximately 90%, but a negative test decreases it to about 15%. In contrast, in a very high or a very low pretest probability of disease, no clinically meaningful diagnostic improvement will be gained by either a positive or negative test result. Symbols: ■ = abnormal; ▲ = posttest probability difference; ● = normal. (Reproduced by permission from Hamilton GW, Trobaugh G, Ritchie JC, Gould KL, DeRouen TA, Williams DL. Myocardial imaging with ^{201}Tl: an analysis of clinical usefulness based on Bayes' theorem. Semin Nucl Med 1978;8:358.)

prevalence of disease, a relatively large number of false-negative results are also obtained and the predictive value of a negative test for absence of coronary artery disease is only 51%. Thus, in a population with a low prevalence of coronary artery disease (such as young, asymptomatic subjects), a positive test is of little practical value, whereas in a population with a high prevalence of coronary artery disease (50–60-year-old males with typical angina pectoris), a negative test is of little practical diagnostic value (281). The difference between pretest probability of disease (276, 278) (determined by patient's age, symptoms, and a stress ECG) and posttest probability (determined by the results of stress myocardial perfusion imaging) directly indicates the practical value of the test (Fig. 25.109). Stress myocardial perfusion imaging has optimal discriminative value in the patient population with a pretest probability of coronary artery disease ranging from about 40–70%. This population includes patients with atypical chest pain and asymptomatic patients with known major risk factors or with a positive stress ECG.

The incremental value of myocardial perfusion imaging in patients with chest pain syndrome and a normal baseline electrocardiogram has been disputed. These patients most likely have normal left ventricular function and a favorable prognosis. In view of the greater awareness of cost-effective patient management, it can be anticipated that optimal patient selection for radionuclide myocardial perfusion imaging will be further defined in the near future.

STRESS MYOCARDIAL PERFUSION IMAGING IN PATIENTS WITH LEFT BUNDLE BRAND BLOCK

In patients with complete left bundle branch block, the electrical conduction abnormality precludes the use of conventional electrocardiographic criteria for the localization of acute infarction or detection of exercise-induced ischemia. Myocardial perfusion imaging should be unaffected by the electrocardiographic abnormality.

In patients without history of myocardial infarction, the *resting* ^{201}Tl images do not show perfusion defects, although frequently the septum was thinner and the left ventricle dilated (Fig. 25.19). In patients with acute or old infarction, resting myocardial perfusion defects were present similar to those seen in infarct patients without conduction abnormalities (Fig. 25.70). Accordingly, we found *resting* ^{201}Tl imaging to be extremely helpful in precisely localizing the site of acute or old infarction (139).

A number of investigators have reported anterior septal myocardial perfusion defects by ^{201}Tl imaging *after exercise* in patients with complete left bundle branch block and *normal coronary arteries* (15, 282–284). In some of these patients, redistribution of anteroseptal defects was observed. In an experimental study, Hirzel, et al. (282), demonstrated in a canine experimental model that right ventricular electrical pacing (left bundle branch block) produced diminished septal blood flow. It was proposed that exercise-induced septal perfusion defects in patients with left bundle branch block does not necessarily indicate coronary artery disease, but may be due to functional hypoperfusion caused by asynchronous septal contraction. We reproduced this study in humans (285). We studied a group of 15 cardiac transplant patients who had angiographically normal coronary arteries. These patients were scheduled for routine right heart catheterization for myocardial biopsy. During two subsequent right heart catheterizations, the patients were paced either in the right atrium or in the right ventricle. At a pacing rate of approximately 150 bpm, ^{201}Tl was injected both times. All patients had normal images with injection during right atrial pacing (normal conduction). None of the patients developed septal defects with right ventricular pacing (electrical left bundle branch block). Thus, it appears that abnormal conduction *alone* does not cause septal myocardial perfusion defects.

It is well-known that many patients with left bundle branch block may have marked left ventricular dilatation. We observed, using quantitative techniques, a relationship between exercise-induced myocardial perfusion defects in patients with left bundle branch block and normal coronary arteries (or low likelihood of coronary artery disease), and the presence of left ventricular dilatation (286). Partial volume effect due to altered geometry of the dilated left ventricle with thinning of the myocardium appears to be a plausible alternative explanation for the defects observed after exercise in patients with electrocardiographic complete left bundle branch block.

The anatomic location of myocardial perfusion in left bundle branch block defects should be considered. Whereas anteroseptal perfusion defects may be nonspecific for coronary artery disease, involvement of the apex contiguous with anteroseptal perfusion defects and inferior location are suggestive of coronary artery disease (287).

Recently, it has been shown that false-positive anteroseptal defects in left bundle branch block can be avoided by using *pharmacologic vasodilation* instead of physical exercise (288). The mechanism of improved specificity is unclear. Nevertheless, most laboratories now use pharmacologic vasodilation in patients with complete left bundle branch block.

THALLIUM-201 STRESS IMAGING IN NONCORONARY ARTERY DISEASE

Syndrome X

Myocardial perfusion stress imaging has been employed in patients with symptoms of angina-like chest pain, but angiographically normal coronary arteries (Syndrome X). We evaluated 31 patients with angiographically normal coronary arteries, chest pain, and an ischemic-appearing exercise ECG (289). In none of the patients was coronary spasm the cause of chest pain. In seven of these patients, ^{201}Tl imaging was abnormal; in five, the defects were exercise-induced; and in two, the defects were also present at rest. Similar observations were reported by other investigators (290–292). Legrand, et al. (292), demonstrated that in patients with Syndrome X, abnormal coronary flow reserve may be present (Fig. 25.110). Additionally, Cannon, et al. (293), and others (289, 294) found that these patients also have abnormal global and regional systolic and diastolic function suggestive of myocardial ischemia. Thus, it appears that at least some of the "false-positive"

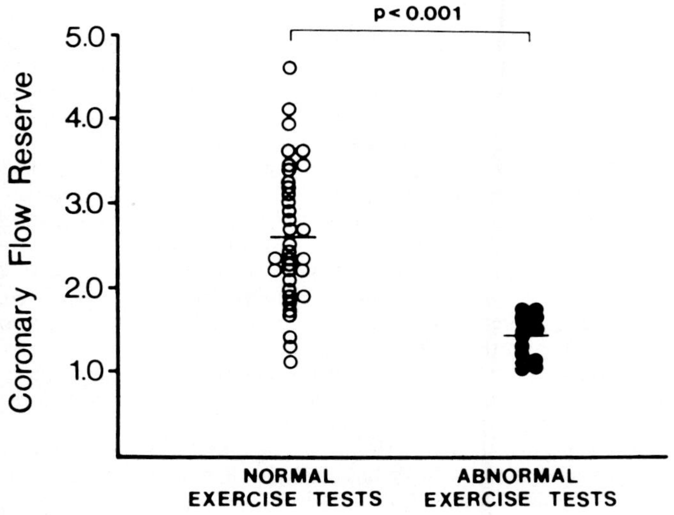

Figure 25.110. Abnormal coronary flow reserve and radionuclide imaging. Coronary flow reserve in distribution of coronary arteries of patients with chest pain and angiographically normal coronary arteries, with (●) and without (○) abnormal radionuclide exercise tests (exercise ^{201}Tl stress imaging, radionuclide stress ventriculography, or both). All patients with abnormal scintigraphic stress test results had low coronary reserve (<1.95 in at least one distribution). Perfusion abnormalities were localized in the arterial distribution with the lowest flow reserve. (Reproduced by permission from Legrand V, Hodgson JM, Bates ER, et al. Abnormal coronary flow reserve and abnormal radionuclide exercise test results in patients with normal coronary angiograms. J Am Coll Cardiol 1985;6:1245.)

^{201}Tl images may reflect true abnormalities in myocardial microvasculature.

Mitral Valve Prolapse

Another group of patients that was studied by ^{201}Tl stress imaging to clarify the occurrence of atypical chest pain, is that of patients with mitral valve prolapse. Klein, et al. (295), and Massie, et al. (296), demonstrated that in patients with mitral valve prolapse, chest pain, and normal coronary arteries, ^{201}Tl stress images were uniformly normal.

Aortic Stenosis

Angina pectoris often occurs in patients with aortic stenosis. Bailey, et al. (297), evaluated the potential of ^{201}Tl stress imaging to predict the presence or absence of coronary artery disease in patients with aortic stenosis. In some of these patients, they observed widespread left ventricular wall thinning on the postexercise ^{201}Tl images, suggesting diffuse subendocardial ischemia, as can be expected in severe aortic stenosis. Additionally, in some patients focal exercise-induced defects occurred, suggesting focal coronary artery disease. However, it was not possible to predict reliably the presence or absence of coronary artery disease in this patient population on the basis of diffuse or focal abnormalities on the images. In general, it is not advisable to submit patients suspected of significant aortic stenosis to a treadmill exercise test. These patients may become hemodynamically unstable and ^{201}Tl stress imaging will, in general, not provide clinically useful information.

Hypertension

In patients with hypertension, ^{201}Tl exercise imaging is an important diagnostic tool because of the increased incidence of coronary artery disease. Exercise function studies have been reported not to be very useful in patients with hypertension and chest pain, because of a significant incidence of false-positive responses in patients with normal coronary arteries (298). Myocardial perfusion imaging could be expected to be a more specific test in this population. No exercise myocardial perfusion data are available in patients with hypertension, with and without angiographic coronary artery disease. We analyzed a group of age-matched normotensive and hypertensive patients who all had ^{201}Tl exercise imaging (299). The patients were categorized according to their likelihood of having coronary artery disease using stepwise probability analysis (265). The prevalence of abnormal ^{201}Tl exercise images was not different in the normotensive and hypertensive group when the likelihood for coronary artery disease was moderate to high (25–100%). However, when the likelihood of coronary artery disease was low (<25%) significantly more abnormal ^{201}Tl stress images were obtained in the hypertensive patients than in the normotensive patients. These results indicate that, at least in hypertensive patients suspected of having coronary artery disease, ^{201}Tl imaging has the same yield as that in the normotensive population. The significance of high prevalence of exercise-induced ^{201}Tl defects in hypertensive patients with low likelihood of coronary artery disease is as yet unclear, and this higher prevalence could be due to either subclinical epicardial coronary artery disease or microvascular disease.

Using SPECT ^{201}Tl imaging in patients with hypertension and left ventricular hypertrophy, the normal ratio of tracer uptake between septum and lateral wall may be reversed; maximal uptake in patients with hypertrophy may be in the septum rather than in the lateral wall. This pattern should not be interpreted as abnormal perfusion of the lateral wall.

Dilated Cardiomyopathy

The distinction between idiopathic and ischemic cardiomyopathy is clinically difficult and myocardial perfusion imaging may be helpful, although not always conclusive. In idiopathic cardiomyopathy, the left ventricle is dilated and shows homogeneous or diffusely inhomogeneous radiotracer uptake. Large, localized defects, involving more than 40% of the circumference of the left ventricle, strongly favor ischemic etiology of cardiomyopathy. However, large, fixed defects have also been reported in patients with idiopathic dilated cardiomyopathy. These are often located at the apex of the left ventricle.

Miscellaneous

Finally, ^{201}Tl exercise-induced defects have been described in a number of diseases where focal myocardial abnormalities are present, such as sarcoidosis (300) and systemic sclerosis (301). Therefore, ^{201}Tl stress images should be interpreted with caution in these patients when coronary artery disease is to be ruled out.

ACKNOWLEDGMENTS

The secretarial assistance of Irene Courtmanche is greatly appreciated. Without the technical expertise and dedication of Jennifer A. Mattera, RTNM, Donna Natale, RTNM, and Robert C. Fetterman, RTNM, B.S., it would not have been possible to collect much of the presented material.

REFERENCES

1. Bradley-Moore PR, Lebowitz E, Greene MW, Atkins HL, Ansari AN. Thallium-201 for medical use. II: Biologic behavior. J Nucl Med 1975:16:156.
2. Wackers FJTh, van der Schoot JB, Busemann Sokole E, et al. Noninvasive visualization of acute myocardial infarction in man with thallium-201. Br Heart J 1975:37:741.
3. Wackers FJTh, Berman DS, Maddahi J, et al. Technetium-99m hexakis 2-methoxyisobutyl isonitrile: human biodistribution, dosimetry, safety, and preliminary comparison to thallium-201 for myocardial perfusion imaging. J Nucl Med 1989:30:301–311.
4. Kiat H, Maddahi J, Roy LT, et al. Comparison of technetium-99m-methoxy isobutyl isonitrile and thallium-201 for evaluation of coronary artery disease by planar and tomographic methods. Am Heart J 1989:117:1–11.
5. Seldin DW, Johnson LL, Blood DK, et al. Myocardial perfusion imaging with technetium-99m SQ30217: comparison with thallium-201 and coronary anatomy. J Nucl Med 1989:30:312–319.
6. Hendel RC, McSherry B, Karimeddini M, Leppo JA. Diagnostic value of a new myocardial perfusion agent, teboroxime (SQ30,217), utilizing a rapid planar imaging protocol: preliminary results. J Am Coll Cardiol 1990:16:855–861.
7. Jain D, Wackers FJTh, Mattera J, McMahon M, Sinusas AJ, Zaret BL. Biokinetics of ^{99m}Tc-tetrofosmin, a new myocardial perfusion a imaging agent: implications for a one-day imaging protocol. J Nucl Med 1993;34:1254–1259.
8. Gerson MC, Millard RW, Roszell NJ, et al. Kinetic properties of ^{99m}Tc-Q12 in canine myocardium. Circulation 1994;89:1291–1300.
9. Strauss HW, Harrison K, Langan JK, Lebowitz E, Pitt B. Thallium-201 for myocardial imaging. Relation of thallium-201 to regional myocardial perfusion. Circulation 1975;51:641.
10. Wackers FJTh, Klay JW, Laks H, Schnitzer J, Zaret BL, Geha AS. Pathophysiologic correlates of right ventricular thallium-201 uptake in a canine model. Circulation 1981;64:1256–1264.
11. Wackers FJTh, Busemann Sokole E, Samson G, van der Schoot JB. Atlas of Tl-201 myocardial scintigraphy. Clin Nucl Med 1977; 2:64.
12. Wackers FJTh. Thallium-201 myocardial imaging. In: Wackers FJTh, ed. Thallium-201 and technetium-99m pyrophosphate myocardial imaging in the coronary care unit. The Hague: Martinus Nijhoff Publishers, 1980:70–104.
13. Dunn RF, Wolff L, Wagner S, Botvinick EH. The inconsistent pattern of thallium-201 defects: a clue to the false positive perfusion scintigram. Am J Cardiol 1981;48:224.
14. Wackers FJTh. Artifacts in planar and SPECT myocardial perfusion imaging. Am J Cardiac Imaging 1992;6:42–58.
15. McGowan RI, Welch TG, Zaret BL, Bryson AL, Martin ND, Flamm MD. Noninvasive myocardial imaging with potassium-43 and rubidium-81 in patients with left bundle branch block. Am J Cardiol 1976;38:422.
16. Johnstone DE, Wackers FJTh, Berger HJ, et al. Effect of patient positioning of left lateral thallium-201 myocardial images. J Nucl Med 1979;20:183.
17. Gordon DG, Pfisterer M, Williams R, Walski S, Ashburn W. The effect of diaphragmatic attenuation of Tl-201 images. Clin Nucl Med 1979;10:150.
18. Esquerre JP, Coca FJ, Martinez SJ, Guiraud RF. Prone decubitus: a solution of inferior wall attenuation in thallium-201 myocardial tomography. J Nucl Med 1989;30:398–401.
19. Barr SA, Shen MYH, Sinusas AJ, et al. Reduced inferior attenuation on rest SPECT myocardial perfusion imaging in the upright position using a rotating chair: comparison with standard supine SPECT imaging. J Nucl Med 1994;35:91P.
20. Friedman J, Van Train K, Maddahi J, et al. "Upward creep" of the heart: a frequent source of false-positive reversible defects during thallium-201 stress-redistribution SPECT. J Nucl Med 1989;30:1718–1722.
21. Maniawski PJ, Morgan HT, Wackers FJTh. Orbit related variation in spatial resolution as a source of artifactual defects in Tl-201 SPECT. J Nucl Med 1991;32:871–875.
22. Civelek AC, Shafique I, Brinker JA, et al. Reduced left ventricular cavitary activity ("black hole sign") in thallium-201 SPECT perfusion images of anteroapical transmural myocardial infarction. Am J Cardiol 1991;68:1132–1137.
23. Germano G, Chua T, Kiat H, Areeda JS, Berman DS. A quantitative phantom analysis of artifacts due to hepatic activity in technetium-99m-myocardial perfusion SPECT studies. J Nucl Med 1994;35:356–359.
24. DePuey EG, Garcia EV. Optimal specific of thallium-201 SPECT through recognition of imaging artifacts. J Nucl Med 1989; 30:441–449.
25. Bulkley BH, Rouleau J, Strauss HW, Pitt B. Idiopathic hypertrophic subaortic stenosis: detection by thallium-201 myocardial perfusion imaging. N Engl J Med 1975;293:1113.
26. Rubin KA, Morrison J, Padnick MB, et al. Idiopathic hypertrophic subaortic stenosis: evaluation of anginal symptoms with thallium-201 myocardial imaging. Am J Cardiol 1979;44:1040.
27. Kronenberg MW, Robertson RM, Bron ML, Steckley RA, Robertson D, Friesinger GC. Thallium-201 uptake in variant angina: probable demonstration of myocardial reactive hyperemia in man. Circulation 1982;66:1332.
28. Cohen HA, Baird MG, Rouleau JR, et al. Thallium-201 myocardial imaging in patients with pulmonary hypertension. Circulation 1976;54:790.
29. Kondo M, Kubo A, Yamazaki H, et al. Thallium-201 myocardial imaging for evaluation of right-ventricular overloading. J Nucl Med 1978;19:1197.
30. Khaja F, Alam M, Goldstein S, Ange DT, Mark KS. Diagnostic value of visualization of the right ventricle using thallium-201 myocardial imaging. Circulation 1979;59:182.
31. Adachi H, Torii Y, Kamide T, Katsume H, Ochiai M, Ijichi H. Visualization of right atrial appendix by thallium-201 myocardial scintigraphy (concise communication). J Nucl Med 1980;21:914.
32. DePuey EG, Jones M, Garcia EV. Evaluation of right ventricular regional perfusion with technetium-99m-sestamibi SPECT. J Nucl Med 1991;32:1199–1205.
33. Hamilton GW, Narahara KA, Trobaugh GB, Ritchie JL, Williams DL. Thallium-201 myocardial imaging: characterization of the ECG-synchronized images. J Nucl Med 1978;19:1103.
34. Alderson PO, Wagner HN Jr, Gomez-Moeiras JJ, et al. Simultaneous detection of myocardial perfusion and wall motion abnormalities by cinematic Tl-201 imaging. Radiology 1978;127:531.
35. McKusick KA, Bingham J, Pohost G, Strauss HW. Comparison of defect detection on ungated vs. gated thallium-201 cardiac images. J Nucl Med 1978;19:725.
36. Parker JA, Markis JE, Royal HD. Assessment of regional wall motion and perfusion by multigated myocardial scintigraphy after intracoronary Tl-201. Radiology 1985;154:783.
37. Marcassa C, Marzullo P, Parodi O, Sambuceti G, L'Abbate A. A new method for noninvasive quantitation of segmental myocar-

dial wall thickening using technetium-99m 2-methoxy-isobutyl-isonitrile scintigraphy—results in normal subjects. J Nucl Med 1990;31:173–177.

38. Camargo E, Hironaka FH, Giorgi M, et al. Amplitude analysis of stress technetium-99m methoxy isobutylisonitrile images in coronary artery disease. Eur J Nucl Med 1992;19:484–491.
39. Sinusas AJ, Shi QX, Vitols PH, et al. Impact of regional ventricular function, geometry and dobutamine stress on quantitative Tc-99m-sestamibi defect size. Circulation 1993;88(Pt 1):2224–2234.
40. Wackers FJTh, Maniawski P, Sinusas AJ. Evaluation of left ventricular wall function by ECG-gated Tc-99m-sestamibi imaging. In: Beller GA, Zaret BL, eds. Nuclear cardiology: state of the art and future direction. St. Louis: Mosby, 1993:85–100.
41. Verzijlbergen JF, Suttorp MJ, Ascoop CAPL, et al. Combined assessment of technetium-99m sestamibi planar myocardial perfusion images at rest and during exercise with rest/exercise left ventricular wall motion studies evaluated from gated myocardial perfusion studies. Am Heart J 1992;123:59–68.
42. Tischler MD, Niggel JB, Battle RW, Fairbank JT, Brown KA. Validation of global and segmental left ventricular contractile function using gated planar technetium-99m sestamibi myocardial perfusion imaging. J Am Coll Cardiol 1994;23:141–145.
43. Clausen M, Henze E, Schmidt A, et al. The contraction fraction (CF) in myocardial studies with technetium-99m-isonitrile (MIBI)—correlations with radionuclide ventriculography and infarct size measured by SPECT. Eur J Nucl Med 1989;15:661–664.
44. Chua T, Kiat H, Germano G, et al. Gated technetium-99m sestamibi for simultaneous assessment of stress myocardial perfusion, postexercise regional ventricular function and myocardial viability. J Am Coll Cardiol 1994;23:1107–1114.
45. Mannting F, Morgan-Mannting MG. Gated SPECT with technetium-99m-sestamibi for assessment of myocardial perfusion abnormalities. J Nucl Med 1993;34:601–608.
46. Takeda T, Toyama H, Ishikawa N, et al. Quantitative phase analysis of wall myocardial wall thickening by technetium-99m 2-methoxy-isobutyl-isonitrile SPECT. Annuals Nucl Med 1992; 6:69–78.
47. Galt JR, Garcia EV, Robbins WL. Effects of myocardial wall thickness on SPECT quantification. IEEE Transactions on Medical Imaging 1990;9:144–150.
48. Ziffer JA, Cooke CD, Folks RD, et al. Quantitative myocardial thickening assessed with sestamibi: clinical evaluation of a count-based method. J Nucl Med 1991;32:1006.
49. Germano G, Kavnangh PB, Kiat H, Chua T, Berman DS. Automated analysis of gated myocardial SPECT: development and initial validation of a method. J Nucl Med 1994;35:816.
50. DePuey EG, Nichols K, Dobrinsky C. Left ventricular ejection fraction assessed from gated technetium-99m-sestamibi SPECT. J Nucl Med 1993;34:1871–1876.
51. Anderson HV, Willerson JT. Thrombolysis in acute myocardial infarction. N Engl J Med 1993;329:703–709.
52. Wackers FJTh, Gibbons RJ, Verani MS, et al. Serial quantitative planar technetium-99m-isonitrile imaging in acute myocardial infarction: efficacy for noninvasive assessment of thrombolytic therapy. J Am Coll Cardiol 1989;14:861–873.
53. Wackers FJTh, Busemann Sokole E, Samson G, van der Schoot JB, Wellens HJJ. Myocardial imaging in coronary heart disease with radionuclides, with emphasis on thallium-201. Eur J Cardiol 1976;4:273.
54. Wackers FJTh, Busemann Sokole E, Samson G, et al. Value and limitations of thallium-201 scintigraphy in acute phase of myocardial infarction. N Engl J Med 1976;295:1.
55. Boucher CA, Wackers FJTh, Zaret BL, Mena IG, and the Multicenter Cardiolite Study Group. Technetium-99m-sestamibi myocardial imaging at rest for the assessment of myocardial infarction and first pass ejection fraction: a multicenter trial. Am J Cardiol 1992;69:22–27.
56. Verani MS, Jeroudi MO, Mahmarian JJ, et al. Quantification of myocardial infarction during coronary occlusion and myocardial salvage after reperfusion using cardiac imaging with technetium-99m hexakis 2-methoxyisobutyl isonitrile. J Am Coll Cardiol 1988;12:1573–1581.
57. Isner JM, Roberts WC. Right ventricular infarction complicating left ventricular infarction secondary to coronary heart disease. Am J Cardiol 1978;42:885.
58. Wackers FJTh, Lie KI, Busemann Sokole E, Res J, van der Schoot JB, Durrer D. Prevalence of right ventricular involvement in inferior wall infarction assessed with myocardial imaging with thallium-201 and technetium-99m pyrophosphate. Am J Cardiol 1978;42:385.
59. Rigo P, Murray M, Taylor DR, et al. Right ventricular dysfunction detected by gated scintiphotography in patients with acute inferior myocardial infarction. Circulation 1975;52:268.
60. Sharpe KN, Botvinick EH, Shames DM, et al. The noninvasive diagnosis of right ventricular infarction. Circulation 1978; 57:483.
61. Mahmarian JJ, Pratt CM, Borges-Neto S, Cashion WR, Roberts R, Verani MS. Quantification of infarct size by ^{201}Tl single-photon emission computed tomography during acute myocardial infarction in humans. Circulation 1988;78:831–839.
62. Kannel WB, Sorlie P, McNamara PM. Prognosis after initial infarction. The Framingham Study. Am J Cardiol 1979;44:53.
63. Shah PK, Maddahi J, Staniloff HM, et al. Variable spectrum and prognostic implications of left and right ventricular ejection fractions in patients with and without clinical heart failure after acute myocardial infarction. Am J Cardiol 1986;58:387.
64. Lie KI, Wellens HJJ, Schuilenburg RM, Becker AE, Durrer D. Factors influencing prognosis of bundle branch block complicating acute anteroseptal infarction. The value of His bundle recordings. Circulation 1974;60:935.
65. Wackers FJTh, Becker AE, Samson G, et al. Location and size of acute transmural myocardial infarction estimated from thallium-201 scintiscans. Circulation 1977;56:71.
66. Nelson AD, Khullar S, Leighton RF, et al. Quantification of thallium-201 scintigrams in acute myocardial infarction. Am J Cardiol 1979;44:664.
67. Page DL, Caulfield JB, Kastor JA, DeSanctis RW, Sanders CA. Myocardial changes associated with cardiogenic shock. N Engl J Med 1971;285:134.
68. Kirchner PT. Infarct sizing with thallium-201 scintigraphy. Am J Cardiac Imaging 1990;4:46–58.
69. O'Connor MK, Hammell T, Gibbons RJ. In vitro validation of a simple tomographic technique for estimation of percentage myocardium at risk using methoxyisobutyl isonitrile technetium-99m (sestamibi). Eur J Nucl Med 1990;17:69–76.
70. Christian TF, O'Connor MK, Hopfenspirger MR, Gibbons RJ. Comparison of reinjection thallium-201 and resting technetium-99m sestamibi tomographic images for the quantification of infarct size after acute myocardial infarction. J Nucl Cardiol 1994; 1:17–28.
71. Liu YH, Sinusas AJ, Shi CQX, et al. An automated approach for quantification of relative regional myocardial blood flow, using SPECT Tc99m-sestamibi: preliminary validation in a canine model. IEEE Transactions on Medical Imaging 1994;16:636–638.
72. Becker LC, Silverman HJ, Bulkley GH, Kallman CH, Mellits ED, Weisfeldt ML. Comparison of early thallium-201 scintigraphy and gated blood pool imaging for predicting mortality in patients with acute myocardial infarction. Circulation 1983;67:1272.
73. Christian TF, Behrenbeck T, Pellikka PA, et al. Mismatch of left ventricular function and infarct size demonstrated by technetium-99m isonitrile imaging after reperfusion therapy for acute

myocardial infarction: identification of myocardial stunning and hyperkinesia. J Am Coll Cardiol 1990;16:1632–1638.
74. Smitherman TC, Osborn RC Jr, Narahara KA. Serial myocardial scintigraphy after a single dose of thallium-201 in men after acute myocardial infarction. Am J Cardiol 1978;42:177.
75. Umbach RE, Lanch RC, Lee JC, Zaret BL. Temporal changes in sequential quantitative thallium-201 imaging following myocardial infarction in dogs: comparison of four- and twenty-four-hour infarct images. Yale J Biol Med 1978;51:597.
76. Dunn RF, Kelly DT, Freedman SB, Uren RF. Serial thallium-201 myocardial perfusion scanning in acute myocardial infarction. Aust NZ J Med 1980;10:629.
77. Schwartz JS, Ponto RA, Forstorm LA, Bache RJ. Decrease in thallium-201 image defect size after permanent coronary occlusion. Am Heart 1983;106:1082.
78. DeWood MA, Spores J, Notske R, et al. Prevalence of total coronary occlusion during the early hours of transmural myocardial infarction. N Engl J Med 1980;303:897.
79. Defeyter PJ, van Eenige MJ, van der Wall EE, et al. Effects of spontaneous and streptokinase-induced recanalization of left ventricular function after myocardial infarction. Circulation 1983;67:1039.
80. Maddahi J, Weiss T, Geft I Shah PK, Berman D, Swan HJC, Ganz W. Coronary thrombolysis with intravenous streptokinase salvages jeopardized myocardium in evolving myocardial infarction: assessment by quantitative Tl-201 imaging. Circulation 1983; 68(Suppl III):III-120.
81. Markis JE, Malagold M, Parker JA, et al. Myocardial salvage after intracoronary thrombolysis with streptokinase in acute myocardial infarction. Assessment by intracoronary thallium-201. N Engl J Med 1981;305:777.
82. Maddahi J, Ganz W, Ninomiya K, et al. Myocardial salvage by intracoronary thrombolysis in evolving acute myocardial infarctions: evaluation using intracoronary injection of thallium-201. Am Heart J 1981;102:664.
83. Schuler G, Schwartz F, Hoffman M, et al. Thrombolysis in acute myocardial infarction using intracoronary streptokinase: assessment by thallium-201 scintigraphy. Circulation 1982; 66:658.
84. Schofer J, Mathey DG, Montz R, Bliefeld W, Stritzke P. Use of dual intracoronary scintigraphy with thallium-201 and technetium-99m pyrophosphate to predict improvement in left ventricular wall motion immediately after intracoronary thrombolysis in acute myocardial infarction. J Am Coll Cardiol 1983; 2:737.
85. Schofer J, Montz R, Mathey DG. Scintigraphic evidence of the "no reflow" phenomenon in human beings after coronary thrombolysis. J Am Coll Cardiol 1985;5:593.
86. Reduto LA, Freund GC, Gaeta J, Killingsworth B, Nussey G, Gould KL. Thallium redistribution following intracoronary streptokinase in acute myocardial infarction: relation to changes in left ventricular performance. Am Heart J 1981;102:1168.
87. Simoons ML, Wijns W, Balakumaran OK, et al. The effect of intracoronary thrombolysis with streptokinase on myocardial thallium distribution and left ventricular function assessed by blood pool scintigraphy. Eur Heart J 1982;3:433.
88. Maddahi J, Ganz W, Fegt I, et al. Intracoronary thrombolysis in acute myocardial infarction: assessment of efficacy by thallium-201 scintigraphy. Am J Cardiol 1982;49:973.
89. Okada RD, Pohost GM. The use of pre- and postintervention thallium imaging for assessing the early and late effects of experimental coronary artery reperfusion in dogs. Circulation 1980;69:1153.
90. DeCoster PM, Melin JA, Detry JR, Brassor LA, Beckers C, Col J. Coronary artery reperfusion in acute myocardial infarction: assessment by pre- and postintervention thallium-201 myocardial perfusion imaging. Am J Cardiol 1985;55:889.
91. Granato JE, Watson DD, Flanagan TL, Gascho JA, Beller GA. Myocardial thallium-201 kinetics during coronary occlusion and reperfusion: influence of method reflow and timing of thallium-201 administration. Circulation 1986;73:150.
92. Melin JA, Becker LC, Bulkley BH. Difference in thallium-201 uptake in reperfused and nonreperfused myocardial infarction. Cir Res 1983;53:414.
93. Kayden DS, Mattera JA, Zaret BL, Wackers FJTh. Demonstration of reperfusion after thrombolysis with technetium-99m isonitrile myocardial imaging. J Nucl Med 1988;29:1869–1867.
94. Gibbons RJ, Verani MS, Behrenbeck T, et al. Feasibility of tomographic ^{99m}Tc-hexakis-2-methoxy-2-methylpropyl-isonitrile imaging for the assessment of myocardia area at risk and the effect of treatment in acute myocardial infarction. Circulation 1989;80:1278–1286.
95. Faraggi M, Assayag P, Messian O, et al. Early isonitrile SPECT in acute myocardial infarction: feasibility and results before and after fibrinolysis. Nucl Med Communications 1989;10:539–549.
96. Santoro GM, Bisi G, Sciagra R, et al. Single photon emission computed tomography with technetium-99m hexakis 2-methoxyisobutyl isonitrile in acute myocardial infarction before and after thrombolytic treatment: assessment of salvaged myocardium and prediction of late functional recovery. J Am Coll Cardiol 1990;15:301–14.
97. Bisi G, Sciagra R, Santoro GM, et al. Comparison of tomography and planar imaging for the evaluation of thrombolytic therapy in acute myocardial infarction using pre- and posttreatment myocardial scintigraphy with technetium-99m sestamibi. Am Heart J 1991;122:13–22.
98. Gibson W, Christian TF, Pellikka PA, Behrenbeck T, Gibbons RJ. Serial tomographic imaging with technetium-99m-sestamibi for the assessment of infarct-related arterial patency following reperfusion therapy. J Nucl Med 1992;33:2080–2085.
99. DeCoster PM, Wijns W, Cauwe F, et al. Area at risk determination by technetium-99m-hexakis-2-methoxyisobutyl isonitrile in experimental reperfused myocardial infarction. Circulation 1990; 82:2152–2162.
100. Christian TF, Behrenbeck T, Gersh BJ, Gibbons RJ. Relation of left ventricular volume and function over one year after acute myocardial infarction to infarct size determined by technetium-99m-sestamibi. Am J Cardiol 1991;68:21–26.
101. Christian TF, Schwartz RS, Gibbons RJ. Determinants of infarct size in reperfusion therapy for acute myocardial infarction. Circulation 1992;86:81–90.
102. Pellikka PA, Behrenbeck R, Verani MS, Mahmarian JJ, Wackers FJTh, Gibbons RJ. Serial changes in myocardial perfusion using tomographic technetium-99m-hexakis-2-methoxy-2-methylpropyl-isonitrile imaging following reperfusion therapy of myocardial infarction. J Nucl Med 1990;31:1269–1275.
103. Maublant JC, Peycelon P, Cardot JC, Verdenet J, Fagret, Comet M. Value of myocardial defect size measured by thallium-201 SPECT: results of a multicenter trial comparing heparin and a new fibrinolytic agent. J Nucl Med 1988;29:1486–1491.
104. Gersh BJ. Noninvasive imaging in acute coronary disease. A clinical perspective. Circulation 1991;84(Suppl I):I-140–I-147.
105. Christian TF, Gibbons FJ, Hopfenspirger MR, Gersh BJ. Severity and response of chest pain during thrombolytic therapy for acute myocardial infarction: a useful indicator of myocardial salvage and infarct size. J Am Coll Cardiol 1993;22:1311–1316.
106. Gibbons RJ, Holmes DR, Reeder GS, et al. Immediate angioplasty compared with the administration of a thrombolytic agent followed by conservative treatment for myocardial infarction. N Engl J Med 1993;328:685–691.
107. Silverman KJ, Becker LC, Bulkley BH, et al. Value of early thallium-201 scintigraphy for predicting mortality in patients with acute myocardial infarction. Circulation 1980;61:996.
108. Perez-Gonzalez J, Botvinick EH, Dunn R, et al. The late prog-

nostic value of acute scintigraphic measurement of myocardial infarction size. Circulation 1982;66:960.
109. Gibson RS, Taylor GJ, Watson DD, et al. Prognostic significance of resting anterior thallium-201 defects in patients with inferior myocardial infarction. J Nucl Med 1980;21:1015.
110. Nestico PE, Hakki A, Felsher J, Heo J, Iskandrian AS. Implication of abnormal right ventricular thallium uptake in acute myocardial infarction. Am J Cardiol 1986;58:230.
111. Cerqueira MD, Maynard C, Ritchie JL, Davis KB, Kennedy JW. Long-term survival in 618 patients from the western Washington streptokinase in myocardial infarction trials. J Am Coll Cardiol 1992;20:1452–1459.
112. Gibson RS, Watson DD, Craddock GB, et al. Prediction of cardiac events after uncomplicated myocardial infarction: a prospective study comparing predischarge exercise thallium-201 scintigraphy and coronary angiography. Circulation 1983;68:321.
113. Leppo JA, O'Brien J, Rothendler JA, Getchell JD, Lee VW. Dipyridamole-thallium-201 scintigraphy in the prediction of future cardiac events after acute myocardial infarction. N Engl J Med 1984;310:1014.
114. Brown KA, O'Meara J, Chambers CE, Plante DA. Ability of dipyridamole-thallium-201 imaging one to four days after acute myocardial infarction to predict in-hospital and late recurrent myocardial ischemic events. Am J Cardiol 1990;65:160–167.
115. Tilkemeier PL, Guiney TE, LaRaia PJ, Boucher CA. Prognostic value of predischarge low-level exercise thallium testing after thrombolytic treatment of a acute myocardial infarction. Am J Cardiol 1990;66:1203–1207.
116. Wackers FJTh, Zaret BL, Chaitman B, Wasserman A, Thompson B. The prognostic significance of reverse redistribution on thallium-201 stress testing after thrombolytic therapy for acute infarction. JACC 1992;19(Suppl A):22A.
117. Gimple LW, Beller GA. Assessing prognosis after acute myocardial infarction in the thrombolytic era. J Nucl Cardiol 1994; 1:198–209.
118. Zaret BL, Wackers FJ, Terrin M, et al. Does left ventricular ejection fraction following thrombolytic therapy have the same prognostic impact described in the prethrombolytic ERA? Results of the TIMI II trial. JACC 1991;17(Suppl II):214A.
119. McCallister BD, Christian TF, Gersh BJ. Prognosis of myocardial infarctions involving more than 40% of the left ventricle after acute reperfusion therapy. Circulation 1993;88(Pt 1):1470–1475.
120. Wackers FJTh, Lie KI, Liem KL, et al. Potential value of thallium-201 scintigraphy as a means of selecting patients for the coronary care unit. Br Heart J 1979;41:111.
121. Van der Wieken LR, Kan G, Belfer AJ, et al. Thallium-201 scanning to decide CCU admissions in patients in the acute phase of myocardial infarction. Int J Cardio 1983;4:285.
122. Varetto T, Cantalupi D, Altiero, Orlandi C. Emergency room technetium-99m-sestamibi imaging to rule out acute myocardial ischemic events in patients with nondiagnostic electrocardiograms. J Am Coll Cardiol 1993;22:1804–1808.
123. Hilton TC, Thompson RC, Williams HJ, et al. Technetium-99m-sestamibi myocardial perfusion imaging in the emergency room evaluation of chest pain. J Am Coll Cardiol 1994;23:1016–1022.
124. Radensky PW, Stowers SA, Hilton TC, Fulmer H, McLaughlin BA. Cost-effectiveness of acute myocardial perfusion imaging with Tc-99m-sestamibi for risk stratification of emergency room patients with acute chest pain. Circulation 1994;90:I528.
125. Weich HF, Strauss HW, Pitt B. The extraction of thallium-201 by the myocardium. Circulation 1977;56:188.
126. Goldhaber SZ, Newell JB, Ingwall JS, Pohost GM, Alpert NM, Fossel ET. Effects of reduced coronary flow on thallium-201 accumulation and release in in vivo and in vitro rate heart preparation. Am J Cardiol 1983;51:891.
127. Leppo JA, Macneil PB, Moring AF, Apstein CS. Separate effects of ischemia, hypoxia, and contractility of thallium-201 kinetics in rabbit myocardium. J Nucl Med 1986;27:66.
128. Pohost GM, Alpert NM, Ingwall JS, Strauss HW. Thallium redistribution: mechanisms and clinical utility. Semin Nucl Med 1980;10:70–93.
129. Okada RD, Glover D, Gaffney T, Williams S. Myocardial kinetics of technetium-99m-hexakis-2-methoxy-2-methylpropyl-isonitrile. Circulation, 1988;2:491–8.
130. Meerdink DJ, Leppo JA. Comparison of hypoxia and ouabain effects on the myocardial uptake kinetics of technetium-99m hexakis 2-methoxyisobutyl isonitrile and thallium-201. J Nucl Med 1989;30:1500–1506.
131. Melon PG, Beanlands RS, DeGrado TR, et al. Comparison of technetium-99m sestamibi and thallium-201 redistribution characteristics in canine myocardium. J Am Coll Cardiol 1992; 20:1277–1283.
132. Piwnica-Worms D, Chiu ML, Kronauge JF. Divergent kinetics of ^{201}Tl and ^{99m}Tc-sestamibi in cultured chick ventricular myocytes during ATP depletion. Circulation 1992;85:1531–1541.
133. Wackers FJTh, Lie KI, Liem KL, et al. Thallium-201 scintigraphy in unstable angina pectoris. Circulation 1978;57:738.
134. Berger BC, Watson DD, Burwell LR, et al. Redistribution of thallium at rest in patients with stable and unstable angina and the effect of coronary artery bypass surgery. Circulation 1979; 60:1114.
135. Maseri A, Parodi O, Severi S, et al. Transient transmural reduction of myocardial blood flow demonstrated by thallium-201 scintigraphy, as a cause of variant angina. Circulation 1976; 54:280.
136. Brown KA, Okada RD, Boucher CA, Phillips HR, Strauss HW, Pohost GM. Serial thallium-201 imaging at rest in patients with stable and unstable angina pectoris: relationship of myocardial perfusion at rest to presenting clinical syndromes. Am Heart J 1983;106:70.
137. Gewirtz H, Beller GA, Strauss HW, et al. Transient defects of resting thallium scans in patients with coronary artery disease. Circulation 1979;59:707.
138. Bilodeau L, Theroux P, Gregoire J, Gagnon D, Arsenault A. Technetium-99m sestamibi tomography in patients with spontaneous chest pain: correlations with clinical, electrocardiographic and angiographic findings. J Am Coll Cardiol 1991;18:1684–1691.
139. Wackers FJTh. Complete left bundle branch block: is the diagnosis of myocardial infarction possible? Int J Cardiol 1983; 2:521.
140. Wackers FJTh, Fetterman RC, Mattera JA, Clements JP. Quantitative planar thallium-201 stress scintigraphy: a critical evaluation of the method. Semin Nucl Med 1985;15:46.
141. DiCola VC, Downing SE, Donabedian RK, Zaret BL. Pathophysiological correlates of thallium-201 myocardial uptake in experimental infarction. Cardiovasc Res 1977;11:141.
142. Nielsen AP, Morris KG, Murdock R, Brune FP, Cobb FR. Linear relationship between the distribution of thallium-201 and blood flow in ischemic and nonischemic myocardium during exercise. Circulation 1980;61:797.
143. Nishiyama H, Adolph RJ, Gabel M, Lukes SJ, Franklin D, Williams CC. Effect of coronary blood flow on thallium-201 uptake and washout. Circulation 1980;61:797.
144. Patterson R, Halgash D, Micelli K, et al. "Steady state" problems in myocardial perfusion imaging to detect transient ischemia: critical role of the duration of the ischemic state after thallium-201 injection. Am J Cardiol 1979;43:357.
145. Wharton TP, Neill WA, Oxendine JM, Painter LN. Effect of duration of regional myocardial ischemia and degree of reactive hyperemia on the magnitude of the initial thallium-201 defect. Circulation 1980;62:516.
146. Lear JL. Effect of exercise position during stress testing on car-

diac and pulmonary thallium kinetics and accuracy in evaluating coronary artery disease. J Nucl Med 1986;27:788.

147. Bruce A. Comparative prevalence of segment ST depression after maximal exercise in healthy men in Seattle and Taipei. In: Simonson E, ed. Physical activity and the heart. Springfield, IL: Charles C Thomas, 1967.

149. Heo J, Kegel J, Iskandrian AS, Cave V, Iskandrian BB. Comparison of same-day protocols using technetium-99m-sestamibi myocardial imaging. J Nucl Med 1992;33:186–191.

150. Chua T, Kiat H, Germano G, et al. Technetium-99m teboroxime regional myocardial washout in subjects with and without coronary artery disease. Am J Cardiol 1993;72:728–734.

151. Berman DS, Kiat H, Friedman JD, et al. Separate acquisitions rest thallium-201/stress technetium-99m sestamibi dual-isotope myocardial perfusion single-photon emission computed tomography: a clinical validation study. J Am Coll Cardiol 1993; 22:1455–1464.

152. Wackers FJTh, Mattera J. Optimizing planar Tl-201 imaging: computer quantification. Cardio 1990;7:103–112.

153. Garcia EV, Cooke CD, Van Train KF, et al. Technical aspects of myocardial SPECT imaging with technetium-99m sestamibi. Am J Cardiol 1990;66:23E-31E.

154. Klein JL, Garcia EV, DePuey EG, et al. Reversibility bull's-eye: a new polar bull's-eye map to quantify reversibility of stress-induced SPECT thallium-201 myocardial perfusion defects. J Nucl Med 1990;31:1240–1246.

155. Beller GA, Watson DD, Pohost GM. Kinetics of thallium distribution and redistribution: clinical applications in sequential myocardial imaging. In: Strauss HW, Pitt B, eds. Cardiovascular nuclear medicine. 2d ed. St Louis: CV Mosby, 1979:225–242.

156. Beller GA, Watson DD, Ackell P, Pohost GM. Time course of thallium-201 redistribution after transient myocardial ischemia. Circulation 1980;61:791.

157. Weiss AT, Maddahi J, Lew AS, et al. Reverse redistribution of thallium-201: a sign of nontransmural myocardial infarction with patency of the infarct-related coronary artery. J Am Coll Cardiol 1986;7:61–67.

158. Boucher CA, Zir LM, Beller GA, et al. Increased lung uptake of thallium-201 during exercise myocardial imaging: clinical, hemodynamic and angiographic implications in patients with coronary artery disease. Am J Cardiol 1980;46:189.

159. Weiss AT, Berman DS, Lew AS, et al. Transient ischemic dilation of the left ventricle on stress thallium-201 scintigraphy: a marker of severe and extensive coronary artery disease. J Am Coll Cardiol 1987;9:752–759.

160. Okada RD, Dai YH, Boucher CA, Pohost GM. Serial thallium-201 imaging after dipyridamole for coronary disease detection: quantitative analysis using myocardial clearance. Am Heart J 1984; 107:475.

161. Okada RD, Leppo JA, Strauss HW, Boucher CA, Pohost GM. Mechanisms and time course of the disappearance of thallium-201 defects at rest in dogs. Am J Cardiol 1982;49:699.

162. Massie BM, Wisneski J, Dramer B, Hollenberg M, Gertz E, Stern D. Comparison of myocardial thallium-201 clearance after maximal and submaximal exercise: implications for diagnosis of coronary disease [Concise Communication]. J Nucl Med 1982; 23:381.

163. Kaul S, Chesler DA, Pohost GM, Strauss HW, Okada RD, Boucher CA. Influence of peak exercise heart rate on normal thallium-201 myocardial clearance. J Nucl Med 1986;27:26.

164. Grunwald AM, Watson DD, Holzgrefe HH, Irving JF, Beller GA. Myocardial thallium-201 kinetics in normal and ischemic myocardium. Circulation 1981;64:610.

165. Pohost GM, Okada RD, O'Keefe DD, et al. Thallium redistribution in dogs with severe coronary artery stenosis of fixed caliber. Circ Res 1981;48:439.

166. Okada RD. Myocardial kinetics of thallium-201 after stress in normal and perfusion-reduced canine myocardium. Am J Cardiol 1985;56:969.

167. Rothendler JA, Okada RD, Wilson RA, et al. Effect of a delay in commencing imaging on the ability to detect transient thallium defects. J Nucl Med 1985;26:880.

168. Okada RD, Glover D, Gaffney T, Williams S. Myocardial kinetics of technetium-99m-hexakis-2-methoxy-2-methylopropyl-isonitrile. Circulation 1988;77(2):491–498.

169. Zaret BL, Wackers FJTh. Medical progress. Nuclear cardiology. N Eng J Med 1993;329:11:773–783, 1993;329:12:855–863.

170. Beck JW, Tatum JL, Cobb FR, Harris CC, Goodrich KL. Myocardial perfusion imaging using thallium-201: a new algorithm for calculation of background activity. J Nucl Med 1979;20:1294.

171. Watson DD, Campbell NP, Read EK, Gibson RS, Teates CD, Beller GA. Spatial and temporal quantitation of plane thallium myocardial images. J Nucl Med 1981;22:577.

172. Garcia E, Maddahi J, Berman DS, Waxman A. Space/time quantitation of thallium-201 myocardial scintigraphy. J Nucl Med 1981;22:309.

173. Garcia EV, van Train K, Maddahi J, et al. Quantification of rotational thallium-201 myocardial tomography. J Nucl Med 1985; 26:17.

174. Liu YH, Sinusas AJ, Shi QX. Quantification of Tc-99m-sestamibi SPECT using mean counts improves accuracy for assessment of relative blood flow: experimental validation. Circulation 1994; 90:I365.

175. Wackers FJTh, Bodenheimer M, Fleiss JL, Brown M, and the MSSMI Tl-201 Investigators. Factors affecting uniformity in interpretation of planar Tl-201 imaging in a multicenter trial. J Am Coll Cardiol 1993;21:1064–1074.

176. Alazaraki NP, Krawczynska EG, DePuey EG, et al. Reproducibility of thallium-201 exercise SPECT studies. J Nucl Med 1994; 35:1237–1244.

177. Ritchie JL, Trobaugh GB, Hamilton GW, et al. Myocardial imaging and thallium-201 at rest and during exercise. Comparison and coronary arteriography and resting and stress electrocardiography. Circulation 1977;56:66.

178. Bailey IK, Griffith LSC, Rouleau J, Strauss HW, Pitt B. Thallium-201 myocardial perfusion imaging at rest and during exercise. Circulation 1977;55:79.

179. Botvinick EH, Taradash MR, Shames DM, Parmley WW. Thallium-201 myocardial perfusion scintigraphy for the clinical clarification of normal, abnormal and equivocal electrocardiographic stress tests. Am J Cardiol 1978;41:43.

180. Ritchie JL, Zaret BL, Strauss HW, et al. Myocardial imaging with thallium-201: a multicenter study in patients with angina pectoris or acute myocardial infarction. Am J Cardiol 1978;42:345.

181. Dunn RF, Freedman B, Bailey IK, Uren F, Kelly DT. Exercise thallium imaging: location of perfusion abnormalities in single vessel coronary disease. J Nucl Med 1980;21:717.

182. Iskandrian AS, Wasserman LA, Anderson GS, Hakki H, Segal BL, Kane S. Merits of stress thallium-201 myocardial perfusion imaging in patients with inconclusive exercise electrocardiograms: correlation with coronary arteriograms. Am J Cardiol 1980; 46:553.

183. Friedman TD, Greene AC, Iskandrian AS, Hakki A, Kane SA, Segal BL. Exercise thallium-201 myocardial scintigraphy in women: correlation with coronary arteriography. Am J Cardiol 1982;49:1632.

184. Maddahi J, Garcia EV, Berman DS, Waxman A, Swan HJC, Forrester J. Improved noninvasive assessment of coronary artery disease by quantitative analysis of regional stress myocardial distribution and washout of thallium-201. Circulation 1981; 64:924.

185. Berger BC, Watson DD, Taylor GJ, et al. Quantitative thallium-201 exercise scintigraphy for detection of coronary artery disease. J Nucl Med 1981;22:585.

186. Kaul S, Boucher CA, Newell JB. Determination of the quantitative thallium imaging variables that optimize detection of coronary artery disease. J Am Coll Cardiol 1986;7:527–537.
187. van Train KF, Berman DS, Garcia EV, et al. Quantitative analysis of stress thallium-201 myocardial scintigrams: a multicenter trial. J Nucl Med 1986;217:17.
188. Maddahi J, Abdulla A, Garcia EV, Swan HJC, Berman DS. Noninvasive identification of left main and triple vessel coronary artery disease: improved accuracy using quantitative analysis of regional myocardial stress distribution and washout of thallium-201. J Am Coll Cardiol 1986;7:53.
189. Dash H, Massie BM, Botvinick EH, Brundage GH. The noninvasive identification of left main and three-vessel coronary artery disease by myocardial stress perfusion scintigraphy and treadmill exercise electrocardiography. Circulation 1979;60:276.
190. Rehn T, Griffith LSC, Achuff SC, et al. Exercise thallium-201 myocardial imaging in left main coronary artery disease: sensitive but not specific. Am J Cardiol 1981;48:217.
191. Nygaard TW, Gibson RS, Ryan JM, Gascho JA, Watson DD, Beller GA. Prevalence of high-risk thallium-201 scintigraphic findings in left main coronary artery stenosis: comparison with patients with multiple- and single-vessel coronary artery disease. Am J Cardiol 1984;53:462.
192. Maddahi J, Van Train K, Prigent F, et al. Quantitative single photon emission computed thallium-201 tomography for detection and localization of coronary artery disease: optimization and prospective validation of a new technique. J Am Coll Cardiol 1989; 14:1689–1699.
193. DePasquale EE, Nody AC, DePuey EG, et al. Quantitative rotational thallium-201 tomography for identifying and localizing coronary artery disease. Circulation 1988;77(2):316–327.
194. Fintel DJ, Links JM, Brinker JA, Frank TL, Parker M, Becker LC. Improved diagnostic performance of exercise thallium-201 single photon emission computed tomography over planar imaging in the diagnosis of coronary artery disease: a receiver operating characteristic analysis. J Am Coll Cardiol 1989;13:600–612.
195. Mahmarian JJ, Boyce, Goldberg RK, Cocanougher MK, Roberts R, Verani MS. Quantitative exercise thallium-201 single photo emission computed tomography for the enhanced diagnosis of ischemic heart disease. J Am Coll Cardiol 1990;15:318–329.
196. Go RT, Marwick TH, MacIntyre WJ, et al. A prospective comparison of rubidium-82 PET and thallium-201 SPECT myocardial perfusion imaging utilizing a single dipyridamole stress in the diagnosis of coronary artery disease. J Nucl Med 1990;31:1899–1905.
197. Tamaki N, Yonekura Y, Mukai T, et al. Stress thallium-201 transaxial emission computed tomography tomography: quantitative versus qualitative analysis for evaluation of coronary artery disease. J Am Coll Cardiol 1984;4:1213–1221.
198. Iskandrian AS, Heo J, Kong B, et al. Effect of exercise level on the ability of thallium-201 tomographic imaging in detecting coronary artery disease: analysis of 461 patients. J Am Coll Cardiol 1989;14:1477–1486.
199. Van Train KF, Maddahi J, Berman DS, et al. Quantitative analysis of tomographic stress thallium-201 myocardial scintigrams: a multicenter trial. J Nucl Med 1990;31:1168–1179.
200. Borges-Neto S, Mahmarian JJ, Jain A, et al. Quantitative thallium-201 single photon emission computed tomography after oral dipyridamole for assessing the presence, anatomic location and severity of coronary artery disease. J Am Coll Cardiol 1988; 11:962–969.
201. Rozanski A, Diamond GA, Forrester JS, Berman D, Morris D, Swan HJC. Comparison of alternative referent standards for cardiac normality. Implications for diagnostic testilng. Ann Intern Med 1984;101:164–171.
202. Taillefer R, Lambert R, Dupras G, et al. Clinical comparison between thallium-201 and Tc-99m-methoxyisobutyl isonitrile (hexamibi) myocardial perfusion imaging for the detection of coronary artery disease. Eur J Nucl Med 1989;15:280–286.
203. Iskandrian A, Heo J, Kong B, Lyons E, Marsch S. Use of technetium-99m isonitrile (RP-30A) in assessing left ventricular perfusion and function at rest and during exercise in coronary artery disease, and comparison with coronary arteriography and exercise thallium-201 SPECT imaging. Am J Cardiol 1989; 64:270–275.
204. Maddahi J, Kiat H, Friedman JD, Berman DS, Van Train KF, Garcia EV. Technetium-99m-sestamibi myocardial perfusion imaging for evaluation of coronary artery disease. In: Zaret BL, Beller GA, eds. Nuclear cardiology. St. Louis: C.V. Mosby, 1993:191–200.
205. Iskandrian AS, Heo J, Nguyen T, et al. Tomographic myocardial perfusion imaging with technetium-99m teboroxime during adenosine-induced coronary hyperemia: correlation with thallium-201 imaging. J Am Coll Cardiol 1992;19:307–312.
206. Serafini AN, Topchik S, Jiminez H, Friden A, Ganz WI, Sfakianakis GN. Clinical comparison of technetium-99m-teboroxime and thallium-201 utilizing a continuous SPECT imaging protocol. J Nucl Med 1992;33:1304–1311.
207. Rigo P, Leclercq B, Itti R, Lahiri A, Braat S. Technetium-99m-tetrofosmin myocardial imaging: a comparison with thallium-201 and angiography. J Nucl Med 1994;35:587–593.
208. Takahashi N, Tamaki N, Tadamura E, et al. Combined assessment of regional perfusion and wall motion in patients with coronary artery disease with technetium-99m-tetrofosmin. J Nucl Cardiol 1994;1:29–38.
209. Heo J, Cave V, Wasserleben V, Iskandrian AS. Planar and tomographic imaging with technetium 99m-labled tetrofosmin: Correlation with thallium 201 and coronary angiographay. J Nucl Cardiol 1994;1:317–324.
210. Hendel RC, Gerson MC, Verani MS, et al. Perfusion imaging with Tc-99m furisfosmin (Q 12): multicenter phase III trial to evaluate safety and comparative efficacy. Circulation 1994;90:I449.
211. Gibson RS, Watson DD, Carabello BA, Holt ND, Beller GA. Clinical implications of increased lung intake of thallium-201 during exercise scintigraphy 2 weeks after myocardial infarction. Am J Cardiol 1982;49:1586.
212. Kushner FG, Okada RD, Kirshenbaum HD, Boucher CA, Strauss HW, Pohost GM. Lung thallium-201 uptake after stress testing in patients with coronary artery disease. Circulation 1981; 63:341.
213. Gill JB, Ruddy TD, Newell JB, Finkelstein DM, Strauss HW, Boucher CA. Prognostic importance of thallium uptake by the lungs during exercise in coronary artery disease. N Engl J Med 1987; 317:1485–1489.
214. Saha M, Farrand TF, Brown KA. Lung uptake of technetium 99m sestamibi: relation to cinical, exercise, hemodynamic, and left ventricular function variables. J Nucl Cardiol 1994;1:52–56.
215. Brown KA, Boucher CA, Okada RD, et al. Prognostic value of exercise thallium-201 imaging in patients presenting for evaluation of chest pain. J Am Coll Cardiol 1983;1:994.
216. Ladenheim ML, Pollock BH, Rozanski A, et al. Extent and severity of myocardial hypoperfusion as predictors of prognosis in patients with suspected coronary artery disease. J Am Coll Cardiol 1986;7:464.
217. Bodenheimer M, Wackers FJTh, Schwartz R, Brown M. Prognostic significance of a fixed thallium defect in patients with stable coronary artery disease. Am J Cardiol 1994;(in press).
218. Abraham RD, Freedman SB, Dunn RF, et al. Prediction of multivessel coronary artery disease and prognosis early after acute myocardial infarction by exercise electrocardiography and thallium-201 myocardial rfusion scanning. Am J Cardiol 1986; 58:423.
219. Candell-Riera J, Permanyer-Miralda G, Castell L, et al. Uncom-

plicated first myocardial infarction: strategy for comprehensive prognostic studies. J Am Coll Cardiol 1991;18:1207–1219.
220. Silva P, Galli M, Campolo L. Prognostic significance of early ischemia after acute myocardial infarction in low-risk patients. Am J Cardiol 1993;71:1142–1147.
221. Freeman MR, Chisholm RJ, Armstrong PW. Usefulness of exercise electrocardiography and thallium scintigraphy in unstable angina pectoris in predicting the extent and severity of coronary artery disease. Am J Cardiol 1988;62:1164–1170.
222. Kaul S, Lilly DR, Gascho JA, et al. Prognostic utility of the exercise thallium-201 test in ambulatory patients with chest pain: comparison with cardiac catheterization. Circulation 1988; 77:745–758.
223. Brown KA. Prognostic value of thallium-201 myocardial perfusion imaging. A diagnostic tool comes of age. Circulation 1991; 83:363–381.
224. Fagan LF, Shaw L, Kong BA, Caralis DG, Wiens RD, Chaitman BR. Prognostic Value of exercise thallium scintigraphy in patients with good exercise tolerance and a normal or abnormal exercise electrocardiogram and suspected or confirmed coronary artery disease. Am J Cardiol 1992;69:607–611.
225. Moss AJ, Goldstein RE, Hall WJ, et al. Detection and significance of myocardial ischemia in stable patients after recovery from an acute coronary event. JAMA 1993;269:2379–2385.
226. Machecourt J, Longere P, Fagret D, et al. Prognostic value of thallium-201 single-photon emission computed tomographic myocardial perfusion imaging according to extent of myocardial defect. J Am Coll Cardiol 1994;23:1096–106.
227. Wackers FJTh, Russo DJ, Russo D, Clements JP. Prognostic significance of normal quantitative planar thallium-201 stress scintigraphy in patients with chest pain. J Am Coll Cardiol 1985; 6:27.
228. Pamelia FX, Gibson RS, Watson DD, Craddock GB, Sirowatka J, Beller GA. Prognosis with chest pain and normal thallium-201 exercise scintigrams. Am J Cardiol 1985;55:920.
229. Wahl J, Hakki AH, Iskandrian AS. Prognostic implications of normal exercise thallium-201 images. Arch Intern Med 1985; 145:253.
230. Staniloff HM, Forrester JS, Berman DS, Swan JHC. Prediction of death, myocardial infarction, and worsening chest pain using thallium scintigraphy and exercise electrocardiography. J Nucl Med 1986;27:1842.
231. Brown KA, Altland E, Rowen M. Prognostic value of normal Tc-99m sestamibi cardiac imaging. J Nucl Med 1994;35:554–557.
232. Raiker K, Sinusas AJ, Zaret BL, Wackers FJTh. One-year prognosis of patients with normal Tc-99m-sestamibi stress imaging. Circulation 1993;88(Suppl):1486.
233. Berman DS, Kiat H, Cohen J, et al. Prognosis of 1044 patients with normal exercise Tc-99m sestamibi myocardial perfusion SPECT. J Am Coll Cardiol 1994;23:1A-63A.
234. Haronian HL, Remetz MS, Sinusas AJ, et al. Myocardial risk area defined by technetium-99m sestamibi imaging during percutaneous transluminal coronary angioplasty: comparison with coronary angiography. J Am Coll Cardiol 1993;22:1033–1043.
235. Pollock SG, Abbott RD, Boucher CA, Beller GA, Kaul S. Independent and incremental prognostic value of tests performed in hierarchical order to evaluate patients with suspected coronary artery disease. Circulation 1992;85:237–248.
236. Melin JA, Robert A, Luwaert R, Beckers C, Detry J-M. Additional prognostic value of exercise testing and thallium-201 scintigraphy in catheterized patients without previous myocardial infarction. Int J Cardiol 1990;27:235–243.
237. Iskandrian AS, Chae SC, Heo J, Stanberry CD, Wasserleben V, Cave V. Independent and incremental prognostic value of exercise single-photon emission computed tomographic (SPECT) thallium imaging in coronary artery disease. J Am Coll Cardiol 1993;22:665–670.
238. Petretta M, Cuocolo A, Carpinelli A, et al. Prognostic value of myocardial hypoperfusion indexes in patients with suspected or known coronary artery disease. J Nucl Cardiol 1994;1:325–337.
239. Miller DD, Stratmann HG, Shaw L, et al. Dipyridamole technetium 99m sestamibi myocardial tomography as an independent predictor of cardiac event-free survival after acute ischemic events. J Nucl Cardiol 1994;1:172–82.
240. Manyari DE, Knudtson M, Kloiber R, Roth D. Sequential thallium-201 myocardial perfusion studies after successful percutaneous transluminal coronary artery angioplasty: delayed resolution of exercise-induced scintigraphic abnormalities. Circulation 1988;77(1):86–95.
241. Hecht HS, Shaw RE, Bruce TR, Ryan C, Stertzer SH, Myler RK. Usefulness of tomographic thallium-201 imaging for detection of restenosis after percutaneous transluminal coronary angioplasty. Am J Cardiol 1990;66:1314–1318.
242. Jain A, Mahmarian JJ, Borges-Neto S, et al. Clinical significance of perfusion defects by thallium-201 single photon emission tomography following oral dipyridamole early after coronary angioplasty. J Am Coll Cardiol 1988;11:970–976.
243. Miller DD, Liu P, Strauss HW, Block PC, Okada RD, Boucher CA. Prognostic value of computer-quantitated exercise thallium imaging early after percutaneous transluminal coronary angioplasty. J Am Coll Cardiol 1987;10:275–283.
244. Gould KL. Noninvasive assessment of coronary stenoses by myocardial perfusion imaging during pharmacologic coronary vasodilatation. I. Physiologic basis and experimental validation. Am J Cardiol 1978;41:267.
245. Gould KL, Westcott RJ, Albro PC, Hamilton GW. Noninvasive assessment of coronary stenoses by myocardial imaging during pharmacologic coronary vasodilatation. II. Clinical methodology and feasibility. Am J Cardiol 1978;41:279.
246. Albro PC, Gould KL, Westcott RJ, Hamilton GW, Ritchie JL, Williams DL. Noninvasive assessment of coronary stenoses by myocardial imaging during pharmacologic coronary vasodilatation. III. Clinical trial. Am J Cardiol 1978;42:751.
247. Sochor H, Pachinger O, Orgris E, Probst P, Kaindl F. Radionuclide imaging after coronary vasodilatation: myocardial scintigraphy with thallium-201 and radionuclide angiography after administration of dipyridamole. Eur Heart J 1984;5:500.
248. Feldman RL, Nichols WW, Pepine CJ, Conti CR. Acute effect of intravenous dipyridamole on regional coronary hemodynamics and metabolism. Circulation 1981;64:333.
249. Iskandrian AS, Verani MS, Heo J. Pharmacologic stress testing: mechanism of action, hemodynamic responses, and results in detection of coronary artery disease. J Nucl Cardiol 1994;1:94–111.
250. Warltier DC, Gross GT, Brooks HL. Coronary steal-induced increase in myocardial infarct size after pharmacologic coronary vasodilatation. Am J Cardiol 1980;46:83.
251. Ranhosky A, Kempthorne-Rawson J. The safety of intravenous dipyridamole thallium myocardial perfusion imaging. Circulation 1990;81:1205–1209.
252. Wackers FJTh. Adenosine-thallium imaging: faster and better? JACC 1990;16(6):1384–1386.
253. Josephson MA, Brown BG, Hecht HS, Hopkins J, Pierce CD, Petersen RB. Noninvasive detection and localization of coronary stenoses in patients: comparison of resting dipyridamole and exercise thallium-201 myocardial perfusion imaging. Am Heart J 1982;103:1008.
254. Santos-O'Campos CD, Herman SD, Travin MI, et al. Comparison of exercise, dipyridamole, and adenosine by use of technetium 99m sestamibi tomographic imaging. J Nucl Cardiol 1994;1:57–64.
255. Francisco DA, Collins SM, Go RT, et al. Tomographic thallium-201 myocardial perfusion scintigrams after maximal coronary artery vasodilation with intravenous dipyridamole: comparison

of qualitative and quantitative approaches. Circulation 1982; 66:370–379.

256. Lam JYT, Chaitman BR, Glaenzer M, et al. Safety and diagnostic accuracy of dipyridamole-thallium imaging in the elderly. J Am Coll Cardiol 1988;11:585–589.

257. Huikuri Hv, Korhonen UR, Airaksinen J, et al. Comparison of dipyridamole-handgrip test and bicycle exercise test for thallium tomographic imaging. Am J Cardiology 1988;61:264–268.

258. Mendelson MA, Spies SM, Spies WG, et al. Usefulness of single-photon emission computed tomography of thallium-201 uptake after dipyridamole infusion for detection of coronary artery disease. Am J Cardiol 1992;69:1150–1155.

259. Kong BA, Shaw L, Miller DD, et al. Comparison of accuracy for detecting coronary artery disease and side-effect profile of dipyridamole thallium-201 myocardial perfusion imaging in women versus men. Am J Cardiol 1992;70:168–173.

260. Verani MS, Mahmarian JJ, Hixson JB, et al. Diagnosis of coronary artery disease by controlled coronary vasodilation with adenosine and thallium-201 scintigraphy in patents unable to exercise. Circulation 1990;82:80–87.

261. Nguyen T, Heo J, Obilby D, et al. Single photon emission computed tomography with thallium-201 during adenosine-induced coronary hyperemia: correlation with coronary anteriography, exercise thallium imaging and two-dimensional echocardiography. J Am Coll Cardiol 1990;16:1375–1383.

262. Iskandrian AS, Heo J, Nguyen T, et al. Assessment of coronary artery disease using single photon emission computed tomography with thallium-201 during adenosine induced coronary hyperemia. Am J Cardiol 1991;67:1190–1194.

263. Coyne EP, Belvedere DA, Vande Streek PR, et al. Thallium-201 scintigraphy after intravenous infusion of adenosine compared with exercise thallium testing in the diagnosis of coronary artery disease. J Am Coll Cardiol 1991;17:1289–1294.

264. Nishimura S, Mahmarian JJ, Boyce TM, et al. Equivalence between adenosine and exercise thallium-201 myocardial tomography: a multicenter, prospective, crossover trial. J Am Coll Cardiol 1992;20:265–275.

265. Gupta NC, Esterbrooks DJ, Hilleman E, et al. Comparison of adenosine and exercise thallium-201 single photon emission computed tomography (SPECT) myocardial perfusion imaging. J Am Coll Cardiol 1992;19:248–257.

266. Boucher CA, Brewster DC, Darling RC, Okada RD, Strauss HW, Pohost GM. Determination of cardiac risk by dipyridamole-thallium imaging before peripheral vascular surgery. N Engl J Med 1985;312:389.

267. Younis L, Stratmann H, Takase B, Byers S, Chaitman BR, Miller DD. Preoperative clinical assessment and dipyridamole thallium-201 scintigraphy for prediction and prevention of cardiac events in patients having major noncardiovascular surgery and known or suspected coronary artery disease. Am J Cardiol 1994; 74:311–317.

268. Stratmann HG, Tamesis BR, Younis LT, Wittry MD, Miller DD. Prognostic value of dipyridamole technetium-99m-sestamibi myocardial tomography in patients with stable chest pain who are unable to exercise. Am J Cardiol 1994;73:647–652.

269. Eagle KA, Singer DE, Brewster DC, Darling RC, Mulley AG, Boucher CA. Dipyridamole-thallium scanning patients undergoing vascular surgery. Optimizing preoperative evaluation of cardiac risk. JAMA 1987;257:2385–2189.

270. Lette J, Waters D, Lapointe J, et al. Usefulness of the severity and extent of reversible, perfusion defects during thallium dipyridamole imaging for cardiac risk assessment before noncardiac surgery. Am J Cardiol 1989;64:276–281.

271. Brown KA, Rowen M. Extent of jeopardized viable myocardium determined by myocardial perfusion imaging best predicts perioperatiive cardiac events in patients undergoing noncardiac surgery. J Am Coll Cardiol 1993;21:335–340.

272. Hendel RC, Whitfield SS, Villegas BJ, Cutler BS, Leppo JA. Prediction of late cardiac events by dipyridamole thallium imaging in patients undergoing elective vascular surgery. Am J Cardiol 1992;70:1243–1249.

273. Pennell DJ, Underwood R, Swanton RH, Walker M, Ell PJ. Dobutamine thallium myocardial perfusion tomography. J Am Coll Cardiol 1991;18:147–149.

274. Eilliot BM, Robison JG, Zellner JL, Hendrix GH. Dobutamine-^{201}Tl imaging assessing cardiac risks associated with vascular surgery. Circulation 1991;84(Suppl III):III-54-III-60.

275. Hays JT, Mahmarian JJ, Cochran AJ, Verani MS. Dobutamine thallium-201 tomography for evaluating patients with suspected coronary artery disease unable to undergo exercise or vasodilator pharmacologic stress testing. J Am Coll Cardiol 1993; 21:1583–1590.

276. Diamond GA, Forrester JS. Analysis of probability as an aid in the clinical diagnosis of coronary artery disease. N Engl J Med 1979;300:1350.

277. Epstein SE. Implications of probability analysis on the strategy used for noninvasive detection of coronary artery disease. Role of single or combined use of exercise electrocardiographic testing, radionuclide cineangiography and myocardial perfusion imaging. Am J Cardiol 1980;46:491.

278. Patterson RE, Horowitz SF, Eng C, et al. Can exercise electrocardiography and thallium-201 myocardial imaging exclude the diagnosis of coronary artery disease? Am J Cardiol 1982; 49:1127.

279. Hlatky M, Botvinick E, Brundage B. Diagnostic accuracy of cardiologists compared with probability calculations using Bayes' rule. J Am Coll Cardiol 1982;49:1927.

280. Diamond GA, Staniloff HM, Forrester JS, Pollock BH, Swan HJC. Computer-assisted diagnosis in the noninvasive evaluation of patients with suspected coronary artery disease. J Am Coll Cardiol 1983;1:444.

281. Melin JA, Piret LJ, Vanbutsele RJM, et al. Diagnostic value of exercise electrocardiography and thallium myocardial scintigraphy in patients without previous myocardial infarction: a Bayesian approach. Circulation 1981;16:1019.

282. Hirzel HO, Senn M, Neusch K, et al. Thallium-201 scintigraphy in complete left bundle branch block. Am J Cardiol 1984;53:764.

283. Braat SH, Brugada P, Bar FW, Gorgels APM, Wellens HJJ. Thallium-201 exercise scintigraphy and left bundle branch block. Am J Cardiol 1985;55:224.

284. Meyer-Pavel MC, Logic JR. Ischemia-induced transient left bundle branch block during exercise documented by thallium-201 perfusion imaging. Eur J Nucl Med 1982;7:44.

286. Hodge J, Mattera J, Fetterman R, Williams B, Wackers FJTh. False-positive Tl-201 defects in left bundle branch block: relationship to left ventricular dilatation [Abstract]. J Am Coll Cardiol 1987;9:139A.

287. Matzer L, Kiat H, Friedman JD, Van Train K, Maddahi J, Berman DS. A new approach to the assessment of tomographic thallium-201 scintigraphy in patients with left bundle branch block. J Am Coll Cardiol 1991;17:1309–1317.

288. Burns RJ, Galligan L, Wright LM, Lawand S, Burke RJ, Gladstone PJ. Improve specificity of myocardial thallium-201 single-photon emission computed tomography in patients with left bundle branch block by dipyridamole. Am J Cardiol 1991; 68:504–508.

289. Berger HJ, Sands MJ, Davies RA, et al. Exercise left ventricular performance in patients with chest pain, ischemic-appearing exercise electrocardiograms, and angiographically normal coronary arteries. Ann Intern Med 1981;94:186.

290. Meller J, Goldsmith SJ, Rudin A, et al. Spectrum of thallium-201 myocardial perfusion imaging in patients with chest pain and normal coronary angiogram. Am J Cardiol 1979; 43:717.

291. Berger BC, Abramowitz R, Park CH, et al. Abnormal thallium-201 scans in patients with chest pain and angiographically normal coronary arteries. Am J Cardiol 1983;52:365.
292. Legrand V, Hodgson JM, Bates ER, et al. Abnormal coronary flow reserve and abnormal radionuclide exercise test results in patients with normal coronary angiograms. J Am Coll Cardiol 1985; 6:1245.
293. Cannon RO, Bonow RO, Bacharach SL, et al. Left ventricular dysfunction in patients with angina pectoris, normal epicardial coronary arteries, and abnormal vasodilator reserve. Circulation 1985;71:218.
294. Gibbons RJ, Lee KL, Cobb FR, Jones RH. Ejection fraction response to exercise in patients with chest pain and normal coronary arteriograms. Circulation 1981;64:952.
295. Klein GJ, Kostuk WJ, Boughner DR, Chamberlain MJ. Stress myocardial imaging in mitral leaflet prolapse syndrome. Am J Cardiol 1978;42:746.
296. Massie B, Botvinick EH, Shames D, Taradash M, Werner J, Schiller N. Myocardial perfusion scintigraphy in patients with mitral valve prolapse. Its advantage over stress electrocardiography in diagnosing associated coronary artery disease and its implications for the etiology of chest pain. Circulation 1978; 57:19.
297. Bailey IK, Come PC, Kelly DT, et al. Thallium-201 myocardial perfusion imaging in aortic valve stenosis. Am J Cardiol 1977; 40:889.
298. Wasserman AG, Katz RJ, Varghese PJ, et al. Exercise radionuclide ventriculographic responses in hypertensive patients with chest pain. N Engl J Med 1984;311:1276.
299. Schulman DS, Francis CK, Black HR, Wackers FJTh. Thallium-201 stress imaging in hypertensive patients. Hypertension 1987; 10:16.
300. Makler PT, Lavine SJ, Denenberg BS, Bove AA, Idell S. Redistribution on the thallium scan in myocardial sarcoidosis [Concise Communication]. J Nucl Med 1981;22:428.
301. Kahan A, Devaux JY, Amor B, et al. Nifedipine and thallium-201 myocardial perfusion in progressive systemic sclerosis. N Engl J Med 1986;314:1397.

26 Cardiac Application of Positron Emission Tomography

M. SCHWAIGER and S. ZIEGLER

Positron emission tomography (PET) was introduced in the late 1970s as a new imaging modality in cardiology by investigators of the Washington University in St. Louis (1, 2). Studies included the use of metabolic tracers such as ^{18}F deoxyglucose and ^{11}C palmitate for the noninvasive characterization of myocardial substrate metabolism. These early studies demonstrated the ability of PET to describe the interaction of various substrates for cardiac energy metabolism, extending previous invasive investigations using arteriovenous sampling across the heart. Studies of myocardial perfusion were followed by introduction of flow markers such as ^{13}N ammonia and ^{15}O water, which aimed at the application of PET in patients with coronary artery disease. These first clinical applications were paralleled by rapid improvement of image technology, which advanced from one-slice tomographs to new multislice instrumentation providing excellent spatial resolution.

Clinical research concentrated primarily on the use of PET in patients with ischemic heart disease. Due to the improved image technology, PET perfusion imaging has been shown to be a superior method for the detection and characterization of coronary artery disease as compared to SPECT. The experimental and clinical experience with metabolic imaging led to the development of ^{18}F-fluorodeoxyglucose (FDG) as a marker of tissue viability in patients with advanced coronary artery disease. Based on these studies, PET became an accepted clinical tool for the detection of coronary artery disease as well as assessment of tissue viability.

This chapter reviews the current state of PET for the noninvasive characterization of coronary artery disease and other cardiovascular disorders. Validated clinical imaging protocols, as well as experimental concepts, are discussed. Finally, the results obtained with PET are compared with those derived from SPECT and other imaging modalities to define the current clinical role of PET in cardiology.

PET INSTRUMENTATION

Any quantitative analysis of tracer uptake requires the accurate measurement of the tracer distribution as well as the application of an appropriate kinetic model to dynamic PET data.

Common to all quantitative cardiac measurements is the procedure of attenuation measurement prior to tracer injection, reconstruction of transversal images, possible realignment according to the long axis of the heart, and region of interest (ROI) analysis to generate circumferential profiles or time-activity-curves. Since the left ventricular wall has a thickness of only about 10 cm, high spatial resolution is necessary for the quantitative analysis of tissue tracer concentration. Myocardial movement and change in wall thickness during the cardiac cycle affects the image resolution. Data quality can be improved by ECG gated acquisitions using state-of-the-art PET instrumentation. However, ECG gating may affect the temporal resolution of data acquisition.

The PET detector system has to perform linearly over a wide range of count rates and be sensitive to allow for short scan time intervals in order to monitor the rapid uptake and release of tracers. Most of the current commercial tomographs employ block detectors made of scintillation crystals (bismuth germanate) that are divided into up to 24 detector rings (3–5). Although cost-effective, this design limits the count rate performance of these scanners. Systems built with fast scintillation materials (barium fluoride) that include the information on the time-of-flight of the annihilation quanta, generally show a better signal-to-noise ratio and excellent high count rate performance (6–8). Their lower sensitivity and increased amount of data handling prohibited the widespread use of these systems in cardiac applications.

Correction of photon attenuation is a prerequisite for tracer distribution measurements in the heart. The attenuation factors are measured with external sources in a transmission scan. Ring or rotating pin sources made of positron emitters are used for this purpose. Several methods have been tested to reduce transmission scan time without loss in data quality. Smoothing of the transmission data increases the accuracy of the correction without any resolution loss in the emission images (9). Other approaches include segmentation of transmission images for classifying different regions as specific tissue types (10). Recent attempts to measure the transmission scans in single data acquisition mode overcome the deadtime problems of coincidence counting with high activity rotating sources and show promising results. Scanning time will be greatly reduced if transmission and emission data are measured simultaneously. This is possible if adequate masking in the sinograms is implemented (11, 12), a method already in use for brain studies and being tested for whole-body applications. The advantages of this method in clinical cardiac studies are obvious.

LIMITATIONS OF PET MEASUREMENTS

Scatter, dead time, counting statistics, and spatial resolution limit quantitative measurements in cardiac PET scanning (3). The effect of scattered radiation is small as long as the myocardial activity is high and lung activity is low. At very high count rates mispositioning of counts and loss of count rate due to dead time of block detector tomographs are noticeable. In current whole-body scanners, correction methods are implemented which compensate for deadtime loss associated with activities of 10–20 mCi in the field-of-view. Since such activity levels are typically encountered in cardiac images, prolonged tracer injection schemes are preferred to avoid high bolus activity during the first pass of the tracer.

The spatial resolution (6–7 mm) of a whole-body scanner results in spillover and partial volume effect which has to be addressed in quantitative cardiac measurements. Myocardial activity contaminates the neighboring blood pool activity in the left ventricle and vice versa. Since the activity concentration in the blood decreases and the myocardial count rate increases over time, the amount of spillover is not a constant. Small regions placed in the tissue of interest minimize the spillover effect. As a consequence of finite resolution, real activity concentration is recovered only in structures which extend over more than twice the FWHM of the tomograph (partial volume effect). Figure 26.1 shows that only with the advent of new, high resolution scanners, can the activity concentration in the 10-cm ventricular wall be fully recovered in the tomographic images. If the actual width of the myocardial wall is known, correction methods can be applied using the information on resolution distortion from phantom measurements. The size can be estimated by edge detection methods or by morphologic imaging modalities like ultrasound or MRI. Another approach determines the extravascular space by subtraction of a blood volume scan from the transmission data and uses this as myocardial tissue fraction in a given region of interest (13).

No further reference measurements are needed if the unknown fraction of blood pool contamination is included in the tracer kinetic model that is used to describe the measured tissue curve (14). In the last frames of the dynamic scan, the tissue ROIs are defined such that they contain some blood pool activity. The input function is generated by placing a very small ROI in the left ventricle, assuming that this region contains pure blood activity. The model parameters are determined by fitting the model equation, including a fourth parameter of tissue/blood fraction, to the measured tissue curves. With this method, spillover and partial volume effect are corrected at the same time, resulting in less biased rate constants (14).

Some of the current limitations in quantitative measurements will be solved when three-dimensional data acquisition is routinely available (15–17). Data are usually acquired in two-dimensional transaxial slices. New scanner developments that work without interplane septa, are aimed at facilitating the three-dimensional acquisition of coincident events. The count rate will increase drastically, allowing lower radiation doses, although the count rate limitations of the detector system must be kept in mind. Although the contribution of scattered events increases in these setups, an improvement by a factor of 3–4 is expected in sensitivity, which leads to a factor of 2 in noise equivalent count rates for cardiac studies (18). New problems might arise from the increased amount of scattered radiation originating in the liver and appropriate correction methods have to be developed.

TRACER KINETIC MODELING

As outlined in previous chapters, PET enables quantification of regional myocardial tracer distribution with high spatial resolution. With current PET instrumentation, scintigraphic data can be obtained with high temporal resolution necessary for the description of tracer kinetics in myocardial and vascular structures. In contrast to other organs, the large blood chambers of the right and left ventricles allow simultaneous measurements of radioactivity in blood and tissue. Several studies have validated the accuracy of this approach for the noninvasive determination

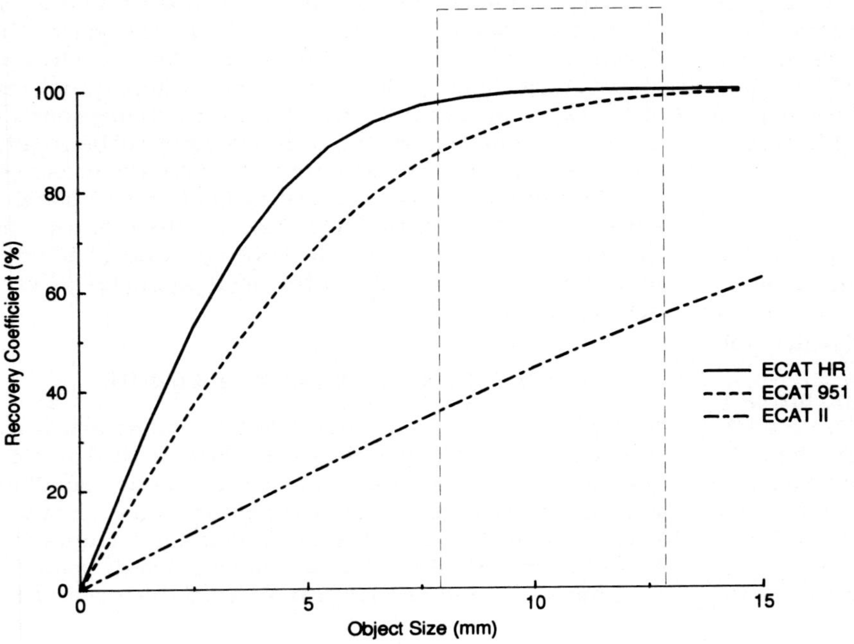

Figure 26.1. Recovery coefficients as a function of object size, according to the resolution of different scanner types. The *vertical dashed lines* delineate the dimensions of the myocardium.

of the arterial input function without the need of arterial blood sampling (19–21).

Combining temporal sequences of activity changes in blood and myocardium, tracer tissue uptake rates, as well as clearance of activity from tissue, can be quantitated. Depending on the radiopharmaceutical used, tracer kinetic models can be employed to derive estimates of myocardial blood flow, metabolic rate, and tissue tracer retention. The most commonly employed kinetic models are two or three compartment models. Although physiologic processes are more complicated than can be described by such simple models, limitations in counting statistics and duration of data acquisition require a simplification of the physiologic process to such models (22).

The use of tracer kinetic models requires an in-depth knowledge of the physiologic process under study, as well as extensive validation of the relationship between tracer and tracee. The advantage of PET tracers using ^{11}C, ^{15}O, ^{13}N, or ^{18}F is that the biologic behavior of most radiotracers is little altered and, thus, physiologic behavior of the tracer is very similar to that of the biologically active compound.

The quantitation of physiologic processes using tracer approaches requires steady-state conditions under which the study is performed. Only under steady-state conditions can the flux of substrates be quantitated using simplified tracer kinetic models. Additionally, PET measurements under various physiologic and pathophysiologic states assume a similar distribution volume of the tracer within the different compartments of the model. For example, the measurement of myocardial oxygen consumption based on ^{11}C acetate kinetics assumes that the distribution of ^{11}C within the various intracellular metabolite pools of ^{11}C acetate (i.e., glutamine, glutamate) remains constant in pathophysiologically altered myocardium. To prove this hypothesis, experimental data are necessary to reproduce a range of pathophysiologic conditions which may alter cardiac acetate metabolism, and to confirm the stability of the relationship between ^{11}C acetate kinetics and myocardial oxygen consumption.

Details of tracer kinetic models and how they apply to the assessment of myocardial blood flow, substrate metabolism, or measurement of receptor density is described later in the text.

Table 26.1.
PET Tracer for the Measurement of Myocardial Perfusion

	Physical Half-life (min)	Tissue Half-life	Energy (MeV)
^{82}Rb	1.3	hrs	3.3
^{81}Rb	276.0	hrs	1.1
^{38}K	7.6	min	2.7
[^{62}Cu]PTSM	9.8	hrs	2.9
[^{13}N]ammonia	10.0	hrs	1.2
[^{15}O]water	2.0	sec	1.7

ASSESSMENT OF MYOCARDIAL BLOOD FLOW

Table 26.1 shows all currently available blood flow tracers used in combination with PET. Based on the production of these radiopharmaceuticals, these tracers can be separated into two groups—one which requires a cyclotron for production, and a second which are generator-produced radiopharmaceuticals (23).

Radiopharmaceuticals can also be classified based on their physiologic behavior. ^{15}O water, for example, represents a freely diffusible tracer which washes in and out from myocardial tissue as a function of blood flow. The first pass extraction of ^{15}O water in the heart is neither diffusion-limited nor affected by any metabolic pathways. Therefore, ^{15}O water represents an ideal tracer for assessment of myocardial blood flow over a wide flow range (24–26). The time-course in the tissue ROI can be modeled by a single tissue compartment using the blood pool activity as an input function (Fig. 26.2).

The second group of flow markers are radiotracers retained in myocardial tissue proportional to myocardial blood flow ("chemical microspheres"). For these radiopharmaceuticals, the initial tracer extraction (first pass extrac-

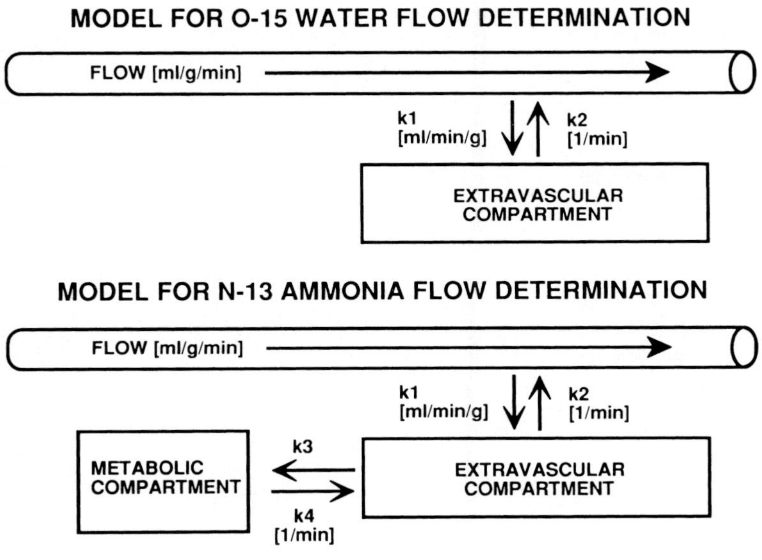

Figure 26.2. Compartmental description of perfusion measurements with [^{15}O]water and [^{13}N]ammonia. The rate constants k1 and k2 describe the exchange of [^{15}O]water between the vascular and extravascular compartment (*top*). The kinetics of [^{13}N]ammonia are described by a three-compartment model (*bottom*) with rate constants for the exchange between vascular and extravascular space (k1, k2) and the trapping in a metabolic compartment (k3, k4). Since metabolism of ^{13}N glutamine is slow, k4 is set to zero.

tion), as well as their tissue retention, are important factors defining their suitability as a blood flow tracer. ^{13}N ammonia is highly extracted by myocardial tissue in form of ^{13}N ammonia (27–29). Within the tissue the tracer can either back diffuse into the vascular space or be trapped in the form of ^{13}N-glutamine (Fig. 26.2). The relative activity retained in myocardial tissue following extraction is about 60–80% depending on the experimental model used (27, 29). The rate limiting step for the tissue retention of ^{13}N-ammonia is the glutamine synthetase reaction. This metabolic pathway is energy dependent and can be altered by extreme pathophysiologic conditions (pH, ischemia) affecting this metabolic pathway, as well as by pharmacologic interventions inhibiting transaminations (27, 29).

Ionic tracers such as ^{82}Rb, ^{81}Rb, or ^{38}K, display similar tracer kinetics as ^{201}Tl (30–34). Initial extraction of these compounds ranges between 60–80%. For both ^{13}N ammonia retention and ionic tracer extraction, a nonlinear relationship exists between blood flow and tissue tracer extraction (Fig. 26.3). With increasing flow rates, the transport of radiopharmaceuticals into the cell or its metabolic trapping (^{13}N-ammonia) becomes rate-limiting, reducing the net tissue retention fraction. Such a nonlinear relationship between tracer tissue uptake and blood flow limits the ability to quantitate myocardial perfusion based on tissue tracer concentration alone (35). However, correction factors or mathematic models can be employed to compensate for the known decrease of tracer extraction fraction at higher flow states (32, 36–38).

Besides the physiologic properties of the radiopharmaceuticals, the physical characteristics have to be considered. The physical half-life of myocardial blood flow tracers varies widely from only 76 seconds for ^{82}Rb to about 4 hours for ^{81}Rb. Short-lived radioisotopes are attractive for repeated blood flow measurements. However, relatively large amounts of radioactivity have to be administered to scintigraphically describe tracer uptake and retention. Most currently available PET scanners cannot cover such a range of activity exposure. For example, the initial bolus application of 60 mCi of ^{82}Rb causes considerable dead time losses in most PET cameras (3). Conversely, due to the rapid decay of activity, high sensitivity for activity detection is required several minutes after tracer injection. Additionally, technical personnel exposure to radiation is high when using a high activity bolus injection (^{15}O water) if an inadequate infusion system is used. This problem has been elegantly solved for the infusion of ^{82}Rb, which can be administered using an automated infusion system (39). Various infusion systems are being tested for the use of ^{15}O water (40).

A physical half-life of 5–20 minutes for ^{13}N-ammonia (10 min), ^{62}Cu (9.8 min), and ^{38}K (7.6 min) appears to provide an acceptable compromise between clinical practicability and image quality. These tracers can be slowly infused without causing considerable dead time losses and imaging protocols of 3–5 minutes provide adequate statistics yielding excellent image quality. Radiopharmaceuticals with a long physical half-life are not suitable for clinical cardiac studies because of the long waiting periods between rest and stress studies, and the relatively high radiation exposure.

The positron energy of the radioisotope is important for intrinsic resolution obtainable with each tracer. ^{82}Rb has a maximal positron energy of 3.3 MeV as compared to 1.2 MeV for ^{13}N. The positron energy determines how far positrons travel in tissue before they interact with electrons. Since PET data acquisition depends on the detection of the location of annihilation, the positron range in tissue affects the resolution of data acquisition. This factor, however, becomes only important if high resolution PET instrumentation, as well as cardiac gating, is employed. The positron range of the tracer is of less importance for image quality in cases where spatial resolution of about 1 cm is used for cardiac imaging.

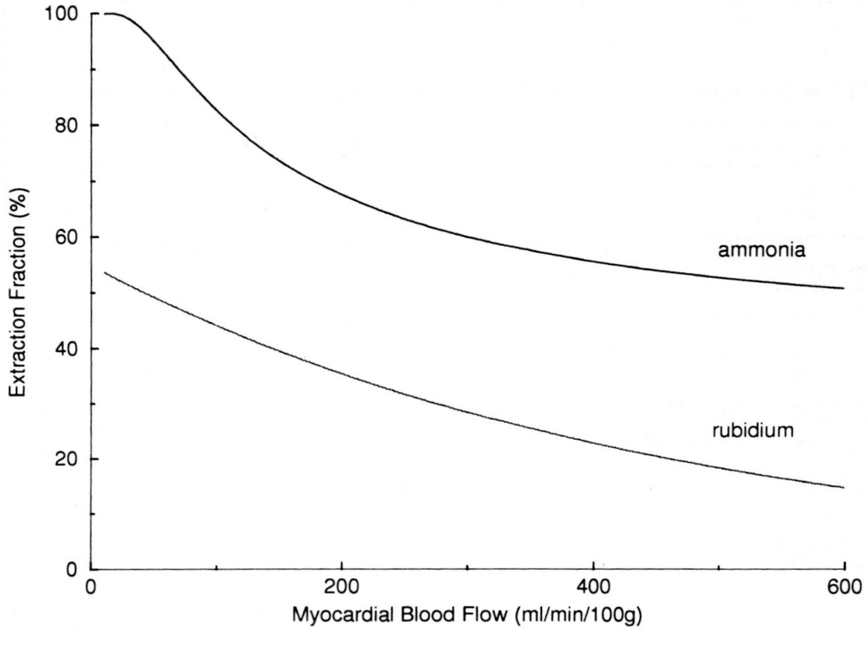

Figure 26.3. Extraction fraction of ammonia and rubidium versus blood flow, empirical values after Schelbert H, Phelps M, Huang S, et al. (27), and Mullani N, et al. (32).

CLINICAL APPLICATION

QUALITATIVE ASSESSMENT OF REGIONAL MYOCARDIAL BLOOD FLOW

First applications of PET for the detection of coronary artery disease consisted of the visual assessment of regional myocardial tracer distribution under rest and stress conditions (41–47). Most commonly, pharmacologic stress testing has been employed in order to assess coronary reserve (41). The advantage of this approach is the standardized stress procedure which can be performed in the PET gantry without moving the patient between rest and stress imaging. The exact positioning of patients is necessary for the attenuation correction of emission data. As discussed earlier, new approaches for simultaneous measurements of emission and transmission may decrease the incidence of motion artifacts and thus allow for stress procedures outside of the scanner gantry (46).

The most commonly used tracers are ^{82}Rb and ^{13}N-ammonia (27, 45). With ^{82}Rb, the rest/stress protocol can be completed in about 1 hour while ^{13}N-ammonia blood flow studies require about 2 hours. Extensive clinical experience exists with both radiopharmaceuticals. Figure 26.4 shows ^{13}N ammonia uptake under rest and stress conditions. Table 26.2 summarizes the reported values of sensitivity and specificity for the detection of coronary artery disease using ^{82}Rb or ^{13}N ammonia. Demer, et al. (47), demonstrated that there is very little difference between the use

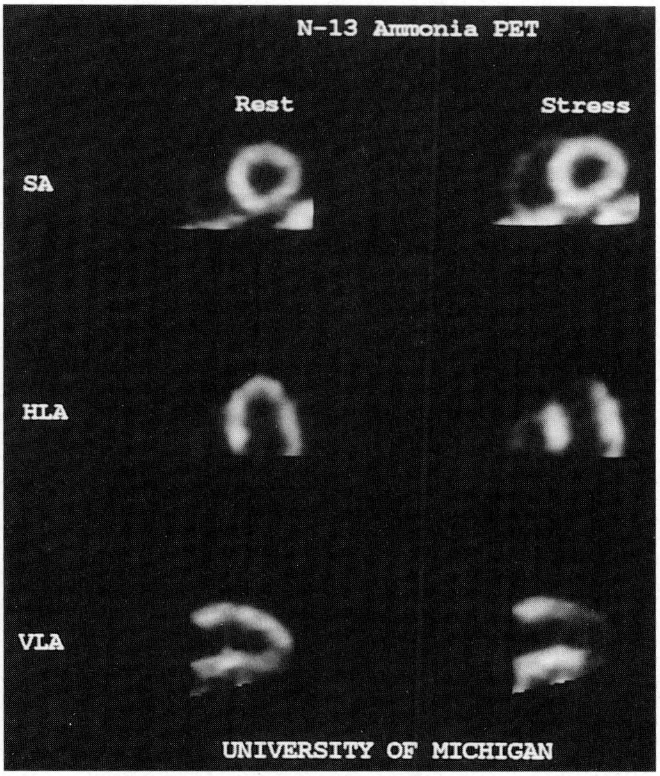

Figure 26.4. PET image of [^{13}N]ammonia uptake in normal myocardium under rest and stress conditions. The apical flow defect under stress is clearly visible in the horizontal long axis (HLA) and the vertical long axis (VLA) slices.

of either tracer for the detection of coronary artery disease. Most studies employed visual data analysis similar to the methods used routinely for ^{201}Tl or technetium-99m sestamibi SPECT imaging (28, 42, 43, 48). Automated approaches for semiquantitative data analysis similar to those used for SPECT imaging have also been developed for PET flow studies (49–51). Using a normal database regional perfusion abnormalities can be quantified in terms of severity as well as extent of perfusion defects (51). Newer approaches employing volumetric data sampling may provide absolute quantification of underperfused myocardial tissue volume based on the quantitative abilities of attenuation corrected PET images. Data are commonly displayed in polar map format, but three-dimensional projection of data on ellipsoids or left ventricular volume-rendered surfaces have been described (49–51) (Fig. 26.5). Initial studies comparing visual with semiquantitative analysis indicate improved inter- and intraobserver variability, as well as high diagnostic accuracy, for the semiquantitative data analysis (51, 52). These analysis approaches have also been applied to the localization of coronary artery disease with excellent results.

Demer, et al. (47), demonstrated that the severity of perfusion abnormalities determined by PET imaging correlated with the angiographically predicted coronary reserve measurements for a given vascular territory. These data demonstrate that PET images can be used not only for the detection of coronary artery disease, but also for the qualitative assessment of stenosis severity. In patients with previous myocardial infarction, the comparison of rest and stress images allows for the detection of reversible perfusion abnormalities. Stewart, et al. (53), demonstrated the superiority of rest/stress ^{82}Rb imaging over stress/redistribution ^{201}Tl SPECT for the definition of reversible stress-induced flow defects.

There are only a few studies comparing the diagnostic accuracy of ^{82}Rb PET or ^{13}N ammonia imaging for detection of CAD with that of ^{201}Tl SPECT imaging in the same patient population (Table 26.3). Combining the results of these studies in about 300 patients suggests that PET improves the diagnostic accuracy of SPECT by about 10%.

Go, et al. (42), from the Cleveland Clinic, used the simultaneous injection of ^{82}Rb and ^{201}Tl following pharmacologic stress testing to avoid variability caused by repeated stress testing. The results in 137 patients indicated a significantly higher sensitivity for PET in the detection of

Table 26.2.
Diagnostic Performance of PET in Combination with ^{13}N-ammonia or ^{82}Rb in Detection of Coronary Artery Disease

Reference	N	Tracer	Sens (%)	Spec (%)	Acc (%)
Gould(45)	50	Rb	95	100	
Yonekura(189)	49	NH_3	97	100	
Williams(190)	146	Rb	98	100	96
Schelbert(191)	32	NH_3	97	100	98
Demer(47)	193	NH_3,Rb	82	95	88
Stewart(43)	81	Rb	84	88	85
Go(42)	135	Rb	95	82	92
Tamaki(48)	48	NH_3	98	—	—

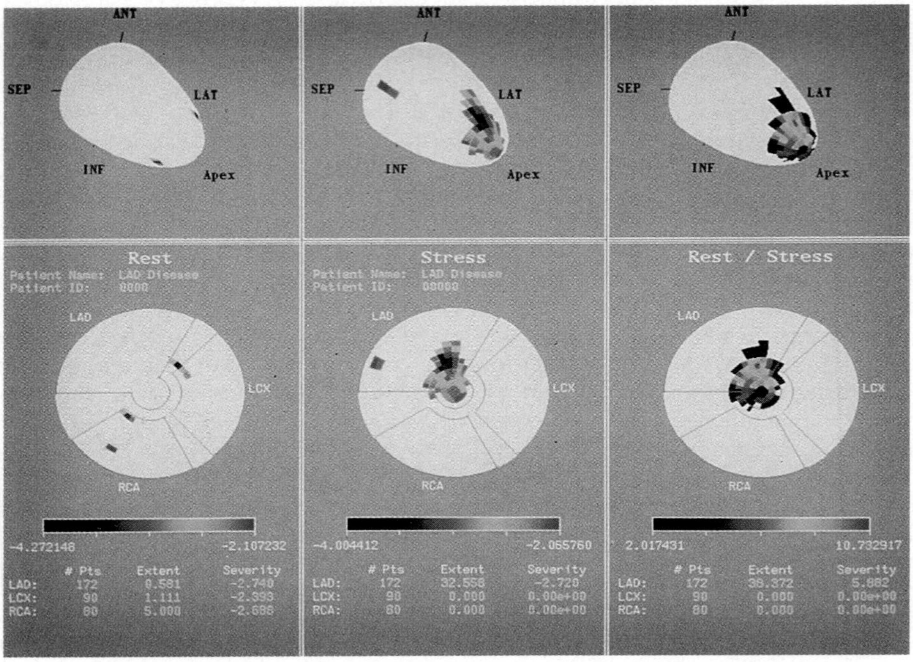

Figure 26.5. Rest and stress polar maps of [^{13}N]ammonia uptake in a patient with 99% narrowing of LAD. The data show the comparison with the normal database, *white areas* correspond to values within 2 standard deviations of the normal population. The *upper panel* shows the same data in three-dimensional display.

Table 26.3.
Diagnostic Performance of PET in Comparison to SPECT

	PET				SPECT			
Reference	N	Sens. (%)	Spec. (%)	Acc. (%)	N	Sens. (%)	Spec. (%)	Acc. (%)
Stewart(43)	81	84	88	85	81	84	53	79
Go(42)	135	95	82	92	135	79	76	78
Tamaki(48)	48	98	—	—	48	96	—	—

significant coronary artery disease as defined by a coronary artery stenosis of more than 50% narrowing of the lumen diameter. The values of specificity were similar for PET and SPECT using visual analysis of color coded images representing normalized regional tracer distribution.

The second study was performed by Stewart, et al. (43), at the University of Michigan, and compared routine ^{201}Tl SPECT stress studies with dipyridamole ^{82}Rb imaging. In this investigation, ^{82}Rb PET demonstrated a significantly higher specificity for exclusion of coronary artery disease. Again, visual analysis was employed for both ^{82}Rb and ^{201}Tl data. The authors concluded that attenuation-corrected images provided by PET reduce the incidence of attenuation artifacts and, thus, increase the specificity of PET imaging.

The differing results of each study with regard to sensitivity and specificity may be explained by the criteria for flow abnormalities employed at each site. Overall diagnostic accuracy, which is less dependent on these criteria, was similar for both studies, yielding about 78% for SPECT imaging and 88% for PET imaging.

QUANTITATIVE ASSESSMENT OF MYOCARDIAL BLOOD FLOW

The potential of PET for the quantitative assessment of myocardial blood flow represents a major advantage over SPECT imaging. Such measurements provide flow estimates in ml/min per 100 g of tissue, which can be used to assess myocardial blood flow under resting and stress conditions, as well as before and after pharmacologic interventions. Regional coronary reserve can be quantitated based on absolute flow values. For such flow measurements, dynamic data acquisition is important to describe arterial input function as well as tissue response. Quality control of data acquisition is necessary to optimize the accuracy and reproducibility of quantitative measurements (54). The tracer administration has to be standardized according to the technical performance of the PET instrumentation used (21). Data processing requires three-dimensional correction for possible displacement of the heart during the dynamic acquisition, as well as automated region assignment for efficient analysis of large data sets (54). The most commonly used radiotracers for quantitation of regional myocardial blood flow are ^{13}N-ammonia and ^{15}O water (55).

^{15}O Water

^{15}O water can be either administered as bolus injection or ^{15}O-labeled CO_2 inhalation (56–58). Radiolabeled CO_2 is rapidly converted to water in lung tissue and transported to the heart in form of ^{15}O water. Both approaches use the uptake, as well as washout, of radioactivity from the myocardium, assuming a constant partition coefficient (0.80–0.90) of water between vascular and tissue space. The water method also assumes homogeneous tissue within the region of interest used for quantitation of myocardial blood flow. To define myocardial tissue boundaries, the blood pool contribution has to be removed from ^{15}O water studies. For this purpose, a separate inhalation of ^{15}O-labeled CO is commonly employed (56, 59). This tracer binds to hemoglobin within the red blood cells allowing specific demarcation of vascular structures. Following the subtraction of blood pool images from ^{15}O water studies, myocardial regions of interest can be identified. The tracer kinetic model approach employed by most institutions also includes a term correcting for the geometric distortion due to limited image resolution provided by PET (partial volume effect, activity cross contamination) (13, 24, 56, 60). The use of ^{15}O water as blood flow water has been extensively validated in various animal models (55, 60, 61). These studies demonstrate an excellent correlation between PET-measured flow values and reference measurements with radioactively labeled microspheres (Table 26.4).

^{13}N-Ammonia

Several approaches have been introduced to describe the myocardial kinetics of ^{13}N-ammonia using tracer kinetic models (38, 62, 63). The most common is the use of a three-compartment model which the ^{13}N activity in the vascular space, the free intercellular space, and the metabolic space (Fig. 26.2). The mathematic configuration of this model can be simplified to a two-compartment model using correction factors for the ^{13}N-ammonia tissue retention fraction (64). Such a correction factor can be derived from animal data comparing ^{13}N-ammonia tissue retention blood flow measurements by the microsphere technique (35, 65). To avoid such correction factors, a model can be used to separate the initial extraction of ^{13}N-ammonia by tissue (K1) from the metabolic retention of the activity in form of ^{13}N-glutamine (K3) (62). Assuming a first transit extraction of ^{13}N-ammonia of approximately 100%, the K1 estimate serves as a quantitative index of perfusion ($F = K_1 \times EF$) (27). Both of these methods have been validated in the animal laboratory comparing ^{13}N-ammonia perfusion measurements with microspheres measurements as the gold standard or with ^{15}O water PET measurements (55, 64). These studies have experimentally demonstrated that regional myocardial blood flow can be quantitated with ^{13}N-ammonia over a wide range.

Table 26.4.
Flow Measurements in Canine Myocardium. Correlation of PET and Microsphere Flow Values

Reference	Tracer	Flow Range (ml/min/100g)	Correlation
Araujo(57)	$H_2[^{15}O]$	50–610	0.91
Bellina(192)	$[^{13}N]H_3$	20–500	0.97
Bergmann(26)	$H_2[^{15}O]$	29–504	0.95
Bol(61)	$H_2[^{15}O]$	37–580	0.97
	$[^{13}N]H_3$	58–548	0.94
Herrero(66)	^{82}Rb	20–200	0.83
Herrero(67)	$[^{62}Cu]$PTSM	23–614	0.95
Kuhle(193)	$[^{13}N]H_3$	20–500	0.93
Muzik(55)	$[^{13}N]H_3$	80–620	0.86
Shah(35)	$[^{13}N]H_3$	50–290	0.94

Other Tracers (Rubidium-82, Copper-62 PTSM, Potassium-38)

Rubidium-82 has been proposed for quantitative flow measurements (66). Preliminary data in the animal model demonstrate the feasibility of using this radiopharmaceutical for quantitative flow measurements. Copper-62 PTSM has also been employed for the assessment of myocardial blood flow (67, 68). Quantitative flow estimates are limited because of the rapid sequestration of activity in red blood cells, thereby altering arterial input function and availability of tracer to tissue. Additionally, its relatively low extraction by the myocardium requires large correction factors at high flow states (68). Future clinical studies using ^{82}Rb, ^{62}Cu-PTSM or ^{38}K (33) have to demonstrate that myocardial blood flow can be as accurately quantitated with these new tracers as with ^{15}O water and ^{13}N-ammonia.

CLINICAL APPLICATION

The quantitation of regional coronary flow reserve has been advocated by Gould, et al. (69), for the functional assessment of the severity of coronary artery stenosis in patients with coronary artery disease. The parameter flow reserve integrates the functional significance of a given coronary lesion, vascular reactivity and collateral blood flow in the poststenotic vascular territories. It has been hypothesized that such functional measurements may complement the anatomic description of coronary artery disease and may be helpful in the selection of patients for revascularization. Limitations of angiographic characterization of coronary artery disease are widely appreciated due to the complex three-dimensional nature of atherosclerotic plaques, as well as considerable interobserver variability in angiographic data interpretation (69–72). Adding functional information to an angiographic description of CAD increases objectivity in the evaluation of disease severity and provides a noninvasive means to follow progression and regression of coronary artery disease (73).

Normal Heart

Quantitative flow measurements allow for the regional assessment of coronary reserve without the need of comparison with other myocardial regions. Qualitative assessment of relative coronary reserve by SPECT and PET imaging relies on the hypothesis that at least one segment of the myocardium displays a normal coronary reserve. This segment serves as an internal standard to which all other segments are normalized. However, this may not be possible in patients with severe triple-vessel disease or other diseases affecting coronary reserve measurements (74).

Table 26.5 summarizes PET blood flow measurements obtained with ^{13}N-ammonia and ^{15}O water in normal volunteers, as well as in patients with coronary artery disease. There is good reproducibility of blood flow measurements under resting, as well as stress, conditions among various

Table 26.5.
Myocardial Blood Flow Estimates in Humans Determined by PET with ^{13}N-ammonia or ^{15}O-water

Reference	Tracer	Rest Flow (ml/min/100g)	Stress Flow (ml/min/100g)	CFR*	Type of Stress
Araujo(25)	$H_2[^{15}O]$	88 ± 8	352 ± 113	4.0 ± 1.6	Dipyridamole
Bergmann(26)	$H_2[^{15}O]$	90 ± 22	355 ± 112	3.9 ± 2.2	Dipyridamole
Camici(194)	$H_2[^{15}O]$	92 ± 13	367 ± 94	4.0 ± 1.6	Dipyridamole
Chan(195)	$[^{13}N]H_3$	110 ± 20	430 ± 13	3.9 ± 0.8	Dipyridamole
		110 ± 20	440 ± 90	4.0 ± 1.5	Adenosine
Czernin(36)	$[^{13}N]H_3$	76 ± 17	300 ± 80	3.9 ± 1.9	Dipyridamole
Geltman(196)	$H_2[^{15}O]$	125 ± 28	462 ± 158	3.7 ± 2.1	Dipyridamole
Hutchins(62)	$[^{13}N]H_3$	88 ± 17	417 ± 112	4.7 ± 2.2	Dipyridamole
Krivokapich(38)	$[^{13}N]H_3$	70 ± 17	135 ± 22	1.9 ± 0.8	Bicycle ergometer
Krivokapich(197)	$[^{13}N]H_3$	77 ± 14	225 ± 25	2.9 ± 0.8	Dobutamine
Sambuceti(198)	$[^{13}N]H_3$	103 ± 25	366 ± 92	3.5 ± 1.7	Dipyridamole

*CFR = coronary flow reserve

imaging laboratories as shown by the consistent measurements of coronary reserve values. The variation of individual resting and maximal flow values suggest that some of the methods may lead to systematic under- or overestimation of "true" myocardial blood flow. In most studies, coronary flow reserve over 2.5 times resting flow can be considered "normal" based on the standard deviation of the measurements in control groups with low likelihood of coronary artery disease (75, 76).

A relationship between coronary reserve measurements and age in subjects without CAD has been demonstrated (36). Considering hemodynamic parameters such as BP and HR, the decreased coronary reserve values in elderly persons may be primarily due to increased resting blood flow as a consequence of higher heart rate and blood pressure in elderly patient populations. However, there are other factors such as left ventricular hypertrophy, hypertension, as well as Syndrome X, which may affect coronary reserve measurements in the absence of vascular abnormalities defined by angiography (74). Animal, as well as clinical, data have indicated that arterial hypertension leads to reduced coronary flow reserve. It has been shown using PET, that therapy of patients with arterial hypertension may improve regional coronary reserve measurements (77).

Coronary Artery Disease

In patients with coronary artery disease, coronary flow reserve measurements are reduced (46, 78–80). Several studies indicated a correlation between the severity of coronary artery disease and severity of flow reserve impairment (55, 77, 79, 81). However, there is a relatively large scatter of data in the range of intermediate coronary artery stenosis (Fig. 26.6). This discrepancy between angiographic and PET results may be best explained by the expected differences in anatomic disease characterization and functional consequences of long-standing coronary artery disease. As discussed earlier, the anatomic description of a coronary lesion relies on relative diameter changes of arterial lumen and does not include overall changes in vascular wall thickness. Additionally, the complex geometric shape of atherosclerotic plaques may be difficult to judge from angiographic views. Finally, collateral blood

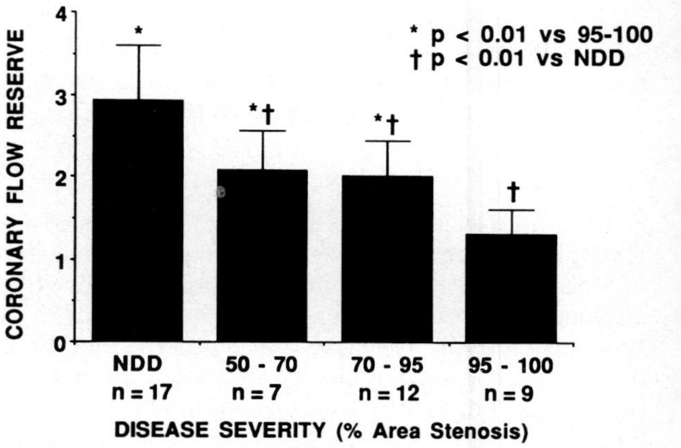

Figure 26.6. Correlation of PET coronary flow reserve ([^{13}N]ammonia) ar severity of coronary artery stenosis as assessed by quantitative angiograph (% area stenosis).

flow may alter the relationship of a coronary stenosis an blood flow measurements to the stenosis site. All these fac tors emphasize the importance of blood flow measure ments to document the functional severity of a given ar giographic lesion, which is necessary for therapeuti decisions.

Comparing the incidence of abnormal coronary flow re serve with the severity of stenosis as defined by quantita tive angiography reveals a very high sensitivity of coronar flow reserve measurements in the detection of severe co onary artery stenosis (Fig. 26.7). Surprising is the high ir cidence (about 30%) of abnormal CFR in territories wit only mild coronary artery disease as defined by angiogra phy (76). These data have been confirmed by several lab oratories, indicating that coronary flow reserve with pha macologic stress agents may provide a more sensitiv means to detect early alterations of coronary arteries tha angiographic criteria alone (82). This hypothesis has bee elaborated by work from Dayanikli, et al. (83), who den onstrated that coronary flow reserve in asymptomatic pa tients without clinical evidence of myocardial ischemia but at high risk for the development of coronary artery dis ease, based on a risk factor profile, was abnormal as com pared to an age-matched group of individuals with low like

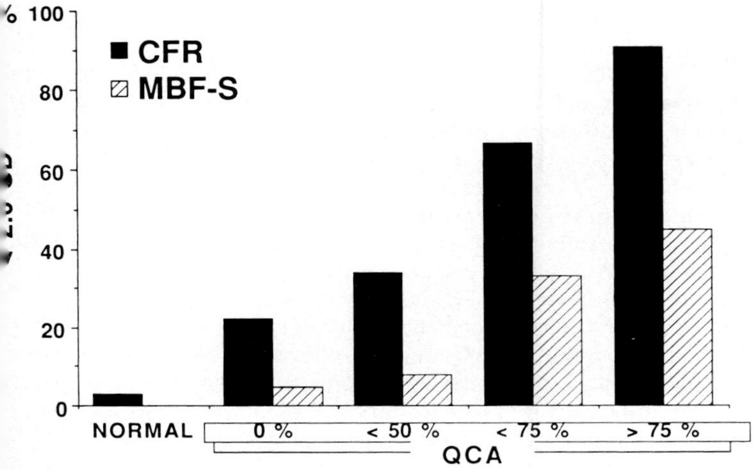

Figure 26.7. Incidence of PET of coronary flow reserve (CFR) and stress myocardial blood flow (MBF-S) below 2 standard deviations of normal values. The severity of stenosis in the territories was determined by quantitative coronary angiography. Note the high incidence (25%) of abnormal flow reserve in angiographically normal territories of patients with CAD.

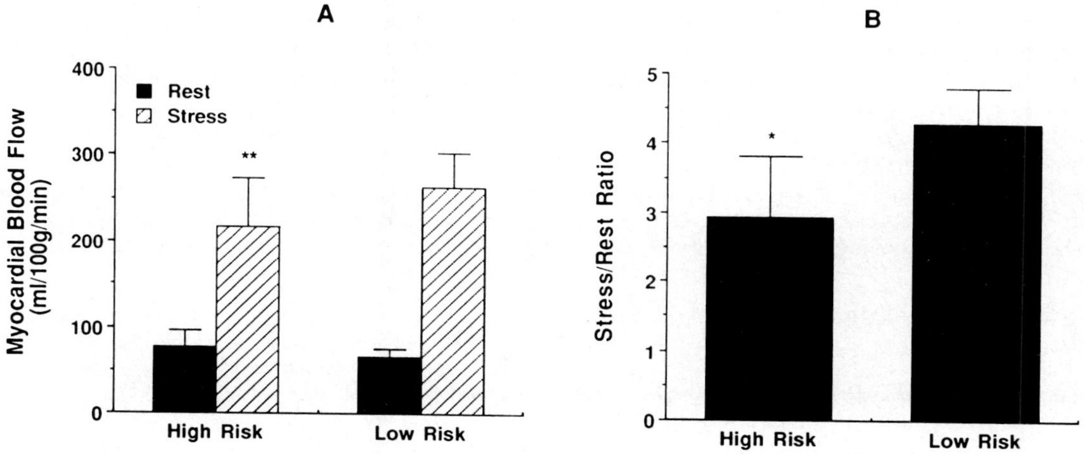

Figure 26.8. Myocardial blood flow (**A**) in stress condition (adenosine) as well as coronary flow reserve (**B**) in age-matched asymptomatic high and low risk populations. (See text for details.) (* $p < 0.001$; ** $p < 0.05$)

hood of coronary artery disease (Fig. 26.8). Additionally, preliminary studies indicated that the coronary flow reserve values are reduced in angiographically normal vascular territories of patients with severe coronary artery disease in other territories (75). The pathophysiologic mechanism of the reduced coronary flow reserve is not yet known, but may represent the interplay of vascular alterations as well as endothelial dysfunction caused by the pharmacologically induced vasodilatation (84). Besides their diagnostic significance, such results also indicate the potential of quantitative flow measurements to provide in vivo assessment of endothelial function and its modification by various therapeutic approaches (85). It is expected that quantitative flow measurements with PET will provide unique noninvasive endpoints for pharmacologic studies aiming for reversal of early atherosclerotic disease in patient populations with high risk.

Noncoronary Artery Disease

Quantitative flow measurements with PET have been employed in patients with cardiac transplantation to study coronary physiology in this patient population. Several studies indicate that coronary reserve is maintained in the cardiac transplant (46, 86). However, resting myocardial perfusion appears to be higher as a consequence of elevated blood pressure and heart rate in these patients. Future studies are necessary to define the clinical role of blood flow measurements in the early detection of transplant vasculopathy since such abnormalities are important limiting factors for the life expectancy of the graft.

First results with quantitative PET flow measurements in patients with cardiomyopathy have been reported (87). Patients with hypertrophic cardiomyopathy display a reduced coronary reserve which affects not only the hypertrophied interventricular septum, but also the free lateral wall (80). These findings indicate that the pathophysiologic process involving patients with hypertrophic cardiomyopathy may not be limited to the hypertrophied interventricular septum (80).

In patients with dilated cardiomyopathy there appears to be a reduction of coronary flow reserve. Studies by Merlet, et al. (87), indicate that PET blood flow measurements are in close agreement with invasive assessment of flow velocity by Doppler methods in this patient population. The physiologic and clinical significance of reduced coronary flow reserve in patients with dilated cardiomyopathy is not defined yet. Future studies are necessary to define the prognostic importance of this finding.

ASSESSMENT OF CARDIAC SUBSTRATE METABOLISM

Myocardial energy metabolism depends on the oxidation of various substrates. Under fasting conditions the majority of cardiac ATP production relies on the oxidation of free fatty acids (88, 89). Free fatty acids are avidly extracted by the myocardium where long-chain acyl-CoA is rapidly formed. Activated fatty acids are used in the synthesis of triglycerides or phospholipids. The majority of acyl-CoA, however, is transported via the carnitine shuttle into the mitochondria where β-oxidation takes place (Fig. 26.9). The end product of β-oxidation is acetyl-CoA which enters the TCA-cycle, the final pathway of oxidative metabolism of all substrates. In the presence of high free fatty acid, as well as low insulin plasma levels, only a little glucose is extracted by the myocardium. However, in the postprandial state, glucose transport into the cell is enhanced and glycolytic rate increased. But even after carbohydrate loading only about 30–50% of overall cardiac substrate metabolism depends on oxidative metabolism of glucose (89). During physical exercise, plasma lactate levels increase and contribute significantly to myocardial energy metabolism (90).

Besides the physiologic increase of glycolysis in the postprandial state, glycolysis plays an important role during and following myocardial ischemia. Experimental studies have shown that myocardial glucose transport and metabolism is upregulated during myocardial ischemia with production and release of lactate (91–94). However, following ischemic episodes, glycolysis remains enhanced with evidence of oxidative and nonoxidative utilization of exogenous glucose (90, 95, 96). There is preliminary evidence that enhanced myocardial oxidative glucose metabolism persists after an ischemic episode, most likely due to an upregulation of glucose transport (97). Biopsy studies in patients with severe coronary artery disease and chronic dysfunction of left ventricular segments have shown increased glycogen storage, as evidence of chronic alterations of glucose metabolism in hibernating myocardium (98). Such metabolic pattern may reflect cell degeneration of repetitively ischemic myocardium with predominant glycolytic metabolism. Several tracers are available to study details of cardiac metabolism (Table 26.6).

^{11}C-PALMITATE

The first radiopharmaceutical used in combination with PET for the assessment of regional cardiac metabolism was ^{11}C-palmitate. ^{11}C-palmitate is avidly taken up by the myo-

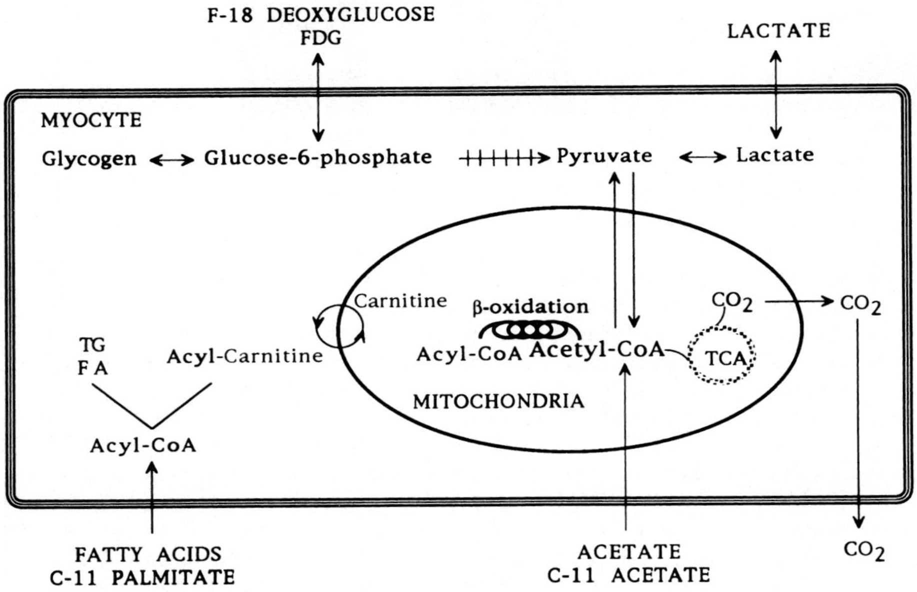

Figure 26.9. Schematic description of myocardial substrate metabolism (*TG* = triglycerides; *FA* = fatty acids; *TCA* = tricarboxic acid cycle).

Table 26.6.
PET Tracer for the Measurement of Myocardial Metabolism

Substance	Physical Half-life (min)	Energy (MeV)	Traced Process	Reference
[^{18}F]FDG	109.7	0.6	exogenous glucose transport and phosphorylation	Gambhir(20)
[^{11}C]palmitate	20.4	1.0	synthesis of triglycerides and β-oxidation	Schoen(99)
[^{18}F]FTHA	109.7	0.6	β-oxidation	Ebert(199)
[^{11}C]leucine	20.4	1.0	protein synthesis	Barrio(200)
[^{11}C]acetate	20.4	1.0	TCA-cycle	Brown(109)

cardium with an extraction fraction of about 50%. ^{11}C activity clears in a biexponential pattern from myocardium. A rapid first-clearance phase is followed by a slow second phase (99). The half-life of the first phase varies between 5 and 10 minutes, while the later phase displays a biologic half-life of about 30–40 minutes. Experimental studies changing cardiac workload or cardiac substrate availability demonstrated changes in the relative contribution of the early and late phase of ^{11}C-palmitate kinetics (100). Based on these studies, a relationship was established between the early clearance phase and the relative contribution of β-oxidation to long-chain fatty acid metabolism (101, 102). The contribution of the early clearance rate was correlated to myocardial oxygen consumption (102, 103).

The slow phase most likely represents the deposition of radioactivity in slow turn-over pools such as triglycerides and phospholipids. The fast phase can be almost completely abolished by blocking the acyl-CoA transferase by pharmacologic means (104). On the other hand, myocardial ischemia also leads to severe impairment of ^{11}C-palmitate oxidation as demonstrated by tracer kinetics (99, 105). Experimental work correlating ^{11}C-palmitate kinetics with ultrastructural tissue analysis in animals with ischemic injury revealed good correlation between lipid droplets and increased deposition of ^{11}C-palmitate into a slow turnover pool (106).

Several studies have indicated the suitability of ^{11}C-palmitate to qualitatively assess myocardial fatty acid metabolism (101, 103). Preliminary data also indicated that ^{11}C-palmitate kinetics can be used for the in vivo estimation of myocardial β-oxidation. However, ^{11}C-palmitate reflects only one of many fatty acids used by myocardium and interpretation of the kinetic data may be limited by the interaction of various substrates regulating long-chain fatty acid metabolism.

^{11}C-ACETATE

To avoid the complexity of substrate interaction defining the relative contribution of long-chain fatty acids and carbohydrates to overall oxidative metabolism, ^{11}C-acetate has been proposed as an alternative probe to describe mitochondrial oxidative metabolism. ^{11}C-acetate is converted to ^{11}C-acetyl-CoA in the mitochondria and enters the TCA-cycle. ^{11}C activity equilibrates within TCA-cycle intermediates and the ^{11}C activity clears from myocardium in the form of $^{11}CO_2$. Several studies indicate that ^{11}C-acetate kinetics, as assessed by dynamic PET imaging, correlate closely with myocardial oxygen consumption as assessed directly in the animal laboratory or by hemodynamic parameters in the clinical setting. Kinetics of ^{11}C-acetate are only a little affected by substrate interactions and thus allow quantification of myocardial oxygen consumption (107–111). Tracer kinetic models have been introduced to quantitate ^{11}C-acetate kinetics (112). However, most clinical studies employ simple determination of clearance rates using monoexponential curve-fitting of regional myocardial ^{11}C myocardial time activity curves.

^{18}F-DEOXYGLUCOSE

^{18}F-deoxyglucose traces transmembraneous transport as well as phosphorylation of exogenous glucose (113, 114). ^{18}F-deoxyglucose-6-phosphate does not enter any further metabolic pathways, but accumulates in myocardium proportional to glucose transport and phosphorylation (115, 116). Very little dephosphorylation of 6-FDG-phosphate occurs in the myocardium. Experimental studies in isolated rabbit septum, as well as canine models, demonstrated a close relationship of FDG-uptake and exogenous glucose metabolism measured by the Fick principle (116, 117). However, FDG molecules display different affinity to glucose transport and phosphorylation than the glucose molecule itself (118). To correct for this discrepancy, a correction term is necessary for the quantification of exogenous glucose utilization of the myocardium by FDG. This correction term (LUMPED-constant) is assumed to be constant under physiologic and most pathophysiologic conditions (119, 120). Recent data indicate that under extreme conditions the LUMPED-constant may actually change as a function of altered affinities to glucose transport as well as hexokinase reaction (121). However, the assumption that FDG-uptake reflects myocardial glucose utilization appears to be valid for most conditions this tracer has been employed clinically (89). The quantitation of glucose metabolism can be performed using a three-compartment model introduced initially by Sokoloff, et al., for assessing cerebral glucose metabolism (113, 114, 122). To simplify quantitation, the Patlak analysis has been employed for myocardial PET studies and validated against this three-compartment quantification (123, 124). A linearization of FDG-kinetics allows pixel-by-pixel quantification of glucose metabolism and thus parametric display of regional glucose utilization rate (125).

CLINICAL APPLICATION

Normal Heart

The use of ^{11}C-palmitate and ^{11}C-acetate in healthy volunteers indicate homogeneous uptake of these tracers within the normal left ventricular myocardium (108, 126, 127) (Fig. 26.10). The high initial extraction of ^{11}C-palmitate and ^{11}C-acetate allow for the qualitative assessment of regional myocardial perfusion (103, 128, 129). Comparison of ^{11}C-acetate uptake and ^{13}N-ammonia blood flow measurements also indicate close correlation of results in patients with coronary artery disease. The kinetics of ^{11}C-palmitate and ^{11}C-acetate can be altered by changing myocardial oxygen demand (103, 130, 131). Intravenous infusion of dobutamine increases the washout of ^{11}C activity following the intravenous injection of ^{11}C-acetate (132, 133).

The comparison of ^{11}C-acetate uptake and clearance with regional FDG-kinetics in normal volunteers demonstrated an inhomogeneity of regional glucose utilization in the heart (134). Regional FDG-uptake is increased in the lateral wall of the left ventricle and slightly decreased in the area of intraventricular septum (135). The relatively small regional changes (8–10%) are more pronounced in the fasting state. The physiologic reason for the heterogeneity of myocardial FDG-uptake in the normal heart is not known and may reflect regional variation in substrate preference by the myocardium. The combined use of ^{11}C-acetate and ^{18}F-deoxyglucose can be employed for the quan-

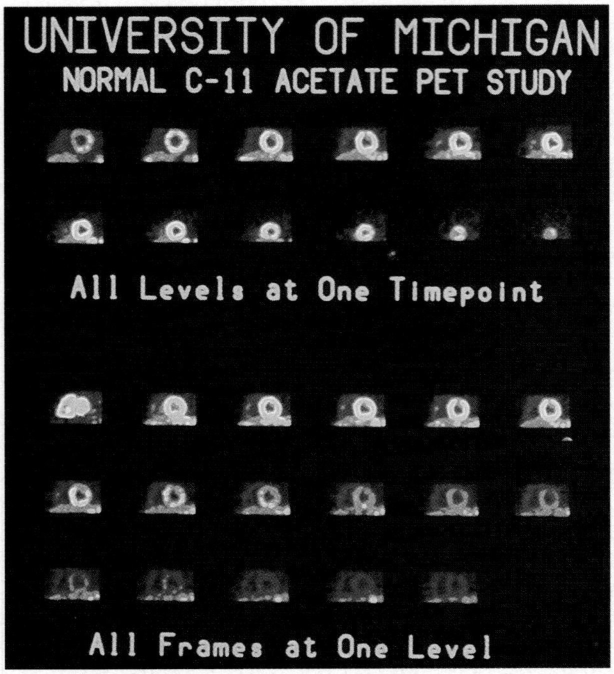

Figure 26.10. PET images of ^{11}C-acetate uptake in the normal myocardium. Displayed are short axis slices of the whole myocardium at one time point (*upper two rows*) and the distribution of ^{11}C-acetate uptake in one midventricular slice at different time points after tracer injection (*lower panel;* time increases from left to right).

tification of myocardial substrate metabolism and determination of the relative contribution of glucose to overall oxidative metabolism (134). Such measurements have been used to evaluate cardiac glucose metabolism in patients with insulin-dependent diabetes mellitus. In this patient population, there was no significant difference in overall glucose utilization as compared to a control population, if insulin was substituted by an euglycemic-insulin clamp (136).

Ischemic Heart Disease

The clinical application of metabolic imaging has been rapidly expanded following the experimental demonstration of specific changes in regional substrate utilization occurring during myocardial ischemia (95, 96, 99, 106, 137). As mentioned earlier, myocardial ischemia results into an impairment of fatty acid oxidation and increased myocardial glucose utilization (94, 99). Comparing regional myocardial FDG-uptake and myocardial blood flow, as assessed by microspheres during acute myocardial ischemia, showed a dissociation of myocardial blood flow and glucose utilization (94). In severe ischemia, however, both blood flow and glucose utilization are reduced, while during moderate ischemia there is evidence for increased glucose utilization. ^{11}C-palmitate studies in patients with coronary artery disease at rest and during pacing-induced stress, demonstrated a reduction of ^{11}C-palmitate turnover in segments distal to a coronary artery stenosis (131). Studies in patients with acute myocardial infarction also confirmed the finding in animal studies, demonstrating impaired ^{11}C-palmitate oxidation in the infarct territory in the presence of increased FDG-uptake (138).

Marshall, et al. (139), were the first to investigate the relationship of increased FDG-uptake in patients with acute myocardial infarction and clinical signs of ongoing ischemia, as well as electrocardiographic changes. This study indicated that in a considerable number of patients with acute myocardial infarction, residual metabolic activity could be demonstrated in the infarct territory, which was associated with postinfarct angina and electrocardiographic signs of recurrent ischemia. Based on this observation, Tillisch, et al. (140), initiated a study comparing relative FDG-uptake in patients with advanced coronary artery disease and impaired regional and global function before and after revascularization. This study demonstrated, for the first time, that maintained FDG-uptake in dysfunctioning segments with reduced flow is associated with functional recovery after revascularization, while segments with concordantly decreased flow and metabolism did not recover after restoration of blood flow. This study was paralleled by other investigations comparing regional FDG-uptake with electrocardiographic criteria of infarction, as well as standard ^{201}Tl stress and redistribution imaging (141–143). All these studies indicated that FDG imaging did provide sensitive means to detect residual tissue viability in myocardial segments with previous ischemic injury. Table 26.7 summarizes clinical PET results, collected from several laboratories, documenting the high predictive value of PET-metabolic imaging for tissue recovery following revascularization.

Early observations of discrepant results between FDG distribution and standard ^{201}Tl redistribution patterns emphasized the limitations of ^{201}Tl redistribution imaging for assessment of tissue viability (144). Such findings led to the reconsideration of ^{201}Tl imaging protocols. Subsequent studies using ^{201}Tl reinjection following the stress procedure revealed considerable increase of sensitivity in the detection of tissue viability (145–147). Using this new ^{201}Tl imaging protocol, similar predictive values for tissue recovery, as previously described with PET FDG imaging, were reported with ^{201}Tl (145–147). However, besides the physiologic signal of regional glucose utilization provided by FDG, the attenuation-corrected PET images avoid imaging artifacts, and thus may be more specific for the assessment of tissue viability (148). This advantage was demonstrated by the comparison of ^{201}Tl reinjection technique and PET FDG imaging in patients undergoing revascularization (148). There was good agreement between PET and SPECT imaging in the anterior and lateral wall of the left ventricle, while there was considerable discrepancy in the inferior wall, most likely reflecting attenuation artifacts.

Recent studies comparing PET FDG imaging and ^{99m}Tc-sestamibi SPECT imaging revealed a considerable underestimation of tissue viability by ^{99m}Tc-sestamibi imaging (149–151). This underestimation depends on the severity of perfusion defects defined by ^{99m}Tc-sestamibi imaging (149). Mild ^{99m}Tc-sestamibi defects are associated with a high likelihood of tissue viability as evidenced by FDG imaging. In contrast, segments with very severe ^{99m}Tc-sestamibi defects displayed a low likelihood of tissue viability. The diagnostic discrepancy between both tests is most ap-

Table 26.7.
Metabolic Imaging and Tissue Recovery Following Revascularization

Reference	Patients	Dysfunctional Segments	Predictive Accuracy (%)	Positive Pred. Accuracy (%)	Negative Pred. Accuracy (%)
Tillisch(140)	17	67	88	85	92
Tamaki(201)	22	46	78	78	78
Tamaki(202)	11	56	82	80	100
Marwick(203)	16	85	74	68	79
Lucignani(204)	14	54	91	95	80
Carrel(205)	21	23	83	84	75
Gropler(158)	16	53	81	79	83
vom Dahl(206)	37	45	80	69	84
Total	154	429	82	82	83

Table 26.8.
Incidence of Cardiovascular Complications in Patients with Decreased Blood Flow

Tissue Type	Therapy	Reference	N	LVEF (%)	Complication
Hibernating	Drug Therapy	Tamaki(154)	31		12 (39%)
		Eitzman(152)	18	33	9 (50%)
		Maddahi(153)	17	24	7 (41%)
Scarred	Drug Therapy	Tamaki(154)	17		1 (6%)
		Eitzman(152)	24	32	3 (13%)
		Maddahi(153)	33	24	3 (9%)
Hibernating	PTCA or CABG	Eitzman(152)	26	36	3 (12%)
		Maddahi(153)	26	25	3 (12%)
Scarred	PTCA or CABG	Eitzman(152)	14	37	1 (7%)
		Maddahi(153)	17	25	1 (6%)

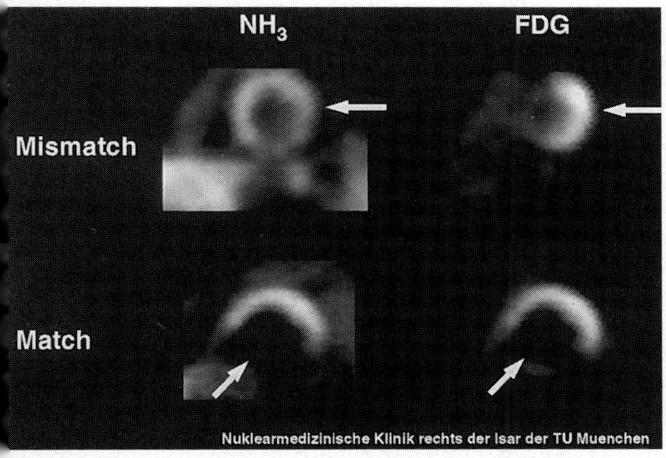

'igure 26.11. Short axis slices of myocardial [^{13}N]ammonia and FDG up-ake. The *top panel* shows corresponding short axis slices with areas of mis-natch between flow (*left*) and metabolism (*right*), whereas the *lower panel* hows an example of matched flow and metabolism.

parent in segments with only intermediate reduction of nyocardial flow as assessed with ^{99m}Tc-sestamibi.

Based on the currently available data comparing PET vith SPECT imaging, we recommend ^{201}Tl reinjection or est redistribution imaging as the first choice to assess re-gional tissue viability. In patients with very high risk re-ascularization procedures or equivocal ^{201}Tl results, an additional PET study may provide important diagnostic in-ormation necessary for the decision of revascularization. Also, PET studies are recommended in CAD patients for whom revascularization may represent an important alternative to cardiac transplant.

Besides the predictive value of FDG for tissue recovery following revascularization, the prognostic information provided by FDG uptake in segments with reduced perfusion as assessed by ^{13}N-ammonia PET has been emphasized by several groups. Retrospective data analysis in a large group of patients (Table 26.8) revealed a high incidence of cardiovascular complications in patients with decreased blood flow but maintained FDG uptake who did not undergo revascularization (152–154). In contrast, the incidence of cardiovascular complications were similar in groups with scintigraphic evidence of scar or normal myocardium, regardless of whether or not they were revascularized. These data indicate that PET patterns of mismatch between flow and metabolism do identify a subset of patients with high risk for cardiovascular complication who may need aggressive therapy in order to improve prognosis (Fig. 26.11).

^{11}C-ACETATE IN THE ASSESSMENT OF TISSUE VIABILITY

Regional FDG uptake is modulated by plasma substrate levels and hormonal milieu. Many patients with coronary artery disease reveal diabetes mellitus or prediabetic conditions affecting glucose tolerance (155). Therefore, the image quality following oral glucose loading and intravenous injection of FDG is limited in some patients undergoing tissue viability studies (156). Aggressive use of insulin to enhance myocardial glucose uptake and, thus, FDG image quality has improved this problem, but diagnostic difficulties remain in some patients (136). As an alternative, ^{11}C-acetate was proposed for the assessment of residual oxidative metabolism in patients with severe coronary artery disease. Gropler, et al. (157), demonstrated this by comparing ^{11}C-acetate and FDG in patients with recent myocardial infarction undergoing revascularization. Tissue viability was defined by ^{11}C-acetate clearance kinetics as well as relative FDG uptake prior to revascularization. There was a significant difference between ^{11}C-acetate kinetics among normal, reversibly dysfunctioning and irreversible dysfunctioning myocardium. There was considerable overlap of regional FDG data in the same segments. As previously described, the variable FDG results may reflect the selection of patients with acute myocardial infarction (138). Schwaiger, et al., have shown that maintained FDG-uptake in the subacute phase of myocardial infarction is associated with functional recovery in only 50% of left ventricular segments. FDG uptake early after ischemic injury may not only reflect myocyte metabolism, but also acute inflammation with leukocyte infiltration. Therefore, the role of FDG uptake in the acute infarcted myocardium may be less diagnostic for tissue viability than in the chronic state of coronary artery disease. However, more recent studies by Gropler, et al. (158), demonstrate that ^{11}C-acetate may be also useful in the assessment of tissue viability in patients with chronic stable coronary artery disease (Fig. 26.12). The advantage of using ^{11}C-acetate is the simultaneous assessment of flow and metabolic studies with only one tracer. As mentioned earlier, the initial uptake of ^{11}C-acetate can be used as a qualitative assessment of regional myocardial perfusion, while the clearance serves as a marker for tissue viability. This tracer approach's advantage is somewhat offset by the requirements of dynamic data acquisition and sophisticated data analysis using regional curve-fitting procedures. Additionally, the relatively short half-life of ^{11}C-acetate requires onsite production of radiopharmaceuticals. In contrast, ^{18}F-deoxyglucose can be transported to PET centers without a cyclotron, allowing a more widespread application of metabolic imaging (148).

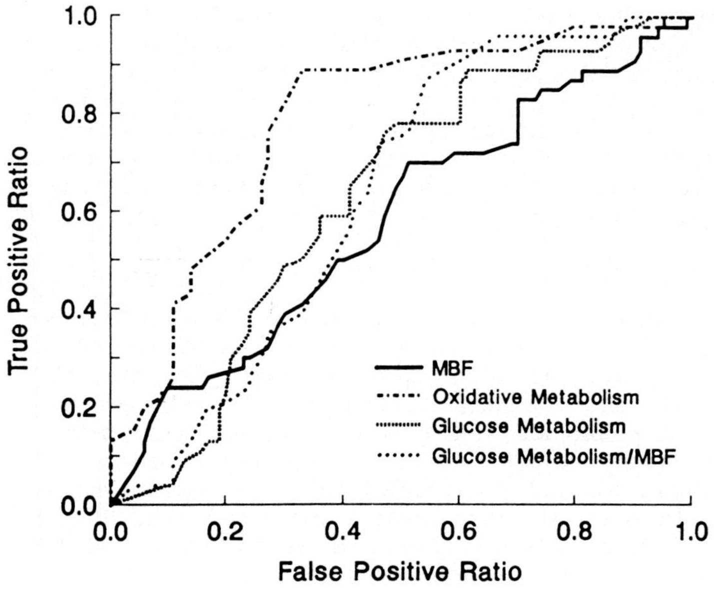

Figure 26.12. Receiver operating characteristic curves for prediction of functional recovery based on measurements of regional myocardial blood flow (*MBF*), oxidative metabolism, glucose metabolism, and glucose metabolism normalized to flow. Measurements of oxidative metabolism were the most accurate, as evidenced by the left and upward shift of the receiver operating characteristics curve for these measurements. (Reproduced by permission from Gropler R, Geltman E, Sampathkumaran K, et al. Comparison of carbon-11-acetate with fluorine-18-fluorodeoxyglucose for delineating viable myocardium by positron emission tomography. JACC 1993; 22(6):1587–1597.)

OTHER APPROACHES TO ASSESS TISSUE VIABILITY

^{82}Rb as a Marker of Tissue Viability

Animal studies indicated that the use of ^{82}Rb kinetics allows differentiation between reversible and irreversible ischemic injury (31). Goldstein, et al., used a model of acute coronary occlusion and evaluated ^{82}Rb kinetics in the infarct territory with postmortem TTC staining. The clearance half-time of activity was significantly shorter in necrotic cell populations as compared to that in reversible injured myocardium. Based on these promising results, Gould, et al. (207), compared two static PET images describing early and late ^{82}Rb distribution following tracer administration in patients with coronary artery disease and compared the results with FDG-imaging. There was a close relationship between the infarct size determined by FDG imaging and the washout pattern of ^{82}Rb. The results of this study have been confirmed subsequently by Dahl, et al., who determined the washout rates for rubidium activity from myocardial segments using regional time-activity curves. The decay corrected time-activity curves demonstrated retention of ^{82}Rb in normal myocardium while segments with low FDG-uptake displayed clearance of activity (159). These data suggest that ^{82}Rb could be used for the assessment of regional myocardial perfusion as well as tissue retention for the identification of tissue viability. Further studies are required to compare ^{82}Rb tissue kinetics with functional recovery after revascularization. However, Yoshida, et al. (160), demonstrated that ^{82}Rb may be useful in the prognostic evaluation of patients considered for revascularization and may improve the selection of patients for high risk intervention.

^{15}O Water Perfusable Tissue Fraction

Since regional myocardial blood flow is related to myocardial oxygen consumption, it can be hypothesized that perfusion of myocardial tissue provides indirect evidence of tissue viability. However, assessment of transmural average perfusion by PET may mask the presence of epicardial layers with maintained flow by a reduced average flow value caused by low flow values in areas of endocardial necrosis. Iida, et al. (13), developed a new method to relate ^{15}O water tissue kinetics to the truly perfused wall segments of the left ventricle. The transmural extent of "perfused tissue fraction" can be used for assessment of tissue viability. Comparing absolute myocardial blood flow measurements with ^{15}O water and the relative tissue perfusion fraction, these investigators demonstrated that the tissue perfusion fraction allows for better differentiation between necrotic and reversible dysfunctioning myocardium as evidenced by postrevascularization wall motion analysis (13, 161). However, this method requires the careful subtraction of blood pool images from transmission images, as well as correction of perfusion images for blood pool activity by ^{15}O CO studies. This sophisticated data analysis may be error sensitive and thus the widespread clinical use is limited (Fig. 26.13).

^{18}F Misonidazole

^{18}F misonidazole is a chemical compound which is retained in severely hypoxic myocardial tissue (162). In the absence of oxygen, misonidazole molecules form a close binding to proteins and other cell structures. Animal experiments have shown that during acute coronary artery ligation an enhanced uptake of ^{18}F misonidazole can be visualized in the affected vascular territory (162, 163). Because of little uptake in normal tissue, the blood clearance rate of this tracer is relatively slow. Therefore, contrast between hypoxic myocardial tissue and blood pool activity is small, requiring correction methods for blood pool activity. Further clinical work is required to validate this approach in patients with acute myocardial infarction. On the other hand, it is unlikely that this tracer can be used to identify viable or dysfunctioning myocardium (hibernating myocardium) in patients with chronic coronary artery disease. As ^{11}C-acetate data demonstrate, residual oxidative metabolism takes place in dysfunctioning myocardium. Such results suggest that hibernating myocardium reflects compromised myocardium, which survives due to decreased metabolic demand without tissue hypoxia.

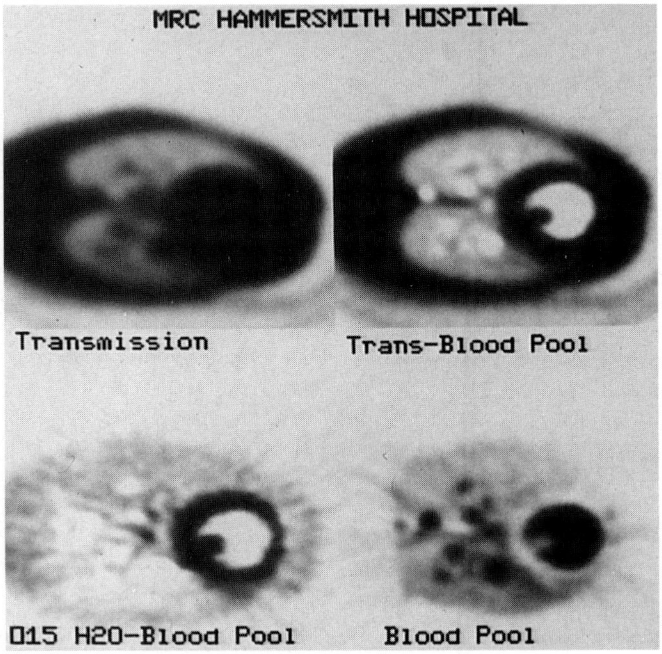

Figure 26.13. Measurement of myocardial blood flow using [^{15}O]water: Transmission image (*upper left*), blood pool image (CO scan) (*lower right*), subtraction images of transmission minus blood pool (*upper right*) (extravascular density), and H_2O image minus blood pool (tissue fraction).

METABOLIC IMAGING IN PATIENTS WITH NONCORONARY ARTERY DISEASE

Dilated Cardiomyopathy

^{11}C-palmitate has been employed to study fatty acid metabolism in patients with dilated cardiomyopathy (164). Observations by Geltman, et al. (132), revealed a heterogeneous fatty acid metabolism in patients with dilated cardiomyopathy in the presence of relatively homogeneous perfusion as measured with ^{201}Tl scintigraphy. Sochor, et al. (164), confirmed the observation of heterogeneous ^{11}C-palmitate kinetics in patients with cardiomyopathy. However, ^{11}C palmitate kinetics in these patients reacted paradoxically to oral glucose loading. Normal myocardium is characterized by delayed ^{11}C activity clearance following oral glucose load, reflecting increased rate of glycolysis competing for the production of acetyl-CoA from β-oxidation. In contrast, patients with dilated cardiomyopathy displayed an increased ^{11}C-activity clearance following oral glucose load, indicating enhanced oxidation of long-chain fatty acids following this metabolic intervention. A biochemical reason for this observation has not been defined and requires further biochemical studies (164).

Kelly (102) addressed the role of ^{11}C-palmitate in probing mitochondrial enzyme defects resulting in an impairment of β-oxidation. These investigators could demonstrate that oxidation of ^{11}C-acetate was dissociated from that of ^{11}C-palmitate in patients affected with this enzyme disorder. These studies indicate the potential of metabolic PET studies for the identification of specific enzyme defects. Furthermore, these techniques can be used to monitor the consequences of genetic enzyme defects, and may be useful in assessing the biochemical results of gene therapy.

As discussed earlier, ^{11}C-acetate allows the noninvasive assessment of myocardial oxygen consumption (165). This tracer approach can be used to probe myocardial oxygen consumption in the normal, as well as diseased, cardiac muscle. Studies by Hicks, et al. (166), demonstrated that ^{11}C-acetate turnover is increased in patients with chronically loaded left ventricles in case of aortic stenosis and aortic insufficiency. Myocardial oxygen consumption was reduced following repair of the valvular lesion by valve replacement. Additionally, this technique can be used to assess right ventricular oxygen consumption as demonstrated by Hicks, et al. (167), who described a close relationship between right ventricular acetate kinetics in patients and pulmonary artery pressure. This work demonstrates the unique ability of imaging approaches to quantitate metabolic rates of the right ventricular myocardium. Similar measurements are not possible by invasive methods due to the complex venous drainage of blood from right ventricular myocardium.

Wolpers, et al. (168), first introduced the concept of noninvasively assessing myocardial efficiency by PET as defined by the external work of the left ventricle divided by oxygen consumption. Such a parameter links mechanical performance and metabolic demand. Animal studies have been used to validate this approach against direct measurements of myocardial oxygen consumption. Cardiac work was defined either by ventricular stroke work index, by hemodynamic measurements, or simultaneous echocardiography. These data indicated that this myocardial work index depends on left ventricular and diastolic volume, as well as vascular resistance (Fig. 26.14).

Beanlands, et al. (133), applied this approach in patients with cardiomyopathy before and after therapy. The aim of this study was to evaluate the possibility that myocardial efficiency can be optimized under given therapeutic intervention. Patients were studied before and after infusion of nitroprusside as well as dobutamine (169). Myocardial efficiency increased following both pharmacologic interventions (Fig. 26.15). In both instances, the improvement of cardiac efficiency was most related to changes in left ventricular afterload. These studies demonstrate the feasability of metabolic imaging to assess noninvasively a work metabolic index which is useful in monitoring therapy in patients with severely impaired left ventricular function. Such imaging approaches may provide objective endpoints in titrating therapy individual in patients with heart failure (133).

Hypertrophic Cardiomyopathy

Few metabolic studies exist describing regional substrate metabolism in patients with hypertrophic cardiomyopathy. Grover, et al. (170), used the ^{11}C-palmitate and FDG to assess fatty acid, as well as glucose metabolism, in the thickened interventricular septum as compared to the free lat-

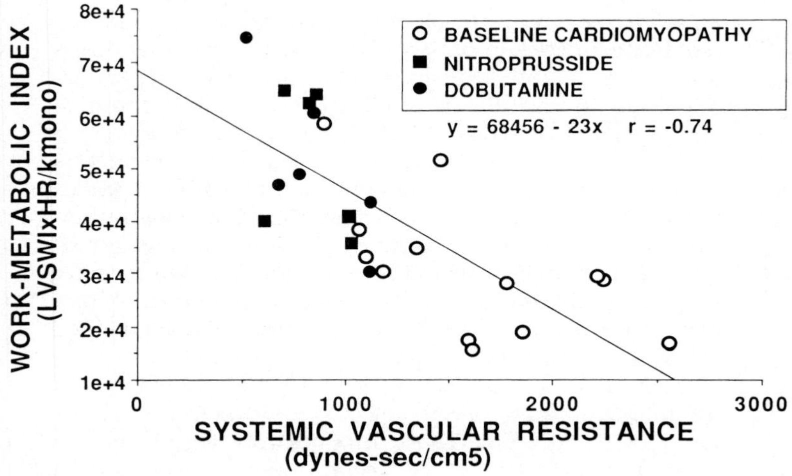

Figure 26.14. Relationship between myocardial work index, as assessed by PET and echocardiography, and systemic vascular resistance, shows a linear decrease of myocardial work index for higher vascular resistance under baseline condition or after therapeutic interventions with dobutamine and nitroprusside. (Reproduced by permission from Wolpers H, Buck A, Nguyen N, et al. An approach to ventricular efficiency in heart failure by use of C-11 acetate and positron emission tomography. J Nucl Cardiol 1994;1:262–269.)

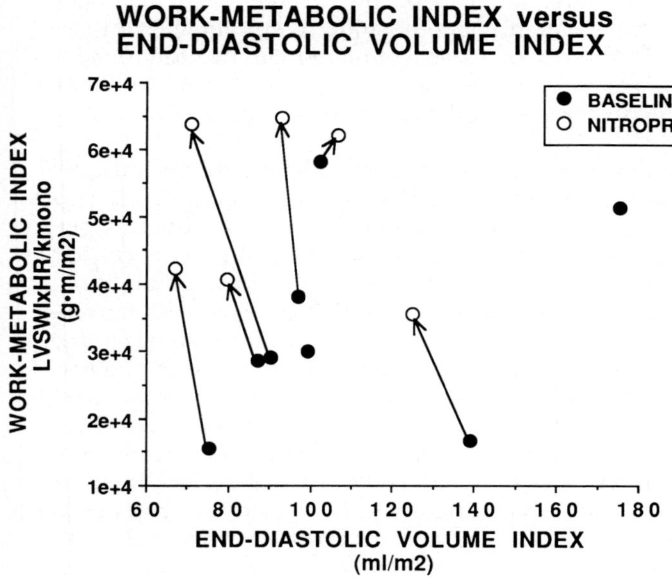

Figure 26.15. Relationship of work metabolic index and endiastolic volume before and after nitroprusside therapy in patients with cardiomyopathy. Work metabolic index increases without major changes of endiastolic volumes. (Reproduced by permission from Beanlands R, Armstrong W, Hicks R, et al. The effects of afterload reduction on myocardial C-11 acetate kinetics and noninvasively estimated mechanical efficiency in patients with dilated cardiomyopathy. J Nucl Cardiol 1994;1:3–13.)

eral wall. They demonstrated no significant difference in ^{11}C-palmitate kinetics within these two regions. Glucose metabolism as measured with regional FDG uptake was altered in some patients, with marked decrease of tracer uptake in the interventricular septum. The physiologic significance of this finding is unclear at this point and requires further biochemical confirmation.

Table 26.9.
Radiopharmaceuticals for the Evalution of the Cardiac Autonomic System

	Sympathetic	Parasympathetic
Presynaptic	MIBG	[11C]Vesamicol
	[^{18}F]Metaraminol	[18F]FEOBV
	[^{18}F]Dopamine	
	[^{18}F]GBR 13119	
	[^{18}F]Norepinephrine	
	[^{11}C]Hydroxyephedrine	
	[^{11}C]Ephedrine	
Postsynaptic	ICYP	[11C]Methyl-QNB
	[^{11}C]Practolol	[11C]Methyl-TRB
	[^{11}C]Propanolol	
	[^{11}C]CGP 12177	
	[^{11}C]Prazosin	

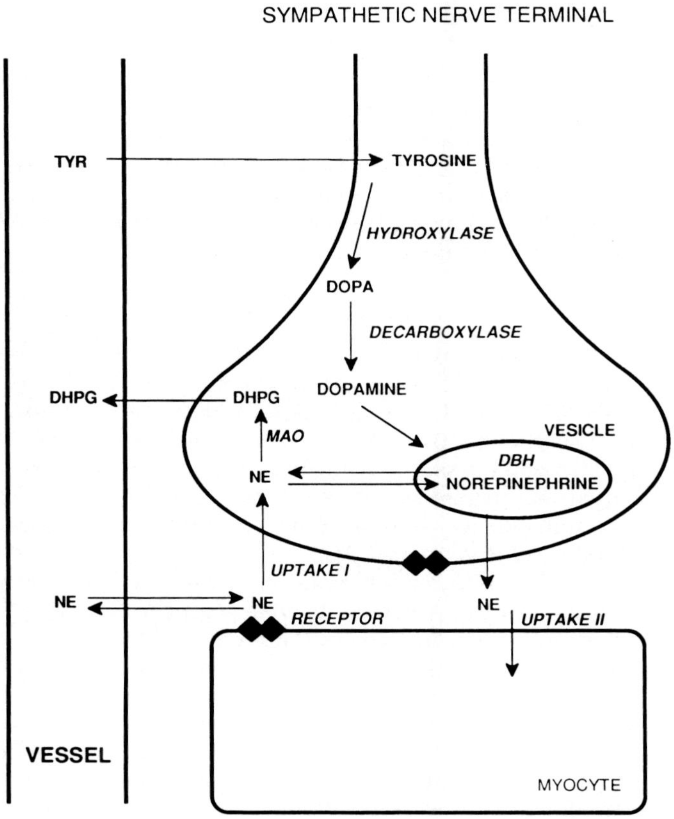

Figure 26.16. Schematic display of sympathetic nerve terminal (*NE* = norepinephrine; *MAO* = monoaminoxidase; *DBH* = dopamin-β-hydroxylase).

ASSESSMENT OF AUTONOMIC INNERVATION

Tracer approaches are uniquely suited for the assessment of specific tissue function. The success of PET in neurology resulted from the specific visualization of neurotransmission processes such as presynaptic neurotransmitter synthesis, storage, and postsynaptic receptor sites. Based on these successes, similar tracer approaches have been employed for the assessment of cardiac autonomic innervation. Table 26.9 summarizes the existing radiopharmaceuticals used to probe both the sympathetic and parasympathetic nervous system, including presynaptic nerve terminals, as well as postsynaptic receptor sites. Although tracers have been developed for the parasympathetic nervous system, especially the postsynaptic muscarinic receptors, the sparse cholinergic innervation of the left ventricle limits the evaluation of this system in vivo. New imaging approaches focus primarily on the scintigraphic delineation of pre- and postsynaptic sympathetic nervous system. Figure 26.16 displays the most important functional unit of the sympathetic nervous system—the sympathetic nerve terminal. The postganglionic sympathetic fibers travel along vascular structures on the surface of the heart. Upon entering the myocardial wall, the fibers branch into multiple sympathetic varicosities. These nerve terminals include vesicles which represent the storage pool for neurotransmitters, enzymes, and other proteins (171). Norepinephrine, the predominant neurotransmitter in cardiac sympathetic nerve terminals, is synthesized from the amino acid tyrosine by several enzymatic steps (Fig. 26.17). Norepinephrine is released upon nerve stimulation by exocytosis. The regulation of neuronal norepinephrine release is complex. Several receptor systems have been postulated to exist on the membrane of the presynaptic nerve terminal modulating norepinephrine release. Activation of these receptors by norepinephrine leads to a negative feedback of the exocytotic process. The reuptake of released norepinephrine by the nerve terminal from the synaptic cleft is an important and efficient mechanism to maintain the stores of neurotransmitters. As much as 80% of the norepinephrine that is released from the nerve terminal is taken up via this mechanism (uptake 1 mechanism). A fraction of the released norepinephrine diffuses back into the vascular space where it can be measured as norepinephrine spillover in the coronary sinus venous blood (172). Only a small amount of norepinephrine in the synaptic cleft is actually available to activate receptors on the surface of the myocytes or to enter cardiac cells directly (uptake 2 mechanism). Norepinephrine undergoes rapid metabolism in neuronal and extraneuronal tissue. Metabolism of the neurotransmitter in the neuronal tissue is mediated by the enzyme monoaminoxidase (MAO), while extraneuronal norepinephrine is metabolized by the catechol-O-methyltransferase (COMT-enzyme system).

ADRENERGIC RECEPTORS

Two general classes of postsynaptic adrenergic receptors are defined as α- and β-receptors. This distinction is based on pharmacologic studies describing specific functional responses of each receptor system. Positive isotropic response to catecholamine stimulation is primarily mediated

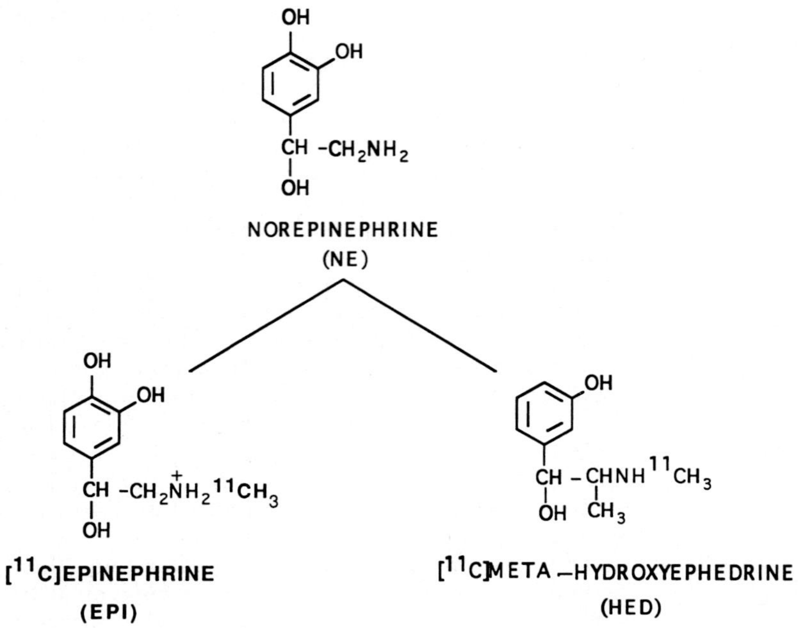

Figure 26.17. Chemical structure of norepinephrine and the tracers [^{11}C]epinephrine and [^{11}C]hydroxyephedrine.

by β-adrenergic receptors. In the normal left and right ventricle the β-1-receptors make up about 80% of the total pool of β-receptors. It has been speculated that β-2-receptors are most prevalent in the atria, and the β-2-cell selective antagonist elicit a more chronotropic response in β-1-selective tracks. Experimental investigations indicate that β-receptors can be translocated from cytosolic sites to cell membranes as well as internalized. Internalization of receptors may be the response to homologous desensitization of β-receptors under various physiologic and pathophysiologic conditions.

PRESYNAPTIC NERVE TERMINALS

The use of radiolabeled norepinephrine or analogues appears to be most promising for the visualization of the sympathetic nerve terminals. ^{11}C-hydroxyephedrine (HED) was recently synthesized at the University of Michigan (Fig. 26.18) (173). This norepinephrine analogue is taken up by the nerve terminal but is not metabolized by the intraneuronal enzyme systems. The myocardial retention of this tracer reflects the activity of the uptake 1 mechanism and, to a lesser degree, the storage of norepinephrine in nerve terminals (174). In contrast, the more recently introduced compound ^{11}C-epinephrine is not only taken up by the nerve terminal, but also stored in the vesicles of nerve terminals (175). ^{11}C-epinephrine cannot be displaced from the nerve terminal following pharmacologic inhibition of uptake 1 after tracer injection (176). A further analogue of epinephrine is phenylephrine, which also was synthesized by Wieland, et al., at the University of Michigan (177). This radiotracer enters the nerve terminal via uptake 1, but is primarily metabolized by the MAO enzyme system. Phenylephrine therefore allows the evaluation of the enzymatic integrity of the nerve terminal. Other radiopharmaceuticals for the characterization of the presynaptic nerve terminal include ^{18}F-dopamine and ^{18}F-norepinephrine, as well as MBBG (178, 179).

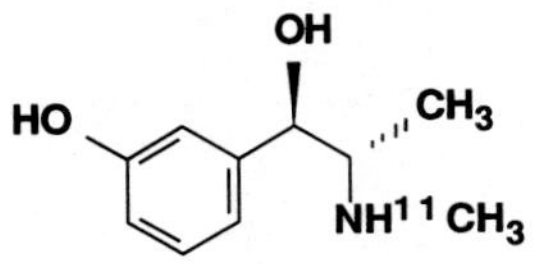

Figure 26.18. Chemical structure of hydroxyephedrine.

The scintigraphic evaluation of nerve terminals requires an in-depth understanding of the kinetic behavior of the radiotracer used. On the other hand, the combination of various tracer approaches may allow for a sophisticated physiologic characterization of neuronal function evaluating catecholamine uptake, metabolism and release rates.

CLINICAL APPLICATION

First clinical applications of ^{11}C HED show excellent image quality with high contrast between myocardial tracer activity and blood pool, as well as lung tissue surrounding the heart (Fig. 26.19). The specificity of the tracer approach for neuronal tissue has been well-documented by studies in cardiac transplant patients, and showed a marked reduction of tracer uptake, suggesting only little nonspecific binding of this tracer (180).

Studies in transplant patients at various time points following surgery indicate partial reinnervation of transplanted myocardium by retention of ^{11}C HED in the anterior septal segments of the left ventricle in transplant recipients several years after operation (181). These data suggested, for the first time, that there is regional reinnervation occurring in the human transplant. The functional significance of these findings is not yet defined, but may be important in the adaptation of the transplanted heart to varying hemodynamic conditions.

Allman, et al. (182), employed ^{11}C HED in the assessment of patients with acute myocardial infarction undergoing thrombolytic therapy. Experimental data indicated that the extent of neuronal damage following transient ischemia is larger than the area of tissue necrosis (183). Wolpers, et al., demonstrated a decreased retention fraction of ^{11}C HED in reperfused canine myocardium, suggesting high sensitivity of neurons to ischemic injury. Similar data have been observed in the clinical setting (182). The area of neuronal dysfunction as evidenced by ^{11}C HED defects was significantly larger than the area of perfusion abnormalities in patients with acute myocardial infarction.

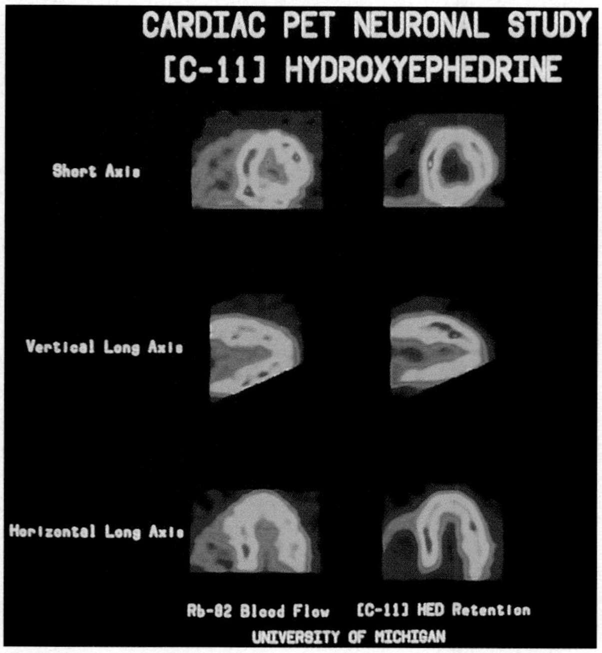

Figure 26.19. PET image of ^{11}C HED tissue retention compared to ^{82}Rb blood flow measurements.

Using semiquantitative data analysis, the discrepancy between defect sizes was larger in patients with non-Q-wave infarction as compared to those with α-wave infarction (Fig. 26.20). Ten patients in this study were restudied more than 6 months after the acute event. There was no change in the relative extent of perfusion abnormalities and HED defects in this small group. These preliminary data, however, suggest that no significant reinnervation occurs following ischemic injury.

Calkins, et al., correlated the scintigraphic distribution of HED with electrophysiologic measurements during open heart surgery in patients undergoing implantation of defibrillators. Relative refractory period as marker of sympathetic tone was regionally evaluated in segments with and without HED uptake determined preoperatively (184). Segments with decreased HED uptake displayed prolonged refractory periods, suggesting an electrophysiologic correlate of decreased sympathetic innervation in these areas (Fig. 26.21).

Although these studies may indicate an association between reduced HED uptake and altered regional electrophysiologic behavior, no prognostic data are currently available supporting the notion that HED scanning may identify patients at high risk for lethal arrhythmias or sudden death.

^{11}C HED PET studies were also performed in patients with diabetic neuropathy. These studies revealed a correlation between the results of autonomic nervous system testing and abnormalities of HED distribution. Surprising was the finding that regional cardiac denervation represents a heterogeneous process in patients with diabetic neuropathy. ^{11}C-hydroxyephedrine defects were most severe in the apical segments of the left ventricle, and least severe in the proximal segments of the left ventricle (185).

Preliminary studies suggest the possible role of HED imaging in patients with congestive heart failure. Schwaiger, et al. (208), demonstrated a decreased HED uptake in patients with severe impairment of left ventricular function, suggesting neuronal damage in this patient population.

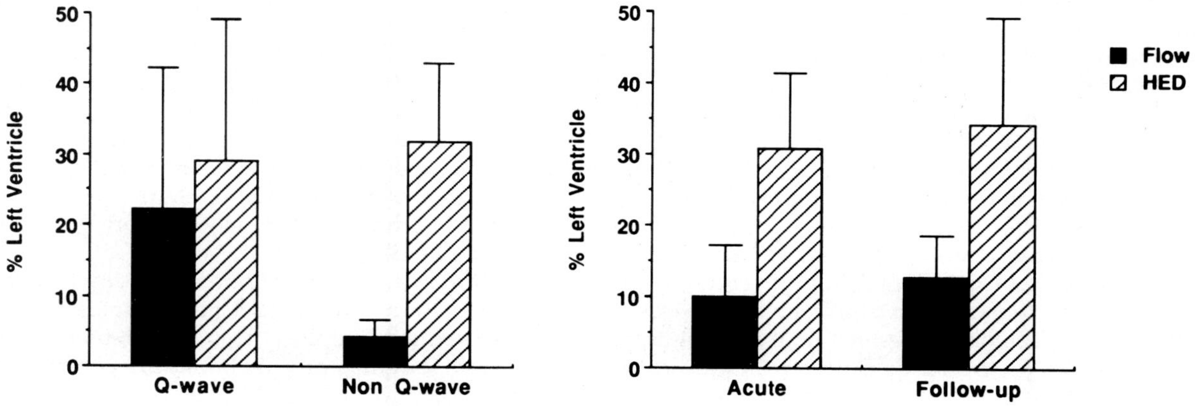

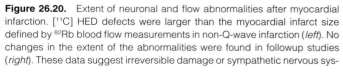

Figure 26.20. Extent of neuronal and flow abnormalities after myocardial infarction. [^{11}C] HED defects were larger than the myocardial infarct size defined by ^{82}Rb blood flow measurements in non-Q-wave infarction (*left*). No changes in the extent of the abnormalities were found in followup studies (*right*). These data suggest irreversible damage or sympathetic nervous system surrounding the infarct territory. (Reproduced by permission from Allman K, Wieland D, Muzik O, DeGrado T, Wolfe E Jr, Schwaiger M. Carbon-11 hydroxyephedrine with positron emission tomography for serial assessment of cardiac adrenergic neuronal function after acute myocardial infarction in humans. JACC 199;22(2):368–375.)

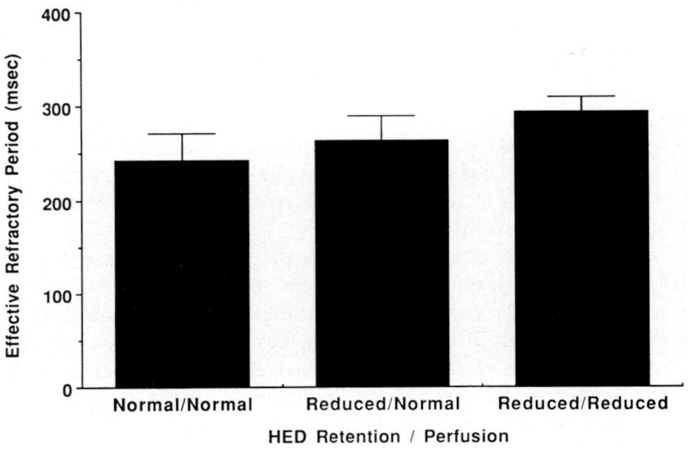

Figure 26.21. Effective refractory period assessed during open heart surgery measured in regions of myocardium according to the pattern of [^{11}C] HED retention and myocardial perfusion. Segments with reduced [^{11}C] HED retention, a prolonged refractory period was observed as compared to those with normal [^{11}C] HED retention. (Reproduced by permission from Calkins H, Allman K, Bolling S, et al. Correlation between scintigraphic evidence of regional sympathetic neuronal dysfunction and ventricular refractoriness in the human heart. Circulation 1993;88(1):173–179.)

Again, this process appears to be heterogeneous with pronounced abnormalities in the apical segments of the left ventricle. Further studies are required to define the prognostic implication of neuronal dysfunction in patients with congestive heart failure as suggested by studies using the single photon tracer MIBG (186). The quantitative imaging approaches provided by PET may improve these qualitative observations.

POSTSYNAPTIC RECEPTOR SITES

The development of radiotracers and the initial clinical validation of tracer methods for the visualization of the adrenergic receptor system has been initiated by the group of Syrota, et al., at Orsay, France. These investigators synthesized radiolabeled β-receptor antagonists such as ^{11}C-propranolol and ^{11}C-practolol (187). They subsequently demonstrated the limitation of these radiopharmaceuticals for cardiac imaging because of their high retention in lung tissue. The specific visualization of cardiac β-receptors became possible by the successful radiosynthesis of a more hydrophilic β-receptor antagonist (CGP-12177). This nonselective ^{11}C-labeled β-receptor antagonist provided excellent image quality of the postsynaptic binding sites in the heart (187). However, the initial uptake of this tracer is primarily determined by delivery of radiotracer and is, therefore, rather flow sensitive. To overcome the effect of high affinity of this tracer for β-receptors, double administration of radiotracer with differing specific activity was advocated for the quantification of myocardial β-receptor density. A new tracer kinetic model approach yielded estimates of receptor densities in agreement with in vitro β-receptor density assessments. The clinical validation of this approach confirmed the in vitro-demonstrated reduction of β-receptor density in patients with congestive heart failure. Thi approach has also been adapted by Camici, et al. (209), a the Hammersmith Hospital, and used in patients with hy pertrophic cardiomyopathy. These PET studies demon strated a reduction in β-receptor density in this patien population. The reduced β-receptor density was nc only limited to the intraventricular septum, but also t the entire left ventricular myocardium, suggesting global change of the β-receptor density. Earlier work b Schwaiger, et al. (188), using ^{11}C HED, supports the hy pothesis, that sympathetic neurotransmission may be a tered in this patient population. These first studies usin β-receptor antagonists for visualization of the adrenergi receptor system indicate the potential of PET imaging i monitoring pathophysiologic alterations in β-receptor der sity and also in probing the effect of various pharmacologi interventions.

SUMMARY

PET imaging of the heart provides important clinical infor mation and exciting new avenues for clinical research. Th improved imaging technology, including attenuation co rection and high spatial resolution, allows for the highl accurate detection of coronary artery disease superior t SPECT imaging. The high costs and complexity of this pro cedure, however, currently limit its widespread clinical us and future cost/benefit studies are needed to define th exact clinical role of PET in the diagnosis of coronary arter disease. Quantitation of regional coronary blood flow an regional coronary reserve may add a new dimension to th noninvasive characterization of coronary artery diseas Coronary reserve measurements may be useful in the ear detection of vascular abnormalities in patients with hig risk for the development of premature coronary artery dis ease. In this patient population, PET could be used to mon itor interventions designed to halt or regress coronary a tery disease.

Assessment of tissue viability has become an importar application of PET in cardiology. Metabolic imaging docu mented the high incidence of hibernating myocardium i patients with severe coronary artery disease. These PE findings resulted in increased diagnostic efforts to identi viable myocardium by various methods. At the curren time, PET has to be considered the most accurate metho for identification of tissue viability, but less expensive tech nologies, such as ^{201}Tl SPECT imaging and dobutamir echocardiography, may be more suitable for widesprea use. In patients with high risk interventions and in trans plant candidates, PET may support the selection proces for revascularization.

Finally, new tracer approaches designed to map cardia innervation may not only prove useful in clinical researc assessing neurophysiology of various cardiovascular dis orders, but also provide important prognostic informatio in patients with congestive heart failure. The future clinic role of PET depends primarily on the development of sin plified PET tomographs and centralized distribution of ra diopharmaceuticals which are necessary to lower the cos of clinical cardiac PET. It is expected that PET and SPEC technology will overlap in the future, and the uniqueness of clinical information provided by each of these modalities will define their place in cardiology.

ACKNOWLEDGMENT

The authors appreciate the excellent secretarial help of Karin Haberl, and are thankful to Ngoc Nguyen for the careful preparation of illustrations.

REFERENCES

1. Sobel B, Breshahan G, Shell W, Yoder R. Estimation of infarct size in man and its retention to prognosis. Circulation 1972; 46:640–648.
2. Hoffman E, Phelps M, Weiss E, et al. Transaxial tomographic imaging of canine myocardium with ^{11}C-palmitic acid. J Nucl Med 1977;18:57–61.
3. Spinks T, Araujo L, Rhodes C, Hutton B. Physical aspects of cardiac scanning with a block detector positron tomograph. J Comput Assist Tomogr 1991;15:893–904.
4. Wienhard K, Eriksson L, Grootoonk S, Casey M, Pietrzyk U, Heiss W. Performance evaluation of the positron scanner ECAT EXACT. J Comput Assist Tomogr 1992;16:804–813.
5. Wienhard K, Dahlbom M, Eriksson L, et al. The ECAT EXACT HR: performance of a new high resolution positron scanner. J Comput Assist Tomogr 1994;18(1):110–118.
6. Ter-Pogossian M, Mullani N, Ficke D, Markham J, Snyder D. Photon time-of-flight-assisted positron emission tomography. J Comput Assist Tomogr 1981;5:227–239.
7. Mazoyer B, Trebossen R, Schoukroun C, et al. Physical evaluation of TTV03, a new high spatial resolution time-of-flight positron tomograph. IEEE Trans Nucl Sci 1990;37:778–782.
8. Lewellen T, Bice A, Harrisson R, Pencke M, Link J. Performance measurements of the SP3000/UW time-of-flight positron emission tomograph. IEEE Trans Nucl Sci 1988;35:665–669.
9. Meikle S, Dahlbom M, Cherry S. Attenuation correction using count-limited transmission data in positron emission tomography. J Nucl Med 1993;34:143–150.
10. Xu E, Mullani N, Gould K, Anderson W. A segmented attenuation correction for PET. J Nucl Med 1991;32:161–165.
11. Thompson C, Ranger N, Evans A. Simultaneous transmission and emission scans in positron emission tomography. IEEE Trans Nucl Sci 1989;36:1011–1016.
12. Thompson C, Ranger N, Evans A, Gjedde A. Validation of simultaneous PET emission and transmission scans. J Nucl Med 1991;32:154–160.
13. Iida H, Rhodes C, deSilva R, et al. Myocardial tissue fraction—correction for partial volume effects and measure of tissue viability. J Nucl Med 1991;32:2169–2175.
14. Hutchins G, Caraher J, Raylman R. A region of interest strategy for minimizing resolution distortions in quantitative myocardial PET studies. J Nucl Med 1992;33:1243–1250.
15. Cherry S, Dahlbom M, Hoffman E. Three-dimensional PET using a conventional multislice tomograph without septa. J Comp Assist Tomogr 1991;15:655–668.
16. Colsher J. Fully three-dimensional positron emission tomography. Phys Med Biol 1980;25:103.
17. Townsend D, Spinks T, Jones T, et al. Three-dimensional reconstruction of PET data from a multiring camera. IEEE Trans Nucl Sci 1989;36:1056–1066.
18. Bailey D, Lee K, Stocks G, Meikle S, Dobko T. Clinical 3D PET for improved patient throughput. J Nucl Med 1993;34:184.
19. Weinberg I, Huang S, Hoffman E, et al. Validation of PET-acquired input functions for cardiac studies. J Nucl Med 1988; 29:241–247.
20. Gambhir S, Schwaiger M, Huang S, et al. Simple noninvasive quantification method for measuring myocardial glucose utilization in humans employing positron emission tomography and fluorine-18 deoxyglucose. J Nucl Med 1989;30:359–366.
21. Raylman R, Caraher J, Hutchins G. Sampling requirements for dynamic cardiac PET studies using image derived input functions. J Nucl Med 1993;34(3):440–447.
22. Huang S, Phelps M. Principles of tracer kinetic modeling in positron emission tomography and autoradiography. In: Phelps M, Mazziotta J, Schelbert H, eds. Positron emission tomography and autoradiography: principles and applications for the brain and heart. New York: Raven Press, 1986:287–346.
23. Schwaiger M, Muzik O. Assessment of myocardial perfusion by positron emission tomography. Am J Cardiol 1991;67:35D-43D.
24. Iida H, Kanno I, Takahashi A, et al. Measurement of absolute myocardial blood flow with $H_2{}^{15}O$ and dynamic positron emission tomography. Strategy for quantification in relation to the partial-volume effect. Circulation 1988;78:104–115.
25. Araujo LI, Lammertsma AA, Rhodes CG, et al. Noninvasive quantification of regional myocardial blood flow in coronary artery disease with oxygen-15-labeled carbon dioxide inhalation and positron emission tomography. Circulation 1991;83:875–885.
26. Bergmann S, Herrero P, Markham J, Weinheimer C, Walsh M. Noninvasive quantitation of myocardial blood flow in human subjects with oxygen-15-labeled water and positron emission tomography. J Am Coll Cardiol 1989;14:639–652.
27. Schelbert H, Phelps M, Huang S, et al. N-13 ammonia as an indicator of myocardial blood flow. Circulation 1981;63:1259–1272.
28. Schelbert HR, Phelps ME, Hoffman EJ, Huang SC, Selin CE, Kuhl DE. Regional myocardial perfusion assessed with N-13-labeled ammonia and positron emission computerized axial tomography. Am J Cardiol 1979;43:209–218.
29. Bergmann S, Hack S, Tewson T, et al. The dependence of accumulation of $^{13}NH_3$ by myocardium on metabolic factors and its implications for quantitative assessment of perfusion. Circulation 1980;61:34–43.
30. Goldstein R, Mullani NA, Fisher DJ, et al. Myocardial perfusion with rubidium-82: II. Effects of metabolic and pharmacologic interventions. J Nucl Med 1983;24:907–915.
31. Goldstein R. Kinetics of rubidium-82 after coronary occlusion and reperfusion. Assessment of patency and viability in open-chested dogs. J Clin Invest 1985;75:1131–1137.
32. Mullani N, Goldstein R, Gould K, et al. Perfusion imaging with rubidium-82: I. Measurement of extraction and flow with external detectors. J Nucl Med 1983;24:898–906.
33. Melon P, Brihaye C, Degueldre C, et al. Myocardial kinetics of potassium-38 in man and comparison with copper-62-PTSM. J Nucl Med 1994;35:1116–1122.
34. Beller G, Cochavi S, Smith T, Brownell G. Positron emission tomographic imaging of the myocardium with Rb-81. J Comput Asst Tomogr 1982;6:341–349.
35. Shah A., Schelbert H, Schwaiger M, et al. Measurement of regional myocardial blood flow with N-13 ammonia and positron emission tomography in intact dogs. J Am Coll Cardiol 1985; 5:92–100.
36. Czernin J, Muller P, Chan S, et al. Influence of age and hemodynamics on myocardial blood flow and flow reserve. Circulation 1993;88(1):62–69.
37. Krivokapich J, Huang S, Phelps M, et al. Dependence of $^{13}NH_3$ myocardial extraction and clearance on flow and metabolism. Am J Physiol 1982;242:536–542.
38. Krivokapich J, Smith GT, Huang SC, et al. ^{13}N ammonia myocardial imaging at rest and with exercise in normal volunteers. Quantification of absolute myocardial perfusion with dynamic positron emission tomography. Circulation 1989;80(5):1328–37.

39. Neirinckx R, Kronauge J, Gennaro G. Evaluation of inorganic absorbents for rubidium-82 generator: I. Hydrous Sno2. J Nucl Med 1982;24:898–906.
40. Hichwa R, Johnston D, Ponto L, Watkins G. Handheld automated injector for O-15 water studies. J Nucl Med 1991;32:109.
41. Gould K. Assessment of coronary stenoses with myocardial perfusion imaging during pharmacologic coronary vasodilation. Am J Cardiol 1978;42:761–768.
42. Go RT, Marwick TH, MacIntyre WJ, et al. A prospective comparison of rubidium-82 PET and thallium-201 SPECT myocardial perfusion imaging utilizing a single dipyridamole stress in the diagnosis of coronary artery disease. J Nucl Med 1990;31:1899–1905.
43. Stewart R, Schwaiger M, Molina E, et al. Comparison of rubidium-82 positron emission tomography and thallium-201 SPECT imaging for detection of coronary artery disease. Am J Cardiol 1991;67:1303–1310.
44. Tamaki N, Yonekura Y, Senda M, et al. Myocardial positron computed tomography with ^{13}N-ammonia at rest and during exercise. Eur J Nucl Med 1985;11:246–251.
45. Gould K, Goldstein R, Mullani N, et al. Noninvasive assessment of coronary stenoses by myocardial perfusion imaging during pharmacologic coronary vasodilation. VIII. Clinical feasibility of positron cardiac imaging without a cyclotron using generator-produced rubidium-82. J Am Coll Cardiol 1986;7:775–789.
46. Krivokapich J, Stevenson LW, Kobashigawa J, Huang SC, Schelbert HR. Quantification of absolute myocardial perfusion at rest and during exercise with positron emission tomography after human cardiac transplantation. J Am Coll Cardiol 1991;18(2):512–517.
47. Demer L, Gould K, Goldstein R, et al. Assessment of coronary artery disease severity by positron emission tomography. Comparison with quantitative arteriography in 193 patients. Circulation 1989;79:825–835.
48. Tamaki N, Yonehura Y, Senda M, et al. Value and limitation of stress thallium-201 single photon positron emission computed tomography: comparison with nitrogen-13 ammonia positron tomography. J Nucl Med 1988;29:1187–1188.
49. Hicks K, Ganti G, Mullani N, Gould K. Automated quantitation of three-dimensional cardiac positron emission tomography for routine clinical use. J Nucl Med 1989;30:1787–1797.
50. Porenta G, Kuhle W, Czernin J, et al. Semiquantitative assessment of myocardial blood flow and viability using polar map displays of cardiac PET images. J Nucl Med 1992;33(9):1628–1636.
51. Laubenbacher C, Rothley J, Sitomer J, et al. An automated analysis program for the evaluation of cardiac PET studies: initial results in the detection and localization of coronary artery disease using nitrogen-13 ammonia. J Nucl Med 1993;34:968–978.
52. Allman C, Rothley J, Yang S, et al. Quantitative analysis of Rb-82 PET images: intra and interobserver variability. J Nucl Med Tech 1992;20(2):101.
53. Stewart R, Popma J, Gacioch G, et al. Comparison of thallium-201 SPECT redistribution patterns and rubidium-82 PET rest-stress myocardial blood flow imaging. Intl J Cardiac Imaging 1994;10:15–23.
54. Muzik O, Beanlands RSB, Wolfe E, Hutchins GD, Schwaiger M. Automated region definition for cardiac nitrogen-13-ammonia PET imaging. J Nucl Med 1993;34(2):336–344.
55. Muzik O, Beanlands RSB, Hutchins GD, Mangner TJ, Nguyen N, Schwaiger M. Validation of nitrogen-13-ammonia tracer kinetic model for quantification of myocardial blood flow using PET. J Nucl Med 1993;34:83–91.
56. Bergmann S, Herrero P, Markham J, Weinheimer C, Walsh M. Noninvasive quantitation of myocardial blood flow in human subjects with oxygen-15-labeled water and positron emission tomography. J Am Coll Cardiol 1989;14:639–652.
57. Araujo L, Lammertsma AA, Rhodes CG, et al. Noninvasive quantification of regional myocardial blood flow in coronary artery disease with oxygen-15-labeled carbon dioxide inhalation and positron emission tomography. Circulation 1991;83(3):875–885.
58. Iida H, Takahashi A, Ono Y, et al. Quantitative and noninvasive measurement of myocardial blood flow using $H_2{}^{15}O$ and dynamic positron emission tomography. J Nucl Med 1986;27:976.
59. Walsh M, Bergmann S, Steele R, et al. Delineation of impaired regional myocardial perfusion by positron emission tomography with $H_2{}^{15}O$. Circulation 1988;78:612–620.
60. Bergmann SR, Fox K, Rand A, et al. Quantification of regional myocardial blood flow with $H_2{}^{15}O$. Circulation 1984;70:724–33.
61. Bol A, Melin JA, Vanoverschelde J-L, et al. Direct comparison of N-13-ammonia and O-15 water estimates of perfusion with quantification of regional myocardial blood flow by microspheres. Circulation 1993;87(2):512–525.
62. Hutchins GD, Schwaiger M, Rosenspire KC, Kripokapich J, Schelbert HR, Kuhl DE. Noninvasive quantification of regional blood flow in the human heart using N-13 ammonia and dynamic PET imaging. J Am Coll Cardiol 1990;15(5):1032–42.
63. Smith G, Huang S, Nienaber C, Krivokapich J, Schelbert H. Noninvasive quantification of regional myocardial blood flow with N-13 ammonia and dynamic PET [Abstract]. J Nucl Med 1988; 29:940.
64. Choi Y, Huang S, Hawkins R, et al. A simplified method for quantification of myocardial blood flow using nitrogen-13-ammonia and dynamic PET. J Nucl Med 1993;34(3):488–497.
65. Nienaber C, Ratib O, Gambhir S, et al. A quantitative index of regional blood flow in canine myocardium derived noninvasively with N-13 ammonia and dynamic positron emission tomography. JACC 1991;17(1):260–269.
66. Herrero P, Markham J, Shelton ME, et al. Noninvasive quantification of regional myocardial perfusion with rubidium-82 and positron emission tomography. Exploration of a mathematical model. Circulation 1990;82:1377–1386.
67. Herrero P, Markham J, Weinheimer C, et al. Quantification of regional myocardial perfusion with generator-produced Cu-PTSM and positron emission tomography. Circulation 1993; 87(1):173–183.
68. Beanlands R, Muzik O, Mintun M, et al. The kinetics of copper-62-PTSM in the normal human heart. J Nucl Med 1992; 33(5):684–690.
69. Gould K, Kirkeeide R, Buchi M. Coronary flow reserve as a physiologic measure of stenosis severity. J Am Coll Cardiol 1990; 15(2):459–474.
70. Mancini JGB, Williamson PR, DeBoe SF. Effect of coronary stenosis severity on variability of quantative arteriography and implications for interventional trials, 1992. Am J Cardiol 1992; 69:806–807.
71. Marcus M, Skorton D, Johnson M, Collins S, Harrison D, Kerber R. Visual estimates of percent diameter coronary stenosis: a battered gold standard. J Am Coll Cardiol 1988;11:882–885.
72. Wilson RF, Marcus ML, White CW. Prediction of the physiologic significance of coronary arterial lesions by quantitative lesion geometry in patients with limited coronary artery disease. Circulation 1987;75(4):723–732.
73. Gould K, Martucci J, Goldberg D, et al. Short-term cholesterol lowering decreases size and severity of perfusion abnormalities by positron emission tomography after dipyridamole in patients with coronary artery disease: a potential noninvasive marker of healing coronary endothelium. Circulation 1994;89(4):1530–1538.
74. L'Abbate A, Camici P, Reisenhofer B. Abnormal coronary flow reserve in syndrome X: a critical view of the concept of vasodilator reserve and its relation to ischemia. Coronary Artery Disease 1992;3:579–585.
75. Beanlands R, Muzik O, Melon P, et al. Noninvasive quantification of regional coronary perfusion reserve in stenosed and angio-

graphically normal vessels of patients with coronary atherosclerosis. Circulation 1994;(in press).
76. Muzik O, Beanlands R, Dayanikli F, Wolfe E, Schwaiger M. Quantification of myocardial blood flow reserve using PET and [N-13]ammonia in patients with angiographically documented CAD. J Nucl Med 1993;34(5):35P.
77. Parodi O, Neglia D, Palombo C, et al. Comparative effect of enalapril and verapamil on myocardial blood flow in systemic hypertension. N Engl J Med 1993; subm.
78. Araujo LI. Myocardial perfusion and metabolis changes associated with transient episodes of ischemia in patients with coronary artery disease as assessed by positron emission tomography. Coronary Artery Disease 1990;1(5):541–546.
79. Beanlands R, Melon P, Muzik O, et al. N-13 ammonia PET identifies reduced perfusion reserve in angiographically normal regions of patients with CAD. Circulation 1992;86(4):I-184.
80. Camici P, Chiriatti G, Lorenzoni R, et al. Coronary Vasodilation is impaired in both hypertrophied and nonhypertrophied myocardium of patients with hypertrophic cardiomyopathy: a study with nitrogen-13 ammonia and positron emission tomography. J Am Coll Cardiol 1991;17:879–886.
81. Picano E, Parodi O, Lattanzi F, et al. Assessment of anatomic and physiological severity of single-vessel coronary artery lesions by dipyridamole echocardiography. Comparison with positron emission tomography and quantitative angiography. Circulation 1994;89(2):753–761.
82. Uren N, Melin J, De Bruyne B, et al. Maximal myocardial flow as a function of stenosis severity in man. Circulation 1993;88(4):I-274.
83. Dayanikli F, Grambow D, Muzik O, Mosca L, Rubenfire M, Schwaiger M. Early detection of abnormal coronary flow reserve in asymptomatic men at high risk for coronary artery disease using positron emission tomography. Circulation 1994; 90(2):808–817.
84. Maseri A, Crea F, Cianflone D. Myocardial ischemia caused by distal coronary vasoconstriction. Am J Cardiol 1992;70:1602–1605.
85. Grambow D, Dayanikli F, Muzik O, et al. Assessment of endothelial function with PET cold pressure test in patients with various degrees of coronary atherosclerosis. J Nucl Med 1993; 34(5):36P.
86. Senneff M, Hartman J, Sobel B, Geltman E, Bergmann S. Persistence of coronary vasodilator responsivity after cardiac transplantation. Am J Cardiol 1993;71:333–338.
87. Merlet P, Mazoyer B, Hittinger L, et al. Assessment of coronary reserve in man: comparison between positron emission tomography with oxygen-15-labeled water and intracoronary Doppler-technique. J Nucl Med 1993;34(10):1–6.
88. Liedtke AJ. Alterations of carbohydrate and lipid metabolism in the acutely ischemic heart. Prog Cardiovasc Dis 1981;23:321–36.
89. Taegtmeyer H. Myocardial metabolism. In: Phelps M, Mazziotta J, Schelbert H, eds. Positron emission tomography and autoradiography: principles and applications for the brain and heart. Ch. 4. New York: Raven Press, 1986:149–195.
90. Gertz EW, Wisneski JA, Stanley WC, Neese RA. Myocardial substrate utilization during exercise in humans. J Clin Invest 1988; 82:2017–2025.
91. Neely J. Metabolic disturbances after coronary occlusion. Hosp Practice 1989;1:81–96.
92. Opie L, Owen P, Riemersma R. Relative rates of oxidation of glucose and free fatty acids by ischemic and nonischemic myocardium after coronary artery ligation in the dog. Eur J Clin Invest 1973;3:419–435.
93. Opie L. Effects of regional ischemia on metabolism of glucose and fatty acids. Circ Res 1976;38(Suppl I):52–74.
94. Kalff V, Schwaiger M, Nguyen N, Mcclanahan TB, Gallagher K. The relationship between myocardial blood flow and glucose uptake in ischemic canine myocardium determined with F-18 deoxyglucose. J Nucl Med 1992;33(7):1346–1353.
95. Schwaiger M, Schelbert HR, Ellison D, et al. Sustained regional abnormalities in cardiac metabolism after transient ischemia in the chronic dog model. J Am Coll Cardiol 1985;6(2):336–347.
96. Camici P, Ferrannini E, Opie L. Myocardial metabolism in ischemic heart disease:basic principles and application to imaging by positron emission tomography. Prog Cardiovasc Dis 1989; 32(3):217–238.
97. Sun D, Nguyen N, DeGrado T, Schwaiger M, Brosius F. Ischemia induces translocation of the insulin-responsive glucose transporter GLUT4 to the plasma membrane of cardiac myocytes. Circulation 1994;89(2):793–798.
98. Borgers M, De-Nollin S, Thone F, Wouters L, Van-Vaeck L, Flameng W. Distribution of calcium in a subset of chronic hibernating myocardium in man. Histochem J 1993;25(4):312–318.
99. Schoen H, Najafi A, Hansen H, et al. C-11-labeled palmitic acid for the noninvasive evaluation of regional myocardial fatty acid metabolism with positron computed tomography. II. Kinetics of C-11 palmitic acid in acutely ischemic myocardium. Am Heart J 1982;1103:548–561.
100. Schelbert HR, Henze E, Schon H, et al. C-11-labeled palmitic acid for the noninvasive evaluation of regional myocardial fatty acid metabolism with positron computed tomography. III. In vivo demonstration of the effects of of substrate availability on myocardial metabolism. Am Heart J 1983;105:492–504.
101. Bergmann S, Nomura H, Rand A, Sobel B, Lange L. Externally detectable changes in fatty acid utilization by perfused hearts from rabbits exposed to alcohol. Circulation 1982;66:II-109.
102. Kelly D, Mendelsohn N, Sobel B, Bergmann S. Detection and assessment by positron emission tomography of a genetically determined defect in myocardial fatty acid utilization (long-chain acyl-CoA dehydrogenase deficiency). Am J Cardiol 1993; 71(8):738–744.
103. Schelbert H, Henze E, Schon H, et al. C-11 palmitic acid for the noninvasive evaluation of regional myocardial fatty acid metabolism with positron computed tomography. IV. In vivo demonstration of impaired fatty acid oxidation in acute myocardial ischemia. Am Heart J 1983;106:736–750.
104. Wijns W, Schwaiger M, Huang S-C, et al. Effects of inhibition of fatty acid oxidation on myocardial kinetics of ^{11}C-labeled palmitate. Circ Res 1989;65:1787–1797.
105. Schwaiger M, Schelbert H, Keen R, et al. Retention and clearance of C-11 palmitic acid in ischemic and reperfused canine myocardium. J Am Coll Cardiol 1985;6:311–320.
106. Schwaiger M, Fishbein M, Block M, et al. Metabolic and ultrastructural abnormalities during ischemia in canine myocardium: noninvasive assessment by positron emission tomography. J Mol Cell Cardiol 1987;19:259–269.
107. Buxton DB, Schwaiger M, Nguyen N, Phelps ME, Schelbert HR. Radiolabeled acetate as a tracer of myocardial tricarboxylic acid cycle flux. Circul Res 1988;63:628–634.
108. Kotzerke J, Hicks RJ, Wolfe E, et al. Three-dimensional assessment of myocardial oxidative metabolism: a new approach for regional determination of PET-derived C-11 acetate kinetics. J Nucl Med 1990;31:1876–1893.
109. Brown M, Marshall D, Sobel B, Bergmann S. Delineation of myocardial oxygen utilization with carbon-11-labeled acetate. Circulation 1987;76:687–696.
110. Brown M, Myears D, Bergmann S. Noninvasive assessment of canine myocardial oxidative metabolism with carbon-11 acetate and positron emission tomography. J Am Coll Cardiol 1988; 12:1054–1063.
111. Brown M, Myears D, Bergmann S. Validity of estimates of myocardial oxidative metabolism with carbon-11 acetate and posi-

tron emission tomography despite altered patterns of substrate utilization. J Nucl Med 1989;30:187–193.

112. Buck A, Wolpers H, Hutchins G, et al. Effect of carbon-11-acetate recirculation on estimates of myocardial oxygen consumption by PET. J Nuc Med 1991;32:1950–1957.
113. Sokoloff L, Reivich M, Kennedy C, et al. The (14C) deoxyglucose method for the measurement local cerebral glucose utilization: theory, procedure and normal values in the conscious and anesthetized albino rat. J Neurochem 1977;28:897–916.
114. Phelps ME, Huang SC, Hoffman EJ, et al. Tomographic measurement of local glucose metabolic rate in humans with (F-18) 2-fluoro-2-deoxy-D-glucose: validation of method. Ann Neurol 1979;6:371–388.
115. Krivokapich J, Huang S, Phelps M, et al. Estimation of rabbit myocardial metabolic rate for glucose using fluorodeoxyglucose. Am J Physiol 1982;243:H884–H895.
116. Krivokapich J, Huang SC, Selin CE, Phelps ME. Fluorodeoxyglucose rate constants, lumped constant, and glucose metabolic rate in rabbit heart. Am J Physiol 1987;252:H777–H787.
117. Ratib O, Phelps ME, Huang SC, Henze E, Selin CE, Schelbert HR. Positron tomography with deoxyglucose for estimating local myocardial glucose metabolism. J Nucl Med 1982;23(7):577–586.
118. Huang SC, Williams BA, Barrio JR, et al. Measurement of glucose and 2-deoxy-2-[18F]fluoro-D-glucose transport and phosphorylation rates in myocardium using dual-tracer kinetic experiments. Febs Lett 1987;216(1):128–132.
119. Marshall R, Nash W, Shine K, Pehlps M, Ricchiuti N. Glucose metabolism during ischemia due to excessive oxygen demand or altered coronary flow in the isolated arterially perfused rabbit septum. Circ Res 1981;49:640–648.
120. Marshall RC, Huang SC, Nash WW, Phelps ME. Assessment of the [18F]fluorodeoxyglucose kinetic model in calculations of myocardial glucose metabolism during ischemia. J Nucl Med 1983;24(11):1060–1064.
121. Ng C, Holden J, DeGrado T, Raffel D, Kornguth M, Gatley S. Sensitivity of myocardial fluorodeoxyglucose lumped constant to glucose insulin. Am J Physiol 1991;260:593–603.
122. Phelps ME, Hoffman EJ, Selin CE, et al. Investigation of 18-F 2-fluoro 2-deoxyglucose for the measure of myocardial glucose metabolism. J Nucl Med 1978;19:1311–1319.
123. Patlak CS, Blasberg RG, Fenstermacher JD. Graphical evaluation of blood-to-brain transfer constants from multiple-time uptake data. J Cereb Blood Flow Metab 1983;3:1–7.
124. Gambhir SS, Schwaiger M, Huang SC, et al. Simple noninvasive quantification method for measuring myocardial glucose utilization in humans employing positron emission tomography and fluorine-18 deoxyglucose. J Nucl Med 1989;30(3):359–366.
125. Choi Y, Hawkins R, Huang S, et al. Parametric images of myocardial metabolic rate of glucose generated from dynamic cardiac PET and 2-[18F]fluoro-2-deoxy-d-glucose studies. J Nucl Med 1991;32(4):733–738.
126. Schelbert H, Schon H, Henze E, Huang S, Barrio J, Phelps M. Effects of substrate availability and acute ischemia on regional myocardial metabolism demonstrated noninvasively with F-18 deoxyglucose, C-11 palmitic acid and positron computed tomography. In: Raynaud C, ed. Nuclear medicine and biology, Proceedings of the Third World Congress of Nuclear Medicine and Biology, 1982. Paris, France: Pergamon Press, 1982:2510–2513.
127. Hicks R, Herman W, Kalff V, et al. Quantitative evaluation of regional substrate metabolism in the human heart by positron emission tomography. JACC 1991;18(1):101–111.
128. Gropler R, Siegel B, Geltman E. Myocardial uptake of carbon-11 acetate as an indirect measurement of regional myocardial blood flow. J Nucl Med 1991;32:245–251.
129. Chan S, Brunken R, Phelps M, Schelbert H. Use of the metabolic tracer carbon-11 acetate for evaluation of regional myocardial perfusion. J Nucl Med 1991;32:665–672.
130. Geltman EM, Smith JL, Beecher D, Ludbrook PA, Ter PMM, Sobel BE. Altered regional myocardial metabolism in congestive cardiomyopathy detected by positron tomography. Am J Med 1983;74(5):773–785.
131. Grover M, Schwaiger M, Sochor H, et al. C-11 palmitic acid kinetics and positron emission tomography detect pacing-induced ischemia in patients with coronary artery disease. Circulation 1984;70(Suppl II):II-340.
132. Geltman E. Metabolic findings in cardiomyopathies. In: Marcus ML, Schelbert HR, Skorton DJ, et al., eds. Cardiac imaging: a companion to Braunwald's heart disease. Ch. 68. Philadelphia: W.B. Saunders Company, Harcourt Brace Jovanovich, Inc., 1991:1244–1255.
133. Beanlands RSB, Bach DS, Raylman R, et al. Acute effects of dobutamine on myocardial oxygen consumption and cardiac efficiency measured using carbon-11 acetate kinetics in patients with dilated cardiomyopathy. JACC 1993;22(5):1389–1398.
134. Hicks RJ, Herman WH, Wolfe E, Kotzerke J, Kuhl DE, Schwaiger M. Regional variation in oxidative and glucose metabolism in the normal heart: comparison of PET-derived C-11 acetate and FDG kinetics [Abstract 279]. J Nucl Med 1990;31(5):774.
135. Gropler R, Lee K, Moerlein S, Siegel B, Geltman E. Regional variation in myocardial accumulation of 18F-fluorodeoxyglucose in fasted normal subjects [Abstract]. JACC 1990;15(2):81A.
136. vom Dahl J, Hermann WH, Hicks RJ, et al. Myocardial glucose uptake in patients with insulin-dependent diabetes mellitus assessed quantitatively by dynamic positron emission tomography. Circulation 1993;88(2):395–404.
137. Schelbert HR, Henze E, Phelps ME, Kuhl DE. Assessment of regional myocardial ischemia by positron-emission computed tomography. Am Heart J 1982;103:588–597.
138. Schwaiger M, Brunken R, Grover-McKay M, et al. Regional myocardial metabolism in patients with acute myocardial infarction assessed by positron emission tomography. J Am Coll Cardiol 1986;8:800–808.
139. Marshall RC, Tillisch JH, Phelps ME, et al. Identification and differentiation of resting myocardial ischemia and infarction in man with positron computed tomography ^{18}F-labeled fluorodeoxyglucose and N-13 ammonia. Circulation 1981;64:766–778.
140. Tillisch J, Brunken R, Marshall R, et al. Reversibility of cardiac wall-motion abnormalities predicted by positron tomography. N Engl J Med 1986;314(14):884–8.
141. Brunken RC, Tillisch JH, Schwaiger M, et al. Detection of viable tissue in myocardial segments with thallium perfusion defects using positron emission tomography. Circulation 1985; 72(Suppl):III-443.
142. Brunken R, Tillisch J, Schwaiger M, et al. Regional perfusion, glucose metabolism, and wall motion in patients with chronic electrocardiographic Q wave infarctions: evidence for persistence of viable tissue in some infarct regions by positron emission tomography. Circulation 1986;73:951–963.
143. Brunken RC, Kottou S, Nienaber CA, et al. PET detection of viable tissue in myocardial segments with persistent defects at T1-201 SPECT. Radiology 1989;172(1):65–73.
144. Brunken RC, Schwaiger M, Grover-McKay M, Phelps ME, Tillisch JH, Schelbert HR. Positron emission tomography detects tissue metabolic activity in myocardial segments with persistent thallium perfusion defects. J Am Coll Cardiol 1987;10:557–567.
145. Dilsizian V, Rocco T, Freeman NMT, Leon MB, Bonow RO. Enhanced detection of ischemic but viable myocardium by the reinjection of thallium after stress-redistribution imaging. N Engl J Med 1990;323:141–146.
146. Ohtani H, Tamaki N, Yonekura Y. Value of thallium-201 reinjec-

tion after delayed SPECT imaging for predicting reversible ischemia after coronary artery bypass grafting. Am J Cardiol 1990; 66:394–399.

147. Bonow RO, Dilsizian V, Cuocolo A, Bacharach SL. Identification of viable myocardium in patients with chronic coronary artery disease and left ventricular dysfunction: comparison of thallium scintigraphy with reinjection and PET imaging with 18-F-fluorodexoyglucose. Circulation 1991;83(1):26–37.

148. Altehoefer C, vom Dahl J, Buell U, Uebis R, Kleinhans E, Hanrath P. Comparison of thallium-201 single-photon emission tomography after rest injection and fluorodeoxyglucose positron emission tomography for assessment of myocardial viability in patients with chronic coronary artery disease. Eur J Nucl Med 1994;21:37–45.

149. Altehoefer C, Kaiser H-J, Doerr R, et al. Fluorine-18 deoxyglucose positron emission tomography for assessment of viable myocardium in perfusion defects found on technetium-99m methoxyisobutylisonitrile single photon emission tomography: a comparative study in patients with coronary artery disease. Eur J Nucl Med 1992;19(5):334–342.

150. Cuocolo A, Pace L, Ricciardelli B, Chiarello M, Trimarco B, Salvatore M. Identification of viable myocardium in patients with chronic coronary artery disease: comparison of thallium-201 scintigraphy with reinjection and technetium-99m-methoxy isobutyl isonitrile. J Nucl Med 1992;33:505–511.

151. Sawada SG, Allman KC, Muzik O, et al. Positron emission tomography detects evidence of viability in rest technetium-99m sestamibi defects. JACC 1994;23(1):92–98.

152. Eitzman D, Al-Aouar ZR, Kanter HL, et al. Clinical outcome of patients with advanced coronary artery disease following positron emission tomography viability studies. J Am Coll Cardiol 1992;20(3):559–565.

153. Maddahi J, DiCarli M, Davidson M, et al. Prognostic significance of PET assessment of myocardial viability in patients with left ventricular dysfunction. JACC 1992;19(3):142A.

154. Tamaki N, Yonekura Y, Yamashita K, et al. Prognostic value of an increase in fluorine-18 deoxyglucose uptake in patients with myocardial infarction: comparison with stress thallium imaging. J Am Coll Cardiol 1993;22:1621–1627.

155. vom Dahl J, Hicks RJ, Lee KS, Eitzman D, Al-Alouar ZR, Schwaiger M. Positron emission tomography myocardial viability studies in patients with diabetes mellitus [Abstract]. J Am Coll Cardiol 1991;17:121A.

156. vom Dahl J, Herman W, Hicks R, et al. Myocardial glucose uptake in patients with insulin-dependent diabetes mellitus assessed quantitatively by dynamic positron emission tomography. Circulation 1993;88(2):395–404.

157. Gropler R, Geltman E, Sampathkumaran K, et al. Functional recovery after coronary revascularization for chronic coronary artery disease is dependent on maintenance of oxidative metabolism. J Am Coll Cardiol 1992;20:569–577.

158. Gropler R, Geltman E, Sampathkumaran K, et al. Comparison of carbon-11-acetate with fluorine-18-fluorodeoxyglucose for delineating viable myocardium by positron emission tomography. JACC 1993;22(6):1587–1597.

159. vom Dahl J, Muzik O, Wolfe E, Schwaiger M. Rubidium-82 (Rb-82) kinetics assessed by positron emission tomography (PET) for characterization of myocardial viability [Abstract]. J Am Coll Cardiol 1992;19(3):142A.

160. Yoshida K, Gould K. Quantitative relation of myocardial infarction size and myocardial viability by positron emission tomography to left ventricular ejection fraction and 3-year mortality with and without revascularization. J Am Coll Cardiol 1993; 22:984–997.

161. Yamamoto Y, de Silva R, Rhodes C, et al. A new strategy for the assessment of viable myocardium and regional myocardial blood flow using 15O-water and dynamic positron emission tomography. Circulation 1992;86:167–178.

162. Martin GV, Caldwell JH, Rasey JS, Grunbaum Z, Cerqueira M, Krohn KA. Enhanced binding of the hypoxic cell marker [H-3] fluoromisonidazole in ischemic myocardium. J Nucl Med 1989; 30:194–201.

163. Shelton M, Dence C, Hwang D-R, Herrero P, Welch M, Bergmann S. In vivo delineation of myocardial hypoxia during coronary occlusion using fluorine-18 fluoromisonidazole and positron emission tomography: a potential approach for identification of jeopardized myocardium. J Am Coll Cardiol 1990;16:477–485.

164. Sochor H, Schelbert HR, Schwaiger M, Henze E, Phelps ME. Studies of fatty acid metabolism with positron emission tomography in patients with cardiomyopathy. Eur J Nucl Med 1986; 12:S66–S69.

165. Buxton DB, Nienaber CA, Luxen A, et al. Noninvasive quantitation of regional myocardial oxygen consumption in vivo with [1-11C] acetate and dynamic positron emission tomography. Circulation 1989;79:134–142.

166. Hicks RJ, Savas V, Currie PJ, et al. Assessment of myocardial oxidative metabolism in aortic valve disease using positron emission tomography with C-11 acetate. Am Heart J 1992; 123(3):653–664.

167. Hicks R, Kalff V, Savas V, Starling M, Schwaiger M. Assessment of right ventricular oxidative metabolism by positron emission tomography with C-11 acetate in aortic valve disease. Am J Cardiol 1991;67:753–757.

168. Wolpers H, Buck A, Nguyen N, et al. An approach to ventricular efficiency in heart failure by use of C-11 acetate and positron emission tomography. J Nucl Cardiol 1994;1:262–269.

169. Beanlands R, Armstrong W, Hicks R, et al. The effects of afterload reduction on myocardial C-11 acetate kinetics and noninvasively estimated mechanical efficiency in patients with dilated cardiomyopathy. J Nucl Cardiol 1994;1:3–13.

170. Grover-McKay M, Schwaiger M, Krivokapich J, Perloff J, Phelps M, Schelbert H. Regional myocardial blood flow and metabolism at rest and during exercise in patients with hypertrophic cardiomyopathy: initial observation. J Am Coll Cardiol 1989; 13(3):745–754.

171. Francis G. Modulation of peripheral sympathetic nerve transmission. J Am Coll Cardiol 1988;12:250–254.

172. Goldstein D, Brush J Jr, Eisenhofer G, Stull R, Esler M. In vivo measurement of neuronal uptake of norepinephrine in the human heart. Circulation 1988;78:41–48.

173. Rosenspire K, Haka M, Jewett D, et al. Synthesis and preliminary evaluation of 11C-meta-hydroxyephedrine: a false transmitter agent for heart neuronal imaging. J Nucl Med 1990;31:1328–1334.

174. DeGrado T, Hutchins G, Toorongian S, Wieland D, Schwaiger M. Myocardial kinetics of carbon-11-meta-hydroxyephedrine: retention mechanisms and effects of norepinephrine. J Nucl Med 1993;34(8):1287–1293.

175. Schwaiger M, Wieland D, Muzik O, et al. Comparison of C-11 epinephrine and C-11 HED for evaluation of sympathetic neurons of the heart. J Nucl Med 1993;34(5):13P.

176. Nguyen N, DeGrado T, Chakraborty P, Stafford K, Wieland D, Schwaiger M. Evaluation of C-11 epinephrine in isolated working rat heart. J Nucl Med 1993;34(5):45P.

177. Corbett J, Chiao P-C, del Rosario R, et al. Mapping neuronal enzyme function of the human heart with C-11 phenylephrine. J Nucl Med 1994;35(5):109P.

178. Goldstein D, Eisenhofer G, Dunn B, et al. Positron emission tomographic imaging of cardiac sympathetic innervation using 6-18F-fluorodopamine: initial findings in humans. J Am Coll Cardiol 1993;22(7):1961–1971.

179. Ding Y, Fowler J, Dewey S, et al. Comparison of high specific

activity (-) and (+)-6-18F-fluoronorepinephrine and 6-18F-fluorodopamine in baboons: heart uptake, metabolism and the effect of desipramine. J Nucl Med 1993;34(4):619–629.
180. Schwaiger M, Kalff V, Rosenspire K, et al. The noninvasive evaluation of the sympathetic nervous system in the human heart by PET. Circulation 1990;82:457–464.
181. Schwaiger M, Hutchins G, Kalff V, et al. Evidence for regional catecholamine uptake and storage sites in the transplanted human heart by positron emission tomography. J Clin Invest 1991; 87:1681–1690.
182. Allman K, Wieland D, Muzik O, DeGrado T, Wolfe E Jr, Schwaiger M. Carbon-11 hydroxyephedrine with positron emission tomography for serial assessment of cardiac adrenergic neuronal function after acute myocardial infarction in humans. JACC 1993; 22(2):368–375.
183. Wolpers H, Nguyen N, Rosenspire K, Haka M, Wieland D, Schwaiger M. C-11 hydroxyephedrine as marker for neuronal dysfunction in reperfused canine myocardium. Coronary Artery Disease 1991;2:923–929.
184. Calkins H, Allman K, Bolling S, et al. Correlation between scintigraphic evidence of regional sympathetic neuronal dysfunction and ventricular refractoriness in the human heart. Circulation 1993;88(1):173–179.
185. Allman K, Stevens M, Wieland D, Wolfe E, Greene D, Schwaiger M. Noninvasive assessment of cardiac diabetic neuropathy by C-11 hydroxyephedrine and positron emission tomography. J Am Coll Cardiol 1993;1425–1432.
186. Merlet P, Valette H, Dubois-Rande J, et al. Prognostic value of cardiac metaiodobenzylguanidine imaging in patients with heart failure. J Nucl Med 1992;33(4):471–477.
187. Syrota A. Positron emission tomography: evaluation of cardiac receptors. In: Marcus M, Scjelbert HR, Skorton DJ, et al., eds. Cardiac imaging: a companion to Braunwalds heart disease. Philadelphia: W.B. Saunders Company, 1991:1256–1270.
188. Schwaiger M, Hutchins G, Das S, Wieland D. C-11 hydroxyephedrine kinetics in patients with hypertrophic cardiomyopathy. J Amer Coll Cardiol 1991;17(2):343A.
189. Yonekura Y, Tamaki N, Senda M, et al. Detection of coronary artery disease with ^{13}N-ammonia and high-resolution positron-emission computed tomography. Am Heart J 1987;113:645–654.
190. Williams B, Jansen D, Wong L, Fiedotin A, Knopf W, Toporoff S. Positron emission tomography for the diagnosis of coronary artery disease: a nonuniversity experience and correlation with coronary angiography. J Nucl Med 1989;30:845.
191. Schelbert H, Wisenberg G, Phelps M, et al. Noninvasive assessment of coronary stenoses by myocardial imaging during pharmacologic coronary vasodilation: VI. Detection of coronary artery disease in man with intravenous 13-NH3 and positron computed tomography. Am J Cardiol 1982;49:1197–1207.
192. Bellina C, Parodi O, Cohnici P, et al. Simultaneous in vitro and in vivo validation of N-13 ammonia for the assessment of regional myocardial blood flow. J Nucl Med 1990;31:1335–1343.
193. Kuhle W, Porenta G, Huang S, et al. Quantification of regional myocardial blood flow using 13N-ammonia and reoriented dynamic positron emission tomographic imaging. Circulation 1992;86(3):1004–1017.
194. Camici P, Marracini P, Marzilli M, et al. Coronary hemodynamics and myocardial metabolism during and after pacing stress in normal humans. Am J Physiol 1989;257:309–317.
195. Chan S, Brunken R, Czernin J, et al. Comparison of maximal myocardial blood flow during adenosine infusion with that of intravenous dipyridamole in normal men. J Am Coll Cardiol 1992; 20:979–985.
196. Geltman E, Henes C, Senneff M, Sobel B, Bergmann S. Increased myocardial perfusion at rest and diminished perfusion reserve in patients with angina and angiographically normal coronary arteries. JACC 1990;16(3):586–595.
197. Krivokapich J, Huang S, Schelbert H. Assessment of the effects of dobutamine on myocardial blood flow and oxidative metabolism in normal human subjects using nitrogen-13 ammonia and carbon-11 acetate. Am J Cardiol 1993;71(15):1351–1356.
198. Sambuceti G, Parodi O, Marcassa C, et al. Alteration in regulation of myocardial blood flow in one-vessel coronary artery disease determined by positron emission tomography. Am J Cardiol 1993;72:538–543.
199. Ebert A, Herzog H, Stöcklin G, et al. Kinetics of 14(R,S)-fluorine-18-fluoro-6-thia-heptadecanoic acid in normal human hearts at rest, during exercise and after dipyridamole injection. J Nucl Med 1994;35:51–56.
200. Barrio JR. Biochemical principles in radiopharmaceutical design and utilization. In: Phelps M, Mazziotta J, Schelbert H, eds. Positron emission tomography and autoradiography: principles and applications for the brain and heart. New York: Raven Press, 1986:451–492.
201. Tamaki N, Yonekura Y, Yamashita K, et al. SPECT thallium-201 tomography and positron tomography using N-13 ammonia and F-18 fluorodeoxyglucose in coronary heart disease. Am J Cardiol Imaging 1989;3:3–9.
202. Tamaki N, Ohtani H, Yamashita K, et al. Metabolic activity in the areas of new fill-in after thallium-201 reinjection: comparison with positron emission tomography using fluorine-18-deoxyglucose. J Nucl Med 1991;32:673–678.
203. Marwick T, MacIntyre W, Lafont A, Nemec J, Salcedo E. Metabolic responses of hibernating and infarcted myocardium to revascularization: a follow-up study of regional perfusion, function and metabolism. Circulation 1992;85:1347–1353.
204. Lucignani G, Paolini G, Landoni C, et al. Presurgical identification of hibernating myocardium by combined use of technetium-99m hexokinase 2-methoxyisobutylisonitrile single photon emission tomography and fluorine-18 fluoro-2-deoxy-d-glucose positron emission tomography in patients with coronary artery disease. Eur J Nucl Med 1992;19:874–881.
205. Carrel T, Jenni R, Haubold-Reuter S, von Schulthess G, Pasic M, Turina M. Improvement of severely reduced left ventricular function after surgical revascularization in patients with preoperative myocardial infarction. Eur J Cardiothorac Surg 1992; 6:479–484.
206. vom Dahl J, Eitzman D, Al-Aouar Z, et al. Relation of regional function, perfusion and metabolism in patients with advanced coronary artery disease undergoing surgical revascularization. Circulation 1994;90:2356–2366.
207. Gould KL, Yoshida K, Hess MJ, Haynie M, Mullani N, Smalling RW. Myocardial metabolism of fluorodeoxyglucose compared to cell membrane integrity for the potassium analogue rubidium-82 for assessing infarct size in man by PET. J Nucl Med 1991; 32(1):1–9.
208. Schwaiger M, Hutchins G, Rosenspire K, Haka M, Wieland DM. Quantitative evaluation of the sympathetic nervous system by PET in patients with cardiomyopathy. J Nucl Med 1990; 31(5):792.
209. Camici P. Unpublished observation.

27 Assessment of Myocardial Viability

ROBERT O. BONOW

In patients with chronic coronary artery disease, left ventricular function is among the most important determinants of long-term prognosis (1–5). In general, patients with normal or near-normal left ventricular systolic function have an excellent outcome whether treated with medical therapy or with revascularization procedures. In contrast, the large subgroup of patients with moderate to severe left ventricular dysfunction are at considerable risk of death during the course of medical therapy (Fig. 27.1). Patients with impaired ventricular function at particular risk are those with inducible myocardial ischemia, poor exercise tolerance, or evidence of complex ventricular ectopic activity. Hence, exercise testing and arrhythmia monitoring are commonly employed in the risk stratification of patients with left ventricular dysfunction.

Testing to evaluate the presence and extent of viable but dysfunctional myocardium in such patients is less well established. Although it was widely believed, as recently as a decade ago, that left ventricular dysfunction at rest in a patient with chronic coronary artery disease was an irreversible process related to previous myocardial infarction, recent findings have proven this is not the case. A substantial subset of patients with left ventricular dysfunction undergoing myocardial revascularization will manifest striking improvement in ventricular function after successful revascularization (6–10), including normalization of ventricular function in some patients. This potentially reversible form of left ventricular dysfunction has been termed "myocardial hibernation," indicating a condition in which myocardial contractility has been reduced in the setting of a sustained reduction in myocardial blood supply (7–9). Importantly, hibernating myocardium will improve in function only if identified and revascularized.

Although the percentage of patients who demonstrate an important reversal of ventricular dysfunction after revascularization varies among reported series (probably related to patient selection factors and revascularization techniques), it is not inconsequential. It has been estimated that up to one-third of patients (Fig. 27.2) with chronic coronary artery disease and left ventricular dysfunction have the potential for significant improvement in ventricular function (11). These findings have several implications. First, given the important relationship between left ventricular function and survival (Fig. 27.1), the improvement in ventricular function after revascularization may translate into an improvement in survival. Although definitive data tying improved function to improved survival are lacking, recent data have begun to establish this point, as discussed subsequently. Second, the decision to proceed with revascularization in patients with moderate to severe left ventricular dysfunction is often very difficult. Such patients undergo coronary artery bypass surgery or coronary angioplasty with considerable risk of procedure-related morbidity and mortality. Hence, accurate methods to detect viable myocardium distal to a coronary stenosis, with the potential for reversal of left ventricular dysfunction, are essential to select in a prospective manner those patients in whom these risks are justified.

At the present time, several clinically reliable physiologic markers of viability can be employed for this purpose. These include indexes of regional coronary blood flow, regional wall motion, and regional systolic wall thickening which are accurate markers of viability only if they are normal or near-normal, but have major limitations in identifying viable myocardium when they are reduced or absent. In the setting of hibernating myocardium, by definition, indexes of regional perfusion and systolic function (regional wall motion and wall thickening) will be severely reduced or absent (7–10) despite maintenance of tissue viability. Thus, these three indexes are imprecise in distinguishing hibernating myocardium from myocardial scar. It should be noted that recent reports indicate that inotropic reserve is maintained in viable, hibernating myocardium, and that this can be assessed using low-dose dobutamine echocardiography (12–14). This is an exciting area of current investigation. However, at the present time, radionuclide tracers that reflect intact cellular metabolic processes or cell membrane integrity have intrinsic advantages over indexes of function and blood flow.

During the past decade, numerous studies have demonstrated that nuclear cardiology techniques, involving single photon methods as well as positron emission tomography (PET), provide critically important viability information in patients with left ventricular dysfunction. This chapter reviews the strengths, applications, and limitations of nuclear cardiology procedures for the assessment of myocardial viability.

THALLIUM-201 IMAGING TO ASSESS MYOCARDIAL VIABILITY

In the setting of reduced blood flow and oxygen availability, tissue viability can be maintained only if persistent metabolic activity is sufficient to meet the energy demands required to maintain a number of fundamental cellular processes. These include, among other processes, sufficient energy to prevent irreversible configurational changes of structural and contractile proteins, to prevent ischemic contracture of myocytes, to prevent disruption of mitochondria, and to maintain sarcolemmal, sarcoplasmic reticulum, and mitochondrial membrane integrity. Maintenance of membrane integrity also implies preservation of electrochemical gradients across the sarcolemma. It is important to note that these processes can persist only if a

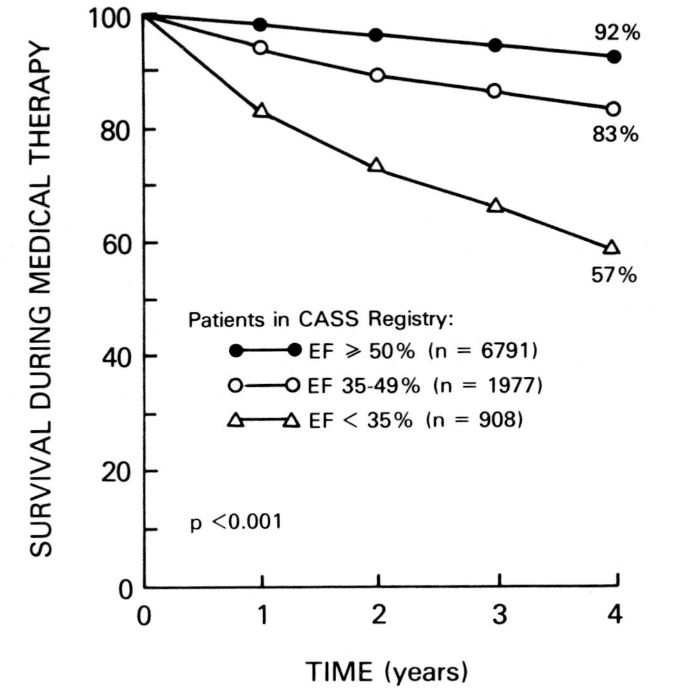

Figure 27.1. Influence of resting left ventricular ejection fraction (EF) on survival during medical therapy in patients in the Coronary Artery Surgery Study (CASS) Registry (4). (Reproduced by permission of the American Heart Association from Bonow RO, Epstein SE. Indications for coronary artery bypass surgery: implications of the multicenter randomized trials. Circulation 1985;72(Suppl V):23–30.)

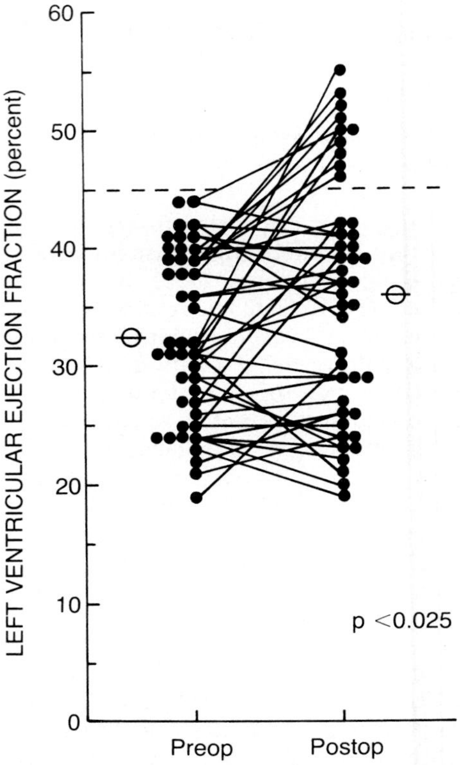

Figure 27.2. Left ventricular ejection fraction at rest by radionuclide ventriculography before (*Preop*) and 6 months after (*Postop*) coronary artery bypass surgery in 43 patients with preoperative left ventricular dysfunction. The *dashed line* at 45% indicates the lower limit of normal resting ejection fraction. Although operation resulted in only a small increase in mean ejection fraction, substantial increases in ejection fraction were observed in 15 patients (35%), and postoperative ejection fraction was normal in 10 patients (23%). (Reproduced with permission of the W.B. Saunders Company from Bonow RO, Dilsizian V. Thallium-201 for assessing myocardial viability. Semin Nucl Med 1991;21:230–241.)

critical level of blood flow is maintained. Sufficient blood flow is necessary both to deliver the substrates for the metabolic processes and to wash out the byproducts of these processes. For example, the metabolites of the glycolytic pathway include lactate and hydrogen ion (15, 16), which have inhibitory effects on glycolytic enzymes. The intracellular accumulation of lactate and hydrogen ion result ultimately in termination of glycolysis, depletion of high energy phosphates, cell membrane disruption, and cell death. The dependence upon a critical level of blood flow for persistence of metabolic activity suggests that, in theory, imaging agents that reflect regional myocardial blood flow and cation flux as an index of membrane integrity should provide excellent information regarding tissue viability. As the retention of ^{201}Tl with time is an active process that is a function of cell viability and cell membrane activity, ^{201}Tl should perform well as a marker of myocardial viability.

THALLIUM REDISTRIBUTION AS A MARKER OF VIABILITY

The single most important index of viability using ^{201}Tl imaging is the demonstration of reversibility of a perfusion defect, that is, net accumulation of ^{201}Tl in a myocardial territory with contractile dysfunction relative to the washout of ^{201}Tl in a normally perfused territory. Myocardial regions that are precariously balanced, with such a marked reduction in flow as to cause contractile dysfunction at rest, are likely to manifest even greater flow inhomogeneity relative to normal regions during either exercise or pharmacologic stress imaging (Fig. 27.3). Hence, a large number (if not the majority) of these regions will manifest reversible ^{201}Tl perfusion defects using a standard exercise-redistribution imaging protocol. The demonstration of reversible ischemia during exercise in regions with con-

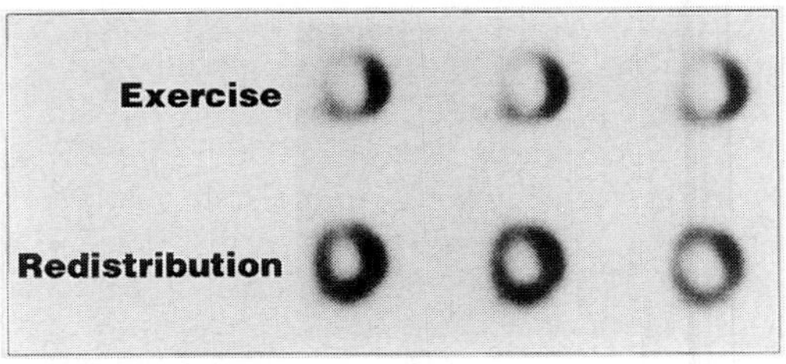

Figure 27.3. Inducible myocardial ischemia with reversible ^{201}Tl defects in a patient with multivessel coronary artery disease, left ventricular dysfunction, and severe anteroseptal hypokinesia at rest. Exercise-induced perfusion defects in the anteroseptal and inferior regions redistribute substantially at 3–4 hours. This identifies the dysfunctional anteroseptal territory as representing viable myocardium with the potential for improvement in function after revascularization.

tractile dysfunction is evidence of viability of these regions, with the potential for substantial improvement in function after revascularization. The positive predictive value of a reversible ^{201}Tl defect, regarding improvement in function after coronary artery bypass surgery or angioplasty, is excellent.

However, the negative predictive value of an irreversible ^{201}Tl defect is relatively poor. Many regions of severely ischemic or hibernating myocardium will not demonstrate appreciable reversibility of ^{201}Tl defects on standard exercise-redistribution imaging. Fifty percent or more of regions with apparently "irreversible" ^{201}Tl defects will improve in function after successful revascularization (17–21). Hence, because of this poor negative predictive accuracy, it is now accepted that standard stress-redistribution ^{201}Tl scintigraphy does not provide satisfactory precision in differentiating hibernating myocardium from fibrotic myocardium in patients with coronary artery disease and left ventricular dysfunction. Recent modifications in imaging protocols with ^{201}Tl have considerably enhanced the ability of ^{201}Tl imaging to detect viable myocardium (11, 22). These include late redistribution imaging and ^{201}Tl reinjection techniques.

LATE THALLIUM REDISTRIBUTION IMAGING

In a considerable number of patients, late imaging at 24–72 hours demonstrates substantial ^{201}Tl redistribution in many defects that appear to be irreversible at 3–4 hours, and this late ^{201}Tl redistribution is consistent with viable myocardium (20, 23–25). As many as 54% of irreversible defects at 3–4 hours will show reversibility at 24 hours, although this number is as low as 22% in some studies. Thallium-201 redistribution is a continual process (26), and a truly irreversible defect on early redistribution images will not reverse at a later time. However, it is also true that in a number of viable regions the magnitude of defect reversal at 3–4 hours may be minimal and poorly detected. Hence, the defect may not reverse appreciably on qualitative interpretation, and the increase in relative tracer activity may also not exceed the reproducibility limit by quantitative analysis. In such regions, late redistribution imaging may enhance the certainty that defect reversibility has occurred.

The positive predictive value of late redistribution is over 90% (24) in predicting improvement after revascularization; thus, defect reversibility with late imaging is an excellent marker of viable myocardium. However, even though 24-hour imaging identifies a greater number of reversible defects than does 3–4-hour imaging, there are important limitations of late redistribution imaging. The negative predictive accuracy of an irreversible defect at 24 hours appears to be little better than that of an irreversible defect at 3–4 hours. It has been shown that 37% of irreversible defects at 24 hours improve after revascularization (24), and 39% of irreversible defects at 24 hours show improvement by quantitative analysis when ^{201}Tl is reinjected at rest (27). Hence, it is apparent that a considerable number of dysfunctional but viable myocardial segments will not demonstrate redistribution after a stress ^{201}Tl study, no matter how lengthy the redistribution period.

THALLIUM REINJECTION IMAGING

^{201}Tl reinjection, either after the standard 3–4-hour redistribution image (28–30) or after a late 24-hour redistribution image (27), facilitates late uptake of ^{201}Tl in many viable regions with apparently irreversible defects, and may be used to distinguish between viable and infarcted myocardium (Fig. 27.4). The available data indicate that the reinjection technique provides greater accuracy in detecting viable myocardium than either early or late redistribution imaging. Up to 49% of "irreversible" defects on 4-hour redistribution images (28) and 39% of such defects on 24-hour redistribution images (27) show improved or normal uptake after ^{201}Tl reinjection (45, 46). In three studies of patients with left ventricular dysfunction and apparently irreversible defects at 3–4 hours, the positive and negative predictive accuracies of ^{201}Tl reinjection for predicting improved wall motion after revascularization has been greater than 85% (21, 28, 31). These studies indicate that ^{201}Tl reinjection is a clinically accurate method with which to identify viable myocardium in patients with chronic coronary artery disease and left ventricular dysfunction.

An imaging protocol that includes stress and redistribution images with ^{201}Tl reinjection as necessary will provide most of the viability information that can be obtained from ^{201}Tl imaging. Rarely do late redistribution images after reinjection provide important additional information not achieved with the earlier three-image acquisitions (32).

On the other hand, a protocol that includes three sets of ^{201}Tl image acquisitions (stress, redistribution, and reinjection) creates logistical constraints for the laboratory and

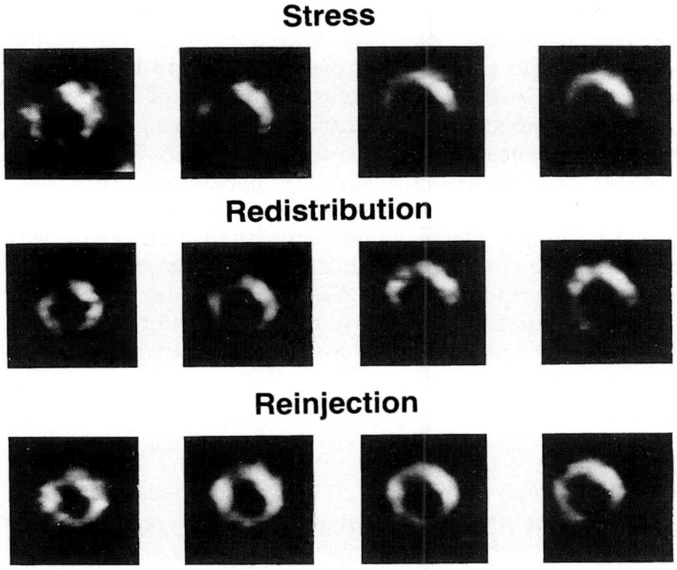

Figure 27.4. Effects of ^{201}Tl reinjection. Short axis ^{201}Tl SPECT images after exercise show extensive abnormalities in anterior, septal, inferior and inferolateral perfusion. The septal defect partially reverses on 4-hour redistribution images, but the other defects persist. All regions improve substantially after reinjection, with the exception only of the inferolateral wall, which remains irreversible. (Reproduced with permission of the W.B. Saunders Company from Bonow RO, Dilsizian V. Thallium-201 for assessing myocardial viability. Semin Nucl Med 1991;21:230–241.)

inconvenience for the patient. Several modifications of the reinjection technique to streamline the imaging protocol are currently in clinical practice, although each requires further investigation before widespread application is advised. The first of these involves the routine reinjection of ^{201}Tl at 3–4 hours without acquiring redistribution images. This approach improves efficiency, and identifies viable myocardium in many patients in whom the redistribution images would have been misleading, by showing persistent defects. However, there is an important limitation of this approach. In a large number of patients with left ventricular dysfunction, regional myocardial perfusion is reduced at rest. Indeed, this is the definition of myocardial hibernation. In a subset of these patients, ^{201}Tl redistribution will occur after exercise or pharmacologic stress. However, the reinjection of ^{201}Tl at rest will increase ^{201}Tl uptake in the normally perfused territories to a greater extent than in the hypoperfused territories, resulting in the appearance of relative ^{201}Tl "washout" compared to the redistribution image. This differential uptake of ^{201}Tl will result in a defect on stress images that improves or normalizes on the redistribution images but then reappears on the reinjection images (28, 33). In such patients, the reinjection images may mirror the stress images, and it is the redistribution image, not the reinjection image, that provides the important information regarding defect reversibility and, hence, viability. Although this effect occurs in only a small subset of patients, the elimination of the redistribution data will create uncertainties regarding the interpretation of an irreversible defect when a stress-reinjection protocol is used (33).

The second modification of the reinjection protocol is the early reinjection of ^{201}Tl immediately after the completion of the stress image acquisition (34–36). Imaging is then repeated 3–4 hours later. This allows both the reinjection ^{201}Tl dose and the initial stress ^{201}Tl dose to redistribute together for several hours before imaging is performed. Although this method is very attractive in concept, the available data indicate mixed results. One study reported favorable results with an early reinjection protocol (35). However, two other studies have shown that defects that persist 3 hours after early reinjection will show later reversal if either 24-hour redistribution imaging or ^{201}Tl reinjection is performed (34, 36). Until further, more definitive data are published, the early reinjection protocol should be considered an investigational, rather than an accepted, imaging protocol.

REST-REDISTRIBUTION THALLIUM IMAGING

As noted earlier, exercise ^{201}Tl imaging creates the uncertainty of whether a defect on stress images represents ischemic myocardium that must be unmasked with further redistribution and/or reinjection images. Exercise imaging also imposes questions regarding which of the many possible imaging protocols to unmask viable myocardium is most efficacious and logistically practical. If the sole clinical issue to be addressed is the viability of one or more left ventricular regions with systolic dysfunction, and not whether there is also inducible ischemia, rest-redistribution ^{201}Tl imaging is a practical approach that can yield accurate viability data. A resting protocol to assess viability must include both initial images (indicating regional perfusion) and subsequent redistribution images (Fig. 27.5). Although the early experience with resting ^{201}Tl protocols yielded mixed results regarding the predictive accuracy of rest-redistribution imaging (37–39), recent studies indicate that a quantitative analysis of regional ^{201}Tl activity in rest-redistribution studies predicts recovery of regional left ventricular function (40) and compares favorably to the results of ^{201}Tl exercise-reinjection imaging and metabolic PET imaging (41).

It should be emphasized that there are cogent reasons to consider exercise ^{201}Tl studies with reinjection rather than rest-redistribution imaging in the majority of patients. The demonstration of exercise-induced ischemia in a patient with left ventricular dysfunction has important prognostic implications that, under most conditions, identifies the patient as a candidate for revascularization therapy. This is especially true in patients with left ventricular dysfunction, in whom evidence of inducible ischemia superimposed on impaired left ventricular function at rest identifies a subgroup of patients at considerable risk of death during medical therapy.

Moreover, many persistent defects on rest-redistribution imaging may have only a mild decrease in relative ^{201}Tl activity, which in itself indicates viability. Although ^{201}Tl uptake in such a region identifies it as being viable, this does not insure improvement in function if revascularization is performed. Only slightly more than 60% of mild persistent defects on rest-redistribution studies improve after revascularization (40). ^{201}Tl defect reversibility is a better predictor of improvement after revascularization than the level of ^{201}Tl activity per se. Importantly, many persistent defects on rest-redistribution imaging demonstrate a greater homogeneous flow with exercise leading to a more severe defect than on the rest study (41). The result is an exercise-induced defect with partial reversibility at rest, which is more convincing evidence of viability than the persistent resting defect. Thus, exercise-redistribution-reinjection ^{201}Tl protocols are attractive, as they provide important information regarding both jeopardized myocardium and viable myocardium. Rest-redistribution

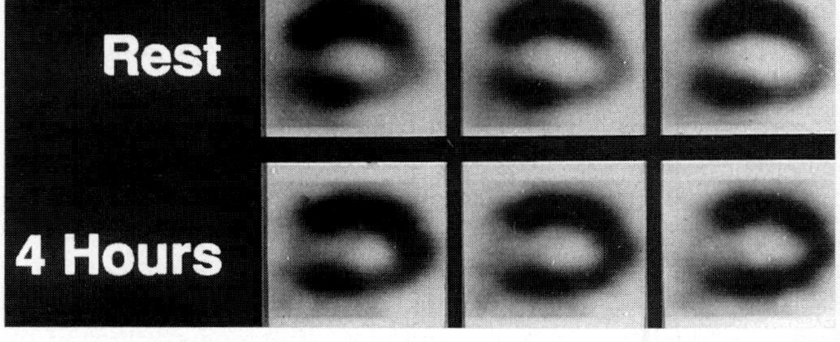

Figure 27.5. Rest-redistribution ^{201}Tl imaging in a patient with left ventricular dysfunction. The resting study demonstrates hypoperfusion at the apex, but redistribution of ^{201}Tl within this defect at 4 hours indicates that this region represents viable myocardium. (Reproduced with permission of the Society of Nuclear Medicine from Hendel RC. Single-photon perfusion imaging for the assessment of myocardial viability. J Nucl Med 1994;35(Suppl):23S–31S.)

protocols should be considered only in patients with known left ventricular dysfunction in whom viability of a ventricular segment distal to a severe coronary artery stenosis is the only clinical question to be addressed.

TECHNETIUM-99M-SESTAMIBI IMAGING TO ASSESS VIABILITY

Technetium-99m-sestamibi, like ^{201}Tl, requires intact sarcolemmal and mitochondrial processes for retention. This agent has been shown to be an excellent marker of cellular viability (42–44). In both experimental and clinical settings in which ^{99m}Tc-sestamibi delivery is adequate to dysfunctional myocardium, such as after reperfusion to previously ischemic or damaged myocardium, the uptake and retention of ^{99m}Tc-sestamibi tracks with markers of myocardial viability rather than with pure markers of perfusion (43,45–47). However, ^{99m}Tc-sestamibi does not redistribute as avidly as ^{201}Tl after its initial uptake, either during exercise or at rest. Thus, compared to ^{201}Tl, ^{99m}Tc-sestamibi has inherent weaknesses for viability assessment in clinical situations in which blood flow is severely impaired and tracer delivery is reduced (48). Several studies comparing rest-exercise ^{99m}Tc-sestamibi imaging to exercise-redistribution-reinjection ^{201}Tl imaging, indicate that ^{99m}Tc-sestamibi underestimates viable myocardium in patients with chronic coronary artery disease and left ventricular dysfunction (49–51). Additionally, a large percentage of ^{99m}Tc-sestamibi defects in patients with left ventricular dysfunction demonstrate ^{18}F-fluorodeoxyglucose (FDG) activity by PET imaging indicating viability (52). However, two recent studies indicate that a quantitative analysis of regional ^{99m}Tc-sestamibi activity after administration at rest substantially increases the accuracy for identifying viable myocardium (53, 54) compared to ^{201}Tl imaging and PET imaging. Additionally, there is evidence that ^{99m}Tc-sestamibi does redistribute in some patients with coronary artery disease (55), and such redistribution on resting ^{99m}Tc-sestamibi studies may be used to advantage for assessing viability (53). These recent findings with ^{99m}Tc-sestamibi should be considered preliminary in nature until confirmed by larger, more definitive studies.

POSITRON EMISSION TOMOGRAPHY

PET has become an exceptional tool for identifying viable myocardium in patients with impaired left ventricular function (56–59). Several PET methods have been developed for this purpose. The method with the greatest cumulative clinical experience and the most extensive documentation in the literature is the use of ^{18}F-fluorodeoxyglucose (FDG) as a marker of regional exogenous glucose utilization in regions of severely underperfused and dysfunctional myocardium (56, 59–64). Thus, PET imaging can be employed to directly assess the persistent metabolic activity that is necessary to maintain cellular viability.

FDG IMAGING FOR VIABILITY ASSESSMENT

A pattern of enhanced FDG uptake relative to blood flow in regions with reduced perfusion, which has been termed the FDG:blood flow "mismatch," indicates viable myocardium in which the metabolic substrate preference has been shifted toward greater glucose utilization rather than utilization of fatty acids or lactate (60–64). The finding of FDG:blood flow mismatch in myocardial regions with impaired systolic function was shown in several studies to be an accurate marker for distinguishing viable from nonviable myocardium (Fig. 27.6). The cumulative experience from six studies, including a total of 146 patients with left ventricular dysfunction undergoing myocardial revascularization procedures, indicates that the finding of FDG:blood flow mismatch has a positive accuracy of 82% and a negative accuracy of 83% in predicting recovery of regional function after myocardial revascularization (61, 64–68).

Recent findings indicate that the identification of viable tissue with FDG:blood flow mismatch has several important, clinically relevant implications. First, the augmentation in regional systolic function after revascularization, as predicted by FDG:blood flow mismatch, results in a tangible and predictable increase in ejection fraction. In four separate reports, involving a total of 94 patients, global left ventricular function significantly increased after revascularization in patients with FDG:blood flow mismatch on prerevascularization PET studies, with the average ejection fraction increasing from 32% before to 45% after revascularization (61, 66, 68, 69). There is also evidence that the extent and magnitude of FDG:blood flow mismatch in a patient with left ventricular dysfunction can be used to predict the magnitude of recovery in global left ventricular function after revascularization (61, 70).

The increase in left ventricular ejection fraction after revascularization in patients with FDG:blood flow mismatch also appears to translate into an improvement in progno-

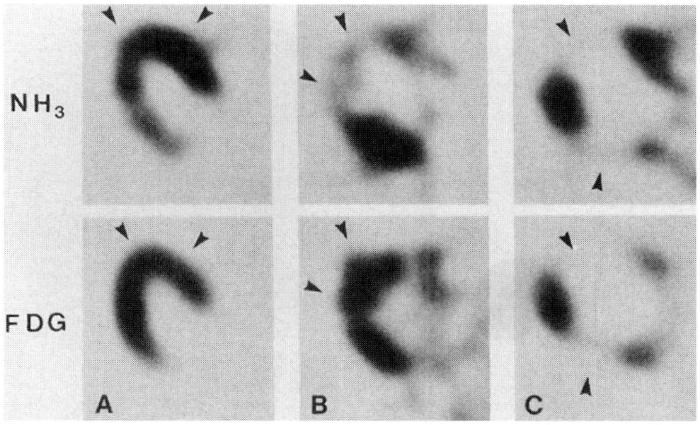

Figure 27.6. Positron emission tomography (PET) assessment of myocardial viability. Transaxial PET images in three patients using ^{13}N-ammonia to assess perfusion and FDG to assess glucose utilization. *Arrows* indicate regions with abnormal wall motion on left ventriculography. Perfusion and FDG uptake are normal in the *left panel*, despite abnormal wall motion. FDG:blood flow mismatch is apparent in the *middle panel*, consistent with viable myocardium, whereas both perfusion and FDG uptake are reduced ("match") in the *right panel*, indicative of myocardial fibrosis. (Reproduced with permission of the New England Journal of Medicine from Tillisch JH, Brunken R, Marshall R, et al. Reversibility of cardiac wall-motion abnormalities predicted by positron tomography. N Engl J Med 1986;314:884–888.)

sis. Recently published data suggest that myocardial revascularization in patients with FDG:blood flow mismatch significantly improves survival compared to the survival results during medical therapy (71, 72). Among 87 patients reported in two separate studies with left ventricular dysfunction (mean ejection fraction 29%) the 1-year mortality was 33% in patients treated medically, but was reduced to only 4% in those patients treated with coronary artery bypass surgery or angioplasty (Fig. 27.7). The limitations of these two studies must be addressed. Both were retrospective, nonrandomized studies that involved relatively small numbers of patients. The factors selecting some patients for revascularization and others for medical therapy are unspecified. However, the overall concordance of the results is remarkable, as identical findings were achieved in these two separate studies (Fig. 27.7). The improvement in left ventricular function after revascularization, as predicted by FDG:blood flow mismatch, is also associated with a significant improvement in symptoms of congestive heart failure (73). Although more definitive data are required before full conclusions can be drawn, these data suggest that patients with impaired left ventricular function and FDG:blood flow mismatch are a subgroup of patients who may have substantial improvement in outcome if identified and treated with myocardial revascularization. These patients appear to have the potential for improved left ventricular function, improved symptoms, and improved survival.

FDG IMAGING COMPARED TO THALLIUM IMAGING

In keeping with the limitations of ^{201}Tl redistribution imaging for assessment of myocardial viability, several studies have shown that metabolic PET imaging with FDG is superior to standard exercise-redistribution ^{201}Tl scintigraphy for this assessment, when both techniques were performed in the same patients (74–77). Between 38% and 47% of irreversible ^{201}Tl defects on 3–4-hour redistribution images in these studies were determined to be metabolically active on the corresponding PET images. Similarly, 51% of persistent defects on late (24-hour) redistribution images were metabolically active with FDG uptake on PET imaging (78). These data provide further evidence that early and late redistribution imaging overestimates the presence and severity of myocardial fibrosis.

A much better concordance between PET and ^{201}Tl imaging is obtained with ^{201}Tl reinjection methods (79–81). Among patients with chronic coronary artery disease and left ventricular dysfunction who were studied by both stress-redistribution-reinjection ^{201}Tl imaging and PET imaging with FDG, the majority of segments with ^{201}Tl defects identified as viable by ^{201}Tl reinjection had FDG uptake (Fig. 27.8) and hence metabolic evidence for myocardial viability (79–81). Although the overall concordance between the ^{201}Tl reinjection and FDG uptake data is excellent, the frequency with which irreversible ^{201}Tl defects (even with reinjection) manifest FDG uptake remains a subject of uncertainty and debate. However, of greater importance, the positive and negative predictive accuracy of ^{201}Tl reinjection for improved wall motion after revascularization (21,

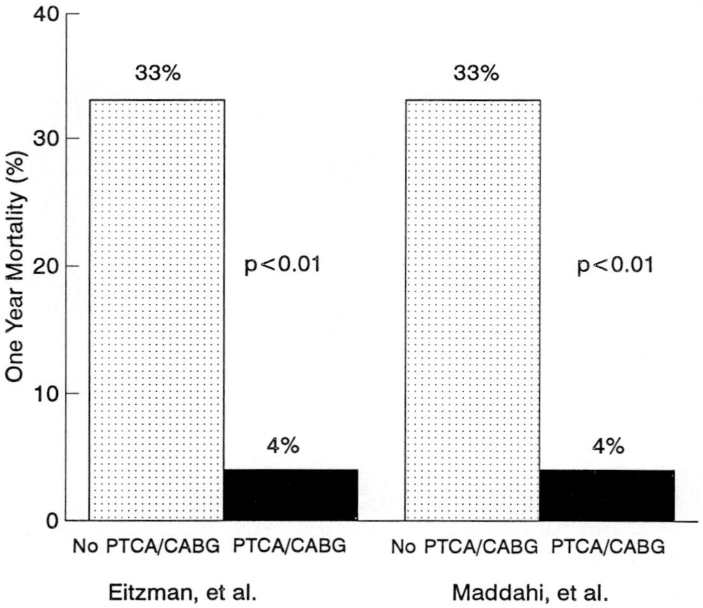

Figure 27.7. One-year survival in patients with left ventricular dysfunction and evidence of viable myocardium, as determined by FDG:blood flow mismatch on PET imaging by Eitzman, et al. (71), and Maddahi, et al. (72). In both series, patients treated medically had a 1-year mortality rate of 33%, compared to only 4% in patients undergoing myocardial revascularization.

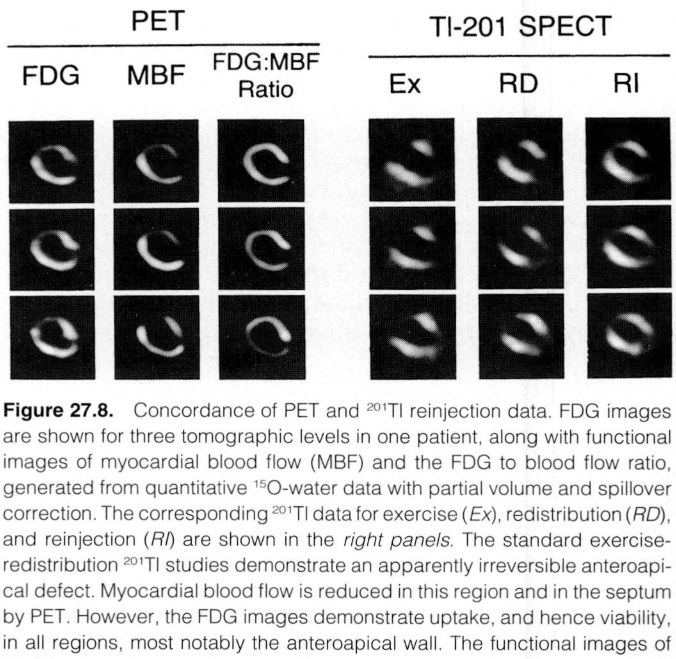

Figure 27.8. Concordance of PET and ^{201}Tl reinjection data. FDG images are shown for three tomographic levels in one patient, along with functional images of myocardial blood flow (MBF) and the FDG to blood flow ratio, generated from quantitative ^{15}O-water data with partial volume and spillover correction. The corresponding ^{201}Tl data for exercise (*Ex*), redistribution (*RD*), and reinjection (*RI*) are shown in the *right panels*. The standard exercise-redistribution ^{201}Tl studies demonstrate an apparently irreversible anteroapical defect. Myocardial blood flow is reduced in this region and in the septum by PET. However, the FDG images demonstrate uptake, and hence viability, in all regions, most notably the anteroapical wall. The functional images of FDG to blood flow ratio demonstrate enhanced FDG uptake relative to blood flow ("mismatch") involving the apex and septum. Thallium reinjection results in enhanced ^{201}Tl uptake in the anteroapical regions, resulting in reinjection images that mirror the FDG images. (Reproduced with permission of the American Heart Association from Bonow RO, Dilsizian V, Cuocolo A, Bacharach SL. Identification of viable myocardium in patients with chronic coronary artery disease and left ventricular dysfunction: comparison of thallium-201 with reinjection and PET imaging with ^{18}F-fluorodeoxyglucose. Circulation 1991;83:26–37.)

28, 31), as noted earlier, is similar to that reported using metabolic PET imaging (61, 64–68).

There is much less information regarding the comparison of rest-redistribution ^{201}Tl imaging to PET imaging in the same patients. However, it was recently demonstrated that a quantitative analysis of regional ^{201}Tl activity in redistribution images of rest-redistribution studies provides viability information that compares favorably to that of metabolic PET imaging (41).

FDG IMAGING COMPARED TO TECHNETIUM-99M-SESTAMIBI IMAGING

Only two studies have compared quantitative regional ^{99m}Tc-sestamibi activity to regional FDG activity in the same patients (52, 53). Unfortunately, these two investigations reached conflicting conclusions regarding the correlation between regional ^{99m}Tc-sestamibi activity as an index of viability compared to FDG activity. These differences could reflect the small numbers of patients studied or differences in methodologies between the two reports. No firm conclusions can be drawn regarding comparisons between ^{99m}Tc-sestamibi and PET imaging until more data are available.

ALTERNATIVE PET TECHNIQUES FOR IDENTIFYING VIABLE MYOCARDIUM

Three methods to assess viability by PET without using FDG were recently reported. The identification of preserved oxidative metabolism, using PET imaging with ^{11}C-acetate, was shown to be an accurate marker for viable myocardium in patients with left ventricular dysfunction and for predicting recovery of regional left ventricular function after revascularization (65). Other PET methods for assessing myocardial viability include the use of ^{15}O-water to determine the amount of perfusable tissue within dysfunctional myocardial segments (82, 83) and the analysis of ^{82}Rb uptake and washout kinetics in regions with impaired systolic function (84). Each of these three PET applications have, thus far, been employed in only a small number of patients, and each has been reported from only a single institution. Greater clinical experience is required before these methods can be recommended for routine purposes.

SINGLE PHOTON EMISSION TOMOGRAPHY VERSUS PET FOR VIABILITY ASSESSMENT

As viability requires both intact membrane function and maintenance of metabolic processes, markers of cell membrane integrity should be, in theory, equally efficacious for assessing myocardial viability as are indicators of metabolic activity. Thus, the relative accuracies of PET or single photon emission tomography (SPECT) methods in identifying viable myocardium are less related to the underlying physiologic processes being measured than to the ability to image these processes with the existing SPECT or PET detectors. In this regard, there are several advantages to PET approaches, including improved image resolution, the ability to correct for photon attenuation, and the ability to assess metabolic activity independent of perfusion. Advantages of SPECT imaging include the ability to assess inducible ischemia along with viability as part of a routine comprehensive imaging protocol. The identification of inducible ischemia provides both prognostic information and viability information (as ischemic myocardium, by definition, is viable myocardium). Additionally, viability can be assessed with ^{201}Tl or ^{99m}Tc-sestamibi imaging in all patients without the standardized and controlled metabolic conditions that are necessary for FDG PET studies. With these considerations in mind, the principal advantage of PET is the availability of routine attenuation correction algorithms (57, 58). Each of the current SPECT protocols shares the limiting feature of photon attenuation of a low energy radioisotope, in which apparently irreversible ^{201}Tl or ^{99m}Tc-sestamibi defects suggesting fibrosis may be merely attenuation artifacts in viable tissue. Thus, it is anticipated that imaging with ^{201}Tl or with ^{99m}Tc based agents will never achieve the accuracy of PET imaging for viability assessment, until techniques to correct for photon attenuation are perfected for SPECT. However, effective attenuation correction algorithms are on the horizon for routine use with multiheaded SPECT systems (85).

SUMMARY

Nuclear cardiology techniques have the rather unique potential to distinguish viable tissue on the basis of perfusion, cell membrane integrity, and metabolic activity, thereby providing greater precision than can be achieved by investigating regional anatomy or function. Despite basic and clinical research in this area for more than a decade, a number of issues regarding the clinical applications of these techniques have not been fully resolved. First, the relative efficacy of PET and ^{201}Tl, using reinjection techniques or resting injections, is a principal issue, and larger scale studies comparing these two methods in patients undergoing revascularization are essential. Although there may be subgroups of patients in whom PET provides more accurate and reliable results than can be accomplished using ^{201}Tl imaging, these subgroups are not fully defined at present. Second, the efficacy of ^{99m}Tc-sestamibi imaging relative to these other modalities in assessing myocardial viability also requires further investigation, and the properties of the newer technetium-based perfusion tracers for viability assessment warrant similar study. Third, single photon approaches for metabolic imaging (such as iodine-123 labeled fatty acids) appear to be very promising (86–87), but further investigation of these agents compared to ^{201}Tl or FDG in the same patient populations are needed.

Above all, the clinical relevance of viability assessment by these and other imaging modalities requires extensive study. Over 80% of dysfunctional myocardial regions identified as viable by these various imaging techniques may improve after revascularization, but the specific patients likely to benefit clinically from this information are not fully delineated. At present, the identification of viable myocardium is only one factor that enters into the equation to recommend or not recommend revascularization in the patient with impaired left ventricular function. As in any other patient with coronary artery disease, this decision should also be based on clinical presentation, coronary anatomy, left ventricular function, and evidence of inducible ischemia. Increasingly, however, determination of the viability of myocardial territories to be revascularized plays a pivotal role in this decisionmaking process. Definitive, accurate, and cost-effective methods are essential to make this determination, and nuclear cardiology techniques will be called upon with increasing frequency in the future for this purpose.

References

1. Bruschke AVG, Proudfit WL, Sones FM. Progress study of 590 consecutive nonsurgical cases of coronary artery diseased followed 5–9 years. II. Ventriculographic and other correlations. Circulation 1973;47:1154–1163.
2. Hammermeister KE, DeRouen TA, Dodge HT. Variables predictive of survival in patients with coronary disease: selection by univariate and multivariate analysis from the clinical, electrocardiographic, exercise, arteriographic, and quantitative angiographic evaluations. Circulation 1979;59:421–430.
3. Harris PJ, Harrel FE, Lee KL, Behar VS, Rosati RA. Survival in medically treated coronary artery disease. Circulation 1979; 60:1259–1269.
4. Mock MB, Ringqvist I, Fisher LD, et al. Survival of medically treated patients in the Coronary Artery Surgery Study (CASS) registry. Circulation 1982;66:562–568.
5. Bonow RO, Epstein SE. Indications for coronary artery bypass surgery: implications of the multicenter randomized trials. Circulation 1985;72(Suppl V):23–30.
6. Rahimtoola SH. Coronary bypass surgery for chronic angina—1981: a perspective. Circulation 1982:65:225–241.
7. Braunwald E, Rutherford JD. Reversible ischemic left ventricular dysfunction: evidence for "hibernating" myocardium. J Am Coll Cardiol 1986;8:1467–1470.
8. Rahimtoola SH. The hibernating myocardium. Am Heart J 1989; 117:211–213.
9. Ross J Jr. Myocardial perfusion-contraction matching: implications for coronary artery disease and hibernation. Circulation 1991;83:1076–1083.
10. Dilsizian V, Bonow RO. Current diagnostic techniques of assessing myocardial viability in hibernating and stunned myocardium. Circulation 1993;87:1–20.
11. Bonow RO, Dilsizian V. Thallium-201 for assessing myocardial viability. Semin Nucl Med 1991;21:230–241.
12. Cigarroa CG, deFilippi CR, Brickner E, Alvarez LG, Wait MA, Grayburn PA. Dobutamine stress echocardiography identifies hibernating myocardium and predicts recovery of left ventricular function after coronary revascularization. Circulation 1993;88:430–436.
13. La Canna G, Alfieri O, Giubbini R, Gargano M, Ferrari R, Visioli O. Echocardiography during infusion of dobutamine for identification of reversible dysfunction in patients with chronic coronary artery disease. J Am Coll Cardiol 1994;23:617–626.
14. Perrone-Filardi P, Prastaro M, Pace L, et al. Dobutamine echocardiography predicts recovery of hypoperfused dysfunctional myocardium in patients with coronary artery disease [Abstract]. J Am Coll Cardiol 1994;23:55A.
15. Opie LH. Effects of regional ischemia on metabolism of glucose and fatty acids: relative rates of aerobic and anaerobic energy production during myocardial infarction and comparison with effects of anoxia. Circ Res 1976;38(Suppl I):52–74.
16. Camici P, Ferrannini E, Opie LH. Myocardial metabolism in ischemic heart disease: basic principles and application to imaging by positron emission tomography. Prog Cardiovasc Dis 1989; 32:217–238.
17. Gibson RS, Watson DD, Taylor GJ, et al. Prospective assessment of regional myocardial perfusion before and after coronary revascularization surgery by quantitative thallium-201 scintigraphy. J Am Coll Cardiol 1983;1:804–815.
18. Liu P, Kiess MC, Okada RD, et al. The persistent defect on exercise thallium imaging and its fate after myocardial revascularization: does it represent scar or ischemia? Am Heart J 1985;110:996–1001.
19. Manyari DE, Knudtson M, Kloiber R, Roth D. Sequential thallium-201 myocardial perfusion studies after successful percutaneous transluminal coronary artery angioplasty: delayed resolution of exercise induced scintigraphic abnormalities. Circulation 1988; 77:86–95.
20. Cloninger KG, DePuey EG, Garcia EV, et al. Incomplete redistribution in delayed thallium-201 single photon emission computed tomographic (SPECT) images: an overestimation of myocardial scarring. J Am Coll Cardiol 1988;12:955–963.
21. Ohtani H, Tamaki N, Yonekura Y, et al. Value of thallium-201 reinjection after delayed SPECT imaging for predicting reversible ischemia after coronary artery bypass grafting. Am J Cardiol 1990;66:394–399.
22. Hendel RC. Single-photon perfusion imaging for the assessment of myocardial viability. J Nucl Med 1994;35(Suppl):23S–31S.
23. Gutman J, Berman DS, Freeman M, et al. Time to completed redistribution of thallium-201 in exercise myocardial scintigraphy: relationship to the degree of coronary artery stenosis. Am Heart J 1983;106:989–995.
24. Kiat H, Berman DS, Maddahi J, et al. Late reversibility of tomographic myocardial thallium-201 defects: an accurate marker of myocardial viability. J Am Coll Cardiol 1988;12:1456–1463.
25. Yang LD, Berman DS, Kiat H, et al. The frequency of late reversibility in SPECT thallium-201 stress-redistribution studies. J Am Coll Cardiol 1990;15:334–340.
26. Watson DD. Methods for detection of myocardial viability and ischemia. In: Zaret BL, Beller GA, eds. Nuclear cardiology. St. Louis: CV Mosby Co., 1992:65–76.
27. Kayden DS, Sigal S, Soufer R, Mattera J, Zaret BL, Wackers FThJ. Thallium-201 for assessment of myocardial viability: quantitative comparison of 24-hour redistribution imaging with imaging after reinjection at rest. J Am Coll Cardiol 1991;18:1480–1486.
28. Dilsizian V, Rocco TP, Freedman NMT, Leon MB, Bonow RO. Enhanced detection of ischemic but viable myocardium by the reinjection of thallium after stress-redistribution imaging. N Engl J Med 1990;323:141–146.
29. Rocco TP, Dilsizian V, McKusick KA, Fischman AJ, Boucher CA, Strauss HW. Comparison of thallium redistribution with rest "reinjection" imaging for detection of viable myocardium. Am J Cardiol 1990;66:158–163.
30. Tamaki N, Ohtani H, Yonekura Y, et al. Significance of fill-in after thallium-201 reinjection following delayed imaging: comparison with regional wall motion and angiographic findings. J Nucl Med 1990;31:1617–1623.
31. Neinaber CA, de la Roche J, Camarius H, Montz R. Impact of ^{201}thallium reinjection imaging to identify myocardial viability after vasodilation-redistribution SPECT [Abstract]. J Am Coll Cardiol 1993;21:283A.
32. Dilsizian V, Smeltzer WR, Freedman NMT, Dextras R, Bacharach SL, Bonow RO. Thallium reinjection after stress-redistribution imaging: does 24-hour delayed imaging following reinjection enhance detection of viable myocardium? Circulation 1991; 83:1247–1255.
33. Dilsizian V, Bonow RO. Differential uptake and apparent thallium-201 "washout" after thallium reinjection: options regarding early redistribution imaging before reinjection or late redistribution imaging after reinjection. Circulation 1992;85:1032–1038.
34. Kiat H, Friedman JD, Wang FP, et al. Frequency of late reversibility in stress-redistribution thallium-201 SPECT using an early reinjection protocol. Am Heart J 1991;122:613–619.
35. van Eck-Smit BLF, van der Wall EE, Kuijper AFM, Zwinderman

AH, Pauwels EKJ. Immediate thallium-201 reinjection following stress imaging: a time-saving approach for detection of myocardial viability. J Nucl Med 1993:34:737–743.
36. Dilsizian V, Bonow RO, Quyyumi AA, Smeltzer WR, Bacharach SL. Is early thallium reinjection after postexercise imaging a satisfactory method to detect defect reversibility? Circulation 1993; 88:1064.
37. Berger BC, Watson DD, Burwell LR, et al. Redistribution of thallium at rest in patients with stable and unstable angina and the effect of coronary artery bypass surgery. Circulation 1979; 60:1114–1125.
38. Iskandrian AS, Hakki A, Kane SA, et al. Rest and redistribution thallium-201 myocardial scintigraphy to predict improvement in left ventricular function after coronary artery bypass grafting. Am J Cardiol 1983;51:1312–1316.
39. Mori T, Minamiji K, Kurogane H, Ogawa K, Yoshida Y. Rest-injected thallium-201 imaging for assessing viability of severe asynergic regions. J Nucl Med 1991;32:1718–1724.
40. Ragosta M, Beller GA, Watson DD, Kaul S, Gimple LW. Quantitative planar rest-redistribution ^{201}Tl imaging in detection of myocardial viability and prediction of improvement in left ventricular function after coronary bypass surgery in patients with severely depressed left ventricular function. Circulation 1993;87:1630–1641.
41. Dilsizian V, Perrone-Filardi P, Arrighi JA, et al. Concordance and discordance between stress-redistribution-reinjection and rest-redistribution thallium imaging for assessing viable myocardium. Circulation 1993;88:941–952.
42. Freeman I, Grunwald AM, Hoory S, Bodenheimer MM. Effect of coronary occlusion and myocardial viability on myocardial activity of technetium-99m-sestamibi. J Nucl Med 1991;32:292–298.
43. Sinusas AJ, Watson DD, Cannon JM, Beller GA. Effect of ischemia and postischemic dysfunction on myocardial uptake of technetium-99m-labeled methoxyisobutyl isonitrile and thallium-201. J Am Coll Cardiol 1989;14:1785–1793.
44. Beanlands RSB, Dawood F, Wen WH, et al. Are the kinetics of technetium-99m methoxyisobutyl isonitrile affected by cell metabolism and viability? Circulation 1990;82:1802–1814.
45. Edwards NC, Ruiz M, Watson DD, Beller GA. Does Tc-99m sestamibi given immediately after coronary reperfusion reflect viability [Abstract]? Circulation 1990;82:III-542.
46. Li QS, Matsumura K, Dannals R, Becker LC. Radionuclide markers of viability in reperfused myocardium: comparison between ^{18}F-2-deoxyglucose, ^{201}Tl, and ^{99m}Tc-sestamibi [Abstract]. Circulation 1990;82:III-542.
47. Christian TF, Behrenbeck T, Pellikka PA, et al. Mismatches of left ventricular function and perfusion with Tc-99m-isonitrile folowing reperfusion therpay for acute myocarial infarctions: identification of myocardial stunning and hyperkinesia. J Am Coll Cardiol 1990;16:1632–1638.
48. Bonow RO, Dilsizian V. Thallium-201 and technetium-99m-sestamibi for assessing viable myocardium. J Nucl Med 1992; 33:815–818.
49. Cuocolo A, Pace L, Ricciardelli B, Chiariello M, Trimarco B, Salvatore M. Identification of viable myocardium in patients with chronic coronary artery disease: comparison of thallium-201 scintigraphy with reinjection and technetium-99m methoxyisobutyl isonitrile. J Nucl Med 1992;33:505–511.
50. Marzullo P, Sambuceti G, Parodi O. The role of sestamibi scintigraphy in the radioisotopic assessment of myocardial viability. J Nucl Med 1992;33:1925–1930.
51. Marzullo P, Parodi O, Reisenhofer B, et al. Value of rest thallium-201/technetium-99m sestamibi scans and dobutamine echocardiography for detecting myocardial viability. Am J Cardiol 1993; 71:166–172.
52. Sawada SG, Allman KC, Muzik O, et al. Positron emission tomography detects evidence pf viability in rest technetium-99m sestamibi defects. J Am Coll Cardiol 1994;23:92–98.
53. Dilsizian V, Arrighi JA, Diodati JG, et al. Myocardial viability in patients with chronic ischemic left ventricular dysfunction: comparison of ^{99m}Tc-sestamibi, ^{201}thallium, and ^{18}F-fluorodeoxyglucose. Circulation 1994;89:578–587.
54. Udelson JE, Coleman PS, Matherall JA, et al. Predicting recovery of severe regional ventricular dysfunction: comparison of resting scintigraphy with thallium-201 and technetium-99m sestamibi. Circulation1994;89:2552–2561.
55. Taillefer R, Primeau M, Costi P, Lambert R, Leveille J, Latour Y. Technetium-99m-sestamibi myocardial perfusion imaging in detection of coronary artery disease: comparison between initial (1-hour) and delayed (3-hour) postexercise images. J Nucl Med 1991; 32:1961–1965.
56. Schelbert HR, Buxton D. Insights into coronary artery disease gained from metabolic imaging. Circulation 1988;78:496–505.
57. Bonow RO, Berman DS, Gibbons RJ, et al. Cardiac positron emission tomography. A report for health professionals from the Committee on Advanced Cardiac Imaging and Technology of the Council on Clinical Cardiology, American Heart Association. Circulation 1991;84:447–454.
58. Schelbert HR, Bonow RO, Geltman E, Maddahi J, Schwaiger M. Clinical use of positron emission tomography. Position paper of the Cardiovascular Council of the Society of Nuclear Medicine. J Nucl Med 1993;34:1385–1388.
59. Schelbert H. Metabolic imaging to assess myocardial viability. J Nucl Med 1994;35(Suppl):8S–14S.
60. Marshall RC, Tillisch JH, Phelps ME, et al. Identification and differentiation of resting myocardial ischemia and infarction in man with positron computed tomography, ^{18}F-labeled fluorodeoxyglucose and N-13 ammonia. Circulation 1983;67:766–778.
61. Tillisch JH, Brunken R, Marshall R, et al. Reversibility of cardiac wall-motion abnormalities predicted by positron tomography. N Engl J Med 1986;314:884–888.
62. Brunken R, Tillisch J, Schwaiger M, et al. Regional perfusion, glucose metabolism, and wall motion in patients with chronic electrocardiographic Q wave infarctions: evidence for persistence of viable tissue in some infarct regions by positron emission tomography. Circulation 1986;73:951–963.
63. Fudo T, Kambara H, Hashimoto T, et al. F-18 deoxyglucose and stress N-13 ammonia positron emission tomography in anterior wall healed myocardial infarction. Am J Cardiol 1988;61:1191–1197.
64. Tamaki N, Yonekura Y, Yamashita K, et al. Positron emission tomography using fluorine-18 deoxyglucose in evaluation of coronary artery bypass grafting. Am J Cardiol 1989;64:860–865.
65. Gropler RJ, Geltman EM, Sampathkumaran K, et al. Functional recovery after coronary revascularization for chronic coronary artery disease is dependent on maintenance of oxidative metabolism. J Am Coll Cardiol 1992;20:569–577.
66. Lucignani G, Paolini G, Landoni C, et al. Presurgical identification of hibernating myocardium by combined use of technetium-99m hexakis 2-methoxyisobutylisonitrile single photon emission tomography and fluorine-18 fluoro-2-deoxy-D-glucose positron emission tomography in patients with coronary artery disease. Eur J Nucl Med 1992;19:874–881.
67. Carrel T, Jenni R, Haubold-Reuter S, Von Schulthess G, Pasic M, Turina M. Improvement in severely reduced left ventricular function after surgical revascularization in patients with preoperative myocardial infarction. Eur J Cardiothorac Surg 1992:6:479–484.
68. vom Dahl J, Altehoefer C, Sheehan FH, et al. Recovery of myocardial function following coronary revascularization: impact of viability and long-term vessel patency as assessed by preoperative F-18 FDG PET and serial angiography [Abstract]. J Nucl Med 1993; 34:23P.
69. Bessozi MC, Brown MD, Hubner KF, et al. Retrospective post-

therapy evaluation of cardiac function in 208 coronary artery disease patients evaluated by positron emission tomography [Abstract]. J Nucl Med 1992;33:885.
70. Nienaber CA, Brunken RC, Sherman CT, et al. Metabolic and functional recovery of ischemic human myocardium after coronary angioplasty. J Am Coll Cardiol 1991;18:966–978.
71. Eitzman D, Al-Aouar Z, Kanter HL, et al. Clinical outcome of patients with advanced coronary artery disease after viability studies with positron emission tomography. J Am Coll Cardiol 1992; 20:559–565.
72. Maddahi J, DiCarli M, Davidson M, et al. Prognostic significance on PET assessment of myocardial viability in patients with left ventricular dysfunction [Abstract]. J Am Coll Cardiol 1992; 19:142A.
73. DiCarli M, Khanna S, Davidson M, et al. The value of PET for predicting improvement in heart failure symptoms in patients with coronary artery disease and severe left ventricular dysfunction [Abstract]. J Am Coll Cardiol 1993;21:129A.
74. Brunken R, Schwaiger M, Grover-McKay M, Phelps ME, Tillisch J, Schelbert HR. Positron emission tomography detects tissue metabolic activity in myocardial segments with persistent thallium perfusion defects. J Am Coll Cardiol 1987;10:557–567.
75. Tamaki N, Yonekura Y, Yamashita K, et al. Relation of left ventricular perfusion and wall motion with metabolic activity in persistent defects on thallium-201 tomography in healed myocardial infarction. Am J Cardiol 1988;62:202–208.
76. Brunken RC, Kottou S, Nienaber CA, et al. PET detection of viable tissue in myocardial segments with persistent defects at Tl-201 SPECT. Radiology 1989;65:65–73.
77. Tamaki N, Yonekura Y, Yamashita K, et al. SPECT thallium-201 tomography and positron tomography using N-13 ammonia and F-18 fluorodeoxyglucose in coronary artery disease. Am J Cardiac Imaging 1989;3:3–9.
78. Brunken RC, Mody FV, Hawkins RA, Neinaber C, Phelps ME, Schelbert HR. Positron emission tomography detects metabolic activity in myocardium with persistent 24-hour single photon emission computed tomography ^{201}Tl defects. Circulation 1992; 86:1357–1369.
79. Bonow RO, Dilsizian V, Cuocolo A, Bacharach SL. Identification of viable myocardium in patients with chronic coronary artery disease and left ventricular dysfunction: comparison of thallium-201 with reinjection and PET imaging with ^{18}F-fluorodeoxyglucose. Circulation 1991;83:26–37.
80. Tamaki N, Ohtani H, Yamashita K, et al. Metabolic activity in the areas of new fill-in after thallium-201 reinjection: comparison with positron emission tomography using fluorine-18-deoxyglucose. J Nucl Med 1991;32:673–678.
81. Perrone-Filardi P, Bacharach SL, Dilsizian V, Maurea S, Frank JA, Bonow RO. Regional left ventricular wall thickening: relation to regional uptake of ^{18}F-fluorodeoxyglucose and thallium-201 in patients with chronic coronary artery disease and left ventricular dysfunction. Circulation 1992;86:1125–1137.
82. Yamamoto Y, de Silva R, Rhodes CG, et al. A new strategy for the assessment of viable myocardium and regional myocardial blood flow using ^{15}O-water and dynamic positron emission tomography. Circulation 1992;86:167–178.
83. de Silva R, Yamamoto Y, Rhodes CG, et al. Preoperative prediction of the outcome of coronary revascularization using positron emission tomography. Circulation 1992;86:1738–1742.
84. Gould KL, Haynie M, Hess MJ, Yoshida K, Mullani N, Smalling RW. Myocardial metabolism of fluorodeoxyglucose compared to cell membrane integrity for the potassium analogue Rb-82 for assessing infarct size in man by PET. J Nucl Med 1991;32:1–9.
85. Garcia EV. Quantitative myocardial perfusion single-photon emission computed tomographic imaging: quo vadis? (Where do we go from here?) J Nucl Cardiol 1994;1:83–93.
86. Tamaki N, Kawamoto M, Yonekura Y, et al. Regional metabolic abnormality in relation to perfusion and wall motion in patients with myocardial infarction: assessment with emission tomography using an iodinated branched fatty acid analog. J Nucl Med 1992;33:659–667.
87. Murray G, Schad N, Ladd W, et al. Metabolic cardiac imaging in coronary artery disease with severe left ventricular dysfunction: assessment of myocardial viability with ^{123}I-iodophenylpentadecanoic acid imaged by a multicrystal camera and correlation with transmural myocardial biopsy. J Nucl Med 1992;33:1269–1277.

28 Myocardial Infarct Imaging

LYNNE L. JOHNSON

To help physicians select appropriate nuclear medicine tests in the management of patients with acute myocardial infarctions, it is necessary to understand the pathophysiology of acute myocardial infarction and, importantly, the relationship between myocardial blood flow and development of myocardial necrosis. The extent of myocardial necrosis measured as both surface area and transmurality resulting from coronary artery occlusion depends on several factors including the duration of vessel occlusion, presence and extent of collaterals, level of coronary flow in a vessel following reperfusion, and presence or absence of local vasoactive substances. A young person without arteriographically defined "critically stenosed" coronary lesions may fissure a plaque on a 50% stenotic lesion with ensuing clot formation and sudden total vessel occlusion. Because of the minor degree of stenosis prior to the ischemic event, the patient will not have developed collaterals. Data from clinical trials suggest that if reperfusion is not achieved early, such a patient will go on to sustain a large infarction with significant left ventricle dysfunction. Alternatively, an older patient with a longstanding severely stenotic left anterior descending lesion has highly developed collaterals (1, 2). In such cases, the left anterior descending may totally occlude asymptomatically without producing any necrosis. The total vessel occlusion may only be identified when coronary arteriography is performed because of clinical angina or a positive stress test.

Wall motion at rest in the distribution of the totally occluded left anterior descending may be normal or hypokinetic. Wall motion abnormalities in the distribution of totally occluded vessels in the absence of prior infarction may represent a form of chronic "stunning" (3). The term "stunning" is generally applied to myocardium that is dysfunctional after a myocardial infarction but which proves to be viable by showing slow return to normal function over time after the acute ischemic event. Stunning probably also occurs in patients with chronic ischemic heart disease who have repeated episodes of ischemia, either symptomatic (angina) or asymptomatic (silent). The alternative explanation for dysfunctional myocardium that is not scarred is the concept of hibernation. This theory proposes that regional dysfunctional myocardium represents a downregulation of function to match flow limitations that are so severe that myocardial blood flow is reduced at rest (4). Because there are no good animal models for hibernation there are no experimental data to prove or disprove this theory. Whether stunning or hibernation is evoked to explain regional myocardial dysfunction, it is important to recognize that dissociation may exist between regional left ventricular wall motion and viability in coronary artery disease, especially in patients with severe coronary artery disease and/or recent myocardial infarction or unstable angina. Even severely dysfunctional myocardium may be viable and recover function either over time following the acute ischemic event or with restoration of blood flow by PTCA or bypass surgery.

LIMITATION OF INFARCT IMAGING WITH PERFUSION TRACERS

It is important to recognize that a perfusion tracer alone will not give the complete picture regarding presence or extent of recent myocardial necrosis in a patient following an acute ischemic event. A perfusion tracer, when injected during coronary occlusion, demarcates the risk region which is larger than the ultimate area of necrosis in the presence of successful thrombolysis (5). Even when injected several days after the infarction, a perfusion tracer may overestimate the scar. Systolic thinning alone may make the counts in viable but stunned myocardium appear reduced because of partial volume effects (6). The perfusion defect size will also overestimate recent necrosis in the presence of additional scarred areas from remote infarctions. A perfusion tracer may be insensitive for detecting non-Q wave infarctions because of the limited resolution of nuclear imaging cameras to detect transmural count differentials. In the thrombolytic era, an increasingly larger percentage of myocardial infarctions are non-Q wave because successful reperfusion therapy converts what would otherwise be a transmural infarction into a subendocardial infarction.

INFARCT AVID IMAGING AGENTS

For all of the foregoing reasons, neither a perfusion tracer alone nor a perfusion tracer combined with assessment of regional wall motion give the complete picture regarding presence or extent of recent myocardial necrosis. Therefore, radiopharmaceuticals that are accumulated in acutely infarcted myocardium ("hot spot" agents) still have a place in cardiovascular nuclear medicine for both diagnosis and for assessing prognosis in patients with recent myocardial infarction. There are two necrosis avid imaging agents in clinical use: technetium-99m (^{99m}Tc) pyrophosphate and indium-111 (^{111}In) antimyosin. Pyrophosphate was developed as a bone imaging agent and was found to show uptake into acutely necrotic myocardium. Antimyosin is a monoclonal antibody fragment targeted against human heavy chain myosin.

TECHNETIUM-99M PYROPHOSPHATE

Twenty years ago, it was observed in some patients undergoing bone scans that there was uptake of ^{99m}Tc pyrophosphate in the region of the heart (7). It turned out that these patients with cardiac uptake of ^{99m}Tc pyrophosphate all had recent myocardial infarctions. Because this radiopharmaceutical binds to calcium in bone it was presumed, and subsequently demonstrated, that the mechanism of uptake into necrotic myocardium is via binding to intracellular calcium in the acute infarction (8). During severe ischemia there is a calcium flux across the sarcolemma. As the intracellular concentration of the electrolyte increases, the cell becomes irreversibly damaged as calcium is deposited in the mitochondria. Because some severely ischemic myocytes that have accumulated intracellular calcium may be capable of recovery, uptake of pyrophosphate is not strictly specific for irreversible myocyte necrosis. In an open chest dog infarct model, maximal uptake of pyrophosphate was observed at the infarct border where flow was only moderately reduced (9). A correlate of these experimental observations, which is seen in patient scans, is a "donut" pattern of tracer uptake in large infarctions. Pyrophosphate uptake is greatest at the borders of the infarction and lowest in the central zone where blood flow and hence tracer delivery is severely limited. Uptake into severely, but reversibly, ischemic myocytes does not decrease the specificity of the radiotracer for detecting necrosis, but it does lead to overestimation of the extent of necrosis.

Another consequence of the mechanism of pyrophosphate uptake is the time lag between infarct vessel occlusion and development of a positive scan. It takes 24–48 hours before the calcium accumulation is sufficient to make the pyrophosphate scans positive. Although some scans may be positive as early as 12 hours, some patients do not become positive until 72 hours. It is important to note that, for this reason, pyrophosphate is not an effective means to rule in or rule out an infarction in a patient who presents to the emergency room with chest pain.

RADIOPHARMACEUTICAL PREPARATION AND IMAGING PROTOCOL

Stannous pyrophosphate is provided commercially in sterile vials to which the ^{99m}Tc-pertechnetate is added. Attention must be paid to proper radiopharmaceutical preparation and administration. Poor scan quality results from in vivo breakdown of the radiopharmaceutical or injection through an indwelling catheter. The radiopharmaceutical is injected intravenously at the bedside. It clears from the blood pool relatively rapidly with a clearance T 1/2 of about 15 minutes. Imaging is usually performed about 2.5 hours after tracer injection to insure low blood-pool levels and optimal target to background count ratios. If the infarction is old or the patient has reduced creatinine clearance, imaging is delayed to 4 hours.

For planar imaging a large or small field of view Anger camera with a low energy-high resolution or all-purpose collimator is used to localize tracer uptake in the heart. Either three or four views are obtained: anterior, shallow LAO and/or steep LAO, and left lateral for 5 minutes per view using a 15% window centered in the 140 keV photopeak of ^{99m}Tc. See Table 28.1 for tomographic acquisition parameters.

INTERPRETATION

In most cases planar imaging is sufficient to establish a diagnosis. A semiquantitative scale is used to score tracer uptake on planar scans for clinical interpretation. A commonly used scoring scale is the following: 0 = negative; 1+ = equivocal; 2+ = tracer uptake in myocardial region less intense than sternal uptake but greater than background; 3+ = tracer uptake in myocardial region equal in intensity to sternal uptake; 4+ = myocardial uptake more intense than sternal uptake (Figs. 28.1 and 28.2). Rib uptake of

Table 28.1.
Tomographic Acquisition Parameters

Acquisition	^{99m}Tc PPi	^{111}In AMA	^{111}In AMA/^{201}Tl
dose	25 mCi	2 mCi ^{111}In	2 mCi ^{111}In 2.5 mCi ^{201}Tl
time interval to imaging scan	4 hours	24–48 hours	24–48 hrs following ^{111}In; immed & 4 hrs following ^{201}Tl
energy window(s)	15% over 140 keV	15% over 171 and 247 keV	15% over 247 keV 20% over 70 keV
collimator	LEHRP	medium energy	medium energy
time/image (planar)	± 3 minutes*	10 minutes	10 minutes
orbit (SPECT)	180° or 360° circular or elliptical	180° circular	180° circular
FOV	128 × 128 planar 64 × 64 SPECT zoom 1–1.4	128× 128 planar 64 × 64 SPECT zoom 1–1.3	64 × 64 zoom 1.3
# projections (SPECT)	30–60 (180°)** 60–120 (360°)**	32	32
time/projection (SPECT)	15–20 seconds	60 seconds	60 seconds
Processing (SPECT)			
filter window	Butterworth	Butterworth	Metz prefilter ramp backprojection
cutoff frequency	0.20–0.35***	0.15	not applicable
order	5	5	not applicable
transaxial or oblique	both	oblique	oblique
slice thickness	1 pixel	2 pixel	2 pixel

*Time for 500,000 counters in anterior projection.
**3° increments preferred.
***Select according to image statistics.

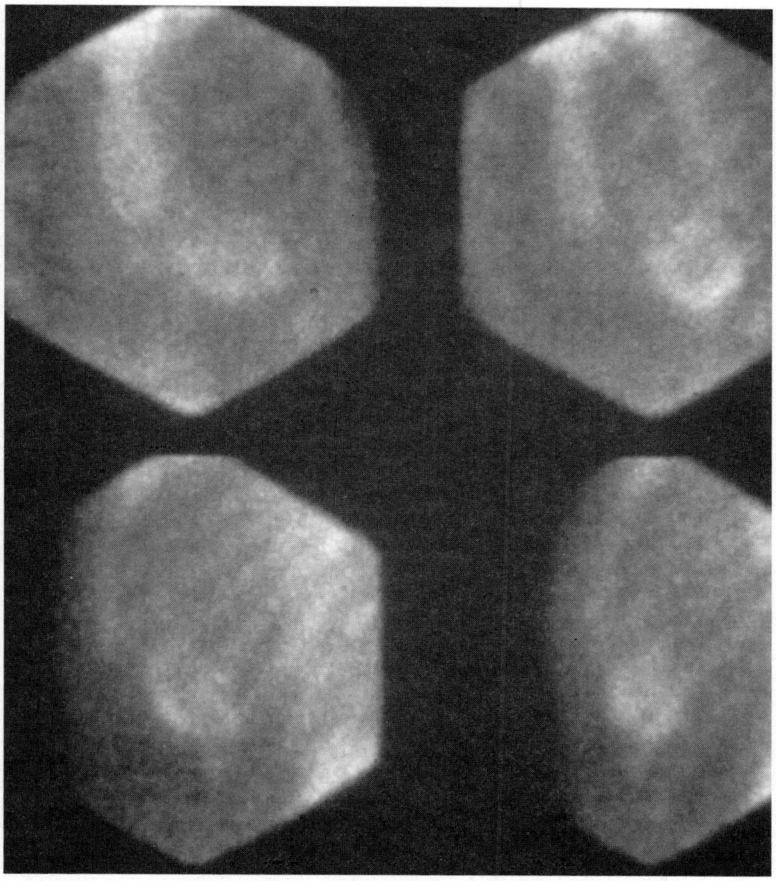

Figure 28.1. Planar ^{99m}Tc pyrophosphate images (anterior, 30°, 70° left anterior oblique and left lateral) from a patient with an acute Q wave anterior wall infarction. In the anterior and shallow oblique projections tracer uptake appears to be in a diffuse myocardial pattern due to visualization of the septum "en face," but in the steep obliques views it is apparent that tracer is localized to the anterior wall and that the inferior and posterior walls are not involved. Tracer uptake is graded 3T. (Figure courtesy of Dr. James Corbett.)

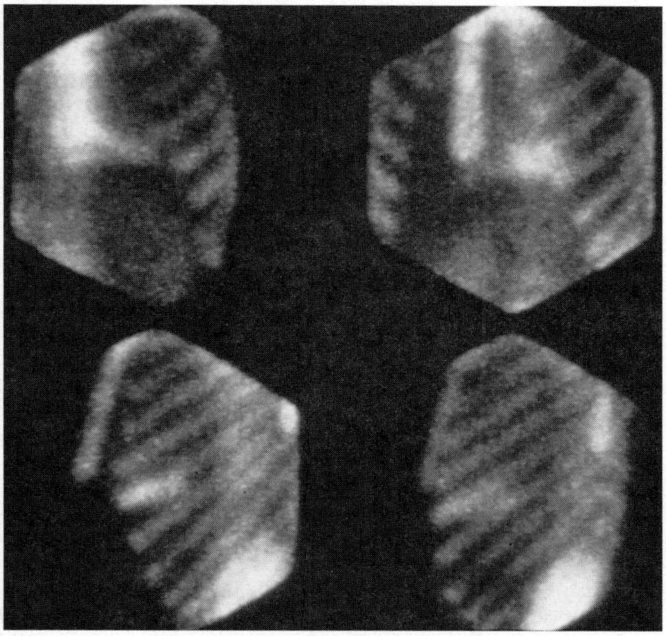

Figure 28.2. Planar ^{99m}Tc pyrophosphate images (anterior, 30°, and 70° left anterior oblique and left lateral) from a patient with an acute Q wave inferior wall infarction. Tracer uptake localized to the diaphragmatic surface of the heart is seen on end in the shallow LAO projection and "en face" in the lateral projection. Tracer uptake is graded 3T. (Figure courtesy of Dr. James Corbett.)

pyrophosphate can interfere with seeing small regions of myocardial uptake of the tracer. Because tomographic imaging provides three-dimensional imaging through the thorax, it offers help in identifying and localizing pyrophosphate uptake. One approach is to acquire planar images and have the interpreting physician look at the scans before the patient leaves the department. If the scans are clearly positive, no further imaging is necessary. If they are clearly negative and the clinical index of suspicion not very high, the study is complete and the scans interpreted as negative. If, however, the scans are equivocal and the index of suspicion fairly high, then tomographic imaging should be acquired.

Even using tomography it may be difficult to resolve small infarcts from blood pool activity. To overcome this problem Corbett and coworkers developed a method for blood pool subtraction (10). At the completion of pyrophosphate tomographic imaging, and without moving the patient, a dose of 20 mCi of ^{99m}Tc-labeled autologous red cells is injected intravenously, and 5 minutes later tomographic images of cardiac blood pool are acquired. The myocardial and blood pool images are overlaid. Blood pool activity is subtracted from the pyrophosphate activity using special computer software and color tables. Although this is an ingenious method and improves the diagnostic accuracy of the technique, it is impractical to perform routinely in the clinical setting.

DIAGNOSTIC YIELD OF ^{99m}Tc PYROPHOSPHATE INFARCT IMAGING

Despite the limitations listed, the one study examining the diagnostic accuracy of pyrophosphate for myocardial infarction reported a high degree of accuracy (11). The report comprised 52 patients who underwent pyrophosphate imaging and subsequently died and underwent necropsy. Predictive indices for the recognition of microscopic or gross myocardial infarction by the radionuclide imaging technique were evaluated. The sensitivity was 89%, the specificity 100%, the predictive value for a positive scan was 100% and for a negative scan 72%. These results correlate fairly well with clinical experience using the radiotracer. The method has trouble identifying small infarctions, especially separating small regions of myocardial uptake from faint but persistent blood pool activity. Unfortunately, the test is not infrequently ordered on patients in whom the diagnosis is in doubt, based on equivocal ECG and enzymes changes. If necrosis has occurred in these patients it is usually small in extent unless the ECG is uninterpretable because of a left bundle branch block and the enzymes are equivocal because they are obtained near the end of their elevation.

Perhaps the best clinical use for this technique is in the patient who presents with an infarct pattern of undetermined age on the ECG, equivocal or flat enzyme elevations, and a history of chest pain 2–7 days earlier. If the scans are clearly negative, the patient does not need to remain in the hospital. If they are positive, the approximate time of the infarction can be determined, remembering that most pyrophosphate scans are positive between 2 and 14 days after the acute event. The clinical importance of dating the approximate time of the infarction also occurs when a patient is scheduled for surgery and is found on ECG to have an infarct pattern which is new since the prior ECG performed more than several months previously. Because of increased risk of general anesthesia in a patient with a recent infarction, surgery should be postponed if the ^{99m}Tc-pyrophosphate scan is positive. In a small number of patients, ^{99m}Tc-pyrophosphate scans can be persistently positive for weeks to months after the acute infarction. This finding usually occurs in patients with large anterior infarctions and the finding implies ongoing ischemia or aneurysm formation.

ANTIMYOSIN ANTIBODY IMAGING

Several murine antimyosin antibodies produced by hybridoma technology have undergone phase I, II, and III clinical trials, and will probably be commercially available soon in Europe and Canada and possibly also in the United States. The antibody which has been evaluated in the greatest number of clinical trials is a Fab fragment of a murine antibody directed against human heavy chain myosin and labeled with ^{111}In. Fragments of the monoclonal antibody have advantages over the whole antibody molecule. The smaller fragments lack the more antigenic Fc moiety, are better able to penetrate the target tissues because they are smaller, and clear from the circulation more rapidly than IgG molecules. Because most of the recently published clinical experience is with ^{111}In labeled antimyosin Fab, the majority of this section describes the clinical experience with this antibody followed by a brief review of ^{99m}Tc-labeled Fab and Fab′ antibodies.

Khaw and coworkers (12) at the Massachusetts General Hospital used the observation that human heavy chain myosin is the least soluble of the myocardial contractile proteins and developed a murine antibody to this highly insoluble protein for in situ infarct labeling. They reasoned that for an antibody to be taken up exclusively into the infarction it cannot bind with components of the myocyte that are released into the circulation. In addition to being highly insoluble, the antigen heavy chain myosin protein, comprises about 10% of the cardiac myocyte. This yields a large number of antibody binding sites, many more than tumor antigenic binding sites. Properties of the antibody include a high specificity for binding to necrotic myocardium (13, 14). The antibody can only bind to the antigen (heavy chain myosin) by passing through holes in the sarcolemmal membrane. The degree of ischemia leading to sarcolemmal disruption usually signifies irreversible cell injury and subsequent cell death. In comparison to pyrophosphate, antimyosin is more specific for myocyte necrosis.

The earliest work with antimyosin antibody used a whole murine, polyclonal IgG antibody and a radioiodine label (^{125}I, ^{133}I) because it is easiest to directly label proteins with radioactive iodine (15). For the reasons cited, antibody fragments are advantageous over whole antibodies. Additionally, ^{131}I and ^{125}I are not convenient radionuclides for γ-camera imaging because their energies are not ideal for imaging range and both have relatively long half-lives. Therefore, Khaw and coworkers (16) used papain digestion to produce Fab fragments of murine monoclonal whole IgG antimyosin antibody. They initially labeled ^{99m}Tc to the Fab fragments using DTPA as the bifunctional chelator but found low target to background ratios on scans performed on patients with acute myocardial infarction. The poor image quality was presumably due to transchelation with loss of the ^{99m}Tc tag to transferrin. Therefore, these investigators further adapted their methods to permit transchelation labeling of DTPA-antibodies with ^{111}In in citrate buffer at pH 5.5. The citrate buffer prevents the indium from forming a colloid and permits the indium to transchelate to the DTPA-coupled antibody at a pH that minimizes damage to the protein and thereby reduces hepatic uptake of radiotracer (17).

RADIOPHARMACEUTICAL PREPARATION AND IMAGING PROTOCOL

The blood pool clearance for ^{111}In antimyosin is relatively slow; the T1/2 for blood pool clearance is 6–12 hours (17). By 24 hours after injection, the blood pool has cleared sufficiently in the majority of patients to yield diagnostic infarct imaging. However, in 12–20% of patients, the blood pool activity precludes obtaining a diagnostic scan at 24 hours and imaging must be repeated at 48 hours (Figs. 28.3–28.5). Although uptake of tracer into necrotic segments occurs immediately after the onset of necrosis, visualization of the antibody in the infarct must wait until blood pool activity clears. A significant extracardiac source

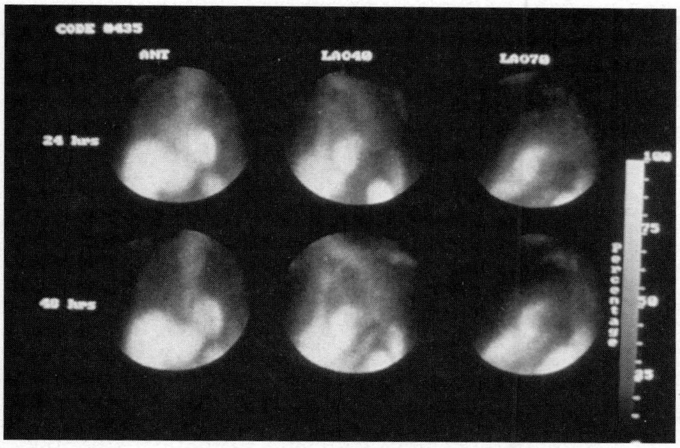

Figure 28.3. Planar ^{111}In antimyosin images (anterior, 40°, and 70° left anterior oblique views) obtained at 24 hours (*top row*) and at 48 hours (*bottom row*) in a patient with acute Q wave anterior wall infarction. There was faint residual blood pool activity present at 24 hours which cleared by 48 hours. Similar to the ^{99m}Tc pyrophosphate planar images in a patient with a large anterior wall infarction shown in Figure 28.1, tracer uptake appears in a diffuse myocardial uptake pattern in the anterior view because the septum is viewed "en face." The oblique views reveal the anteroseptal and apical localization of the tracer.

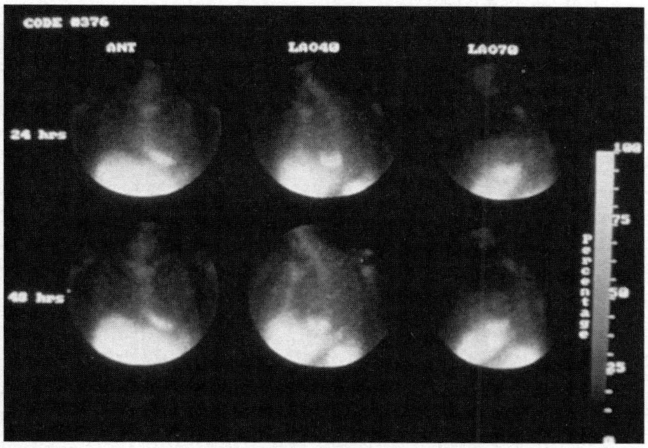

Figure 28.4. Planar ^{111}In antimyosin images (anterior, 40°, and 70° left anterior oblique views) obtained at 24 hours (*top row*) and at 48 hours (*bottom row*) in a patient with acute Q wave inferior wall infarction. There is very faint residual blood pool activity on the 24-hour images. Tracer uptake is seen in the inferior, inferoseptal (in shallow LAO) and posterior (in steep LAO) walls. Although there is tracer uptake in the liver, uptake in the inferior wall of the left ventricle is quite clearly separable from liver activity.

of ^{111}In activity includes the kidneys which are the target organs receiving a dose of 9.5 mRads (95.3 mGy) for 2 mCi (74 mBq) of ^{111}In antimyosin. Additionally, the liver accumulates ^{111}In presumably due to transchelation of the ^{111}In from the chelate antibody complex to transferrin and subsequent uptake of ^{111}In into the reticuloendothelial system.

For planar imaging of ^{111}In antimyosin, a large or small field of view Anger camera with a medium energy collimator is used. Fifteen percent windows are set over the 171 and 247 keV photopeaks of ^{111}In. The number of images, angle per image, and time per image are the same as they are for

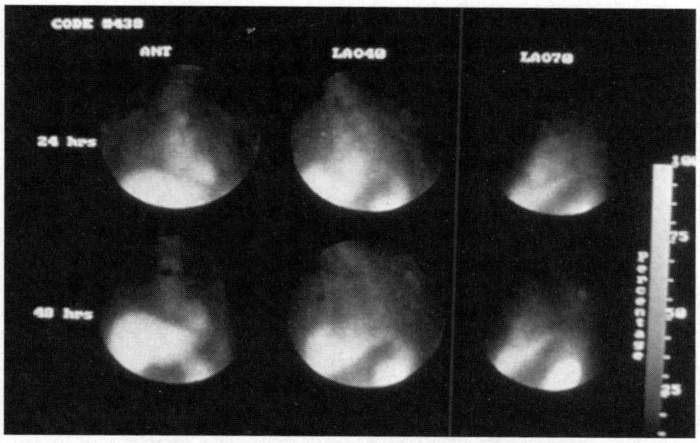

Figure 28.5. Planar ^{111}In antimyosin images (anterior, 40°, and 70° left anterior oblique views) obtained at 24 hours (*top row*) and at 48 hours (*bottom row*) in a patient with acute unstable angina. There is prominent blood pool activity at 24 hours. By 48 hours the blood pool has cleared sufficiently to show localization of tracer to the apex of the LV.

^{99m}Tc pyrophosphate imaging. Tomographic imaging parameters are listed in Table 28.1.

The scoring of antimyosin uptake on planar scans can be performed using a schema similar to that described for pyrophosphate with intensity of cardiac uptake compared to liver activity instead of being compared to sternal activity.

DIAGNOSTIC YIELD

Uptake of the antibody into infarctions varies with the degree of necrosis and can approach 1–3% of the injected doses into large infarctions. Uptake is also dependent on antibody delivery and infarct location. In a dog infarct model, intensity of antimyosin uptake on planar scans was found to be greater in infarctions reperfused following 2 hours of occlusion than in infarctions reperfused following 6 hours of balloon occlusion (close to no reflow) despite the infarctions being larger in the 6 hour occlusion group (18) (Fig. 28.6). In a more recent nonimaging experimental study, it was found that ^{111}In antimyosin activity in infarct zones increases with increasing ischemic injury, as measured by TTC for both early reperfused and nonreperfused infarctions, but that this relationship is attenuated in the nonreperfused infarctions (19). This difference in ratios of ^{111}In activity to TTC grade between reperfused and nonreperfused infarction was abolished when the indium activity was corrected for residual blood flow. Correlates of these observations made in laboratory experiments have been observed in a clinical study. Faint uptake of ^{111}In antimyosin or a false-negative scan correlated with both posterior infarct location and total occlusion of the infarct-related vessel with absent collaterals, suggesting that in patients it is necessary for the antibody to be delivered to the site of necrosis for the scans to be positive (20).

The safety and diagnostic accuracy of planar antimyosin imaging was evaluated in a multicenter clinical trial in which 497 patients with chest pain were enrolled in 25 sites in the US and Europe (21). There was no reported incidence of allergic reaction or serum sickness to the mu-

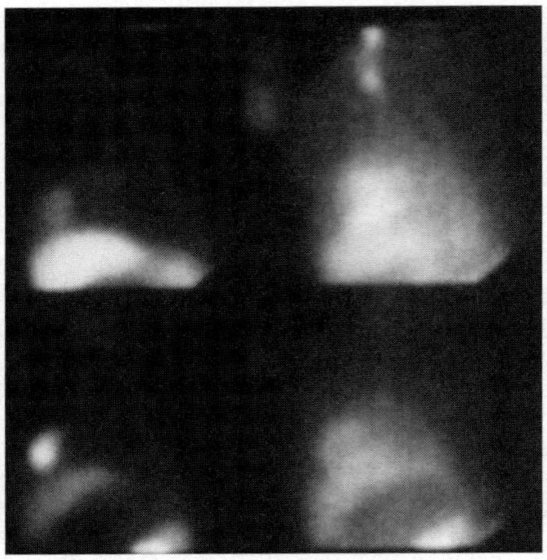

Figure 28.6. Left lateral planar images in two dogs showing ^{111}In antimyosin uptake in anteroapical infarctions created by a 2-hour occlusion (early reflow) infarction on the left and by a 6-hour occlusion (no reflow) infarction on the right. In addition to tracer uptake in the heart there is also uptake in the liver and kidney (seen on the *left image*). When comparing the intensity of tracer uptake in the infarction to the intensity in the liver, the early reflow infarction shows more intense uptake than the late reflow infarction.

rine protein. Additionally, elevations in the titers of human antimouse antibody were not detected in any patients. This lack of response to the foreign protein is probably due to the use of the antibody fragment which is less antigenic than the whole antibody. This multicenter clinical trial used electrocardiographic and enzyme criteria as the "gold standard" for myocardial infarction. These parameters have limited sensitivity but are the only feasible comparisons since few patients died and provided pathologic confirmation. From this study, the overall sensitivity for detecting myocardial necrosis was 89% with a higher sensitivity for detecting Q wave infarctions (94%) than non-Q infarctions (82%). Specificity was 95% as assessed from patients admitted to the hospital with chest pain syndromes determined clinically not to be ischemic in origin at hospital discharge. These sensitivity and specificity values are similar to those reported in two smaller series. The few "false-positive" scans reported in all series appear to occur in patients who subsequently are diagnosed to have acute viral myocarditis. The false-negative scans are found to occur in patients with inferoposterior infarctions. This finding is explained by several factors. Hepatic activity may, in some cases, make it difficult to detect small and faint areas of uptake on the diaphragmatic surface of the heart. Other factors relate to tracer delivery and attenuation. The posterior wall of the heart is farthest from the detector and attenuation of photons would affect small regions of faint tracer uptake in the posterior wall more than it would affect faint uptake in the anterior wall which is closest to the detector. Therefore, faint tracer uptake occurring in patients with inferoposterior infarctions due to total vessel occlusion with absent collaterals would be far less likely to be picked up on imaging than would faint anterior wall uptake.

The diagnostic accuracy of tomographic antimyosin imaging has not been reported. From the 87 patients with acute ischemic syndromes (61 Q wave MI, 17 non-Q wave MI, 6 unstable angina, 3 with LBBB) undergoing tomographic imaging at Columbia Presbyterian Medical Center from 1986–1991, 79 of 87 (91%) had positive scans. Specificity could not be calculated from this population.

UNSTABLE ANGINA

An interesting additional finding from the multicenter trial is that 37% of scans performed in patients with the clinical diagnosis of unstable angina showed uptake of antimyosin in the heart. At the beginning of this chapter, it was noted that the duration of vessel occlusion is one of the major factors determining the extent of necrosis. The pathophysiology of unstable angina involves an unstable atherosclerotic plaque that develops transient thrombus with spontaneous lysis. Local vasospasm may also play a role. Spontaneous reductions in resting flow leading to angina and transient ST segment changes may not produce detectible myocardial necrosis based on CK-MB enzyme elevation, but necrosis may actually ensue although undetected because of the limitations in the sensitivity of the enzymatic markers. The prognostic importance of a positive antimyosin scan in patients with unstable angina has not been evaluated.

DELAYED AND PERSISTENTLY POSITIVE ^{111}In ANTIMYOSIN IMAGING

While the duration of ^{99m}Tc-pyrophosphate scan positivity gives a fairly narrow window for pinpointing the time of infarction, the window for ^{111}In antimyosin scan positivity is wider. As a follow-up to the large multicenter trial, 182 patients received either delayed injection or reinjection up to 68 weeks after the acute event with the following results: 65% were positive at 2–4 months, 62% at 4–6 months, 51% at 6–8 months, 46% at 8–10 months, and 29% at 10–12 months. No study has reported a positive antimyosin scan occurring in a patient with an infarction occurring at 1 year or greater before the time of injection and imaging. Several smaller studies have also reported persistently positive scans, but the time intervals postinfarction were not as long as those investigated in the multicenter trial (22, 23). The presumed mechanism for late positivity is antimyosin binding to strands of myosin imbedded in the scar. In all the late injection studies, it has been observed that the antimyosin uptake late after infarction is always fainter and that tracer appears to wash out more rapidly from the myocardium.

Similar to ^{99m}Tc-pyrophosphate, the clinical use of ^{111}In antimyosin to confirm the presence of myocardial necrosis in a patient in whom other clinical parameters are diagnostic is unnecessary and not cost effective. As a diagnostic modality, the use of this technology should be reserved for patients in whom the clinical history and routine diagnostic tests are equivocal and in whom confirming or excluding the diagnosis will aid in planning further care. Because of the higher percentage of positive scans and the longer period of scan positivity postinfarction, the value of a negative antimyosin scan in a patient with an infarct pattern on the ECG of indeterminate age, would be even more valuable than a negative pyrophosphate scan for excluding a recent event.

TECHNETIUM-99M ANTIMYOSIN AND OTHER ANTIBODY MODIFICATIONS

As mentioned earlier, ^{99m}Tc has been used as a radiolabel of monoclonal Fab antimyosin using DTPA as the transchelator. However, due to high background activity and suboptimal target to background ratios, it was abandoned for ^{111}In DTPA antimyosin Fab. ^{111}In has several disadvantages when compared to ^{99m}Tc, including a relatively long half-life of 67 hours, which limits the dose of ^{111}In antimyosin in man to 2.0 mCi. ^{111}In is cyclotron produced and supply is limited compared with ^{99m}Tc which is generator produced and readily available. Additionally, because of the high energy of the two photopeaks of ^{111}In (167 and 247 keV) a medium energy collimator must be used for imaging. Because of these disadvantages of ^{111}In, renewed efforts have been made to develop other methods for radiolabeling the monoclonal antimyosin Fab or Fab′ fragments with ^{99m}Tc. Because of the relatively short half-life of ^{99m}Tc, the blood pool clearance of the radiolabeled antibody complex must be shorter than it is for ^{111}In antimyosin so that the blood pool clears while there is sufficient residual tracer activity present at the antigenic site to produce good quality images.

Another bifunctional chelator (RP-1) was developed to label Fab′ fragments of monoclonal antimyosin with ^{99m}Tc (24). These chelators are attached to the sulfhydryls of the C-terminus region of the antibody Fab′ fragments using an ester linkage. The ester linkage facilitates breakdown of the antibody complex in the kidney and subsequent excretion, and shortens intravascular clearance times. This ^{99m}Tc labeled antibody has undergone phase I and II clinical trials in Europe.

There are two other methods besides the use of transchelators for labeling ^{99m}Tc to antibody fragments: a direct labeling method via the native cysteine residues and by conjugating a preformed ^{99m}Tc complex to the protein. Another monoclonal antimyosin antibody has been developed in Canada (25). This antibody, which is also directed against heavy chain human antimyosin, is a mixture of Fab′ and F(ab′)2 fragments which are labeled with ^{99m}Tc by reducing both the protein sulfhydryl groups and the technetium thereby allowing the two to bind.

These ^{99m}Tc labeled antimyosin fragments show more rapid blood pool clearance and earlier scan positivity after injection than ^{111}In antimyosin (26). The one disadvantage of the ^{99m}Tc labeled antimyosin antibodies is that it may not be feasible to perform simultaneous dual isotope imaging with ^{201}Tl to map simultaneously perfusion and necrosis, as described later in this chapter, because of the large dose differential between ^{99m}Tc and ^{201}Tl and scatter of photons from the ^{99mTc} window into the ^{201} Tl window.

Several other antibody modifications have been pursued to improve image quality and dosimetry. To decrease the transchelation of ^{111}In from the antibody complex to transferrin, a new bifunctional chelating agent, SCN-DPTA was developed and appears to show less hepatic uptake of radiotracer and higher specific activity (27). All cells possess a global negative charge to their surfaces which contributes to nonselective protein binding and decreases the specificity of antibody imaging. Khaw and coworkers (28, 29) have developed a polylysine antimyosin which is an antibody that has been modified by a negatively charged low molecular polylysine. This modification gives the antibody molecule a negative charge, decreases nonspecific binding, and increases the number of radiotracer/chelator molecules that can be linked to each antibody, thus increasing the specific activity and decreasing the administered dose needed to deliver the same activity at the site of myocyte necrosis. Finally, the greatest advance in antibody technology is the development of the sFv fragment of the antimyosin antibody. This small fragment contains only the antigenic binding sites. Because of its small size it clears rapidly from the blood pool and in experimental animals, infarct uptake can be discerned from blood pool activity as early as 1 hour following injection (30). Obviously, a radiotracer with this kind of specificity for myocyte necrosis and rapidity of positivity would be of great potential clinical value, but at present it is too costly to produce in large quantities because it is a fusion protein produced in E Coli. One final note is that the positron emitter, ^{18}F, has been labeled to antimyosin for positron imaging of myocardial necrosis (31).

INFARCT AVID TRACERS TO DETERMINE PROGNOSIS POSTINFARCTION

There are two time periods following acute myocardial infarction when risk stratification of patients is performed: early (up to 4 days) and at the time of hospital discharge. At the time of hospital discharge, noninvasive tests to assess left ventricular function and to identify myocardium at further jeopardy are recommended. These tests can be a gated blood pool scan or an echocardiogram plus a treadmill stress test with or without a radionuclide perfusion study. The extent of necrosis is inversely related to the resting left ventricular ejection fraction when the latter is measured sufficiently late after the acute event so that myocardial stunning has reversed. A reduced left ventricular ejection fraction resulting from either a large anterior infarction or from multiple infarctions is associated with reduced survival (32). Mortality among these patients is due to events associated with a large scar or aneurysm such as heart failure or to ventricular arrhythmia. Defect extent and/or reversibility on stress perfusion imaging performed at hospital discharge correlate with reduced event-free survival. Cardiac events in this latter group of patients include predominantly ischemic events (33).

Thrombolytic therapy is only about 80% successful in opening vessels. Additionally, some vessels opened with thrombolytic therapy are left with tight residual stenoses, and some patients, especially the elderly, have contraindications to receiving thrombolytic therapy. When a perfusion tracer is used alone to assess ischemic potential in these patients, it is necessary to provoke a flow differential in the coronary vascular bed. In the early infarction period, most patients cannot, and probably should not, perform even low level exercise stress and, therefore, in this patient population pharmacologic stress using coronary vasodilators has been used. If performed early after infarction, pharmacologic stress perfusion imaging can identify patients at increased risk early in their hospital courses for interventional treatment, thereby reducing hospital stays and preventing inhospital ischemic events. Although studies to date report that pharmacologic stress in the early postinfarction period is safe, the numbers of patients studied remains relatively small (34, 35).

SIMULTANEOUS DUAL ISOTOPE IMAGING

An alternative method to risk stratify patients in the early postinfarction period which does not require any stress at all, and only a single tomographic acquisition, is simultaneous dual isotope imaging using a perfusion tracer (^{201}Tl) and an infarct avid tracer (^{111}In antimyosin). The physiologic basis for this approach to imaging was described at the beginning of this chapter. When a flow/viability tracer such as ^{201}Tl is injected at rest in the early postinfarction period, there are several different underlying mechanisms which may lead to reduced tracer uptake, including recent transmural scar, recent nontransmural scar, myocardial stunning where the severity of regional contraction abnormalities may affect apparent tracer uptake on ungated images due to a partial volume effect, and myocardial ischemia at rest when resting flow is limited. Quantitating the level of ^{201}Tl uptake may help to some extent to distinguish among these possible causes, but the addition of an infarct avid tracer helps to a great degree.

^{111}In and ^{201}Tl can be imaged together with minimal cross-talk between the energies of the two tracers. The half-lives and, therefore, the doses of the two are almost equivalent. The high photopeak of ^{111}In (247 keV) is well-separated from the major photopeak of ^{201}Tl (70 keV). The lower photopeak of ^{111}In (171 keV) is not used because it is close to the high photopeak of ^{201}Tl. Although the percentage of ^{201}Tl counts in this photopeak is small, the relative percentage of ^{201}Tl to ^{111}In counts is high.

In an experimental infarct study, 26 dogs underwent balloon occlusion of the LAD (18). In 14 animals, the balloon was deflated after 2 hours (early reperfused) and in 12 the balloon was deflated after 6 hours, which, because of the length of occlusion, is considered to produce a close to "no reflow" state. ^{111}In antimyosin was injected 1 hour after balloon deflation and the animals underwent planar and tomographic imaging 24 hours later. The animals were then sacrificed, the hearts excised, sliced into transverse sections, and stained with TTC. The infarctions resulting from 6 hours of occlusion were predominantly transmural while the infarctions resulting from 2 hours of occlusion were predominantly nontransmural. In this experimental model there was no residual myocardium at ischemic risk because the infarct-related vessels were all open and no other vessels were diseased. In the late reflow group, the location and extent of antimyosin uptake correlated well with the location and extent of the ^{201}Tl defect on both planar and tomographic scans (Fig. 28.7). In the early reflow group, the ^{201}Tl defect was not as severe and there was some overlap between the two tracers in the infarct zone. A more recent study using a dog model and ^{99m}Tc-sestamibi as the perfusion agent, documented overlap of the two tracers in myocardial segments of infarctions demonstrated histopathologically to be nontransmural (36).

In the earlier animal study, it was also observed that the early reflow infarctions showed more intense antimyosin uptake than did the late reflow infarctions (18) (Fig. 28.8). Although the infarct-related vessels were open in these animals, late reperfused infarctions are known to show limitations to flow at the microvascular level due to cell swelling. Presumably it was these microvascular changes which limited antimyosin delivery to the central infarct zone. The early reflow infarctions showed intense antimyosin uptake, which probably aided in the detection of small amounts of necrosis (infarct size down to 2 g).

A dog infarct model cannot reproduce all the variables seen in patients with acute myocardial infarctions. These variables include differences in collateral flow among patients, differences in the severity of disease in other vessels,

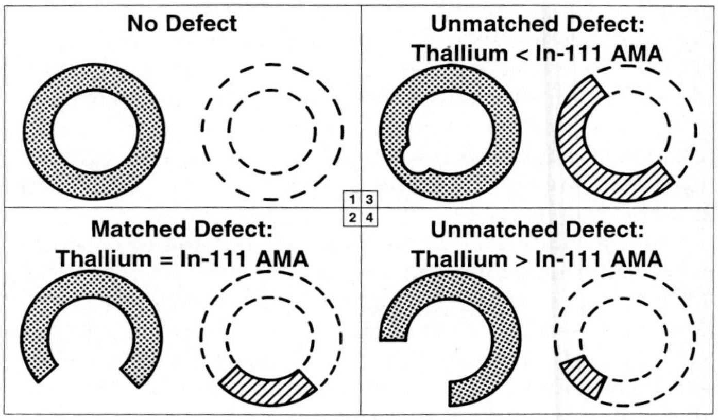

Figure 28.7. Schematic representation of the patterns of uptake of ^{111}In antimyosin and ^{201}Tl on simultaneous dual isotope tomographic acquisition.

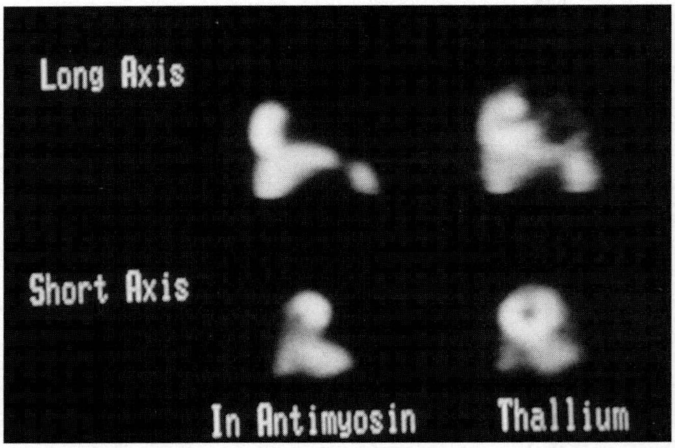

Figure 28.8. Display of simultaneous ^{111}In antimyosin and ^{201}Tl mid-vertical long axis and short axis tomographic slices from dog balloon occlusion infarct study. The location of the anteroapical ^{111}In antimyosin uptake corresponds to the ^{201}Tl defect. There is some tracer overlap at the infarct borders. (Reproduced by permission from Johnson LL, Lerrick KS, Coromilas J, et al. Measurement of infarct size and percentage myocardium infarcted in a dog preparation with single photon emission computed tomography, thallium-201 and indium-111 monoclonal antimyosin Fab. Circulation 1987;76:186.)

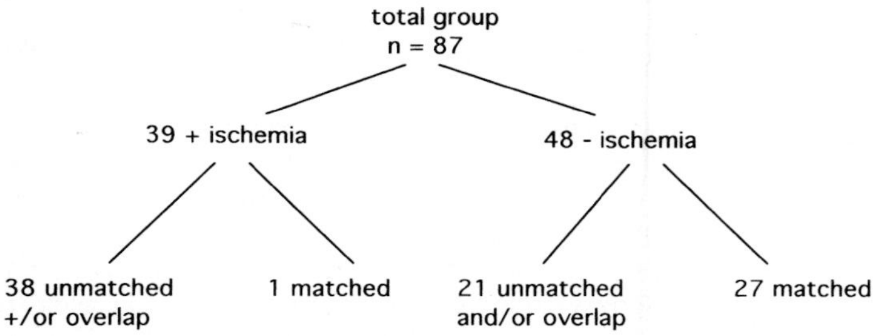

Figure 28.9. Ischemic events related to dual isotope scan patterns in 87 patients with acute ischemic syndromes.

and differences in the severity of residual stenoses in the infarct-related vessels. All of these variables contribute to the presence and extent of residual myocardium at further ischemic jeopardy postinfarction.

To investigate the ability of simultaneous dual isotope imaging (^{111}In antimyosin antibody and ^{201}Tl) to identify patients with myocardium at further ischemic risk postinfarction, 87 patients underwent dual isotope imaging over a 4-year period at Columbia Presbyterian Medical Center (37). Included were 81 patients with necrosis confirmed by CK-MB fractions and 6 with unstable angina. Results in the first 42 were reported (37). There were 54 men and 33 women with a mean age of 59 $\pm$ 12 years. Sixty-one patients had Q wave infarctions (anterior in 27, inferoposterior in 34), 17 had non-Q infarctions, 3 had infarctions that could not be localized by ECG. Only 10 of the 87 received thrombolytic therapy.

Patients were injected with 2 mCi of ^{111}In antimyosin at bedside within 48 hours of the onset of chest pain and imaged 48 hours later. The imaging protocol is described in Table 28.1. The raw ^{201}Tl tomographic data were reconstructed first and the same angles used to reconstruct the ^{111}In antimyosin data. Hepatic uptake of ^{111}In is almost always in the reconstructed images and may be greater in intensity than myocardial uptake, thereby downscaling cardiac uptake. The ^{111}In antimyosin images were rescaled to the hottest pixel in the heart.

Images with two different tracers were interpreted and matched as follows: corresponding short axis, vertical long axis, and horizontal long axis slices from the simultaneously acquired tomograms were lined up on a color video display for qualitative interpretation. ^{201}Tl defects with ^{111}In antimyosin uptake corresponding in size and location were classified as matches. ^{201}Tl defects without corresponding ^{111}In antimyosin uptake were classified as mismatches and regions of uptake of both ^{201}Tl and ^{111}In antimyosin in the same segments were classified as overlap (Fig. 28.8). During 6 weeks of follow-up, 39 patients had further ischemic endpoints (Figs. 28.9 and 28.10). Thirty-eight of these 39 patients had dual isotope scan patterns interpreted as either mismatches and/or overlap, giving this scanning method a very high sensitivity (97%). The majority of these patients showed multiple patterns of uptake of the two tracers in their hearts, for instance a matched or unmatched pattern in one vascular territory and an overlap pattern in another vascular territory.

While these scan patterns were sensitive for detecting patients at risk, the scan patterns were not very specific. Of the 48 patients who were event-free up to 6 weeks, the

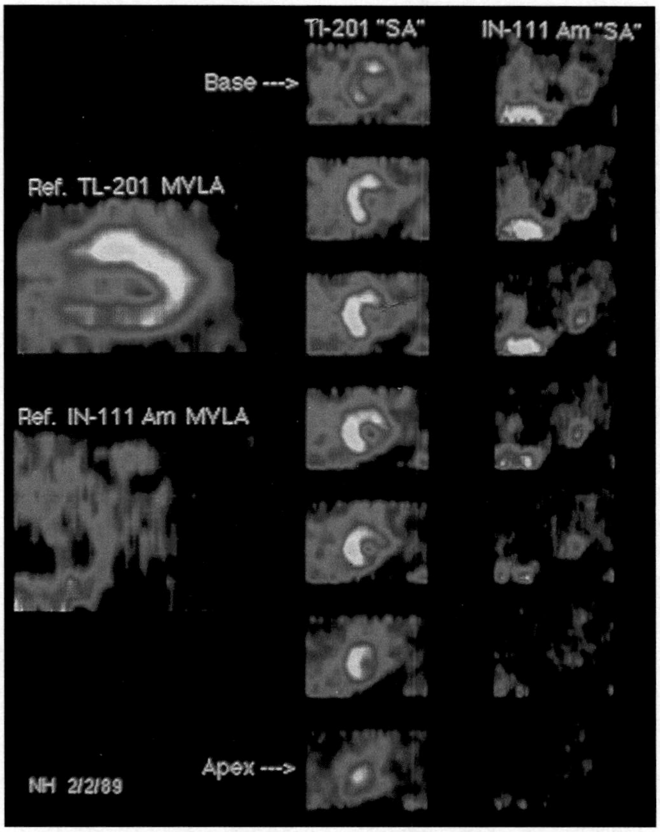

Figure 28.10. Display of simultaneous ^{111}In antimyosin/^{201}Tl SPECT imaging performed in a patient with an acute non-Q lateral wall MI who underwent thrombolytic therapy. Within 24 hours of the acquisition of these scans, the patient had recurrent chest pain and underwent angiography which showed a severe proximal stenosis of the left circumflex artery. Short axis slices show a fairly extensive ^{201}Tl defect of the inferior and lateral walls. There is a small region of ^{111}In antimyosin uptake in the midlateral wall. Because the ^{201}Tl defect is greater in extent than the ^{111}In antimyosin uptake, this scan pattern was classified a mismatch.

dual isotope scan patterns were almost evenly divided between matched and unmatched and/or overlap patterns, yielding a specificity of only 56%. Reasons for "false-positive" scans include old infarctions producing unmatched ^{201}Tl defects, poor ^{111}In antimyosin tracer delivery into a transmural infarction associated with total infarct vessel occlusion and absent or inadequate collaterals, or true stunned or hibernating myocardium not associated with further events in the 6-week follow-up period. In this last category, 9 patients had anterior infarctions and moderate to intense ^{111}In antimyosin uptake in part, but not all, of the risk zone as delineated by the ^{201}Tl defect. These patients underwent coronary angiography which revealed total occlusion of the LAD. It could be hypothesized that these patients have myocardium at further risk and should undergo rescue angioplasty, but more research needs to be performed in this area.

NECROSIS AVID TRACERS TO DIAGNOSE ACUTE RIGHT VENTRICULAR INFARCTION

Right ventricular infarction may occur in the setting of inferior wall infarction when the occlusion to the right coronary artery occurs proximal to the take-off of the acute marginal branch which is the major source of blood supply to the right ventricular free wall. Because the right ventricular mass is much less than the left ventricular mass, when infarction of the right ventricle does occur it is small in size compared to infarctions of the left ventricle. Additionally, the right ventricle is extremely resilient to ischemic insults, and even in the absence of reperfusion, right ventricular function usually returns to normal or near normal over time. The only clinical situation in which making the diagnosis of right ventricular infarction is helpful in patient management is in the patient with acute inferior wall infarction and hypotension. The differential diagnoses include hypovolemia, right ventricular infarction, or incipient cardiogenic shock. The treatment for the first two conditions is to increase intravenous fluids, while the treatment for the last is to administer pressors and consider emergency angiography. The routine use of pulmonary artery catheters, which yield data that can distinguish among these three diagnostic possibilities and two-dimensional echocardiographic imaging in the coronary care unit, no longer make it clinically important to use radionuclide imaging to diagnose acute right ventricular infarctions in coronary care unit patients. The following brief discussion of the scan patterns of technetium-99m pyrophosphate and ^{111}In antimyosin in acute right ventricular infarctions will help the physician interpreting scans performed for other reasons on patients with recent myocardial infarctions to recognize coexisting right ventricle infarction.

Several investigators have evaluated the efficacy of ^{99m}Tc pyrophosphate imaging to diagnose right ventricular infarction. Right ventricular uptake of ^{99m}Tc pyrophosphate occurred in 33–37% of patients with acute inferior infarctions. Myocardial uptake of ^{99m}Tc pyrophosphate also correlated with evidence of right ventricular dysfunction on either gated blood pool scans or on first pass studies (38, 39). The percentage of positivity in these reported series is slightly lower than the reported incidence in autopsy studies. As mentioned, because of the small size of right ventricular infarctions, it is frequently difficult to resolve right ventricular uptake of pyrophosphate from background activity or to separate it from adjacent sternal uptake.

It is even more difficult to see right ventricular uptake of ^{111}In antimyosin on planar scans than it is to see uptake of ^{99m}Tc pyrophosphate on planar scans because the dose of ^{111}In antimyosin is much smaller than the dose of ^{99m}Tc pyrophosphate. Although there is no appreciable sternal uptake of ^{111}In antimyosin to interfere with visualizing right ventricular uptake, hepatic uptake can interfere with seeing small areas of right ventricular uptake on planar scans. Tomographic imaging improves image contrast over planar imaging and dual isotope imaging technique provides anatomic landmarks to aid in localizing antimyosin uptake to the region of the right ventricle. Of the 87 patients undergoing simultaneous dual isotope (^{111}In antimyosin/^{201}Tl) imaging at Columbia Presbyterian Medical Center, 30 had ECG documented inferoposterior Q wave infarctions. Scans from these 30 patients were evaluated for presence of right ventricular uptake of ^{111}In antimyosin (40). Right ventricular necrosis was defined as uptake of ^{111}In anterior and to the right of septal thallium uptake. Twenty-nine of 30 (97%) patients had ^{111}In antimyosin uptake in the inferior, posterior, and/or lateral wall of the left ventricle, and 14 of 30 (47%) had additional right ventricular antimyosin uptake. Three patterns of right ventricular antimyosin uptake were identified. Antimyosin uptake appeared either as a "crescent" shape on the short axis slices corresponding anatomically to the free wall of the right ventricle, or it appeared as focal uptake either in the free wall of the right ventricle on short axis slices or localized to the apex of the right ventricle best visualized on vertical long axis slices taken to the right of the septum (Figs. 28.11 and 28.12).

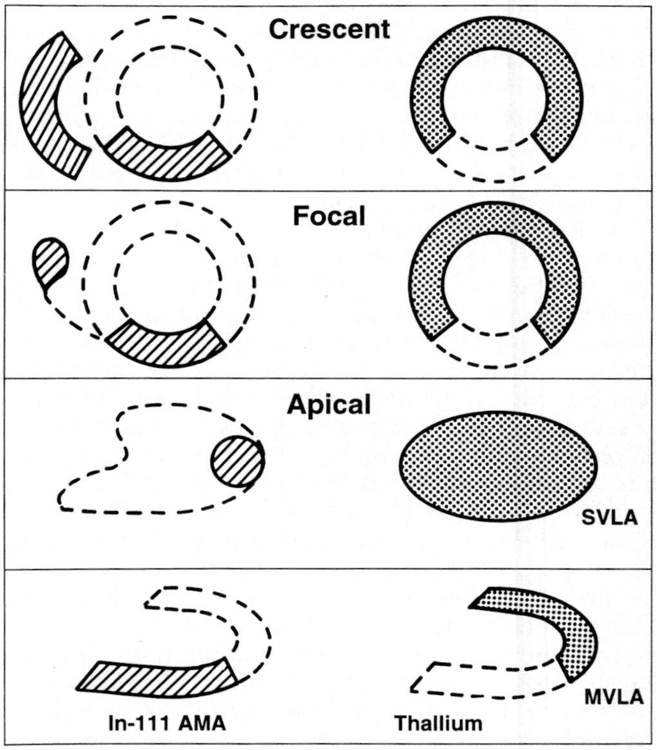

Figure 28.11. Schematic representation of the patterns of uptake of ^{111}In antimyosin in right ventricular infarctions.

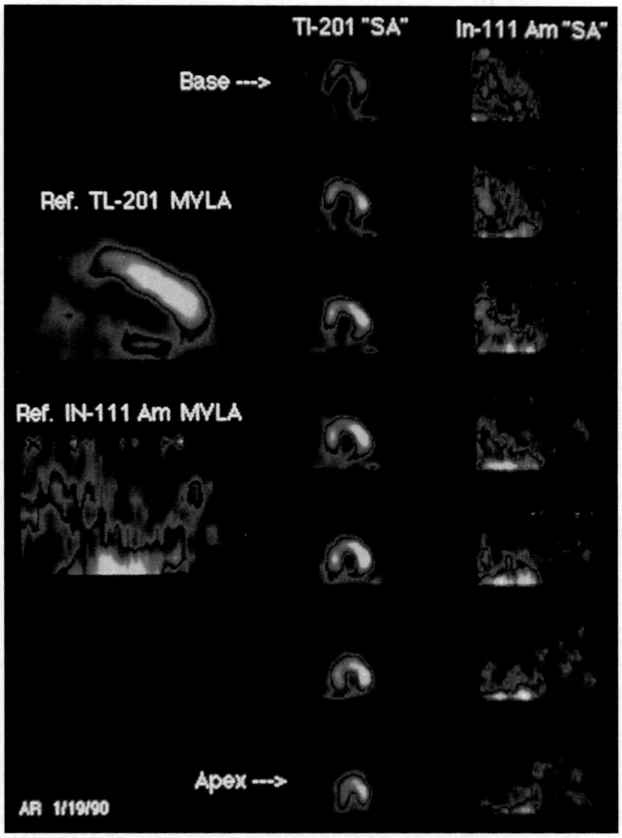

Figure 28.12. Display of simultaneous ^{111}In antimyosin/^{201}Tl SPECT imaging in a patient with an acute Q wave inferior MI by ECG. The short axis slices show decreased ^{201}Tl uptake in the segments from base to apex. The corresponding ^{111}In antimyosin slices show tracer uptake in a "crescent" shaped pattern to the right of the intraventricular septum. The reference mid-ventricular vertical long axis slices from the two tomograms show decreased ^{201}Tl uptake in the inferior wall of the left ventricle with ^{111}In antimyosin uptake in the inferior wall, but difficult to distinguish from hepatic uptake.

INFARCT SIZING

Several approaches to measuring infarct size from tomographic reconstructions have been reported. These approaches include applying a threshold technique to size the defect from perfusion tracer uptake (either ^{201}Tl of ^{99m}Tc-sestamibi) (41–43), applying a count-based method to quantitate count reduction on ^{201}Tl tomograms (44), and applying a threshold technique to size the uptake of either ^{99m}Tc pyrophosphate or ^{111}In antimyosin. In theory, sizing the uptake of an infarct avid tracer can be anticipated to be more accurate than sizing a defect since the latter may be due not only to recent necrosis but old scar, or stunned or hibernating myocardium.

In the balloon occlusion infarction experimental study noted earlier, both early and late reperfused infarctions were sized from the tomographic slices using a single threshold value that was determined prospectively from the first few experiments. To see whether a single threshold value could be applied to infarcts with varying intensity of tracer uptake, phantom experiments were performed using different sized balls filled with different concentrations of ^{111}In placed in baths with varying concentrations of ^{111}In activity. These experiments demonstrated that the indium filled objects of varying count intensity could be accurately sized by applying a single threshold if background activity was subtracted before the threshold value was applied. Performing background subtraction and applying a threshold to all tomographic slices with ^{111}In antimyosin uptake in the dogs with early and late reperfused infarctions, infarcts were sized in vivo. There was an excellent correlation between infarct size calculated from the reconstructed tomographic slices and infarct size determined by TTC (Fig. 28.13).

Using a similar method, infarct size was measured in 27 patients who had undergone simultaneous dual isotope ^{111}In antimyosin ^{201}Tl tomographic imaging (45). Patients with overlap of the two tracers were not included for infarct sizing because a threshold technique would overestimate the extent of necrosis in these nontransmural infarctions.

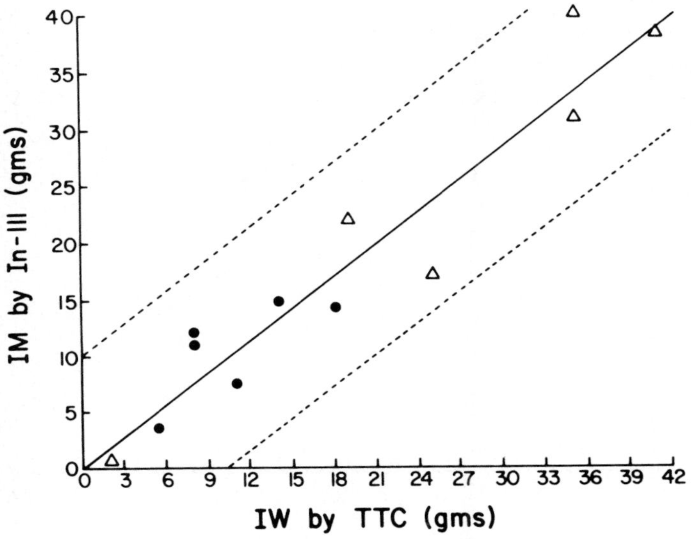

Figure 28.13. Infarct mass calculated from tomographic scans versus infarct weight by TTC in 12 dogs. *Closed circles* represent 4-hour reperfused infarctions and *open triangles* represent 6-hour reperfused infarctions. (Reproduced by permission from Johnson LL, Lerrick KS, Coromilas J, et al. Measurement of infarct size and percentage myocardium infarcted in a dog preparation with single photon emission computed tomography, thallium-201 and indium-111 monoclonal antimyosin Fab. Circulation 1987;76:185.)

Hepatic activity was masked out of the short axis slices. Myocardial ^{111}In antimyosin activity was normalized to the short axis slice with maximum activity. Background activity was subtracted by the operator by increasing the lower level cutoff percentage until extracardiac activity disappeared. The pixel value corresponding to this percentage was uniformly subtracted from the entire study. For these patient studies, the threshold value applied to find the infarct borders was determined using a torso phantom. This threshold value was applied to the tomographic slices that had undergone liver masking and background subtraction and the number of voxel elements in each slice determined (Fig. 28.14). All voxel elements from slices with antimyosin uptake were then summed to obtain the infarct volume, which was then multiplied by the specific gravity of heart muscle to obtain infarct mass. Infarct size obtained using these methods ranged from 11–87 g and was higher in anterior (60 ± 20 g) than inferior (34 ± 21 g) infarctions. There was an excellent inverse correlation between infarct size in grams and left ventricular ejection fraction measured from the predischarge gated blood pool scan (Fig. 28.15).

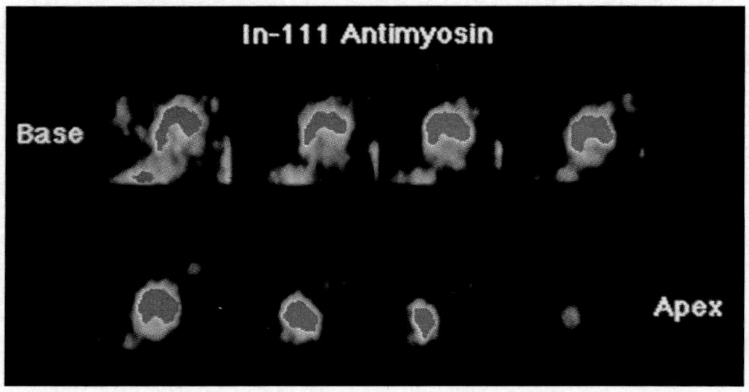

Figure 28.14. Short axis slices with ^{111}In antimyosin from patient with acute Q wave anterior wall infarction. Background has been subtracted and a threshold value (determined from phantom studies) applied. All voxels comprised in these slices were summed and multiplied by the specific gravity of heart muscle to yield infarct size in grams.

Large infarct size determined using this method did identify patients with cardiac events potentially related to large myocardial scars (left ventricular failure, malignant ventricular arrhythmias, death). Among these 27 patients, 2 died inhospital and 6 of the 25 survivors had cardiac events over a follow-up period of 5–32 months. Four of 5 patients with a first infarction and an infarct size greater than 60 g had cardiac events, while only 1 of 13 with first infarctions and an infarct size less than 60 g had further events. The remaining 3 patients with events and an infarct size less than 60 g had multiple infarctions.

A similar method was used to size infarctions from ^{99m}Tc pyrophosphate tomograms in 46 patients (46). Patients were injected with both Tc-99m pyrophosphate and Tc-99m labeled autologous blood cells. Thresholds were applied to both the blood pool and myocardial activity, and the blood pool was subtracted to better delineate the endocardial infarct border. Infarct size ranged from 2.5–81.2 g and correlated with CK-MB values (47). Patients with prior infarction and acute infarctions that weighed more than 40 g had an increased frequency of death and myocardial infarction.

SUMMARY

This chapter focuses on the infarct avid imaging agents, ^{99m}Tc pyrophosphate and ^{111}In antimyosin. ^{99m}Tc pyrophosphate is a bone imaging agent which is also accumulated in severely ischemic and necrotic myocardium. Limitations to using this agent include the window of positivity which does not begin until about 48 hours after the onset of necrosis, bone uptake which can interfere with visualizing cardiac uptake on planar imaging, and blood pool

Figure 28.15. Correlation of ^{111}In antimyosin infarct size and left ventricular ejection fraction in 18 patients. (Reproduced by permission from Antunes ML, Seldin DW, Wall RM, Johnson LL. Measurement of acute Q wave myocardial infarct size with single photon emission computed tomography imaging of indium-111 antimyosin. J Am Coll Cardiol 1991;18:1267.)

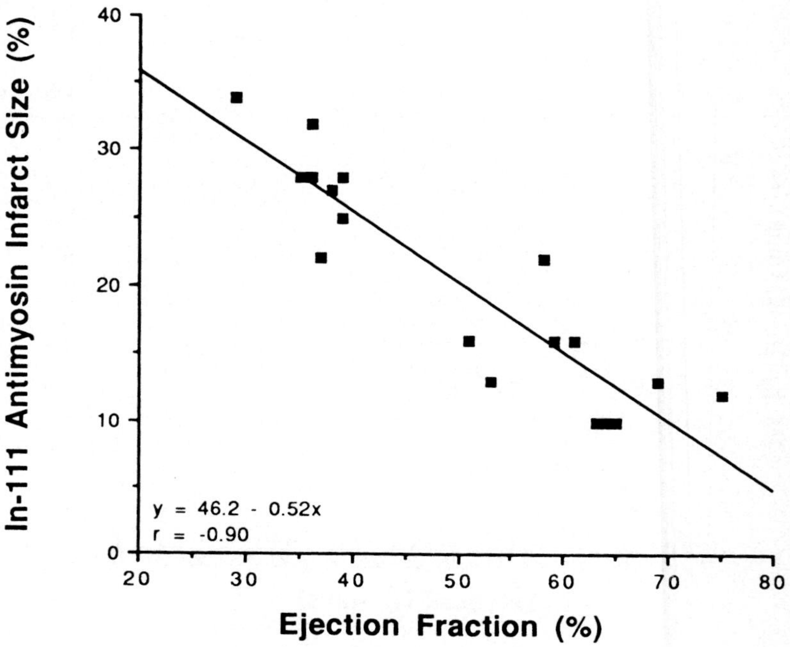

activity which can make it difficult to distinguish small areas of cardiac uptake. ^{111}In antimyosin is a Fab fragment of a monoclonal antibody directed against human heavy chain myosin. Limitations to using this agent include the relatively high energy, long half-life, and the relatively slow blood pool clearance of the Fab fragment, delaying imaging to 24–48 hours after injection. Several radiochemical techniques are now available to bind ^{99m}Tc to antimyosin fragments and ^{99m}Tc labeled antimyosin fragments may be available for clinical use in the future. Despite the limitations enumerated, infarct avid imaging has several clinical uses, including diagnosis of recent infarction in the patient who is first seen with an infarct pattern on the ECG, equivocal enzymes, and a history of chest pain 5–10 days previously. The best use of these tracers may be to determine prognosis in patients postinfarction by combining imaging of a tracer specific for myocyte necrosis with a perfusion imaging agent. Infarctions may be sized using a threshold technique applied either to ^{99m}Tc pyrophosphate uptake or ^{111}In antimyosin uptake. Acute infarction of the right ventricle can be diagnosed in patients with acute inferoposterior myocardial infarctions based on uptake of either ^{99m}Tc pyrophosphate of ^{111}In antimyosin in the region of the right ventricle.

REFERENCES

1. Ambrose JA, Tannenbaum MA, Alexopoulos D, et al. Angiographic progression of coronary artery disease and the development of myocardial infarction. J Am Coll Cardiol 1988;12:56–62.
2. Little WC, Constantinescu M, Applegate RJ, et al. Can coronary angiography predict the site of a subsequent myocardial infarction in patients with mild-to-moderate coronary artery disease? Circulation 1988;78:1157–1166.
3. Vanoverschelde JLJ, Wijns W, Depré C, et al. Mechanisms of chronic regional postischemic dysfunction in humans: new insights from the study of noninfarcted collateral-dependent myocardium. Circulation 1993;87:1513–1523.
4. Braunwald E, Rutherford JD. Reversible ischemic left ventricular dysfunction: evidence for the "hibernating myocardium." J Am Coll Cardiol 1986;8:1467–1470.
5. Wackers FJT, Gibbons RJ, Verani MS, et al. Serial quantitative planar technetium-99m isonitrile imaging in acute myocardial infarction: efficacy for noninvasive assessment of thrombolytic therapy. J Am Coll Cardiol 1989;4:861–873.
6. Sinusas AJ, Qing XS, Vitols PJ, et al. Impact of regional ventricular function, geometry, and dobutamine stress on quantitative ^{99m}Tc-sestamibi defect size. Circulation 1993;88:2224–2234.
7. Parkey RW, Bonte FJ, Meyer SL, Atkins JM, Curry GC, Willerson JT. A new method for radionuclide imaging of acute myocardial infarction in humans. Circulation 1974;50:540–546.
8. Buja M, Tofe A, Kulkarni PV, et al. Sites and mechanisms of localization of technetium-99m phosphorous radiopharmaceuticals in acute myocardial infarcts and other tissues. J Clin Invest 1977; 60:724–740.
9. Beller GA, Chow BA, Haber E, Smith TW. Localization of radiolabeled cardiac myosin-specific antibody in myocardial infarcts-comparison with technetium-99m stannous pyrophosphate. Circulation 1977;55:74–78.
10. Corbett JR, Lewis M, Willerson JT, et al. Technetium-99m pyrophosphate imaging in patients with acute myocardial infarction: comparison of planar images with single photon tomography with and without blood pool overlay. Circulation 1984;69:1120–1128.
11. Poliner LR, Buja LM, Parkey RW, Bonte FJ, Willerson JT. Clinicopathologic findings in 52 patients studied by technetium-99m stannous pyrophosphate myocardial scintigraphy. Circulation 1979;59:257–267.
12. Khaw BA, Beller GA, Haber E, Smith TW. Localization of cardiac myosin-specific antibody in myocardial infarction. J Clin Invest 1976;58:439–446.
13. Khaw BA, Fallon JT, Beller GA, et al. Specificity of localization of myosin-specific antibody fragments in experimental myocardial infarction, histologic, histochemical, autoradiographic and scintigraphic studies. Circulation 1979;60:1527–1531.
14. Khaw BA, Scott J, Fallon JT, et al. Myocardial injury: quantification by cell sorting initiated with antimyosin fluorescent spheres. Science 1982;217:1050–1053.
15. Khaw BA, Beller GA, Haber E. Experimental myocardial infarct imaging following intravenous administration of iodine-131 labeled antibody $(Fab)_2$ fragments specific for cardiac myosin. Circulation 1978;57:743–750.
16. Khaw BA, Gold HK, Yasuda T, et al. Scintigraphic quantification of myocardial necrosis in patients after intravenous injection of myosin-specific antibody. Circulation 1986;74:501–508.
17. Khaw B, Yasuda T, Gold HK, et al. Acute myocardial infarct imaging with indium-111-labeled monoclonal Fab. J Nucl Med 1987; 28:1671–1678.
18. Johnson LL, Lerrick KS, Coromilas J, et al. Measurement of infarct size and percentage myocardium infarcted in a dog preparation with single photon emission computed tomography, thallium-201 and indium-111 monoclonal antimyosin Fab. Circulation 1987;76:181–190.
19. Vaghaiwalla F, Buxton DB, Araujo LI, et al. Blood flow dependent uptake of indium-111 monoclonal antimyosin antibody in canine acute myocardial infarction. J Am Coll Cardiol 1993;21:233–239.
20. Johnson LL, Seldin DW, Becker LC, et al. Antimyosin Imaging in acute transmural myocardial infarctions: results of a multicenter clinical trial. J Am Coll Cardiol 1989;13:27–35.
21. Berger H, Lahiri A, Leppo J, et al. Antimyosin imaging in patients with ischemic chest pain: initial results of phase III multicenter trial [Abstract]. J Nuc Med 1988;29:805–806.
22. Matsumori A, Yamada T, Tamaki N, et al. Persistent uptake of indium-111-antimyosin monoclonal antibody in patients with myocardial infarction. Am Heart J 1990;120:1026–1030.
23. Tamaki N, Yamada T, Matsumori A, et al. Indium-111-antimyosin antibody imaging for detecting different stages of myocardial infarction: comparison with technetium-99m-pyrophosphate imaging. J Nucl Med 1990;31:136–142.
24. Weber RW, Boutin RH, Nedelman MA, Lister-James J, Dean RT. Enhanced kidney clearance with an ester-linked ^{99m}Tc-radiolabeled antibody Fab′-chelator conjugate. Bioconjugate Chemistry 1990;2:431–437.
25. Rhodes BA, Zamora PO, Newell KD, Valdez EF. Technetium-99m labeling of murine monoclonal antibody fragments. J Nucl Med 1986;27:685–693.
26. Senior R, Bhattacharya S, Manspeaker P, Liu XJ, Leppo JA, Lahiri A. ^{99m}Tc-antimyosin antibody imaging for the detection of acute myocardial infarction in human beings. Am Heart J 1993; 126:536–542.
27. Khaw, BA, Gansow O, Brechbiel MW, O'Donnell SM, Nossiff N. Use of isothiocyanatobenzyl-DTPA derivatized monoclonal antimyosin Fab for enhanced in vivo target localization. J Nucl Med 1990; 31:211–217.
28. Khaw BA, Torchilin VP, Klibanov AL, et al. Modification of monoclonal antimyosin antibody: enhanced specificity of localization and scintigraphic visualization in acute experimental myocardial infarction. J Mol Cell Cardiol 1989;21(Suppl 1):31–35.
29. Torchilin VP, Klibanov AL, Nossiff ND, et al. Monoclonal antibody modification with chelate-linked high-molecular-weight polymers: major increases in polyvalent cation binding without loss of antigen binding. Hybridoma 1987;6:229–240.
30. Nedelman MA, Shealy DJ, Boulin R, et al. Rapid infarct imaging

with a technetium-99m-labeled antimyosin recombinant single-chain Fv: evaluation in a canine model of acute myocardial infarction. J Nucl Med 1993;34:234–241.
31. Zalutsky MR, Garg PK, Johnson SH, Utsonomiya H, Coleman RE. Fluorine-18-antimyosin monoclonal antibody fragments: preliminary investigations in a canine myocardial infarct model. J Nucl Med 1992;33:575–580.
32. Multicenter Post Infarction Research Group. Risk stratification and survival after myocardial infarction. N Eng J Med 1983; 309:331–336.
33. Epstein SE, Palmari ST, Patterson RE. Evaluation of patients after myocardial infarction: indications for cardiac catheterization and surgical intervention. N Eng J Med 1982;307:1487–1492.
34. Brown KA, O'Meara J, Chambers CE, Plante DA. Ability of dipyridamole-thallium-201 imaging 1 to 4 days after acute myocardial infarction to predict inhospital and late recurrent myocardial ischemic events. J Am Coll Cardiol 1990;65:160–167.
35. Mahmarian JJ, Pratt CM, Nishimura S, Abreu A, Verani MS. Quantitative adenosine Tl-201 single-photon emission computed tomography for the early assessment of patients surviving acute myocardial infarction. Circulation 1993;87:1197–1210.
36. Tobinick E, Shelbert HR, Henning H, et al. Right ventricular ejection fraction in patients with acute anterior and inferior myocardial infarction assessed by radionuclide angiography. Circulation 1978;57:1078–1084.
37. Johnson LL, Seldin DW, Keller AM, et al. Dual isotope thallium and indium antimyosin SPECT imaging to identify acute infarct patients at further ischemic risk. Circulation 1990;81:37–45.
38. Wackers FJT, Lie KI, Sokole EB, Res J, Van Der Shoot JB, Durrer D. Prevalence of right ventricular involvement in inferior wall infarction assessed with myocardial imaging with thallium-201 and technetium-99m pyrophosphate. J Am Coll Cardiol 1978;42:358–362.
39. Sharpe DV, Botvinick EH, Shames DM, et al. The noninvasive diagnosis of right ventricular infarction. Circulation 1978;57:483–490.
40. Antunes ML, Johnson LL, Seldin DW, et al. Diagnosis of right ventricular acute myocardial infarction by dual isotope thallium-201 and indium-111 antimyosin SPECT imaging. J Am Coll Cardiol 1992;70:426–431.
41. Holman ML, Moore SC, Shulkin PM, Kirsch CM, English RJ, Hill TC. Quantitation of perfused myocardial mass through thallium-201 and emission computed tomography. Invest Radiol 1983; 4:322–326.
42. Christian TF, Clements IP, Gibbrons RJ. Noninvasive identification of myocardium at risk in patients with acute myocardial infarctions and nondiagnostic electrocardiograms with technetium-99m sestamibi. Circulation 1991;83:1615–1620.
43. Holman BL, Goldhaber SZ, Kirsch L, et al. Measurement of infarct size using single photon emission computed tomography and technetium-99m pyrophosphate: a description of the method and comparison with patient prognosis. J Am Coll Cardiol 1982; 50:503–511.
44. Prigent F, Maddahi J, Garcia EV, Resser K, Lew AS, Berman DS. Comparative methods for quantifying myocardial infarct size by thallium-201 SPECT. J Nucl Med 1987;28:325–333.
45. Antunes ML, Seldin DW, Wall RM, Johnson LL. Measurement of acute Q wave myocardial infarct size with single photon emission computed tomography imaging of indium-111 antimyosin. J Am Coll Cardiol 1989;63:777–783.
46. Corbett JR, Lewis SE, Wolfe CL, et al. Measurement of myocardial infarct size by technetium pyrophosphate single photon tomography. J Am Coll Cardiol 1984;54:1231–1236.
47. Jansen DE, Corbett J, Wolfe CL, et al. Quantification of myocardial infarction: a comparison of single photon emission computed tomography with pyrophosphate to serial plasma MB-creatine kinase measurement. Circulation 1985;72:327–333.

29 Peripheral Vascular Imaging

GEORGE A. WILSON and ROBERT E. O'MARA

Techniques for evaluation of the cardiovascular system are among the oldest in nuclear medicine. Arm-to-arm circulation times were determined in humans using the naturally occurring radioactivity of radium and reported by Blumert and Yens in 1924 (1). In 1948, Prinzmetal, et al. (2), used artificially produced radioactive sodium to evaluate the circulation time through the heart in both normal subjects and patients with heart disease. This technique utilized an intravenous injection of ^{24}Na into the antecubital vein of one arm and the generation of a graph of the count rate with Geiger-Muller tube placed over the precordium as the radiolabeled blood passed through the chambers of the heart. This simple measurement had many components to it: a venous phase, a pulmonary circulation phase, and a phase for the cardiac chambers. Since this early work, the development of short-lived radiopharmaceuticals, advances in detection devices, and the introduction of computers into clinical nuclear medicine have permitted us to separate these various components, allowing the study of venous, pulmonary, intracardiac, arterial, and capillary phases. The use of tracer techniques in the evaluation of heart disease and for the detection of venous thrombosis are covered in separate chapters elsewhere in this text.

RADIONUCLIDE VENOGRAM AND ANGIOGRAM

Many different radioisotopes may be used for obtaining dynamic studies of the vascular system. The ideal isotope for these studies will (a) have a relatively short half-life, because most angiograms are completed in less than a minute; (b) be readily available; and (c) have an energy that is efficiently detected by an imaging system. Because it is readily available and partially meetings the other criteria, ^{99m}Tc pertechnetate is the most common isotope used, although other isotopes may be utilized (Table 29.1). When an ultrashort half-life isotope is chosen, background activity is not a problem when repeat studies are desired. However, if an isotope with a half-life greater than 15 minutes is used, there will be significant residual background activity introduced by the first injection. Therefore, if repeat studies are desired or if the contralateral side is to be studied, a method that results in the rapid removal of the tracer from the circulation and a lower background is necessary. Radiolabeled macroaggregated albumin may be used because the particles are removed from circulation on their first pass through a capillary bed, usually the lung, resulting in a rapid decrease in background activity at sites that are distant to the capillary bed. This technique is useful when evaluating venous structures distant to the lungs. When repeat studies of thoracic structures are necessary, the use of a colloid that is primarily removed by the reticuloendothelial cells of the liver and spleen will result in a sufficiently low background within 15 minutes following injection. When it is anticipated that the study will not need to be repeated in a very short time interval, a compound with rapid renal clearance, such as DTPA or glucoheptonate, may be utilized to reduce background activity. The development of the ability to label red cells efficiently both in vivo and vitro with ^{99m}Tc also will allow assessment of arterial and venous anatomy, flow, and patency.

Table 29.1.
Isotopes Used in Vascular Studies

	$t\frac{1}{2}$	γ Energy
^{191m}Ir	4.9 sec	127
^{195m}Au	30.6	261
^{137m}Ba	2.6 min	662
^{178}Ta	9.5	93
^{113m}In	100 min	393
^{99m}Tc	6 hr	140
Gases		
^{81m}Kr	13 sec	190
^{133}Xe	5 day	81
^{127}Xe	36 day	203 plus others

Some method of obtaining rapid serial images is necessary for adequate data collection. A standard Anger-type camera or multicrystal imagining device coupled to a multiformatter is usually adequate. Additionally, the information may be stored on videotape or by digital computer on one of the magnetic media for later evaluation and data manipulation. The computer system digitizes the signal from the nuclear imaging device and the data may be stored either in list or frame mode. The resolution, both temporal and spatial, is dependent upon the memory and storage capacity of the computer system. The addition of a computer to the imaging system offers the capability of being able to develop histograms from selected areas of interest and is of value in the detection of shunts, determination of circulation times, and evaluation of the quality of the injection bolus. The development of the ability to label red cells efficiently both in vivo and vitro with ^{99m}Tc will allow assessment of arterial and venous anatomy, flow, and patency.

VENOUS PHASE

The superior vena cava may be evaluated by injecting a bolus of a suitable radioisotpe into one of the antecubital veins. Usually, the basilic vein is chosen because it has a more direct route to the superior vena cava. Different techniques have been utilized for the administration of an adequate bolus of activity. Olendorf, et al. (3), described the technique utilizing a blood pressure cuff that is inflated to 100 mm Hg for 1 minute, distending the veins. A small-gauge needle is inserted into the vein and, prior to injection, the cuff is inflated to above systolic blood pressure. Injection is made and the cuff is rapidly released, resulting in a rapid propulsion of the bolus toward the central venous system by the blood in the distended distal veins. Other techniques have been described, including flushing the activity in with a bolus of saline through a three-way stopcock, or using an intravenous tube that has a volume greater than the radiopharmaceutical dose and, after filling the tubing with the tracer dose, attaching a syringe of saline and rapidly injecting, propelling the bolus of activity to the central venous stem. Serial images should demonstrate a rapid progression of activity through the veins toward the heart. Following injection into the basilic vein, visualization of the basilic, axillary, subclavian, and innominate veins occurs before the activity enters the superior vena cava and the chambers of the right heart (Fig. 29.1). Frequently, the cephalic vein is also visualized (Fig. 29.2). A study of the opposite side should be performed to function as a control or to demonstrate bilateral pathology. This may also be accomplished by bilateral simultaneous injection, a technique that is more complex to perform and may lead to problems in interpretation.

The superior vena cava syndrome presents with swelling and cyanosis of the head, neck, and upper extremities with prominence of the superficial veins of the neck due to distention resulting from obstruction of the superior vena cava and the development of collateral pathways. In over 80% of these cases, the obstruction is secondary to a malignant neoplasm (4–6), usually carcinoma of the lung or a lymphoma, but may be seen with metastatic carcinoma. Less common are obstructions due to aneurysms (7), hematomas, infections, and masses in the mediastinum. Such benign masses include multinodular goiters (8, 9), cystic parathyroid adenomas (10), and mediastinal granulomas. The clinical findings of superior vena caval syndrome may be present when obstruction of only one of the innominate veins has occurred (Figs. 29.3 and 29.4). Indwelling catheters placed in one of the major veins may lead to thrombophlebitis of the vessel, resulting in the clinical syndrome (Fig. 29.5). The syndrome has been reported in patients with catheters placed for cardiac pacing (11), hyperalimentation (12), or prolonged central venous monitoring. In many patients with known malignancy who present with the superior vena caval syndrome, the treatment of choice is emergency radiation therapy. In these patients, accurate localization of the site of obstruction not only aids the radiotherapist in portal planning, but serves as a prognosticator of the success of therapy. However, the site of obstruction demonstrated may not represent the extent of tumor only, but may include the lesion plus any clot formed as a result of the obstruction. In one study of 60 patients (13), those patients who had developed collateral circulation received less benefit from radiation therapy than those without collateral circulation (Fig 29.6). The demonstration of collateral routes indicates that chronic obstruction is present. The clinical syndrome may not de-

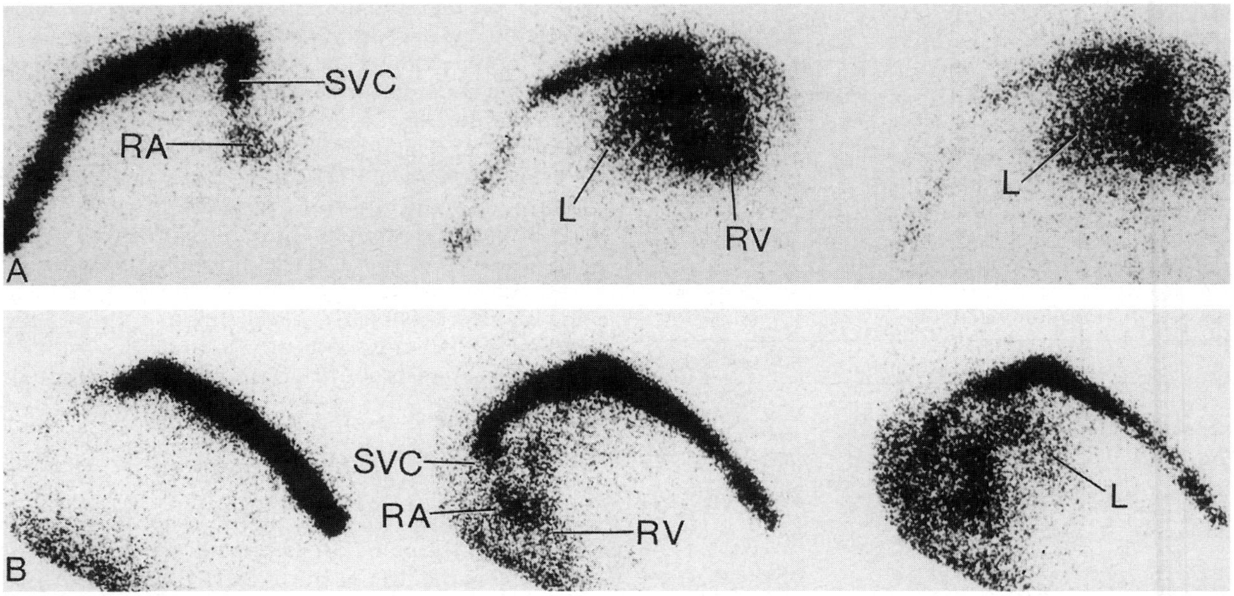

Figure 29.1. Evaluation of superior vena cava. Normal upper venogram following injection of ^{99m}Tc sulfur colloid into (**A**) right basilic vein, and ^{99m}Tc pertechnetate into (**B**) left basilic vein. *SVC* = superior vena cava, *RA* = right atrium, *RV* = right ventricle, *L* = lungs.

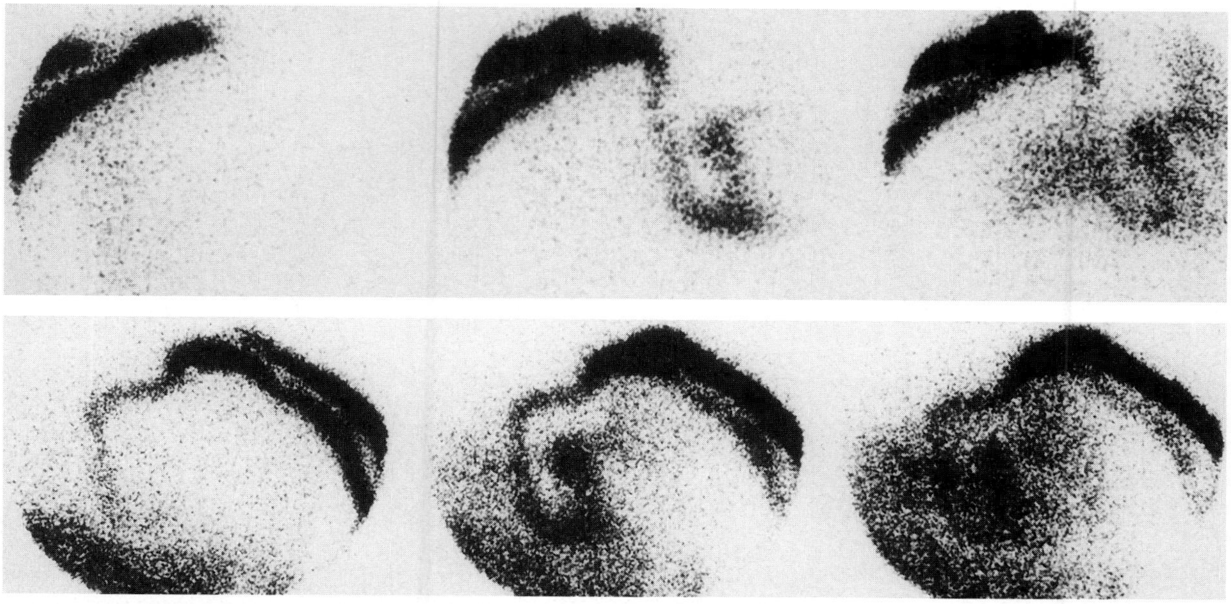

Figure 29.2. Venogram in 55-year-old male with small cell carcinoma of the lung. Note basilic and cephalic veins demonstrated bilaterally and lack of perfusion to the right upper lung caused by the tumor.

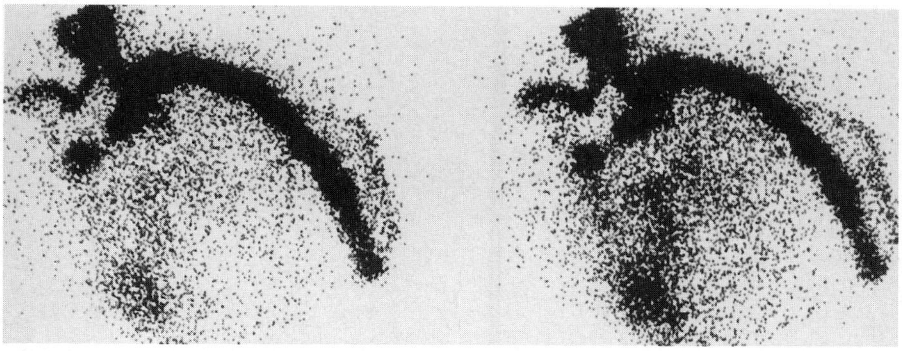

Figure 29.3. Obstruction of left innominate vein. Abnormal venogram in an 86-year-old male with lung carcinoma demonstrates complete obstruction of left innominate vein with collateralization through the thyroidal veins and incomplete obstruction of the superior vena cava.

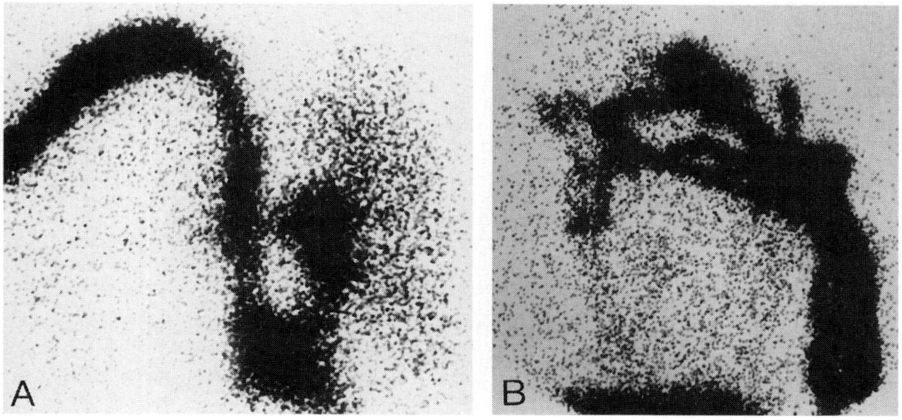

Figure 29.4. Left innominate obstruction with patent superior vena cava. A 45-year-old female presented with metastatic adenocarcinoma to the mediastinum. The right-sided injection demonstrated a patent superior vena cava (**A**), whereas an obstruction of the innominate vein is seen following injection from the left (**B**). Note the absence of perfusion to the right lung due to compression of the right pulmonary artery by the tumor.

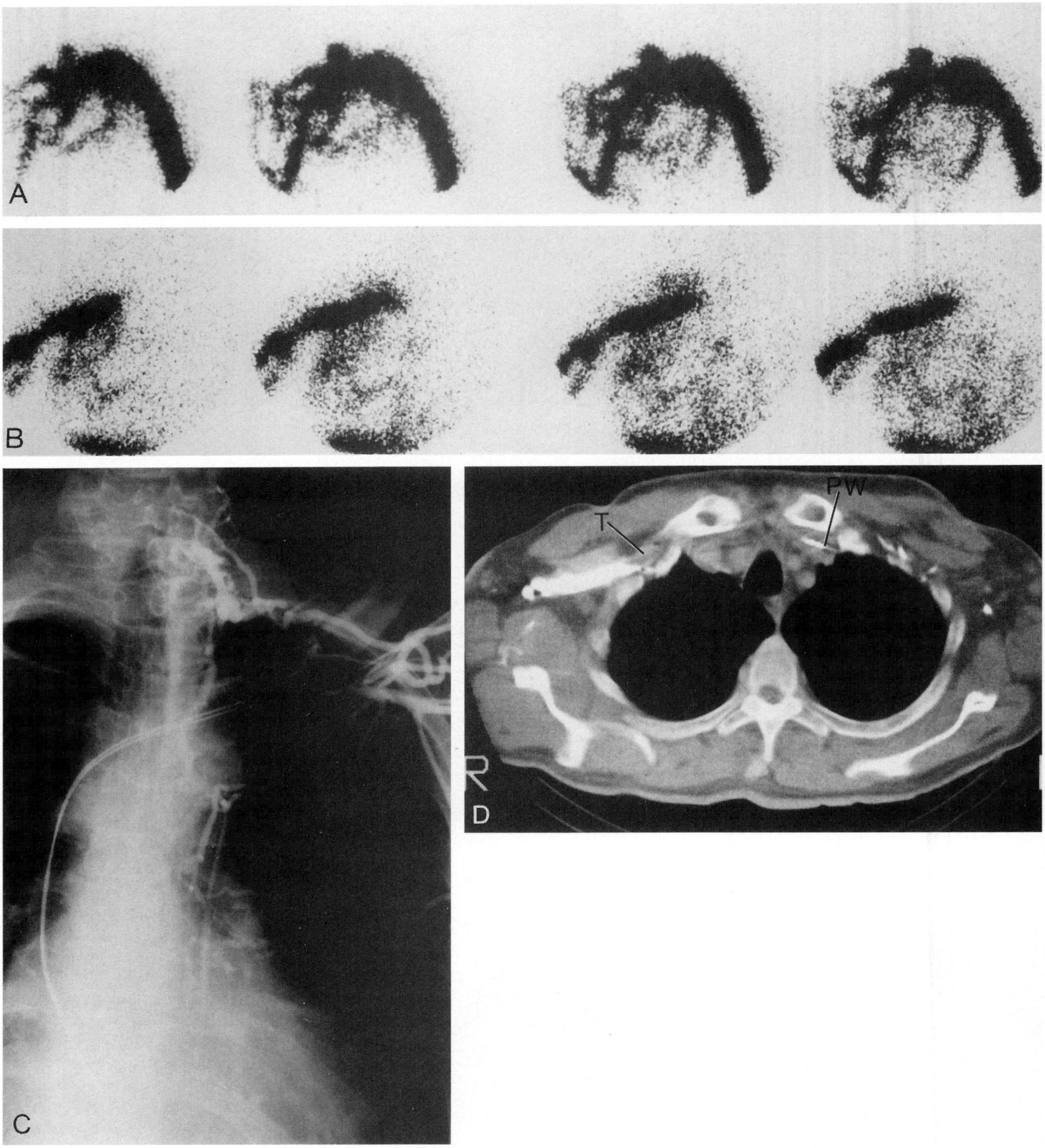

Figure 29.5. Superior vena caval syndrome. A 50-year-old male with superior vena caval obstruction resulting from thrombosis caused by transvenous cardiac pacemaker wire (**A**, **B**). **C**. Left-sided contrast venogram demonstrating obstruction. **D.** Contrast computed tomography study showing pacing wire (*PW*) and thrombosis *(T)*.

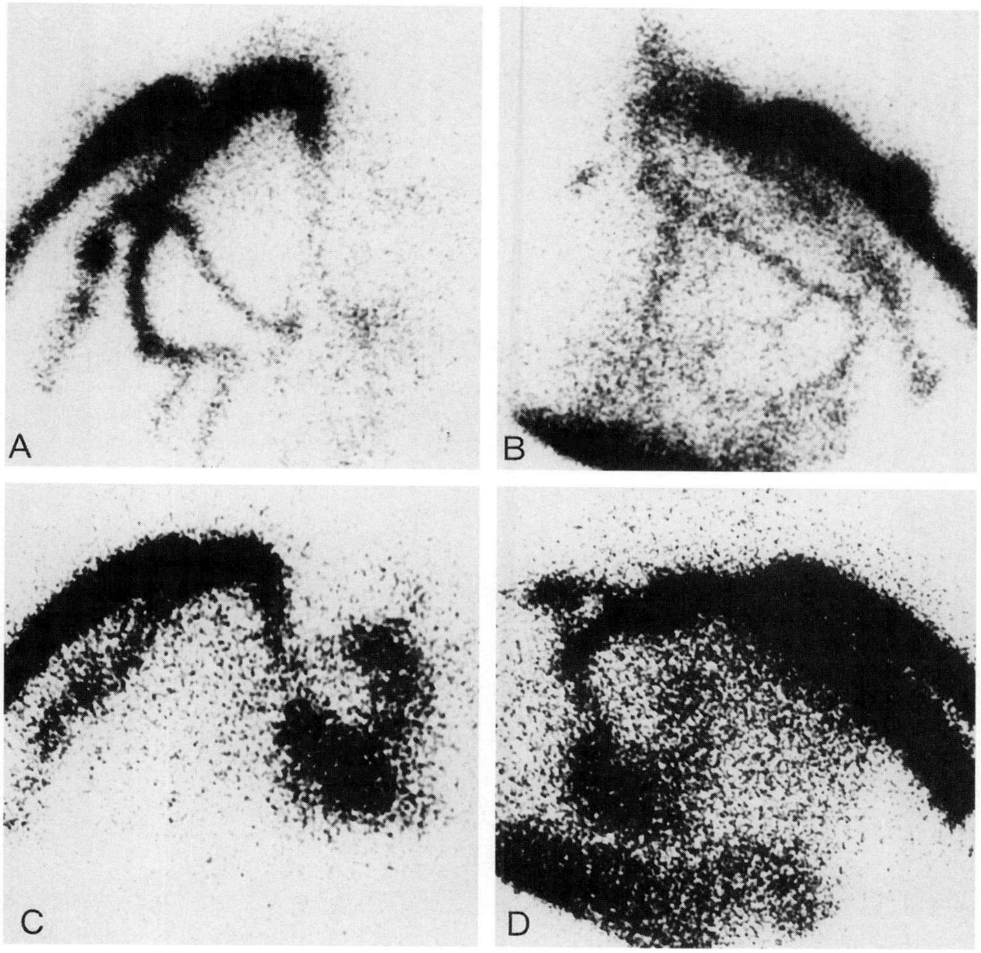

Figure 29.6. Degree of collateralization and radiation therapy benefit. A 59-year-old female with mediastinal lymphoma causing obstruction of the superior vena cava with early collateralization (**A**, **B**). Superior venal caval study performed 4 weeks after, following radiation therapy (**C**, **D**), demonstrates patency of the superior vena cava with loss of prior collateralization.

velop if the obstruction has taken place over a prolonged period of time which permits ample collateral circulation to develop. Persistent activity in the subclavian vein, 42 seconds or longer after injection, should be considered as evidence of superior vena caval obstruction (14). If sulfur colloid has been utilized as the radiopharmaceutical and the route of collateralization is through the liver, a "hot spot" within the liver, which is detected on delayed images, may be present (Figs. 29.7 and 29.8). This occurs at the site of entry into the liver of the collateral circulation. In the patient with known malignancy who is receiving radiation or chemotherapy, repeated studies offer an effective method of evaluating the response to therapy (13, 15).

The presence of an unusual shadow in the mediastinum on chest x-ray may be the result of a congenital vascular malformation. Persistent left superior vena cava (16), double inferior vena cavas (17), and congenital saccular aneurysms of the superior vena cava (18) are readily detected using a bolus of radioactivity. The obstruction to the superior vena cava caused by a substernal goiter may be intermittent. To detect the presence of significant obstruction, the patient should be imaged with his or her neck flexed during the injection of the bolus of activity (19). A greater number of patients with potential superior vena caval obstruction by the goiter will be detected by this simple maneuver. In the patient in whom substernal goiter is suspected, subsequent imaging with ^{99m}Tc pertechnetate, or, preferably, radioiodine will aid in establishing this diagnosis.

The inferior vena cava is usually studied by the injection of the tracer into one of the dorsal veins of the foot. Tourniquets placed at the ankles and knees help direct the activity into the deep venous systems. Multiple images obtained over the lower abdomen demonstrate the femoral vein, iliac veins, and the formation of the inferior vena cava. When a timed injection is used in conjunction with a moving imaging system, the entire venous system from feet to heart may be visualized (20).

In the study of the lower venous system, the intensity of the activity normally decreases as a result of dilution of the bolus with blood that does not contain radioactive material. This phenomenon may be seen where the internal iliac vein joins the external iliac vein (Fig. 29.9) to form the common iliac vein, where the right and left iliac veins join to form the inferior vena cava, and at the entry of the renal veins. The presence of this dilution effect may be used as indirect evidence of perfusion of the organ that is draining into the vessel. When the dilution effect occurs at the site

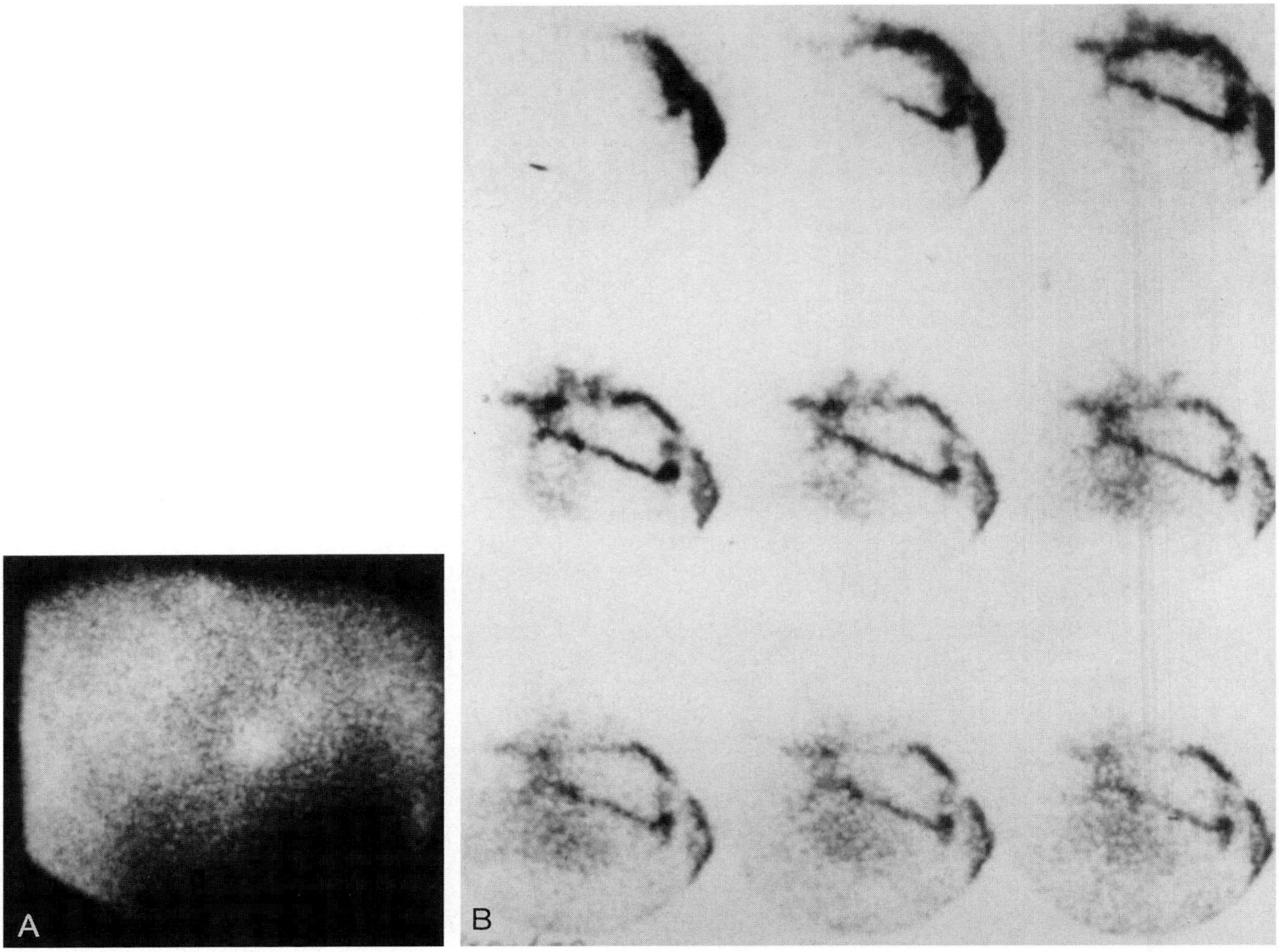

Figure 29.7. "Hot spot" in liver due to collateral circulation. **A**. Static image of the liver in a 22-year-old male with lymphoma showing focal "hot spot" of increased activity caused by blood flow into the liver via collateral circulation. **B**. Left-sided superior vena caval study demonstrating obstruction with extensive collateralization in same patient.

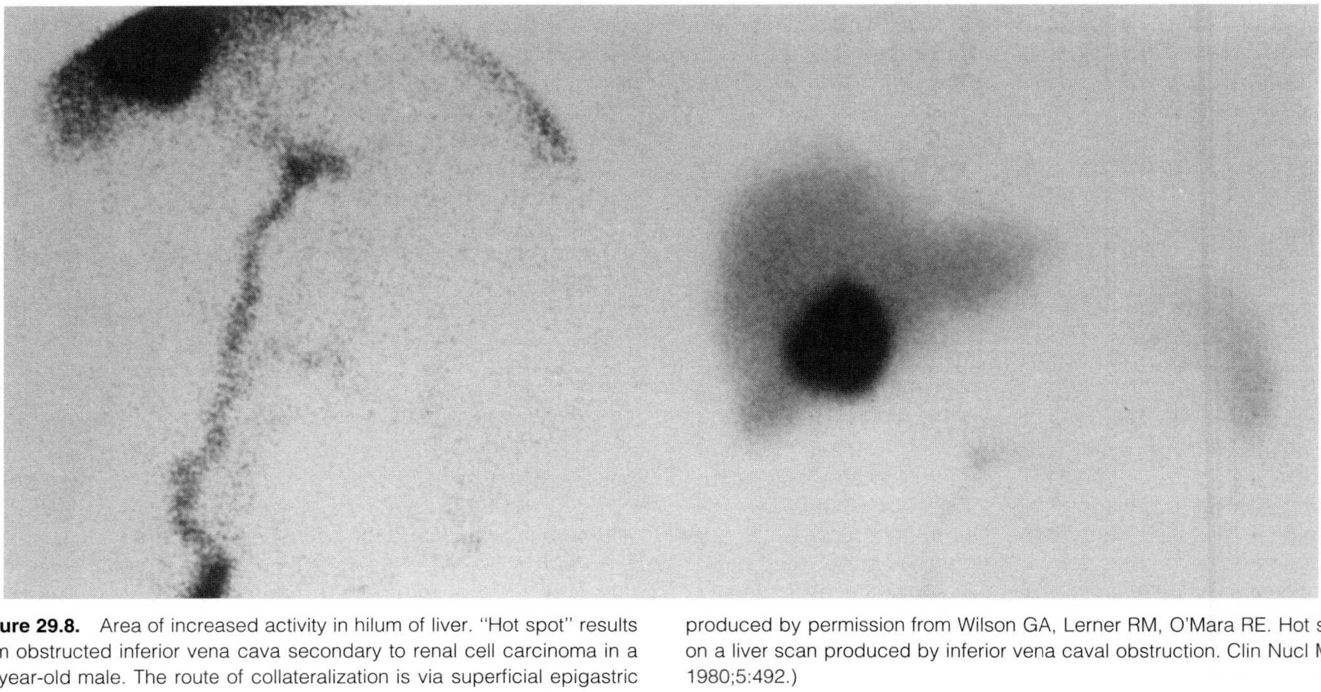

Figure 29.8. Area of increased activity in hilum of liver. "Hot spot" results from obstructed inferior vena cava secondary to renal cell carcinoma in a 52-year-old male. The route of collateralization is via superficial epigastric veins and the paraumbilical veins that accompany the round ligament. (Reproduced by permission from Wilson GA, Lerner RM, O'Mara RE. Hot spot on a liver scan produced by inferior vena caval obstruction. Clin Nucl Med 1980;5:492.)

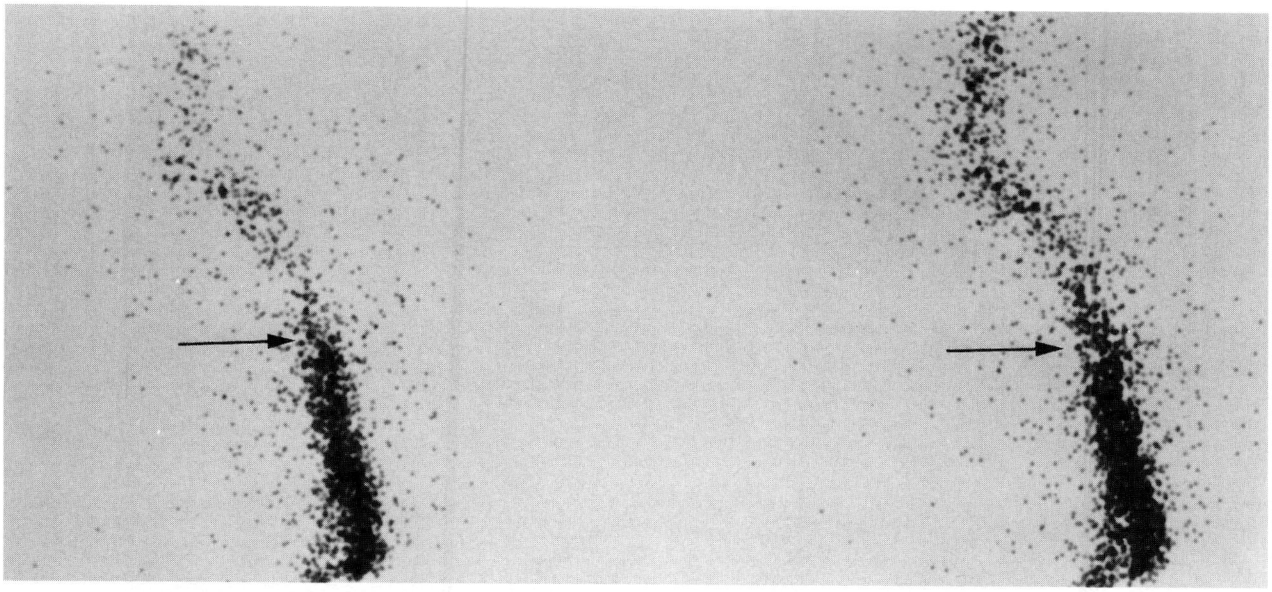

Figure 29.9. Dilution of radioactive bolus in lower venous system study. Pelvic portion of an inferior vena cavagram demonstrating normally decreased activity in the common iliac vein after the junction of internal iliac and external iliac veins *(arrow)*. This results in the reduction of the radioactive column of blood because of the addition of the nonradioactive blood from the internal iliac vein.

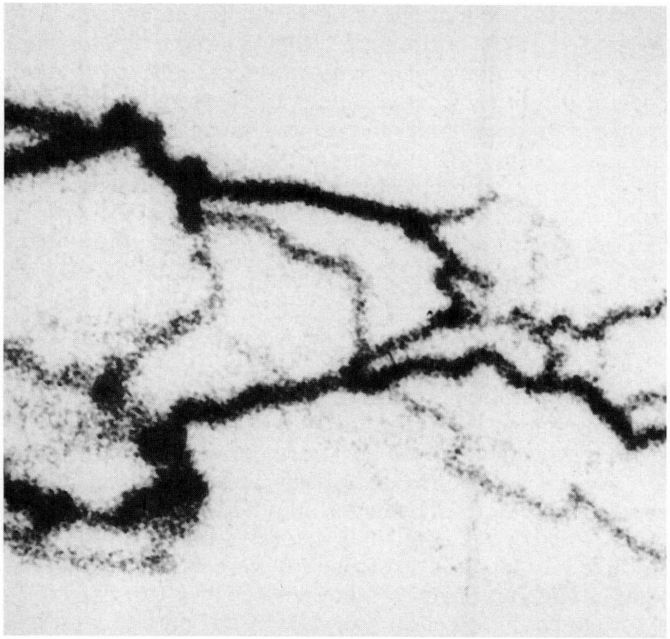

Figure 29.10. Epigastric vein collateralization in inferior vena cava obstruction. Collateral pathways involving deep and superficial epigastric veins in 62-year-old patient 2 years after inferior vena caval ligation for recurrent pulmonary emboli.

of the venous anastomosis of a renal transplant, it is an indication that there is perfusion of the transplant (21).

Obstruction of the inferior vena cava may result in peripheral edema, ascites, and venous distension over the abdomen. Thrombophlebitis is the most common cause of inferior vena caval obstruction. However, tumors, including renal cell carcinoma, carcinoma of the cervix, and plasmacytomas, have been demonstrated to have the ability to compress the inferior vena cava, producing significant obstruction (22, 23). Surgical ligation of the inferior vena cava for the prevention of pulmonary embolus may also produce the syndrome, but in this situation the cause is obvious. Since other conditions besides inferior vena cava obstruction may result in ascites, peripheral edema, and venous distensions, the determination of patency of the inferior vena cava is helpful in establishing a diagnosis. Obstruction of the inferior vena cava will result in collateral circulation via the deep and superficial epigastric veins in the abdominal wall (Fig. 29.10), through the portal circulation, and via the ascending lumbar veins. Any or all of these routes may be visualized depending upon the cause and site of obstruction and the hemodynamics of the various collateral routes. Similar findings of obstruction with or without collateralization may be demonstrated in any portion of the peripheral venous system (24) (Fig. 29.11).

Obstruction of the venous return at the level of the iliac veins may result in collateralization with return via the contralateral iliac or superficial epigastrics (Fig. 29.12). Collateralization may also be via the portal system and, if ^{99m}Tc sulfur colloid is used for imaging, this may result in a persistent "hot spot" in the liver. In addition to being simple, the radioisotope venogram offers an advantage over the conventional radiographic contrast venogram, because the flow pressures with the former are physiologic. Different patterns of collateral flow may be demonstrated by each

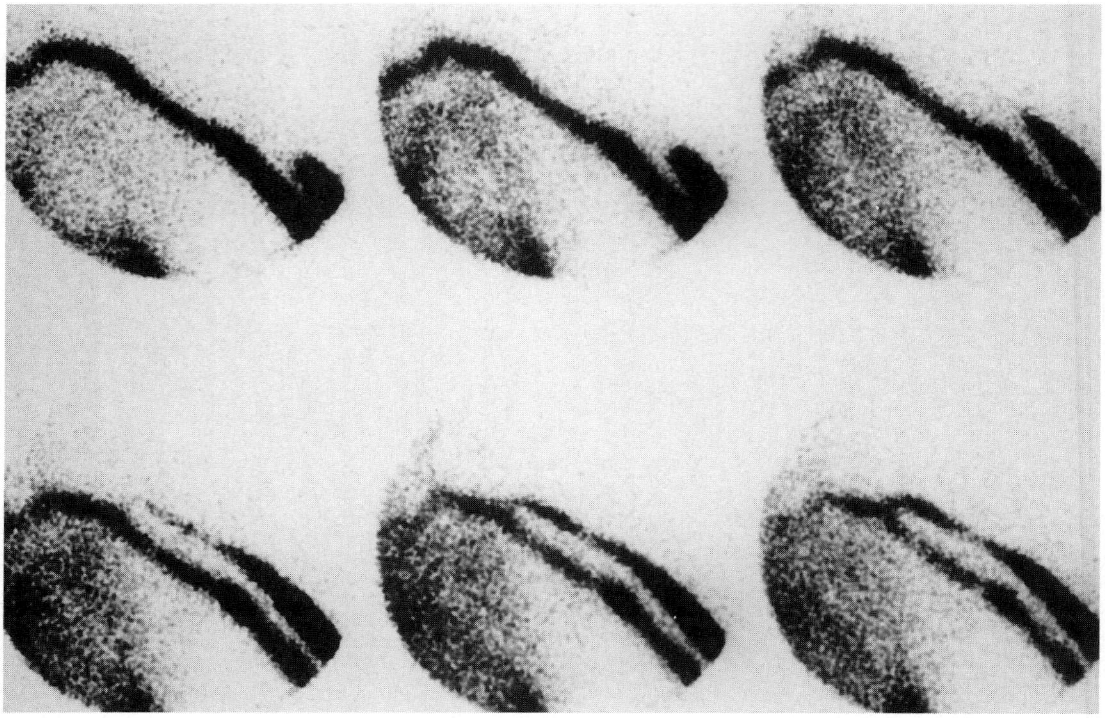

Figure 29.11. Peripheral venous system obstruction. Incomplete obstruction of basilic and cephalic veins in 58-year-old male with extensive cellulitis of the left arm.

technique as a result of the intrinsic difference in the flow pressure (22). Accurate assessment of the patency of the vein grafts performed for obstructive venous disease may easily be obtained with a bolus injection peripheral to the graft (25).

Most venography is performed with a ^{99m}Tc-labeled radiopharmaceutical. However, other short-lived radiopharmaceuticals may be used. High-quality images of the venous system in the extremities have been obtained through the use of infusion of ^{81m}Kr in saline (26). The 15-second half-life of this radioisotope and its short biologic half-life, due to elimination through the lungs, virtually eliminates all radioactivity from the arterial system, providing excellent resolution of the veins. By constant infusion of this short-lived isotope, or other short-lived isotopes such as ^{195m}Au (27), multiple images may be obtained of the entire venous system from the site of injection to the right heart.

PULMONARY PHASE

Careful observation of the bolus as it passes through the pulmonary vasculature may reveal abnormalities of the pulmonary arterial system. Many of these are covered in Chapter 31. When a radiopharmaceutical that is not trapped in the capillary bed is administered, defects in pulmonary perfusion may be observed. These defects may be readily seen in the late phases of the superior or inferior vena caval study. In patients with tumor, perfusion defects may be present as the result of tumor compressing the pulmonary artery (Figs. 29.2 and 29.4). Prolonged progression of the bolus of activity through the pulmonary circulation with dilation of the pulmonary arteries may indicate pulmonary hypertension (28). Aortic aneurysms have been reported to compress the pulmonary vasculature (7), producing a relative perfusion defect. With careful timing of images, pulmonary sequestration may be demonstrated by observing a secondary peak of activity passing through an isolated segment of the lung (29). This second peak coincides with the arrival of activity in the systemic circulation. Careful attention must be paid to the technical performance of this examination, because the bolus must remain compact so that drainage from the lung occurs before a significant amount of activity arrives in the systemic circulation. This examination may be performed with any radiopharmaceutical that is not trapped in the pulmonary bed.

ARTERIAL PHASE

Abnormalities of the arterial system may be detected if multiple images are obtained as a bolus of activity progresses through the system. The major vessels of the head, the neck, the abdomen, and the extremities (Fig. 29.13) may be evaluated with images obtained at the appropriate times. Aneurysms and atherosclerotic manifestations, including stenosis and tuberosity of vessels, as well as fistula, emboli, and arterial patency, are easily defined with a simple bolus injection (30, 31). In the patient who has undergone aortic or arterial reconstruction with the insertion of a graft or some other surgical procedure, the patency of the vessel may be questioned (Figs. 29.14 and

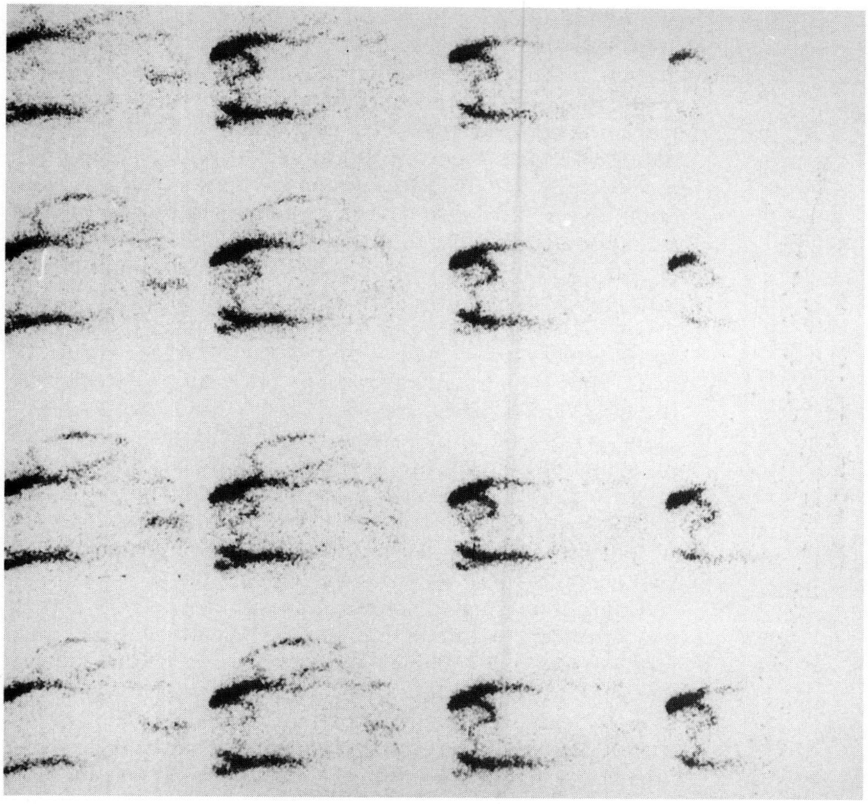

Figure 29.12. Collateralization in obstruction of venous return at level of iliac veins. Collateral pattern in a patient with right common iliac vein thrombosis, demonstrating flow through right and left superior external pudendal veins to left femoral vein, as well as flow via the right superficial epigastric veins.

29.15). The status of the lumen may be ascertained with a radionuclide angiogram (32). This technique offers several advantages: (a) a small amount of material is injected, (b) it is noninvasive, and (c) it does not compromise renal function as may occur after the administration of iodinated contrast material for standard radiographic angiography and digital subtraction angiography, but is adequate for the determination of patency (Fig. 29.16) (33). In the patient with compromised renal function, it may be the only imaging modality that is feasible. Aneurysms of the aorta or major arterial vessels may present on the dynamic flow image as an area of increased activity resulting from increased vessel size (34). The increase in the diameter of the vessel may also be detected by a persistence of activity at the site of the aneurysm as a result of turbulence and slow flow (35, 36). Not all aneurysms are detected, because clot formation within the aneurysmal sac may ablate it, thus producing an apparent normal flow pattern. When active bleeding from an abdominal aneurysm occurs, persistence of activity outside of the vascular channel on the radionuclide angiogram demonstrates and confirms the site of extravasation (37). Abdominal masses may displace or compress the aorta and may be inferred when significant displacement of the aorta is noted. Pseudocysts of the pancreas (38) and periaortic lymph node enlargement have been noted to produce displacement and/or compression of the aorta and the inferior vena cava on radionuclide angiography. Disease of the major abdominal arteries may be detected by carefully observing the progression of the flow throughout the abdomen. In the normal situation, activity is identified almost simultaneously in the spleen and the kidneys. This is followed by a diffuse blush over the general abdomen with a delayed but progressive increase in activity in the liver, the result of the circuitous route through the portal system that most of the hepatic blood supply takes prior to reaching the liver. Mesenteric thrombosis has been correctly diagnosed when the usual abdominal blush is not visualized and there has been premature arrival of activity in the liver as a result of a shift in hepatic perfusion from the portal system to the hepatic artery (39). The hypervascularity of many tumors may result in an abnormal blush in an unusual location during the perfusion imaging sequence (40) (Fig. 29.17). In the abdomen, such blushes have been noted in hypernephromas (41), leiomyosarcomas of the stomach (42), and over tumors and metastases.

In the evaluation of the patient who has sustained injury adjacent to an artery but in whom there is no significant evidence of arterial injury, such as occlusion or excessive ground bleeding, and in whom conservative therapy is considered, the radionuclide angiogram offers a rapid, simple method of ascertaining the integrity of the arterial structures (43, 44). A normal radionuclide study has been demonstrated in several series (45, 46) to virtually eliminate the possibility of significant arterial trauma. Abnormal radionuclide angiograms have demonstrated the presence of pseudoaneurysms, lacerations with hemorrhage, and occlusion of the vessels. The absence of activity in a peripheral vessel may suggest complete occlusion, which can occur from a variety of causes. If the onset of occlusive

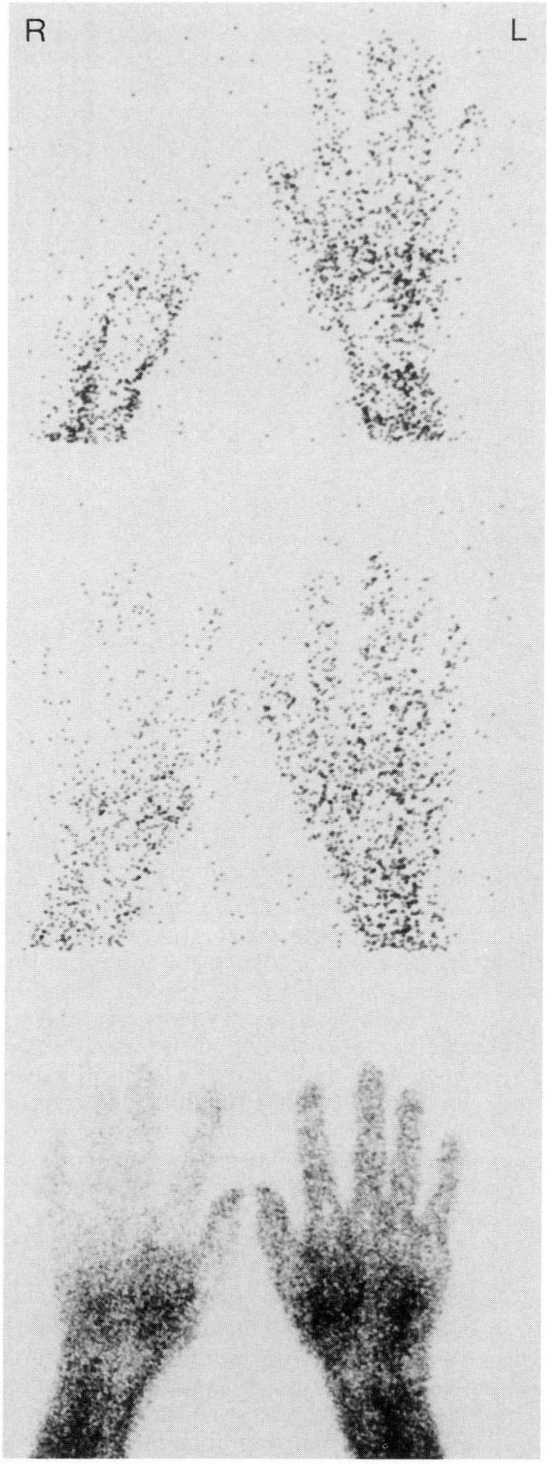

Figure 29.13. Decreased perfusion of right hand after trauma in 50-year-old male with symptoms of vascular insufficiency. Note the excellent delineation of the radial and ulnar arteries and the palmar arcade.

symptomatology is sudden, embolus should be considered. Because the actual site of occlusion may not be known, peripheral radionuclide angiography may be indicated and, although resolution is not as good as with contrast angiography, the level of obstruction may be well enough defined to permit therapy (47, 48). This technique is especially useful in that patient with severe cardiovascular or renal disease who is at increased risk from contrast angiography. When the occlusion is complete, the lesion is usually readily discernible; however, when there is only significant stenosis, this may not be as evident. Small areas of active peripheral bleeding resulting from a ruptured aneurysm or laceration might not be seen with an agent that remains intravascular, but may be detected by the intravenous administration of ^{99m}Tc sulfur colloid. Imaging is delayed until background activity decreases. The presence of peripheral extravascular activity on the delayed images confirms the presence and location of active hemorrhage. Slow arterial or intermittent hemorrhage may be localized with serial images with a radiopharmaceutical that remains intravascular (49) (Fig. 29.18).

Computer-assisted construction of time-activity curves over the involved site, compared to the contralateral area, may demonstrate delayed arrival of the activity or a total decrease in the amount of activity present, suggesting a stenotic lesion. Detection of premature arrival of activity in the venous system suggests some type of shunt is present. Aortocaval fistulas have been demonstrated by the premature arrival of activity in the venous phase. Hemangiomas located in the skin, subcutaneous tissues, joints, or other locations, may present with a variety of symptoms depending upon their location. On the flow images there may be a premature blush that subsequently fades. When imaged with an intravascular agent, such as technetium-labeled red blood cells, there is a persistence of activity at the site of the hemangioma, confirming the higher vascular component of this pathologic condition (51–53). This technique may also be used to image the major vessels when they are separated anatomically from other major vessels (Fig. 29.19).

MICROCIRCULATION PHASE

Many disease processes have little effect on the major vessels but do involve the smaller vessels affecting the microcirculation, resulting in decreased perfusion to an organ. Image resolution is not sufficient for visualization of the microcirculation using a bolus technique. However, various alternate techniques have been developed to evaluate organ perfusion. In 1949, Kety (54) described a method of isotope clearance from a peripheral organ utilizing radioactive sodium. Subsequent investigators used many different diffusible isotopes, including ^{24}Na, ^{131}I (55, 56), ^{85}Kr, ^{133}Xe (57, 58), and ^{99m}Tc (59). To determine perfusion rate using the isotope clearance method, the tracer must be concentrated in the organ to be studied. Usually this is by direct injection into the organ or its blood supply. In determining the organ perfusion by the isotope clearance method, the assumption is made that the isotope leaves only via the venous blood, making the rate at which the isotope is removed a function for the rate of organ perfu-

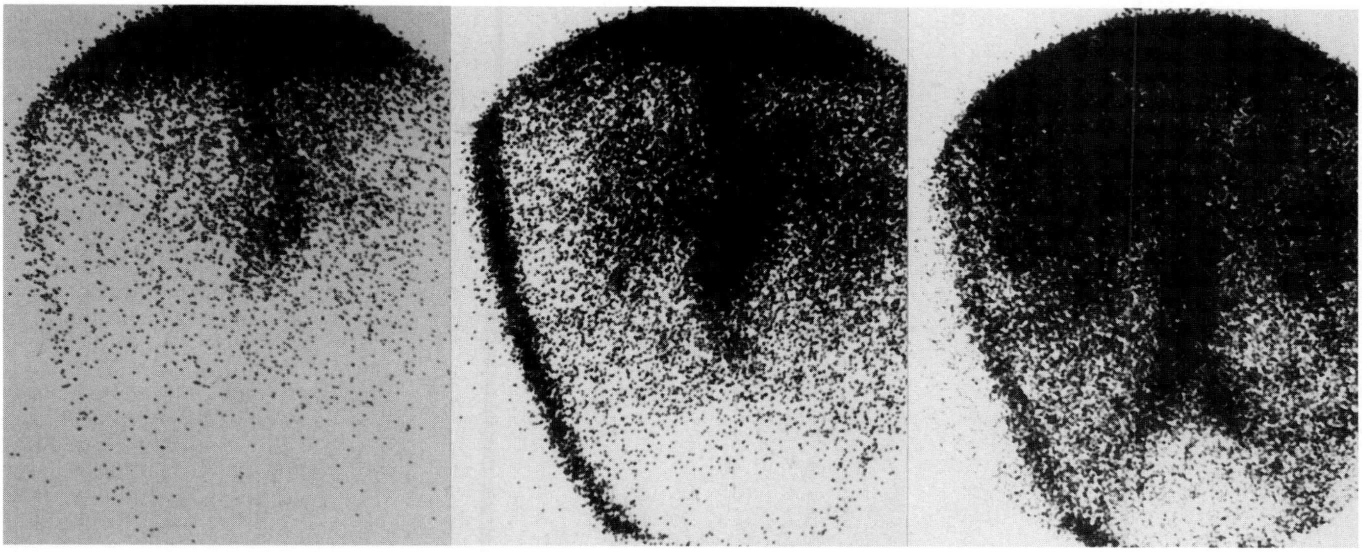

Figure 29.14. Patency of brachiofemoral arterial bypass graft. Graft patency is demonstrated in 79-year-old male following ligation of abdominal aorta for unresectable aneurysm.

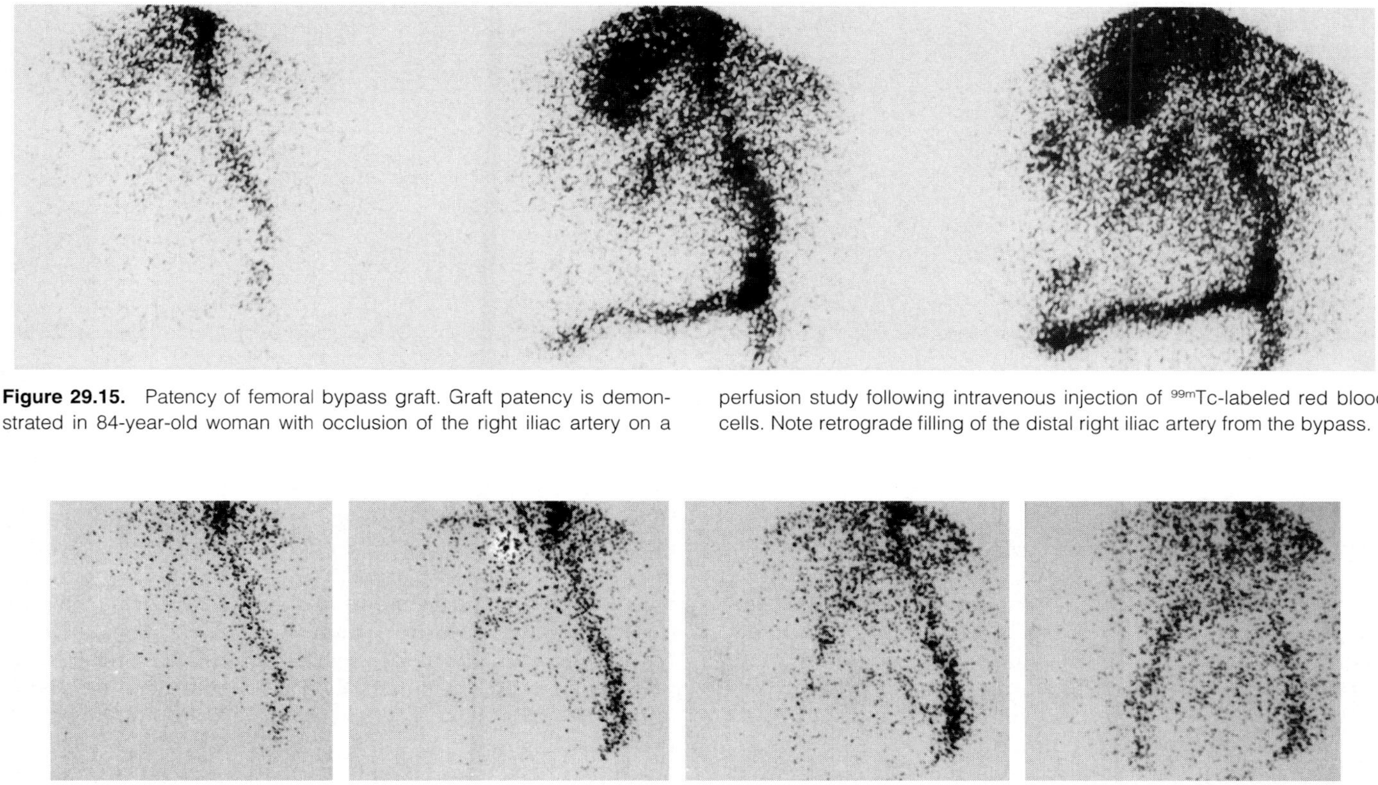

Figure 29.15. Patency of femoral bypass graft. Graft patency is demonstrated in 84-year-old woman with occlusion of the right iliac artery on a perfusion study following intravenous injection of ^{99m}Tc-labeled red blood cells. Note retrograde filling of the distal right iliac artery from the bypass.

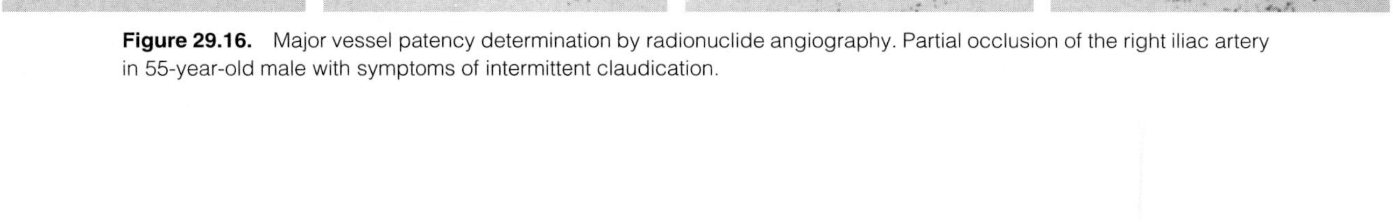

Figure 29.16. Major vessel patency determination by radionuclide angiography. Partial occlusion of the right iliac artery in 55-year-old male with symptoms of intermittent claudication.

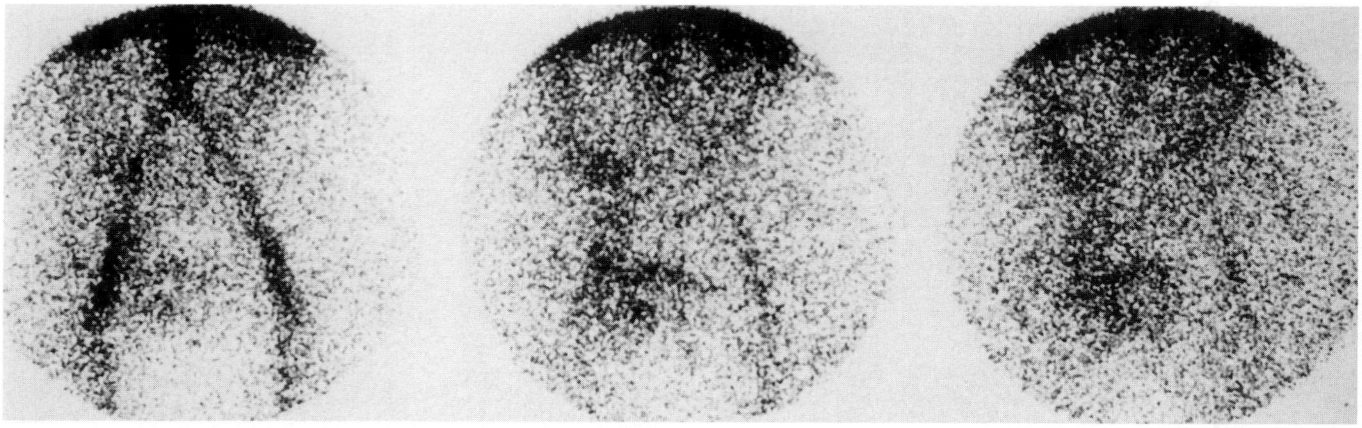

Figure 29.17. Radioactivity blush due to hypervascularity of tumor. Vascular undifferentiated sarcoma demonstrated during the vascular phase of a "three-phase" bone scan in a 59-year-old woman with right leg pain.

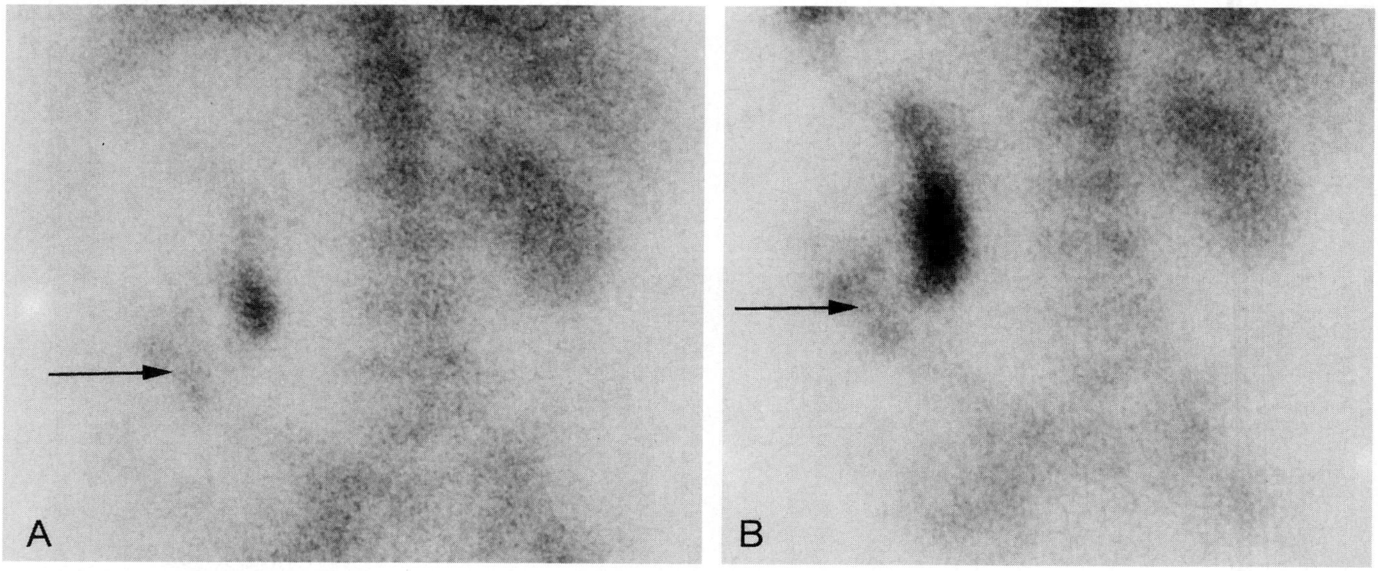

Figure 29.18. Localization of hemorrhage by serial imaging. A 68-year-old male with history of renal trauma. **A**. Image 15-minutes after labeling of red blood cells with ^{99m}Tc demonstrates bleeding site (*arrow*). **B**. A 45-minute image demonstrates increase in amount of extravasation (*arrow*).

sion. Organ flow may be calculated from the Schmidt-Kety equation:

$$F = \frac{\lambda \times K \times 100}{p}$$

where F equals the perfusion in milliliters of blood per minute per 100 g of tissue; λ is the blood-organ partition coefficient of the tracer; K is the slope constant of the tracer washout, which is calculated from 0.693 divided by the t1/2 of the washout curve; and p equals the specific gravity of the organ. When this equation is used, the following assumptions are made: (a) the tracer leaves the organ by venous flow only, (b) the tissue is homogeneously perfused, (c) the tracer reaches a rapid diffusion equilibrium between blood and the organ tissue, and (d) arterial concentration of the tracer is negligible. The fourth assumption implies there will be no recirculation of the tracer. Of the various tracers that have been used for this technique, the noble gases appear most attractive because of their lack of significant recirculation. With gases currently used (Krypton and Xenon), the majority of activity is eliminated with the first pass through the lungs. A small residual remains in solution within the bloodstream, usually less than 5% of the initial concentration, which for most clinical procedures can be considered negligible. Xenon has become the preferred isotope because of its high solubility in blood, and is the most widely used isotope for this technique at the present time.

The pain of intermittent claudication results from ischemic changes that are a consequence of inadequate blood flow to muscle during exercise. Pain frequently occurs in the calf on walking but subsides with rest. In these patients, perfusion rates at rest are essentially the same as in normal controls. However, when these patients are

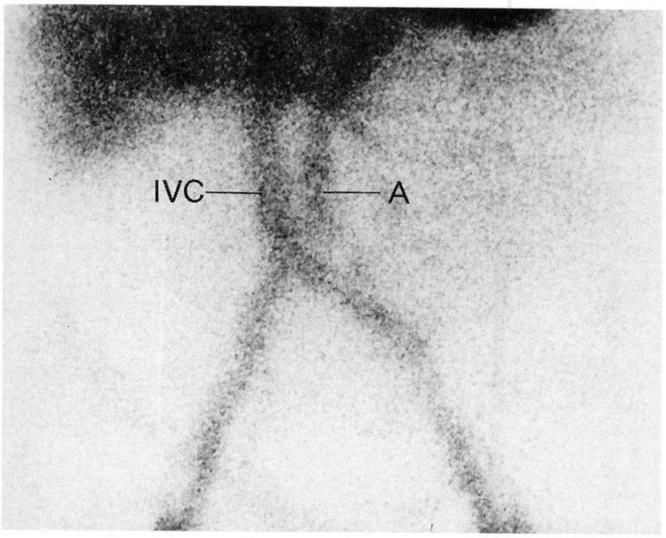

Figure 29.19. Imaging with labeled red blood cells. Aorta *(A)* and inferior vena cava (*IVC*) demonstrated with ^{99m}Tc-labeled red blood cells. Insufficient anatomic separation prevents individual evaluation of the iliac vessels.

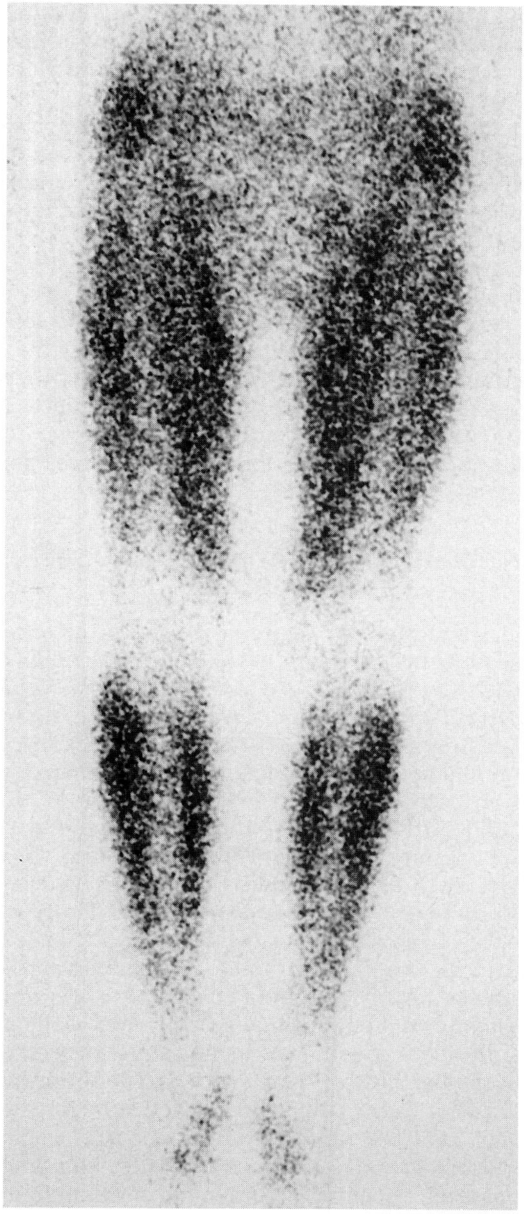

Figure 29.20. Radionuclide determination of peripheral distribution of cardiac output. Normal distribution of ^{201}Tl in the lower extremities of a 48-year-old male following exercise.

exercised, a marked decrease in perfusion to the involved muscle is noted when compared with controls. Many different exercise protocols (60, 61) have been devised to evaluate muscle perfusion under stress. When such protocols are used and strictly adhered to, serial determinations may be obtained that are of value in determining response to therapeutic procedures such as sympathectomy, vasodilator drug therapy, or reconstructive arterial surgery. Standardization of the protocol for the individual laboratory is essential, because perfusion not only depends on the amount of exercise but may vary with the position of the patient and extremity, because of the effects of gravity on circulation (60). Impediments to the circulation, whether arterial or venous, may result in a prolonged washout and reflect decreased perfusion. To overcome some of the difficulties in exercising elderly, debilitated, or uncooperative patients, the phenomenon of reactive hyperemia may be used. To produce vasodilatation, a tourniquet is applied to the extremity and the extremity is exercised under ischemic conditions. The tracer is injected into the organ of interest, and the tourniquet is then released, producing reactive hyperemia in the extremity. Using this technique, reproducible results may be obtained for the evaluation of occlusive vascular disease. The method of administration of the tracer may be by intraarterial injection, inhalation, or direct injection into the organ to be studied. A modification of this technique, using ^{131}I-labeled serum albumin or ^{99m}Tc-labeled red blood cells injected systemically during tourniquet occlusion (62), measures the rate of increase in activity in the organ under study after release of the tourniquet. In this modification, the rate at which the nonradioactive blood is washed out is actually determined. This method offers an advantage over techniques involving Xenon in that there is no significant tailing off of the curve generated as a result of the greater solubility of xenon in fat compartment. Such muscle perfusion rates have been found useful in determining the viability of muscle following flame or electrical energy burns (63) and in planning reconstructive surgery.

Perfusion to the skin is of critical importance to wound healing. Once the decision to perform an amputation as a result of vascular disease is made, the surgeon is faced with the problem as to the level of amputation. Roon, et al. (64), have reported, and other authors (65) confirmed, that amputation stump healing will occur when skin blood flow is equal to or greater than 2.4 ml/min/100 g. Accurate assessment of skin blood flow may be made by an intradermal injection of Xenon in saline (66). Multiple sites at different levels may be injected and the washout curve for each site determined to permit selection of the level with adequate flow. This technique not only is useful in selecting the level for successful amputation, but is helpful in determining the prognosis of ischemic leg ulcers and the perfusion to pedicular skin grafts.

The relative perfusion of peripheral organs such as muscle may be determined by observing the localization of a freely diffusible indicator. Utilizing the principles described by Sapirstein (67), ^{201}Tl may be injected intravenously and the initial localization will reflect the relative distribution of the cardiac output at the time of injection (Fig. 29.20) (68). Areas with relative decreased perfusion are seen to have a lesser amount of activity. This method offers the advantage of being simple and usable under a wide variety of conditions, including stress or following drug therapy. It also offers several advantages over previous methods that utilize the intra-arterial injection of particular matter, because it is noninvasive and redistribution images may be obtained (43, 69–71).

INTRA-ARTERIAL CATHETER PLACEMENT DISTRIBUTION

Regional chemotherapy administered intra-arterially has been used for the treatment of localized neoplasms for two decades (72). In theory, this technique delivers higher concentrations of chemotherapeutic agents to the tumor without increasing systemic toxicity. The greatest use of this approach has been in the treatment of neoplasm localized in the liver, with significant improvement in survival reported (73). Other tumors, including head and neck, breast, pelvic, neoplasms, and those localized to one extremity, have also responded to intra-arterial therapy. Proper catheter placement is critical for the adequate delivery of the chemotherapeutic agent. Variations in the arterial patterns, partial or complete obstruction of the blood flow by the catheter, streaming effects, or inadequate mixing may result in a suboptimal distribution of the chemotherapeutic agent. Contrast angiography has been used to ascertain proper catheter placement and determine the relative perfusion to the tumor. The amount of contrast material used, and the rapid rate at which it is injected for adequate radiographic visualization, alter the flow characteristics from those present during normal chemotherapeutic administration, and may result in an incorrect assessment of the actual tumor perfusion. With the use of a radiotracer, flow rates that approximate those of the therapeutic agent may be achieved and reflect the true distribution of the chemotherapeutic agent. This is essential when one deals with low flow rates such as those produced by subcutaneously implanted pump reservoir systems. ^{99m}Tc sulfur colloid has been utilized for imaging liver perfusion. However, not all of the colloid is removed on the first passage through the abnormal liver, and delayed images are not a true reflection of the distribution of this agent following administration into the hepatic artery. Macroaggregated albumin labeled with ^{99m}Tc or ^{113m}In, administered through the intra-arterial catheter, is trapped in the sinusoids of the liver and capillaries of the tumor, and more accurately reflects the distribution of the administered chemotherapeutic agent (Fig. 29.21) (74–77). Inappropriate catheter placement or occlusion of the catheter is detectable and permits correction prior to commencement of chemotherapy (Fig. 29.22). In many neoplastic conditions, significant arteriovenous shunting may be present within the tumor, and the appearance of microaggregated albumin particles within the lung indicates that such shunting occurred. Estimations of the degree of shunting may be

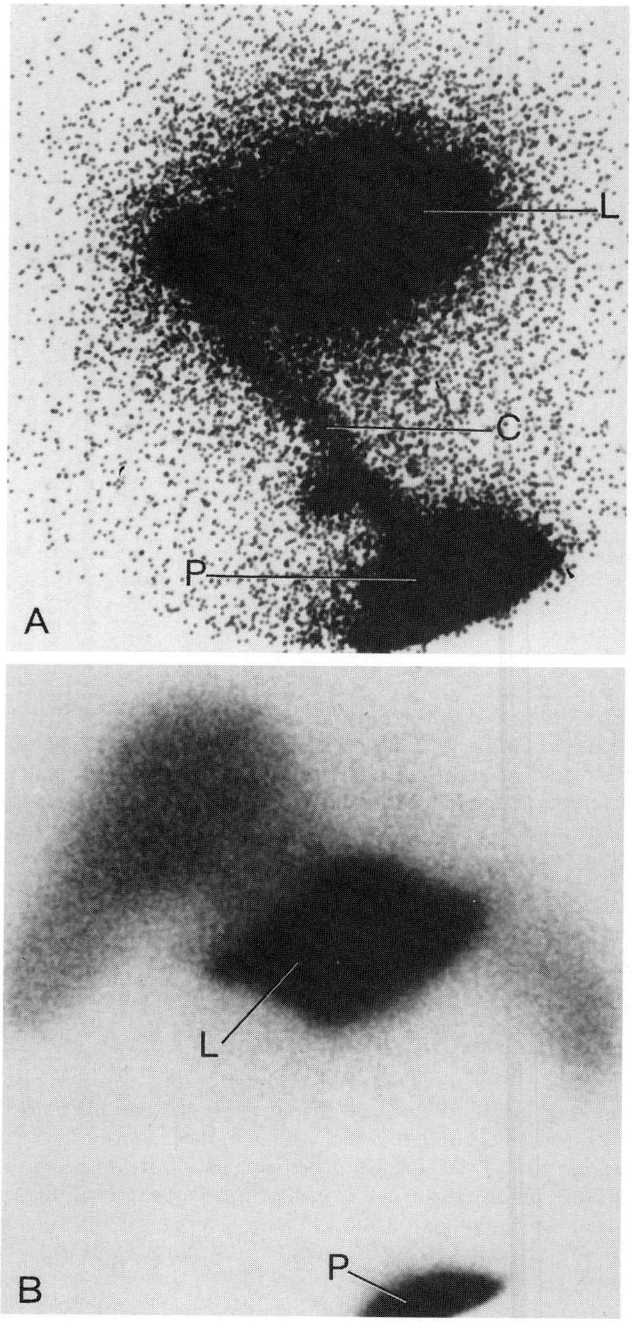

Figure 29.21. Radionuclide determination of distribution of chemotherapeutic agent. **A**. ^{99m}Tc-labeled macroaggregated albumin has been injected into a subcutaneously implanted liver perfusion pump (*P*), demonstrating catheter (*C*) and portion of the liver (*L*) perfused. **B**. Following intravenous injection of ^{99m}Tc sulfur colloid, the liver image demonstrates that only the left lobe of the liver (*L*) is being perfused by the chemotherapy pump system (*P*).

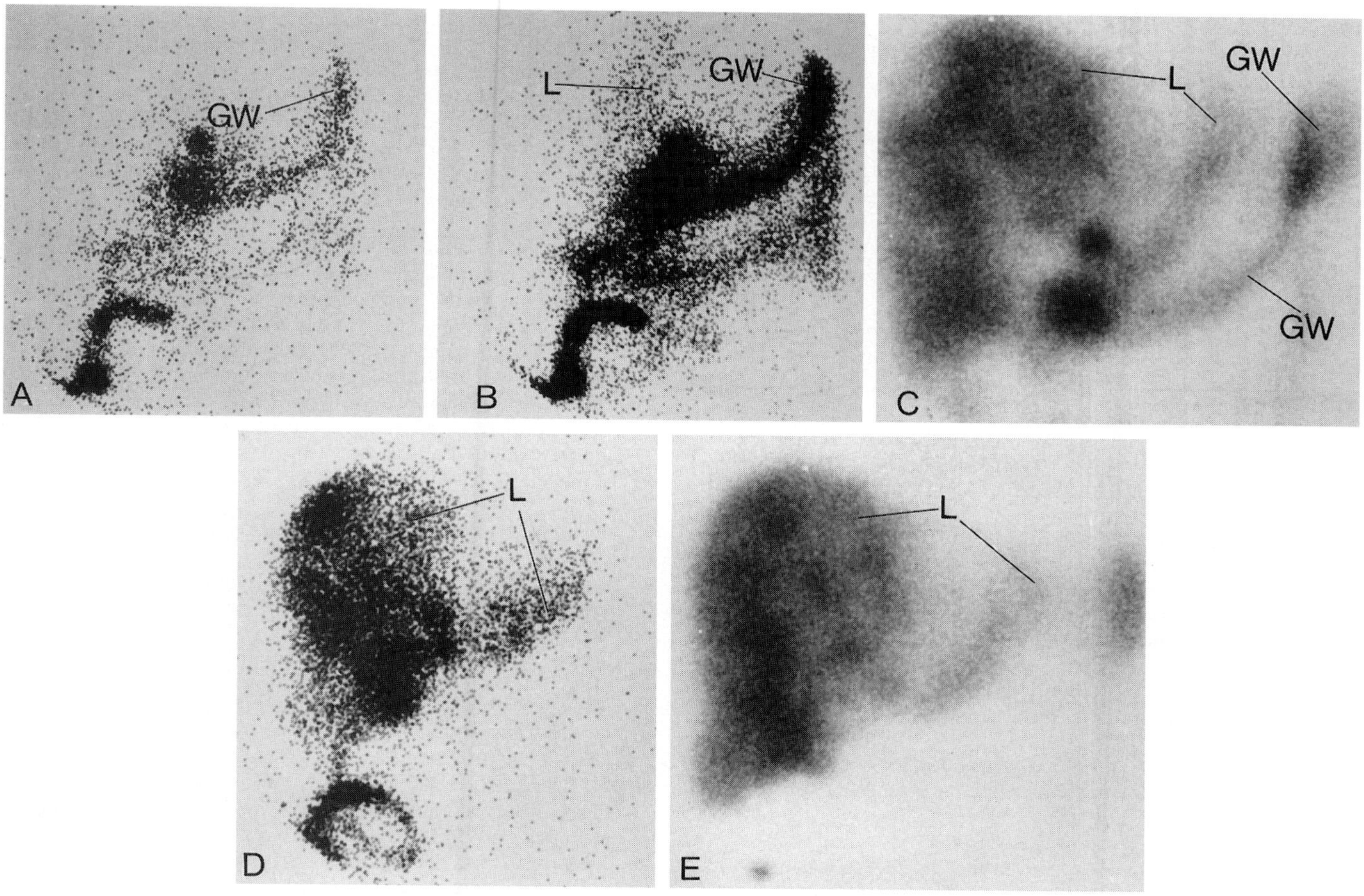

Figure 29.22. Radionuclide determination of intra-arterial catheter placement. **A**, **B**. Perfusion pump study with ^{99m}Tc-labeled macroaggregated albumin demonstrates perfusion of the gastric wall (*GW*). **C**. ^{99m}Tc sulfur colloid image demonstrates that very little of the liver (*L*) is perfused by pump system. **D**. Pump study with ^{99m}Tc-labeled macroaggregated albumin demonstrating improved perfusion to the liver (*L*) after repositioning of the catheter. **E**. Sulfur colloid study confirming appropriate placement of chemotherapy perfusion pump catheter.

made and, if shunting is great, may warrant reducing the amount of chemotherapeutic agent being administered, because an increase in systemic toxic symptoms can be anticipated with increased shunting.

In patients in whom the malignancy is confined to an extremity, an isolated perfusion of the chemotherapeutic agent to the extremity may be performed. The inclusion of a radiopharmaceutical that remains within the intravascular compartment may be added to the isolated circulation setup. The detection of radioactivity within systemic circulation indicates escape of the chemotherapeutic agent from the isolated circulation. The amount detected may be used as an indicator of the degree of cross-circulation, permitting calculation of the maximal amount of chemotherapy that may be administered to the extremity before toxic levels appear in the systemic circulation.

SUMMARY

Radionuclide vascular studies will not provide the resolution of vessel anatomy that can be obtained with standard radiographic contrast angiography or digital subtraction angiography, but do provide an alternate method for answering the clinical question of vessel patency, vascular integrity, perfusion rates, and the effects on intervention. These methods are noninvasive, relatively simple, and rapid to perform. They are safe and, at times, may be the only feasible method for evaluating the seriously ill patient with a compromised renal or cardiovascular system.

However, these studies have fallen into the status of valuable but infrequently performed radionuclide procedures. The development of vascular imaging techniques such as color flow, Doppler, either by itself or as part of a duplex ultrasound study, and magnetic resonance angiography and venography (MRA/MRV), however, have caused a reduction in the utilization of radionuclide techniques. Although more costly, both color Doppler and MRA/MRV offer anatomic information and functional information about the state of the arteries and veins. Additionally, these procedures do not involve the use of contrast or radiation. They offer the great advantage of being able to image the tissues surrounding the vessels in question, thereby giving information about the anatomic cause of flow change as well as the pathophysiology resulting from alterations in the blood flow dynamics. Finally, they can rapidly produce images in multiple projections, including three-dimension. As a result, these modalities have become the procedures of choice in the evaluation of peripheral vascular problems.

ACKNOWLEDGMENTS

This chapter is dedicated to the memory of George A. Wilson, M.D. I would like to thank Johanna Uncur for her patience and assistance.

REFERENCES

1. Blumert HL, Yens OC. Studies on the velocity of blood flow. I. The method utilized. J Clin Invest 1927;4:1.
2. Prinzmetal M, Corday E, Bergman HC, Schwartz L, Spritzler RJ. Radiocardiography: a new method for studying the blood flow through the chambers of the heart in human beings. Science 1948;108:340.
3. Oldendorf, WH, Kitano M, Shimizu S. Evaluation of a simple technique for abrupt intravenous injection of radioisotope. J Nucl Med 1965;6:205.
4. Gollub S, Hirose T, Klauber J. Scintigraphic sequelae of superior vena caval obstruction. Clin Nucl Med 1980;5:89.
5. Sy WM, Lao RS. Collateral pathways in superior vena caval obstruction as seen on gamma images. Br J Radiol 1982;55:294.
6. Harris ME. Superior vena caval obstruction demonstrated on the dynamic perfusion study of the liver in a patient with carcinoma of the lung. Clin Nucl Med 1977;2:431.
7. Farrer PA, Kloiber R. Combined superior vena cava and pulmonary artery obstruction by an ascending aortic aneurysm. Clin Nucl Med 1979;4:495.
8. Sy WM, Lao RS, Seo IS. Scintigraphic features of superior vena caval obstruction due to substernal non-toxic goitre. Br J Radiol 1982;55:301.
9. Puri S, Spencer RP, Moskowitz H, Kendall EM. Partial obstruction of left brachiocephalic vein by a goiter. Clin Nucl Med 1976;1:246.
10. DeLong JF, Davis HG Jr. Bone scan findings in a patient with hyper-parathyroidism and a large cystic parathyroid adenoma in the mediastinum. Clin Nucl Med 1977;2:114.
11. Fritz T, Richeson JF, Fitzpatrick P, Wilson GA. Venous obstruction. A potential complication of transvenous pacemaker electrodes. Chest 1983;83:534.
12. Baiocchi L, Cohen A. Superior vena cava thrombosis following subclavian vein catheterization. J Cardiovasc Surg 1981;22:190.
13. Scrantino C. Salazar OM, Rubin P, Wilson GA, MacIntosh P. The optimum radiation schedule in treatment of superior vena caval obstruction: importance of ^{99m}Tc scintiangiograms. Int J Radiat Oncol Biol Phys 1979;5:1987.
14. Van Houtte P, Fruhling J. Radionuclide venography in the evaluation of superior vena cava syndrome. Clin Nucl Med 1981; 6:177.
15. Struse TB. Demonstration of a progressive superior vena caval obstruction reversed following radiation therapy. Clin Nucl Med 1976;1:247.
16. Sheikh Al, Pavel DG, Rosen KM. Demonstration of persistant left superior vena cava by radionuclide angiography. Cardiovasc Rev Rep 1982;3:1637.
17. Rivera JV, Ficek MA. Double inferior vena cava and anomalous venous drainage from the left arm demonstration by radionuclide angiogram. Clin Nucl Med 1983;8:306.
18. Modry DL, Hidvegi RS, LaFleche LR. Congenital saccular aneurysm of the superior vena cava. Ann Thorac Surg 1980;29:258.
19. Vincken W, Roels P, Sonstabo R, DeGreve J, Bossuyt A, Jonckheer M. Effect of neck position during radionuclide superior cavography. Clin Nucl Med 1983;8:424.
20. Hayt DB, Reedy K, Patel H, Freeman LM. Radionuclide venography of the lower extremities and inferior vena cava by continuous injection and moving bed gamma-camera technique. Radiology 1976;121:748.
21. Barnes RW, McDonald GB, Hamilton GW, Rudd TG, Nelp WB, Strandness DE Jr. Radionuclide venography for rapid dynamic evaluation of venous disease. Surgery 1973;73:706.
22. Dhekne RD, Moore WH, Long SE. Radionuclide venography in iliac and inferior vena caval obstruction. Radiology 1982;144:597.
23. McDaniel MM, Coleman JM, Morton ME: Inferior vena cava obstruction due to plasmacytoma demonstrated on phlebography using ^{99m}Tc macroaggregated albumin. Clin Nucl Med 1977; 2:135.
24. Greenwald LV, Rodrigo R. Radionuclide venographic demonstration of portal and systemic collaterals in a case of complete IVC obstruction. Clin Nucl Med 1984;9:156.
25. Volarich DT, Duong RB, Fernandez-Ulloa M. Demonstration of saphenous vein bypass graft patency on radionuclide venogram. Clin Nucl Med 1983;8:223.
26. Ham HR, Van Devivere J, Guillaume M, Niethammer R, Sergeysels R. Radionuclide venography using continuous ^{81m}Kr infusion: preliminary note. Clin Nucl Med 1981;6:461.
27. Brihaye C, Guillaume M, Lavi N, Cogneau M. Development of a reliable ^{195m}Hg-^{195m}Au generator for the production of ^{195m}Au, a short-lived nuclide for vascular imaging. J Nucl Med 1982; 23:1114.
28. Baum S, d'Avignon MB, Latshaw RF. Radionuclide pulmonary arteriography. Clin Nucl Med 1979;4:461.
29. Gooneratne N, Conway JJ. Radionuclide angiographic diagnosis of bronchopulmonary sequestration. J Nucl Med 1976;17:1035.
30. Moss CM, Rudavsky AZ, Veith FJ. The value of scintiangiography in arterial disease. Arch Surg 1976;111:1235.
31. Matin P, Glass EC, Villarica J. Peripheral radionuclide angiography. JAMA 1979;242:1781.
32. Moss CM, Rudavsky AZ, Veith FJ. Isotope angiography: technique, validation and value in the assessment of arterial reconstruction. Ann Surg 1976;184:116.
33. Shelley BE Jr, Vujic I, Schabel SI, Gordon L. Supraceliac aortic occlusion demonstrated by radionuclide aortography. Clin Nucl Med 1981;6:581.
34. Bergan JJ, Yao JST, Henkin RE, Quinn JL III. Radionuclide aortography in detection of arterial aneurysms. Arch Surg 1974; 109:80.
35. Powers TA, Harolds JA, Kadir S, Grove RB. Pseudoaneurysm of the profunda femoris artery diagnosed on angiographic phase of bone scan. Clin Nucl Med 1979;4:422.
36. Baron RL, Bannmer MP, Pollack HM. Isolated internal iliac artery aneurysms presenting as giant pelvic masses. AJR 1983;140:784.
37. Bunko H, Seto H, Tonami N, Hisada K. Detection of active bleeding from ruptured aortic aneurysm by emergency radionuclide angiography. Clin Nucl Med 1978;3:276.
38. Makhija MC, Schultz S. Displacement of the abdominal aorta by a pseudocyst of the pancreas. Clin Nucl Med 1979;4:476.
39. Sty JR, Asimacopoulos PJ. Scintiangiographic diagnosis of acute mesenteric vascular occlusion. Clin Nucl Med 1980;5:170.
40. Pearlman AW. Preoperative evaluation of liposarcoma by nuclear imaging. Clin Nucl Med 1977;2:47.
41. Simon H. Metastatic and recurrent hypernephroma demonstrated by isotope angiography. Clin Nucl Med 1977;2:214.
42. Oliver TW, Fajman WA. Leiomyosarcoma of the stomach demonstrated on radionuclide angiogram. Clin Nucl Med 1982;7:227.
43. Diamond AB, Meg C-H, Wolsanske AC, Freeman LM. Radionuclide demonstration of traumatic arterial injury. Radiology 1973; 109:623.
44. A simple test for arterial trauma [Editorial]. Emerg Med 1980; 12:83.
45. Suarez CA, Bernstein DM, Goldberger JH, Hourani MH, Rodman GH Jr, Colletta J. The role of nuclear scanning in the evaluation of arterial injuries. Am Surg 1983;49:209.
46. Moss CM, Veith FJ, Jason R, Rudavsky A. Screening isotope angiography in arterial trauma. Surgery 1979;86:881.

47. Moss CM, Delany HM, Rudavsky AZ. Isotope angiography for detection of embolic arterial occlusion. Surg Gynecol Obstet 1976; 142:57.
48. Salimi Z, Vas W, Tang-Barton P, Eachempati RG, Morris L, Carron M. Assessment of tissue viability in frostbite by ^{99m}Tc pertechnetate scintigraphy. AJR 1984;142:415.
49. Rosenbaum RC, Johnston GS, Whitley NO. Scintigraphic detection of occult hemorrhage in a patient receiving anticoagulants. J Nucl Med 1986;27:223.
50. Birnholz JC. Radionuclide angiography in the diagnosis of aortacaval fistula. J Thorac Cardiovasc Surg 1973;65:292.
51. Sty J, Simons G, Becker D. Radionuclide angiography and blood pool imaging: synovial hemangioma. Clin Nucl Med 1980; 5:517.
52. Front D, Isreal O, Kleinhaus U, Gdal-On M. ^{99m}Tc-labeled red blood cells in the evaluation of hemangiomas of the skull and orbit [Concise communication]. J Nucl Med 1982;23:1080.
53. Gordon L, Vujic I, Spicer KM. Visualization of cutaneous hemangioma with ^{99m}Tc tagged red blood cells. Clin Nucl Med 1981; 6:468.
54. Kety SS. Measurement of regional circulation by the local clearance of radioactive sodium. Am Heart J 1949;38:321.
55. Coffman JD, Mannick JA. A simple, objective test for arteriosclerosis obliterans. N Engl J Med 1965;273:1297.
56. Cuypers Y, Steels P. Clinical significance of the radioisotope test using ^{131}I-labeled serum albumin for evaluating the peripheral circulation in the foot during a period of reactive hyperemia. Angiology 1983;34:91.
57. Lassen NA. Muscle blood flow in normal man and in patients with intermittent claudication evaluated by simultaneous ^{133}Xe and ^{24}Na clearances. J Clin Invest 1964;43:1805.
58. Marcus ML, Bischof CJ, Heistad DD. Comparison of microsphere and xenon-133 clearance method in measuring skeletal muscle and cerebral blood flow. Circ Res 1981;48:748.
59. Angelides NS, Nicolaides AN. Simultaneous isotope clearance from the muscles of the calf and thigh. Br J Surg 1980;67:220.
60. Hinsenkamp M, d'Hollander A, Coussaert E, Rasquin C, Schoutens A. Measurement of blood flow in peripheral muscles using ^{133}Xe. Angiology 1980;31:58.
61. Davies WT. Blood flow measurement in patients with intermittent claudication. Angiology 1980;31:164.
62. Parkin A, Robinson PJ, Wiggins PA, et al. The measurement of limb blood flow using technetium-labelled red blood cells. Br J Radiol 1986;59:493.
63. Clayton JM, Hayes AC, Hammel J, Boyd WC, Hartford CE, Barnes RW. Xenon-133 determination of muscle blood flow in electrical injury. J Trauma 1977;17:293.
64. Roon AJ, Moore WS, Goldstone H. Below-knee amputation: a modern approach. Am J Surg 1977;134:153.
65. Silberstein EB, Thomas S, Cline J, Kempczinski R, Gottesman L. Predictive value of intracutaneous xenon clearance for healing of amputation and cutaneous ulcer sites. Radiology 1983;147:227.
66. Moore WS, Henry RE, Malone JM, Daly MJ, Patton D, Childers SJ. Prospective use of xenon-133 clearance for amputation level selection. Arch Surg 1991;116:86.
67. Sapirstein LA. Fractionation of the cardiac output of rats with isotopic potassium. Circ Res 1956;4:689.
68. Siegel ME, Stewart CA. Thallium-201 peripheral perfusion scans: feasibility of single-dose, single-day, rest and stress study. AJR 1981;136:1179.
69. Siegel ME, Giargiana FA Jr, Rhodes BA, Williams GM, Wagner HN Jr. Perfusion of ischemic ulcers of the extremity. Arch Surg 1975; 110:265.
70. Seder JS, Botvinick EH, Rahimtoola SH, Goldstone J, Price DC. Detecting and localizing peripheral arterial disease: assessment of ^{201}Tl scintigraphy. AJR 1981;137:373.
71. Burt RW, Mullinix FM, Schauwecker DS, Richmond BD. Leg perfusion evaluated by delayed administration of thallium-201. Radiology 1984;151:219.
72. Freckman HA. Chemotherapy for metastatic colorectal liver carcinoma by intraaortic infusion. Cancer 1971;28:1152.
73. Petrek JA, Minton JP. Treatment of hepatic metastases by percutaneous hepatic arterial infusion. Cancer 1979;43:2182.
74. Kim EE, Bledin AG, Kavanagh J, Haynie TP, Chuang VP. Chemotherapy of cervical carcinoma: use of ^{99m}Tc-MAA infusion to predict drug distribution. Radiology 1984;150:677.
75. Ensminger W, Niederhuber J, Dakhll S, Thrall J, Wheeler R. Totally implanted drug delivery system for hepatic arterial chemotherapy. Cancer Treat Rep 1981;65:393.
76. Kantarjian HM, Bledin AG, Kim EE, Cogan BM, Chuang VP, Wallace S, Haynie TP. Arterial perfusion with ^{99m}Tc-macroaggregated albumin (MAAAP) in monitoring intra-arterial chemotherapy of sarcomas. J Nucl Med 1983;24:297.
77. Ziessman HA, Thrall JH, Yang PJ, et al. Hepatic arterial perfusion scintigraphy with ^{99m}Tc-MAA. Radiology 1984;152:167.

30 Evaluation of Patients with Suspected Venous Thromboembolism

H. DIRK SOSTMAN, RONALD D. NEUMANN, and ALEXANDER GOTTSCHALK

Pulmonary embolism (PE) is not itself a *disease*. Rather, it is a potentially fatal *complication* of deep vein thrombosis (DVT). Accordingly, these two processes must be considered together. Although effective therapy is available for venous thromboembolism, the therapy itself can produce significant morbidity. Thus, an accurate diagnosis is mandatory. The clinical presentation and laboratory findings in pulmonary embolism are nonspecific, requiring additional evaluation with imaging studies is essential. However, accurate imaging tests are invasive and noninvasive imaging tests still are imperfectly accurate.

These simple facts are at the center of diagnostic evaluation and clinical management of patients who are suspected of having PE. Despite this underlying simplicity, the attendant details can be problematic. Many of the issues in diagnosis and management of suspected PE revolve around the appropriate performance, interpretation, and utilization of imaging tests, the subjects of this chapter.

PRETEST PROBABILITY

EPIDEMIOLOGY

Subclinical pulmonary emboli may be extremely common if the autopsy data represent the true picture, because pathologic studies have shown PE to be present in up to 70% of autopsies when they are searched for zealously (1). However, the occurrence of *clinically significant* pulmonary embolism probably depends upon several factors including the degree of vascular occlusion produced by the emboli, the pulmonary vascular reserve, the age of the embolized thrombus, and the presence of associated medical or surgical conditions affecting cardiac function, pulmonary vascular smooth muscle function, and fibrinolytic activity.

There is uncertainty about patient selection and the accuracy of diagnostic tests as applied in clinical studies defining the frequency of pulmonary emboli. Therefore, interpretation of their results is not straightforward. The prevalence of PE in large series of patients who were suspected clinically of having PE and referred for ventilation-perfusion (V/Q) scans has ranged from 25–50%. A reasonable point estimate would be about 33%, which was the frequency observed in the PIOPED study (2). However, it should be recalled that most of the prevalence data in the literature emanates from academic, tertiary care hospitals and associated clinics. The prevalence of pulmonary embolism in other types of inpatient and outpatient settings may be quite different (consider, for example, the possible differences between private suburban family practice offices and inner city public hospitals).

For clinical practice, we would like to know the actual pretest probability in an individual patient. If this and the operating characteristics of the diagnostic test (e.g., the likelihood ratios for positive and negative results) are known, a reasonable estimate of the probability of the disease in an individual patient can be derived. The starting point for the assessment of pretest probability is the *relative* risk of venous thrombosis in certain groups to which individual patients may belong.

The clinical groups at high-risk for venous thrombosis and PE are well-known. Certain discrete coagulopathies, such as antithrombin III, protein C, and protein S deficiencies, are associated with a high risk of thrombosis. A variety of clinical conditions in which venous stasis or intimal injury is present, place the patient at high-risk of DVT and PE. Such conditions, which may be transient, include pelvic and lower extremity trauma (including surgery), prolonged general anesthesia, burns, pregnancy and the postpartum state, venous obstruction (prior DVT, extrinsic mass or fibrosis), occupational venous stasis, congestive heart failure, immobility (long automobile and airplane trips are notorious risk factors), obesity, cancer, advanced age, and certain drugs (e.g., estrogens). These risk factors may be additive.

The approximate prevalence, therefore, of PE in a particular population may or may not be known, but it usually is possible for the clinician to have an initial estimate of the relative risk of venous thromboembolism in an individual patient before a detailed clinical and imaging evaluation begins.

NATURAL HISTORY

Dalen and Alpert (3) estimated that in 11% of patients with PE there is sudden death. They further estimated that the diagnosis of PE is not made in 63% of patients, and no treatment is given. In this group there is an estimated 30% mortality, presumably due to recurrent emboli. In the other 26% of patients, the diagnosis is made and treatment is given; in this group the mortality is thought to be reduced to 8%. Thus, proper diagnosis and therapy are believed to reduce mortality significantly. However, Dalen and Alpert based their estimates of the consequences of not treating on series in which the diagnosis of PE was made on clinical grounds alone (4). Because the clinical diagnosis of PE is inaccurate, the 30% death rate ascribed to PE in patients not anticoagulated is likely also to be inaccurate. Thus, we must recognize that we do not know precisely the efficacy of anticoagulant therapy.

Only limited data are available concerning the long-term outcome for the patients who survive the initial episode of PE. Owing to the interplay between fibrinolysis and organization, the degree of net residual vascular obstruction is variable. Resolution of acute PE has not been documented to occur in less than 24 hours. The documented rates of resolution vary from a day or two to several weeks or months. At a 4-month follow-up, 60% or more of all patients with PE will show at least improvement in pulmonary blood flow, and 40 per cent will show complete recovery. However, 35% of patients may have incomplete resolution of scintigraphic abnormalities. Older patients, patients with larger emboli, and patients with coexisting CHF are more likely to show incomplete resolution and residual perfusion defects on V/Q scans. Accordingly, follow-up scans are highly useful in defining the new baseline for the patient for possible future diagnostic encounters (5).

CLINICAL ASSESSMENT

The clinical presentations which may be seen in patients with PE are variable and relatively nonspecific (6, 7). Although numerous signs and symptoms have been touted as diagnostic, none have been found truly discriminatory after objective assessment. The "classic" triad of dyspnea, pleurisy, and hemoptysis, for example, was present in only a small minority of patients with confirmed pulmonary emboli in the Urokinase Pulmonary Embolism Trial. However, some characteristic clinical features do occur in many patients. In patients with confirmed pulmonary emboli without preexisting cardiac or pulmonary disease, either dyspnea or tachypnea occurred in 96%. When the clinical diagnosis of deep venous thrombosis was also present, 99% of patients with a positive diagnosis of pulmonary embolism were included. Unfortunately, dyspnea and tachypnea may be seen in a wide variety of both serious and trivial clinical disorders and thus these findings are not specific for PE.

Reliable exclusion or confirmation of acute PE by the ECG or by any blood chemistry is not currently possible. pCO_2 and pO_2 lack sensitivity and specificity, although they can serve to assess the severity of the acute event. pO_2 cannot, be used to exclude an embolus, as up to 15% of patients with PE may have pO_2 tensions greater than 80 torr when breathing ambient air. The use of blood markers for coagulation has been studied extensively and some (such as D-dimer levels) may have an adjunctive role in clinical evaluation, but low specificity vitiates their usefulness (8).

The clinical examination also has been shown to be inaccurate for deep vein thrombosis (DVT). The signs and symptoms used to make a clinical diagnosis of DVT (calf pain and tenderness, unilateral lower limb swelling, positive Homan sign) occur with equal frequency in patients with and without confirmed thrombi. In about 50% of cases with clinically suspected deep vein thrombosis, no thrombus is demonstrated on further testing. Autopsy series demonstrate the poor sensitivity of the clinical exam. In only 11–25% of patients with autopsy-proven deep vein thrombi will the diagnosis have been suspected prior to death. However, if the clinical picture suggests DVT, there is a greater chance that a thrombus will be present than in patients having a normal clinical examination. More recent analysis has suggested that a limited number of clinical findings can predict the occurrence of DVT with relative accuracy (9), but this remains to be confirmed by independent evaluations.

The low sensitivity of symptoms, signs, and clinical laboratory testing implies that a significant number of silent pulmonary emboli and deep vein thrombi occur. In high-risk patients, an unremarkable clinical examination does not reliably exclude thromboembolic disease. Conversely, the diagnosis needs confirmation even when the clinical picture is classic for DVT or PE, because of the low specificity of the clinical and laboratory evaluation.

OVERALL ASSESSMENT OF PRETEST PROBABILITY

Although objective testing is obviously crucial to the diagnosis of venous thromboembolism, the population under a particular physician's care is probably well-defined experientially, and the clinical assessment of disease probability is probably much more useful than has been suggested. In the PIOPED study, the pretest estimate as to the likelihood of PE by experienced clinicians was almost as accurate as the V/Q scan categorization of patients (Table 30.1). These clinical estimates were not made according to set criteria and thus it is impossible for them to be tested or improved upon by other studies. In addition to the overall assessment, recent analyses suggest that V/Q scan interpretive criteria may usefully be adjusted according to the patient's history (see "Diagnostic Criteria—Newer Data").

APPROACH TO THE IMAGING EVALUATION

The goal of diagnostic imaging is to direct therapy. Since anticoagulation will be appropriate for patients who have either pulmonary emboli or deep vein thrombi, the demonstration of either a venous thrombus or a pulmonary embolus is sufficient to begin heparin therapy.

When considering venous thrombus, note that some physicians normally only treat thrombi which are located in the popliteal vein or deep veins more proximally, while some will selectively or always treat calf thrombus or superficial thrombus. Calf vein thrombosis without proximal extension is unlikely to result in pulmonary embolism.

Table 30.1.
Positive predictive value in the PIOPED study for PE of the pretest clinical assessment (which was given as 80–100%, 20–79% and 0–19%) and the V/Q scan categories of high, intermediate, and low-through-normal. (Data from The PIOPED Investigators. Value of the ventilation/perfusion scan in acute pulmonary embolism. JAMA 1990; 263:2753–2759.)

V/Q Scintigraphy		Clinical Assessment	
Category	PPV	Category	PPV
High	87%	80–100%	74%
Intermediate	29%	20–79%	31%
Low-Normal	11%	0–19%	9%

When examining the lungs to establish the diagnosis of acute pulmonary embolism, the demonstration of a single embolus is sufficient. The therapeutic effort is rarely directed toward treating the event which has already occurred, but rather at preventing a subsequent event (10). Thus, demonstrating the disease process is sufficient and quantification of the size or number of emboli normally is not required. However, when clinical concern relates to possibly recurrent embolism or evaluating clot burden for possible lytic therapy, the quantification of disease may be useful.

VENOUS IMAGING

ROLE IN THE DIAGNOSTIC WORKUP

In some patients it may be more appropriate to look for thrombus in the venous system than for a pulmonary embolus, particularly if venous interruption is contemplated. There is, of course, a strong correlation between pulmonary embolism and venous thrombosis. In one study, 71% of patients with positive pulmonary angiograms and 33% of patients with negative pulmonary angiograms had DVT on bilateral venography (11). Conversely, in another study, 76% of patients with proven DVT had abnormal lung scans, including 35% who had "high probability of PE" interpretations (12). Proximal vein thrombosis appears to carry by far the greatest risk for PE.

In a patient with respiratory symptoms that may result from PE, imaging evaluation should be directed to the chest. A lung scan and a chest radiograph should be obtained. If a diagnosis of PE is established, venous imaging should be considered if there is reason to believe that recurrent venous disease could develop or that venous thrombosis could persist despite therapy, because venous imaging would be important in follow-up and venous interruption may be considered as therapy. If the diagnosis remains in doubt after the scintigraphic study, venous imaging can be considered as an alternative to pulmonary angiography (see "Patient Management After the V/Q Scan"). Venous imaging is generally safer and more pleasant for the patient than arteriography, requires less technical expertise than arteriography, is more widely available, and is generally less expensive than arteriography. However, there is a substantial negative rate in venous studies of patients with PE, as indicated earlier, and arteriography may still be needed if the venous imaging is negative. Finally, if arteriography is negative but venous thrombosis is still suspected clinically, venous imaging is indicated.

RADIOLOGIC VENOUS IMAGING TECHNIQUES

Contrast venography is the diagnostic "gold standard" for DVT. Extensive experience has shown that identification of well-defined filling defects in fully opacified veins is accurate for detection of DVT, while negative conventional venography has been shown to exclude clinically significant DVT (13). However, venography does have limitations including difficulties in venous cannulation, incomplete filling of the venous system, and other technical problems in as much as 5% of cases (14); discomfort in up to 18% of patients even with nonionic contrast (15, 16); and a variety of local and systemic reactions to contrast material, including induced DVT in as much as 8% of cases even with nonionic contrast (15, 16).

Such limitations of conventional venography have led to development of alternative, noninvasive tests for DVT. Compression ultrasound has been investigated extensively in patients with documentations by either venography (17) or outcome analysis (18). The sensitivity and specificity of ultrasound for femoropopliteal DVT have been shown in these and many other studies to exceed 90%. Accordingly, ultrasound has been widely adopted as a cost-effective, noninvasive method for screening patients suspected of having DVT. However, ultrasound also has limitations. Its accuracy in calf DVT is variable (17, 19); it is less accurate in recurrent DVT (20–22), although follow-up studies after acute episodes can improve accuracy in subsequent diagnostic encounters; it is operator-dependent; and its accuracy in pelvic DVT has not been investigated extensively. Of concern, it appears that asymptomatic DVT is detected by ultrasound with significantly reduced sensitivity (23). A recent meta-analysis (24) found a sensitivity in asymptomatic patients of only 39% in a study of six publications (including 1015 patients) when compared with sensitivity of 97% for detecting DVT in symptomatic patients. Moreover, it is physically impossible to examine the peripheral pulmonary arteries with ultrasound to detect PE.

Preliminary reports described the use of venous imaging with MR for detecting DVT (25–27) in a total of 111 patients with correlative conventional venograms. In two series (62 patients with conventional venogram correlation), sensitivities of 90% and 100% and specificities of 100% and 93% were reported (25, 26). We recently performed two prospective trials of MR for DVT in a total of 136 patients. In a prospective blinded trial comparing MR and venography in 61 patients (28), MR was better (sensitivity 100%, specificity 95%) in the pelvis than venography (sensitivity 78%, specificity 100%); the two tests were completely concordant in the thigh (the sensitivity and specificity of both determined to be 100%), and venography was better than MR (sensitivity 87%, specificity 97%) in the calf. In a second study (unpublished, 1993), 75 patients referred clinically for ultrasound were imaged on a research basis with MR. When there was disagreement between ultrasound and MR, either repeat ultrasound or venography was performed. Although it was not possible to document the true status of the patient in all cases of minor disagreement, almost all cases with major disagreement (one test showing DVT and the other negative) could be resolved. Preliminary analysis of the results shows MR to be more sensitive than ultrasound in areas which are known to be difficult to image with ultrasound (pelvis, adductor canal, calf), while the specificity of the two techniques appears to be equivalent. For detection of proximal (above-knee) DVT, we found that MR (sensitivity 96%, specificity 100%) was more accurate than ultrasound (sensitivity 70%, specificity 98%). Other reports have indicated that MR can detect venous thrombi accurately in other body regions (29). The current clinical role of MR for DVT at Duke is: MR is recommended as the best test for DVT in: (a) asymptomatic patients being screened for DVT because of suspected PE;

(b) suspected pelvic DVT; (c) nondiagnostic ultrasound or conventional venography; (d) clinical suspicion of DVT versus nonvascular disease (e.g., cellulitis or ruptured Baker cyst). About 250 MR exams are done for suspected DVT per year at Duke (with routine on-call coverage), compared to about 750 ultrasound studies and 50 venograms.

RADIONUCLIDE VENOUS IMAGING TECHNIQUES

Several radionuclide techniques have been studied for the detection of DVT, including radionuclide venography and radiolabeled fibrinogen (either alone or in combination with impedance plethysmography), platelets, and monoclonal antibodies.

The combination of impedance plethysmography (IPG) and ^{125}I-fibrinogen uptake measurements has been proposed for the detection of DVT. Proximal DVT has been accurately detected by IPG (11, 30, 31), and ^{125}I-fibrinogen has been effective for detection of DVT in the calf (30, 31). However, although good results have been reported in well-designed studies, IPG is clearly operator-dependent and good results (even when combined with ^{125}I-fibrinogen) have not been reported by all investigators (32–34). Our clinical experience with IPG also has been less favorable than that in some reported studies. The ^{125}I-fibrinogen uptake test is also operator-dependent and the radiopharmaceutical is no longer available commercially in the United States. Thus, the combined test is no longer feasible to routinely perform.

Radionuclide venography (35–38) is still used in some hospitals and requires pedal or bipedal injection of ^{99m}Tc-MAA and imaging during and immediately following the administration of the radiopharmaceutical. Thus, multiple images are required to visualize the calf, thigh, and pelvic regions. Obstruction to the flow of radiopharmaceutical through the deep venous system and the presence of collateral veins are interpreted as positive for DVT. The attractive feature of this technique is that the deep veins can be studied for DVT, followed by a perfusion lung scan to evaluate for PE. However, there are a number of interpretive pitfalls (35, 37, 38) and the technique is quite cumbersome when incorporated into the V/Q examination. Accordingly, it is used in a minority of clinical practices today and is becoming of mostly historical interest. Blood pool scintigraphy using ^{99m}Tc red blood cells is also advocated for detecting DVT, but this technique is not widely used.

The idea of utilizing a radiopharmaceutical which preferentially adheres to thrombi is theoretically attractive and has been pursued for many years. The potential advantages of examination with a radiolabeled thrombus-detecting agent are that such an examination would likely be relatively inexpensive compared to CT or MR, that the entire body could be surveyed for thromboembolic disease in a single examination, that nuclear medicine imaging equipment is widely available, and potentially that "active" thrombi and chronic thrombi could be distinguished, aiding selection of treatment. A number of candidate agents have been investigated, including fibrin and fibrin lytic products, platelets, components of the fibrinolytic system, and a variety of monoclonal antibodies and derivatives. To date, none of these agents has proven useful enough for widespread clinical use, but the powerful rationale for them has prompted continued investigations, which are yielding increasingly promising results (39–43).

PULMONARY IMAGING

ROLE IN THE DIAGNOSTIC WORKUP

The recent emphasis which has been placed upon venous imaging in the evaluation of patients with suspected venous thromboembolism should not obscure the central role of pulmonary imaging in patients who present with respiratory or thoracic symptoms. In these patients, the diagnostic investigations should be directed first to the thorax (see, however, "Patient Management After the V/Q Scan" for a more complete discussion).

CHEST RADIOGRAPH

The chest radiograph is not an accurate means of diagnosing PE (44), although it may, on occasion, be suggestive. Most patients with PE, and many patients who undergo a negative workup for PE, have abnormal chest radiographs. The radiographic changes are nonspecific. The common findings include consolidation, various manifestations of atelectasis, pleural effusion (usually small), and diaphragmatic elevation. Less common findings include nodules, focal oligemia, proximal pulmonary artery enlargement, and acute congestive heart failure. Some of the previously described "diagnostic" signs (particularly focal oligemia or changes in proximal pulmonary artery size) can be extremely subtle and difficult to interpret unless good comparison films are available. Resolution of the parenchymal abnormalities usually occurs within 1–4 weeks; residual abnormalities may include pleural reaction and linear scars. Cavitation may occur in bland infarcts, but is uncommon in the absence of secondary infection.

However, the chest radiograph is an essential component in the imaging evaluation of a patient clinically suspected of having PE. Its primary importance in evaluation of suspected PE, however, is twofold. The chest film is needed to establish or exclude some of the clinical simulators of PE such as pneumonia, rib fracture, and pneumothorax. It is also essential for adequate evaluation of the lung scintigram, which is interpreted by comparing the chest radiographic, ventilation scan, and perfusion scan findings in the same areas of the lung. One should obtain a high quality PA and lateral examination at the same time as the lung scan. Portable AP films are a poor substitute, and films more than a few hours old should not be used for interpretation of lung scans. If a portable film must be used, the patient's position should be accurately recorded so that account may be made for layering of pleural fluid.

VENTILATION-PERFUSION SCINTIGRAPHY: IMAGE ACQUISITION

Normal scintigraphic studies of the lungs demonstrate homogenous patterns of evenly matched ventilation (V) and perfusion (Q) which correlate precisely with the aerated lung seen on the chest radiograph. Pathophysiologic states commonly are associated with scintigraphically detectable perturbations of ventilation and perfusion. These perturbations generally result in regional heterogeneity of pulmonary perfusion and ventilation rather than overall changes.

Vascular occlusive processes include PE, extrinsic vascular compression, pulmonary vasculitis, and congenital abnormalities. These processes usually leave alveoli structurally intact, and thus ventilation usually is preserved in regions of vascular occlusion. Accordingly, V/Q mismatch is the hallmark of this type of pathophysiology. *Airspace occlusion* may be associated with pneumonia, pulmonary infarction, and other airspace disorders. The degree of ventilation and perfusion loss can vary independently, but both usually are reduced concomitantly. Therefore, a V/Q match typically is present, usually associated with a radiographic opacity. *Obstructive physiology* is seen in disorders such as emphysema, bronchitis, bronchiectasis, and asthma, which predominately affect the conducting and exchanging air spaces. Alveolar hypoxia results, and the corresponding pulmonary arteries constrict, thus redistributing blood to better ventilated alveoli and preserving the matching of ventilation and blood flow. Matched V/Q abnormalities are seen in this type of physiology as well, but corresponding radiographic opacities are less common. In *restrictive lung disease*, chronic inflammation and fibrosis may eventually obliterate alveoli and capillaries. However, the airways remain functional and regional ventilation may be increased relative to perfusion. The configuration and pattern of perfusion abnormalities is usually different from the vascular occlusive state. Of course, mixtures of these pathophysiologic states are extremely common in individual patients.

Perfusion Imaging

Perfusion scintigraphy of the lung is accomplished by inducing microembolization of radiolabeled particles in the pulmonary arterioles. The number of particles which impact in a particular volume of the lung is proportional to the pulmonary arterial blood flow to that region. Perfusion scintigraphy provides a visual representation of the regional distribution of pulmonary blood flow at the time of radiopharmaceutical injection.

Particulate embolization does cause a minor degree of obstruction of pulmonary blood flow, but this effect is almost never physiologically significant. An even distribution of radioactivity in the vascular bed requires injection of 60,000 or more particles. The usual 2–4 mCi ^{99m}Tc (140 keV photon) MAA patient dose contains approximately 500,000 particles, so injections of a low number of particles and statistically invalid scans are rarely a problem. Freshly prepared macroaggregated albumin (MAA) should be used, because breakdown products in the preparation such as ^{99m}Tc pertechnetate can cause spurious extrapulmonary uptake. The intravenous injection of labeled particles should be performed with the patient supine, and the radiopharmaceutical should be injected slowly over 5–10 seconds while the patient takes moderately deep breaths. This method ensures that pulmonary blood flow is evenly distributed, which is important for adequate visualization of the upper lung and other physiologically hypoperfused regions. The syringe containing the radiopharmaceutical should be agitated immediately prior to the injection to ensure a homogeneous suspension of the labeled particles. One must not allow blood to clot within the syringe, because clots will adsorb the radioactive aggregates and cause an uneven distribution of activity (Fig. 30.1). If the radiopharmaceutical must be injected through intravenous tubing, the fluid must be flowing rapidly. Even so, a portion of the dose may adhere to the tubing and injections through tubing are discouraged. Injection into central venous or pulmonary artery catheters should be avoided, because streaming or selective catheter position may result in uneven distribution of the injected particles.

Imaging for perfusion scintigraphy is done with a wide-field-of-view γ camera equipped with a low-energy, all-purpose collimator. Eight views of the thorax (anterior, posterior, right and left posterior and anterior oblique, and right and left lateral) are obtained routinely (Fig. 30.2). In each view, 750,000 counts are obtained, except that for the lateral views in which one view is imaged for 500,000 counts, the time noted, and the second lateral view acquired for the same length of time.

Perfusion scintigraphy is sensitive but not specific. As discussed earlier in the description of physiologic patterns, nearly all pulmonary diseases can produce significantly decreased pulmonary artery blood flow to affected lung zones (45, 46).

Ventilation Imaging

Abnormalities in the perfusion scan that are *matched* by zones of abnormal ventilation are less likely to represent PE, while mismatched abnormalities (reduced perfusion with preserved ventilation, i.e., the vascular occlusive state) have a high correspondence with PE, given a normal

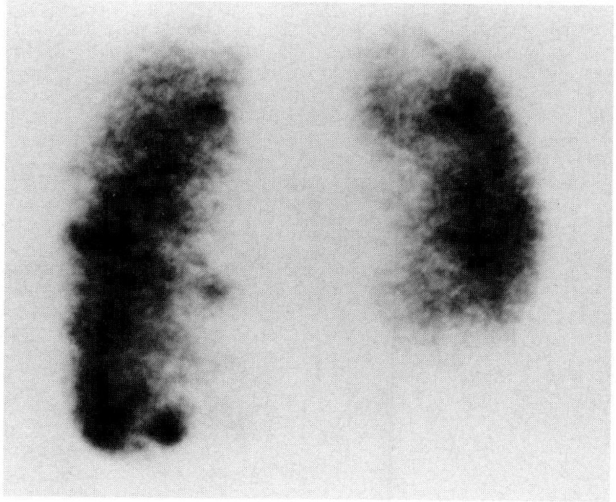

Figure 30.1. Radionuclide Absorption by Clotted Blood Within Syringe. This is an old case showing "hot clots" due to absorption of ^{99m}Tc-MAA to blood that has clotted in the syringe used for injecting the radiopharmaceutical (we are happy to say we do not have any recent examples). Note the cutoff of the left costophrenic angle on this posterior view, due to the use of a small-field-of-view camera. There is marked inhomogeneity of lung activity, as a result of the small number of free particles remaining (note, for example, the spurious right upper lobe defect). Such a study should not be interpreted. A repeat perfusion examination 18 hr later was normal.

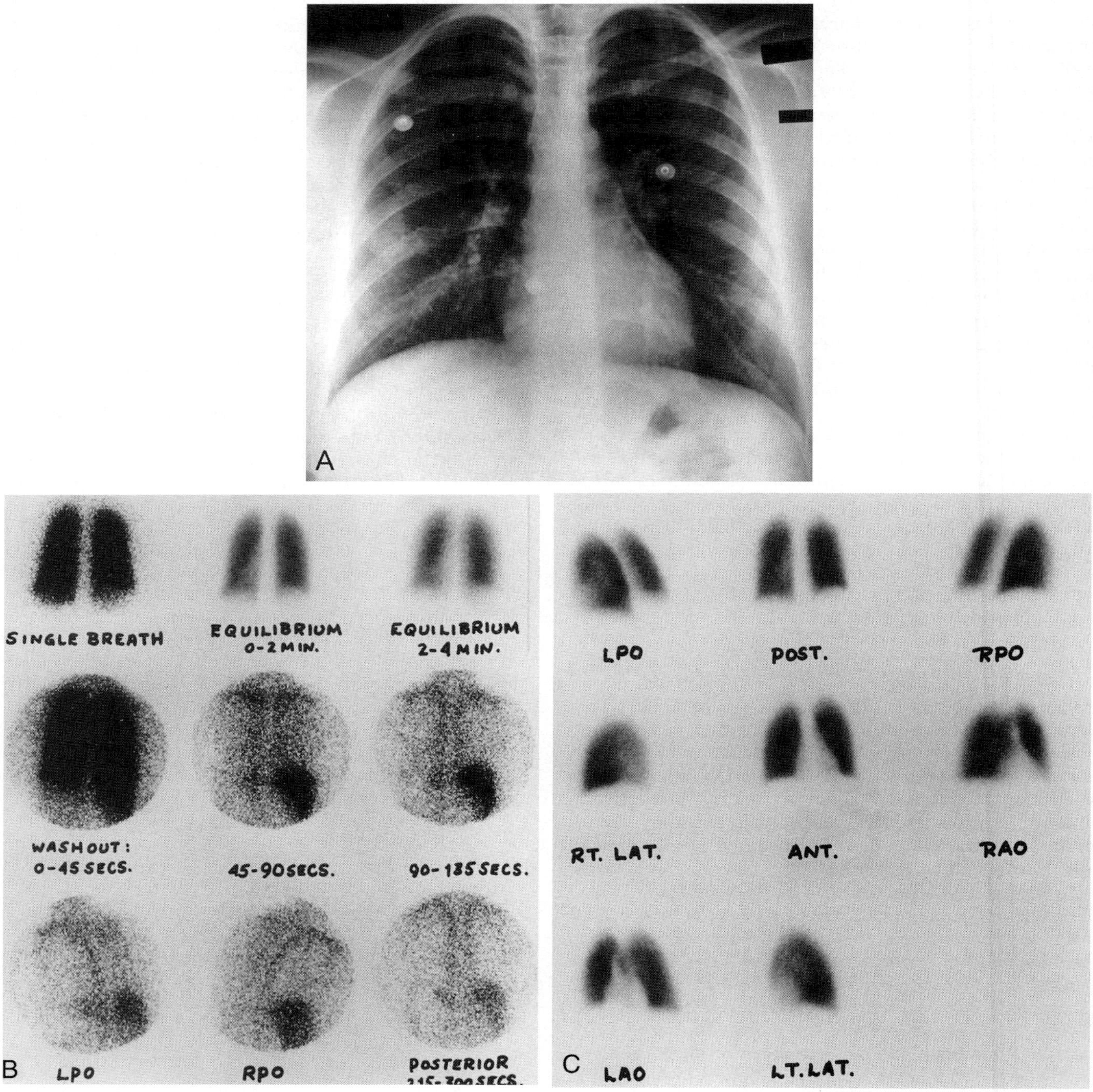

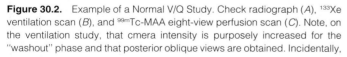

Figure 30.2. Example of a Normal V/Q Study. Check radiograph (*A*), ^{133}Xe ventilation scan (*B*), and ^{99m}Tc-MAA eight-view perfusion scan (*C*). Note, on the ventilation study, that cmera intensity is purposely increased for the "washout" phase and that posterior oblique views are obtained. Incidentally, note on this study (*B*) the ^{133}Xe uptake in subcutaneous and hepatic fat. *LPO* = left posterior oblique, *PRO* = right posterior oblique, *POST.* = posterior, *LAT.* = lateral, *ANT.* = anterior, *RAO* = right anterior oblique, *LAO* = left anterior oblique.

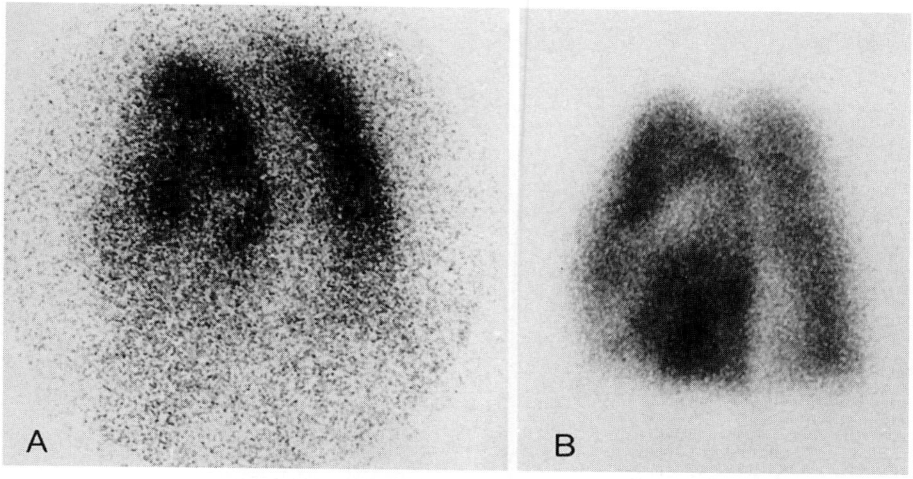

Figure 30.3. Use of Posterior Oblique "Washout" View to Help Localize Areas of Abnormal Ventilation on ^{133}Xe Study. The left posterior oblique view of the ^{133}Xe scan (*A*) shows abnormal areas of ^{133}Xe retention that correspond well to perfusion deficits on the LPO view of the ^{99m}Tc-MAA scan (*B*).

chest radiograph in the same lung region (45). Therefore, most nuclear physicians consider it essential to obtain both ventilation and perfusion images to ensure accurate categorization when perfusion scans are abnormal.

^{133}Xe (80-keV photon) gas has been used for many years and is still the radionuclide used for most routine ventilation studies. Its use requires apparatus for administering the gas and for trapping exhaled gas. This ventilation apparatus includes a tightly sealing face mask or mouthpiece, a spirometer, tubing with intake and exhaust valves, and a shielded charcoal trap.

A wide-field-of-view scintillation camera and an all-purpose collimator are used to obtain a ventilation study *before the perfusion imaging is done.* We recommend the following technique: A "first breath" image of 100,000 counts or 10–15 seconds is obtained after administration of 15–20 mCi (550–770 MBq) of ^{133}Xe into the intake port as the patient inspires maximally. Then the patient rebreathes gas in a closed spirometer system while three 75-second "equilibrium" images are made in posterior, RPO and LPO projections. The intake valves of the system are then readjusted so that the patient breathes ambient air, and "washout" images are obtained at 45-second intervals. The first three washout images are standard posterior views. Next, right and left posterior oblique images are made, followed by a final posterior image. The posterior oblique equilibrium and washout views are obtained to better localize zones of abnormal lung volume and xenon retention with respect to their anterior-posterior location (Fig. 30.3).

The equilibrium image has a radioactivity distribution corresponding to the aerated lung volume. Images made during washout from normal lungs show rapid and symmetrical clearance of activity from the lungs (usually within 90 seconds). In contrast to the first-breath image, which indicates ventilatory abnormality as a deficit in radioactivity in the lung, zones with abnormal ventilation become apparent as "hot spots" on washout images, as delayed clearance of ^{133}Xe produces areas of focal retained activity on a background of decreasing activity from normal lung regions. To obtain maximum information from the washout images, one first must use a sufficiently long (>3 minutes) rebreathing period, in order to permit the radionuclide to enter abnormal lung zones by collateral air drift.

Obtaining the ventilation study before the perfusion is the most accurate technique to use with ^{133}Xe. It allows optimum images in the washout portion of the ventilation study since there is no ^{99m}Tc present in the lungs to produce scatter; this scatter occurs in the same energy window as ^{133}Xe primary photons and can obscure ^{133}Xe retention. The postperfusion ^{133}Xe ventilation technique is less reliable diagnostically, although it is more efficient, because the ventilation study is not needed if the perfusion study is normal.

^{81m}Kr is another commonly used radiogas for ventilation studies. It is expensive and has a very short half-life (13 seconds). Therefore, washout images are not obtained. ^{81m}Kr is obtained from a generation which has ^{81}Rb (T 1/2 = 4.7 minutes) as the parent radionuclide. The generation is thus limited to the day of delivery. However, the higher photon energy (190 keV) of ^{81m}Kr allows it to be used after the perfusion study, permitting selection of the optimal imaging view(s), and its short half-life enables multiple views to be obtained. There are some data to suggest that ^{81m}Kr is not as sensitive as ^{133}Xe in detecting all ventilation abnormalities because the washout phase cannot be obtained. Nevertheless, some larger hospitals with a large volume of V/Q studies consider the advantages to outweigh the corresponding disadvantages, and preferentially use ^{81m}Kr for ventilation scintigraphy.

Radioaerosols also provide a means for imaging regional ventilation and are available commercially in the form of small and efficient aerosol nebulizers. Radioaerosols are small particles, rather than gases. The usual radioaerosol agent is ^{99m}Tc-labeled DTPA (Fig. 30.4). Typically, 30 mCi (1110 MBq) of ^{99m}Tc DTPA is placed in the nebulizer and inhalation of the aerosol continues until 1 mCi (37 MBq) is in the lungs. The radioaerosol inhalation study usually is performed before the perfusion scintigram. To yield uniform apex-to-base deposition, the inhalation study should be performed with the patient in the supine position. However, if postperfusion aerosol images are obtained, and the perfusion defects are in the bases, the erect position may

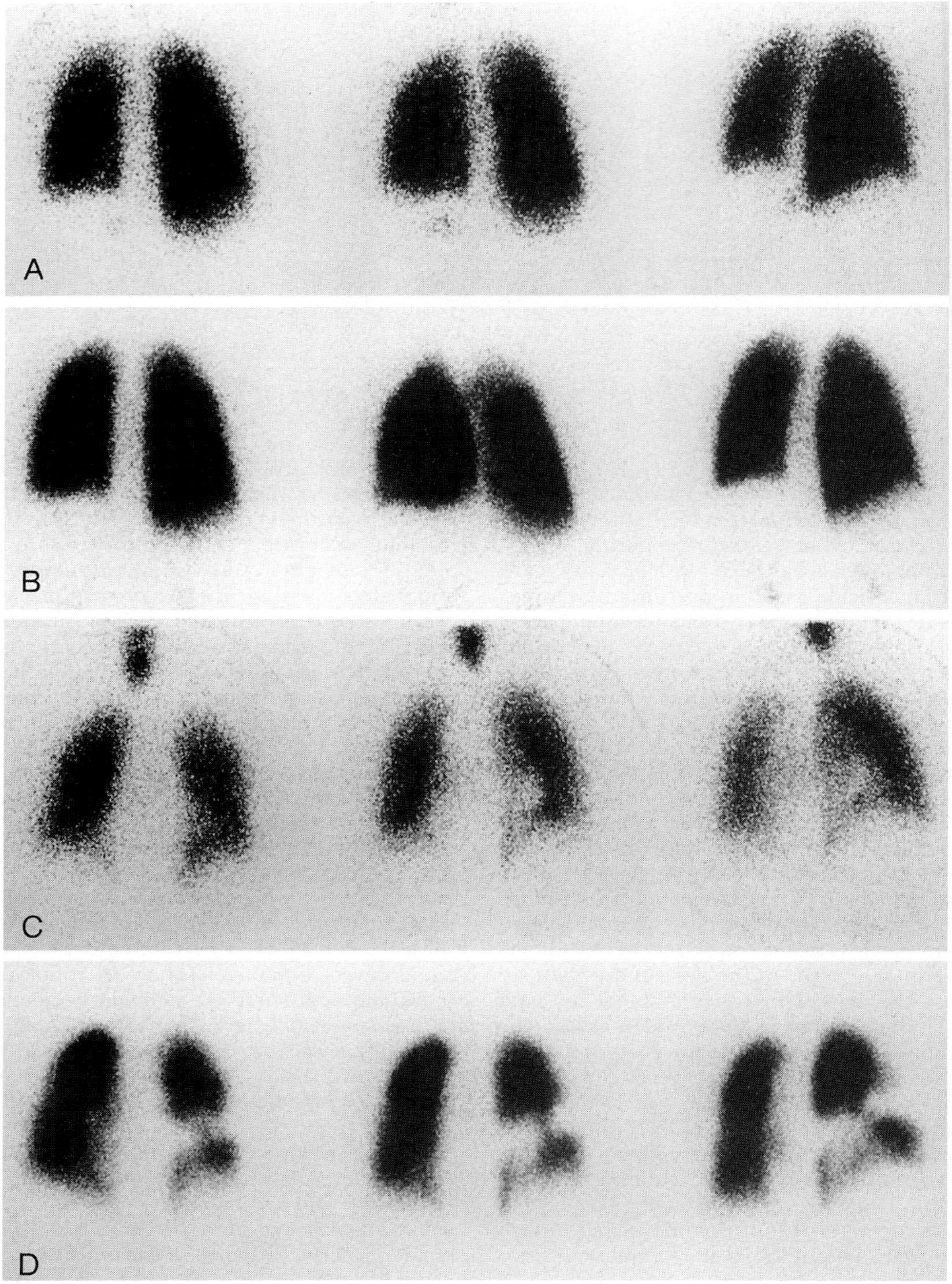

Figure 30.4. Two Examples of Aerosolized ^{99m}Tc-DTPA/^{99m}Tc-MAA V/Q Studies. Normal (*A*) and abnormal (*C*) ventilation scans with corresponding normal (*B*) and abnormal (*D*) perfusion scans. In both examples, posterior and both posterior oblique views are shown in each panel. *A,* A normal ^{99m}Tc-DTPA aerosol ventilation study. *B,* A normal ^{99m}Tc-MAA perfusion study. Note the faint gastric (*A*) and renal (*B*) activity from the ^{99m}Tc-DPTA, and the precise correspondence of the lung images of ventilation (*A*) and perfusion (*B*). *C,* A deficit in activity in the right lower lobe on the aerosol ventilation images; recall that aerosol ventilation imaging, like ^{81m}Kr and early phases ("first breath" and "equilibrium") of ^{133}Xe studies, shows abnormal ventilation as a deficit in activity. *D,* Corresponding ^{99m}Tc-MAA perfusion images. There are perfusion deficits in the right lower lobe (matched by abnormal ventilation) and in the right upper lobe anterior segment (a "mismatched" deficit). Note how simple comparison of the two studies is made by the ability to obtain multiple-view ventilation images.

be used. The use of ^{99m}Tc-pyrophosphate aerosols yields a longer residence time, which is important in smokers (46). Recently, in Europe and Australia an ultrafine dry dispersion of ^{99m}Tc-labeled carbon particles ("Technegas") has become popular. It provides speed and ease of administration, deep peripheral penetration with minimal bronchial deposition, and prolonged pulmonary retention. Comparison with radioactive gases has generally been very favorable. This agent is not yet generally available in the United States.

At the present time, it is not obvious that any one of these agents is ideal for ventilation studies. Comparisons between the various techniques are limited, but suggest that there is no major diagnostic difference (47, 48). Indeed, it is common for many institutions to use more than one agent at different times. An institution which employs one of the radioactive gases for routine V/Q scintigraphy might use the convenient aerosols for portable examinations in the intensive care unit. Accordingly, considerations such as cost, patient logistics, and referral patterns will determine which of these ventilation agents is best suited for a specific institution.

VENTILATION-PERFUSION SCINTIGRAPHY: IMAGE INTERPRETATION

Diagnostic Criteria—Older Data

A truly normal perfusion scan has long been accepted to exclude PE for practical purposes (that is, the morbidity and mortality of missed PE has been thought to be less than that from pulmonary arteriography or anticoagulant therapy). It is the perfusion portion of the examination that is important in consideration of possible PE—as long as perfusion is normal, the ventilation images or chest radiograph can be abnormal and the scan is still read as normal in the sense of being negative for PE (Fig. 30.5). Theoretic reasons for PE with a "normal" perfusion scan are central, nonobstructing PE which cause subtle decrease in whole lung perfusion or minimal defects on scan that are not appreciated. However, perfusion scans should be interpreted *very conservatively*, and a "normal" diagnosis reserved for *unequivocally normal perfusion studies* (Fig. 30.2) because (a) it has been demonstrated experimentally that perfusion scintigraphy *is not perfectly sensitive* and (b) great weight is placed upon normal scan interpretations in clinical management. In dogs, the sensitivity of the perfusion scan is about 80% for emboli that completely occlude pulmonary vessels, but only about 30% for partially occluding emboli (49). The high sensitivity of perfusion scintigraphy for PE in the *patient*, as opposed to an individual *site* in the patient, results from the occurrence of multiple emboli in the great majority of patients. Usually, a normal scan result stops the workup for PE and diverts attention to other possibilities.

Although it is sensitive, perfusion scintigraphy is not specific for pulmonary embolism. Nearly all pulmonary diseases, including neoplasms, infections, and chronic obstructive pulmonary disease (COPD), can produce decreased pulmonary blood flow to affected regions (50). To overcome this problem, Wagner (51) and DeNardo (52) suggested combined ventilation-perfusion lung imaging. McNeil, et al. (45), highlighted the findings of numerous investigators by pointing out that abnormalities in the perfusion scan that are matched by abnormal ventilation usually are not due to pulmonary embolism, but that mismatched abnormalities, coexisting with a normal chest radiograph, have a high correlation with angiographically demonstrated pulmonary embolism. Alderson and coworkers (53) later showed that the overall diagnostic accuracy for scintigraphic detection of pulmonary emboli was significantly improved when ^{133}Xe ventilation studies were added to the perfusion scan and chest radiograph.

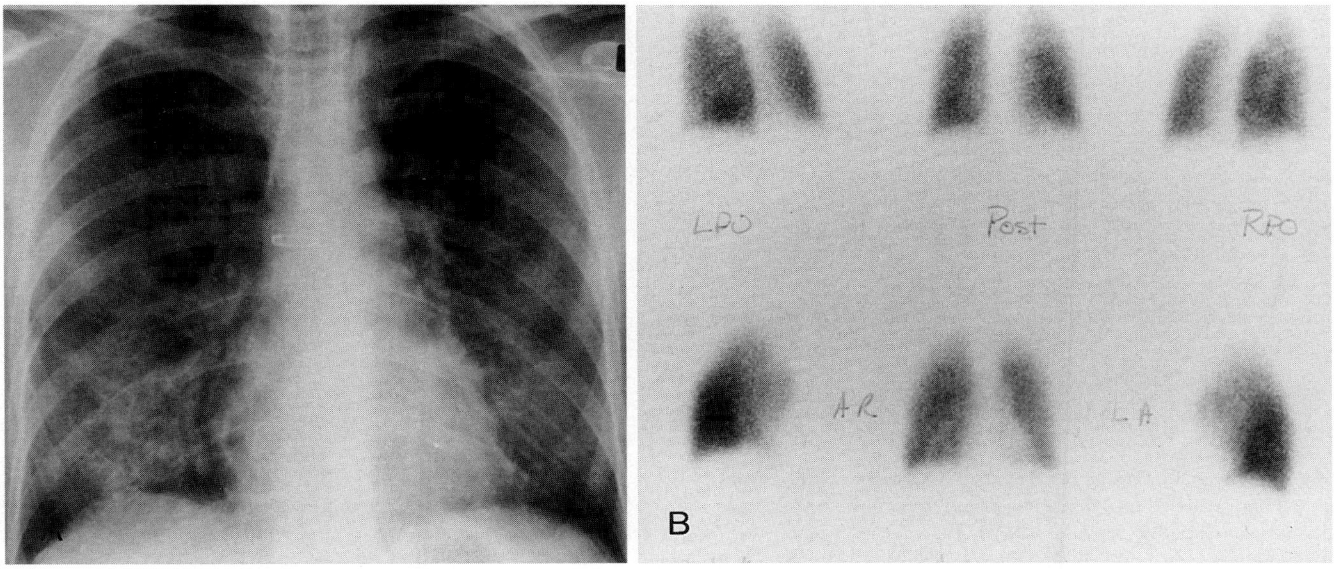

Figure 30.5. The perfusion scintigram can be normal or nearly normal despite the presence of significant pulmonary disease. It is the perfusion scan findings which govern the categorization of the study as to likelihood of PE. In this patient with resolving ARDS, the chest radiograph (**A**) shows diffuse opacities but the perfusion scan (**B**) is essentially normal. The study is therefore correctly interpreted as negative for PE.

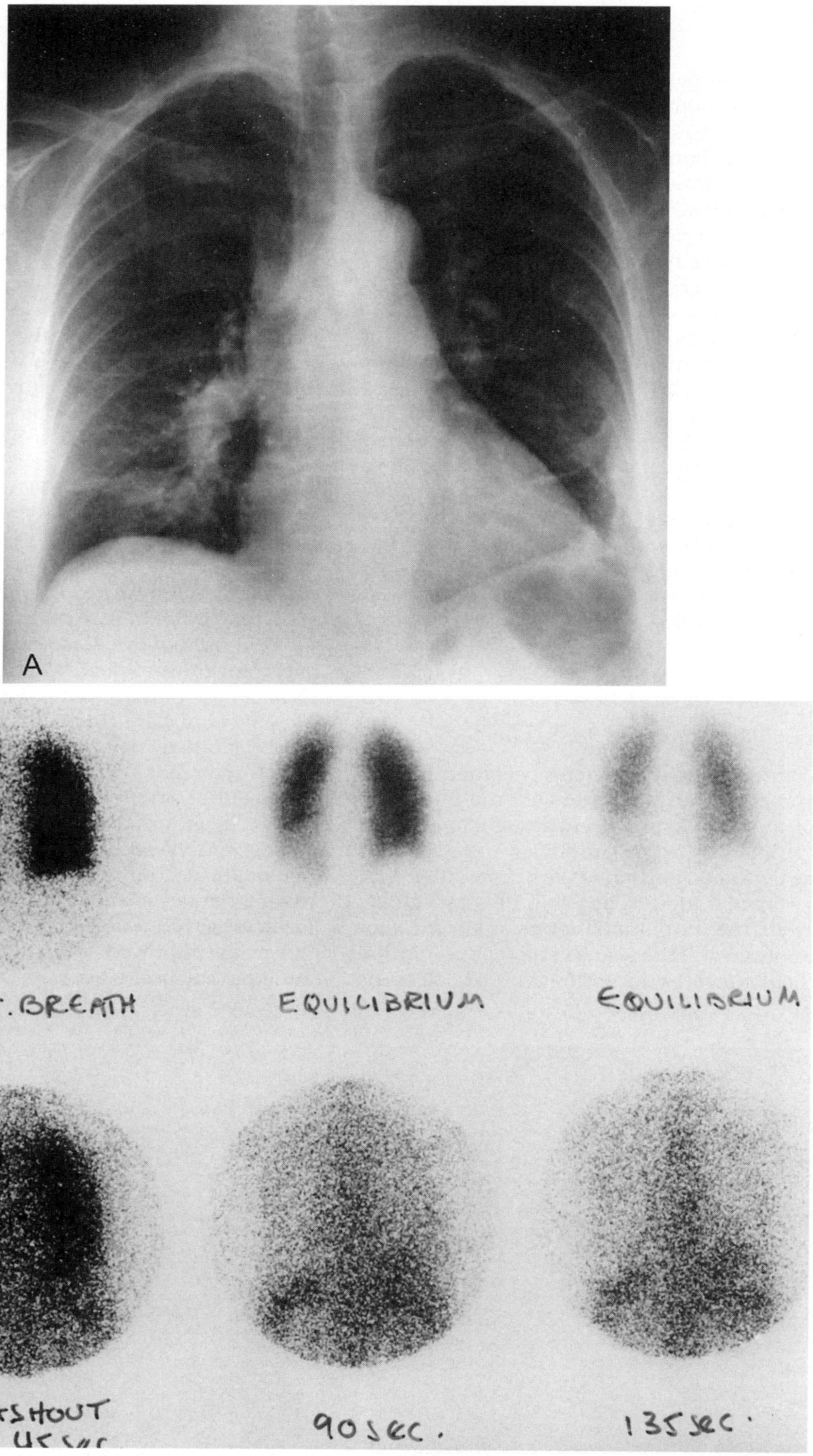

Figure 30.6. High Probability of Pulmonary Embolism. The chest radiograph (*A*) demonstrates pleuroparenchymal scarring at both bases and a wide mediastinum due to vascular ectasia. The ^{133}Xe ventilation scan (*B*) shows normal ventilation. Note that on the "washout" phase (remember that camera intensity is purposely increased here) there is residual bone, liver, and spleen activity from a prior ^{67}Ga scan and that consequently a high-energy collimator was used for both the ventilation and perfusion images. The perfusion study (*C*) shows large mismatched defects bilaterally. This case also points out that when a low-energy (^{99m}Tc) examination is done in a patient with higher energy tracer "on board" (^{67}Ga), it is imperative to collimate for the high-energy photons.

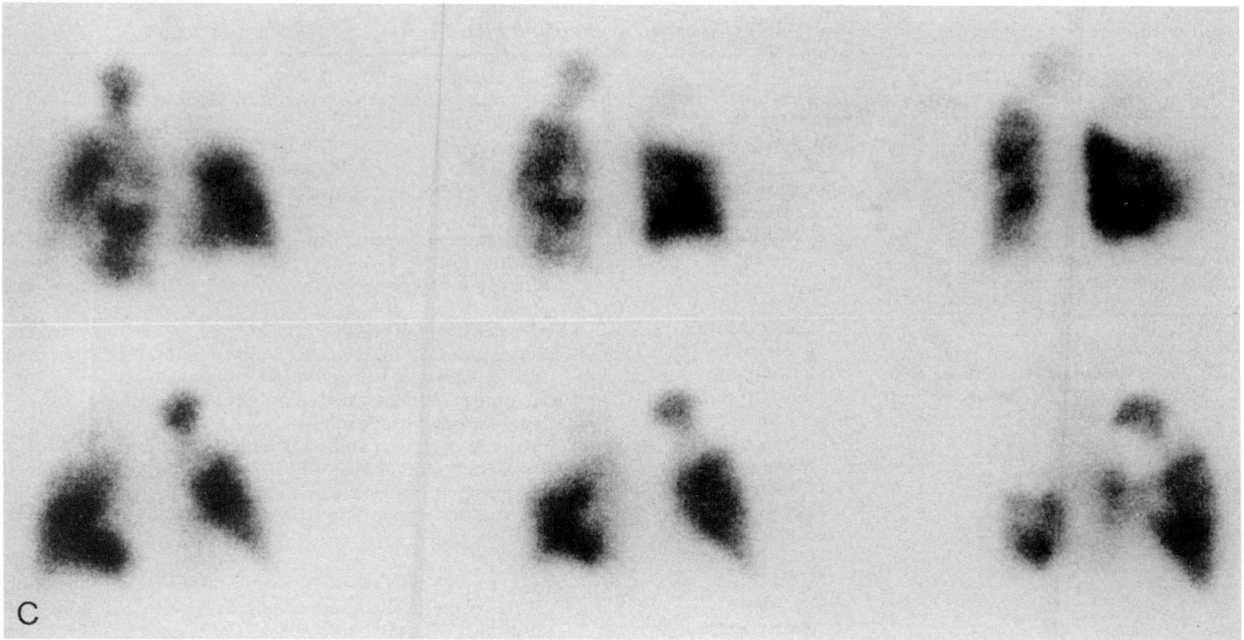

Figure 30.6—*Continued*

Neumann and colleagues (54) introduced the concept of "segmental equivalents"—that two subsegmental perfusion defects may be added to produce the same diagnostic significance as a single segmental defect. A subsequent retrospective study by Kotlyarov and Reba (55) supported the usefulness of this approach.

Extensive work by Biello and collaborators (56, 57) further categorized perfusion defects matched by ventilatory or radiographic abnormalities and provided grounds for reducing the number of "indeterminate" diagnoses. Further evaluation of this work (58) indicated that this diagnostic scheme provides improved interobserver consistency and a 30% reduction in "indeterminate" readings compared with the results from an older scheme.

Experience has clearly shown that a scintigraphic study demonstrating multiple large, wedge-shaped, pleural-based perfusion defects with normal ventilation and a clear chest radiograph in the corresponding areas has a high correspondence with PE (Fig. 30.6). The major cause of error in this situation is prior, unresolved PE (see "Pulmonary Embolism Mimics"). Normally, a scan pattern of this type is read as "high probability of PE" and results in a clinical diagnosis of PE, followed by appropriate therapy.

Intermediate patterns on the V/Q scan are less diagnostic, and must be interpreted with care. As discussed later, the degree of pretest clinical probability of PE must be taken into account strongly in deciding upon management of patients in this group. Often another study such as pulmonary angiography is required.

Table 30.2 shows two sets of commonly used diagnostic criteria: the "Biello" criteria and the PIOPED criteria, while Table 30.3 shows the revised PIOPED criteria, with modifications based upon retrospective review of the database of proven cases provided by the PIOPED study (59, 60).

Certain definitions are important to understanding and proper use of these criteria. In all these criteria, "small" is defined as a defect involving less than 25% of the area of an average-sized pulmonary arterial segment; "moderate" is equivalent to 25–75% of the area of a segment; and "large" means more than 75% of a segment. Figure 30.7 shows examples of different sizes of perfusion defects. Note that different bronchopulmonary segments typically are of different sizes (Fig. 30.8). In principle, one could attempt to individualize the rating of defect size to the particular segment in which the defect is thought to be located, but in practice most readers, including experts in the field, simply use an average, idealized segment and apply this size template to evaluation of defects in any location. A chest x-ray (CXR) defect indicates a radiographic opacity in the *region* related to the Q or V lesion. When CXR is called "normal" this also alludes to the CXR appearance in the same *region* as the V or Q defect. Finally, a lung zone is one-third of a lung divided craniocaudally (i.e., upper, middle, and lower zones).

An example of a classic high probability scan is shown in Figure 30.6. Examples of scans that should be interpreted as showing low or intermediate probability of PE are shown in Figures 30.9–30.12.

Diagnostic Criteria—Newer Data

Interestingly, there are data to indicate that some experienced individuals can achieve more accurate results using their own experience than the reference criteria cited here (60, 61). Nevertheless, diagnostic reference criteria can be extremely useful, particularly for observers who do not have extensive and ongoing experience in interpreting V/Q studies. Use of reference criteria has been shown to re-

Table 30.2.
Scintigraphic Reference Criteria for Pulmonary Emboli

Probability of PE	Washington U/ Columbia (40-43)	PIOPED/Yale
Normal	Normal perfusion	Normal perfusion
Low	1. Small V/Q mismatches	1. Small Q defects regardless of number, V or CXR findings
	2. Q defect substantially smaller than CXR opacity	2. Q defect substantially smaller than CXR defect (V irrelevant)
	3. V/Q match no more than 50% of one lung field	3. V/Q match in no more than 50% of one lung *or* no more than 75% of one lung zone; CXR normal *or* nearly normal
		4. Single moderate Q with normal CXR (V irrelevant)
		5. Nonsegmental Q defects
Intermediate	1. Diffuse V/Q match 2. Matched Q and CXR 3. Single moderate V/Q mismatch (one segment or smaller) with CXR normal in area	Abnormality that is not defined by either "High" *or* "Low"
High	1. Q substantially larger than CXR opacity, which shows some area of mismatch	1. Two or more Q; V and CXR normal
	2. Two or more large or moderate-sized V/Q mismatches; CXR normal in corresponding area	2. Two or more large Q where Q substantially larger than either matching V or CXR
		3. Two or more moderate Q and one large Q; V and CXR normal
		4. Four or more moderate Q; V and CXR normal

duce the number of indeterminate readings. Additionally, if all the physicians in a group practice use the same reference criteria, standardization of V/Q scan interpretations is likely to improve. In the PIOPED study, pairs of independent readers achieved high levels of prospective agreement (90–95%) for high probability and normal-near normal diagnoses, but lesser agreement (70–75%) for intermediate and low probability. The implications of these findings for clinical interpretations are obvious. It is worth noting that *the good agreement between scan readers was only achieved after several practice sessions* in which the description of findings and assignment of diagnostic categories was standardized.

This discussion suggests that further refinement of diagnostic criteria is possible and there have been several

Table 30.3.
Revised PIOPED V/Q Scan Criteria

High Probability (≥ 80%)
- ≥ 2 Large mismatched segmental perfusion defects or the arithmetic equivalent in moderate or large + moderate defects*

Intermediate Probability (20–79%)
- 1 moderate to 2 large mismatched segmental perfusion defects or the arithmetic equivalent in moderate or large + moderate defects*
- Single matched ventilation-perfusion defect with clear chest radiograph**
- Difficult to categorize as low or high, or not described as low or high

Low Probability (≤ 19%)
- Nonsegmental perfusion defects (e.g., cardiomegaly, enlarged aorta, enlarged hila, elevated diaphragm)
- Any perfusion defect with a substantially larger chest radiographic abnormality
- Perfusion defects matched by ventilation abnormality** provided that there are (a) clear chest radiograph and (b) some areas of normal perfusion in the lungs
- Any number of small perfusion defects with a normal chest radiograph

Normal
- No perfusion defects—perfusion outlines exactly the shape of the lungs seen on the chest radiograph (note that hilar and aortic impressions may be seen, and the chest radiograph and/or ventilation study may be abnormal)

*Two large mismatched perfusion defects are borderline for "high probability." Individual readers may correctly interpret individual scans with this pattern as "high probability." In general, it is recommended that more than this degree of mismatch be present for the "high probability" category.

**Very extensive matched defects can be categorized as "low probability." Single V/Q matches are borderline for "low probability" and should be considered for "intermediate" in most cases by most readers, although individual readers may correctly interpret individual scans with this pattern as "low probability."

recent attempts to do this. The PIOPED Nuclear Medicine Working Group revised the PIOPED criteria as described earlier and in Tables 30.2 and 30.3. A recent prospective trial done at Duke tested the revised PIOPED criteria (Table 30.3) and found that they were more accurate than the original PIOPED criteria, but that the "gestalt" impression of experienced readers remains the most accurate diagnostic impression (Table 30.4). The V/Q scans of 104 consecutive patients who underwent clinically motivated pulmonary angiography were reviewed by two experienced readers who had participated in the PIOPED study. The scans were described using the PIOPED scan description method. The scans were categorized according to the original PIOPED and the revised PIOPED criteria and a "gestalt" percent probability estimate was made. Additionally, the official clinical reading (original PIOPED criteria, by one of a larger group of nuclear medicine physicians) was recorded. The "gestalt" percent probability estimate was the most accurate for assessing the likelihood of PE from the scan (Mann-Whitney roc curve area = 0.836). The revised PIOPED criteria (area = 0.753) were more accurate than the original PIOPED criteria used either by the two study investigators (area = 0.650) or by the clinical nuclear medicine physicians (area = 0.584).

Recent papers by Stein, et al. (62, 63), help to make the criteria for high probability easier to apply and more sensitive. A subset of their data is shown in Tables 30.5 and

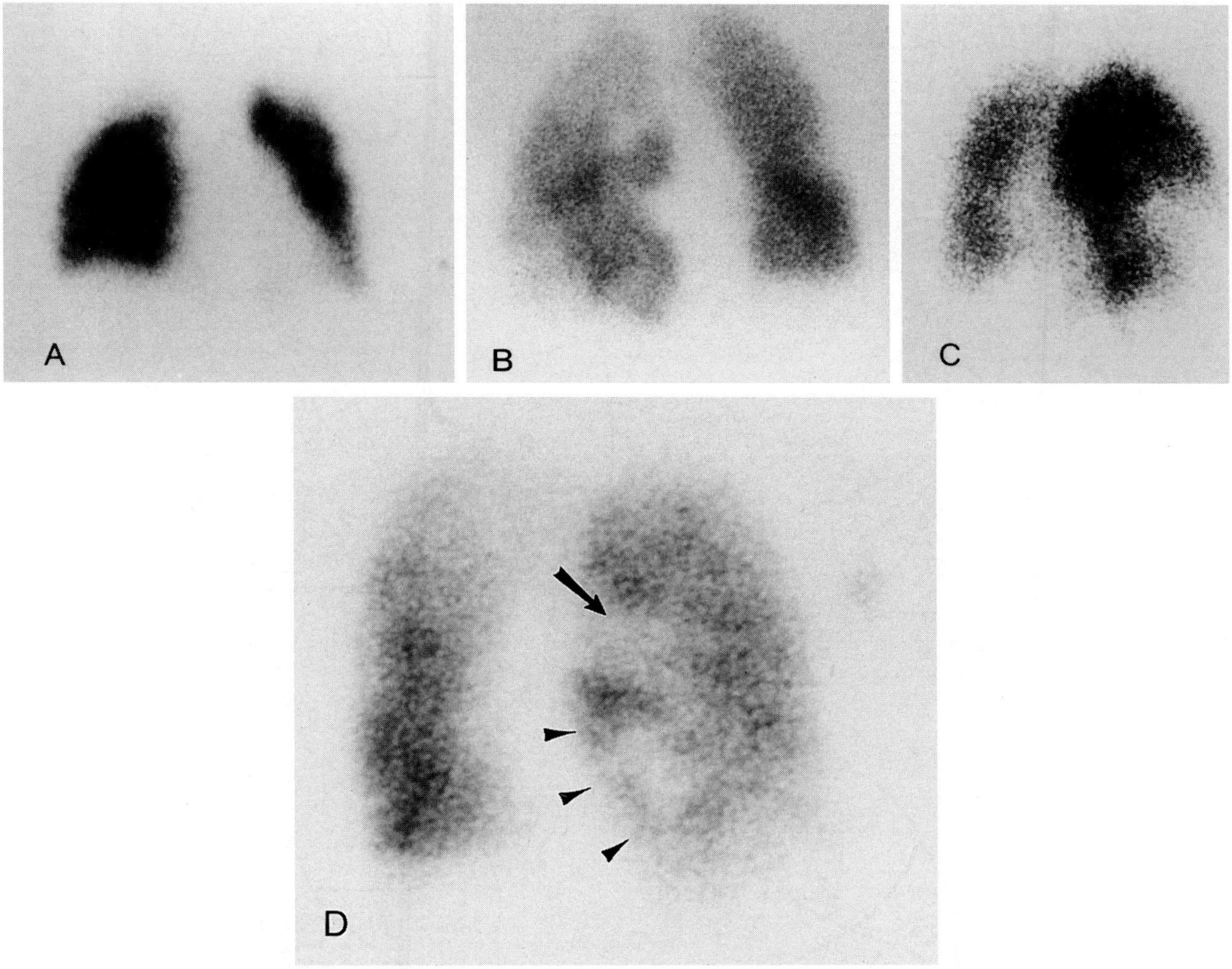

Figure 30.7. Examples of small (**A**), moderate (**B**), and large (**C**) perfusion defects. Additionally, in (**D**) two perfusion defects are shown to illustrate the difference between a segmental, pleural based large defect (*arrow*) and a defect (*arrows*) which exhibits the "stripe sign." (Reproduced with permission from Sostman HD, Gottschalk A. Prospective validation of the stripe sign in ventilation-perfusion scintigraphy. Radiology 1992;184:455–459.)

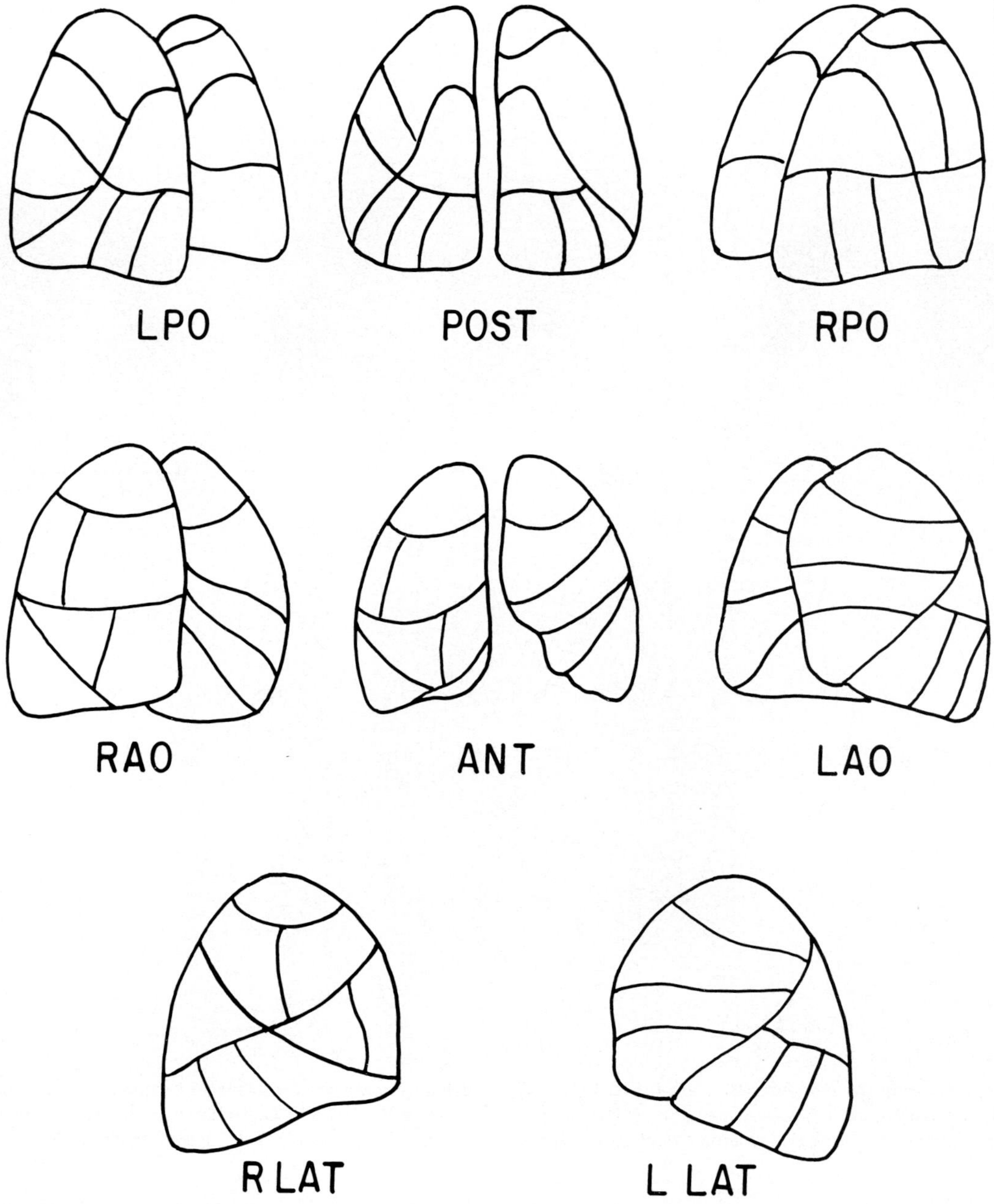

Figure 30.8. Diagrammatic Depiction of Pulmonary Segments. We use this as a reference for localizing perfusion defects. *LPO* = left posterior oblique, *POST* = posterior, *RPO* = right posterior oblique, *RAO* = right anterior oblique, *ANT* = anterior, *LAO* = left anterior oblique, *R LAT* = right lateral, *L LAT* = left lateral.

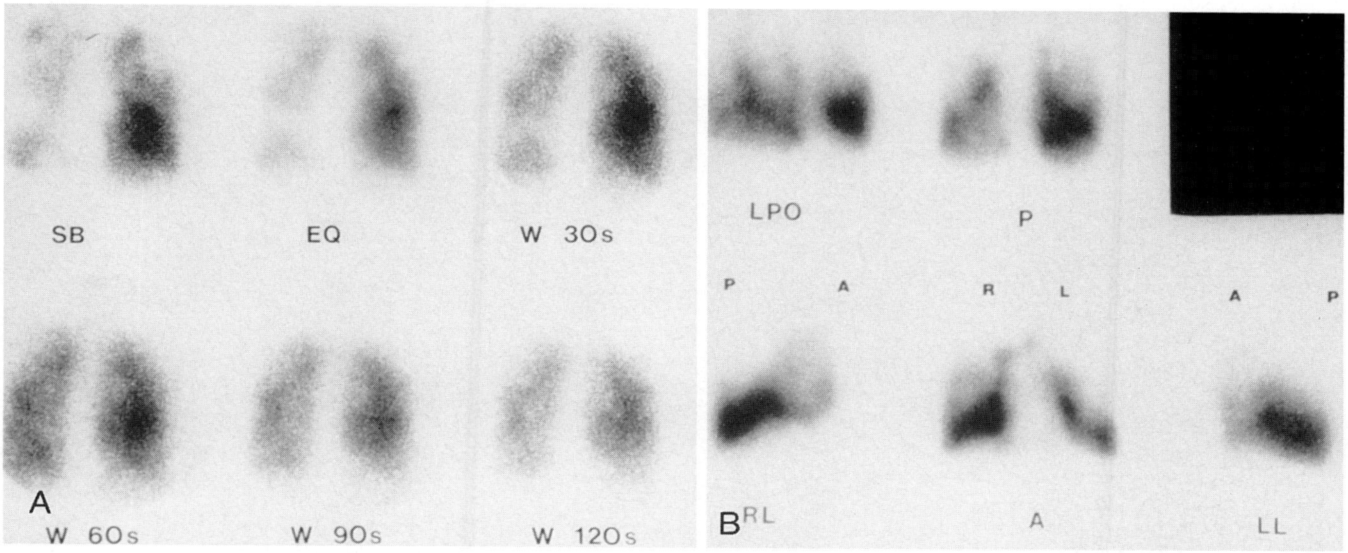

Figure 30.9. The ventilation images (**A**) and perfusion images (**B**) in this patient with COPD both show extensive abnormality, involving most of the lungs but without areas of mismatch. Most older diagnostic criteria would categorize this case as intermediate, but the PIOPED data and the revised PIOPED criteria (60) indicate that it is correctly categorized as having a low probability for PE. Pulmonary angiography was negative for PE in this case.

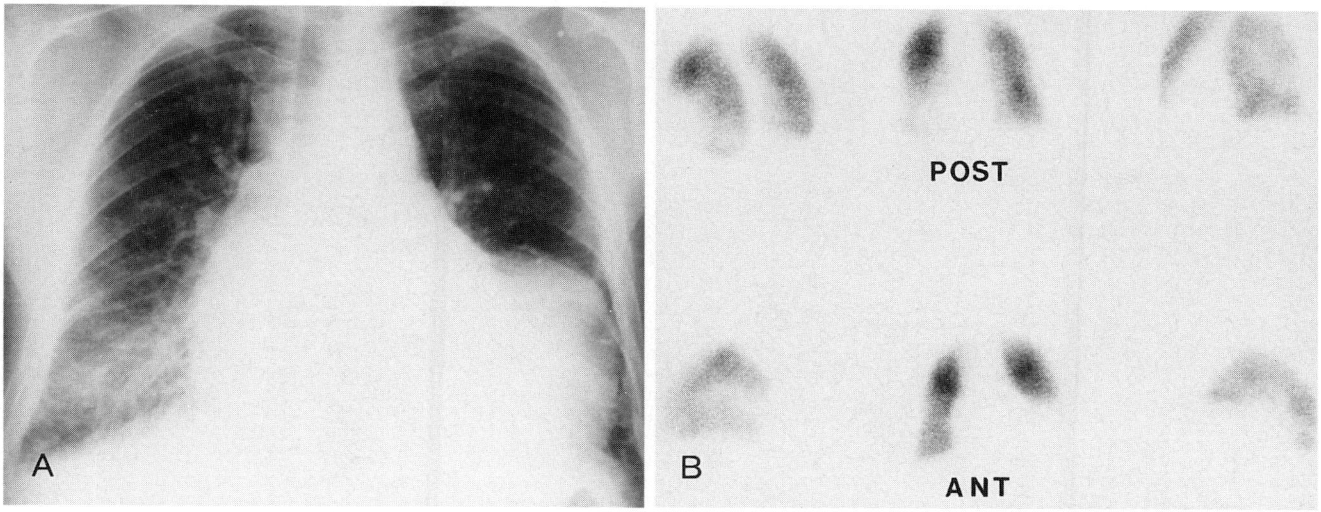

Figure 30.10. The massive cardiomegaly and left ventricular aneurysm shown on the radiograph (**A**) account for the large perfusion defect in the left lung seen on the perfusion scintigram (**B**). This defect is properly classified as nonsegmental. Overall, the study is low probability for PE. This patient did not have pulmonary embolism.

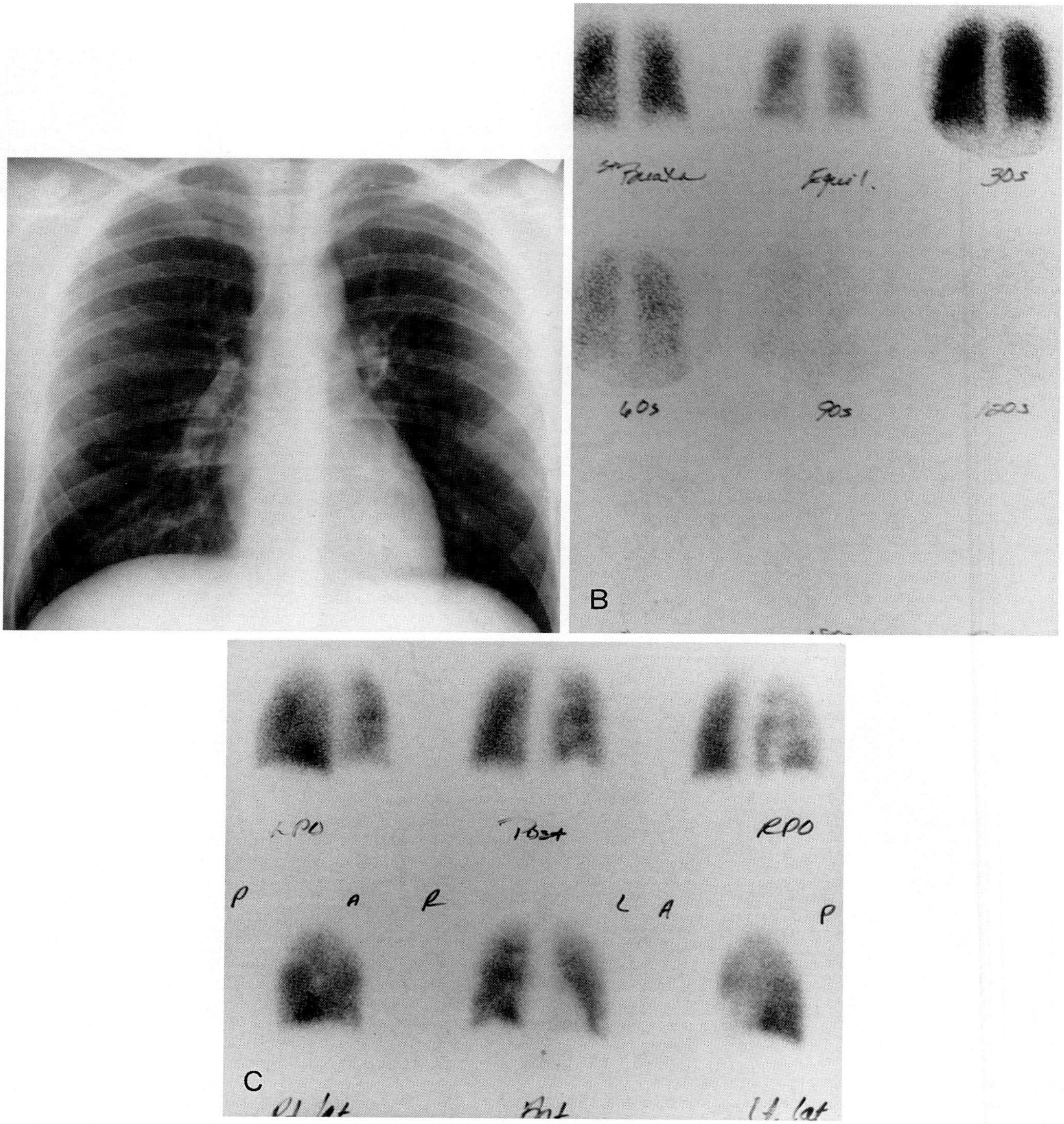

Figure 30.11. The chest radiograph (**A**) is normal except for prominence of the right descending pulmonary artery. The ventilation images (**B**) are normal. The perfusion images (**C**) demonstrate multiple small perfusion defects, particularly notable in the right lung. This scan is correctly classified as low probability. However, this patient had a large embolus in the posterior basal segment of the right lower lobe.

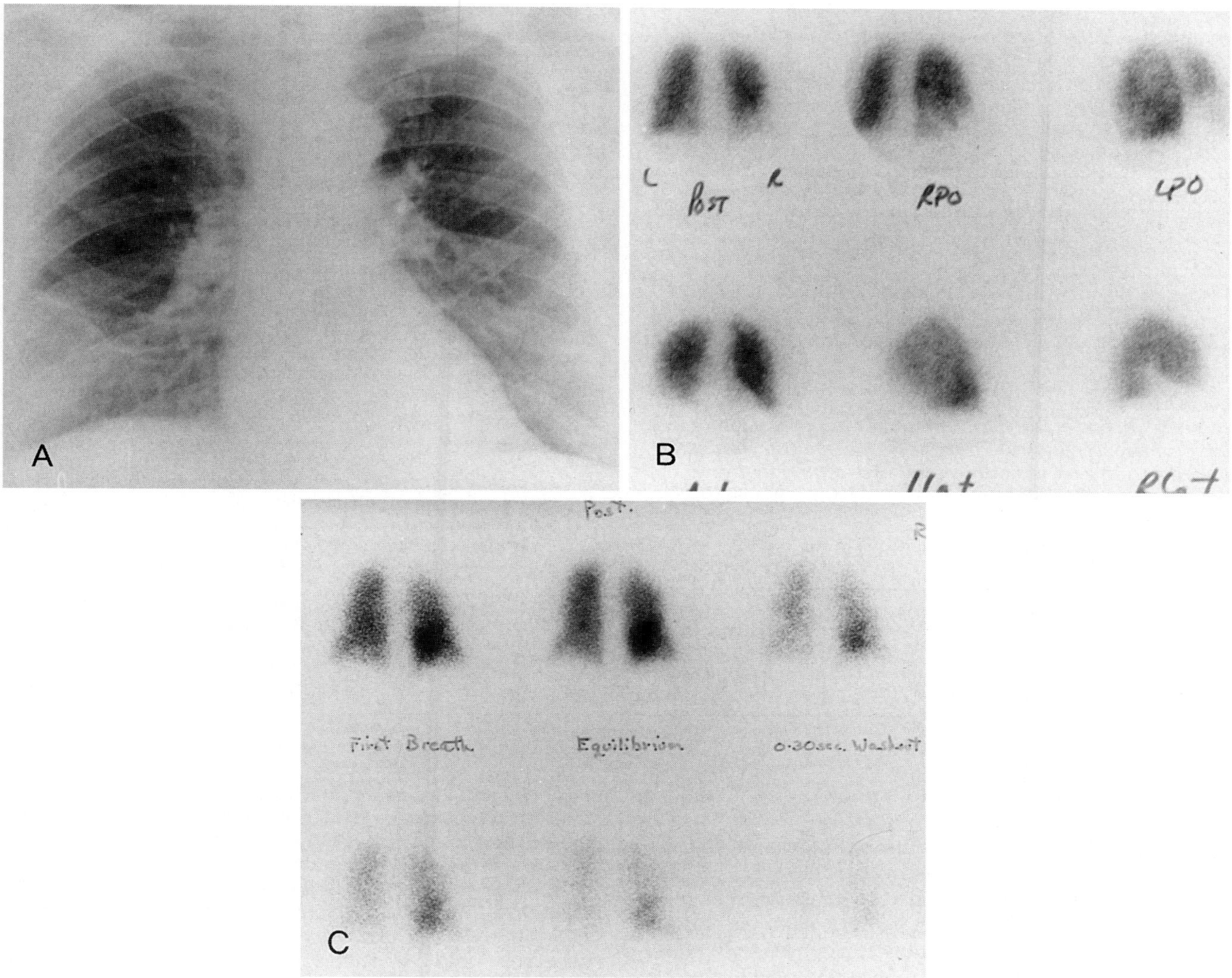

Figure 30.12. There is an opacity at the right base on the chest radiograph (**A**), matching a perfusion defect on the perfusion scintigram (**B**). Additionally, there is a single area of ^{133}Xe retention (**C**) medial to the radiographic opacity, also matched by a perfusion defect. This scan is properly classified as intermediate probability of PE. Angiography showed embolism in multiple basilar segments of the right lower lobe.

Table 30.4.
Accuracy (area under the roc curve) in 104 patients at Duke for the original PIOPED criteria (as used in the official hospital report and as used by two experienced observers) and for the revised PIOPED criteria (two experienced observers) are compared with the "gestalt" probability estimates of two experienced observers. The differences are statistically significant. (Sostman HD, Coleman RE, DeLong DM, Newman GB, Paine S. Evaluation of revised criteria for ventilation-perfusion scintigraphy in patients with suspected pulmonary embolism. Radiology 1994; 193:103–107.)

Category	Area Under ROC Curve
Hospital Report	0.584
Original PIOPED	0.650
Revised PIOPED	0.753
Gestalt	0.836

Table 30.5.
Cumulative number of mismatched moderate or large-size perfusion defects compared with sensitivity, specificity, and positive predictive value for PE in patients with no history of prior cardiopulmonary disease. (Data from Stein PD, Henry JW, Gottschalk A. Mismatched vascular defects. Chest 1993; 104:1468–1472.)

Number of Defects	Sensitivity	Specificity	PPV (95% C.I.)
≥ 1	71%	88%	80% (74–86)
≥ 2	54%	95%	89% (83–95)
≥ 3	46%	97%	91% (85–97)
≥ 4	39%	97%	89% (81–97)
> 5	32%	98%	92% (84–100)

Table 30.6.
Cumulative number of mismatched moderate or large-size perfusion defects compared with sensitivity, specificity, and positive predictive value for PE in patients who did have history of prior cardiopulmonary disease. (Data from Stein PD, Henry JW, Gottschalk A. Mismatched vascular defects. Chest 1993; 104:1468–1472.)

Number of Defects	Sensitivity	Specificity	PPV (95% C.I.)
≥ 1	63%	86%	68% (62–74)
≥ 2	51%	93%	77% (69–85)
≥ 3	44%	95%	80% (72–88)
≥ 4	40%	96%	84% (76–92)
≥ 5	37%	98%	89% (83–95)

Table 30.7.
Positive predictive value for PE in individual perfusion defects *when perfusion defects are matched by ventilation defects and radiographic abnormalities and are located with the upper, middle, or lower lung zones. (Data from Worsley DF, Kim CK, Alavia A, Palevsky HI. Detailed analysis of patients with matched ventilation-perfusion defects and chest radiographic opacities. J Nucl Med 1993; 34:1851–1853.)*

Zone	Percent of Defects Due to PE	95% C.I.
Upper	11%	3%–26%
Middle	12%	4%–23%
Lower	33%	27%–41%

30.6. Their contribution has been to indicate (a) that the segmental equivalent concept (60) does not really add to diagnostic accuracy and that the total number of large or moderate defects is the important finding and (b) that patients who have had cardiopulmonary disease previously need to have more mismatched perfusion defects to achieve the same positive predictive value as those patients who have no history of cardiopulmonary disease.

A study by Worsley, et al. (64), investigated whether the location of matched perfusion-radiographic abnormalities could be used to reduce the number of intermediate probability categorizations. Their data suggests that perfusion-radiographic matches in the upper and middle lung zones have a low likelihood (11–12%) of being associated with PE in the same zone, while those in the lower zones have a higher likelihood (33%). The data are shown in Table 30.7. Although the differences in frequency of PE between different zones are statistically significant, because of the small number of cases the confidence intervals are quite large and we do not yet feel comfortable incorporating this promising work into clinical diagnosis.

In Table 30.8 we list the criteria which we currently use for interpretation of V/Q scans in patients suspected of having pulmonary embolism. Among many issues which still need to be resolved, we mention only two. First, the significance of a single matched V/Q defect with clear chest radiograph is still not clear. The data from the PIOPED study suggests that this should be intermediate probability; however, this finding is without a physiologic rationale and a small prospective study at Duke did not necessarily confirm the PIOPED data (Table 30.9). However, in both instances the confidence intervals are very wide. Second, it is not clear whether to recommend use of the "stripe sign" in routine V/Q scan interpretation. The data shown in Table 30.10 seems to support its use, but one should note that the stripe sign is more accurate when used by experienced observers (65).

Table 30.8.
Current Duke/PIOPED V/Q Scan Criteria

High Probability (> 80%)
- No prior cardiopulmonary disease: ≥ 2 mismatched moderate or large perfusion defects
- Prior cardiopulmonary disease or uncertain: ≥ 4 mismatched moderate or large perfusion defects

Intermediate Probability (20–80%)
- Difficult to categorize or not described as low or high
- Single perfusion defect matched by ventilation abnormality

Low Probability (< 20%)
- Nonsegmental perfusion defects (e.g., cardiomegaly, enlarged hila, elevated diaphragm)
- Perfusion defect with a substantially larger chest radiographic abnormality
- Perfusion defects matched by ventilation abnormality of equal or larger size provided that there are (a) clear chest radiograph and (b) some areas of normal perfusion in the lungs
- Any number of small perfusion defects with a normal chest radiograph

Normal
- No perfusion defects—perfusion outlines exactly the shape of the lungs seen on the chest radiograph (normal hilar and aortic impressions may be seen, and the chest radiograph and/or ventilation study may be abnormal)

Notes:
1. Single perfusion defect matched by ventilation abnormality requires more investigation and is likely appropriate for low probability—may depend on coexisting factors
2. Presence of "stripe sign" (65) can be used to eliminate a perfusion defect from consideration (essentially relegating it from the "segmental" to the "nonsegmental" category)

Table 30.9.
Positive predictive value for PE in individual perfusion defects *when single perfusion defects are matched by ventilation defects in zones which are radiographically normal. (Data from The PIOPED Investigators. Value of the ventilation/perfusion scan in acute pulmonary embolism. JAMA 1990; 263:2753–2759, and Sostman HD, Coleman RE, DeLong DM, Newman GE, Paine S. Evaluation of revised criteria for ventilation-perfusion scintigraphy in patients with suspected pulmonary embolism. Radiology 1994; 193:103–107.)*

Study	N of Patients	Percent of Defects Due to PE (95% C.I.)
PIOPED	23	26% (8%–44%)
Duke	8	0% (0%–37%)

Table 30.10.
Positive predictive value for PE in individual perfusion defects *when perfusion defects exhibit the "stripe sign," (Data from Sostman HD, Gottschalk A. Prospective validation of the stripe sign in ventilation-perfusion scintigraphy. Radiology 1992; 184:455–459, and reference 1 therein.)*

Study	N of Defects	Percent of Defects Due to PE (95% C.I.)
Yale	17	6% (0%–20%)
PIOPED	85	7% (3%–15%)

Pulmonary Embolism Mimics

Numerous disease processes can result in V/Q mismatch, but fortunately most of them are quite uncommon (10). The pathology of these lesions involves the pulmonary vessels, whether in the lumen, the vessel wall, or the perivascular tissues, to produce *vascular occlusive* physiology.

The most common cause of V/Q mismatch not due to acute PE is unresolved prior PE (Fig. 30.13). One study (66) showed that as many as 35% of patients with acute pulmonary embolism have incomplete scintigraphic resolution. Data from the PIOPED study implies that prior PE is one of the most common causes of false-positive "high-probability" scans (the positive predictive value of a "high probability" scan was 91% in patients with no history of prior PE and only 74% in those with that history, $p < 0.05$). Other processes occurring in the pulmonary arterial lumen (embolism of material other than thrombus, in situ throm-

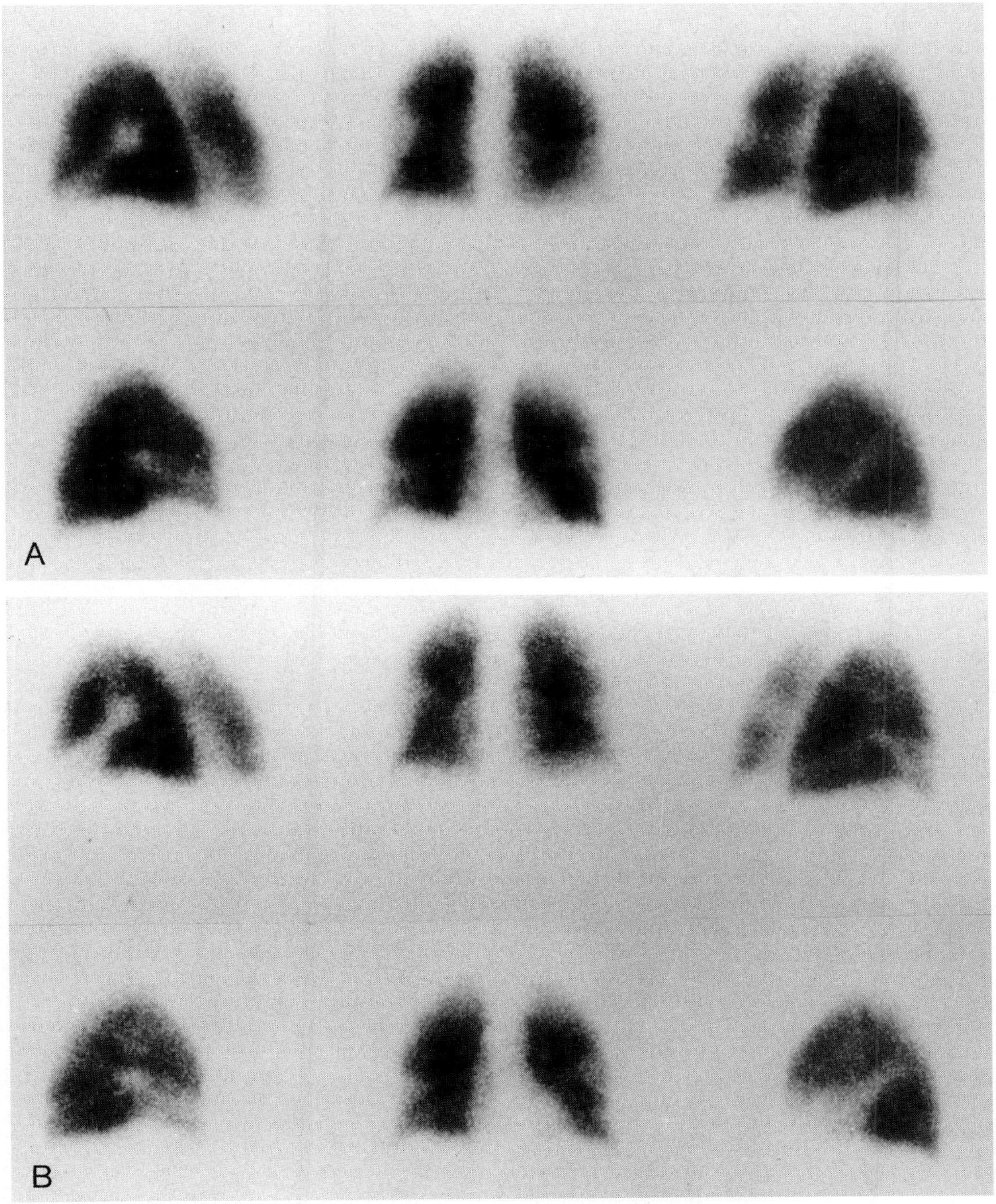

Figure 30.13. Chronic Unresolved Perfusion Defect from Previous PE. This patient has a massive embolus with significant but incomplete resolution (*A*). A subsequent study 18 months later (*B*) shows no change (except for lower display intensity). Chest radiograph and ventilation study at this time were entirely normal.

bosis or pulmonary artery tumor), processes involving the arterial wall (vasculitis, connective tissue disorder (Fig. 30.14), tuberculosis, or irradiation), vascular anomalies (pulmonary artery agenesis, peripheral coarctations (Fig. 30.15), arteriovenous malformations, or surgical pulmonic-systemic shunts) and extrinsic compression of pulmonary arteries or veins (mediastinal or hilar carcinomas or fibrosis) can result in segmental or lobar perfusion deficits. In some of these pathologic entities, the perfusion deficits may be matched by ventilatory or radiographic abnormalities, but V/Q mismatch mimicking acute pulmonary embolism can be seen in all of them.

In spite of the extensive list of possibilities, we have found that most pulmonary embolism mimics are due to one of three etiologies: (a) unresolved pulmonary embolism, (b) intravenous drug abuse, or (c) hilar or mediastinal involvement (usually by bronchogenic carcinoma). Clues to the correct diagnosis often can be found on the chest ra-

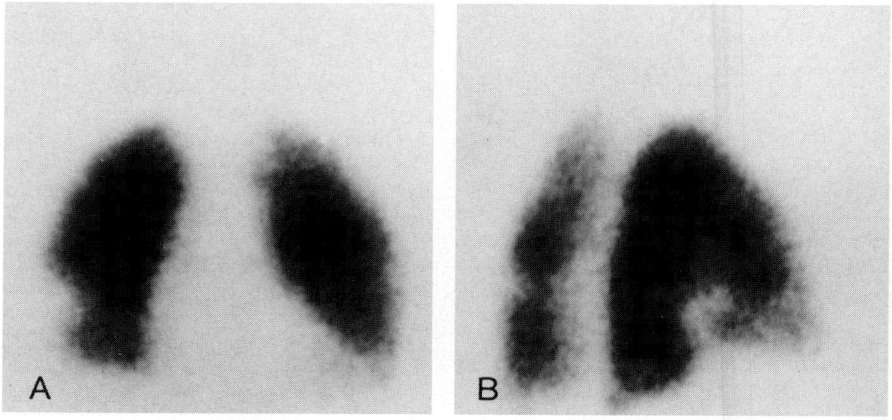

Figure 30.14. Pulmonary Emoblism Mimic. These are anterior (*A*) and right posterior oblique (*B*) perfusion images of a patient with active systemic lupus erythematois. The chest radiography showed only linear atelectasis and small pleural effusions, and the ^{133}Xe ventilation study was normal. Multiple segmental perfusion defects are obvious. The study is a nice example of a "high-probability" scan, but the pulmonary angiogram (done because of the possibility of a PE mimic) was negative. Fortunately, this is a very uncommon diagnostic problem.

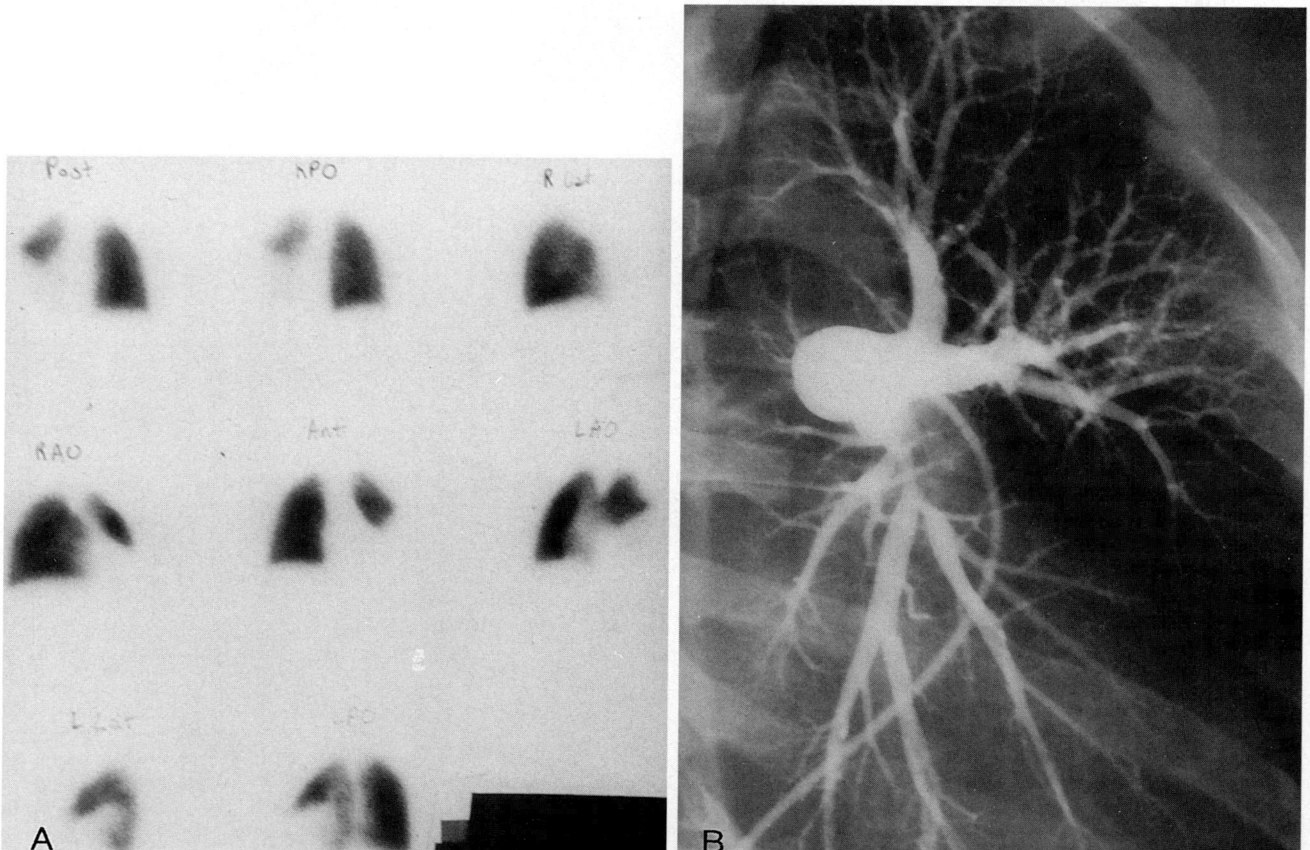

Figure 30.15. The perfusion images (**A**) demonstrate a large defect involving multiple segments of the left lung. Perfusion to the right lung is normal. On angiography (**B**) peripheral pulmonary artery coarctation is seen, which accounts for the perfusion defect. There is no evidence of acute PE.

diograph, and the patient's history is of paramount importance, since unresolved PE appears to be the most common cause of false-positive scans.

If the possibility of a PE mimic is present, it is essential to alert the referring physician of this fact, and one should obtain a baseline V/Q scan on all patients with PE about 3 months after the acute episode to avoid confusion in future interpretations.

Interpretive Pitfalls

Some physicians who interpret V/Q scans have considered perfusion defects as large or segmental only if perfusion was completely *absent*. This requirement will lead to erroneous results in the application of modern diagnostic criteria, in which only the *area* of the perfusion deficit is considered (Fig. 30.16). The rationale for using decreased or absent perfusion as abnormal is that a partially occluding embolus often produces diminished rather than absent perfusion in the involved segments.

We caution against interpreting a lesion which is visible on only a single view of the perfusion series as abnormal. It is our experience that using this finding as abnormal results in overcalling perfusion defects. The most common mistakes of this type are interpreting the defects caused by prominent aortic arch or pulmonary hila as due to PE. With an eight-view lung scan, virtually any real lesion can be identified on at least two of the eight views.

It is worth reemphasizing that the chest radiograph may become a serious pitfall in the interpretation of the V/Q scintigram. A poor quality radiograph may not show parenchymal opacities or pleural effusions which correspond to perfusion defects. Whenever possible, a standard chest radiograph should be obtained.

Finally, it is difficult to make a diagnosis of *recurrent* PE utilizing the V/Q scan alone. If a central embolus is present, it has the potential to fragment over the course of its resolution time (probably weeks), potentially causing a variety of different perfusion scan patterns. Furthermore, differential clot lysis and varying pulmonary arterial pressures may cause changing scan patterns (67). Only when the lung scan has been stable for at least 3 months before an acute change can the diagnosis of recurrent PE be considered (Fig. 30.13).

OTHER NONINVASIVE TECHNIQUES FOR IMAGING PE

Thrombus-specific scintigraphy (39), dynamic high-speed CT (68, 69), and MRI (70, 71) have been investigated extensively for their accuracy in diagnosing PE. None of them has produced results sufficiently good and sufficiently well-validated to be generally applicable to clinical work, although PE can be demonstrated in patients by all of them. Perhaps the most theoretically attractive of these methods are thrombus-specific radiopharmaceuticals and MRI because of their ability to scan the whole body. However, experience with these modalities for detecting PE is quite limited and it is too early to predict whether they will become clinically useful or whether they will join the large number of initially promising but ultimately discredited noninvasive tests for detecting PE. Even if such methods

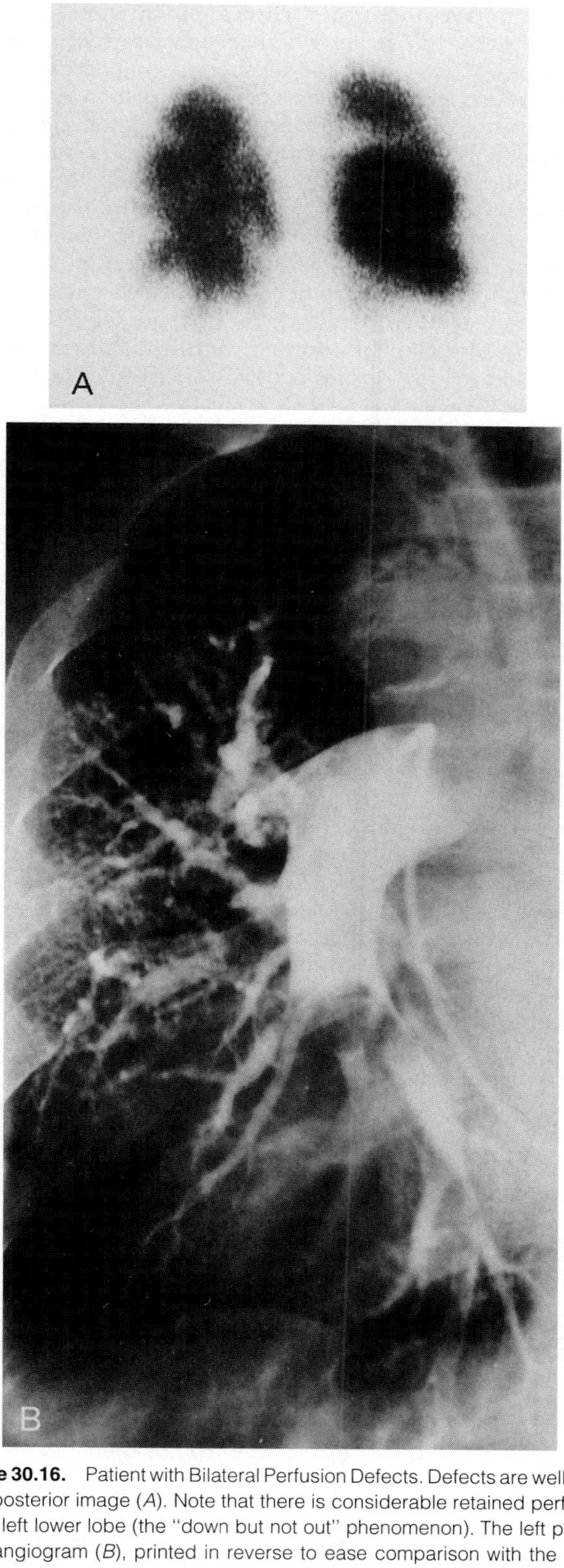

Figure 30.16. Patient with Bilateral Perfusion Defects. Defects are well seen on a posterior image (*A*). Note that there is considerable retained perfusion in the left lower lobe (the "down but not out" phenomenon). The left pulmonary angiogram (*B*), printed in reverse to ease comparison with the scan, shows extensive embolic occlusion of the lower lobe arteries. Residual diminished perfusion does *not* excluse embolic occlusion in the segment(s) involved.

prove to be accurate under clinical conditions, it is probably too early to predict whether they are more likely to replace the V/Q scan or the pulmonary angiogram in clinical management. In research experience to date, high speed (helical or electron beam) CT has yielded the highest accuracy for detecting PE and is probably the most clinically applicable. It has the potential drawback that it is not likely to be easy to use to evaluate the venous system in addition to the pulmonary arteries in a single examination.

Only when the costs, accuracy, and patient management implications of such new tests are well-characterized will it be possible to formulate rational guidelines for their use in routine clinical practice. Until that time, the V/Q scan is likely to retain its central role in the diagnosis of PE.

PATIENT MANAGEMENT AFTER THE V/Q SCAN

DIAGNOSTIC ALGORITHMS

In the PIOPED study, the combined clinical and scintigraphic diagnosis could identify subgroups of patients in whom the predictive value of the combined diagnosis was over 90% (see Table 30.11). This level of accuracy should often be sufficient for clinical management. Unfortunately, the groups of patients in whom this relatively accurate performance was possible only comprised 20% of the total population. Therefore, in the majority of patients, even after clinical evaluation and a V/Q scan, further decisions about diagnosis are necessary.

The classic diagnostic algorithms (see Fig. 30.17 for an example) have combined pretest and post-test clinical judgments of disease likelihood with liberal recommendations for arteriography. More recently, the PIOPED results have been used to recommend a more frequent use of pulmonary angiography. Other investigators have suggested that noninvasive venous imaging studies can substitute for angiography in many patients (see Fig. 30.18 for an example of this type of algorithm). This approach is based on data from the study by Hull, et al. (11). In that study, pulmonary angiography alone would have detected 77% of patients with abnormal perfusion lung scans who required anticoagulant therapy, while venous imaging alone would have identified 71%. A recent publication (72) by authors representing both the PIOPED and the Canadian prospective trials has extensively summarized the available data and provided the most detailed management algorithms yet proposed (Fig. 30.19). Some authorities (73) suggest a more radical approach, beginning the workup for PE with a venous ultrasound study rather than a V/Q scan. Recently, it has been suggested, based upon retrospective data, that evaluation of patients with low or intermediate probability V/Q scans by performing lower extremity ultrasound is more cost-effective than performing pulmonary angiography (74) when the V/Q scan result is low or intermediate probability for PE. Further, prospective, evaluation of the cost-benefit performance of newer work-up algorithms when compared to the "classic" model should yield new approaches to the diagnostic workup.

Table 30.11.
Positive predictive value of combined scan category and clinical assessment in the PIOPED study is shown together with (number of patients in category). (Data from The PIOPED Investigators. Value of the ventilation/perfusion scan in acute pulmonary embolism. JAMA 1990; 263:2753–2759, and Sostman HD, Coleman RE, DeLong DM, Newman GE, Paine S. Evaluation of revised criteria for ventilation-perfusion scintigraphy in patients with suspected pulmonary embolism. Radiology 1994; 193:103–107.)

	Clinical Probability		
Scan Category	80–100%	20–79%	0–19%
High	95% (29)	85% (80)	83% (9)
Intermediate	71% (41)	29% (236)	14% (68)
Low	43% (15)	16% (191)	4% (90)
N-NN	0% (5)	7% (62)	2% (61)

PULMONARY ANGIOGRAPHY FOR ACUTE PULMONARY EMBOLISM

Indications

In general, pulmonary arteriography is selected on the basis both of clinical probability and of V/Q scan probability rating. The potential settings in which angiography is indicated based upon the interplay of these two assessments are shown in Figures 30.17–30.19. Additionally, a pulmonary arteriogram is indicated when the treatment of pulmonary embolism would have a particularly high risk that includes patients who are at risk for complications of anticoagulant therapy (such as peptic ulcer, intracranial neoplasm, recent major surgery, or even previous heparin induced thrombocytopenia). Consideration of vena caval interruption often requires performance of arteriography. If the therapeutic consideration involves thrombolytic therapy, the embolic disease normally should be documented by an arteriogram.

An indication for emergent pulmonary angiography is in the acutely ill patient with hemodynamic compromise, in whom massive pulmonary embolism is considered and who may be a candidate for percutaneous embolectomy or emergency surgical embolectomy. Aside from this situation, there are few compelling reasons to perform pulmonary arteriography at night.

Contraindications

There are many relative contraindications to pulmonary angiography (10, 75). Appropriate recognition and management of these can reduce the risk of the subsequent angiographic procedure. These relative contraindications include a history of a previous allergic reaction to radiographic contrast material, elevated right ventricular and pulmonary artery pressures, bleeding diatheses, renal insufficiency, and left bundle branch block.

Complications of Pulmonary Angiography

The PIOPED study established pulmonary angiography as a relatively safe, but not trivial, procedure (2). The death rate was 0.3%, the minor complication rate was 4.5%, and the major nonfatal complication rate was 1.6%.

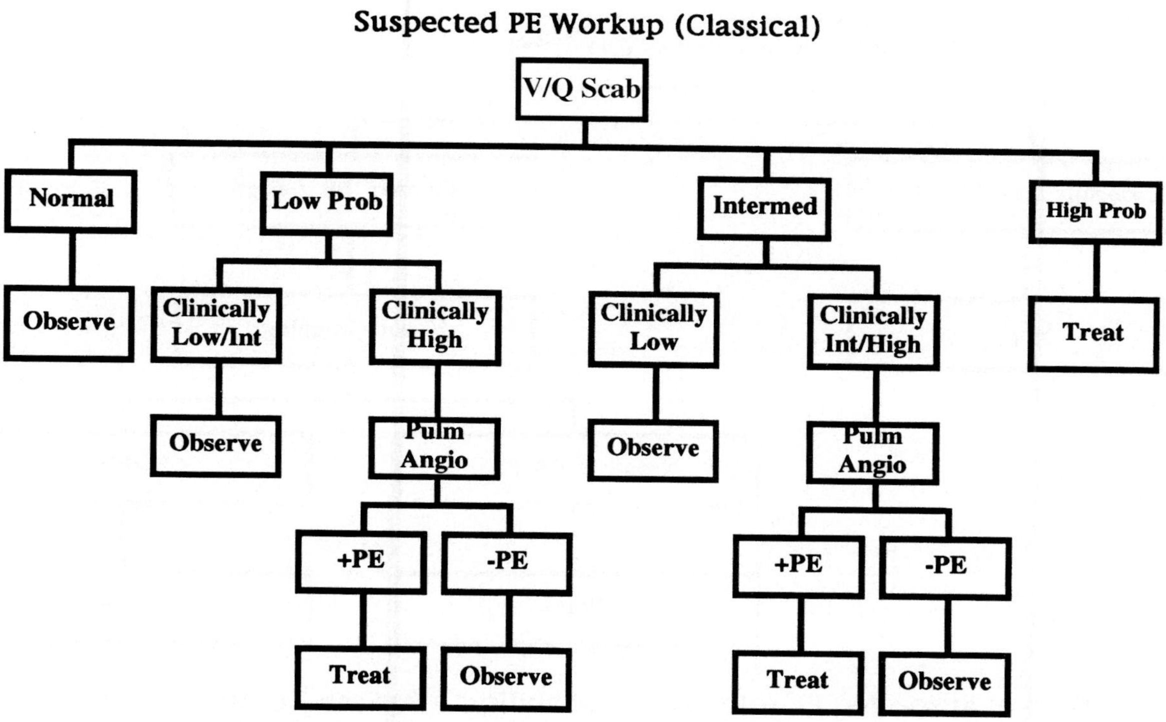

Figure 30.17. This flow chart diagrams the classical algorithm for the workup of patients with respiratory symptoms and suspected PE.

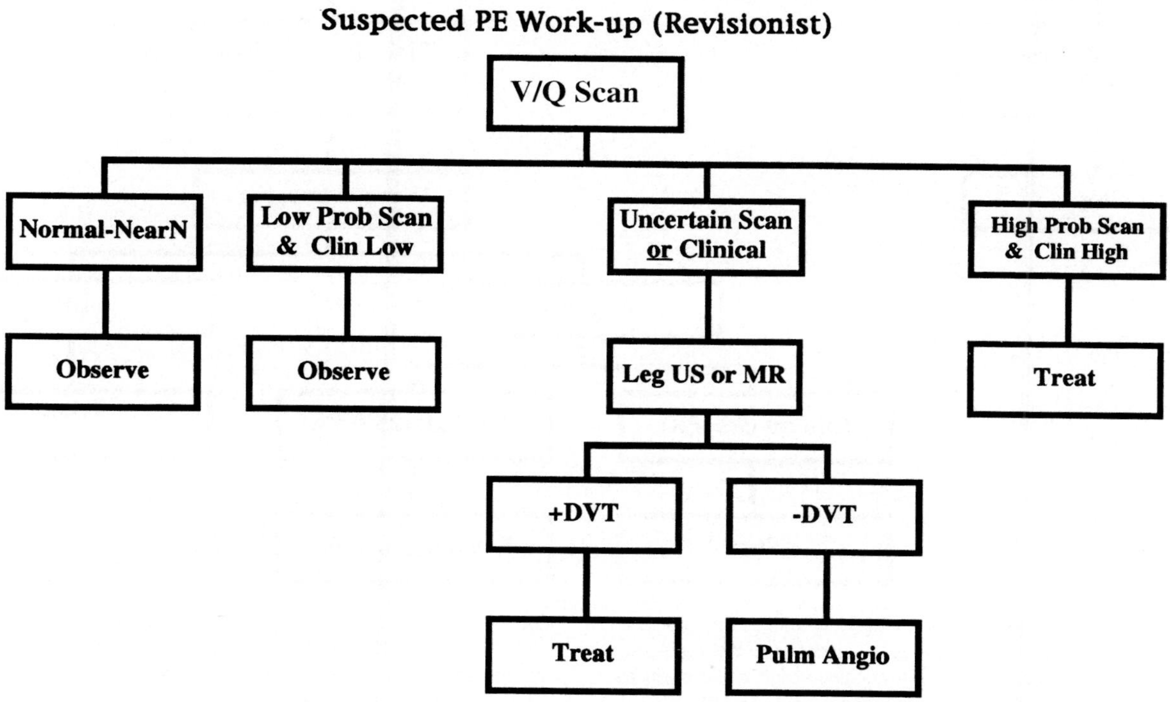

Figure 30.18. This flow chart diagrams one recently proposed algorithm for the workup of patients with respiratory symptoms and suspected PE. It differs from the classical approach by incorporating noninvasive lower extremity venous imaging into the diagnostic workup.

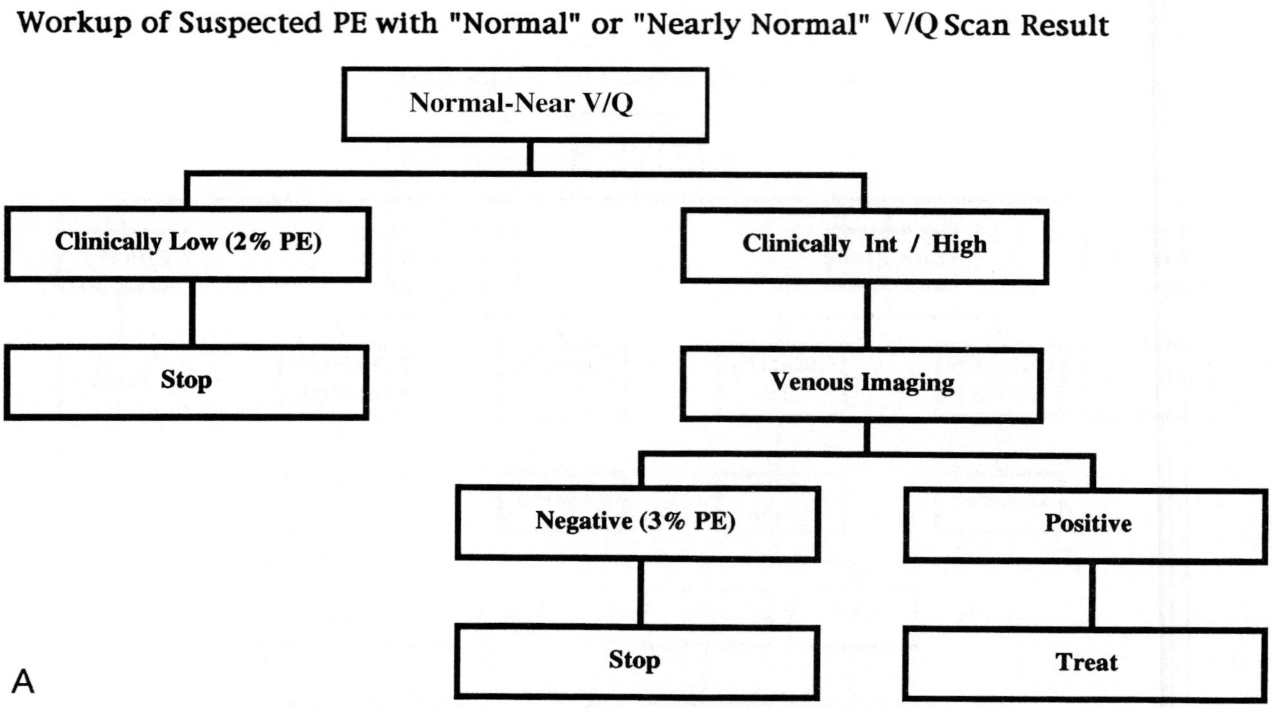

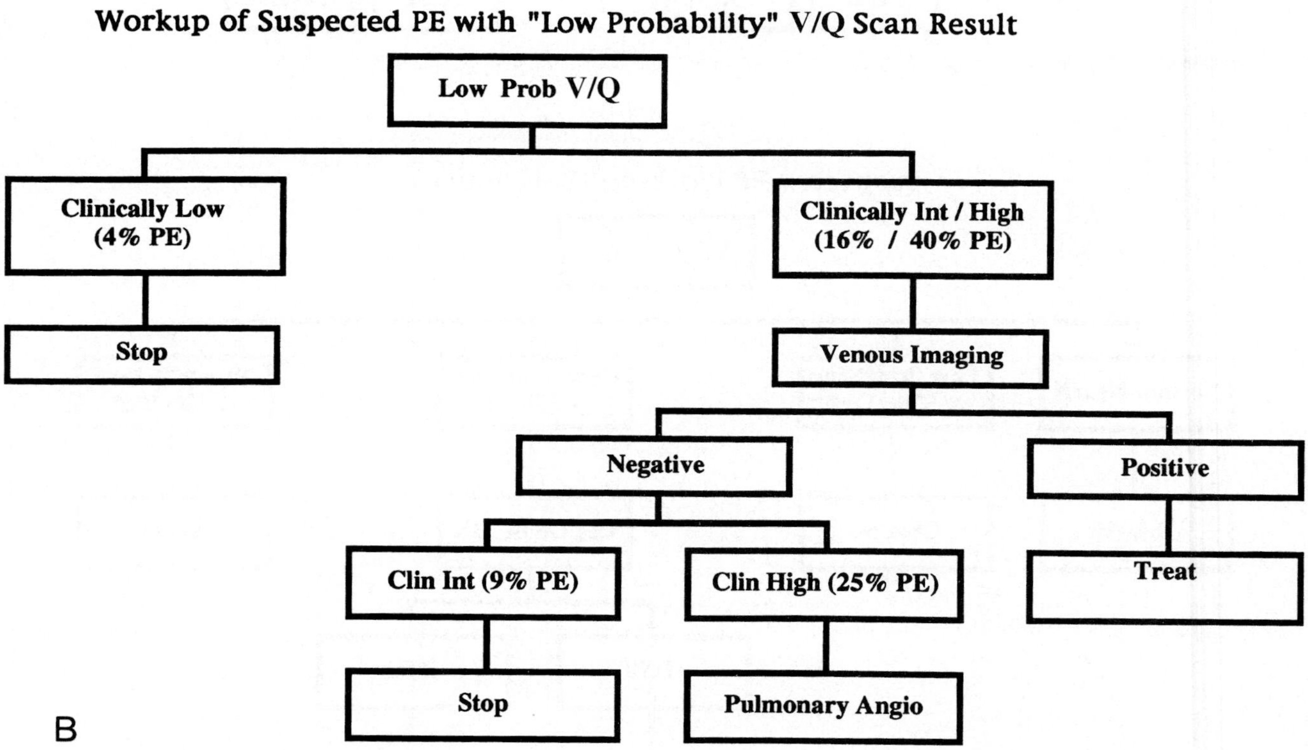

Figure 30.19. This flow chart (modified from reference 72) diagrams an extensively detailed algorithm for the workup of patients with respiratory symptoms and suspected PE. It incorporates detailed clinical probability assessments, V/Q scan results, lower extremity venous diagnostic studies, and pulmonary angiography into an overall strategy for diagnostic management of patients and relies upon prevalence data generated in the Canadian (11) and PIOPED (2) studies. **A**, **B**, **C**, and **D** show the recommended pathways following a normal or near-normal, low probability, intermediate probability, and high probability V/Q scan results.

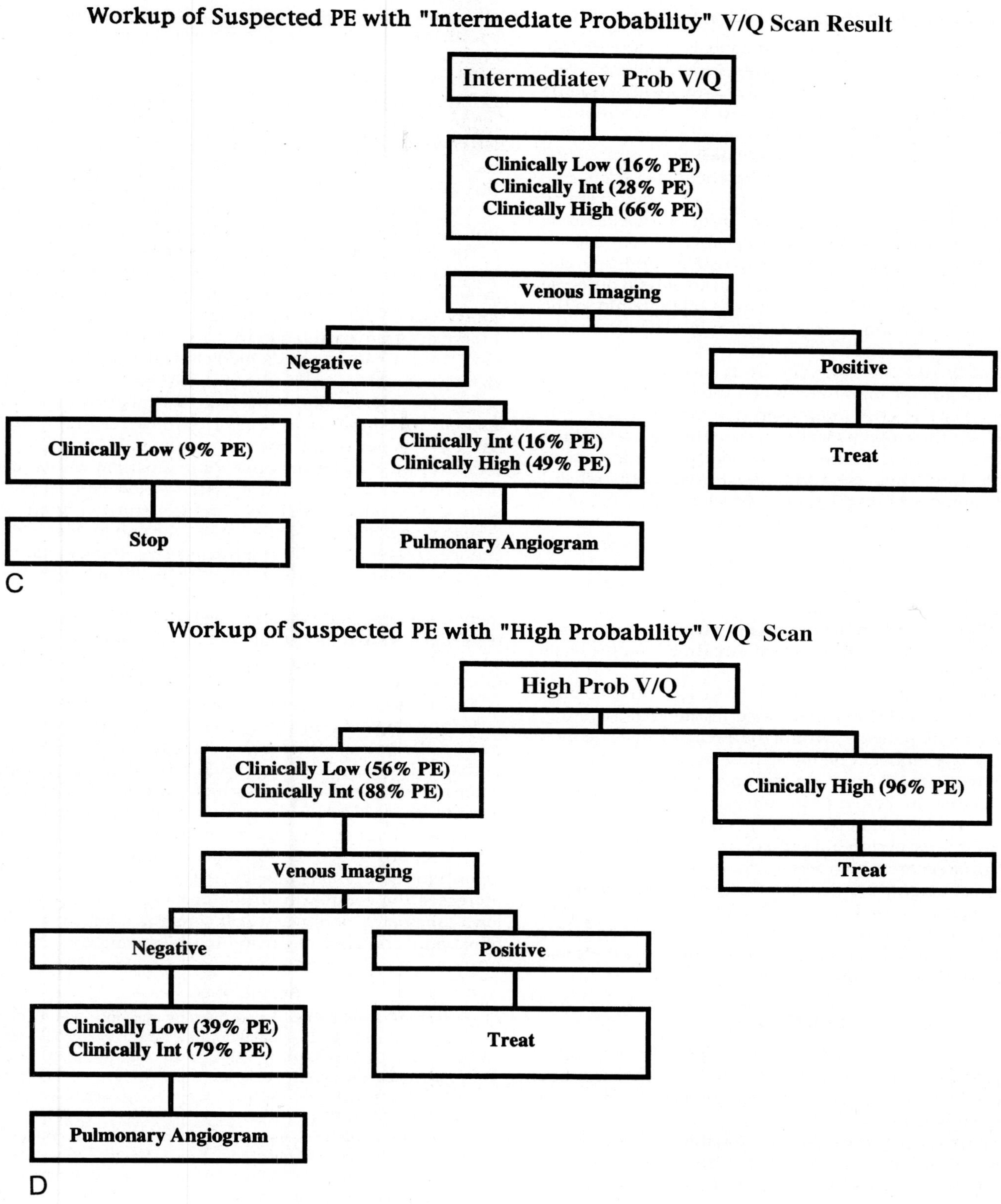

Figure 30.19—*Continued*

Diagnostic Results of Pulmonary Angiography

The angiographic criteria for the diagnosis of acute PE (10, 75) include demonstration of an intraluminal filling defect and/or demonstration of an occluded artery with a trailing edge of clot (Figs. 30.11, 30.12, and 30.16). Other findings, which are nonspecific and may be seen in many different pulmonary diseases, include diminished flow, diminished perfusion, abnormal pulmonary parenchymal stain, tortuous peripheral vasculature, and delayed venous return.

In the PIOPED study (2), the accuracy of arteriography for the diagnosis of acute PE was not investigated specifically. However, the interobserver variability and the relationship of the arteriographic diagnosis to patient outcome were investigated and bear an obvious relationship to the clinical value of pulmonary arteriography. The agreement between pairs of blinded observers as to the presence of emboli in the main pulmonary artery or lobar pulmonary artery was greater than 97%. When the embolus was in a segmental artery, the interobserver agreement was only 80%. When the embolus was in a more peripheral pulmonary arterial segment, the independent reader agreement was only 40%. Thus, even with the superb spatial resolution of pulmonary angiography, small peripheral emboli are difficult to diagnose with confidence even for acknowledged experts. However, review of clinical outcomes rarely changed angiographic diagnoses in this study. Thus, it is unlikely that clinically significant pulmonary emboli will be missed by good quality pulmonary arteriography. How many clinically insignificant, small emboli or normal patients are subjected to unnecessary treatment on the basis of angiography is unknown.

Additionally, the occurrence and distribution of solitary pulmonary emboli was investigated in the PIOPED study (2). Fifty-eight patients within the PIOPED investigation had only one embolus demonstrated by pulmonary arteriography. Four (7%) were in the main pulmonary artery, 10 (17%) were in a lobar pulmonary artery, 30 (52%) were in a segmental pulmonary artery, and an additional 14 (24%) were in a peripheral pulmonary artery. This distribution underscores the necessity for excellent quality pulmonary arteriography, including magnification technique. It also suggests a mechanism by which some patients with PE could be missed by V/Q scanning. Fortunately, in the overall study only 14 of 251 (5.6%) of patients with PE had only a solitary peripheral embolus.

SUMMARY

Since the clinical diagnosis of pulmonary embolism is elusive, imaging evaluation is necessary. The V/Q scan has been used for many years to assess the likelihood of pulmonary embolism.

Previous retrospective series, probably skewed toward problem cases, have shown patients with a high probability V/Q scan to have a 65–90% chance of having an embolus demonstrated on a pulmonary arteriogram. A large multi-institutional prospective study (PIOPED) examined all patients referred for V/Q imaging for suspected PE. Among patients with a high probability V/Q scan, 87% were confirmed to have an embolus by pulmonary arteriography. Pulmonary arteriography demonstrated pulmonary embolism in 10–35% of patients with a low probability V/Q scan in previous retrospective reviews. It is likely that these studies included patients with a high clinical suspicion of PE despite a low probability V/Q scan. The prospective PIOPED study found only 13% of patients with low probability scans to have PE. Patients with intermediate (indeterminate) scans are found to have a pulmonary embolus in approximately one-third of angiograms in both retrospective and prospective studies. Twenty-nine percent of these patients had angiographic evidence of pulmonary embolism in the PIOPED study.

The likelihood of pulmonary embolism being present can also be estimated using clinical criteria. In the PIOPED study, the clinical likelihood of pulmonary embolism, when added to the V/Q scan interpretation sometimes provided a more accurate correlation with the results of arteriography. Thus, a patient with a high clinical probability had a 43% chance of having PE when the V/Q scan was low probability, but a 4% chance when the clinical probability was also low. In certain scan categories, however, the clinical index of suspicion was not very influential. For example, there was an 83% likelihood of PE in a patient with a high probability V/Q scans even if there is a low clinical probability, although if both the clinical assessment and the V/Q scan reveal high probability of PE, the patient had a 95% chance of having PE. In other categories, the clinical impression could help to influence the likelihood of PE, but the predictive values were still not adequate for management decisions. For example, when the V/Q scan was intermediate probability, a high clinical suspicion was associated with a 71% occurrence of PE while a low clinical probability was associated with a 14% likelihood.

The decision whether or not to perform a pulmonary arteriogram depends on the degree of diagnostic certainty needed. Patients in whom the clinical and scintigraphic probabilities are concordant seldom require angiographic confirmation. The categories which most often need angiography are patients with an intermediate probability radionuclide examination and those with a low probability V/Q scan but a high clinical suspicion. Newer diagnostic algorithms add venous imaging to the decision tree, which increases the complexity of the decision process, but allows conclusive, noninvasive diagnosis in a larger number of patients and also may result in cost savings.

REFERENCES

1. Morrell MT, Dunnill MS. The postmortem incidence of pulmonary embolism in a hospital population. Br J Surg 1968;55:347–352.
2. The PIOPED Investigators. Value of the ventilation/perfusion scan in acute pulmonary embolism. JAMA 1990;263:2753–2759.
3. Dalen JE, Alpert JS. Natural history of pulmonary embolism. Prog Cardiovas Dis 1975;17:259–270.
4. Barritt DW, Jordan SC. Anticoagulant drugs in treatment of pulmonary embolism: controlled trial. Lancet 1960;1:1309–1312.
5. Moser KM, Fedullo PF, LitteJohn JK, Crawford R. Frequent asymptomatic pulmonary embolism in patients with deep venous thrombosis. JAMA 1994;271:223–225.
6. Humphries JO, Bell WR, White RI. Criteria for the recognition of pulmonary emboli. JAMA 1976;235(18):2011–2012.
7. Bell WR, Simon TL, DeMets DS. The clinical features of submassive and massive pulmonary emboli. Am J Med 1977;62:355–359.
8. Goldhaber SZ, Simons GR, Elliott CG, et al. Quantitative plasma

D-dimer levels among patients undergoing pulmonary angiography for suspected pulmonary embolism. JAMA 1993;270:2819–2822.
9. Landefeld CS, McGuire E, Cohen AM. Clinical findings associated with acute proximal deep venous thrombosis: a basis for quantifying clinical judgement. Am J Med 1990;88:382–388.
10. Pope CF, Sostman HD. Venous thrombosis and pulmonary embolism. In: Putman CE and Ravin CE, eds. Textbook of diagnostic imaging. Philadelphia: W.B. Saunders, 1983:584–604.
11. Hull RD, Hirsch J, et al. Pulmonary angiography, ventilation lung scanning and venography for clinically suspected pulmonary embolism with abnormal perfusion lung scan. Ann Intern Med 1983; 98:891–899.
12. Dorfman GS, Cronan JJ, Tupper TB, et al. Occult pulmonary emoblism: a common occurrence in deep venous thrombosis. AJR 1987;148:263–266.
13. Hull R, Hirsh J, Sackett DL, et al. Clinical validity of a negative venogram in patients with clinically suspected venous thrombosis. Circulation 1981;64:622–625.
14. Redman HC. Deep venous thrombosis: is contrast venography still the diagnostic "gold standard"? Radiology 1988;168:277–278.
15. Bettmann MA, Robbins A, Braun SD, Wetzner S, Dunnick NR, Finkelstein J. Contrast venography of the leg: diagnostic efficacy, tolerance and complication rates with ionic and nonionic contrast media. Radiology 1987;165:113–116.
16. Lensing AWA, Prandoni P, Buller HR, Casara D, Cogo A, Wouter ten Cate J. Lower extremity venography with iohexol: results and complications. Radiology 1990;177:503–505.
17. Lensing AWA, Prandoni P, Brandjes D, et al. Detection of deep-vein thrombosis by real-time B-mode ultrasonography. N Engl J Med 1989;320:342–345.
18. Vaccaro JP, Cronan JC, Dorfman GS. Outcome analysis of patients with normal compression US examinations. Radiology 1990;175:645–649.
19. Yucel EK, Fisher JS, Egglin TK, Geller SC, Waltman AC. Isolated calf venous thrombosis: diagnosis with compression US. Radiology 1991;179:443–446.
20. Murphy TP, Cronan JJ. Evolution of deep venous thrombosis: a prospective evaluation with US. Radiology 1990;177:543–548.
21. Cronan JJ, Leen V. Recurrent deep venous thrombosis: limitations of US. Radiology 1989;170:739–742.
22. Murphy TP, Cronan JJ. Evolution of deep venous thrombosis: a prospective evaluation with US. Radiology 1990;177:543–548.
23. Ginsberg JS, Caco CC, Brill-Edwards PA, et al. Venous thrombosis in patients who have undergone major hip or knee surgery: detection with compression US and impedance plethysmography. Radiology 1991;181:651–654.
24. Khaitan L, Midgette AS, Taylor CL, Zwolak RM, Stukel TA. A meta-analysis of the use of color-flow Doppler ultrasound in assessing proximal deep vein thrombosis in symptomatic compared to asymptomatic high-risk patients. Presented at the 15th Annual Meeting, Society for Medical Decision Making, Research Triangle, NC, 1993.
25. Spritzer CE, Sostman HD, Wilkes DC, Coleman RE. Deep venous thrombosis: experience with gradient-echo MR imaging in 66 patients. Radiology 1990;177:235–241.
26. Erdman WA, Jayson HT, Redman HC, Miller GL, Parkey RW, Peshock RW. Deep venous thrombosis of the extremities role of MR imaging in the diagnosis. Radiology 1990;174:425–431.
27. Vukov LF, Berquist TH, King BF. Magnetic resonance imaging for calf deep venous thrombosis. Ann Emerg Med 1991;20:497–499.
28. Evans AJ, Sostman HD, Knelson MH, et al. Detection of deep venous thrombosis: prospective comparison of MR imaging with contrast venography. AJR 1993;161:131–139.
29. Hansen ME, Spritzer CE, Sostman HD. Assessing the patency of mediastinal and thoracic inlet veins: value of MR imaging. AJR 1990;155:1177–1182.
30. Hull R, Hirsh J, Sackett DL, Stoddard G. Cost effectiveness of clinical diagnosis, venography and noninvasive testing in patients with symptomatic deep vein thrombosis. N Engl J Med 1986; 314:823–828.
31. Hull R, Hirsh J, Sackett DL, et al. Replacement of venography in suspected venous thrombosis by impedance plethysmography and 125I-fibrinogen leg scanning. Ann Int Med 1981;94:12–15.
32. Agnelli G, Cosmi B, Ranucci V, et al. Impedance plethysmography in the diagnosis of asymptomatic deep vein thrombosis in hip surgery. Arch Int Med 1991;151:2167–2171.
33. Moser KM, Brach CB, Dolan GF. Clinically suspected deep venous thrombosis of the lower extremities. A comparison of venography, impedance plethysmography and radiolabeled fibrinogen. JAMA 1977;237:2195–2198.
34. Sandler DA, Duncan JS, Ward P, et al. Diagnosis of deep vein thrombosis: comparison of clinical evaluation, ultrasound, plethysmography and venoscan with x-ray venogram. Lancet 1984;2; 716–719.
35. Gomes AS, Webber MM, Buffkin D. Contrast venography vs. radionuclide venography: a study of discrepancies and their possible significance. Radiology 1982;142:719–728.
36. Secker-Walker R, Potchen EJ. Radiology of venous thrombosis-current status. Radiology 1971;101:449–452.
37. Ryo UI, Srikantswam YS, Pinsky S. Radionuclide venography: correlation with contrast venography. J Nucl Med 1977;18:11.
38. Henkin RE. Radionuclide venography. In: Gottschalk A, Hoffer PB, Potchen EJ, eds. Diagnostic nuclear medicine. Baltimore: Williams & Wilkins, 1988:475–481.
39. Knight LC. Scintigraphic methods for detecting vascular thrombus. J Nucl Med 1993;34:554–561.
40. Knight LC, Olexa SA, Malmud LS, Budzynski AZ. Specific uptake of radioiodinated fragment El by venous thrombi in pigs. J Clin Invest 1983;72:2007–2013.
41. Alavi A, Palevsky HI, Gupta N, et al. Radiolabeled antifibrin antibody in the detection of venous thrombosis: preliminary results. Radiology 1990;175:79–85.
42. Ezekowitz MD, Pope CF, Sostman HD, et al. In-111 platelet scintigraphy for the diagnosis of deep venous thrombosis. Circulation 1986;73:668–674.
43. Palabrica TM, Furie BC, Konstam MA, et al. Thrombus imaging in a primate model with antibodies specific for an external membrane protein of activated platelets. PNAS USA 1989;86:1036–1040.
44. Greenspan RH, Ravin CE, Polansky SM, McLoud TC. Accuracy of the chest radiograph in diagnosis of pulmonary embolism. Invest Radiol 1982;17:539543.
45. McNeil BJ, Holman L, Adelstein J. The scintigraphic definition of pulmonary embolism. JAMA 1974;227:753–756.
46. Krasnow AZ, Isitman AT, Collier BD, et al. Diagnostic applications of radioaerosols in nuclear medicine. In: Freeman LM, ed. Nuclear medicine annual 1993. New York: Raven Press, 1993:123–193.
47. Alderson PO, Biello DR, Gottschalk A, et al. Tc-99m-DTPA aerosol and radioactive gases compared as adjuncts to perfusion scintigraphy in patients with suspected pulmonary embolism. Radiology 1984;153:515–521.
48. Ramanna L, Alderson PO, Berman D, et al. Comparison of Tc-99m-DTPA aerosol and radioactive gas ventilation studies in patients with suspected pulmonary embolism. J Nucl Med 1986; 27:1391–1396.
49. Alderson PO, Doppman JL, Diamond SS, Mendenhall KG, Barron EL, Girton M. Ventilation-perfusion lung imaging and selective pulmonary angiography in dogs with experimental pulmonary embolism. J Nucl Med 1978;19:164–171.
50. Secker-Walker RH, Siegel BA. The use of nuclear medicine in the diagnosis of lung disease. Radiol Clin North Am 1973;11:215–241.
51. Wagner HN Jr, Lopez-Majano V, Langan JK, et al. Radioactive xe-

non in the differential diagnosis of pulmonary embolism. Radiology 1968;91:1168–1174.
52. DeNardo GL, Goodwin DA, Ravasini R, et al. The ventilatory lung scan in the diagnosis of pulmonary embolism. N Engl J Med 1970; 282:1334–1336.
53. Alderson PO, Rujanavech N, Secker-Walker RH, et al. The role of 133-xenon ventilation studies in the scintigraphic detection of pulmonary embolism. Radiology 1976;120:633–640.
54. Neumann RD, Sostman HD, Gottschalk A. Current status of ventilation-perfusion imaging. Semin Nucl Med 1980;10:198–217.
55. Kotlyarov EV, Reba RC. The concept of using abnormal V/Q segment equivalents to refine the diagnosis of pulmonary embolism [Abstract]. Invest Radiol 1981;16:383.
56. Alderson PO, Biello DR, Sachariah KG, et al. Scintigraphic detection of pulmonary embolism in patients with obstructive pulmonary disease. Radiology 1981;138:661–666.
57. Biello DR, Mattar AG, McKnight RC, et al. Ventilation-perfusion studies in suspected pulmonary embolism. AJR 1979;133:1033–1037.
58. Carter WD, Brady TM, Keyes JW, et al. Relative accuracy of two diagnostic schemes for detection of pulmonary embolism by ventilation-perfusion scintigraphy. Radiology 1982;145:447–451.
59. Gottschalk A, Juni JE, Sostman HD, et al. Ventilation-perfusion scintigraphy in the PIOPED study. Data collection and tabulation. J Nucl Med 1993;34:1109–1118.
60. Gottschalk A, Sostman HD, Juni JE, et al. Ventilation-perfusion scintigraphy in the PIOPED study. Evaluation of the scintigraphic criteria and interpretations. J Nucl Med 1993;34:1119–1126.
61. Sullivan DC, Coleman RE, Mills SR, Ravin CE, Hedlund LW. Lung scan interpretation: effect of different observers and different criteria. Radiology 1983;149:803–807.
62. Stein PD, Gottschalk A, Henry JW, Shivkumar K. Stratification of patients according to prior cardiopulmonary disease and probability assessment based on the number of mismatched segmental equivalaent perfusion defects. Chest 1993;104:1461–1467.
63. Stein PD, Henry JW, Gottschalk A. Mismatched vascular defects. Chest 1993;104:1468–1472.
64. Worsley DF, Kim CK, Alavia A, Palevsky HI. Detailed analysis of patients with matched ventilation-perfusion defects and chest radiographic opacities. J Nucl Med 1993;34:1851–1853.
65. Sostman HD, Gottschalk A. Prospective validation of the stripe sign in ventilation-perfusion scintigraphy. Radiology 1992; 184:455–459.
66. Paraskos VA, Adelstein SJ, Smith RE, et al. Late prognosis of acute pulmonary embolism. N Engl J Med 1973;289:55–58.
67. Alderson PO, Dzebolo NN, Biello DR, Seldin DW, Martin EC, Siegel BA. Serial lung scintigraphy: utility in diagnosis of pulmonary embolism. Radiology 1983;149:797–802.
68. Remy-Jardin M, Remy J, Wattine L, Giraud F. Central pulmonary thromboembolism: diagnosis with spiral volumetric CT with the single-breath-hold technique—comparison with pulmonary angiography. Radiology 1992;185:381–387.
69. Chintapolli K, Thorsen MK, Olsen DL, Goodman LR, Gurney J. Computed tomography of pulmonary thromboembolism and infarction. JCAT 1988;12:553–559.
70. Grist TM, Sostman HD, MacFall JR, et al. Pulmonary angiography using MRI: initial clinical experience. Radiology 1993;189:528–530.
71. Schiebler ML, Holland GA, Hatabu H, et al. Suspected pulmonary embolism: prospective evaluation with pulmonary MR angiography. Radiology 1993;189:125–131.
72. Stein PD, Hull RD, Saltzman HA, Pineo G. Strategy for diagnosis of patients with suspected acute pulmonary embolism. Chest 1993;103:1553–1559.
73. Murray JF. Pulmonary embolism. Clinical evaluation and treatment. Fleischner Society. Proceedings, 21st Annual Symposium on Chest Disease, 1991:41–45.
74. Beecham RP, Dorfman GS, Cronan JJ, Spearman MP, Murphy TP, Scola FH. Is bilateral lower extremity compression sonography useful and cost-effective in the evaluation of suspected pulmonary embolism? AJR 1993;161:1289–1292.
75. Sostman HD, Rapoport S, Gottschalk A, Greenspan RH. Imaging of pulmonary embolism. Invest Radiol 1986;21:443–454.

31 Scintigraphic Studies of Nonembolic Lung Disease

BRUCE R. LINE

Although the use of scintigraphy in nonembolic disease is much less frequent than that for thromboembolic disease, the diagnostic and technical challenges in nonembolic disease are far greater for the practitioner of Nuclear Medicine. Over the past decades, scintigraphic evaluations of pulmonary function, inflammation, infection, and metabolic disorders were developed and applied clinically. The initial portion of this chapter discusses the functional, technical, metabolic, and molecular principles that underlie these scintigraphic studies. This introduction is followed by a review of the clinical experience gained from applying these scintigraphic studies to nonembolic lung disease.

SCINTIGRAPHIC METHODS OF LUNG FUNCTION ASSESSMENT

SCINTIGRAPHIC PATTERNS OF PULMONARY DYSFUNCTION

Respiratory gas transfer occurs under optimum conditions when the rates of capillary perfusion and alveolar ventilation are nearly matched. With mismatch, the ability of the alveolar-capillary unit to maintain its function declines. Thus, the presence of parenchymal disease can be detected by local abnormalities in the distribution of ventilation or perfusion. Scintigraphic studies of the normal lung demonstrate homogeneous patterns of matched ventilation and perfusion, a pattern that is disturbed in the presence of lung disease. For the sake of simplicity, the myriad of pathologic conditions affecting the lung may be divided into four functional categories: vascular occlusive, consolidative, obstructive, and restrictive states (Fig. 31.1). Each of these pathophysiologic conditions is associated with scintigraphically detectable distortions of ventilation and perfusion.

Vascular occlusive conditions include those caused by pulmonary emboli, neoplastic vascular compression, or pulmonary vasculitis. Ventilation is unaffected because occlusions in the pulmonary arterial tree usually leave alveoli structurally intact (Fig. 31.1**A**). Nonetheless, airway constriction may be caused either by substances released from emboli or by reduced alveolar carbon dioxide, a potent airway dilator. This response usually is transient and is not commonly observed in scintigraphic studies (1). In the absence of this effect, ventilation is preserved in regions of vascular occlusion; that is, a functional ventilation-perfusion mismatch is seen.

The consolidative state (Fig. 31.1**B**) is found when pulmonary infarction occurs with pulmonary embolism (2), as well as in many types of infection and inflammatory lung disease. With inadequate supplies of oxygen for alveolar metabolism, pulmonary surfactant production may be inhibited, leading to alveolar collapse and atelectasis. Injury to the capillary bed causes increased capillary permeability and a leak of intravascular fluid into the alveolar space, worsening the abnormalities. Although the degree of ventilation or perfusion loss can vary, both are usually markedly reduced.

The obstructive state (Fig. 31.1**C**) is found in chronic lung diseases such as emphysema, bronchitis, or bronchiectasis, and in acute asthmatic exacerbations. Destructive loss of alveolar walls and the capillary bed in emphysema increases alveolar volume and decreases the surface area for gas exchange. Partial airway obstruction can occur either from loss of structural support or from excessive bronchial secretions, bronchospasm, or foreign bodies, all of which serve to increase resistance to airflow and decrease alveolar oxygen tension. The precapillary sphincters respond to alveolar hypoxia by constricting, protecting the patient from large shunts of unoxygenated blood. This state is associated with increased regional lung volumes, reduced ventilation, and matched perfusion abnormalities. Reduced perfusion results from either loss of capillary bed or hypoxic vasoconstriction (Fig. 31.2).

The morphologic features of restrictive lung disease (Fig. 31.1**D**) are caused by chronic inflammation and fibrosis, which may eventually obliterate alveoli (3). Fibrotic alveolar stiffening, however, helps to keep the airways from collapsing. Furthermore, because secretions are not excessive in this state, ventilation may be preserved or even increased through decreases in alveolar compliance. Because capillaries become entrapped by thickened and inflamed alveolar walls, regional ventilation usually is increased relative to perfusion (3).

VENTILATION AND PERFUSION SCANS IN ASSESSMENT OF REGIONAL FUNCTION

Physiologic Factors Affecting Lung Images

Perfusion Images. Pulmonary blood flow increases toward the bottom of the upright lung. Its gradient of change is determined by the relationships between alveolar, capillary arterial, and capillary venous pressures (4). The upright lung may be divided into four contiguous physiologic zones (Fig. 31.3), beginning with the most apical (zone 1), and progressing to the most basal (zone 4). In zone 1, there is little blood flow because the alveolar pressure in the apex exceeds both capillary arterial and venous pressures. Slightly lower, in zone 2, the capillary arterial pressure gradually increases above the alveolar pressure, and blood flow increases in proportion to the difference. Lower still, in zone 3, both capillary arterial and venous pressures are greater than the alveolar pressure, causing full distention of the capillary. Here flow is dependent on the difference

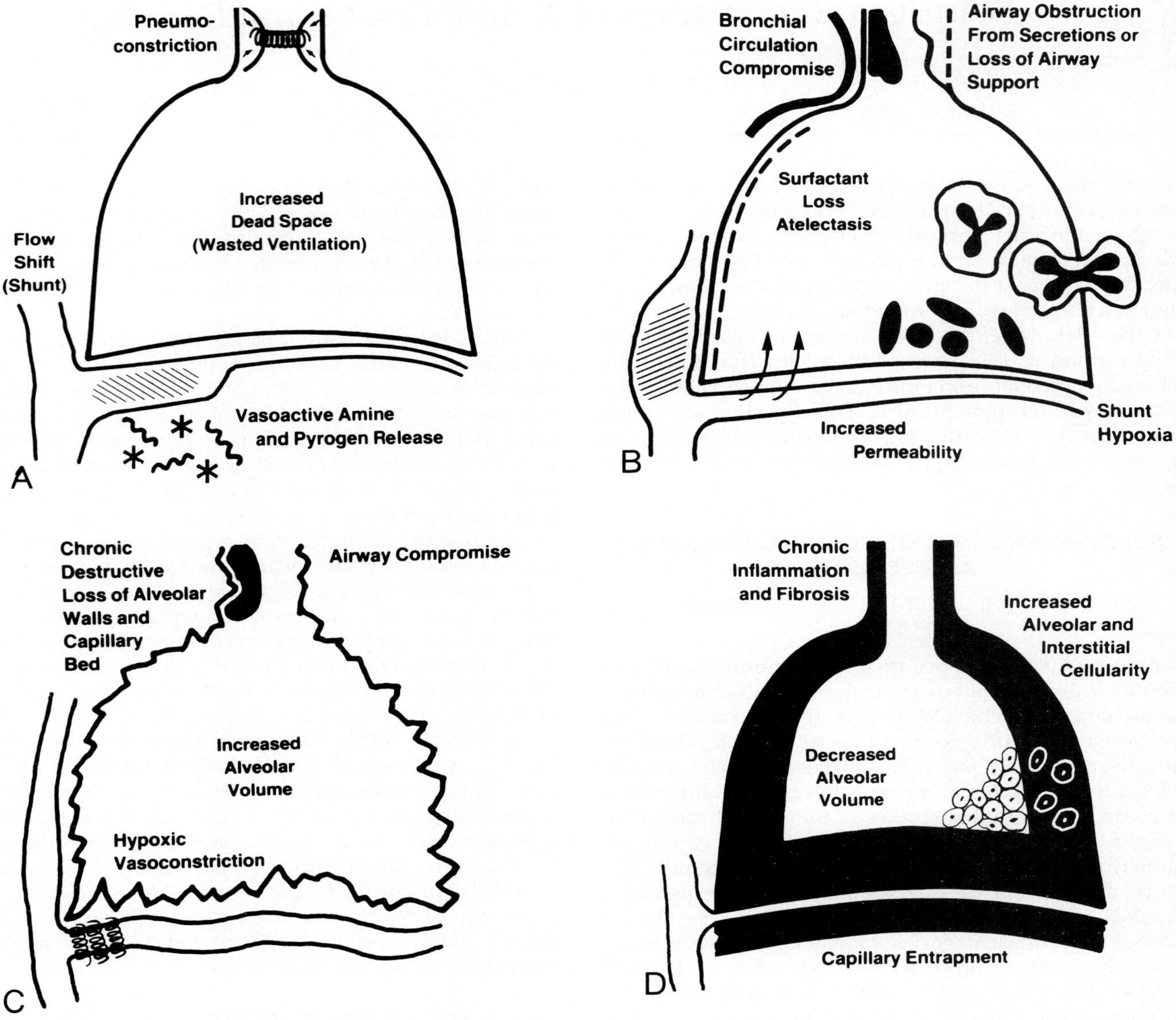

Figure 31.1. Four functional categories of pulmonary pathology. **A.** Vascular occlusive disease, here represented by pulmonary embolism, produces mechanical obstruction to blood flow and increased ventilatory dead space. **B.** Consolidative disease as caused by either pulmonary infection or embolic infarction. Rarely, bronchoconstriction may occur. **C.** Obstructive disease as found in pulmonary emphysema associated with increased lung volumes, reduced ventilation, and perfusion abnormalities from loss of capillary bed or hypoxic vasoconstriction. **D.** Restrictive disease characterized by capillary entrapment and reduced alveolar volume secindary to chronic inflammation and fibrosis.

between the arterial and venous pressures alone. At the bottom of the lung, in zone 4, flow may be reduced by compression of the lung from abdominal viscera or perivascular fluid.

Gravitational effects on the lung cause the apex to base perfusion gradient to be nearly homogeneous horizontally. Although nearly every disease condition affecting the lung will disturb regional perfusion, normal subjects have homogeneous blood flow patterns well into middle age. Fedullo and coworkers (5, 6) found that it was very uncommon for either smokers or nonsmokers between the ages of 30 and 49 to have abnormal perfusion scans.

Ventilation Images. The distribution of ventilation is altered by abnormal airway resistance and/or abnormal alveolar compliance. These abnormalities are important scintigraphically, because they determine the local rates of arrival or elimination of gases like xenon or krypton, as well as the extent of aerosol deposition (Fig. 31.4). For example, the regional clearance time of xenon is roughly proportional to the product of local compliance and airway resistance.

Compliance is expressed as the ratio of the change in lung volume to a change in distending pressure. Alveoli with low compliance due to stiffening by interstitial fluid or

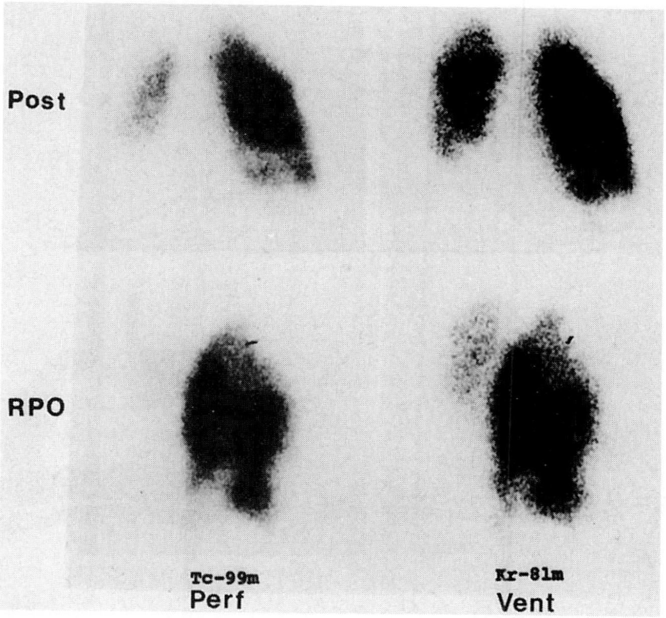

Figure 31.2. Obstructive airway disease. Selected ^{99m}Tc perfusion (*Perf*) and ^{81m}Kr ventilation (*Vent*) images illustrate the pattern of matching ventilation-perfusion abnormalities seen in obstructive airway disease. ^{81m}Kr studies show the regional distribution of tidal ventilation. In patients with airway disease, ^{81m}Kr images often reveal distributions of activity that are virtually identical to those seen in the same perfusion view. Such close similarity is illustrated in this patient, who had obstructive airway disease. The likelihood for such similarity is enhanced by the fact that the ^{81m}Kr image is obtained immediately after each perfusion image by having the patient inhale ^{81m}Kr in the same position in which the perfusion view was obtained (i.e., without moving the patient). *Post* = posterior; *RPO* = right posterior oblique.

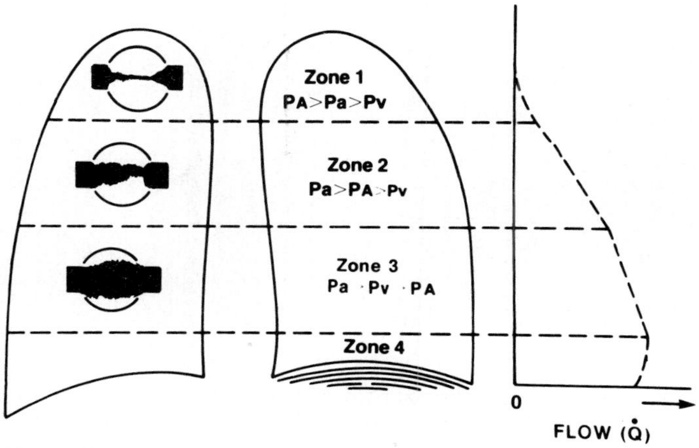

Figure 31.3. Effect of gravitational gradients on the distribution of pulmonary perfusion. Zones of perfusion in upright patients. The gradient of perfusion is determined by the relationships between alveolar, arterial capillary, and venous capillary pressures.

fibrosis have small volumes and exchange a large fraction of their volume with each respiration. Alveoli with increased compliance, as found in chronic obstructive pulmonary disease, usually have reduced wall integrity. They are larger than normal for a given transpulmonary pressure and exchange a smaller fraction of their internal volume during respiration. This fractional exchange (i.e., flow per unit alveolar volume) is an important physiologic determinant of the oxygen-carbon dioxide exchanging capability and affects the rate of tracer arrival and clearance in ventilation images.

Regional airway resistance is the second major factor determining the distribution of lung ventilation. For a given change in inflation pressure, gas flow is inversely related to airway resistance (i.e., the higher the resistance, the lower the flow). Increased airway resistance can be caused by any process that reduces the airway diameter. Increased airway secretions, bronchospasm, the presence of foreign bodies, extrinsic airway compression, parenchymal strictures, and loss of supporting lung tissue that normally keeps the airway patent, all can increase resistance to airflow.

The combined influences of regional compliance and resistance affect the rate of tracer localization and removal. The product of a region's resistance and compliance is its time constant. This time constant or "clearance time" is simply the time required to exchange the volume of gas in the region once. It also is equal to 1.44 times the effective tracer half-life in the region. Time constants of 200 seconds or longer are common in regions of severe obstructive airway disease where both the airway resistance and alveolar compliance are increased due to alveolar wall damage which causes an increase in the time required for gas turnover or tracer clearance (Fig. 31.5). In the restrictive state, the resistance of the airway is slightly increased, but the overwhelming decrease in compliance due to alveolar stiffening causes the clearance time to fall. The normal or vascular occlusive states are characterized by normal airflow kinetics.

Regional ventilation normally increases gradually toward the bottom of the lung, following the influence of the intrapleural pressure gradient (Fig. 31.6). This gradient is formed by three factors: (a) the outward pull of the chest wall, (b) the opposing inward pull of the lung, and (c) the weight of the lung. Intrapleural pressure is most negative at the top of the lung and least negative at the bottom, where the weight of the lung is the greatest. Because alveoli at the top of the lung experience a greater distending pressure, they are larger at end-expiration than those at the bottom of the lung. Therefore, the alveoli at the top of the lung fill to a lesser extent during inspiration than those at the bottom. This causes the ventilatory flow to increase toward the lung base in a smooth pattern that is horizontally homogeneous. However, ventilatory flow is no longer homogeneous where alveolar morphology is changed by alveolar disease.

Patient positioning has an important effect on the distribution of pulmonary function. In the upright position, intrapleural pressure becomes progressively more subatmospheric from the lung base (about -2.5 cm H_2O), where the lung is compressed by its own weight, to the apex (-10 cm H_2O), where the lung's weight actually tends to pull the lung down and away from the parietal pleural surface. This apical negative pressure stretches the alveoli outward, making them larger and less compliant. These alveoli ventilate inefficiently compared to the less distended alveoli in the lung base. These regional differences can be altered by changing the patient's position. In normal upright patients, the bases ventilate better than the apices, but in the

Figure 31.4. Morphologic factors affecting clearance time. The product of regional airway resistance (*R*) and alveolar compliance (*C*) is the clearance rate (*t*). The normal or vascular occlusive states are characterized by normal xenon washout kinetics. In the obstructive state, however, the resistance and compliance of the alveous is increased due to alveolar wall damage. This causes an increase in the time required for xenon clearance. In the restrictive state, the resistance of the airway is slightly increased, but the overwhelming decrease in compliance due to alveolar stiffening causes the clearance time to fall.

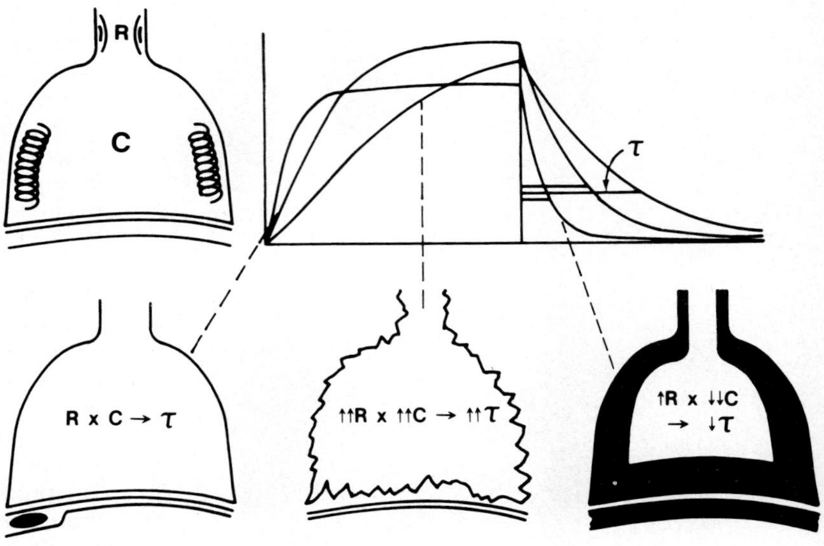

Figure 31.5. Xenon clearance in obstructive airway disease. Posterior washin (*top left*) and sequential (1 minute, 3 minutes, and 5 minutes) washout ^{133}Xe images are shown in a patient who had obstructive airway disease. In patients with obstructive airway disease, the clearance of xenon is slow and inhomogeneous. The inhomogeneity of clearance is the most reliable hallmark of obstructive airway disease because changes in minute ventilation and other variables affect overall clearance times more than the regional pattern of clearance.

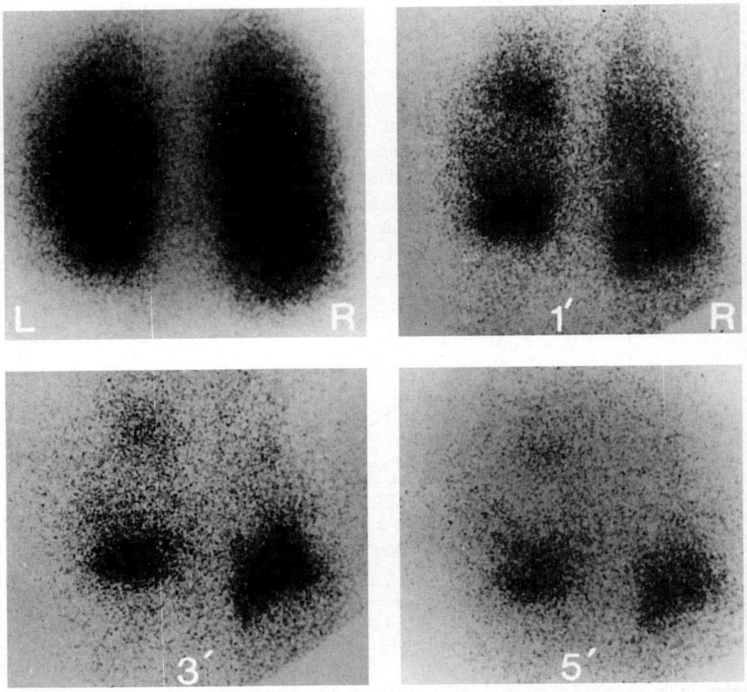

lateral decubitus position, the lower lung shows greater ventilation per unit volume than the upper lung. When a patient is studied in the supine position there is little apex-to-base gradient in alveolar size, but there is an anterior-posterior lung gradient, with the lowermost alveoli being less distended and ventilating more efficiently.

Ventilation-perfusion mismatch occurs physiologically because capillary perfusion tends to be greater than the alveolar ventilation in dependent lung zones and it falls more rapidly than ventilation toward the top of the lung. In the upright lung, for example, the V/Q ratio approximates values of 0.5–1 in the lower lobes and increases to about 3.5 in the apical zones. Because the gradients of these two flow rates tend to change smoothly and are homogeneous along horizontal planes, the V/Q ratio increases smoothly toward the top of the lung. As with ventilatory or perfusion distributions, pulmonary dysfunction is reflected by regionally inhomogeneous V/Q ratios.

Xenon Ventilation Studies

In a typical ^{133}Xe ventilation study, patients are positioned with their back to the gamma-camera, and inhale from a closed loop lead-shielded delivery system that contains 10–20 mCi ^{133}Xe and a CO_2 absorber. The patient initially breathes room air until comfortable with the device. Care is taken toensure that there are no loose tubing connections or avenues of gas escape at the system-patient inter-

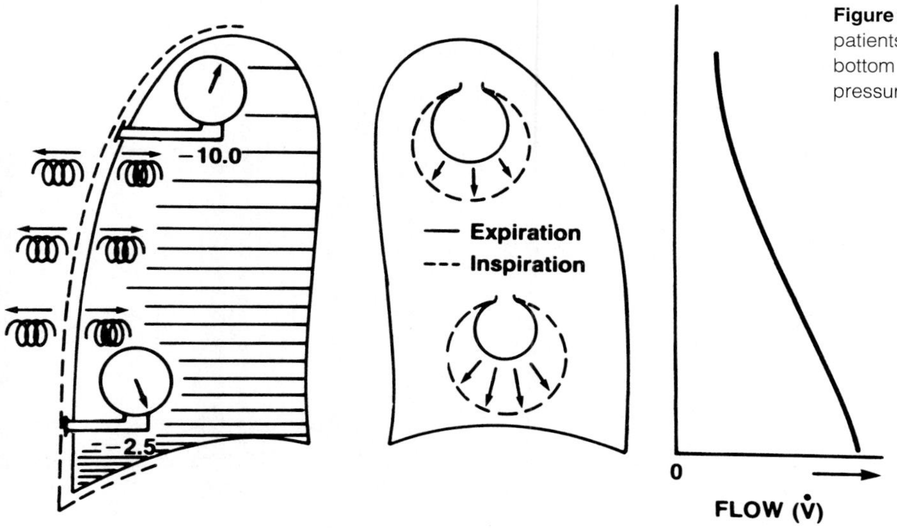

Figure 31.6. Gravity-induced gradient of ventilation in upright patients. Regional ventilation increases gradually toward the bottom of the lung following the influence of the intrapleural pressure gradient.

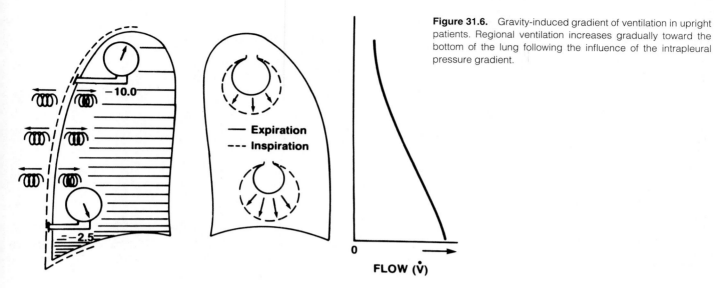

face. Once xenon rebreathing is begun, an initial "first breath" image of 50,000 counts is obtained. Although some patients with obstructive airway disease will fail to reach equilibrium, a 5-minute xenon rebreathing (i.e., washin phase) will allow regions with time constants of 100 seconds or less to achieve at least 95% of their equilibrium value (7). During the course of the washin, two 400,000-count equilibrium images are obtained. The patient then begins to breathe room air (i.e., washout phase). The room air is inhaled and expired into an exhaust system or through a charcoal trap. During washout, a sequence of 50,000-count images are obtained, each 30–60 seconds, for a total of 5–8 minutes. Collection of washout images for a preset count ensures that the intensity of the images will be proper and that regions with mild to moderate clearance abnormalities will be evident in the later washout frames.

Ventilation compromise is manifest by slow xenon clearance. Prolonged retention of xenon suggests obstructive airway disease. There is no absolute normal range of clearance times because the time required to clear a region of lung is dependent on the local lung volume and air flow. For example, increasing air flow by a change in either rate or depth of respiration decreases pulmonary clearance time (Fig. 31.7). Although it may be difficult to pick a clearance time that distinguishes normal and abnormal regions, the normal lung appears homogeneous horizontally in regional volume, ventilation, and xenon clearance rate. Inhomogeneity of lung clearance during xenon washout is an indicator of dysfunctional lung (see Fig. 31.5).

Quantitative procedures may be used to derive images of regional ventilation and V/Q ratios that help characterize nonembolic disorders by differentiating the functional patterns associated with the obstructive, consolidative, and restrictive disease categories.

Functional Images of Xenon Clearance Time and Ventilation/Perfusion Ratio. Quantitative estimates of regional clearance times may be used to assess the nature and degree of ventilatory dysfunction in regions of the lung. A simple lung model may be used to extract clearance rate constants from regional xenon activity curves. Typically, each

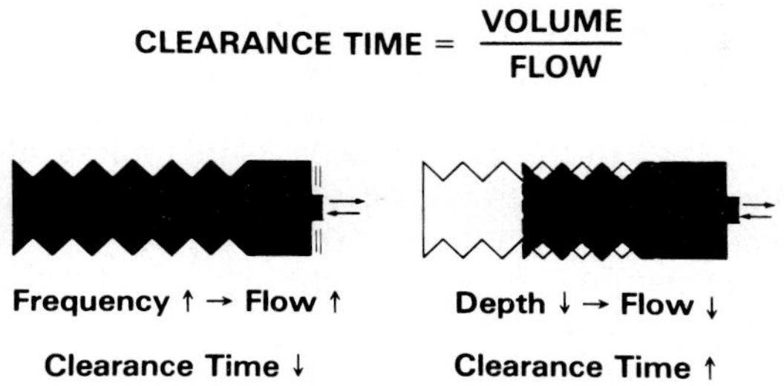

Figure 31.7. Patient factors affecting clearance time estimates. Clearance time is related to regional volume and flow rates and can be modified by changes in frequency or depth of respiration. For example, increasing air flow either by changes in rate or depth of respiration decreases pulmonary clearance time.

element of a 64×64 picture matrix is considered an independent compartment characterized by a volume and a time constant for tracer clearance (Fig. 31.8). A clearance time may be estimated for each image pixel using a modified Stewart-Hamilton equation (7, 8) and assembled into an image of regional clearance time (Fig. 31.9). A functional image of regional ventilation then may be produced by dividing an equilibrium volume image by the clearance time map. Patients with ventilatory dysfunction show wide distributions of clearance time with higher intensities in the clearance time image in regions associated with reduced airflow. The ventilation image may be used to assess the effect of clearance time abnormalities on regional tidal airflow, and may be compared directly to the static perfusion scan to evaluate regional V/Q matching.

Quantitative V/Q ratio images are obtained by dividing the parametric image of ventilation produced from the clearance time analysis by the static posterior perfusion image. Prior to the division, both images are masked to exclude data from regions outside the lung. Since only the relative distribution of these functions is available scintigraphically, both images are scaled so that global pulmonary ventilation and perfusion are equal. The point-by-point ratios of the resulting images are reassembled into a topographic map of regional V/Q ratios.

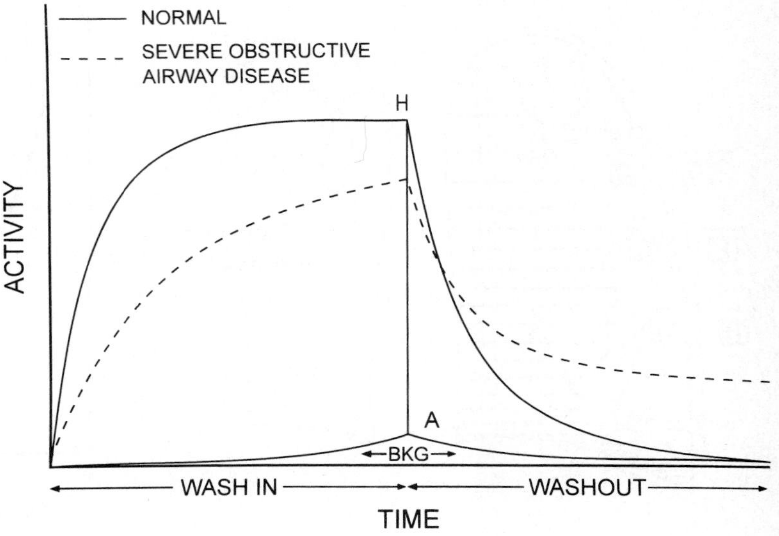

Figure 31.8. Schematic illustrations of xenon time-activity curves from lung regions with theoretically normal and abnormal ventilation. Regions of normal ventilation (*solid lines*) are characterized by an exponential rise of activity during washin that eventually plateaus when equilibrium is reached (i.e., when the amount of activity entering the region with each breath is the same as that leaving the region). This represents the height (*H*) in the diagram. During normal washout, there is a rapid exponential decline of activity that becomes somewhat slower during the later phases of clearance. Regional clearance can be quantified by dividing the counts at *H* by the area (*A*) under the washout curve. In abnormal patients (*dashed lines*) the rate of rise of activity during washin is slower, and equilibrium is not reached by the time that washout begins. The washout is slower and the area under the washout curve is greater. Since the H reached at the end of the time allowed for washin is lower and the A is greater, the calculation of H/A indicates that regional air exchange is lower. If a patient with abnormal regions were allowed to continue breathing for many minutes, the regions might eventually come to equilibrium, but the radiation dose to the patient would be greatly increased. Therefore, washin sequences usually are terminated after 3–5 minutes of breathing.

Clearly, the computed V/Q values are very crude estimates of alveolar physiology. They reflect the macroscopic V/Q relationships from poorly defined cylinders of lung perpendicular to the camera face. Nonetheless, the V/Q ratio image represents a logical endpoint of scintigraphic assessments of ventilation-to-perfusion matching and provides information useful in evaluating the relative function of various portions of the lung.

Krypton Ventilation Studies

^{81m}Kr is a relatively insoluble inert gas with a 13.4-second half-life. It decays to ^{81}Kr by isomeric transition, emitting 190-keV γ-rays (65%) and internal conversion electrons. The gas is obtained by eluting a generator containing its 4.7-hour half-life parent ^{81}Rb. During ^{81m}Kr ventilation studies, patients breathe at their own rate from a reservoir that stores the ^{81m}Kr being eluted from the generator. The higher photon keV of ^{81m}Kr allows ^{81m}Kr ventilation studies to follow ^{99m}Tc MAA perfusion scans. Given its short, 13.4 second half-life, ^{81m}Kr can be administered intermittently, so that ventilation images can be interdigitated with each of the 6–8 view perfusion study images (Fig. 31.2). ^{81m}Kr studies can be easily performed on infants, children, uncooperative patients, or patients being mechanically ventilated. The rapid disappearance of the tracer from the lungs also allows ventilation studies to be performed before and after medications or exercise. The gas does not require expensive delivery systems, room monitors, ventilation ducts, fans, or charcoal traps. Its low dosimetry and absence of gas waste disposal problems make it a very attractive alternative to ^{133}Xe or ^{127}Xe.

Perhaps most important, the static distribution of ^{81m}Kr reflects the pattern of lung ventilation (*V*). It is therefore directly comparable to the distribution of ^{99m}Tc MAA perfusion (*Q*) to evaluate the regional ventilation-perfusion ratio (*V/Q*) (9–11).

Static ^{81m}Kr images reflect ventilation because of the mechanics of respiration and bulk air flow in the lung airways. Beyond the gases in the deadspace, a significant fraction of the molecules inhaled into the alveoli with each breath are also exhaled. This means that the radioactive species of ^{81m}Kr is primarily concentrated in the deadspace, in the terminal conducting airways, and in the proximal respiratory zone. The molecules that occupy the more distal alveolar regions (90% of lung volume) have a much longer residence and a correspondingly lower specific activity. Hence, the total count rate in the static ^{81m}Kr lung image is due predominantly to ^{81m}Kr that is in the tidal volume. The faster the tidal volume is refreshed, the higher its mean activity, and the higher the lung image intensity.

Experimental evidence suggests that ^{81m}Kr reflects ventilation at all flow rates, even at the ventilatory turnover rates found in infants and children (12). Based on gated lung studies of ^{81m}Kr distributions over a range of respiratory frequencies, tidal volumes and alveolar turnover rates, Modell and Graham (12) found that both end-expiration and end-inspiration activities were linearly related to ventialtionlation for ventilatory turnover rates up to and exceeding 10 per minute (12).

Radioaerosol Inhalation Studies

Radioaerosols are very small droplets that deposit in the lung by impaction in central airways, sedimentation in more distal airways, and random contact with alveolar walls during diffusion in the air sacs (13). Radioaerosols have become widely used for investigating regional ventilation, largely because of the introduction of small and efficient aerosol nebulizers. Nebulizers produce submicron aerosols that penetrate to the lung periphery, except where there is excessive airway turbulence from rapid shallow breathing or partial airways obstruction. In these circumstances, there may be substantial degrees of central lung deposition that can lead to poor images of peripheral ventilation.

The radioaerosol most commonly employed is ^{99m}Tc-diethylenetriaminepentaacetic acid (DTPA), due in part to its rapid renal clearance. DTPA is a small, water soluble chelate, that is chemically inert and is able to clear the lung

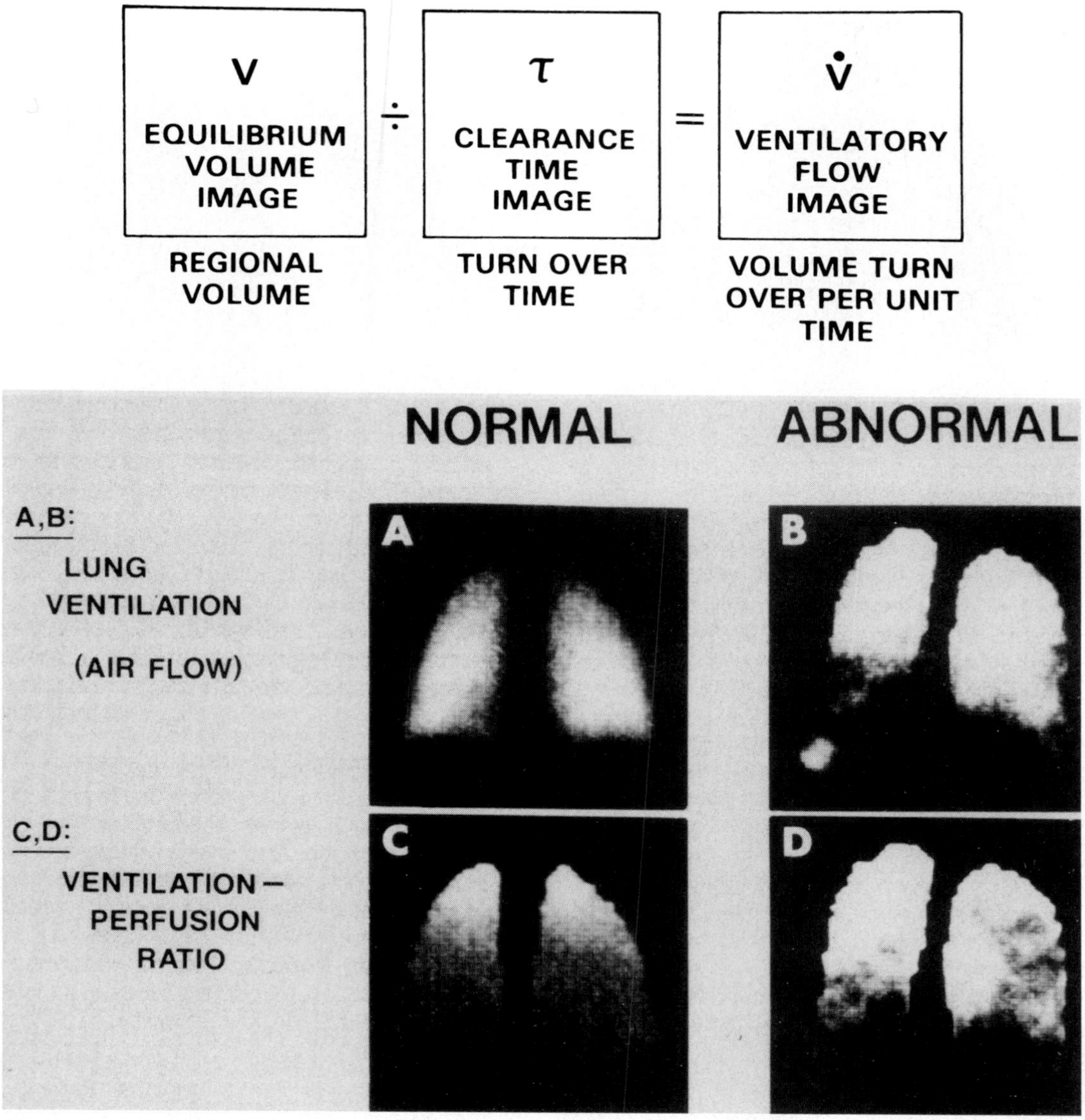

Figure 31.9. **A.** Regional clearance time and ventilation analysis. The equilibrium volume image is combined with the clearance time image to obtain the ventilation flow image, i.e., the volume turnover per unit time. **B.** Functional images of lung ventilation and ventilation-perfusion ratios. The normal patient shows the typical increase of V/Q ratios in the apices, and an even decrease in the V/Q ratios through the lung bases. The abnormal patient had pulmonary fibrosis and shows several areas of elevated V/Q ratios (the bright areas in the functional images). These areas indicate regions where ventilation exceeds perfusion by an abnormal amount (i.e., areas of so-called deadspace ventilation). In the lung bases and midzones of the abnormal patient, the dark areas indicate regions of low V/Q ratios (i.e., areas with V/Q ratios much less than 1.0). These zones represents regions of so-called intrapulmonary shunting. (Reproduced by permission from Alderson PO, Line BR. Scintigraphic evaluation of regional pulmonary ventilation. Semin Nucl Med 1980;10:218–242.)

through the alveolar-capillary membrane (14). Because of the low amounts deposited in the lung and the short pulmonary half-time (55 minutes) the radiation dose to patients from preperfusion DTPA aerosol scintigraphy is lower than that of either ^{81m}Kr or ^{133}Xe. ^{99m}Tc aerosol studies (Fig. 31.10) have proven to be a satisfactory alternative to ^{81m}Kr in the setting of pulmonary embolism screening (15–17) but are less accurate than ^{81m}Kr in defining regional ventilation (18). Aerosol activity is usually absent or diminished in areas of obstructive airway disease. Airway deposition patterns ("central hot spots") are found in areas of nonlaminar airflow or turbulence due to mucous secretions, airway narrowing, or collapse. For example, aerosols will accumulate at sites of obstructive bronchospasm, such as those present in active asthma. Aerosols are not commonly used to study regional ventilation in nonembolic lung disease because of the relatively nonlinear relationship between ventilation, flow rate, and aerosol deposition.

ASSESSMENT OF ALVEOLAR-CAPILLARY MEMBRANE PERMEABILITY

The primary use of radioaerosols in nonembolic lung disease is to evaluate alveolar-capillary membrane perme-

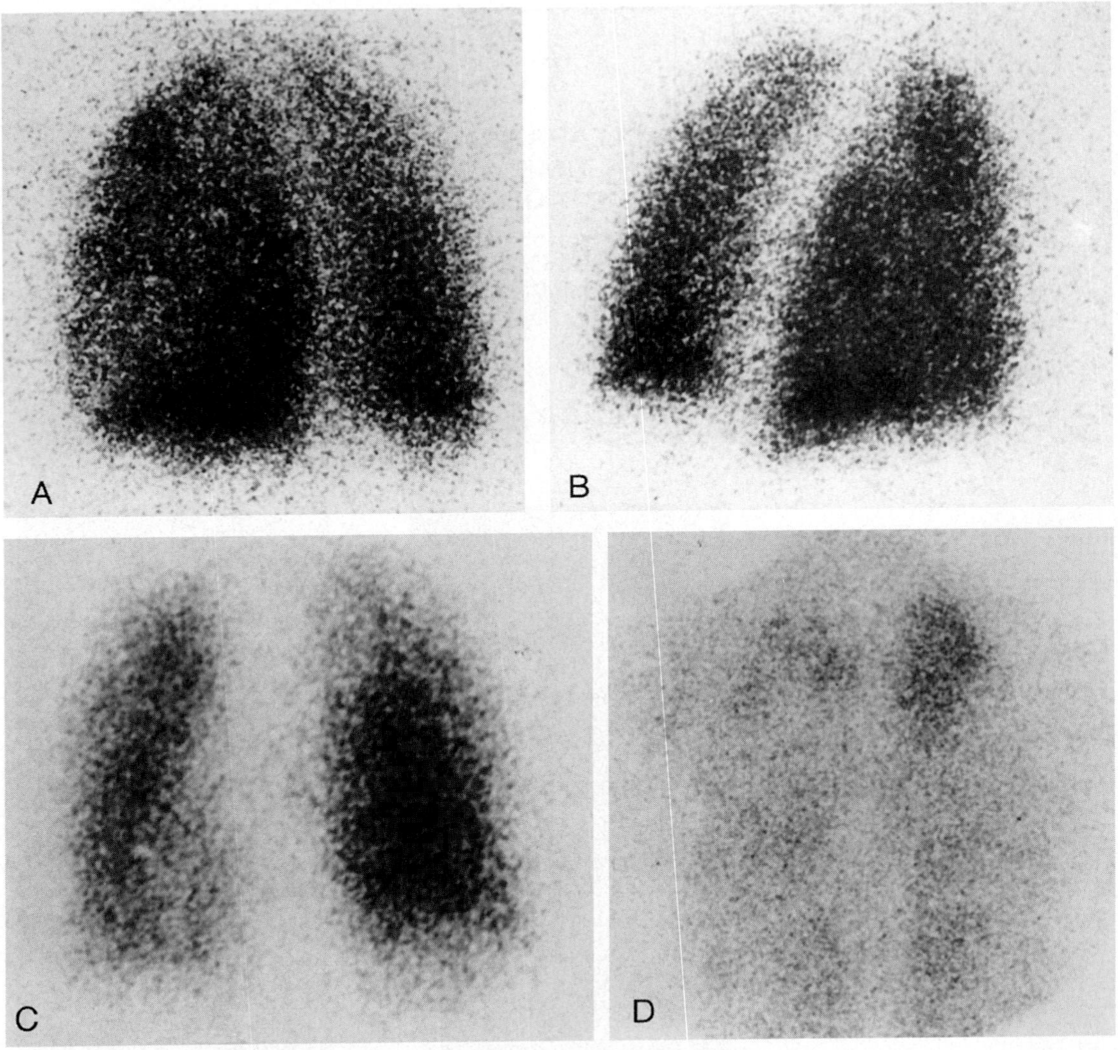

Figure 31.10. Radioaerosol detection of regional airway abnormality. Left **A** and right **B** posterior oblique ^{99m}Tc-DTPA aerosol images and a ^{133}Xe study with single-breath **C** and a 3-minute washout image **D** are illustrated. Note the mild ^{133}Xe retention in both upper lobes. These mild airways abnormalities are detected as small deficits of aerosol deposition in the posterior aspects of both upper lobes (A, B). Radioaerosol studies are nearly as sensitive as ^{133}Xe washout studies in detecting airway disease, and regions with especially mild airway abnormalities detected only by ^{133}Xe usually are associated with small or absent perfusion abnormalities. (Reproduced by permission from Alderson PO, Biello DR, Gottschalk A, et al. Comparison of Tc-99m DTPA aerosol and radioactive gases as adjuncts to perfusion scintigraphy in patients with suspected pulmonary embolism. Radiology 1984;153:515–521.)

ability (19–21). The rate of aerosol clearance from the lung is accelerated in the presence of epithelial alveolar injury (Fig. 31.11). Furthermore, pulmonary capillary protein leaks can be evaluated by serial determinations of the lung-heart radioactivity ratio (22, 23).

Normally, the alveolar epithelium and capillary endothelium are separated by the connective tissue of the interstitial space (24). DTPA clearance is modulated primarily by alveolar epithelial permeability because the alveolar epithelium is the chief barrier to diffusion of solutes between the alveolar surface and the pulmonary capillaries (21). There are several factors, however, that influence the rate at which solutes leave the lung. One of the most important is determined by the site of aerosol deposition. Relatively rapid clearance occurs by transepithelial absorption if the aerosol lands on small airways or alveolar surfaces. Much slower clearance by mucociliary transport removes aerosol impacting on large airways. Where the aerosol lands is determined by regional air flow, aerosol particle size, and the rate and depth of ventilation (25). Larger aerosols have greater inertia and are more likely to impact on proximal airway walls. The submicron-sized aerosols used clinically deposit primarily in small airways and alveoli (80% or more) (26). Maximum peripheral deposition occurs during quiet breathing, whereas rapid inhalation causes turbulent flow and more central deposition at airway bifurcations (Fig. 31.12). Although DTPA is removed from the lung by the pulmonary circulation, increasing

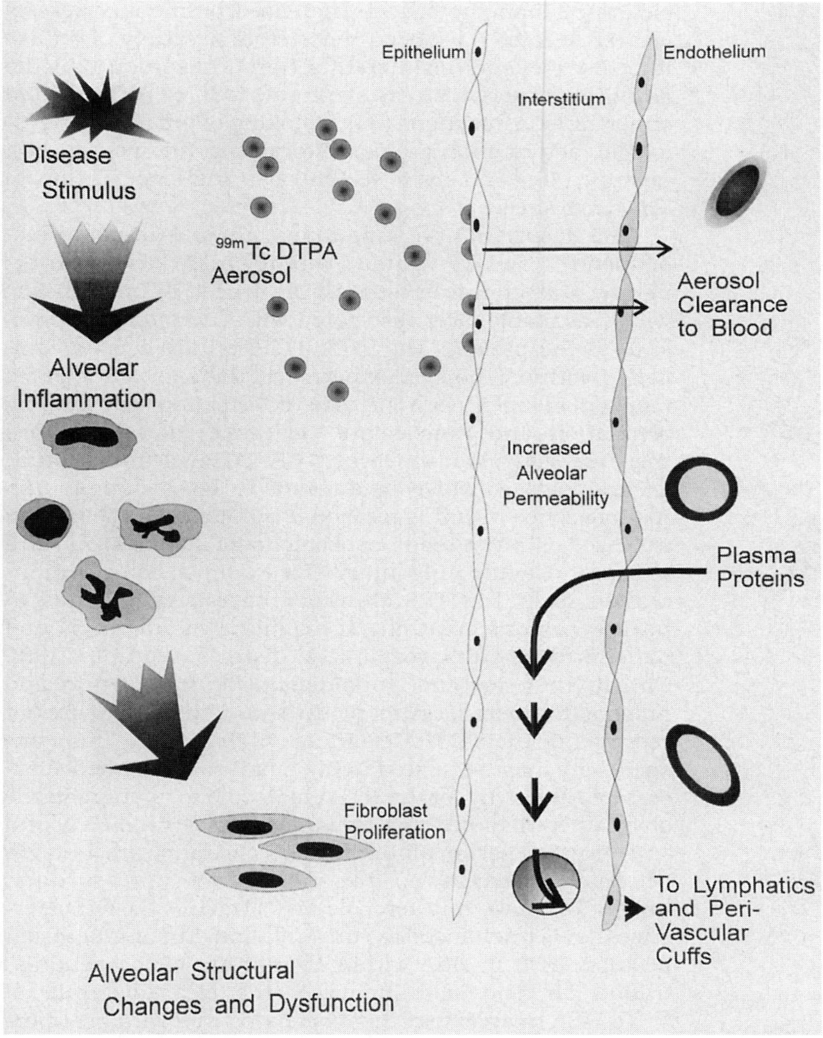

Figure 31.11. Clearance of ^{99m}Tc-DTPA aerosol. Submicron-sized ^{99m}Tc-labeled aerosols enter the alveolus and settle onto the epithelial surface. The rate at which solutes pass into the interstitium and then into the blood depends on the alveolar epithelial wall integrity. Diffuse lung diseases that cause alveolar inflammation and loss of epithelial integrity result in increased clearance of aerosol. The epithelium is normally less permeable than the endothelium. Plasma proteins that leave the lung capillaries normally do not enter the alveoli but pass down the interstitial space to the lymphatics and perivascular cuff. (Reproduced by permission from Line BR. Scintigraphic studies of inflammation in diffuse lung disease. Rad Clin No Am 1991;29:1095–1114.)

pulmonary blood flow does not increase the DTPA clearance significantly (27) because DTPA diffusion is slow in comparison with blood flow. The rate of diffusion is directly dependent on both the permeability of the epithelial wall as well as on the surface area available for diffusional transfer. For example, exercise increases pulmonary clearance (28), probably by recruitment of the pulmonary microvascular bed and through the unfolding of alveolar septa. These factors serve to increase the surface area for diffusion. Pulmonary clearance of DTPA has been found to increase during rapid shallow ventilation with increased positive end-expiratory pressure (29). Egan and others (30) have also shown that the alveolar epithelium becomes more permeable as inflation volume increases. The mechanism for the increase in DTPA clearance at a high lung volume may be due to increased surface area for diffusion-increased permeability of the epithelium or changes in the functional integrity of the alveolar surfactant layer (31). Another determinant of solute transfer across the alveolar epithelial barrier relates to the size of the tracer molecule. As a first approximation, the rate of diffusion of a small molecule is inversely proportional to the square root of its molecular weight—the smaller the molecule, the faster it diffuses.

Procedure to Determine Aerosol Clearance

To measure the pulmonary clearance rate of DTPA aerosol, it is breathed quietly for 1–2 minutes. Submicron-sized aerosols are generated by commercially available jet nebulizers that are loaded with 30–50 mCi of ^{99m}Tc-DTPA in 2 ml of saline. The nebulizer is driven by a compressed oxygen tank that delivers a flow rate of 10 l/min (31). Although a dose of 30–50 mCi of ^{99m}Tc-DTPA is administered as an aerosol, only 2 mCi of radionuclide is typically retained in the lungs. At this level, the lungs receive between 2 and 8 mrad; the average radiation exposure to the whole body is about 40 mrad (20).

The rate of pulmonary ^{99m}Tc-DTPA clearance can be measured with either a sodium iodide probe or gamma-camera. Care must be taken to properly prepare the patient for measurement. The patient should avoid deep breathing

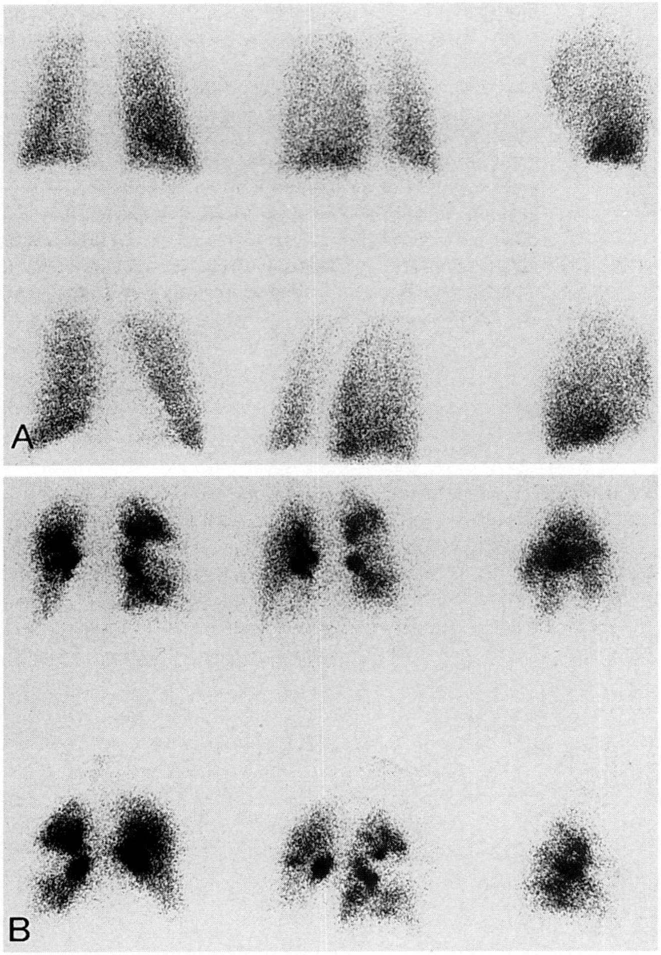

Figure 31.12. ^{99m}Tc-DTPA aerosol pulmonary deposition patterns related in part to respiratory rate and tidal volume. **A.** Normal six-view ^{99m}Tc-DTPA aerosol deposition pattern in a 59-year-old man who did not smoke and who had radiographically normal lungs. **B.** Images obtained from a 26-year-old man with AIDS who had a normal ^{67}Ga scan 3 weeks earlier and a normal chest radiograph at the time of the study. He was breathing rapidly and had a small tidal volume during the aerosol administration. Note the irregular peripheral distribution and intense central foci that are most likely sites of highly turbulent flow at airway bifurcations. (Reproduced by permission from Line BR. Scintigraphic studies of inflammation in diffuse lung disease. Rad Clin No Am 1991;29:1095–1114.)

or vital capacity maneuvers prior to and during aerosol administration and scanning. The more rapid curvilinear clearance produced by several deep breaths may be due to transiently increased epithelial permeability or reduced volume of liquid in the alveoli in some lung regions. Resting for 20 minutes prior to inhaling the aerosol of ^{99m}Tc-DTPA is recommended to avoid alterations in clearance rates from deep breathing (32). During the first 30 minutes, the normal ^{99m}Tc-DTPA pulmonary clearance curve can be modeled as a single compartment emptying exponentially with a mean half-time of 86±26 minutes (31). Multicompartmental curves may occur when there are two or more populations of alveoli, one having significantly greater clearance than the others. Increased pulmonary aerosol clearance rates have been reported in a variety of diffuse lung diseases such as interstitial fibrotic disorders (20), the adult respiratory distress syndrome (33), or AIDS-related opportunistic infections (34). Smoking of tobacco or physiologic factors such as inspiratory lung volume (32, 35), posture (36), and exercise (28) also influence epithelial lung clearance.

As a determinant of lung injury, there is much to recommend ^{99m}Tc-DTPA studies with regard to ease of performance and noninvasiveness. The tracer is inexpensive, widely available, and associated with low radiation exposure to the patient. The ^{99m}Tc-DTPA study can be completed within 1 hour. Furthermore, the same radiopharmaceutical agent can provide information on regional ventilation and mucociliary clearance rates. However, there are several reasons why ^{99m}Tc-DTPA clearance studies are not used widely as a means to assess lung injury. As experience with this method has increased, it has been criticized as being too nonspecific to be a clinically useful indicator of acute lung injury. For example, equivalent increases in ^{99m}Tc-DTPA clearance have been reported in healthy persons breathing at high lung volumes (35), and patients with adult respiratory distress syndrome (33). Clearly, there are enormous diagnostic, therapeutic, and prognostic differences among these conditions that are not reflected in their DTPA clearance (37). In part, this nonspecificity may be related to the small size, and hence excessive sensitivity, of the DTPA molecule to changes in the alveolar epithelium. For example, both ^{99m}Tc-DTPA and ^{99m}Tc-human serum albumin (HSA) clearance are found to be equally affected by positive end-expiratory pressure and lung injury (38), but aerosols of ^{99m}Tc-HSA have a clearance that is unchanged by lung inflation. Furthermore, deposition of ^{99m}Tc-HSA within 15 minutes of the administration of oleic acid increases the clearance rate of ^{99m}Tc-HSA to an extent that correlated well with postmortem lung water volume. It is possible that in the future, non-DTPA aerosols may be used in procedures that are simple, noninvasive, have a low radiation dose, and provide a way to assess lung injury rapidly in the diffuse lung diseases.

ASSESSMENT OF MUCOCILIARY CLEARANCE

^{99m}Tc radiolabeled macroaggregated albumin and sulfur colloid are inert and nonpermeable substances that can be delivered to the tracheobronchial surfaces as aerosols and used noninvasively to determine mucociliary clearance rates. During imaging studies spanning 60–120 minutes, subjects are asked to refrain from coughing and maintain a normal pattern of breathing. Clearance of the aerosolized particulates are then assessed visually and by quantitative curve fitting. Time activity curves obtained over each lung are fit to two compartment models to determine the fast and slow component of the clearance process. The half-time of the fast compartment is used as a measure of the mucociliary clearance (39).

Mucociliary transport depends on several factors, the most important being ciliary activity, mucous production, and differential airflow. Mucociliary impairment may be a reflection of airways inflammation, chronic obstructive pulmonary disease, and exacerbations of asthma (40). Even stable asthmatic subjects have impaired mucociliary clearance compared to normal subjects (41). Reduced mucociliary clearance can also be demonstrated in patients with bronchial surgery, tracheobronchoplasty, and pulmonary irradiation (39).

Unfortunately, there are a number of practical difficulties that have limited the application of this technology to the research laboratory. To meaningfully compare mucociliary clearance on serial studies, it is necessary to ensure similar initial deposition patterns. The more central the deposition pattern, the more rapidly the deposited particles are cleared due to the shorter path of these particles to the pharynx. Changing breathing patterns also complicate the assessments of changes in mucociliary clearance.

ASSESSMENT OF INFLAMMATION

Inflammation, Injury, and ^{67}Ga Uptake in the Lung

In most of the diffuse lung diseases, injury is associated with an inflammatory infiltration of the alveolar and interstitial spaces. Acute inflammation is primarily exudative and is characterized by vasodilatation, increased vascular permeability, and emigration of polymorphonuclear leukocytes. Chronic inflammation is characterized by a predominantly mononuclear cell infiltrate (macrophages, lymphocytes, and plasma cells), and by a fibroblastic proliferative response that usually leads to parenchymal derangement and pulmonary dysfunction.

In many of the diffuse lung diseases (Table 31.1), ^{67}Ga scintigraphy is useful in evaluating the presence and extent of acute and chronic pulmonary inflammation. Whereas normal lung accumulates little ^{67}Ga, patients who have alveolitis localize the radionuclide in their pulmonary parenchyma. Using techniques that evaluate the amount of localization, several investigators have suggested that the quantity and intensity of gallium uptake reflect the degree of inflammatory change in the lung. Others assert that gallium scintigraphy is helpful for identifying subclinical disease and for evaluating the response to treatment (42–44).

There are important assumptions implicit in the use of ^{67}Ga scanning to stage the alveolitis of diffuse lung disease. First, it is assumed that ^{67}Ga is localized by a mechanism that is related to inflammation and the process of lung injury (Fig. 31.13). Furthermore, it is assumed that the amount of gallium localized in the lung is proportional to the degree of pulmonary injury. Finally, for localization to be of clinical significance, it is assumed that the associated lung injury will cause permanent dysfunction if left untreated. It is unlikely that these assumptions are valid for all of the diffuse lung diseases, but for some there is sufficient evidence to accept these premises as true.

The mechanisms of ^{67}Ga localization in regions of inflammation are not clearly defined. Many factors contribute to ^{67}Ga uptake, and it is likely that their influence depends on the disease and the extent of injury (45). One important factor is that ^{67}Ga behaves like iron in vivo, being bound by transferrin after intravenous administration. The subsequent distribution of ^{67}Ga depends on its migration from the plasma to tissue proteins and cells that have a stronger affinity for the radionuclide (46). Thus, erythema, hyperpermeability of the capillary endothelium, and the presence of gallium-binding cells in areas of inflammation may partially explain the localization of ^{67}Ga in the lung. The transferrin receptor on the surface of cells appears to be important in the localization of ^{67}Ga in lung cancer and in some of the diffuse lung diseases (47). Transferrin receptors have been identified in the membrane of alveolar macrophages in idiopathic pulmonary fibrosis and in epithelioid cells of granuloma in sarcoidosis and pneumoconiosis (47).

The character of the injurious process in each of the diffuse lung diseases is dependent on both the numbers and types of inflammatory cells, as well as on their state of ac-

Table 31.1.
Diffuse Nonmalignant, Lung Diseases Showing ^{67}Ga Lung Uptake.

Disease Process	Author
Infections	
Tuberculosis	van Der Schoot, et al.[169]
Atypical Mycobacterium	Ganz and Serafini[198]
Pneumocystis carinii	Levenson, et al.[208]
Cytomegalovirus	Ganz and Serafini[198]
Actinomycoses	Ganz and Serafini[198]
Cryptococcus	Fineman, et al.[209]
Aspergillosis	Fogh, et al.[210]
Blastmycosis	Rosen, et al.[211]
Filariasis	van Der Schoot, et al.[169]
Drug reactions	
Amiodarone	Moinuddin, et al.[212]
Bleomycin	Richman, et al.[168]
Busulfan	Manning, et al.[213]
Cyclophosphamide	Laven, et al.[214]
Methotrexate	Laven, et al.[214]
Nitrofurantoin	Laven, et al.[214]
Procarbizine	Garbes, et al.[215]
Vincristine	Laven, et al.[214]
Disorders of unknown origin	
Sarcoidosis	Heshiki, et al.[175]
Idiopathic pulmonary fibrosis	Line, et al.[53]
Histiocytosis X	Javaheri, et al.[216]
Progressive systemic sclerosis	Rossi, et al.[186]
Polymyosistis-dermatomyositis	Greene, et al.[187]
Mixed connective tissue disease	Greene, et al.[187]
Systemic lupus erythematosis	Teates, et al.[217]
Rheumatoid arthritis	Greene, et al.[187]
Lymphocytic interstitial pneumonitis	Zuckler, et al.[207]
Lymphomatoid granulomatosis	Tien, et al.[218]
Wegener's granulomatosis	Crystal, et al.[165]
Organic and inorganic dusts	
Coal workers' pneumoconiosis	Siemsen, et al.[189]
Silicosis	Siemsen, et al.[55]
Asbestosis	Siemsen, et al.[189]
Berylliosis	Deseran, et al.[219]
Talc granulomatosis	Bekerman, et al.[167]
Miscellaneous injuries	
Adult respiratory distress syndrome	Hooper and Kearl[220]
Postcardiopulmonary pump syndrome	Specht, et al.[60]
Radiation (direct or scatter)	Gibson, et al.[221]

(Reproduced by permission from Line BR. Scintigraphic studies of inflammation in diffuse lung disease. Rad Clin No Am 1991;29:1095–1114.)

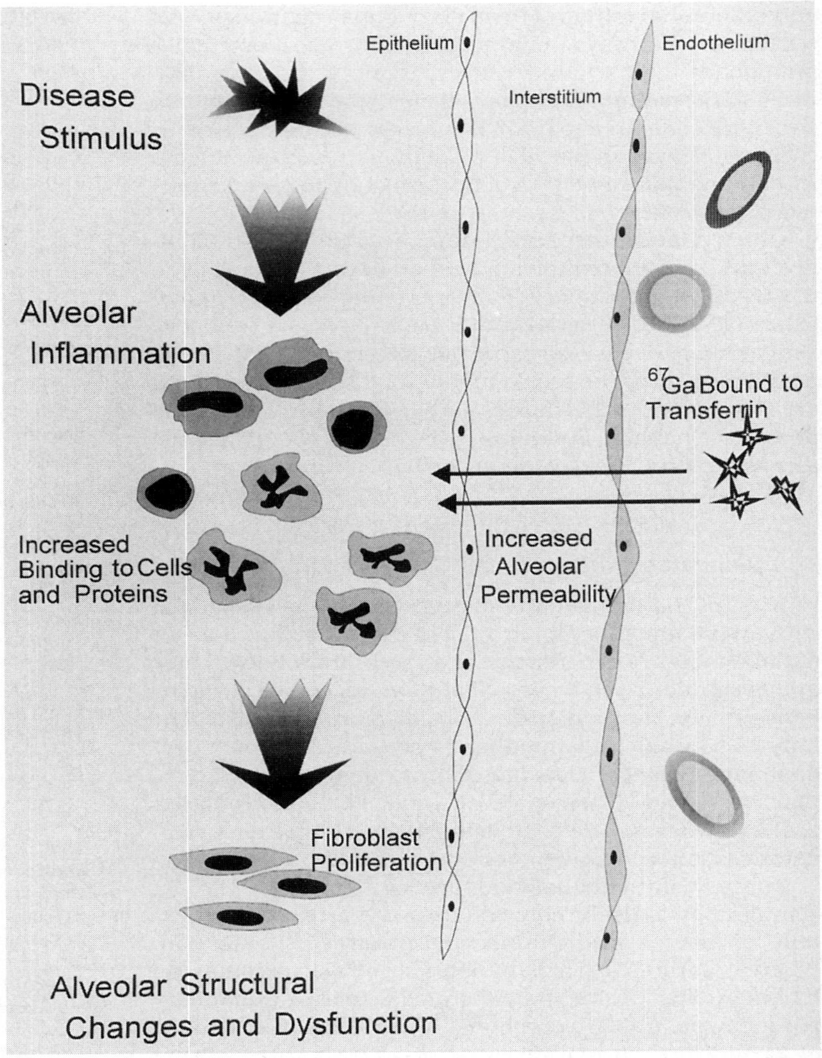

Figure 31.13. Possible factors influencing ^{67}Ga uptake. Where a disease stimulus leads to alveolar inflammation, populations of activated alveolar effector cells release substances that increase alveolar permeability. The serum protein transferrin, which carries ^{67}Ga, leaks into the interstitial and alveolar spaces where the isotope becomes localized by cells or other alveolar protein substances. ^{67}Ga does not localize in lung fibroblasts and does not reflect the degree of alveolar dysfunction due to alveolar structural changes. (Reproduced by permission from Line BR. Scintigraphic studies of inflammation in diffuse lung disease. Rad Clin No Am 1991;29:1095–1114.)

tivation (48). Activated alveolar macrophages, for example, play an important role in perpetuating lung injury, including the release of neutrophil chemotactic factor, a mediator that attracts neutrophils with their potent oxidants and proteases. In other circumstances, macrophages may contribute to the formation of granulomata by their role in activating T lymphocytes (48). Thus, a positive ^{67}Ga scan probably reflects, at least in part, the density of activated inflammatory cells in the lung parenchyma and, for some diseases, the numbers of activated macrophages in the lower respiratory tract. It is also of interest that 60–70% of inhaled ^{67}Ga aerosol is retained in the lungs for more than 96 hours by healthy nonsmokers (49). The predominant site of this localization was the alveolar macrophage. This finding suggests that lung injury may expose the population of resident alveolar macrophages to sufficient ^{67}Ga for external detection even in disease conditions that are not associated with increased numbers of activated macrophages. Thus, increased permeability of the lung microvasculature and alveoli to ^{67}Ga-laden serum proteins in association with injury may be crucial to achieving detectable pulmonary tracer localization.

Imaging Technique and Quantification of Gallium Lung Uptake

^{67}Ga is a cyclotron-produced radionuclide that decays by electron capture and it generates γ-emissions in three principal energy peaks at 93 keV (41%), 185 keV (23%), and 300 keV (18%). Hence, ^{67}Ga scintigraphy commonly is performed with a large field-of-view gamma-camera that has a multiple energy peak acquisition capability and medium energy collimation (50). Imaging routinely begins 48–72 hours after intravenous injection of 3–5 mCi of ^{67}Ga citrate. ^{67}Ga is slowly removed from the blood stream. Hence, pulmonary images obtained within the first 24 hours after injection may be clouded by a high blood pool background which may result in diffusely increased lung activity even in healthy individuals.

Although normal lung tissue does not accumulate appreciable levels of ^{67}Ga, localization does occur normally in other thoracic sites. Faint bronchial activity is common and in children, ^{67}Ga activity may be seen in normal thymic tissue (51). ^{67}Ga is physiologically absorbed by bone matrix and can be localized to a small extent by marrow. Localization is usually evident in the sternum, ribs, vertebral bodies, and scapulae. The lower end of each scapula may show a prominent concentration of activity because of the thickness of the bone at this site. In women, the normal faint localization of ^{67}Ga in normal breast tissue may be enhanced during pregnancy and menarche, during administration of cyclic estrogen or progestational agents, and can be particularly prominent in postpartum women (52).

Investigators began to estimate the degree of lung uptake of ^{67}Ga soon after it was recognized that ^{67}Ga localization might reflect the extent of pulmonary inflammatory disease (53–55). The procedures used to estimate ^{67}Ga lung uptake have been refined continuously to better stage pulmonary alveolitis and to allow correlation with other tests such as bronchoalveolar lavage. Regardless of whether the procedure is primarily qualitative (54, 56, 57), semiquantitative (53, 58), or computer-based quantitative (59–61), each method must establish a background level and a scale for pulmonary uptake intensity.

The simplest, albeit binary, means to detect increased gallium lung localization is to note if the heart is silhouetted against the lung (62). A graded qualitative approach used by several investigators classifies scans as negative when the pulmonary uptake does not exceed soft tissue background (proximal upper limb), 1+ when soft-tissue uptake and lung uptake are equal, 2+ when lung uptake is greater than soft-tissue uptake but less than liver uptake, 3+ when lung uptake is equal to liver uptake, and 4+ when lung uptake is greater than liver uptake. Qualitative evaluations are simple to make and usually are adequate to gauge disease activity. Unfortunately, the grades they produce do not reflect regional variation or heterogeneous patterns of uptake. Furthermore, they do not take into account the size of localizations and depend on reference sites such as the liver, where uptake may vary because of nonpulmonary disease (e.g., cirrhosis or hepatitis) (59).

Semiquantitative procedures also rely on internal reference regions to estimate the degree of uptake but extend the power of qualitative estimates because these procedures consider localization size and intensity to generate an "index" of lung activity. One of the original semiquantitative procedures (53) estimates the area of each region of increased ^{67}Ga uptake as a percentage of the total lung area. The intensity of gallium uptake within each of these areas is graded on a scale of 0 to 4. The area and intensity factors from each different area are multiplied, and the sum of these products yields the gallium lung index (Fig. 31.14).

Duffy, et al. (63), compared the mean parenchymal lung activity of ^{67}Ga to that at three remote sites: the liver, the abdomen, and the thigh. The best correlation with bronchoalveolar lavage data was found when the lung activity was compared to thigh uptake measurements. In another approach that does not rely on an internal standard for background activity, Van Unnick, et al. (61), assessed pulmonary and mediastinal activity recorded in regions imaged on anterior and posterior chest scintigrams. They then compared the recorded activity with external standards and the injected dose to achieve a measurement of the absolute amount of tracer localized in the lung.

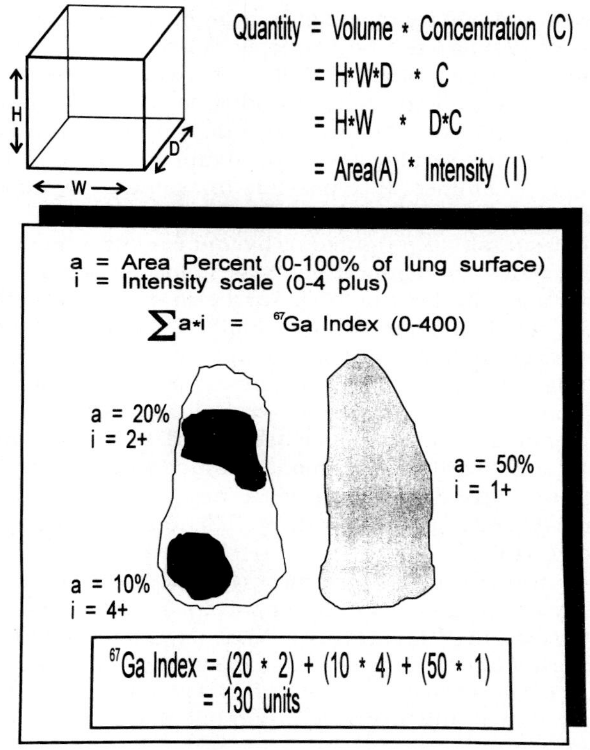

Figure 31.14. Semiquantitative assessment of ^{67}Ga uptake. The quantity of ^{67}Ga localization is estimated based on the simple model of a container from which volume and concentration estimates can be derived. For scintigraphic images, volume and concentration are represented by image area and intensity estimates. The ^{67}Ga index is obtained by adding the products of area and intensity for each region of abnormal ^{67}Ga uptake. The area index is expressed as a percentage of the entire lung surface area; the intensity index is determined against a scale of 0 to 4+ where 0 represents the background and 4+ is equivalent to the most intense body region. In the example shown schematically, three areas of uptake with intensities above background are assigned area (*a*) and intensity (*I*) index values. The sum of the products of area and intensity yeilds a ^{67}Ga index of 130 index units. (Reproduced by permission from Line BR. Scintigraphic studies of inflammation in diffuse lung disease. Rad Clin No Am 1991;29:1095–1114.)

Unfortunately, there are nearly as many methods to evaluate gallium localization in the lungs as there are investigators. The methods vary sufficiently that it is difficult to compare results from different institutions, but it appears that computerized procedures generate indices that are more closely related, are more reproducible, and are more sensitive to lower levels of abnormal localization (60, 64, 65).

ASSESSMENT OF METABOLIC AND NEOPLASTIC DISORDERS

Evaluation of Metabolic Properties of the Lung

In addition to its function as an organ of external gas exchange, the lung serves as a metabolic regulator of substances circulating in the blood. The lung has been shown to modify many circulating vasoactive substances either by activation, deactivation, or removal and storage for subsequent metabolism and release (66, 67). The relationship between pulmonary metabolism of amines and other disease entities has not been clearly defined, primarily because studies of amine metabolism have been invasive. By using single photon emitting radiopharmaceuticals that have potential for evaluation of lung amine metabolism (e.g., ^{123}I amphetamine (68, 69) or diamine (70)), or by employing ^{11}C amines, it is possible to evaluate pulmonary amine metabolism on a regional basis.

For example, the uptake of bioamines and kinetics of psychoactive compounds such as chlorpromazine have been imaged in the lung (71). Furthermore, the saturable nature of ^{123}I-iodoamphetamine (IMP) (69) and ^{123}I-metaiodobenzylguanidine (MIBG) (72) uptake in the lung has been demonstrated. Metaiodobenzylguanidine, which accumulates via active transport-dependent mechanisms in neuroendocrine tissue, has been used to depict early, short-term disorders of pulmonary amine metabolism (70). Large and rapid decreases in MIBG lung activity have been demonstrated in endotoxic sheep (73) and with bleomycin toxicity (74).

Positron emission tomography can be used to quantitatively evaluate biologically important radiotracers containing carbon (^{11}C), nitrogen (^{13}N), or oxygen (^{15}O). Studies measuring amine clearance, glucose metabolism, and receptor localization can be quantified regionally with an accuracy that is unrivaled by any other noninvasive technique (75).

Radionuclides in Detection of Lung Neoplasia

Several tracers have been used to assess neoplastic diseases of the lung. These tracers take advantage of features of the disease such as pathologic changes in tumor cell metabolism, increased tumor blood flow, and enhanced permeability of the tumor capillaries. They may also target specific cell surface receptors, uptake mechanisms, and intracellular binding sites (76).

^{67}Ga-citrate was one of the first tracers used to stage lung cancer. In early studies, it was reported to show high sensitivity and specificity in detection of primary lung tumors and mediastinal disease (77), but subsequent investigations in larger populations were unable to substantiate its initial success. Confounding results because of the localization of ^{67}Ga in inflammatory diseases, its high blood pool background, and limited image resolution have caused it to no longer be used. Unfortunately, ^{67}Ga scintigraphy has been found to be too nonspecific. It may show localization due to tissue injury in patients following radiotherapy or chemotherapy, it may localize in benign mediastinal processes such as with thymic hyperplasia, and it is positive in a broad cross-section of acute and chronic infections.

Other tracers, such as ^{201}Tl chloride and ^{18}F-fluorodeoxyglucose, localize due to the increased metabolism of tumor tissue. ^{201}Tl is a potassium analog that enters cells through the sodium-potassium pump and it accumulates in a high percentage of primary lung cancer lesions (78). Initial tumor localization is likely due to a combination of increased relative blood flow and high metabolic activity. There is also a longer ^{201}Tl residence time in neoplastic tissue relative to normal or inflamed cells (78). Slower clearance of ^{201}Tl in adenocarcinoma and small cell carcinoma relative to squamous cell carcinoma has been described (78), but these differences have not been shown to be of clinical utility.

The glucose analog, 2-[fluorine-18]-fluoro-2-deoxy-D-glucose (FDG) and positron emission tomography (PET) are highly successful in imaging all lung cancer cell types (Fig. 31.15) (79). Relative to normal tissue, tumor cells express more messenger RNA for the glucose transporter molecule which subsequently results in increased glucose uptake and metabolism. FDG behaves similarly to D-glucose in its transport through the cell membrane and phosphorylation by hexokinase in the glycolytic pathway. However, once FDG is phosphorylated, structural changes created by a hexose-phosphate bond largely prevent FDG from being catabolized or transported back into the extracellular space. Thus, increased uptake and accumulation of FDG occur within highly metabolic tumor cells (80).

Neoplastic cells also demonstrate increased amino acid utilization. Methionine labeled with ^{75}Se was initially studied in patients with lung cancer, but has high β-emissions, so only microcurie quantities can be used for imaging. The positron-emitting radiopharmaceutical L-[methyl ^{11}C] methionine (MET) has far superior imaging characteristics, and its short half-life of 20 minutes allows it to be used in relatively large doses (81). Although both FDG and MET uptake vary with tumor type (82), the reproducibility and utility of this finding is controversial (83, 84). Selection of treatment based on the specific histologic type of the tumor per se has not been justified, because survival depends on resectability in toto and not on histology.

Another important property of tumor growth is neoplastic cell DNA replication. ^{57}Co-bleomycin binds firmly to DNA like Fe-bleomycin, the cytotoxic form of bleomycin (85, 86). The initial uptake of ^{57}Co-bleomycin depends on tumor blood flow, tumor capillary permeability, and extracellular volume. Eight hours later, however, after blood and extracellular space concentrations are decreased, tumor activity appears to reflect DNA binding and tumor cell kinetics (76, 87). Rapidly growing tumors that have poor prognosis also have a large proportion of cells engaged in DNA synthesis (87, 88). These tumors also appear to show high ^{57}Co-bleomycin uptake (87).

Other radiopharmaceuticals developed to target receptors and cell surface antigens are beginning to appear in clinical practice. Although most of these tracers are based on antibodies or their derivatives, radiolabeled peptides have been used successfully to image high affinity somatostatin receptors on small cell lung tumors (Fig. 31.16) (89, 90). Among the lung cancers, small cell tumors are relatively unique in this regard in that they stem from cells that express high affinity somatostatin receptors and have the ability to synthesize peptide hormones through amine precursor uptake and decarboxylation (APUD cells).

Radiolabeled monoclonal antibodies and fragments have been evaluated in lung cancer in several multicenter trials. These biologics are likely to become widely used in the future, but have been slow to achieve clinical application. Limiting factors include high background uptake by normal tissues, in addition to tumor and the inherent problems of detecting and localizing small lesions (91). Im-

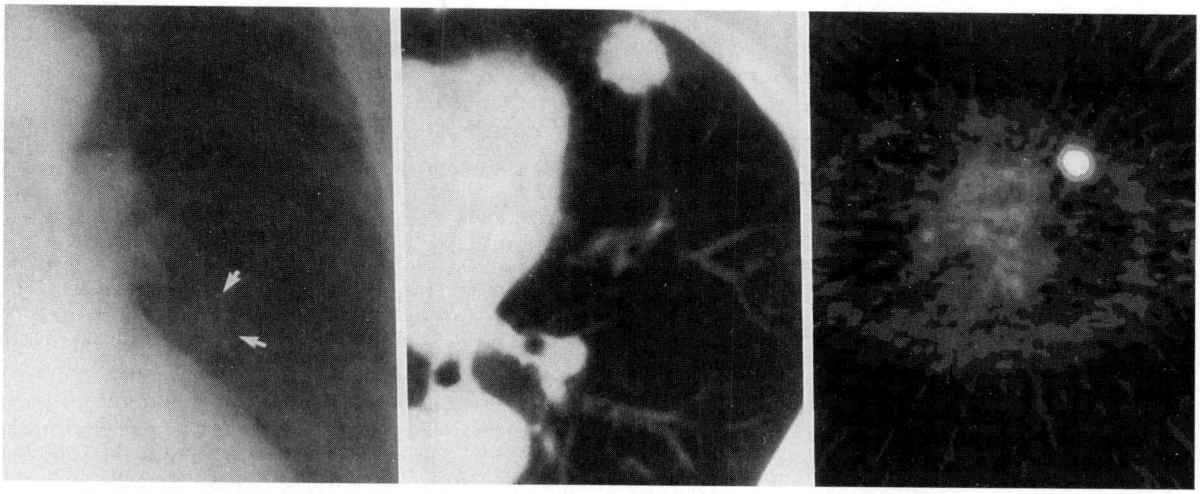

Figure 31.15. Adenocarcinoma in an asymptomatic 72-year-old woman. **A.** Posterior chest radiograph demonstrates a 1.5 cm lingular nodule adjacent to the left heart border. Radiographs obtained previously were not available. **B.** CT scan of the nodule demonstrates a homogeneous, irregularly marginated lesion. **C.** Axial FDG PET scan demonstrates substantial uptake in the nodule. Biopsy revealed adenocarcinoma. (Reproduced by permission from Patz EF Jr, Lowe VJ, Hoffman JM, et al. Focal pulmonary abnormalities: evaluation with F-18 fluorodeoxyglucose PET scanning. Radiology 1993; 188:487–490.)

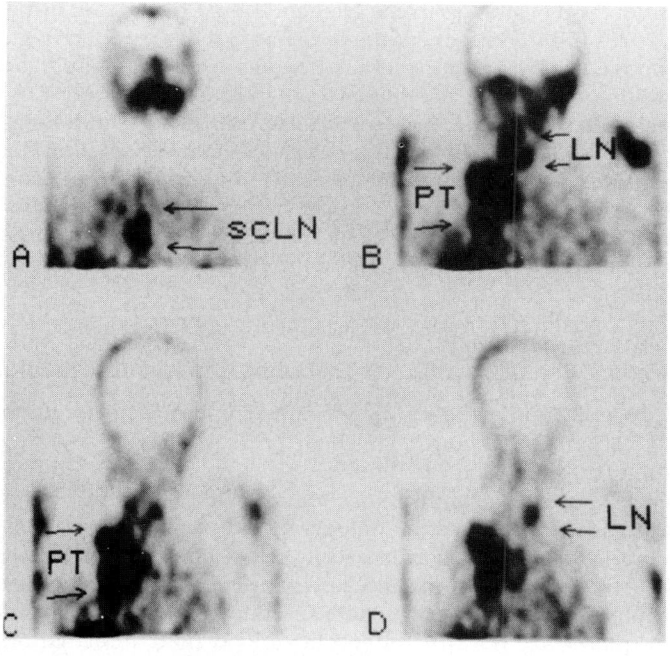

Figure 31.16. Localization of ^{123}I-Tyr-3-octriotide accumulation in small cell lung cancer. The coronal SPECT images of the head and thorax show positive image of the primary tumor and lymph node metastases. The subcarinal lymph node metastasis (scLN) is seen in image **A**. The primary tumor (PT, diameter 8 cm) in the right upper lobe is delineated best in images **B** and **C**. Lymph node metastases (*LN*) in the superior mediastinum are best seen in images **B**, **C**, and **D**. Activity in the lower left part of all images represents physiologic tracer uptake by the liver. (Reproduced by permission from Leitha T, Meghdadi S, Studnicka M, et al. The role of iodine-123-Tyr-3-octreotide scintigraphy in the staging of small cell lung cancer. J Nucl Med 1993; 34:1397–1402.)

proved accuracy may result from image fusion or registration techniques that allow correlation with CT and MRI. For example, "fused" radiolabeled antibody SPECT with CT in patients with lung cancer has been shown to decrease SPECT false-positives and CT false-negatives (92).

SPECIFIC DISEASE APPLICATIONS

DESTRUCTIVE LUNG DISEASE

There have been many studies that have applied V/Q scanning to nonembolic lung disorders. ^{133}Xe has been used to evaluate the extent of air trapping following smoke inhalation injury (93) or exposure to airway toxins. ^{81m}Kr and radioaerosols have been used to evaluate the restrictive lung disease of radiation fibrosis (94). Both perfusion and ventilation have been shown to be reduced within minutes of pulmonary contusion (95), an example of posttraumatic consolidative lung disease.

Nonetheless, ventilation and perfusion (V/Q) lung studies have not achieved routine use in nonembolic lung disease. Despite evidence to suggest that regional ventilation studies can be more sensitive to the presence of lung disease than pulmonary function studies or radiographic assessments (96, 97), there is little clinical enthusiasm for routine scanning. In part, this is due to the nonspecific nature of V/Q scintigraphic abnormalities. VQ scans are not a satisfactory means to define disease etiology, or the local cause for ventilation abnormalities, i.e., similar findings may accompany airway secretions, atelectasis, bronchial obstruction, invasion or collapse, parenchymal destruction, inflammation or edema. Abnormal study findings may also have little pathophysiologic importance (98). For example, diffuse ventilation abnormalities are found in 41% of middle-age smokers with either mild or no respiratory symptoms. There is only a weak relationship between an abnormal ventilation scan and the deterioration of overall lung function (reduced FEV1, VC, increased single breath N2 slope, and closing volume) and there is no relationship between the presence of chronic expectoration and an abnormal scan (99). Although ventilatory dysfunction may be an early sign of disease, the extent of scintigraphic findings due to age-related "normal" dysfunction is unknown. Other reasons for the lack of a routine application of V/Q scintigraphy are logistical and economic, but the most important is the general utility of standard pulmonary function studies and the chest radiograph.

What about the staging and follow-up of lung disease? With the exception of studies performed before lung resection to predict postoperative lung reserve (100), V/Q scans are rarely used in staging pulmonary disease (101). This lack of use is due to the pulmonologist's reliance on pulmonary function tests and to the relative (nonabsolute) nature of pulmonary scintigraphy. Unlike ^{67}Ga lung scans or aerosol clearance studies that can detect the acute process, ventilation studies are unable to separate acute and treatable disease from chronic parenchymal processes. Similar arguments hold for serial assessments of pulmonary disease. As an indicator of overall change, there are too many circumstances where regional function is either unreliable or misleading to be useful in following disease progression or response to therapy. The standard chest radiograph and pulmonary functions are not likely to be displaced by routine scintigraphy in such assessments. Nonetheless, ventilation studies do have an important role in certain patient populations, e.g., the small child or infant, where lack of cooperation is an issue, and where accurate pulmonary function tests are difficult to obtain (102–104).

SCINTIGRAPHIC STUDIES IN CHILDREN

Radioactive gases provide a simple, safe, and unique method for evaluating regional lung function in children with pulmonary disease. Inert gases, such as ^{81m}Kr provide high quality images with low radiation exposure, and require little cooperation from the child. ^{81m}Kr ventilation and ^{99m}Tc perfusion scanning are particularly useful in small children in whom tests of overall pulmonary function cannot be carried out because of lack of cooperation (104).

^{133}Xe scans have been used to screen children before bronchoscopic examination with the aim of obtaining a more exact indication for bronchography (105). Another inhalation scintigraphic agent, ^{99m}Tc technegas has also been found to be a reliable, nonhazardous procedure to preselect young patients for directed bronchoscopy (106).

Bronchopleural Fistula and Foreign Body Aspiration

Fistulas following pneumonectomy and in the setting of empyema have been imaged by ^{133}Xe ventilation lung scanning (107, 108). Because of its ease and simplicity, the ventilation study should be one of the first diagnostic tests performed when bronchopleural fistula is suspected.

Aspiration of a foreign body into the lower respiratory tract is an emergency that occurs mainly in young children, 70% of whom are below 4 years of age, and is a main cause of accidental death in children under 1 year of age. Although complete obstruction is relatively rare, foreign bodies can cause radiographic signs of obstructive emphysema, atelectasis, or elevation of the diaphragm. More commonly, the radiograph is of limited help and fluoroscopy may be insensitive to the presence of small foreign bodies. In this setting, ^{133}Xe ventilation scanning is useful in the selection of patients for bronchoscopy (109) because it is rapidly performed and requires little patient cooperation.

Hyperlucent Lung

The Swyer-James syndrome is thought of result from insults to the lung occurring during childhood. These include radiation therapy (110), measles, pertussis, tuberculosis, adenoviral infection, and after aspiration of a foreign body. These initiate an inflammatory process that proceeds to bronchiolitis obliterans with eventual destruction of the lung parenchyma. The reduction in the pulmonary capillary bed causes significant reduction in the major pulmonary arteries and, ultimately, hypoplastic vasculature (111). Radiographically, these pathologic changes result in a small hyperlucent lung with an ipsilateral small hilum, diffuse air trapping, and segmental bronchiectasis.

Careful assessment of the ventilation and perfusion scan findings can reliably differentiate primary ventilatory causes of unilateral hyperlucent lung from the Swyer-James syndrome (111). Swyer-James syndrome is usually associated with significantly reduced and irregular ventilation and perfusion to the affected lung. Primary acquired causes of hyperlucency due to bronchial obstruction (e.g., foreign body, intrabronchial neoplasm, mucus plug) or pulmonary artery occlusion (e.g., pulmonary artery stenosis, pulmonary arteritis, massive pulmonary embolism) can be differentiated by the nearly complete loss of either airflow or blood flow to the affected lung on the scan. The ventilation perfusion scan can be of importance to patients who present acutely where accurate assessment can preclude more invasive diagnostic procedures.

PULMONARY VASCULAR DISORDERS

Evaluation of Pulmonary Vascular Abnormality/Shunt

Congenital or postoperative lung perfusion abnormalities in patients with congenital heart defects may be asymptomatic and difficult to detect, especially if they are unilateral. These abnormalities are often amenable to correction with surgery or balloon angioplasty. Fewer than half of patients with these disorders show chest x-ray findings that correspond to abnormalities evident by perfusion scintigraphy (112). Additionally, radionuclide studies can be used to quantitate relative pulmonary blood flow, information important in planning interventions that is not available from chest x-rays or two-dimensional echocardiography (112). Over 80% of patients have perfusion abnormalities involving up to an entire lung following operation for transposition of the great arteries (113). In patients like these, scans may be used in the postoperative period to assess capillary perfusion reserve. Scintigraphy may also be used to determine the severity of pulmonary parenchymal damage in patients with atrial septal defect. Patients with apically redistributed and mottled perfusion show a significant increase in pulmonary arteriolar resistance and a significant decrease in pulmonary to systemic blood flow ratio (114).

Severe hypoxia is often due to intrapulmonary shunts through pulmonary arteriovenous fistulas. These abnormalities are tiny and are difficult to demonstrate angiographically. Hypoxemia induced by intrapulmonary shunts is associated with significant intraoperative and postoperative risk and is a relative contraindication to liver transplantation (115). Thus, calculation of the right-to-left shunt through pulmonary arteriovenous malformations is important in assessing surgical risk. It is also used to gauge the potential benefit from therapeutic embolization or surgical resection.

^{99m}Tc macroaggregates of albumin and human albumin microspheres have been used for determination of cardiac output or its distribution among various organs, study of right to left intracardiac shunts, and the diagnosis of great vein abnormalities (115). The systemic distribution of labeled albumin particles can be used to determine shunt fraction because they do not normally traverse the pulmonary capillary bed. The right-to-left shunt fraction can be obtained by comparing radioactive counts in the right kidney (an index of systemic activity) to counts in the injected dose (or total lung counts) (116). Whole-body scanning has also been used to calculate the right-to-left shunt fraction, but extrapulmonary activity may be falsely elevated due to unbound ^{99m}Tc or scatter from the lung region. (115)

An index based upon brain and pulmonary activity may also be used to quantify intrathoracic shunt (Fig. 31.17). Determination of brain activity avoids pulmonary scattering and possible salivary or thyroid activity. Cerebral activity is not increased by unbound ^{99m}Tc (115).

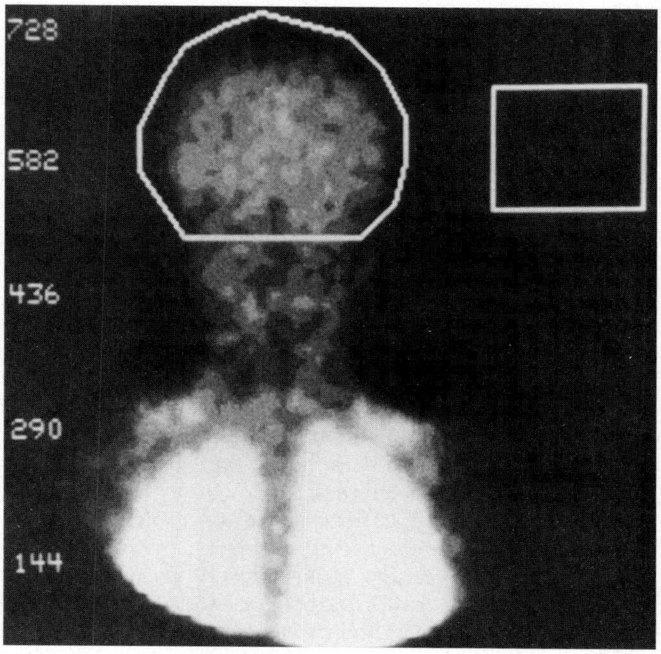

Figure 31.17. Calculation of intrapulmonary shunt index in a patient with high intrapulmonary shunting and localization of ^{99m}Tc macroaggregated albumin in the brain. Brain and background regions of interest are shown. Shunt index is determined by the background corrected percentage of activity in the brain relative to the lung. (Reproduced by permission from Grimon G, Andre L, Bernard O, Raffestin B, Desgrez A. Early radionuclide detection of intrapulmonary shunts in children with liver disease. J Nucl Med 1994; 35:1328–1332.)

Evaluation of Hemoptysis/Hemorrhage

^{99m}Tc-sulfur colloid and ^{99m}Tc red blood cells have been used to identify sites of hemoptysis using techniques primarily developed to locate gastrointestinal tract bleeding (117). The minimum detectable rate of bleeding appears to be about 50 ml/24 hr. In patients with massive pulmonary hemorrhage, localized deposition of radionuclide can be demonstrated rapidly and confirmed via bronchoscopy. In this setting, lung scans provide clinically useful information regarding the bleeding site that is not available from the medical history, physical examination, or chest x-ray (118).

Pulmonary Hypertension

The diagnosis of primary pulmonary hypertension is made by exclusion and must be differentiated from thromboembolic pulmonary hypertension which is potentially surgically correctable. Unfortunately, patients with chronic thromboembolic pulmonary hypertension commonly present with progressive dyspnea, evidence of cor pulmonale, and no clear prior history of acute thromboembolism. While perfusion scans in primary pulmonary hypertension may show certain abnormalities, such as nonsegmental, patchy defects of perfusion, the presence of segmental or larger perfusion defects should suggest the diagnosis of potentially correctable, large-vessel thromboembolic pulmonary hypertension rather than small-vessel, obliterative (primary, idiopathic) pulmonary hypertension (119). A retrospective review of 15 patients with angiographically or biopsy documented primary pulmonary hypertension showed that none demonstrated a segmental or larger perfusion defect whereas such defects have been uniformly present in patients with large-vessel thromboembolic pulmonary hypertension (120).

NEOPLASTIC LUNG DISEASE

Lung cancer is now the most frequent cause of cancer deaths among both men and women in the United States. Its overall incidence is rising. Bronchogenic carcinoma now accounts for approximately 25% of all deaths from cancer and has an overall 5-year survival of only 13%. The diagnosis, staging, and therapeutic monitoring of lung cancer present a variety of radiographic challenges (121).

It is likely that all bronchogenic carcinomas are derived from a pleuripotential stem cell of epithelial origin. The term bronchogenic carcinoma, literally meaning a carcinoma of the bronchus, now represents any of the major cell types of lung cancer comprising squamous cell, small cell, large cell, adenosquamous, and adenocarcinoma. Together these account for more than 90% of all lung cancers. Other, relatively rare, primary lung neoplasms include the sarcomas, mesotheliomas, carcinoids, and mucoepidermoid cancers.

For clinical purposes, bronchogenic carcinoma is usually subdivided into two categories; small cell and nonsmall cell lung cancer. Twenty percent of lung malignancies are small cell lung cancers (SCLC). These tumors are rapidly dividing and metabolically active tumors that are relatively sensitive to chemotherapy and radiation therapy. Unfortunately, they also are often widely disseminated at the time of patient presentation. With systemic therapy, mean survival is less than 1 year, and 5-year survival is an abysmal 10% (122). Small cell cancers express the entire range of neuroendocrine cell markers and are believed to arise from pulmonary endocrine cells that are scattered throughout the tracheobronchial tree. In contrast to small cell cancers, nonsmall cell cancers (NSCLC) are less metabolically active, less disseminated, and less responsive to chemotherapy or radiotherapy.

Chest radiography, with or without supplemental sputum cytology, can detect lung cancer at an earlier stage than controls, but chest x-ray screening has not been found to reduce overall lung cancer mortality. Radiologic detection of lung cancer occurs relatively late in the course of the disease process. Given that the smallest detectable lesion is about 10 mm in size, by the time diagnosis can be made, the tumor has gone through about 30 doublings in cell mass and has achieved a population of more than a billion cells. Depending on cell type, each doubling requires 30–180 days, so that by the time of detection, the average cancer has been present for nearly 9 years. It is little surprise, therefore, that none of the current clinical, laboratory, radiographic, or scintigraphic technologies has been shown to have any impact on survival when used as a screening test for lung cancer (123). The utility of a cancer screening test depends ultimately on its ability to detect early disease, but the cost of a program depends both on the expense of the test itself and the added cost and morbidity of false-positive tests that lead to other unnecessary procedures. The requirement of adequate sensitivity and very high specificity is beyond the capabilities of current imaging technologies (124). Thus, the role of imaging procedures is only relevant to cancer staging and posttherapy follow-up studies.

Staging of Lung Cancer

A bronchogenic carcinoma is staged to estimate the anatomic extent of the cancer and thereby define the therapeutic approach and patient prognosis. The most broadly accepted staging system is that proposed by the 1986 American Joint Commission on Cancer. This system uses TNM notation which codifies cancer stage (I-IV) from the degree and distribution of disease at the tumor primary (T), in thoracic nodes (N), and at metastatic sites (M). Five-year survival for stage I and II disease is 50–70% and 30–50% respectively, provided that the tumor does not extend beyond the lung and that the mediastinal nodes are uninvolved. In stage IIIa, i.e., with extension beyond the lung parenchyma or ipsilateral mediastinal lymph nodes, 5-year survival falls to less than 20%. Stages IIIb (contralateral mediastinal or hilar node involvement) or stage IV (distant metastasis) have much poorer outcomes with 5-year survival less than 5% (125).

The TNM lung cancer staging system has had its greatest impact in NSCLC. Small cell lung cancer, however, is distinguished from other bronchopleural neoplasms by its great likelihood of covert and overt metastatic tumor at the time of presentation. For SCLC, the clinical performance status and the extent of tumor dissemination are the most important prognostic factors. A clinical, two-stage system proposed by the Veteran's Administration Lung Group, distinguishes between limited and extensive disease and has a higher prognostic strength than the TNM stage (126). Limited disease is defined as confined to the hemithorax, mediastinum, and ipsilateral supraclavicular space, whereas extensive disease has escaped these boundaries.

Positron Emission Tomography and Monoclonal Antibody Studies

Although CT and MRI remain the primary means to stage lung cancer, radionuclide studies using monoclonal antibodies and positron emission tomography are beginning to challenge the anatomic procedures in clinical practice. A number of studies have shown the clinical utility of monoclonal antibody (MoAb) imaging and report accuracies that compare favorably with CT. Positron emission tomography (PET) scanners are becoming widely available and are establishing an important clinical role because (a) the labeled compounds are biologically important, (b) the radionuclide half-life is usually short, and (c) the radionuclide tissue concentration can be determined quantitatively, accurately, and, in many cases, noninvasively (75).

MoAb and PET radionuclide imaging studies are of greatest practical importance in identifying patients with pulmonary tumors, staging the patient's hilum and mediastinal nodes, and following the treated patient for recurrence of disease.

Solitary Pulmonary Nodules. Many lung carcinomas are initially encountered as solitary pulmonary nodules (SPN). SPN are parenchymal lung lesions that are usually well-defined and less than 4 cm in diameter. An estimated 130,000 new, benign, or malignant SPN are discovered each year in the United States. Primary bronchogenic carcinoma and benign granulomas constitute over 80% of pulmonary nodules, with about equal distribution in both categories (127). Less common diagnoses include hamartoma (6%), solitary metastases from nonlung primaries (5%), and bronchial adenoma (2%) (127, 128).

The goal of evaluation of a SPN is to distinguish between benign and malignant disease. Factors that increase the probability of malignancy include cigarette smoking, patient age greater than 35 years, irregular nodule margins, absence of calcification, and the size of the nodule (129). In a recent study of lung nodules larger than 3 cm, 98% of the nodules were malignant (130). The only two definite radiographic criteria for benign solitary pulmonary nodules are the presence of central, concentric, or stippled calcification as seen on chest radiographs or computed tomographic CT scan, and stability of the nodule for more than 2 years (130). Currently, plain radiography and CT are most commonly used to evaluate SPN, but most noncalcified SPN remain indeterminate (84). The typical pattern of dense central, laminated, or diffuse calcification, which virtually excludes malignancy, is only seen in a minority of SPNs (84).

Positron emission tomography with FDG was found to be highly accurate in differentiating benign from malignant focal pulmonary abnormalities seen on chest radiographs (Fig. 31.18) (80, 84, 130). In one series of 51 well-characterized pulmonary nodules, malignant lesions all exceeded a threshold value of FDG localization (standardized uptake ratio of 2.5), while nodules falling below the threshold were all found to be benign disease (80). In a prospective study of 30 patients presenting with indeterminate solitary pulmonary nodules less than 3 cm in size, FDG differential uptake ratios produced positive and negative predictive values of about 90% (130). Analogous results separating benign and malignant SPN were found in studies comparing FDG and L-[methyl ^{11}C]methionine (131, 132).

These studies suggest that PET-FDG imaging has a high degree of accuracy in differentiating benign from malignant pulmonary nodules greater than 1–1.5 cm in size. Quantitation is difficult, however, for lesions less than 1–1.5 cm in diameter due to limits in PET resolution, respiratory motion, and partial volume effects (80, 132). Occasional false-positive studies were found in highly metabolic benign diseases such as tuberculosis, histoplasmosis, aspergilloma, and abscesses (80, 83, 130).

Studies of pulmonary lesions using radiolabeled antibodies show sensitivities ranging from 68–100%, depending on the antigen targeted, the radiolabel, and the antibody form. Lower sensitivities are generally found with tracers that clear the blood slowly, or decay rapidly, due to lower tumor target to blood background ratios (133, 134). For example, blood pool activity in pulmonary vessels was more intense than the lung tumors at 6–8 hours for an anti-CEA ^{99m}Tc Fab′ antibody fragment in patients with NSCLC (134). Better imaging results were evident with a CEA-specific ^{111}In F(ab′)$_2$ (Fig. 31.19) (135). Monoclonal antibody imaging has compared well with CT in staging primary tumors. In a study comparing CT to ^{111}In F(ab′)$_2$ fragments of an anti-CEA antibody, the MoAb study showed accuracies of 78% and 86% for T3 and T4 disease, respectively, as compared to CT accuracies of 78% and 84%, respectively (136).

The target antigen in most of the recent studies was the carcinoembryonic antigen (CEA) (Table 31.2), but milk fat globule (137), epidermal growth factor receptors (138), and cell surface glycoproteins (139) were also studied in clinical trials. Sensitivities reported for antibodies targeting these antigens have ranged from 86–100%. For the primary NSCLC tumors reported in these studies, small size or central location was the usual cause for nonvisualization of tumors. Typically, to avoid high blood pool background activity, images were obtained at approximately two blood half-lives after antibody administration (134).

It is recognized that nonspecific factors may play a supportive role in tumor detection. For example, in one study, the target antigen was present in only 89% of the tumors where the antibody localized (135). Nonspecific antibody

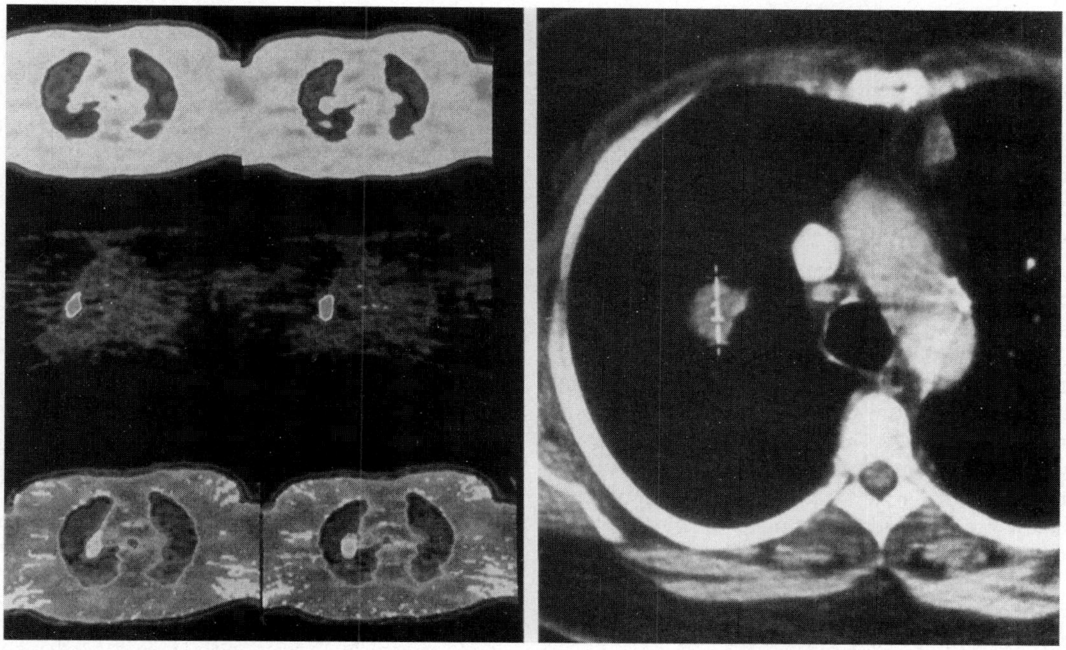

Figure 31.18. PET-FDG (**A**) and CT scans (**B**) in a 50-year-old woman with a 2.0×1.5 cm nodule in her right lung that was adenocarcinoma at thoracotomy. Intense metabolic activity is present in the nodule on the emission scans (*middle images in A*) obtained in the transaxial projection. *Top images in A* are transmission scans, *bottom images in A* are overlays. (Reproduced by permission from Gupta NC, Frank AR, Dewan NA, et al. Solitary pulmonary nodules: detection of malignancy with PET with 2-[F-18]-fluoro-2-deoxy-D-glucose. Radiology 1992;184:441–444.)

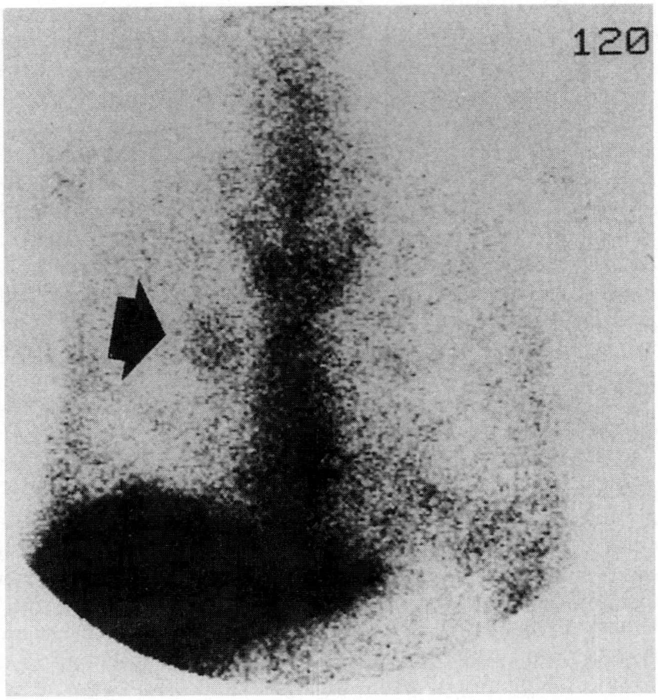

Figure 31.19. Squamous-cell carcinoma of the right anterior bronchus as demonstrated by ^{111}In-anti-CEA MoAb imaging. Anterior view of the thorax at 120 hours after intravenous injection, shows circumscribed uptake in the right hilar region. Left lower lobe activity is due to the cardiac blood pool. Tumor/heart ratio was 1.02▲mor/lung ratio was 1.6. (Reproduced by permission from Biggi A, Buccheri G, Ferrigno D, et al. Detection of suspected primary lung cancer by scintigraphy with indium-111-anticarcinoembryonic antigen monoclonal antibodies (type F023C5). J Nucl Med 1991;32:2064–2068.)

uptake in histologically nonreactive tumors may be due to anomalies in tumor angioarchitecture, enhanced transvascular leak in neoplastic capillaries, cross-reactivity with nontarget antigens, and nonspecific ^{111}In uptake by transferrin receptors of tumor cells (136).

Evaluation of Mediastinal Lymph Nodes and Metastasis. Preoperative assessment of the mediastinal lymph nodes is mandatory because if mediastinal lymph node metastases are present at the time of diagnosis, 5-year survival after surgery falls to less than 10% (79). Unfortunately, with regard to diagnostic imaging accuracy in presurgical staging, prospective data from the multi-institutional Radiologic Diagnostic Oncology Group trial showed that in NSCLC, CT was only 52% sensitive and 69% specific, whereas MR imaging was 48% sensitive and 64% specific (140). The accuracy of CT also varies according to the mediastinal region examined. For example, the aortopulmonary window region is less accurately assessed than the peritracheal, subcarinal, and anterior mediastinal regions (123). The location of the primary cancer is one of the factors that can decrease anatomic staging accuracy. Squamous cell cancers, which are often centrally located, can cause postobstructive, reactive lymph node enlargement and false-positive nodal assessments. Furthermore, it is often difficult to determine the size/extent of the primary tumor within the density caused by postobstructive collapse and reactive inflammation (134).

FDG PET imaging can provide information to enhance the accuracy of presurgical staging (79, 141). A prospective trial to compare FDG PET and CT in surgically confirmed patients, having a high percentage of mediastinal disease, showed that PET (82% sensitive, 81% specific, and 81% accurate) was significantly better than CT (64% sensitive, 44% specific, and 52% accurate) in staging mediastinal disease (Fig. 31.20) (79). It is likely that the greater utility of PET imaging relative to more conventional whole-body or planar scintigraphy is related to its high sensitivity (20–

Table 31.2.
Monoclonal Antibodies in Human Clinical Trials.

Antibody Name	Isotope	Form	Target	Reference
NR-LU-10	^{99m}Tc	Fab′	Pan CA	91, 139, 222–225
	^{111}In	Fab′	Pan CA	135
BW 431/26	^{99m}Tc	IgG1	CEA	226–231
BW 431/31	^{111}In	F(ab′)2	CEA	228, 231
	^{131}I	F(ab′)2	CEA	228
IMACIS-1	^{131}I	MoAb	CEA	228
ZCE025	^{111}In	MoAb	CEA	133, 232, 233
FO23C5	^{111}In	F(ab′)2	CEA	136, 234, 235
IMMU-4	^{99m}Tc	Fab′	CEA	134
KC-4G3	^{111}In	MoAb	Milk fat globule antigens	137
HMFG1	^{111}In	F(ab′)2	Milk fat globule antigens	236, 237
MAb 225	^{111}In	IgG1	EGF	138

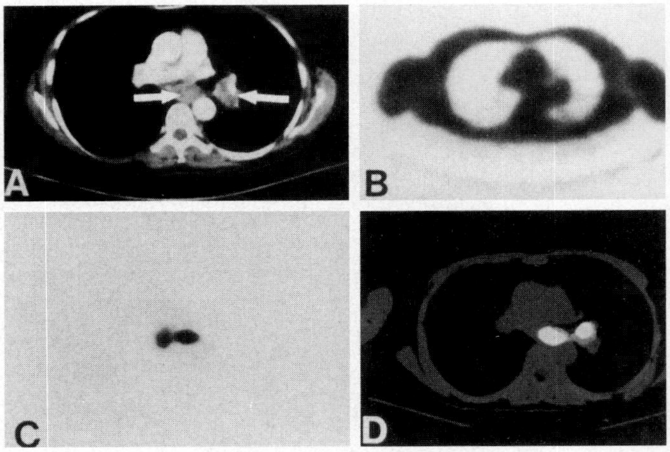

Figure 31.20. FDG-PET scans in a patient with mediastinal node involvement from nonsmall cell lung cancer. **A.** Enlarged mediastinal lymph nodes (*arrows* are present on diagnostic contrast-enhanced CT scan. **B.** Transmission PET scan provides low-resolution anatomic image of thorax. **C.** Emission PET can shows intense FDG uptake by mediastinum 50–60 minutes after tracer injection. **D.** Anatometabolic fusion image shows intense FDG uptake by enlarged nodes. Metastatic (poorly differentiated) cancer was proved present in mediastinal nodes in this patient. (Reproduced by permission from Wahl RL, Quint LE, Greenough RL, Meyer CR, White RI, Orringer MB. Staging of mediastinal nonsmall cell lung cancer with FDG PET, CT, and fusion images: preliminary prospective evaluation. Radiology 1994;191:371–377.)

50 times more sensitive than a standard gamma-camera) and tumor-blood background ratios that are often more than 10:1 (79). Like other radionuclides (^{67}Ga, ^{201}Tl), however, FDG uptake is not specific for malignancy, false-positives being mainly due to inflammatory disease. Nonetheless, the ability of PET to quantitate FDG uptake may provide greater specificity than can be achieved from the more qualitative gamma emission studies.

^{111}In F(ab′)$_2$ fragments of an anti-CEA antibody have also performed well in all regional assessments of nodal disease. Accuracies of 65%, 76%, and 92% for N1, N2, and N3 disease, respectively, were found for the antibody, as compared to CT accuracies of 62%, 68%, and 42%, respectively (136). Similarly, a ^{99m}Tc Fab fragment that recognizes a 40 kD glycoprotein (NR-LU-10) was as accurate as CT in assessing mediastinal nodal involvement (Fig. 31.21). Both imaging modalities tended to have false-positive rather than false-negative findings, but not necessarily in the same patients (91). Another study using the same antibody in 52 patients with nonsmall cell lung carcinoma, compared antibody imaging to CT and histologic confirmation (139). CT detected 88% of confirmed lung lesions and nodal regions, but only 44–57% of patients with N2 disease. The antibody study detected 91% of lesions and identified 86–89% of patients with N2 disease. The combined utility of both CT and antibody imaging was very high, with an overall sensitivity of 100% and a 100% negative predictive value (139).

The role of MoAb imaging in SCLC addresses whether the patient has extensive disease. In 89 evaluable patients with SCLC, MoAb imaging was accurate in 82–86% of patients with extensive disease, with a positive predictive value of 95–100% (139).

Cancer Therapy Follow-up. The therapeutic effectiveness of cancer treatment by radiotherapy and chemotherapy is usually evaluated by morphologic changes in tumor size. However, it is well-known that changes in tumor size do not necessarily indicate a therapeutic effect (142). Furthermore, anatomic imaging modalities provide important morphologic information but often do not distinguish between recurrent tumor and benign posttreatment inflammation or fibrosis (121).

FDG PET has been used to evaluate lung cancer after therapy, in an effort to predict treatment response (142, 143). Unfortunately, a decreased FDG uptake with treatment does not necessarily indicate a good prognosis (142). Similar findings were noted in a study using MET (132).

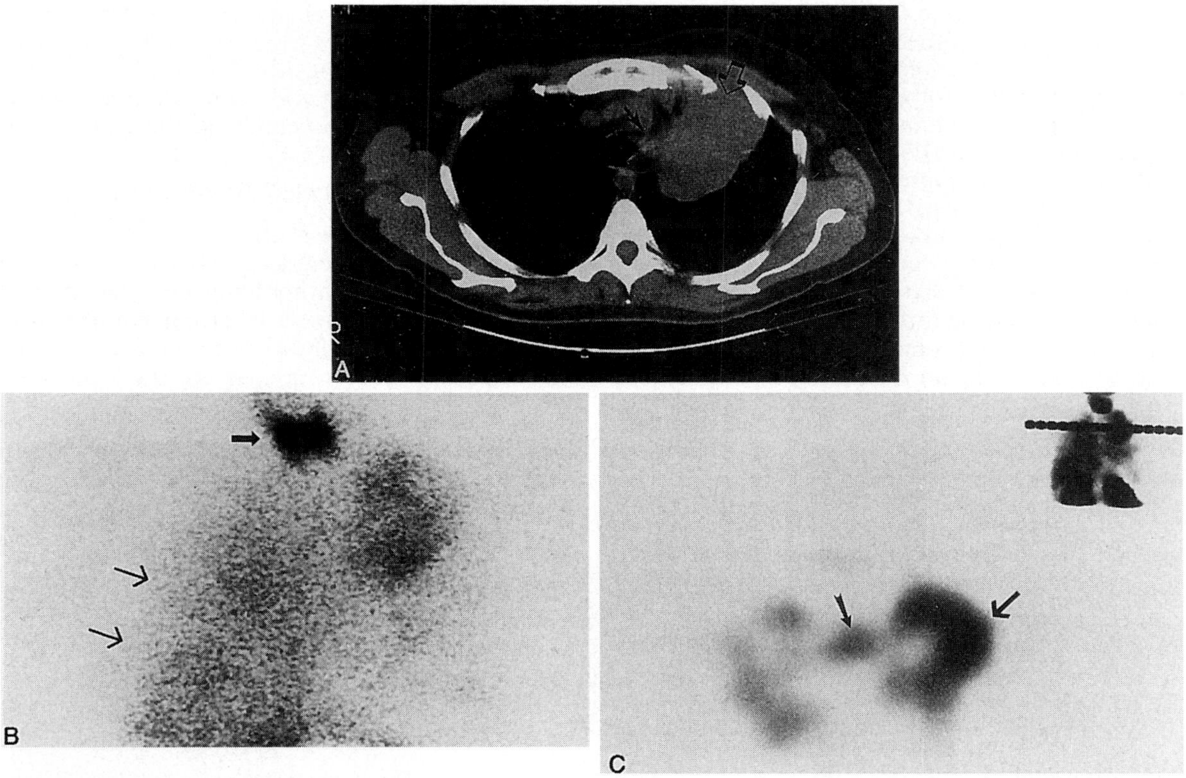

Figure 31.21. Monoclonal antibody imaging in a patient with mediastinal nodal disease in nonsmall cell lung carcinoma. **A.** CT scan of chest showing large mass in left lung (*open arrow*) and enlarged left paratracheal node (*closed arrow*). **B.** Anterior planar view from NR-LU-10 monoclonal antibody scan of patient in A. There is minimal background activity in right lung (*thin arrows*) and intense uptake in thyroid gland (*wide arrow*) and in primary left upper lobe tumor. Left paratracheal lymph node cannot be appreciated on this scan. **C.** Transaxial SPECT image of chest from antibody scan of same patient. Coronal SPECT image (*upper right-hand corner*) is shown as a reference for location of transaxial cut. SPECT shows intense antibody uptake in primary tumor (*large arrow*) and demonstrates paratracheal node found to be positive at operation (*small arrow*). (Reproduced by permission from Rusch V, Macapinlac H, Heelan R, et al. NR-LU-10 monoclonal antibody scanning. A helpful new adjunct to computed tomography in evaluating nonsmall cell lung cancer. J Thorac Cardiovasc Surg 1993;106:200–204.)

Indeed, it is probably too much to expect that uptake of FDG or MET can define tumor biology sufficiently to characterize prognosis. There are a host of factors beyond metabolic activity that are important in this regard.

FDG PET imaging can be used to distinguish persistent or recurrent bronchogenic carcinoma from posttherapy fibrosis. Quantitative analysis of FDG uptake is highly successful in separating these patient groups (Fig. 31.22) (121). Thus, patients with residual abnormalities on radiographs greater than 1 cm in size, but normal findings on PET scans, will very likely be free of disease. However, apparent FDG activity in lesions smaller than 1 cm may be falsely low because of partial volume effects on PET images (121). False-positive studies in this setting may be the result of inflammation due to infection or radiation therapy within the prior 12 months (144).

Gallium-67 and Thallium-201 Scans

^{67}Ga scans have been evaluated with regard to uptake in the primary tumor, mediastinal uptake, and localization in distant metastatic disease. Over 90% of NSCLC take up ^{67}Ga. The overall accuracy for detecting a suspected primary tumor is 89% (145). The overall accuracy for mediastinal staging in patients with peripheral lung cancers is 80%. The presence of a centrally located primary tumor causes the accuracy to drop to 61% because of the difficulty in separating uptake of the primary from that of mediastinal lymph nodes (145, 146). Although ^{67}Ga scans can identify mediastinal node involvement, there is considerable controversy over the relationship between the sensitivity and specificity of the method. Two main factors limit the sensitivity of ^{67}Ga scintigraphy. Microscopic intranodal metastases may fail to increase the size of a node into the range (1.5–2.0 cm) which can be successfully resolved by ^{67}Ga scintigraphy. Secondly, in patients with primary paramediastinal tumors, ^{67}Ga uptake by adjacent mediastinal nodes may not be separately identifiable owing to their close proximity to the primary tumor.

The accuracy of scanning for distant organ metastases exceeds 90% and otherwise occult metastatic disease is identified in about 10% of patients(123). By detecting distant extrathoracic metastases, the ^{67}Ga scan may identify a small group of patients who can be spared a needless operation. ^{67}Ga scanning fails specifically for metastases within the brain; thus, it does not supplant CT scans of the brain and it is less sensitive than bone scans in detecting osseous metastases. Since CT scanning is currently used in staging of most patients with lung cancer, the additional yield from ^{67}Ga scintigraphy has proven to be relatively low. Fewer than 10% of patients will have significant findings on ^{67}Ga scintigraphy that were unsuspected by CT, and most of those individuals have clinical findings suggesting the presence of metastatic disease (147). Thus, ^{67}Ga scintigraphy is no longer considered a primary imaging modality in the staging of pulmonary tumors (123).

^{201}Tl has also been shown to localize in pulmonary malignancies. Tonami and associates (78) studied 170 patients who had a malignant pulmonary lesion greater than 20 mm in diameter on surgical specimens. Single photon emission computed tomography performed at 3 hours after injection was positive in all of the 147 malignant pulmonary lesions and 16 of 23 (69.6%) benign pulmonary foci. ^{201}Tl residence in malignant tumors was shown to be significantly longer than in benign disease. Although mediastinal blood pool activity clouded early images, mediastinal lymph node metastases were detected on delayed scans, the smallest of which was 1.5 cm in diameter (78). Although ^{201}Tl imaging provides insight as to the metabolic nature of pulmonary and mediastinal masses, it remains unclear whether it can challenge the utility of CT imaging.

Other Radionuclide Studies in Lung Cancer

Radionuclide studies of the brain, liver, and bones have been used to detect metastatic disease, but are rarely abnormal in patients without suggestive symptoms or signs of metastasis. Conversely, when clinical signs of metastatic disease are present, liver scintigraphy is often false-negative (123). Given their greater accuracy and anatomic de-

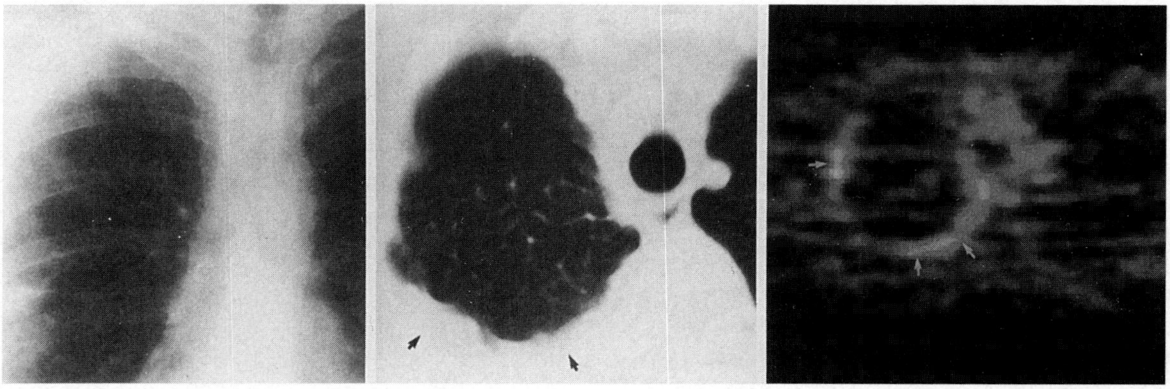

Figure 31.22. FDG-PET imaging in a patient with recurrent bronchogenic carcinoma. **A.** Posteroanterior chest radiograph demonstrates minimal right apical pleural thickening 12 months after right lower lobe resection for bronchoalveolar cell carcinoma. **B.** CT scan of the right apex shows thickening of the pleura, which is suggestive of recurrent tumor (*arrows*). **C.** Axial FDG-PET image in the right apex demonstrates several small areas of distinctly increased FDG uptake (*arrows*). Percutaneous biopsy results revealed recurrent tumor. (Reproduced by permission from Patz EF Jr, Lowe VJ, Hoffman JM, Paine SS, Harris LK, Goodman PC. Persistent or recurrent bronchogenic carcinoma: detection with PET and 2-[F-18]-2-deoxy-D-glucose. Radiology 1994;191:379–382).

tail, CT scans of the brain and liver have essentially replaced the corresponding radionuclide studies. Bone scans have been shown to detect clinically unsuspected metastases in as many as 8% of patients and are useful for confirming metastatic disease in patients with clinical findings (123).

Ventilation/perfusion studies have not been useful in tumor detection or in predicting the likelihood of resectability (148). Pulmonary scintigraphy is generally too nonspecific to assess the presence or extent of lung carcinoma. Mediastinal or hilar involvement, for example, are unsuspected scintigraphically in 50% of affected patients (149). Although V/Q studies may allow tumor localization in a small number of patients with abnormal sputum cytology and normal chest radiographs, no specific patterns have been found (150). The frequency of tumor nonresectability may increase when the affected lung perfusion falls to one-third or less of the total pulmonary blood flow (151), but this finding is too unreliable to be considered a contraindication to surgical therapy (149, 152).

Despite the limitations of scintigraphy in evaluating resectability, quantitative studies have an important role in determining patient operability. Considerable disability may result from hypercarbia and chronic ventilatory insufficiency if the patient's postoperative forced expiratory volume in 1 second (FEV1) is less than 0.8 liter (153, 154). To avoid crippling surgery, the contribution of the involved lung to the overall function must be known (155). The good correlation between differential bronchospirometry and ^{133}Xe radiospirometry (156, 157) prompted the use of ^{133}Xe in predictions of postoperative FEV1 and forced vital capacity (FVC) in patients undergoing pneumonectomy (158). Subsequently, the quantitative differential perfusion scan was found to be as accurate in predicting postoperative lung function (155), presumably because of a close relationship between unilateral ventilation and perfusion in patients with lung cancer. Thus, the "split field" perfusion scan rapidly became the procedure of choice because it was simple to perform and widely available (Fig. 31.23).

It has been suggested that for a patient undergoing lung

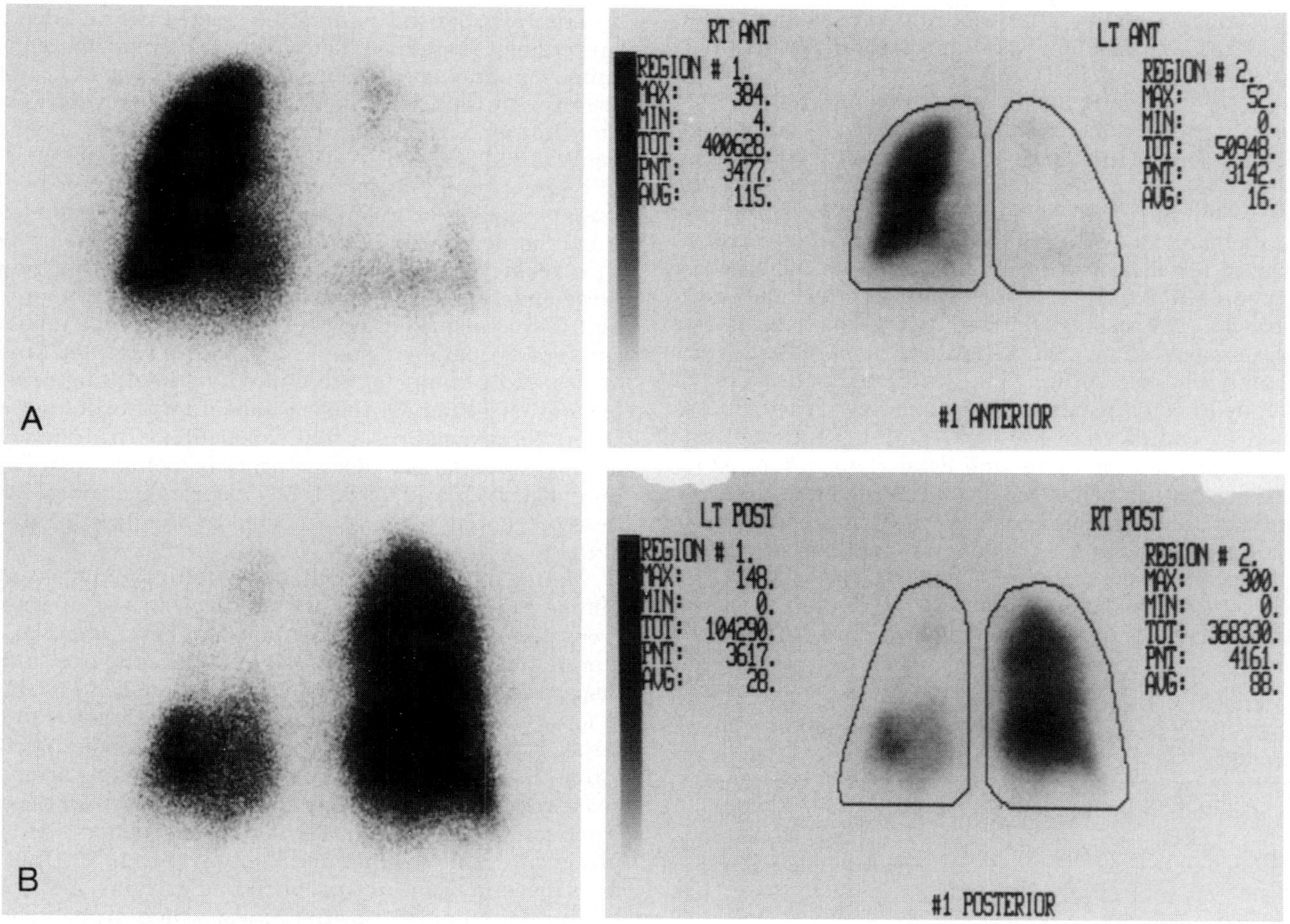

Figure 31.23. Radionuclide Split Function Study Before Lung Resection. Anterior (**A**) and posterior (**B**) perfusion images (*left*) and quantitative analyses (*right*) in a patient with a central left lung carcinoma. The importance of obtaining both anterior and posterior quantitative studies is illustrated by the fact that in the anterior view the relatively normal right lung contains nearly eight times as many total counts as the left lung. In the posterior projection, however, the right lung contains only between three and four times as many counts. Quantitative data from both projections must be combined to allow accurate predictions of postoperative relative lung function. (Reproduced by permissioin from Alderson PO, Biello DR. Radionuclide studies of the pulmonary vasculature. In: Taveras JM, Ferucci JT, eds. Radiology—diagnosis, imaging, intervention. Vol. 1. Philadelphia: JB Lippincott, 1986:11.)

resection, preoperative evaluation should include total pulmonary function measurements. It is highly likely that the patient will tolerate removal of a whole lung if preoperative studies meet these criteria:

- FEV1 is greater than 50% of FVC and is greater than 2 liters.
- The maximum voluntary ventilation is greater than 50% of predicted.
- The ratio of residual volume to total lung capacity is less than 50%.

If these criteria are not satisfied, radionuclide split-function studies are appropriate. Surgery usually is not performed if a postoperative FEV1 of less than 0.8 liter is predicted (159). Split-function studies are done by summing the activity of each lung in anterior and posterior views. The postoperative FEV1 is predicted by multiplying the preoperative value by the ratio of the counts in the lung that will remain to the total lung activity (Table 31.3) (160).

Where pneumonectomy is avoidable, segmental resection or lobectomy has become the surgical procedure of choice. The operative mortality of lobectomy is approximately the same as for pneumonectomy, but the 5-year survival rate is higher after lobectomy, presumably because of a lower incidence of respiratory disability (161, 162).

Because of the difficulty of obtaining quantitative ^{133}Xe ventilation measurements in multiple views, ^{81m}Kr scintigraphy and aerosol inhalation studies provide attractive alternatives for estimating lobar ventilation. ^{81m}Kr imaging has been found to permit quantification of both regional ventilation and lobar V/Q ratios (163). Appropriate regions of interest are drawn to separate lung lobes using either ^{81m}Kr ventilation or ^{99m}Tc perfusion images. Regional quantitation may be best performed using the lateral and oblique images, since lobar separation is more readily defined in these views. Although the interlobar planes are not as well-defined in the posterior oblique views, they are less affected by counts from the opposite lung. Although the optimum method for extracting lobar data is not established, an average of the lobar counts obtained from the lateral and oblique views may be a reasonable compromise between the conflicting goals of optimum lobar separation and avoidance of contralateral activity.

The percentage of global function contributed by the selected lobe is determined as the ratio of counts in that lobe to total counts in the lung. The predicted postlobectomy FEV1 may be determined as in the split-function study, i.e., by multiplying the preoperative FEV1 by the lobar percentages of the ventilation or perfusion of the lung regions that will remain.

Table 31.3.
Ventilation and Perfusion Scintigraphy for Estimating Lobar Ventilation[a].

	^{81m}Kr Ventilation (V) (%)	^{99m}Tc MAA[b] Perfusion (Q) (%)	V/Q
Right Lung	59.5	52.3	1.14
Left Lung	40.5	47.7	.85
Left upper lobe (LUL)	8.6	7.2	1.19
Left lower lobe (LLL)	31.9	40.5	.79
Predicted FEV_1 (ml)	1.49	1.52	

[a]The preoperative FEV_1 was 1.64 liters. Prior to left upper lobectomy the predicted postoperative FEV_1 was calculated as follows:

$$\text{PreOp } FEV_1 \times (100\% - V\%_{LUL}) \text{ or preOp } FEV_1 \times (100\% - Q\%_{LUL})$$

[b]MAA = macroaggregated albumin

INFLAMMATORY LUNG DISEASE

The diffuse lung diseases encompass more than 150 etiologies that are disseminated throughout the lung parenchyma (164). Although some of these diseases develop rapidly because of the action of infectious or toxic agents, most of the disorders are chronic, taking months to years to be manifest clinically.

The delay is probably due to the functional reserve of the lung, which allows it to sustain significant injury before symptoms arise. Because of the potential disparity between injury and symptoms, it is useful to conceptualize each of the diffuse lung diseases as two overlapping processes. One of these is the active injurious process and the other, a more static condition that represents the dysfunction resulting from injury. This distinction is important, because alveolar injury must be treated before it leads to irreversible structural deterioration. Unfortunately, results of pulmonary function tests and chest radiographs are strongly influenced by derangements of alveolar structure that may have little relation to the extent of ongoing injury (165).

To determine the appropriate therapy it is necessary to characterize the cellular nature of the inflammation and to stage the degree of alveolar injury. Lung biopsy or bronchoalveolar lavage studies are essential tools that achieve these ends. Subsequent monitoring of the nature and extent of this alveolitis, however, has been problematic because of the patients' poor acceptance of repeated lung biopsies and because of the limited value of lung function tests or chest radiographs as indicators of ongoing injury (166). Noninvasive tests that can evaluate the "activity" of a diffuse pulmonary disease process include ^{67}Ga-citrate lung scanning and ^{99m}Tc-DTPA clearance studies. These tests are not significantly affected by the functional state of the lung parenchyma.

Uptake of ^{67}Ga in the lungs of patients who have active diffuse lung disease is common, even in the absence of gross radiographic changes. Abnormal ^{67}Ga pulmonary accumulation has been observed in both acute and chronic diseases across a broad range of etiologies (Table 31.1) and is found in patients with acute disease secondary to bacterial, fungal, mycoplasmic, and opportunistic infections (167). ^{67}Ga uptake also occurs in pulmonary toxicity associated with chemotherapy and was proposed for the early detection of interstitial pneumonitis associated with bleomycin or cyclophosphamide therapy (44, 168). Drug addicts also may have normal chest radiographs and intense accumulation of ^{67}Ga in the lungs, which probably is related to hypersensitivity to the talc associated with long-term intravenous injection of addictive drugs (167). Patients who have lung or mediastinal neoplasms and are scanned immediately after receiving radiation therapy, may show diffuse ^{67}Ga lung uptake caused by a transient radiation pneumonitis (169). Several disorders representative of granulomatous, infectious, toxic, idiopathic, and connective tissue diseases are discussed briefly to illustrate the variety of disease etiologies in which ^{67}Ga scanning has been useful clinically.

Open lung biopsy, bronchoalveolar lavage, and ^{67}Ga lung scanning are the three most widely used tests to monitor pulmonary inflammation in the diffuse lung diseases. Lung biopsy is the most sensitive and specific among these procedures, but it samples only a small area of the lung and is usually limited to a single use during the course of the disease. Bronchoalveolar lavage may be performed repeatedly, and provides an assessment of the types, relative numbers, and activation of the effector cells present in the lower respiratory tract. ^{67}Ga scanning is the least invasive study and is capable of assessing the activity of the disease in the entire lung, as well as in extrapulmonary sites.

Many studies show a relatively good correlation among these three assessments of disease activity in the diffuse lung diseases, but results may vary depending on the disease and study design. The reasons for agreement and disagreement are poorly understood, but several factors may contribute to the findings. These factors include differences in the amount of lung sampled, differences in the timing or frequency of sampling, and differences in the aspect of the injury and inflammatory process that each test samples. For example, comparisons between ^{67}Ga scanning and either lavage or lung biopsy may suffer from differences in the site or the amount of lung examined. The cellular material obtained from a saline lavage is derived from a relatively limited region of lung parenchyma. As the distribution of disease lesions is not always diffuse and homogeneous, such a sample may not be representative (170). Another situation wherein ^{67}Ga scanning and lavage differ is that associated with airway disease. Lavage analyses are difficult to interpret in the presence of bronchitis (i.e., the cell samples recovered are contaminated by airway cells), and ^{67}Ga are generally insensitive to inflammation that is limited to major airway tissue.

^{67}Ga localization is likely to be an early event in pulmonary inflammation and should be strongly influenced by factors that increase endothelial permeability and less strongly influenced by the cellularity of the inflammatory process. Furthermore, ^{67}Ga localization is not a measure of pulmonary fibrosis and is unlikely to be highly predictive of disease outcome or prognosis. In combination with bronchoalveolar lavage or biopsy, it appears to be useful as a tool to initially stage the alveolitis of many of the inflammatory diffuse lung diseases (48, 53, 171, 172). During the course of therapy, ^{67}Ga imaging may be valuable to determine the effectiveness of treatment in reducing alveolar inflammation. It may be of limited use, however, as a measure of the impact of therapy on the population of effector cells in the lower respiratory tract.

Sarcoidosis and Other Granulomatous Diseases

Sarcoidosis is a multisystem granulomatous disorder of unknown cause that frequently occurs with mediastinal or hilar adenopathy and pulmonary infiltration. The lower respiratory tract is the site most commonly associated with morbidity and mortality. At least 90% of the patients who have sarcoidosis have pulmonary manifestations, 20–25% have a permanent loss of lung function, and 5–10% die of complications related to sarcoidosis (173).

^{67}Ga lung scanning is abnormal in most patients who have sarcoidosis and may be observed in both intrathoracic and extrathoracic lymph nodes, and in other organs where there is active disease (Fig. 31.24) (172, 174). In addition to being useful in assessing the magnitude of the alveolitis of the disease (54, 175–177), ^{67}Ga scans are of use in guiding the lung biopsy and in choosing pulmonary segments for bronchoalveolar lavage (178). ^{67}Ga scanning appears to be valuable in follow-up studies of sarcoidosis patients who are on steroid therapy, and it may be a more sensitive indicator of treatment response than clinical symptoms, chest radiographs, and pulmonary function tests (178).

In the lung, the pattern is generally diffuse and often intense, but, like the disease itself, uptake can have a highly variable presentation. Several patterns of ^{67}Ga localization have been reported to be highly specific for sarcoidosis. In 605 consecutive ^{67}Ga scans, right peritracheal with para- and infrahilar lymph node uptake was noted only in those patients who had sarcoidosis (179). These authors also found that the combination of symmetric parotid, lacrimal, and submandibular salivary gland localization also was strongly associated with patients having sarcoidosis.

The limitations of chest radiography in detecting sarcoid parenchymal disease are well-recognized (180). It is clear that the classic radiograph groups of sarcoidosis do not necessarily represent sequential progression or activity of the disease. In a large combined study of untreated patients with sarcoidosis (178), ^{67}Ga lung uptake was found in 20% of group 1 patients despite roentgenographically clear lung. Nearly half (44%) of the patients with normal radiographs (group 0) had positive scans. In 42% of untreated patients and 46% of treated patients who were studied 3–9 months later, the ^{67}Ga lung scan was more sensitive to altered disease status than the chest radiograph. No patient on therapy showed a worsened radiograph with an unchanged scan. In 154 patients who had three to nine scans at intervals of 2–12 months, the ^{67}Ga lung scan was far more sensitive than the chest radiograph, both in detecting improvement and in foreseeing relapses (178). In 20% of 481 untreated patients, the ^{67}Ga lung scan appeared to be the only noninvasive method with which clinical activity could be detected. In contrast, in a group of 179 untreated patients who had negative ^{67}Ga lung scans, other signs of clinical activity (i.e., fever, weight loss, arthralgia, extrathoracic involvement) could be shown in 51 (30%) (178).

The use of ^{67}Ga scans to monitor the progress of sarcoidosis was judged to be impractical because the radiation exposure to the patient makes repetition more often than twice yearly undesirable, and because prednisone therapy inhibits ^{67}Ga uptake (181). Because positive scans recur in many patients as therapy is withdrawn (178), however, ^{67}Ga scintigraphy may be valuable in defining a subset of patients at risk for continued alveolitis and in separating them from patients whose inflammatory stimulus has abated (Fig. 31.25). For example, there is a rebound

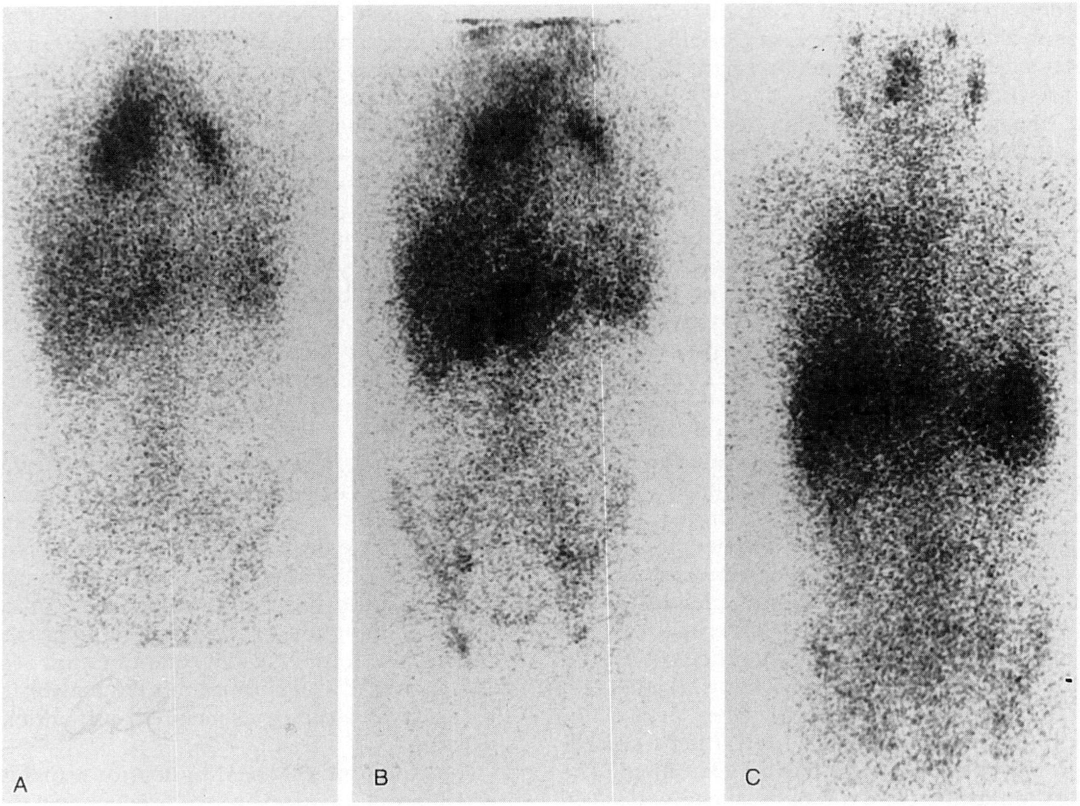

Figure 31.24. Scintigraphic pattern variation in a patient with sarcoidosis over a 16-month period. **A.** Anterior scintiscan in a 24-year-old woman showing uptake suggesting right peritracheal, hilar, and early para-aortic disease. **B.** Scintiscan obtained 5 months later showing a similar mediastinal pattern but also increased activity in the parenchyma of the right lower lobe and greater abdominal disease involving nodal sites in the para-aortic, inguinal, and femoral regions. **C.** Scintiscan obtained at 16 months. The nodal uptake pattern has disappeared in all sites, but there is now significant involvement of the right pulmonary parenchyma. Parotid localization is also noted. (Reproduced by permission from Line BR. Scintigraphic studies of inflammation in diffuse lung disease. Rad Clin No Am 1991;29:1095–1114.)

positivity of the ^{67}Ga lung scan in about 40% of patients after steroid discontinuation and in about 20% of patients after reduction of steroid therapy (178). The time of discovery of rebounds ranged from 1 month to 3 years. When used to monitor therapy, it is recommended that the ^{67}Ga dose may be reduced from 3–5 mCi to 1.5 mCi, especially when the subjective scoring method is used. This serves to reduce the cost and the radiation burden of follow-up imaging studies (178).

The relationship between the degree of ^{67}Ga localization and disease prognosis is controversial. Observation of 32 patients with sarcoidosis who were studied 3 or more years after the initial ^{67}Ga scans were done, showed no correlation between initial findings and later course (181). In another study, patients with sarcoidosis who had 28% or more T cells in the lavage analysis and a positive ^{67}Ga scan had clear deterioration in lung function over a 6-month period, unlike those patients who had less than 28% T cells or a negative ^{67}Ga scan or both (43).

Fibrotic Lung Diseases

Idiopathic Pulmonary Fibrosis. Idiopathic pulmonary fibrosis (IPF) is a fatal disorder characterized by parenchymal inflammation and interstitial fibrosis. ^{67}Ga scans are positive in about 70% of all patients who have IPF (53, 182). The pattern is usually diffuse and confined to the lung parenchyma. Quantitative ^{67}Ga scan evaluations have been useful in staging of the activity of IPF and in evaluating response to therapy. Therapeutic intervention can suppress alveolar inflammation as measured by ^{67}Ga lung uptake and the number of inflammatory cells in lavage samples (53, 183). The level of ^{67}Ga, however, has not consistently predicted which patients will deteriorate. In one study, for example, there were patients with normal levels of uptake who deteriorated and patients with high uptake who were unchanged or improved (166). Others found that patients deteriorated when they had higher ^{67}Ga lung uptake, especially when there was an associated increase in lavage neutrophil count (184).

Collagen Vascular Diseases. The interstitial process in many collagen vascular diseases (e.g., rheumatoid arthritis, systemic lupus erythematosus, polymyositis/dermatomyositis, and the overlap syndrome) is associated with an alveolitis in which inflammatory and immune effector cells are thought to mediate much of the lung parenchymal injury (165). ^{67}Ga scanning and bronchoalveolar lavage may be useful in assessing progressive pulmonary fibrosis

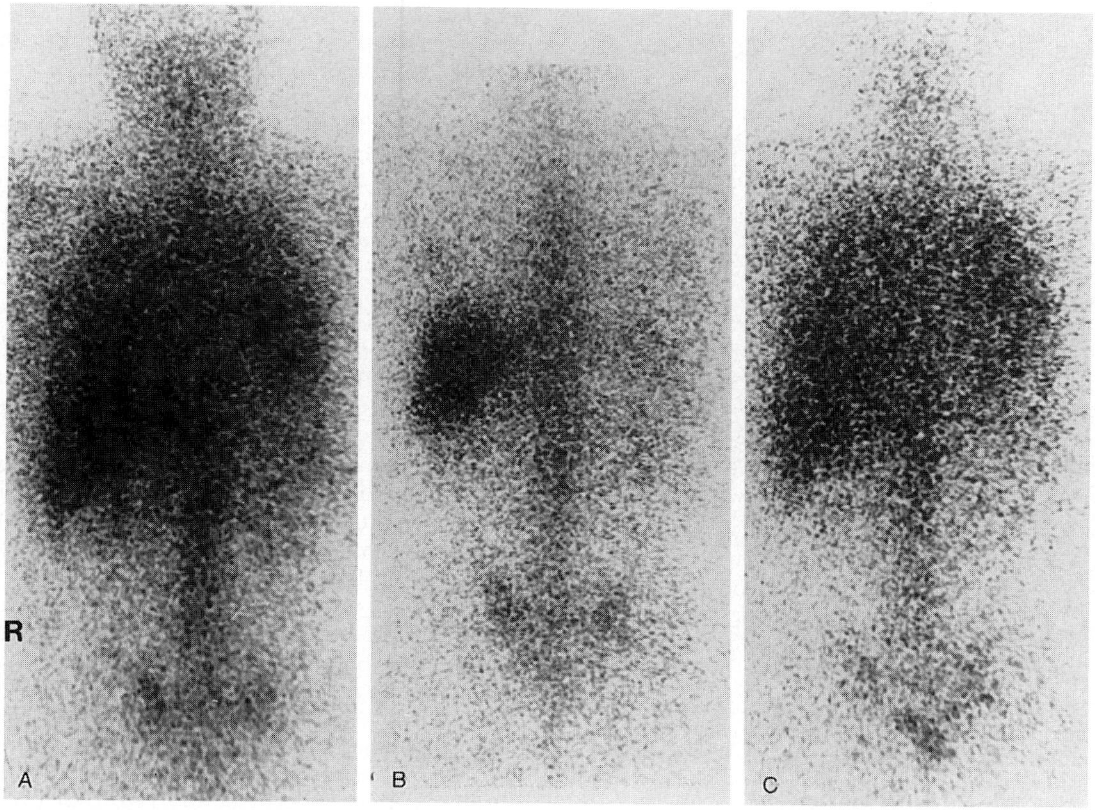

Figure 31.25. ^{67}Ga scans spanning a period of corticosteroid therapy for sarcoidosis in a 47-year-old man. **A.** Posterior whole-body scintiscan showing diffuse pulmonary localization of ^{67}Ga that is nearly equivalent to that of the liver in intensity. **B.** Scintiscan obtained 7 months later while the patient was receiving corticosteriod therapy. The spine and liver localizations are clearly more intense than that of the lung, which shows a normal uptake pattern. **C.** Scintiscan obtained 4 months after the end of therapy. Study shows diffuse intense localization consistent with reactivation of sarcoid alveolitis. (Reproduced by permission from Line BR. Scintigraphic studies of inflammation in diffuse lung disease. Rad Clin No Am 1991;29:1095–1114.)

in the collagen vascular diseases (Fig. 31.26). For example, progressive systemic sclerosis (PSS), or scleroderma, is a disorder in which fibrous connective tissue is deposited in many organs. Respiratory insufficiency is a major cause of death in patients who have PSS. ^{67}Ga scans are positive in three-fourths of patients, showing diffuse, primarily lower zone, uptake that is often independent of the pattern on the chest film (185, 186). In one study of a small group of patients with PSS, there was no consistent effect of corticosteroid therapy on the result of the ^{67}Ga scan or proportions of cells in lavage fluid (186). In another study of patients who had various collagen vascular diseases, ^{67}Ga uptake was seen in the lung in 17 of 20 progressively dyspneic patients, but in none of 16 patients without progressive symptoms (187).

Pneumoconiosis

The pneumoconioses are chronic diseases of the lower respiratory tract that result from prolonged exposure to high concentrations of airborne inorganic dusts, such as dusts of asbestos, coal, and silica. Studies of the diseases caused by these three dusts show that individuals who do not smoke but who have such disorders, have ongoing, active inflammation in their lower respiratory tracts (188). Although ^{67}Ga uptake does not appear to be associated with increased lavage cell subpopulation percentages, it appears to be localized in the lung through enhanced protein-bound leakage into the bronchoalveolar milieu and through accumulation by macrophages at disease sites (171).

^{67}Ga scanning can be used to detect the early stages of pneumoconiosis and to gauge the activity and progression of the disease (189). Siemsen, et al. (189), reported a high incidence of positive ^{67}Ga lung scans among 98 patients with silicosis, and found that in 25% of their patients ^{67}Ga accumulation was intense and more extensive than expected from the radiographic abnormalities. Nearly 90% of crocidolite-exposed workers who have asbestosis show increased ^{67}Ga uptake in their lungs (56). Additionally, pulmonary ^{67}Ga uptake is increased in almost one-half of the crocidolite-exposed workers who do not have definite chest film evidence of asbestosis, suggesting the presence of subclinical pulmonary inflammation (171). Although the disease findings in these workers do not meet the criteria for asbestosis, 85% of these patients have increased rigidity of the lung pressure volume curve, and in several there is evidence of macrophage alveolitis as demonstrated by lung biopsy and lavage (171). Follow-up studies show that most of these workers develop asbestosis within 5 years (190). Asbestos-exposed individuals with equivocal or normal chest radiographs who have increased pulmonary ^{67}Ga up-

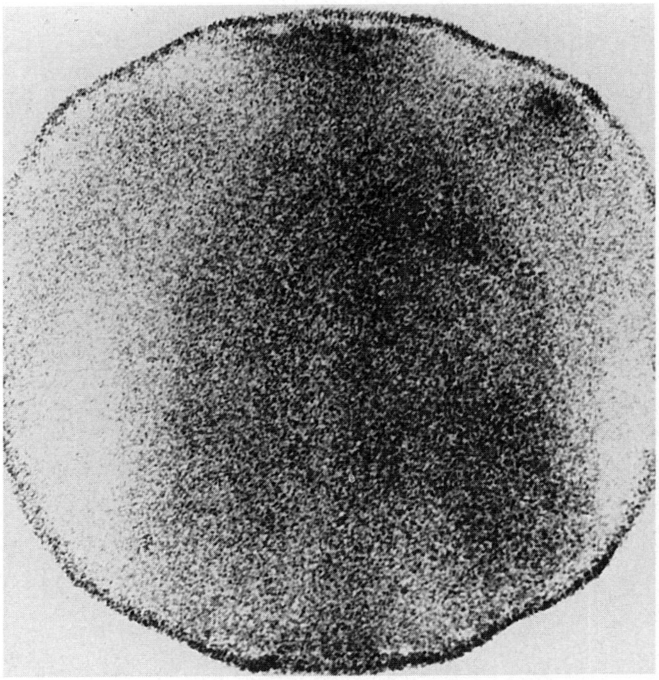

Figure 31.26. Diffuse pulmonary uptake in progressive rheumatoid lung in a 68-year-old woman. Posterior scan of the thorax showing homogeneous 2–3+ intensity in the left lung and a more heterogeneous pattern on the right. The intensity of the lung approximates that of the liver. A focus of intense activity is evident in the right shoulder that was associated with acute symptoms of rheumatoid disease. (Reproduced by permission from Line BR. Scintigraphic studies of inflammation in diffuse lung disease. Rad Clin No Am 1991;29:1095–1114.)

take or an abnormal lavage appear to be at risk of developing future asbestosis (56, 190).

Pulmonary Drug Toxicity

There has been a rapid growth of the list of drugs and their injurious metabolites implicated in lung injury (191). Reactive oxygen metabolites, for example, appear to play an important role in the adult respiratory distress syndrome, emphysema, pulmonary oxygen toxicity, and radiation-induced pulmonary damage. Oxidant species include the superoxide anion, hydrogen peroxide, the hydroxyl radical, singlet oxygen, and hypochlorous acid. These molecules are formed within polymorphonuclear cells and phagocytic cells, including macrophages and monocytes. Toxic effects appear to occur through participation of these molecules in oxidation-reduction reactions and subsequent fatty acid oxidation that may lead to membrane instability and inflammatory reactions (192).

Localization of ^{67}Ga in the pulmonary inflammation associated with cytotoxic or hypersensitivity injury has been reported for a large number of drugs. Amiodarone toxicity is a reasonable example of the use of ^{67}Ga in these disorders. A potentially lethal pulmonary toxicity may occur in 5–10% of patients receiving a daily dose of 400–800 mg of amiodarone for refractory arrhythmias. ^{67}Ga scintigraphy is reported to be sensitive to the presence of amiodarone pulmonary toxicity. Scan abnormalities are often intense, even when radiographic changes are subtle or nonspecific (193, 194).Pulmonary toxicity and related ^{67}Ga uptake appear to be dose related, and resolution of scintigraphic and radiographic findings is observed when amiodarone is withheld (195). ^{67}Ga image abnormalities parallel the development of amiodarone pulmonary toxicity and may help to establish a diagnosis, especially when the chest radiograph is normal or ambiguous (195).

Adult Respiratory Distress Syndrome

Adult respiratory distress syndrome (ARDS) is estimated to affect 150,000 persons each year and to be fatal in approximately half (196). Radionuclide techniques used for the diagnosis and study of ARDS include the routine clinical procedures of perfusion lung scanning,^{67}Ga and white-cell imaging, as well as PET based indicator dilution methods for measuring extravascular lung water, and means of measuring protein accumulation, protein flux, and solute transfer (75). The techniques that reflect the rate of protein leak from the microvasculature and sensitive measures of rapidly reversible alveolar injury appear most promising. While clinical usefulness remains to be documented, these methods may ultimately assist with the diagnosis of ARDS and with the evaluation of prognosis and therapy (197).

Aerosol studies may be useful for evaluating patients with ARDS because ARDS is associated with changes in alveolar-capillary permeability (19) that occur before radiographs and other forms of common clinical assessment are able to detect the abnormality.

INFECTIOUS LUNG DISEASE AND ACQUIRED IMMUNODEFICIENCY SYNDROME

Although ^{67}Ga has been described in association with all types of infectious etiologies, now its primary use is in the evaluation of patients who have the acquired immunodeficiency syndrome (AIDS) and associated pneumonias. Worldwide, approximately 10 million individuals are estimated to be infected with the human immunodeficiency virus (HIV). In the next decade, up to 50% of these individuals will present with maladies related to HIV infection (198). Characteristically, patients who have AIDS also have lymphocytopenia and are predisposed to opportunistic infections. The most common of these are Pneumocystis carinii pneumonia (PCP), disseminated Mycobacterium avium-intracellulare (MAI), Candida esophagitis, toxoplasmosis, cytomegalovirus (CMV), Cryptococcus, and herpes simplex infections.

^{67}Ga-citrate scans play an important role in the clinical management of the patient with AIDS who has a fever or respiratory symptoms. In part, this is due to the high prevalence of PCP in AIDS patients and the high sensitivity (90–96%) of ^{67}Ga scans for PCP (199–201). Although diffuse interstitial infiltrates on chest radiographs may be present in early cases of PCP, subtle prolonged symptoms and normal chest radiographs frequently occur. Unfortunately, chest radiographs have relatively low sensitivity for detecting early lung disease in patients who have AIDS. Kramer and coworkers (200) found that 27 of 57 abnormal ^{67}Ga lung scans were associated with normal chest radiographs. Conversely, a negative ^{67}Ga scan with a positive chest radiograph is often associated with pulmonary Kaposi's sarcoma (201). Kaposi's sarcoma is a major manifestation of AIDS, and in one review was present (either with or without other manifestations of the syndrome) in one-third of the patients who had AIDS (202).

PCP has a variable presentation on ^{67}Ga lung scans, ranging from negative to total lung involvement, and from minimal above background activity to greater than hepatic uptake (Fig. 31.27). Diffuse pulmonary uptake is the most common ^{67}Ga scan pattern associated with PCP. Perihilar or nodal uptake is much less common but has been reported (200). In a study of 180 HIV seropositive patients who had suspected pulmonary infections, the presence of a heterogeneous diffuse uptake pattern had an 87% positive predictive value for PCP, which was higher than that of any other pattern. The negative predictive value of a normal ^{67}Ga lung scan for PCP was 96% (203). When scans with only nodal lung uptake also were considered to be negative for PCP, the negative predictive value rose to 98% (203). Kramer, et al. (203), found a positive ^{67}Ga lung scan to have a 93% positive predictive value for any pulmonary disease, but commented that this value was probably low because of the difficulty in verifying disease in some patients (203). In another study, 20 patients with suspected PCP were evaluated by ^{67}Ga scans and fiberoptic bronchoscopy for initial diagnosis and response to therapy. ^{67}Ga localization was demonstrated in 100% of patients who had PCP, including those who had subclinical infection. Fiberoptic bronchoscopy identified P. carinii in the bronchial washings of 100% of patients (19 patients), whereas only 13 of 16 patients (81%) were found to have P. carinii in lung tissue obtained by transbronchial biopsy (57).

As ^{67}Ga scanning is relatively expensive and requires 48–72 hours to be completed, its use in the initial diagnosis of PCP generally should be restricted to those who have normal or atypical chest roentgenograms but suggestive clinical symptoms. The patient who has AIDS or is at risk for AIDS, and presents with typical symptoms and chest roentgenographic abnormalities suggestive of PCP, should not require ^{67}Ga scanning in addition to fiberoptic bronchoscopy to confirm the diagnosis (57). Because of the slow response to therapy and the high rate of recurrence, Ganz and Serafini (198) suggest that a baseline and follow-up ^{67}Ga scan may be useful to demonstrate successful response to treatment and to detect early recurrences. PCP recurs in more than half of patients within 18 months.

The effectiveness of ^{67}Ga scanning in the HIV seropositive population is due not only to its sensitivity for PCP, but also to its utility in the detection of other opportunistic infections, inflammatory processes, and lymphomas that occur in these patients. When PCP is not present, other disease processes usually are documented. MAI, for example, causes widespread disease in 25–50% of AIDS patients (204). Other granulomatous diseases that may mimic MAI include coccidioidomycosis, histoplasmosis, and tuberculosis. In mycobacterial lung infections, the ^{67}Ga scintigraphy pattern may demonstrate increased activity associated with tuberculous pleural effusion or tuberculous lobar pneumonias or show patchy low-grade uptake along with hilar and nonhilar nodal uptake. The atypical mycobacterial infections present more frequently with extrahilar nodes, whereas tuberculosis tends to be more commonly limited to hilar uptake (198). In one study, the positive predictive value of ^{67}Ga accumulation in intrathoracic regional lymph nodes for MAI infections was 90%(200). Only one patient had lymphadenopathy appreciated on the plain film. Because MAI is a common infection in AIDS patients,

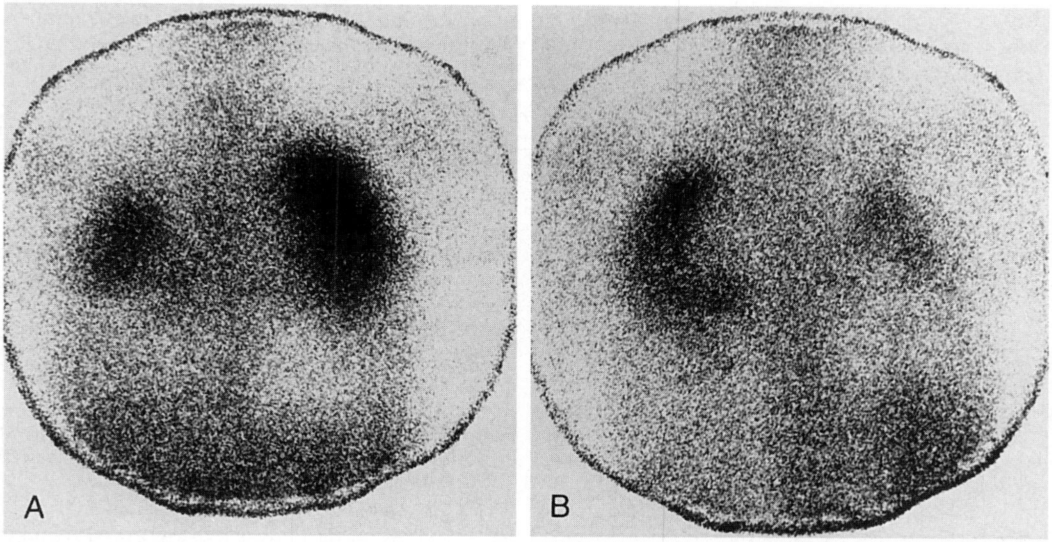

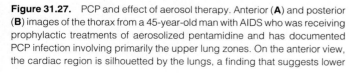

Figure 31.27. PCP and effect of aerosol therapy. Anterior (**A**) and posterior (**B**) images of the thorax from a 45-year-old man with AIDS who was receiving prophylactic treatments of aerosolized pentamidine and has documented PCP infection involving primarily the upper lung zones. On the anterior view, the cardiac region is silhouetted by the lungs, a finding that suggests lower intensity alveolitis in the lower lobes as well. The localization pattern is presumably due to better delivery of aerosolized drug prophylaxis to the lower lung regions. (Reproduced by permission from Line BR. Scintigraphic studies of inflammation in diffuse lung disease. Rad Clin No Am 1991;29:1095–1114.)

the finding of focal lymph node ^{67}Ga uptake (Fig. 31.28) should suggest MAI lymphadenitis (200), but nodal ^{67}Ga uptake along with normal lung activity has been seen in patients who have lymphoma (203, 205), and possibly in those who have AIDS-related complex lymphadenopathies (205).

Siemsen and colleagues (177) report high intensity ^{67}Ga pulmonary uptake in 97% of patients with active tuberculosis. They found a positive correlation between the extent of ^{67}Ga accumulation and the extent of radiographic abnormalities. All patients with active disease and a positive baseline ^{67}Ga scan who were rescanned 3–9 months after tuberculostatic chemotherapy, showed disappearance or marked regression of ^{67}Ga concentration (177). Although active disease is difficult to diagnose when extensive fibrotic areas appear on chest radiographs, reactivated tuberculous foci can be demonstrated by ^{67}Ga imaging (177). Whole-body scanning appears to be a simple, useful means to locate active foci of extrapulmonary tuberculosis and can demonstrate the response to effective therapy (206).

Of the bacterial infections in those patients who have AIDS, streptococcal pneumonia is the most common, but Hemophilus influenzae and Salmonella typhi also are seen. The ^{67}Ga scintigraphic pattern of localized lobar uptake without nodal uptake suggests bacterial infection rather than PCP or mycobacterial infection. When ^{67}Ga is localized in multiple pulmonary lobes as well as in bone, an aggressive infection such as actinomycosis or nocardia should be considered (207). In these aggressive infections, the results of a needle biopsy are often negative.

Clinically significant pulmonary CMV infection is uncommon and usually occurs in conjunction with more aggressive PCP infections. Because of the difficulty in diagnosing CMV infection, the pattern of uptake seen on the whole-body ^{67}Ga scan may be important. CMV infection is suggested by a pattern of low grade lung uptake with perihilar prominence (203) associated with eye (retinitis), adrenal, and renal uptake at 48 hours and/or persistent colonic uptake when diarrheal symptoms persist and there are not any obvious pathogens in multiple stool specimens (198).

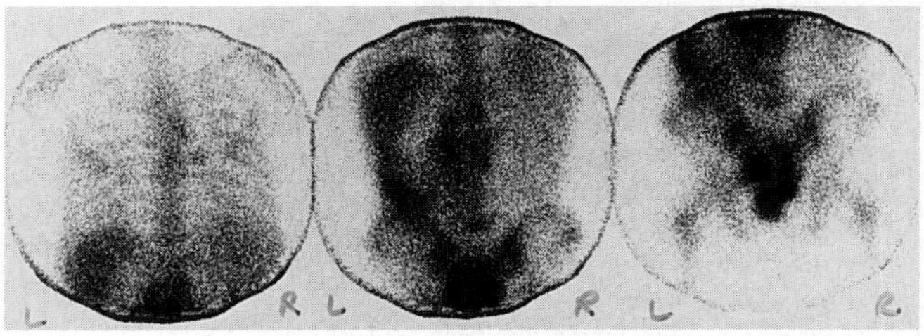

Figure 31.28. Nodal disease pattern in patient with Mycobacterium avium-intracellulare infection. Posterior ^{67}Ga scans of the chest, abdomen, and pelvis of a 37-year-old man with AIDS. He had a prior history of PCP, but shows nodal uptake in the hilar zones and para-aortic region, as well as splenic and marrow space prominence. The patient was subsequently documented to have a disseminated Mycobacterium avium-intracellulare infection. (Reproduced by permission from Line BR. Scintigraphic studies of inflammation in diffuse lung disease. Rad Clin No Am 1991;29:1095–1114.)

FUTURE APPLICATIONS OF RADIONUCLIDE LUNG STUDIES

In the past, pulmonary nuclear medicine was dominated by techniques that depict the distribution of pulmonary perfusion and ventilation, or V/Q balance, and these techniques were used to detect pulmonary embolism, obstructive airway diseases, lung carcinoma, and other pulmonary disorders in humans. With the development of emission tomography and the potential for new, function-oriented radiopharmaceuticals, nuclear medicine investigators are developing techniques for assessing alveolar-capillary permeability to specific molecules, for evaluation of pulmonary cell kinetics and the role of these cells in pulmonary disorders, and for evaluating various aspects of lung metabolism. The years ahead are likely to see major improvements in our ability to diagnose nonembolic pulmonary disorders.

REFERENCES

1. Kessler RM, McNeil BJ. Impaired ventilation in a patient with angiographically demonstrated pulmonary emboli. Radiology 1975;114:111–112.
2. Moser KM. Pulmonary embolism. Am Rev Respir Dis 1977; 115:829–852.
3. Scadding JG. Diffuse pulmonary alveolar fibrosis. Thorax 1974; 29:271–281.
4. West JB. Pulmonary function studies with radioactive gases. Annu Rev Med 1967;18:459–470.
5. Fedullo PF, Moser KM, Hartman MT, Ashburn WL. Patterns of pulmonary perfusion scans in normal subjects. III. The prevalence of abnormal scans in nonsmokers 30 to 49 years of age. Am Rev Respir Dis 1983;127:776–779.
6. Fedullo PF, Kapitan KS, Brewer NS, Ashburn WL, Hartman MT, Moser KM. Patterns of pulmonary perfusion scans in normal subjects. IV. The prevalence of abnormal scans in smokers 30 to 49 years of age. Am Rev Respir Dis 1989;139:1155–1157.
7. Bunow B, Line BR, Horton MR, Weiss GH. Regional ventilatory clearance by xenon scintigraphy: a critical evaluation of two estimation procedures. J Nucl Med 1979;20:703–710.
8. Secker-Walker RH, Hill RI, Markham J, et al. The measurement of regional ventilation in man: a new method of quantitation. J Nucl Med 1973;14:725–732.
9. Harf A, Pratt T, Hughes JMB. Regional distribution of Va/Q in man at rest and with exercise measured with Krypton-81m. J Appl Physiol 1978;44:115–123.
10. Hughes JM. Short-life radionuclides and regional lung function. Br J Radiol 1979;52:353–370.
11. Meignan M, Simonneau G, Oliveira L, et al. Computation of ventilation-perfusion ratio with Kr-81m in pulmonary embolism. J Nucl Med 1984;25:149–155.
12. Modell HI, Graham MM. Limitations of Kr-81m for quantitation of ventilation scans. J Nucl Med 1982;23:301–305.
13. Stuart BO. Deposition of inhaled aerosols. Arch Intern Med 1973;131:60–73.
14. Coates G, Dolovich M, Koehler D, Newhouse MT. Ventilation scanning with technetium-labeled aerosols. DTPA or sulfur colloid? Clin Nucl Med 1985;10:835–838.
15. Alderson PO, Biello DR, Gottschalk A, et al. Tc-99m-DTPA aerosol and radioactive gases compared as adjuncts to perfusion scintigraphy in patients with suspected pulmonary embolism. Radiology 1984;153:515–521.
16. Peltier P, De-Faucal P, Chetanneau A, Chatal JF. Comparison of technetium-99m aerosol and krypton-81m in ventilation studies

for the diagnosis of pulmonary embolism. Nucl Med Commun 1990;11:631–638.

17. White PG, Hayward MW, Cooper T. Ventilation agents—what agents are currently used? Nucl Med Commun 1991;12:349–352.
18. Susskind H, Brill AB, Harold WH. Quantitative comparison of regional distributions of inhaled Tc-99m DTPA aerosol and Kr-81m gas in coal miners' lungs. Am J Physiol Imaging 1986;1:67–76.
19. Huchon GJ, Little JW, Murray JF. Assessment of alveolar-capillary membrane permeability of dogs by aerosolization. J Appl Physiol 1981;51:955–962.
20. Rinderknecht J, Shapiro L, Krauthammer M, et al. Accelerated clearance of small solutes from the lungs in interstitial lung disease. Am Rev Respir Dis 1980;121:105–117.
21. Jones JG, Minty BD, Lawler P, Hulands G, Crawley JC, Veall N. Increased alveolar epithelial permeability in cigarette smokers. Lancet 1980;1:66–68.
22. Sugerman HJ, Strash AM, Hirsch JI, et al. Sensitivity of scintigraphy for detection of pulmonary capillary albumin leak in canine oleic acid ARDS. J Trauma 1981;21:520–527.
23. Anderson RR, Holliday RL, Driedger AA, Lefcoe M, Reid B, Sibbald WJ. Documentation of pulmonary capillary permeability in the adult respiratory distress syndrome accompanying human sepsis. Am Rev Respir Dis 1979;119:869–877.
24. Gorin AB, Stewart PA. Differential permeability of endothelial and epithelial barriers to albumin flux. J Appl Physiol 1979; 47:1315–1324.
25. Brain JD, Valberg PA. Deposition of aerosol in the respiratory tract. Am Rev Respir Dis 1979;120:1325–1373.
26. Chamberlain MJ, Morgan WK, Vinitski S. Factors influencing the regional deposition of inhaled particles in man. Clin Sci 1983; 64:69–78.
27. Rizk NW, Luce JM, Hoeffel JM, Price DC, Murray JF. Site of deposition and factors affecting clearance of aerosolized solute from canine lungs. J Appl Physiol 1984;56:723–729.
28. Meignan M, Rosso J, Leveau J, et al. Exercise increases the lung clearance of inhaled technetium-99m DTPA. J Nucl Med 1986; 27:274–280.
29. Evander E, Wollmer P, Jonson B. Pulmonary clearance of inhaled [99Tcm]DTPA: effects of ventilation pattern. Clin Physiol 1990;10:189–199.
30. Egan EA, Nelson RM, Olver RE. Lung inflation and alveolar permeability to nonelectrolytes in the adult sheep in vivo. J Physiol Lond 1976;260:409–424.
31. Coates G, O'Brodovich H. Measurement of pulmonary epithelial permeability with 99mTc-DTPA aerosol. Semin Nucl Med 1986; 16:275–284.
32. Smith RJ, Hyde RW, Waldman DL, et al. Effect of pattern of aerosol inhalation on clearance of technetium-99m-labeled diethylenetriamine penta-acetic acid from the lungs of normal humans. Am Rev Respir Dis 1992;145:1109–1116.
33. Mason GR, Effros RM, Uszler JM, Mena I. Small solute clearance from the lungs of patients with cardiogenic and noncardiogenic pulmonary edema. Chest 1985;88:327–334.
34. Mason GR, Duane GB, Mena I, Effros RM. Accelerated solute clearance in Pneumocystis carinii pneumonia. Am Rev Respir Dis 1987;135:864–868.
35. Marks JD, Luce JM, Lazar NM, Wu JN, Lipavsky A, Murray JF. Effect of increases in lung volume on clearance of aerosolized solute from human lungs. J Appl Physiol 1985;59:1242–1248.
36. Dusser DJ, Minty BD, Collignon MA, Hinge D, Barritault LG, Huchon GJ. Regional respiratory clearance of aerosolized 99mTc-DTPA: posture and smoking effects. J Appl Physiol 1986; 60:2000–2006.
37. Huchon GJ, Montgomery AB, Lipavsky A, Hoeffel JM, Murray JF. Respiratory clearance of aerosolized radioactive solutes of varying molecular weight. J Nucl Med 1987;28:894–902.
38. Peterson BT, Dickerson KD, James HL, Miller EJ, McLarty JW, Holiday DB. Comparison of three tracers for detecting lung epithelial injury in anesthetized sheep. J Appl Physiol 1989; 66:2374–2383.
39. Kosuda S, Kubo A, Sanmiya T, et al. Assessment of mucociliary clearance in patients with tracheobronchoplasty using radioaerosol. J Nucl Med 1986;27:1397–1402.
40. Messina MS, O'Riordan TG, Smaldone GC. Changes in mucociliary clearance during acute exacerbations of asthma. Am Rev Respir Dis 1991;143:993–997.
41. O'Riordan TG, Zwang J, Smaldone GC. Mucociliary clearance in adult asthma. Am Rev Respir Dis 1992;146:598–603.
42. Beaumont D, Herry JY, le-Cloirec J, le-Jeune JJ, de-Labarthe B. Sensitivity of ^{67}Ga-scanning in sarcoidosis: detection of biopsy proven pulmonary lesions radiographically undetectable. Eur J Nucl Med 1982;7:41–43.
43. Keogh BA, Hunninghake GW, Line BR, Crystal RG. The alveolitis of pulmonary sarcoidosis. Evaluation of natural history and alveolitis-dependent changes in lung function. Am Rev Respir Dis 1983;128:256–265.
44. MacMahon H, Bekerman C. The diagnostic significance of gallium lung uptake in patients with normal chest radiographs. Radiology 1978;127:189–193.
45. Tsan MF. Mechanism of gallium-67 accumulation in inflammatory lesions. J Nucl Med 1985;26:88–92.
46. Hoffer PB, Huberty J, Khayam-Bashi H. The association of Ga-67 and lactoferrin. J Nucl Med 1977;18:713–717.
47. Tsuchiya Y, Nakao A, Komatsu T, Yamamoto M, Shimokata K. Relationship between gallium-67 citrate scanning and transferrin receptor expression in lung diseases. Chest 1992;102:530–534.
48. Crystal RG, Bitterman PB, Rennard SI, Hance AJ, Keogh BA. Interstitial lung diseases of unknown cause. Disorders characterized by chronic inflammation of the lower respiratory tract. N Engl J Med 1984;310:235–244.
49. Kennedy SM, Walker DC, Belzberg AS, Hogg JC. Macrophage accumulation of inhaled gallium-67 citrate in normal lungs. J Nucl Med 1985;26:1195–1201.
50. Bekerman C, Caride VJ, Hoffer PB, Boles CA. Noninvasive staging of lung cancer. Indications and limitations of gallium-67 citrate imaging. Radiol Clin North Am 1990;28:497–510.
51. Johnson PM, Berdon WE, Baker DH, Fawwaz RA. Thymic uptake of gallium-67 citrate in a healthy 4-year-old boy. Pediatr Radiol 1978;7:243–244.
52. Larson SM, Schall GL. Gallium-67 concentration in human breast milk. JAMA 1971;218:257.
53. Line BR, Fulmer JD, Reynolds HY, et al. Gallium-67 citrate scanning in the staging of idiopathic pulmonary fibrosis: correlation and physiologic and morphologic features and bronchoalveolar lavage. Am Rev Respir Dis 1978;118:355–365.
54. Nosal A, Schleissner LA, Mishkin FS, Lieberman J. Angiotensin-I-converting enzyme and gallium scan in noninvasive evaluation of sarcoidosis. Ann Intern Med 1979;90:328–331.
55. Siemsen JK, Grebe SF, Sargent EN, Wentz D. Gallium-67 scintigraphy of pulmonary diseases as a complement to radiography. Radiology 1976;118:371–375.
56. Hayes AA, Mullan B, Lovegrove FT, Rose AH, Musk AW, Robinson BW. Gallium lung scanning and bronchoalveolar lavage in crocidolite-exposed workers. Chest 1989;96:22–26.
57. Tuazon CU, Delaney MD, Simon GL, Witorsch P, Varma VM. Utility of gallium-67 scintigraphy and bronchial washings in the diagnosis and treatment of Pneumocystis carinii pneumonia in patients with the acquired immune deficiency syndrome. Am Rev Respir Dis 1985;132:1087–1092.

58. Schoenberger CI, Line BR, Keogh BA, Hunninghake GW, Crystal RG. Lung inflammation in sarcoidosis: comparison of serum angiotensin-converting enzyme levels with bronchoalveolar lavage and gallium-67 scanning assessment of the T lymphocyte alveolitis. Thorax 1982;37:19–25.
59. Bourguet P, Delaval P, Herry JY. Direct quantitation of thoracic gallium-67 uptake in sarcoidosis. J Nucl Med 1986;27:1550–1556.
60. Specht HD, Brown PH, Haines JE, McNeill M. Gallium-67 lung index computerization in interstitial pneumonitis. J Nucl Med 1987;28:1826–1830.
61. van-Unnik JG, van-Royen EA, Alberts C, van-der-Schoot JB. A method of quantitative ^{67}Ga scintigraphy in the evaluation of pulmonary sarcoidosis. Eur J Nucl Med 1983;8:351–353.
62. Cooke SG, Goddard PR. Interpretation of gallium scans using the "negative heart " sign. Br J Radiol 1988;61:424.
63. Duffy GJ, Thirumurthi K, Casey M, et al. Semiquantitative gallium-67 lung scanning as a measure of the intensity of alveolitis in pulmonary sarcoidosis. Eur J Nucl Med 1986;12:187–191.
64. Alberts C, van-der-Schoot JB. Standardized quantitative ^{67}Ga scintigraphy in pulmonary sarcoidosis. Sarcoidosis 1988;5:111–118.
65. Bisson G, Lamoureux G, Begin R. Quantitative gallium-67 lung scan to assess the inflammatory activity in the pneumoconioses. Semin Nucl Med 1987;17:72–80.
66. Gillis CN. Metabolism of vasoactive hormones by lung. Anesthesiology 1973;39:626–632.
67. Gillis CN, Cronau LH, Greene NM, Hammond GL. Removal of 5-hydroxytryptamine and norepinephrine from the pulmonary vascular space of man: influence of cardiopulmonary bypass and pulmonary arterial pressure on these processes. Surgery 1974; 76:608–616.
68. Rahimian J, Glass EC, Touya JJ, Akber SF, Graham LS, Bennett LR. Measurement of metabolic extraction of tracers in the lung using a multiple indicator dilution technique. J Nucl Med 1984; 25:31–37.
69. Touya JJ, Rahimian J, Grubbs DE, Corbus HF, Bennett LR. A noninvasive procedure for in vivo assay of a lung amine endothelial receptor. J Nucl Med 1985;26:1302–1307.
70. Slosman DO, Brill AB, Polla BS, Alderson PO. Evaluation of [iodine-125]N,N,N′-trimethyl-N′-[2-hydroxy-3-methyl-5-iodo benzyl]-1,3-propanediamine lung uptake using an isolated-perfused lung model. J Nucl Med 1987;28:203–208.
71. Fowler JS, Gallagher BM, MacGregor RR, et al. Radiopharmaceuticals. XIX. ^{11}C-labeled octylamine, a potential diagnostic agent for lung structure and function. J Nucl Med 1976;17:752–754.
72. Slosman DO, Donath A, Alderson PO. ^{131}I-metaiodobenzylguanidine and ^{125}I-iodoamphetamine. Parameters of lung endothelial cell function and pulmonary vascular area. Eur J Nucl Med 1989;15:207–210.
73. Slosman DO, Morel DR, Mo-Costabella PM, Donath A. Lung uptake of ^{131}I-metaiodobenzylguanidine in sheep. An in vivo measurement of pulmonary metabolic function. Eur J Nucl Med 1988;14:65–70.
74. Slosman DO, Polla BS, Donath A. ^{123}I-MIBG pulmonary removal: a biochemical marker of minimal lung endothelial cell lesions. Eur J Nucl Med 1990;16:633–637.
75. Schuster DP. Positron emission tomography: theory and its application to the study of lung disease. Am Rev Respir Dis 1989; 139:818–840.
76. Front D, Israel O, Even-Sapir E, et al. The concentration of bleomycin labeled with Co-57 in primary and metastatic tumors. Cancer 1989;64:988–993.
77. Alazraki NP, Ramsdell JW, Taylor A, Friedman PJ, Peters RM, Tisi GM. Reliability of gallium scan chest radiography compared to mediastinoscopy for evaluating mediastinal spread in lung cancer. Am Rev Respir Dis 1978;117:415–420.
78. Tonami N, Yokoyama K, Shuke N, et al. Evaluation of suspected malignant pulmonary lesions with ^{201}Tl single photon emission computed tomography. Nucl Med Commun 1993;14:602–610.
79. Wahl RL, Quint LE, Greenough RL, Meyer CR, White RI, Orringer MB. Staging of mediastinal nonsmall cell lung cancer with FDG PET, CT, and fusion images: preliminary prospective evaluation. Radiology 1994;191:371–377.
80. Patz EF Jr, Lowe VJ, Hoffman JM, et al. Focal pulmonary abnormalities: evaluation with F-18 fluorodeoxyglucose PET scanning. Radiology 1993;188:487–490.
81. Waxman AD. The role of nuclear medicine in pulmonary neoplastic processes. Semin Nucl Med 1986;16:285–295.
82. Fujiwara T, Matsuzawa T, Kubota K, et al. Relationship between histologic type of primary lung cancer and carbon-11-L-methionine uptake with positron emission tomography. J Nucl Med 1989;30:33–37.
83. Strauss LG, Conti PS. The applications of PET in clinical oncology. J Nucl Med 1991;32:623–648; discussion 649–650.
84. Gupta NC, Frank AR, Dewan NA, et al. Solitary pulmonary nodules: detection of malignancy with PET with 2-[F-18]-fluoro-2-deoxy-D-glucose. Radiology 1992;184:441–444.
85. Fujimoto J. Radioautographic studies on the intracellular distribution of bleomycin-^{14}C in mouse tumor cells. Cancer Res 1974;34:2969–2974.
86. Kakinuma J, Orii H. DNA interaction with ^{57}Co-bleomycin. Nuklearmedizin 1982;21:232–235.
87. Even-Sapir E, Bettman L, Iosilevsky G, et al. SPECT quantitation of cobalt-57-bleomycin to predict treatment response and outcome of patients with lung cancer. J Nucl Med 1994;35:1129–1133.
88. Abe S, Makimura S, Itabashi K, Nagai T, Tsuneta Y, Kawakami Y. Prognostic significance of nuclear DNA content in small cell carcinoma of the lung. Cancer 1985;56:2025–2030.
89. Krenning EP, Bakker WH, Breeman WA, et al. Localisation of endocrine-related tumours with radioiodinated analogue of somatostatin. Lancet 1989;1:242–244.
90. Bakker WH, Krenning EP, Breeman WA, et al. Receptor scintigraphy with a radioiodinated somatostatin analogue: radiolabeling, purification, biologic activity, and in vivo application in animals. J Nucl Med 1990;31:1501–1509.
91. Rusch V, Macapinlac H, Heelan R, et al. NR-LU-10 monoclonal antibody scanning. A helpful new adjunct to computed tomography in evaluating nonsmall cell lung cancer. J Thorac Cardiovasc Surg 1993;106:200–204.
92. Kramer EL, Noz ME. CT-SPECT fusion for analysis of radiolabeled antibodies: applications in gastrointestinal and lung carcinoma. Int J Rad Appl Instrum B 1991;18:27–42.
93. Robinson NB, Hudson LD, Robertson HT, Thorning DR, Carrico CJ, Heimbach DM. Ventilation and perfusion alterations after smoke inhalation injury. Surgery 1981;90:352–363.
94. Alderson PO, Bradley EW, Mendenhall KG, et al. Radionuclide evaluation of pulmonary function following hemithorax irradiation of normal dogs with ^{60}Co or fast neutrons. Radiology 1979; 130:425–433.
95. Oppenheimer L, Craven KD, Forkert L, Wood LD. Pathophysiology of pulmonary contusion in dogs. J Appl Physiol 1979; 47:718–728.
96. Fazio F, Lavender JP, Steiner RE. ^{81m}Kr ventilation and ^{99m}Tc perfusion scans in chest disease: comparison with standard radiographs. AJR Am J Roentgenol 1978;130:421–428.
97. Susskind H, Atkins HL, Goldman AG, et al. Sensitivity of Kr-81m and Xe-127 in evaluating nonembolic pulmonary disease. J Nucl Med 1981;22:781–786.
98. Cunningham DA, Lavender JP. Krypton-81m ventilation scan-

ning in chronic obstructive airways disease. Br J Radiol 1981; 54:110–116.
99. Barter SJ, Cunningham DA, Lavender JP, Gibellino F, Connellan SJ, Pride NB. Abnormal ventilation scans in middle-aged smokers. Comparison with tests of overall lung function. Am Rev Respir Dis 1985;132:148–151.
100. Narabayashi I, Otsuka N. Pulmonary ventilation and perfusion studies in lung cancer. Clin Nucl Med 1984;9:97–102.
101. Ellis DA, Hawkins T, Gibson GJ, Nariman S. Role of lung scanning in assessing the resectability of bronchial carcinoma. Thorax 1983;38:261–266.
102. Treves S, AhnBerg DS, Laguarda R, Strieder DJ. Radionuclide evaluation of regional lung function in children. J Nuc Med 1974; 15:582–587.
103. Li DK, Treves S, Heyman S, et al. Krypton-81m: a better radiopharmaceutical for assessment of regional lung function in children. Radiology 1979;130:741–747.
104. Gordon I, Helms P, Fazio F. Clinical applications of radionuclide lung scanning in infants and children. Br J Radiol 1981;54:576–585.
105. Fein R, Thal W, Otto HJ, Gunkel H. Combined ^{113}Xe/^{99m}TC human serum albumin microspheres lung scintigraphy in children with recurrent and chronic bronchitis. Z Erkr Atmungsorgane 1988;171:135–142.
106. Kropp J, Overbeck B, Klumpp J, Hotze A, Biersack HJ. Inhalation scintigraphy with an ultrafine aerosol in infants with functional bronchial stenoses. Clin Nucl Med 1993;18:223–226.
107. Moote D, Ehrlich L, Martin RH. Postpneumonectomy bronchopleural fistula imaged by ventilation lung scanning. Clin Nucl Med 1987;12:337–338.
108. Lowe RE, Siddiqui AR. Scintimaging of bronchopleural fistula. A simple method of diagnosis. Clin Nucl Med 1984;9:10–12.
109. Samuel J, Houlder AE. Use of Xe-133 gas in the detection of foreign bodies in the lower respiratory tract. Clin Otolaryngol 1987; 12:115–117.
110. Wencel ML, Sitrin RG. Unilateral lung hyperlucency after mediastinal irradiation. Am Rev Respir Dis 1988;137:955–957.
111. Miller MB, Caride VJ. Ventilation-perfusion scan in the acutely ill patient with unilateral hyperlucent lung. J Nucl Med 1988; 29:114–117.
112. Tamir A, Melloul M, Berant M, et al. Lung perfusion scans in patients with congenital heart defects. J Am Coll Cardiol 1992; 19:383–388.
113. Houzard C, Andre M, Guilhen S, Thivolle P, Berger M. Perfusion lung scan in patients operated for transposition of the great arteries. Clin Nucl Med 1989;14:268–270.
114. Hayashida K, Nishimura T, Kumita S, Uehara T. Scintigraphic determination of severity in pulmonary parenchymal damage in patients with atrial septal defect. Eur J Nucl Med 1990;16:713–716.
115. Grimon G, Andre L, Bernard O, Raffestin B, Desgrez A. Early radionuclide detection of intrapulmonary shunts in children with liver disease. J Nucl Med 1994;35:1328–1332.
116. Chilvers ER, Peters AM, George P, Hughes JM, Allison DJ. Quantification of right to left shunt through pulmonary arteriovenous malformations using ^{99m}Tc albumin microspheres. Clin Radiol 1988;39:611–614.
117. Winzelberg GG, Wholey MH, Jarmolowski CA, Sachs M, Weinberg JH. Patients with hemoptysis examined by Tc-99m sulfur colloid and Tc-99m-labeled red blood cells: a preliminary appraisal. Radiology 1984;153:523–526.
118. Haponik EF, Rothfeld B, Britt EJ, Bleecker ER. Radionuclide localization of massive pulmonary hemorrhage. Chest 1984; 86:208–212.
119. Fishman AJ, Moser KM, Fedullo PF. Perfusion lung scans vs. pulmonary angiography in evaluation of suspected primary pulmonary hypertension. Chest 1983;84:679–683.
120. Lisbona R, Kreisman H, Novales-Diaz J, Derbekyan V. Perfusion lung scanning: differentiation of primary from thromboembolic pulmonary hypertension. AJR Am J Roentgenol 1985;144:27–30.
121. Patz EF Jr, Lowe VJ, Hoffman JM, Paine SS, Harris LK, Goodman PC. Persistent or recurrent bronchogenic carcinoma: detection with PET and 2-[F-18]-2-deoxy-D-glucose. Radiology 1994; 191:379–382.
122. Boring CC, Squires TS, Tong T, Montgomery S. Cancer statistics, 1994. CA Cancer J Clin 1994;44:7–26.
123. Ferguson MK. Diagnosing and staging of nonsmall cell lung cancer. Hematol Oncol Clin North Am 1990;4:1053–1068.
124. Greene R. Immunoscintigraphy for lung cancer detection: reality testing [Editorial]. J Nucl Med 1991;32:2069–2070.
125. Mountain CF. A new international staging system for lung cancer. Chest 1986;89:225S–233S.
126. Leitha T, Meghdadi S, Studnicka M, et al. The role of iodine-123-Tyr-3-octreotide scintigraphy in the staging of small cell lung cancer. J Nucl Med 1993;34:1397–1402.
127. Caskey CI, Zerhouni EA. The solitary pulmonary nodule. Semin Roentgenol 1990;25:85–95.
128. Swensen SJ, Jett JR, Payne WS, Viggiano RW, Pairolero PC, Trastek VF. An integrated approach to evaluation of the solitary pulmonary nodule. Mayo Clin Proc 1990;65:173–186.
129. Lillington GA. Management of solitary pulmonary nodules. Dis Mon 1991;37:271–318.
130. Dewan NA, Gupta NC, Redepenning LS, Phalen JJ, Frick MP. Diagnostic efficacy of PET-FDG imaging in solitary pulmonary nodules. Potential role in evaluation and management. Chest 1993;104:997–1002.
131. Kubota K, Matsuzawa T, Fujiwara T, et al. Differential diagnosis of lung tumor with positron emission tomography: a prospective study. J Nucl Med 1990;31:1927–1932.
132. Kubota K, Yamada S, Ishiwata K, et al. Evaluation of the treatment response of lung cancer with positron emission tomography and L-[methyl-^{11}C]methionine: a preliminary study. Eur J Nucl Med 1993;20:495–501.
133. Krishnamurthy S, Morris JF, Antonovic R, et al. Evaluation of primary lung cancer with indium-111 anticarcinoembryonic antigen (type ZCE-025) monoclonal antibody scintigraphy. Cancer 1990;65:458–465.
134. Kramer EL, Noz ME, Liebes L, Murthy S, Tiu S, Goldenberg DM. Radioimmunodetection of nonsmall cell lung cancer using technetium-99m-anticarcinoembryonic antigen IMMU-4 Fab′ fragment. Preliminary results. Cancer 1994;73:890–895.
135. Biggi A, Buccheri G, Ferrigno D, et al. Detection of suspected primary lung cancer by scintigraphy with indium-111-anticarcinoembryonic antigen monoclonal antibodies (type F023C5) J Nucl Med 1991;32:2064–2068.
136. Buccheri G, Biggi A, Ferrigno D, Leone A, Taviani M, Quaranta M. Anti-CEA immunoscintigraphy might be more useful than computed tomography in the preoperative thoracic evaluation of lung cancer. A comparison between planar immunoscintigraphy, single photon emission computed tomography (SPECT), and computed tomography. Chest 1993;104:734–742.
137. Dienhart DG, Schmelter RF, Lear JL, et al. Imaging of nonsmall cell lung cancers with a monoclonal antibody, KC-4G3, which recognizes a human milk fat globule antigen. Cancer Res 1990; 50:7068–7076.
138. Divgi CR, Welt S, Kris M, et al. Phase I and imaging trial of indium-111-labeled antiepidermal growth factor receptor monoclonal antibody 225 in patients with squamous cell lung carcinoma. J Natl Cancer Inst 1991;83:97–104.
139. Friedman S, Sullivan K, Salk D, et al. Staging nonsmall cell carcinoma of the lung using technetium-99m-labeled monoclonal antibodies. Hematol Oncol Clin North Am 1990;4:1069–1078.
140. Webb WR, Gatsonis C, Zerhouni EA, et al. CT and MR imaging

in staging nonsmall cell bronchogenic carcinoma: report of the Radiologic Diagnostic Oncology Group. Radiology 1991; 178:705–713.
141. Pounds TR, Valk PE, Hopkins DM, Myers RA, Haseman MK, Lutrin CL. Staging of lung cancer by positron emission tomography [Abstract]. J Nucl Med 1994;36:76P.
142. Ichiya Y, Kuwabara Y, Otsuka M, et al. Assessment of response to cancer therapy using fluorine-18-fluorodeoxyglucose and positron emission tomography. J Nucl Med 1991;32:1655–1660.
143. Kim EE, Chung SK, Haynie TP, et al. Differentiation of residual or recurrent tumors from posttreatment changes with F-18 FDG PET. Radiographics 1992;12:269–279.
144. Lowe VJ, Hebert ME, Hawk TC, Anscher MS, Coleman RE. Chest wall FDG accumulation in serial FDG-PET images in patients being treated for bronchogenic carcinoma with radiation [Abstract]. J Nucl Med 1994;36:76P.
145. Pannier R, Verlinde I, Puspowidjono I, Willemot JP. Role of gallium-67 thoracic scintigraphy in the diagnosis and staging of patients suspected of bronchial carcinoma. Thorax 1982;37:264–269.
146. Fosburg RG, Hopkins GB, Kan MK. Evaluation of the mediastinum by gallium-67 scintigraphy in lung cancer. J Thorac Cardiovasc Surg 1979;77:76–82.
147. MacMahon H, Scott W, Ryan JW, et al. Efficacy of computed tomography of the thorax and upper abdomen and whole-body gallium scintigraphy for staging of lung cancer. Cancer 1989; 64:1404–1408.
148. Cooper WR, Guerrant JL, Teates CD. Prediction of postoperative respiratory function in patients undergoing lung resection. Va Med 1980;107:264–268.
149. Lipscomb DJ, Pride NB. Ventilation and perfusion scans in the preoperative assessment of bronchial carcinoma. Thorax 1977; 32:720–725.
150. Katz RD, Alderson PO, Tockman MS, et al. Ventilation-perfusion lung scanning in patients detected by a screening program for early lung carcinoma. Radiology 1981;141:171–178.
151. Secker-Walker RH, Alderson PO, Wilhelm J, Hill RL, Markham J, Kinzie J. Ventilation-perfusion scanning in carcinoma of the bronchus. Chest 1974;65:660–663.
152. Lefrak SS. Preoperative evaluation for pulmonary resection. The role of radionuclide lung screening [Editorial]. Chest 1977; 72:419–420.
153. Olsen GN, Block AJ, Swenson EW, Castle JR, Wynne JW. Pulmonary function evaluation of the lung resection candidate: a prospective study. Am Rev Respir Dis 1975;111:379–387.
154. Williams CD, Brenowitz JB. dures. Am J Surg 1976;132:763–766.
155. Wernly JA, DeMeester TR, Kirchner PT, Myerowitz PD, Oxford DE, Golomb HM. Clinical value of quantitative ventilation-perfusion lung scans in the surgical management of bronchogenic carcinoma. J Thorac Cardiovasc Surg 1980;80:535–543.
156. Miorner G. ^{133}Xe-radiospirometry. A clinical method for studying regional lung function. Scand J Respir Dis Suppl 1968;64:1–84.
157. DeMeester TR, Van-Heertum RL, Karas JR, Watson RL, Hansen JE. Preoperative evaluation with differential pulmonary function. Ann Thorac Surg 1974;18:61–71.
158. Kristersson S, Lindell SE, Svanberg L. Prediction of pulmonary function loss due to pneumonectomy using ^{133}Xe-radiospirometry. Chest 1972;62:694–698.
159. Block AJ, Olsen GN. Preoperative pulmonary function testing. JAMA 1976;235:257–258.
160. Boysen PG, Block AJ, Olsen GN, Moulder PV, Harris JO, Rawitscher RE. Prospective evaluation for pneumonectomy using the technetium-99m quantitative perfusion lung scan. Chest 1977;72:422–425.
161. Kirsh MM, Rotman H, Bove E, et al. Major pulmonary resection for bronchogenic carcinoma in the elderly. Ann Thorac Surg 1976;22:369–373.
162. Weiss W, Cooper DA, Boucot KR. Operative mortality and 5-year survival rates in men with bronchogenic carcinoma. Ann Intern Med 1969;71:59–65.
163. Ciofetta G, Silverman M, Hughes JM. Quantitative approach to the study of regional lung function in children using krypton-81m. Br J Radiol 1980;53:950–959.
164. Krumpe PE, Lum CC, Cross CE. Approach to the patient with diffuse lung disease. Med Clin North Am 1988;72:1225–1246.
165. Crystal RG, Gadek JE, Ferrans VJ, Fulmer JD, Line BR, Hunninghake GW. Interstitial lung disease: current concepts of pathogenesis, staging and therapy. Am J Med 1981;70:542–568.
166. Pantin CF, Valind SO, Sweatman M, et al. Measures of the inflammatory response in cryptogenic fibrosing alveolitis. Am Rev Respir Dis 1988;138:1234–1241.
167. Bekerman C, Hoffer PB, Bitran JD, Gupta RG. Gallium-67 citrate imaging studies of the lung. Semin Nucl Med 1980;10:286–301.
168. Richman SD, Levenson SM, Bunn PA, Flinn GS, Johnston GS, DeVita VT. ^{67}Ga accumulation in pulmonary lesions associated with bleomycin toxicity. Cancer 1975;36:1966–1972.
169. van-Der-Schoot JB, Gruen AS, Dejong J. Gallium-67 scintigraphy in lung diseases. Thorax 1972;27:543–547.
170. Perrin-Fayolle M, Gindre D, Azzar D, et al. Pulmonary sarcoidosis. Study of the distribution of active alveolitis assessed by comparison of data from radiological examination, gallium-67 scintigraphy and double bronchoalveolar lavage. Rev Pneumol Clin 1985;41:31–37.
171. Begin R, Cantin A, Drapeau G, et al. Pulmonary uptake of gallium-67 in asbestos-exposed humans and sheep. Am Rev Respir Dis 1983;127:623–630.
172. Line BR, Hunninghake GW, Keogh BA, Jones AE, Johnston GS, Crystal RG. Gallium-67 scanning to stage the alveolitis of sarcoidosis: correlation with clinical studies, pulmonary function studies, and bronchoalveolar lavage. Am Rev Respir Dis 1981; 123:440–446.
173. Israel HL. Prognosis of sarcoidosis. Ann Intern Med 1970; 73:1038–1039.
174. Wallaert B, Ramon P, Fournier E, Tonnel AB, Voisin C. Bronchoalveolar lavage, serum angiotensin-converting enzyme, and gallium-67 scanning in extrathoracic sarcoidosis. Chest 1982; 82:553–555.
175. Heshiki A, Schatz SL, McKusick KA, Bowersox DW, Soin JS, Wagner HN Jr. Gallium-67 citrate scanning in patients with pulmonary sarcoidosis. Am J Roentgenol Radium Ther Nucl Med 1974;122:744–749.
176. McKusick KA, Soin JS, Ghiladi A, Wagner HN. Gallium-67 accumulation in pulmonary sarcoidosis. JAMA 1973;223:688.
177. Siemsen JK, Grebe SF, Waxman AD. The use of gallium-67 in pulmonary disorders. Semin Nucl Med 1978;8:235–249.
178. Rizzato G, Blasi A. A European survey on the usefulness of ^{67}Ga lung scans in assessing sarcoidosis. Experience in 14 research centers in seven different countries. Ann NY Acad Sci 1986; 465:463–478.
179. Sulavik SB, Spencer RP, Weed DA, Shapiro HR, Shiue ST, Castriotta RJ. Recognition of distinctive patterns of gallium-67 distribution in sarcoidosis. J Nucl Med 1990;31:1909–1914.
180. Young RL, Krumholz RA, Harkleroad LE. A physiologic roentgenographic disparity in sarcoidosis. Dis Chest 1966;50:81–86.
181. Israel HL, Gushue GF, Park CH. Assessment of gallium-67 scanning in pulmonary and extrapulmonary sarcoidosis. Ann NY Acad Sci 1986;465:455–462.
182. Crystal RG, Fulmer JD, Roberts WC, Moss ML, Line BR, Reynolds HY. Idiopathic pulmonary fibrosis. Clinical, histologic, radiographic, physiologic, scintigraphic, cytologic, and biochemical aspects. Ann Intern Med 1976;85:769–788.
183. Turner-Warwick M, Haslam PL. The value of serial bronchoal-

veolar lavages in assessing the clinical progress of patients with cryptogenic fibrosing alveolitis. Am Rev Respir Dis 1987;135:26–34.

184. Vanderstappen M, Mornex JF, Lahneche B, et al. Gallium-67 scanning in the staging of cryptogenetic fibrosing alveolitis and hypersensitivity pneumonitis. Eur Respir J 1988;1:517–522.

185. Baron M, Feiglin D, Hyland R, Urowitz MB, Shiff B. Gallium-67 lung scans in progressive systemic sclerosis. Arthritis Rheum 1983;26:969–974.

186. Rossi GA, Bitterman PB, Rennard SI, Ferrans VJ, Crystal RG. Evidence for chronic inflammation as a component of the interstitial lung disease associated with progressive systemic sclerosis. Am Rev Respir Dis 1985;131:612–617.

187. Greene NB, Solinger AM, Baughman RP. Patients with collagen vascular disease and dyspnea. The value of gallium scanning and bronchoalveolar lavage in predicting response to steroid therapy and clinical outcome. Chest 1987;91:698–703.

188. Rom WN, Bitterman PB, Rennard SI, Cantin A, Crystal RG. Characterization of the lower respiratory tract inflammation of nonsmoking individuals with interstitial lung disease associated with chronic inhalation of inorganic dusts. Am Rev Respir Dis 1987;136:1429–1434.

189. Siemsen JK, Sargent EN, Grebe SF, Winsor DW, Wentz D, Jacobson G. Pulmonary concentration of Ga67 in pneumoconiosis. Am J Roentgenol Radium Ther Nucl Med 1974;120:815–820.

190. Begin R, Cantin A, Berthiaume Y, et al. Clinical features to stage alveolitis in asbestos workers. Am J Ind Med 1985;8:521–536.

191. Cooper JA Jr, White DA, Matthay RA. Drug-induced pulmonary disease. Part 1: cytotoxic drugs. Am Rev Respir Dis 1986; 133:321–340.

192. Freeman BA, Crapo JD. Biology of disease: free radicals and tissue injury. Lab Invest 1982;47:412–426.

193. Dake MD, Hattner R, Warnock ML, Golden JA. Gallium-67 lung uptake associated with amiodarone pulmonary toxicity. Am Heart J 1985;109:1114–1116.

194. van-Rooij WJ, van-der-Meer SC, van-Royen EA, van-Zandwijk N, Darmanata JI. Pulmonary gallium-67 uptake in amiodarone pneumonitis. J Nucl Med 1984;25:211–213.

195. Zhu YY, Botvinick E, Dae M, Golden J, Hattner R, Scheinman M. Gallium lung scintigraphy in amiodarone pulmonary toxicity. Chest 1988;93:1126–1131.

196. Rinaldo JE, Rogers RM. Adult respiratory-distress syndrome: changing concepts of lung injury and repair. N Engl J Med 1982; 306:900–909.

197. Mishkin FS, Mason GR. Application of nuclear medicine techniques to the study of ARDS. J Thorac Imaging 1990;5:1–8.

198. Ganz WI, Serafini AN. The diagnostic role of nuclear medicine in the acquired immunodeficiency syndrome. J Nucl Med 1989; 30:1935–1945.

199. Barron TF, Birnbaum NS, Shane LB, Goldsmith SJ, Rosen MJ. Pneumocystis carinii pneumonia studied by gallium-67 scanning. Radiology 1985;154:791–793.

200. Kramer EL, Sanger JJ, Garay SM, et al. Gallium-67 scans of the chest in patients with acquired immunodeficiency syndrome. J Nucl Med 1987;28:1107–1114.

201. Woolfenden JM, Carrasquillo JA, Larson SM, et al. Acquired immunodeficiency syndrome: Ga-67 citrate imaging. Radiology 1987;162:383–387.

202. Fauci AS, Macher AM, Longo DL, et al. NIH conference. Acquired immunodeficiency syndrome: epidemiologic, clinical, immunologic, and therapeutic considerations. Ann Intern Med 1984; 100:92–106.

203. Kramer EL, Sanger JH, Garay SM, Grossman RJ, Tiu S, Banner H. Diagnostic implications of Ga-67 chest-scan patterns in human immunodeficiency virus-seropositive patients. Radiology 1989;170:671–676.

204. Hawkins CC, Gold JW, Whimbey E, et al. Mycobacterium avium complex infections in patients with the acquired immunodeficiency syndrome. Ann Intern Med 1986;105:184–188.

205. Bitran J, Bekerman C, Weinstein R, Bennett C, Ryo U, Pinsky S. Patterns of gallium-67 scintigraphy in patients with acquired immunodeficiency syndrome and the AIDS-related complex. J Nucl Med 1987;28:1103–1106.

206. Sarkar SD, Ravikrishnan KP, Woodbury DH, Carson JJ, Daley K. Gallium-67 citrate scanning—a new adjunct in the detection and follow-up of extrapulmonary tuberculosis: concise communication. J Nucl Med 1979;20:833–836.

207. Zuckier LS, Ongseng F, Goldfarb CR. Lymphocytic interstitial pneumonitis: a cause of pulmonary gallium-67 uptake in a child with acquired immunodeficiency syndrome. J Nucl Med 1988; 29:707–711.

208. Levenson SM, Warren RD, Richman SD, Johnston GS, Chabner BA. Abnormal pulmonary gallium accumulation in P. carinii pneumonia. Radiology 1976;119:395–398.

209. Fineman DS, Palestro CJ, Kim CK, et al. Detection of abnormalities in febrile AIDS patients with In-111-labeled leukocyte and Ga-67 scintigraphy. Radiology 1989;170:677–680.

210. Fogh J, Bertelsen S, Schmidt A. Diagnostic value of ^{67}Ga-scintigraphy in chest surgery. Thorax 1974;29:26–31.

211. Rosen Y, Athanassiades TJ, Moon S, Lyons HA. Nongranulomatous interstitial pneumonitis in sarcoidosis. Relationship to development of epithelioid granulomas. Chest 1978;74:122–125.

212. Moinuddin M, Rockett J. Gallium scintigraphy in the detection of amiodarone lung toxicity. AJR Am J Roentgenol 1986; 147:607–609.

213. Manning DM, Strimlan CV, Turbiner EH. Early detection of busulfan lung: report of a case. Clin Nucl Med 1980;5:412–414.

214. Laven DL, Shaw SM. Detection of drug interactions involving radiopharmaceuticals: a professional responsibility of the clinical pharmacist. J Pharm Pract 1989;2:287–291.

215. Garbes ID, Henderson ES, Gomez GA, Bakshi SP, Parthasarathy KL, Castillo NB. Procarbazine-induced interstitial pneumonitis with a normal chest x-ray: a case report. Med Pediatr Oncol 1986;14:238–241.

216. Javaheri S, Levine BW, McKusick KA. Serial ^{67}Ga lung scanning in pulmonary eosinophilic granuloma. Thorax 1979;34:822–823.

217. Teates CD, Hunter JG Jr. Gallium scanning as a screening test for inflammatory lesions. Radiology 1975;116:383–387.

218. Tien R, Moore WH, Glasser LM, Dhekne RD, Long SE. Thoracic gallium uptake in patients with lymphomatoid granulomatosis. Clin Nucl Med 1988;13:886–888.

219. Deseran MW, Colletti PM, Ratto D, Ansari AN, Siegel ME. Chronic berylliosis. Demonstration by gallium-67 imaging and magnetic resonance imaging. Clin Nucl Med 1988;13:509–511.

220. Hooper RG, Kearl RA. Established ARDS treated with a sustained course of adrenocortical steroids. Chest 1990;97:138–143.

221. Gibson PG, Bryant DH, Morgan GW, et al. Radiation-induced lung injury: a hypersensitivity pneumonitis? Ann Intern Med 1988;109:288–291.

222. Balaban EP, Walker BS, Cox JV, et al. Radionuclide imaging of bone marrow metastases with a Tc-99m-labeled monoclonal antibody to small cell lung carcinoma. Clin Nucl Med 1991;16:732–736.

223. Balaban EP, Walker BS, Cox JV, et al. Detection and staging of small cell lung carcinoma with a technetium-labeled monoclonal antibody. A comparison with standard staging methods. Clin Nucl Med 1992;17:439–445.

224. Morris JF, Krishnamurthy S, Antonovic R, Duncan C, Turner FE, Krishnamurthy GT. Technetium-99m monoclonal antibody fragment (Fab) scintigraphy in the evaluation of small cell lung can-

cer: a preliminary report. Int J Rad Appl Instrum B 1991;18:613–620.
225. Vansant JP, Johnson DH, O'Donnell DM, et al. Staging lung carcinoma with a Tc-99m-labeled monoclonal antibody. Clin Nucl Med 1992;17:431–438.
226. Baum RP, Lorenz M, Hertel A, Baew-Christow T, Schwarz A, Hor G. Successful immunoscintigraphic tumor detection with technetium-99m-marked monoclonal anti-CEA antibodies. Onkologie 1989;12(Suppl 1):26–29.
227. Kroiss A, Tuchmann A, Schuller J, et al. Tumor diagnosis by immunoscintigraphy with anti-CEA antibodies (Tc-99m MAK BW 431/26). Wien Klin Wochenschr 1989;101:621–626.
228. Leitha T, Baur M, Steger G, Dudczak R. Anti-CEA immunoscintigraphy in postoperative follow-up of tumor patients. Differentiated use of various monoclonal antibody preparations. Wien Klin Wochenschr 1990;102:503–509.
229. Leitha T, Walter R, Schlick W, Dudczak R. ^{99m}Tc-anti-CEA radioimmunoscintigraphy of lung adenocarcinoma. Chest 1991; 99:14–19.
230. Macmillan CH, Perkins AC, Wastie ML, Leach IH, Morgan DA. Immunoscintigraphy of small cell lung cancer: a study using technetium and indium labelled anti-carcinoembryonic antigen monoclonal antibody preparations. Br J Cancer 1993;67:1391–1394.
231. Kairemo KJ, Aronen HJ, Liewendahl K, et al. Radioimmunoimaging of nonsmall cell lung cancer with ^{111}In- and ^{99m}Tc-labeled monoclonal anti-CEA-antibodies. Acta Oncol 1993;32:771–778.
232. Brown PH, Krishnamurthy GT, Turner FE, Denney RK, Gilbert SA, Slauson ME. Primary lung cancer: biodistribution and dosimetry of two In-111-labeled monoclonal antibodies. Radiology 1989;173:701–705.
233. Saleh MN, Wheeler RH, Lee JY, et al. In-111-labeled monoclonal anticarcinoembryonic antigen antibody (ZCE025) in the immunoscintigraphic imaging of metastatic antigen-producing adenocarcinomas. Clin Nucl Med 1991;16:110–116.
234. Riva P, Moscatelli G, Paganelli G, Benini S, Siccardi A. Antibody-guided diagnosis: an Italian experience on CEA-expressing tumours. Int J Cancer Suppl 1988;2:114–120.
235. Riva P, Paganelli G, Callegaro L, et al. Immunoscintigraphy of adenocarcinomas by means of 111In-labeled F(ab')2 fragments of anti-CEA monoclonal antibody F023C5. Nucl Med Commun 1988;9:577–589.
236. Kalofonos HP, Sivolapenko GB, Courtenay-Luck NS, et al. Antibody guided targeting of nonsmall cell lung cancer using 111In-labeled HMFG1 F(ab')2 fragments. Cancer Res 1988;48:1977–1984.
237. Kalofonos HP, Rusckowski M, Siebecker DA, et al. Imaging of tumor in patients with indium-111-labeled biotin and streptavidin-conjugated antibodies: preliminary communication. J Nucl Med 1990;31:1791–1796.

32 Primary and Metastatic Bone Disease

MARTIN CHARRON and MANUEL L. BROWN

Bone scintigraphy is one of the most commonly performed nuclear medicine studies. The bone scan has been used for over 30 years in evaluating primary bone tumors, metastatic bone tumors, and primary soft tissue tumors. This chapter reviews the common scintigraphic findings in benign and malignant primary bone tumors and in metastatic disease, and the efficacy of bone scintigraphy in the work-up of common malignancies.

Conventional radiographic examinations can often reveal the anatomic location of a lesion and its effect on normal bone and can lead to a suggestion as to its histologic type. Bone scintigraphy with ^{99m}Tc-methylene diphosphonate (MDP) is a very sensitive, widely available, and safe procedure. Because of its high degree of sensitivity, bone scintigraphy provides for the early detection of metastatic disease in the entire skeleton and involves a radiation dose to the patient that is comparable to than a conventional radiographic procedures.

Whole body bone scintigraphy provides an excellent method for evaluating patients with suspected metastatic disease because most metastatic lesions are manifest as areas of increased activity. When evaluating patients with primary bone tumors or patients who have malignancies that result in lytic lesions, greater attention to detail is important to optimize the bone scan. In these cases, the diagnostic accuracy of bone scintigraphy is highly dependent on the technical quality of the study.

PATTERNS

There are several patterns of abnormality which one should be aware of in neoplastic diseases. In benign osseous neoplasms, uptake may vary from being quite faint if present at all, such as in fibrocortical defects or nongrowing bone islands, to markedly intense lesions such as in giant cell tumors. Relatively intense focal uptake may be seen in osteoid osteomas, sometimes with a double density sign, and several tumors can show a doughnut pattern of uptake with moderately increased uptake in the periphery of the lesion surrounding a relatively photopenic area centrally.

Another pattern that can be seen in both benign and malignant disease is the extended pattern of abnormally increased radiopharmaceutical accumulation in the bones of an extremity, either in the bones adjacent to the primary lesion or more distally throughout the extremity (Fig. 32.1). This pattern was described by Thrall and colleagues (1) and probably results from a combination of increased blood flow about the primary lesion and/or a change in the way the patient ambulates, and, therefore, a change in the stresses on the involved extremity.

The patterns of uptake of benign tumors are shown in Table 32.1. Osseous metastatic disease usually occurs in sites of relatively increased blood flow such as in areas of active bone marrow. In a survey of the pattern of metastatic disease, Krishnamurthy (2) noted that metastatic lesions occur in the axial skeleton in approximately 80% of cases. The remainder of lesions occurred in the extremities and skull. This distribution is similar for most soft tissue tumors that metastasize to bone via venous or lymphatic routes. However, in lung tumors that can metastasize via an arterial route, isolated solitary lesions may appear in distal extremities.

The most common presentation for widespread metastatic disease is multiple asymmetric areas of increased uptake throughout the axial skeleton and, to a lesser extent, the appendicular skeleton (Fig. 32.2).

Boxer and colleagues (3) reviewed a large series of patients with breast cancer who were eventually found to have metastatic disease to bone. In their series, 21% of the cases initially presented with a solitary bone metastasis, the most common site being in a vertebra. In patients with known soft tissue or primary bone tumors, the likelihood that any solitary area of increased uptake on a bone scan represents metastatic disease varies on a site by site basis. There are several articles that discuss the solitary lesion (4–11). By combining the results of these articles, one can make some general statements concerning the significance of a solitary lesion. In a patient with a known soft tissue or osseous malignancy, a solitary lesion in the pelvis or a vertebra will be due to metastatic disease 60–70% of the time, whereas, lesions in the extremities or in the skull would be due to metastatic disease between 40–50% of the time. It is much less likely for a solitary rib lesion to be due to metastatic disease. In a study by Tumeh (11), a single lesion in the rib was due to metastatic disease in only 10% of cases. An isolated sternal lesion in a patient with a known breast carcinoma has a much higher likelihood of being due to metastatic disease (Fig. 32.3). In a study by Kwai (7), almost 80% of these lesions were due to metastatic disease. This high likelihood of malignancy probably results from the lymphatic drainage from breast carcinoma and the internal mammary lymph nodes. When a bone scan demonstrates a solitary lesion in a patient with a known malignancy, especially one that is new and cannot be related to benign causes such as recent trauma, it is important to assess the finding with plain film radiography. If the plain film does not show a benign cause for the uptake, and there is a need to accurately assess the lesion, plain film tomography, CT, or MRI, and, where appropriate, a biopsy, may be needed.

Another pattern that results from metastatic disease is generalized increased uptake throughout the skeleton, a pattern that is called a superscan. The superscan occurs

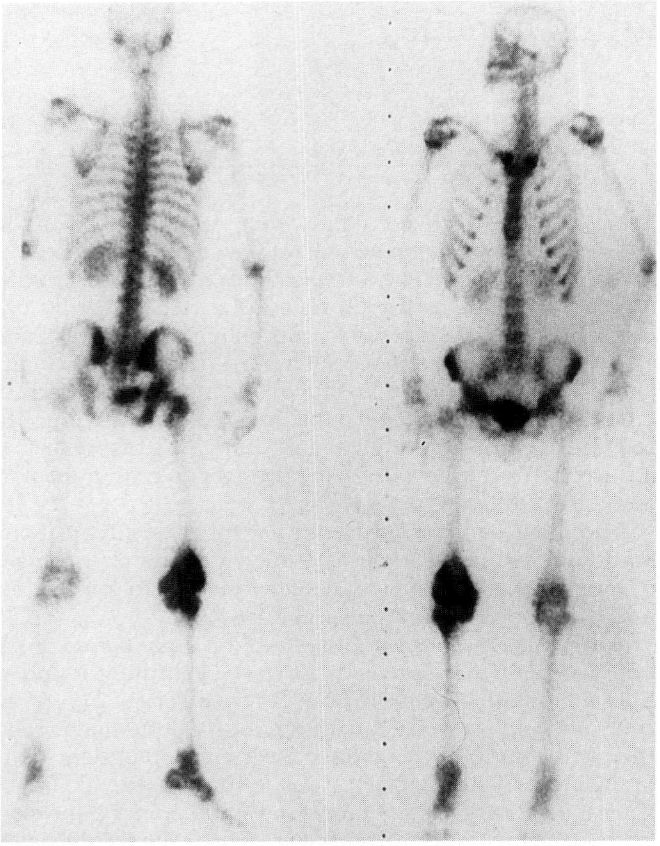

Figure 32.1. Giant cell tumor. 18-year-old with intense uptake in a giant cell tumor of the distal right femur. Note the extended pattern of the abnormality with moderately increased uptake in the proximal tibia and mildly increased uptake in the proximal femur and mildly increased uptake throughout the remainder of the right leg and the right ischium.

when there is diffuse metastatic disease and it is often associated with relatively little, if any, radiopharmaceutical accumulation in the kidneys. With modern gamma-cameras, the bladder is often seen in patients with superscans.

Greenberg and colleagues (12) described the pattern of the flare phenomenon in metastatic disease. This phenomenon occurs following a therapeutic intervention that results in improvement in the patient's clinical condition but a worsening of the bone scan. Serial bone scintigraphy may show increasing intensity in lesions and new lesions. This finding of increasing intensity indicates a healing of the metastatic lesions. Repeat bone scintigraphy in several months will show a marked improvement. The flare phenomenon has been described to occur in up to 20% of patients, but the frequency of occurrence clearly depends on the type of tumor, the therapy employed, and the interval between the therapy and the bone scan (13–17). One study, in fact, has demonstrated that the flare phenomenon is a good prognostic sign (18).

A pattern that can be seen in patients with metastatic disease to the lung is that of increased activity in the long bones and flat bones in various locations throughout the skeleton. This pattern results from hypertrophic pulmonary osteoarthropathy (HPO) and demonstrates diffusely

Table 32.1.
The Appearance of Benign Tumors on Bone Scintigraphy.

Adamantinoma	++
Aneurysmal bone cyst	+++
Bone cyst	−/o/+
Bone island	o/+
Chondroblastoma	+++
Cortical desmoid	o/+
Enchondroma	o/+
Fibrous cortical defect	o/+
Fibrous dysplasia	+++
Giant cell tumor	+++
Hemangioma	▲
Hereditary multiple exostoses	▲
Multiple enchondromatosis	▲
Myosites ossificans	▲
Nonossifying fibroma	+
Osteoblastoma	+++
Osteoid osteoma	+++
Osteoma	▲
Solitary osteochondroma	▲

+, ++, +++ mild, moderate, intense
− "cold"
▲ variable
o isointense
(Modified from Kech G, Christie JH, Mettler FA. Benign bone tumors and tumorlike conditions: In Mettler FA Jr, ed. Radionuclide bone imaging and densitometry. New York: Churchill-Livingstone, 1988:32.)

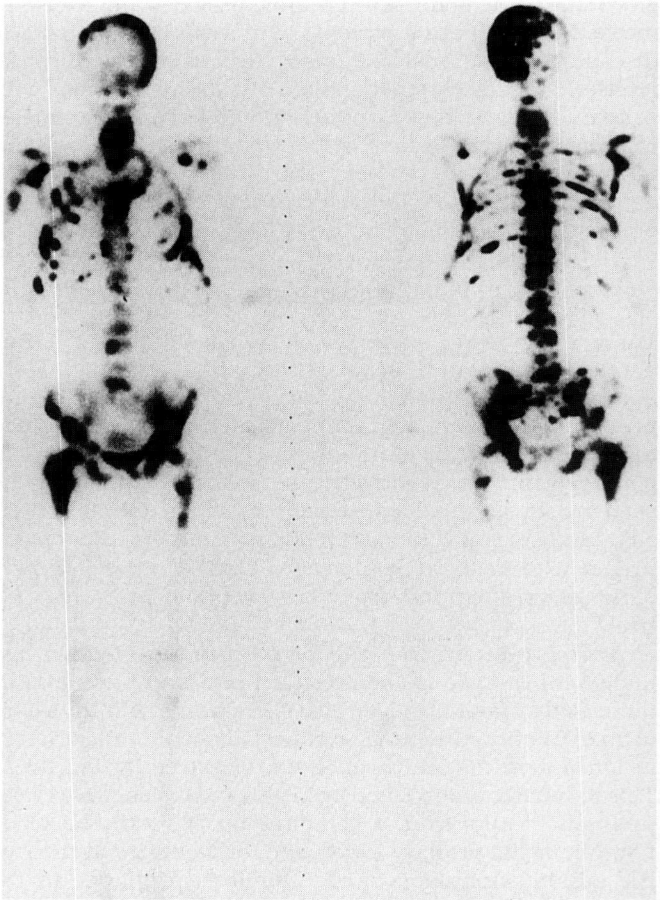

Figure 32.2. Prostate cancer. Multiple sites of markedly increased uptake throughout the axial skeleton, proximal appendicular skeleton, and skull in a patient with metastatic prostate cancer.

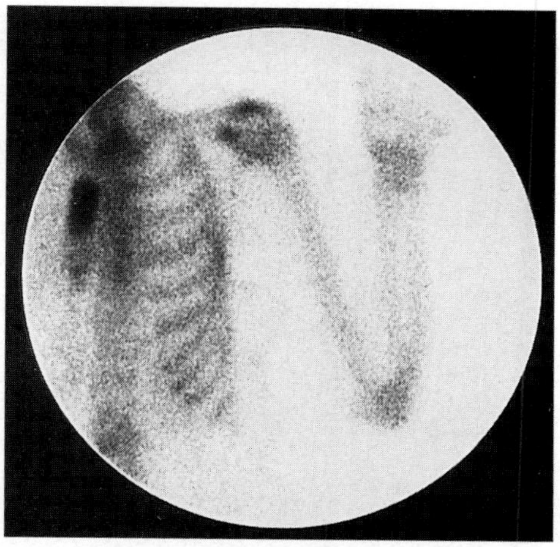

Figure 32.3. Breast cancer. Solitary site of intense uptake in the sternum representing metastatic disease in a patient with breast cancer.

and symmetrically increased uptake in the diaphysis and metaphysis of tubular bones along their cortical margins creating distinctive parallel tracks. Ali (19) reported the following distribution of HPO involvement in 48 patients: tibia and fibula 95%, femur 88%, hands and wrists 88%, radius and ulna 85%, feet 81%, scapula 67%, mandible 42%, clavicle 33%, ribs 2%, and pelvis 2%. Of note, none of these 48 patients had increased spinal uptake. The scintigraphic findings of HPO frequently appear before radiographic abnormalities, correspond well with clinical manifestations, and may decrease after treatment.

BENIGN BONE TUMORS

One cannot differentiate a benign from a malignant bone tumor on the basis of scintigraphic findings. Samuels (20) stated that with strontium-87 bone scans, benign bone lesions often appear only slightly more intense than surrounding bone, whereas malignant lesions often show intense radionuclide concentration. Although this characterization is a reasonable generalization, the intensity of a lesion on the bone scan is not predictive of a histopathologic outcome. Osteoid osteomas and benign giant cell (Fig. 32.1) tumors may have uptake as intense as any primary malignant bone tumor or metastatic lesion.

The uptake on bone scintigraphy in benign tumors was well-described by Keck and colleagues (21) (Table 32.1). A benign bone tumor is usually discovered when the bone scan is ordered to assess musculoskeletal pain or when it is ordered to assess metastatic disease for a lesion that is initially thought to be malignant.

ADAMANTINOMA (AMELOBLASTOMA)

Adamantinoma is a rare tumor of unknown cell origin. Radiographically these appear as large radiolucent lesions, and the most common location involves the midshaft of the tibia. Adamantinoma may occur in association with fibrous dysplasia or osteofibrous dysplasia. It is an uncommon, pluripotential neoplasia. The bone scan shows moderate uptake.

ANEURYSMAL BONE CYST

Aneurysmal bone cysts are uncommon benign tumors of unknown etiology. One-half of cases involve the long bones. Most cases occur in children and adolescents. The cyst contains anastomosing cavernous spaces filled with unclotted blood and walls that are not typical of blood vessels. In some cases, the histologic differentiation from a simple bone cyst is impossible. The radiographic appearance can mimic a malignant process. Up to one-third of these lesions are linked to other benign or malignant processes. The imaging algorithm includes plain film and MRI or CT. The bone scan typically reveals a doughnut pattern. Hyperemia may be absent despite the presence of increased uptake on the delayed image. Hudson (22) reported that 64% of aneurysmal bone cysts have the doughnut pattern of uptake (Fig. 32.4).

BONE ISLAND

Bone islands are focal areas of mature lamellar bone located within normal cancellous bone. This common lesion may enlarge after puberty. It is devoid of malignant potential. Bone islands can have increased uptake (23, 24) or normal uptake (25) on the bone scan.

CHONDROBLASTOMA

Chondroblastoma is an uncommon benign tumor that originates from cartilage and often involves the epiphysis of the lower extremities. Flat bones that can be involved include the talus and calcaneus. They are highly cellular and composed of chondroblast—like cells with distinct outlines. Most exhibit intense uptake on bone scans (26–29).

DESMOPLASTIC FIBROMA

Desmoplastic fibroma of bone is a very rare, benign, but locally aggressive, tumor and is characterized by small fibroblasts, fibers of collagen, and absence of new bone. The location is usually in the long bones, vertebrae, and pelvis (30). They occur most often during the first three decades of life and demonstrate no sex predilection. Plain films reveal an expansible radiolucent lesion that can extend into the soft tissue. The bone scan shows increased uptake.

ENCHONDROMA

Enchondroma is a common, benign, asymptomatic tumor located in the metaphyses, frequently of the hand (50%), and is composed of lobules of mature hyaline cartilage. Enchondroma accounts for about 10% of benign bone tumors and occurs in an age group ranging from 5–50 years. Plain radiographs show circumscribed areas of rarified bone with thinning and often bulging of the cortex and stippled calcification. Lesions in the large long bone and in membranous bone have malignant potential and can be difficult to differentiate from malignant lesions. The bone scan

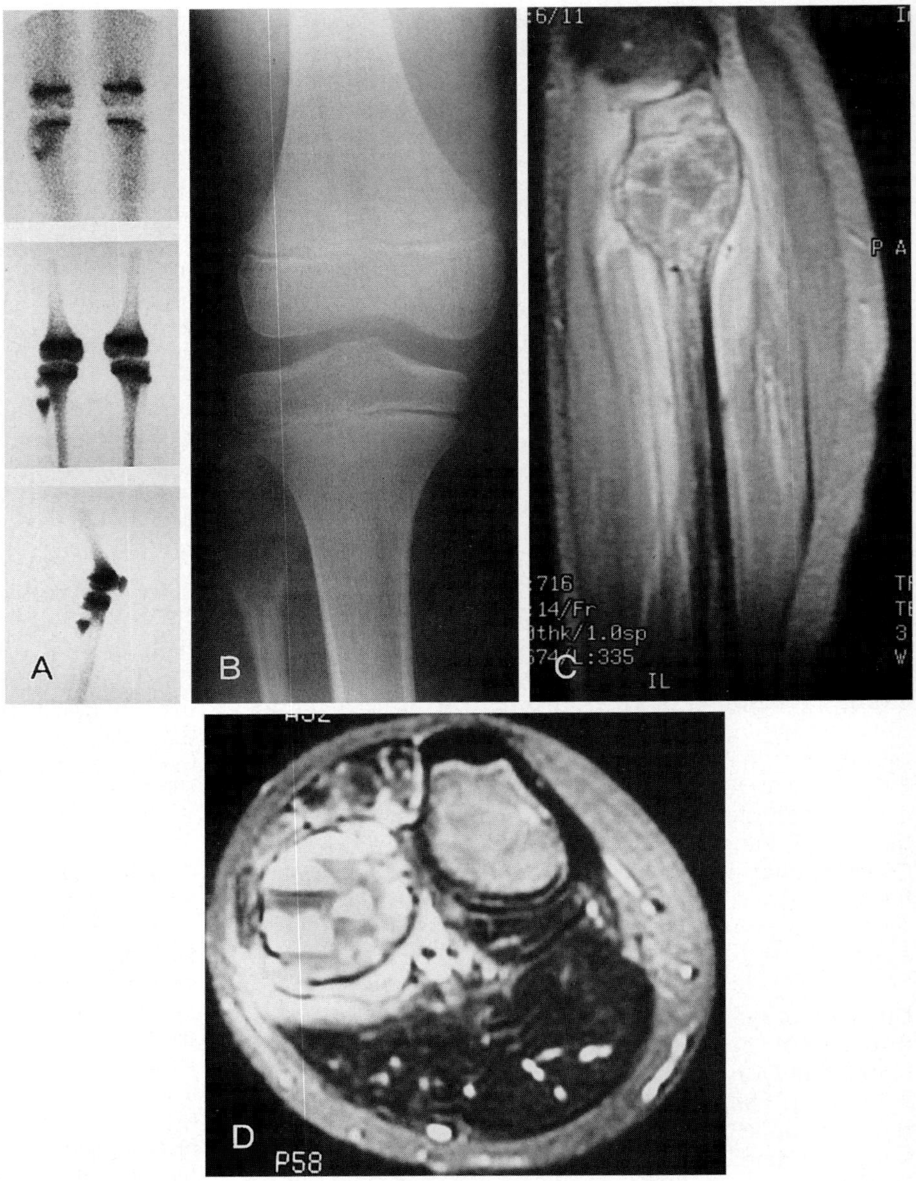

Figure 32.4. Aneurysmal bone cyst. **A.** The blood pool image (*top image*) shows a photopenic region surrounded by a rim of increased activity involving the proximal aspect of the right fibula. The delayed anterior (*middle image*) and right lateral projection (*bottom image*) also reveal a doughnut pattern. **B.** The plain x-ray of the right knee shows a lytic expansile lesion of the proximal end of the shaft of the right fibula with a pathological fracture. **C** and **D.** MRI reveals a proximal fibular lesion consisting of multiple cavernous spaces containing fluid which has an appearance most suggestive of an aneurysmal bone cyst.

shows normal or mildly increased uptake. A rapid change with increased uptake should be considered suspicious for malignant transformation. A bone scan is recommended in the initial evaluation to search for other lesions and as a baseline. Enchondromas produce a relatively distinctive appearance on MRI that is explainable by the presence of hyaline cartilage in the lesion.

Enchondromatosis or multiple enchondroma is a sporadic condition. It is usually first identified in infancy. These multiple enchondromas originate in the metaphyseal regions of tubular bones and in flat bones. When one side of the body is affected more than the other, the condition is termed Ollier's disease; when associated with soft tissue hemangioma and/or lymphangioma, it is called Maffucci syndrome. Sixteen to 18% of endochondromas degenerate into chondrosarcomas in this latter syndrome.

EPIDERMOID CYST

An epidermoid cyst is a sharply delineated cystic tumor which has a lining of squamous epithelium filled with a mushy material. If large enough, the center of the lesion will be photopenic on the bone scan.

FIBROCORTICAL DEFECT

Fibrocortical defect (FCD) is small, eccentric in location, and a pure cortical rest of fibrous tissue. It originates from the periosteum and invades the underlying cortex. Sites of predilection are the long bone, primarily the femur and tibia. The detection of FCD is often incidental. The lesion is seen in both children and adolescents and is rarely seen below the age of 2 years and almost never after the age of 14. Rare complaints consist of pain and swelling that are commonly attributed to some previous trauma. One-third of the pediatric population may have one or more of these lesions (31).

Plain films are usually distinctive and reveal a round, oval, or multiloculated lucency, often with sclerotic edges. This common benign tumor rarely shows uptake of ^{99m}Tc-MDP unless fractured (31).

FIBROUS DYSPLASIA

This benign tumor of fibrous tissue involves either one or more bones and usually does not cause any symptoms. There is a less than 1% incidence of malignant transformation. Seventy-five percent of solitary lesions are seen in ribs, femurs, and skull. It is usually recognized before 20 years of age. The lesions consist of fibroblasts, poorly oriented trabeculae, and islands of cartilage, and tend to stabilize at puberty. The association of fibrous dysplasia with multiple endocrine neoplasia (MEN) syndromes and skin hyperpigmentation is termed Albright syndrome. The bone scan shows markedly intense increased activity in all three phases. As many as 15% of lesions depicted by plain film may not be detected on the bone scan (33). In one series, 85% of patients with polyostotic fibrous dysplasia developed a pathologic fracture. Additionally, a bone scan cannot be used to diagnose a pathologic fracture at the site of active fibrous dysplasia because of the intense uptake in the lesion.

GIANT CELL TUMOR (OSTEOCLASTOMA)

Giant cell tumors comprise less than 5% of all primary bone tumors. Most of them are benign (90%) and have a high predilection to recurrence (~50%). One-half of the lesions are epiphyseal-metaphyseal in location and are found in the lower extremities. Almost all giant cell tumors reveal increased uptake of ^{99m}Tc-MDP (34), although minimal uptake may be seen (35–37). The lesion's hypervascularity can be identified on the angiographic phase, and a doughnut sign is seen about 50% of the time (38). This pattern is caused by an area of accelerated osteoblastic activity around a relatively photopenic tumor. Often, the abnormal uptake is noted beyond the tumor margin, in the bone adjacent to the joint, and in other joints of the same extremity (Fig. 32.1).

HEMANGIOMA

Hemangiomas of bone are composed of many vascular channels of different sizes, and can be cavernous, capillary, or venous. The common sites of involvement are the vertebrae and calvarium. Hemangiomas may reveal increased perfusion on the angiogram phase while photopenic on the delayed images (39). Radiographically, hemangiomas, when they involve the spine, show exaggerated vertical trabeculae or collapse of the vertebral body.

OSTEOBLASTOMA

Osteoblastoma is closely related to osteoid osteoma, and there is considerable debate about whether the origin is infectious or neoplastic. The differentiation between osteoblastoma and osteoid osteoma is not histologic, but rather based upon size. When the nidus is greater than 2 cm, the lesion is called an osteoblastoma; and when the nidus is less than 2 cm, it is called an osteoid osteoma. Osteoblastoma primarily affects patients between the ages of 10 and 30, the median age at diagnosis is approximately 18 years, and the male to female ratio is approximately 2:1. Osteoblastoma accounts for approximately 0.8% of all bone tumors and 3% of all benign bone tumors. Osteoid osteomas are four times more common than osteoblastomas. Forty to 60% of osteoblastomas are noted in the spine in comparison to 7% of osteoid osteomas. Another frequent location is long tubular bones, usually in the metadiaphyseal region. Osteoblastoma does not regress spontaneously, but usually involutes following radiation therapy. Unlike the symptoms related to osteoid osteoma, the pain does not abate with aspirin. The lesion can cause systemic toxicity and should be differentiated from osteomyelitis. The most characteristic manifestation of osteoblastoma on plain radiograph is that of a lytic expansile lesion with a variable quantity of dense amorphous bone or stippled ring-like calcification. CT scans provide evaluation of the tumor morphology and the effects on adjacent structures; the lesion has well-marginated borders and is relatively lucent and expansile. Typically, the bone scans reveal intense accretion on the blood pool and delayed imaging (40). Bone scans are especially useful in detecting obscure lesions on plain radiographs such as lesions that appear in the sacrum or small lesions in the spine (41–45).

OSTEOCHONDROMA

Osteochondroma is a osseous projection protruding from the surface of normal bone in areas where cartilage is found, is not true neoplasm, and is a developmental defect of unknown etiology. Solitary osteochondromas are the most common bone tumors in children, with the lesion being detected most commonly between the ages of 10 and 20. The lesion is usually located in the metaphyseal area and any bone preformed in cartilage may be affected. The lesion is not tender and is usually discovered incidentally. Occasionally, osteochondroma is found in association with previous local trauma or following irradiation. In children, osteochondroma should be expected to grow. The most common clinical presentation is the presence of a painless mass. Malignant degeneration of chondrosarcoma is rare and occurs in less than 0.25% of lesions. The bone scan cannot differentiate these benign and malignant enchondromas although the intensity on the bone scan generally increases as a lesion undergoes malignant degeneration. Absent uptake of ^{99m}Tc-MDP virtually excludes the possibility of malignant transformation of an osteochondroma (46). The CT appearance of an osteochondroma is that of a lobulated bony mass with a well-defined cortical margin, but MRI is the imaging modality of choice. These lesions are very well demonstrated on MRI and the most useful role is the accurate depiction of the cartilage cap.

Heredity multiple exostoses are similar to that of a solitary osteochondroma, except that the cartilage cap is

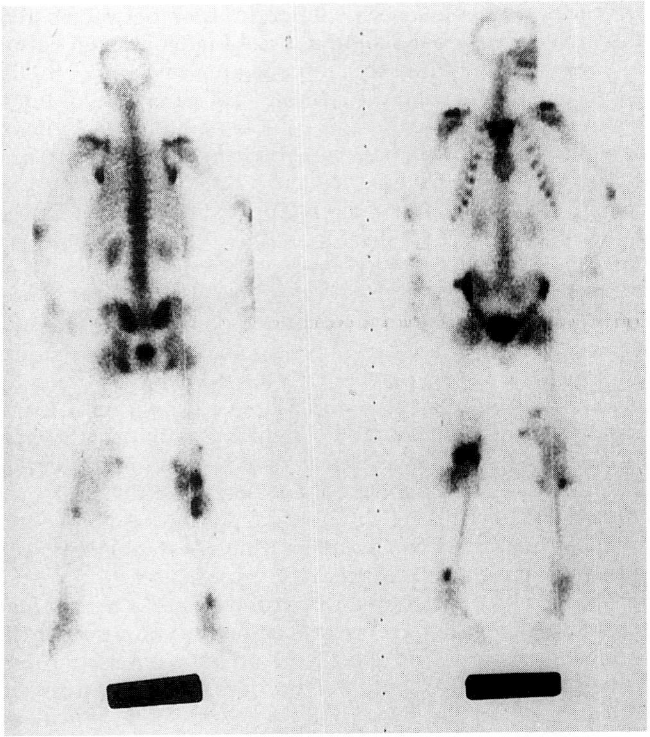

Figure 32.5. Osteochondromatosis. Young adult with multiple hereditary osteochondromatosis. Prominent lesions can been seen about the knee, right pelvis, and right ankle.

thicker, the frequency of malignant transformation is higher, and inheritance is autosomal dominant. The lesions may appear anywhere in the skeleton, although they are more frequently located around the knee and wrist (Fig. 32.5).

OSTEOID OSTEOMA

First described by Jaffe (47), osteoid osteoma is a painful, benign bone lesion that is characterized by a small nidus (usually <1 cm) of calcified osteoid tissue in a stroma of loose vascular connective tissue surrounded by a margin of dense sclerotic bone. One-half of osteoid osteomas are found in the femur or tibia, accounting for approximately 10% of all benign bone tumors. Osteoid osteomas are most frequently found in male patients between the ages of 7 and 25 years and cause pain that is worse at night, accentuated by weight bearing or ingestion of alcohol, and relieved by salicylates. After weeks or months of increasing pain there may be localized tenderness, but signs of inflammation are unusual.

The classic radiographic appearance of osteoid osteoma is that of a round radiolucent nidus, less than 1 cm in diameter, surrounded by a zone of uniform bone sclerosis. The nidus may have varying degree of calcification. If the nidus is located near the hip joint, secondary inflammation can lead to chronic synovitis and cartilage damage. Because of overlying bony structure and paucity of sclerosis, lesions in the spine, hip, and small bones of the hand and feet, are often difficult to detect radiographically. When located in the spine, osteoid osteomas are virtually always located in the posterior element of the vertebral body and often are associated with a painful scoliosis. The convexity of the curve is usually oriented away from the site of the tumor. The sensitivity of conventional skeletal radiographs in the diagnosis of osteoid osteoma ranges from 55–90% (48–50). Forty percent of osteoid osteomas occur in the femur and tibia, and 10% in the spine. Conversely, osteoblastomas are more frequent in the spine.

Bone scanning is of great value in identification of the lesion, especially in the spine and pelvis. Plain radiographs should be obtained first, and then the bone scan should be performed before any further imaging workup. Demonstration of the presence of the nidus by either plain radiograph or CT is a sine qua non to confirm the diagnosis. With very rare exception, osteoid osteoma avidly accumulates ^{99m}Tc-MDP on the three phases of the bone scan. Thus, the sensitivity of the bone scan is excellent. In a series of 20 patients with symptomatic osteoid osteoma, all 20 were positive on the bone scan while only 11 were positive by radiography (51, 52). Some patients present with referred pain, and imaging should include at least one joint above and below the site of pain; i.e., an osteoid osteoma in the intratrochanteric region can result in pain referred to the knee or back. Helms (53) described a double density sign that is purportedly specific for osteoid osteoma. This sign consists of intense uptake centrally with less uptake in the sclerotic bone, findings that are not noted in cases of osteomyelitis or abscess. Pinhole imaging may be helpful, especially if the planar images are nondiagnostic.

Surgical excision of the nidus will cause cessation of pain. The surgical resection may be aided with scintigraphic guidance to ensure complete resection of the nidus. When the lesion is located in the spine or hip, scintigraphic guidance will limit the amount of bone needed to be removed. ^{99m}Tc-MDP is injected prior to surgery. A mobile camera is used in the operating room to identify the nidus. Images of the resected specimen are obtained. Lee, et al., recently reported their experience (54) with radionuclide imaging, tetracycline fluorescence, and thermography in the preoperative staging of osteoid osteoma and concluded that intraoperative radionuclide imaging is a reliable technique in confirming complete removal of the nidus with no increase in operating time.

OSTEOMA

Osteomas are benign tumors that are usually found in the calvaria, paranasal sinuses, and mandible. They are usually asymptomatic and do not undergo malignant degeneration. These lesions are radiographically extremely sclerotic and measure approximately 2 cm in diameter. Gilday (55) reported one case of osteoma with intense accumulation of MDP.

SIMPLE (UNICAMERAL) BONE CYST

A unicameral bone cyst is a true fluid filled cyst, walled off by fibrous tissue, with varying amounts of hemosiderin. Simple cysts, more frequent in male patients, are typically found between the ages of 3 and 14 years, and are usually asymptomatic. The etiology of a simple cyst is unknown. It is not a true neoplasm and the most frequent location is in the metaphysis of the humerus or femur. These cysts are rarely present in adults, and thus they are thought to involute. The lesions are almost always solitary.

Radiographically the appearance is fairly typical with a large radiolucent lesion, broad at the metaphyseal end and narrow at the shaft end, that does not cross the epiphyseal plate. These lesions may resolve spontaneously. Those located in the lower extremity, contrary to those in the upper extremity, are at greater risk of fracture.

The recommended imaging approach is to obtain first a plain film and then, if needed, CT or MRI to define the content of the lesion. Bone scintigraphy is recommended if trauma is suspected; these lesions typically demonstrate abnormally increased activity following a fracture. An untraumatized cyst can be undetectable, but typically the bone scan discloses a slightly reactive margin surrounding a photopenic center, i.e., the doughnut sign.

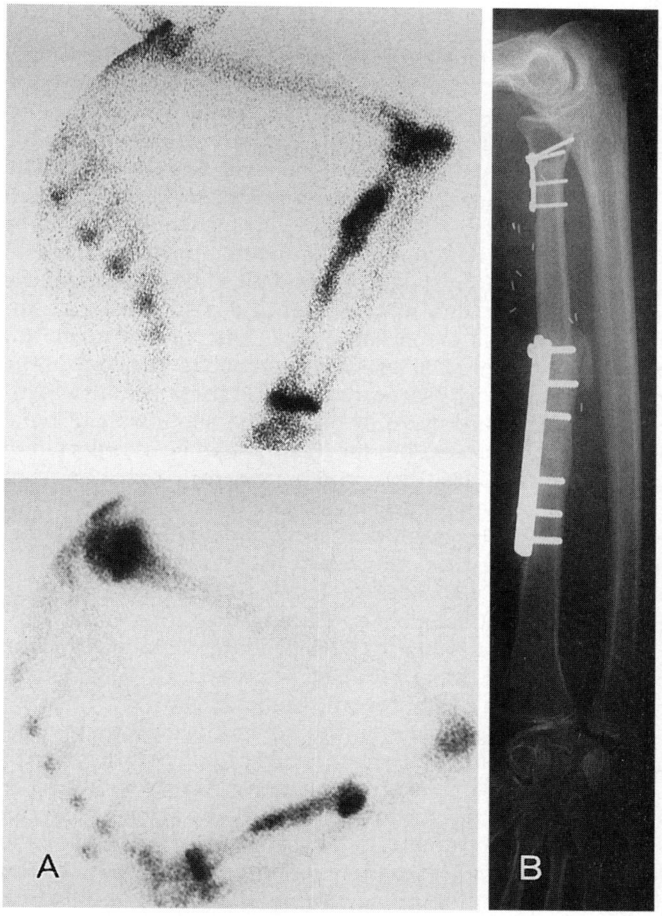

Figure 32.6. Ewing's sarcoma. **A.** Bone scan (*top image*) shows primary uptake in the Ewing's sarcoma involving the left radius. Two years later, the bone scan (*bottom image*) reveals a similar uptake; however, this was secondary to postsurgical change. **B.** Plain radiograph reveals two orthopedic fixation devices with evidence of callous formation and orthotopic ossification.

PRIMARY MALIGNANT LESIONS

CHONDROSARCOMA

Chondrosarcoma is a tumor of cartilaginous origin. The typical radiographic appearance is that of a radiolucent expansile irregular lesion. The margin of the tumor with time can become ill-defined with cortical destruction and invasion of the adjacent soft tissue. CT and MRI are useful to define the extent of the tumor, both in the bone and the soft tissue. The medullary form of chondrosarcoma shows patchy areas of moderately increased activity on the bone scan; the exostotic form of chondrosarcoma reveals high uptake focally. Chondrosarcomas occurring in the spine are detected more easily with bone scintigraphy than with routine radiography (56).

EWING'S SARCOMA

Ewing's sarcoma often arises in the femur or pelvis and is the second most common malignant bone tumor of children and young adults. Ewing's sarcoma, myeloma, primary osteocytic lymphoma of bone, and metastatic neuroblastoma are all members of an heterogeneous group of lesions termed small round-cell tumors. Ewing's sarcoma is believed to originate from a primary mesenchymal cell. One-half of the cases occur between the ages of 10 and 20. Common sites of involvement are the long tubular bones and are dependent on the marrow distribution. The primary symptom is pain which may be accompanied by fever and tenderness. The differential diagnosis often includes eosinophilic granuloma and osteomyelitis. The recommended approach for imaging involves obtaining plain radiographs, MRI for tumor extent, and bone scan for evaluating metastatic sites. Some authors advocate obtaining a bone marrow scan if the bone scan is negative. Lung metastases may be solitary, multiple, or diffuse, and CT should be used to detect these.

This tumor in a long bone typically arises in a metaphyseal-diaphyseal location with a mottled moth-eaten appearance of the bone. Multiple layers of periosteal reaction can be noted. Often Ewing's sarcoma will reveal very intense activity on the three phases of the bone scan. These findings of this very vascular tumor can be similar to osteomyelitis. The uptake is usually homogeneous and has been contrasted to the patchy uptake noted in osteosarcoma (57) (Fig. 32.6). Uptake in the soft tissue is less common in patients with Ewing's sarcoma than in patients with osteosarcoma because of the lack of production of osteoid. Following radiation therapy, decreased uptake in the primary tumor will be noted after 3–4 months (58). If increased uptake persists after treatment, it is suggestive of tumor recurrence, infection, or fracture. Bone marrow involvement can be evaluated with ^{99m}Tc sulfur colloid. However, bone marrow imaging is unreliable following chemotherapy or radiation therapy (59).

Metastatic bone disease is present at diagnosis in 10% of patients and indicates a poor prognosis. The usual sites of metastases are the lungs and bones, and up to 50% of patients will eventually have bone metastases.

HISTIOCYTOSIS X

Histiocytosis X can express itself through the abnormal proliferation of histiocytes that ranges from isolated bone involvement (eosinophilic granuloma) to a benign disseminated disease (Hand-Schüler-Christian disease), and includes a highly malignant form (Letterer-Siwe disease). The etiology is unknown and trauma has been suggested as a predisposing factor. The disease can involve bone and/or soft tissue. The recommended imaging approach consists of obtaining plain radiographs and a CT scan to detect the soft tissue extension of vertebral and pelvic lesions. Approximately 80% of patients have lytic bone lesions on plain radiographs. The lesion is destructive, the edge of the lesion is usually well-demarcated, and there is minimal increase in the deposition of bone. The sensitivity of bone scintigraphy to detect histiocytosis X has been reported to range from 35–94%; thus, the bone scan cannot be used reliably for screening purposes. One report suggests that bone scintigraphy is more reliable for detection of recurrence on follow-up examination (60). Additionally, there are occasional instances of lesions discovered on bone scan that are not detected on plain radiographs and, therefore, the greatest sensitivity is probably achieved by the combination of radiographs and bone scans (61–64). Large lytic lesions can be photopenic on bone scan.

Eosinophilic granuloma, the benign form of histiocytosis can express itself monostotically or polyostotically. Approximately 70% are found in the flat bones such as the skull, mandible, pelvis, and ribs, and 30% are found in the long bones. Involvement of the sacrum or small bones is rare. Many of the lesions heal spontaneously. CT has the potential to reveal more accurately the extent of bone destruction than the plain radiograph. The bone scan can demonstrate decreased, normal or increased uptake (Fig. 32.7). Kumar (65) reported a series of 24 lesions in seven patients of which the radiography detected 92% and the bone scan detected 67% of the lesions.

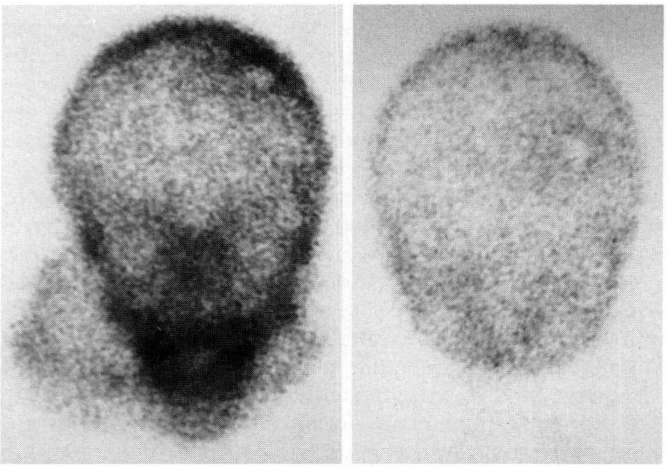

Figure 32.7. Eosinophilic granuloma. These vertex images (*left image without lead shielding*) reveal a photopenic region in the skull surrounded by a rim of faint increase activity (*arrowheads*).

MULTIPLE MYELOMA

Multiple myeloma is the most common primary bone tumor in adults. Several articles in the last decade have reviewed the role of bone scintigraphy (66–69) in multiple myeloma, and all demonstrate that plain film radiography remains the primary method of evaluating skeletal involvement by myeloma. Although bone scintigraphy may show many of the lesions seen on radiographs, radiographs are more likely to show more extensive disease than the bone scan (68, 69). Feggie and colleagues (70) did demonstrate that occasionally bone scintigraphy is helpful in patients with multiple myeloma in areas that are difficult to evaluate with routine radiography such as in the ribs and sternum. A bone scan should also be considered when patients with multiple myeloma have bone pain and negative radiographs.

Feggie and colleagues (70) also evaluated the role of bone marrow scintigraphy in multiple myeloma. In their series, they documented marrow expansion; however, bone marrow scintigraphy did not improve diagnostic accuracy.

OSTEOSARCOMA

This tumor constitutes one-fifth of all primary malignant bone tumors, and the peak incidence is during the second or third decade of life with a second peak in the sixth decade. Osteosarcomas are believed not to arise from the cortex, but rather to arise from an intramedullary location where they then invade the Haversian canals of the cortex, interfere with the blood supply, and eventually destroy the cortex. Often the lesion involves the metaphysis of a long bone, commonly the distal femur, proximal tibia, or proximal humerus. This tumor is more common in male subjects.

The most common initial finding is pain at the site of the tumor that the patient often ascribes to trauma. Osteosarcoma is also known to occur following radiation therapy or chemotherapy (71). Certain diseases of bone may be predisposed to develop osteosarcoma and include osteochondromatosis (Ollier's disease), Maffucci's syndrome, multiple hereditary exostosis, osteogenesis imperfecta, and Paget's disease.

The recommended approach for the evaluation of patients with osteosarcoma involves obtaining plain radiographs, bone scintigraphy to detect metastasis, and MRI to establish the extent of the primary lesion. Typically, on plain radiography, two-thirds of the patients present with advanced disease and the lesion consists of mixed lytic and blastic changes accompanied by a varying amount of extraosseous soft tissue mass containing calcified osteoid matrix. Often periosteal reaction is present. Typically the bone scan will reveal intense and expanded uptake (Fig. 32.8) and occasionally photopenic areas are noted in the tumor. The extended pattern of increased uptake noted on bone scan limits its uselessness for determination or the local extent of involvement.

Osteosarcoma that occurs in Paget's disease presents a very different pattern on bone scan than primary osteosar-

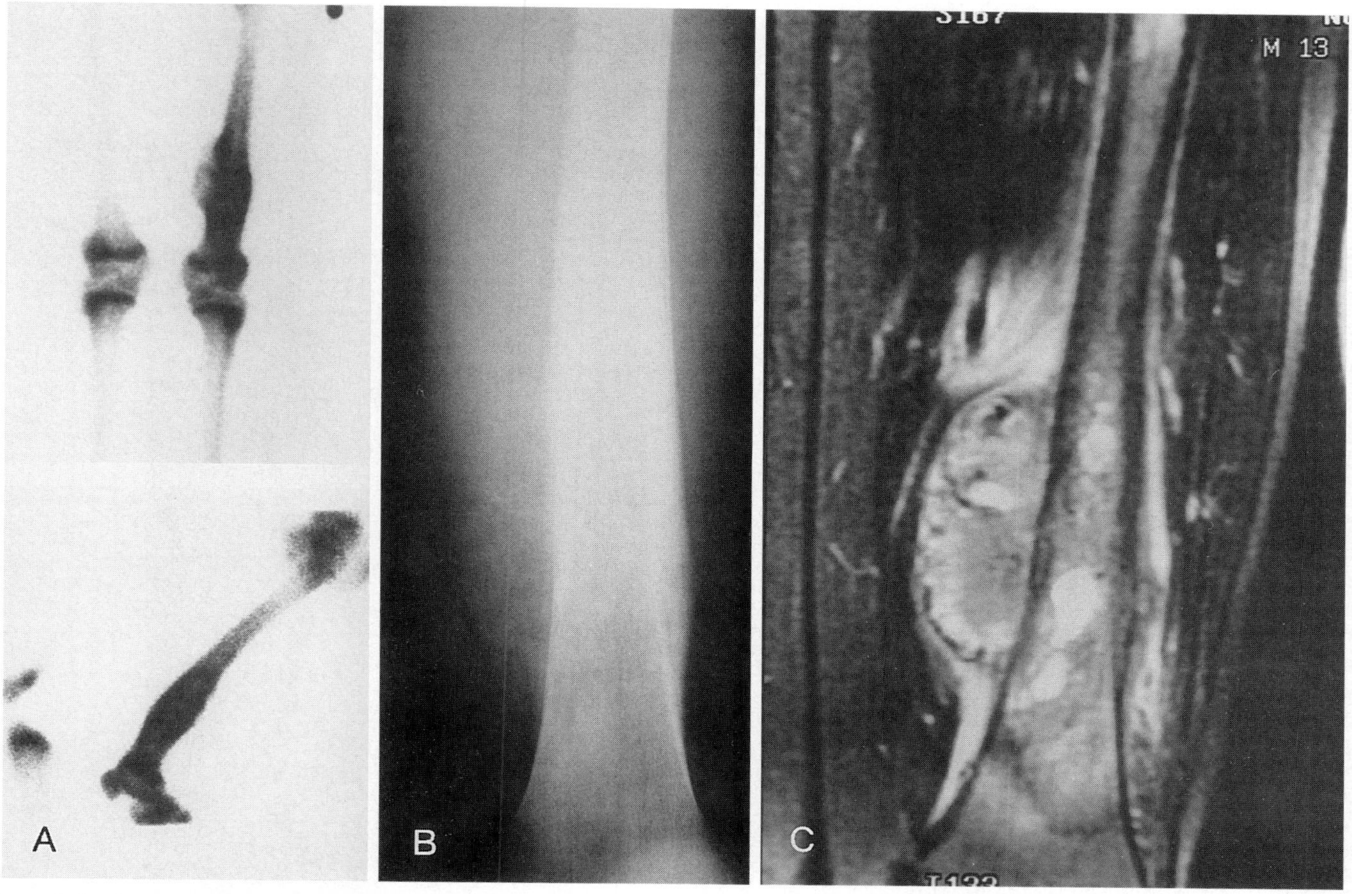

Figure 32.8. Osteosarcoma. **A.** The bone scan of a 13-year-old boy with osteosarcoma demonstrates on the anterior (*top image*) and lateral (*bottom image*) images of the left femur intense uptake that extends into the soft tissue. **B.** The plain radiograph of the femur shows the lesion with a soft tissue mass. **C.** The MRI of the left femur shows extensive marrow abnormality and a large mass extending into the soft tissue.

coma. A photopenic lesion will be noted in the pagetic bone that has diffusely increased activity. The cold area represents the osteosarcoma and the surrounding area is the Paget's disease. This pattern was noted in 13 out of 17 patients with osteosarcoma arising in pagetic bone (72). The cold area of primary osteosarcoma tends to have abnormally increased radioactivity.

Following amputation, patients may demonstrate abnormal areas of uptake in the lower extremities secondary to weight-bearing changes. Increased activity in the ipsilateral acetabulum, sacroiliac joint, and remaining articulations of the joint should not be assumed to represent tumor.

Distant osseous metastases are found at initial staging in only approximately 2% of cases (73, 74). Nevertheless, an initial bone scan may be important because the presence of metastatic disease greatly alters the choice of therapy. Osseous metastases have been noted to occur at a rate of 1% per month between 5 and 29 months after diagnosis, with a decrease in the rate thereafter (75). Follow-up bone scans at intervals of approximately 6 months are, therefore, recommended. With the routine use of chemotherapy in the treatment of osteosarcoma, approximately 20% of patients will have bone metastases before lung metastases (76–78) Additionally, bone scans can detect soft tissue metastases before they appear on chest x-ray (79–84). However, CT has the highest sensitivity for detection of pulmonary metastases. The main purpose of bone scintigraphy is to detect osseous metastatic involvement.

Edeline, et al. (85), recently reported the usefulness of bone scans in 19 cases of pediatric osteosarcoma. Bone scans were performed before chemotherapy and were repeated half-way through the course of chemotherapy at 6 weeks. Using factor analysis they were able to detect poor histologic responders to neoadjuvant chemotherapy. Similarly, Knop, et al. (86), studied the effect of preoperative chemotherapy on the uptake of ^{99m}Tc-MDP in 30 osteosarcomas and correlated this with the surgical specimen. The overall accuracy in presurgical prediction of tumor regression was found to be above 90%, and it was found possible to localize areas of viable tumor if greater than 1 cm in diameter. These authors concluded that ^{99m}Tc-MDP bone scanning was a highly sensitive and specific modality for the accurate evaluation of tumor regression following treatment.

Recently, Menendez, et al. (87), evaluated thallium-201

scans in 16 patients with high grade osteosarcoma or soft tissue sarcoma to determine whether this technique could be used to ascertain accurately the amount of viable tumor, as well as to predict the response to chemotherapy. They concluded that thallium-201 scintigraphy should be used concomitantly with other radiographic procedures in the diagnosis, planning of treatment, and follow-up of patients with sarcoma, because this technique appears to be able to predict the response of high-grade osteosarcoma to preoperative chemotherapy. Similarly, Rosen, et al. (19), reported, in 24 osteosarcomas, that a decreased uptake of thallium-201 correlated with a good response to preoperative chemotherapy. An excellent, thorough review is available for the reader interested in the use of thallium-201 in oncologic imaging (89).

RHABDOMYOSARCOMA

Rhabdomyosarcoma is a malignant soft tissue tumor of muscle origin and frequently involves the head and neck, the genitourinary tract, and extremities. This tumor metastasizes to the lungs, lymph nodes, bone, liver, and brain. The recommended diagnostic approach includes obtaining plain radiographs, ultrasonography, and MRI. Bone scanning is useful to define bone metastases (Fig. 32.9) and, occasionally, soft tissue uptake of the primary tumor.

METASTATIC LESIONS

BREAST CANCER

The bone scan is more sensitive for the early detection of metastatic disease in breast cancer than routine skeletal surveys (90–92). Abnormalities on the bone scan will precede radiographic findings by 4–6 months (91, 93). Although this increased sensitivity is well-documented, the exact role of bone scintigraphy in patients with breast carcinoma remains controversial.

The role of the bone scan in staging breast carcinoma has been studied in a number of centers (94–97). These studies report a very low true positive yield in stage I and II breast cancer. The true positive yield increases to approximately 14% in stage III disease. In a retrospective study of almost 400 patients, Ahmed (98) showed a frequency of true positive bone scans increasing from 2.5% for Stage I disease to 16% for Stage II disease. Coleman, et al. (18), reported a true positive yield of zero in stage I, 3% in stage II, 7% in stage III, and 47% in stage IV breast cancer. The efficacious use of bone scintigraphy must be considered in the initial staging of breast cancer patients. Patients with relatively small primary tumors (i.e., less than 2cm) should only have preoperative scans when they are symptomatic or have laboratory values worrisome for metastatic disease. Coleman and colleagues (18) recommend a baseline bone scan for all patients with stage II through IV disease.

There are also conflicting results regarding the utility of the bone scan in the routine follow-up of patients with breast cancer. Front and colleagues (99) demonstrated metastatic disease on the bone scan in 32 patients without bone pain, and a similar result was shown in a study by Chaudary (100). There are at least two studies (101, 102) that showed a much closer correlation between musculoskeletal pain and documented metastatic disease. In the study by Ahmed (98), 27 patients had bone scans at the time of the initial evaluation, but only eight of those had scans that were felt to be positive for metastatic disease.

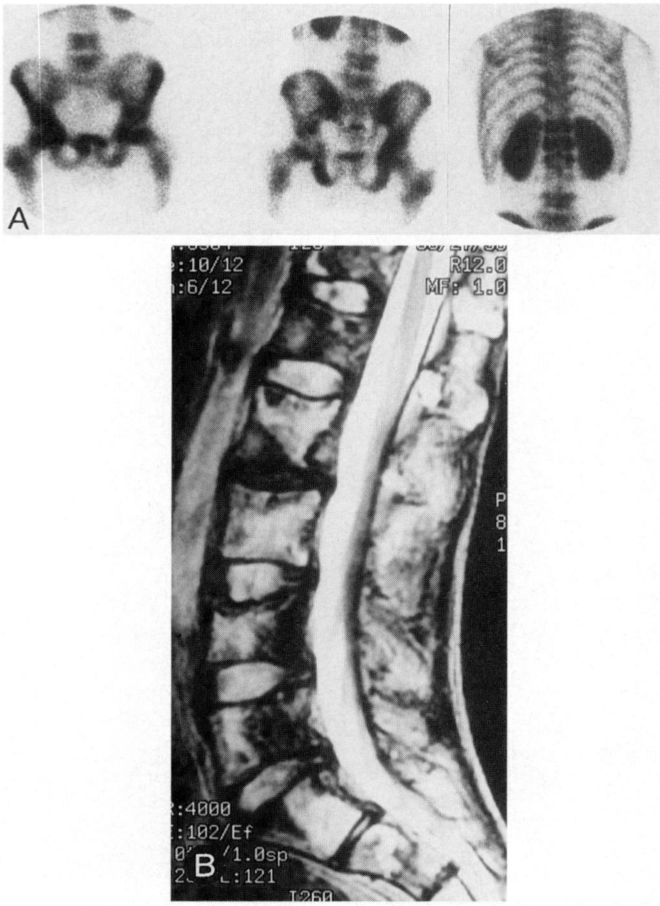

Figure 32.9. Rhabdomyosarcoma. **A.** The selected images from a bone scan of an 8-year-old with rhabdomyosarcoma show extensive abnormal uptake in the pelvis and spine. The inhomogeneous uptake in the spine may be related to tumor or previous radiation therapy. Chemotherapy caused the increased renal activity. **B.** MRI shows diffuse abnormality of the bone marrow within the spine most likely secondary to diffuse bone marrow involvement by malignancy.

A substantial number of patients will develop metastatic disease as a solitary lesion (3). Patients with known breast cancer who develop an isolated sternal lesion (Fig. 32.3) have a very high likelihood (approximately 80%) that the lesion is due to metastatic disease (7).

The flare phenomenon can occur in patients who have breast cancer. In a study by Coleman, et al. (18), 12 out of 16 patients with lytic metastatic disease showed a worsening on the bone scan, which later showed improvement after successful therapy. This flare response was seen in patients who responded to therapy compared to nonresponders, and, therefore, Coleman concluded that the flare response was a rule rather than an exception when there had been successful systemic therapy.

Metastatic disease from breast carcinoma often starts in the marrow. Imaging tests that can evaluate marrow as opposed to osseous involvement should be more sensitive for detecting early metastatic disease. This has been the case in several reports in the MRI literature. Duncker and colleagues (103), using a marrow scanning technique which utilized a radiolabeled antigranulocyte monoclonal antibody (with a normal marrow distribution), were able to detect metastatic disease as defects in the bone marrow in 25 out of 32 patients. The bone scan performed at approximately the same time showed metastatic disease in only 53% of patients. In the majority (approximately 70%) of patients who had positive bone scans and positive marrow scans, the marrow scans demonstrated more lesions. They concluded that marrow scintigraphy was a better test for the early detection of metastatic disease in breast cancer patients than standard bone scintigraphy.

HEAD AND NECK TUMORS

An early study by Wolfe and colleagues (104) showed that there was a very low prevalence of bone metastases at the time of initial staging in their series of 118 patients. Sham and colleagues (105) studied 132 patients who had nasopharyngeal carcinoma and no clinical evidence of distant metastatic disease. Their results showed a relatively low sensitivity and specificity for bone scanning, and they did not recommend the routine use of bone scintigraphy for the staging of nasopharyngeal carcinoma.

Baker and colleagues (106) showed in a relatively small series that the bone scan was useful as it demonstrated abnormal uptake, later proven to be due to involvement by tumor, where panorex films were negative.

Yui and associates (107) studied patients with bone scanning and single photon emission computed tomography to assess the skull base involvement by nasopharyngeal carcinoma. In this relatively small series, eight patients had bone involvement by SPECT, whereas the CT identified involvement in only three cases. In the five cases that were originally negative by CT, three later developed positive findings.

Although Wolfe and colleagues (104) and Sham (105) showed a relatively low yield for bone scintigraphy in head and neck cancers, Sundram, et al. (108), had different results. In their study, which included 143 patients at the time of staging and an additional 162 patients who had follow-up care with either bone pain or other suggestions of metastases, they showed a relatively high yield for the bone scan. In the patients who had bone scans as part of initial staging of nasopharyngeal carcinoma, 23% had evidence of bony metastases. The bone scans obtained as part of the follow-up examinations demonstrated a 59% true positive yield. The authors concluded that in their population, which does not seem to be typical, bone scanning was useful both in staging and in follow-up of symptomatic patients. A more reasonable recommendation would be that bone scans are indicated at initial staging or follow-up only in symptomatic patients. The exact role of bone scintigraphy in the initial evaluation of patients with head and neck tumors to evaluate local bone involvement may prove to be useful although this is not yet well documented in the literature.

LEUKEMIA

In the United States, leukemias constitute the most common pediatric malignancy and account for about one-third of new cases of cancer diagnosed each year. Involvement of the skeletal system occurs in the form of bone marrow infiltration. The most frequent finding on plain radiography in acute lymphocytic leukemia is the presence of transverse radiolucent bands in the metaphysis of long bones. Destructive bone lesions are more likely to be found in patients who have experienced bone pain for a period of longer than 3 weeks. Bone scans may be ordered to differentiate bone pain secondary to infiltrative process from osteomyelitis, although these two entities can both demonstrate increased uptake on the bone scan. The proliferation of leukemic cells in the marrow space may interfere with the blood supply, and thus bone infarctions may occur that can be seen as areas of decreased uptake. If the bone marrow scan shows an area of decreased activity in correspondence with a normal bone scan, leukemic infiltration rather than infection should be considered. The bone scan is rarely performed as part of the routine evaluation of leukemia.

LUNG CARCINOMA

The routine use of bone scintigraphy is not required as a preoperative test in patients with newly diagnosed lung cancer because of its relatively low yield (109). This low yield is especially true when history, physical examination, and laboratory values are normal. Ramsdell and colleagues (109) showed that bone scintigraphy and clinical evaluation agreed in 37 out of 51 cases and that there were 14 out of 23 cases where the bone scan was falsely positive. When bone scanning is performed, the finding of a positive bone scan is a very poor prognostic indicator in patients with bronchogenic carcinoma. In a study by Gravenstein, et al. (110), 46 patients had abnormal bone scans. In this group of patients with positive bone scintigraphy, 40 were dead within 6 months and another four died within 1 year. Similar results were found by Merric and Merric (111) who followed almost 600 patients with lung cancer. Their results showed that bone scintigraphy had a sensitivity of 89% and an accuracy of 78%. They also found that bone pain and an abnormal bone scan were independently associated with a significant reduction in survival for all cell types of lung cancer (111).

Bone scintigraphy in patients with lung cancer can also show the findings of hypertropic pulmonary osteoarthropathy. When performing bone scans in patients with lung cancer, it is important to image the entire body including the distal extremities as isolated peripheral lesions can be seen in the hands and feet (112, 113).

LYMPHOMA

Lymphoma is the third most common neoplasm in children. Hodgkin's disease represents about 5% of cases of childhood malignancy and four histologic types are described and relate to prognosis. The clinical presentation consists of localized pain with or without a palpable mass. The systemic signs of childhood lymphoma include fever, malaise, weight loss, and pallor. One-third of patients present with painless lymph node enlargement, which is usually in the cervical area. The recommended diagnostic algorithm should include obtaining plain radiographs, CT, or MRI to evaluate the characteristics of individual lesions, and bone scan or gallium scans to evaluate for metastatic disease. The radiographic appearance of primary skeletal lymphoma is that of a destructive lesion with permeative lytic changes. Periosteal reaction may include speculated and lamellated components that can mimic Ewing's sarcoma. The most frequent sites of bony involvement in Hodgkin's lymphoma are the spine and pelvis. In non-Hodgkin's lymphoma, the most frequent sites are the spine, the sacrum, and the facial bones. The bone scan in one series reported an average of 3.5 lesions per study in patients with Hodgkins and non-Hodgkins lymphoma; however, the bone scan was considered positive in only 4% of the cases. Skeletal pain, although specific, was very insensitive. Another interesting finding was that Hodgkin's disease had more frequent extremity lesions and fewer axial lesions than non-Hodgkin's lymphoma (114). Schecter, et al. (115), reported that bone scanning was very useful in the initial staging of Hodgkin's lymphoma, with a 45% increase in detection of osseous involvement compared to conventional radiographs. Gallium scintigraphy is essential to evaluate soft tissue involvement.

NEUROBLASTOMA

Neuroblastoma is a highly malignant neural crest tumor and is the second most common solid malignancy of childhood. Neuroblastoma in children under the age of 15 years occurs at a rate of about 1/100,000/year, with a median age at the time of diagnosis of about 2 years old. The tumor may arise in any site where neural crest cells are present, i.e., the adrenal medulla or any segment of the sympathetic ganglia of the neck, thorax, abdomen, and pelvis. Approximately 50% of the primary tumors arise in the adrenal glands, 25% in the abdominal sympathetic ganglia, and 15% in the posterior mediastinum. They are locally invasive and metastasize to liver, skin, bone, and bone marrow. Although they secrete catecholamines (mainly dopamine), these are extensively metabolized within the tumor itself, so that urinary levels of VMA and HVA are disproportionately elevated and hypertension is unusual. The more common presentations include abdominal mass, fever of unknown origin, anemia, hematuria, cord compression, and pathologic fracture. At presentation, 50% of patients have disseminated disease. The liver is more frequently involved in infancy and afterwards metastases occur more commonly in the bone.

Bone Scan

Bone scans are used in neuroblastoma to detect bone metastases and often will reveal primary uptake in the soft tissue tumor because of micro- and/or macrocalcifications. Heisel (116) reported that 91% of primary tumors were diagnosed by bone scan compared to 72% by radiographic examination (Fig. 32.10). Metastases often involve the calvarium. False-negative bone scans are possible if the lesions involve the metaphysis close to the growth plate. Thus, careful attention must be given in performing high quality imaging that includes magnification images with a pinhole collimator, especially of the knees. When the growth plate is blurred and nonlinear in shape, metastatic involvement should be suspected. Photopenic lesions (Fig. 32.11) may occur on the bone scan and are explainable by the impairment of blood flow or the extensive destruction. Recently, MacDonald (117) demonstrated that the scintigraphic appearance at diagnosis does not confer any prognostic information in children with advanced neuroblastoma.

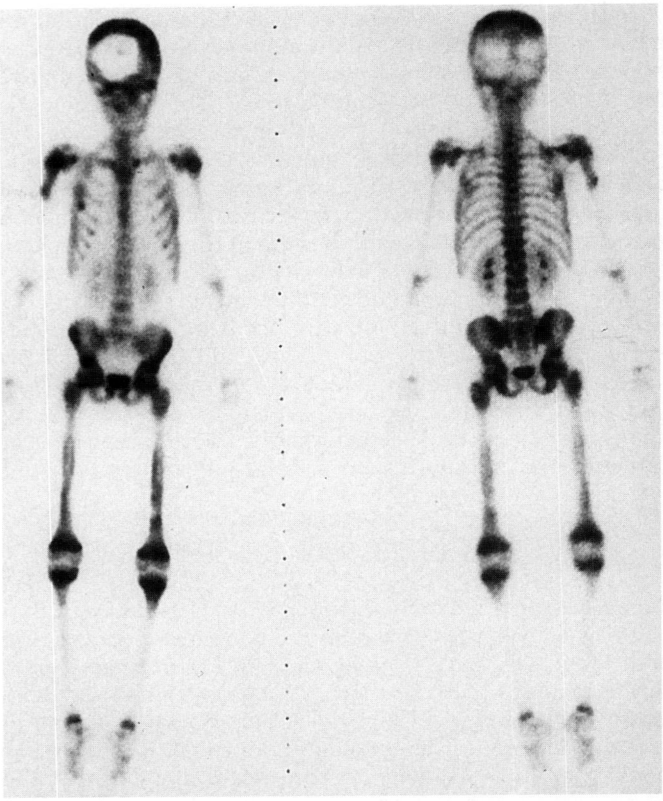

Figure 32.10. Neuroblastoma. The bone scan of an 8-year-old with stage IV neuroblastoma disclosed multiple areas of metastatic involvement of the bone and postsurgical change in the skull.

Metaiodobenzylguanidine

Metaiodobenzylguanidine (MIBG) imaging offers the ability to directly image the tumor. Metaiodobenzylguanidine structurally resembles the endogenous neurotransmitter hormone, norepinephrine, and the ganglion blocking drug guanethidine. MIBG enters the neuroendocrine cell, is recognized by the uptake-1 mechanism, and is stored in the catecholamine storage vesicles. Metaiodobenzylguanidine and norepinephrine share similar specific, active, energy, and sodium-dependent uptake mechanisms. Tricyclic antidepressants, phenylpropanolamine, and labetalol,

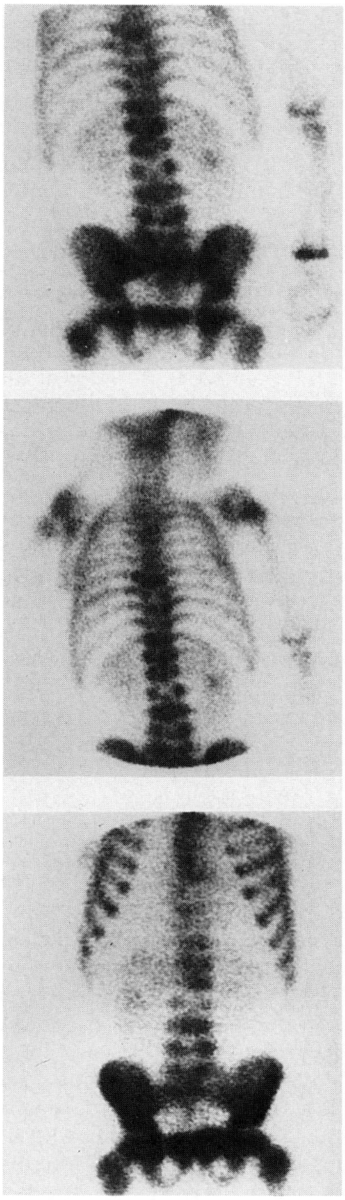

Figure 32.11. Neuroblastoma. The posterior bone images of the chest (*top image*) and spine (*middle image*) and the anterior image of the pelvis (*bottom image*) reveal widespread metastatic disease in a 5-year-old with neuroblastoma. The pelvis is involved diffusely and the spine shows metastatic disease as areas of increased and decreased uptake.

amongst other medications, reduce MIBG uptake by inhibiting the tissue catecholamine uptake and, therefore, should be avoided.

A supersaturated solution of potassium iodine (SSKI), at a dose of 1 drop in water or juice three times a day, is given 1 day before the study and up to 10 days after the administration of ^{131}I-MIBG. One-half a millicurie of ^{131}I-MIBG is used and imaging is obtained at 24 and 48 hours, and occasionally at 72 hours. A high-energy collimator should be used. Images of 20-minute duration are obtained of the chest, abdomen, and pelvis are obtained.

^{123}I-MIBG labeled with ^{123}I has advantages compared to ^{123}I-MIBG that include the low photon energy, which is better suited to modern gamma-cameras and provides far higher detection efficiency, and the radiation dosimetry, which is far more favorable. Ten mCi of ^{123}I-MIBG delivers approximately the same radiation absorbed dose as 0.5 mCi of ^{131}I-MIBG. The twentyfold larger administered dose yields sufficiently high counting statistics to improve spatial resolution, permit SPECT imaging, and improve lesion detectability. The disadvantages of ^{123}I-MIBG are its cost, limited availability, and limited shelf-life.

With ^{131}I-MIBG, the normal adrenal medulla is not usually visualized; however, faint uptake can be seen in up to 16% of cases. Colonic uptake is seen in 15–20% of cases and may mimic or obscure abdominal tumor activity. The salivary glands are normally visualized. Cardiac uptake is variable. Splenic uptake is variable and increases between 24 and 48 hours. Approximately one-half the dose is excreted in the urine by 24 hours and 70–90% is recovered within 4 days. Adequate hydration and frequent bladder voiding will reduce the bladder, gonadal, and whole-body radiation absorbed doses. Thyroid uptake of liberated radioiodide will occur unless the thyroid is blocked.

Any focus of activity not conforming to the normal scintigraphic distribution of ^{131}I-MIBG must be considered abnormal. Most tumors are demonstrated on the 24-hour images, and the depiction becomes clearer with time in most cases because uptake declines more slowly in tumors than in normal organs. Rarely, delayed visualization of tumor can occur up to 7 days after injection. Normally, in the lower limb, there is only diffuse, faint tracer uptake. Caution must be exercised in evaluating the urinary tract because an abnormality, such as a dilated renal pelvis, may demonstrate ^{131}I-MIBG activity and may be confused with tumorous foci of MIBG uptake.

The accumulation of MIBG is noted in many APUD tumors and has been reported to occur in pheochromocytoma, neuroblastoma, carcinoid, medullary thyroid carcinoma, nonfunctioning paraganglioma, adrenal metastases of choriocarcinoma, oat cell carcinoma, schwannoma, and Merkel cell tumor (see chapter 54).

In staging a patient with known neuroblastoma, MIBG scintigraphy can provide more information than CT or MRI. Following treatment, an abnormal focus of uptake represents evidence of viable tumor. Trocone, et al. (118), studied 158 patients with different APUD tumors. Sensitivity was above 80% in both pheochromocytoma and neuroblastoma. The specificity was greater than 95%, and no false-positive results were noted in tumors not originating from the neural crest. They compared MIBG with the CT and concluded that the former allowed the screening of the whole body, gave fewer false-positive results, had exquisite specificity, and allowed the nature of the neoplastic lesion to be identified. It was found to be reliable in the initial staging, in the postoperative phase, and in the monitoring of the response to different treatments. Its outstanding feature was found not to be to reveal morphologic details, but rather to image the functional aspect of the neoplastic lesions.

Schmiegelow, et al. (119), evaluated 145 MIBG scans performed on 96 children, including 71 with neuroblastoma and 25 with other neoplastic or nonneoplastic diseases. The MIBG studies had a sensitivity of 94% and a specificity of 88%.

Bone Scan versus MIBG

Because the bone scan and MIBG scan both provide information in the evaluation of patients with neuroblastoma, the accuracy of the two techniques have been compared in the same patients. Lumbroso, et al. (120), obtained 115 whole body MIBG and bone scans in 70 children. The scans were interpreted as positive if there was the presence of any nonphysiologic uptake. The uptake of MIBG was compared to the combination of available results from the ultrasound, radiograph, CT, MRI, surgery, cytology, and histology. The sensitivity of MIBG for detection of a primary tumor was 73%. For involvement of the bone marrow, the sensitivity was 90%, and the specificity was 100%. In comparison, the bone scans had a sensitivity of 78% and a specificity of 51%, when compared to the cytology. In their opinion, the best application of MIBG scintigraphy was to evaluate the viability of posttherapeutic tumor following surgery, chemotherapy, and/or radiation therapy. Metaiodobenzylguanidine imaging should be used in close relation to CT and can provide functional information on equivocal abnormalities depicted by CT. The sensitivity of MIBG for detection of liver metastases was lower than the other modalities available. The sensitivity of MIBG was 10% greater than bone scan for bone and bone marrow metastases. However, in patients with negative MIBG scans, the use of bone scans is still recommended. These authors (120) concluded that a sufficient amount of data has been accumulated to accept MIBG as a major modality in neuroblastoma staging.

Shulkin, et al. (121), recently reported a study in which they performed bone scans and MIBG scans within 1 month of each other in 77 patients. Both modalities were concordant for the presence or absence of skeletal metastases in all patients. However, there was a twofold greater number of skeletal lesions detected with MIBG. No patient with a normal bone scan had an MIBG scan indicating bone involvement. In patients with extraskeletal disease as shown by CT, there was soft-tissue uptake of MIBG in 80% of lesions. They concluded that both MIBG and bone scans were useful in the detection of metastatic skeletal disease. Metaiodobenzylguanidine was felt to be a better agent to characterize the extent of disease and was clearly superior for the detection of extraskeletal neuroblastoma.

Parisi, et al. (122), studied 26 patients who had both MIBG and bone scans that were performed less than a month apart. These studies were evaluated independently by six observers. There were seven false-positive bone scans. Metaiodobenzylguanidine scans were all true-positive and true-negative. The conclusion was that there was a higher specificity and sensitivity with MIBG scans compared with bone scans and that MIBG was the more efficacious agent for the evaluation of neuroblastoma.

Englaro, et al. (123), studied 31 patients who had both MIBG and bone scans. Twenty-six prebone marrow transplant and 90 postbone marrow transplant studies were reviewed. In patients who had undergone bone marrow transplantation, the MIBG scan reverted to normal more rapidly than the bone scan, and, compared with the bone scan, appeared to reflect more accurately tumor involvement in bone and bone marrow. In their experience, both ^{131}I-MIBG and bone scintigraphy occasionally demonstrated some lesions that the other missed. The specificity of MIBG was 100%. Small CT lesions, less than 1 cm, remain a diagnostic problem. These authors recommend a multiple modality approach that includes CT, bone scan, and MIBG studies.

Gordon, et al. (124), studied 44 children with MIBG and bone scans performed within 4 weeks. Bone marrow aspirations were obtained. There were eight false-negative MIBG scans with a positive bone scan at diagnosis. These authors felt that underassessment of skeletal involvement occurred with MIBG. A persistent abnormality on bone scan cannot be considered as evidence of viable tumor; only a bone scan revealing new lesions can be considered as likely true-positive.

Gilday and Greenberg (125), in the editorial to Gordon's study, emphasized that soft-tissue involvement is best detected by MIBG scintigraphy. Therefore, all children with a diagnosis of neuroblastoma should have both the MIBG and ^{99m}Tc-MDP scans to stage and monitor their neuroblastoma involvement.

Summary

The advantages of the bone scan over MIBG imaging for the evaluation of neuroblastoma are that (a) some cases are positive on the bone scan despite a normal MIBG, (b) imaging is completed at 3 hours, and (c) the radiation exposure is lower. The disadvantages of the bone scan are that (a) it has poor specificity for a single lesion, (b) its sensitivity is somewhat lower in the growth plate area, and (c) the study is technically demanding in order to obtain the best results. Conversely, the advantages of the MIBG scan over the bone scan are that (a) it has a high intraobserver consistency, (b) some cases are positive despite a normal bone scan, (c) it provides accurate assessment of the viability of the tumor posttreatment, and (d) it provides evaluation of extraosseous involvement. The disadvantages of the MIBG study are that (a) the study takes 2–3 days, (b) it results in higher radiation dose, and (c) there is poor sensitivity for the evaluation of metastatic liver disease. Metaiodobenzylguanidine was approved by the FDA in 1994. Based on the data currently available, our recommendation is (a)if there is a question of sensitivity, namely, "Is there any lesion in the whole body?" use both the MIBG and bone scan, or (b)if the clinical question is "Is there a lesion locally?," then the CT or MR is probably more sensitive. If the clinical question is one of specificity, namely, "Is a finding on plain film/CT/MRI viable tumor?," then the MIBG is the proper study.

PROSTATE CANCER

One of the major indications for bone scintigraphy in the past has been the staging and the early detection of metastatic disease in prostate carcinoma. A study in the 1970s by Schaffer and Pendergrass (126) demonstrated that the bone scan was more sensitive for the detection of early metastatic disease than radiographs, clinical evaluation, and the laboratory studies that were available at that time. Their study of 219 patients with adenocarcinoma of the prostate showed that 47% of patients without pain had positive bone scans, 39% of patients with normal acid phosphatase had positive bone scans, and 23% of patients with normal alkaline phosphatase had positive bone scans. In 15% of patients with positive bone scans, there was no bone pain and both alkaline and acid phosphatase were within the normal range. Their study also showed that patients who had pain, or elevated acid phosphatase, or elevated alkaline phosphatase, but normal bone scans, had other causes for those findings (126). Other studies have also demonstrated the high sensitivity of bone scintigraphy (127, 128).

Bone scans have value as a means of prognostic stratification. Soloway and colleagues (129) performed a semiquantitative grading of the bone scan, using an estimate of the number of vertebral bodies involved and showed a good correlation with survival. With their classification, the two year survival rates for extent of disease classes I–IV were 94%, 74%, 68%, and 40%, respectively. This prognostic value was also seen in a European study (130). The bone scan is also of use for prognosis following treatment (17, 130). However, as noted earlier, in patients treated for cancer of the prostate, the flare phenomena may be seen (14, 17, 131).

Since the introduction of prostate-specific antigen (PSA) the role of bone scintigraphy in the initial evaluation of patients with prostate cancer, the follow-up and evaluation of early metastatic disease, and the following of these patients during therapy has changed dramatically. PSA is a 33,000 dalton glycoprotein produced by epithelial cells in the normal prostate, hyperplastic tissue, and prostate cancer. It has been shown to be a very useful serum marker for the detection of prostate cancer, and it is also used in following response to therapy. Prostate specific antigen levels are more specific than prostatic acid phosphatase in the detection of early prostate cancer (132), but as noted earlier, the serum level is also elevated in benign prostatic hyperplasia. In a large study from the Mayo Clinic, Chybowski and colleagues (133) showed that the PSA level correlated well with the bone scan, clinical staging, tumor grade, and acid phosphatase. However, the PSA level had the best overall correlation with bone scintigraphy. This study showed that in the initial evaluation of patients, those who had a low PSA level had a very low likelihood of having a bone scan positive for metastatic disease (133). In approximately 300 men with PSA levels of 20nanograms per ml or less, only one patient had a positive bone scan, yielding a negative predictive value of 99.7%. Similar results were reported by Freitas, et al. (134), where in patients who had a PSA level of less than or equal to 8nanograms per ml there were rarely positive bone scan results. Their negative predictive value with this level of PSA was 98.5%. In another study from the Mayo Clinic, Osterling, et al. (135), did a retrospective review of 2064 consecutive patients with prostate cancer. For that study they used a PSA level of 10mg/l or less and, in patients who met this criteria and had no skeletal symptoms, a bone scan did not appear to be necessary as part of the initial staging. From this large series, the criteria of a low PSA and no skeletal symptoms occur in only 39% of patients presenting with newly diagnosed prostate cancer. In this time of cost containment, it is reasonable to conclude that bone scanning is not indicated in the evaluation of patients with newly diagnosed prostate cancer if the serum PSA levels are in the lower range of abnormal (10–20mg/ml) and if they do not have pain suggestive of metastatic disease.

The routine use of bone scintigraphy in following patients with prostate cancer is also declining because of the use of PSA. A study by Miller, et al. (136), showed that in patients who developed bone metastases, all had PSA levels of 20 nanograms/ml or greater. However, Sissons (137) concluded that although PSA levels are the appropriate way to follow patients, bone scans were still useful for the evaluation of symptomatic patients or when a change in management is contemplated. The use of PSA in evaluating progression of metastatic disease, although valuable in most cases, may not be as valuable in patients who have had hormonal treatment. Leo and colleagues (138) studied a group of patients who had been hormonally treated with antiandrogen therapy and compared them to a group of patients with no prior treatment for prostate cancer. The groups were matched for grade, symptoms, and bone scan findings. In the untreated patients, elevations of PSA levels were routinely found. However, in a substantial percentage (35%) of patients on the antiandrogen therapy, with definite metastatic disease, there were normal levels of PSA. They concluded that a serum PSA level in the normal range in prostate cancer patients who have been treated hormonally does not necessarily mean that the patient is free of disease nor that the disease is stable (138).

In patients who have had a radical prostatectomy, PSA levels will go to zero and these patients do not need evaluation with bone scintigraphy until they either become symptomatic or show a rising PSA level (139).

Therefore, although the bone scan remains an important study in the initial staging, the detection of early metastatic disease, and the evaluation during and following therapy in prostate cancer patients, the introduction of prostate-specific antigen changes the appropriate use of bone scintigraphy. The bone scan should be limited to patients who have either elevation of the PSA level, patients who are symptomatic, patients who have been hormonally treated or where the results of the bone scan will alter patient care.

RENAL CELL CARCINOMA

Kim and associates (140) showed that bone scanning was more sensitive than plain films for the detection of renal cell carcinoma metastatic to bone. In 18 patients with 68 proven lesions, the sensitivity of the bone scan was approximately 90% compared to a sensitivity for plain films of only 33%. Fifty-five of the lesions in this series had increased activity and another seven showed a photon-deficient pattern. But Steinbacher (141) had 16% of 91 osteolytic lesions showing no radiopharmaceutical accumulation. If photon-deficient lesions are to be detected, much greater care must be taken to perform the bone scan using high resolution collimation and longer imaging times to obtain a higher information density.

Bone scintigraphy has only limited value in patients with renal cell carcinoma. In a study by Lindner, et al. (142), in which they reviewed 231 charts, they found 71 patients who had metastases at first presentation. In that study there was no case where the first diagnosis of metastatic disease was made on the bone scan. Their data indicated that routine bone scintigraphy in the absence of clinical or laboratory findings suggestive of metastatic disease was not indicated. A recent study by Atlas (143) demonstrated that the bone scan was not as good a prognostic indicator as preoperative serum alkaline phosphatase levels.

With the relatively low yield in the preoperative setting (142, 144) and the difficulties in detecting some lesions in the postoperative setting, bone scintigraphy should not be performed routinely in patients with renal cell carcinoma. Bone scans should be used when patients are symptomatic and plain films are negative or where a change in therapy will depend on the results of the bone scan.

THYROID CANCER

Tenenbaum, et al. (145), reported their experience with bone scan in localizing bone metastases from thyroid cancer and concluded that bone scintigraphy in thyroid cancer should not be performed routinely. When bone lesions take up radioiodine, the addition of bone scan to the radioiodine posttherapy whole-body scan provides more accurate localization of tumor sites.

REFERENCES

1. Thrall JH, Geslien GE, Corcoron RJ, et al. Abnormal radionuclide deposition patterns adjacent to focal skeletal lesions. Radiology 1975;115:659.
2. Krishnamurthy GT, Tubis M, Hiss J, et al. Distribution pattern of metastatic bone disease. A need for total body skeletal image. JAMA 1977;237:2504.
3. Boxer DI, Todd CEC, Coleman R, et al. Bone secondaries in breast cancer: the solitary metastasis. J Nucl Med 1989; 30:1318–1320.
4. Boyd CM, Ridout RG, Angtuaco TL, et al. Significance of the solitary lesion on bone scans of adults with primary extraosseeous cancer [Abstract]. Radiology 1984;153:119.
5. Brown ML. The role of radionuclides in the patient with osteogenic sarcoma. Seminars in Roentgenology 1989;24:185.
6. Corcoran RJ, Thrall JH, Kyle RW, et al. Solitary abnormalities in bone scans of patients with extraosseous malignancies. Radiology 1976;121:663.
7. Kwai AH, Stomper PC, Kaplan WD. Clinical significance of isolated scintigraphic sternal lesions in patients with breast cancer. J Nucl Med 1988;29:324.
8. Rappaport AH, Hoffer PB, Genant HK. Unifocal bone findings by scintigraphy. Clinical significance in patients with known primary cancer. West J Med 1978;129:188–192.
9. Robey EL, Schellhammer F. Solitary lesions on bone scan in genitourinary malignancy. J Urol 1984;132:1000–1002.
10. Shirazi PH, Rayudu GVS, Fordham EW. Review of solitary ^{18}F bone scan lesions. Radiology 1974;112:369.
11. Tumeh SS, Beadle G, Kaplan WD. Clinical significance of solitary rib lesions in patients with extraskeletal malignancy. J Nucl Med 1985;26:1140.
12. Greenberg EJ, Chu FCH, Dwyer AJ, et al. Effects of radiation therapy on bone lesions as measured by ^{67}Ga and ^{85}Sr local kinetics. J Nucl Med 1972;13:747.
13. Gillespie PJ, Alexander JL, Edelstyn GA. Changes in ^{87m}Sr concenetrations in skeletal metastases in patients responding to cyclical combination chemotherapy for advanced breast cancer. J Nucl Med 1975;16:191.
14. Pollen JJ, Witztum KF, Ashburn WL. The flare phenomenon on radionuclide bone scan in metastatic prostate cancer. AJR 1984; 142:773–776.
15. Rossleigh MA, Lovegrove FTA, Reynolds PM, et al. Serial bone scans in the assessment of response to therapy in advanced breast carcinoma. Clin Nucl Med 1982;7:397–402.
16. Rossleigh MA, Lovegrove FTA, Reynolds PM, et al. The assessment of response to therapy of bone metastases in breast cancer. Aust NZ J Med 1984;14:19–22.
17. Levenson RM, Sauerbrunn BJL, Bates HR, Newman RD, Edy JL, Ihde DC. Comparative value of bone scintigraphy and radiography in monitoring tumor response in systemically treated prostatic carcinoma. Radiology 1983;146:513–518.
18. Coleman RE, Rubens RD, Fogelman I. Reappraisal of the baseline bone scan in breast cancer. J Nucl Med 1988;29:1045–1049.
19. Ali A, Tetalman MR, Fordham EW. Distribution of hypertrophic pulmonary osteoarthropathy. Am J Roentgenology 1980; 134:771–780.
20. Samuels LD. Diagnosis of malignant bone disease with strontium-87m scans. Can Med Assoc J 1971;104:411–413.
21. Keck G, Christie JH, Mettler FA. Benign bone tumors and tumorlike conditions. In: Mettler FA Jr, ed. Radionuclide bone imaging and densitometry. New York: Churchill-Livingstone, 1988.
22. Hudson TM. Scintigraphy of aneurysmal bone cysts. AJR 1984; 142:761.
23. Sickles EA, Genant HK, Hoffer PB. Increased localization of ^{99m}Tc-pyrophosphate in a bone island: a case report. J Nucl Med 1976;17:113–115.
24. Raback DL. Tc-99m-MDP bone scintigraphy and "growing" bone islands. Clin Nucl Med 1980;5:98–101.
25. Hall FM, Goldberg, RP, Davies, JA, et al. Scintigraphic assessment of bone island. Radiology 1980;135:737–742.
26. Murray IPC. Bone scanning in the child and young adult. Skeletal Radiol 1980;5:1.
27. Simon M, Kirchner PT. Scintigraphic evaluation of primary bone tumors. Comparison of technetium-99m phosphonate and gallium citrate imaging. J Bone Joint Surg 1980;62A:758–764.
28. Humphry A, Gilday DL, Brown RG. Bone scintigraphy in chondroblastoma. Radiology 1980;13:497–499.
29. Ulreich S, Swartz G, Stier SA, Philips E. Benign chondroblastoma of talus demonstrated by skeletal scanning. Clin Nucl Med 1978;3:62.
30. Giannestras NJ, Diamond JR. Benign osteoblastomas of the talus. JBJS 1958;40:469.
31. Blau RA, Kwick DL, Westphal RA. Multiple non-ossifying fibromas: a case report. JBJS 1988;70A:299–304.
32. Gilday DC, Ash JM. Benign bone tumor. Sem Nuc Med 1976; 1:33–46.
33. Machida K, Makita K, Nishikawa J, et al. Scintigraphic manifestation of fibrous dysplasia. CNM 1986;11:426–429.
34. Levine E, De Smett AA, Neff JR. Role of radiologic imaging in management planning of GCT of bone. Skel Radiol 1984;12:79–89.
35. Simon MA, Kirchner PT. Scintigraphic evaluation of primary bone tumors. Comparison of technetium-99m phosphonate and gallium citrate imaging. J Bone Joint Surg 1980;62(5):758–764.
36. Goodgold HM, Chen DCP, Majd M, et al. Scintigraphic features of giant cell tumor. Clin Nucl Med 1984;9:526–530.
37. Veluvolu P, Collier BD, Isitman AT. Scintigraphic skeletal

"doughnut" sign due to giant cell tumor of the fibula. Clin Nucl Med 1984;9:631–634.
38. Van NonstrandD., Madewell JE, McNiesh LM, et al. Radionuclide bone scanning in giant cell tumor. JNM 1986;27:329–338.
39. Williams AG, Mettler FA. Vertebral hemangioma, radionuclide, radiographic and CT correlation. Clin Nucl Med 1985;10:598.
40. Martin NL, Preston DF, Robinson RG. Osteoblastomas of the axial skeleton shown by skeletal scanning. J Nucl Med 1976; 17:187.
41. Pettine KA, Klassen RA. Osteoid osteoma and osteoblastoma of the spine. J Bone Joint Surg Am. 1986;68:354–361.
42. Wells RG, Miller JH, Sty JR. Scintigraphic patterns in osteoid osteoma and spondylolysis. Clin Nucl Med 1987;12:39–44.
43. Dahlin DC. Bone tumors. 3rd ed. Springfield: Thomas, 1978:28–42.
44. Kroon HM, Schurmans J. Osteoblastoma: clinical and radiologic findings in 98 new cases. Radiology 1990;175:783–790.
45. Kenan S, Floman Y, Robin GC, Laufer A. Aggressive osteoblastoma. A case report and review of the literature. Clin Orthop 1985;195:294–298.
46. Lange RH, Lange TH, Rao BK. Correlative radiographic, scintigraphic and histological evaluation of exostoses. JBJS 1984; 66:1454–1459.
47. Jaffe HL. Osteoid osteoma a benign osteoblastic tumor composed of osteoid and atypical bone. Arch Surg 1935;31:709–728.
48. Swee RG McLeod RA, Beabout JW. Osteoid osteoma: detection, diagnosis, and localization. Radiology 1979;130:117–123.
49. Smith FW, Gilday DL. Scintigraphic appearances of osteoid osteoma. Radiology 1980;137:191–195.
50. Omojola MF, Cockshott WP, Beatty EG. Osteoid osteoma: an evaluation of diagnostic modalities. Clin Radiol 1981;32:199–204.
51. Lisbona R, Rosenthall L. Role of radionuclide imaging in osteoid osteoma. Am J Roentgenol 1979;132:77–80.
52. Rosenthall L, Lisbona R. Role of radionuclide imaging in benign bone and joint disease of orthopedic interest. In: Freeman LM, Weissmann HS, eds. Nuclear medicine annual 1980. New York: Raven Press, 1980:267–306.
53. Helms C, Hattner R, Vogler J. Osteoid osteoma, radionuclide diagnosis. Radiology 1984;151:779.
54. Lee DH, Malawer MN. Staging and treatment of primary and persistent (recurrent) osteoid osteoma. Evaluation of intraoperative nuclear scanning, tetracycline fluorescence, and tomography. Clinical Orthopaedics & Related Research 1992;281:229–38.
55. Gilday DL, Ash JM. Benign bone tumors. Semin Nucl Med 1976; 6:33.
56. Smith FW, Nandi MB, Mils K. Spinal chondrosarcoma demonstrated by Tc-99m-MDP bone scan. Clin Nuc Med 1980;7:111–112.
57. Nair N. Bone scanning in Ewing's sarcoma. J Nucl Med 1985; 26:349–52.
58. McNeil BJ, Cassady JR, Geiser CF, et al. Fluorine-18 bone scintigraphy in children with osteosarcoma or Ewing's sarcoma. Radiology 1973;109:27–31.
59. Siddiqui AR, Oseas RS, Wellman HN, et al. Evaluation of bone marrow scanning with technetium-99m sulfur colloid in pediatric oncology. J Nucl Med 1979;20:379–386.
60. Crone-Munzebrock W, Brassow F. A comparison of radiographic and bone scan findings in histiocytosis X. Skeletal Radiol 1983; 9:170–173.
61. Parker BR, Pinckney L, Etcubanas E. Relative efficacy of radiographic and radionuclide bone surveys in the detection of the skeletal lesions of histiocytosis X. Radiology 1980;134:377–380.
62. Siddiqui AR, Tashjian JH, Lazarus K, Wellman HN, Baehner RL. Nuclear medicine studies in evaluation of skeletal lesions in children with histiocytosis X. Radiology 1981;140:787–789.
63. Crone-Munzebrock W, Brassow F. A comparison of radiographic and bone scan findings in histiocytosis X. Skeletal Radiol 1983; 9:170–173.
64. Schaub T, Ash JM, Gilday DL. Radionuclide imaging in histiocytosis X. Pediatr Radiol 1987;17:397–404.
65. Kumar R, Balachandran S. Relative roles of radionuclide scanning and radiographic imaging in eosinophilic granuloma. Clin Nucl Med 1980;5:538.
66. Ludwig H, Kumpan W, Sinzinger H. Radiography and bone scintigraphy in multiple myeloma: a comparative analysis. Br J Radiol 1982;55:173.
67. Nilsson-Ehle H, Holmdahl C, Suurkiula M, et al. Bone scintigraphy in the diagnosis of skeletal involvement and metastatic calcification in multiple myeloma. ACTA Med Scand 1982; 211:427.
68. Woolfenden JM, Pitt MJ, Durie BGM, et al. Comparison of bone scintigraphy in radiography in multiple myeloma. Radiology 1980;134:723.
69. Wahner HW, Kyle RA, Beabout JW. Scintigraphic evaluation of the skeleton in multiple myeloma. Mayo Clin Proc 1980;55:739–746.
70. Feggie LM, Spanedda R, Scutellari PN, et al. Bone marrow scintigraphy in multiple myeloma. A comparison with bone scintigraphy and skeletal radiology. Radiol Med (Torino) 1988;76:311–315.
71. Freeman CRK, Gledhill R, Chevalier LM, et al. Osteogenic sarcoma following treatment with megavoltage radiation and chemotherapy for bone tumors in children. Med Pediatr Oncol 1980; 8:35–382.
72. Smith J, Botet JF, Yeh SD. Bone sarcomas in Paget disease: a study of 85 patients. Radiology 1984;152:583.
73. Goldstein H, McNeil BJ, Zuall E, et al. Changing indications for bone scintigraphy in patients with osteosarcoma. Radiology 1980;135:177–180.
74. McKillop JH, Etcubnas E, Goris ML. The indications for and limitations of bone scintigraphy in osteogenic sarcoma. Cancer 1981;48:1133–1138.
75. McNeil BJ, Hanley J. Analysis of serial radionuclide bone images in osteosarcoma and breast carcinoma. Radiology 1980; 135:171–176.
76. Goldstein H, McNeil BJ, Zufall E, et al. Changing indications for bone scintigraphy in patients with osteosarcoma. Radiology 1980;135:177.
77. McNeil BJ. Value of bone scanning in neoplastic disease. Semin Nucl Med 1984;14:277.
78. McKillop JH, Elcubanas E, Goris ML. The indications for and limitations of bone scintigraphy in osteosarcoma. Cancer 1981; 48:1133.
79. Teates CD, Brpwer AC, Williamson BJR. Osteosarcoma extraosseous metastases demonstrated on bone scans and radiographs. Clin Nucl Med 1977;2:298–302.
80. Samuels LD. Lung scanning with ^{87m}Sr in metastatic osteosarcoma. Am J Roentgenol 1968;104:766–769.
81. Flowers WM. ^{99m}Tc-polyphosphate uptake within pulmonary and soft-tissue metastases from osteosarcoma. Radiology 1974; 112:377–378.
82. Ghaed N, Thrall JH, Pinsky SM, et al. Detection of extraosseous metastases from osteosarcoma with ^{99m}Tc-polyphosphate bone scanning. Radiology 1974;112:373–375.
83. Hughes S. Radionuclides in orthopaedic surgery. J Bone Joint Surg 1980;62B:141–150.
84. Siddiqui AR, Wellman HN, Weetman RM, et al. Bone scanning in management of metastatic osteogenic sarcoma. Clin Nucl Med 1979;4:6–11.
85. Edeline V, Frouin F, Bazin JP, et al. Factor analysis as a means of determining response to chemotherapy in patients

with osteogenic sarcoma. Eur J Nucl Med 1993;20(12):1175–1185.

86. Sommer HJ, Knop J, Heise U, Winkler K, Delling F. Histomorphometric changes of osteosarcoma after chemotherapy. Correlation with ^{99m}Tc methylene diphosphonate functional imaging. Cancer 1987;59(2):252–8.
87. Menendez LR, Fideler BM, Mirra J. Thallium-201 scanning for the evaluation of osteosarcoma and soft-tissue sarcoma. A study of the evaluation and predictability of the histological response to chemotherapy. Am J Bone & Joint Surgery 1993;75(4)526–31.
88. Rosen G, Loren GJ, Brien EW, et al. Serial thallium-201 scintigraphy in osteosarcoma. Correlation with tumor necrosis after preoperative chemotherapy. Clin Orthop 1993;293:302–306.
89. Nadel HR. Thallium-201 for oncological imaging in children. Seminars in Nuclear Medicine 1993;23:243–254.
90. Citrin DL, Tormey DC, Carbone PP. Implications of the ^{99m}Tc diphosphonate bone scan on treatment of primary breast cancer. Cancer Treat Rep 1977;61:1249.
91. Galasko CSB. The detection of skeletal metastases from carcinoma of the breast. Surg Gynecol Obstet 1971;132:1019.
92. Sklaroff DM, Charkes ND. Bone metastases from breast cancer at the time of radical mastectomy. Surg Gynecol Obstet 1968; 127:763.
93. Joo KG, Parthasarathy KL, Bakshi SP, et al. Bone scintigrams: their clinical usefulness in patients with breast carcinoma. Oncology 1979;36:94.
94. Hahn P, Vikterlof KJ, Rydman H, et al. The value of whole body bone scan in the preoperative assessment of carcinoma of the breast. Eur J Nucl Med 1979;4:207.
95. McNeil BJ, Pace PD, Gray EB, et al. Preoperative and follow-up bone scans in patients with primary carcinoma of the breast. Surg Gynecol Obstet 1978;147:745.
96. O'Connell MJ, Wahner HW, Ahmann DL, et al. Value of preoperative radionuclide bone scan in suspected primary breast carcinoma. Mayo Clin Proc 1978;53:221.
97. Wilson GS, Rich MA, Brennan MJ. Evaluation of bone scan in preoperative clinical staging of breast cancer. Arch Surg 1980; 115:415.
98. Ahmed A, Glynne-Jones R, Ell PJ. Skeletal scintigraphy in carcinoma of the breast—a 10-year retrospective study of 389 patients. Nuc Med Comm 1990;11:421.
99. Front D, Schneck SO, Frankel A, et al. Bone metastases and bone pain in breast cancer. Are they closely associated? JAMA 1979;242:1747.
100. Chaudary MA, Maisey MN, Shaw PJ, et al. Sequential bone scans and chest radiographs in the postoperative management of early breast cancer. Br J Surg 1983;70:517.
101. Brand WN. Clinical value of bone scanning with fluorine-18. In: Goswitz FA, Andrew GA, Viamonte, eds. Clinical uses of radionuclides: critical comparison with other techniques. AEC Symposium Series. Vol. 27. Oakridge, TN: US Atomic Energy Commission, 1972:156.
102. Schutte HE. The influence of bone pain on the results of bone scan. Cancer 1979;44:2039.
103. Duncker CM, Carrio I, Berna L, et al. Radioimmune imaging of bone marrow in patients with suspected bone metastases from primary breast cancer. J Nucl Med 1990;31:1450–1455.
104. Wolfe JA, Rowe LD, Lowry LT. The value of radionucleotide scanning in the staging of head and neck carcinoma. Ann Otol 1979; 88:832–836.
105. Sham JS, Tong CM, Choy D, et al. Role of bone scanning in detection of subclinical bone meteastases in nasopharyngeal carcinoma. Clin Nucl Med 1991;16:27–29.
106. Baker HL, Woodbury DH, Krause CJ, Saxon KG, Stewart RC. Evaluation of bone scan by scintigraphy to detect subclinical invasion of the mandible by squamous cell carcinoma of the oral cavity. Otolaryngol Head Neck Surg 1982;90:327–336.
107. Yui N, Togawa T, Kinoshita F, et al. Assessment of skull-based involvement of nasopharyngeal carcinoma by bone SPECT using three detectors system. Japanese J Nucl Med 1992;29:37–47.
108. Sundram FX, Chua ET, Goh AS, et al. Bone scintigraphy in nasopharyngeal carcinoma. Clin Radiol 1990;42:166–169.
109. Ramsdell JW, Peters RM, Taylor AT, et al. Multiorgan scans for staging lung cancer: correlation with clinical evaluation. J Thorac Cardiovasc Surg 1977;73:653.
110. Gravenstein S, Pelta MA, Pories W. How ominous is an abnormal scan in bronchogenic carcinoma. JAMA 1979;241:2523.
111. Merric MV, Merric JM. Bone scintigraphy in lung cancer: a reappraisal. Br J Rad 1986;59:1185.
112. Kosuda S, Gokan T, Tamura K, et al. Radionuclide imaging of two patients with metastases to a distal phalanx of the hand. Clin Nucl Med 1986;11:659–660.
113. Lederer A, Fluckiger F, Wildling R, et al. A solitary metastasis in the trapezium bone. Radiologe 1990;30:79–80.
114. Orzel JA, Sawaf NW, Richardson ML. Lymphoma of the skeleton: scintigraphic evaluation. Am J Roentgenol 1988;150:1095–1099.
115. Schecter JP, Jones SE, Woolfended JM, et al. Bone scanning in lymphoma. Cancer 1976;38;1142–1148.
116. Heisel MA, Miller JH, Reid BS, et al. Radionuclide scan in neuroblastoma. Pediatrics 1983;71:206–209.
117. MacDonald WB, Stevens MM, Dalla Pozza L, et al. Gallium-67 and technetium-99m-methylene diphosphonate skeletal scintigraphy in determining prognosis for children with stage IV neuroblastoma. J Nucl Med 1993;34(7):1082–1086.
118. Troncone L, Rufini V, Montemaggi P, Danza FM, Lasorella A, Mastrangelo R. The diagnostic and therapeutic utility of radiodinated metaiodobenzylguanidine (MIBG). Eur J Nucl Med 1990;16:325–335.
119. Schmiegelow K, Simes MA, Agertoft L, et al. Radio-iodobenzylguanidine scintigraphy of neuroblastoma: conflicting results, when compared with standard investigations. Med and Pediatr Oncol 1989;17:127–130.
120. Lumbroso JD, Guermazi F, Hartmann O, et al. Meta-iodobenzylguanidine (MIBG) scans in neuroblastoma: sensitivity and specificity, a review of 115 scans. Advances in Neuroblastoma Research 2. New York: Alan R. Liss, Inc., 1988:689–705.
121. Shulkin BL, Shapiro B, Hutchinson RJ. Iodine-131-metaiodobenzylguanidine and bone scintigraphy for the detection of neuroblastoma. J Nucl Med 1992;33:1735–1740.
122. Parisi MT, Greene MK, Dykes TM, Moraldo TV, Sandler ED, Hattner RS. Efficacy of metaiodobenzylguanidine as a scintigraphic agent for the detection of neuroblastoma. Invest Radiol 1992; 27:768–773.
123. Englaro EE, Gelfand MJ, Harris RE, Smith HS. I-131 MIBG imaging after bone marrow transplantation for neuroblastoma. Radiology 1992;182:515–520.
124. Gordon I, Peters AM, Gutman A, Morony S, Dicks-Mireaux C, Pritchard J. Skeletal assessment in neuroblastoma—the pitfalls of iodine-123-MIBG scans. J Nucl Med 1990;31:129–134.
125. Gilday DL, Greenberg M. The controversy about the nuclear medicine investigation of neuroblastoma [Editorial]. J Nucl Med 1990;31:135.
126. Schaffer DL, Pendergrass HP. Comparison of enzyme, clinical, radiographic, and radionuclide methods of detecting bone metastases from carcinoma of the prostate. Radiology 1976; 121:431.
127. McGregor B, Tulloch AGS, Quinlan MF, et al. The role of bone scanning in the assessment of prostataic carcinoma. Br J Urol 1978;50:178.
128. O'Donogue EPN, Constable AR, Sherwood T, et al. Bone scanning

and plasma phosphatases in carcinoma of the prostate. Br J Urol 1978;50:172.
129. Soloway MS, Hardeman SW, Hickey D, et al. Stratification of patients with metastatic prostate cancer based on extent of disease on initial bone scan. Cancer 1988;61:195–202.
130. Lund F, Smith PH, Suciu S, EORTC Urological Group. Do bone scans predict prognosis in prostatic cancer? A report of the EORTC Protocol 30762. Br J Urol 1984;56:58–63.
131. Johns WD, Garnick MB, Kaplan WD. Leuprolide therapy for prostate cancer. An association with scintigraphic "flare" on bone scan. Clin Nucl Med 1990;15:485–487.
132. Stamey TA, Yang N, Hay AR, et al. Prostate-specific antigen as a serum marker for adenocarcinoma of the prostate. N Engl J Med 1987;317:909–916.
133. Chybowski FM, Keller JL, Bergstralh EJ, et al. Predicting radionuclide bone scan findings in patients with newly diagnosed, untreated prostate cancer: prostate specific antigen is superior to all other clinical parameters. J Urol 1991;145:313.
134. Freitas JE, Gilvydas R, Ferry JD, et al. The clinical utility of prostate-specific antigen and bone scintigraphy in prostate cancer follow-up. J Nucl Med 1991;32:1387–1390.
135. Oesterling JE, Martin SK, Bergstralh EJ, Lowe FC. The use of prostate-specific antigen in staging patients with newly diagnosed prostate cancer. JAMA 1993;269:57–60.
136. Miller PD, Eardley I, Kirby RS. Prostate specific antigen and bone scan correlation in the staging and monitoring of patients with prostate cancer. Br J Urol 1992;70:295–298.
137. Sissons GRJ, Clements R, Peeling WB, Penney MD. Can serum prostate-specific antigen replace bone scintigraphy in the follow-up of metastatic prostate cancer. Br J Urology 1992;65:861–864.
138. Leo ME, Bilhart DL, Bergstralh EJ, et al. Prostate-specific antigen in hormonally treated stage D2 prostate cancer: Is it always an accurate indicator of disease status? J Urol 1991;145:802.
139. Terris MK, Kilnecke AS, McDougall IR, et al. Utilization of bone scans in conjunction with prostate-specific antigen levels in the surveillance for recurrence of adenocarcinoma after radical prostatectomy. J Nucl Med 1991;32:1713.
140. Kim EE, Bledin AG, Gutierrez C, Haynie TP. Comparison of radionuclide images and radiographs for skeletal metastases from renal cell carcinoma. Oncology 1983;40:284–286.
141. Steinbacher M, Rieden K, Bihl H, et al. Uptake behavior of bone metastases of hypernephroma in the 99mTc-MDP bone scintigram. A comparison with x-ray findings. Rofo: Fortschritte Auf Dem Gebiete Der Rontgenstrahlen Und Der Nuklearmedizin 1987:146:555.
142. Lindner A, Goldman DG, deKernion JB. Cost effective analysis of prenephrectomy radioisotope scans in renal cell carcinoma. Urology 1983;22(2):127–129.
143. Atlas I, Kwan D, Stone N. Value of serum alkaline phosphatase and radionuclide bone scans in patients with renal cell carcinoma. Urology 1991;38(3):220–222.
144. Rosen PR, Murphy KG. Bone scintigraphy in the initial staging of patients with renal cell carcinoma: concise communication. J Nucl Med 1984;25:289–291.
145. Tenenbaum F, Schlumberger M, Bonnin F, et al. Usefulness of technetium-99m hydroxymethylene diphosphonate scans in localizing bone metastases of differentiated thyroid carcinoma. Eur J Nucl Med 1993;20(12):1168–1170.

33 Benign Bone Disease

ROBERT E. O'MARA

The study of the skeleton by nuclear medicine techniques has advanced steadily over the years to the point where skeletal scintigraphy is one of the most frequently performed procedures in nuclear medicine departments. Marked improvement in instrumentation, including increased resolution of gamma-camera systems, the addition of single photon emission computed tomography (SPECT), and positron emission tomography (PET), has contributed to this advance. Additionally, the improvements in radiopharmaceuticals such as the introduction of labeled phosphate and diphosphonate compounds, ^{99m}Tc-HMPAO and ^{111}In-oxine-labeled leukocytes (^{99m}Tc-WBC, ^{111}In-WBC), ^{67}Ga citrate, and radiolabeled antibodies also contributed to this advance. Finally, the ability to view the entire skeleton in an economical manner involving low radiation dose has also been a major factor in the increased utilization of skeletal scintigraphy. Nuclear medicine bone imaging remains a highly sensitive, noninvasive method of detecting a wide variety of skeletal diseases. Unfortunately, in most cases, it still lacks high specificity. However, in addition to the developments of the technical factors mentioned, the ability of the nuclear physician to develop pattern recognition has resulted in some increase in specificity. Much of this advance has been related to the study of neoplastic disease, both benign and malignant, and in trauma. These applications are discussed elsewhere in this text as is the role of PET imaging in evaluation of skeletal disease. This chapter deals predominantly with benign disease in which skeletal imaging may play a significant role, including infection, metabolic disease, avascular necrosis (osteonecrosis), arthritides, and irradiated bone. In applying skeletal imagining techniques to the study of benign disease, one must be aware of the relationship between the radionuclide imagining appearance and the timed course of the disease process. Other conditions, such as soft tissue uptake of bone seeking agents, other underlying bone disease processes, or surgical intervention, may cause confusion. Broadly, radionuclide bone imagining applications are used for early recognition of the disease process, assessment of the extent of disease, differential diagnosis of the disease, assessment of the activity status of the condition, identification of sites for further evaluation with other radiographic techniques or by closed or open biopsy, and to assess the efficacy of therapeutic regimens.

The nuclear physician must also be aware of the complementary and sometimes competing roles of radiographic evaluation. The standard radiographic evaluations of bone still excel in the demonstration of osseous structural detail. However, such changes usually occur late in the disease process reflecting a slow rate of bone mineral loss or accumulation. Standard roentgenologic exams usually contribute little to the evaluation of function, an area where bone scintigraphy excels. Nevertheless, radiographs are exceptional in demonstrating radiodense or radiolucent, but metabolically inactive, lesions that may not be visualized on the radionuclide bone study. The development of the ability to visualize bone well on computerized tomography (CT) has increased its utilization in defining bony involvement by disease. Magnetic resonance imagining (MRI) has developed to give the best resolution of soft tissue versus bone involvement of any imagining technique. Additionally, the ability to visualize marrow changes in bone that contains marrow, and the ability to visualize disease that causes increased tissue water has enhanced the role of this modality to where, in most institutions, it has replaced CT in the evaluation of focal bony disease, especially in the young, since it gives no radiation to the patient. Finally, as more rapid imaging systems in both modalities develop, the ability to visualize large parts or all of the skeletal system has become real. How this development impacts utilization of skeletal scintigraphy remains a subject of ongoing study. In our institution, an algorithmic approach was developed in conjunction with members of the orthopedic department for localized bony symptomatologoy. The standard radiograph is utilized first, despite its somewhat low sensitivity. It is cheap, quick, and readily available at all times. If it is noncontributory, then other imaging modality approaches come into play (Table 33.1). In diseases that can afflict changes in the entire skeletal system or in many places in the skeletal system, such as Paget's disease, other metabolic diseases, and metastases, the approach is to start with a total body skeletal image and, if necessary, investigate specific areas with either standard radiographs, CT, or MRI exams (Table 33.2).

Table 33.1.
Focal Symptoms.

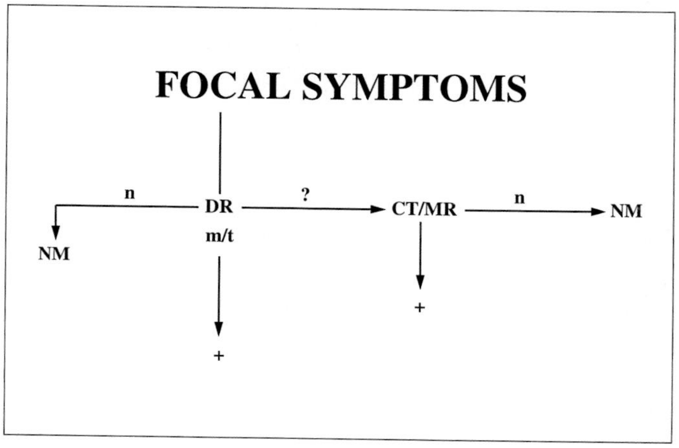

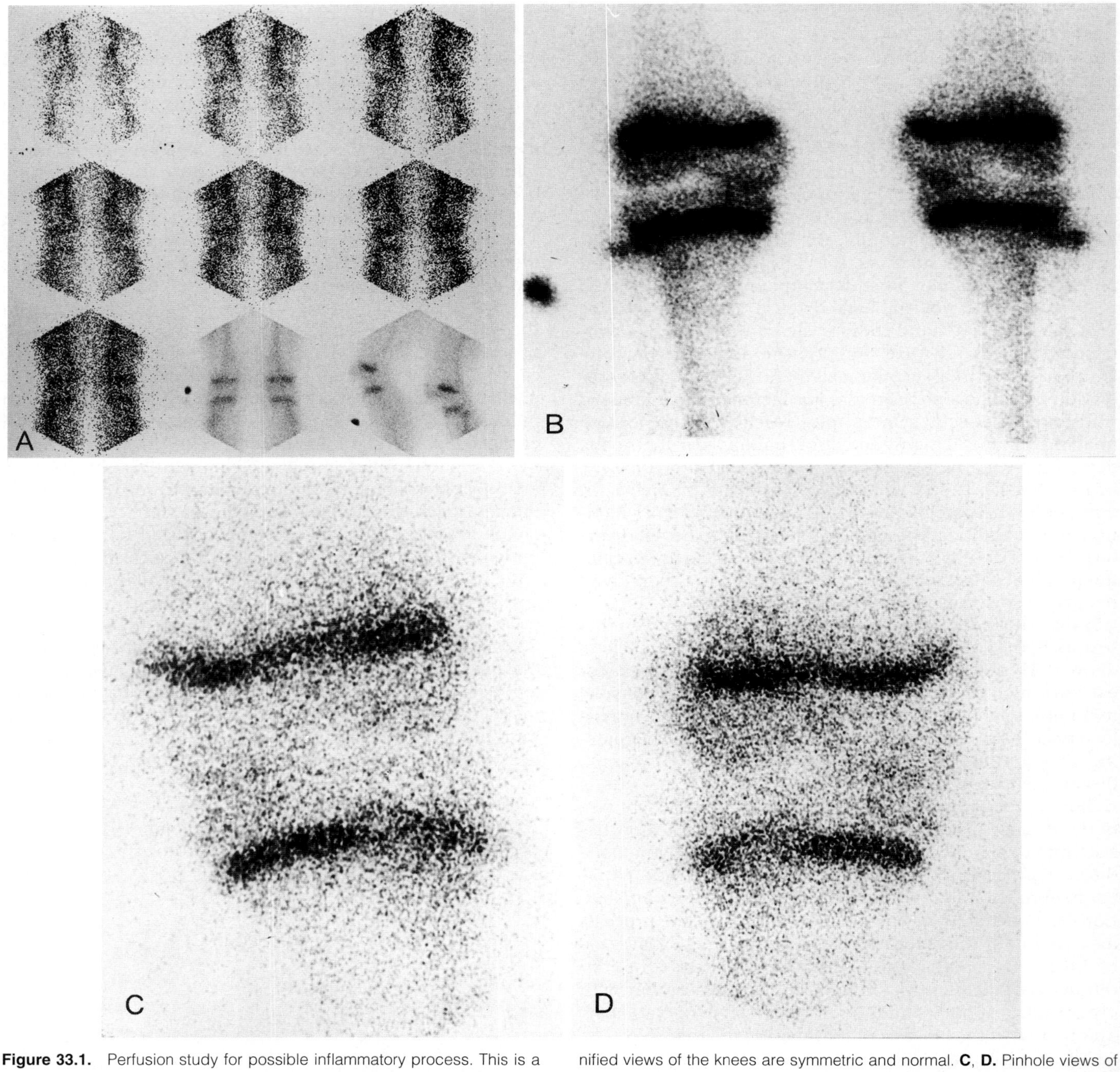

Figure 33.1. Perfusion study for possible inflammatory process. This is a normal three-phase study in a 10-year-old male who was being evaluated for possible osteomyelitis of the right knee. He had fever and complaints of pain in the right knee for 4 days. Radiographs were normal. **A.** Perfusion and immediate soft tissue views show no abnormal changes. **B.** Delayed magnified views of the knees are symmetric and normal. **C**, **D.** Pinhole views of the knees are also normal. The lack of perfusion change indicates that no infectious or inflammatory process is taking place in this child's leg. Detailed views, such as these, and multiple projections must be performed if the bone scan is to be properly utilized.

One must always remember such decision trees are guidelines only. They will change as advances in imaging and diagnostic techniques occur. Furthermore, they must be adapted to each institution, recognizing differences in available equipment, imaging times, and personnel availability.

INFECTION

Radionuclide skeletal imaging plays an important role in the workup of patients suspected of having acute osteomyelitis. As with most osseous lesions, bone imaging is frequently positive in acute osteomyelitis while standard radiographic images are still negative or equivocal. In infectious disease, in particular, radiographs tend to demonstrate osseous abnormalities late in the course of the disease. Abnormal bone scans occur early in the process and allow early institution of therapy. If the diagnosis of infection is in doubt, the imaging procedure may point to the area to be considered for biopsy and subsequent microbiologic studies. Satisfactory results are obtained only when the nuclear medicine physician is willing to pay great attention to technique. This includes the willingness to tailor the study to the particular patient problem, the use of multiple projections and magnification views to adequately assess questionable areas, especially in the young, and the use of SPECT to provide an alternative approach to obtaining maximum information from imaging studies in such patients.

Table 33.2.
Diffuse Search.

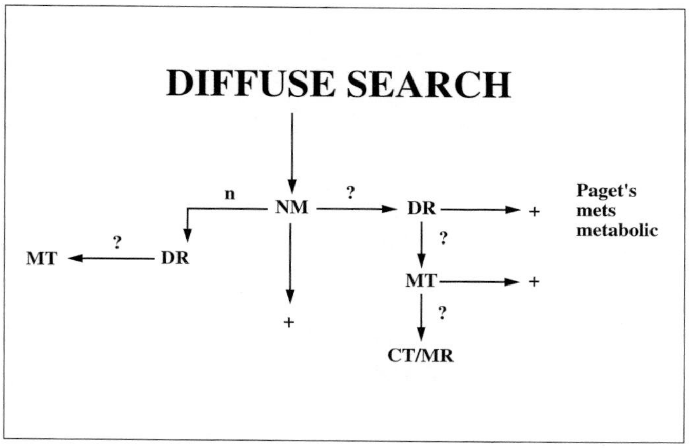

In most laboratories, the standard approach to the question of osteomyelitis is to perform the three-phase bone imaging procedure to examine perfusion, immediate soft tissue blood pool, and bone uptake as reflected in the 2–4 hour delay images. It must be remembered that virtually any pathologic condition affecting bone will result in increased perfusion in that area. The main advantage of performing the perfusion study in such cases is that a normal perfusion pattern in an extremity or other area of bone usually excludes the presence of an acute inflammatory process (Fig. 33.1). Increased soft tissue activity in the initial imaging phase is seen with cellulitis. Clearing of this activity to normal or slightly increased activity levels in the same areas on the delayed images is the usual pattern when cellulitis alone is present. When soft tissue inflammation and infection are present together, the resulting increased perfusion to an affected limb will cause increased activity in that limb (Fig. 33.2). When soft tissue infection alone is present, no focal abnormally increased areas of activity are present in the bone but diffuse increase in the osseous structures may be observed. Osteomyelitis is usu-

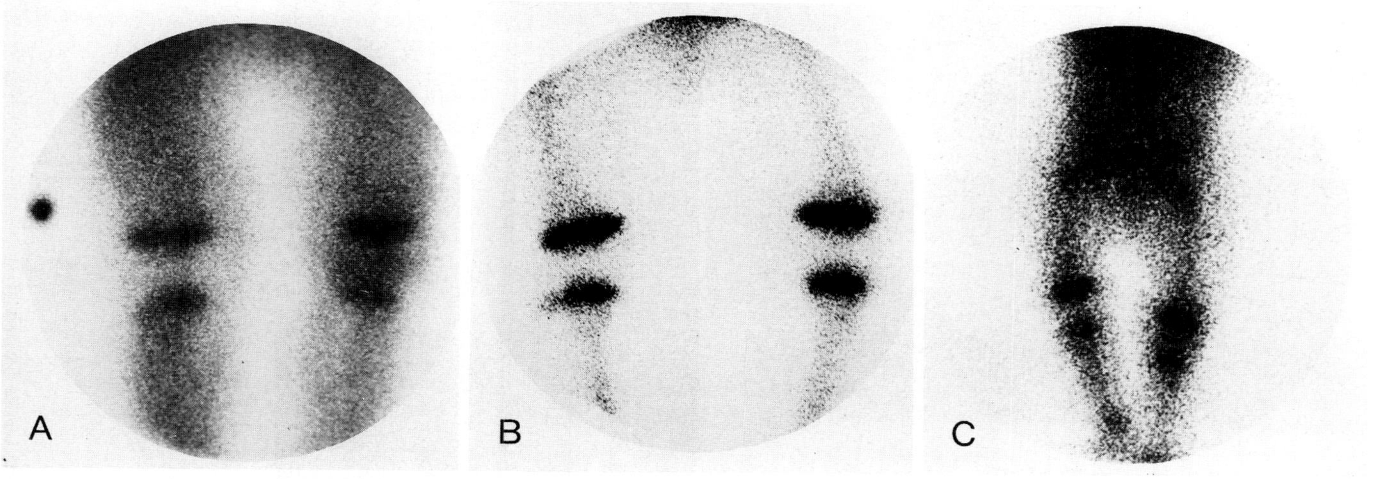

Figure 33.2. Soft tissue infection. Bone scan images of a 6-year-old boy with fever for 3 days and complaints of pain and swelling in the left knee for 2 days prior to the study. There is increased perfusion to the left leg and knee. **A.** Immediate soft tissue views show increased soft tissue activity in and about the knee joint. **B.** The 2-hour delayed views of the knees demonstrate no focal changes of increased activity in the bones of the joint. At this time, the findings were considered to be consistent with cellulitis or septic arthritis of the knee rather than osteomyelitis. **C.** A 24-hour gallium study shows diffusely increased activity about the soft tissues of the joint with no abnormal osseous localization. Culture of the joint aspirate revealed Staphylococcus aureus.

ally demonstrated as an area of focally increased activity on the routine delayed images (Fig. 33.3). At times, a further delay past the usual 2–4 hour interval for delayed static imaging will accentuate the difference between focal areas of increased activity and diffuse activity seen as a result of increased perfusion. These (4th and 5th phase) studies are usually performed at 6–8 hours postinjection and 24 hours postinjection (Fig. 33.4). When utilized in this fashion, the routine skeletal imaging procedure exhibits both high sensitivity and high specificity in the workup of osteomyelitis (1). In most situations, the sensitivity of bone scintigraphy for the detection of osteomyelitis approaches 90% with a likewise high specificity and overall accuracy. Despite this, diagnostic radiography is the initial procedure of choice in cases in which osteomyelitis is suspected. Radiographs are inexpensive, rapid to perform, and do not submit the patient to a total-body radiation dose. When the radiograph is negative or equivocal in the face of significant clinical suspicion, radionuclide imaging is indicated.

It must be recognized that routine bone imaging will not be positive in all cases of osteomyelitis. Difficulty may be encountered at both ends of the age spectrum. Some regard the use of routine skeletal scintigraphy in neonates as futile, while others report results similar to that stated earlier (2–5). Again, difficulty in diagnosis may be met at the other end of the age spectrum, with the elderly, especially those with peripheral vascular disease such as seen in diabetics. In these patients, the poor blood flow may make abnormal findings at best equivocal, particularly when superimposed upon degenerative diseases in the joints or other underlying bone conditions, such as Charcot-type joints in the foot of diabetic patients (Fig. 33.5).

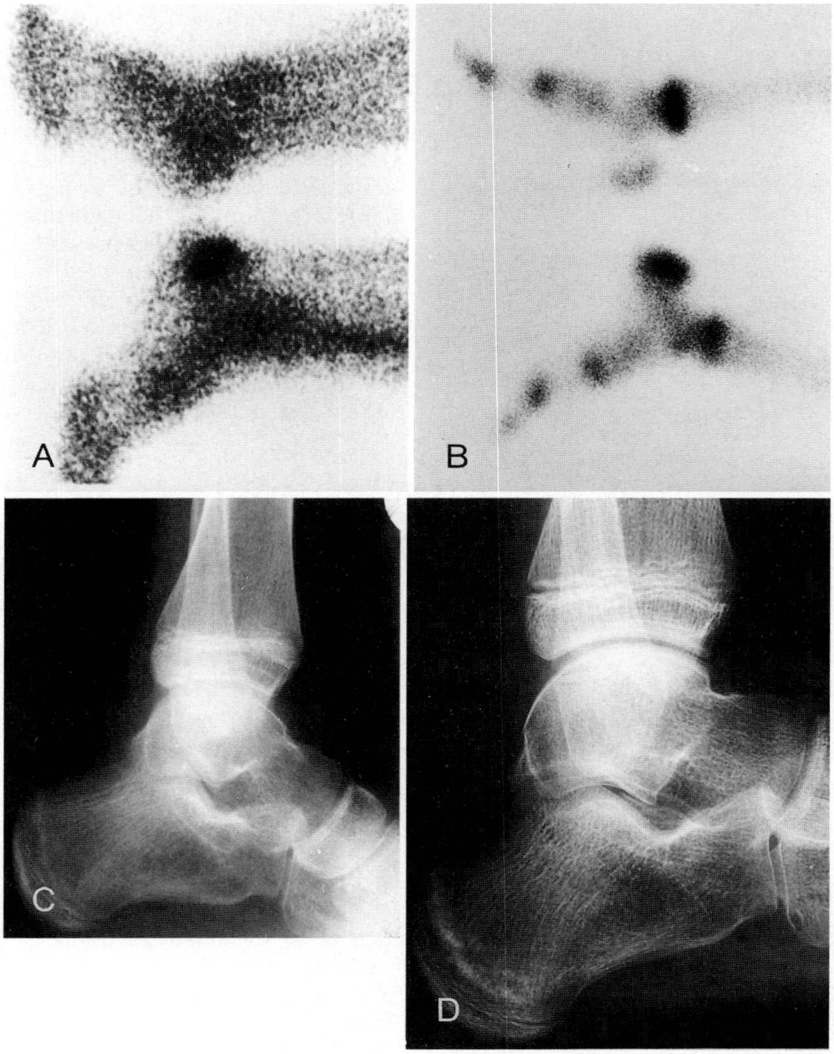

Figure 33.3. Osteomyelitis. This patient is an 11-year-old male with hypogammaglobinemia who had developed a painful foot and ankle over a period of 3 days. Increased perfusion to the ankle is seen. **A.** The immediate soft tissue portion of the study demonstrates focal increased activity at the left os calcis. **B.** Delayed views of the feet reveal focal increased activity in this bone. This was believed to represent osteomyelitis, and Klebsiella aerobacter was found at biopsy. The initial radiograph (**C**) was interpreted as normal, whereas a magnified view obtained 10 days after the bone imaging study (**D**) demonstrates radiographic evidence of osteomyelitis.

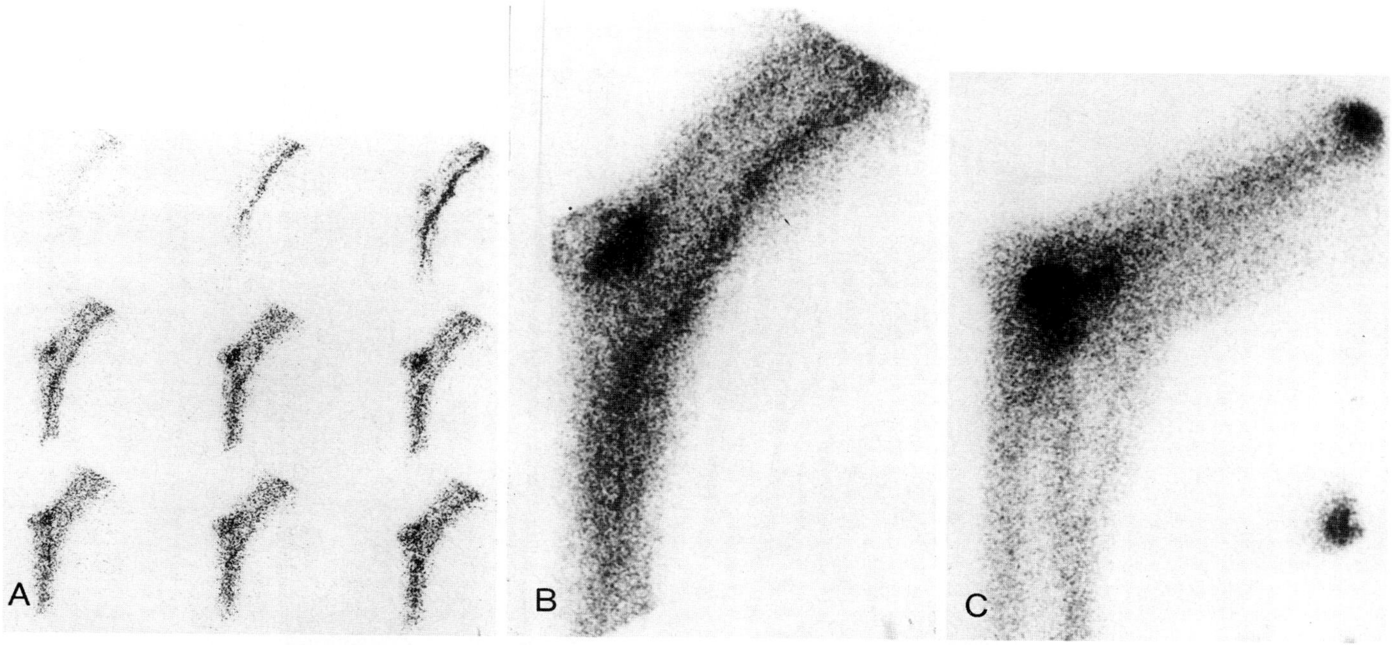

Figure 33.4. Osteomyelitis cellulitis. A 47-year-old male who presented with a 2-day history of fever and left elbow swelling and pain without trauma. Radiographs were normal. **A.** Perfusion phase showing increased perfusion to the elbow including the bursa. **B.** Blood pool phase demonstrates increased activity in the bursae indicating olecranon bursitis. **C.** Six-hour delayed view shows clearing of the bursal soft tissue activity with focal increase in the olecranon. Staphylococcus aureus was cultured from a needle biopsy of the olecranon.

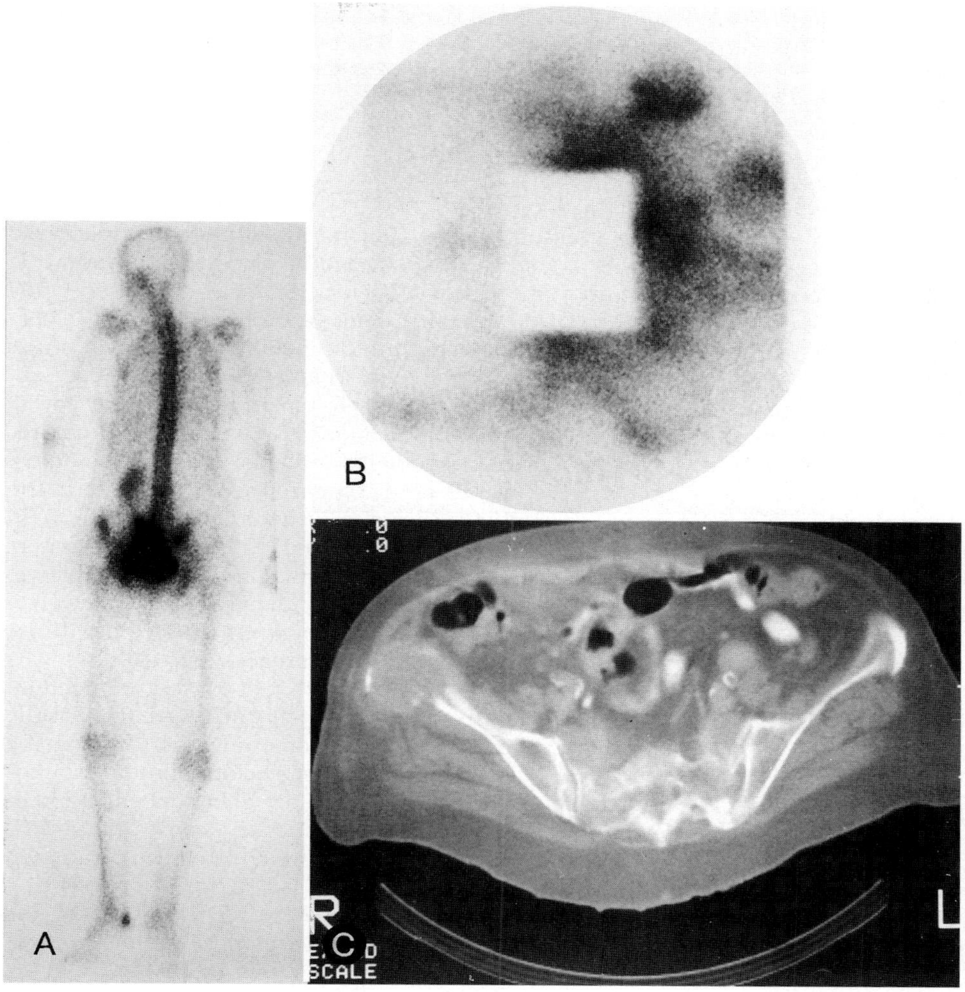

Figure 33.5. Metastases resembling osteomyelitis pattern. Radiographs were normal in a 63-year-old female diabetic with pain in the left heel for 1-week's duration. On the bone imaging study there was increased perfusion and soft tissue activity in the os calcis. More importantly, the posterior total body image (**A**) revealed multiple lesions in the spine, pelvis (**B**), and femur, more compatible with metastatic process. Note also the absent right kidney, which, upon further investigation, turned out to have been removed 15 years before. The pelvic lesions were confirmed on computed tomography (**C**). Needle biopsy of the iliac wing and left os calcis revealed metastatic renal cell carcinoma.

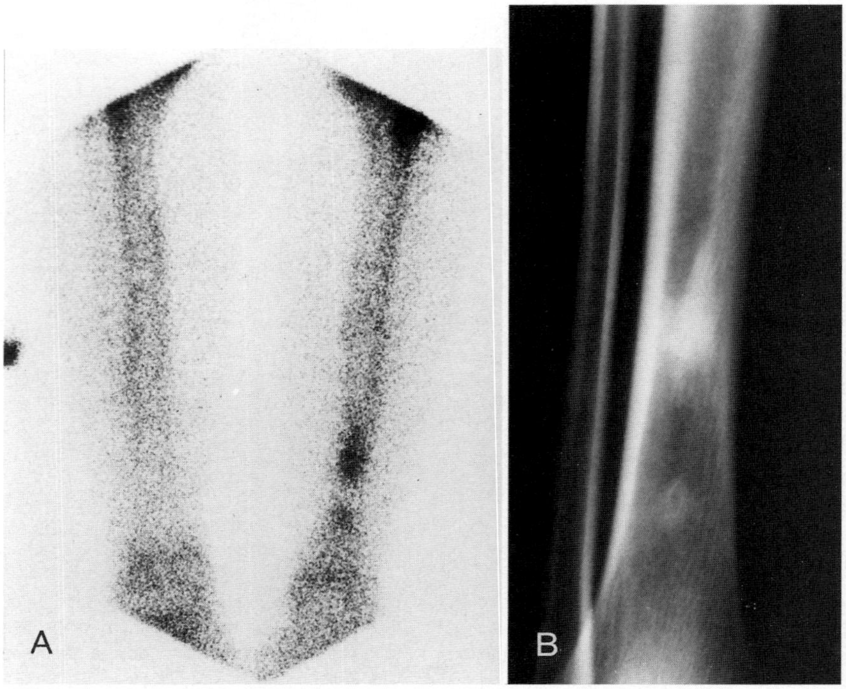

Figure 33.6. Chronic osteomyelitis. A 16-year-old female athlete had complained of pain in the left lower leg 4 months prior to examination. Radiographs at that time revealed a poorly defined density believed to represent stress fracture. The patient was placed at rest for 6 weeks with some relief of pain. Upon resuming activity, the pain returned and increased. There was no radiographic change and the patient was placed in a cast for 4 weeks. Upon removal of the cast, the pain immediately returned and the bone imaging study was ordered. The perfusion study was normal. **A.** Delayed view of the leg revealed two sites of low-grade abnormally increased activity in the tibia. This was considered to be more consistent with a chronic osteomyelitis rather than fracture. **B.** Radiographic tomography confirmed the presence of these two lesions. Biopsy revealed changes consistent with chronic, indolent osteomyelitis. This condition may be difficult to diagnose with routine bone imaging or secondary studies such as ^{67}Ga-citrate or ^{111}In-labeled leukocytes.

Frequently, osteomyelitis in such patients may not be acute but of a chronic nature, which results in a rather poor uptake of the bone-seeking radiopharmaceutical, even in the young (Fig. 33.6). In some instances, especially in the pediatric age group, the early increased pressure involving the marrow space may result in decreased radionuclide accumulation and the appearance of a photon deficient lesion at the site of infection. This is usually seen very early in the disease process. Serial studies with routine bone imaging agents or with secondary agents such as ^{67}Ga-citrate or radiolabeled leukocytes may help achieve the diagnosis (6–9) (Fig. 33.7). Multifocal abnormal sites may be seen when osteomyelitis is caused by organisms such as Salmonella typhi, or they may be the result of viral infection (10) (Fig. 33.8). Finally, the addition of intervening antibiotic therapeutic regimens, whether complete or incomplete, may result in lessened activity patterns in patients being studied for osteomyelitis by standard bone imaging.

OTHER RADIOPHARMACEUTICALS

^{67}Ga-citrate has been used to study both acute and chronic osteomyelitis especially as backup in cases where osteomyelitis is under clinical suspicion and routine bone scans/radiographs are normal or equivocal. Early imaging at 24 hours may demonstrate abnormally increased activity at the site of suspected involvement. However it is still important to do a delay for a 48-hour image, especially in the axial skeleton and before reporting the study as normal. Nonetheless, one must remember that a ^{67}Ga study will show increased activity in areas of increased bone remodeling such as fractures, postsurgery, neuropathic changes, arthritis, and pseudoarthrosis. One method proposed to increase sensitivity and specificity for the detection of osteomyelitis is to compare the ^{67}Ga uptake in the suspect lesion with that of routine bone scan (Fig. 33.9). The mismatch of greater increased ^{67}Ga uptake versus normal or increased routine bone imagining agent activity is an important finding that does indicate infectious involvement, especially if bone has not been interfered with by prior trauma, surgery, or other process (11, 12).

^{111}In-WBC has been utilized to study bone infection. Multiple studies indicated sensitivity and specificity in the high 80% to low 90% range. Some authors feel that the ^{111}In-WBC scan will be abnormal before standard radionuclide bone imaging and show a higher concentration in experimental joint inflammation than does ^{67}Ga (13–17). However, chronic infection and prior antibiotic therapy will reduce sensitivity (18).

Recently, several techniques for labeling leukocytes with ^{99m}Tc have been proposed: The most common proce-

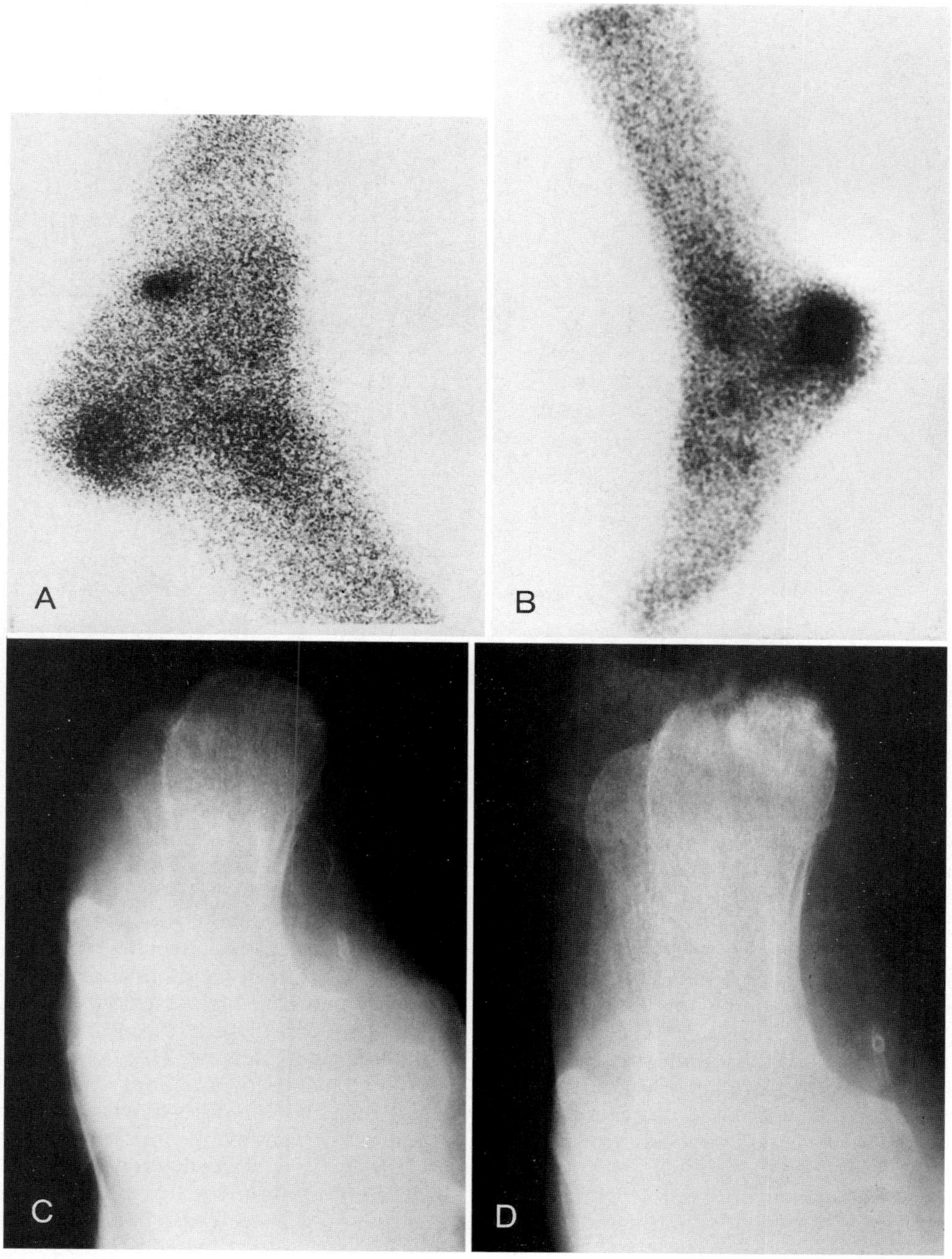

Figure 33.7. Serial study of osteomyelitis. A 27-year-old drug addict complained of pain in her right heel for 2 days. At initial study, perfusion was slightly increased to this area. **A.** The delayed images revealed faint but definite abnormal increase in the os calcis and in the cuneiform bone. **B.** A repeat study 3 days later shows marked increased activity in the os calcis, confirming the impression of osteomyelitis. **C.** The initial radiograph was interpreted as normal. **D.** A radiograph obtained 12 days later revealed marked destruction of the os calcis.

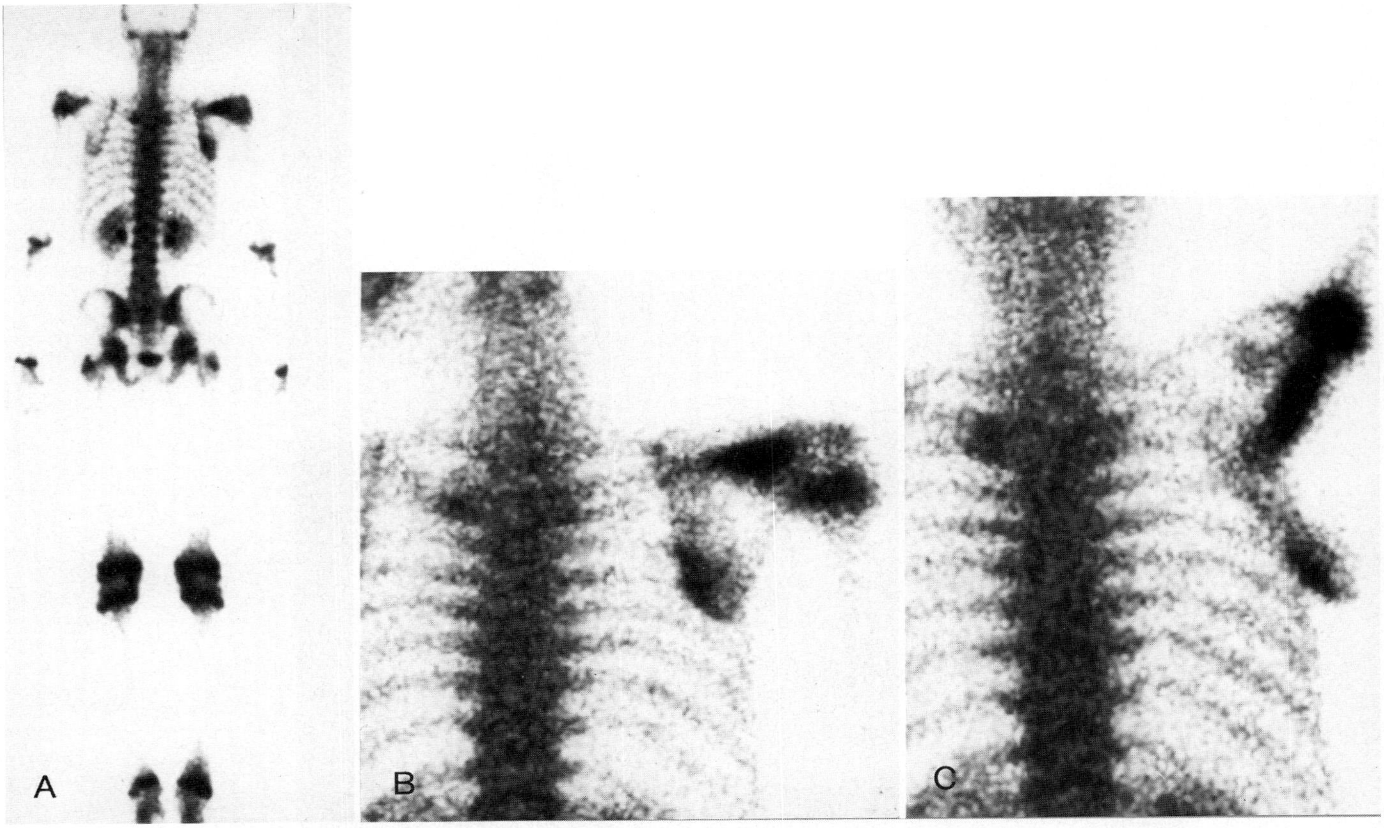

Figure 33.8. Multifocal osteomyelitis. This patient is an 11-year-old boy who developed upper back, shoulder, and ankle pain during a viral pulmonary infection. **A.** Posterior total body view demonstrating abnormally increased activity in the right distal tibia, right scapula, and third left costovertebral junction. **B, C.** Spot views of the posterior chest with the arms neutral and elevated confirm the abnormal sites in the left third rib and right scapula.

dure at present is to label the leukocytes with ^{99m}Tc-HMPAO-labeled-WBCs. The sensitivity and specificity for ^{99m}Tc-WBC is similar to ^{111}In-WBC. It is to be expected that both would have similar false-positive and false-negative results since both procedures use leukocytes to carry the radionuclide to the site of infection. Nonetheless, ^{99m}Tc-WBC offers advantages. The higher dose administered allows for superior technical imagining including SPECT. Additionally, the possibility of labeling leukocytes with ^{99m}Tc-HMPAO is more prevalent than that with ^{111}In. Virtually all hospitals have technetium generators available on a routine basis, whereas ^{111}In must be ordered for a specific patient study. However, it must be remembered that both ^{111}In and ^{99m}Tc-WBC's suffer the drawback of requiring extensive cell separation and cell labeling techniques. The procedure may take up to 2 hours and it must be ensured that the white cells are separated with considerable skill to avoid cell damage and red cell labeling, especially with the ^{99m}Tc-WBC technique. Newer kits are online which may allow more rapid labeling.

It must also be remembered that labeled leukocytes are not totally specific for acute infection. It must be recognized that both sensitivity and specificity are reduced in the face of chronic infection, the presence of soft tissue sepsis (Fig. 33.10), especially adjacent to bones, the presence of prior conditions such as fractures and tumors that will localize leukocytes to a certain extent, and by prior treatment with antibiotics and/or steroids. Nonetheless, labeled leukocyte imaging plays a strong role as either a primary or secondary skeletal imaging agent in infectious disease (19–20).

Early results using radiolabeled antibodies offer some promise in the study of infected bone. The first reports concern technetium- or iodine-labeled antigranulocyte antibodies which have high sensitivity and specificity reported (21–23). Unfortunately, these are produced from mouse antibodies and adverse HAMA reactions have been reported. Recently, ^{111}In- and ^{99m}Tc-labeled human polyconal immunoglobulin-g have been introduced (24–26). Again, early results appear promising with high sensitivity and specificity. As this class of agents is a human antibody, it does not produce the human antimouse antibody reaction that may be seen with the antigranulocyte antibodies. This group of agents remains of considerable interest and promise depending on the outcome of ongoing studies.

OTHER MODALITIES

CT can be a valuable tool in the attempt to diagnose osteomyelitis. CT with bone windows gives excellent images of the bony cortex. It may well be used in many cases to determine extent of bone infection and to guide biopsy for specimen retrieval and study.

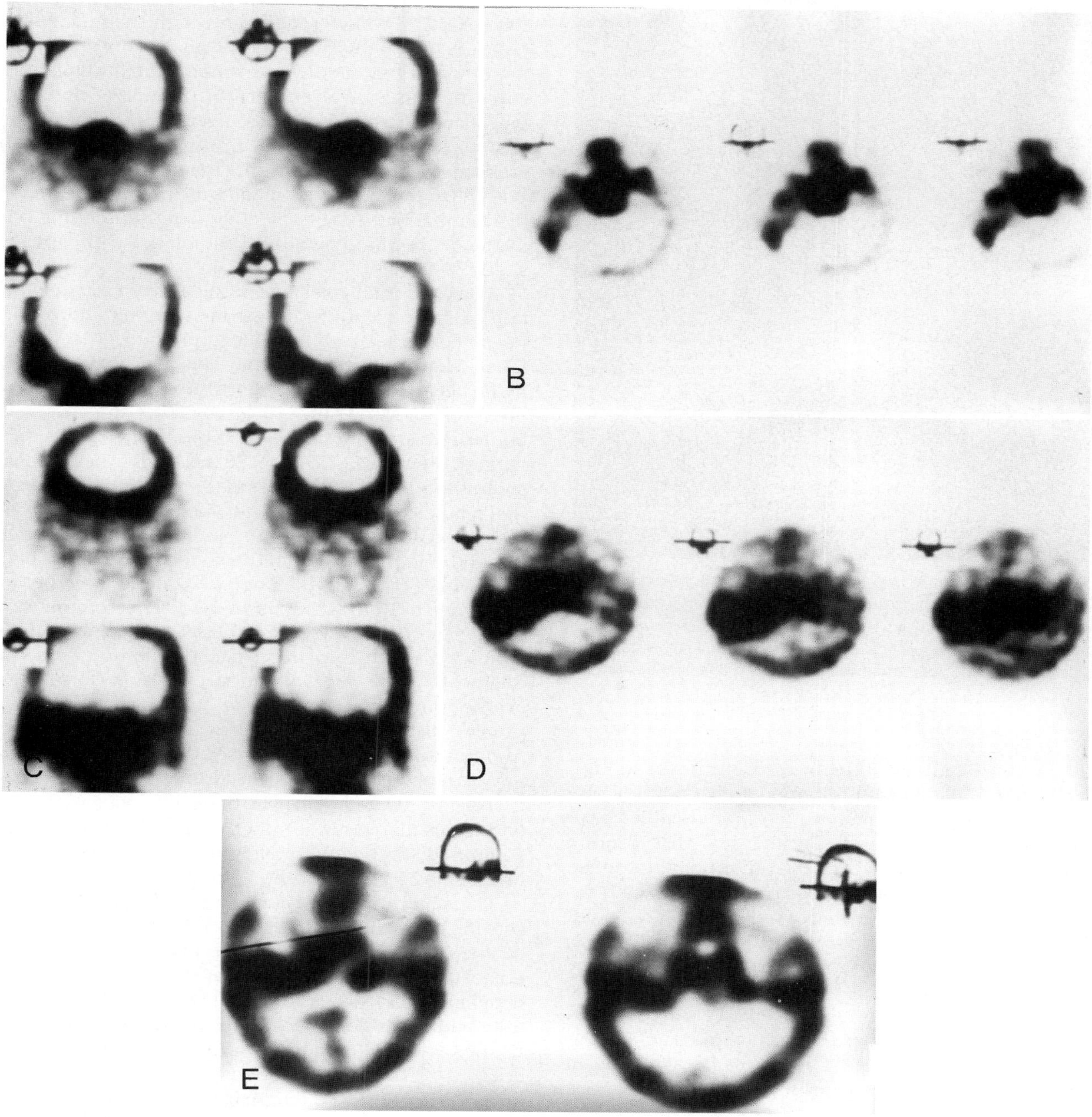

Figure 33.9. Malignant otitis externa. Patient is a 57-year-old male with a history of prior drainage procedure for mastoiditis 2 1/2 years before. He now presents with headache, hearing loss, and fever for 1 week. Routine bone imaging demonstrates abnormal increase in temporal mastoid bones on coronal and axial SPECT (**A**, **B**). ^{67}Ga-citrate study 48 hours later shows marked increase and greater area of involvement (**C**, **D**). Repeat ^{67}Ga study after 7 weeks of antibiotic therapy shows marked improvement, but is still abnormal (**E**).

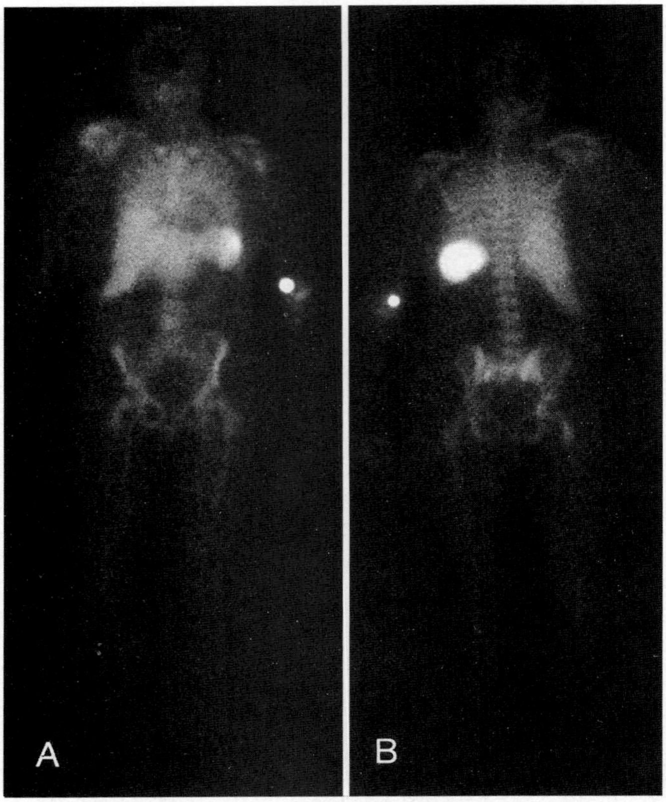

Figure 33.10. Septic arthritis. (**A**) Anterior and (**B**) posterior views in a 56-year-old female on hemodialysis with a documented infection in the right arm (note marked swelling) and septicemia. The ^{99m}Tc-WBC study shows abnormal activity in the right shoulder joint but not in the bones. No other abnormal areas are seen. Klebsiella aer. was cultured by needle aspiration from the joint.

MRI has the advantage of the best resolution of soft tissue involvement, as opposed to bone involvement, of any of the current radiographic techniques. Many studies have indicated that sensitivity and specificity of MRI is quite high and may even exceed that of radionuclide studies. However, we must remember that any process which replaces bone marrow or causes increased tissue water, such as healing fractures, metabolic conditions, and tumors, may resemble osteomyelitis. Finally, artifacts produced by orthopedic insertion of prosthetic devices may degrade the images and reduce the diagnostic accuracy. Also, MRI is considerably more expensive than the radionuclide approach, and time on MRI units may not be available to study the patient in an emergency setting.

IMAGING STRATEGIES

The plethora of radionuclide and radiologic imaging techniques simply demonstrates that, except in very simple cases of acute peripheral osteomyelitis, the diagnosis of bone infection may be difficult to achieve without surgical intervention that may include bone biopsy, joint aspiration, and the like. Nonetheless, protocols have been developed which may assist in the more complex cases of bone infection either directly or through pattern recognition. Following are descriptions of some that are currently in use in the author's institution.

Evaluation of the diabetic foot remains a vexing problem (27). Osteomyelitis may be the result of direct extension of a chronic soft tissue infection in these patients. In our laboratory, we have obtained our best results using combined ^{67}Ga and ^{99m}Tc-MDP studies in which the mismatch of increased ^{67}Ga activity versus normal or increased routine bone imagining agent is an important finding that indicates infectious involvement (28). (It must be noted that the use of combined radionuclide agent approaches raises our cost to the point that the argument concerning the increased expense of CT or MRI imaging is no longer valid.) With ^{67}Ga or leukocyte imaging it may not be possible to distinguish soft tissue infection from underlying bone infection without a good quality radiolabeled phosphate bone scan (29, 30).

Axial, especially vertebral, infections may also be difficult to diagnose on routine bone imaging and require the use of combined radionuclide approaches (31, 32). Radiolabeled leukocyte imaging may give poor results when used alone because it normally distributes in marrow as well as areas of infection. Indeed, 10–30% of infected vertebral bodies may demonstrate as a photon deficient lesion on the leukocyte scan (33–35) (Fig. 33.11). It may be best to utilize a combination of leukocyte imaging with an agent such as ^{99m}Tc-labeled nanocolloid for demonstration of normal marrow distribution and any interruption in this pattern (36, 37). When this technique is used, one must, of course use ^{111}In-WBC if dual isotope imaging is to be performed, otherwise a 2-day study is needed. The demonstration of incongruent leukocyte and colloid images with increased leukocyte activity and decreased colloid uptake is virtually diagnostic. Our general practice is to perform an initial evaluation with MRI and then, if necessary, utilize radionuclide techniques for the detection of vertebral infection. Another approach for demonstrating incongruous marrow and leukocyte activity is to double-label leukocytes with ^{99m}Tc-HMPAO and ^{111}In. The bone marrow may be detected on images at 1-hour obtained on the ^{99m}Tc photopeak and compared (both qualitatively and quantitatively) against images at 24 hours on the ^{111}In photopeak.

The separation of septic arthritis from osteomyelitis by routine bone skeletal imaging alone may present a difficult problem (38). In most cases of septic arthritis, diffusely increased activity in the bones of the joint may be seen on delayed images, while the perfusion in early soft tissue uptake and early blood pool images may be limited to the soft tissues only (Fig. 33.10). If a focal area of abnormally increased ^{99m}Tc-phosphate activity is not seen in the bones around the joint, the diagnosis of osteomyelitis cannot be established. Here, again, ^{67}Ga-citrate imaging or, more commonly, radiolabeled white blood cell imaging may be quite helpful. In septic arthritis, these agents demonstrate activity patterns of a diffuse nature in the soft tissue in and about the joint with no focal abnormality in the bone. However, this may be very difficult to ascertain without a demonstration of exactly where the bone lies in relation to the soft tissue infection and may require a combined imaging, such as ^{99m}Tc-MDP/^{111}In-WBC imaging. The ^{111}In-WBC/^{99m}-MDP combined study is more specific than the ^{67}Ga/

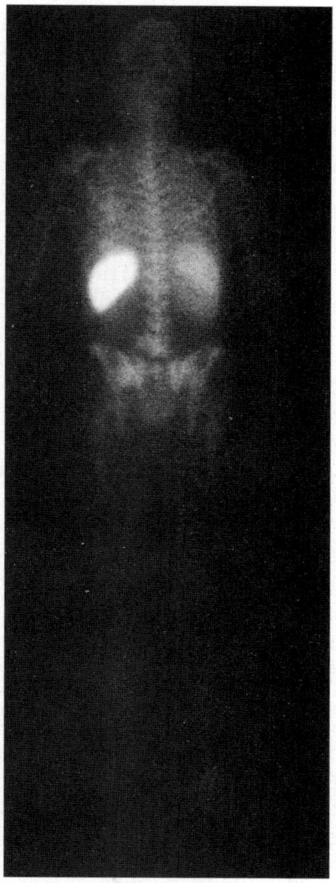

Figure 33.11. Photon deficient lesion. This is a 48-year-old HIV positive female who presents with a 1-week history of low back pain. Standard radiographs of the spine are normal. The posterior ^{99m}Tc-WBC study demonstrates abnormal activity in the left lung pneumonia seen on chest x-ray and a photon deficient area on the left at L5-S1. CT guided needle biopsy recovered purulent material which cultured staph aureus.

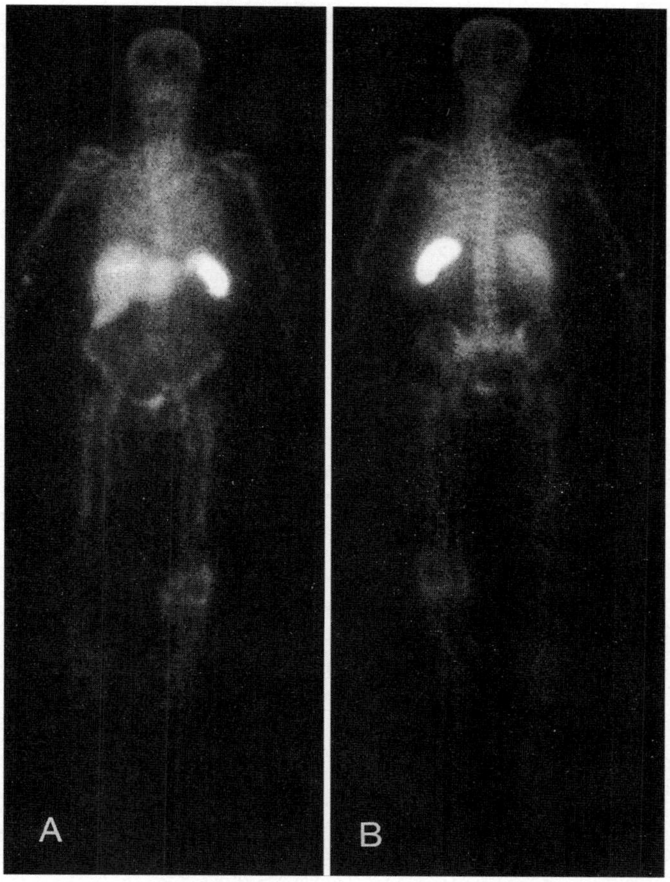

Figure 33.12. Infected prosthesis. ^{99m}Tc-WBC scan in an 81-year-old woman with a history of bilateral total knee replacements 6 years before and increasing left knee pain. Radiographs were not helpful. The ^{99m}Tc-WBC study demonstrates abnormal accumulations across the bone and prosthesis on the left and in adjacent soft tissue (**A**, anterior; **B**, posterior). An infected prosthesis was removed at surgery.

^{99}Tc-MDP method and produces fewer equivocal results. One must remember that although the ^{111}In-WBC/^{99m}-MDP combination will decrease the number of false-positive studies, abnormal findings still may be seen in patients with neuropathic joint disease, rheumatoid arthritis, gout, and even metastatic disease. Finally, even with such combined efforts differentiation may still be difficult. Aspiration of the joint and culture of the contents remains an advantageous and rapid tool in this diagnosis.

In the pediatric age group, especially in the neonate, we will utilize ^{99m}Tc-MDP in the 3- or 4-phase mode for whole-body imaging. Others have recommended ^{99m}Tc-WBC as the procedure of choice for the detection of osteomyelitis (39). The advent of whole-body MRI capability may prove to be the procedure of choice since it does not involve any radiation exposure of a child, although young infants may require sedation to prevent motion artifacts.

When a bone has had prior surgical insertion of a prosthesis, we usually evaluate this with ^{99m}Tc-WBC as the first step, especially when the question is one of infection versus loosening (40–41) (Fig. 33.12). The routine phosphate imaging techniques are rarely helpful in these situations as they remain abnormally increased following the surgical intervention. The newer types of prostheses may demonstrate scintigraphic appearances that are different from the older prostheses. Increased activity at the stem of a porous prosthesis may be seen as a normal change for as long as 2–3 years postsurgery. Abnormal activity from loosening is usually located along the lateral border of the tip. One must remember that some leukocyte accumulation may occur postoperatively and that this may lead to some difficulty.

At times, combined procedures such as ^{99m}Tc-MDP imaging and indium chloride or ^{111}In-DPTA arthrography may be necessary. The results of these approaches are not strikingly different from that of contrast arthrography, although the radionuclide arthrogram may give better definition of the location of the metallic prosthesis. Finally, a combined ^{111}In-WBC and ^{99m}Tc-MDP bone scan may be performed in which the leukocyte label will show relatively greater uptake in infected bone than in noninfective, reactive bone (42). A similar approach for concordant or discordant pattern formation may be performed with a labeled white cell and radiocolloid combination in which the discordant pattern is increased ^{111}In-WBC uptake greater than the radiocolloid uptake. These techniques do lead to higher specificity for the presence of infection in these complicated patterns (43).

Individuals suffering from sickle cell disease often present with acute bone pain. Although this is usually a result of infarction, it may represent osteomyelitis. This clinical dilemma may be difficult to solve on a routine basis. Early in infarction, the routine phosphate complex bone study may present as photon deficient lesion. A similar photon deficient lesion will be found with colloid marrow imaging in the early phase of infarction (44). As a result, increased activity on a routine phosphate bone imaging study performed within days, or at most a week, of the onset symptom will suggest infection. Likewise, normal colloid marrow distribution during this initial week after onset increases the likelihood of infection. However, phosphate imaging activity rapidly increases in a nonuniform fashion in infarcts as the bone tries to repair itself and the infarct is revascularized. As a result, the increased phosphate complex activity after the first week will not distinguish osteomyelitis from infarction. Therefore, at this time, interval imaging with radiolabeled white blood cells becomes an important tool to increase the sensitivity of diagnosis of infection (45).

Finally, both ^{111}In- and ^{99m}Tc-WBC's as well as ^{67}Ga-citrate may be used to assess the effects of therapy (Fig. 33.9). The pretherapy abnormally increased uptake of these agents will return to normal after definitive antibiotic therapy (46–48). ^{99m}Tc-phosphate complex uptake is not useful to monitor therapy since these will remain abnormal as a result of reparative bone formation even after definitive therapy has been completed and the infection eliminated. With the newer therapeutic administration advances, the patient no longer needs prolonged hospitalization. As a result, these procedures are much less frequently performed than a few years ago.

OSTEONECROSIS

Osteonecrosis (formally called avascular or aseptic necrosis) involves the death of both the osseous and marrow components of bone. Skeletal scintigraphy will demonstrate photon-deficient lesions early at sites of osteonecrosis well in advance of radiographic changes (49, 50). Although osteonecrosis may be detected in numerous skeletal locations, the greatest clinical experience has been gained in evaluation of lesions of the femoral head (51). In addition to idiopathic osteonecrosis (Legg-Calve-Perthes disease), interruption of blood supply to the femoral head, or other bone area, may be seen in conditions such as trauma, slipped capital femoral epiphysis, septic joint, and leukemia. Additionally, other causes may include such conditions as vasculitis, infarction (sickle cell disease, Gaucher's disease), neoplasm, alcoholism, caisson disease, lupus erythematosus, steroid therapy, and impaired circulation such as found in diabetes and frostbite. When skeletal scintigraphy is used as the primary diagnostic modality, correlation with the clinical condition is vital. Studies performed extremely early after the onset of clinical symptoms may demonstrate a photon-deficient or "cold" lesion while examinations at a later interval after onset of symptoms may demonstrate increased activity around and through the site of necrosis, the sequelae of revascularization, and/or bone remodeling. If the bone is one that contains marrow, both ^{99m}Tc-phosphate complex and ^{99m}Tc-sulfur colloid (Sc) imaging of the marrow may be used to diagnose osteonecrosis. Skeletal scintigraphy is usually preferred since many adults may not have sufficient active marrow in the bone area to be studied to provide adequate uptake of the colloidal agents. Attention to technique is vital here, as it is everywhere in skeletal scintigraphy. The study should be tailored to the individual case and should include magnification or pinhole views of the affected and contralateral site in the frog-leg position, or, preferably, SPECT images of the hip or other bones under consideration (52–55). Some investigators believe the changes noted due to steroid therapy are the result of microfracture and may not be associated with initial decreased femoral head activity. This has not been this author's experience nor that of others. Once again it is important to note the findings on skeletal scintigraphy in relationship to the onset of symptomatology. When such patients are imaged very early after the advent of pain, a photon-deficient lesion in the femoral head may be seen. However, the advancement to microfracture and revascularization is more rapid than in the usual idiopathic case.

In idiopathic osteonecrosis or Legg-Calve-Perthes disease, the earliest sign is the absence of activity most commonly seen in the superior lateral portion of the femoral head and associated with normal radiographs (56, 57). The appearance of disease may then go through stages which include early revascularization within 4 months post-onset. At this time, early radiographic changes may be seen, while the radionuclide study will demonstrate a lateral column of revascularization. The third stage after onset in uncomplicated cases is generally represented by diffuse zones of increased activity, while the last stage will show a return to normal activity with no area of activity greater than that in the epiphysis (Fig. 33.13). In severe cases, the femoral head may never return to normal activity, but as remodeling occurs increased tracer uptake may be seen for a prolonged time. MRI and CT may also be used to study osteonecrosis with somewhat higher sensitivity for femoral osteonecrosis achieved in the adult for MRI (Fig. 33.14). With pediatric cases the relationship is similar, with MRI offering the advantage in the child of having no radiation exposure despite having greater expense (58).

Spontaneous osteonecrosis is an idiopathic disorder of knee that occurs in elderly patients with a rapid onset of pain. While it usually involves the medial femoral condyle, multifocal involvement may be seen. Abnormally increased ^{99m}Tc-phosphate activity will precede radiographic abnormality. This condition may be related to nontraumatic osteonecrosis of underlying conditions as described earlier. This disorder, and a similar rare disorder, regional migratory osteoporosis, may involve multiple sites, most commonly the medial lateral femoral condyle, the femoral or humeral head, and the talus.

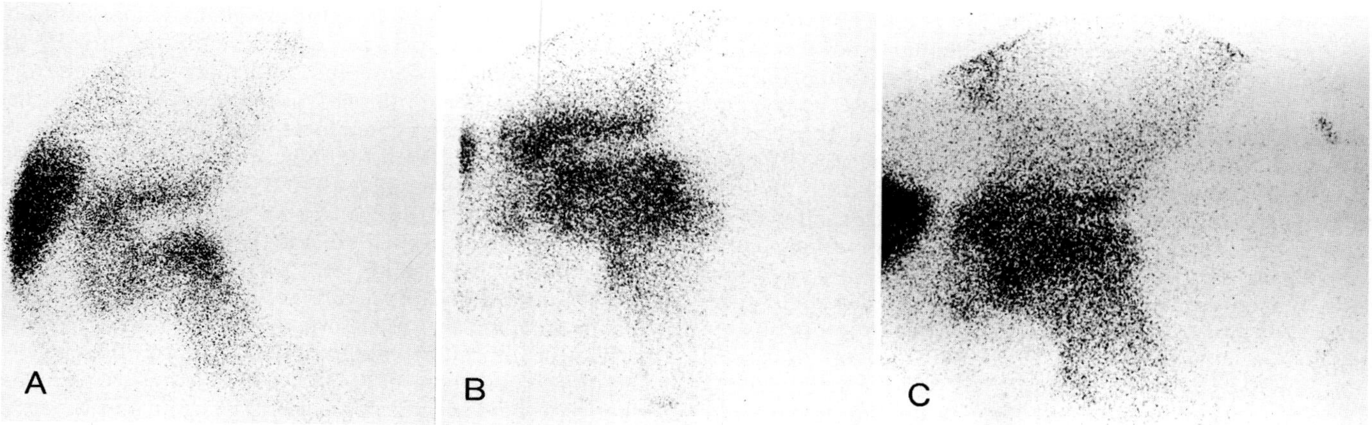

Figure 33.13. Legg-Calve-Perthes disease. Pinhole views of a 9-year-old male with Legg-Calve-Perthes disease of the left hip. **A.** This study was obtained 2 weeks after the onset of pain in this child's hip and demonstrates lack of activity in the superior lateral portion of the femoral head. **B.** This study was obtained 10 months after the initial study and shows base filling. **C.** Images obtained 26 months following onset of symptoms shows revascularization and remodeling of the femoral head. This is the common pattern seen in the disease process.

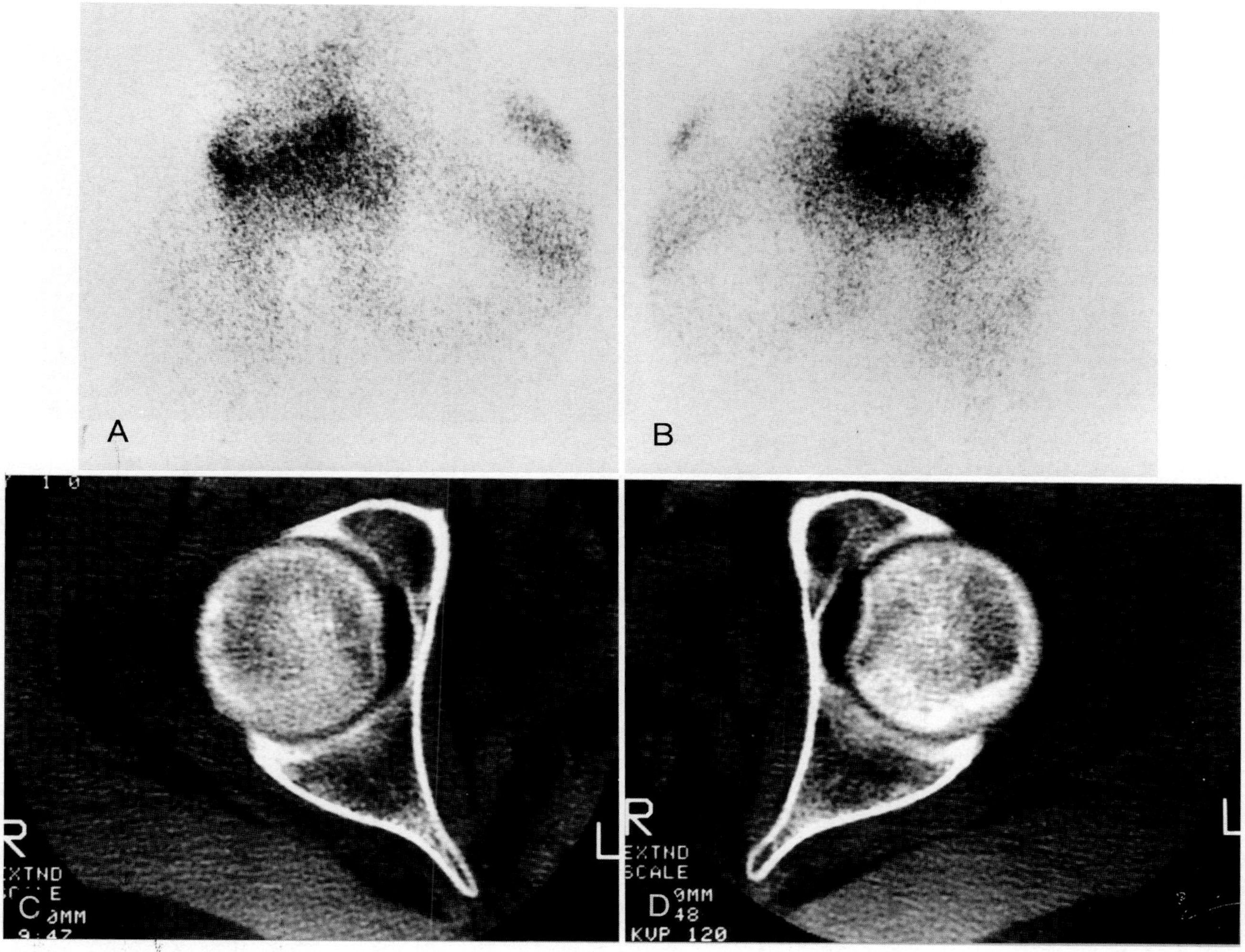

Figure 33.14. Avascular necrosis. Avascular necrosis with steroid-therapy in a 36-year-old male with chronic renal disease, renal transplantation, and long-standing steroid therapy who developed pain in both hips beginning 2 months before study. **A**. Pinhole collimator views of the right hip demonstrate a mixed pattern with photon-deficient activity and increased activity along the base of the femoral head. **B**. Similar views show generalized increased activity about the left femoral head. Similar findings are demonstrated on computed tomographic studies of the right hip joint (**C**) and left femoral head (**D**).

Osteochondritidities will include ischemic necrosis and repair of many bones including the medial femoral condyle (osteochondritis dessecans), the talus, the humerus, the carpal and tarsal navicular bones, the lunate bones, the tibial tubercle, and the heads of the second and third metatarsals. Although skeletal radiographs frequently will have diagnostic findings evident at the time of clinical presentation, skeletal scintigraphy may show increased activity prior to the appearance of the radiographic abnormality (59). These entities almost invariably present as a focus of increased activity even when imaged early after onset of symptoms when one might expect focal photopenic defects.

Unfortunately bone imaging has not been shown to be an accurate indicator of complete healing in patients with osteonecrosis (60). Studies of resolving femoral neck fractures indicate that imaging may provide a means for discriminating between those individuals who heal normally and those who will have avascular aseptic necrotic complications and require prosthetic insertion (Fig. 33.15). The findings on skeletal imaging are again dependent upon when the study is performed after initiating insult, the quality of repair mechanisms, and morphologic changes present in the bone or joint. Traumatic osteonecrosis may be occasionally found when located next to a fracture, and may prove to be difficult to image completely without specialized techniques such as SPECT imaging, as the activity related to healing at the fracture site may obscure adjacent findings in planar projections (39, 61, 62).

In patients with sickle cell anemia as the underlying cause of infarction, it is again important to relate the time of bone imaging to the chronology of the clinical events. Early after infarction, one may find a photon deficient lesion on the bone scan (Fig. 33.16). (Bone marrow imaging will give a similar finding if the insult occurs in a part of the skeleton containing marrow.) Later, as the bone repairs itself, increased activity will be found. Since osteomyelitis may be a frequent complication at these sites, radiolabeled leukocyte imaging may also be necessary to distinguish between the two entities (Fig. 33.17). MRI of symptomatic ar-

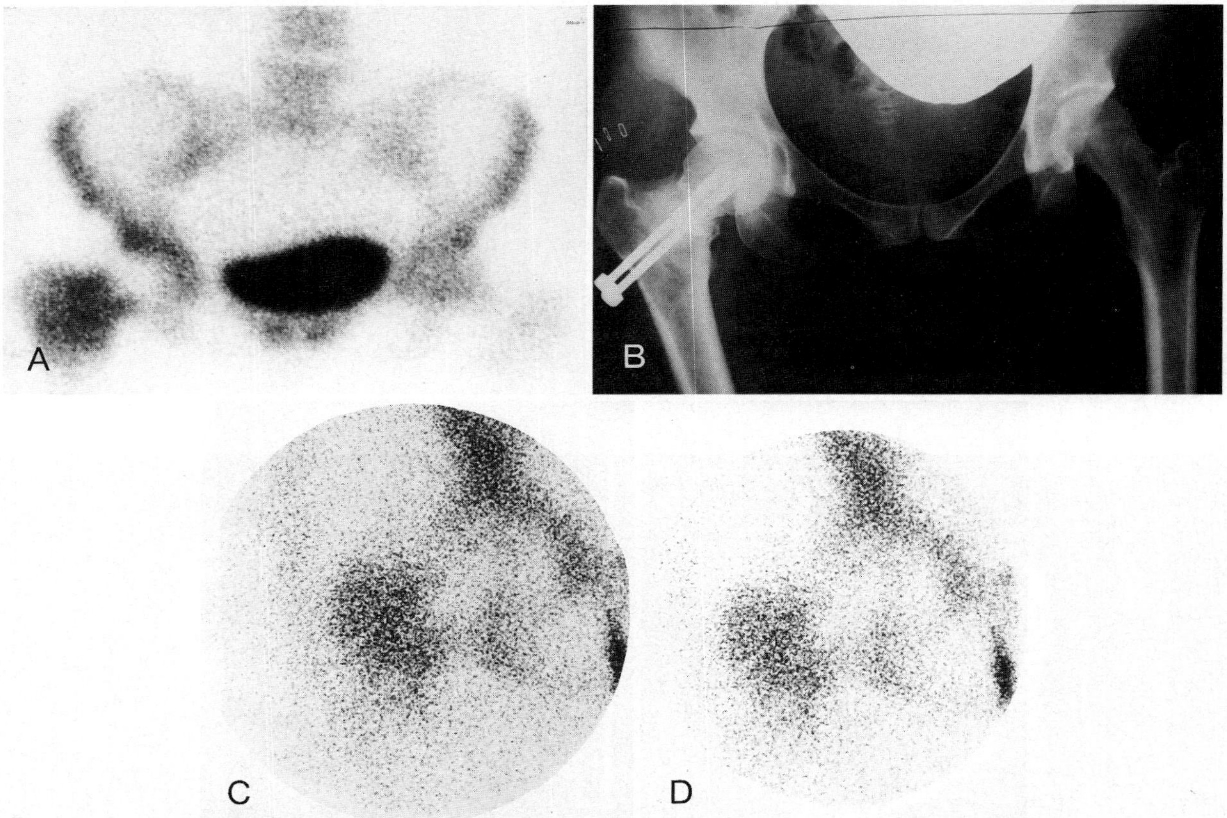

Figure 33.15. Fracture of femoral neck. **A.** Anterior view of the pelvis obtained in a 22-year-old female approximately 7 hours following fracture of the femoral neck in a car accident. The photopenic area in the head is a sign of interruption of the vascular supply to the femoral head. Although such photon-deficient areas may also be seen with the pressure effect of intracapsular hemorrhage, infection, and the like, it is important to alert the surgeon so that he or she may better plan the operative repair. **B.** Frontal radiographs of the pelvis, 1 week later, demonstrating hip pinning. A pedicle flap graft was performed in an attempt to restore vascularity to the femoral head in this patient. **C.** Pinhole magnification views of the right hip, taken at the time of the radiograph in **B**, demonstrate some activity in the superior lateral portion that is presumed to be in the flap and not in the femoral head. **D.** Unfortunately, repeat views 2 months later again revealed a nonviable femoral head. At this time, a prosthesis was installed.

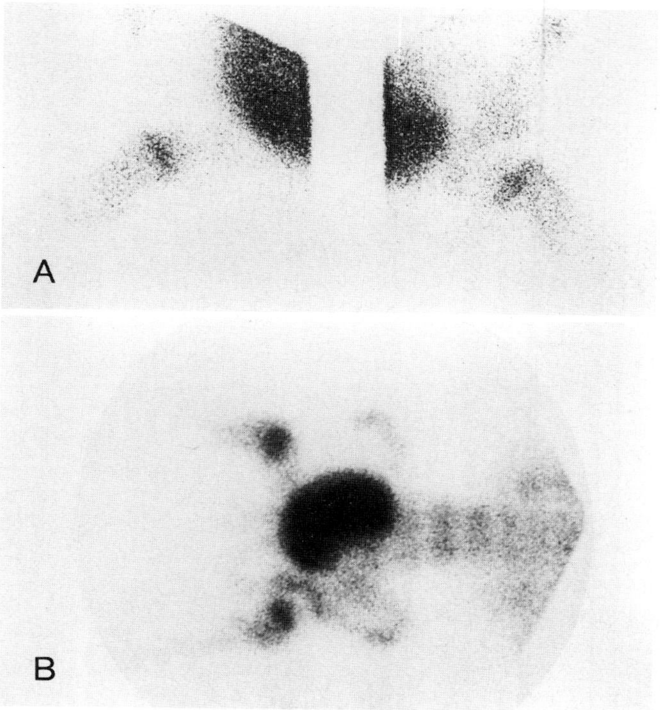

Figure 33.16. Sickle cell anemia bone infarction. **A.** Anterior pinhole collimator views of the hips in an 18-month-old child who had been irritable for 3 days and had refused to move her right leg for 4 days. Note absence of activity in both femoral heads. However, this is one time when relying on pinhole views alone, without scout views of the skeleton, might lead one astray. **B.** An anterior view of the lower spine and pelvis reveal a large photon-deficient area in the right hemipelvis that is difficult to appreciate on the pinhole magnification views. This represents bone infarction as a result of the patient's sickle cell crisis.

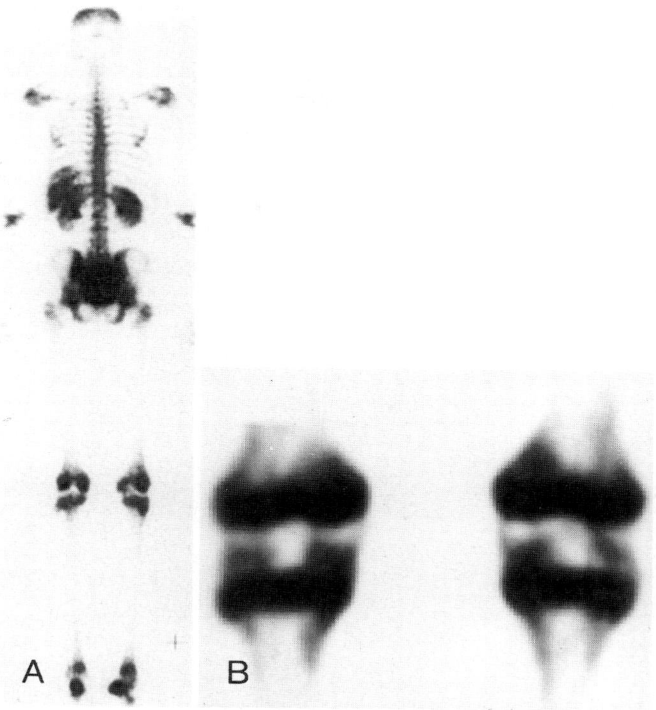

Figure 33.17. Sickle cell anemia with healing infarct. This is a 22-year-old male with a history of sickle cell anemia for several years. He presented with complaint of pain in the right knee and ankle for 10 days duration. Note the increased activity in the spleen and the right distal femur and tibia (**A**). Coronal SPECT views of the knee show the abnormal activity in the right femur (**B**). A ^{99m}Tc-WBC study, performed to exclude possible osteomyelitis, was normal.

eas is playing an increasing role in the evaluation of these patients, especially in the pediatric age group.

Bone imaging techniques may be utilized to assist the surgeon in delineating the level of the loss of vascularity and viability of bone in conditions such as frostbite and diabetes (Fig. 33.18). In such instances, routine bone imaging may be combined with (a) the marking of the patient's skin at the level of reasonable bone activity by using external radioactive markers and the persistence scope when imaging the patient, or (b) a transmission image of the leg associated with dermal marking at that time (Fig. 33.19). Both techniques greatly assist the surgeon if amputation is planned.

ARTHRITIDES

Although it is not commonly used, skeletal imaging may be of assistance in the diagnosis of arthritis (63–65). However, since bone scanning is a nonspecific procedure (Fig. 33.20), pattern recognition (Fig. 33.21), as well as interpretation in the clinical context, plays an important role in allowing differentiation among the variety of causes of arthritis such as rheumatoid, degenerative or osteoarthritis, inflammatory, psoriatic, gouty arthritis, Reiter's syndrome, ankylosing spondylitis, lupus erythematosus, sarcoidosis, and regional migratory osteoporosis (Figs. 33.22–33.24). The ability to perform total body views allows rapid and more economical multiple joint evaluation than standard radiographic evaluation. Skeletal scintigraphy may show diffuse periarticular increase reflecting the increased perfusion of the soft tissues in arthritides that affect soft tissue and cartilage. It also represents osteoblastic activity in subchondral bone and will, on occasion, show focal abnormal findings before the patient complains of joint pain or radiographic changes are present. The routine bone scan may be combined with studies performed after the injection of ^{99m}Tc-pertechnetate or albumin to allow the differentiation between inflammatory, proliferative arthropathies such as rheumatoid arthritis and degenerative osteoarthritis. The latter is not associated with increased soft tissue uptake of ^{99m}Tc-pertechnetate or albumin. It must be remembered that although abnormal ^{99m}Tc-pertechnetate uptake is sensitive and specific for the presence of synovitis, it says nothing about the etiology. Other forms of inflammatory arthritis, including gout and sacroidosis, may show dramatic uptake with radiolabeled leukocytes, antibodies, and ^{67}Ga-citrate.

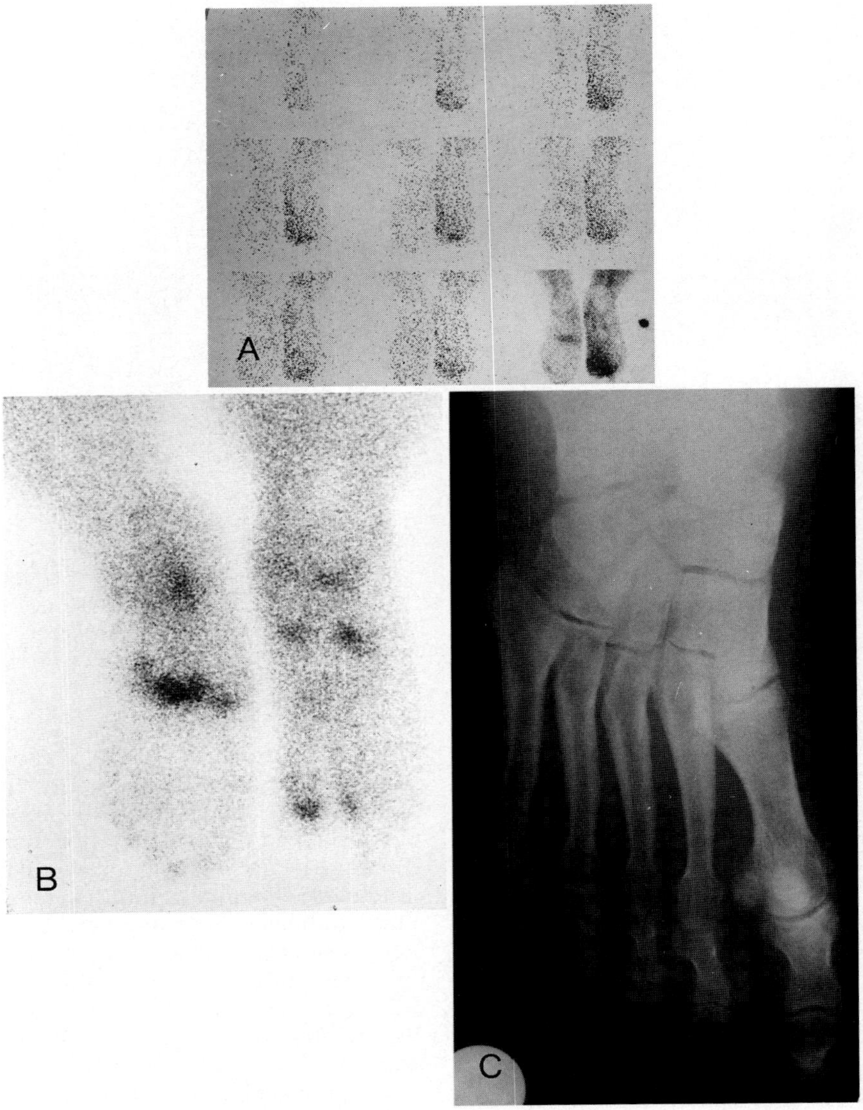

Figure 33.18. Loss of bone vascularity in diabetes. **A.** Plantar perfusion of both feet in a 57-year-old male diabetic with a painful right toe and fever. Note the overall decreased perfusion in both lower legs and feet as a result of the patient's vascular problems. Despite this, there is increased perfusion to the right foot but a lack of perfusion to the right toe. **B.** Delayed plantar views of the feet demonstrating multiple sites of increased activity from the patient's diabetic arthropathy. However, no activity at all is seen in the distal right great toe, despite knowledge that it is indeed present on the radiograph (**C**). This represents avascular necrosis of the toe. Gangrene of the distal great toe became evident within a few days and amputation was carried out using the line of vascular demarcation marked on the skin at the time of imaging.

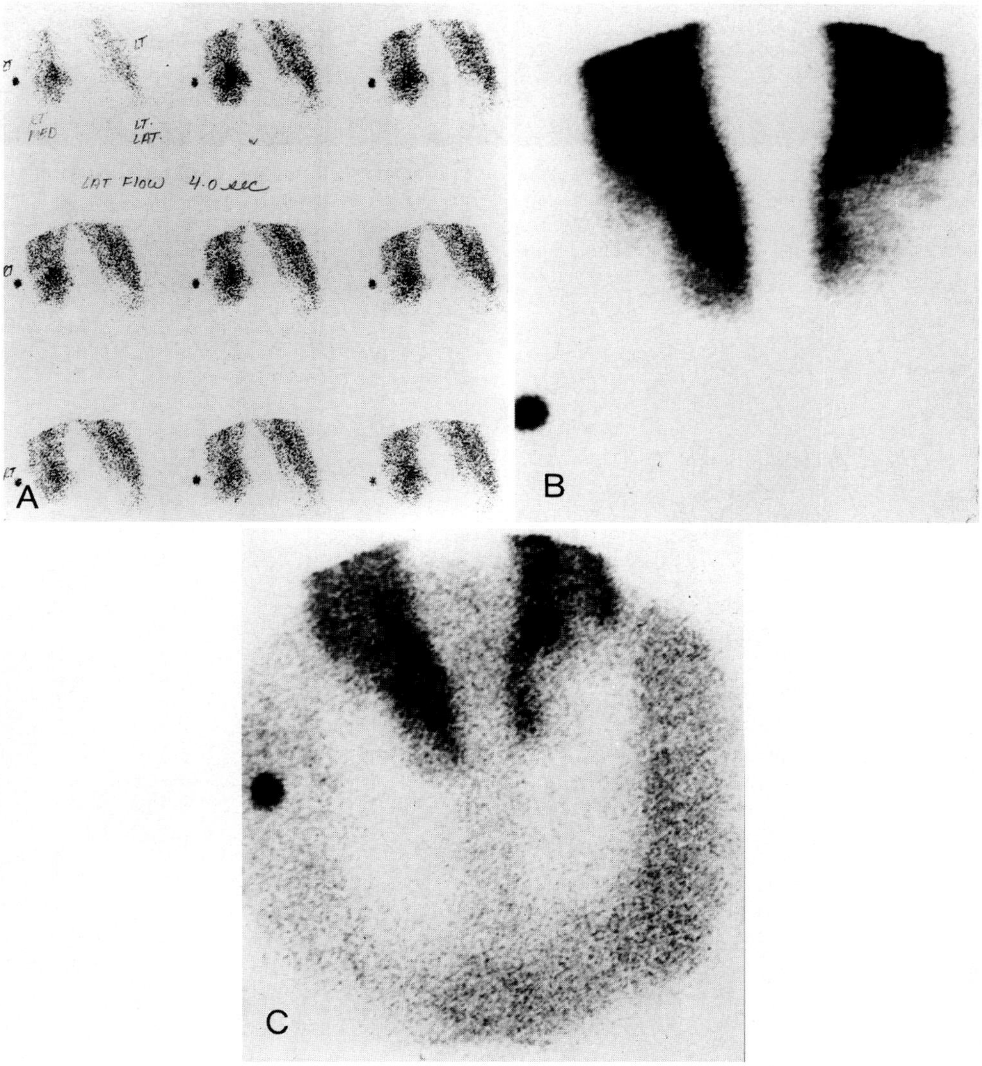

Figure 33.19. Infarction of bone from frostbite. A 27-year-old male was brought to the emergency room after spending a night exposed to a northern climate. **A.** Perfusion study demonstrating lack of perfusion on the ankle and feet bilaterally. **B.** Delayed static images in the plantar projection demonstrating lack of osseous activity. **C.** Outline of the feet allowing determination of the level of activity using a transmission scan with the source behind the feet and face of the collimator. (Case courtesy of Dr. Herman Wallinga, The Genesee Hospital, Rochester, NY.)

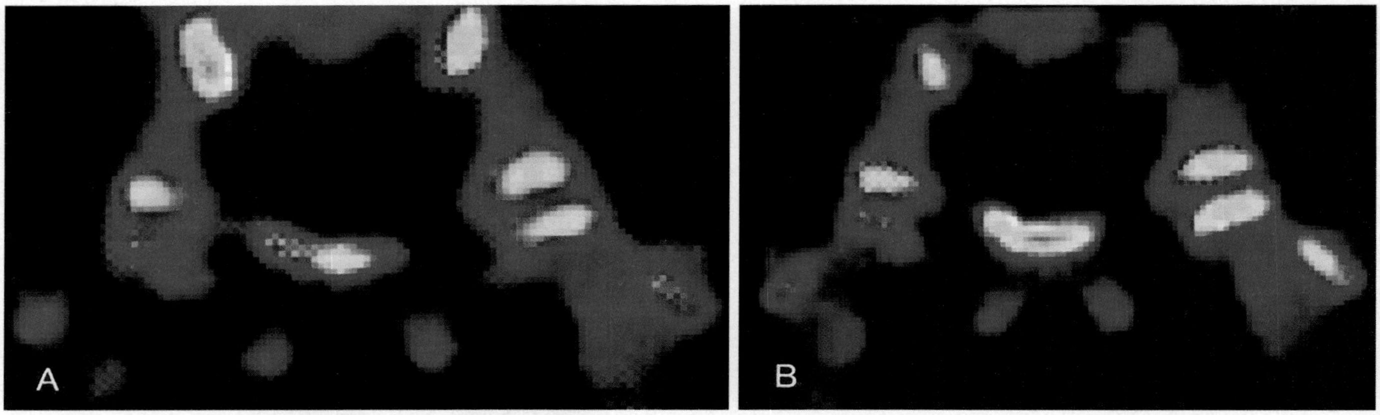

Figure 33.20. Rheumatoid arthritis. Coronal SPECT views (**A** and **B**) of the hips in an 18-year-old female with known rheumatoid arthritis. She complained of pain in the left hip. Standard radiographs were normal. Despite the abnormally increased activity in the left hip including greater trochanter (also abnormal on the perfusion and blood pool phases), this case illustrates the problem of nonspecificity in skeletal scintigraphy. Similar findings could be found with trauma, tumor, infection, and trochanteric bursitis.

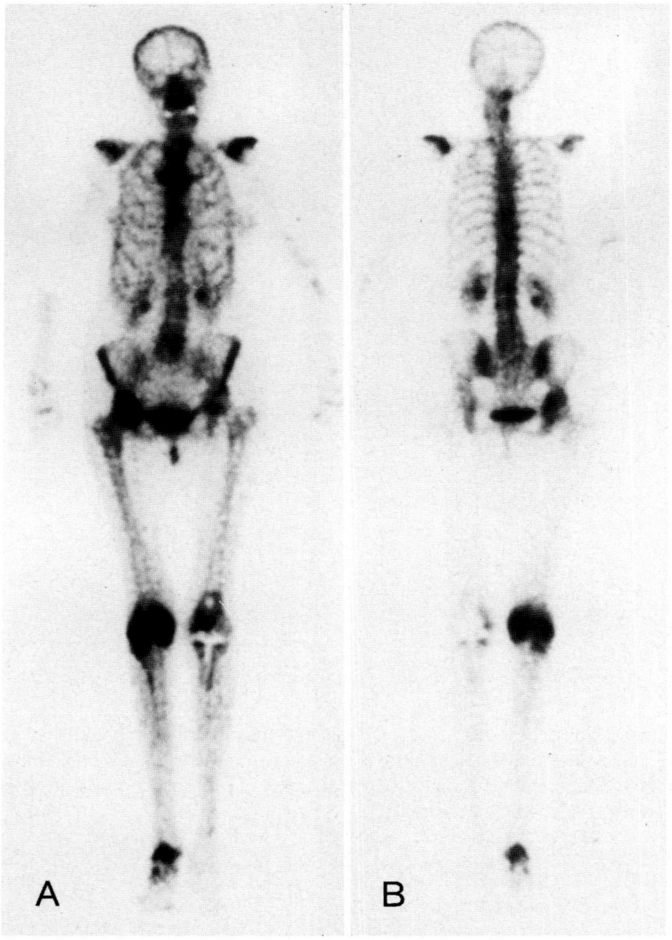

Figure 33.21. Degenerative arthritis. Total body anterior (**A**) and posterior (**B**) views in a 67-year-old female with complaints of pain in multiple joints for years. Note the nonsymmetric, diffuse joint involvement, especially in weight bearing or motion stressed joints. The patient had undergone prosthetic knee replacement 4 years earlier.

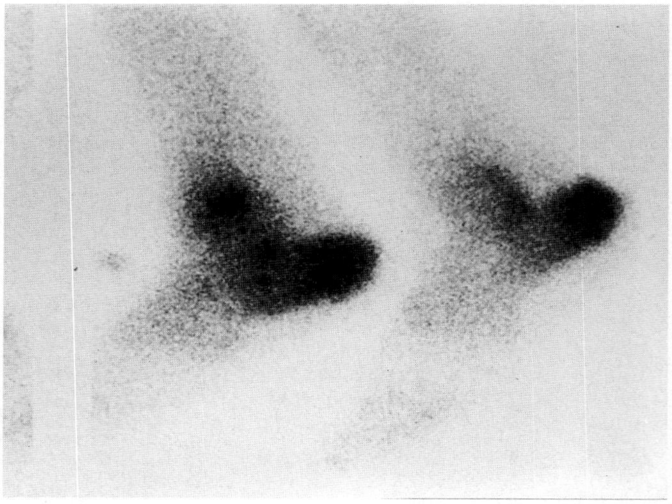

Figure 33.22. Reiter's syndrome. Lateral and medial views of the left and right ankle and feet in a 30-year-old male suffering from uveitis and prostatitis. He complained of pain in the left heel and back. This study exhibited a heel inflammation index (ratio of activity over the rear of the calcaneus to an equal sized area at the junction of the mid and lower third of the tibia) of 14.8. Diffusely abnormal activity was also found in the back. These findings are consistent with the diagnosis of Reiter's syndrome.

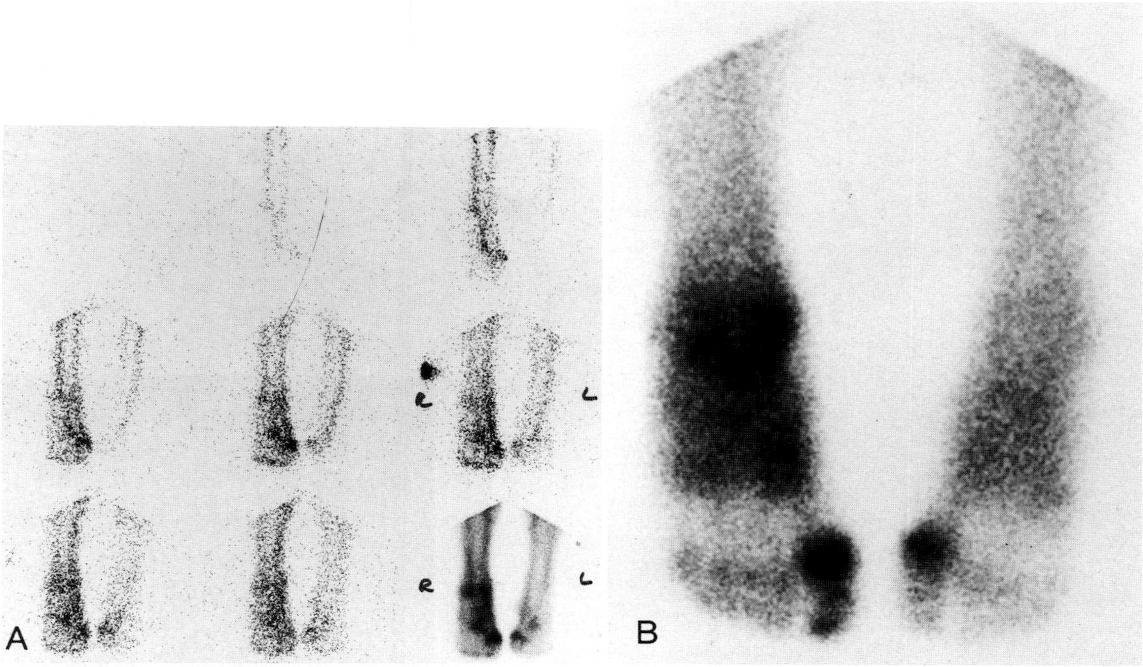

Figure 33.23. Gouty arthritis. This 60-year-old male had been admitted to the hospital following a myocardial infarction. On the fifth day of hospitalization, he began to complain of severe pain in both great toes, much worse on the right. A bone scan was performed to investigate the possibility of vascular compromise in the lower extremities. **A.** The perfusion and immediate soft tissue phases demonstrate marked increased perfusion to the right ankle and foot with focal increased perfusion to the hallux valgus deformity in the left foot. **B.** The delayed skeletal image revealed abnormal foci of activity about the great toes and right ankle. Serum urate levels were markedly elevated in this gentleman, leading to the final diagnosis of gouty arthritis.

As a result, differentiation from osteomyelitis in periarticular bone may be difficult or impossible by scintigraphy alone (Fig. 33.25).

When patients are studied for peripheral arthritic problems, the three-phase bone procedure is usually used. Perfusion and early blood pool images of this technique may allow identification of synovial involvement and avoid the need for a combined ^{99m}Tc-pertechnetate/albumin study. Individual joints must be studied with high-resolution views and/or SPECT and complex joints. The pattern of distribution of abnormality on the delayed images may be typical of the arthritic type involved and allow for diagnostic separation. Normal skeletal imaging indicates lack of active arthritic involvement. Despite the sensitivity of skeletal scintigraphy, most rheumatologists will workup their patients with only a combination of clinical history, physical exams, laboratory and standard radiograph findings.

Quantitative methods of studying individual joints have met with mixed success and none has become widely accepted (66–68). Little is known about normal and abnormal quantitative values for regions other than the sacroiliac and temporomandibular joints (69, 70). The quantitative indices usually are calculated as the ratio of activity in such areas as the sacroiliac joint compared to the normal sacrolumbar or iliac bone activity. The technique is quite dependent upon the imaging position of the patient as well as patient age and chronologic status of the disease (Fig. 33.26). This approach remains somewhat controversial, with mixed results from a variety of investigators. Profile slice counting and separate regions of interest have been proposed. The author prefers the region of interest method since the pattern of sacroilitis will range from focal involvement early to later involvement of the whole joint. Another reason for preferring separate regions of interest is the difficulty that can be met when counting over the sacral tubercle when it appears as an anatomic variant. Similar applications have been made to other regions such as the temporomandibular joint. Here SPECT imaging improves the sensitivity of detection and quantification of bony involvement.

Ankylosing spondylitis is a chronic soft tissue inflammatory process that usually involves the sacroiliac and vertebral joints, but may also involve peripheral joints, sternum, and costochondral junctions. When peripheral joints are involved it is frequently confused with rheumatoid arthritis. Progression of the disease can lead to debilitating conditions with osseous ankylosis and fusion of the vertebral bodies, resulting in a rigid spine that is subject to fracture. Bone imaging will be successful in early detection of such spinal fractures (71). This condition is usually manifested by a pattern of focal increased activity in a vertebral body superimposed upon the more diffusely in-

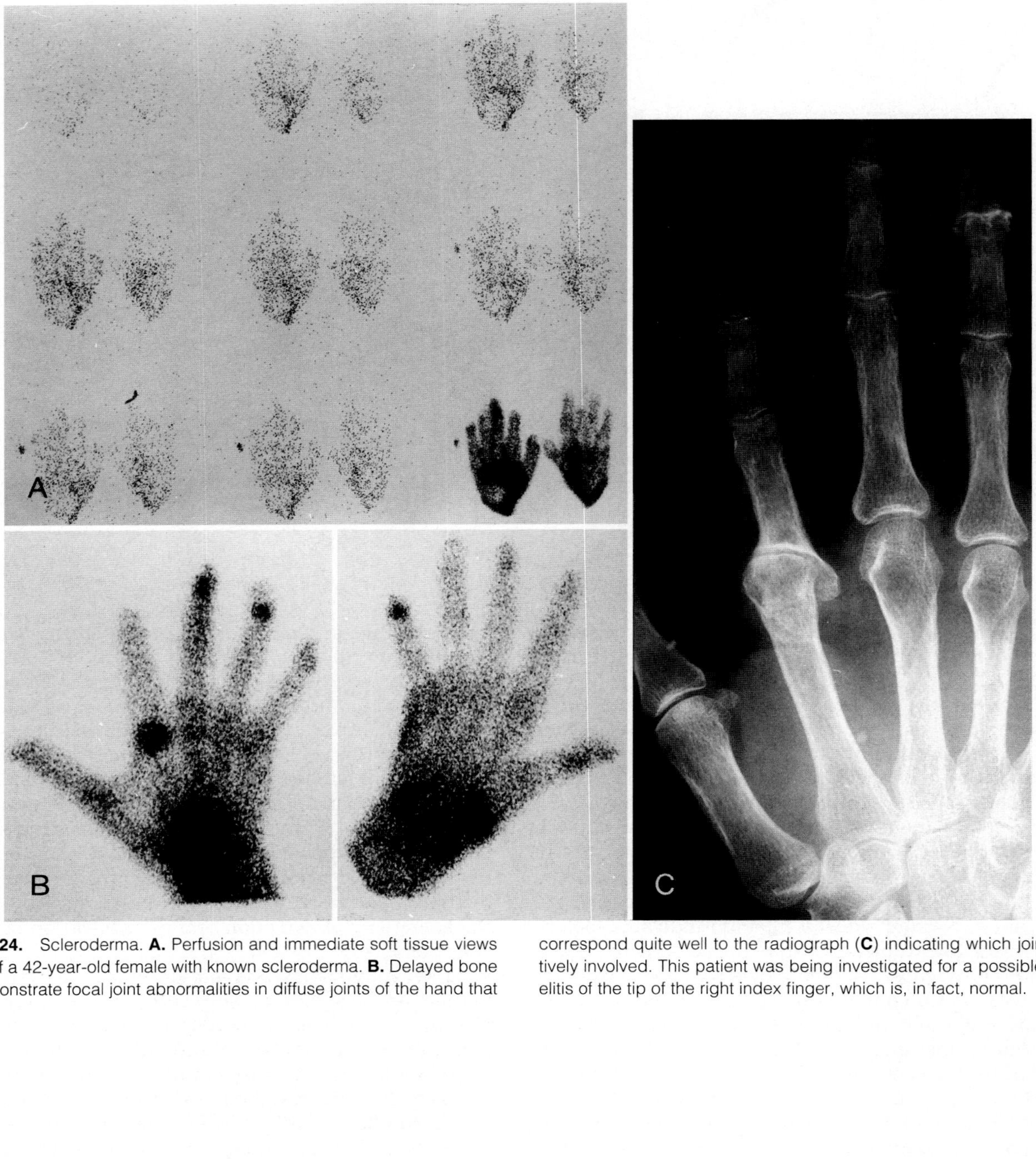

Figure 33.24. Scleroderma. **A.** Perfusion and immediate soft tissue views of hands of a 42-year-old female with known scleroderma. **B.** Delayed bone views demonstrate focal joint abnormalities in diffuse joints of the hand that correspond quite well to the radiograph (**C**) indicating which joints are actively involved. This patient was being investigated for a possible osteomyelitis of the tip of the right index finger, which is, in fact, normal.

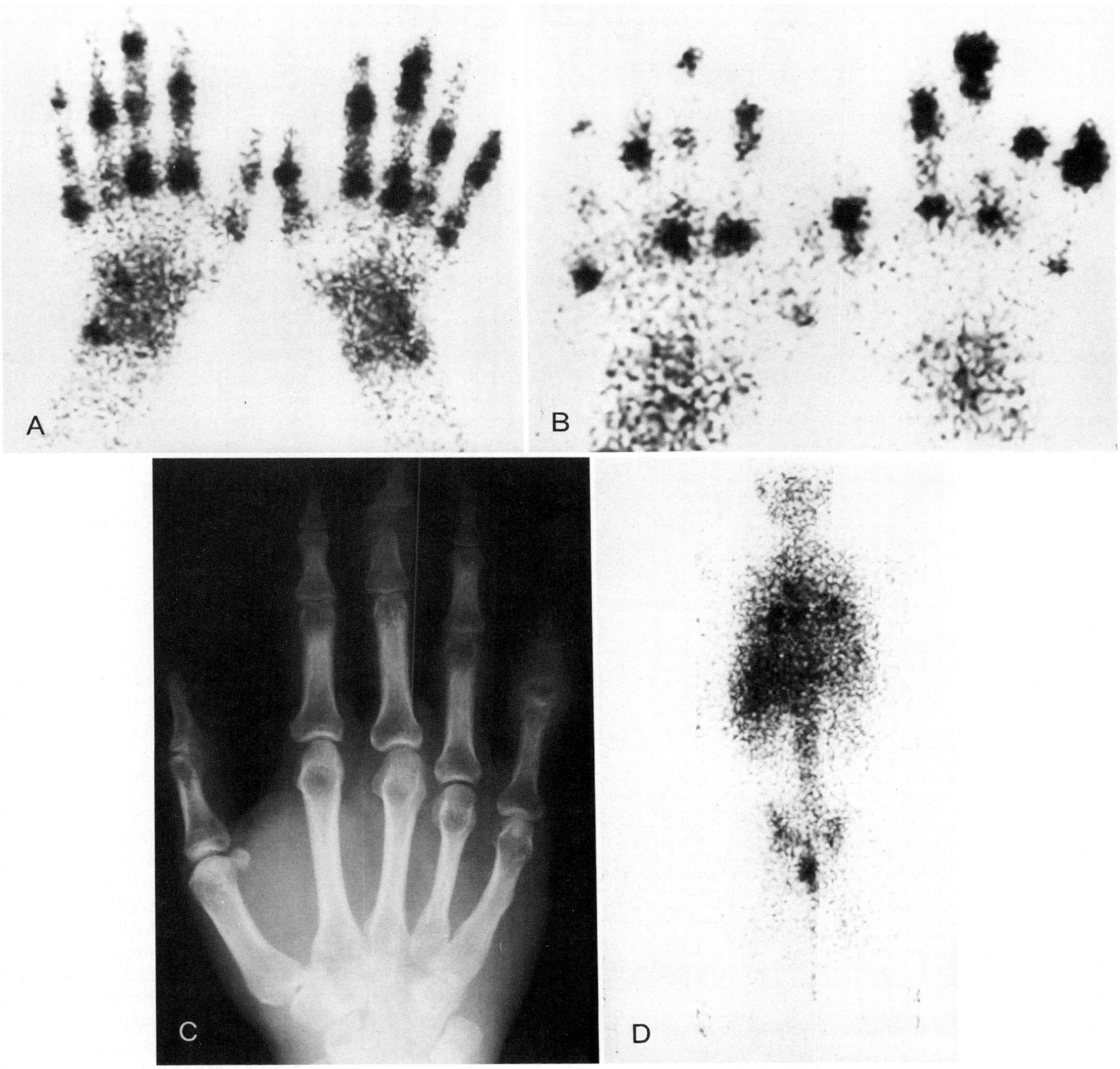

Figure 33.25. Sarcoidosis. **A.** Delayed views from three-phase bone scan in a 32-year-old male who complained of increasing weakness and pain in his fingers for 2 months. A similar pattern was seen during the perfusion and immediate phases. **B.** Similar projection from a ^{67}Ga-citrate study 72 hours later. **C.** Magnification x-ray of right hand which demonstrates destruction of the 3rd and 5th DIP joints. **D.** Anterior total body views from 72-hour ^{67}Ga study which shows diffuse pulmonary activity increased and abnormal activity in hilar and mediastinal nodes. Sarcoid was confirmed by biopsy of the 5th DIP joint.

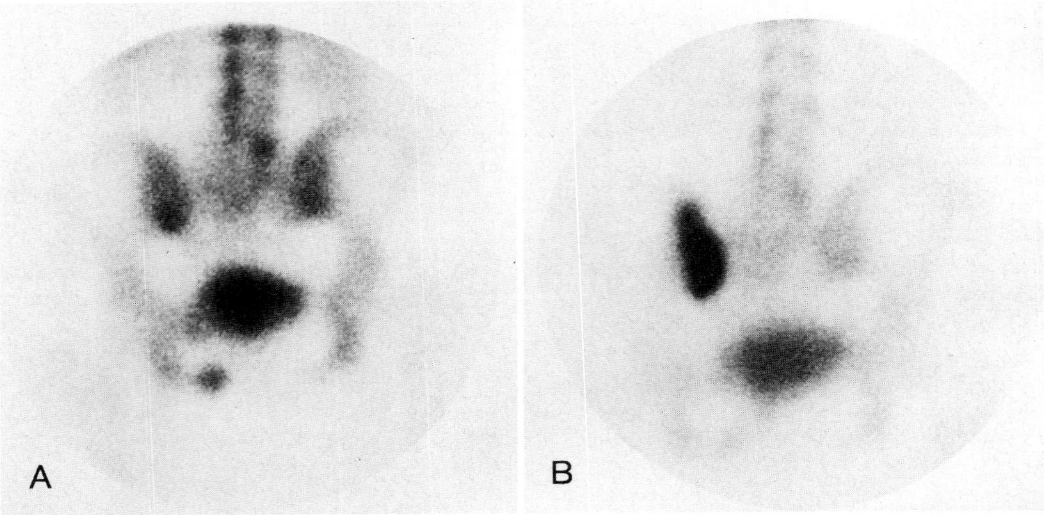

Figure 33.26. Sacroiliitis. Posterior views of the lower lumbar spine and pelvis in a 37-year-old female with complaints suggesting sacroiliitis. **A.** The initial study demonstrates diffuse abnormal activity throughout the thoracolumbar spine as a result of the patient's severe scoliosis. Note the focal area of increased uptake inferiorly in the left sacroiliac joint, a sign of early sacroiliitis. **B.** Six months later, the patient's pain had worsened despite therapy. Skeletal imaging at that time reveals involvement of the entire sacroiliac area. This pattern illustrates the usual development of sacroiliitis.

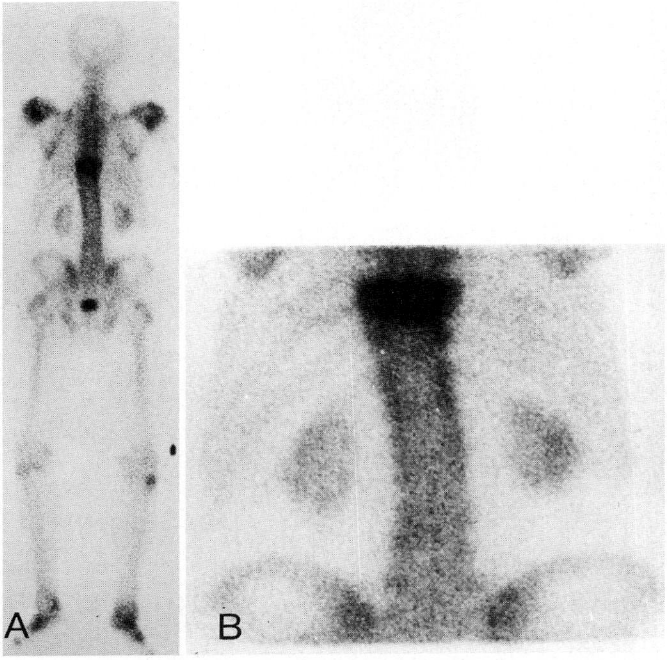

Figure 33.27. Ankylosing spondylitis. Posterior total body view (**A**) and magnified spot view (**B**) of the thoracolumbar spine in a 47-year-old male suffering from ankylosing spondylitis. Note the diffuse activity throughout the thoracolumbar spine and other joints, with focal increased activity noted at the ninth thoracic vertebra. This patient had a recent exacerbation of his back pain localized to the midback. Radiographs of this area did not reveal fracture. However, the focal increase superimposed upon the diffuse changes caused by the spondylitis indicates recent fracture.

creased activity resulting from ankylosing spondylitis (Fig. 33.27).

When joint replacement is considered to be necessary, bone imaging may be utilized to show the areas of greatest involvement. SPECT imaging will correctly predict compartmental involvement in cases of arthritis involving the knees (72, 73). Contrast arthrography or routine radiographic study is far less accurate in predicting compartmental involvement.

METABOLIC DISEASE

The exact role of bone imaging in evaluating metabolic bone disease is still unclear as many varieties of such disease share similar scintigraphic findings (74, 75). A wide variety of quantification techniques have been suggested that do offer useful information (76–80). These range from highly technical total body calculations involving sophisticated whole-body counting equipment, to more practical approaches for the smaller, clinically oriented community hospital involving the determination of the percentage of injected dose of ^{99m}Tc-MDP that is retained in the skeletal system based on calculations derived from simple scintillation detectors or the gamma-camera. Bone absorption studies that involve single or dual energy approaches have been used, as well as computed tomography and neutron activation analysis. More focal quantifications, such as the 24-hour/4-hour ratio of ^{99m}Tc-MDP uptake over lesions versus nonlesions, or SPECT calculations of skull ^{99m}Tc-MDP uptake, have been proposed. All of these techniques have been used with reasonable success in the study of patients with acromegaly, hyperthyroidism, primary hyperparathyroidism, renal osteodystrophy, osteonecrosis, osteoporosis, osteomalacia, and other diseases of calcium metabolism (81–83). However, the lack of full acceptance of such procedures in the study of these conditions is the result of present technical difficulties. The variety of quantification techniques already introduced produces different numerical values for normal and abnormal subjects depending on the laboratory in which they are used. Some techniques measure trabecular bone, some measure cancellous bone, and some measure both. Additionally, they require exact standardization of the application among patients within the individual laboratory. Many technical factors affect the quality of the results, including choice of radiopharmaceutical, choice of collimator/camera system, time of imaging after injection, information density on the images, computer and display options, matrix size, region of interest, profile selections, total body counting, standard background subtraction techniques, and calculation of normal ranges determined by age and sex.

The routine radionuclide bone scan does not give a good measure of absolute bone uptake. Abnormally increased uptake may be suggested by an increase in the bone to soft tissue ratio, but only when this ratio is marked. One of the two best measures that have achieved some clinical use is quantitation of retained phosphate complex skeletal activity after 24 hours (84). Such measurements will improve the detection of metabolic disease over qualitative or visual evaluation of total body scans. Of the many metabolic disorders only osteoporosis will show normal levels of retention. All others show increased retention.

The second quantification method for evaluation is that of bone densitometry as used in the study of osteoporosis. This condition increases with normal aging but may also be found as a component of many diseases. An accurate and early diagnosis of it is essential in order to involve the patient with therapy to prevent fractures. Multiple techniques for the measurement of bone density are utilized but all rely on measuring the difference in attenuation of photons of a specific energy by soft tissue and bone in comparison to standards (85–89). The most commonly used measurement of the bone mineral mass is single photon absorptiometry with scanning across the radius, calcaneus, or even hip. Other techniques include dual photon absorptiometry, dedicated x-ray absorptiometry, or quantitative computerized tomography involving both single and dual energy techniques (see Chapter 53).

Qualitative imaging of the variety of metabolic diseases may suggest their presence. The degree of activity between bone and soft tissues is changed with increased activity in the bone. Scan findings may range from increased uptake at the costochondral junction ("beading"), mandible, skull, sternum, ribs, and the juxta-articular are particular areas of the long bones (Fig. 33.28).

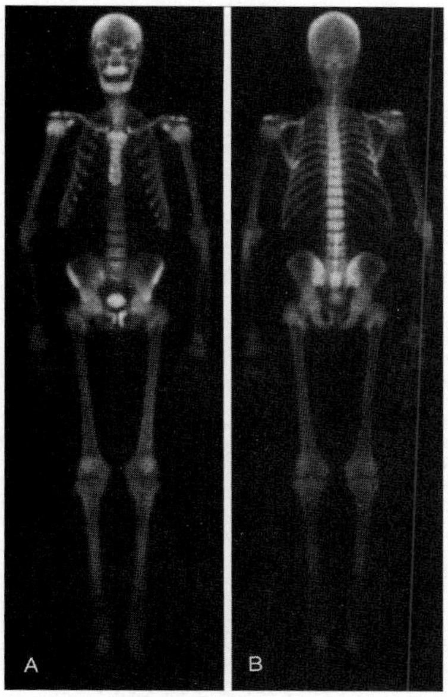

Figure 33.28. Hyperparathyroidism. Anterior (**A**) and posterior (**B**) total body images in a 39-year-old male renal transplant patient complaining of back and right shoulder pain. Note the diffusely increased activity in bones and the lack of soft tissue and renal activity.

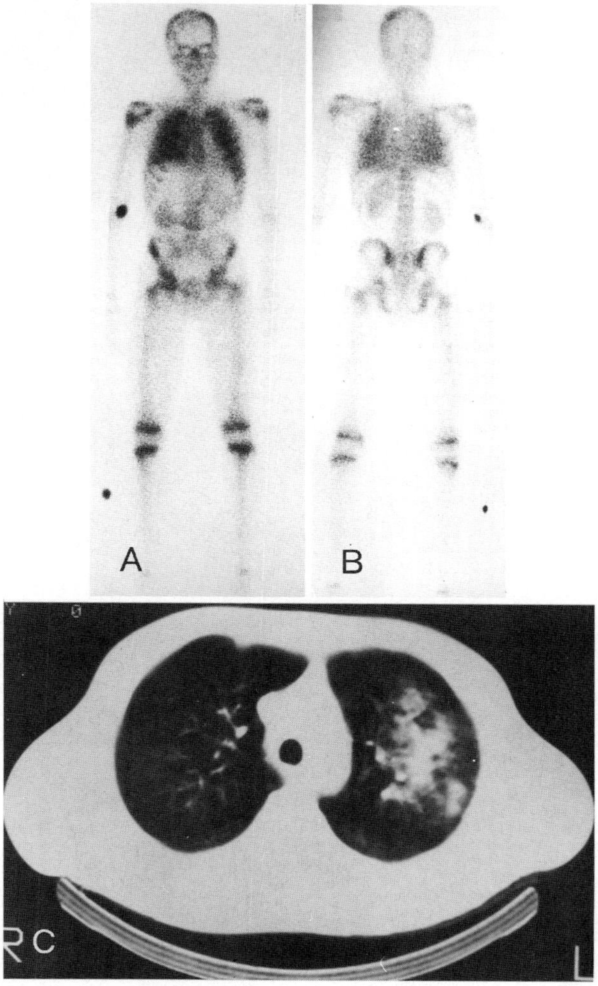

Figure 33.29. Renal osteodystrophy. Anterior (**A**) and posterior (**B**) total body views in a 17-year-old male with renal osteodystrophy. Note the diffuse increase in soft tissue activity seen most markedly in the lungs and in the stomach wall. Although the chest radiograph at this time was normal, computed axial tomographic examination of the chest (**C**) performed 3 days after the skeletal images revealed diffuse calcification in both lung fields.

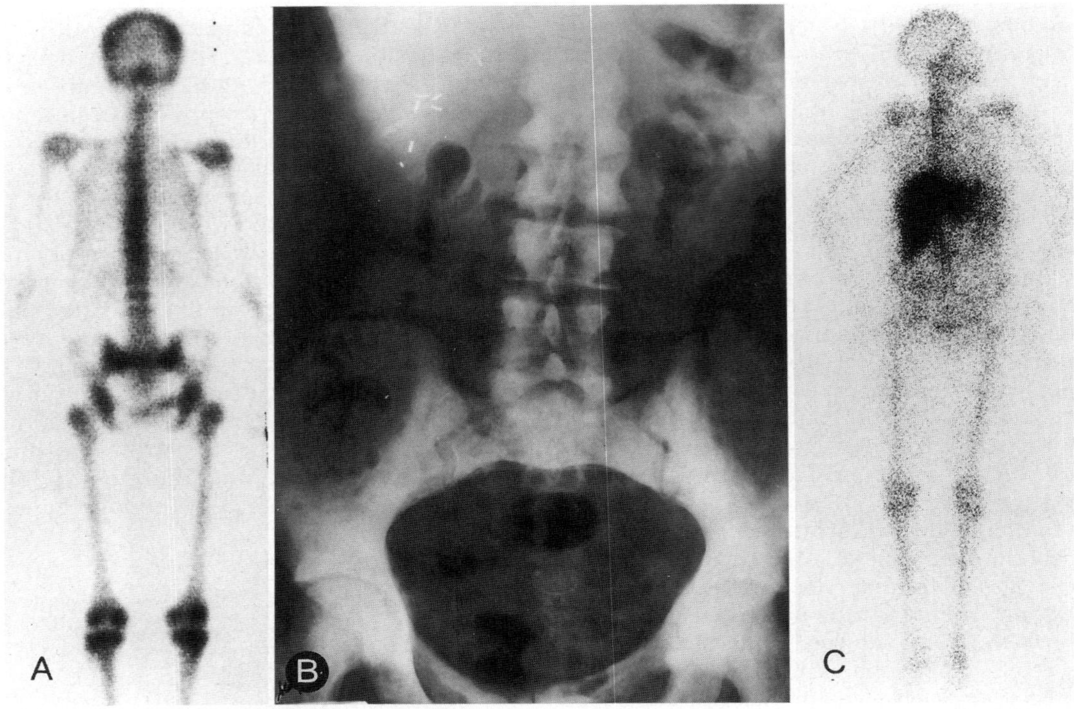

Figure 33.30. Progressive osteosclerosis. **A.** Posterior total body view of a 64-year-old woman with an 8-year history of progressive osteosclerosis and myelofibrosis of unknown etiology. Note the marked increase in activity in the skeleton, the decreased renal function, and the lack of soft tissue activity on this rectilinear scan. The skeletal uptake corresponds quite nicely with the radiograph of the lumbar spine and pelvis (**B**), illustrating the marked generalized sclerosis of this patient's osseous structures. **C.** An ^{111}In-chloride bone marrow study obtained at the same time demonstrates decreased marrow function in the spine and proximal extremities.

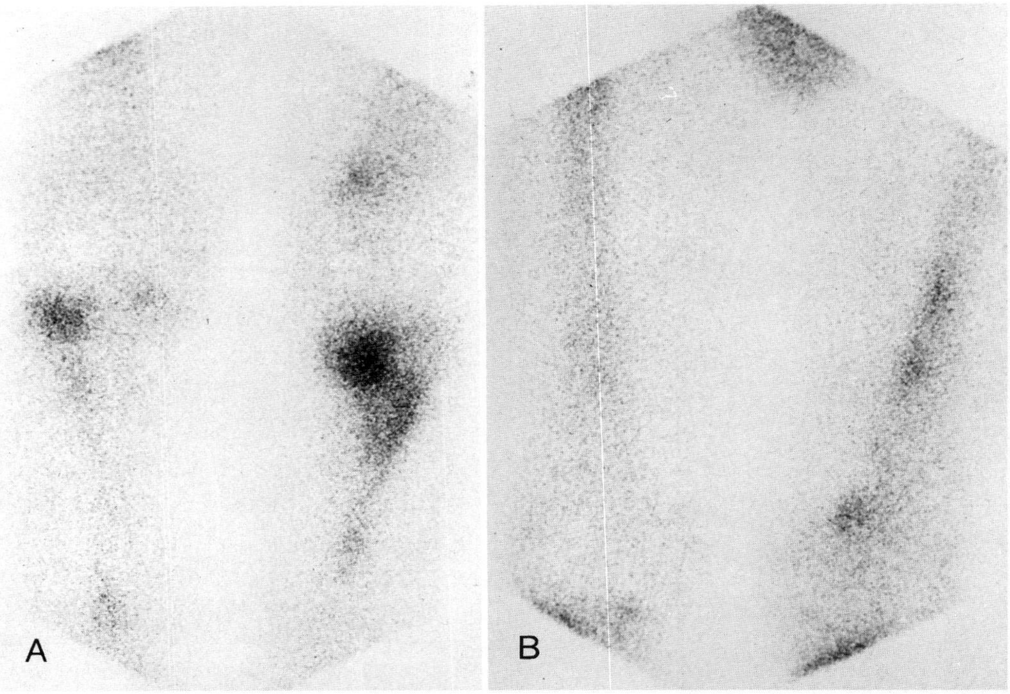

Figure 33.31. Hypertrophic pulmonary osteoarthropathy. Anterior views of the tibias (**A**) and femurs (**B**) demonstrating hypertrophic pulmonary osteoarthropathy in a 67-year-old male with degenerative arthritis (note changes about the knees). The scan was requested to investigate the patient's complaint of increasing pain in his lower extremity. A carcinoma of the lung was found on chest radiography obtained after bone scan.

Renal activity may be decreased or absent resulting in a superscan appearance. In hyperparathyroidism, soft tissue activity may be found in the lungs, stomach, and elsewhere as a result of metastatic calcifications, while focal areas of increased osseous activity may be seen at the sites of brown "tumors" (Fig. 33.29). Focal increases may also be seen at the pseudofractures (of osteomalacia) and fractures of osteogenesis imperfecta. Multiple benign compression fractures of the spine are commonly seen in osteoporotic patients.

Imaging techniques may still be useful in assessing a variety of conditions such as renal migratory osteoporosis, hypertropic pulmonary osteoarthropathy, reflex sympathetic dystrophy, Paget's disease, or any osteosclerotic condition with increased bone metabolism (melorheostosis, poikilocytosis, etc.). (90–94) (Fig. 33.30).

Hypertrophic osteoarthropathy, which is usually caused by pulmonary disease, is evident before radiographic changes may be seen (95) (Fig. 33.31). It usually produces a fairly characteristic appearance on scintigraphic studies consisting of a generalized increase in the cortical activity in the long bones and focal sites of increased activity in the periarticular regions of the long bones, phalanges, scapula, and clavicle.

Reflex sympathetic dystrophy is another condition in which skeletal scintigraphy changes are seen before radiographic evidence of the condition is found. This is true whether the sympathetic dystrophy is the result of trauma or vascular compromise, or one in which no specific cause can be determined. It is also important to relate study findings to the duration of symptoms. Increased perfusion and early blood pool activity is usually evident only in the first 2–3 months after onset of the process. Delayed static images may reveal diffuse periarticular activity in the affected extremity for no more than a year after symptomatology begins (Fig. 33.32). After this radionuclide diagnosis is less accurate as the images may return to normal or may even show reduced activity.

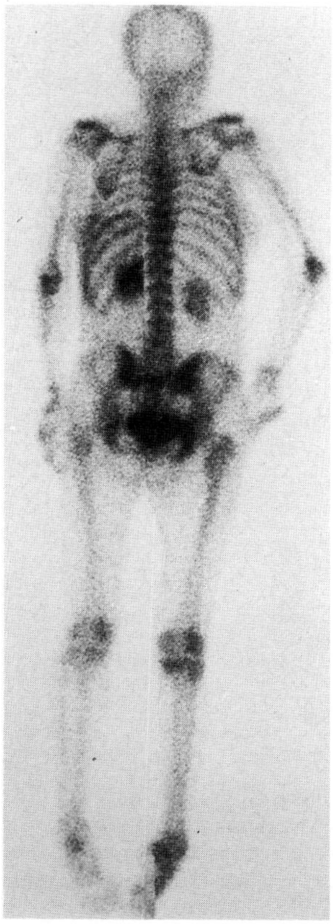

Figure 33.32. Reflex sympathetic dystrophy. Posterior total body view demonstrating diffuse increased activity in the lower extremity on the right in a 51-year-old female with adult-onset diabetes.

Paget's disease (osteitis deformans) is seen frequently in individuals who are middle-aged and older. Again, it is a condition in which the bone scan changes usually precede radiographic abnormalities (96). It is more common to be polyostotic in nature with only 20–30% of early cases being monostotic. Increased activity may be present in the early osteolytic phase as well as in the later osteoblastic phase (97). In the early osteolytic stage (circumscripta), perfusion and blood pool images may precede changes in the delayed static bone imaging (98). Additionally, the uptake is most intense at the edge of the lytic lesion (99). In the later osteoblastic phase, one may see diffuse multiple bony site involvement which may be unilateral and with apparent expansion in the size of the bone when seen in the extremities, ribs, and clavicle. In long bones, the abnormal activity pattern will invariably extend to at least one end of the bone. Calvarial activity may be intense and range from focal to diffuse involvement (100) (Fig. 33.33).

At times the polyostotic nature of Paget's disease may make it difficult to differentiate from metastases, whether on scan or radiographs. Although scan patterns as described earlier may make Paget's disease more likely, one may eventually have to resort to biopsy for this differentiation. Serial studies of the activity pattern in Paget's disease may allow for the differentiation of the development of sarcomas which occurs in about 1% of patients (101). Early sarcomatous degeneration usually results as an even further increase in the already dramatically focal activity changes. Later changes may present as photon deficient lesions, presumably as a result of interruption of blood supply and bone necrosis.

A diphosphonate, disodium etidronate, is a commonly used drug for the therapy of Paget's disease. Serial bone scans may be utilized to monitor the effectiveness of the therapeutic regimen, an important finding since the therapeutic doses of this drug may be toxic. Successful therapy is usually seen as a decrease in activity (102, 103) (Fig. 33.34).

This is another area in which quantitative study may be utilized for assessing the effect of this therapy in Paget's disease, as well as in treatment for fibrous dysplasia, eosinophilic granuloma, and histiocytosis x (when abnormal) (Fig. 33.35). Fibrous dysplasia and other bone dysplasias are conditions in which the scan may be quite abnormal in the face of normal radiographic findings. It is important to demonstrate whether the condition is polyostotic or mon-

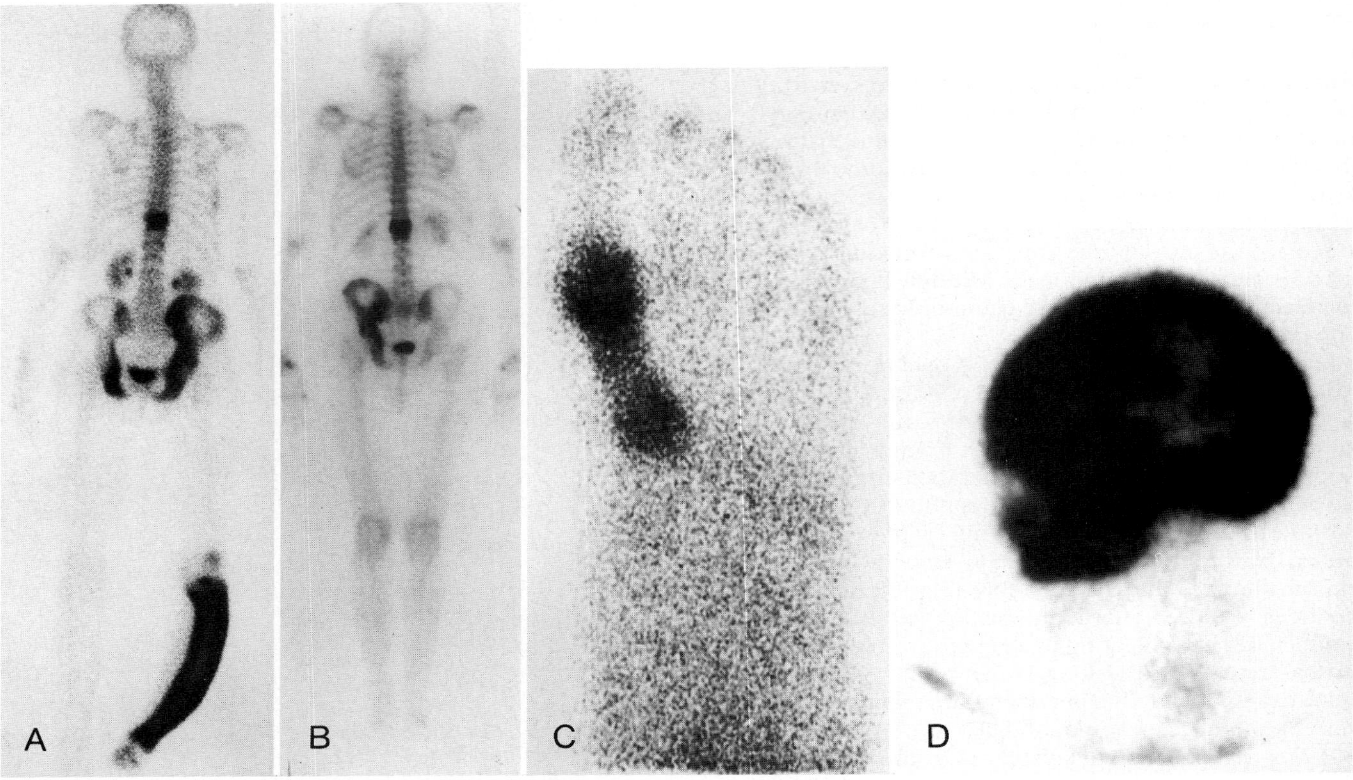

Figure 33.33. Paget's disease. This entity has many faces. It may be mono static or polyostatic, deforming of bone or not, and of uneven uptake as in circumscripta. **A.** Posterior view in a 54-year-old female with marked increased activity in multiple bones. **B.** Posterior projection in a 68-year-old male with much less deformity in spine and pelvis. **C.** Plantar view in a 57-year-old male with pain in left leg and foot. This was the only site of abnormality in this patient. **D.** Lateral view of skull in a 57-year-old female with diffuse but uneven activity in the skull with sparing of the mandible. This also was the only abnormal site in this patient.

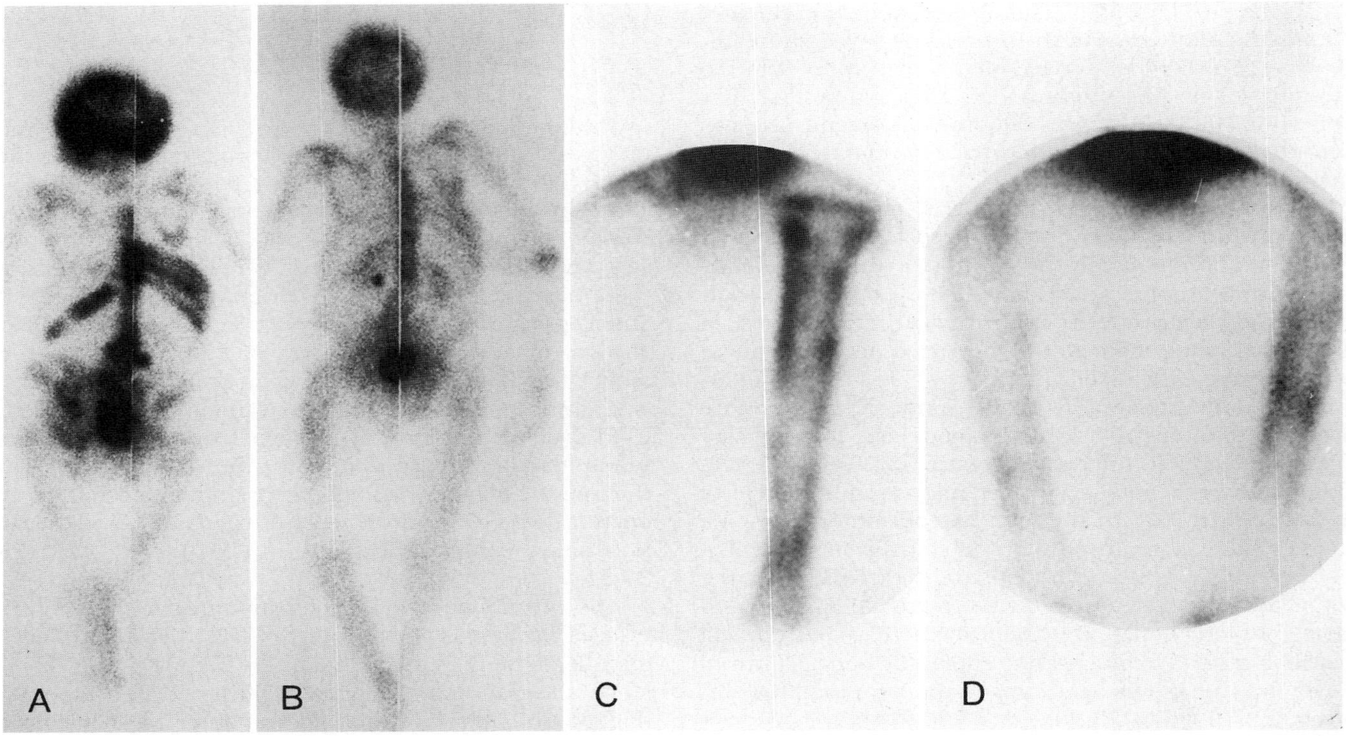

Figure 33.34. Assessment of therapy in paget disease. Total body posterior views (**A** and **B**) in a 41-year-old male with Paget's disease. At the time of the first study (**A**), he was experiencing severe bone pain. The second study (**B**) was obtained 2 years later following an intensive course of diphosphonate therapy. There had been marked improvement in the patient's clinical status, which is marked by the loss of avidity of the bones for the bone-seeking agent. Similar findings are seen in the spot views of the femurs (**C** and **D**).

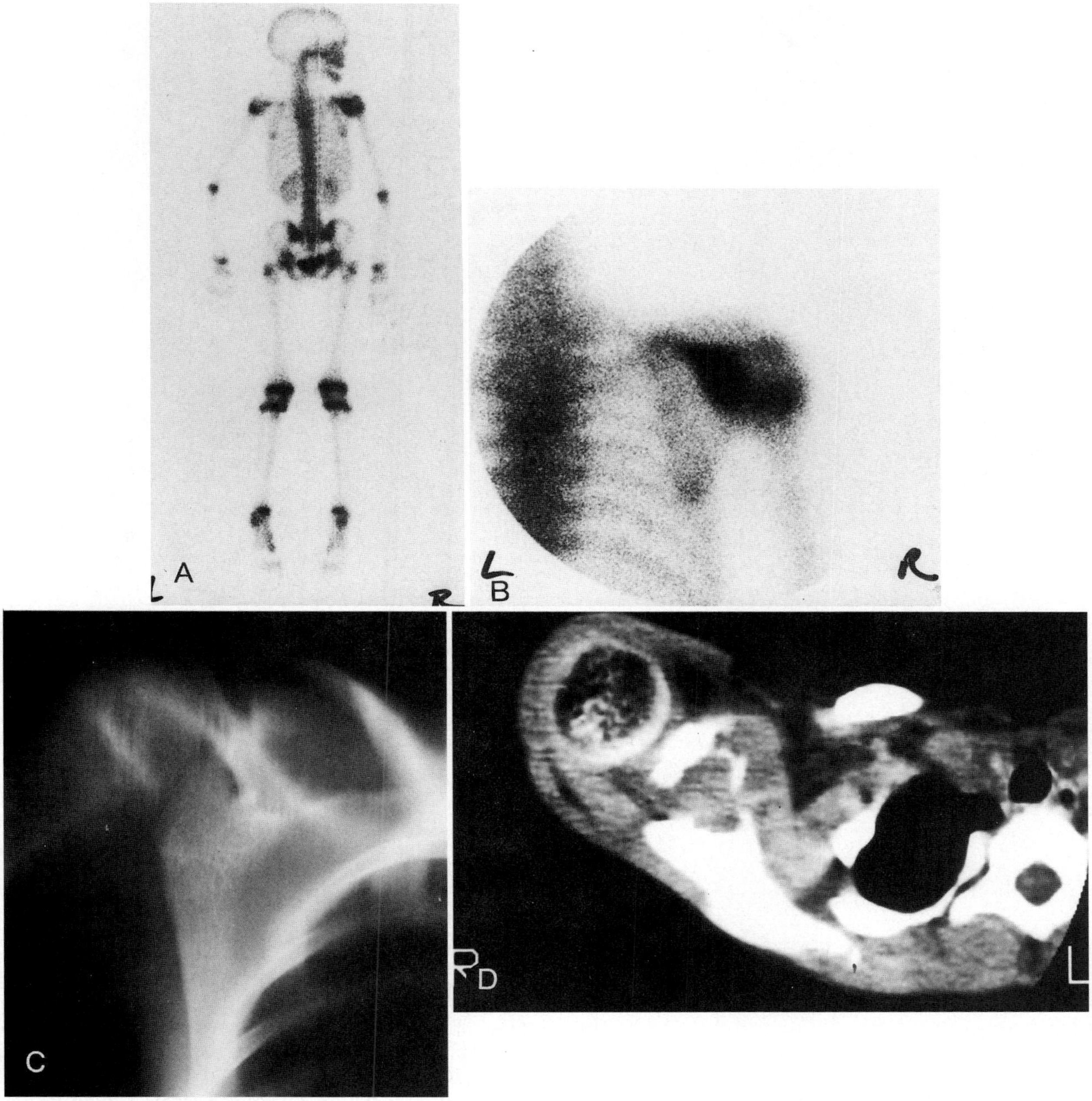

Figure 33.35. Histocytosis X. Posterior total body view (**A**) and spot view of the right shoulder (**B**) in an 11-year-old male who had been treated 5 years before for histocytosis X of the femur. He had felt well until he developed complaints of pain in the right upper arm. Outside radiographs of the humerus were normal. Histocytosis X is one of the disease entities in which the radionuclide bone imaging study may not be rewarding because many lesions do not take up ^{99m}Tc-phosphate. However, when abnormal, as in this case, they can direct further radiographic study. Tomograms of the scapula (**C**) and computed tomography of the shoulder (**D**) demonstrate the lesion quite well.

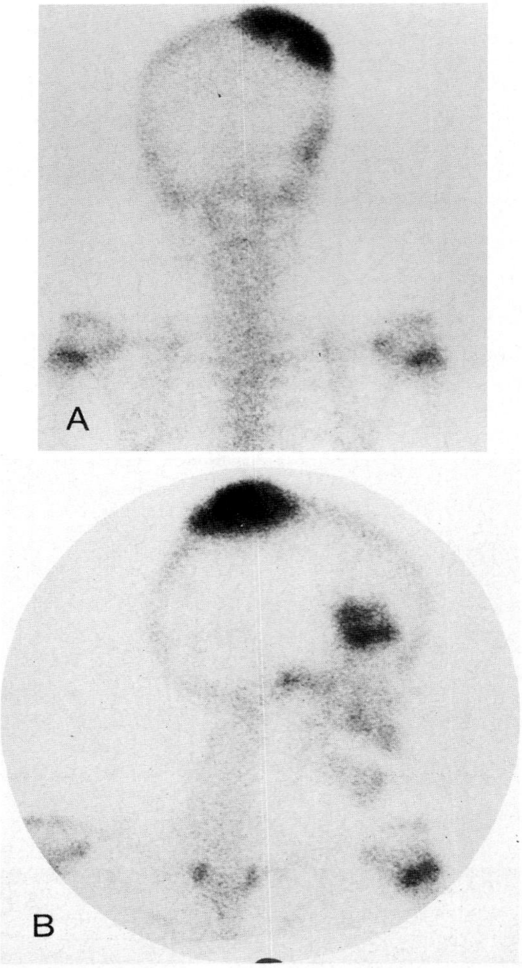

Figure 33.36. Polyostotic fibrous dysplasia. **A.** Posterior view of the skull showing markedly increased activity at the site of what was thought to be monostotic fibrous dysplasia in the posterior parietal region in an 11-year-old male. However, lateral views of the skull (**B**) reveal a second site in the skull that may be faintly visualized in the posterior view. This places the child into the category of polyostotic fibrous dysplasia.

ostotic for therapeutic regimens to be installed (Fig. 33.36). Again, skeletal scintigraphy allows a rapid, safe, reliable, and economical study of the entire skeleton in such patients. As opposed to Paget's disease, fibrous dysplasia in a long bone will frequently not reach the end of the bone, a minor differentiating point.

Other dysplastic conditions of bone may present in a variety of patterns. Such patterns range from the dense and uneven distribution in a single bone, usually the femur, that will be seen with melorheostosis to the widespread punctate-increased activity in poikilocytosis to the marked skeletal deformity and multiple fractures of osteogenesis imperfecta (104–106).[1]

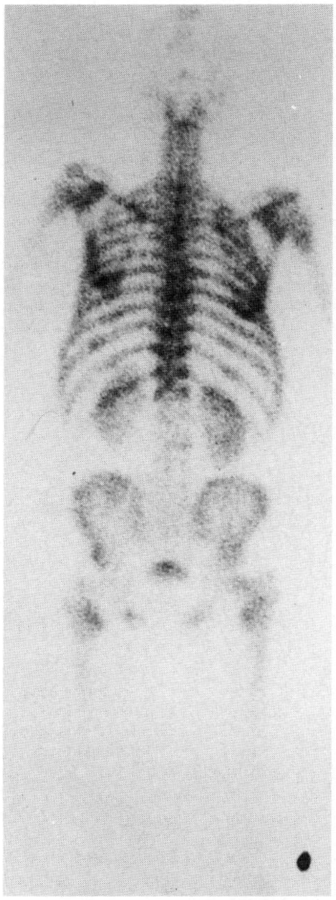

Figure 33.37. Decreased activity at radiation therapy portal. Posterior image in a 23-year-old male with testicular seminoma who had been treated with a radiotherapy portal 7 months before. His recent complaint was of back pain. Photon-deficient regions in the lumbar spine, corresponding to the portal, can be seen. The activity in the remainder of the thoracic spine and rib case pose a problem. Quantitation of this activity by rationing selected areas of interest to the tibia may frequently assist in determining if this is due to sparing or actual increased uptake. In this case, uptake was within normal limits. The patient's back pain disappeared without any further therapy.

MISCELLANEOUS CONDITIONS

IRRADIATED BONE

Radiation therapy portals usually result in decreased localization of bone-seeking radiopharmaceuticals (Fig. 33.37). However, increased activity may be seen if bone imaging is carried out shortly after completion of the radiation therapy (107, 108). Numerous factors influence the localization of bone-seeking radiopharmaceuticals in irradiated portions of bone. These include the amount and rate of delivery of the radiation, the time between the treatment and the imaging study, and the type of irradiated tissue. In animal experiments and some clinical situations, bone imaging reveals increased activity over the treatment portal for the first few weeks following cessation of radiotherapy. Within 2–3 months, the activity pattern in the treated area will decrease, giving a photopenic pattern at the site of irradiation. In one clinical study,

14 of 20 patients examined 4–6 months after treatment had such photopenic defects on their bone images (109). No changes were seen in regions that received less than 2000 rad, and the mean dose delivered was 3750 rad. The cause of such defects is unclear, but they are usually assumed to be the result of vasculitis and hyalinization of small vessels (osteonecrosis). A return to normal activity pattern may occur within 12 months but, more commonly, takes several years. Increase in radionuclide uptake may be observed in soft tissue included in the radiation port.

Because of the presence of a photopenic area in bone within the radiation port, it is often difficult to decide if activity in bones next to the port is normal or abnormal. Quantification techniques involving the calculation of abnormal to normal bone ratios can aid in solving this perplexing clinical problem.

GRAFTED BONE

The use of bone grafting has increased with the development of better surgical techniques and the ability to preserve viable bone. The three-phase bone scan is an excellent noninvasive method of monitoring viability in grafts. Autologous grafts with accompanying microvascularization result in a pattern that shows uniform perfusion, blood pool, and delayed activity throughout the graft immediately following graft surgery (110). Early in the postsurgical condition this activity pattern may be increased over the surrounding bone, but will become uniform with the surrounding bone within 12–18 months as the graft is assimilated into surrounding bone and healing is completed (38).

Most allografts are not well microvascularized at the time of surgical insertion and rely upon reestablishment of blood flow from surrounding vessel attachment (111, 112). In the immediate postsurgical phase, the graft may appear as a photon-deficient area. Repetitive examinations are necessary for full evaluation. These will demonstrate progressively increased perfusion, blood pool, and delayed uptake that will begin at the edges of the graft and migrate centrally as revascularization progresses. This sequential change follows the time curve in which osteoblastic cells repopulate the graft from the peripheral portions. Nonetheless, skeletal scintigraphy is more sensitive than plain radiographs, CT, or MRI in monitoring this revascularization process. Magnification and SPECT images may be necessary to separate the peripheral osseous activity from the adjacent normal bone and soft tissue activity for full evaluation.

SOFT TISSUE ACCUMULATION

In the normal patient, the only soft tissue structures visualized are usually the kidney and bladder. Soft tissue background is usually slight, especially in younger patients who not only have good renal function and thereby excrete a large portion (40–50%) of the injected dose, resulting in efficient clearance of activity from soft tissues, but also high blood flow and metabolic activity in bone. As the patient population ages, generalized soft tissue background often increases, presumably as a result of the reduction in bone metabolism, osseous blood flow, and increasingly poor renal function. Diminished renal uptake may also be seen in the so-called superscan, but this is associated with low soft tissue background activity and increased skeletal uptake which reduced the amount of tracer available for renal excretion. The genitourinary system should be inspected on every bone imaging procedure to rule out the presence of space-occupying disease in the kidney or bladder, as well as distortion or displacement of these structures by extrarenal and extravesicular masses. A rough estimate of renal function can also be made on

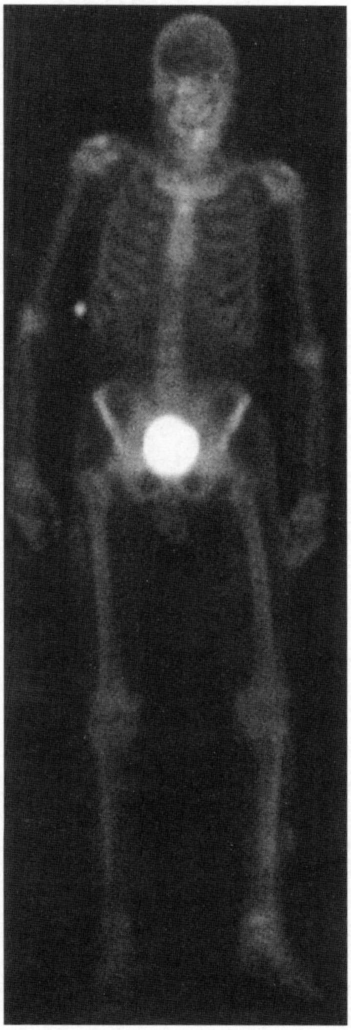

Figure 33.38. Bone graft. Anterior total body view in a 42-year-old male who is 3 months postradiotherapy and surgical excision of a squamous cell carcinoma of the mouth which involved the left mandible. An autograft from the left fibula was used to reconstruct the mandible. Note the activity in the left mandibular graft indicating viability and the activity in the left fibula at the site from which the graft was removed.

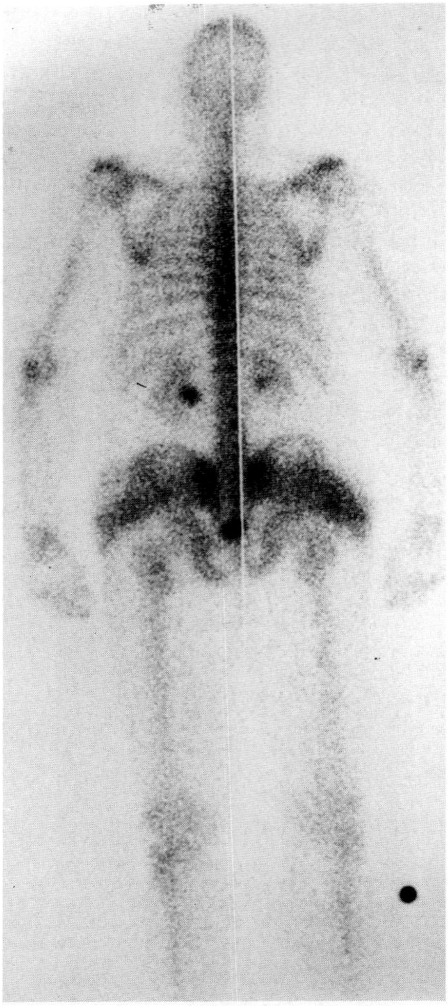

Figure 33.39. Soft tissue activity with iron dextran injection. Posterior total body view from ^{99m}Tc-MDP study performed in a 57-year-old male with iron-deficiency anemia and back pain. He had been receiving intramuscular injections of iron dextran in both buttocks. Note the soft tissue activity in the buttocks corresponding to the injection sites.

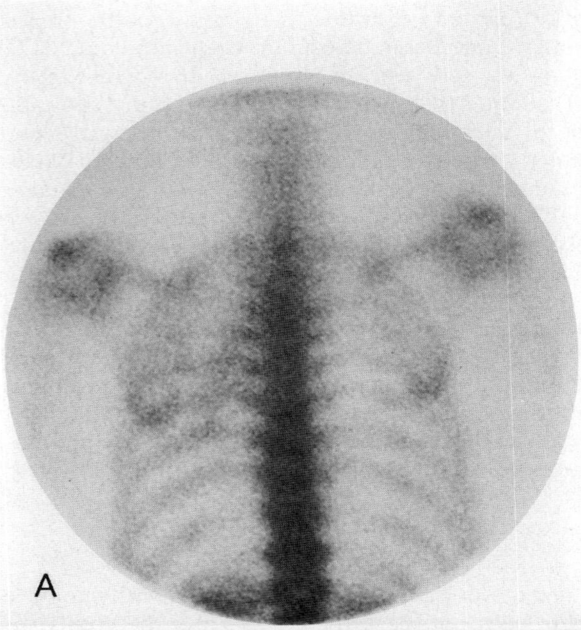

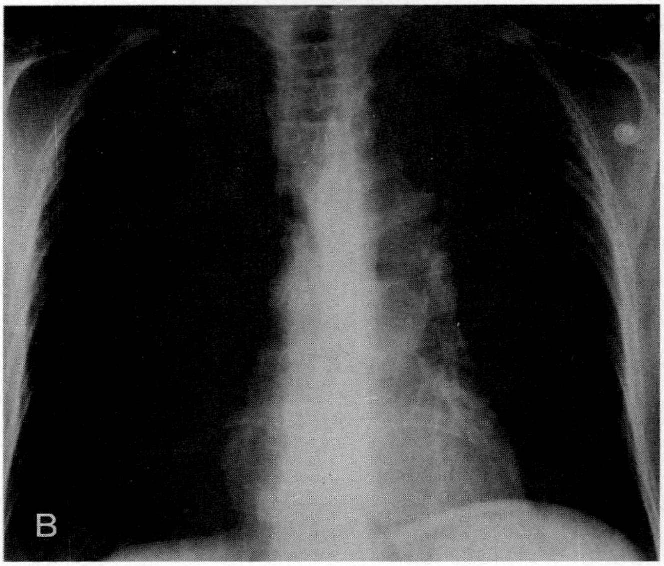

Figure 33.40. Soft tissue activity with carcinoma of lung. Posterior view of the thorax (**A**) in a 47-year-old male demonstrating abnormal activity in the left hilum corresponding to the radiographic demonstration of this patient's carcinoma of the lung (**B**).

these studies. Diffusely increased activity within the kidneys may be seen in conditions such as obstruction, amyloidosis, and sacroidosis, as well as after radiotherapy and/or chemotherapy.

The presence of abnormal activity in soft tissue is usually the result of either increased blood flow, calcification, irradiation, enzyme interaction, changes in endocrine function, tissue necrosis, or direct interaction with injectable pharmaceuticals such as iron dextran (Fig. 33.39). Tumors such as neuroblastoma, lymphoma, and lung carcinoma frequently show soft tissue accumulation (Fig. 33.40). Occasional soft tissue activity patterns may be seen in other tumors, but this is a much less common event (Fig. 33.41). Nonosseous uptake may be seen in soft tissues resulting from infarction or other vascular insult including heart, brain, gut, and muscle. Bone imaging is one of the most sensitive indicators of rhabdomyolysis (Fig. 33.42). The etiology of rhabdomyolysis includes trauma (runners), frostbite, and alcohol abuse. Intense increased perfusion of blood pool and delayed accumulation may also be seen in myositis ossificans (heterotopic bone formation) long before radiographic evidence of this process is found (Fig. 33.43). The three-phase bone scan may be used to assist the surgeon in planning when to surgically excise sites of heterotopic bone formation. The surgeons at our institu-

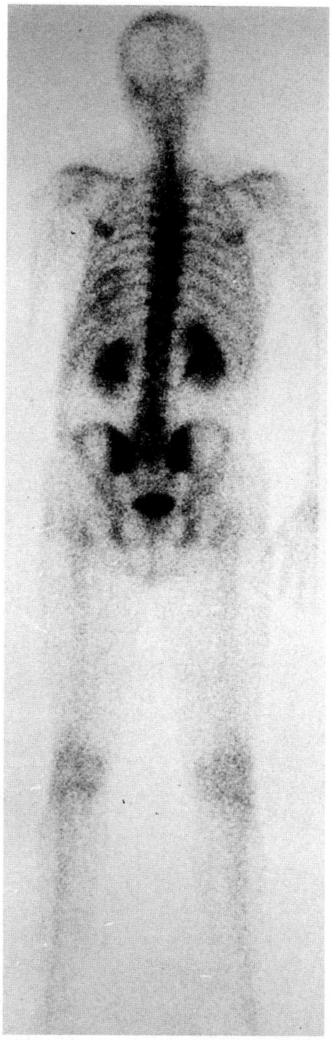

Figure 33.41. Soft tissue activity with colon carcinoma. Posterior total body image from study performed in a 46-year-old male with known carcinoma of the colon, now being evaluated for back pain. Note the abnormal increased activity in the liver. Routine liver imaging revealed multiple defects. Biopsy demonstrated metastatic adenocarcinoma of the colon.

tion usually wait until these areas have lost increased perfusion and delayed avidity for bone-seeking radiopharmaceuticals. Attempts at surgical removal before this usually results in recurrence of the process (Fig. 33.44). Increased amounts of bone-seeking radionuclides may be found in areas of inflammation and abscesses (Fig. 33.45). Increased activity in the breast may be seen in the normal female patient but may also be noted in patients with carcinoma of the breast, mastitis, trauma, or fibrocystic disease. In the male patient, breast activity is usually associated with gynecomastia. Diffuse abnormal activity may be seen in body cavities, such as the thorax, with pleural effusions, and in the abdomen and ascites (Fig. 33.46).

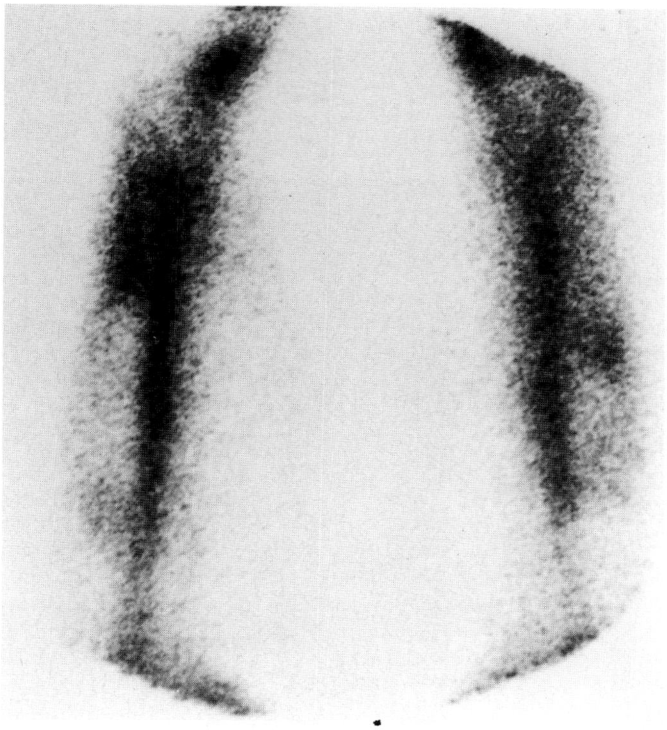

Figure 33.42. Rhabdomyolysis due to frostbite. Posterior views of the lower legs from routine bone imaging study demonstrates rhabdomyolysis of the calf muscles caused by exposure and frostbite. (Case courtesy of Dr. Herman Wallinga, The Genesee Hospital, Rochester, NY).

As discussed earlier, diffusely abnormal soft tissue activity may be seen in disease states such as hypo/hyperparathyroidism, scleroderma, polymyositis, and sickle cell long before they are evident on radiographs. Activity within the stomach may be the result of improper formulation of the bone-seeking complexes or a delay between preparation and patient injection as a result of oxidation of the radiopharmaceutical, but may also be the result of sacroidosis, amyloidosis, trauma, excessive use of antacids, hyperparathyroidism, patients on dialysis, and Retin A toxicity. Finally, one must always assure themselves that prior nuclear medicine procedures are not causing apparent soft tissue uptake on the bone scan.

A listing of conditions that will result in soft tissue localization is given in Table 33.3. This is, at best, a partial listing. It is constantly being enlarged. However, it is important that these causes of soft tissue localization of bone-seeking radiopharmaceuticals be kept in mind when bone imaging studies are reviewed so that mistakes in interpretation are not made. Additionally, proper attention to soft tissue activity patterns may result in a diagnosis being made.

SUMMARY

The use of bone imaging in benign disease has advanced rapidly in the past few years. However, in many instances,

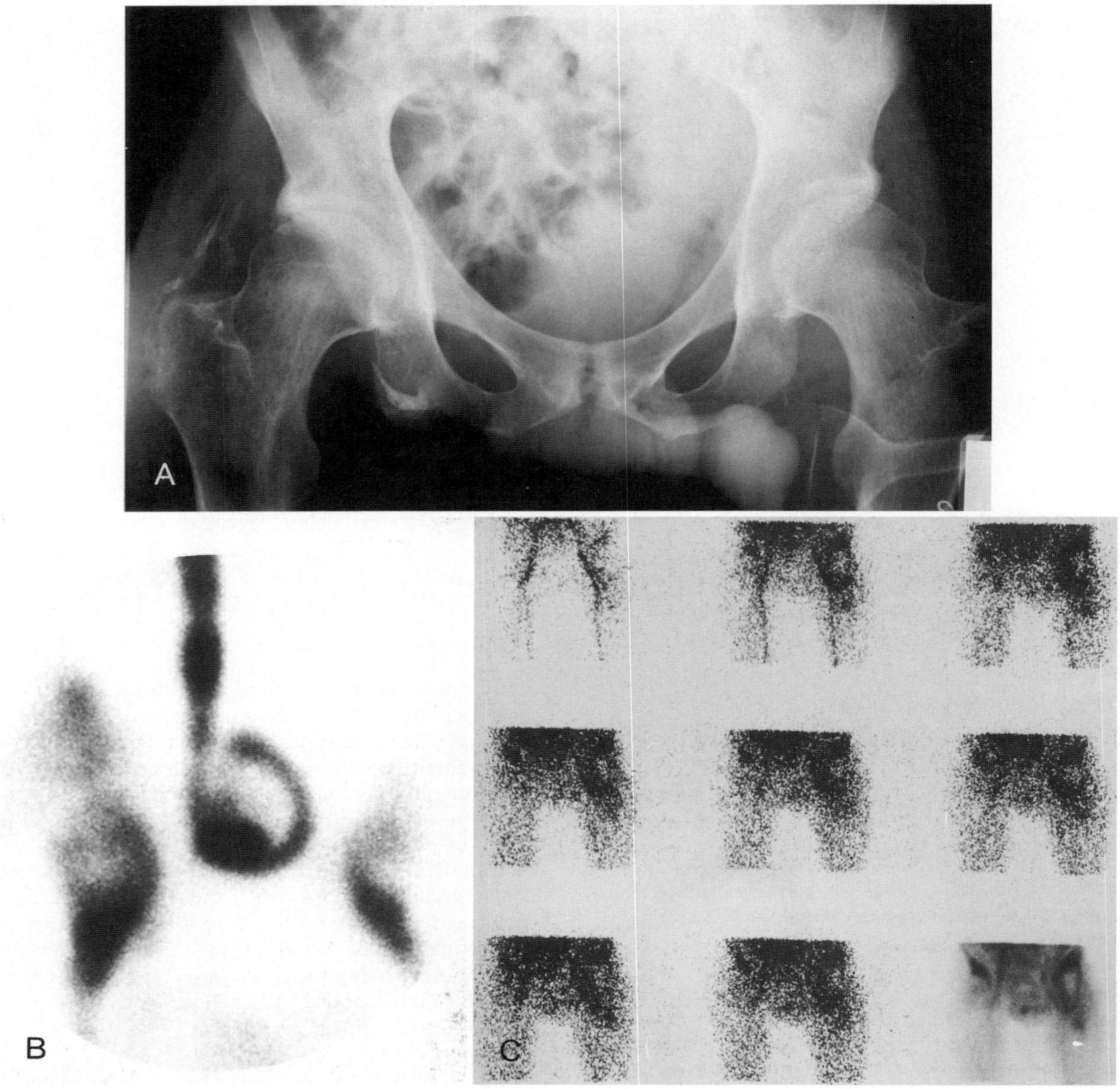

Figure 33.43. Soft tissue activity with myositis ossificans. A 21-year-old male with a 3-year history of paraplegia following cervical vertebral fracture. He recently complained of increased pain in both hips. **A.** The radiograph demonstrates myositis ossificans (PAO) about the right hip but nothing is seen in the soft tissues of the left hip. **B.** A perfusion study done during the administration of ^{99m}Tc-MDP demonstrates markedly increased perfusion to the soft tissues about the left hip and slight increased perfusion to the muscles of the right hip. **C.** Delayed image reveals markedly increased activity in the muscle and soft tissue of the left hip with much slighter amounts on the right. Despite radiotherapy this process continued and within 6 months muscular calcification was demonstrable on radiographs.

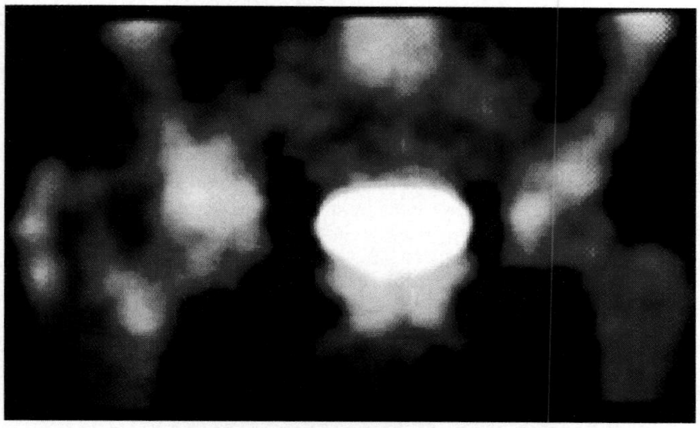

Figure 33.44. Heterotopic bone. Coronal reconstruction of SPECT exam of the pelvis in a 68-year-old male who suffered a femoral neck fracture 5 months before. He had undergone pinning but now complained of increasing pain. Note the increased soft tissue activity about the right hip which still exhibits osseous increase from the trauma and surgery. Note the bladder activity—the patient suffered bladder outlet obstruction from an enlarged prostate.

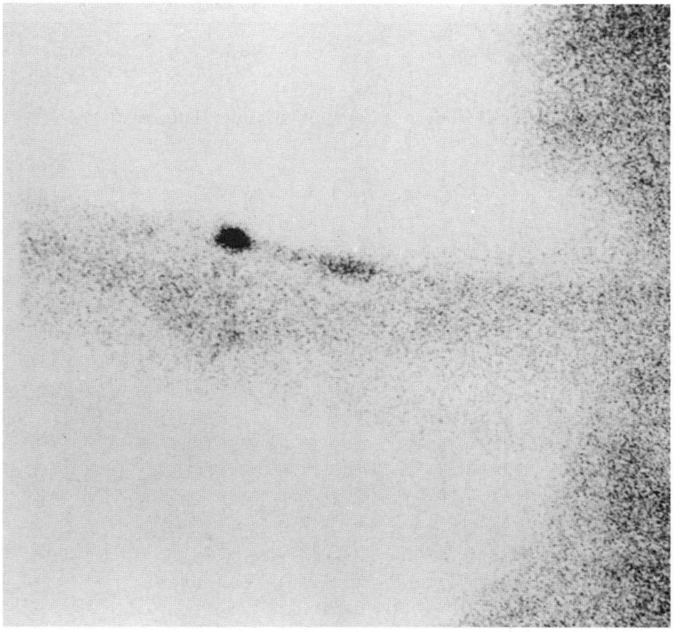

Figure 33.45. Soft tissue activity in thrombophlebitis. The left arm 1 hour after the injection of ^{99m}Tc-MDP into the antecubital fossa in a 51-year-old female. Note the slight extravasation in the injection site, followed by the linear activity along the basilic vein. This is the result of thrombophlebitis of this vein following placement and removal of a central venous pressure catheter.

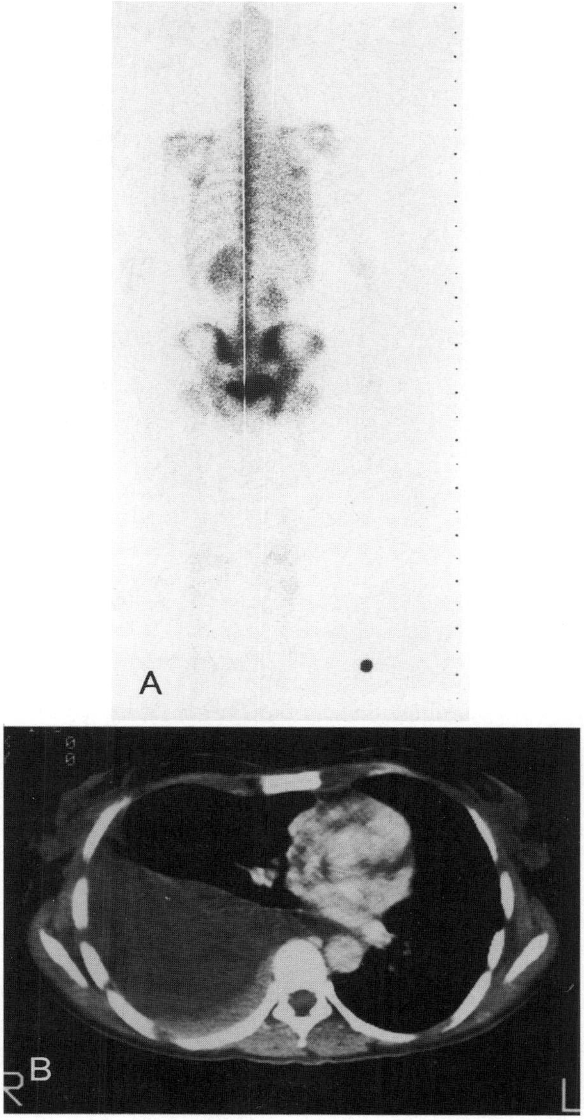

Figure 33.46. Activity in pleural effusion. **A.** Posterior total body view performed in a 51-year-old female being evaluated for possible metastatic carcinoma of the breast. Note the hazy density over the right hemithorax, a sign of pleural effusion. The patient's upright chest x-ray was normal. However, computed tomography of the chest revealed the large subpulmonic pleural effusion (**B**). (This probably could have been demonstrated more economically by the use of lateral decubitus views in chest radiography.)

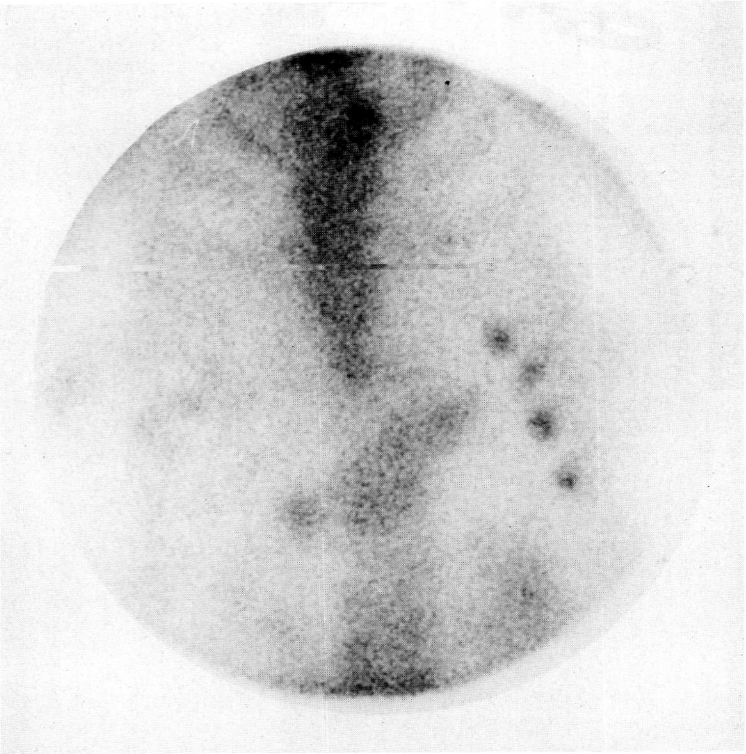

Figure 33.47. Gastric activity from trauma. 58-Year-old female who received a crushing injury to the chest from the steering wheel in a motor vehicle accident. Radiographs of the ribs were normal. The patient continued to complain of severe deep-seated lower back thoracic pain. This anterior view of the chest and abdomen was obtained 2 hours after injection of ^{99m}Tc pyrophosphate performed to evaluate possible myocardial damage. Note the increased activity at the anterior ends of the left rib cage and the diffuse activity seen throughout the stomach wall as a result of the blunt trauma.

Table 33.3.
Soft Tissue Accumulation of Bone Seeking Radiopharmaceuticals

Locations of normal accumulation
- Kidney
- Ureter
- Bladder
- Breast
- Cartilage-rib, thyroid cricoid
- Urine and salivary contamination

Abnormal accumulation
- Granuloma/fungal infections
- Inflammation/cellulitis
- Abscess
- Thrombophlebitis/vasculitis
- Tumors
  - Lung, lymphoma, neuroblastoma, breast, ovary, hemangioma, osteosarcoma, thyroid, fibroid, etc.
  - Soft tissue metastases from colon, pancreas, ovary, etc.
- Radiation treatment ports
- Infarction-heart, cerebral, muscle, gastrointestinal, splenic
- Fluid collections-effusions, ascites, edema, lymphedema
- Myositis ossificans, heterotopic bone formation
- Rhabdomyolysis, polymyositis, muscle trauma
- Healing wound
- Amyloidosis-heart, liver, kidneys, para-articular stomach
- Hyperthyroidism
- Scleroderma
- Dermatomyositis
- Sickle cell disease
- Uremia
- Fat necrosis
- Hepatic necrosis
- Hematoma
- Paraplelgic states
- Pseudogout
- Hypervitaminosis D; Retin A toxicity
- Heterotopic calcification and bone formation postoperatively
- Hypercalcemia
- Hemochromatosis
- Sarcoid
- Obesity
- Pulmonary microlithiasis
- Renal microlithiasis
- Calcified aneurysms
- Pseudoxanthoma elasticum
- Heart valve calcification
- Cutaneous calcinosis universalis
- Venous stasis or obstruction
- Adriamycin toxicity
- Congestive heart failure
- Dehydration
- Postsympathectomy
- Lymphedema
- Fibrocystic disease
- Iron dextran injection sites

Artifactual accumulation due to faculty preparation
- Thyroid, gut, salivary glands with free pertechnetate
- Liver/spleen with colloid formation
- Biliary system
- Renal
- Excess iron and blood (multiple transfusions)

Intra-arterial injection, injection sites, and lymph nodes following extravasation we are still only feeling our way in finding the advantages and disadvantages of this procedure in evaluating benign disease. It is to be expected that this process will continue to evolve. Nonetheless, skeletal imaging remains a valuable tool in the study of benign diseases provided good communication is established between the referring clinician and nuclear medicine physician to tailor the procedure to answer the clinical question. The exact role of radionuclide bone imaging in relationship to other imaging procedures such as standard radiography, CT, and MRI continues to evolve as progress is made in the development and application of all these modalities. It is imperative that the nuclear medicine physician remain knowledgeable about the advantages and disadvantages of the wide variety of imaging processes in the individual type of patients so that the best clinical and most economical decisions can be reached for the good of the patient. Attention to technical factors remains all important, as does continuing efforts to increase knowledge concerning the patterns of benign disease that may be presented by bone imaging.

ACKNOWLEDGMENT

I would like to thank Ms. Johanna Uncur for her valuable assistance and patience with me during the preparation of this manuscript.

REFERENCES

1. O'Mara RE, Wilson GA, Burke AM. The role of nuclear imaging in osteomyelitis. In: Raynaud C, ed. Nuclear medicine and biology. Proceedings of the Third World Congress of nuclear medicine and biology. Vol. I. Paris: Pergamon Press, 1982: 1094.
2. Ash JM, Gilday DL. Futility of bone scanning in neonatal osteomyelitis. Concise communication. J Nucl Med 1980;21:417.
3. Gilday DL, Paul DJ, Paterson J. Diagnosis of osteomyelitis in children by combined blood pool and bone imaging. Radiology 1975;117:331.
4. Bressler EL, Conway JJ. Bone scintigraphy in neonatal osteomyelitis. Radiology 1983;149:35, 291.
5. Bressler EL, Conway JJ, Weiss SC. Neonatal osteomyelitis examined by bone scintigraphy. Radiology 1984;152:65.
6. Graham GD, Lundy MM, Frederick RJ, et al. Scintigraphic detection of osteomyelitis with 99m-Tc MDP and 67-Ga citrate. J Nucl Med 1983;24:1019.
7. Handmaker H, Giammona ST. Improved early diagnosis of acute inflammatory skeletal articular diseases in children: a two radiopharmaceutical approach. Pediatrics 1984;73:661.
8. Rosenthall L. Radionuclide investigation of osteomyelitis. Curr Opin Radiol 1992;4:62.
9. Keenan AM, Tindel NL, Alavi A. Diagnois of pedal osteomyelitis in diabetic patients using current scintigraphic techniques. Arch Inter Med 1989;149:2262.
10. Howman-Giles R, Uren R. Multifocal osteomyelitis in childhood. Review by radionuclide bone scan. Clin Nucl Med 1992; 17:274.
11. Rosenthall L, Kloiber R, Damtew B, Al-Majid H. Sequential use of radiophosphate and radiogallium imaging in the differential diagnosis of bone, joint and soft tissue infection: quantitative analysis. Diagn Imaging 1982;51:249–258.
12. Wellman HN, Siddiqui AR, Mail JT, Georgi P. Choice of radiotracer in the study of bone or joint infection in children. Ann Radiol (Paris) 1983;26:411–420.
13. Wellman HN, Georgi P, Sinn H, Scheer. Scintimaging of keletal infectious processes with a new leukocyte labeling technique utilizing In-111 acetylacetone. J Nucl Med 1981;22:27.
14. Raptopoulis V, Doherty PW, Goss TP, King MA, Johnson K, Gantz NM. Acute osteomyelitis: advantage of white cell scans in early detection. AJR 1982;139:1077.
15. McDougall IR, Raumert JE, Lantieri RL. Evaluation of 111-In leukocyte whole-body scanning. AJR 1979;133:849.
16. Guze BH, Webber MM, Hawkins, RA, Sinha K. Indium-111 white blood cell scans: sensitivity, specificity, acuracy, and normal patterns of distribution. Clin Nucl Med 1990;5:8.
17. Schauwecker DS. Osteomyelitis. Diagnosis with In-111 labeled leukocytes. Rad 1989;171:141.
18. Datz FL, Thorne DA. Effect of antibiotic therapy on the sensitivity of indium-111 labeled leukocyte scans. J Nucl Med 1986; 27:1849–1953.
19. Peters AM. The utility of ^{99m}TcHMPAO-leukocytes for imaging infection. Semin Nucl Med 1994;24:2:110.
20. Schauwecker DS. The scintigraphic diagnosis of osteomyelitis. AJR 1992;158:9.
21. Lind P, Langsteger W, Koltringer P, Diami HP, Passl R, Eber O. Immunoscintigraphy of inflammatory process with a technetium-99m-labeled monoclonal antigranulocyte antibody (Mab BW 250/183). J Nucl Med 1990;31:417–423.
22. Seybold K, Locher JT, Cossemans C, Andres, RY, Schubiger PA, Blauenstein P. Immunoscintigraphic localization of inflammatory lesions: clinical experience. Eur J Nucl Med 1988;13:587–593.
23. Kroiss A, Bock F,Perneczyk G, Auinger C, Weidlich G, Kleinpeter G, et al. Clinical application of Tc-99m-labeled granulocytes antibody in bone and joint disease. Prog Clin Biol Res 1990; 355:337.
24. Hotze AL, Briele B, Overbeck B, et al. Technetium-99m-labeled anti-granulocyte antibodies in suspected bone infections. J Nucl Med 1992;33:526.
25. Oyen WJ, Claessens RA, van Horn JR, vander Meer JW. Scintigraphic detection of bone and joint infections with indium-111-labeled nonspecific polyclonal human immunoglobulin G. J Nucl Med 1990;31:403.
26. Fischman AJ, Rubin RH, Khaw BA, et al. Detection of acute inflammation with In-111 labeled nonspecific polyclonal IgG. Semin Nucl Med 1988;18:335–334.
27. Littenberg B, Mushlin AI. Technetium bone scanning in the diagnosis of osteomyelitis: a meta-analysis of test performance. Diagnostic technology assessment consortium. J Gen Intern Med 1992;7:158–164.
28. Splittgerber GF, Spiegelhoff DR, Buggy BP. Combined leukocyte and bone imaging used to evaluate diabetic osteoarthropathy and osteomyelitis. Clin Nucl Med 1989;14:156–60.
29. Gandsman EJ, Deutsch SD, Kahn CB, McCullough RW. Differentiation of Charcot joint from osteomyelitis through dynamic bone imaging. Nucl Med Commun 1990;11:45–53.
30. Zeiger LA, Fox IM. Use of indium-111-labeled white blood cells in the diagnosis of diabetic foot infections. J Foot Surg 1990; 29:46–51.
31. Choong K, Monaghan P, McGaigan L, McLean, R, Department of Nuclear Medicine, St. George Hospital, Kogarah, NSW, Australia. Role of bone scintigraphy in the early diagnosis of discitis. Ann Rheum Dis 1990;49:932–934.
32. Nolla-Sole JM, Mateo-Soria L, Rozadilla-Sacanall A, Mora-Salvador J, Valverde-Garcia J, Roig-Escofet D. Role of technetium-99m diphosphonate and gallium-67 citrate bone scanning in the early diagnosis of infectious spondylodiscitis. A comparative study. Ann Rheum Dis 1992;51:665–657.
33. Whalen JJL, Brown ML, McLeod R, Fitzgerald RH Jr. Limitations of indium leukocyte imaging for the diagnosis of spine infections. Spine 1991;16:193–197.

34. Eisenberg B, Powe JE, Alavi A. Cold defects in In-111-labeled leukocyte imaging of osteomyelitis in the axial skeleton. Clin Nucl Med 1991;16:103–106.
35. Jacobson AF, Gilles CP, Cerqueira MD. Photopenic defects in marrow containing skeleton on indium-111 leukocyte scintigraphy: prevalance at sites suspected of osteomyelitis and as an incidental findings. E J Nucl Med 1992;19:858–864.
36. King AD, Peters AM, Stuttle AW, Lavender JP. Imaging of bone infection with labelled white blood cells: role of contemporaneous bone marrow imaging. E J Nucl Med 1990;17:148–151.
37. Palestrao CJ, Roumanas P, Swyer AJ, Kim CK, Goldsmith SJ. Diagnosis of musculoskeletal infection using combined In-111 labeled leukocyte and Tc-99m SC marrow imaging. Clin Nucl Med 1992;17:269–273.
38. Kim EE, Haynie TP, Podoloff DA, Lowry PA, Harle TS. Radionuclide imaging in the evaluation of osteomyelitis and septic arthritis. Crit Rev Diagn Imaging 1989;29:257–305.
39. Lantoo T, Kaukonen JP, Kokkola A, Laitinen R, Vorne M. Tc-99m HMPAO labeled leukocytes superior to bone scan in the detection of osteomyelitis in children. Clin Nucl Med 1992;17:7–10.
40. Copping C, Dalgiesh SM, Dudley NJ, et al. The role of ^{99m}Tc-HMPAO white cell imaging in suspected orthopaedic infection. Br J Radiol 1992;65:309–12.
41. Verlooy H, Mortelmans L, Verbruggen A, Stuyck J, Boogaerts M, DeRoo M. Tc-99m HM-PAO labelled leucocyte scanning for detection of infection in orthopedic surgery. Prog Clin Biol Res 1990;355:181–187.
42. Bessette PR, Hanson MJ, Czarnicki DJ, Yuille DL, Rankin JJ. Evaluation of postoperative osteomyelitis of the sternum comparing CT and dual Tc-99m MDP bone and In-111 WBC SPECT. Clin Nucl Med 1993;18:197–202.
43. Al-Sheikh W, Sfakianakis GN, Hourani M, et al. A prospective comparative study of the sensitivity and specificity in In-111 leukocyte, gallium 67-citrate and bone scintigraphy and roentgenograms in the diagnosis of osteomyelitis with and without orthopedic prosthesis. J Nucl Med 1982;23:29.
44. Kim HC, Alavi A, Russell MD, Schwartz E. Differentiation of bone and bone marrow infarcts from osteomyelitis in sickle cell disorders. Clin Nucl Med 1989;14:249–254.
45. Fernandez-Ulloa M, Vasavada PJ, Black RR. Detection of acute osteomyelitis with indium-111-labeled white blood cells ina patient with sickle cell disease. Clin Nucl Med 1989;14:97–100.
46. Kolyoas E, Rosenthal L, Ahronheim GA, et al. Serial 67-Ga-citrate imaging during treatment of acute osteomyelitis in childhood. Clin Nucl Med 1978;3:461.
47. Graham GD, Lundy MM, Moreno AJ, Frederick RJ. The role of Tc-99m MDP and Ga-67 citrate in predicting the cure of osteomyeliltis. Clin Nucl Med 1983;8:344.
48. Newman, LG, Waller J, Palestro CJ, Schwartz M, Klein MJ, Hermann G, et al. Unsuspected osteomyelitis in diabetic foot ulcers. Diagnosis and monitoring by leukocyte scanning with indium-111 oxyquinoline. JAMA 1991;266:1246–1251.
49. Bauer G, Weber DA, Ceder L, et al. Dynamics of Tc-99m methylenediphosphonate imaging of the femoral head following hip fracture. Clin Orthop 1980;152:85.
50. Gregg PJ, Walder DN. Scintigraphy versus radiography in early diagnosis of experimental bone necrosis with special reference to Caisson disease of bone. J Bone Joint Surg 1980; 62B:214.
51. Uren RF, Howman-Giles R. The cold hip sign on bone scan. A retrospective review. Clin Nucl Med 1991;16:553–556.
52. Danigelis JA. Pinhole imaging in Legg-Perthes disease: further observations. Semin Nucl Med 1976;17:184.
53. Murray IP, Dixon J. The role of single photon emission computed tomography in bone scintigraphy. Skeletal Radiol 1989;18:493.
54. Krasnow AZ, Collier SD, Peck DC, et al. The value of oblique angle reorientation in SPECT bone scintigraphy of the hips. Clin Nucl Med 1990;15:287.
55. Kim KY, Lee SH, Moon DH, Nah HY. The diagnostic value of the triple-head single photon emission computed tomography (3H-SPECT) in avascular necrosis of the femoral head. Int Orthop 1993;17:132–138.
56. Conway JJ, Weiss SC, Maldonadov U. Scintigraphic patterns in Legg-Calve-Perthes disease. Radiology 1983;149P:102.
57. Lausten GA, Christensen SB, Distribution of 99mTc-phosphate compounds in osteonecrotic femoral heads. Acta Orthop Scand 1989;60:419–423.
58. Alavia A, Mitchell M, Kundelh H, et al. Comparison of RN, MRI, and XCT imaging in the diagnosis of avascular necrosis of the femoral head. J Nucl Med 1986;27:1952.
59. Cahill BR, Phillips MR, Navarro R. The results of conservative management of juvenile osteochondritis dissecans using joint scintigraphy. A prospective study. Am J Sports Med 1989; 17:601–605.
60. Sutherland AD, Savage JP, Paterson DC, et al. The nuclide bone scan in the diagnosis and management of Perthes' disease. J Bone Joint Surg 1980;147:221.
61. Mortensson W, Rosenborg M, Gretzer H. The role of bone scintigraphy in predicting femoral head collapse following cervical fractures in children. Acta Radiol 1990;31:291–292.
62. Stromquist B. Femoral head vitality after intracapsular hip fracture. 490 cases studied by intravital tetracycline labeling and Tc-MDP radionuclide imaging. Acta Orthop Scan 1983;54(Suppl 200).
63. Hoffer PB, Genant HK. Radionuclide joint imaging. Semin Nucl Med 1976;6:121.
64. Weissberg DL, Resnick D, Taylor A, et al. Rheumatoid arthritis and its variants: anaysis of scintiphotographic, radiographic and clinical examinations. Am J Roentgenol 1978;131:665.
65. Greyson ND. Radionuclide bone and joint imaging in rheumatology. Bull Rheumat Dis 1980;30:1034.
66. Khalkhali I, Stadalnik RC, Weisner KB, et al. Bone imaging of the heel in Reiter's syndrome. Am J Roentgenol 1979;132:110.
67. Sewell JR, Balck CM, Chapman AH, Stratham J, Hughes GRD, Lavender JP. Quantitative scintigraphy in diagnosis and management of plantar fasciitis. J Nucl Med 1980;21:633.
68. Ho G Jr, Sadovnikoff N, Malhotra CM, et al. Quantitative sacroiliac joint scintigraphy: clinical assessment. Arthritis Rheum 1979;22:837.
69. Domeij-Nyberg B, Kjallman M, Nylen O, et al. The reliability of quantitative bone scanning in sacroiliitis. Scand J Rheumatol 1980;9:77.
70. Katzberg RW, O'Mara RE, Tallent RH, Weber DA, Miller TL, Wilson GA. Radionuclide skeletal imaging and single photon emission computed tomography in suspected internal derangements of the temporomandibular joint. J Oral Maxillofac Surg 1984; 42:782.
71. Resnick D, Williamson S, Alazraki N. Focal spinal abnormalities on bone scans in ankylosing spondylitis. Clin Nucl Med 1981; 6:213.
72. Thomas RH, Resnick D, Alazraki NP, et al. Compartmental evaluation of osteoarthritis of the knee. Radiology 1975; 116:585.
73. Collier BD, Johnson RP, Carrera GF, et al. Chronic knee pain assessed by SPECT: comparison with other modalities. Radiology 1985;157:795.
74. McAfee JG. Radionuclide imaging in metabolic and systemic skeletal diseases. Semin Nucl Med 1987;17:334.
75. Clarke SE, Fogelman I. Bone scanning in metabolic and endocrine bone disease. Endocrinol Metab Clin North Am 1989; 18(4):977–993.

76. Fogelman I, Bessent RG, Gordon D. A critical assessment of bone scan quantitation (bone to soft tissue ratios) in the diagnosis of metabolic bone disease. Eur J Nucl Med 1981;6:93.
77. Fogelman I, Hay ID, Citrin DL, et al. Semiquantitative analysis of the bone scan in acromegaly: correlation with human growth hormone values. Br J Radiol 1980;53:974.
78. Worth DP, Smye SW, Robinson PJ, Davison AM, Will EJ. Quantiative bone scanning in the diagnosis of aluminum osteomalacia. Nephrol Dial Transplant 1989;4:721–724.
79. Rubini G, Lauriero F, Rubini D, D'Addabbo A. ^{99m}Tc-MDP global skeletal uptake and markers of bone metabolism in patients with bone diseases. Nucl Med Commun 1993;14:567–572.
80. Reschini E, Ulivieri FM, Ortolani S. Clinical experience with two simple methods of measurement of ^{99m}Tc-methylene diphosphonate body retention in bone disease. J Nucl Biol Med 1991; 35:123–130.
81. Novikov AI, Ermolenko AE, Ermakova IP, Baeva LB, Levitskii ER. Dynamic scintigraphy with sodium 1-hydroxy-ethane-1,1 diphosphonate for the differential diagnosis of osteomalacia in patients in the terminal stage of chronic kidney failure. Urol Nefrol 1990;11–15.
82. Ohashi K, Smith HS, Jacobs MP. "Superscan" appearance in distal renal tubular acidosis. Clin Nucl Med 1991;16:318–320.
83. Kitamura N, Wada S, Hayama K, et al. Study on renal osteodystrophy using 2-compartment model analysis of bone scintigraphy. Clincial significance of K index. Shigaku-Odontology 1989; 77:983–995.
84. Israel O, Kleinhaus U, Keren R, Frankel A, Front D. The 24 hour/ 4 hour ratio (T/F ratio) of Tc-99m MDP uptake in patients with bone metastases and degenerative changes. J Nucl Med 1984; 25:77.
85. Isaia GC, Salamano G, Mussetta M, Molinatti GM. Photon densitometry in the diagnosis of osteoporosis. Minerva Endocrinol 1991;16:93–99.
86. Valkema R, Verheij LF, Blokland JA, et al. Limited precision of lumbar spine dual-photon absorptiometry by variations in the soft-tissue background. J Nucl Med 1990;31:1774–1781.
87. Fogelman I. An evaluation of the contribution of bone mass measurements to clinical practice. Semin Nucl Med 1989;19:62–68.
88. Ryan PJ, Evans P, Gibson T, Fogelman I. Osteoporosis and chronic back pain: a study with single-photon emission computed tomography bone scintigraphy. J Bone Miner Res 1992; 7:1455–1460.
89. Bergot C, Laval-Jeantet AM, Laval-Jeantet MH, Kuntz D. Measurement of vertebral bone density. Quantitative tomodensitometry or dual-photon absorptiometry? J Radiol 1993;74:195–204.
90. Iancu TC, Almagor G, Friedman E, et al. Chronic familial hyperphosphatasemia. Radiology 1978;129:669.
91. O'Mara RE, Pinals RS. Bone scanning in regional migratory osteoporosis. Radiology 1970;97:579.
92. Bray ST, Partain CL, Teates CD, et al. The value of the bone scan in idiopathic regional migratory osteoporosis. J Nucl Med 1979; 20:1268.
93. Kozin F. Soin JS, Ryan LM, et al. Bone scintigraphy in the reflex sympathetic dystrophy syndrome. Radiology 1981;138:437.
94. Ali A, Tetalmin MR, Fordham EW, et al. Distribution of hypertrophic pulmonary osteoarthropathy. Am J Roentgenol 1980; 134:771.
95. Vaquer RA, Dunn EK, Bhat S, Heurich AE, Kamholz SL, Strashun AM. Reversible pulmonary uptake and hypertrophic pulmonary osteoarthropathic distribution of technetium-99m methylene diphosphonate in a case of Pneumocystis carinii pneumonia. J Nucl Med 1989;30:1563–1567.
96. Lavendar JP, Evans MA, Arnot R, et al. A comparison of radiography and radioisotope scanning in the detection of Paget's disease and in the assessment of response to human calcitonin. Br J Radiol 1977;50:243.
97. Wioland M. Bonnerot V. Diagnosis of partial and total physeal arrest by bone single-photon emission computed tomography. J Nucl Med 1993;34:1410–1415.
98. Chaudhuri TK, Fink S. Radionuclide imaging in osteitis deformans. Am J Physiol Imaging 1990;5:42–45.
99. Boudreau RJ, Llisbona R, Hadjiipavlou A. Observations on serial radionuclide blood flow studies in Paget's disease. J Nucl Med 1981;22:510.
100. Brixen K, Hansen HH, Mosekilde L, Halaburt H. SPECT bone scintigraphy in assessment of cranial Paget's disease. Acta Radiologica 1990;31:549–550.
101. Patel U, Gallacher SJ, Boyle IT, McKillop JH. Serial bone scans in Paget's disease: development of new lesions, natural variation in lesion intensity and nature of changes seen after treatment. Nucl Med Commun 1990;11:747–760.
102. Ryan PJ, Gibson T, Fogelman I. Bone scintigraphy following intravenous pamidronate for Paget's disease of bone. J Nucl Med 1992;33:1589–1593.
103. Weber DA. The quantitative measurement of the response to treatment. Int J Rad Oncol Biol Phys 1976;1:1221.
104. Davis DC, Skylawer R, Cole RL. Melorheostosis on three-phase bone scintigraphy. Case report. Clin Nucl Med 1992;17:561–564.
105. Mahoney J. Acong DM. Demonstration of increased bone metabolism in melorheostosis by multiphase bone scanning. Clin Nucl Med 1991;16:847–848.
106. Adams BK, Smuta NA. The detection of extramedullary hematopoiesis in a patient with osteopetrosis. Eur J Nucl Med 1989; 15:803–804.
107. King MA, Weber DA, Casarett GW, et al. A study of irradiated bone. Part II: Changes in Tc-99m pyrophosphate bone imaging. J Nucl Med 1980;21:22.
108. King MA, Casarett GW, Weber DA, et al. A study of irradiated bone. Part III: Scintigraphic and radiographic detection of radiation induced osteosarcomas. J Nucl Med 1980;21:426.
109. Hattner RS, Hartmeyer J, Wara WM. Characterization of radiation-induced photopenic abnormalities on bone scans. Radiology 1982;145:161.
110. Dee P, Lambruschi PG, Hiebert JM. Use of ^{99m}Tc-MDP bone scanning in the study of vascularized bone implants. J Nucl Med 1981;22:522.
111. Stevenson JS, Bright RW, Dunson GL, et al. Technetium-99m phosphate bone imaging: a method of assessing bone graft healing. Radiology 1974;110:391.
112. Velasco JG, Vega A, Leisorek A. The early detection of free bone graft viability with ^{99m}Tc: a preliminary report. Br J Plast Surg 1976;29:344.

34 Athletic Injuries

LAWRENCE E. HOLDER

Insults to the skeletal system result in repair and remodeling which are generic and generally etiologically indistinguishable. Similarly, the movement and accumulation of tracer following the intravenous administration of ^{99m}Tc-labeled methylenediphosphonate or other similar radiopharmaceutical, reflects blood flow to bone (radionuclide angiogram or phase I), passive diffusion of tracer into the extravascular and extracellular spaces (blood pool, tissue phase, extracellular phase, or phase II), and the initial active accumulation of tracer thought to be associated with the hydration shell surrounding bone crystal (delayed images, metabolic images, or phase III), rather than the specific etiology which leads to the observed changes (1).

Athletic injuries are often separated as a subset of traumatic injury. Understanding the mechanisms of injury, which are often related to the actions and activities of a particular sport, allows for a more specific differential diagnosis. Placing the demonstrated blood flow, relative vascularity, and metabolic activity into the context of the athlete's training regimen, the level of his or her participation (professional, college, high school, recreational), and the athlete's short- and long-term goals, allows the nuclear physician to participate with the treating physician in patient care. Even if a specific diagnosis cannot be made, therapy can often be started if the site of increased bone turnover can be precisely located, and its degree of metabolic activity estimated. Appropriate additional anatomic imaging correlation can then be suggested (1–3).

Although correlative imaging is extremely important in routine practice, there are other sources for obtaining information about the use of plain radiography, CT scanning, and MR imaging in the sports medicine setting (3). This chapter emphasizes the indications for scintigraphy and the interpretation of scintigraphic images. Although three-phase bone imaging (TPBI) is primarily utilized when the clinical questions involve pain or symptoms of potentially osseous origin, those soft tissue components of injury which are encountered are also briefly discussed.

PATHOPHYSIOLOGIC AND BIOMECHANICAL CONSIDERATIONS

THREE-PHASE BONE IMAGING

Some controversy exists as to the appropriate indications for TPBI. Little disagreement remains in such areas as the differential diagnosis of cellulitis versus osteomyelitis (4), but when other problems that can be diagnosed with great sensitivity and specificity with the delayed image only, such as reflex sympathetic dystrophy (RSD), are suspected (5), the value of routine TPBI has been called into question (6, 7). TPBI in the sports medicine setting is important, because usually there is clinical uncertainty as to the etiology of the symptoms. Information about blood flow, vascularity, and metabolic activity allows for differential diagnosis as well as for the provision of physiologic information which, even without a specific diagnosis, can direct appropriate therapy (1, 8, 9). Rupani, et al. (9), and others (10) utilized the three phases to help date the injury. They expanded the earlier observations of Matin (11) regarding the relationship of fracture healing demonstrated on delayed bone imaging to the time after injury when imaging was performed.

Although the technical details of TPBI were described in Chapter 32, it is important to emphasize that, in general, spatial resolution should take precedence over temporal resolution in choosing acquisition parameters for the radionuclide angiogram, and that spatial resolution considerations demand the use of the highest resolution collimators possible for delayed images. The location of an abnormal focus of increased tracer is important in the effort to determine a specific etiology.

PERIOSTITIS/SHIN SPLINTS

Shin splints, or the medial tibial stress syndrome (12–14), have been defined as disruption of the Sharpey fiber-periosteum interface and result from abnormal excursion of the musculotendon complex, with pathologic and scintigraphic changes representing a periostitis. Other periosteal lesions, such as periostitis resulting from a direct blow to the shin by a lacrosse stick, for example, should not be confused with the shin splint lesion causing pain in the lower leg.

BIOMECHANICAL STRESS LESIONS

These are sports medicine's equivalents of the repetitive stress syndromes, such as the carpal tunnel syndrome, which affect the musculoskeletal system secondary to a wide range of activities (2, 15). In some cases, these lesions may represent enthesopathies or other more generic type stress responses of bones and joints, simply with a sports activity related etiology. An enthesis is the site of insertion of a tendon, ligament, or articular capsule into bone, with Resnik (16) suggesting that an alteration at these sites be termed enthesopathy.

AVULSION FRACTURE

Avulsion fractures are caused by the pull of a muscle or tendon and usually occur in younger, skeletally immature patients whose apophyseal attachments are less strong than their tendon-bone interfaces. Even after the physis appears closed radiographically, there is a relative weakness at this site for several years and avulsion fractures are occasionally seen after fusion of the apophysis. In the athletic setting, avulsion injuries also occur in the mature skeleton because of very strong concentrations of force associated with overstretched musculotendon complexes.

AVASCULAR NECROSIS

Sudden disruption of the blood supply to areas of bone without adequate collateral blood supply is an obvious etiology for avascular necrosis, as illustrated by the football injury sustained by Heisman trophy winner Bo Jackson. Less obvious, often repetitive microtraumatic episodes, also result in avascular injuries to bone (17). This topic is covered in Chapter 33.

BONE BRUISE

This is a nonspecific term most often used in the athletic setting to describe a focal, traumatic painful injury to bone, which does not have the clinical or imaging findings associated with more established or accepted lesions or syndromes, such as shin splints or stress fracture. Initially, a tiny focal area of increased tracer accumulation on a delayed bone scan image was postulated to represent some repair associated with minimal intraosseous bleeding or periosteal elevation (8). During MRI, a geographic, nonlinear area of marrow signal loss involving subcortical bone on T1-weighted images has also been termed a bone bruise (18). Postulations regarding underlying pathophysiology have included blood, edema, hyperemia, or microfractures. The radionuclide bone scan is used to determine the physiologic significance of nonspecific anatomic findings seen with other imaging modalities, and to detect foci of abnormal metabolism when such anatomic imaging modalities do not show lesions.

STRESS FRACTURES

Stress fractures in the athletic setting are most often fatigue fractures, associated with cyclic loading of normal bone. As the biomechanics become more understood, older, more situational subcategorizations, such as the novice syndrome or the overuse syndrome, are less often used (8). Damage to a small number of osteonal units can occur acutely as the applied stress exceeds the bone's inherent strength or when loading initiates appropriate remodeling, but continues or increases before remodeling is complete, with fatigue fracture occurring during the process.

TENDINITIS/STRAINS/MYOSITIS/BURSITIS

Primary soft tissue processes are occasionally demonstrated during TPBI when they are associated with increased perfusion or vascularity, which can be seen on Phase I or Phase II images, but most often are detected because of secondary changes to associated or underlying bone which lead to focal areas of increased tracer uptake on delayed images. The exact etiology of such uptake is uncertain (2). Some authors suggest that more intense diffuse uptake about the lateral ligaments of the ankle is related to more severe injury and might warrant more aggressive therapy (19). Direct localization of labeled bone tracers in injured muscle, whether in the process of resolving or progressing to myositis ossificans or heterotopic bone formation (HBF), is not an uncommon finding when evaluating athletes for pain. Baker (20) reviewed clinical concepts in the diagnosis and treatment of musculotendinous injuries. He defined strain as a stretch or tear of a musculotendinous unit. A first degree strain involves minimal stretching; second degree strain indicates partial tearing; and a third degree strain indicates complete disruption of a portion of this unit. The bleeding and pathophysiologic sequela underlie tracer uptake in the injured muscle. Early work by Siegel, et al. (21), which still appears valid, suggested that uptake of ^{99m}Tc-diphosphonate in acutely damaged skeletal muscle is directly related to the deposition of calcium salts within the injured muscle fibers.

A bursa is a synovial membrane sac located about a joint or at a bony prominence where muscle or tendon movement occurs. When inflamed, the bursa is a source of pain. Most episodes of bursitis are not imaged acutely, but when bursitis is detected on delayed bone scan images as a focus of abnormal increased activity in the subadjacent bone, it can be implicated as a source of the patient's pain. The mechanism of tracer uptake in calcific bursitis is probably similar to that in lesions like myositis or calcifying hematomas, while the pathophysiology of direct bone uptake is not understood but is probably similar to the increased delayed activity which is seen in association with tendinitis (3).

ANKLE AND FOOT

NAVICULAR STRESS FRACTURE

All types of injury involving the tarsal navicular, but especially stress fractures, are often symptomatic for months before the diagnosis is considered (22, 23). Running with abrupt stopping and starting, which occurs in athletes such as basketball players and racket sports participants, directs posterior to anterior force through the navicular. On delayed images, intense focal uptake involving the entire navicular is very characteristic (Fig. 34.1). Increased radionuclide angiogram and blood pool activity, in more acute cases reflecting the stage of healing, or, paradoxically, in later cases, reflecting nonunion and inflammatory stress change, are also often present. Plain radiographs taken in the anatomic AP projection (24) can be helpful, but CT scanning is more sensitive in confirming the fracture (25).

CALCANEAL STRESS FRACTURE

Calcaneal stress fractures are relatively uncommon in athletes when compared to the number of fractures in the long bones of the legs. As with other fractures which occur in in cancellous bone, the initial radiographic appearance of minimal increased bone density, with an appearance which is often described as fluffy coalescence, is subtle. This fracture is often first diagnosed when the foot is imaged for unexplained pain. Focal linear increased tracer accumulation is most often located in the superior mid-

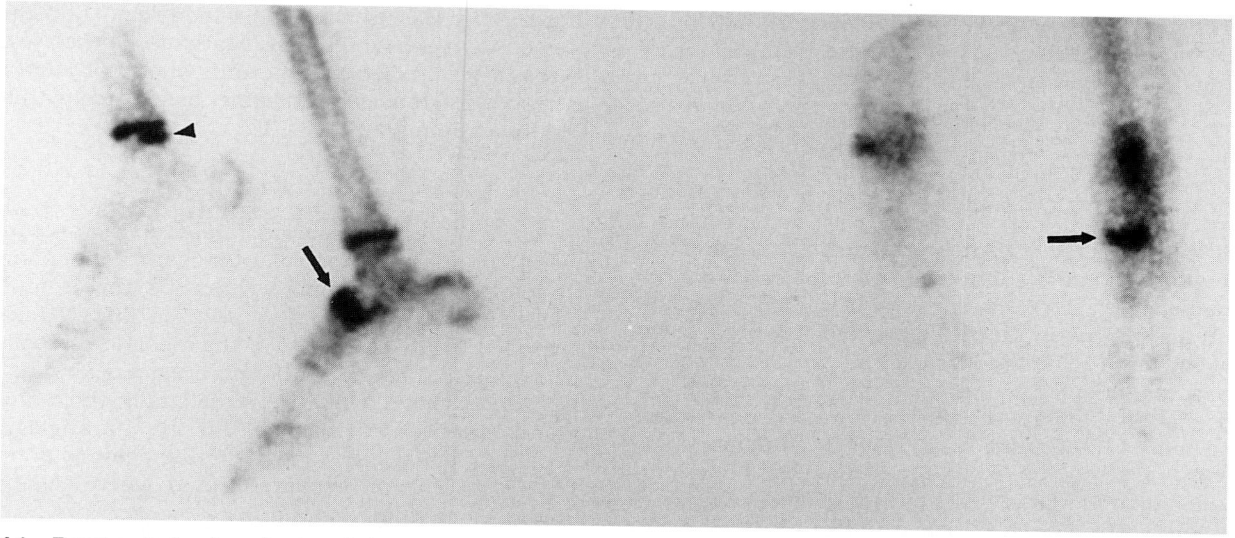

Figure 34.1. Tarsal navicular stress fracture. Delayed plantar (*right*) and right medial, left lateral (*left*) images. Moderately intense, focal increased tracer accumulation defines the entire tarsal navicular (*short arrows*). Physeal activity in the distal fibula is best seen on the left lateral view (*arrowhead*).

portion of the calcaneus. Because standard acquisition techniques often result in intense activity involving the entire bone, computer manipulated images are particularly important to illustrate the focal and more linear pattern of tracer uptake which would strongly suggest the diagnosis (2, 8, 26). Pain with calcaneal stress fractures is often medial or lateral rather than on the plantar surface, with physical examination producing pain when the heel is squeezed from the sides (27).

METATARSAL STRESS FRACTURE

The distribution of metatarsal stress fractures in athletes is similar to those reported in military recruits (28). Most commonly occurring in the second, third, and fourth metatarsals, these stress fractures are similar to those in other long cortical bones. Particularly when background-subtracted delayed images are obtained, the uptake is focal and fusiform. In the first metatarsal, where much of the weight bearing affects cancellous bone rather than cortical bone, the abnormal activity on the bone scan image is often more horizontal or perpendicular to the direction of stress (8, 29). Morton originally discussed foot problems in association with shortness and hypermobility of the first metatarsal segment, which resulted in the second distal phalanx projecting more distally than the first. A statistical analysis of metatarsal stress fractures by Drez, et al. (30), did not support the contention that a short first metatarsal is associated with metatarsal stress fractures. Because of differences in treatment between fractures of the tuberosity of the fifth metatarsal and of the metatarsal shaft within 1.5 cm of the tuberosity (31), it is important to use background-subtracted images to precisely locate the site of the fracture and to communicate its specific location to the clinician.

STUBBING INJURIES TO THE HALLUX

Stubbing injuries to the hallux, as reported by Jahss (32) in 1981, are less common than capsular and tendon injuries of the metatarsophalangeal joint, which are commonly associated with sports. These injuries are often termed turf-toe, referring to a sprain of the metatarsophalangeal joint occurring as a result of an injury on one of the newer artificial playing surfaces (33). The turf-toe will be swollen and tender but is usually stable to stress. The stubbing fracture tends to occur more often when a youngster is running barefoot. As emphasized by Pinckney, et al. (34), when Salter I type fractures do occur, they should be considered compound and prophylactically treated with antibiotics. TPBI, which confirms active bone disease, may have to be supplemented by ^{67}Ga-citrate imaging for further differential diagnosis if there is a reason not to give antibiotics (34).

OS TRIGONUM SYNDROME

The os trigonum is an accessory ossicle located at the posterior aspect of the talus (35). When posterior ankle pain is present, especially if the pain is increased with flexion of the great toe, the diagnostic considerations of the visualized ossicle are a normal os trigonum, a fracture of the posterior process of the talus, a bruised ossicle, and disruption of fibrous fusion of the ossicle. Focal increased tracer on delayed images suggests that whatever the underlying etiology, this ossicle is the source of pain (2). Surgical removal is often necessary for relief of pain.

TIBIOTALAR IMPINGEMENT SYNDROME

As described by Black and Brand (36), repetitive trauma occurs when the athlete "drives" off his planted foot and the anterior edge of the distal tibia impinges against the neck of the talus. O'Donoghue (37) originally described the biomechanics of this area. He pointed out that there actually is no true ligamentous attachment at either the anterior lip of the tibia or the sulcus into which it articulates at the top of the talus between the body and the head. He postulated, therefore, that spur formation was the result of direct trauma during forcible dorsiflexion of the foot on the leg. Abnormal increased tracer on delayed images localized to the osseous spurs, indicates that active repair is taking place and indirectly implies that the spur is the source of pain (Fig. 34.2).

RETROCALCANEAL BURSITIS

The retrocalcaneal recess is the radiolucent triangle at the inferior end of the preachilles fat pad located between the posterior aspect of the calcaneus and the achilles tendon. This bursa is also often called the preachilles bursa. Scintigraphically, on the delayed image increased activity can be seen in the inflamed bursa itself, possibly due to calcification, or, more commonly, in the adjacent posterosuperior aspect of the calcaneus (8) (Fig. 34.3). When combined with inflammation of the superficial bursa dorsal to the achilles tendon and achilles tendinitis itself, the diagnosis of Haglund's disease can be considered (3, 38).

ACHILLES TENDINITIS

The achilles tendon is formed from the fusion of the aponeurosis of the gastrocnemius muscle and the tendon of the soleus muscle. It is the thickest and strongest tendon in the body. It is anatomically called the calcaneal tendon and inserts into the middle part of the posterior surface of the calcaneus. Most often this insertion is visualized on delayed images as a focal area of increased tracer accumulation involving the bone (8). Occasionally posttraumatic calcification within the substance of the achilles tendon at the site of prior rupture may show some mildly increased tracer accumulation. Calcifications seen on radiographs at the insertion site, which do not take up tracer, are common in asymptomatic patients. These are thought to result from prior trauma and, when not metabolically active, by inference are no longer associated with the production of pain (8) (Fig. 34.3).

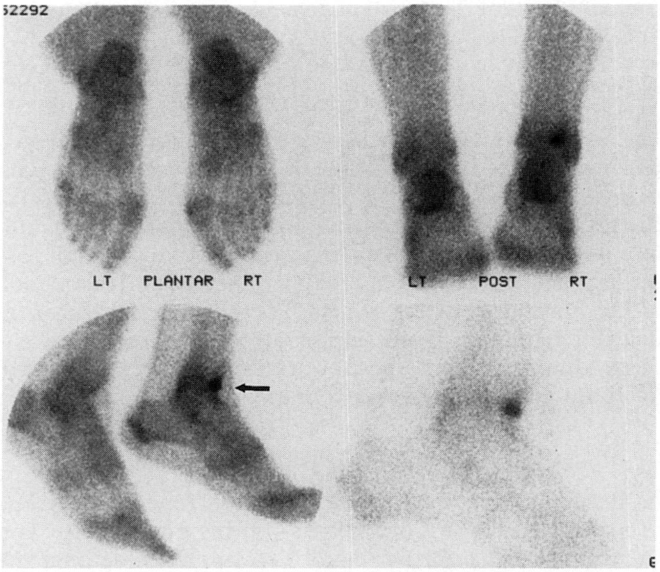

Figure 34.2. Tibiotalar impingement syndrome. Delayed images including a magnified right lateral view (*lower right*) demonstrate a tiny focus of moderately increased tracer accumulation associated with a hypertrophic spur at the anterior lip of the right tibia (*arrow*). (Reproduced by permission from Holder LE. Bone scintigraphy in skeletal trauma. RCNA 1993;31:739–781.)

PLANTAR FASCIITIS

Plantar fasciitis is a traumatic inflammation secondary to a strain or tear of the long plantar ligament or aponeurosis. The more typical pain, as well as the abnormal focal increased tracer accumulation seen on delayed images, is located at the fascial origin at the medial tuberosity of the calcaneus (Fig. 34.3). Although a calcaneal spur can be present, it is not diagnostic. Occasionally, the radionuclide bone scan will show abnormal tracer on the angiogram and blood pool phases, but most often imaging is done in patients with chronic symptoms and where the first two phases are normal (8).

MEDIAL MALLEOLAR STRESS FRACTURE

Another consideration in the athlete with pain over the medial malleolus, especially with an associated ankle effusion and a history of running, is a medial malleolar stress fracture (39). Because this diagnosis is based on focal abnormal tracer accumulation on delayed images without radiographic confirmation of fracture, the underlying process in some patients may be a bone bruise. Because successful nonsurgical therapy for this group has been described, further differential diagnostic efforts do not appear necessary. Schils, et al. (40), demonstrated intra-articular extension of the fracture into the tibial plafond in 7 patients with intense increased tracer accumulation.

OSTEOCHONDRAL FRACTURE OF THE TALAR DOME

As a not uncommon associated lesion in athletes who continue to complain of pain and disability after a "routine ankle sprain," osteochondral fractures of the talar dome can be suspected. Focal increased tracer accumulation, often subarticular, but also involving all of the posterior half of the talus is seen on delayed imaging (41). Confirmation and fracture staging can be provided by MR imaging in patients whose plain radiographs, even in retrospect, are normal (42).

LISFRANC FRACTURE

The original descriptions of fracture/dislocation of the tarsometatarsal (TMT) joint were reported in cavalry officers and subsequently in patients involved in motor vehicle and industrial accidents. Curtis, et al. (43), studied 20 patients who injured TMT joints during athletic activity. In most patients, the injuries occurred as a result of combined forced plantar flexion and rotation, with or without adduction of the forefoot. The injury is primarily a soft tissue disruption of the ligamentous support for the articulation but may include a fracture. Radionuclide bone imaging is important because in many of these patients the fracture is not seen during the initial workup and they are evaluated

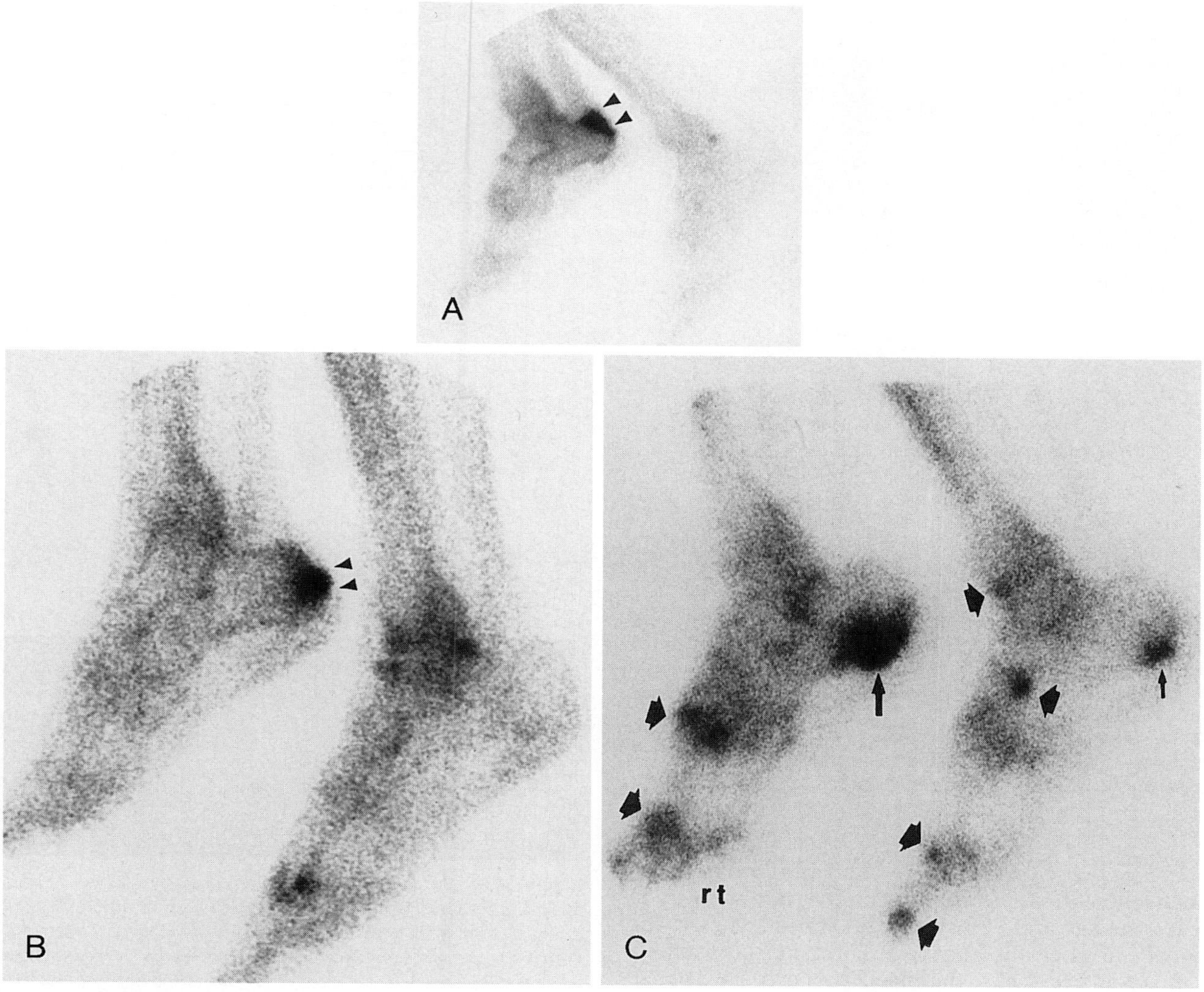

Figure 34.3. Retrocalcaneal bursitis, achilles tendinitis, and plantar fasciitis. **A.** Retrocalcaneal bursitis. Delayed lateral view demonstrates focally intense tracer accumulation in the retrocalcaneal bursa and underlying bone surface of the calcaneus (*arrowheads*). **B.** Lateral achilles tendinitis. Delayed lateral view demonstrates round, focally increased tracer accumulation in the posterior calcaneus at the junction of the middle and lower third at the insertion of the achilles tendon (*arrowheads*). **C.** Plantar fasciitis. Delayed lateral views demonstrate focally increased tracer accumulation in the posteroinferior portion of the calcaneus at the level of the medial tuberosity, right foot (*larger arrow*) greater than left foot (*smaller arrow*). *Small arrows* point to areas of nonspecific stress changes. (Reproduced by permission from Holder LE. Bone scintigraphy in skeletal trauma. RCNA 1993;31:739–781.)

later for pain of potentially osseous origin which is of uncertain etiology.

CUNEIFORM AND FIRST METATARSAL BASE STRESS FRACTURES

Because a large proportion of body weight passes through the base of the first metatarsal, this bone is susceptible to stress fractures of the compression type. Meurman and Elfing (44) suggest that the same biomechanical factors affect the first and largest cuneiform which is in the same axis and exposed to similar muscular forces. These types of injuries were common in a group of military recruits they reviewed, but they have also been noted in athletes and ballet dancers (44, 45). Although abnormal activity on routine delayed images can usually be localized to the specific tarsal bone or metatarsal base, because of the intensity of activity present in acute fractures, background subtracted images may be necessary for precise localization.

LOWER LEG

TIBIAL STRESS FRACTURE

Tibial stress fractures are most commonly detected on delayed bone scan images as solitary, focal, fusiform, longitudinally oriented areas of increased uptake involving the posterior medial cortex (Fig. 34.4). The original scintigraphic criteria for the diagnosis of stress fractures were based on descriptions published in the literature (46) and the results of TPBI in a highly selected subset of patients who were believed to have classic stress fractures by phys-

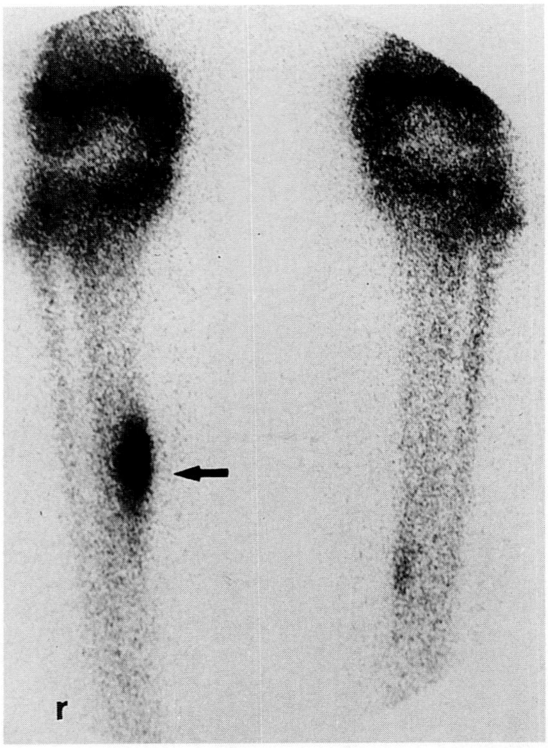

Figure 34.4. Tibial stress fracture. Delayed anterior image. Focal fusiform increased tracer in the middle third of the medial tibial cortex (*arrow*). The medial view (not shown) demonstrated a posterior cortical location of activity.

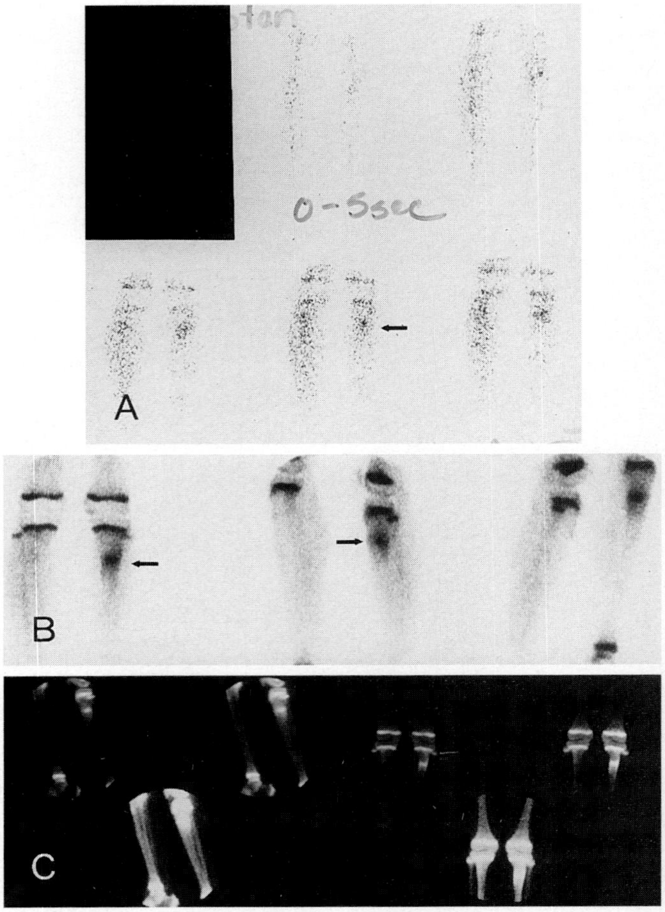

Figure 34.5. Proximal tibial stress fracture. **A.** Radionuclide angiogram. Minimal increased tracer in the proximal left tibia (*arrow*). **B.** Blood pool images, anterior, left lateral, right medial views. Moderately intense focal, increased tracer in the proximal left tibia (*arrow*). **C.** Delayed images, triple lens polaroid display. Anterior (*on right*) and left lateral, right medial (*on left*). Linear intense increased activity in the proximal tibia somewhat posteromedially. Blood pool and delayed images demonstrate increased vascularity and metabolic activity associated with the normal physes activity of the femur, tibia, and fibula. (Reproduced by permission from Holder LE. Bone scintigraphy in skeletal trauma. RCNA 1993;31:739–781.)

ical examination, clinical course, and abnormal radiographs on follow-up (9). Depending on the time of injury in relation to the age and severity of the stress fracture, the radionuclide angiograms may be abnormal for 2–4 weeks, with a mean of 2.9 weeks, the blood pool or tissue phase images abnormal for 1–8 weeks, with a mean of 5.2 weeks, and the delayed images abnormal for 3–36 weeks, with a mean of 11 weeks (9). Although there has been intermittent controversy about the specific scintigraphic pattern and its relationship to other bone stress lesions (47, 48), most authors agree with this classification (49, 50). The specific location of the stress fracture is certainly related to the biomechanics in the individual patient. Daffner, et al. (51), and Pilgaard, et al. (52), both reported stress fractures in the more proximal tibia, including the area along the popliteal-soleal line. Pilgaard, et al. (52), described bilateral stress fractures in the upper third of the tibia and emphasized, as did Devas (53) earlier that in children, stress fractures in the upper third of the tibia are relatively common (Fig. 34.5). In the reporting by Rupani, et al. (9), 42 were at the junction of the middle and distal third, 26 in the distal tibia, and 11 at the junction of the proximal and middle tibia. Transverse tibial stress fractures in adults are a special problem, because they have a tendency to result in nonunion (54).

Hulkko and Orava (55) emphasized that competitive athletes had stress fractures in the tibia significantly more often than recreational athletes, who had metatarsal bone and pelvic areas affected. In our view, recreational "joggers" who run many miles each day also fall into the competitive athlete category. Rosen, et al. (56), and Rupani, et al. (9), have emphasized the multiplicity of lesions, with both noting that many of the second and third lesions were asymptomatic.

FIBULAR STRESS FRACTURE

Fibular stress fractures are much less common than tibial stress fractures. They occur most often in the lower third of the bone, possibly secondary to stress resulting from the powerful contraction of the flexor muscles of the ankle and foot which approximate the fibula to the tibia. Devas and Symeoindes (57, 58) agree that excessive muscular force on the proximal fibula is the underlying mechanism. The focal fusiform increased tracer on delayed images does most often involve the posterior cortex, although even with good imaging technique, the smaller size of the fibula does not always allow separation of the anterior and posterior cortices as seen in tibial stress fractures (9) (Fig. 34.6). Fibular stress fractures are most often in the middle portion of the bone in athletes who run, whereas those involved in jumping sports show lesions higher in the fibula (58). Kottmeier, et al. (59), reported a fibular stress fracture associated with distal tibiofibular synostosis in a collegiate football player and emphasized the concept of dynamic fibular function which in this case was altered by the synostosis.

SHIN SPLINTS

The clinical entity shin splint is characterized by the findings of exercise-induced pain and tenderness to palpation along the posteromedial border of the tibia (12, 13). Mubarak, et al. (14), suggested the term "medial tibial stress syndrome." Radionuclide angiograms and blood pool images are almost always normal in these patients. On delayed images, tibial lesions involve the posterior cortex, are longitudinally oriented, and usually long, involving one-third of the length of the bone. They most often show varying tracer uptake along their length (12) (Fig. 34.7). Cadaver, EMG, and muscle stimulation studies emphasized the relationship of this syndrome to the soleus muscle and its investing fascia (13).

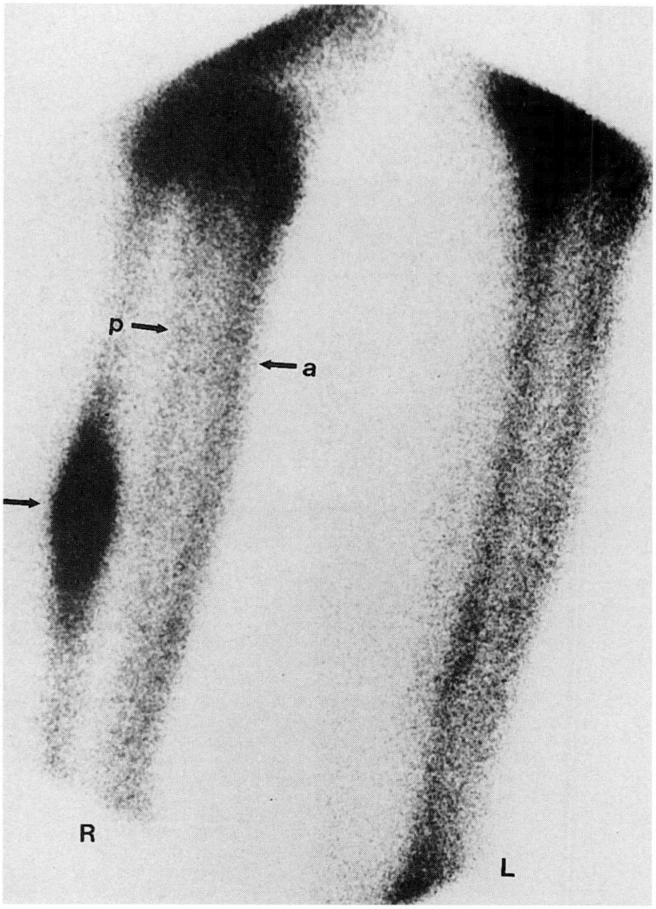

Figure 34.6. Fibular stress fracture. Lateral view of right leg (*R*) and simultaneously obtained medial view of left leg (*L*). Focal fusiform area of increased tracer in fibula (*straight arrow*). Note the definition of the anterior (*a*) and posterior (*p*) tibial cortices. (Reproduced by permission from Holder LE, Matthews LS. The nuclear physician and sports medicine. In: Freeman LM, Weissman HS, eds. Nuclear medicine annual 1984. New York: Raven Press, 1984:81–140.)

MYOSITIS OSSIFICANS

Traumatic myositis ossificans usually results from blunt trauma to large muscle groups (60). The process is usually self-limited because the calcific deposits in the soft tissues eventually mature. Pain may persist, however, secondary to mechanical irritation and/or increased compartmental pressure. Radionuclide bone imaging is utilized to assess and confirm maturation of these masses. When mature, the metabolic activity associated with them on delayed images is similar in intensity to normal bone.

INTEROSSEOUS MEMBRANE HEMORRHAGE

Patients with severe rotational ankle trauma can also injure the interosseous membrane between the tibia and fibula, with the development of hemorrhage (61). The clinical findings in the distal lower leg can be similar to compartment syndrome, and this tightness and lack of motility can

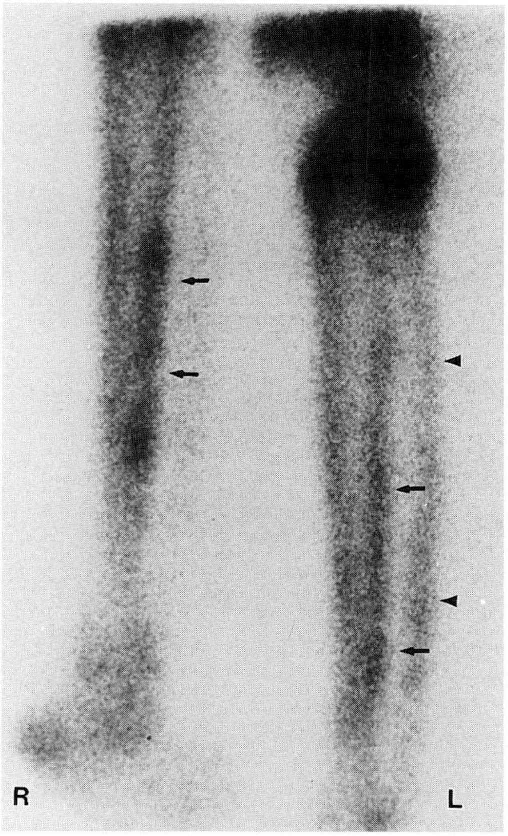

Figure 34.7. Shin splints. Delayed images left lateral and right medial views. Abnormality is longer than in a stress fracture and often demonstrates varying intensity of tracer accumulation along its length. A shin splint is particularly well seen on the right medial view (*arrows*). The fibular shin splint is particularly well seen in the left lateral view (*arrowheads*).

be incapacitating for several months. Also usually a self-limiting injury, calcification of the interosseous membrane can be identified and occasionally tibiofibular syndesmosis can occur (62). Increased radiotracer activity on all three phases of the study again demonstrates the degree of metabolic activity and/or maturation present (61).

KNEE AND THIGH

QUADRICEPS MECHANISM INJURY

Common to all quadriceps mechanism injuries is strong contraction of the quadriceps muscle opposed by forced flexion of the knee. As elegantly described by Nance and Kaye (63), the site and severity depend on the age of the patient and on underlying weakness at a specific level of the extensor mechanism. Consisting of the quadriceps femoris muscle and tendon, the patella, and the patellar tendon, the site of injury is also often related to patient age. In adults, focal increased activity on delayed images at the origin at the inferior pole of the patella is termed patellar tendinitis (Fig. 34.8). In children, focal increased activity on delayed images at the tibial tubercle insertion of the patellar tendon is most often seen. True avulsions of the tibial tubercle and transverse fractures of the patella are more obvious clinically and are not usually imaged (64).

ANTERIOR KNEE PAIN

Dye and his colleagues (65, 66) use radionuclide bone imaging as part of the routine evaluation of patients with unexplained knee pain. Their patients' complaints were not exclusively or specifically related to athletic activities, but their study provides a good overview of this complaint which is commonly encountered in athletes. Focal uptake seen on delayed images can be associated with abnormal cartilage and subarticular bone, but the findings in general remain nonspecific. In 142 patients with pain that was primarily patellar, 77 (54%) had increased patellar uptake. In 86 patients with chronically symptomatic tears of the anterior cruciate ligament, 73 (85%) had increased subchondral activity on delayed bone images. Kohn, et al. (67), performed RNBI on 100 adult sports medicine patients with clinical findings suggesting chondromalacia of the patella. They reported that the intensity of abnormal patellar tracer uptake correlated with the Metcalf grade for severity of chondromalacia seen at arthroscopy. Marymount, et al.

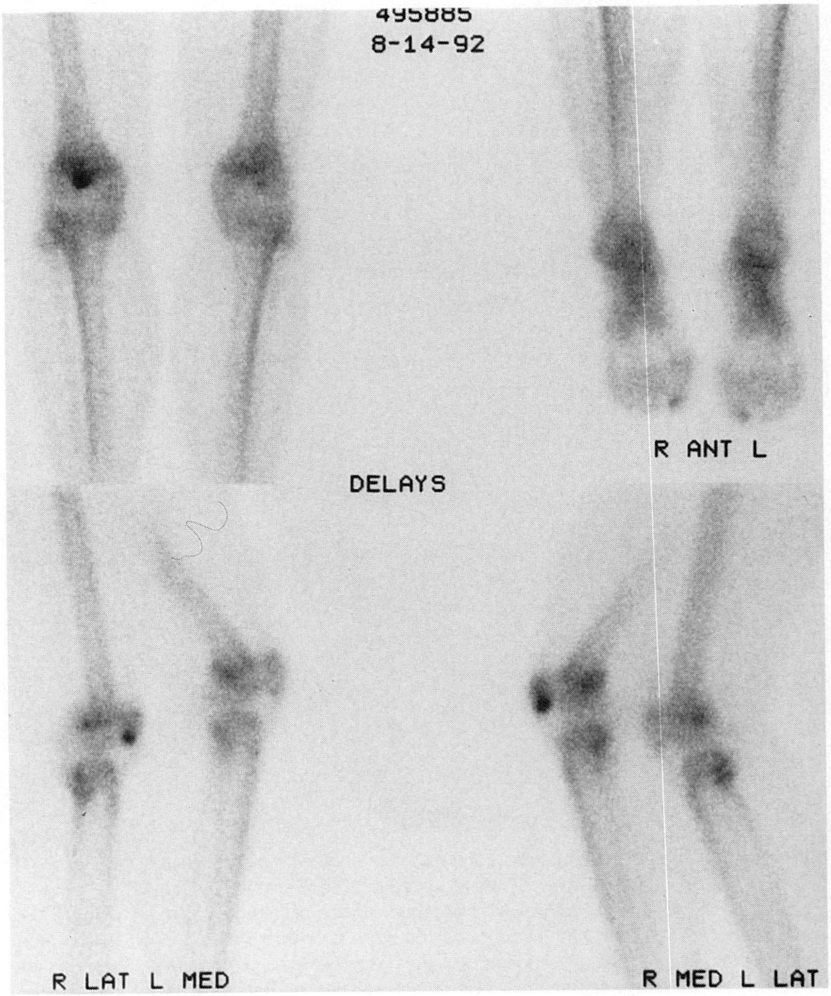

Figure 34.8. Patellar tendinitis, delayed images. Very focal, mild to moderately intense increased tracer in the inferior pole of the right patella. Note that when simultaneously obtaining a medial view of one knee and the contralateral-lateral view, it is difficult to get true anatomic position of both knees. (Reproduced by permission from Holder LE. Bone scintigraphy in skeletal trauma. RCNA 1993;31:739–781.)

(68), also demonstrated increased subchondral activity in the involved compartment of patients with a symptomatic menisceal tear. Collier and his group utilized SPECT (Single Photon Emission Computed Tomography) techniques to exam the knee, and speculated that altered joint mechanics and degenerative changes secondary to a longstanding meniscus tear eventually leads to increased uptake of the scanning agent in the subchondral bone adjacent to the torn meniscus (69). SPECT has also been utilized for imaging patients who have acute knee pain to provide delineation and siting of abnormalities immediately preceding arthroscopy (70). Butler-Manuel and colleagues (71) evaluated a variety of entities and defined the anterior knee pain syndrome as anterior pain of greater than 6 months duration exacerbated by activity, particularly climbing stairs, and associated with weakness, giving way, and pain on sitting. The postpatellectomy syndrome is defined as chronic anterior knee pain with weakness and giving way following patellectomy. For the diagnosis of RSD of the knee, they used the International Association for the Study of Pain, Subcommittee on Taxonomy 1986 definition which states: "continuous pain in a portion of the extremity after trauma which may include fracture but does not involve a major nerve, associated with sympathetic hyperactivity" (72). In the knee, it is characterized by continuous burning pain, increased sweating, and alteration in skin temperature and color. They found that although many of these patients had abnormal scans, their work was neither sensitive nor specific. They suggest that RSD had diffuse increased uptake in all three compartments. In the postpatellectomy syndrome, patients had more focal increased uptake in the femoral groove. They postulated that this uptake was due to increased stress from continued maltracking or subluxation of the patellar tendon, or from chondromalacia of the femoral groove itself. They also noted a lack of sensitivity, specificity, or correlation between the severity of chondromalacia and the scan appearance of focal uptake in the patella. Although other authors have investigated patients purported to have RSD and have demonstrated many with diffuse abnormal uptake on bone scans (73, 74), the criteria for the diagnosis of RSD was not as strict as has been reported for other areas (75, 76). RSD is discussed in more detail in Chapter 33.

PAINFUL BIPARTITE PATELLA

One of the more common indications for TPBI in the athletic setting is to evaluate the physiologic significance of an anatomic lesion identified on x-ray. The bipartite patella, with the accessory ossification center located at the supralateral pole, is not an uncommon radiologic finding in the adolescent. Ogden, et al. (77), reviewed this topic from both developmental and pathophysiologic viewpoints. In both of the new patients with painful knees following athletic trauma that they added to the literature, the delayed images on the radionuclide bone scan were abnormal, demonstrating focal increased tracer accumulation at the site of the osseous fragmentation. The cause of pain in these patients is assumed to be mobility in the abnormal synchondrosis.

LUCENT ARTICULAR LESION LATERAL FEMORAL CONDYLE

Trauma to the lateral femoral condyle at the point where it contacts the lateral facet of the patella has been postulated as the etiology for a lucent articular lesion occasionally seen in adolescent athletes (78). Delayed bone scan images demonstrate a focal area of increased tracer accumulation. In those patients, arthrography and arthrotomography can be used to demonstrate an intact overlying cartilage.

FEMORAL SHAFT STRESS FRACTURE

Although femoral neck fractures are well-known and are discussed subsequently, it is not as often appreciated that stress fractures of the proximal medial shaft of the femur also occur in runners (79–81). Butler, et al. (81), described them as more subtrochanteric and felt they were related to an exercise called bounding which consists of repetitive jumps with or without weights. All were members of a university track team ranging in age from 18–22 years. Activity on bone scan was focal and fusiform involving the medial cortex of the femur (Fig. 34.9). We think it is difficult scintigraphically to differentiate true femoral shaft stress fractures from adductor avulsion-type injuries, although stress fractures early in their course tend to have increased flow and blood pool activity on the first two phases of the radionuclide angiogram.

ADDUCTOR AVULSION FRACTURE

Adductor avulsion injuries tend to occur when the groin muscles are being stretched and patients can very often remember exactly when the first pain occurred. In an avulsion injury related to the pectineus muscle described by Rockett and Freeman (82), their 45-year-old runner's symptoms were initially more severe when he took longer strides, which would stretch the adductor muscles more than would shorter running strides. Activity on delayed images can be more focal and less fusiform than is often seen with the femoral shaft stress fracture, but it is really the mechanism of injury and anatomic localization which helps relate the focus of uptake to a particular muscle or tendon, and allows the characteristic of the uptake to be related to the mechanism of injury (82) (Fig. 34.9). Charkes, et al. (83), also discussed avulsion injuries of the adductor muscles. Because in some of their patients abnormal tracer activity was more linear than focal and fusiform, they suggested a potential periostitis type injury. An avulsion-type injury should become asymptomatic more rapidly than a stress fracture. Rockett and Freeman (82) reported complete relief of pain in their patient upon compression and support of the injured muscle.

SOFT TISSUE INJURY

Soft tissue injuries are usually clinically obvious or suspected and are evaluated by ultrasound or MR imaging. If located in deeper structures, however, they are often encountered incidentally when imaging is performed to evaluate nonspecific pain of potentially osseous origin. He-

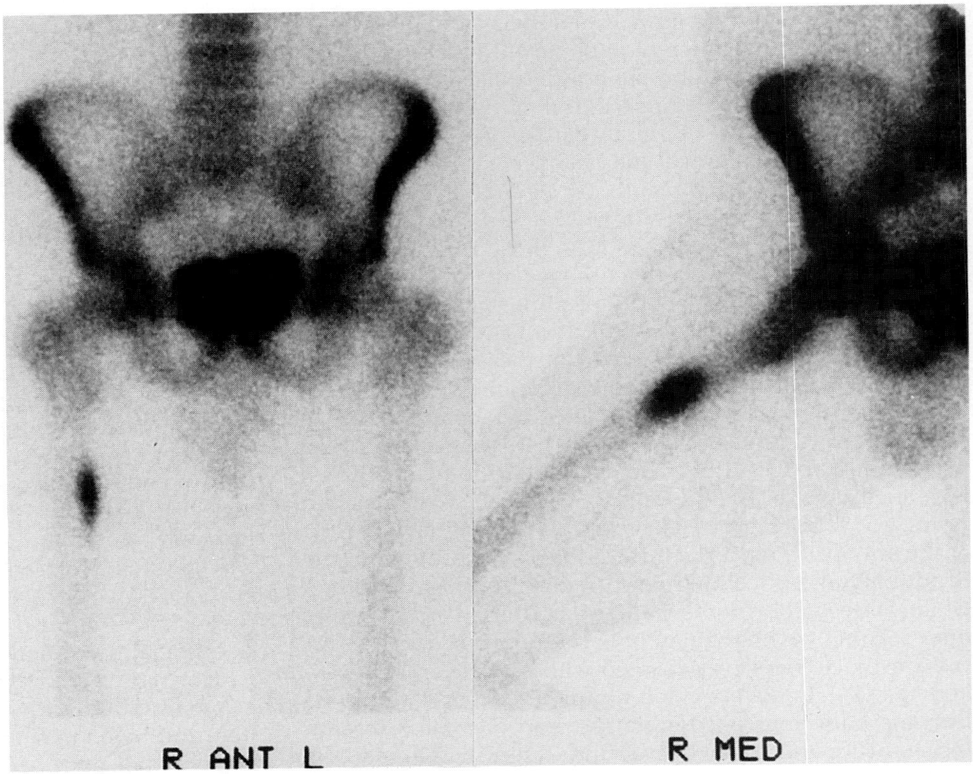

Figure 34.9. Adductor avulsion versus femoral shaft stress fracture. Delayed images. Abnormal tracer located medially is not as linear as seen in a typical shin splint-type lesion, nor is it quite as fusiform as normally seen in stress fractures. The history in this 16-year-old strongly suggested an adductor avulsion. (Reproduced by permission from Holder LE. Bone scintigraphy in skeletal trauma. RCNA 1993;31:739–781.)

matomas prior to any calcification can appear as a photon deficient area on both blood pool and delayed imaging with a rim of increased vascularity on the blood pool images, as well as occasional activity surrounding the hematoma on delayed images. Martire (61) reported a long-distance runner with right calf pain who had a ruptured popliteal cyst which was also identified on delayed imaging as a photon deficient area with a rim of slight increased activity.

PELVIS AND HIPS

PUBIC SYMPHYSITIS

Pubic symphysitis is commonly found in runners. Koch and Jackson (84) postulated that avulsions associated with the adductor and rectus abdominal muscles are the cause. The symptoms are often vague and referred to the lower abdomen or groin, occasionally with perineal radiation. When the appropriate athletic history is present, the diagnosis is most often confirmed by finding pain over the pubis. Delayed radionuclide images demonstrate increased activity involving varying portions of one or both pubic bones at the symphysis. This increased activity most often obliterates the area of relative photon deficiency centrally, which in the normal situation represents the fibrocartilaginous symphysis (8).

STRESS FRACTURES OF THE PUBIC RAMUS

Stress fractures of the pubic ramus are thought to be produced by the tensile forces resulting from strong muscle pulls on the lateral part of the pubic ramus and ischium as the hip is extended (85). In our experience, fractures in the pubis and entire pelvic ring area occur primarily in distance runners, but are not confined to the inferior pubic ramus. Since pain can often be diffuse and referred to the groin, buttock, or thigh, the delayed bone images with increased activity demonstrated at the fracture site can be very valuable in differential diagnosis. Combined fractures of the pelvis, in the medial aspect of the right pubis for example, and avulsion of the adductus longus have been reported (86).

AVULSION INJURIES

Fernbach and Wilkinson (87) discussed the entire range of **apophyseal avulsion fractures** of the pelvis and proximal femur which occur in adolescents engaged in active sports (Fig. 34.10). Because most imagers and clinicians are now aware of these lesions, they are rarely mistaken for bone-producing tumors. Although more acute and larger avulsions may have increased flow and blood pool activity, the delayed image activity is usually much more focal and less extensive than one would see, for example, in an osteogenic sarcoma. Rockett (88) reviewed TPBI in stress injuries of the anterior iliac crest. The external oblique abdominal muscle, transversus abdominis, gluteus medius, and tensor fasciae latae all originate or insert on the anterior iliac crest. Athletes who swing their arms across their bodies as they run are thought to be especially likely to suffer this injury. In this area, symmetric patient positioning for imaging is most important because even slight rotation can create asymmetric anterior iliac crest activity. Clancy and Foltz (89) used the term iliac crest apophysitis as a less severe variant of avulsion or stress fracture. Degenerative

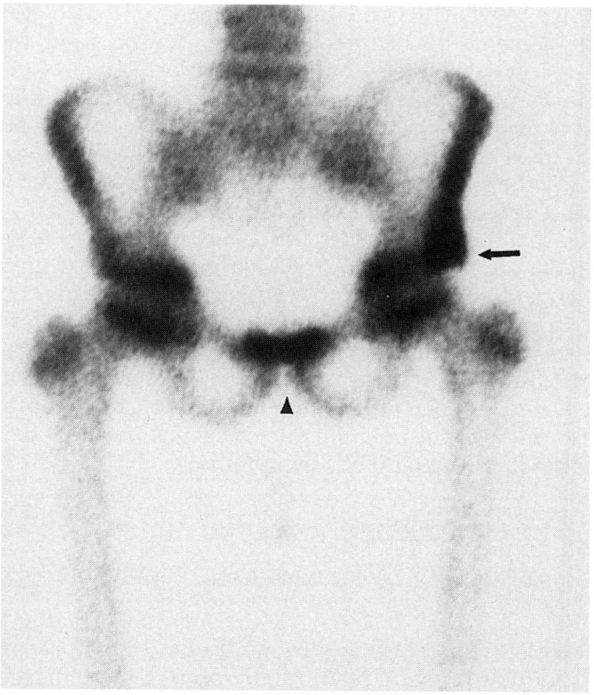

Figure 34.10. Avulsion fracture, left rectus femoris. Delayed anterior image. Very intense focal activity associated with the apophysis for the rectus femoris muscle at the anteroinferior iliac spine (*arrow*). Note the normal photon deficiency associated with the fibrocartilage at the symphysis (*arrowhead*). (Reproduced by permission from Holder LE. Bone scintigraphy in skeletal trauma. RCNA 1993;31:739–781.)

hypertrophic proliferative spurs may cause mechanical obstruction and limitation of motion in many areas. The degree of metabolic activity associated with **enesthopathies**, and by inference their role as the site or origin of the patient's pain production, can be ascertained by TPBI. The abnormality is demonstrated by focal tracer accumulation on delayed images. One of the most dramatic symptomatic traction-type spurs we have encountered was at the supralateral aspect of the acetabulum in a kick boxer. Focal activity on delayed images gave objective proof of involvement in this area and following surgery the patient could again fully hyperextend his hip.

EPIPHYSEAL AND PHYSEAL INJURIES

Epiphyseal and physeal injuries which tend to occur in the adolescent athlete were well-reviewed by Resnik (90). Although MR imaging has the ability to visualize unossified cartilage in the immature skeleton, radionuclide bone imaging still has an important place in differential diagnosis. The few anecdotal reports indicated similar sensitivities for these two modalities in early detection of abnormal movement at the physis (91). In patients with slipped capital femoral epiphysis, which occurs predominantly during the adolescent growth spurt, both the physeal activity on blood pool, but especially delayed images, is more intense, broader, and thicker than the normal side (8). Pain, which is often referred to the thigh or knee in these patients, is the common clinical complaint and is often associated with a limp (92).

FEMORAL NECK STRESS FRACTURE

Femoral neck stress fractures in athletes are usually seen in the medial neck at the point of maximum compression stress. Although many, particularly prescintigraphic, reports describe vague or uncharacteristic symptoms with referred pain to the groin or knee, most of the patients we see are specifically referred because the patient complains of pain in the hip region, has a normal plain radiograph, and the clinician has a high degree of suspicion (8, 93, 94). Because athletes tend to play through what they consider minor pain, many patients with femoral neck stress fractures already present with x-ray evidence of femoral neck stress fractures, with bone scintigraphy performed to document the age of the lesion so that appropriate therapeutic advice can be provided. As with other stress fractures, the earlier and larger the lesion, the more likely there is increased flow and blood pool activity, whereas a small lesion with only a few osteons involved, has only increased tracer on delayed images present (Fig. 34.11). Most authors report essentially 100% sensitivity in detecting symptomatic femoral neck and other stress fractures (8, 9). A single case report of a patient with pain in the hip with a normal bone scan performed 12 days after the onset of pain, who had continued pain and 5 weeks later was subsequently shown to have a femoral neck stress fracture with MR imaging, is of uncertain significance (95). Details of the imaging technique were not provided nor were the SPECT images that were obtained illustrated.

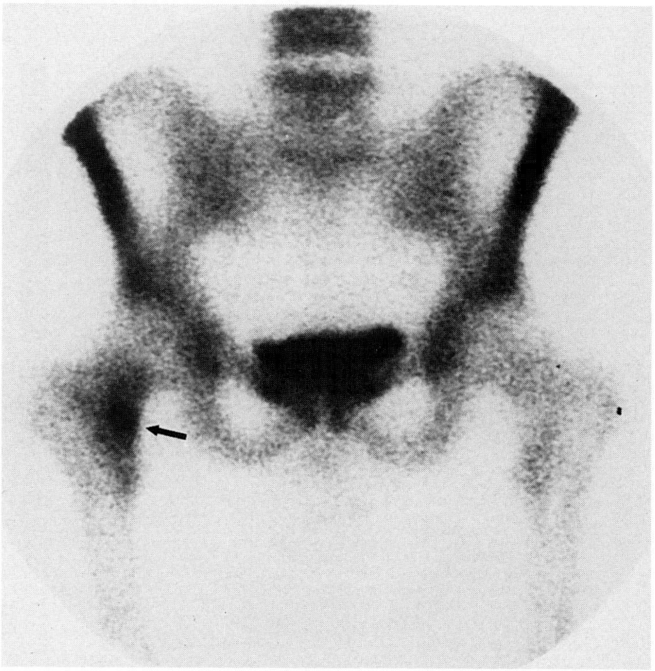

Figure 34.11. Femoral neck stress fracture. Delayed anterior image. Intense round focal area of increased tracer in the distal medial femoral neck region. (Reproduced by permission from Holder LE. Bone scintigraphy in skeletal trauma. RCNA 1993;31:739–781.)

SPINE

Low back pain is one of the most common symptoms associated with all types of athletic endeavor. Although in most cases the etiology will be muscular, or potentially radicular and demonstrated on CT or MR imaging, in many patients the etiology is uncertain. When potentially osseous in origin, TPBI with planar and SPECT techniques is usually performed (2, 8, 96–100). Often a radiographic lesion such as a **pars interarticularis defect** is identified and the radionuclide bone scan is performed to evaluate the metabolic activity or physiologic significance of the anatomic lesion.

Jackson, et al. (98, 101), first emphasized that persistent lumbar pain in the young athlete that interferes with performance and does not have associated nerve root signs should raise the possibility of a stress-type reaction in the pars interarticularis region. A focal abnormality associated with an anatomic defect suggests that it is metabolically active and most likely in the process of healing. If the lesion appears to be nonunited roentgenographically, abnormal activity can be associated with nonunion. Alternatively, an old nonunited or malunited pars defect can be associated with **contralateral stress**, the metabolic activity of which can also be evaluated by radionuclide bone imaging. Collier, et al. (99), and Bellah, et al. (96), discussed the place of SPECT imaging in this condition and both concluded that lesions could be detected by this technique which were not seen with radiography or planar bone imaging (Fig. 34.12). Most authors consider bone scintigraphy valuable in the athletic population with low back pain (9, 97). There has been some question as to the value of bone scintigraphy in nonathletic patients with very long-standing low back pain and normal radiographs and normal laboratory findings (102). The common etiologic factor in athletic injuries appears to be the hyperextended position which places increased stress on the posterior elements of the spine. Tennis players, lacrosse players, gymnasts, hockey players, soccer players, and interior linemen in football seem most affected. **Pedicle stress fractures, stress lesions** of the **spinous processes**, and stress associated with **lamina defects** have all been reported and seen.

Sports related injuries in the thoracic and cervical spine are most often related to direct trauma and are evaluated and considered similarly to traumatic lesions in other areas. In many of these situations, the radionuclide bone scan is used to determine if a lesion demonstrated radiographically is acute, with focal increased tracer accumulation, and etiologically related to the patient's symptoms, or chronic, without significant tracer accumulation, and not related to the patient's symptoms.

SHOULDER, ARM, AND CHEST

ACROMIOCLAVICULAR JOINT PROBLEMS

Various degrees of separation of the acromioclavicular (AC) joint are usually recognized from the clinical history, physical examination, and plain radiographs. When imaged as part of the workup for unexplained shoulder pain, delayed images will show increased tracer accumulation on both the acromion and clavicular side with obliteration of the normal photon deficiency of the joint space. This finding is nonspecific but provides objective evidence that the pain is probably coming from the AC joint. The appearance of the uptake in middle-aged racket sport participants is no different than that seen in acromioclavicular arthritis secondary to nonsports related etiologies.

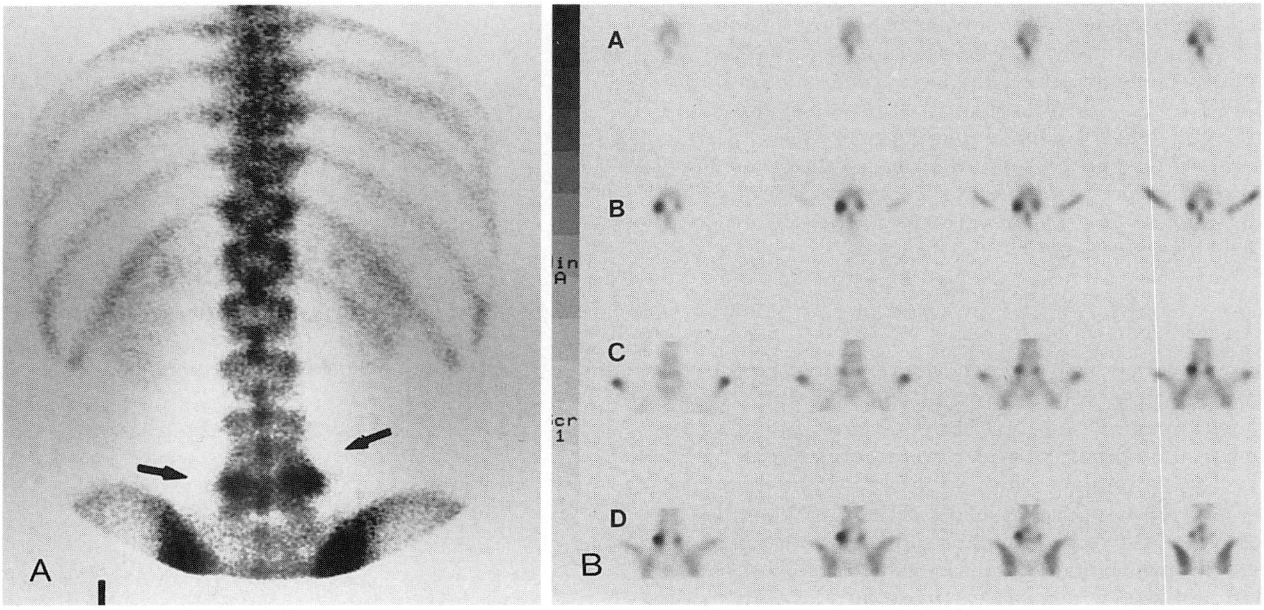

Figure 34.12. Bilateral spondylolisthesis. **A.** Posterior planar image. Bilateral increased activity (*arrows*), is greater on the right than the left (*L*). Posterior oblique views (not shown) were highly suggestive of pars interarticularis location. **B.** SPECT images. Sequential reconstructed 1-pixel 6-mm thick transaxial (*rows A and B*) and coronal (*rows C and D*) sections with increased contrast, further localized abnormal tracer uptake. (Reproduced by permission from Holder LE. Clinical radionuclide bone imaging. Radiology 1990; 176:607–614.)

OSTEOLYSIS DISTAL CLAVICLE

Osteolysis of the distal clavicle is associated with any type of acute trauma and can be seen in association with contusions, clavicular fractures, or AC joint separations. Cahill (103) discussed this condition specifically in relation to male athletes, 45 of whom were weight lifters, reporting that all 46 of his patients had increased uptake of ^{99m}Tc-labeled phosphate tracer in the distal part of the clavicle and occasionally in the adjacent acromion process. More recently, Matthews, et al. (104), reviewed this entire topic while reporting the first case of osteolysis in a female weight lifter. In their patient, the asymmetric increased activity on delayed images was similar to that seen in nonspecific arthritis or stress remodeling change.

STRESS FRACTURES

Kaye, et al. (105), reported a **fatigue fracture** of the medial aspect of the clavicle in a healthy 12-year-old athletically active boy being evaluated because of a 2-week history of vague pain in his shoulder. Although they traced the etiology of that fracture to a recent spurt of academic activity—he was carrying a large number of books under his left arm each day—their description of the biomechanical forces acting about the clavicle is instructive as is the observation that any unusual repetitive activity may result in a fatigue fracture.

Stress fractures of the first rib have been reported in a variety of athletes and the entire topic is reviewed by Gurtler, et al. (106), who added an ipsilateral first rib stress fracture in a 17-year-old pitcher to the literature. They emphasized that the deep groove for the subclavian artery forms the weakest point in the first rib and lies between the scalenes forces pulling up and the intercostal and serratus anterior forces pulling down.

HUMERAL STRESS FRACTURE

Stress injuries to the humerus are less common than in any other long bone. Fulton, et al. (107), reported a cortical desmoid-like lesion in the proximal humerus in gymnasts, terming this a Ringman's shoulder lesion. We have seen avulsion and or periostitis type stress responses in the humerus at the insertion of the pectoralis major (61), but have not felt these were confined to gymnasts. This activity is located on the anteromedial cortical border. A normal stress response with mildly increased tracer accumulation on delayed images at the insertion of the deltoid muscle on the lateral aspect of the proximal humerus should not be mistaken for a more significant lesion.

MYOSITIS

Myositis ossificans of the upper arm is less common than in the thigh. The classical triad of local pain, a hard palpable mass in the muscle, and a flexion contracture of the muscle, is only present occasionally (108).

Tondeur, et al. (109), reported bilateral upper arm muscle accumulation of tracer in an 11-year-old karate student. Standard x-rays were normal except for soft tissue swelling. There were no signs of infection, but after the positive bone scan an increase in overall CPK and MB isoenzyme were both abnormal. A follow-up scan 10 days after cessation of activity had returned to normal. **Tackler's exostosis** results from contusions and strains of the outer aspect of the midhumerus with the development of a myositis mass. When heterotopic bone formation (HBF) results, and surgical removal is contemplated for relief of pain, radionuclide bone imaging is utilized to document maturation of the process (8, 108). Oblique and lateral views are often necessary to demonstrate the soft tissue location of the activity (Fig. 34.13). Uptake in mature heterotopic bone formation on delayed images is similar in intensity to uptake in other portions of the humerus (normometabolic).

ELBOW AND FOREARM

Slocum (110) initially categorized elbow injuries based on precipitating stress. These were recently reviewed by Gore, et al. (111), who described both the anatomy and pathophysiology of the osseous manifestations of elbow stress associated with a variety of sports activities, not just with baseball. These categories include diffuse generalized stress, rotational humeral shaft forces, medial tension forces, lateral compression forces, and extensor stress. The resultant osseous changes may include bony hypertrophy, loose bodies, traction spur formation, osteochondral irregularities, and epiphyseal and apophyseal changes which are often seen on plain radiographs (2, 9, 111). TPBI was utilized to demonstrate abnormal increased metabolic activity and, by implication, the physiologic significance of these changes. About the elbow, computer manipulated, background-subtracted images, as well as creative positioning such as the acute flexion view (112), are often necessary to define the precise focus of greatest activity.

Medial epicondylitis (little league elbow) and **lateral epicondylitis** (tennis elbow) are usually obvious clinically. Other traction spurs have been described. When the degree of inflammation is marked from any cause, there is the potential for the radionuclide angiogram and blood pool phases of the study to be positive (2). When imaged, the most sensitive indicator of abnormality is focal uptake on delayed images. In children with normal activity present in the growth plate regions, meticulous positioning and high resolution imaging are required to compare the symptomatic and asymptomatic sides.

Torg and Moyer (113) described a **stress fracture through the epiphyseal plate** in an adolescent baseball pitcher and discussed King's original description of the mechanics of pitching. They felt that during repetitive forceful pitching, traction to the olecranon epiphysis was exerted, allowing it to separate from its adjacent epiphyseal plate. Epiphyseal uptake on blood pool or delayed images, recognized by asymmetric size and intensity compared to the normal side, is usually the result of healing, or in the case of a slipped epiphysis as the result of abnormal movement (8).

STRESS FRACTURE

Stress fractures in the diaphysis of the ulna have been reported by a variety of authors. Most postulate repeated

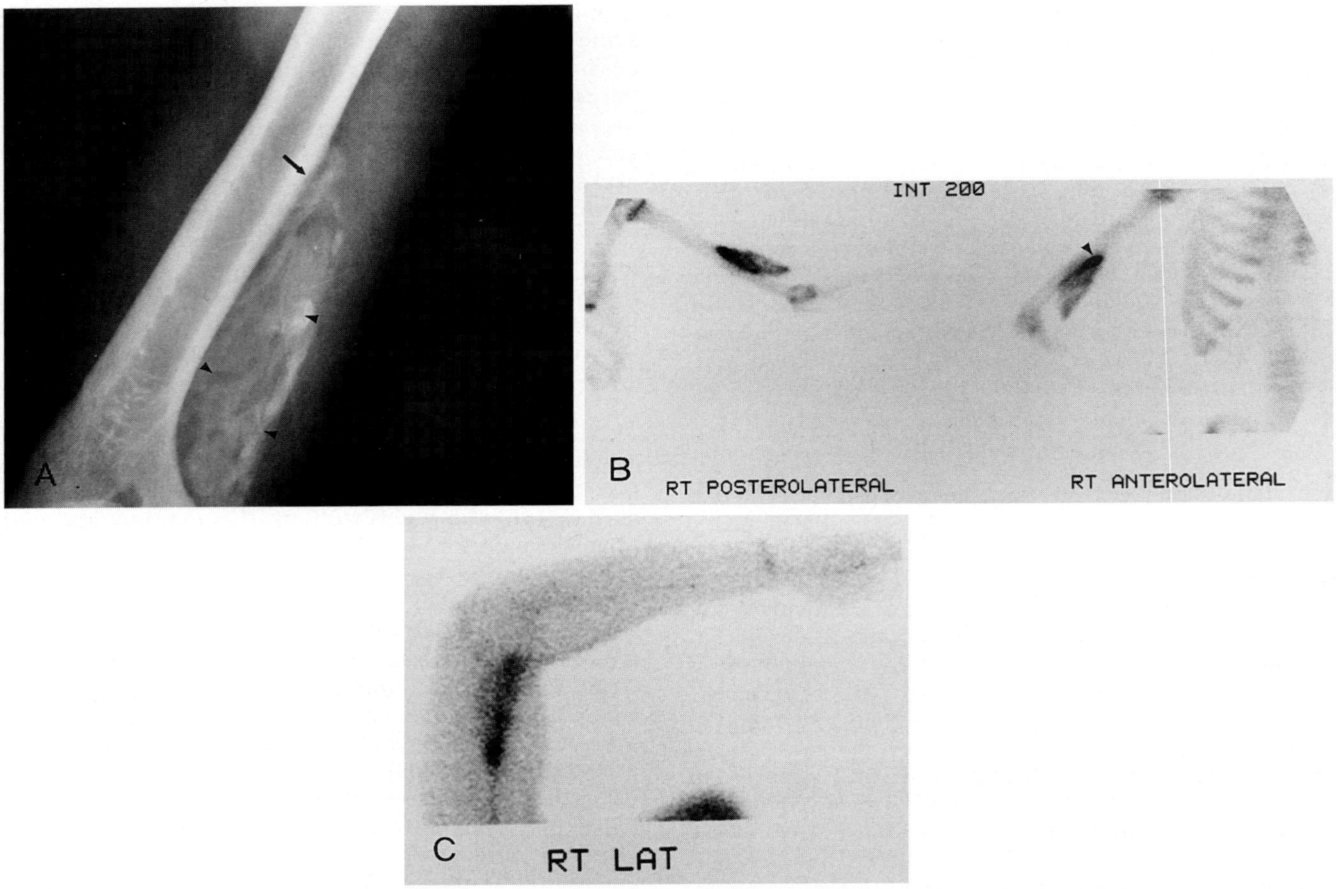

Figure 34.13. Myositis ossificans of the upper arm. **A.** Plain radiograph. Ossification in the anteromedial muscle of the lower arm is identified (*arrowheads*). At the upper portion of the mass, there is a tiny focus of periosteal new bone (*arrow*). **B.** Delayed images. Oblique images demonstrate the separation of most of this activity from the bone and its shape which corresponds to the ossification seen on the radiograph. The upper area, which is more focally intense, may represent an associated avulsion (*arrowhead*). **C.** Blood pool image. Blood pool lateral view demonstrating increased vascularity of the heterotopic bone formation, suggests further that the lesion is not mature.

flexor muscle activity as the etiology (114–116). Lesions in tennis players, weight lifters, as well as baseball and softball players have been identified. Delayed images demonstrate focal fusiform increased tracer occasionally localized to one portion of the cortex, but more often the activity tends to be circumferential.

WRIST AND HAND

Athletic injuries to the wrist and hand are commonly encountered in sports medicine practice. Linscheid and Dobyns (117) discussed the clinical and biomechanical aspects and noted that in addition to acute falls, dorsiflexion injuries and repetitive stress syndromes are the most common. The scintigraphic finding of focal increased tracer accumulation on delayed images in the distal radius, carpal bones, or about the joints of the hand, is extremely nonspecific. Occult fracture, stress fracture, bone bruise, or even less specific subchondral or periosteal injury can result in focal uptake. Location of uptake, clinical symptoms, and therapeutic considerations dictate the need for additional anatomic imaging. Some authors have described focal uptake in the areas such as the distal radius as a stress fracture even without plain radiograph or CT confirmation (118). We prefer to use the term bone bruise or nonspecific stress response if the history is longer than 2 weeks and there is no plain radiographic correlation (1, 2, 119). Other authors have reported that fractures can usually be found if more advanced imaging modalities such as computed tomography are utilized to evaluate regions of focal abnormal tracer uptake on bone scans (120). The scaphoid, lunate, trapezium, and distal radius are most commonly involved.

Stark, et al. (121), described tennis players, golfers, and baseball players who fractured the hook of the hamate by the butt end of the racket, club, or bat striking it during a swing. Although they described carpal tunnel radiographs as being extremely sensitive, it has been our experience that radionuclide bone imaging to identify the site of injury, supplemented by CT scanning for anatomic detail, is necessary for some hook and most base of the hamate fractures. Delayed images demonstrate intense focal increased tracer accumulation. Acutely, the radionuclide angiogram and/or blood pool images may also be abnormal (Fig. 34.14).

Suspected **vascular injuries** are primarily evaluated by Doppler ultrasound or magnetic resonance angiography,

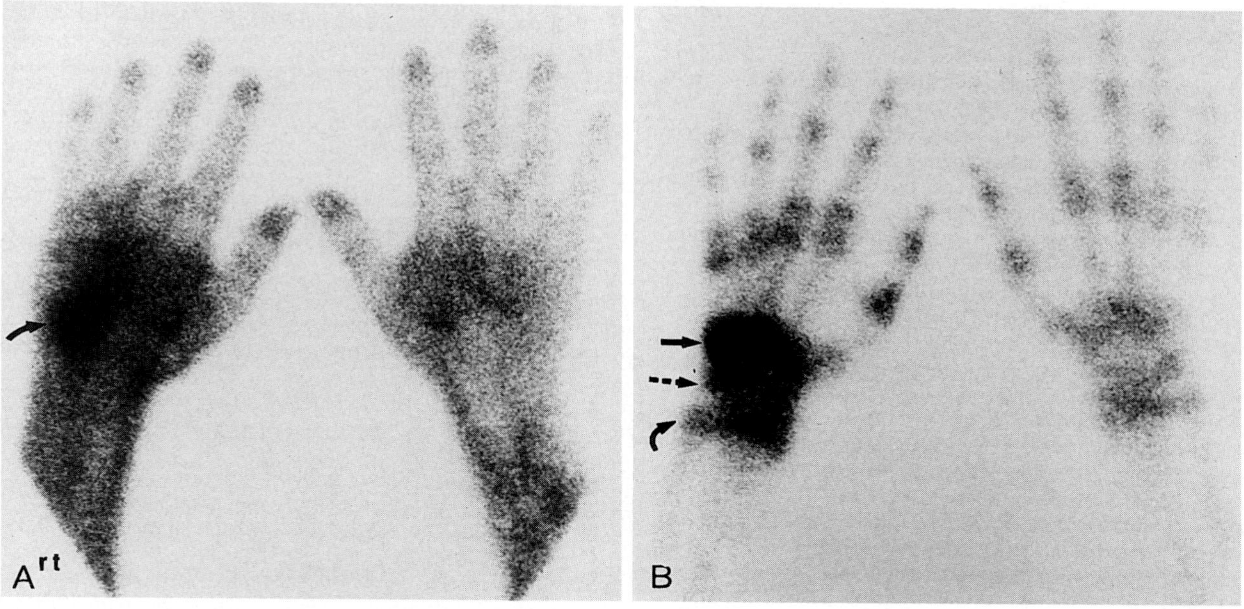

Figure 34.14. Hook of the hamate fracture. **A.** Blood pool. Focal area of increased tracer accumulation in general area of hamate (*arrow*). **B.** Delayed image. Focal increased tracer accumulation can be localized to the hamate (*short, straight arrow*) by recognizing the distal ulna (*curved arrow*) and pisiform (*broken arrow*) on the ulnar side of the proximal carpal row. In this relatively acute fracture, the intensity of activity blurs the margins of the individual carpal bone. (Reproduced by permission from Holder LE, Matthews LS. The nuclear physician and sports medicine. In: Freeman LM, Weissman HS, eds. Nuclear medicine annual 1984. New York: Raven Press, 1984:81–140.)

although such lesions in the hand are readily identified when TPBI is performed. Ho, et al. (122), reported two cases of true **aneurysms** arising in the vasculature of the hand after blunt athletic trauma. Diagnosis in one of those patients was confirmed on radionuclide bone imaging with a focal round area of increased activity in the blood pool phase corresponding to a 7 mm clinically palpable mass. **Reflex sympathetic dystrophy** as a posttraumatic sequela of athletic injury is less common than after work-related injury (5, 75). This syndrome is discussed in Chapter 33. **Avascular necrosis** of the **lunate** is also a common lesion which can occur in the athletic setting (123).

REFERENCES

1. Holder LE. Clinical radionuclide bone imaging. Radiology 1990; 176:607–614.
2. Holder LE. Bone scintigraphy in skeletal trauma. RCNA 1993; 31:739–781.
3. Pavlov H. Athletic injuries. RCNA 1990;28:435–443.
4. Maurer AH, Chen DCP, Camargo EE, Wong DF, Wagner HN Jr, Alderson PO. Utility of three-phase skeletal scintigraphy in suspected osteomyelitis: concise communication. J Nucl Med 1981; 22:941–949.
5. Holder LE, Mackinnon SE. Reflex sympathetic dystrophy in the hands: clinical and scintigraphic criteria. Radiology 1984; 152:517–522.
6. Wehbe MW. Reflex sympathetic dystrophy [Letter]. J Hand Surg 1994;19A:884–885.
7. Holder LE, Kline SC. Reflex sympathetic dystrophy [Letter]. J Hand Surg 1994;19A:8845–8856.
8. Holder LE, Matthews LS. The nuclear physician and sports medicine. In: Freeman LM, Weissman HS, eds. Nuclear medicine annual: 1984. New York: Raven Press, 1984:81–140.
9. Rupani HD, Holder LE, Espinola DA, Engin SI. Three-phase radionuclide bone imaging in sports medicine. Radiology 1985; 156:187–196.
10. Deutsch SD, Gandsman EJ. The use of bone scanning for the diagnosis and management of musculoskeletal trauma. SCNA 1983;63:567–583.
11. Matin P. The appearance of bone scans following fractures, including immediate and long-term studies. J Nucl Med 1979; 20:1227–1231.
12. Holder LE, Michael RH. The specific scintigraphic pattern of "shin splints in the lower leg": concise communication. J Nucl Med 1984;24:865–869.
13. Michael RH, Holder LE. The soleus syndrome. A cause of medial tibial stress (shin splints). Am J Sports Med 1985;13:87–94.
14. Mubarak SJ, Gould RN, Lee YF, et al. The medial tibial stress syndrome (a cause of shin splints). Am J Sport Med 1982; 10:201–205.
15. Lawson JP. Not-so-normal variants. Orthop Clin North Am 1990; 21:483–495.
16. Resnick D, Niwayama G. Entheses and Enthesopathy. Radiology 1983;146:1–9.
17. Brower AC. The osteochondroses. Orthop Clin North Am 1983; 14:99–117.
18. Mink JH, Deutsch AL. Occult cartilage and bone injuries of the knee: detection, classification and assessment with MR imaging. Radiology 1989;170:823–829.
19. Maurice H, Watt I. Technetium-99m hydroxymethylene diphosphonate scanning of acute injuries to the lateral ligaments of the ankle. Br J Radiol 1989;62:31–34.
20. Baker BE. Current concepts in the diagnosis and treatment of musculotendinous injuries. Med Sci Sports 1984;16:323–327.
21. Siegel BA, Engel WK, Derrer EC. Localization of technetium-99m diphosphonate in acutely injured muscle. Neurology 1977; 27:230–238.
22. Goergen TG, Venn-Watson EA, Rossman DJ, Resnick D, Gerber

KH. Tarsal navicular stress fractures in runners. AJR 1981; 136:201–203.
23. Torg JS, Pavlov H, Cooley LH, Bryant MH, Arnoczky SP, Bergfield J, Hunter LY. Stress fractures of the tarsal navicular. JBJS 1982;64A:700–712.
24. Pavlov H, Torg JS, Freiberger RH. Tarsal navicular stress fractures: radiographic evaluation. Radiology 1983;148:641–645.
25. Kiss ZS, Khan KM, Fuller PJ. Stress fractures of the tarsal navicular bone: CT findings in 55 cases. AJR 1993;160:111–115.
26. Weissman BNW, Sledge CB, eds. Orthopedic radiology. Philadelphia: W.B. Saunders, 1986:50–54.
27. Berquist TH, Johnson KA. Trauma. In: Berquist TH, ed. Radiology of the foot and ankle. New York: Raven Press, 1989:204.
28. Rupani HD, Holder LE, Espinola DA, Engin SI. Three-phase radionuclide bone imaging in sports medicine. Radiology 1985; 156:187–196.
29. Levy JM. Stress fractures of the first metatarsal. AJR 1978; 130:679–681.
30. Drez D Jr, Young JC, Johnston RD, Parker WD. Metatarsal stress fractures. Am J Sports Med 1980;8:123–125.
31. Delee JC, Evans JP, Julian J. Stress fracture of the fifth metatarsal. Am J Sports Med 1983;11:349–353.
32. Jahss MH. Stubbing injuries to the hallux. Foot Ankle 1981; 1:327–332.
33. Coker TP, Arnold JA, Weber DL. Traumatic lesions of the metatarsophalangeal joint of the great toe in athletes. Am J Sports Med 1978;6:326–335.
34. Pinckney LE, Currarino G, Kennedy LA. The stubbed great toe: a cause of occult compound fracture and infection. Radiology 1981;138:375–377.
35. Johnson RP, Collier BD, Carrera GF. The os trigonum syndrome: use of bone scan in the diagnosis. J Trauma 1984;8:761–764.
36. Black HM, Brand RL. Injuries of the foot and ankle. In: Scott WN, Missonson W, Nicholas JA, eds. Principles of sports medicine. Baltimore: Williams and Wilkins, 1984:356–358.
37. O'Donoghue DH. Impingement exostoses of the talus and tibia. JBJS 1957;39A:835–852.
38. Pavlov H, Heneghan MA, Hersh A, Goldman AB, Vigorita V. The haglund syndrome: initial and differential diagnosis. Radiology 1982;144:83–88.
39. Shelbourne KD, Fisher DA, Rettig AC, McCarroll JR. Stress fractures of the medial malleolus. Am J Sports Med 1988;16:60–63.
40. Schils JP, Andrish JT, Piraino DW, et al. Medial malleolar stress fractures in seven patients: review of the clinical and imaging features. Radiology 1992;185:219–221.
41. Urman M, Ammann W, Sisler J, et al. The role of bone scintigraphy in the evaluation of talar dome fractures. J Nucl Med 1991; 32:2241–2244.
42. Anderson IF, Crichton KJ, Grattan-Smith T, Cooper RA, Brazier D. Osteochondral fractures of the dome of the talus. JBJS 1989; 71A:1143–1152.
43. Curtis MJ, Myerson M, Szura B. Tarsometatarsal joint injuries in the athlete. Am J Sports Med 1993;21:497–502.
44. Meurman KOA, Elfving S. Stress fracture of the cuneiform bones. Br J Radiol 1980;53:157–160.
45. Marymont JH Jr, Mills GQ, Merritt WD III. Fracture of the lateral cuneiform bone in the absence of severe direct trauma. Am J Sports Med 1980;8:135–136.
46. Roub LW, Gumerman LW, Hanley EN, et al. Bone stress: a radionuclide imaging perspective. Radiology 1979;132:431–438.
47. Zwas ST, Elkanovitch R, Frank G. Interpretation and classification of bone scintigraphic findings in stress fractures. J Nucl Med 1987;28:452–457.
48. Matheson GO, Clement DB, McKenzie DC, Taunton JE, Lloyd-Smith DR, Macintyre JG. Stress fractures in athletes: a study of 320 cases. Am J Sports Med 1987;15:46–58.
49. Matin P. Bone scintigraphy in the diagnosis and management of traumatic injury. Sem Nucl Med 1983;13:104–122.
50. Goldfarb CF. Interpretation and classification of bone scintigraphic findings in stress fractures [Letter]. J Nucl Med 1988; 29:1150–1151.
51. Daffner RH, Martinez S, Gehweiler JA Jr, Harrelson JM. Stress fractures of the proximal tibia in runners. Radiology 1982; 142:63–65.
52. Pilgaard S, Poulsen JO, Christensen JH. Stress fractures. Acta Orthop Scan 1976;47:167–169.
53. Devas MD. Stress fractures in children. JBJS(B) 1963;45B:528–541.
54. Blank S. Transverse tibial stress fractures: a special problem. Am J Sports Med 1987;15:597–602.
55. Hulkko A, Orava S. Stress fractures in athletes. J Sports Med 1987;8:221–226.
56. Rosen PR, Micheli LJ, Treves S. Early scintigraphic diagnosis of bone stress and fractures in athletic adolescents. Pediatrics 1987;70:11–15.
57. Devas MB, Sweetnam R. Stress fractures of the fibula—a review of 50 cases in athletes. JBJS 1956;59A:869–874.
58. Symeonides PP. High stress fractures of the fibula. JBJS 1980; 62B:192–193.
59. Kottmeier SA, Hanks GA, Kalenak A. Fibular stress fracture associated with distal tibiofibular synostosis in an athlete: a case report and literature review. Clin Orthop 1992;281:195–198.
60. Lipscomb AB, Thomas ED, Johnston RK. Treatment of myositis ossificans in athletes. Am J Sports Med 1976;4:111–120.
61. Martire JR. The role of nuclear medicine bone scans in evaluating pain in athletic injuries. Clinics Sports Med 1987;6:713–737.
62. Whiteside LA, Reynolds FC, Ellsasser JC. Tibulo-fibular syostosis and recurrent ankle sprains in high performance athletes. Am J Sports Med 1978;6:204–208.
63. Nance EP Jr., Kaye JJ. Injuries of the quadriceps mechanism. Radiology 1982;142:301–307.
64. Mitchell MJ, Ho C, Resnick D, et al. Diagnostic imaging of lower extremity trauma. Radiol Clin North Am 1989;27:909–928.
65. Dye SF, Chew MH. The use of scintigraphy to detect increased osseous metabolic activity about the knee. JBJS 1993; 75A:1388–1406.
66. Dye SF, Boll DA. Radionuclide imaging of the patellofemoral joint in young adults with anterior knee pain. Orthop Clin North America 1986;17:249–262.
67. Kohn HS, Guten GN, Collier BD, Veluvolu P, Whalen JP. Chondromalacia of the patella: bone imaging correlated with arthroscopic findings. Clin Nucl Med 1988;13:96–98.
68. Marymont JV, Lynch MA, Henning CE. Evaluation of meniscus tears of the knee by radionuclide imaging. Am J Sports Med 1983;11:432–435.
69. Collier BD, Johnson RP, Carrera GF, et al. Chronic knee pain assessed by SPECT: comparison with other modalities. Radiology 1985;157:795.
70. Murray IPC, Dixon J, Kohan L. SPECT for acute knee pain. Clin Nucl Med 1990;11:828–840.
71. Butler-Manuel PA, Guy RL, Heatley FW, Nunan TO. Scintigraphy in the assessment of anterior knee pain. Acta Orthop Scand 1990;61(5):438–442.
72. International Association for the Study of Pain, Subcommittee on Taxonomy. Classification of chronic pain. Pain 1987; 3(Suppl):29–30.
73. Katz MM, Hungerford DS. Reflex sympathetic dystrophy affecting the knee. JBJS 1987;69B:797–803.
74. Ogilvie-Harris DJ, Roscoe M. Reflex sympathetic dystrophy of the knee JBJS (Br) 1987;69:804–806.
75. Mackinnon SE, Holder LE. The use of three-phase radionuclide scanning in the diagnosis of reflex sympathetic dystrophy. J Hand Surg (Am) 1984;9:556–563.

76. Holder LE, Cole LA, Myerson MS. Reflex sympathetic dystrophy in the foot: clinical and scintigraphic criteria. Radiology 1992; 184:531–535.
77. Ogden JA, McCarthy SM, Jokl P. The painful bipartite patella. J Pediatr Orthop 1982;2:263–269.
78. Cayea PD, Pavlov H, Sherman MF, Goldman AB. Lucent articular lesion in the lateral femoral condyle: source of patellar femoral pain in the athletic adolescent. AJR 1981;137:1145–1149.
79. Lombardo SJ, Benson DW. Stress fractures of the femur in runners. Am J Sports Med 1982;10:219–227.
80. Blatz DJ. Bilateral femoral and tibial shaft stress fractures in a runner. Am J Sports Med 1981;322–325.
81. Butler JE, Brown SL, McConnell BG. Subtrochanteric stress fractures in runners. Am J Sports Med 1982;10:228–232.
82. Rockett JF, Freeman BL. Scintigraphic demonstration of pectineus muscle avulsion injury. Clin Nucl Med 1990;15:800–803.
83. Charkes ND, Siddhivarn N, Schneck CD. Bone scanning in the adductor insertion avulsion syndrome ("thigh splints"). J Nucl Med 1987;28:1835–1838.
84. Koch RA, Jackson DW. Pubic symphysitis in runners: a report of two cases. Am J Sports Med 1981;9:62–63.
85. Pavlov H, Nelson TL, Warren RF, Torg JS, Burstein AH. Stress fractures of the pubic ramus: a report of twelve cases. JBJS 1982;64A:1020–1025.
86. Tehranzadeh J, Kurth LA, Elyaderani MK, Bowers KD. Combined pelvic stress fracture and avulsion of the adductor longus in a middle-distance runner: a case report. Am J Sports Med 1982; 10:108–111.
87. Fernbach SK, Wilkinson RH. Avulsion injuries of the pelvis and proximal femur. AJR 1981;137:581–584.
88. Rockett JF. Three-phase radionuclide bone imaging in stress injury of the anterior iliac crest. J Nucl Med 1990;31:1554–1556.
89. Clancy WG, Foltz AS. Iliac apophysitis and stress fractures in adolescent runners. Am J Sports Med 1976;4:214–218.
90. Resnik C. Diagnostic imaging of pediatric skeletal trauma. RCNA 1989;27:1013–1022.
91. Yang A, Yang SS, Holder LE, Bright RW. MR imaging of physeal and epiphyseal abnormalities. 78th Scientific Assembly and Annual Meeting, Radiological Society of North America, November 29-December 2, 1992. (Video disc production of scientific exhibit from 1992 RSNA meeting.)
92. Apple DF Jr, Cantwell JD. Medicine for sport. Chicago: Yearbook Medical Publishers, 1979.
93. Erne P, Burckhardt A. Femoral neck fatigue fracture. Arch Orthop Traumat Surg 1980;97:213–220.
94. El-Khoury GY, Wehbe MA, Bonfiglio M, Chow KC. Stress fractures of the femoral neck: a scintigraphic sign for early diagnosis. Skeletal Radiol 1981;6:271–273.
95. Keene JS, Lash EG. Negative bone scan in a femoral neck stress fracture: a case report. Am J Sports Med 1992;20:234–236.
96. Bellah RD, Summerville DA, Treves ST, Micheli LJ. Low-back pain in adolescent athletes: detection of stress injury to the pars interarticularis with SPECT. Radiology 1991;180:509–512.
97. Papanicolaou N, Wilkinson RH, Emans JB, Treves S, Micheli LJ. Bone scintigraphy and radiography in young athletes with low back pain. AJR 1985;145:1039–1044.
98. Jackson DW, Wiltse LL, Dingeman RD, Hayes M. Stress reactions involving the pars interarticularis in young athletes. Am J Sports Med 1981;9:304–312.
99. Collier BD, Johnson RP, Carrera GF, et al. Painful spondylolysis or spondylolisthesis studied by radiography and single-photon emission computed tomography. Radiology 1985;154:207–211.
100. Traughber PD, Havlina JM Jr. Bilateral pedicle stress fractures: SPECT and CT features. J Comp Assis Tomog 1991;15:338–340.
101. Jackson DW, Wiltse LL, Cirincione RJ. Spondylolysis in the female gymnast. Clin Orthop 1976;117:68–73.
102. Schutte HE, Park WM. The diagnostic value of bone scintigraphy in patients with low back pain. Skeletal Radiol 1983;10:1–4.
103. Cahill BR. Osteolysis of the distal part of the clavicle in male athletes. JBJS 1982;64–A:1053–1058.
104. Matthews LS, Simonson BG, Wolock BS. Osteolysis of the distal clavicle in a female body builder: a case report. Am J Sports Med 1993;21:150–152.
105. Kaye JJ, Nance EP Jr, Green NE. Fatigue fracture of the medial aspect of the clavicle. Radiology 1982;144:89–90.
106. Gurtler R, Pavlov H, Torg JS. Stress fracture of the ipsilateral first rib in a pitcher. Am J Sports Med 1985;13:277–279.
107. Fulton MN, Albright JP, El-Khoury GY. Cortical desmoid-like lesion of the proximal humerus and its occurrence in gymnasts (ringman's shoulder lesion). Am J Sports Med 1979;7:57–61.
108. Huss CD, Puhl JJ. Myositis ossificans of the upper arm. Am J Sports Med 1980;8:419–424.
109. Tondeur M, Haentjens M, Piepsz A, Ham HR. Muscular injury in a child diagnosed by ^{99m}Tc-MDP bone scan. Eur J Nucl Med 1989;15:328–329.
110. Slocum DB. Classification of elbow injuries from baseball pitching. Tex Med 1968;64:48–53.
111. Gore RM, Rogers LF, Bowerman J, Suker J, Compere CL. Osseous manifestations of elbow stress associated with sports activities. AJR 1980;134:971–977.
112. Fink-Bennett D, Carichner S. Acute flexion of the elbow: optimal imaging position for visualization of the capitellum. Clin Nucl Med 1986;11:667–668.
113. Torg JS, Moyer RA. Non-union of a stress fracture through the olecranon epiphyseal plate observed in an adolescent baseball pitcher. JBJS 1977;59A:264–265.
114. Mutoh Y, More T, Suzuki Y. Stress fractures of the ulna in athletes. Am J Sports Med 1982;10:365–367.
115. Hamilton HK. Stress fracture of the diaphysis of the ulna in a body builder. Am J Sports Med 1984;12:405–406.
116. Rettig AC. Stress fracture of the ulna in an adolescent tournament tennis player. Am J Sports Med 1983;11:103–106.
117. Linscheid RL, Dobyns JH. Athletic injuries of the wrist. Clin Orthop 1985;198:141–151.
118. Loosli AR, Leslie M. Stress fractures of the distal radius: a case report. Am J Sports Med 1991;19:523–524.
119. Pin PG, Semenkovich JW, Young VL, Bartell T, Crandall RE, Gilula LA, Reed K, Weeks PM, Siegel BA. Role of radionuclide imaging in the evaluation of wrist pain. J Hand Surg 1988; 13A:810–814.
120. Tiel-van Buul MM, vanBeek EJ, Dijkstra PF, et al. Significance of a hot spot on the bone scan after carpal injury—evaluation by computed tomography. Eur J Nucl Med 1993;20:159–164.
121. Stark HH, Jobe FW, Boyes JH, Ashworth CR. Fracture of the Hook of hamate in athletes. JBJS 1977;59–A:575–582.
122. Ho PK, Dellon AL, Wilgis EFS. True aneurysms of the hand resulting from athletic injury: report of two cases. Am J Sports Med 1985;13:136–137.
123. Sowa DT, Holder LE, Patt PG, et al. Application of magnetic resonance imaging to ischemic necrosis of the lunate. J Hand Surg 1989;14:1008–1016.

35 Pet Imaging of the Skeletal System

RANDALL A. HAWKINS, CARL K. HOH, and MICHAEL E. PHELPS

Imaging bone metabolic activity with gamma-camera systems and ^{99m}Tc-methylene diphosphonate (MDP) and related radiopharmaceuticals is one of the most common and important techniques employed in nuclear medicine. Other chapters deal extensively with the various methods and techniques employed in the scintigraphic evaluation of the skeletal system. In addition to single photon emitters, positron emitting radiopharmaceutics, including [^{18}F]fluoride ion, and other radiopharmaceuticals including 2-[^{18}F]fluoro-2-deoxy-D-glucose (FDG), have been employed for evaluation of the skeletal system (1–3). In fact, [^{18}F]fluoride ion was at one time the standard bone scanning agent (4–9), but it was replaced for routine clinical use in the 1970s by ^{99m}Tc-labeled bone seeking radiopharmaceutics, because of the more optimal physical characteristics of ^{99m}Tc for gamma-camera systems.

Positron emission tomography (PET), like single photon emission computed tomography (SPECT) produces tomographic images reflective of the tissue distribution of administered radiopharmaceutics. Because of the more physically precise methods for photon attenuation correction with PET, compared to single photon gamma-camera techniques, one potential advantage of PET bone imaging is greater quantitative precision. Additionally, because PET systems in general have better resolution than most gamma-camera or SPECT systems (10), it is possible to obtain images of the skeletal system of higher resolution with PET than with SPECT.

With modern PET systems, however, there is a relatively limited amount of experience with PET bone imaging. Most of the reported investigations have focused on evaluation of musculoskeletal malignancies with the PET FDG technique, but some studies have also been performed with [^{18}F]fluoride ion (1–3).

RADIOPHARMACEUTICALS AND KINETIC MODELS

The fundamental biologic information produced by PET, like other nuclear medicine methods, is dependent on the radiopharmaceutical employed. Reviews of PET radiopharmaceuticals are available (1, 11), but to date the positron emitting radiopharmaceuticals of most relevance to bone are [^{18}F]fluoride ion and FDG.

Blau, et al. (8), were the first to perform bone imaging with [^{18}F]fluoride ion. Following their initial work, [^{18}F]fluoride ion became the standard nuclear medicine bone scanning agent (4–9).

Because of interest in fluoride as a potential therapeutic agent for osteoporosis and because of the role of fluoride in preventing dental caries, there is a large literature on the metabolism and pharmakokinetics of fluoride (12). In vitro studies have demonstrated that fluoride ion exchanges with the hydroxyl ion in the bone mineral hydroxyapatite crystal $Ca_{10}(PO_4)_6(OH)_2$ to form fluoroapatite: $Ca_{10}(PO_4)_6(F)_2$ (13). Because PET studies of bone with [^{18}F]fluoride ion utilize tracer quantities of fluoride ion, the direct pharmacologic effects of macroscopic (as opposed to tracer) quantities of fluoride ion on both bone cells and bone crystals (12) do not have to be considered when interpreting PET [^{18}F]fluoride ion studies. However, kinetic PET [^{18}F]fluoride ion studies are an excellent way to map the distribution of fluoride ion transport and trapping in bone, based on the tracer principle.

Studies have shown that there is a high initial extraction fraction of [^{18}F]fluoride ion in its transit through bone (14, 15). Based on the assumption that the initial extraction fraction approximated 100%, Reeve, et al. (16), estimated skeletal blood flow in humans with a plasma clearance method alone (i.e., without PET imaging) with [^{18}F]fluoride ion. Utilizing this clearance method, Wooton, et al. (17), found a positive correlation between decreases in skeletal blood flow and decreases in alkaline phosphatase in patients with Paget's disease treated with calcitonin.

Charkes, et al. (18–20), were the first to develop an in vivo pharmakokinetic model of [^{18}F]fluoride ion distribution using compartmental modeling techniques and animal tissue sampling data. The kinetic approaches described later for PET studies of [^{18}F]fluoride ion distribution are similar in concept to those originally developed by Charkes, et al., but are based on direct imaging of the kinetics of bone uptake of [^{18}F]fluoride ion with a PET system. While many elegant studies of in vivo pharmakokinetics of compounds have been performed with plasma and tissue sampling methods alone (21), PET and other imaging methods make it possible to "sample" (image) tissue noninvasively. When coupled with plasma measurements of radionuclide concentrations as a function of time, it becomes possible to apply a wide variety of mathematic models to PET data (10).

In addition to [^{18}F]fluoride ion, the other primary positron emitting radiopharmaceutical used in PET bone imaging applications is FDG (1). FDG, like glucose, is transported across capillary membranes via a carrier mediated transport process, in the direction of a concentration gradient (facilitated diffusion). Both FDG and glucose are then phosphorylated by hexokinase, but because the phosphorylation product FDG-6-PO_4 cannot be metabolized further through the glycolytic cycle (22), it accumulates in cells, unlike glucose-6-PO_4, which undergoes further metabolism through the glycolytic and Krebs cycle to be eventually metabolized to CO_2 and H_2O. Because deoxyglucose competes with glucose for both capillary transport and phosphorylation by hexokinase, Sokoloff, et al. (23), were able to develop a mathematic model relating the net transport of ^{14}C deoxyglucose (DG) and accumulation of DG-6-PO_4 in tissue to glucose transport and metabolism based upon Michaelis Menten kinetics. The original Sokoloff deoxyglucose method, developed in rats for autoradiography, was extended to humans utilizing PET and FDG by Reivich, Phelps, and colleagues (24–26).

The intent of the FDG (and DG) model is to produce a measurement of tissue glucose metabolic rates with a single time measurement of tissue radionuclide concentration (i.e., ^{18}F, distributed between unphosphorylated FDG and FDG-6-PO_4) (Fig. 35.1). It is also necessary to measure the time course of FDG in the plasma space (the input function). Additionally, if one desires an absolute measurement of tissue glucose metabolism in μmol/min/g of tissue, it is necessary to also measure or arbitrarily assign a numerical value to a term in the FDG model known as the "lumped constant" (LC) (24–26). The LC is in essence a calibration term related to the fact that glucose and FDG have differential affinities (K_m and V_{max} values) for both the glucose transporter protein and for hexokinase. While numerical values for these affinity terms are available for glucose and FDG in some tissues, such as mammalian brain, in most human tissue, including bone and tumor tissues, the values are either unknown, or approximations from related tissues are used.

Because the total amount of ^{18}F in tissue at any point in time (distributed between FDG and FDG-6-PO_4) is approximately linearly related to tissue glucose utilization, semiquantitative PET methods using ratios of tissue uptake are often employed (27).

As an alternative to the classic autoradiographic FDG model, it is also possible to perform kinetic FDG studies in order to directly measure FDG transport (forward, K_1 and reverse, k_2) and phosphorylation (k_3) and dephosphorylation (k_4) rate constants, as opposed to assuming population values for these rate constants in single time imaging studies with the autoradiographic model. The units most commonly used for these rate constants are ml/min/g for K_1, and min^{-1} for k_2, k_3, and k_4, respectively. While this results in a simple expression for tissue glucose metabolic rates (equation 1), it is still necessary to assign a value to the LC if an absolute value (in units of μmol/min/g tissue) is desired.

$$\text{Metabolic Rate Glucose} = \frac{K_1 \times k_3}{k_2 + k_3} \times (C_p/LC)$$

where K_1, k_2, and k_3 are the rate constants described above, Cp is the plasma glucose concentration, and LC is

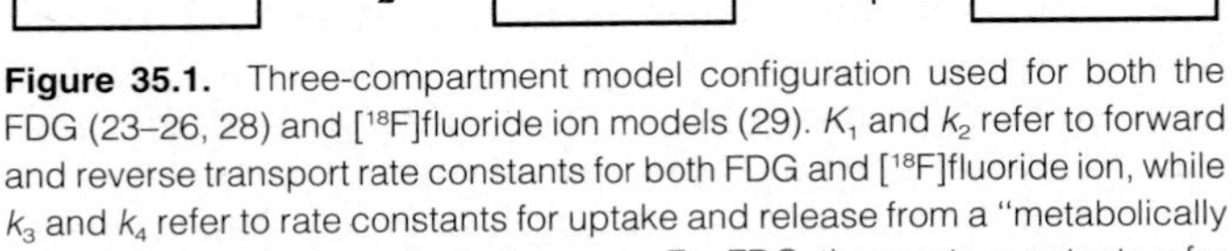

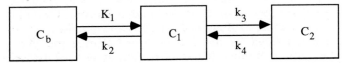

Figure 35.1. Three-compartment model configuration used for both the FDG (23–26, 28) and [^{18}F]fluoride ion models (29). K_1 and k_2 refer to forward and reverse transport rate constants for both FDG and [^{18}F]fluoride ion, while k_3 and k_4 refer to rate constants for uptake and release from a "metabolically trapped" space in tissue for both agents. For FDG, these rate constants refer to the hexokinase and phosphatase catalyzed phosphorylation and dephosphorytion of FDG and FDG-6-PO_4, respectively, while for [^{18}F]fluoride ion k_3 and k_4 are rate constants for uptake and release from hydroxyapatite crystal related binding space in bone (29).

the lumped constant. The reader is referred to more detailed discussions in the literature for a full discussion of the assumptions and methods used to measure tissue glucose metabolic rates with this method (1, 23–28).

Most quantitative studies with the FDG method have been performed in brain and heart studies. Because of the potential to better biochemically characterize neoplasms based on numeric estimates of metabolism, and because of interest in monitoring interventions in cancer, such as chemotherapy by serially measuring changes in metabolic parameters, as opposed to relying on the more delayed end point of tumor volume changes, there is increasing interest in developing appropriately validated methods for quantitative PET FDG imaging in many tumor systems, including primary and metastatic bone tumors.

While the mechanism of [^{18}F]fluoride ion uptake in bone, described earlier, is different than the biochemical mechanisms underlying FDG transport and phosphorylation, both processes have in common a tissue phase distributed between two kinetically discrete compartments—for FDG: (a) free FDG and (b)"metabolically trapped" FDG-6-PO_4; for [^{18}F]fluoride ion: (a) "unbound" and (b) hydroxyapatite crystal related "bound" [^{18}F]fluoride ion. Based on this similarity in tissue distribution kinetics, Hawkins, et al. (29), employed the same three compartment model configuration illustrated in Figure 35.1 to evaluate the kinetics of [^{18}F]fluoride ion uptake in bone with PET. These methods again illustrate that with PET, as with other digital tomographic imaging techniques such as SPECT, MRI, and CT, the "output" of the studies fall into two categories: images and numeric results. A valuable characteristic of PET is the high resolution and quantitative precision of the method. This characteristic facilitates development of appropriate numeric descriptions of the results that may have practical clinical significance, as well as producing better insight into biochemical processes.

PET METHODS FOR BONE IMAGING

With both [^{18}F]fluoride ion and FDG, there are several methods one may use for acquiring PET bone images, including:

1. Standard transaxial attenuation corrected images at a preselected time after injection of [^{18}F]fluoride ion or FDG;
2. Serial transaxial attenuation corrected images beginning simultaneously with injection of [^{18}F]fluoride ion or FDG (kinetic studies);
3. Whole-body images.

Most PET systems contain rings of detectors, analogous to CT scanners in design (10). The axial field of view of such devices is defined by the number of detector rings and by the axial field of view of each ring, as well as by the acquisition and image reconstruction strategy employed. Some PET systems utilize two-dimensional detector systems similar to gamma-camera designs, but all PET systems, like other imaging devices, have a defined axial field of view.

If a patient is imaged in a given bed position within a PET scanner, the data may be corrected for tissue attenuation with a transmission scan method using a $^{68}Ga/^{68}Ge$ transmission source, and a set of transaxial images generated either in static mode (method 1) or kinetic mode (method 2). These acquisition sequences are the "gold standard" for PET acquisitions. Because a strength of PET, as compared to SPECT, is a more accurate retrieval of voxel count density based on more accurate attenuation correction methods (30), both methods 1 and 2 produce images of high resolution and quantitative precision.

A relative limitation of methods 1 and 2, however, is the axial field of view of the methods. The situation is very much analogous to SPECT. While SPECT bone imaging is a very useful method for generating more anatomically precise cross-sectional bone scan images than planar gamma-camera methods, SPECT is not convenient for total skeletal surveys, because the acquisition time for serial SPECT image sets that include the whole body are inconveniently long.

Because many potential applications of [^{18}F]fluoride ion and FDG PET bone imaging involve patients with malignancies and potentially widespread skeletal and nonskeletal metastases, Dahlbom, et al. (30), developed a whole-body PET imaging method that produces tomographic and nontomographic (projection) image sets of the whole body. The method is based on sequential acquisitions of standard transaxial PET image data sets at discrete locations in the body, followed by acquisitions at other body locations until the entire body (or more limited regions of interest) have been included in the data set. Standard transaxial images are reconstructed with filtered backprojection methods, and coronal and sagittal tomographic images are extracted from the stack of transaxial images via a sorting operation. Additionally, two-dimensional "projection" images, analogous to two-dimensional raw data sets with SPECT, are generated by appropriate sampling and sorting of the raw sinograhic data. The end result is a whole-body image set consisting of transaxial, coronal and sagittal tomographic images, together with two-dimensional projection images at various angles around the body.

There are two fundamental limitations to the whole-body PET method as it is usually currently employed: (a) The individual transaxial data sets are usually acquired for relatively short intervals (e.g., approximately 2–4 minutes) to permit acquisition of the whole-body data set in a reasonable time period (e.g., about 60 minutes). This method results in transaxial image quality inferior to what is generated with longer (e.g., 10–30 minute) acquisitions over given body locations. (b) Whole-body PET images are usually acquired without attenuation correction because standard transaxial transmission scanning at each bed position to generate an attenuation correction matrix would prohibitively lengthen the total time of the study. For this reason, whole-body skeletal PET images are primarily useful as qualitative maps of the whole-body distribution of [^{18}F]fluoride ion, FDG, or other compounds. However, in appropriate clinical contexts, such qualitative whole-body image sets can be very useful in mapping disease extent.

Refinements of the whole-body PET method, that should increase both its quantitative precision and clinical utility, include development of practical attenuation correction approaches (31) and application of alternative reconstruction methods such as the three-dimensional method (32). The three-dimensional reconstruction method makes it possible to utilize a much higher fraction of coincident events in the image reconstruction process, essentially by including coincident events between detector planes, as well as within individual or directly adjacent detector planes. This technique has the effect of significantly increasing the count rate efficiency of the PET system, with a potential result being a decrease in acquisition time by up to a factor of 4 or more. While both the whole-body attenuation correction and three-dimensional reconstruction methods remain to be validated in clinical applications, they promise to make whole-body PET skeletal imaging increasingly practical and quantitative.

CLINICAL EXAMPLES OF PET BONE IMAGING

Normal Patterns

Figure 35.2 includes examples of [^{18}F]fluoride ion images acquired with the whole-body PET method. Selected two-dimensional projection, as well as transaxial, coronal, and sagittal images, are included. Note that the relative body distribution of the [^{18}F]fluoride ion is very similar to the distribution of ^{99m}Tc MDP compounds, as expected based on the distribution and metabolism of the agent as discussed earlier.

While the impact of the lack of attenuation correction on whole-body [^{18}F]fluoride ion images is evident (Fig. 35.2), it tends to be less apparent on selected tomographic images compared to FDG whole-body images for two reasons: (a) the bone/tissue contrast of [^{18}F]fluoride ion is high and the relative uptake of [^{18}F]fluoride ion in bone, adjusted for bone size and partial volume effects, is relatively uniform, and (b) many bony structures are relatively near the body surface. Nevertheless, tissue attenuation effects are still visible on these images, as illustrated in Figure 35.2.

Additionally, because a single whole-body PET study can produce a large number of tomographic and projection images, it is very helpful to view such images on a workstation equipped with appropriate volume viewing software. Such display options are available on a variety of nuclear medicine workstations and, with the standardization of image file formats into DICOM3 and other standard file formats, display and viewing of such data sets on workstations designed for general imaging environments as part of larger PACS (Picture Archival Communication Systems), will become progressively easier and more routine.

Another advantage of workstation viewing strategies for whole-body PET [^{18}F]fluoride ion and FDG bone studies is the ease of appropriate contrast adjustment (windowing) of images. While FDG uptake in normal bone is low, normal bone marrow uptake produces a visible signal on appropriately windowed FDG images. This uptake will be most evident in hematopoietically active marrow spaces, such as the vertebral bodies and proximal femoral shafts.

Pathologic Conditions

PET bone imaging with [^{18}F]fluoride ion produces the expected findings of increased tracer uptake in the range of pathologic conditions known to also cause increased uptake of ^{99m}Tc MDP and related compounds: neoplastic, inflammatory, traumatic, and other processes known to re-

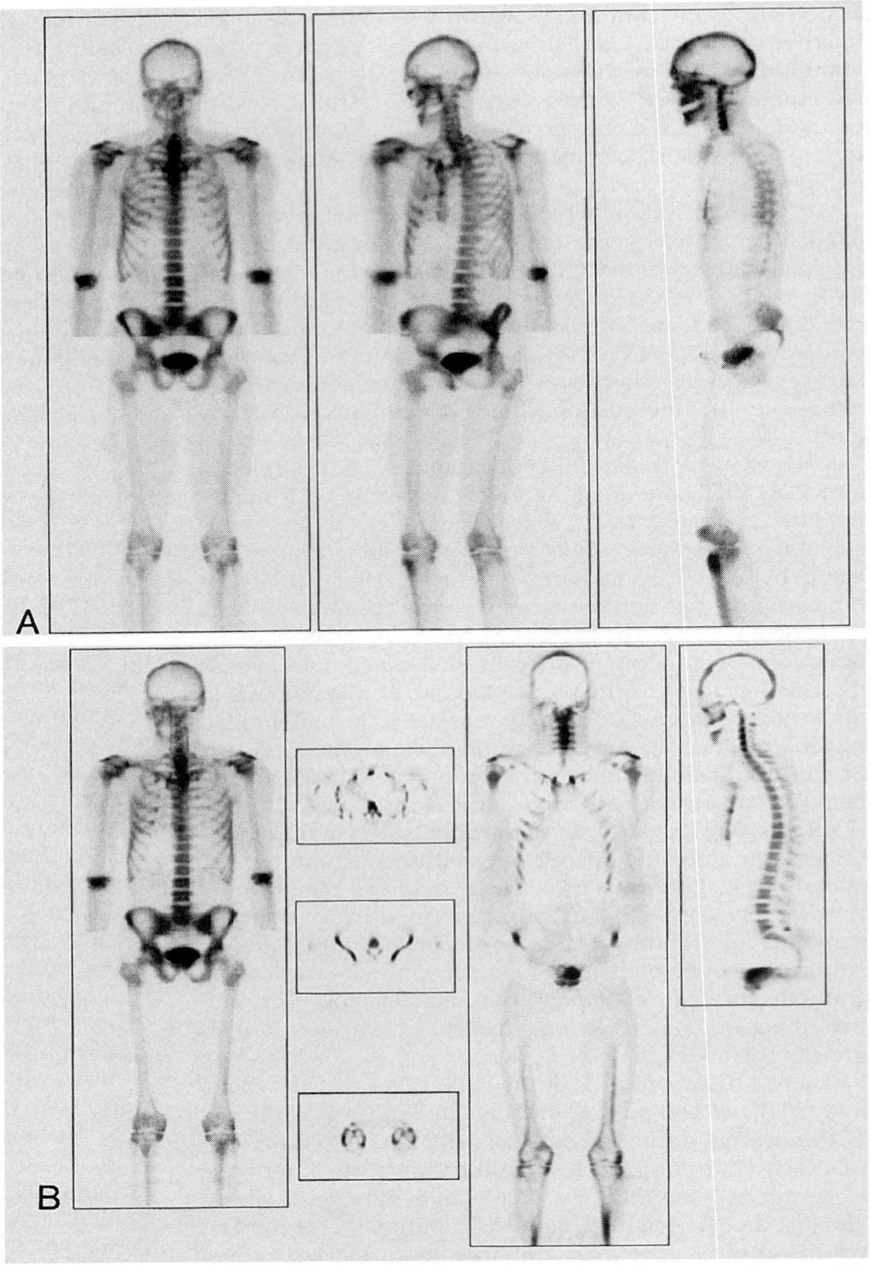

Figure 35.2. A. Projection images of [18F]fluoride ion using whole-body PET technique in a normal volunteer. Illustrated are three different angular views of [18F]fluoride ion distribution (*anterior on left, left anterior oblique in center,* and *lateral on right*). Note that the lack of attenuation correction produces differential relative attenuation in the femurs and spine, most evident in the lumbar region, on the lateral as opposed to the anterior views. There is physiologic excretion of [18F]fluoride ion into the bladder. The hands were not included in the acquisition sequence acquired over the upper body; acquisitions over the upper and lower body were photographically combined for this illustration. This image and other illustrations in this chapter were acquired on a Siemens 931–08 tomograph. This device has eight detector rings, and produces 15 simultaneous transaxial images, spaced at 6.75 mm per plane (2). (Reproduced by permission from Hoh CK, Hawkins RA, Dahlbom M, et al. Whole-body skeletal imaging with [18F]fluoride ion and PET. J Comp Asst Tomogr 1993;17(1):34–41.) **B.** Projection (*left*) and tomographic images (*right three columns*) of [18F]fluoride ion distribution in a normal volunteer, illustrating the range of tomographic display options available with this technique. The second column of images includes three transaxial images at the approximate levels of the midthoracic spine, pelvis, and knees respectively. Single coronal (*second from right*) and sagittal (*far right*) tomographic image sections are also included. Note the excellent delineation of the vertebral bodies and spinous processes, the tibila plateaus, and other bone structures.

sult in an acceleration of osteoblastic activity and bone blood flow.

In a series of 19 patients, with a range of malignant and benign skeletal conditions, Hoh, et al. (2), found that the tomographic (transaxial, coronal, and sagittal) [18F]fluoride ion images had a 13% higher sensitivity for lesion detection than did the projection image set. Given that a fundamental advantage of any form of tomography is higher in-plane contrast (10), this result is not surprising. The primary utility of projection whole-body images, both [18F]fluoride ion and FDG, is to help the observer become appropriately oriented in three dimensions relative to the distribution of abnormalities. Specific lesions may only be visible, however, on the tomographic image set. Figure 35.3, which contains [18F]fluoride ion images of a patient with polyostotic fibrous dysplasia and metastatic osteogenic sarcoma, illustrates better delineation of a pathologic focus on a tomographic, as compared to projection, image (33).

Because accelerated osteoblastic activity and bone blood flow are sensitive, but nonspecific, indicators of pathology, it is logical to expect that images of a different process, such as tissue glucose utilization mapped with FDG, should produce a different view of bone pathology. A feature shared by many aggressive neoplasms is an acceleration of their glycolytic rates (34). Because bone (cortical and trabecular) has relatively low glucose utilization rates, compared to tissues such as the brain, heart, and striated muscle, whole-body PET FDG images in patients with skeletal primary or metastatic neoplasms frequently illustrate dramatic focal abnormalities that have very high contrast compared to the background normal bone FDG uptake pattern. This finding is illustrated in Figure 35.4, in which skeletal metastases from a patient with primary carcinoma of the breast were detected with this method.

Whole-body and standard transaxial PET FDG imaging for cancer detection, staging, and treatment monitoring is becoming a major focus of both research and clinical use of PET. Review articles on this subject are available in the literature (1, 35, 36). Specifically related to skeletal disease, several investigators have demonstrated that PET FDG imaging is useful for detecting and characterizing various types of primary and metastatic disease. A fundamental potential utility of the method is differentiating benign from malignant causes of increased uptake on "osteoblastic" bone scans, either PET [^{18}F]fluoride ion or gamma-camera MDP studies. While increased FDG uptake in bone is not pathognomonic for cancer (inflammatory processes may also produce increased FDG uptake and subcutane-

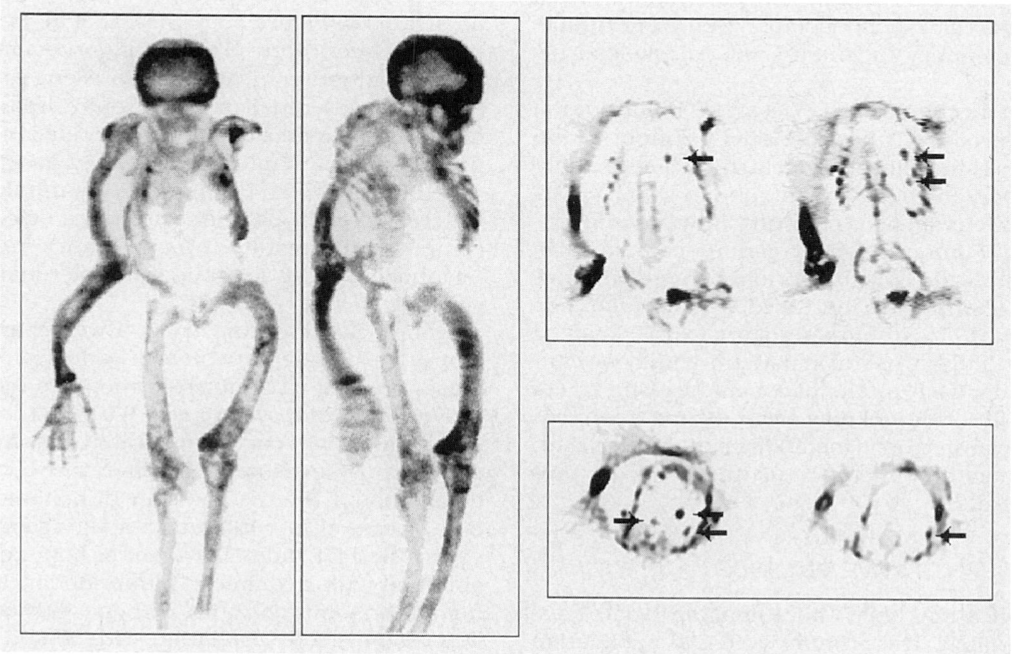

Figure 35.3. Projection [^{18}F]fluoride ion bone images (*left two images*), coronal tomographic (*upper right images*), and transaxial tomographic (*lower right images*) in a patient with polyostotic fibrous dysplasia who had previously undergone an amputation of the left upper extremity for an osteosarcoma. *Arrows* on the tomographic images identify foci uptake in the lung fields consistent with metastatic osteogenic sarcoma deposits. These foci are more evident on the tomographic, as opposed to the projection planar, images. Note the dramatic distortion of skeletal anatomy and diffusely increased uptake of [^{18}F]fluoride ion consistent with widespread fibrous dysplasia. (Reproduced by permission from Tse N, Hoh C, Hawkins R, Phelps M, Glaspy J. Positron emission tomography diagnosis of pulmonary metastases in osteogenic sarcoma. Am J Clin Oncol 1994;17(1):22–25.)

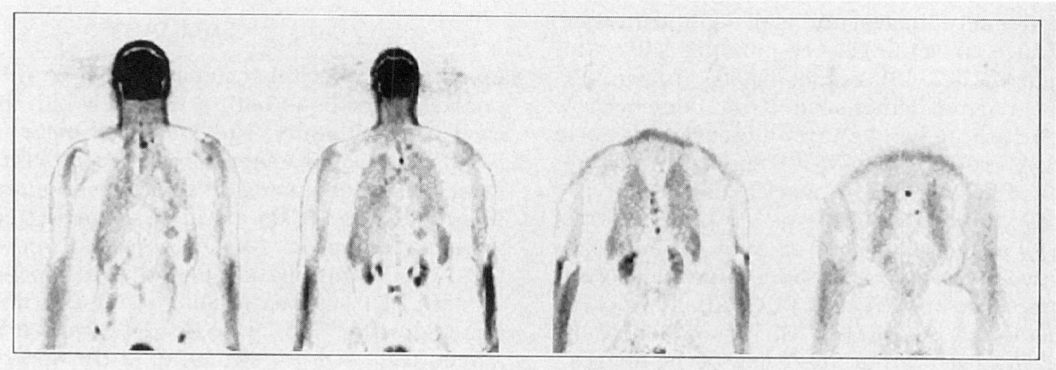

Figure 35.4. Four separate coronal PET FDG whole-body images (upper body region) in a patient with metastatic breast carcinoma. Note scattered areas of increased FDG uptake in the upper and midthoracic spine on all four images. Appropriate correlation of such images with plain films, as well as interactive windowing of images (see text), facilitates localization of individual lesions on images sets such as this. Note the very intense uptake of FDG in the brain (*left two images*) that, because of contrast setting, exceeds the upper limit of the gray scale. Note also the physiologic uptake of FDG in muscles, kidney, and bladder. There is only minimal FDG uptake in the heart on this study, because it was acquired in a fasting state.

ous injections of FDG may result in significantly increased uptake in normal lymph nodes (37, 38)), it is likely that the specificity of FDG will be higher than MDP or [^{18}F]fluoride ion for bone cancer detection, as indicated by initial studies. By using FDG, one is changing the primary cellular focus of the images from the osteoblastic system with [^{18}F]fluoride ion and MDP, to cells with high glycolytic rates (i.e., cancer) with FDG. In a study of 25 patients with various types of musculoskeletal disorders, Adler, et al. (39), found that by quantifying FDG uptake in lesions, they could more accurately differentiate benign from malignant processes. Kern, et al. (40), in an earlier preliminary study, also found a good correspondence between FDG uptake and grade of malignancy in human musculoskeletal tumors.

These different mechanisms of FDG and [^{18}F]fluoride ion uptake also can produce "uncoupling" of [^{18}F]fluoride ion and FDG uptake (1) in primary or metastatic bone tumors successfully responding to treatment, and in which a persistent osteoblastic response, resulting in increased uptake on a PET [^{18}F]fluoride ion or gamma-camera MDP bone scan, may indicate ongoing normal bone repair once the tumor, characterized by increased FDG uptake, has become suppressed. This characteristic of FDG imaging could make it particularly useful in patients with bone cancers in whom increased uptake of a bone-seeking tracer (e.g., MDP or [^{18}F]fluoride ion) may occur during treatment secondary to accelerated bone metabolism and repair that, in some cases, may be difficult to distinguish from progression of cancer itself.

QUANTITATIVE METHODS

Quantitative applications of PET bone imaging to date have been relatively limited. The primary potential application of quantitative PET FDG imaging in bone relates to disease characterization and treatment monitoring, as discussed in previous reviews (1, 27). Additionally, quantitative PET FDG kinetic studies can help elucidate normal metabolic processes, such as bone marrow-stimulating growth factors (GMCSF) effects on hematopoietically active marrow uptake of FDG (41). GMCSF is one of a family of glycoprotein cytokines that stimulates bone marrow production of granulocytes and macrophages, and is of significant therapeutic importance in some cancer patients with suppressed bone marrow (42, 43). Yao, et al. (41), utilizing dynamic PET FDG imaging, demonstrated that bone marrow FDG uptake (glucose metabolic rate) increased by up to threefold during 3–10 days of GMCSF therapy, and progressively declined following therapy. Because these types of therapeutically-induced alterations in bone marrow metabolic activity occur relatively uniformly in the hematopoietically active marrow spaces, differentiating such effects from discrete foci in increased FDG uptake in bone, secondary to metastatic disease (Fig. 35.4), should usually be straightforward with appropriate review of the images.

An additional form of quantification in bone for which there is a potential role for PET is in better defining and noninvasively measuring trabecular and cortical bone metabolic activity. Single photon emitters, such as ^{99m}Tc MDP, were previously used to evaluate generalized bone metabolism and were applied to specific disorders such as hyperparathyroidism, both with planar and SPECT methods (44–47). Such methods have not been widely utilized, partially because the challenge of absolute voxel quantification of signal secondary to accurate correction for tissue attenuation effects remains to be accurately solved. New generation SPECT systems, equipped with transmission sources for attenuation correction, may result in renewed interest in utilization of single photon bone-seeking tracers for quantitative bone metabolic studies.

Utilizing a kinetic PET acquisition sequence with [^{18}F]fluoride ion and the three compartment kinetic model illustrated in Figure 35.1, Messa, et al. (48), evaluated the utility of quantitative PET [^{18}F]fluoride ion kinetic studies in the evaluation of patients with one form of metabolic bone disease—renal osteodystrophy. Using kinetically determined estimates of net [^{18}F]fluoride ion transport (K (in units of ml/min/ml tissue) defined as $k_1^*k_3/(k_2+k_3)$) (29, 48), they measured [^{18}F]fluoride ion uptake in normal volunteers, in eight patients with renal osteodystrophy, and compared the results to bone biopsy indicators of bone metabolic activity acquired from the renal osteodystrophy group.

Bone histomorphometry is a well-characterized tissue biopsy technique in which a variety of indices of bone mass, growth, and mineralization are measured quantitatively from biopsy samples. With oral tetracycline labeling, bone growth can be accurately measured with appropriate biopsy specimens. The literature contains additional details about the methodology of histomorphometry (49–51). Messa, et al. (48), found a very good correlation between the PET index (K value) of bone metabolic activity obtained with dynamic [^{18}F]fluoride ion imaging and the histomorphometric index of bone formation rate. There was also a good correlation with K and serum alkaline phosphatase and parathyroid hormone levels ($r > 0.8$ in each case). While this initial series requires validation in larger groups of patients, it illustrates the potential of quantitative PET bone imaging to better define metabolic characteristics of bone, some of which, such as bone formation rate, may otherwise be available only from direct tissue assay techniques.

SUMMARY

Imaging the skeletal system with positron emitting radiopharmaceuticals is both a relatively old and also a new, evolving technique. While clinical bone scanning with [^{18}F]fluoride ion was appropriately supplanted by gamma-camera methods using ^{99m}Tc diphosphonate-related compounds in the 1970s, because of the better sensitivity of gamma-cameras for 140 keV photons from ^{99m}Tc compared to 511 KeV annihilation photons from positron emitters, modern PET scanners make qualitative and quantitative imaging with [^{18}F]fluoride ion, FDG, and other radiopharmaceutics, both practical and, in the appropriate setting, clinically useful.

Gamma-camera and SPECT methods are becoming progressively more sophisticated and precise. It is, therefore, unlikely that [^{18}F]fluoride ion PET bone imaging will become a serious competitor to gamma-camera bone scans for routine clinical surveys, but in situations where the higher resolution and better quantitative precision of PET are required, [^{18}F]fluoride ion imaging and quantitative studies should have a role. These situations include both quantitative metabolic studies, such as the renal osteodystrophy work of Messa, et al. (48), and qualitative studies in patients, where the resolution of a state-of-the-art PET system is needed to definitively detect or localize a lesion.

The major clinical role of PET bone imaging will probably be in the field of oncology, because of the greater specificity of FDG and other agents for mapping and detecting cancers than the highly sensitive, but nonspecific, bone scanning methods based on osteoblastic tracers MDP and [^{18}F]fluoride ion. While in the future the range of processes evaluated with PET will increase, transaxial and whole-body methods with existing agents FDG and [^{18}F]fluoride ion indicate that it already has an appropriate role to play in clinical medicine.

REFERENCES

1. Hawkins RA, Hoh C, Glaspy J, et al. The role of positron emission tomography in oncology and other whole-body applications. Sem Nucl Med 1992;22(4):268–284.
2. Hoh CK, Hawkins RA, Dahlbom M, et al. Whole body skeletal imaging with [^{18}F]fluoride ion and PET. J Comp Asst Tomogr 1993; 17(1):34–41.
3. Hoh CK, Hawkins RA, Glaspy JA, et al. Cancer detection with whole-body PET using 2-[^{18}F]fluoro-2-deoxy-D-glucose. J Comp Asst Tomogr 1993;17(4):582–589.
4. French RJ, McCready VR. The use of ^{18}F for bone scanning. Br J Radiol 1967;40:655–661.
5. Spencer R, Herbert R, Rish MW, Little WA. Bone scanning with ^{85}Sr, ^{87m}Sr and ^{18}F. Physical and radiopharmaceutical considerations and clinical experience in 50 cases. Br J Radiol 1967; 40:641–654.
6. Moon NF, Dworkin HJ, LaFluer PD. The clinical use of sodium fluoride F-18 in bone photoscanning. JAMA 1968;204:974–980.
7. Harmer CL, Burns JE, Sams A, Spittle M. the value of fluorine-18 for scanning bone tumours. Clin Radiol 1969;20:204–212.
8. Blau M, Nagler W, Bender MA. Fluorine-18: a new isotope for bone scanning. J Nucl Med 1962;3:332–334.
9. Weber DA, Keyes JW Jr, Landman S, Wilson GA. Comparison of Tc-99m polyphosphate and F-18 for bone imaging. Am J Roentgenol Radium Ther Nucl Med 1974;121:184–190.
10. Sorenson JA, Phelps ME, eds. Physics in nuclear medicine. 2nd ed. Orlando, FL: Grune & Stratton, 1987.
11. Fowler JS, Wolf AP. Positron emitter-labeled compounds: priorities and problems. In: Phelps M, Mazziotta J, Schelbert H, eds. Positron emission tomography and autoradiography: principles and applications for the brain and heart. New York: Raven Press, 1986:391–450.
12. Murray TM, Singer FR, eds. Journal of bone and mineral research: proceedings of the international workshop on fluoride and bone. New York: Mary Ann Liebert, Inc., 1990;5(Suppl 1).
13. Grynpas MD. Fluoride effects on bone crystals. In: Murray TM, Singer FR, eds. Journal of bone and mineral research: proceedings of the international workshop on fluoride and bone. New York: Mary Ann Liebert, Inc., 1990;5(Suppl 1):S169–S175.
14. Van Dyke D, Anger HO, Yano Y, Bozzini C. Bone blood flow shown with ^{18}F and the positron camera. Am J Physiol 1965;209(1):65–70.
15. Wooton R, Dore C. The single-passage extraction of ^{18}F in rabbit bone. Clin Phys Physiol Meas 1986;7:333–343.
16. Reeve J, Arlot M, Wooton R, et al. Skeletal blood flow, iliac histomorphometry, and strontium kinetics in osteoporosis: a relationship between blood flow and corrected apposition rate. J Clin Endocrinol Metab 1988;66:1124–1131.
17. Wooton R, Reeve J, Spellacy E, Tellez-Yudilevich M. Skeletal blood flow in Paget's disease of bone and its response to calcitonin therapy. Clin Sci Molec Med 1978;54:69–74.
18. Charkes ND, Brookes M, Makler PT. Studies of skeletal tracer kinetics. II. Evaluation of a five-compartment model of [^{18}F]fluoride kinetics in rats. J Nucl Med 1979;121:1150–1157.
19. Charkes ND, Makler PT Jr, Phillips C. Studies of skeletal tracer kinetics. I. Digital computer solution of a five-compartment model of [^{18}F]fluoride kinetics in humans. J Nucl Med 1978;19:1301–1309.
20. Charkes ND. Skeletal blood flow: implications of bone-scan interpretation. J Nucl Med 1980;21:91–98.
21. Lassen NA, Perl W. Tracer kinetic methods in medical physiology. New York: Raven Press, 1979.
22. Gallagher BM, Fowler JS, Gutterson NI, et al. Metabolic trapping as a principle of radiopharmaceutical design: some factors responsible for the biodistribution of [^{18}F]2-deoxyglucose. J Nucl Med 1980;19:1154–1161.
23. Sokoloff L, Reivich M, Kennedy C, et al. The [^{14}C]deoxyglucose method for the measurement of local cerebral glucose utilization: theory, procedure, and normal values in the conscious and anesthetized albino rat. J Neurochem 1977;28:897–916.
24. Phelps ME, Huang SC, Hoffman EJ, et al. Tomographic measurements of local cerebral glucose metabolic rate in humans with (F-18)-2-fluoro-2-deoxy-D-glucose: validation of method. Ann Neurol 1979;6:371–388.
25. Reivich M, Kuhl D, Wolf A, et al. The [^{18}F]fluorodeoxyglucose method for the measurement of local cerebral glucose utilization in man. Circ Res 1979;44:127–137.
26. Huang SC, Phelps ME, Hoffman EJ, Sideris K, Selin CJ, Kuhl DE. Noninvasive determination of local cerebral metabolic rate of glucose in man. Am J Physiol 1980;238:E69–E82.
27. Hawkins RA, Choi Y, Huang SC, Messa C, Hoh CK, Phelps ME. Quantitating tumor glucose metabolism with FDG and PET. J Nucl Med 1992;33:339–344.
28. Hawkins RA, Phelps ME, Huang SC. Effects of temporal sampling, glucose metabolic rate and disruptions of the blood brain barrier (BBB) on the FDG model with and without a vascular compartment: studies in human brain tumors with PET. J Cereb Blood Flow Metab 1986;6:170–183.
29. Hawkins RA, Choi Y, Huang SC, et al. Evaluation of the skeletal kinetics of fluorine-18-fluoride ion with PET. J Nucl Med 1992; 33:633–642.
30. Dahlbom M, Hoffman EJ, Hoh CK, et al. Evaluation of a positron emission tomography scanner for whole body imaging. J Nucl Med 1992;33:1191–1199.
31. Meikle SR, Dahlbom M, Cherry SR, et al. Attenuation correction in whole body PET [Abstract]. J Nucl Med 1992;33:826.
32. Cherry SR, Dahlbom M, Hoffman EJ. High sensitivity, total body PET scanning using 3-D data acquisition and reconstruction. IEEE Transactions Nucl Sci 1992;39(4):1088–1092.
33. Tse N, Hoh C, Hawkins R, Phelps M, Glaspy J. Positron emission tomography diagnosis of pulmonary metastases in osteogenic sarcoma. Am J Clin Oncol 1994;17(1):22–25.
34. Warburg O. On the origin of cancer cells. Science 1956;123:309–314.
35. Ott RJ. The applications of positron emission tomography to oncology [Editorial]. Br J Cancer 1991;63:343–345.
36. Strauss LG, Conti PS. The applications of PET in clinical oncology. J Nucl Med 1991;32:623–648.
37. Gold RH, Hawkins RA, Katz RD. Imaging osteomyelitis—from plain films to MRI: a pictorial essay. AJR 1991;157:365–370.
38. Wahl RL, Kaminski MS, Ethier SP, et al. The potential of 2-deoxy-2[^{18}F]fluoro-d-glucose (FDG) for the detection of tumor involvement in lymph nodes. J Nucl Med 1990;31:1831–1835.

39. Adler LP, Blair HF, Makley JT. Noninvasive grading of musculoskeletal tumors using PET. J Nucl Med 1991;32:1508–1512.
40. Kern KA, Brunetti A, Norton JA, et al. Metabolic imaging of human extremity musculoskeletal tumors by PET. J Nucl Med 1988; 29:181–186.
41. Yao WJ, Hoh CK, Hawkins RA, et al. Bone marrow glucose metabolic response to GMCSF by quantitative FDG PET imaging [Abstract]. J Nucl Med 1994;35(5):8P.
42. Gasson JC. Molecular physiology of granulocyte-macrophage colony stimulating factor. Blood 1991;7:1131–1145.
43. Demetri GD, Antman KH. Granulocyte-macrophage colony-stimulating factor (GM-CSF): preclinical and clinical investigations. Sem Oncol 1992;19:362–385.
44. Fogelman I, Bessent RG, Turner JG, et al. The use of whole-body retention of ^{99m}Tc-diphosphonate in the diagnosis of metabolic bone disease. J Nucl Med 1978;19:270–275.
45. Fogelman I, Bessent RG, Beastall G, et al. Estimation of skeletal involvement in primary hyperparathyroidism. Ann Intern Med 1980;92:65–67.
46. Front D, Israel O, Jerushalmi J, et al. Quantitative bone scintigraphy using SPECT. J Nucl Med 1989;30:240–245.
47. Israel O, Front D, Hardoff R, et al. In vivo SPECT quantitation of bone metabolism in hyperparathyroidism. J Nucl Med 1991; 32:1157–1161.
48. Messa C, Goodman WG, Hoh CK, et al. Bone metabolic activity measured with positron emission tomography and [^{18}F]fluoride ion in renal osteodystrophy: correlation with bone histomorphometry. J Clin Endocrinol Metab 1993;77(4):949–955.
49. Parfitt AM, Drezner MK, Glorieux FH, et al. Bone histomorphometry: standardization of nomenclature, symbols and units: report of the ASBMR histomorphometry nomenclature committee. J Bone Mine Res 1987;2:595–610.
50. Goodman WG, Coburn JW, Slatopolsky E, Saluski IB. Renal osteodystrophy in adults and children. In: Favus MJ, ed. Primer on the bone metabolic diseases and disorders of mineral metabolism. 1st ed. Kelseyville, CA: American Society of Bone and Mineral Research, 1990:200–212.
51. Recker RR. Bone biopsy and histomorphometry in clinical practice. In: Favus MJ, ed. Primer on the bone metabolic diseases and disorders of mineral metabolism. 1st ed. Kelseyville, CA: American Society of Bone and Mineral Research, 1990:101–104.

36 Esophageal Transit, Gastroesophageal Reflux, and Gastric Emptying

JEAN-LUC C. URBAIN, MARIE-CHRISTIANE M. VEKEMANS, and LEON S. MALMUD

SCINTIGRAPHIC EVALUATION OF ESOPHAGEAL TRANSIT

The esophagus is a 20 cm long muscular tube which extends from the cricoid cartilage to the stomach. Histologically, the proximal third of the esophagus consists of striated muscle, the distal third is composed of smooth muscle, and the middle portion is a transitional mixture of the two. Anatomically, three areas can be identified: the upper esophageal sphincter, the body, and the lower esophageal sphincter. The coordinated function of these structures conveys swallowed material from the mouth to the stomach and clears residual substances.

Esophageal motility follows a precisely coordinated pattern. First, a pharyngeal contraction transfers the bolus through a relaxed upper esophageal sphincter into the esophagus. The sphincter then contracts, and a primary peristaltic wave propels the food bolus aborally into the stomach through a relaxed lower esophageal sphincter. Secondary peristaltic waves occur in the esophageal body in response to residual food or refluxed gastric content. Tertiary nonperistaltic contractions induced by intramural reflex mechanisms can also be seen as a variant phenomenon. The so-called deglutitive inhibition phenomenon refers to the complete inhibition of the contractile activity induced by a first swallow when a second swallow is initiated and inversely. This effect can last for 20–30 seconds and must be taken into account if performing a multiple swallow acquisition test.

TEST PROCEDURE

Test procedures vary depending upon the radionuclide used, the type of bolus and its consistency, the position of the subject, the acquisition protocol, and the method of data processing and analysis.

Acquisition Protocol

The esophageal transit test should be performed after a 4–6 hour fast (1) and after withdrawal of any medication likely to interfere with esophageal motility.

Bolus Material. Solid food boluses are theoretically more physiologic in the assessment of esophageal transit (2–6); however, they usually disperse along the length of the esophagus and are practically inadequate for esophageal transit studies. In contrast, liquid boluses are homogeneous and provide more reproducible results. Water is the most common medium employed. It is usually given in the form of a bolus of 10–20 ml. Gelatin, a semisolid nutrient containing mainly water, is occasionally used as an alternative (7).

Radiopharmaceuticals. ^{99m}Tc sulfur colloid is usually preferred to label boluses, because it is inexpensive, easy to prepare, neither absorbed nor secreted by the esophageal mucosa (8), and has optimal physical characteristics for imaging. Limitations to the use of ^{99m}Tc tracers include the radiation exposure and scattered activity from the stomach, particularly when using multiple radiolabeled boluses.

^{81m}Kr has been used as an alternative in water or glucose solution. Its short half-life of 13 seconds permits the use of several millicuries per test, while keeping a low radiation burden. It produces a better counting statistic, but cannot adequately visualize esophageal retention in patients with stasis.

Patient Positioning. The supine position is preferred for the early characterization of the esophageal motor disorders because it eliminates the effect of gravity (9). The erect position, however, is more physiologic and is used to evaluate the effectiveness of medical or surgical treatment of achalasia or scleroderma (10). When performing the test in both positions sequentially, the upright position is performed first in anticipation of more rapid clearance of the radioactivity from the esophagus (11).

A ^{57}Co marker is placed over the cricoid cartilage to facilitate the identification of the upper esophageal sphincter. The patient is then positioned to visualize the mouth, esophagus, and gastric fundus in the same field of view. Anterior imaging is usually performed with the assumption that the attenuation along the length of the esophagus is uniform (12). The advantage of a more constant attenuation in posterior imaging has never really been proven (13, 14).

Acquisition Procedure. When gelatin or a solid food is used, a spoon with ±10 g of medium is administered. Liquid is usually given under the form of a 10 ml bolus labeled with 150–500 μCi of ^{99m}Tc-sulfur colloid or albumin colloid, or, alternatively, up to 8 mCi of ^{81m}Kr, and given to the patient with a syringe or a straw. Patients are instructed to retain the bolus in the mouth and to swallow the entire bolus in one gulp; two or three practice swallows with unlabeled material help the patient to understand the procedure. The multiple-swallow technique is preferred over the single swallow test because of the considerable intra-individual variations in esophageal emptying in normals (15–17) and patients (18). Four to six swallows followed by multiple dry swallows at 20–30 second intervals are usually adequate (19).

Acquisition Parameters. A high-speed framing rate is required to image esophageal transit. Typically, two sets of 64×64 matrix dynamic images are acquired for a total of ±2 minutes. During the first step, 0.25 second images are obtained to evaluate the oropharyngeal transit; for the second step, images of 1 second each are acquired to characterize the esophageal transit. Delayed images at 5, 10, and 15 minutes are useful in patients with significant stasis of radioactivity in the esophagus.

Data Processing—Data Analysis

The basic analysis of esophageal transit resides in the generation of time-activity curves using either a global esophageal region of interest, ranging from the cricoid to the gastroesophageal junction, and/or separate regions outlined around the hypopharynx, the total esophagus, the proximal, middle, and distal esophagus, and the stomach.

Global esophageal transit is determined based on the amount of residual activity in the esophagus using the formula $C(t) = E\,max - E(t)/E\,max$, where $C(t)$ represents the percentage of esophageal emptying at time t, $E\,max$, the maximal count rate in the esophagus, and $E(t)$, the esophageal count rate at time t (20).

Four parameters can be derived from the segmental time-activity curves (Fig. 36.1) (11): (a) the esophageal transit time is the time interval between the peak activity of the proximal esophageal curve and the peak activity of the distal esophageal curve; (b) the segmental emptying time characterizes the time required for more than an arbitrary percentage of the maximal radioactivity in each region of interest to be eliminated; (c) the global esophageal emptying time represents the time from entry of the bolus in the proximal esophagus to the clearance of more than 90% from the entire esophagus; and (d) the esophagogastric transit time is defined as the time interval between peak activity of the proximal esophageal curve and maximal gastric activity (11).

Condensed Images

Summing all computer frames during the transit of the bolus, Kjellen and Svedberg (21) introduced the concept of a "topographic picture" of the esophagus. A refined approach was proposed by Svedberg (22) and Klein (23) using the "condensed picture."

The condensed image consists of the summation of the activity in the pixel rows into a single column for each frame of the swallowing test data series, and the creation of a single image where the vertical axis shows the spatial distribution of the radioactivity from the mouth to the stomach and the horizontal axis is temporal (Fig. 36.2). With this approach, a complete dynamic sequence is displayed in one single image, facilitating qualitative assessment of radionuclide esophageal transit and improving diagnostic ability (24). To integrate the dynamic sequences after each bolus swallow, Tatsch, in 1991 (18), introduced the "pseudogating" technique of condensed esophageal images (Fig. 36.3). This technique has the advantage of displaying into one single image the average esophageal transit of multiple boluses and dry swallows. Its major built-in disadvantage resides in the sum of dynamic sequences which are not necessarily in phase with the swallows.

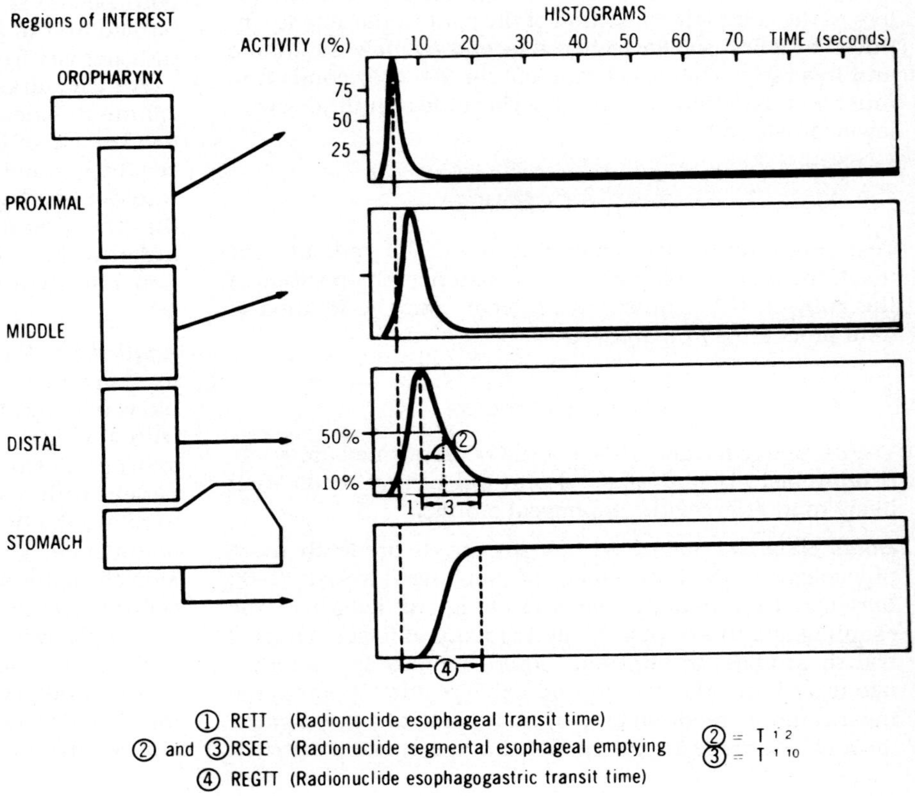

Figure 36.1. Parameters which can be derived from an esophageal transit study. Regions of interest around the entire esophagus, its proximal, middle, and distal segments, and the stomach, allow for the determination of the esophageal transit time, the segmental emptying time, the global esophageal emptying time, and the esophagogastric transit time (Reproduced by permission from Taillefer R, Beauchamp G. Radionuclide esophagogram. Clin Nucl Med 1984;9:465–483.)

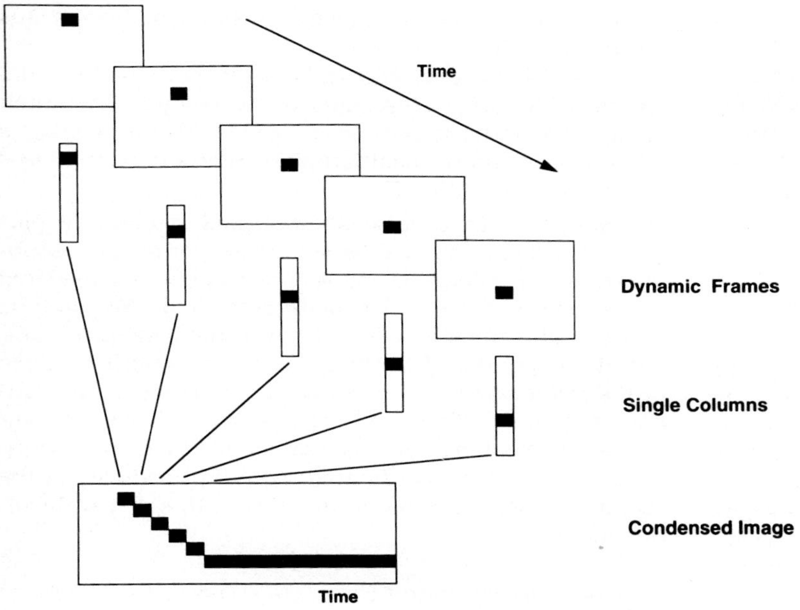

Figure 36.2. Condensed image representation. For each dynamic frame of the swallow set, the esophagus is represented by a single column. Columns are then added together to generate a single condensed image. On the condensed image, the spatial distribution of the radioactivity in the esophagus over time is represented by the vertical axis.

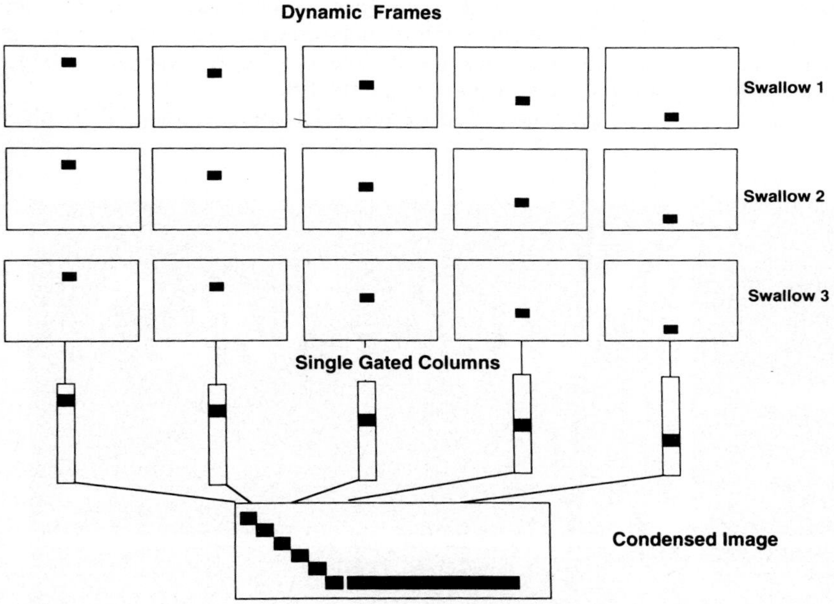

Figure 36.3. Gated esophageal condensed image. In the gated technique, columns of the same numbered frame of the swallow sets are added together and a single composite condensed image is generated.

INTERPRETATION

Visual inspection of dynamic sequences allows for the assessment of the completeness of bolus ingestion, for the assessment of progression of the bolus through the esophagus, and for the identification of bolus stasis in any portion of the esophagus. Episodes of reflux or any abnormal extraluminal focus of activity can also be detected.

In normal subjects, passage of the bolus from the pharynx into the esophagus takes less than 0.5–1 second. Esophageal transit time for water or semisolid boluses varies from 5.5 ± 1.1 to 9.5 ± 1.5 seconds, depending on the definition and calculation methods used (3, 17, 25–27). Because of the compression by the aortic arch or tracheal bifurcation, a slowing of bolus progression can be observed at the midportion of the esophagus. Abnormal esophageal motility caused by aging (the so-called "presbyesophagus") and delayed esophageal transit in obese patients with reflux (28) have been described.

Esophageal motility disturbances are classically categorized into primary or secondary disorders depending on the pathophysiologic mechanisms. Disruption of the anatomy of the esophageal tube can also result in transit abnormalities. In this chapter, we review the most common diseases which affect esophageal transit.

Primary Esophageal Motility Disorders

Achalasia. Achalasia is characterized by a loss of peristalsis in the esophageal body and a failure of the lower esophageal sphincter to relax. The esophageal transit test shows a marked and prolonged retention of the radioactive bolus in the distal segment of the esophagus with very little activity in the stomach. The condensed image may also demonstrate a chaotic movement of the activity (Fig. 36.4**B**).

Although the sensitivity of the test is high (2, 20, 30–32), endoscopy or radiographic techniques are the primary diagnostic tests of this disease because they permit exclusion of anatomic abnomalities or obstructive lesions, such as cancer. Quantitative evaluation of the effectiveness of pneumatic dilatation is the principal indication for esophageal transit scintigraphy.

Diffuse Esophageal Spasm. Diffuse esophageal spasm syndrome is characterized by spastic activity of the lower two-thirds of the esophagus with intermittent chest pain and/or dysphagia. Typically, the radionuclide transit test demonstrates a prolonged transit time associated with decreased segmental esophageal emptying, periods of esophrageal retrograde movements, and fragmentation of the radioactive bolus. Time-activity curves show multiple peaks of activity in all esophageal segments. Sensitivity of esophageal transit in this disorder is about 77% (33, 34).

Nutcracker Esophagus. The nutcracker esophagus is characterized by high amplitude peristaltic contractions in the esophageal body occurring simultaneously with noncardiac chest pain and/or dysphagia (35). Typical scintigraphic findings consist in a prolonged retention of activity in the distal esophagus and a mild distal to midesophagus esophageal reflux.

The sensitivity of esophageal transit scintigraphy in detecting nutcracker esophagus depends upon the cutoff value used for the amplitude of the mean distal esophagus contractions and the scintigraphic criteria used to assess the transit delay (36, 37).

Nonspecific Motor Disorders. Abnormal manometric patterns that do not fit established criteria for diffuse esophageal spasm, achalasia, or scleroderma, are considered nonspecific motor disorders of the esophagus. Manometric abnormalities include peristaltic contractions of low amplitude or prolonged duration, waveforms with multiple peaks or followed by repetitive waves, and/or sustained increase in the baseline esophageal pressure. The most common scintigraphic finding is a prolonged esophageal transit time with an incoordinated pattern. Sensitivity of the esophageal scintigraphic transit test in this disparate entity is variable.

Neuromuscular and Connective Tissue Disorders

Abnormal esophageal motility has been described in all connective tissue disorders, which involve either the smooth muscle, such as scleroderma, systemic lupus erythematosus, Raynaud's disease, or the striated muscle, such as dermatopolymyositis (38).

In progressive systemic sclerosis, esophageal involve-

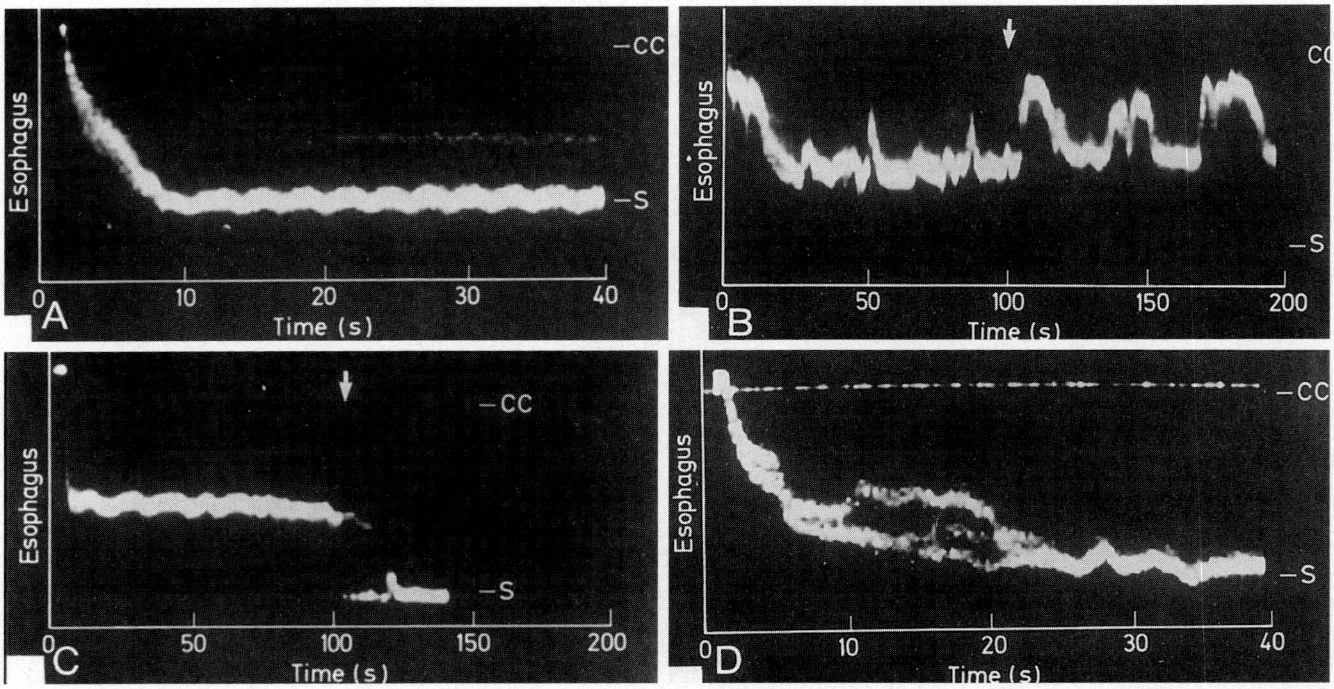

Figure 36.4. Esophageal condensed images. **A.** In normal subjects, the bolus transit quickly and smoothly through all segments. **B.** In achalasia, there is a marked and prolonged retention of the bolus in the distal segment of the esophagus with very little activity in the stomach. Episodes of retrograde motion are frequently observed. **C.** In patients with scleroderma a stagnation of the bolus in the lower portion of the esophagus is characteristic. The administration of water (*arrow*) can clear out the activity into the stomach by forcing the bolus through the hypokinetic segment. **D.** Patients with gastroesophageal reflux demonstrate retrograde movements of activity from the stomach into the esophagus. (Reproduced by permission from O'Connor MK, Byrne PJ, Keeling P, Hennessy TP. Esophageal scintigraphy: applications and limitations in the study of esophageal disorders. Eur J Nucl Med 1988;14:131–136.)

ment is frequent, but often asymptomatic, in early stages of the disease. Esophageal transit scintigraphy has been employed both to detect early involvement of the esophagus and to evaluate the impairment of the esophageal function.

The esophageal transit pattern is characteristic and demonstrates stagnation of the bolus in the lower two-thirds of the esophagus (Fig. 36.4**C**). The sensitivity of scintigraphy in this disease is approximately 88% (39–43). Excellent correlation exists between scintigraphy, manometry, and the patient's symptoms (43). Abnormal esophageal motility has also been described in neuromuscular diseases such as myotonic dystrophy or myasthenia gravis.

Other Conditions

Hiatal Hernia. Qualitative visualization of persistent radioactivity along the distal esophagus is often found in hiatal hernia and should not be confused with esophageal stasis of other etiology.

Tumors of the Esophagus. Evaluation by endoscopy is mandatory in patients with suspicion of tumors of the esophagus. Scintigraphically, tumors appear as areas of decreased radioactivity with stenotic lesions and are associated with delayed esophageal transit. In some instances, the esophageal lumen is enlarged above the stenosis. Esophageal transit scintigraphy is the only available tool for the quantitative evaluation of therapeutic approaches such as laser therapy or prosthesis placement (44).

Zenker's Diverticulum. Zenker's diverticulum is an acquired pharyngoesophageal outpouch located above the upper esophageal sphincter. Classically, scintigraphic findings consist of an ovoid or spheric area of persistent esophageal retention of radioactivity at the level of the upper esophagus.

Esophageal Surgery. Radionuclide esophageal transit is the only test which allows for the physiologic quantitative evaluation of esophageal transit before and after surgical treatment for hiatal hernia and reflux.

Miscellaneous. An abnormal esophageal transit test is observed in about 50% of patients with gastroesophageal reflux (8, 20, 25). Diabetes mellitus and chronic alcoholism (45), infection, systemic illnesses, and trauma may also lead to secondary motor disorders of the esophagus.

SCINTIGRAPHIC EVALUATION OF ESOPHAGEAL REFLUX

Gastroesophageal reflux scintigraphy was introduced in 1976 by Fisher and Malmud (46) to quantitate gastroesophageal reflux and to assess the effectiveness of medical and surgical treatment (47–53). The availability and accuracy of endoscopy, the Bernstein test, esophageal manometry, and 24-hour pH monitoring has resulted in gastroesophageal reflux scintigraphy being almost obsolete in adults. However, because of its physiologic and noninvasive character, scintigraphy has gained wide acceptance in the detection and evaluation of gastroesophageal reflux in infants and children.

TEST PROCEDURE

Acquisition Protocol

The patient is studied after an overnight fast and positioned supine under the camera to avoid the counterreflux effect of gravity. Two additional aggravants of reflux are used to enhance the sensitivity of the test: (a) an acid load to the stomach can be given to decrease the tone of the lower esophageal sphincter, and (b) an inflatable abdominal binder placed around the lower abdomen is used to increase the pressure gradient across the lower esophageal sphincter.

Three hundred ml of acidified orange juice containing 300 μCi of ^{99m}Tc-sulfur colloid and consisting of 150 ml orange juice and 150 ml 0.1N hydrochloric acid are administrated orally to the patient in the upright position, and a first static 30-second exposure image is acquired to assure complete clearance of the radiolabeled material from the esophagus. If needed, 30 ml of water are given to clear any residual activity. Dynamic images are then acquired in the supine position, at baseline and at each 20 mm Hg pressure gradient from 0–100 mm Hg.

In infants and children, the study is performed using the infant's formula, milk, or pudding, and the examiner's hand is used to create pressure on the abdomen. Positions and circumstances during which reflux occurs can be determined scintigraphically as can the rate of gastric emptying (54, 55). A possible relationship between gastroesophageal reflux and sudden infant death syndrome (56, 57), as well as various respiratory diseases (58–60), has been evoked.

Giving ^{99m}Tc-sulfur colloid or, preferably, ^{111}In-DTPA in a liquid meal to the child at bedtime, and scanning the lungs the next day, can provide objective and direct evidence of pulmonary aspiration of refluxed gastric material (61).

Visual Description, Data Processing, and Interpretation

In normal subjects, gastroesophageal reflux of radioactivity cannot be seen even by increasing pressure up to 100 mm Hg. In patients with reflux, an increase in the amount of reflux material is observed as the gradient across the lower esophageal sphincter is increased.

Reflux can be quantified at each step, using regions of interest over the esophagus and stomach using the formula $R = E(t) - E(b) \times 100/Go$, where R is the percentage of reflux material into the esophagus; $E(t)$, the esophageal counts at time t; $E(b)$, the paraesophageal background counts; and Go, the gastric counts at the beginning of the study. In practice, reflux $\geq$4% is considered abnormal. This value coincides with the visibility of refluxed radioactivity on the gamma-camera screen. Overall sensitivity of the technique is in the range of 88–91%.

Reflux is also nicely documented on condensed images by a rebound of activity above the gastroesophageal junction line (Fig. 36.4**D**).

GASTRIC EMPTYING SCINTIGRAPHY

Anatomically, the stomach can be divided into three regions: the fundus, the corpus, and the antrum.

Physiologically, the human stomach consists of two functionally integrated, but electromechanically distinct, portions. The proximal stomach, which encompasses the fundus and the proximal corpus, functions as a reservoir for solid and liquid food and controls the emptying of liquids. The distal stomach, which includes the mid and distal corpus and the antrum, is characterized by peristaltic contractions at a rate of 3 per minute. These contractions break down solid food into small particles, mix them with gastric secretions to form a semiliquid juice which is then emptied into the duodenum. The rate of gastric emptying is determined by many factors, including the volume, physical state, caloric content, caloric density, concentration of the nutrients, the meal distribution, and its salinity, acidity, and viscosity.

Emptying of Liquids. Saline, neutral, isosmolar, and calorically inert solutions empty in a single exponential manner as a function of volume (62, 63). When the stomach is filled with a nutrient solution, the shape of the emptying curve becomes more linear (64) or may even consist of two linear phases: an initial rapid and a slower late phase (65). Osmolytes, acids, fatty acids (particularly medium-chains), carbohydrates, and proteins activate receptors along the small bowel and control gastric emptying by feedback mechanisms (66–70).

Emptying of Solids. Emptying-time course for solid food is sigmoidal in shape and characterized by an initial lag phase during which no or little solid emptying occurs, followed by a linear phase with a constant emptying rate, and a late, much slower phase. Physical characteristics of solid food, antral contractions, and antroduodenal coordination determine the lag phase duration and emptying rate. Both the lag phase and emptying time are increased by high caloric meals (71, 72). Increasing the volume of solid food speeds up gastric emptying. This effect is overridden by intestinal inhibition, as additional calories enter the small intestine (73).

Emptying of a Solid-Liquid Test Meal. Liquids, in presence of solids, empty much more rapidly than solids, but at a slower rate than if given alone (71, 74). The "solid-liquid discrimination" appellation refers to the rapid emptying of water from the stomach while solids are retained; it is predominantly related to the sieving effect of solid particles by the pylorus (75).

Emptying of Fat. Fat relaxes the fundus, lowers the intragastric pressure, increases the reservoir capacity, inhibits antral motility, and increases pyloric contraction (76). Fat slows the emptying of all constituents of a mixed meal (77) and is emptied at a slower rate than solids (78).

TEST PROCEDURE

Acquisition Protocol

Gastric emptying should to be evaluated following at least a 12-hour overnight fast (79, 80). Subjects should refrain from smoking (81) and no medication likely to interfere with gastric emptying should be taken before the test. Diabetic patients should be studied early in the morning following administration of their insulin dose.

Test Meal—Test Meal Labeling. Among the various radionuclides and radiopharmaceuticals which have been used for labeling meals, both ^{99m}Tc-sulfur colloid and ^{111}In-DTPA have emerged as the tracers of choice because of their short half-lives, better imaging characteristics, low radiation burdens, and strong binding to food.

The first meal used to evaluate gastric emptying consisted of porridge, milk, bread and butter, and scrambled eggs, mixed with ^{51}Cr (Griffith (82)). Chicken liver, labeled in vivo with ^{99m}Tc-sulfur colloid, was introduced in 1976 to insure radiotracer binding to the solid food (83); it is the most stable test meal in gastric juice (84, 85).

The dual-isotope scanning method, introduced in 1976 by Heading (74), for the simultaneous measurement of ^{99m}Tc solid and ^{111}In DTPA liquid emptying, has rapidly gained widespread clinical and investigational acceptance. With time however, it appeared that the liquid constituent of a test meal is less sensitive than the solid phase to detect gastric emptying impairment (65, 86–87).

Numerous solid foods, including whole eggs, egg whites, chicken liver, liver paté, hamburgers, fibers, and nondigestible particles, have been used with or without a liquid component, usually water. Because of the availability, low cost, and stability of ^{99m}Tc-sulfur colloid in gastric juice and the ready availability of eggs, radiolabeled eggs are now preferred by most authors. Our standardized test meal consists of 1 scrambled egg, 2 slices of regular white bread (weighing ±50 g each), and 150 ml of tap water, and contains approximately 230 calories with 35% fat, 47% carbohydrate, and 18% protein. The egg is mixed with 0.5–1.0 mCi ^{99m}Tc-sulfur colloid, cooked until firm in a Teflon-coated pan, and given to the patient as an egg sandwich. For dual-isotope solid-liquid emptying studies, water is labeled with 75 μCi of ^{111}In-DTPA. Ingestion of the radiolabeled test meal should optimally be completed within 10 minutes.

Acquisition Procedure. To reproduce physiologic conditions, the patient is positioned sitting or standing in front of the gamma-camera. A ^{99m}Tc or ^{57}Co marker taped over the xyphoid process or the iliac crest helps to reposition the subject for imaging.

Dual Phase Emptying Test Meal

Immediately after ingestion of the ^{99m}Tc-radiolabeled solid phase of the meal, an initial 1 minute image of the stomach is acquired in the 140 keV ±20% ^{99m}Tc window using a medium-energy parallel hole collimator. The patient then ingests the liquid phase, labeled with ^{111}In-DTPA, and a second 1 minute picture is taken in the ^{99m}Tc window to calculate the downscatter percentage of ^{111}In into the ^{99m}Tc window. A third 1 minute picture is subsequently acquired on the 247 keV ^{111}In peak ±20% window. Pictures of the stomach are then taken in both windows every 10 minutes for 1 hour, and every 15–20 minutes for up to 2 hours, if needed, until 50% emptying. Since exercise accelerates gastric emptying, the patient should remain seated between images.

Single Label Test Meal

When using a single radionuclide to label either the liquid or solid component of the meal, images are taken using the appropriate radionuclide peak and collimator, following similar time intervals as for the dual-labeled meal.

Imaging

To allow for the correction of the increase of counts as the food moves from the more posterior fundus to the more anterior antrum, geometric mean data are obtained from simultaneous anterior and posterior static images (dual-headed system), or from anterior, immediately followed by posterior views (single-head system), using a 64×64 or 128×128 pixel matrix (88–91). Other correction methods have been advocated, and use either an additional lateral view of the stomach (62), a left anterior oblique (LAO) projection (92–95), or the peak-to-scatter ratio (96).

To obtain information on antral motility, 64×64 pixel matrix dynamic images are taken at a rate of 1 frame per second for 4 minutes after each set of static images (97–100).

Visual Description—Data Processing

Visual Description. Immediately after meal completion, the test meal is usually retained in the proximal stomach. The water component of the meal distributes uniformly throughout the stomach before being emptied into the duodenum. In contrast, solid food moves progressively from the proximal to the distal stomach where it is ground into small particles before emptying (Fig. 36.5**A**).

Data Processing. The geometric mean of the gastric counts, i.e., the square root of the product of the anterior activity multiplied by the posterior activity in the stomach, is calculated at each imaging interval. Counts are corrected for radionuclide decay and normalized to 100% based on total gastric counts obtained immediately following ingestion of the meal. This is defined as $t = 0$ minutes. Data are then plotted as percentage retention versus time.

Liquid emptying typically follows a single exponential pattern, while solid emptying is sigmoidal in shape and characterized by an initial shoulder with little emptying called the lag phase (Tlag), followed by a linear phase and a much slower phase when the stomach is almost emptied (Fig. 36.6).

Data Analysis

The simplest method to evaluate gastric emptying is the determination on the gastric emptying curve of the time required for 50% emptying (half emptying time or $T_{1/2}$). This parameter does not fully characterize gastric emptying. Gastric emptying data are more completely analyzed using mathematic functions which reflect the time course of emptying and, eventually, gastric emptying physiology.

Two functions have been shown to adequately fit biphasic solid gastric emptying data: the power exponential function $y = (e^{-kt})^{\beta}$ (101) and a modified power exponential function ($y(t) = 1-(1-e^{-kt})^{\beta}$) (102). In both, $y(t)$ is the fractional meal retention at time t, k is the gastric emptying rate in minutes^{-1} and β is the extrapolated y-intercept from the terminal portion of the curve. Four parameters can be derived from these two functions: the β value,

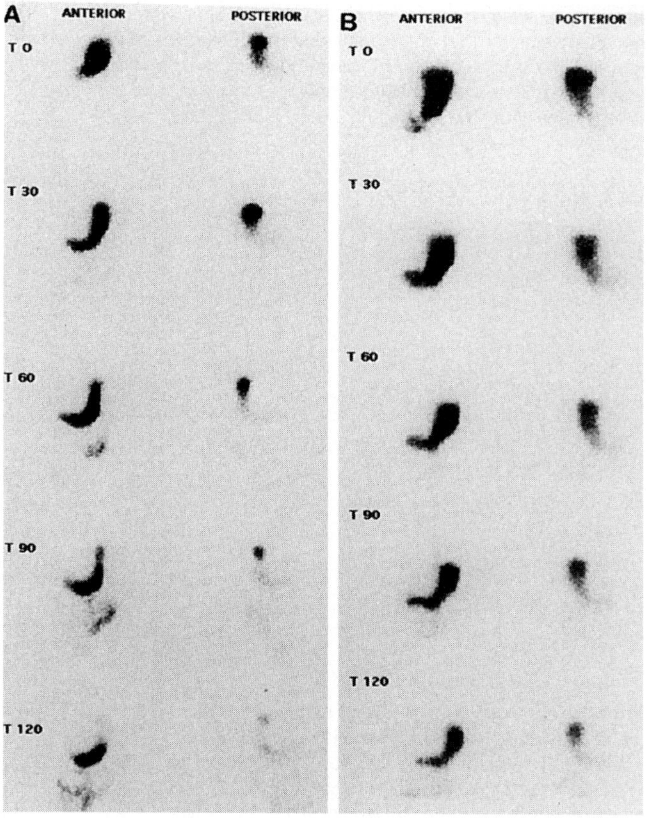

Figure 36.5. Gastric emptying study of solids. Anterior and posterior images of the stomach are shown 0, 30, 60, 90, and 120 minutes after meal completion (*T0*) in a normal subject (**A**) and in a patient with diabetic gastroparesis (**B**). In normal subjects, the test meal is initially retained in the proximal stomach and then moves progressively to the distal stomach where it is ground into small particles before emptying. In patients with diabetic gastroparesis, a significant retention of food is observed in the proximal portion of the stomach and the filling of the distal stomach is delayed.

the Tlag (in minutes), the emptying rate (in percent of emptying per minute) and the half emptying time ($T_{1/2}$)(in minutes). The β parameter determines the shape of the curve. Solid curves have usually an initial lag phase and β is >1. A value of $\beta < 1$ indicates initial rapid emptying followed by a second slower emptying phase. This is the pattern often seen in patients after antrectomy or following ingestion of some liquid meals. Numerically, the lag phase, Tlag, is equal to Ir β/k (modified power exponential function) and to $((\beta - 1)/\beta)^{1/\beta}/k$ (Elashoff function). Mathematically, it represents the time at which the second derivative of the function equals zero and coincides with the antral filling peak (Fig. 36.7). Liquid emptying curves are described by the single exponential function ($y(t) = e^{-kt}$), where $y(t)$ is the fractional meal retention at time t, and k is the emptying rate in minutes^{-1}.

Gastric Motility and Scintigraphy

Time activity curves generated from antral regions of interest display a sinusoid pattern which reflects the rhythmic mechanical activity of the antrum. Antral activity

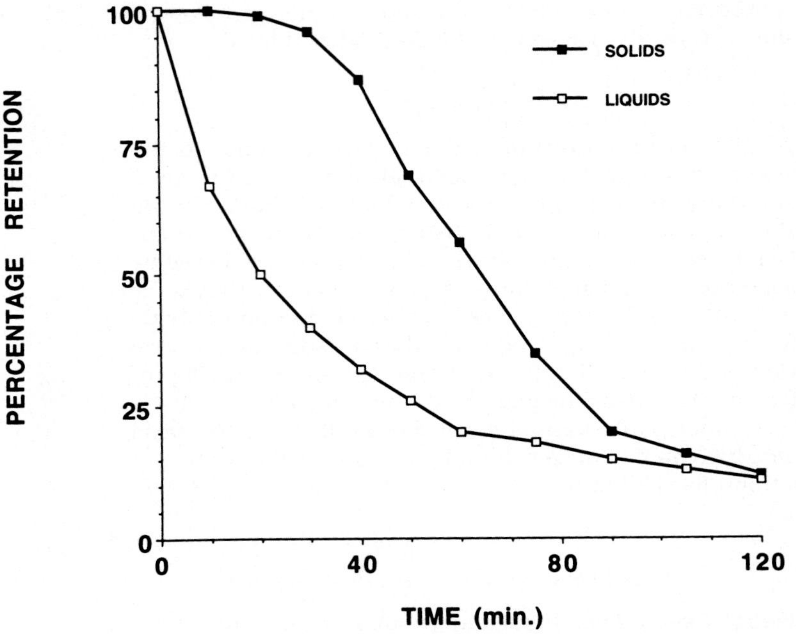

Figure 36.6. Gastric emptying curves for solids and liquids. In normal subjects, solid emptying is sigmoidal in shape with an initial shoulder with no or little emptying (the lag phase), followed by a linear phase with constant emptying rate, and a much slower phase when the stomach is nearly empty. Liquid curve follows an exponential pattern.

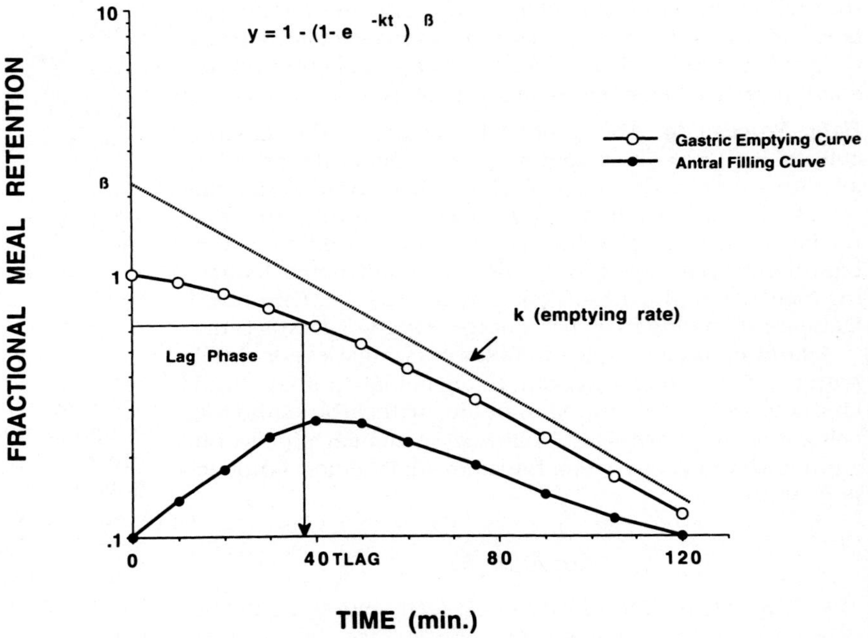

Figure 36.7. Modified power exponential fitting function. The modified power exponential function characterizes the three portions of a solid emptying curve: the lag phase (TLAG), which is numerically equal to ln β/k and corresponds to the inflection point of the total gastric emptying curve, and to the peak antral filling, the emptying rate (*k*), and half-emptying time.

curves can be analyzed using the autocorrelation technique (97) and the Fourier transform function (97–100, 103) to determine the frequency and the amplitude of gastric contractions (Fig. 36.8**A**).

In normal subjects, gastric contractions occur at a rate of 3 per minute and both the frequency and amplitude of those contractions can be correlated with the emptying of food (103). In diabetic gastroparesis, delayed gastric emptying is related to a retention of food in the proximal stomach, as well as a decrease in the amplitude of antral contractions (97) (Fig. 36.8**B**). In functional dyspepsia, the amplitude of gastric contractions is increased regardless of the emptying rate (98, 100) (Fig. 36.8**C**).

Reproducibility

Inter- and intraindividual variations of gastric half-emptying time can be significant in normal subjects and patients with gastroparesis (62, 65, 104–107). This explains the broad range usually observed in normal subject, and emphasizes the need to carefully standardize the acquisition parameters, especially when the effects of a drug are being assessed.

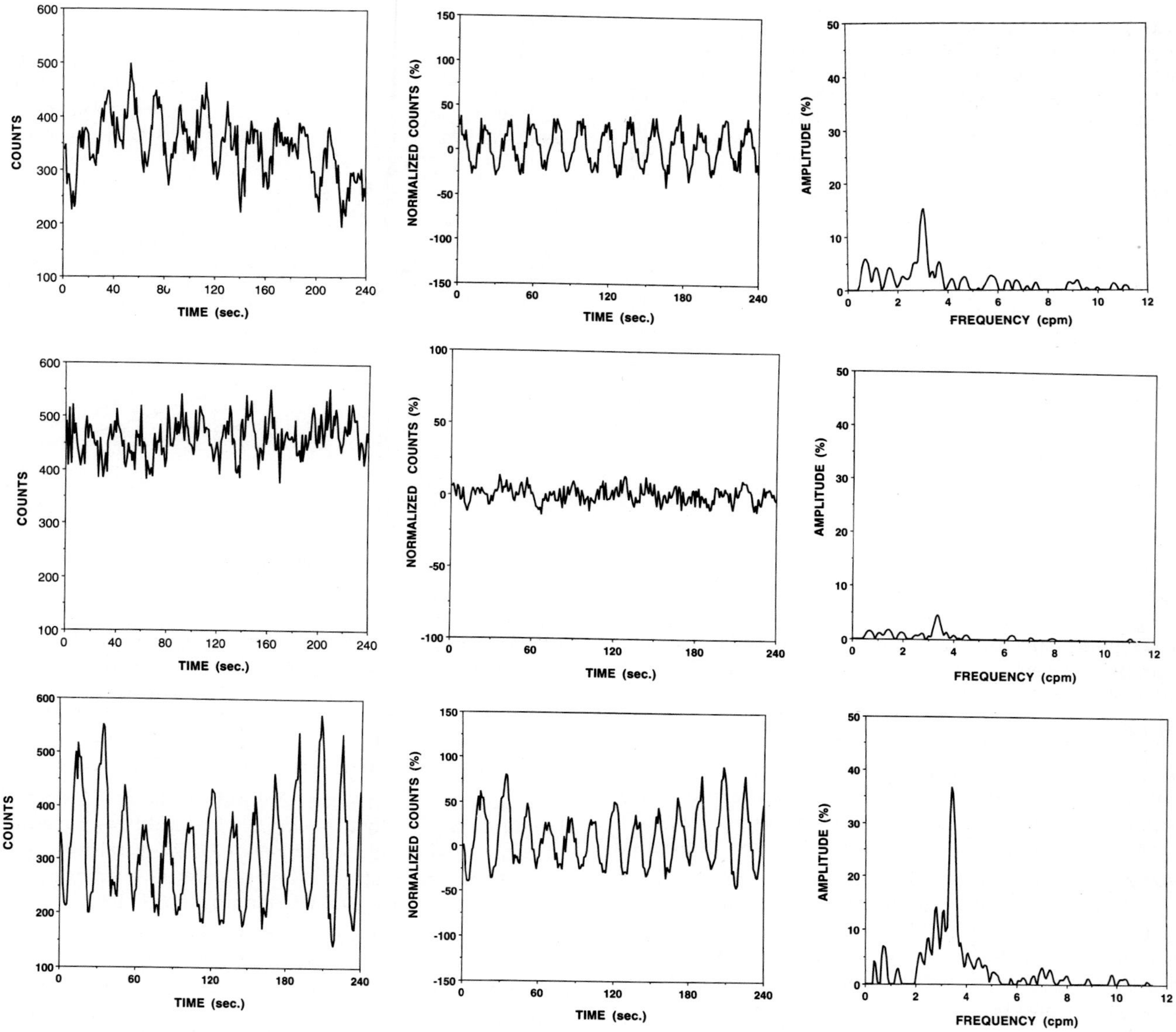

Figure 36.8. Antral time activity curves processing. The processing of dynamic antral time activity curves is shown in this figure for a healthy control (*top row*), a patient with diabetic gastroparesis (*middle row*) and a patient with functional dyspepsia (*lower row*). *Left column:* Four-minute raw antral time-activity curves. *Middle column:* Curves are normalized to their respective mean count. *Right column:* The autocorrelation function and the Fourier transform are then applied to determine the dominant frequency and the amplitude. In all subjects, the dominant frequency of the antral contractions is about 3 cycles per minute. The amplitude is the variable parameter of the contraction with a decrease in diabetic gastroparesis and an increase in functional dyspepsia.

INTERPRETATION

In this section, we review the most frequent causes of gastric motility impairment and describe their gastric emptying pattern.

Medical Disorders and Diseases

Diabetes. Delayed gastric emptying in symptomatic and asymptomatic diabetics (65, 108–112) is mainly accounted for by a prolonged lag phase (65, 113), an impairment of the proximal stomach function and a reduction in the antral motor activity (97, 110) (Fig. 36.9**B**). A markedly prolonged linear gastric emptying of solids (up to several hours) and a delayed emptying of liquids characterize advanced diabetic gastroparesis (65, 111, 112, 114, 115). In patients with type II diabetes of recent onset, an accelerated gastric emptying for solids was recently described (116).

Functional Dyspepsia. The clinical description of functional dyspepsia includes a constellation of symptoms such as abdominal pain or discomfort, early satiety, fullness, distension, bloating, nausea, vomiting, belching, and epigastric or retrosternal burning. Dyspepsia is categorized as either organic or functional (idiopathic), based on the presence or the absence of underlying structural and/or biochemical abnormalities. Idiopathic dyspepsia occurs

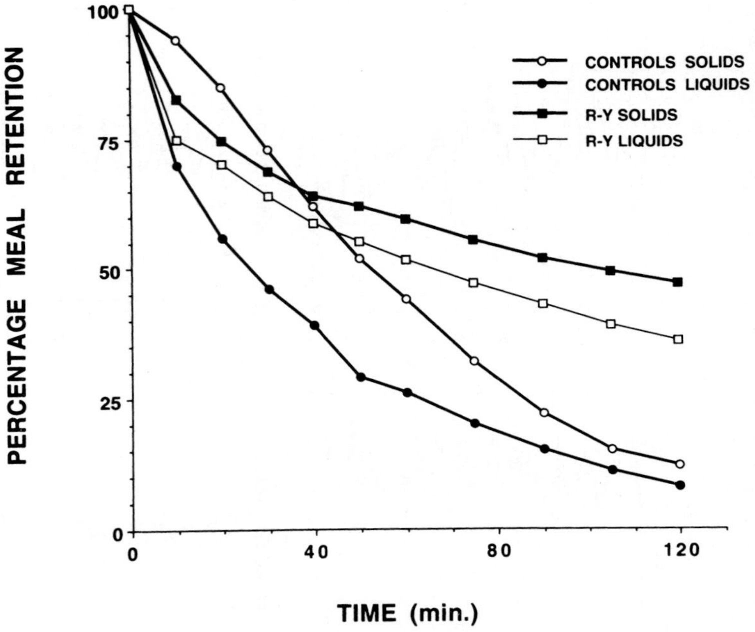

Figure 36.9. Gastric emptying curves in patients Roux-en-Y diversion. In the Roux-en-Y gastrojejunostomy with vagotomy, both solid and liquid emptying follow a biexponential pattern with an early rapid emptying of the food from the stomach pouch and a slower emptying phase. No lag phase is observed for solids.

more commonly in women under the age of 50, but no correlation between the occurrence of symptoms and the menstrual cycle has been found. The pathophysiology of functional dyspepsia remains unclear. Antral hypomotility is observed in 25–70% of patients (117–119). However, a hypermotility pattern has also been described. In this case, an antropyloric dyscoordination motility pattern could be responsible for the delay in solid food emptying (98, 100). Liquid emptying appears to be normal in these patients.

Anorexia Nervosa. About 80% of anorectic patients display a delayed gastric emptying for solids, while liquid emptying remains normal (120). Hypersensitivity of small intestinal nutrient receptors resulting from chronic food deprivation might explain the persistent delay in gastric emptying after oral renutrition of these patients.

Gastritis. In chronic gastritis, emptying of liquids is usually normal, while emptying of solids is delayed. Stasis of both liquids and solids has been described in atrophic gastritis, while in pernicious anaemia delayed gastric emptying for solids only is observed (121, 122).

Gastroesophageal Reflux. Gastric retention of acid and food favor gastroesophageal reflux in adults (123, 124). More than 60% of patients with gastroesophageal reflux have delayed gastric emptying of solids. Liquids may be emptied normally or with a delay, depending on the test meal (123, 125–127).

In infants, a fundic disorder producing a rapid rise in the intragastric pressure is responsible for gastroesophageal reflux and gastric retention (128, 129).

Acid-Peptic Diseases. *Gastric Ulcer.* Transient slow emptying has been observed in patients with an ulcer of the proximal stomach (82, 127–129). Antral hypomotility, abnormalities of the interdigestive migrating motor complex and increased concentration of bile salts are possible causes of gastric stasis.

Duodenal Ulcer. No definite conclusion can be found in the literature on gastric emptying in this disorder. Solid emptying has been found delayed by some authors (130, 131) while others have reported a faster solid (81, 132, 133) or liquid emptying (134, 135). Normal solid and liquid emptying has also been described (136, 137).

Zollinger-Ellison Disease. Zollinger-Ellison disease has been unequivocally associated with rapid gastric emptying of both solids and liquids. A defective inhibitory mechanism of gastric emptying due to extensive inflammation of gastric mucosa may be responsible (138, 139).

Connective Tissue Disorders. Delayed gastric emptying of solids and liquids is present in 50% of patients with progressive systemic sclerosis (4, 140). In systemic lupus erythematosus, polymyositis, and dermatomyositis, delayed gastric emptying, when present, may be asymptomatic. Antral hypomotility and impaired fasting motor activity are possible pathophysiologic factors (38).

Surgical Procedures

Gastric emptying pattern may be affected in several different ways, depending on the type of operation. As a rule of thumb, proximal gastric vagotomy impairs the reservoir function and the emptying of liquids, while truncal or selective vagotomy affects both proximal and distal stomach and alters emptying of both solids and liquids. Antral removal suppresses the grinding and sieving of solid food which is emptied faster into the small bowel.

Vagotomy. *Highly Selective or Proximal Gastric Vagotomy.* Following proximal gastric vagotomy, liquid emptying shows a biexponential pattern with an initial rapid emptying with up to 50% emptied within the first 10 minutes followed by a normal rate (141, 142). Solid gastric emptying, which may be slightly delayed initially, usually returns to normal within a few weeks or months (131, 143, 144). In some instances, prolongation of the solid lag phase persists for many months after surgery (145, 146).

Truncal and Selective Vagotomy. Solid food emptying is transiently delayed, but this delay may persist in 20–25% of the patients (147–149). Liquid hypertonic solutions empty in an accelerated fashion, because of the loss of fundal relaxation and weakened duodenal feedback mechanisms (150–152).

Drainage Procedures. Pyloroplasty accelerates gastric emptying of solids and allows the passage of larger size particles in the small bowel (153). Following vagotomy and pyloroplasty, liquids empty precipitously, particularly in the erect position, and solid emptying is moderately delayed (154).

Gastrectomy. Proximal gastrectomy accelerates gastric emptying (155). After distal gastrectomy, solid emptying is accelerated and larger particles are allowed to pass into the small bowel (153, 156–158). Liquid emptying is usually normal or rapid in this instance (141, 156, 159). The combination of truncal vagotomy and distal gastrectomy accelerates gastric emptying of liquids (150, 152), while solid emptying is retarded (157, 160). Total or subtotal gastrectomy associated with truncal vagotomy results in an initial precipitous emptying followed by an exponential course for solids (161). In the Roux-en-Y diversion with vagotomy, gastric emptying of solids and liquids follows a biexponential curve characterized by an early rapid emptying of the remnant gastric pouch, followed by a very slow evacuation phase (146, 157, 162) (Fig. 36.9).

Intrathoracic Stomach. Emptying of the intrathoracic stomach is much slower than normal esophageal transit, and is characterized by an early phase of rapid gastric evacuation (within the first 10 minutes after the meal), followed by a later slower phase (163, 164). Gastroesophageal reflux may also occur with a high incidence, especially if the stomach is entirely intrathoracic (165–167).

Gastrokinetic Compounds

The increased interest in gastric emptying procedures over the past two decades is partially explained by the availability of specific and effective gastrokinetic compounds. Numerous therapeutic trials have been conducted using scintigraphy to assess their effects on gastric emptying.

Metoclopramide increases both the frequency and amplitude of antral contractions and accelerates emptying of solids and liquids (110, 168–171).

Domperidone inhibits the stomach's receptive relaxation reflex, increases antral motility, and improves antroduodenal coordination, and, as a result, accelerates gastric emptying (120, 172).

Cisapride is a prokinetic agent without antidopaminergic properties, which improves gastric emptying of solids and liquids in diabetics (111), in patients after gastric surgery, and in patients with idiopathic gastroparesis (173).

Erythromycin, a macrolide antibiotic, abolishes the solid-liquid discrimination in normals, in diabetics with gastroparesis and functional dyspepsia, and dramatically increases gastric emptying of both solids and liquids (112, 174). Erythromycin is a motilin agonist (175–177), which initiates Phase III of the interdigestive motor complex (178–181) and generates powerful antral contractions (182).

Recently, the gastrointestinal peptide motilin has been used successfully to improve gastric emptying of solids and liquids in diabetic gastroparesis (183), opening the avenue for the endocrine treatment of gastric stasis with physiologic compounds.

REFERENCES

1. Diamant NE, Akin AN. Effect of gastric contractions on the lower esophageal sphincter. Gastroenterology 1972;63:38–44.
2. Gross R, Johnson LF, Kaminski RJ. Esophageal emptying in achalasia quantitated by a radioisotope technique. Dig Dis Sci 1979;24:945–949.
3. DeVincentis N, Lenti R, Pona C, et al. Scintigraphic evaluation of the esophageal transit time for the noninvasive assessment of esophageal motor disorders. J Nucl Med 1984;28:137–142.
4. Maddern GJ, Horowitz M, Jamieson GG, Chatterton BE, Collins PJ, Roberts-Thomson P. Abnormalities of esophageal and gastric emptying in progressive systemic sclerosis. Gastroenterology 1984;87:922–926.
5. Eriksen CA, Holdsworth RJ, Sutton D, Kennedy N, Cuschieri A. The solid bolus esophageal transit test: its manometric interpretation and usefulness as a screening test. Br J Surg 1987; 74:1130–1133.
6. Sutton D, Eriksen C, Kennedy N, Millar B, Cuschieri A. Investigation of esophageal motility using a solid bolus egg transit technique: results of two studies. Nucl Med Commun 1988;9:158–159.
7. Bosch A, Dietrich R, Lanaro AE, Frias Z. Modified scintigraphic technique for the dynamic study of the esophagus. Int J Nucl Med Biol 1977;4:195–199.
8. Taillefer R, Beauchamp G, Devito M, Levasseur A. Radionuclide esophagogram (Tc-99m-sulfur colloid) in experimental esophagitis: manometric and histopathologic correlations [Abstract]. J Nucl Med 1983;24:100.
9. Hellemans J, Vantrappen G. Physiology. In: Van Trappen G, Hellemans J, eds. Diseases of the esophagus. Berlin: Springer-Verlag, 1974:40–102.
10. Lamki L. Radionuclide esophageal transit (RET) study. The effect of body posture. Clin Nucl Med 1985;10:108–110.
11. Taillefer R, Beauchamp G. Radionuclide esophagogram. Clin Nucl Med 1984;9:465–483.
12. Klein HA, Wald A. Esophageal transit scintigraphy. In: Freeman LM, Weissmann HS, eds. Nuclear medicine annual. New York: Raven Press, 1988:79–124.
13. O'Sullivan G, Ryan J, Brundsen B, DeMeester T, Winans C, Skinner D. Quantitation of esophageal transit: a scintigraphic and manometric analysis [Abstract]. Gastroenterology 1982; 82:A1143.
14. Klein HA. The effect of projection in esophageal transit scintigraphy. Clin Nucl Med 1990;15:157–162.
15. Ham HR, Georges B, Froideville JL, Piepsz A. Oesophageal transit of liquid: effects of single or multiple swallows. Nucl Med Commun 1985;6:263–267.
16. Sand A, Ham H, Piepsz A. Oesophageal transit patterns in healthy subjects. Nucl Med Commun 1986;7:741–745.
17. Klein HA, Wald A. Normal variation in radionuclide esophageal transit studies. Eur J Nucl Med 1987;13:115–120.
18. Tatsch K, Schroettle W, Kirsch CM. Multiple swallow test for the

quantitative and qualitative evaluation of esophageal motility disorders. J Nucl Med 1991;32:1365–1370.
19. Bartlett RJV, Parkin A, Ware FW, Riley A, Robinson PJA. Reproducibility of oesophageal transit studies: several "single swallows" must be performed. Nucl Med Commun 1987;8:317–326.
20. Tolin RD, Malmud LS, Reillely J, Fisher RS. Esophageal scintigraphy to quantitate esophageal transit (quantitation of esophageal transit). Gastroenterology 1979;76:1402–1408.
21. Kjellén G, Svedberg JB, Tibbling L. Computerized scintigraphy of oesophageal bolus transit in asthmatics. Int J Nucl Med Biol 1981;8:153–158.
22. Svedberg JB. The bolus transport diagram: a functional display method applied to oesophageal studies. Clin Phys Physiol Meas 1982;3:267–272.
23. Klein HA, Wald A. Computer analysis of radionuclide esophageal transit studies. J Nucl Med 1984;25:957–964.
24. Klein HA. Applications of condensed dynamic images. Clin Nucl Med 1986;11:178–182.
25. Russell COH, Hill LD, Holmes ER III, Hull DA, Gannon R, Pope CE II. Radionuclide transit: a sensitive screening test for esophageal dysfunction. Gastroenterology 1981;80:887–892.
26. Kjellén G, Svedberg JB. Solid-bolus passage in patients with pathological oesophageal acid clearing. Scand J Gastroenterol 1983;18:183–187.
27. Llamas-Elvira JM, Martinez-Parades M, Sopena-Monforte R, Garrigues V, Cano-Terol C, Velasco-Lajo T. Value of radionuclide oesophageal transit in studies of functional dysphagia. Br J Radiol 1986;59:1073–1078.
28. Mercer CD, Rue C, Hanelin L, Hill LD. Effect of obesity on esophageal transit. Am J Surg 1985;149:177–181.
29. O'Connor MK, Byrne PJ, Keeling P, Hennessy TP. Esophageal scintigraphy: applications and limitations in the study of esophageal disorders. Eur J Nucl Med 1988;14:131–136.
30. Rozen P, Gelfond M, Zaltzman S, Baron J, Gilat T. Dynamic, diagnostic, and pharmacological radionuclide studies of the esophagus in achalasia: correlation with manometric measurements. Radiology 1982;144:587–590.
31. Holloway RH, Krosin G, Lange RC, Baue AE, McCallum RW. Radionuclide esophageal emptying of a solid meal to quantitate results of therapy in achalasia. Gastroenterology 1983;84:771–776.
32. Netscher D, Larson GM, Polk HC. Radionuclide esophageal transit. Arch Surg 1986;121:843–848.
33. Blackwell JN, Hannan WJ, Adam RD, Heading RC. Radionuclide transit studies in the detection of oesophageal dysmotility. Gut 1983;24:421–426.
34. DeCaestecker JS, Blackwell JN, Adam RD, Hannan WJ, Brown J, Heading RC. Clinical value of radionuclide oesophageal transit measurement. Gut 1986;27:659–666.
35. Benjamin SB, Gerhardt DC, Castell DO. High amplitude, peristaltic esophageal contractions associated with chest pain and/or dysphagia. Gastroenterology 1979;77:478–483.
36. Benjamin SB, O'Donnell JK, Hancock J, Nielsen P, Castell DO. Prolonged radionuclide transit in "Nutcracker esophagus." Dig Dis Sci 1983;28:775–779.
37. Drane WE, Johnson DA, Hagan DP, Cattau EL. "Nutcracker" esophagus: diagnosis with radionuclide esophageal scintigraphy versus manometry. Radiology 1987;163:33–37.
38. Horowitz M, McNeil JD, Collins GJ, Shearman DJC. Abnormalities of gastric and esophageal emptying in polymyositis and dermatomyositis. Gastroenterology 1986a;90:434–439.
39. Garg A, Prakash K, Gopinath PG, Malaviya AN. Radionuclide oesophageal transit time in progressive systemic sclerosis. Indian J Med Res 1984;79:110–113.
40. Carette S, Lacourciere Y, Lavoie S, Hallé P. Radionuclide esophageal transit in progressive systemic sclerosis. J Rheumatol 1985;12:478–481.
41. Davidson A, Russell C, Littlejohn GO. Assessment of esophageal abnormalities in progressive systemic sclerosis using radionuclide transit. J Rheumatol 1985;12:72–477.
42. Drane WE, Karvelis K, Johnson DA, Curran JJ, Silverman ED. Progressive systemic sclerosis: radionuclide esophageal scintigraphy and manometry. Radiology 1986;160:73–76.
43. Akesson A, Gustafson T, Wollheim F, Brismar J. Esophageal dysfunction and radionuclide transit in progressive systemic sclerosis. Scand J Rheumatol 1987;16:291– 299.
44. Kazem I. A new scintigraphic technique for the study of the esophagus. Am J Roentgenol Rad Ther Nucl Med 1972;115(4):681–688.
45. Russell CO, Gannan FR, Coatsworth J, et al. Relationship among esophageal dysfunction, diabetic gastroenteropathy, and peripheral neuropathy. Dig Dis Sci 1983;28:289–293.
46. Fisher RS, Malmud LS, Roberts GS, Lobis IF. Gastroesophageal (GE) scintiscanning to detect and quantitate GE reflux. Gastroenterology 1976;70:301–308.
47. Malmud LS, Fisher RS. Quantitation of gastroesophageal reflux before and after therapy using the gastroesophageal scintiscan. South Med J 1978;71(Suppl 1):10–15.
48. Devos PG, Forget P, DeRoo M, Eggermont E. Scintigraphic evaluation of gastroesophageal reflux (GER) in children. J Nucl Med 1979;20:636.
49. Malmud LS, Charkes ND, Littlefield J, Reilley J, Stern H, Fischer RS. The mode of action of alginic acid compound in the reduction of gastroesophageal reflux. J Nucl Med 1979;20:1023–1028.
50. Menin RA, Malmud LS, Petersen RP, Maier WP, Fisher RS. Gastroesophageal scintigraphy to assess the severity of gastroesophageal reflux disease. Ann Surg 1980;191:66–71.
51. Malmud LS, Fisher RS. The evaluation of gastroesophageal reflux before and after medical therapies. Semin Nuc Med 1981;11:205–215.
52. Malmud LS, Fisher RS. Radionuclide studies of esophageal transit and gastroesophageal reflux. Semin Nucl Med 1982;12:104–115.
53. Malmud LS, Fisher RS. Scintigraphic evaluation of gastroesophageal reflux. In: Wahner HW, ed. Nuclear medicine: quantitative procedures. Boston: Little, Brown & Co., 1983:147–170.
54. Hillemeier AC, Lange R, McCallum RW. Delayed gastric emptying in infants with gastroesophageal reflux. J Pediatr 1981;98:190–193.
55. DiLorenzo C, Piepz A, Ham A, Cadranel S. Gastric emptying with gastroesophageal reflux. Arch Dis Child 1987;62:449–453.
56. Leape LL, Holder TM, Franklin JD, Amoury RA, Ashcraft KW. Respiratory arrest in infants secondary to gastroesophageal reflux. Pediatrics 1977;60:924–928.
57. Herbst JJ, Book LS, Bray PF. Gastroesophageal reflux in the "near miss" sudden infant death syndrome. J Pediatr 1978;92:73–75.
58. Davis MV. Relationship between pulmonary disease, hiatal hernia and gastroesophageal reflux. NYS J Med 1972;72:935–938.
59. Euler AP, Byrne WJ, Ament ME, et al. Recurrent pulmonary disease in children: a complication of gastroesophageal reflux. Pediatrics 1979;63:47–51.
60. Foglia RP, Fonkalsrud EW, Ament ME, et al. Gastroesophageal fundoplication for the management of chronic pulmonary disease in children. Am J Surg 1980;140:72–77.
61. Ghaed N, Stein MR. Assessment of a technique for scintigraphic monitoring of pulmonary aspiration of gastric contents in asthmatics with gastroesophageal reflux. Ann Allergy 1979;42:306–308.
62. Collins PJ, Horowitz M, Cook DJ, Harding PE, Shearman DJC. Gastric emptying in normal subjects: a reproducible technique using a single scintillation camera and computer system. Gut 1983;24:1117–1125.
63. Smith JL, Jiang CL, Hunt JN. Intrinsic emptying pattern of the human stomach. Am J Physiol 1984;246:R959–R962.

64. McHugh PR, Moran TH. Calories and gastric emptying: a regulatory capacity with implications for feeding. Am J Physiol 1979; 236(5):R254–R260.
65. Loo FD, Palmer DW, Soergel KH, Kalbfleisch JH, Wood CM. Gastric emptying in patients with diabetes mellitus. Gastroenterology 1984;86:485–494.
66. Hunt JN. The site of receptors slowing gastric emptying in response to starch in test meals. J Physiol 1960;134:270–276.
67. Hunt JN, Knox MTA. A relation between the chain length of fatty acids and the slowing of gastric emptying. J Physiol 1968; 194:327–336.
68. Burn-Murdoch RA, Fisher MA, Hunt JN. The slowing of gastric emptying by proteins in test meals. J Physiol 1978;274:477–483.
69. Gulsrud PO, Taylor IL, Watts HD, Cohen MB, Meyer JH. How gastric emptying affects glucose tolerance and symptoms after truncal vagotomy with pyloroplasty. Gastroenterology 1980; 78:1463–1471.
70. Brener W, Hendrix TR, McHugh PR. Regulation of the gastric emptying of glucose. Gastroenterology 1983;85:76–82.
71. Moore JG, Christian PE, Coleman RE. Gastric emptying of varying meal weight and composition in man. Evaluation by dual liquid and solid phase isotopic method. Dig Dis Sci 1981;26:16–22.
72. Urbain JL, Siegel JA, Mortelmans L, VanCutsem E, VanDen-Maegdenbergh V, DeRoo M. Effect of solid-meal caloric content on gastric emptying kinetics of solids and liquids. Nuklear-Medizin 1989a;28:120–123.
73. Moore JG, Christian PE, Brown JA, et al. Influence of meal weight and caloric content on gastric emptying of meals in man. Dig Dis Sci 1984;29:513–519.
74. Heading RC, Tothill P, McLoughlin GP, Shearman DJG. Gastric emptying rate measurement in man. A double isotope scanning technique for simultaneous study of liquid and solid component of a meal. Gastroenterology 1976;71:45–50.
75. Meyer JH. Motility of the stomach and gastroduodenal junction. In: Johnson LR, ed. Physiology of the gastrointestinal tract. New York: Raven Press, 1987:613–629.
76. Keinke O, Ehrlein HJ. Effect of oleic acid on canine gastroduodenal motility, pyloric diameter and gastric emptying. Q J Exp Physiol 1983;68:675–686.
77. Cortot A, Phillips SF, Malagelada J-R. Parallel gastric emptying of nonhydrolyzable fat and water after a solid-liquid meal in humans. Gastroenterology 1982;82:877–881.
78. Jian R, Vigneron N, Najean Y, Bernier J-J. Gastric emptying and intragastric distribution of lipids in man. A new scintigraphic method of study. Dig Dis Sci 1982;27:705–711.
79. Goo RH, Moore JG, Greenberg E, Alazaraki N. Circadian variation in gastric emptying of meals in man. Gastroenterology 1987; 93:515–518.
80. Trout DL, King SA, Bernstein PA, Halberg F, Cornelissen G. Circadian variation in the gastric emptying response to eating in rats previously fed once or twice daily. Chronobiol Int 1991;8:14–24.
81. Johnson RD, Horowitz M, Maddox AF, Wishart JM, Shearman DJC. Cigarette smoking and rate of gastric emptying: effect on alcohol absorption. Br Med J 1991;302:20–23.
82. Griffith GH, Owen GM, Kirkman S, Shields R. Measurement of rate of gastric emptying using Chromium-51. Lancet 1966; 1:1244–1245.
83. Meyer JH, MacGregor IL, Gueller R, Martin P, Cavalieri R. ^{99m}Tc-tagged chicken liver as a marker of solid food in the human stomach. Am J Dig Dis 1976;21(4):296–304.
84. Knight LC, Malmud LS. Tc-99m-ovalbumin labeled eggs: comparison with other solid food markers in vitro. J Nucl Med 1981; 22:P28.
85. Knight LC, Fisher RS, Malmud LS. Comparison of solid food markers in gastric emptying studies. In: Nuclear medicine and biology advances: proceedings of the Third World Congress of nuclear medicine and biology. Paris, New York: Pergamon Press, 1982;2407–2410(3).
86. Urbain J-LC, Siegel JA, Charkes ND, Maurer AH, Malmud LS, Fisher RS. The two-component stomach: effects of meal particle size on fundal and antral emptying. Eur J Nucl Med 1989b; 15:254–259.
87. Urbain J-LC, VanDenMaegdenbergh V, Siegel JA, Mortelmans L, Vandecruys A, DeRoo M. The dual phase gastric emptying: is labeling of liquid useful? Eur J Nucl Med 1989c;8:A532–533.
88. Tothill P, McLoughlin GP, Heading RC. Techniques and errors in scintigraphic measurements of gastric emptying. J Nucl Med 1978;19:256–261.
89. Tothill P, McLoughlin GP, Holt S, Heading RC. The effect of posture on errors in gastric emptying measurements. Phys Med Biol 1980;25:1071–1077.
90. Christian PE, Moore JG, Sorenson JA, Coleman RE, Weich DM. Effects of meal size and correction technique on gastric emptying time: studies with two tracers and opposed detectors. J Nucl Med 1980;21:883–885.
91. Moore JG, Christian PE, Taylor AT, Alazraki N. Gastric emptying measurements: delayed and complex emptying patterns without appropriate correction. J Nucl Med 1985;26:1206–1210.
92. Collins PJ, Horowitz M, Shearman DJC, Chatterton BE. Correction for tissue attenuation in radionuclide gastric emptying studies: a comparison of a lateral image method and a geometric mean method. Br J Radiol 1984;57:689–695.
93. Fahey FH, Ziessman HA, Collen MJ, Eggli DF. Left anterior oblique projection and peak-to-scatter ratio for attenuation compensation of gastric emptying studies. J Nucl Med 1989;30:233–239.
94. Roland J, Dobbeleir A, Ham HR, Vandevivere J. Continuous anterior acquisitions in gastric emptying: comparison with the mean. Clin Nucl Med 1989;14:881–884.
95. Maurer AH, Knight LC, Krevsky B. Proper definitions for lag phase in gastric emptying of solid foods. J Nucl Med 1992; 33:466–467.
96. Meyer JH, VanDeventer G, Graham LS, Thomson J, Thomasson D. Error and corrections with scintigraphic measurement of gastric emptying of solid foods. J Nucl Med 1983;24:197–203.
97. Urbain J-LC, Vekemans M-C, Bouillon R, et al. Characterization of gastric antral motility disturbances in diabetes using the scintigraphic technique. J Nucl Med 1993a;34(4):576–581.
98. Urbain J-LC, et al. Characterization of gastric emptying pathophysiology in idiopathic dyspepsia using scintigraphy. J Nucl Med 1993b;34:10P.
99. Urbain J-LC, Vekemans MC, Parkman H, et al. Evaluation of the effect of gastrokinetic compounds on antral motor activity and gastric emptying using the radiogastrogram technique. J Nucl Med 1994a;35(5):A684.
100. Urbain J-LC, Vekemans MC, Parkman H, et al. Characterization of gastric antral motility in functional dyspepsia using digital antral scintigraphy. J Nucl Med (in press).
101. Elashoff JD, Reedy TJ, Meyer JH. Analysis of gastric emptying data. Gastroenterology 1982;83:1306–1312.
102. Siegel JA, Wu RK, Knight LC, Zelac RE, Stern HS, Malmud LS. Radiation dose estimates for oral agents used in upper gastrointestinal disease. J Nucl Med 1983;24:835–837.
103. Urbain J-LC, VanCutsem E, Siegel JA, et al. Visualization and characterization of gastric contractions using a radionuclide technique. Am J Physiol 1990a;259:G1062–G1067.
104. Chaudhuri TK, Greenwald AJ, Heading RC, Chaudhuri TK. A new radioisotopic technic for the measurement of gastric emptying time of solid meal. Am J Gastroenterol 1976;65:46–51.
105. Scarpello JHB, Barber DC, Hague RV, Cullen DR, Sladen GE. Gastric emptying of solid meals in diabetics. Br Med J 1976; 2:671–673.
106. Carryer PW, Brown ML, Malagelada J-R, Carlson GL, McCall JT.

Quantification of the fate of dietary fibers in humans by a newly developed radiolabeled fiber marker. Gastroenterology 1982; 82:1389–1394.
107. Brophy CM, Moore JG, Christian PE, Egger MJ, Taylor AT. Variability of gastric emptying measurements in man employing standardized radiolabeled meals. Dig Dis Sci 1986;31:799–806.
108. Campbell IW, Heading RC, Tothill P, Buist TAS, Ewing DJ, Clarke BF. Gastric emptying in diabetic autonomic neuropathy. Gut 1977;18:462–467.
109. Fox S, Behar J. Pathogenesis of diabetic gastroparesis: a pharmacologic study. Gastroenterology 1980;78:757–763.
110. Malagelada J-R, Rees WDW, Mazzotta LJ, Go VLW. Gastric motor abnormalities in diabetic and postvagotomy gastroparesis: effect of metoclopramide and bethanechol. Gastroenterology 1980; 78:286–293.
111. Horowitz M, Maddox A, Harding PE, et al. Effect of cisapride on gastric and esophageal emptying in insulin-dependent diabetes mellitus. Gastroenterology 1987;92:1899–1907.
112. Urbain J-LC, Vantrappen G, Janssens J, VanCutsem E, Peeters T, DeRoo M. Intravenous erythromycin dramatically accelerates gastric emptying in gastroparesis diabeticorum and normals and abolishes the emptying discrimination between solids and liquids. J Nucl Med 1990b;31:1490–1493.
113. Urbain J-L, Siegel JA, Buysschaert M, Pauwels S. Characterization of the early pathophysiology of diabetic gastroparesis. Dig Dis Sci 1987;32:930(A31).
114. Wright RA, Clemente R, Wathen R. Diabetic gastroparesis: an abnormality of gastric emptying of solids. Am J Med Sci 1985; 289:240–242.
115. Horowitz M, Harding PE, Maddox A. Gastric and esophageal emptying in insulin-dependent diabetes mellitus. J Gastroenterol Hepatol 1986b;1:97–113.
116. Phillips WT, Schwartz JG, McMahan CA. Rapid gastric emptying in patients with early non-insulin dependent diabetes mellitus. N Engl J Med 1991;324:130–131.
117. Narducci F, Bassotti G, Granata MT, et al. Functional dyspepsia and chronic idiopathic gastric stasis. Role of endogenous opiates. Arch Int Med 1986;146:716–720.
118. Kerlin P. Postprandial antral hypomotility in patients with idiopathic nausea and vomiting. Gut 1989;30:54–59.
119. Malagelada JR. Where do we stand on gastric motility? Scand J Gastroenterol 1991;175P:42–51.
120. McCallum RW, Grill BB, Lange RC, Planckey M, Glass E, Greenfield DG. Definition of a gastric emptying abnormality in patients with anorexia nervosa. Dig Dis Sci 1985;30:713–722.
121. Halvorsen L, Dotevall G, Walan A. Gastric emptying in patients with achlorhydria or hyposecretion of hydrochloric acid. Scand J Gastroenterol 1973;8(5):395–399.
122. Frank EB, Lange R, McCallum RW. Abnormal gastric emptying in patients with atrophic gastritis with or without pernicious anemia. Gastroenterology 1981;80:1151.
123. McCallum RW, Berkowitz DM, Lerner E. Gastric emptying in patients with gastroesophageal reflux. Gastroenterology 1981; 80:285–291.
124. Holloway RH, Hongo M, Berger K, McCallum RW. Gastric distention: a mechanism for postprandial gastroesophageal reflux. Gastroenterology 1985;89:779– 784.
125. Behar J, Ramsby G. Gastric emptying and antral motility in reflux esophagitis. Gastroenterology 1978;74:253–256.
126. Csendes A, Henriquez A. Gastric emptying in patients with reflux esophagitis or benign strictures of the esophagus secondary to reflux compared to controls. Scand J Gastroenterol 1978; 13:205–207.
127. Maddern GJ, Chaterton BE, Collins PJ, Horowitz M, Shearman DJ, Jamieson GG. Solid and liquid gastric emptying in patients with gastro-oesophageal reflux. Br J Surg 1985;72:344–347.
128. Rock E, Malmud L, Fisher RS. Motor disorders of the stomach. Med Clin North Am 1981;65:1269–1289.
129. Minami H, McCallum RW. The physiology and pathophysiology of gastric emptying in humans. Gastroenterology 1984;86:1592–1610.
130. Lin DS. Abnormal rates of gastric emptying. Semin Nucl Med 1985;15:70–71.
131. Mistiaen W, VanHee R, Blockx P, Hubens A. Gastric emptying for solids in patients with duodenal ulcer before and after highly selective vagotomy. Dig Dis Sci 1990;35:310–316.
132. Fordtran JS, Walsh JH. Gastric acid secretion rate and buffer content of the stomach after eating. Results in normal subjects and in patients with duodenal ulcer. J Clin Invest 1973;52:645–657.
133. Geurts WJC, Winckers EKA, Wittebol P. The effects of highly selective vagotomy on secretion and emptying of the stomach. Surgery 1977;145:826–836.
134. Rotter JI, Rubin R, Meyer JH. Rapid gastric emptying—an inherited physiologic defect in duodenal ulcer [Abstract]. Gastroenterology 1979;76:1229.
135. Parr NJ, Grime S, Critchley M, Baxter JN, Mackie CR. Abnormal pattern of gastric emptying of liquid in chronic duodenal ulcer. Digestion 1988;40:237–243.
136. George JD. Gastric acidity and motility. Am J Dig Dis 1968; 13:376–383.
137. Cobb JS, Bank S, Marks IN. Gastric emptying after vagotomy and pyloroplasty: relation to some postoperative sequelae. Am J Dig Dis 1971;16:207–215.
138. Dubois A, VanEerdewegh P, Gardner JD. Gastric emptying and secretion in Zollinger-Ellison syndrome. J Clin Invest 1977; 59:255–263.
139. Harrison A, Ippoliti A, Cullison R. Rapid gastric emptying in Zollinger-Ellison syndrome (ZES) [Abstract]. Gastroenterology 1980;78:A1180.
140. Peachey RD, Creamer B, Pierce JN. Sclerodermatous involvement of the stomach and small and large bowel. Gut 1969; 10:285–292.
141. Wilbur BG, Kelly KA. Effect of proximal gastric, complete gastric, and truncal vagotomy on canine gastric electric activity, motility and emptying. Ann Surg 1973;178:295–303.
142. Lavigne ME, Wiley ZD, Martin P, et al. Gastric, pancreatic and biliary secretion and the rate of gastric emptying after parietal cell vagotomy. Am J Surg 1979;138:644–651.
143. Lopasso FP, BrunodeMello J, Meneguetti J, Gama-Rodrigues J, Pinotti HW. Study of gastric emptying in patients with duodenal ulcer before and after proximal gastric vagotomy. The use of solid and digestible particles labeled with Tc-99m. Surg Gastroenterol 1982;1:321–326.
144. Wilkinson AR, Johnston D. Effect of truncal, selective and highly selective vagotomy on gastric emptying and intestinal transit of food-barium meal in man. Ann Surg 1973;178:190–193.
145. Sheiner HJ, Quinlan MF, Thompson IJ. Gastric motility and emptying in normal and post-vagotomy subjects. Gut 1980; 21:753–759.
146. Urbain JL, Penninckx F, Siegel JA, et al. Effect of proximal vagotomy and Roux-en-Y diversion on gastric emptying kinetics in asymptomatic patients. Clin Nucl Med 1990c;15:688–691.
147. Dragstedt LR, Schafer PW. Removal of the vagus innervation of the stomach in gastroduodenal ulcer. Surgery 1945;17:742–749.
148. Edwards LW, Herrington J. Vagotomy and gastroenterostomy—vagotomy and conservative gastrectomy: a comparative study. Ann Surg 1952;137:873–883.
149. Roman C, Gonella J. Extrinsic control of digestive tract motility. In: Johnson LR, ed. Physiology of the gastrointestinal tract. New York: Raven Press, 1981:289–334.

150. McKelvey STD. Gastric incontinence and postvagotomy diarrhoea. Br J Surg 1970;57:741–747.
151. Hinder RA, Horn BKP, Bremner CG. The volumetric measurement of gastric emptying and gastric secretion by a radioisotope method. Dig Dis Sci 1976;21:940–945.
152. Kelly KA. Effect of gastric surgery on gastric motility and emptying. In: Akkermans LMA, Johnson AG, Read NW, eds. Gastric and gastroduodenal motility. East Sussex, UK: Praeger, 1984:241–262.
153. Meyer JH, Thomson JB, Cohen MB, Shadchehr A, Mandiola SA. Sieving of solid food by the canine stomach and sieving after gastric surgery. Gastroenterology 1979;76:804–813.
154. Wittebol P, Haarman HJ, Hoekstra A. Gastric emptying after gastric surgery. Dig Surg 1988;5:160–166.
155. Gustavsson S, Kelly KA. Effect of gastric and small bowel operations. In: Kummar D, Gustavsson S, eds. Gastrointestinal motility. London: John Wiley and Sons, 1988;291–310.
156. Hinder RA, San-Garde BA. Individual and combined roles of the pylorus and the antrum in the canine gastric emptying of a liquid and a digestible solid. Gastroenterology 1983;84:281–286.
157. Vogel SB, Vair DB, Woodward ER. Alterations in gastrointestinal emptying of 99m-Technetium labeled solids following sequential antrectomy, truncal vagotomy and Roux-en-Y gastroenterostomy. Ann Surg 1983;198:506–515.
158. Pasma FG, Akkermans LMA, Oei HY. Gastric emptying in asymptomatic partial gastrectomy (BII) patients. In: Roman C, ed. Gastrointestinal motility: proceedings of the 9th International Symposium on gastrointestinal motility. Lancaster: MTP Press, 1984:143–148.
159. Dozois RR, Kelly KA, Code CF. Effect of distal antrectomy on gastric emptying of liquids and solids. Gastroenterology 1971; 61:675–681.
160. Yamagishi T, Debas HT. Control of gastric emptying: interaction of the vagus and pyloric antrum. Ann Surg 1978;187:91–94.
161. MacGregor IL, Martin P, Meyer JH. Gastric emptying of solid food in normal man and after subtotal gastrectomy and truncal vagotomy with pyloroplasty. Gastroenterology 1977;72:206–211.
162. Hocking MP, Vogel SB, Falasca CA, Woodward ER. Delayed gastric emptying of liquids and solids following Roux-en-Y biliary diversion. Ann Surg 1981;194:494–501.
163. Mannell A, Hinder RA, Sun-Garde DA. The thoracic stomach: a study of gastric emptying, bile reflux and mucosal change. Br J Surg 1984;71:438–441.
164. Hölscher AH, Voit H, Buttermann G, Siewert JR. Function of the intrathoracic stomach as esophageal replacement. World J Surg 1988;12:835–844.
165. Borst HG, Dragojevic D, Stegmann T, Hetzer R. Anastomotic leakage, stenosis, and reflux after esophageal replacement. World J Surg 1978;2:861–866.
166. Pichlmaier H, Müller JM, Wintzer G. Oesophagusersatz. Chirurg 1978;49:65–71.
167. Skinner DB. Invited commentary to complications following esophageal resection. World J Surg 1978;2:865–866.
168. Hancock BD, Bowen-Jones E, Dixon R, Dymock IW, Cowley DJ. The effect of metoclopramide on gastric emptying of solid meals. Gut 1974;15:462–467.
169. Metzger WH, Cano R, Sturdevant RAL. Effect of metoclopramide in chronic gastric retention after gastric surgery. Gastroenterology 1976;71:30–32.
170. Snape WJ, Battle WM, Schwartz SS, Braunstein SN, Goldstein HA, Alavi A. Metoclopramide to treat gastroparesis due to diabetes mellitus. A double-blind, controlled trial. Ann Int Med 1982;96:444–446.
171. McCallum RW, Ricci DA, Rakatansky H, et al. A multicenter placebo-controlled clinical trial of oral metoclopramide in diabetic gastroparesis. Diabetes Care 1983;6:463–467.
172. Horowitz M, Harding PE, Chatterton BE, Collins PJ, Shearman DJ. Acute and chronic effects of domperidone on gastric emptying in diabetes autonomic neuropathy. Dig Dis Sci 1985;30:1–9.
173. Urbain J-LC, Siegel JA, Debie N, Pauwels SP. Effect of Cisapride on gastric emptying in dyspeptic patients. Dig Dis Sci 1988; 33:779–783.
174. Urbain J-LC, Bouillon M, Muls E, et al. Effect of long-term oral erythromycin on gastric emptying and blood glucose control in patients with diabetic gastroparesis. J Nucl Med 1991;32:931.
175. Kondo Y, Torii K, Omura S, Itoh Z. Erythromycin and its derivatives with motilin-like biological activities inhibit the specific binding of ^{125}I-motilin to duodenal muscle. Bioch Biophys Res Commun 1988;150:877–882.
176. Depoortere I, Peeters TL, Matthijs G, Vantrappen G. Macrolide antibiotics are motilin receptor agonists. Hepato-Gastroenterol 1988;35:198.
177. Peeters T, Matthijs G, Depoortere I, Cachet T, Hoogmartens J, Vantrappen G. Erythromycin is a motilin receptor agonist. Am J Physiol 1989;257:G470–G474.
178. Itoh Z, Honda R, Hiwatashi K, et al. Motilin-induced mechanical activity in the canine alimentary tract. Scand J Gastroent 1976; 11(Suppl 39):93–110.
179. Itoh Z, Nakaya M, Suzuki T, Arai H, Wakabayashi K. Erythromycin mimics exogenous motilin in gastrointestinal contractile activity in the dog. Am J Physiol 1984;247:G688–G694.
180. Zara GP, Thompson HH, Pilot MA, Ritchie HD. Effects of erythromycin on gastrointestinal tract motility. J Antimicrob Chemoth 1985;16:A175–A179.
181. Tomomasa T, Kuroume T, Arai H, Wakabayashi K, Itoh Z. Erythromycin induces migrating motor complex in human gastrointestinal tract. Dig Dis Sci 1986;31:157–161.
182. Annese V, Janssens J, Vantrappen G. Erythromycin accelerates gastric emptying by inducing antral contractions and improving antroduodenal coordination. Gastroenterology 1992;102:823–828.
183. Peeters TL, Muls E, Janssens J, et al. Effect of motilin on gastric emptying in patients with diabetic gastroparesis. Gastroenterology 1992;102:97–101.

37 Liver Imaging

BERNARD E. OPPENHEIM

Since the previous edition of this book, the clinical use of radionuclide studies of the liver has waned drastically. Computed tomography (CT), which provides better spatial resolution and the ability to examine structures outside the liver, and ultrasound, which is cheaper, more readily available, and often more specific, have become the preferred modalities in most instances. This discussion is limited to those conditions for which radionuclide imaging of the liver appears to be warranted.

RADIOPHARMACEUTICALS

The liver consists of two dominant cell populations. The parenchymal (polygonal) cells perform the metabolic functions of the liver and account for about 85% of the cell population, whereas the other 15% are the reticuloendothelial (Kupffer) cells, which phagocytize foreign particles (1). The polygonal cells selectively extract iminodiacetic acid (IDA) derivatives from the circulating blood and can be imaged using technetium-labeled IDA compounds. The Kupffer cells remove colloids from the blood and are imaged using ^{99m}Tc sulfur colloid. While images of either cell population can demonstrate liver morphology, the IDA agents are excreted into the biliary tract over time and hence have a changing distribution within the liver, while the distribution of sulfur colloid remains fixed, allowing more time for imaging the liver parenchyma. In particular, tomographic imaging (SPECT) of the liver requires a fixed distribution of tracer during data acquisition. This chapter will not discuss the use of the IDA agents, which are dealt with in Chapter 38. Other agents that are dealt with in this chapter are ^{99m}Tc-labeled red blood cells (RBCs) for blood pool imaging of the liver, and ^{67}Ga for tumor imaging.

INSTRUMENTATION

Planar liver imaging with the stationary scintillation camera is generally adequate, but greater accuracy in lesion detection is achieved with tomographic imaging performed with a rotating camera (2). The newer multiple detector SPECT systems are preferred if available, because the higher photon sensitivity permits the detection of smaller lesions than can be detected with a rotating single detector (3).

PROCEDURE

For planar imaging of the liver, a dose of 4–6 mCi (148–222 mBq) of ^{99m}Tc sulfur colloid is typically used and results in a radiation dose to the liver of approximately 1.5–2 rads. For SPECT imaging of the liver, a dose of 8–10 mCi (296–370 mBq) is recommended. The dose for children is 50 μCi (18,500 kBq) per kilogram, with a minimum dose of 500 μCi (18,500 kBq).

The study is performed with a scintillation camera using a low-energy high-resolution parallel-hole collimator. Dynamic blood flow imaging at the time of injection can be performed. Static imaging is begun 3–5 minutes after radiopharmaceutical administration. An anterior image is obtained with lead markers along the lower margins of the rib cage and a 10-cm lead strip over the liver for size calibration. Four additional views are then obtained: anterior liver/spleen, posterior liver/spleen, right lateral liver, and left lateral spleen. The anterior and posterior views should be acquired to contain 1 million counts. The patient is supine for all views with the camera under the table for the posterior view because the liver shape can change if the patient's position is changed. The patient's body should be as close to the collimator as possible, as spatial resolution falls off rapidly with increasing distance.

Following the examination, the physician in charge palpates the abdomen and notes all findings. If a mass is palpated, an additional view should be obtained in which the mass is outlined during imaging using a small ^{99m}Tc source, such as a syringe or cotton applicator with radioactive material in the tip, covered with a needle cap.

SPECT IMAGING

Successful tomographic imaging of the liver with the scintillation camera requires meticulous attention to technical details. The camera must be well-tuned with good intrinsic uniformity, but all images should always be uniformity-corrected with a high count flood source because nonuniformities of only 1% can produce significant artifacts (4). The center of rotation must be determined accurately. Some form of attenuation correction should always be applied. Finally, one must attempt to keep the camera head as close to the patient as possible because of significant loss of resolution with increasing distance.

DYNAMIC BLOOD FLOW IMAGING

A rapid sequence of images of liver blood flow immediately following injection of tracer can produce valuable information (5, 6) and can be performed as a standard component of the ^{99m}Tc sulfur colloid study. Anterior images are obtained every 4 seconds during the first minute following injection. Vascular lesions of the liver, including most hepatomas and metastases, have early flow because they are supplied by the hepatic artery, in contrast to normal liver parenchyma which has somewhat delayed flow because it

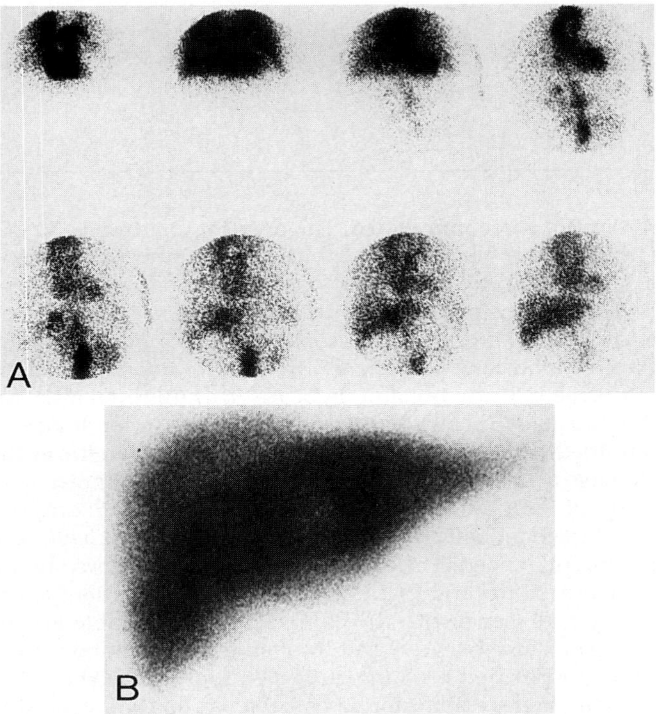

Figure 37.1. Dynamic blood flow study with vascular tumor. **A.** Serial 4-second images show gradual liver uptake which occurs after the appearance of the aorta, kidneys, and spleen. There is an abnormal focus of early uptake in the region of the porta hepatis (*frame 4*). The lower abdominal aorta is abnormally wide. **B.** The anterior image demonstrates a prominent porta hepatis defect. On angiography, a vascular mass was demonstrated in the region of the porta hepatis, as well as an aneurysm of the abdominal aorta.

receives 75% of its blood supply from the portal vein (Fig. 37.1).

INTERPRETATION

A knowledge of normal anatomy, normal variants, and artifacts as they appear on each view is essential for proper interpretation of the liver study. The wide variation in liver shape, the appearance of normal structures such as the superior wedge defect produced by the hepatic vein, the central defect produced by the porta hepatis, the inferior indentations produced by the round ligament and the gallbladder fossa, the lateral indentation produced by the rib cage, and the posterior indentation produced by the right kidney, must be appreciated when interpreting the images. On SPECT imaging, the vasculature and biliary tree may appear as multiple focal defects (7). Artifacts such as overlying breast, skin lesions, buttons or other external objects can produce defects whose cause must be recognized.

DISEASES OF THE LIVER

For the purpose of discussion, it is helpful to group liver diseases according to whether they produce focal abnormalities or involve the liver diffusely. Biliary tract disease is discussed in Chapter 38.

DISEASES PRODUCING FOCAL DEFECTS

Radionuclide imaging is no longer a primary method for detecting the presence of focal liver defects. Some lesions, because of their physiological behavior, can have findings on radionuclide imaging that clarify their nature.

Hepatocellular Carcinoma

Primary hepatocellular carcinoma is uncommon in the United States. It is much more frequent among cirrhotics than noncirrhotics; about two-thirds of the patients who have this carcinoma are cirrhotic (8). While CT is generally the study obtained to make the diagnosis, its specificity is very poor in cirrhotic patients, as the great majority of cases will have regenerative nodules or fatty infiltration (8). Combined radionuclide studies consisting of sulfur colloid scintigraphy (including dynamic blood flow imaging) and ^{67}Ga scintigraphy are highly specific for this diagnosis (9). Most hepatocellular carcinomas have increased vascular flow while regenerative nodules nearly always have decreased flow. About 75–90% of hepatocellular carcinomas are ^{67}Ga avid and show either increased uptake or filling of defects seen on the colloid images (10–13) (Fig. 37.2). Regenerative nodules, conversely, do not take up ^{67}Ga and the defects on the colloid images remain as defects on the gallium images.

Hemangioma

Hemangiomas are the most frequent benign tumor of the liver, with a reported prevalence ranging from 0.5% to 7% (14). These lesions are usually asymptomatic and are detected as incidental findings on ultrasound or CT studies. If extremely large they can produce compressive symptoms and may also be associated with pain if spontaneous thrombosis or hemorrhage occurs. The characteristic pathologic feature of these lesions is their large blood volume. Although the dynamic radionuclide study can be variable depending on the filling rate, hemangiomas have a typical appearance of increased activity on the delayed blood pool image (15, 16).

The imaging study is performed following an intraveous administration of 20 mCi of autologous ^{99m}Tc-labeled red cells. Some investigators consider a dynamic flow study to be essential in order to distinguish hemangiomas from hepatocellular carcinomas because large hepatocellular carcinomas occasionally have increased uptake on the delayed blood pool image, but they will always have increased flow on the dynamic flow study, whereas increased flow is unusual for hemangiomas (17, 18). Other investigators have found the dynamic flow study to be unnecessary, because the findings do not contribute to the specificity of the studies (3, 19, 20). One of these investigators (19) reported that among 45 hepatocellular carcinomas, all smaller than 5 cm, none had increased uptake on the delayed blood pool study.

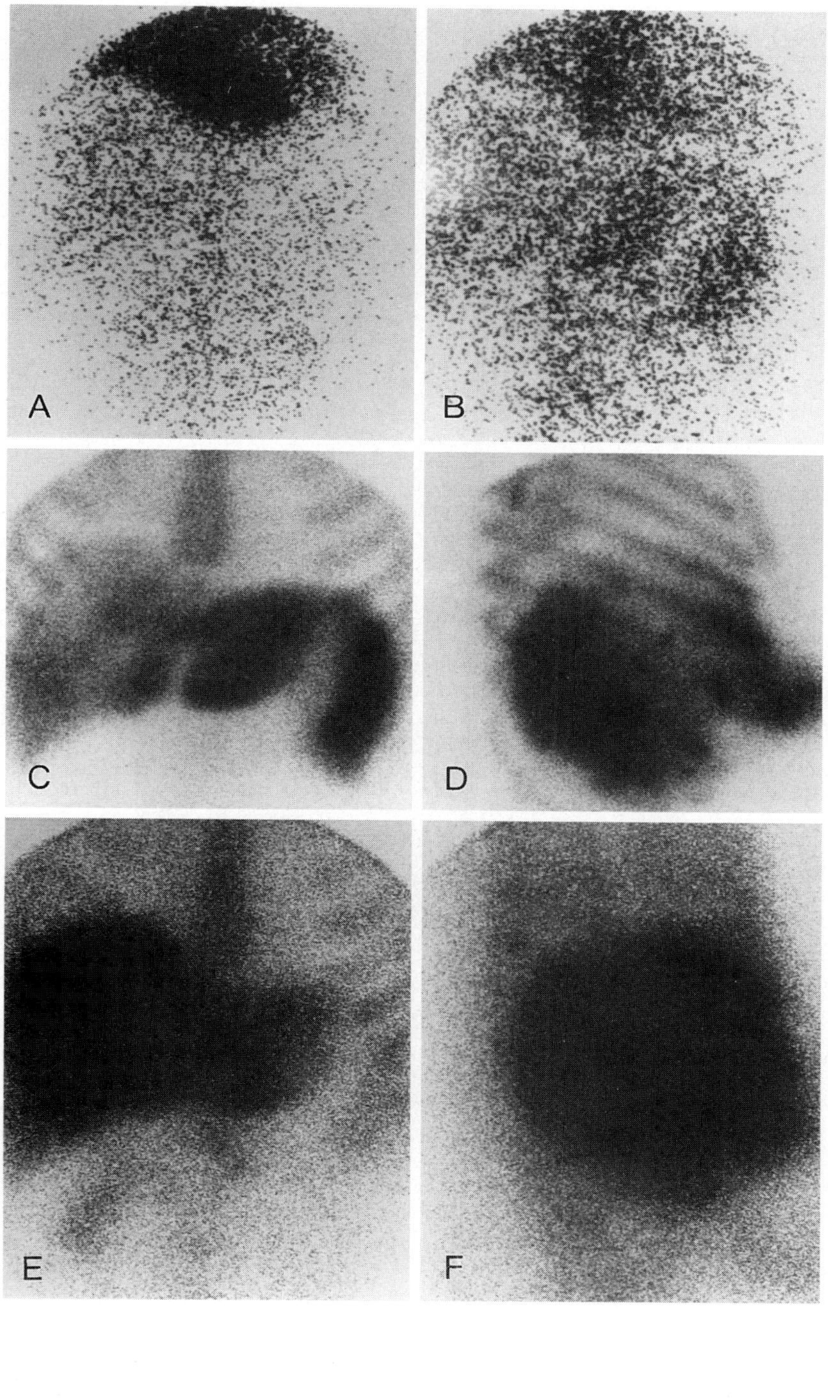

Figure 37.2. Hepatoma in cirrhosis. Thirty-two-year-old nonalcoholic man with history of hepatitis developed progressive liver failure. **A.** Early anterior dynamic blood flow image and **B** image 60 seconds later. Early flow is primarily to the right lobe, with later accumulation of tracer in the left lobe and spleen. These findings are consistent with a vascular mass in the right lobe. **C** and **D.** Anterior and right lateral liver, ^{99m}Tc sulfur colloid images. A large defect is present in the anterior half of the right lobe and colloid shift to the spleen and bone marrow are noted. **E** and **F.** Anterior and right lateral liver, ^{67}Ga. There is increased uptake of ^{67}Ga corresponding to the liver defect in the colloid images. Liver biopsy revealed hepatocellular carcinoma and cirrhosis.

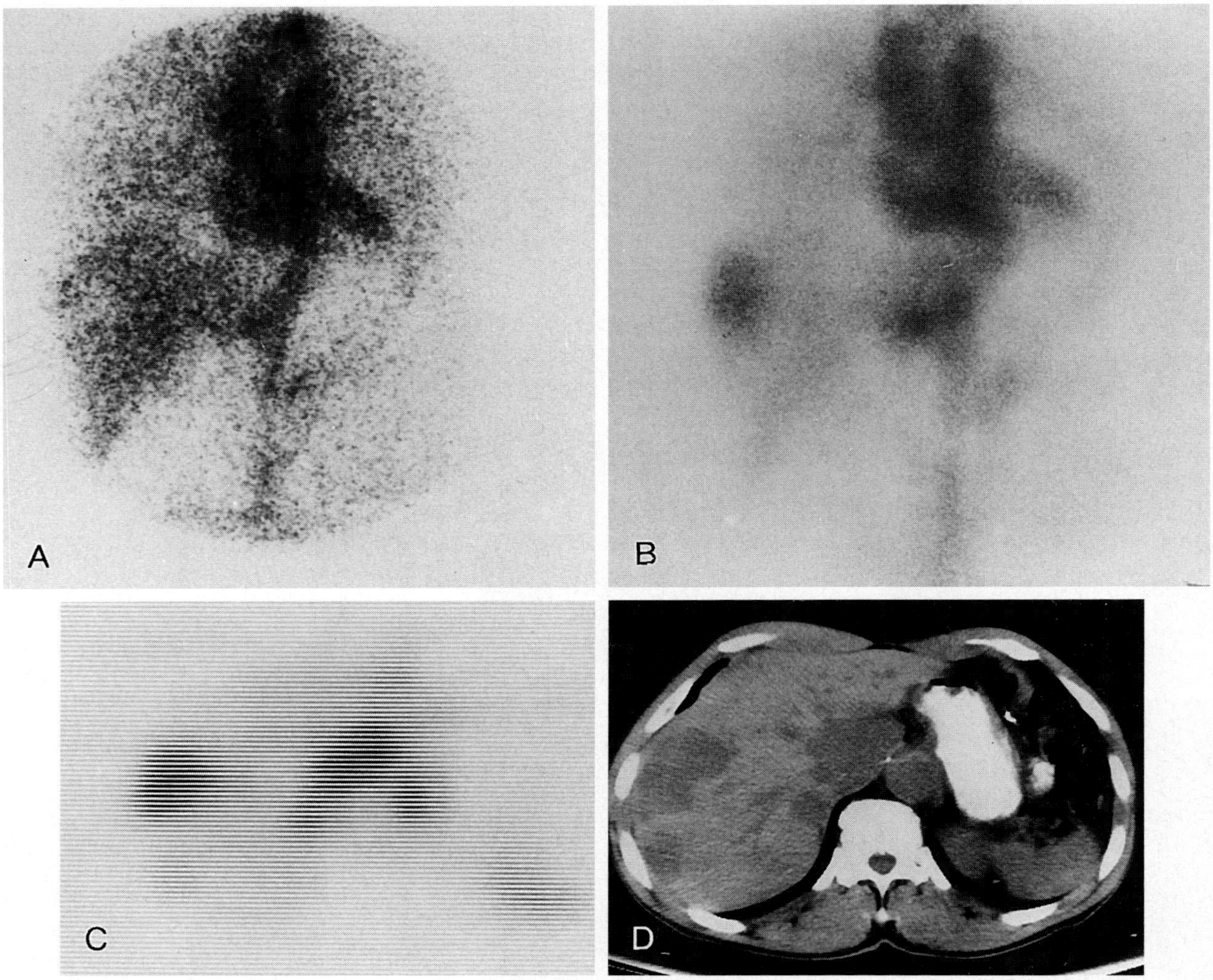

Figure 37.3. Hemangioma. **A.** ^{99m}Tc-labeled red cell study, anterior flow image. A defect is present at the lateral margin of the right lobe. **B.** Anterior 30-minute image. Increased uptake, corresponding to the perfusion defect on the flow image, is demonstrated and represents a hemangioma. **C.** Transverse SPECT image, and **D** corresponding CT image. Two areas of increased uptake are noted in the lateral right lobe on the SPECT image, as well as increased uptake in the periportal region, corresponding to low attenuation regions on the CT image. These represent hemangiomas.

After a 2-hour delay, planar images are acquired in multiple projections and then SPECT images are acquired. The SPECT images are clearly superior to the planar images in identifying small hemangiomas (18, 19, 21). The three-headed SPECT system is quite sensitive in detecting hemangiomas larger than 1.3 cm (3). It is helpful to compare transverse SPECT images with corresponding CT images to evaluate suspicious lesions seen on the CT study (Fig. 37.3). Foci of increased uptake on the SPECT images can be considered to be hemangiomas if their uptake is equal to or greater than that of nearby blood vessels, and if by tracing them in serial tomographic images along all three axes they can be shown to lack the contiguity of blood vessels (20).

Increased uptake on the delayed blood pool image is quite specific for hemangioma, although this finding has been seen in hepatocellular carcinoma (17), hemangiosarcoma (22, 23), and metastatic neuroendocrine carcinoma (24). Rarely, a large hemangioma will not have increased uptake on the delayed blood pool image because of extensive thrombosis or fibrosis (25, 26).

Focal Nodular Hyperplasia and Hepatic Adenoma

These benign liver tumors are being diagnosed with increased frequency and are associated in most instances with use of oral contraceptives. Resection of hepatic adenoma is indicated because of the frequent occurrence of hemorrhage, which is sometimes fatal (27), and the rare transformation to hepatocellular carcinoma (28). Focal nodular hyperplasia (FNH) needs not be resected because hemorrhage is rare and malignant degeneration has not been reported. Unfortunately, it is difficult to distinguish these two conditions through diagnostic imaging, and the sulfur colloid liver study often aids in making this distinction. Focal nodular hyperplasia is nearly always hypervascular (29), while hepatic adenoma frequently has avascular regions due to hemorrhage and infarction. About two-thirds of FNH lesions will accumulate sulfur colloid that is greater or equal to that of normal liver parenchyma (29) (Fig. 37.4). Adenomas have been described as never having sulfur colloid uptake, but such uptake does occur not infrequently (30). A tumor that has sulfur colloid uptake greater than normal liver parenchyma is probably FNH (30). Because adenomas usually contain foci of hemorrhage which would produce focal defects if there were sulfur colloid uptake, a tumor with uniform uptake equal to normal liver parenchyma is most likely FNH, though rarely one may see uniform uptake in adenoma (31) or hepatoblastoma (32). SPECT should be helpful in assessing colloid uptake in these tumors (33).

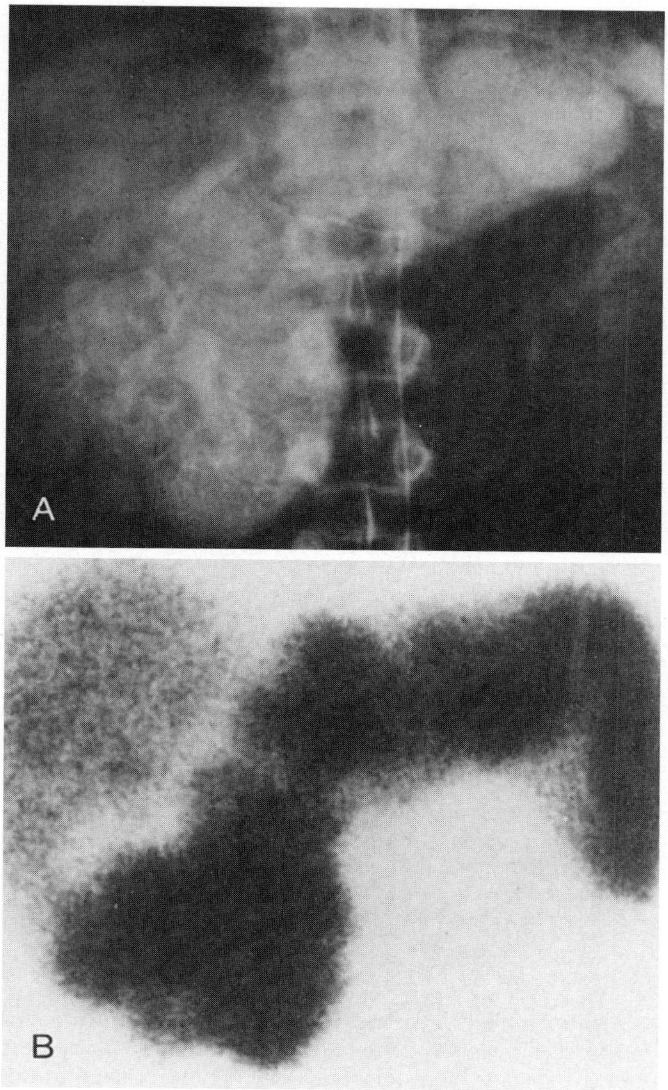

Figure 37.4. Focal nodular hyperplasia. Seventeen-year-old man with right upper quadrant mass. The entire left lobe of the liver has been removed. **A.** Capillary phase of selective hepatic angiography. Intense, homogeneous capillary staining is evident, indicating that the mass is hypervascular. **B.** Anterior view, ^{99m}Tc sulfur colloid study. The hypervascular lesion has prominently increased sulfur colloid uptake. (Reproduced by permission from Welch TJ, Sheedy PF, Johnson CM, et al. Focal nodular hyperplasia and hepatic adenoma: comparison of angiography, CT, US, and scintigraphy. Radiology 1985;156:593–595.)

Focal Fatty Infiltration

Focal areas of infiltration with fat in the liver can produce focal low attenuation lesions on CT that can be misinterpreted as metastases. This condition is most frequently associated with alcohol abuse, but can also be seen in diabetes, malabsorption, exogenous obesity, or intravenous hyperalimentation (34). The correct diagnosis can usually be made when CT demonstrates the typical findings of a nonspherical mass with indistinct margins that does not produce a mass effect (34). In one study, however, a third of these lesions were spherical or oval with well-defined margins, and one-half produced a mass effect (35). Ultrasound demonstrates these lesions to be hyperechoic, but this finding is nonspecific. In alcoholics, the diagnosis can be confirmed by a repeat CT study which will demonstrate resolution of the lesions after 3–6 weeks of total abstinence

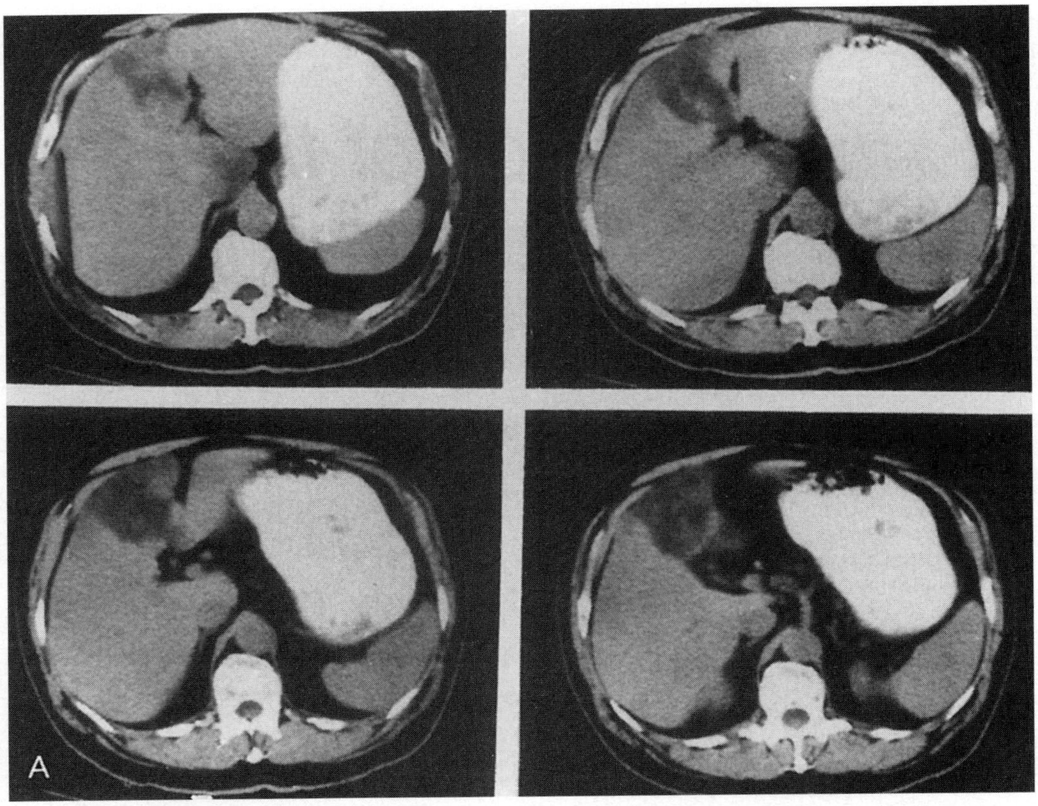

Figure 37.5. Focal fatty infiltration. **A.** Four consecutive slices from CT study of abdomen in 61-year-old man reveal a low density lesion in the liver. **B.** Anterior, RAO, right lateral, and RPO planar images from a ^{99m}Tc sulfur colloid study of the liver show no abnormality. **C.** Four consecutive transaxial views from a SPECT study show a focal defect in the liver that corresponds with the lesion seen on the CT study. Biopsy revealed only fat. (Reproduced by permission from Schauwecker DS, Wass J. Focal fatty infiltration of the liver: evaluation by planar and SPECT images. Clin Nucl Med 1991;16:449–451.)

(35). Alternatively, radionuclide imaging with sulfur colloid will nearly always indicate the correct diagnosis by demonstrating that the lesions seen on CT have normal uptake of colloid (36). Focal fatty infiltration can sometimes produce defects on the sulfur colloid study (37–39), especially if SPECT is performed (40) (Fig. 37.5). ^{133}Xe uptake by the lesion also confirms the diagnosis, since its high partition coefficient causes xenon to be taken up by fat; however, xenon uptake occurs much less consistently than sulfur colloid defects (41).

DIFFUSE LIVER DISEASE

Radionuclide liver imaging complements other procedures (liver function tests, needle biopsy, etc.) in the diagnosis and management of diseases that diffusely involve the liver. The study is helpful in distinguishing between localized and diffuse disease, demonstrating the coexistence of both types of disease, documenting liver size and shape, and following the clinical course of diffuse disease.

Hepatomegaly is often an early sign of diffuse hepatic disease. A rough estimate of liver size can be obtained from an anterior image made with a 10-cm lead strip overlying the liver for size calibration. A vertical dimension greater than 15.5 cm in the right midclavicular line probably indicates abnormality (42). Attempts have been made to quantify liver volume from dimensions on planar images (43), but these volume measurements have been much less accurate than measurements from SPECT images (44–47).

Colloid shift (increase in splenic and/or marrow uptake of colloid relative to liver uptake) is an important sign of impaired liver function. This finding may be assessed from the posterior liver/spleen view. Splenic uptake is abnormally increased if the spleen appears more intense than the liver. Marrow uptake is increased if most of the spine is clearly visible. Assessment of the spleen to liver uptake ratio is much more accurate for quantitative SPECT methods than for planar imaging (45–48).

In alcoholics, imaging procedures usually have little role in the evaluation of liver disease. Instead, the physician will rely on clinical findings, liver function tests, and liver biopsy. Liver biopsy is expensive, occasionally leads to complications, and is subject to sampling error and, therefore, not totally accurate (49). Radionuclide imaging of the liver with sulfur colloid has been proposed as a screening procedure prior to biopsy (47, 49). One might forego biopsy in patients found to have little or no abnormality on liver imaging. For those patients found to have severe disease,

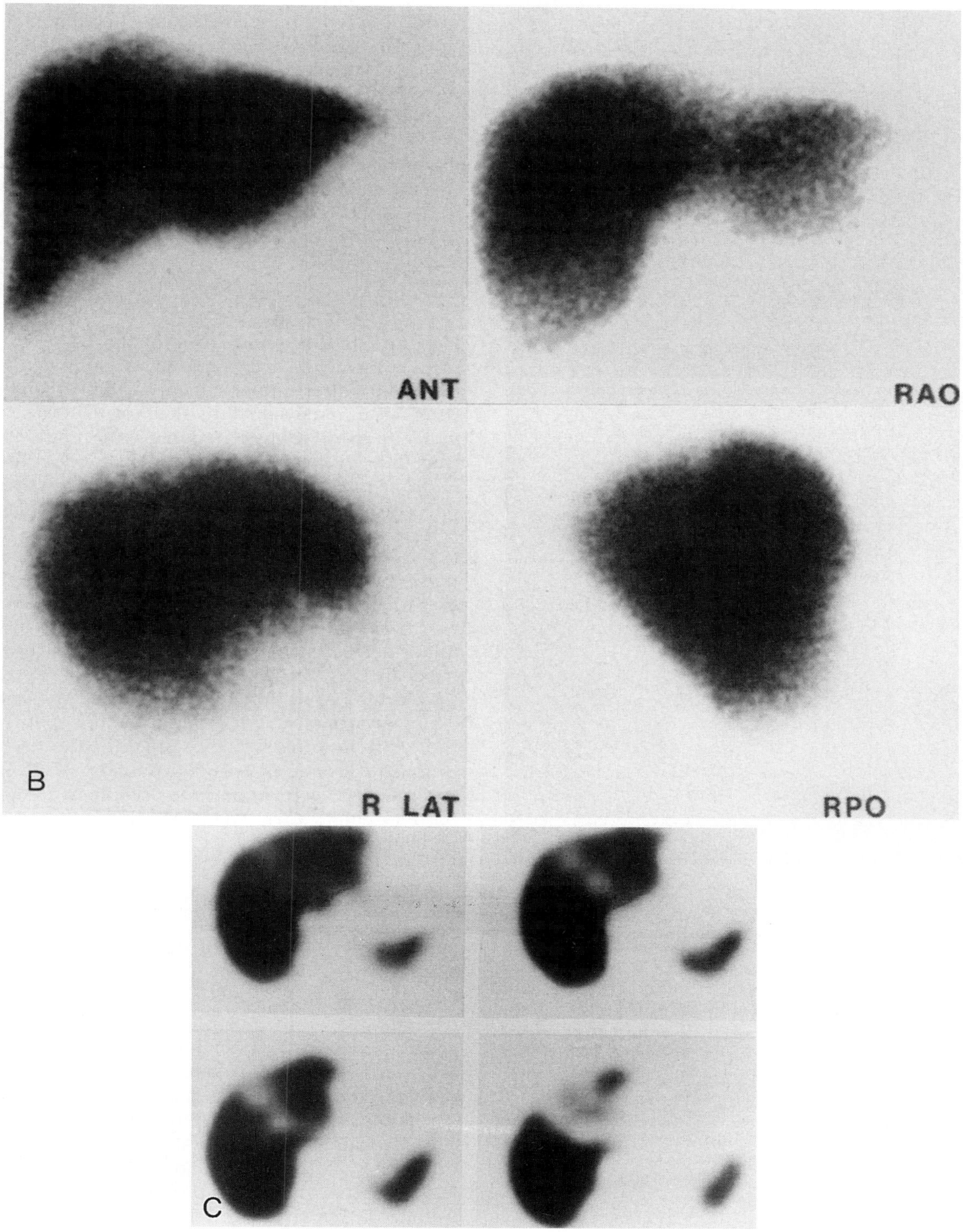
ANT
RAO
B
R LAT
RPO
C

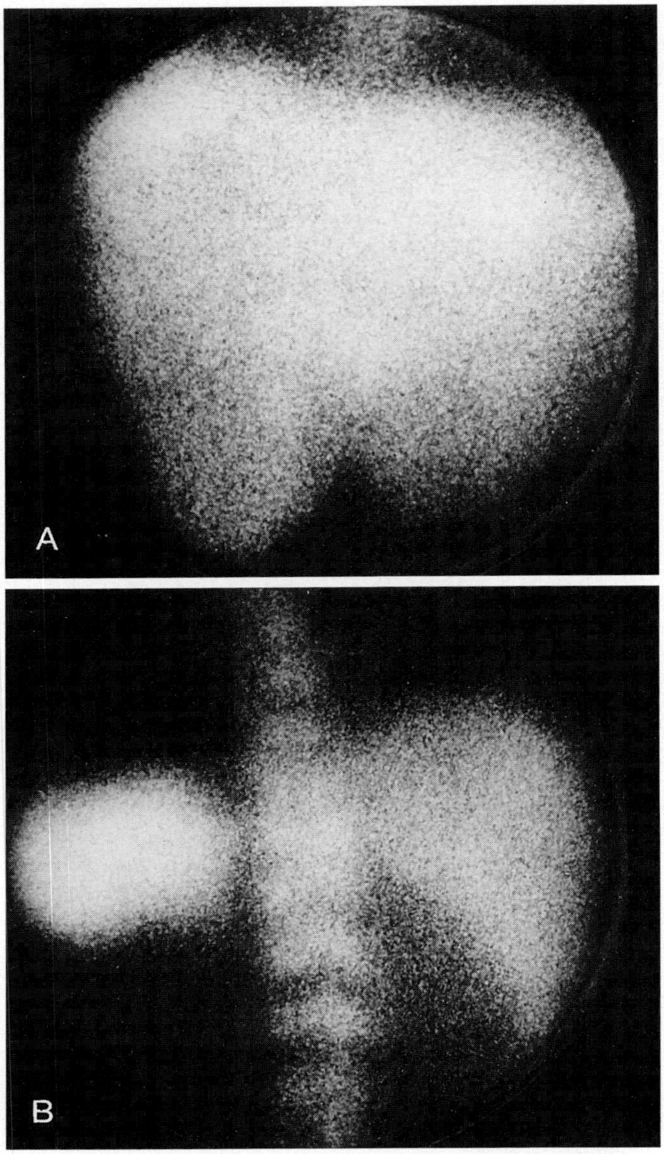

Figure 37.6. Cirrhosis. **A.** Anterior liver. Hepatomegaly is present. **B.** Posterior liver and spleen. The spleen is brighter than the liver, and the spine is prominent, indicating increased spleen and marrow uptake.

one might proceed without biopsy to a full workup for the complications of cirrhosis. It should be noted that in the detection of diffuse disease of the liver, radionuclide imaging has been shown to be more sensitive than CT or ultrasound (50, 51), especially when SPECT is performed (47, 52).

Cirrhosis

Mild cirrhosis may produce only minimally decreased liver uptake and minimally increased spleen uptake. A fairly good correlation between splenic and marrow uptake and the degree of liver decompensation has been demonstrated (53–57). These findings are not specific for cirrhosis, however, because they may also be seen in anemia (58), hepatitis, chronic passive congestion (59), fatty infiltrate of the liver (59), cancer chemotherapy (60), and a number of other conditions.

Moderate to advanced cirrhosis has a characteristic appearance on radionuclide imaging (61) (Fig. 37.6). The liver is large with decreased colloid uptake that is heterogeneous in its distribution. Splenic and marrow uptake are increased, often markedly, and the ribs may be clearly visualized. The spleen is often enlarged. Ascites may be present, as indicated by a separation between the lateral margin of the liver and the rib cage (Fig. 37.1**C** and **D**). If a focal defect is present it may represent a regenerative nodule or a hepatocellular carcinoma (see "Hepatocellular Carcinoma").

Hepatic Vein Thrombosis

Hepatic vein thrombosis (Budd-Chiari syndrome) can produce a variety of liver patterns on sulfur colloid imaging (62). The pattern most typical of the disease is a diffuse decrease in radiocolloid uptake except for the caudate lobe, which is relatively hypertrophic with increased colloid uptake (62). In these cases, there is generally thrombosis of all three main branches of the hepatic vein with preserved patency of the accessory veins draining the caudate lobe. SPECT can be helpful in demonstrating this distribution (63). Occasionally, a main branch of the hepatic vein remains patent, in which case the region drained by it retains its function. Other patterns that may be seen are hepatomegaly with nonhomogeneous colloid uptake, or multiple filling defects suggestive of mass lesions, but these patterns are nonspecific (62). Frequently, there is extrahepatic uptake similar to that seen in cirrhosis; however, the tendency toward a central distribution of hepatic uptake and the relatively rapid progression of the disease help to distinguish it from cirrhosis (64, 65) (Fig. 37.7). Hepatic vein thrombosis has been noted especially in conjunction with paroxysmal nocturnal hemoglobinuria (64) and polycythemia rubra vera (65).

Diffuse Fatty Infiltration

Diffuse fatty infiltration is a more generalized form of the same process described under "Focal Fatty Infiltration." Occasionally, this condition coexists with focal liver lesions demonstrated on CT or ultrasound (66, 67). One is then confronted with the question of whether the focal lesions represent tumors or other masses, or are merely regions of normal liver parenchyma embedded within the fatty infiltration. The sulfur colloid study, preferably performed with SPECT, will demonstrate a defect if the focal lesion was a mass, but will show normal or even increased uptake if the lesion represents normal parenchyma (66, 67). Increased uptake in this situation reflects the higher concentration of Kupffer cells in the normal parenchyma relative to the surrounding fatty infiltration (67). ^{133}Xe studies have been recommended to confirm the presence of the fatty infiltration, but are of little value since they will not distinguish between normal parenchyma and liver mass.

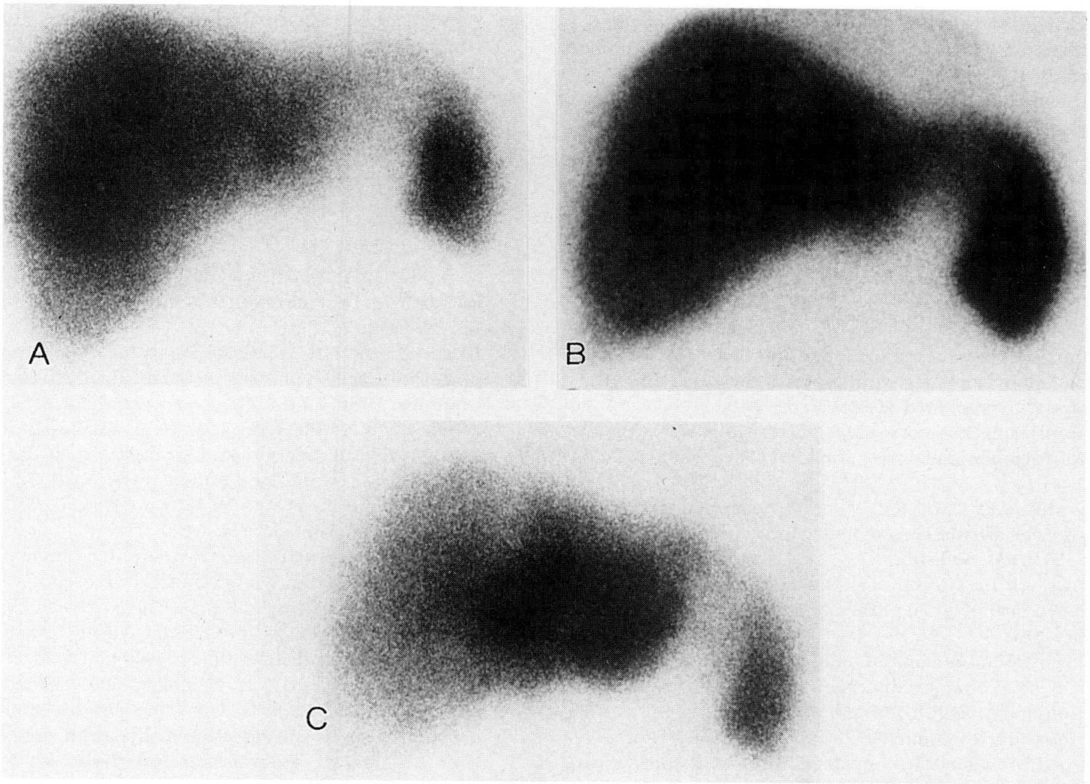

Figure 37.7. Hepatic vein thrombosis. Thirty-year-old nonalcoholic female with antithrombin III deficiency and clotting tendency developed liver failure over a 3-year interval. **A.** Original study was considered normal. **B.** Study 2 months later shows some colloid shift to the spleen. **C.** Study 3 years later shows decreased liver size with relatively increased uptake centrally. Hepatic venogram showed a narrowed inferior vena cava and occlusion of hepatic veins. The preservation of function in the central region of the liver in hepatic vein thrombosis is attributed to the separate venous drainage of the caudate lobe.

REFERENCES

1. Gates GA, Henley KS, Pollard HM, et al. The cell population of the human liver. J Lab Clin Med 1961;57:182–184.
2. Coleman RE, Russell AB, Jaszczak RJ. Single photon emission computed tomography (SPECT). Part II: Clinical applications. Invest Radiol 1986;21:1–11.
3. Ziessman HA, Silverman PM, Patterson J, et al. Improved detection of small cavernous hemangiomas of the liver with high-resolution three-headed SPECT. J Nucl Med 1991;32:2086–2091.
4. Rogers WL, Clinthorne NH, Harkness BA, et al. Field-flood requirements for emission computed tomography with an Anger camera. J Nucl Med 1982;23:162–168.
5. Waxman AD, Apau R, Siemsen JK. Rapid sequential liver imaging. J Nucl Med 1972;13:522–527.
6. DeNardo GL, Stadalnik RC, DeNardo SJ, et al. Hepatic scintiangiographic patterns. Radiology 1974;111:135–141.
7. Pettigrew RI, Witztum KF, Perkins GC, et al. Single photon emission computed tomograms of the liver: normal vascular intrahepatic structures. Radiology 1984;150:219–223.
8. Henderson JM, Campbell JD, Olson R, et al. Role of computed tomography in screening for hepatocellular carcinoma in patients with cirrhosis. Gastrointest Radiol 1988;13:129–134.
9. Lee VW, O'Brien MJ, Morris PM, et al. The specific diagnosis of hepatocellular carcinoma by scintigraphy: multiple radiotracer approach. Cancer 1985;56:25–36.
10. Lomas F, Dibos PE, Wagner HN. Increased specificity of liver scanning with the use of ^{67}Gallium citrate. N Engl J Med 1972; 286:1323–1329.
11. Suzuki T, Honjo I, Hamamoto K, et al. Positive scintiphotography of cancer of the liver with Ga-67 citrate. AJR 1971;113:92–103.
12. James O, Wood EJ, Sherlock S. ^{67}Gallium scanning in the diagnosis of liver disease. Gut 1974;15:404–410.
13. Nagasue N. Gallium scanning in the diagnosis of hepatocellular carcinoma: a clinicopathological study of 45 patients. Clin Radiol 1983;34:139–142.
14. Ishak KG, Rabin L. Benign tumors of the liver. Med Clin North Am 1975;59:995–1013.
15. Front D, Royal H, Israel O, et al. Scintigraphy of hepatic hemangiomas: value of 99m-technetium labeled red blood cells. J Nucl Med 1981;22:684–687.
16. Engel MA, Marks DS, Sandler MA, et al. Differentiation of focal intrahepatic lesions with 99m-technetium red blood cell imaging. Radiology 1983;146:777–782.
17. Rabinowitz SA, McKusick KA, Strauss HW. ^{99m}Tc red blood cell scintigraphy in evaluating focal liver lesions. AJR 1984;143:63–68.
18. Brodsky RI, Friedman AC, Maurer AH, et al. Hepatic cavernous hemangioma: diagnosis with ^{99m}Tc-labeled red cells and single-photon emission CT. AJR 1987;148:125–129.
19. Kudo M, Ikekubo K, Yamamoto K, et al. Distinction between hemangioma of the liver and hepatocellular carcinoma: value of labeled RBC-SPECT scanning. AJR 1989;152:977–983.
20. Krause T, Hauenstein K, Studier-Fischer B, et al. Improved evaluation of technetium-99m-red blood cell SPECT in hemangioma of the liver. J Nucl Med 1993;34:375–380.

21. Tumeh SS, Benson C, Nagel JS, et al. Cavernous hemangioma of the liver: detection with single-photon emission computed tomography. Radiology 1987;164:353–356.
22. Ginsberg F, Slavin JD, Spencer RP. Hepatic angiosarcoma: mimicking of angioma on three-phase technetium-99m red blood cell scintigraphy. J Nucl Med 1986;27:1861–1863.
23. Hardoff R, Aghai E, Bitterman H. Scintigraphic evaluation of a patient with hemangiosarcoma: labeled red blood cell imaging is nondiagnostic. Clin Nucl Med 1993;18:986–988.
24. Farlow DC, Little JM, Gruenewald SM, et al. A case of metastatic malignancy masquerading as a hepatic hemangioma on labeled red blood cell scintigraphy. J Nucl Med 1993;34:1172–1174.
25. Intenzo C, Kim S, Madsen M, et al. Planar and SPECT Tc-99m red blood cell imaging in hepatic cavernous hemangiomas and other hepatic lesions. Clin Nucl Med 1988;13:237–240.
26. Groshar D, Ben-Haim S, Gips S, et al. Spectrum of scintigraphic appearance of liver hemangiomas. Clin Nucl Med 1992;17:294–299.
27. Casarella WJ, Knowles DM, Wolff M, et al. Focal nodular hyperplasia and liver cell adenoma: radiologic and pathologic differentiation. AJR 1978;131:393–402.
28. Tesluk H, Lawrie J. Hepatocellular adenoma: its transformation to carcinoma in a user of oral contraceptives. Arch Pathol Lab Med 1981;105:296–299.
29. Welch TJ, Sheedy PF, Johnson CM, et al. Focal nodular hyperplasia and hepatic adenoma: comparison of angiography, CT, US, and scintigraphy. Radiology 1985;156:593–595.
30. Lubbers PR, Ros PR, Goodman ZD, et al. Accumulation of technetium-99m sulfur colloid by hepatocellular adenoma: scintigraphic-pathologic correlation. AJR 1987;148:1105–1108.
31. Lerona PT, Go RT, Cornell SH. Limitations of angiography and scanning in diagnosis of liver masses. Radiology 1974;112:139–145.
32. Tanasescu DE, Waxman AD, Hurvitz C. Scintigraphic findings mimicking focal nodular hyperplasia in a case of hepatoblastoma. Clin Nucl Med 1991;16:236–238.
33. Park CH, Kim SM, Intenzo C, et al. Focal nodular hyperplasia of the liver: diagnosis by dynamic and SPECT scintigraphy. Clin Nucl Med 1993;18:701–703.
34. Halvorsen RA, Korobkin M, Ram PC, et al. CT appearance of focal fatty infiltration of the liver. AJR 1982;139:277–281.
35. Tang-Barton P, Vas W, Weissman J, et al. Focal fatty liver lesions in alcoholic liver disease: a broadened spectrum of CT appearances. Gastrointest Radiol 1985;10:133–137.
36. Lisbona R, Mishkin S, Derbekyan V, et al. Role of scintigraphy in focally abnormal sonograms of fatty livers. J Nucl Med 1988; 29:1050–1056.
37. Black RR, Winfield DF, Fernandez-Ulloa M. Solitary defect on liver sulfur colloid imaging secondary to focal fatty infiltration. Clin Nucl Med 1989;14:603–605.
38. Khedkar N, Pestika B, Rosenblate H, et al. Large focal defect on liver/spleen scan caused by fatty liver and masquerading as neoplasm. J Nucl Med 1992;33:258–259.
39. Marmolya GA, Miron SD, Eckhauser M, et al. Focal fatty infiltration of the liver appearing as a defect on a liver-spleen scintigram: case report. Clin Nucl Med 1992;17:300–302.
40. Schauwecker DS, Wass JL. Focal fatty infiltration of the liver: evaluation by planar and SPECT images. Clin Nucl Med 1991;16:449–451.
41. Baker MK, Schauwecker DS, Wenker JC, et al. Nuclear medicine evaluation of focal fatty infiltration of the liver. Clin Nucl Med 1986;11:503–506.
42. Rosenfield AT, Schneider PB. Rapid evaluation of hepatic size on radioisotope scan. J Nucl Med 1974;15:237–240.
43. Rollo FD, DeLand FH. The determination of liver mass from radionuclide images. Radiology 1968;91:1191–1194.
44. Kan MK, Hopkins GB. Measurement of liver volume by emission computed tomography. J Nucl Med 1979;20:514–520.
45. Chandler ST. A comparison of liver-spleen ratios and uptakes obtained using planar and tomographic techniques. Nucl Med Commun 1989;10:297–307.
46. Kodama T, Watanabe K, Hoshi H, et al. Diagnosis of diffuse hepatocellular diseases using SPECT. J Nucl Med 1986;27:616–619.
47. Delcourt E, Vanhaeverbeek M, Binon JP, et al. Emission tomography for assessment of diffuse alcoholic liver disease. J Nucl Med 1992;33:1337–1345.
48. Jago JR, Gibson CJ, Diffey BL. Evaluation of subjective assessment of liver function from radionuclide images. Br J Radiol 1987; 60:127–132.
49. Baudouin SV, Grey H, Hall-Craggs M, et al. Liver scintiscanning as a screening test in the detection of alcoholic cirrhosis. Nucl Med Commun 1986;7:71–75.
50. Meek DR, Mills PR, Gray HW, et al. A comparison of computed tomography, ultrasound and scintigraphy in the diagnosis of alcoholic liver disease. Br J Radiol 1984;57:23–27.
51. Drane WE, VanNess MM. Hepatic imaging in diffuse liver disease. Clin Nucl Med 1988;13:182–185.
52. Yudd AP, Van Heertum RL, Brunetti JC. Single photon emission computed tomography and transmission computed tomography in the evaluation of liver disease. Clin Nucl Med 1988;13:397–401.
53. Christie JH, Gomez Crespo G, Koch-Weser D, et al. The correlation of clearance and distribution of colloidal gold in the liver as an index of hepatic cirrhosis. Radiology 1967;88:334–341.
54. Gheorghescu B, Jovin G, Pavel D, et al. Interpretation of scintigraphic changes during chronic hepatitis and cirrhosis of the liver. In: Medical radiosotope scintigraphy. Vol 2. Vienna: International Atomic Energy Agency, 1969:517–532.
55. Whang KS, Fish MB, Pollycove M. Evaluation of hepatic photoscanning with radioactive colloidal gold. J Nucl Med 1965;6:494–505.
56. Prakash V, Lin MS, Kriss JP. Liver scintigraphy in alcoholic ilver disease. Clin Nucl Med 1977;2:308–309.
57. Wasnich R, Glober G, Hayashi T, et al. Simple computer quantitation of spleen-to-liver ratios in the diagnosis of hepatocellular disease. J Nucl Med 1979;20:149–154.
58. Bekerman C, Gottschalk A. Diagnostic significance of the relative uptake of liver compared with spleen in ^{99m}Tc-sulfur colloid scintiphotography. J Nucl Med 1971;12:237–240.
59. Wilson GA, Keyes JW. The significance of the liver-spleen uptake ratio in liver scanning. J Nucl Med 1974;15:593–597.
60. Kaplan WD, Drum DE, Lokich JJ. The effect of cancer chemotherapeutic agents on the liver-spleen scan. J Nucl Med 1980; 21:84–87.
61. Drum DE, Beard JO. Liver scintigraphic features associated with alcoholism. J Nucl Med 1978;19:154–160.
62. Picard M, Carrier L, Chartrand R, et al. Budd-Chiari syndrome: typical and atypical scintigraphic aspects. J Nucl Med 1987; 28:803–809.
63. Kim CK, Palestro CJ, Goldsmith SJ. SPECT imaging in the diagnosis of Budd-Chiari syndrome. J Nucl Med 1990;31:109–111.
64. Staab EV, Hartman RC, Parrott JA. LIver imaging in the diagnosis of hepatic venous thrombosis in paroxysmal nocturnal hemoglobinuria. Radiology 1975;117:341–348.
65. Tavill AS, Wood EJ, Kreel L, et al. The Budd-Chiari syndrome: correlation between hepatic scintigraphy and the clinical, radiological, and pathological findings in nineteen cases of hepatic venous outflow obstruction. Gastroenterology 1975;68:509–518.
66. Lipman JC, Stomper PC, Kaplan WD, et al. Detection of hepatic metastases in diffuse fatty infiltration by CT: the complementary role of imaging. Clin Nucl Med 1988;13:602–605.
67. Newman JS, Oates E, Arora S, et al. Focal spared area in fatty liver simulating a mass: scintigraphic evaluation. Dig Dis Sci 1991; 36:1019–1022.

38 Hepatobiliary Imaging

DARLENE FINK-BENNETT

ACUTE CHOLECYSTITIS

It is estimated that approximately 10–15% of Americans have gallstones. Of these 20 million Americans, 20–25% will develop a cystic duct obstruction and signs and symptoms indicative of an acutely inflamed hemorrhagic gallbladder wall. Of these 16 million women and 4 million men, 20–35% will develop symptoms of chronic cholecystitis while the remainder will be asymptomatic (1).

Gallstones occur more frequently in women than in men, as the ingestion of estrogens, progesterone, and pregnancy increase the production of lithogenic bile and the formation of nucleation sites, i.e., substances which precipitate or permit gallstone formation. Additionally, estrogens, progesterone, and pregnancy result in decreased gallbladder motility, another factor that contributes to gallstone formation. Obesity and rapid weight loss also increase cholesterol supersaturation and decrease gallbladder motility. These conditions are not unique to women, but are more often seen in them than men. In fact, of the 1 million newly diagnosed patients with cholelithiasis per year, the majority are female (1–3).

Gallstones are comprised principally of cholesterol though pigmented stones do occur. Gallstones increase in size over a 2–3 year period then stabilize. Most are small and less than 2 cm in diameter. Unless one obstructs the cystic duct, their presence may go undetected. If, however, one becomes impacted in the cystic duct, acute cholecystitis develops and can be life-threatening (3).

In 95% of patients with an acutely inflamed hemorrhagic gallbladder, a gallstone or gallstones are responsible for the cystic duct obstruction. In 5% of patients with acute cholecystitis, the obstruction is caused by inflammation, edema, gallbladder mucous, or a tumor (1, 2).

The signs and symptoms of acute cholecystitis include severe epigastric or right upper quadrant pain, fever, nausea, and vomiting. A mild-to-moderate leukocytosis and abnormal liver function tests are also usually present. If the pain radiates to the back in the region of the scapula or there is rebound tenderness, the clinical diagnosis of acute cholecystitis is strengthened (4).

If a stone has become impacted in the common bile duct, hyperbilirubinemia is present (greater than 5 mg/dl). If the latter has occurred, a dilated common bile duct can be identified sonographically 3 days post its impaction. The patient may also relate a prior history of pancreatitis (1, 2, 4).

Choledocholithiasis is not uncommon. It is estimated that 8–15% of patients under the age of 6 and 15–60% of patients over the age of 6 will have stones in their common bile duct in conjunction with one in their cystic duct (3).

If the serum amylase is elevated, concomitant pancreatitis is present (1, 2).

The diagnosis of acute cholecystitis is not always an easy one as other conditions have signs and symptoms, as well as biochemical abnormalities, that are similar to acute cholecystitis. These include, but are not necessarily limited to, coronary artery disease, chronic passive congestion of the liver, pneumonia, an intestinal obstruction, renal colic, herpes zoster, and phlegmonous gastritis (4).

Most patients with an obstructed cystic duct and acute cholecystitis do not require urgent surgery. Surgery is usually delayed for up to 72 hours to stabilize the patient, correct electrolyte imbalances if present, and begin antibiotic therapy. Elderly patients, however, and up to 10–15% of patients with a prior history of acute cholecystitis which resolved spontaneously, do require early surgery, as gangrenous changes with or without perforation, gallstone ileus, or cholangitis, occur in up to 25% of them if the proper diagnosis is not made, and treatment instituted within the first 72 hours of symptoms (1–3). Since history, physical examination, and laboratory tests alone cannot always establish the diagnosis, numerous imaging modalities have evolved to confirm the clinical impression of acute cholecystitis. These include hepatobiliary scintigraphy, realtime ultrasonography of the gallbladder, and gallbladder computed tomography.

The pathogenesis of acute cholecystitis is still not completely understood but is believed to occur when the obstructed gallbladder becomes distended and its mucosa irritated and inflamed by retained lithogenic bile. Vascular congestion, mural edema, leukocytic infiltration, and ultimately hemorrhagic necrosis of the gallbladder wall then results (2).

The sensitivity and specificity of hepatobiliary scintigraphy in confirming the clinical impression of a cystic duct obstruction and acute cholecystitis, is superior to realtime ultrasonography and CT of the gallbladder. The sensitivity of cholescintigraphy in detecting acute cholecystitis is greater than 95%, whereas liberal criteria, realtime ultrasonography of the gallbladder is only 80–86%; strict criteria, 24%. Liberal realtime gallbladder ultrasonography criteria are findings indicative of but no pathognomonic for acute cholecystitis. They include the demonstration of stones, a thick gallbladder wall, nonshadowing echoes, and the Murphy sign. In the absence of cirrhosis, ascites, and hypoalbuminemia, strict realtime sonographic findings of acute cholecystitis are pericholecystic fluid and wall edema (5).

The sensitivity of gallbladder computed tomography is similar to realtime gallbladder ultrasonography, as the only pathognomonic finding of acute cholecystitis tomographically is gas bubbles within the gallbladder wall (6, 7).

The specificity of hepatobiliary imaging is also superior to realtime ultrasonography and computed tomography of the gallbladder in excluding the presence of a cystic duct obstruction and acute cholecystitis. Gallbladder realtime ultrasonography's specificity in negating the diagnosis ranges from 60% to 64%, whereas hepatobiliary imaging specificity is 93–96%. Gallbladder computed tomography's specificity is similar to realtime cholosonography's acute cholecystitis specificity as both modalities are subject to, and limited by, a high false positive rate; i.e., the presence of sludge, stones, or a thick gallbladder wall being interpreted as a sign or signs of acute cholecystitis in the absence of an occluded cystic duct and hemorrhagic gallbladder wall. In fact, in several studies, more than one-third of patients with acute epigastric and right upper quadrant pain would have been misdiagnosed as having acute cholecystitis had they simply undergone gallbladder sonography (7–9).

The positive predictive value of an abnormal hepatobiliary scan in confirming the diagnosis of acute cholecystitis is as high as 92.1%, whereas realtime gallbladder ultrasonography's positive predictive value is only 40–50%. Cholescintigraphy's negative predictive value is 99% (8, 10, 11).

Hepatobiliary imaging is also a highly accurate modality for detecting a high grade or a total common bile duct obstruction. Hepatobiliary scintigraphy's sensitivity in identifying a total or high grade common bile duct obstruction is over 95% and its presence can be detected immediately following stone impaction. Realtime ultrasonography of the biliary tree, on the other hand, requires greater than 72 hours from the time of impaction before ductal dilatation is demonstrable sonographically (12–15).

For hepatobiliary imaging to achieve its high degree of accuracy in acute cholecystitis detection, images have to be obtained up to 4 hours following the intravenous administration of ^{99m}Tc-labeled immunodiacetic acid derivative (IDA). If imaging is ceased sooner, i.e., at 1 hour, the specificity of the procedure is reduced from 93–96% to 80–88% (9, 11, 12). This occurs in up to 20% of individuals with chronic cholecystitis in whom there is increased intraluminal gallbladder pressure from highly viscus/stagnant bile and/or from sludge, and can require up to 4 hours of imaging time for enough radiotracer to enter the gallbladder to permit its visualization (12).

To eliminate the need for prolonged imaging time, patients clinically suspected of acute cholecystitis can either be premedicated with cholecystokinin (CCK) 30 minutes prior to the administration of ^{99m}Tc-IDA, or be given morphine sulfate if their gallbladder does not visualize within 60 minutes and if radiotracer is seen within the small intestine (16, 17).

If a patient is pretreated with CCK, the CCK causes the gallbladder to contract, ejecting any viscus bile/sludge from it. Thus, the potential source of increased resistance to bile flow is eliminated and the need for delayed imaging unnecessary. After contraction, the gallbladder relaxes, creating an optimal state for the accumulation of ^{99m}Tc-IDA if the cystic duct is patent. In fact, it is this "low resistance to bile flow state" that accounts for preferential gallbladder filling and delayed biliary to bowel transit in patients who have been pretreated with 0.01–0.02 mg/kg of cholecystokinin 30 minutes prior the administration of ^{99m}Tc-IDA (18).

The sensitivity and specificity of pretreatment CCK cholescintigraphy in detecting and excluding acute cholecystitis is identical to conventional hepatobiliary scintigraphy. Why then do most laboratories not employ CCK as a premedicate in patients undergoing hepatobiliary scintigraphy for the detection of acute cholecystitis? The reason is and was that Freeman, et al., were concerned that (a) patients with chronic cholecystitis would not be differentiated from normal individuals, (b) patients would be exposed unnecessarily to a pharmacologic agent that, although it has not been associated with significant side effects, can cause nausea, cramping, and, in some, an exacerbation of gallbladder pain, and, occasionally, (c) patients with acute cholecystitis exhibiting delayed gallbladder visualization would be totally missed, a situation that occurred in 5/143 patients with proven acute cholecystitis. Additionally, Freeman, et al., were concerned that if delayed views were not obtained, serendipitous findings of malrotation, enterogastric reflux, and/or masses displacing or inflammatory processes affecting the small bowel would go undetected (19).

The use of pretreatment CCK to diminish the time required to establish the diagnosis of a cystic duct obstruction and acute cholecystitis scintigraphically is now rarely, if ever, considered, as morphine-augmented cholescintigraphy is as accurate, timely, and without pretreatment CCK hepatobiliary scintigraphy's potential pitfalls and complications.

Morphine sulfate enhances sphincter of oddi tone. This results in increased pressure within the lumen of the common bile duct. The pressure within the common bile duct following the administration of as little as 0.04 mg/kg morphine sulfate intravenously, is increased by approximately 50%, from 12.7 $\pm$2.4 to 20 $\pm$2.4 cm of saline. It is this pharmacologically induced increased intraluminal common bile duct pressure that diverts bile away from the sphincter of oddi to and into a functionally obstructed sludge filled gallbladder if the cystic duct is patent (17, 20–23).

Hepatobiliary scintigraphy is performed following the intravenous administration of a ^{99m}Tc-IDA derivative. There are two immunodiacetic acid derivatives that are commercially available. One is disofenin (Hepatolite; Dupont-Merck) and the other is mebrofenin (Choletec; Squibb Inc.). Both compounds are extracted by the hepatocytes, secreted into the bile cuniculi and transported via the intra- and extrahepatic biliary radicals to the gallbladder and small bowel.

The hepatic uptake of ^{99m}Tc-IDA derivatives, be it disofenin or mebrofenin, is accomplished by the same carrier-mediated nonsodium-dependent organic anion path as bilirubin. The degree of hepatic uptake of these compounds and their rate of excretion is dependent upon their structural configuration. Approximately 85% of disofenin and 98% of mebrofenin is extracted by the hepatocytes. Mebrofenin's rate of clearance is 6–28 minutes, disofenin 6–32 minutes (24).

Hepatic extraction of ^{99m}Tc-IDA derivatives decreases

with increasing serum bilirubin levels and thus, in the presence of hyperbilirubinemia (greater than 8 ng/dl), common bile duct and gallbladder visualization is best achieved with mebrofenin as opposed to disofenin. Mebrofenin is useful to bilirubin levels of up to 30 ng/dl. In the absence of hyperbilirubinemia, either agent provides excellent visualization of the hepatobiliary tree. Mebrofenin does, however, have a rapid biliary to bowel transit time. This is a characteristic that must be taken into consideration when evaluating patients with possible acute cholecystitis for if little tracer remains within the intrahepatic biliary tree at 1 hour, none will be available to enter the gallbladder postmorphine administration or following delayed imaging (9, 25, 26).

Conventional hepatobiliary scintigraphy is performed after a 2–4 hour fast and following the intravenous administration of 5 mCi of either ^{99m}Tc-disofenin (Hepatolite) or ^{99m}Tc-mebrofenin (Choletec). If a patient has fasted for greater than 24–48 hours, he or she is given 0.02 mg/kg of cholecystokinin 30 minutes prior to the intravenous administration of the radiotracer. If cholecystokinin is utilized, it should be injected slowly over a 5-minute period. This will minimize abdominal cramping, one of the potential side effects of CCK administration (14). An anterior, 1 million count, large field of view gamma-camera image, or 500,000 count, small field of view gamma-camera image, of the liver and biliary tree is then obtained at 5 minutes with a low-energy medium-resolution all-purpose collimator and a 20% window centered on the 140 keV ^{99m}Tc photopeak. Images are then obtained every 10 minutes for a set time, that time being determined from the number of seconds required to obtain the initial anterior 1 million or 500,000 count hepatobiliary image. Right lateral views are obtained at 30 and 60 minutes postradiotracer administration. Oblique views are obtained if necessary to separate gallbladder from small bowel activity. If there is nonvisualization of the gallbladder at 60 minutes, delayed images are obtained up to 4 hours after the intravenous administration of either the ^{99m}Tc-disofenin or ^{99m}Tc-mebrofenin.

On occasion, gallbladder visualization is difficult to distinguish from duodenal activity. Should this occur, 5–10 cc of water should be ingested to distinguish transient duodenal activity from activity within the gallbladder (9, 27). Viewing the cholescintiscan in cine mode or having the patient assume an upright position can also help differentiate intraluminal gallbladder activity from activity within a loop of small bowel. Seeing the radiotracer leave the area of the gallbladder fossa assures that its location is within a loop of small bowel and not within the gallbladder itself (27–29).

In patients in whom a conventional hepatobiliary scan is being performed to confirm the clinical impression of acute cholecystitis, one of six scan patterns are usually seen: (a) gallbladder visualization within 1 hour following the intravenous administration of a ^{99m}Tc-IDA derivative, (b) nonvisualization of the gallbladder up to 4 hours postradiotracer administration, (c) delayed gallbladder visualization between 1 and 4 hours post-^{99m}Tc-disofenin or mebrofenin administration, (d) persistent (up to 24 hours) nonvisualization of the intra- and extrahepatic biliary tree in a patient with a normal hepatic extraction efficiency, (e) preferential gallbladder filling with delayed visualization of the small bowel or, (f) the presence of a nubbin of activity (focus of ^{99m}Tc-IDA accumulation) adjacent to the common bile duct and medial to the gallbladder fossa which persists up to 4 hours postradiotracer administration.

A normal hepatobiliary scan is one in which the gallbladder and small bowel are visualized within 1 hour of the intravenous administration of ^{99m}Tc-IDA (Fig. 38.1). Failure to visualize the gallbladder up to 4 hours postradiotracer administration in conjunction with a normal ^{99m}Tc-IDA hepatic extraction efficiency and normal biliary to bowel transit time, is consistent with a cystic duct obstruction and, in an appropriate clinical setting, acute cholecystitis (12) (Fig. 38.2). If a band or rim of increased ^{99m}Tc-disofenin or mebrofenin is located adjacent to the gallbladder fossa, a "rim" sign is present. Pericholecystic activity is indicative not only of a cystic duct obstruction and acute cholecystitis, but often is a manifestation of the inflammatory changes resulting from a gangrenous gallbladder wall (30) (Fig. 38.3).

Delayed gallbladder visualization between 1 and 4 hours following the intravenous administration of ^{99m}Tc-IDA, is most often the result of increased intraluminal gallbladder pressure resulting from viscus bile/sludge in patients with chronic cholecystitis (Fig. 38.4). Delayed gallbladder visualization, however, may also be seen in patients with hepatocellular disease if their hepatic extraction efficiency is less than 80%. The slow biliary transit which results when there is reduced or delayed hepatic extraction of ^{99m}Tc-IDA prolonging gallbladder visualiza-

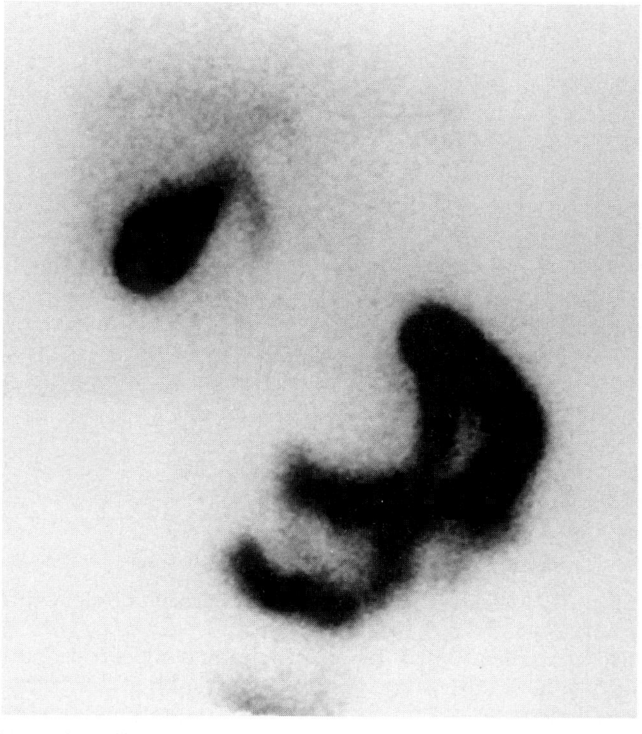

Figure 38.1. Normal anterior hepatobiliary scan as ^{99m}Tc-IDA is identified within the gallbladder, common bile duct, and small intestine within 60 minutes of radiotracer administration.

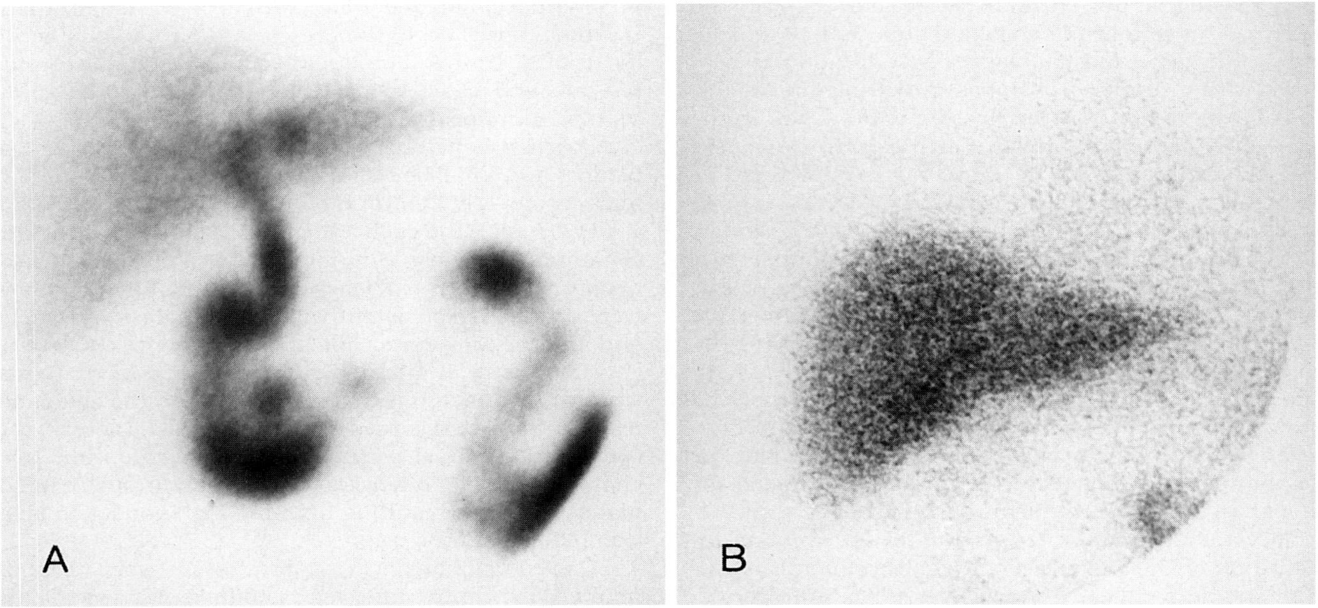

Figure 38.2. The anterior (**A**) 60-minute and (**B**) 4-hour delayed hepatobiliary scan reveals persistent nonvisualization of the gallbladder in a patient with a complete cystic duct obstruction and acute cholecystitis. (From Nuclear Medicine: Principles and practices.)

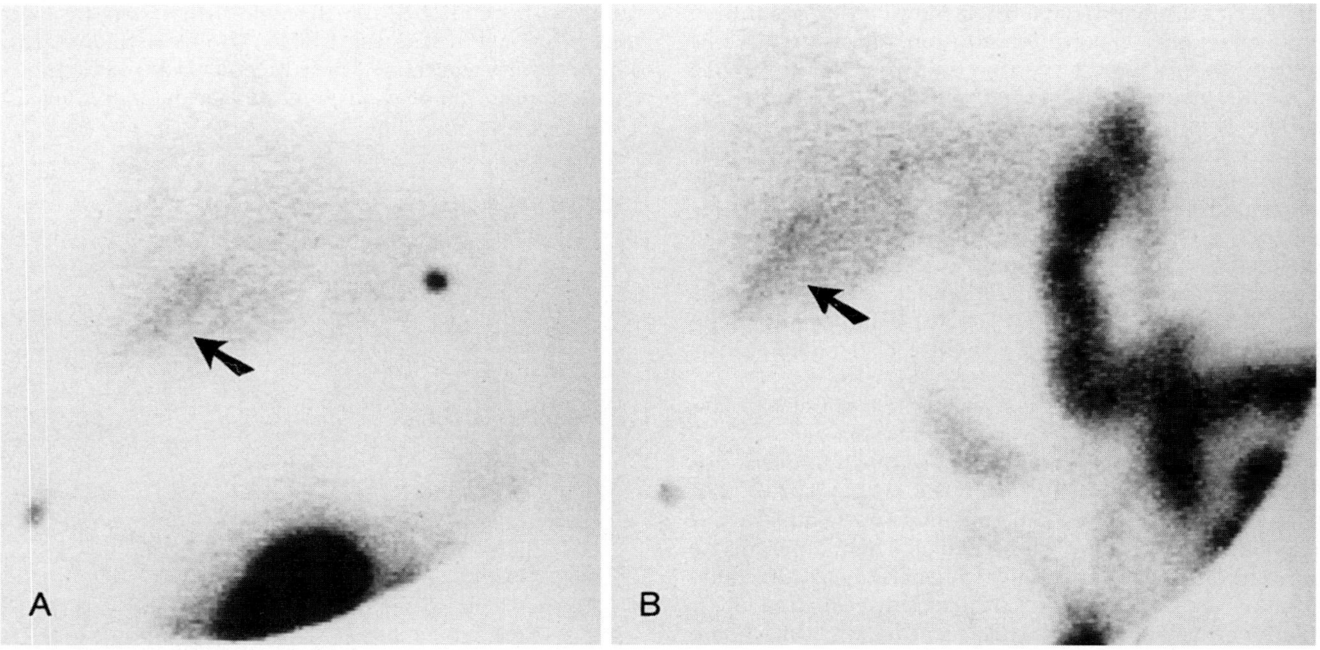

Figure 38.3. The (**A**) anterior 60-minute and (**B**) 4-hour delayed hepatobiliary scan revealed persistent nonvisualization of the gallbladder in conjunction with pericholecystic activity (*arrow*) consistent with this individual's surgically confirmed gangrenous gallbladder. (From Henkin R.)

tion and does not necessarily imply chronic cholecystitis (9, 12).

Nonvisualization of the intrahepatic and extrahepatic biliary tree in patients who have a normal hepatic extraction efficiency 6–24 hours post-^{99m}Tc-IDA administration is indicative of a high grade or total common bile duct obstruction. The presence or absence of a concomitant cystic duct obstruction and acute cholecystitis, however, cannot be determined scintigraphically, as choledocholithiasis in conjunction with a cystic duct obstruction and acute cholecystitis occurred in 14–93% of patients in whom only hepatocyte activity was demonstrable at 24 hours (Fig. 38.5). In situations where radiotracer is identified between 6 and 24 hours post-^{99m}Tc-IDA administration, an ERCP is often required to determine the underlying etiology of the partially occluded common bile duct (9, 12).

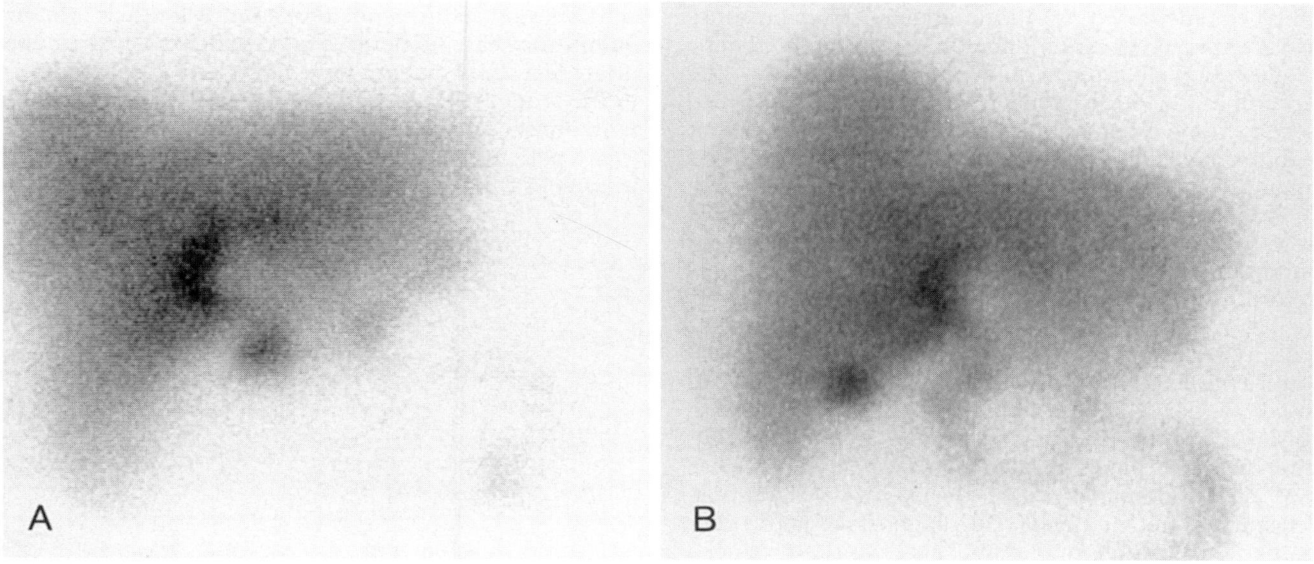

Figure 38.4. The (**A**) anterior 60-minute hepatobiliary scan reveals nonvisualization of the gallbladder. The (**B**) 3-hour delayed anterior scan, however, demonstrates ^{99m}Tc-IDA within a chronically inflamed sludge filled gallbladder in a patient with chronic cholecystitis. (From Hepatobiliary imaging.)

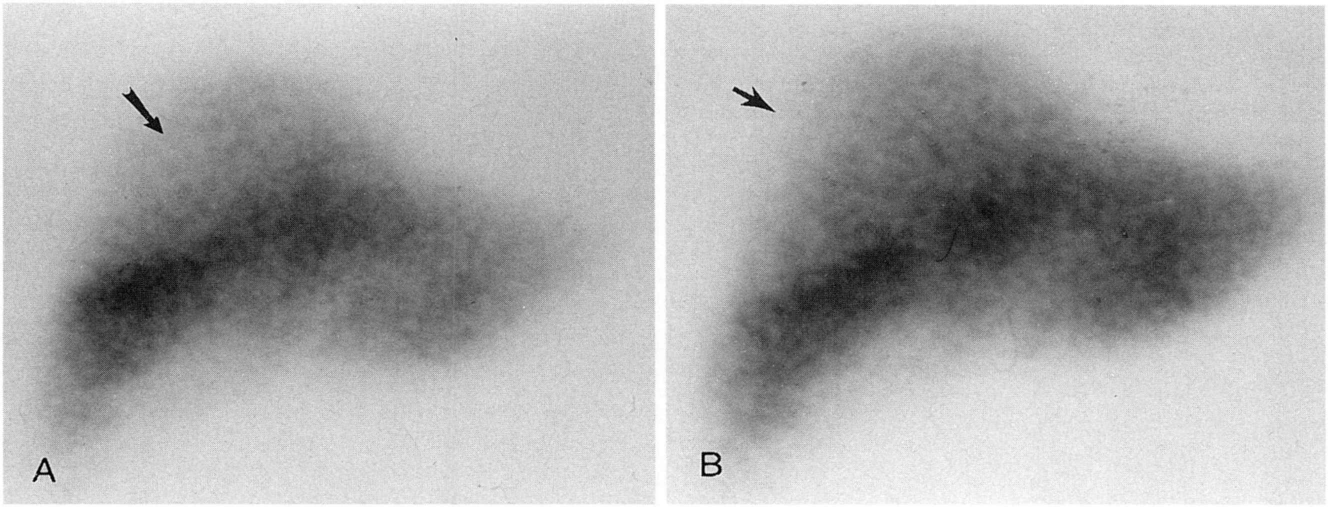

Figure 38.5. The (**A**) anterior 60-minute and (**B**) 4-hour anterior delayed hepatobiliary scan reveals radiotracer only within hepatocytes. None is present within the intrahepatic or extrahepatic biliary tree or small intestine in a patient with a total common bile duct obstruction. The hepatic extraction fraction = 100%. A breast attenuation artifact is demonstrated (*arrow*).

The presence of a nubbin of activity located adjacent to the common bile duct and medial to the gallbladder fossa which persists up to 4 hours postradiotracer administration is a manifestation of a "dilated cystic duct sign" and acute cholecystitis. The nubbin of activity represents radiotracer within a patent cystic duct proximal to its site of obstruction, e.g., calculous (31) (Fig. 38.6).

Preferential gallbladder filling is present when radiotracer is located in the lumen of a dilated gallbladder and within a nondilated common bile duct up to its site of termination at the sphincter of Oddi 60 minutes post-^{99m}Tc-IDA administration. No ^{99m}Tc-IDA is present within the small bowel (Fig. 38.7).

Preferential gallbladder filling occurs when the common bile duct is functionally obstructed as the result of enhanced tone of the sphincter of Oddi due to sphincter of Oddi dyskinesia or from the ingestion or injection of an opiate. Increased pressure within the common bile duct can also result from ampullitis secondary to the repeated passage of small stones through the ampulla of vater in patients with chronic calculous cholecystitis. Greater than 50% of patients pretreated with CCK will also demonstrate preferential gallbladder filling, as there is less resistance to bile flow within the gallbladder 30 minutes post CCK administration than at the sphincter of Oddi (12, 18).

If the gallbladder is visualized after ^{99m}Tc enters the small bowel, increased intraluminal gallbladder pressure is probably present, a finding that has been reported to be a manifestation of chronic cholecystitis (32).

Morphine-augmented cholescintigraphy is performed as is conventional hepatobiliary scintigraphy, except that 0.04 mg/kg morphine sulfate diluted in 10 ml of saline is administered intravenously over a 3-minute period when there is nonvisualization of the gallbladder at 60 minutes post-^{99m}Tc-IDA administration, provided radiotracer is demonstrated within the small bowel. Five-minute serial postmorphine images are then obtained for 30 minutes for the same time as the premorphine images. Persistent nonvisualization of the gallbladder is indicative of acute cholecystitis, whereas chronic cholecystitis is deemed present if the gallbladder visualizes within the 30 minutes following morphine administration (Figs. 38.8 and 38.9). By administering morphine at 60 minutes instead of 30–40 minutes post-^{99m}Tc-IDA administration, the diagnosis of chronic cholecystitis is not sacrificed, the diagnosis of acute cholecystitis is accurately made, and imaging time reduced from 4 to 1 1/2 hours (17, 18, 20, 21, 23, 26).

False-positive and false-negative hepatobiliary scans can occur whether one employs conventional 3–4 hour hepatobiliary scintigraphy or one reduces the time required to make the diagnosis by using morphine sulfate.

Patients must be fasted for at least 2–4 hours prior to the intravenous administration of ^{99m}Tc disofenin or mebrofenin, or a false-positive study may occur as up to 64% of patients who have eaten within 4 hours of their study will not have their gallbladder visualized despite a patent cystic duct. The presence of endogenously produced cholecystokinin ($T_{1/2}$ 45 minutes) causes the gallbladder to contract and reduces bile flow to it. It is, therefore, mandatory that each patient be screened to assure an appropriate fast. If the patient has not fasted for 2–4 hours prior to the study, postpone it or a false-positive study will potentially occur (9, 26).

If a patient has fasted for greater than 24 hours but less than 48–72 hours prior to the intravenous administration

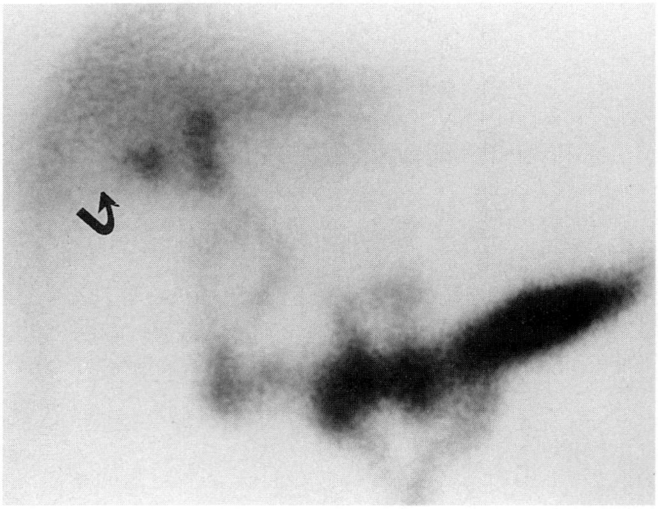

Figure 38.6. The 3-hour anterior hepatobiliary scan reveals a nubbin (focus) of ^{99m}Tc-IDA adjacent to the common bile duct and proximal to its site of obstruction in the cystic duct (the cystic duct sign) in a patient with surgically confirmed acute cholecystitis. The photon deficient area (*arrow*) represents the gallbladder fossa.

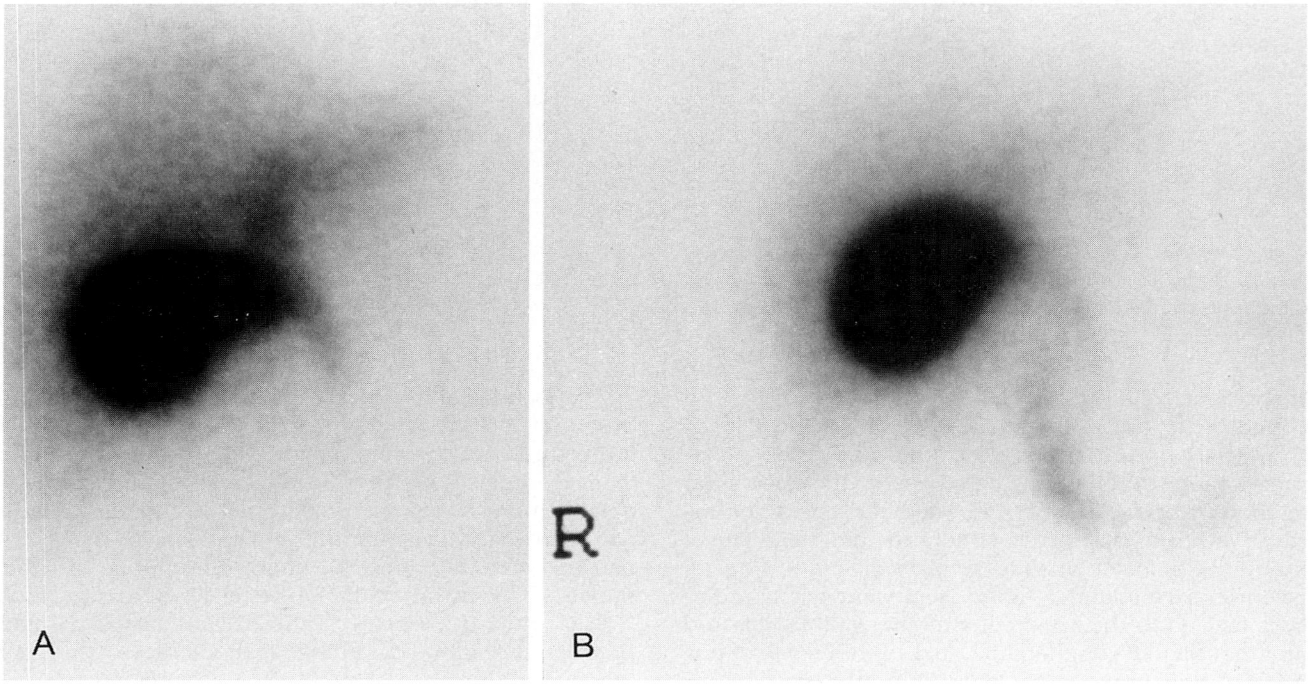

Figure 38.7. The (**A**) anterior 60-minute hepatobiliary scan reveals preferential gallbladder filling in a patient who was pretreated with CCK 30 minutes prior to the intravenous administration of ^{99m}Tc-IDA. The (**B**) 2-hour anterior hepatobiliary scan demonstrates some radiotracer in the small bowel.

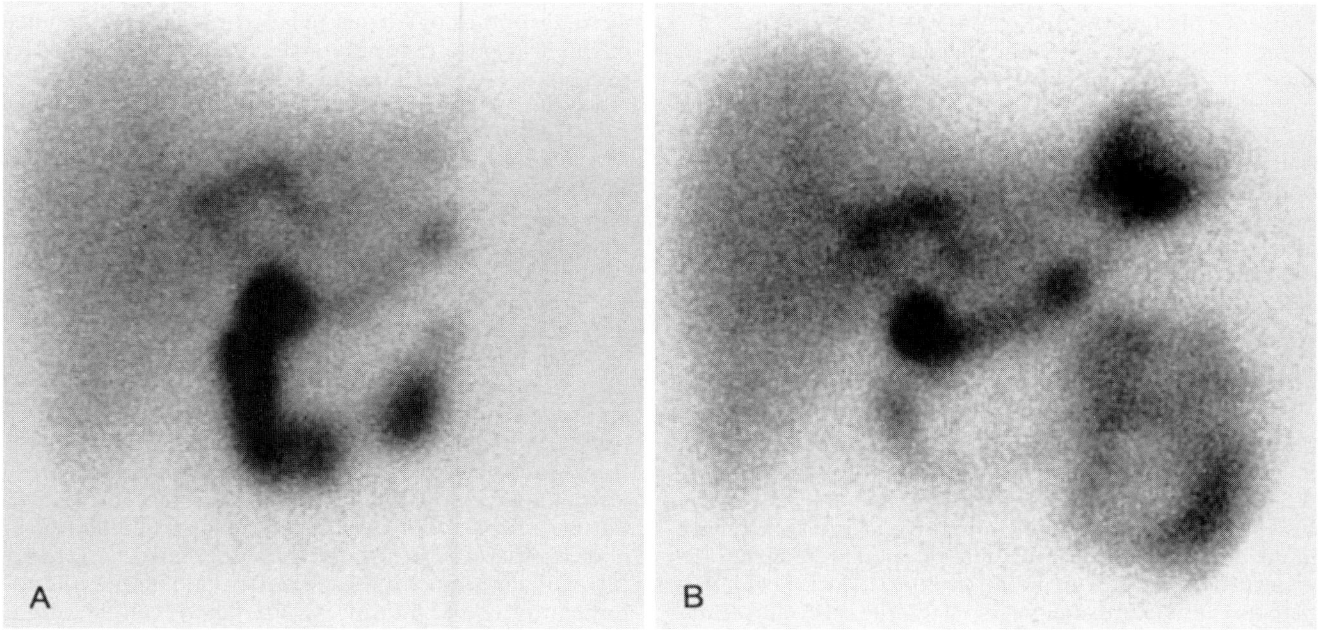

Figure 38.8. The (**A**) anterior 60-minute hepatobiliary scan reveals no radiotracer within the gallbladder. Enterogastric reflux, however, is present. The (**B**) 30-minute postmorphine anterior hepatobiliary scan demonstrates persistent nonvisualization of the gallbladder, a finding consistent with this patient's cystic duct obstruction and surgically confirmed acute cholecystitis. Enterogastric reflux is again demonstrated. It has increased postmorphine administration.

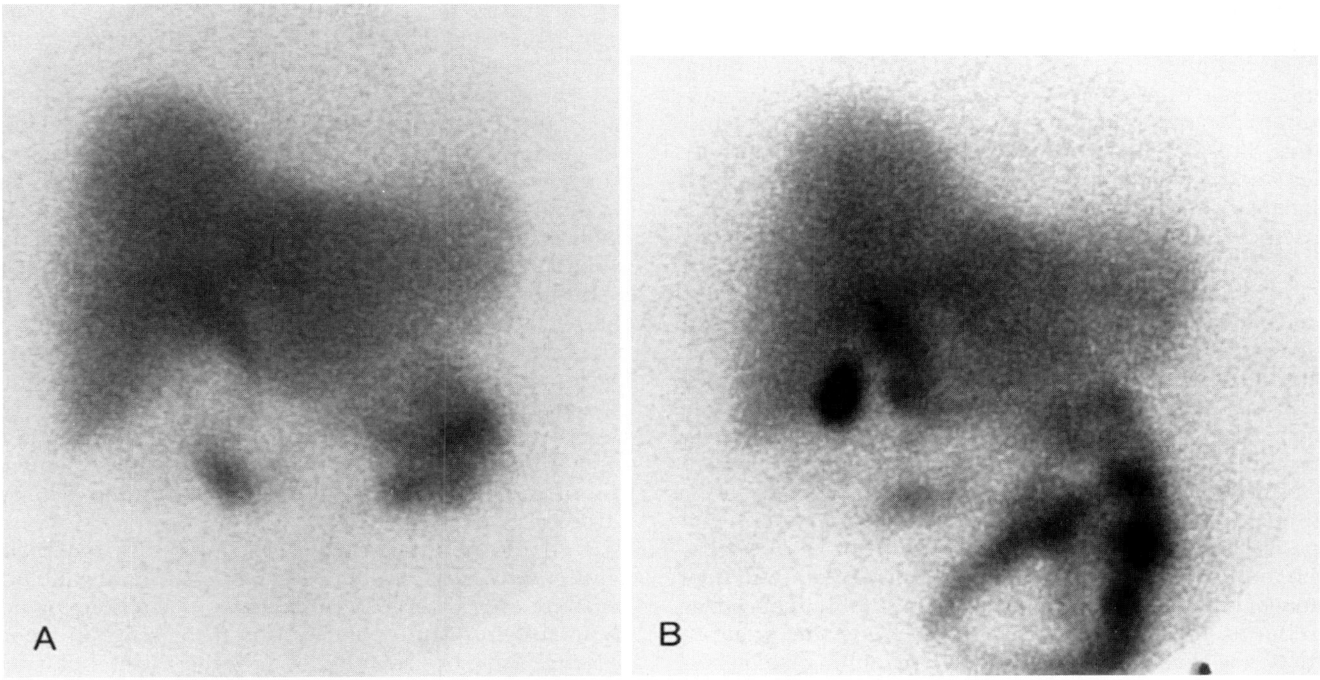

Figure 38.9. The (**A**) anterior 60-minute hepatobiliary scan reveals nonvisualization of the gallbladder. The (**B**) 15-minute postmorphine anterior hepatobiliary scan, however, demonstrates radiotracer within a sludge-filled, chronically inflamed gallbladder in a patient with chronic cholecystitis.

of ^{99m}Tc-IDA, another false-positive study may occur. In the absence of endogenously produced CCK, increased intraluminal gallbladder pressure develops and can result in reduced or absent tracer flow to the gallbladder even though the cystic duct is patent. In this situation, as well as for situations where patients have fasted for a prolonged period of time, an intravenous administration of CCK should be given 30 minutes prior to the performance of either their morphine-augmented or conventional hepatobiliary scan. The CCK will cause the gallbladder to contract, eject the source of increased intraluminal gallbladder pressure (retained bile and sludge), and eliminate the source of increased resistance to bile flow (12, 16, 33, 34).

Care must always be taken to assure that adequate amounts of radiotracer are present within the hepatobiliary tree to permit gallbladder visualization after morphine administration or following a 3–4 hour delay. If not, a false-positive study will occur. This is especially true if using ^{99m}Tc-mebrofenin as it has a very rapid biliary to bowel transit time. If only residual amounts of radiotracer are present in the liver and intrahepatic biliary tree, reinject (booster) the patient with an additional 2–3 mCi of ^{99m}Tc-IDA to prevent a misdiagnosis. If employing morphine-augmented cholescintigraphy to confirm the clinical impression of acute cholecystitis, the morphine should be administered as soon as "the booster" activity is seen within the hepatocytes and intrahepatic biliary tree. If then there is gallbladder nonvisualization up to 30 minutes postmorphine administration, a cystic duct obstruction is confirmed. If morphine is not used, a cystic duct obstruction is confirmed by the presence of nonvisualization of the gallbladder at 4 hours postbooster dosing (20, 26, 34).

Patients who demonstrate the "dilated cystic duct sign" of acute cholecystitis should not be given morphine to reduce the time required to detect a cystic duct obstruction, but should be evaluated with conventional hepatobiliary scintigraphy, i.e., images obtained up to 4 hours postradiotracer administration. If not, the increased intraluminal common bile duct pressure created postmorphine administration can result in dislodging a cystic duct stone. Thus, in this situation, it is probably best to simply obtain delayed images to confirm that the radiotracer demonstrated adjacent to the common bile duct is indeed located in a dilated cystic duct proximal to its site of obstruction (20, 26, 31, 34).

The dilated cystic duct sign is not a common manifestation of acute cholecystitis but has been reported to occur in 7% of patients with acute cholecystitis (31).

Insufficient conventional or postmorphine imaging time in patients with severe chronic cholecystitis in whom there is marked increased intraluminal gallbladder pressure can also result in false-positive hepatobiliary scans. To prevent them from occurring, additional delayed images must be obtained, whether morphine-augmented or conventional hepatobiliary scintigraphy is employed. If the patient was given morphine sulfate, wait an additional 1 hour and then reimage. If no morphine sulfate was used, obtain an image at 5 hours. If the gallbladder visualizes, a cystic duct obstruction is excluded. Delayed imaging should also be performed when a small amount of radiotracer is present in the region of the gallbladder fossa on 30-minute postmorphine or on 3–4-hour delayed conventional hepatobiliary scan. By obtaining further delayed images, the significance of this tracer activity can be ascertained, i.e., is it located in a small chronically inflamed gallbladder or in a loop of bowel. If the latter, it will dissipate or change in position (9, 21, 26, 34).

Other conditions that can create a false-positive hepatobiliary scan include hepatocellular disease, sepsis, total parental hyperalimentation, and prolonged fasting. In these situations, the use of realtime ultrasonography of the gallbladder, CT imaging and ^{111}In white blood cell (^{111}In WBC) scintigraphy should help to prevent a misdiagnosis (26, 34–36).

False-negative scans can also occur and, in particular, in patients with acute acalculous cholecystitis if the increased intraluminal pressure within the edematous cystic duct and gallbladder is insufficient to prevent radiotracer from entering it either postmorphine administration or following delayed imaging. In this situation, and in any situation where there is a high pretest likelihood of acute cholecystitis and a negative hepatobiliary scan, real time ultrasonography of the gallbladder, gallbladder computed tomography, or Indium white blood cell scintigraphy should be employed to confirm the presence or absence of an acutely inflamed hemorrhagic gallbladder wall. In the absence of hypoalbuminemia, cirrhosis, and ascites, the pathognomonic realtime ultrasonographic findings of acute cholecystitis are pericholecystic fluid and gallbladder wall edema. The characteristic findings of acute cholecystitis on computed tomography of the gallbladder are gas bubbles within the gallbladder wall. An ^{111}In WBC scan that confirms the presence of an acutely inflamed hemorrhagic gallbladder wall is one in which ^{111}In WBCs are present within the gallbladder wall (34, 35) (Fig. 38.10).

^{111}In WBC gallbladder scintigraphy is performed following the intravenous administration of 500 mg Ci of autologously labeled ^{111}In WBCs. White blood cells are a mixed population and are labeled using the method described in the Amersham package insert for ^{111}In oxyquinolone solution for the radiolabeling of autologous leukocytes, except that ACD is used as an anticoagulant, hetastarch is employed in all sedimentation steps, and centrifugation is accomplished at 300 g $\times$ 5 minutes. Images of the gallbladder are performed at 6 and 24 hours after intravenous administration of the autologously labeled ^{111}In WBCs. A medium energy collimator with a 20% window centered on the 175 and 247 keV ^{111}In photopeaks is used. Images are obtained in the anterior projection. Twenty-four-hour delayed images are required, for without them, the sensitivity of Indium white blood cell scintigraphy in identifying an acutely inflamed gallbladder wall is reduced from 85% to 66%. An acutely inflamed hemorrhagic gallbladder wall is one in which Indium white blood cell uptake is present within it (35).

It should be remembered that ^{111}In WBC gallbladder scintigraphy is not influenced by intraluminal gallbladder pressure and, thus, ^{111}In WBCs is an ideal imaging agent for identifying acute cholecystitis in patients in whom a potential false-positive or false-negative hepatobiliary scan is clinically suspected.

Fortunately, acute acalculous cholecystitis accounts for

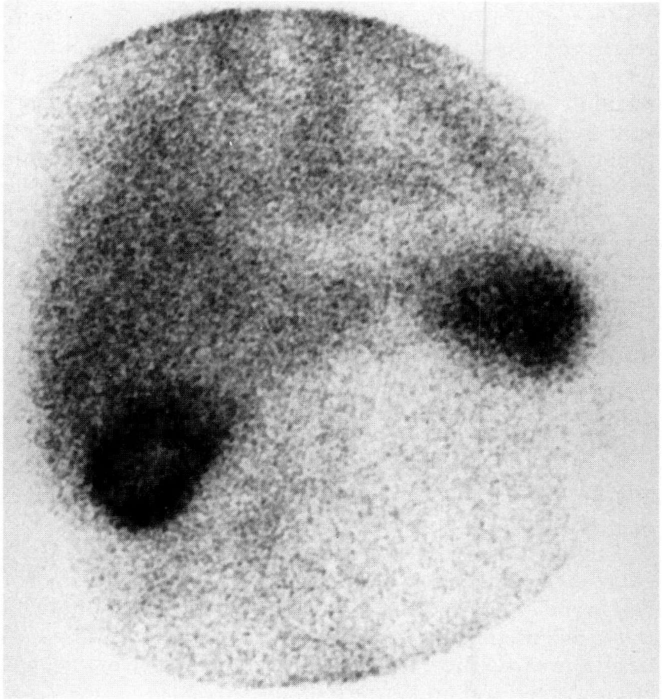

Figure 38.10. The 24-hour ^{111}In WBC abdominal scan reveals ^{111}In WBC uptake within an acutely inflamed hemorrhagic gallbladder wall. (Reproduced by persmission from "The dialated common bile duct sign" a potential indicator of the sphincter of Oddi dysjkinesia. J Nucl Med 1984;59(95):262–263.)

only 5–6% of all patients with an acutely inflamed hemorrhagic gallbladder wall; it does not account for a large portion of the population evaluated for a cystic duct obstruction and acute cholecystitis. Additionally, the majority of patients with acute acalculous cholecystitis do have a sufficient degree of increased intraluminal gallbladder and cystic duct pressure to prevent radiotracer from entering it either postmorphine augmentation or following 3–4-hour delayed imaging (9).

Even though there are many potential false-positive and false-negative conventional or morphine-augmented hepatobiliary scans, cholescintigraphy's accuracy still remains superior to any other imaging modality for the detection of an acutely inflamed hemorrhagic gallbladder wall.

ACALCULOUS DISORDERS OF THE HEPATOBILIARY TREE

Cholecystokinin (CCK) cholescintigraphy can be utilized to confirm the clinical diagnosis of symptomatic chronic acalculous biliary disease. The sensitivity and specificity of CCK cholescintigraphy in confirming the presence of symptomatic chronic acalculous cholecystitis, the cystic duct syndrome, and gallbladder dyskinesia ranges from 89–100% and 80–100%, respectively (37–45).

Cholecystokinin cholescintigrams have been performed in over 800 patients with symptoms indicative of impaired gallbladder motor function. It has not only been found to be a highly accurate method of detecting impaired gallbladder motor contraction or evacuation, but a highly accurate predictor of which patient with abnormal gallbladder motility will benefit from a cholecystectomy. Ninety-five percent of patients' whose symptoms were clinically believed to be a manifestation of one of the chronic acalculous disorders of the hepatobiliary tree, in whom reduced gallbladder motor function was identified, had their symptoms relieved postcholecystectomy (41–45).

The chronic acalculous disorders of the hepatobiliary tree include chronic acalculous cholecystitis, the cystic duct syndrome, gallbladder dyskinesia, and sphincter of Oddi dyskinesia.

Chronic acalculous cholecystitis is a disorder caused by a chronic inflammation of the gallbladder wall. It accounts for up to 20% of all chronic gallbladder disorders. It also accounts for 5–20% of all elective surgery treated gallbladder disorders (43).

Chronic acalculous cholecystitis has been reported to occur more frequently in men than women. It is precipitated by conditions that result in gallbladder atony, a state that occurs when there is decreased production of endogenous cholecystokinin. Thus, patients who are critically ill, burn victims, postoperative patients, etc., who require total parenteral hyperalimentation are prime candidates for developing a chronic inflammation of their gallbladder wall (46–48).

Histologically, chronic acalculous cholecystitis is characterized by hypertrophy of the gallbladder wall (greater than 1.5–2.0 mm), hypertrophy of the muscularis propria in conjunction with or without a monocellular infiltrate, the presence of Aschoff Rokitansky sinuses, foamy macrophages filling the tips of mucosal folds, or by the presence of yellow papillary nodules (cholesterolosis) (46–48).

The cystic duct syndrome, described in 1963 by Cozzolini, et al., is a condition that results in a constellation of signs and symptoms that result from a partial noncalculous obstruction of the cystic duct due to fibrosis, kinking, or from adhesions constricting it. The cystic duct syndrome may occur in conjunction with chronic acalculous cholecystitis or without it (49, 50).

European and South American synonyms for the cystic duct syndrome are infidibullar cervicocystic dyskinesia, mechanical dyskinesia, cystic cholecystic syndrome, and gallbladder siphopathy (51, 52).

Gallbladder dyskinesia is a disorder that occurs when the gallbladder wall responds abnormally to endogenously produced CCK. This occurs when the CCK or neurotransmitter mediated contractor receptor cells located within the gallbladder wall are abnormally or nonhomogeneously distributed throughout it (53, 54).

Sphincter of Oddi dyskinesia is caused by a paradoxical response of the sphincter of Oddi to CCK or by spontaneous spasms of the sphincter of Oddi itself (54, 55). Sphincter of Oddi dyskinesia occurs in pre- and postcholecystectomy patients and is one of the commonest causes of the postcholecystectomy syndrome (56).

The clinical signs and symptoms of chronic acalculous cholecystitis, the cystic duct syndrome, and gallbladder dyskinesia are similar—recurrent postprandial right upper quadrant pain, fatty food intolerance, heart burn, flatulence, epigastric fullness, and upper abdominal discomfort. All result from increased intraluminal gallbladder pressure due to impaired gallbladder contraction (gallbladder dyskinesia, chronic acalculous cholecystitis) or evacuation (the cystic duct syndrome) (34, 40, 53, 57).

Patients with chronic recurrent postprandial right upper quadrant pain and biliary colic resulting from impaired gallbladder motor function require a cholecystectomy to alleviate their symptoms. If not performed, their symptoms can become so severe that anorexia nervosa develops. Surgeons, however, are reluctant to perform a cholecystectomy on patients whose gallbladder is reported to be functioning normally on an oral cholecystogram and morphologically intact sonographically without objective evidence to support their and the gastroenterologist's clinical/subjective impression that the patient's symptoms are due to abnormal gallbladder motor function from a chronically inflamed, partially obstructed, or dysfunctional gallbladder (34, 40).

A normal gallbladder sonogram and a normal oral cholecystogram should not be surprising as oral cholecystography evaluates the gallbladder's ability to concentrate bile, and gallbladder sonography evaluates its morphology. Neither evaluates the gallbladder's ability to contract or eject bile, the impairment of which is the underlying etiology of chronic acalculous cholecystitis, the cystic duct syndrome, and gallbladder dyskinesia. Thus, only if one monitors the gallbladder's ejection fraction response to CCK can individual's with impaired gallbladder motor function/motility be objectively identified.

Cholecystokinin cholescintigraphy is a simple procedure to perform. The study, however, is a confirmatory one and must be utilized in patients with a history of chronic recurrent postprandial right upper quadrant pain, in whom a biliary sonogram, oral cholecystogram, or ERCP is normal. Patients must be thoroughly screened to assure that their symptoms are from abnormal gallbladder motor function and not a manifestation of another disorder which can mimic gallbladder dysfunction, such as Crohn's disease, irritable bowel syndrome, bile gastritis, inflammatory bowel disease, etc. If, and only if, performed in this select patient group, will the efficacy and clinical utility of CCK cholescintigraphy be attained/maintained.

Cholecystokinin cholescintigraphy's rationale is based upon the hypothesis that individuals with a partially obstructed, chronically inflamed, or functionally impaired gallbladder will respond differently to exogenous cholecystokinin than individuals with normal gallbladder motor function and evacuation, i.e., have a reduced (less than 35%) maximal gallbladder ejection fraction response to exogenous CCK (58–60) (Figs. 38.11 and 38.12).

Endogenous or exogenous cholecystokinin have identical effects on the gastrointestinal and biliary system. Both cause the gallbladder to contract, the sphincter of Oddi to relax, augment pyloric sphincter tone, enhance small and large bowel motility, and increase the secretion of bile, pancreatic enzymes, and enterokinase (57, 61).

Endogenous cholecystokinin is a 33-amino acid polypeptide hormone released from the duodenal mucosa in response to lipolytic products, fats, amino acids, and small polypeptides. The cholecystokinetic or active portion of this endogenously produced hormone resides in its C terminal octapeptide (last 8 amino acids) fragment. Cholecystokinin was discovered by Ivy and Oldberg in 1928, and isolated

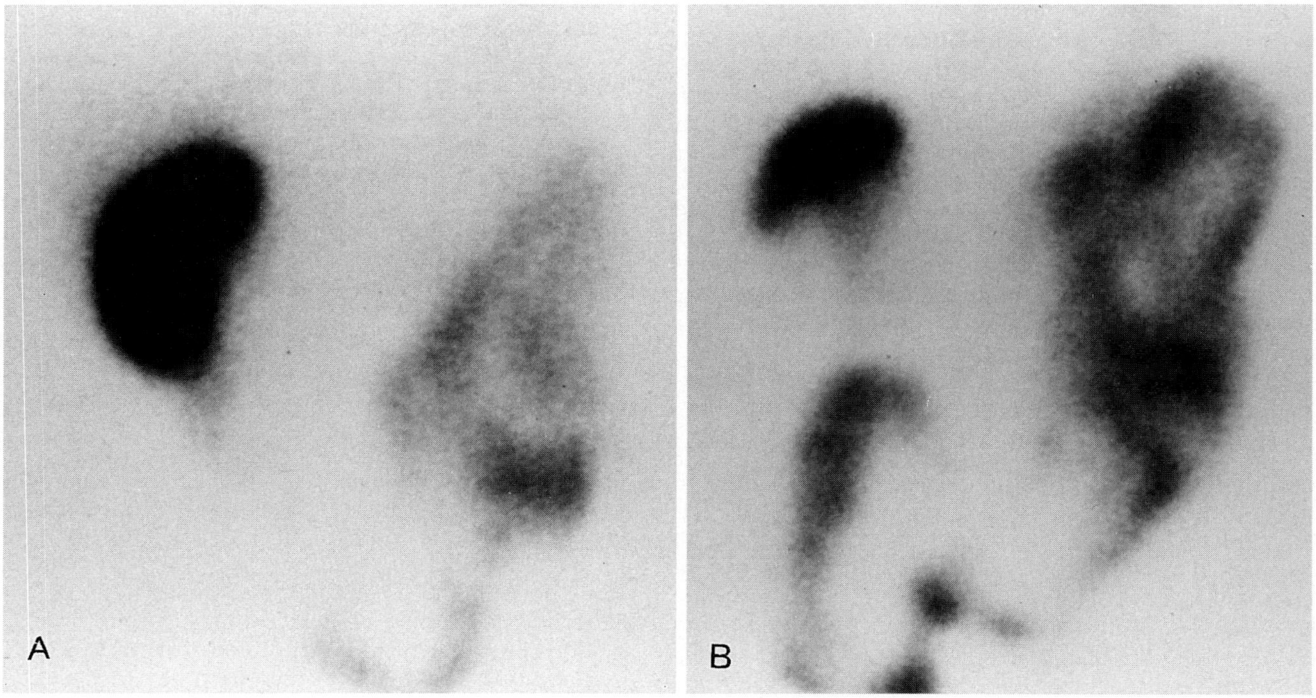

Figure 38.11. The (**A**) anterior pre-CCK hepatobiliary scan reveals maximal gallbladder filling. The (**B**) 20-minute post-CCK anterior hepatobiliary scan reveals normal gallbladder motor function. The calculated maximal gallbladder ejection fraction response to CCK = 79%.

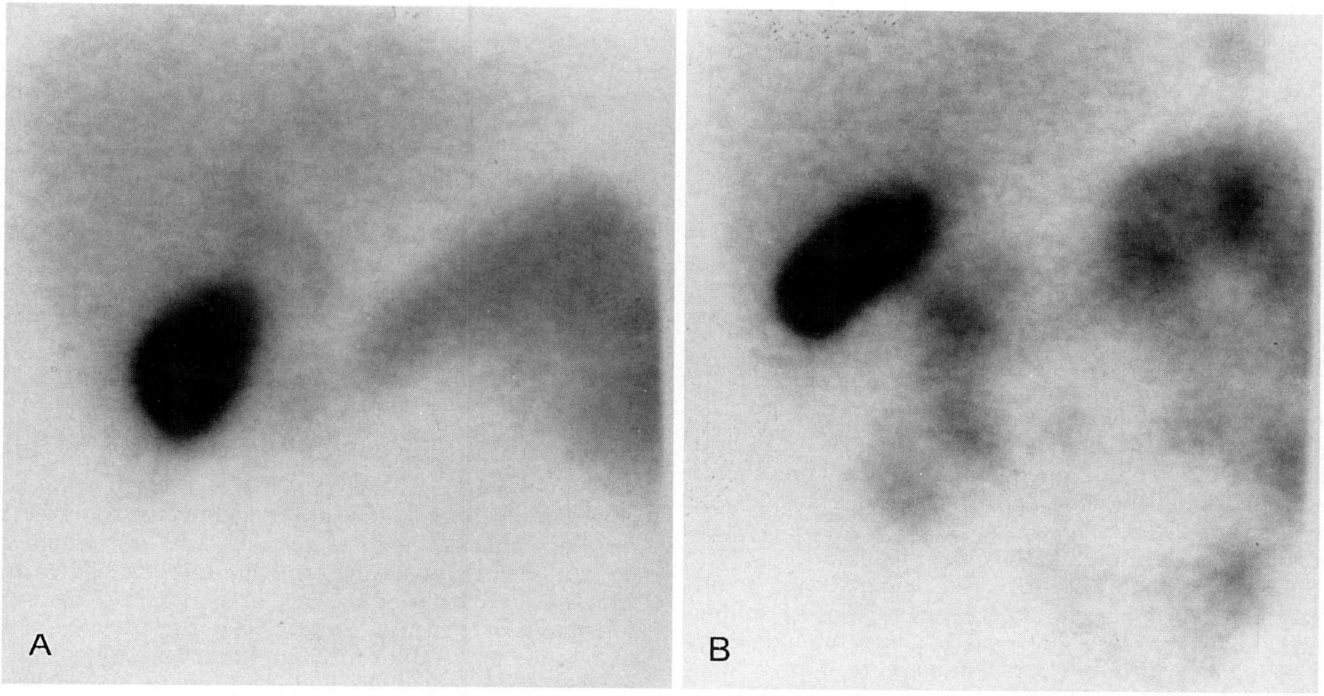

Figure 38.12. The (**A**) anterior pre-CCK 60-minute baseline hepatobiliary scan reveals ^{99m}Tc-IDA in a maximally filled gallbladder. The (**B**) 20-minute post-CCK anterior hepatobiliary scan demonstrates reduced gallbladder motor function as the calculated maximal gallbladder ejection fraction response to CCK is only 17%.

from the porcine GI tract in 1968 by Jobes and Mutt (62, 63).

Cholecystokinin can be purchased in its entirety as a 33-amino acid polypeptide from the Karlinsky Institute, Stockholm, Sweden, or from Boots Company LTD, Nottingham, England, as Cholecystokinin or Pancreazymin respectively. Sincalide (Kinovac) is the C terminal octapeptide of the 33-amino acid polypeptide cholecystokinin. Sincalide can be purchased from ER Squibb, Princeton, NJ, and is the routinely employed cholecystagogue used in conjunction with hepatobiliary scintigraphy to perform CCK cholescintiscans.

CCK cholescintiscans are performed after an overnight fast and following the intravenous administration of either 5 mCi of ^{99m}Tc-disofenin (Hepatolite) or ^{99m}Tc-mebrofenin (Choletec). Utilizing a large field of view gamma-camera, a low energy resolution all-purpose collimator, and a 20% window centered at 140 keV, anterior 500,000 count hepatobiliary images are obtained every 10 minutes for 1 hour or until the gallbladder is maximally filled. Maximal gallbladder filling is manifested when little to no activity is present within the major hepatic radicals, most within the gallbladder itself. Normal biliary-to-bowel transit must be identified prior to performing/interpreting a CCK cholescintigram or a potential false-positive study (misinterpretation) may occur as the etiology of an abnormal gallbladder ejection response to CCK in an individual with delayed biliary-to-bowel transit is either due to reduced gallbladder motor function or the normal gallbladder's inability to contract against increased pressure at the sphincter of Oddi. Once the gallbladder is maximally filled and normal biliary-to-bowel transit identified, the infusion of 0.02 mg/kg of Sincalide is begun. It is administered over a 3-minute duration. The CCK can be administered manually by diluting it in 10 ml of normal saline or given via an infusion pump. Most importantly, it must not be given as a bolus injection. If bolused, spasm of the neck of the gallbladder may occur and result in a spuriously reduced maximal gallbladder ejection fraction response to cholecystokinin.

Following the 3-minute infusion of CCK, anterior post-CCK analogue hepatobiliary images are obtained every 5 minutes for 20 minutes. Post-CCK analogue images are obtained for equal time intervals, not counts, and the time for each image is determined by the number of seconds required to obtain the pre-CCK anterior 500,000 count biliary scintiscan.

Gallbladder ejection fractions are determined from data simultaneously acquired on a computer at 1 frame/minute for 20 minutes. The data is stored on a 64×64×16 computer matrix. Acquisition is begun 1 minute prior to and continues for 20 minutes following the 3-minute infusion of CCK. Ejection fractions are determined manually by assigning areas of interest around the gallbladder and an adjacent background area on the pre-CCK, 5, 10, 15, and 20-minute post-CCK digital images. The background area (region of interest (ROI)) is selected adjacent and to the right of the gallbladder with a width measuring approximately 5 pixels and a length equal to the anterior maximal height of the gallbladder itself. Background activity is subtracted from both pre- and post-CCK images. Total counts and the number of pixels within each ROI are determined and the ejection fraction calculated according the following formula:

$$\text{GBEF(I)} = \frac{\text{Net pre-CCK-GB cts} - \text{Net post-CCK GB cts (at t = min)}}{\text{Net pre-CCK GB cts}}$$

Where *I* equals the time post-CCK administration and for each observation

$$\text{Net GB cts} = \text{Total GB cts} - (\text{background Cts/pixel} \times \# \text{ of GB pixels})$$

Gallbladder motor function can also be assessed by evaluating the gallbladder's ejection fraction response to a 45-minute continuous infusion of cholecystokinin. If employing this methodology, a gallbladder ejection fraction of greater than 40% is deemed normal. The efficacy of 3- or 45-minute infusion CCK cholescintigraphy is similar. Both accurately identify patients with abnormal gallbladder motility either as the result of a chronically inflamed, partially obstructed, or dyskinetic gallbladder (40–42).

Sphincter of Oddi dyskinesia is demonstrated scintigraphically if there is a paradoxical response of the sphincter of Oddi to CCK. Scintigraphically, this is manifested by a delay in biliary to bowel transit and failure of the sphincter of Oddi to relax post-CCK administration, i.e., the common duct becomes dilated (the dilated common duct sign) (64) (Fig. 38.13).

Patients in whom the etiology of the postcholecystectomy syndrome is believed to be secondary to sphincter of Oddi dysfunction can be detected noninvasively by performing a ^{99m}Tc-IDA "scintigraphic score." To obtain this, patients are pretreated with CCK 15 minutes prior to the injection of 5 mCi of ^{99m}Tc-IDA. Hepatobiliary scans are then obtained in the anterior projection over a 60-minute period. Simultaneously, a dynamic study is acquired at a rate of 1 frame/minute and stored on a computer. Regions of interest are placed over the liver and common bile duct from which a time activity curve is created. From this, a time to peak hepatic uptake is calculated, as is the percent common bile duct emptying. These values, in conjunction with qualitative indices obtained from the 60-minute analogue hepatobiliary images, permit the identification of individuals whose postcholecystectomy pain is due to sphincter of Oddi dysfunction. The qualitative indices evaluated include time to biliary visualization, the presence or absence of prominent intrahepatic ducts, time to bowel visualization, and a common bile duct to liver ratio. The percent common bile duct emptying is calculated by determining the peak common bile duct counts then subtracting them from the counts within the common bile duct at 60 minutes. This value is then divided by the peak common bile duct counts multiplied by 100 to obtain the percent common bile duct emptying. A score is assigned to each assessed qualitative and quantitative indice from which the presence or absence of sphincter of Oddi dysfunction is determined. Scores of 0–4 are indicative of normal sphincter of Oddi function, whereas scores ranging from 5–12 are indicative of either sphincter of Oddi dyskinesia, a common bile duct stricture, sphincter of Oddi stenosis, or the presence of a retained common bile duct stone. The sensitivity and specificity of this noninvasive test for detecting or excluding a sphincter of Oddi abnormality in a pilot study conducted on 26 symptomatic and 14 asymptomatic postcholecystectomy patients was 100% (56).

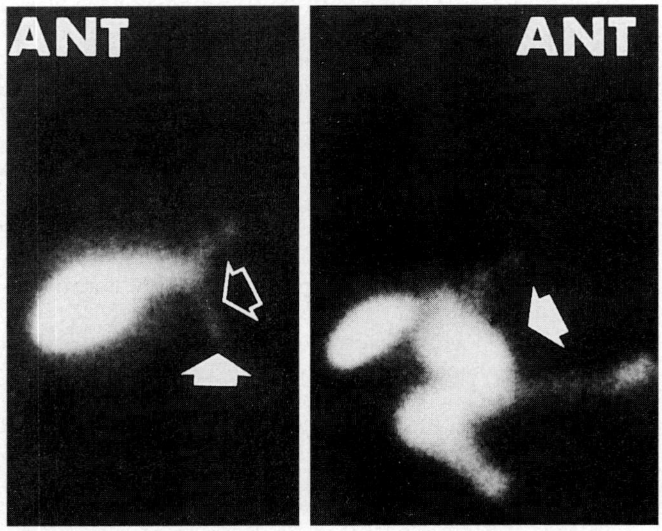

Figure 38.13. The (**A**) anterior 75-minute cholescintiscan demonstrates normal visualization of the gallbladder. There is, however, delayed biliary to bowel transit. The common bile duct is visualized (*arrow*). The (**B**) anterior 5-minute post-CCK hepatobiliary scan demonstrates normal gallbladder motor function but an abnormal (paradoxical) response of the sphincter of Oddi (the dilated common duct sign) to CCK in this patient with sphincter of Oddi dyskinesia. (Reproduced by permission from Leukocycte imaging in acute cholecystitis. J Nucl Med 1991; 32(5): 803–804.)

ACKNOWLEDGMENT

The author would like to thank Maureen Rotarius for her secretarial support.

REFERENCES

1. Anderson WHD. Pathology. St. Louis: C.V. Mosby Co., 1971:1261–1265.
2. Hardy JD. Hardy's textbook of surgery. 2d ed. Philadelphia: J.B. Lippincott Co., 1988:677–690.
3. Anonymous. Gallstones and laproscopic cholecystectomy [NIH consensus conference]. JAMA 1993;29:1018–1024.
4. Rhoads JE, Allen JG, Harkins HN, Moyer CA. Surgery, principles and practice. Philadelphia: W.B. Saunders Co., 1970:887–890.
5. Fink-Bennett D, Freitas JE, Ripley SD, Bree RL. The sensitivity of hepatobiliary imaging and real-time ultrasonography in the detection of acute cholecystitis. Arch Surg 1985b;120:904–906.
6. Kane RA, Costello P, Duszlak E. Computed tomography in acute cholecystitis: new observations. AJR 1983;141:697–701.
7. Moss AA, Gamsu G, Genant HK. Computed tomography of the body. Philadelphia: W.B. Saunders Co., 1983:14–18, 691–697.
8. Samuels BI, Freitas JE, Bree RL, Schwab RE, Heller ST. A comparison of radionuclide hepatobiliary imaging and real-time ultrasound for the detection of acute cholecystitis. Radiology 1983; 147:207–210.
9. Freitas JE. Cholescintigraphy in acute and chronic cholecystitis. Semin Nucl Med 1982;12(1):18–26.
10. Freitas JE, Coleman RE, Nagle CE, Bree RL, Krewer KD. Influence of scan pathologic criteria on the specificity of cholescintigraphy. Concise Communication. J Nucl Med 1983;24:876–879.

11. Freitas JE, Rajinder M, Gulati MD. Rapid evaluation of acute abdominal pain by hepatobiliary scanning. JAMA 1980;244(14):1585–1587.
12. Weissman H. The clinical role of technetium-99m iminodiacetic acid cholescintigraphy. In: Freeman LM, Weissman HS, eds. Nuclear medicine annual. New York: Raven Press, 1981:35–90.
13. Kaplun L, Weissman HS, Rosenblatt RR, Freeman LM. The early diagnosis of common bile duct obstruction using cholescintigraphy. JAMA 1985;254:2431–2434.
14. Zeissman H, Fahey F, Hilson, D. Calculation of a gallbladder ejection fraction: advantage of continuous sincalide infusion over the three-minute infusion method. J Nuc Med 1992;33(1):537–541.
15. Miller DR, Egbert RM, Braunstein P. Comparison of ultrasound and hepatobiliary imaging in the early detection of acute total common bile duct obstruction. Arch Surg 1984;119:1233–1237.
16. Eikman EA, Cameron JL, Coleman M, Natarajan TK, Dugal P, Wagner HN Jr. A test for patency of cystic duct in acute cholecystitis. Ann Int Med 1975;82:318–322.
17. Choy D, Shi EC, McLean RG, Hoschl R, Murry IPC, Ham JM. Cholescintigraphy in acute cholecystitis: use of intravenous morphine. Radiology 1984;151:203–207.
18. Kim CK, Palestro CJ, Solomon RW, et al. Delayed biliary-to-bowel transit in cholescintigraphy after cholecystokinin treatment. Radiology 1990;176(2):553–556.
19. Freeman L, Sugarman L, Weissman H. Role of cholecystokinetic agents in 99m-Tc-IDA cholescintigraphy. Semin Nucl Med 1981; 11:186–193.
20. Fink-Bennett D, Balon H, Robbins T, Tsai D. Morphine augmented cholescintigraphy: its efficacy in detecting acute cholecystitis. J Nucl Med 1991b;32:1231–1233.
21. Keslar PJ, Turbiner EH. Hepatobiliary imaging and the use of intravenous morphine. Clin Nucl Med 1987;12:592–596.
22. Kim EE, Pjura G, Lowry P, Nguyen M, Pollack M. Morphine-augmented cholescintigraphy in the diagnosis of acute cholecystitis. AJR 1986;147:1177–1179.
23. Vasques TE, Greenspan G, Evans DG, Halpern SE, Ashburn WL. Clinical efficacy of intravenous morphine administration in hepatobiliary imaging for acute cholecystitis. Clin Nucl Med 1988; 13:4–6.
24. Krishnamurthy S, Krishnamurthy K. Quantitative assessment of hepatobiliary diseases with Tc-99m-IDA scintigraphy. In: Freeman LM, Weissman HS, eds. Nuclear medicine annual. New York: Raven Press, 1988:309–313.
25. Datz F. Handbook in radiology, nuclear medicine. St. Louis: Mosby Yearbook, 1988:154–155.
26. Fink-Bennett D, Balon H. The role of morphine-augmented cholescintigraphy in the detection of acute cholecystitis. Clin Nucl Med 1993;18(10):891–897.
27. Keller IA, Weissman HS, Kaplan LL, et al. The use of water ingestion to distinguish the gallbladder and duodenum on cholescintigrams. Radiology 1984;152:151.
28. Lette J, Morin M, Heyen F, Paquet A, Levasseur A. Standing views to differentiate gallbladder or bile leak from duodenal activity on cholescintigrams. Clin Nucl Med 1990;15(4)231–236.
29. Shaffer PB, Olsen JO. Differentiation of the gallbladder from the duodenum on cholescintigrams by dynamic display. Radiology 1982;145:217.
30. Bushnell DL, Perlman SC, Wilson MA, Polycr, RD. The RIM sign: association with acute cholecystitis. J Nucl Med 1986;27:353–356.
31. Coleman RE, Freitas JE, Fink-Bennett D, Bree RL. The dilated cystic duct sign—a potential cause of false-negative cholescintigraphy. Clin Nucl Med 1984;9(3):134–136.
32. Achong DM, Oates E. A reversed sequence of gallbladder and small bowel visualization during cholescintigraphy: its relationship to chronic cholecystitis. Clin Nucl Med 1994;19(2);89–92.
33. Fink-Bennett D. The role of cholecystogogues in the evaluation of biliary tract disorders. In: Freeman LM, Weissman HS, eds. Nuclear medical annual. New York: Raven Press, 1985a.
34. Fink-Bennett D. Augmented cholescintigraphy: its role in detecting acute and chronic disorders of the hepatobiliary tree. Semin Nucl Med 1991c;21(2):128–139.
35. Fink-Bennett D, Clark K, Tsai D, Nuechterlein P. Indium-111 WBC imaging in acute cholecystitis. J Nucl Med 1991a;32:803–804.
36. Datz FL. Utility of indium-111 labeled leukocyte imaging in acute acalculous cholecystitis. AJR 1986;147:813–814.
37. Topper TE, Ryerson TW, Nora PF. Quantitative gallbladder imaging following cholecystokinin. J Nucl Med 1980;21:694–696.
38. Newman P, Browne MK, Mowat W. A simple technique for quantitative cholecystokinin-HIDA scanning. Br J Radiol 1983;56:500–502.
39. Pickelman J, Peiss RL, Henkin R, et al. The role of Sincalide cholescintigraphy in the evaluation of patients with acalculous gallbladder disease. Arch Surg 1985;120:693–697.
40. Fink-Bennett D, DeRidder P, Kolozsi W, Gordon R, Jaros R. Cholecystokinin cholescintigraphy: detection of abnormal gallbladder motor function in patients with chronic acalculous gallbladder disease. J Nucl Med 1991d;32:1695–1699.
41. Halverson JD, Garner BA, Siegel BA, et al. The use of hepatobiliary scintigraphy in patients with acalculous biliary colic. Arch Int Med 1992;152(6):1305–1307.
42. Yap L, Wycherley AG, Morphett AD, Toouli J. Acalculous biliary pain: cholecystectomy alleviates symptoms in patients with abnormal cholescintigraphy. Gastroenterology 1991;101;786–793.
43. Zech ER, Simmons LB, Kendrick RR, et al. Cholecystokinin enhanced hepatobiliary scanning with ejection fraction calculation an an indicator of disease of the gallbladder. Surgery Gyn/Ob 1991;172:21–22.
44. Brugge W, Brand D, Atkins H, Lane B, Abel W. Gallbladder dyskinesia in chronic acalculous cholecystitis. Dig Dis Sci 1986; 31:(5)461–467.
45. Mishra DC, Blooson GB, Fink-Bennett DF, Glover JJ. Results of surgical therapy for biliary dyskinesia. Arch Surg 1991;26;957–959.
46. Anderson WHD. Pathology. St. Louis: C.V. Mosby Co., 1971:1261–1265.
47. Harrison TR, Adams RD, Bennett IL, et al. Principles of internal medicine. New York: McGraw-Hill, 1966:1088–1093.
48. Cecil B. Textbook of medicine. Philadelphia: W.B. Saunders, 1979:1624–1628.
49. Fink-Bennett D, DeRidder P, Kolozsi W, Gordon RM, Rapp J. Cholecystokinin cholescintigraphic findings in the cystic duct syndrome. J Nucl Med 1985c;26:1123–1128.
50. Cozzolino HJ, Goldstein F, Greening RR, Wirts CW. The cystic duct syndrome. JAMA 1963;185:100–104.
51. McFarland JO, Currin J. Cholecystokinin and the cystic duct syndrome. Clinical experience in a community hospital. Amer J Gastorent 1965;515–522.
52. Camishion RD, Goldstein F. Partial, noncalculous cystic duct obstruction (cystic duct syndrome). Surg Clin NA 1967;47:1107–1114.
53. Bolen G, Javitt NB. Biliary dyskinesia: mechanisms and management. Hosp Prac 1982;17:115–130.
54. Lechin F, Van Der Dijs B, Bentolila A, Pena F. Adrenergic influences on the gallbladder emptying. Am J Gastroent 1978;69:662–668.
55. Hogan W, Green J, Dodds I, et al. Paradoxical response to cholecystokinin (CCK-OP) in patients with suspected sphincter-of-Oddi dysfunction [Abstract]. Gastroentology 1982;82:1085.
56. Sostre S, Kalloo A, Speigler E, Camaigo E, Wagner H. A noninvasive test of sphincter of Oddi dysfunction in postcholecystectomy patients: the scintigraphic score. J Nucl Med 1992;33(6):1216–1222.

57. Harvey RF, Oliver JM. Cholecystokinins and the gallbladder. Gastroenterology 1980;78:1117–1119.
58. Krishnamurthy GT, Bobba VR, McConnell D, et al. Quantitative biliary dynamics: introduction of a new noninvasive scintigraphic technique. J Nucl Med 1983;24(3):217–213.
59. Krishnamurthy GT, Bubba VR, Kingston E. Radionuclide ejection fraction: a technique for quantitative analysis of motor function of the human gallbladder. Gastroenterology 1981;80:482–90.
60. Bobba VR, Krishnamurthy GT, Kingston E, et al. Gallbladder dynamics induced by a fatty meal in normal subjects and patients with gallstones: Concise communication. J Nucl Med 1984; 25(1):21–24.
61. Morley JE. The ascent of cholecystokinin (CCK)—from gut to brain. Life Sciences 1982;30:479–493.
62. Ivy AC, Oldbert E. A hormone mechanism for gallbladder contraction and evacuation. Am J Physiol 1982;86:599–613.
63. Jopes JE, Mutt V. The gastrointestinal hormones, secretin and cholecystokinin—pancreomyzin. Ann Intern Med 1961;55:395–405.
64. DeRidder P, Fink-Bennett D. The dilated common duct sign: a potential indicator of a sphincter of Oddi dyskinesia. Clin Nucl Med 1984;9(5):262–263.

INDEX

Page numbers in *italics* denote figures; those followed by a "t" denote tables.